BRAIN
TUMORS

An Encyclopedic Approach

THIRD EDITION

Andrew H. Kaye MB BS, MD, FRACS

Head of Department and
James Stewart Professor of Surgery,
Department of Surgery,
The University of Melbourne;
Director, Department of Neurosurgery,
The Royal Melbourne Hospital,
Melbourne, Victoria, Australia

Edward R. Laws Jr MD, FACS

Professor of Surgery,
Harvard Medical School;
Director, Pituitary and Neuroendocrine Center,
Brigham and Women's Hospital,
Boston, Massachusetts, USA

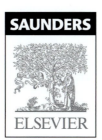

SAUNDERS

ELSEVIER

Edinburgh   London   New York   Oxford   Philadelphia   St Louis   Sydney   Toronto

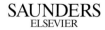

An imprint of Elsevier Limited.

First edition 1995
Second edition 2001

Notices

Knowledge and best practice in this field are constantly changing. As new research and experience broaden our understanding, changes in research methods, professional practices, or medical treatment may become necessary. Practitioners and researchers must always rely on their own experience and knowledge in evaluating and using any information, methods, compounds, or experiments described herein. In using such information or methods they should be mindful of their own safety and the safety of others, including parties for whom they have a professional responsibility.

With respect to any drug or pharmaceutical products identified, readers are advised to check the most current information provided (i) on procedures featured or (ii) by the manufacturer of each product to be administered, to verify the recommended dose or formula, the method and duration of administration, and contraindications. It is the responsibility of practitioners, relying on their own experience and knowledge of their patients, to make diagnoses, to determine dosages and the best treatment for each individual patient, and to take all appropriate safety precautions.

To the fullest extent of the law, neither the Publisher nor the authors, contributors, or editors, assume any liability for any injury and/or damage to persons or property as a matter of products liability, negligence or otherwise, or from any use or operation of any methods, products, instructions, or ideas contained in the material herein.

British Library Cataloguing in Publication Data
Brain tumors : an encyclopedic approach. – 3rd ed.
1. Brain–Tumors.
I. Kaye, Andrew H.   II. Laws, Edward R.
616.9′9481 – dc22

ISBN-13: 9780443069673

A catalogue record for this book is available from the British Library

Library of Congress Cataloging in Publication Data
A catalog record for this book is available from the Library of Congress

Printed in China
Last digit is the print number: 9 8 7 6 5 4 3 2 1

CONTENTS

When I began specializing in neuro-oncology, *Brain Tumors: An Encyclopedic Approach* was the textbook I turned to for a comprehensive overview of the field. Edited by the preeminent neurosurgeons Edward Laws and Andrew Kaye, the third edition is updated to highlight the changes in diagnosis and management that are rapidly occurring as a result of advances in our understanding of tumor biology and etiology. During my career, I have been fortunate enough to collaborate with Dr. Laws, who has been on the front lines of brain tumor treatment and research since the 1970s – he is not only a brilliant physician, but also a generous educator and esteemed scholar.

As with the previous editions, the third edition contains excellent illustrations and clear, coherent descriptions of all central nervous system tumors, including those that are very rare. However, the most important aspect of the third edition is the attention given to the explosion of research into the cellular origins of brain tumors, as well as an understanding of the aberrant biologic pathways and the rational use of targeted therapies. It is critical to understand the development of these treatment strategies as we advance towards personalized medicine.

Over fifteen years since the original publication of the first edition, *Brain Tumors: An Encyclopedic Approach* is an outstanding, comprehensive reference guide for the diagnosis and management of brain tumors. It is an invaluable resource for all medical professionals who treat patients with this disease, especially for residents and fellows who are contemplating careers in neuro-oncology.

SUSAN M. CHANG MD
Director, Division of Neuro-Oncology
Department of Neurological Surgery
University of California, San Francisco

PREFACE TO THE FIRST EDITION

The management of brain tumors is the single most important role of the present day neurosurgeon. The chilling diagnosis of a brain tumor quite reasonably strikes fear into patients, their friends, and relatives. The consequences of the diagnosis include the implication of an erosion of the faculties of the mind combined with physical disablility and death. The appropriate diagnosis and management requires the very best skills a neurosurgeon has learned, a culmination of all the knowledge that has been gleaned from his or her first days in medical school to the most recent clinical experience practising the art of neurosurgery, along with the insight that has been obtained into human nature and frailty. Treatment involves the very best of both technical skills and human interaction. Throughout the often protracted management of a patient with a brain tumor the surgeon must constantly strive to utilize the very latest in scientific advancement, whilst maintaining a sympathetic and guiding influence on the patient and the family. The treatment of brain tumors has expanded rapidly over the past decades. It was the discovery of the cell by Schleiden and Schwann in 1838 and 1839 and the description of neuroglia by Virchow in 1846 that formed the basis for the neuropathology of brain tumors. The concept of cerebral localization of neurological function developed through the nineteenth century and the first scientifically performed brain tumor operation took place on 25 November 1884 by Rickman Godlee in London. That patient died from the glioma twenty five days after surgery. The subsequent pioneers in brain tumor surgery, including Cushing, Dandy, Keen, MacEwen, and Horsley demonstrated not only the possibilities of brain tumor surgery, but also at times, the seemingly insurmountable difficulties that had to be overcome for the patient to be treated effectively and safely. The last two decades have, in particular, provided the technological advancement necessary for the understanding of the many varied facets of brain tumors, including their intricate biology, the molecular events that are at the basis of their development, and the equipment necessary for effective treatment. We now know that the ideal management involves a wide range of skills and techniques, utilizing all the best technical and human resources of a hospital and community.

In the past the mystique of brain tumors has, at times, inadvertently restricted the full understanding of these tumors. This book aims to provide a complete coverage of brain tumors, including their biological basis, diagnosis and management techniques. Aiming to be the ultimate reference on all the technical facets of brain tumor management, this book describes the present concepts of the treatment and the management of all brain tumors, although we realise that social values vary from region to region and in many countries facilities are less than optimal. In general, references have been chosen for their general coverage of the topics, ease of access, historical interest, and, in some cases, because they will provide thought-provoking alternatives to give a different perspective to the subject. It is not possible to list and acknowledge all the many people who have helped in the preparation of this volume both knowingly and as the result of their influences on our own neurosurgical practices. We particularly acknowledge our many colleagues, both past and present, who by their influence and example have made this type of book possible. This work would not have come to fruition without the guidance and stimulation initially from Peter Richardson and then from his colleagues, Michael Parkinson, Dilys Jones, and Janice Urquhart at Churchill Livingstone. We are especially grateful for the encouragement and patience of our wives, Judy and Peggy.

ANDREW H. KAYE
EDWARD R. LAWS JR
1995

PREFACE TO THE THIRD EDITION

It is a real pleasure to see this comprehensive, encyclopedic treatise on the ever-fascinating subject of Brain Tumors reach its Third Edition. The recognition of the problems posed by the diagnosis, treatment and pathogenesis of brain tumors has steadily increased among scientists, physicians and surgeons, and the public in general. As health care access and expertise increase, and with the mixed blessing of information from the internet, more and more brain tumors are being diagnosed, and their treatment has steadily improved, particularly regarding the quality of life of our patients.

This edition continues to be divided into segments on Basic Principles and Individual Tumor Types. Each chapter has been assiduously updated, key points have been emphasized and pertinent references have been highlighted. Many new chapters have been included, along with many new authors, all reflecting the continuous change in concepts,

techniques and outcomes for our patients. Novel insights into molecular neuropathology, the role of cancer stem cells, changes in tumor classification, new models of brain tumors, and avenues for future progress are included. The goal of making each chapter authoritative, comprehensive and interesting to a variety of readers has been achieved, and hopefully will be widely appreciated.

As always, we are indebted to the hard work of all the contributors, and of the editorial and production staff at Elsevier who have seen this impressive volume through to final publication. We are continually grateful to our colleagues, trainees, patients, and to our wives, families and others who have supported this endeavor.

ANDREW H. KAYE
EDWARD R. LAWS JR.

LIST OF CONTRIBUTORS

Ossama Al-Mefty, MD, FACS
Department of Neurosurgery, Brigham & Women's Hospital,
Harvard Medical School, Boston, MA, USA
31   Meningiomas
33   Meningeal Sarcomas

Ashok R. Asthagiri, MD
Staff Neurosurgeon, National Institutes of Health,
Bethesda, MD, USA
30   Brain Tumors Associated with Neurofibromatosis

Samer Ayoubi, MD
Consultant Neurosurgeon, Damascus, Syria
31   Meningiomas

Mitchel S. Berger, MD
Professor and Chairman, Department of Neurological Surgery;
Director of the Brain Tumor Research Center, UCSF,
San Francisco, CA, USA
20   Low-Grade Astrocytomas

Rajesh K. Bindal, MD
Clinical Assistant Professor, Department of Neurosurgery,
Baylor College of Medicine, Houston, TX, USA
45   Metastatic brain tumors

Robert J. S. Briggs, MBBS, FRACS
Clinical Associate Professor,
Department of Otolaryngology,
The University of Melbourne,
Melbourne, VIC, Australia
28   Acoustic Neurinoma (Vestibular Schwannoma)

Jeffrey N. Bruce, MD
Edgar M. Housepian Professor of Neurological Surgery;
Vice-Chairman of Neurosurgery,
Columbia University College of Physicians and Surgeons;
Attending Neurosurgeon,
Neurological Institute of New York,
New York Presbyterian Medical Center,
New York, NY, USA
34   Pineal Cell and Germ Cell Tumors

Jan C. Buckner, MD
Professor of Oncology,
Mayo Clinic,
Rochester, MN, USA
40   Esthesioneuroblastoma: Management and Outcome

Ronil V. Chandra, MBBS (HON), FRANZCR
Department of Radiology, The Royal Melbourne Hospital,
University of Melbourne, Melbourne, VIC, Australia
10   Advanced Imaging of Brain Tumors

Susan M. Chang, MD
Director, Division of Neuro-Oncology, Department of
Neurological Surgery, University of California,
San Francisco, CA, USA
6   Biologic Therapy for Malignant Glioma

Nikki Charles, PHD
Department of Cancer Biology & Genetics and the Brain
Tumor Center; Memorial Sloan-Kettering Cancer Center,
New York, NY, USA
17   Mouse Models for Brain Tumor Therapy

Thomas C. Chen, MD, PHD
Director, Neuro-Oncology Program;
Associate Professor of Neurosurgery and Pathology,
University of Southern California,
Los Angeles, CA, USA
26   Uncommon Glial Tumors

Antonio Chiocca, MD, PHD
Professor and Chairman, Dardinger Center for
Neuro-oncology and Neurosciences,
and Department of Neurological Surgery, James Cancer
Hospital/Solove Research Institute,
The Ohio State University Medical Center,
Columbus, OH, USA
21   Glioblastoma and Malignant Astrocytoma

Christopher P. Cifarelli, MD, PHD
Department of Neurosurgery,
University of Arkansas for Medical Sciences,
Little Rock, AR, USA
16   Clinical Trials and Chemotherapy

David A. Clump, MD, PHD
University of Pittsburgh, and the Center for
Image-Guided Neurosurgery,
UPMC Presbyterian, Pittsburgh, PA, USA
15   Radiosurgery and Radiotherapy for Brain Tumors

Charles S. Cobbs, MD
Attending Neurosurgeon, California Pacific Medical Center,
San Francisco, CA, USA
32   Meningeal Hemangiopericytomas

E. Sander Connolly JR, MD, FACS
Professor of Neurological Surgery;
Vice Chairman of Neurosurgery;
Director, Cerebrovascular Research Laboratory,
Surgical Director, Neuro-Intensive Care Unit,
Neurological Institute, Columbia University Medical Center,
New York, NY, USA
34   Pineal Cell and Germ Cell Tumors

Shlomi Constantini, MD, MSc
Director, Department of Pediatric Neurosurgery;
Director, The Gilbert Neurofibromatosis Center,
Dana Children's Hospital,
Tel-Aviv Medical Center, Tel Aviv University,
Tel Aviv, Israel
18 *Management of Brain Tumors in the Pediatric Patient*

Douglas J. Cook, MD, PhD
Division of Neurosurgery, Department of Surgery,
Faculty of Medicine, Toronto Western Hospital,
University of Toronto, Toronto, ON, Canada
7 *Gene Therapy for Human Brain Tumors*

Helen V. Danesh-Meyer, MBChB, MD, FRANZCO
Sir William and Lady Stevenson Professor of Ophthalmology,
NZ National Eye Centre, Department of Ophthalmology,
University of Auckland, New Zealand
11 *Neuro-ophthalmology of Brain Tumors*

R. Andrew Danks, MD
Department of Neurosurgery, Monash Medical Center, Clayton,
VIC, Australia
39 *Carcinoma of the Paranasal Sinuses*

Ryan DeMarchi, BSc, MD
Division of Neurosurgery, Department of Surgery,
University of Toronto,
University Hospital Network Toronto Western Hospital,
Division of Neurosurgery, Toronto, ON, Canada
27 *Medulloblastoma and Primitive Neuroectodermal Tumors*

Katharine J. Drummond, MD, FRACS
Department of Surgery, University of Melbourne;
Department of Neurosurgery, The Royal Melbourne Hospital,
Melbourne, VIC, Australia
14 *Surgical Principles in the Management of Brain Tumors*
22 *Oligodendroglioma*

Ian F. Dunn, MD
Attending Neurosurgeon, Department of Neurosurgery,
Brigham & Women's Hospital,
Harvard Medical School, Boston, MA, USA
31 *Meningiomas*
33 *Meningeal Sarcomas*

James B. Elder, MD
Assistant Professor, Department of Neurological Surgery,
The Ohio State University Medical Center, Columbus, OH, USA
26 *Uncommon Glial Tumors*

Richard G. Ellenbogen, MD, FACS
Professor and Chairman, Department of Neurological Surgery,
Theodore S. Roberts Endowed Chair, University of
Washington, School of Medicine Seattle, Washington,
Seattle, WA, USA
25 *Choroid Plexus Tumors*

Michael Ellis, MD
Division of Neurosurgery, Department of Surgery,
The Hospital for Sick Children, The University of Toronto,
Toronto, ON, Canada
27 *Medulloblastoma and Primitive Neuroectodermal Tumors*

Rudolf Fahlbusch, MD, PhD
Director, Endocrine Neurosurgery,
International Neuroscience Institute, Hannover, Germany
35 *Non-functional Pituitary Tumors*

John C. Flickinger, MD, FACR
Departments of Neurological Surgery and Radiation Oncology,
University of Pittsburgh, and the Center for Image-Guided
Neurosurgery, UPMC Presbyterian, Pittsburgh, PA, USA
15 *Radiosurgery and Radiotherapy for Brain Tumors*

Jeremy L. Fogelson, MD
Department of Neurosurgery,
Mayo Clinic, Rochester, MN, USA
40 *Esthesioneuroblastoma: Management and Outcome*

Robert L. Foote, MD
Professor of Radiation Oncology, Mayo Clinic,
Rochester, MN, USA
40 *Esthesioneuroblastoma: Management and Outcome*

Venelin M. Gerganov, MD, PhD
Associate Neurosurgeon, Department of Neurosurgery,
International Neuroscience Institute, Hannover, Germany
35 *Non-Functional Pituitary Tumors*

Caterina Giannini, MD, PhD
Professor of Laboratory Medicine and Pathology, Mayo Clinic,
Rochester, MN, USA
40 *Esthesioneuroblastoma: Management and Outcome*

Graham G. Giles, BSc, MSc, PhD
Professor, School of Population Health, University of
Melbourne; Director, Cancer Epidemiology Centre,
Cancer Council Victoria, Carlton, VIC, Australia
4 *Epidemiology of Brain Tumors*

Michael Gonzales, MBBS, FRCPA
Associate Professor, Department of Pathology;
University of Melbourne; Senior Pathologist,
Department of Anatomical Pathology,
The Royal Melbourne Hospital, Melbourne, Australia
3 *Classification and Pathogenesis of Brain Tumors*

Ignacio Gonzalez-Gomez, MD
Department of Pathology and Laboratory Medicine,
All Children's Hospital, Saint Petersburg, FL, USA
26 *Uncommon Glial Tumors*

Abhijit Guha, MSc, MD, FRCS(C), FACS
Professor, Surgery (Neurosurgery), Western Hospital,
University of Toronto, Co- Dir. & Sr. Scientist: Arthur & Sonia
Labatt Brain Tumor Center, Hospital for Sick Children,
University of Toronto, Alan & Susan Hudson Chair in
Neurooncology, Toronto, ON, Canada
5 *Neurogenetics and the Molecular Biology of Human Brain Tumors*

Barton L. Guthrie, MD
Professor of Neurosurgery,
University of Alabama at Birmingham (UAB),
Birmingham, AL, USA
32 *Meningeal Hemangiopericytomas*

Georges F. Haddad, MD, FRCS(C)

Clinical Associate Professor of Neurosurgery, Department of Surgery, American University of Beirut, Beirut, Lebanon

33   Meningeal Sarcomas

Griffith R. Harsh IV, MD, MA, MBA

Professor and Vice-Chairman, Department of Neurosurgery, Stanford University School of Medicine, Stanford, CA, USA

19   Management of Recurrent Gliomas and Menigiomas
37   Chordomas and Chondrosarcomas of the Skull Base

Cynthia Hawkins, MD

Division of Neurosurgery, Department of Surgery, The Hospital for Sick Children, The University of Toronto, Toronto, ON, Canada

27   Medulloblastoma and Primitive Neuroectodermal Tumors

Eric C. Holland, MD, PhD

Attending Surgeon, Memorial Sloan Kettering Cancer Center, New York, NY, USA

17   Mouse Models for Brain Tumor Therapy

Lewis Hou, MD

Stanford Medical School, Stanford, CA, USA

19   Management of Recurrent Gliomas and Meningiomas

Kathryn Howe, MD, PhD

Division of Neurosurgery, Department of Surgery, University of Toronto, Division of Neurosurgery, University Hospital Network, Toronto Western Hospital, University of Toronto, Toronto, ON, Canada

7   Gene Therapy for Human Brain Tumors

Samar Issa, FRACP, FRCPA

Consultant Haematologist, Clinical Head, Lymphoma Service, Middlemore Hospital, Auckland, New Zealand

41   Primary Central Nervous System Lymphoma

John A. Jane, Jr, MD

Associate Professor of Neurosurgery and Pediatrics, Department of Neurosurgery, University of Virginia Health System, Charlottesville, VA, USA

36   Diagnostic Considerations and Surgical Results for Hyperfunctioning Pituitary Adenomas

Rashid M. Janjua, MD

Fellow Skull Base/Cerebrovascular Neurosurgery, University of South Florida, Tampa, FL, USA

38   Glomus Jugulare Tumors

Derek R. Johnson, MD

Neuro-oncologist, Department of Neurology, Mayo Clinic, Rochester, MN, USA

6   Biologic Therapy for Malignant Glioma

Bhadrakant Kavar, MBChB, FCS, FRACS

Neurosurgeon, The Royal Melbourne Hospital, Melbourne, VIC, Australia

43   Dermoid, Epidermoid and Neurenteric Cysts

Andrew H. Kaye, MB BS, MD, FRACS

Head of Department and James Stewart Professor of Surgery, Department of Surgery, The University of Melbourne; Director, Department of Neurosurgery, The Royal Melbourne Hospital, VIC, Australia

1   Historical Perspective
28   Acoustic Neurinoma (Vestibular Schwannoma)
39   Carcinoma of the Paranasal Sinuses
42   Craniopharyngioma
43   Dermoid, Epidermoid and Neurenteric Cysts
44   Colloid Cysts

James A. J. King, MB BS, PhD, FRACS

Neurosurgeon, The Royal Melbourne Hospital; Neurosurgeon, The Royal Children's Hospital; Senior Lecturer, Department of Surgery, The University of Melbourne, Melbourne, VIC, Australia

10   Advanced Imaging of Brain Tumors
24   Intracranial Ependymomas

Douglas Kondziolka, MD, MSc, FRCSC, FACS

Peter J. Jannetta Professor and Vice-Chairman of Neurological Surgery; Professor of Radiation Oncology; Director, Center for Brain Function and Behavior; Co-Director, Center for Image-Guided Neurosurgery, University of Pittsburgh, Pittsburgh, PA, USA

15   Radiosurgery and Radiotherapy for Brain Tumors

Abhaya V. Kulkarni, MD, PhD, FRCS(C)

Division of Neurosurgery, Hospital for Sick Children, Toronto, ON, Canada

24   Intracranial Ependymomas

John Laidlaw, MBBS, FRACS

Deputy Director, Department of Neurosurgery; Director Cerebrovascular Neurosurgery The Royal Melbourne Hospital, Melbourne, VIC, Australia

44   Colloid Cysts

Frederick F. Lang, MD

Professor and Director of Clinical Research, Department of Neurosurgery, The University of Texas M. D. Anderson Cancer Center, Houston, TX, USA

45   Metastatic Brain Tumors

Andrew B. Lassman, MD

Director, Fellowship Program in Neuro-oncology, Memorial Sloan-Kettering Cancer Center; Assistant Attending Neurologist, Memorial Hospital for Cancer & Allied Diseases, New York, NY, USA

17   Mouse Models for Brain Tumor Therapy

Edward R. Laws Jr, MD, FACS

Professor of Surgery, Harvard Medical School; Director, Pituitary and Neuroendocrine Center, Brigham and Women's Hospital, Boston, MA, USA

1   Historical Perspective
36   Diagnostic Considerations and Surgical Results for Hyperfunctioning Pituitary Adenomas

Commissioning Editor: Julie Goolsby
Development Editor: Alexandra Mortimer
Editorial Assistant: Poppy Garraway / Rachael Harrison
Project Manager: Mahalakshmi Nithyanand
Design: Lou Forgione
Illustration Manager: Merlyn Harvey
Illustrator: Philip Wilson and Ethan Danielson
Marketing Manager: Helena Mutak

BRAIN
TUMORS

An Encyclopedic Approach

THIRD EDITION

Michael J. Link, MD
Professor of Neurologic Surgery, Mayo Clinic,
Rochester, MN, USA
40 Esthesioneuroblastoma - Management and Outcome

Russell R. Lonser, MD
Chief, Surgical Neurology Branch,
National Institute of Neurological Disorders and Stroke,
National Institutes of Health, Bethesda, MD, USA
23 Brainstem Tumors
30 Brain Tumors Associated with Neurofibromatosis

M. Beatriz S. Lopes, MD, PhD
Professor of Pathology and Neurological Surgery,
University of Virginia School of Medicine;
Director of Neuropathology, University of Virginia Health
Systems, Charlottesville, VA, USA
9 Histopathology of Brain Tumors

L. Dade Lunsford, MD, FACS
Department of Neurological Surgery,
University of Pittsburgh, and the Center for Image-Guided
Neurosurgery, UPMC Presbyterian, Pittsburgh, PA, USA
15 Radiosurgery and Radiotherapy for Brain Tumors

Nicholas F. Maartens, MBChB, FRACS, FRCS, FRCS
Neurosurgeon, The Royal Melbourne Hospital, Parkville, VIC,
Australia
42 Craniopharyngiomas

J. Gordon McComb, MD
Professor and Chief, Division of Neurosurgery,
Children's Hospital of Los Angeles;
Department of Neurological Surgery, Keck School of Medicine,
University of Southern California, Los Angeles, CA, USA
26 Uncommon Glial Tumors

Scott A. Meyer, MD
Atlantic Neurosurgery Group,
Overlook Hospital, Summit,
NJ, USA
29 Other Schwannomas of Cranial Nerves

Eric J. Moore, MD
Associate Professor of Otorhinolaryngology,
Mayo Clinic, Rochester, MN, USA
40 Esthesioneuroblastoma: Management and Outcome

Andrew P. Morokoff, MBBS, PhD, FRACS
Senior Lecturer/Neurosurgeon, Department of Surgery,
The Royal Melbourne Hospital, The University of Melbourne,
Parkville, VIC, Australia
12 Epilepsy Associated with Brain Tumors
28 Acoustic Neurinoma (Vestibular Schwannoma)
39 Carcinoma of the Paranasal Sinuses

Edward C. Nemergut, MD
Associate Professor of Anesthesiology and Neurosurgery,
University of Virginia, Charlottesville, VA, USA
*13 Anesthesia and Intensive Care Management of Patients with
Brain Tumors*

Ajay Niranjan, MCh, MBA
Departments of Neurological Surgery and Radiation Oncology,
University of Pittsburgh, and the Center for Image-Guided
Neurosurgery, UPMC Presbyterian, Pittsburgh, PA, USA
15 Radiosurgery and Radiotherapy for Brain Tumors

Terence J. O'Brien, MBBS, MD, FRACP
James Stewart Professor of Medicine and Head of Department,
Department of Medicine, The Royal Melbourne Hospital;
University of Melbourne, Parkville, VIC, Australia
12 Epilepsy Associated with Brain Tumors

Kerry D. Olsen, MD
Professor of Otolaryngology,
Mayo Clinic, Rochester, MN, USA
40 Esthesioneuroblastoma: Management and Outcome

Robert G. Ojemann, MD
(Deceased), Professor of Surgery (Neurosurgery),
Harvard Medical School,
Senior Attending Neurosurgeon, Massachusetts General
Hospital, Boston, MA, USA
14 Surgical Principles in the Management of Brain Tumors

Claudia Petritsch, PhD
Assistant Adjunct Professor of Neurological Surgery,
University of California, San Francisco, CA, USA
*2 Stem Cells and Progenitor Cell Lineages as Targets for Neoplastic
Transformation in the Central Nervous System*

Kalmon D. Post, MD
Professor and Chairman Emeritus, Department of
Neurosurgery, Mount Sinai School of Medicine,
New York, NY, USA
29 Other Schwannomas of Cranial Nerves

Nader Pouratian, MD, PhD
Neurosurgeon, University of California, Los Angeles, CA, USA
16 Clinical Trials and Chemotherapy

Ivan Radovanovic, MD, PhD
Division of Neurosurgery, University Hospitals of Geneva,
Geneva, Switzerland
5 Neurogenetics and the Molecular Biology of Human Brain Tumors

Jesse Raiten, MD
Assistant Professor,
Department of Anesthesiology and Critical Care,
University of Pennsylvania, Philadelphia, PA, USA
*13 Anesthesia and Intensive Care Management of Patients with
Brain Tumors*

Jeffrey V. Rosenfeld, MD, MS, FRACS, FRCS(Ed), FACS
Professor and Head, Department of Surgery,
Monash University;
Director, Department of Neurosurgery,
The Alfred Hospital,
Melbourne, VIC, Australia
18 Management of Brain Tumors in the Pediatric Patient

Mark A. Rosenthal, MD, PhD

Director, Department of Medical Oncology,
The Royal Melbourne Hospital, Parkville, VIC, Australia

41   Primary Central Nervous System Lymphoma

Jonathan Roth, MD

Department of Pediatric Neurosurgery,
Dana Children's Hospital,
Tel-Aviv Medical Center, Tel Aviv, Israel

18   Management of Brain Tumors in the Pediatric Patient

James T. Rutka, MD, PhD, FRCSC

RS McLaughlin Professor and Chair of Surgery, University of
Toronto, Toronto, ON, Canada

7   Gene Therapy for Human Brain Tumors
27   Medulloblastoma and Primitive Neuroectodermal Tumors

Nader Sanai, MD

Department of Neurological Surgery,
University of California at San Francisco,
San Francisco, CA, USA

20   Low-Grade Astrocytomas

Atom Sarkar, MD, PhD

Department of Neurological Surgery,
The Ohio State University Medical Center, Columbus, OH, USA

21   Glioblastoma and Malignant Astrocytoma

Raymond Sawaya, MD

Professor and Chairman, Department of Neurosurgery,
Baylor College of Medicine;
Professor and Chairman, Department of Neurosurgery,
The University of Texas M.D. Anderson Cancer Center,
Houston, TX, USA

45   Metastatic Brain Tumors

Bernd W. Scheithauer, MD

Consultant in Pathology, Professor of Pathology,
Mayo Clinic, Rochester, MN, USA

9   Histopathology of Brain Tumors

David Schiff, MD

Harrison Distinguished Professor, Neuro-Oncology Center,
Departments of Neurology, Neurological Surgery and
Medicine, University of Virginia, Charlottesville, VA, USA

16   Clinical Trials and Chemotherapy

R. Michael Scott, MD

Director of Clinical Pediatric Neurosurgery,
Children's Hospital; Professor of Neurosurgery,
Harvard Medical School, Boston, MA, USA

25   Choroid Plexus Tumors

Mark E. Shaffrey, MD

David D. Weaver Professor and Chairman, Department of
Neurological Surgery, University of Virginia Health System,
Charlottesville, VA, USA

16   Clinical Trials and Chemotherapy

Adam M. Sonabend, MD

Neurological Surgery, Columbia University Medical Center,
New York, NY, USA

34   Pineal Cell and Germ Cell Tumors

Dima Suki, PhD

Associate Professor, Department of Neurosurgery,
The University of Texas M. D. Anderson Cancer Center,
Houston, TX, USA

45   Metastatic Brain Tumors

Kamal Thapar, MD, PhD, FRCSC

Neurosurgeon, Marshfield Clinic;
Medical Director, Department of Neurosurgery;
Chairman, Tertiary Care Services,
Sacred Heart Hospital, Eau Claire, WI, USA

*36   Diagnostic Considerations and Surgical Results for
Hyperfunctioning Pituitary Adenomas*

Robert H. Thiele, MD, FRCSC

Department of Anesthesiology,
University of Virginia, Charlottesville, VA, USA

*13   Anesthesia and Intensive Care Management of Patients with
Brain Tumors*

Harry R. van Loveren, MD

David W. Cahill Professor and Chairman of Neurosurgery,
Department of Neurosurgery and Brain Repair,
University of South Florida, Tampa, FL, USA

38   Glomus Jugulare Tumors

Scott R. VandenBerg, MD, PhD

Professor of Pathology; Director, Division of Neuropathology,
Department of Pathology, School of Medicine,
University of California, San Diego, La Jolla, CA, USA

*2   Stem Cells and Progenitor Cell Lineages as Targets for Neoplastic
Transformation in the Central Nervous System*

David G. Walker, MBBS(Hon), PhD, FRACS

Associate Professor, University of Queensland,
Briz Brain and Spine Neurosurgery, Brisbane, QLD, Australia

8   Immunology of Brain Tumors and Implications for Immunotherapy

Katherine E. Warren, MD

Head, Neuro-Oncology Section, Pediatric Oncology Branch,
National Cancer Institute, Bethesda, MD, USA

23   Brainstem Tumors
30   Brain Tumors Associated with Neurofibromatosis

Tanya Yuen, MBBS

Department of Neurosurgery, The Royal Melbourne Hospital;
Department of Surgery, The University of Melbourne,
Melbourne, VIC, Australia

12   Epilepsy Associated with Brain Tumors

Historical perspective

1

Andrew H. Kaye and Edward R. Laws Jr

The concept of a tumor of the brain is, for most individuals and many physicians as well, one of the most dramatic forms of human illness. Virtually every family has had some exposure to an individual suffering from a tumor of the brain, either within the family proper or within a circle of friends, relatives, and acquaintances. Brain tumors occur as the second most common form of malignancy in children and have a dramatic effect on the families involved. Among adults, primary tumors of the brain rank from 6th to 8th in frequency of all neoplasms, and tumors metastatic to the brain affect more and more individuals as methods for control of primary cancers become even more effective. The advent of AIDS and immunosuppression associated with organ transplants has led to an increased incidence of lymphomas of the brain.

Primary brain tumors account for about 2% of cancer deaths, but are responsible for 7% of the years of life lost from cancer before the age of 70. They are responsible for 20% of malignant tumors diagnosed before the age of 15. About 30% of deaths are due to cancer in western society, and one in five of these will have intracranial metastatic deposits at autopsy.

The revolutionary advances that have occurred in the diagnosis of brain tumors have led to an increased detection rate and a major increase in efficacy of surgical management. This is based on the exquisite detail of anatomic relationships afforded by modern imaging techniques. Additionally, there is evidence from epidemiologic studies that brain tumors are becoming increasingly more prevalent, especially as the population ages, and this increase appears to be in excess of the improvement in detection rates.

There has been an explosion in neuroscience related to the molecular biology and genetics of brain tumors, which should stimulate major advances in neurooncology. The characterization of genes and gene products related to neurofibromatosis has been a major advance. The identification of other promoter and suppressor genes operative in brain tumor pathogenesis has also occurred and has done much to elucidate basic mechanisms of tumorigenesis. The advent of gene therapy is an exciting therapeutic frontier with major possibilities. Other areas of intense research interest are monoclonal antibodies peculiar to various types of brain tumors and receptors characteristic of certain tumors that may be manipulated for diagnostic and therapeutic purposes.

Despite some earlier reports of surgical success, modern brain tumor surgery is generally thought to have commenced on November 25, 1884, when a London surgeon, Rickman Godlee, operated on a 25-year-old patient who suffered from focal motor epilepsy and progressive hemiparesis. The operation was performed at the Hospital for Paralysis, Regent's Park, London (Fig. 1.1) and the patient died 28 days after surgery, from meningitis. There has been some confusion regarding the name of this patient, and although the patient was thought to have been a 25-year-old Scottish farmer named Alexander Henderson, it is now considered it was most likely a John Mitchell who died on December 23, 1884. The patient had been under the care of Hughes Bennett, a neurologist on the staff of the hospital, who had diagnosed that the patient had a brain tumor which involved the cortical substance, was of limited size and situated in the neighborhood of the upper-third of the fissure of Rolando. The tumor had the histological characteristics of an oligodendroglioma 'about the size of a walnut'. Present at the operation were Hughlings Jackson, David Ferrier, Victor Horsley, and perhaps Joseph Lister himself. Rickman Godlee was the nephew of Lister, and Hughes Bennett's father was a well-known Professor of Medicine in Edinburgh who died following a lithotomy in 1875. At autopsy, a benign parietal lobe tumor was discovered and it is speculative whether this influenced Hughes Bennett's decision to suggest surgery for his patient.

Modern brain tumor surgery was made possible by three discoveries of the nineteenth century: anesthesia, asepsis and neurologic localization of cerebral lesions. Rickman Godlee's operation in 1884 was not the first time that a tumor had been removed, but it was the first occasion that a tumor had been localized solely by neurologic methods, and antiseptic surgical techniques had been utilized. Previously, tumors of the brain had been removed from time to time when they had deformed the skull, or when the skull had been trephined, usually for epilepsy or intractable headache, or where a scar or depressed fracture indicated the probable site of a lesion. Archeologists have found skulls with holes bored in them dating from the mesolithic or middle Stone Age period, as well as from neolithic times (Fig. 1.2). There is evidence that patients survived these operations as the holes in the bone are healed by new formation of bone tissue, and the sharp edges of the bored or hacked holes have become rounded off. Trephination was carried out by primitive peoples as late as the beginning of the

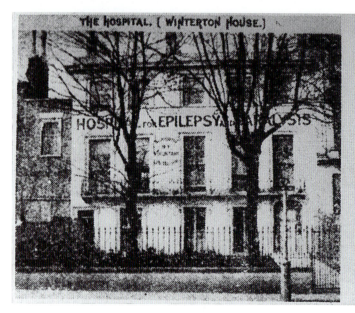

Figure 1.1 The Hospital for Epilepsy and Paralysis, Regent's Park, London, site of the first modern brain tumor operation in 1884. (From Spillane J, Doctrine of the Nerves: Chapters in the History of Neurology. Oxford University Press.)

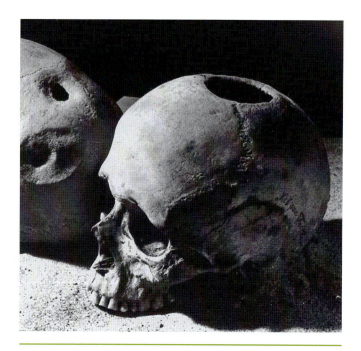

Figure 1.2 Trephined neolithic skull with evidence of new bone formation, indicating that the patient had survived the procedure. (From Lyons A S, Petrucelli J R II, Petrucelli R J, Medicine: An Illustrated History. Abradale Press, Australia.)

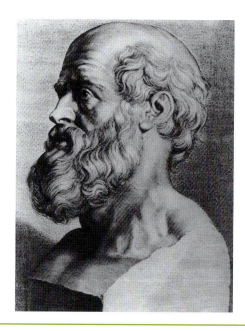

Figure 1.3 Hippocrates, who described trephination. (From K. Haeger, The Illustrated History of Surgery. Harold Starke Publishers.)

twentieth century. The Serbs of Albania and Montenegro trephined for neuralgia, migraine, psychosis, and other maladies, using a crude wire saw. In the South Sea Islands of the Pacific, trephining was relatively common, playing an important role in native custom. In the Bismarck Archipelago, the surgical instruments consisted of a tooth of a shark and a sharp shell. It is evident that although there may have been a medical basis to some of the cranial procedures,

many were performed for magical rather than medical reasons.

Hippocrates described trephination in detail, and advised it for headaches, epilepsy, fractures, and blindness (Fig. 1.3). The famous second century Chinese neurosurgeon Hua To performed trephination (Fig. 1.4). Hua To's most notorious patient was the warlord Kuan Yun, whose bitter enemy Tsao Tsao consulted Hua To with a headache. Hua To decided to trephine, but the patient thought that Hua To had been bribed by Kuan Yun to murder him. On this suspicion, Hua To was summarily executed.

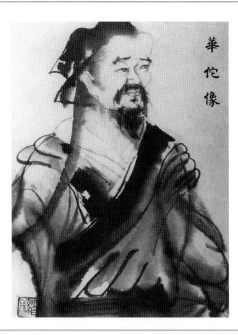

Figure 1.4 Hua To, the second century Chinese surgeon who practiced trephination.

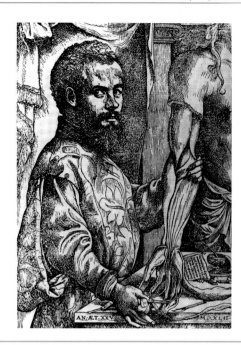

Figure 1.5 Andreas Vesalius, the 'patron saint' of Harvey Cushing. (From Lyons A S, Petrucelli J R II, Petrucelli R J, Medicine: An Illustrated History. Abradale Press.)

The foundation of modern neurology, which underpins neurosurgical practice, and especially brain tumor surgery, rests on the accomplishments of three men: Galen, Vesalius, and Willis. Galen (AD 130–200) was born in Pergamon on the shores of Asia Minor. It was in Pergamon that parchment was first used as a writing material and it was also famous for its medical temple of Asklepios. Often described as the first 'experimental physiologist', Galen became the personal physician to Marcus Aurelius. Many believe that Galen's neurology was the best feature of his medical system. His major works of neurologic interest include *De usu partium, De anatomicis administrationibus, De locis affectis*, and *De facultatibus naturabilus*. Galen described the corpus callosum, ventricles, sympathetic nerves, pituitary, infundibulum, and seven pairs of cranial nerves. His anatomy was based on dissection of animals, as at that time autopsy was forbidden. Galen's views dominated European medicine for 1500 years, and although it is a longstanding conventional belief that Galen shackled medical thought, he is unjustly blamed for the blind dependence on his writings, which were sanctified to the extent that any adverse opinion was regarded as heresy.

Andreas Vesalius (1514–1564; Fig. 1.5), known as the 'founder of anatomy', was appointed to the Chair of Surgery and Anatomy in Padua. His famous *De Fabrica* (*De Humani Corporis fabrica libri septem*) was published in Basle in 1543, when he was only 28 years old. The books are superbly illustrated by Jan Stephan Van Calcar, a favorite disciple of Titian. Book 7, on the brain, surpassed anything previously published and provide the foundations for much of modern neuroanatomy. Vesalius was Harvey Cushing's 'patron saint', and Cushing suffered his fatal anginal attack after lifting a heavy Vesalius portfolio.

Thomas Willis (1621–1675; Fig. 1.6) was the first 'inventor of the nervous system' and coined the word 'neurologie'. He is often described as the 'Harvey of the nervous system'.

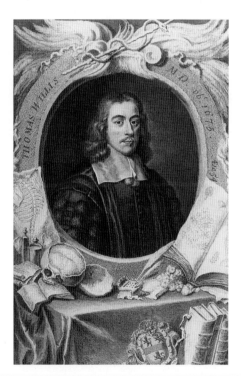

Figure 1.6 Thomas Willis, a portrait by Vertue, 1742, based on an engraving made in 1666. (From Thomas Willis, Anatomy of the Brain and Nerves. Classics of Neurology & Neurosurgery, Gryphon Editions.)

He was born in the village of Great Bedwyn, Wiltshire, and studied medicine at Oxford, graduating in 1646. He obtained the Chair in Natural Philosophy at Oxford, and his *Cerebri Anatomi* was published in 1664. His contributions to the knowledge of the anatomy of the brain are well established.

He suggested such terms as hemisphere, lobe, pyramid, corpus striatum, and peduncle; however, many believe that Willis's main contribution was that he realized that neurologic function depended primarily on the brain itself, its stuff and substance and not the hollows within it.

The concept of cerebral localization, which forms the basis of brain tumor surgery, was still in dispute up until the middle of the nineteenth century. Although these great men and others raised the possibility of some form of cerebral localization, the concept was still doubted by authorities no less brilliant than Brown-Séquard.

Broca's description of two patients with pure motor aphasia, in whom he had defined the pathologic findings, was confirmed by the experimental studies in animals by Fritsch and Hitzig in 1870 in Germany and by Ferrier in 1873 in London. The experimental results were reproduced in a human by Bartholow of Cincinnati in 1874. The opportunity for this remarkable experiment was afforded by a patient whose parietal bones had been destroyed by osteomyelitis caused by an ill-fitting wig that had eroded the skin and bone. Bartholow stimulated the rolandic areas of the brain by puncturing the dura with an electrode, inducing contralateral, local, and spreading contractions and even convulsions.

Suppuration, putrefaction, and infection had haunted surgeons up to and during the nineteenth century and prohibited any realistic possibility of intracranial, and especially intradural surgery for brain tumors. Following Pasteur's and Koch's proof of the bacterial origin of putrefaction, and a demonstration by Semmelweiss that sepsis could be controlled by hygienic means, hospitals gradually rid themselves of the unsanitary practices which fomented infection. Lister (Fig. 1.7), however, deserves the credit for developing the technique to prevent bacterial contamination of wounds during surgical procedures. He introduced carbolic acid 'initially in the form of creosote' on wounds and first reported on the treatment in *The Lancet* in 1867. This is regarded as the birthdate of antisepsis; intracranial surgery could henceforth be undertaken without the previous high likelihood of infection.

The introduction of anesthesia was a potent influence on surgery in general and neurosurgery in particular. William Morton demonstrated the use of ether on October 16, 1846, which is still celebrated as 'ether day' in the original operating room at the Massachusetts General Hospital in Boston. With the patient asleep, it became possible to perform long delicate operations, such as neurosurgical procedures.

An understanding of the pathology of brain tumors was essential before intracranial surgery for these tumors could advance. A new period of rapid advance in knowledge is often consequent upon the discovery of a novel approach or development of a new instrument. The grinding of improved lenses by Amici in 1827 led directly to the development of a well-corrected compound microscope that made possible the recognition of the cell as a basic unit of living matter. Shortly after, Schleiden and Schwann developed the cell theory, and Virchow enunciated the concept that the fundamental changes in human disease can be traced to alterations in cells. Virchow, known during his time as the 'Pope of medicine', was the first to describe the neuroglia and to classify brain tumors, with 'gliomas' as a separate entity (Fig. 1.8).

By the end of the nineteenth century, the development of neurology, neurologic localization of cerebral tumors, anesthesia, antisepsis, and a basic understanding of the histology of brain tumors had laid the groundwork for the successful operations for cerebral tumors. By 1900, however, the initial enthusiasm over the pioneering operations had waned and at the turn of the century, cerebral tumors were only operated on as a last resort. Until the 1920s there was little knowledge of the varied histologic appearance of the gliomas and their correlated clinical course. In an attempt

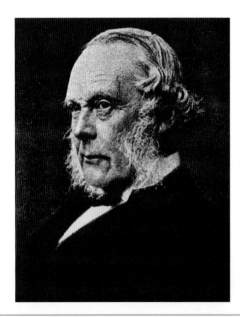

Figure 1.7 Lord Joseph Lister, who introduced antiseptic techniques in 1867.

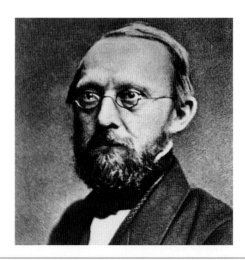

Figure 1.8 Rudolph Virchow. (From the World Health Organization, Geneva.)

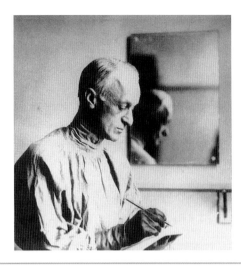

Figure 1.9 Harvey Cushing. (From A Bibliography of the Writings of Harvey Cushing, 1939. Kessinger Publishing.)

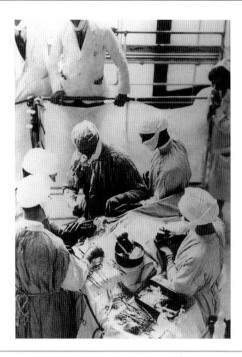

Figure 1.10 Cushing's 2000th brain tumor operation. (From A Bibliography of the Writings of Harvey Cushing, 1939. Kessinger Publishing.)

to improve the surgical treatment of brain tumors, and to determine if treatment should vary with the type of tumor, Bailey and Cushing studied the histologic appearance of gliomas and classified them on a histogenetic basis. It was Harvey Cushing (Figs 1.9, 1.10) who introduced the methodical (although at times slow), meticulous technique of Halsted to neurosurgical operations. William Macewen, in 1879, was the first to successfully remove an intracranial neoplasm, a meningioma invading the frontal bone, and the first successfully treated meningioma in the USA was removed by William W. Keen in December 1887. It was Cushing who coined the term 'meningioma' in 1922, describing the tumor identified by Virchow in 1854 as 'fungus of the dura mater', which he had called a sarcoma.

The improvement in the treatment of patients with brain tumors since the operation by Godlee in November 1884 has been related to the advances in surgical techniques, the introduction of adjuvant therapies, the revolution in imaging brain tumors, and an improved understanding of the biology of these tumors. More recently, brain tumor research has concentrated on understanding the pathogenesis of the tumors, investigating the multiple facets of biology of the tumors, and studying new treatment methods. Investigations using molecular biology and cell biology techniques have focused on the intricate and complex orchestra of activities in the normal cells and what disturbances are necessary to produce the cascade of events that results in the development of a tumor cell.

Advances in surgical techniques now usually allow a safe and atraumatic excision of a brain tumor. Standard neurosurgical equipment includes ultrasonic aspiration devices and lasers of a wide range of wavelengths, which enable their ablative properties to be tailored to the particular tumor type. Stereotactic equipment has enabled a safer and more accurate exposure of deep intracranial tumors, and when combined with the laser, allows a precise excision of deep cerebral tumors in eloquent and dangerous positions. By 1920, radiation therapy was being used for the treatment of cerebral gliomas. This first adjuvant therapy is still the mainstay of treatment for cerebral glioma, the most common type of brain tumor. During the twentieth century, many other adjuvant therapies such as chemotherapy, immunotherapy, hyperthermia, and photodynamic therapy have been introduced with varying degrees of success. Although in some circumstances the therapy may help control the tumor for a while, none has been shown to be curative. There is now cause for cautious optimism with a better understanding of the pathogenesis and biology of brain tumors, improvements in imaging and surgical techniques, and especially the development of gene therapies.

FURTHER READING

Greenblatt, **S.H.**, 1997. A history of neurosurgery. American Association of Neurological Surgeons, Park Ridge, IL.

Walker, **A.E.**, 1951. A history of neurological surgery. Williams & Wilkins, Baltimore, MD.

Walker, **A.E.**, 1998. The genesis of neuroscience. American Association of Neurological Surgeons, Park Ridge, IL.

2

Stem cells and progenitor cell lineages as targets for neoplastic transformation in the central nervous system

Claudia Petritsch and Scott R. VandenBerg

Introduction

The conceptual link between immature neural cells arising during development and the parenchymal CNS tumors was an implicit hypothesis in the 'histogenetic' basis for the classification of gliomas published over 75 years ago by Bailey and Cushing (Bailey & Cushing 1926; Bailey 1948). Parenchymal tumors arising from the neuroepithelium of the CNS were assigned to groups that were organized by the histologic cell type constituting the neoplasm, and these cell populations were typically defined in terms of presumptive developmental origins within the brain. Nearly 25 years ago, Rubinstein hypothesized that a combination of factors contributed to the development and progression of parenchymal CNS tumors, including (1) the existence of a reserve population of neural stem cells; (2) the capability of differentiated neural cells to proliferate; (3) the number of replicating cells at risk for transforming events and the duration of that 'window of neoplastic vulnerability'; (4) the state of differentiation and differentiation potential of that population; and (5) the plasticity of differentiation manifested by successive cell generations (Rubinstein 1987). This concept is even more relevant in the current discussion of the role for neural stem and progenitor cell lineages in the development and growth of parenchymal CNS tumors in the adult. For the primitive or embryonal-type of neoplasms arising in the CNS, Rubinstein suggested a cytogenetic scheme to serve as a frame of reference for a classification of embryonal CNS tumors that would account for the different histological entities and for the range of and the restrictions on their differentiating capabilities with the implicit assumption that these tumors, by their association with a developing and immature nervous system, arose from neural stem cells or multiple progenitor cell lineages with varying capacities for cellular differentiation (Rubinstein 1972, 1985). Significant progress has been made from the formulation of these insightful, but largely hypothetical, conceptual frameworks to a better understanding of the biology of stem cells and the differentiation of proliferative progenitor cell lineages in the developing and adult brain. More recently, similar techniques have been applied to both experimental murine and human CNS tumors. The availability of defined growth factor supplements applied to the widespread use of non-adherent neurosphere cultures; high resolution morphologic techniques using more precise biomarkers and cell lineage tracking applied to intact tissue; and cell-specific conditional gene expression using mouse models have played important roles in these advances.

Neural stem cells and stem cells in CNS tumors

General considerations

The specific properties of neural stem cells with respect to proliferative activity, cellular populations and location are highly regulated in both a temporal and spatial fashion throughout the neuraxis (Corbin et al 2008; Emmenegger & Wechsler-Reya 2008). However, neural stem cells are defined by a set of generic features: (1) self-renewing (symmetric cell division) with a capacity to undergo lineage commitment and generate progenitor cell populations (asymmetric cell divisions) that have variable potentials to differentiate into cells with neuronal, astrocytic, oligodendroglial and possibly ependymal phenotypes; (2) expression of specific sets of neural biomarkers (Table 2.1); and (3) distinct *in vitro* growth requirements, including non-adherent conditions. Implicit in these generic features would be that (1) different intrinsic signaling pathways that would regulate these properties, depending on the specific neural stem cell or progenitor cell populations and (2) neural stem cells are highly regulated by their niche or microenvironment (Kim & Dirks 2008), and may be slowly proliferating with a prolonged cycling time, depending on the location and age. Several similarities and distinctions can be made when considering stem cells in CNS tumors. First, the brain tumor stem cells would also be capable of self-renewal and variable asymmetric cell divisions to produce the cell populations which comprise the specific phenotypes within a specific tumor type. In addition, the brain tumor stem cells, while capable of self-renewal may not be the most rapidly proliferating cell population within the tumors, analogous to adult neural stem cells in specific niches. However, an important distinction must be made between the stem cell(s) which initiate tumor development and the stem cells that can essentially propagate the tumors. The first type of tumor stem cell (i.e., the initiating cells) can only be studied in experimental animal models, whereas the self-renewing stem cells that can be isolated from growing tumors can be studied in both experimental models and in human tumors. These tumor propagating cells may vary in their degree of lineage commitment from multipotent stem cells to more committed progenitor cells. The properties of the tumor-initiating cells in human brain tumors can only be inferred from experimental animal models and from the properties of the self-renewing, primitive cells isolated from human tumor tissue. Therefore in this chapter, the phrase 'brain tumor stem cell'

Table 2.1 Biomarkers associated with specific central neural cell types

Cell type	Biomarker expression
Multipotential neural stem cells	Nestin, GFAP, LeX/CD15, MSI1&2, Hes1&5, PDGFRα, CD133/PROM1, SOX2, MCM2, OLIG2
Transit amplifying cells	LeX/CD15, OLIG2, DLX2, EGFR++, NG2 (?), absence of GFAP
Radial glia	GLAST, RC2 ,PAX6, BLBP
Ependymal cells	CD24
Oligodendroglial progenitors	OLIG2, NG2, PDGFRα, O4 (late progenitor, after NG2), GT3 ganglioside/A$_2$B$_5$ (bi-potential glial progenitor)
Neuroblasts/neuronal progenitors	PSA-NCAM (migrating neuroblasts), DCX (Type A cells and migrating neuroblasts), β-III tubulin and MAP2 (committed progenitors)
Mature astrocytes	GLAST, GFAP
Mature oligodendrocytes	MBP, GalC, Rip/CNP, PLP
Mature neurons	NeuN, NFP H/M (SMI-31/33); NSE

BLBP, brain lipid-binding protein; CD133/PROM1, prominin-1; DCX, doublecortin; DLX2, distal-less homeobox 2; EGFR, epidermal growth factor receptor; GalC, galactosylceramidase; GFAP, glial fibrillary acidic protein; GLAST, glial high affinity glutamate transporter; LeX/CD15, LewisX glycosphingolipid/3-fucosyl-N-acetyl-lactosamine; MAP2, microtubuleassociated protein 2; MBP, myelin basic protein; MCM2, minichromosome maintenance complex component 2; MSI1 & 2, Musashi homolog1 & 2; NFP H/M, neurofilament protein; NG2, chondroitin sulfate proteoglycan (CSPG); NSE, neuron-specific enolase; OLIG2, oligodendrocyte lineage transcription factor 2; PAX6, paired box 6; PDGFRα, platelet-derived growth factor receptor, alpha polypeptide; PLP, proteolipid protein 1; PSA-NCAM, neural cell adhesion molecule; RC2, intermediate filament associated protein (Mus musculus); Rip/CNP, 2′,3′-cyclic nucleotide 3′ phosphodiesterase; SOX2, SRY (sex determining region Y)-box 2.

is intended to connote the tumor-initiating and the brain tumor-propagating stem cells and these cells may specifically differ among the various types of intrinsic brain tumors.

Isolation of brain tumor stem cells in tumorspheres

Brain tumor stem cells were first isolated by their ability to grow spheroid structures called tumorspheres under non-adhesive conditions. This technique was originally used to isolate neural stem cells from several areas of the developing and adult brain based on their formation of large adherent clones and non-adherent spheroid structures that are neurospheres. In response to serum-free, epidermal growth factor (EGF) and basic fibroblastic growth factor (bFGF) conditions (Reynolds & Weiss 1992, 1996; Vescovi et al 1993), embryonic and adult neural stem cells when grown as neurospheres retain their ability to undergo extensive self-renewal and to differentiate into multiple brain cells. Clonal neurosphere assays proved to be very useful in isolating and characterizing brain tumor stem cells retrospectively from pediatric anaplastic astrocytoma and glioblastoma and from adult anaplastic astrocytoma, glioblastoma and oligodendroglioma.

A sub-population of cells within dissociated high-grade glioma formed tumorspheres, whereas the remaining bulk of tumor cells exhibited adherence, loss of proliferation, and subsequent differentiation under neurosphere-forming conditions. Importantly, tumorspheres showed extensive self-renewal and proliferation compared with control neurospheres (Singh et al 2003) and generate a sufficiently large number of progeny that can differentiate upon growth factor withdrawal into astrocytes, oligodendrocytes and neurons (Galli et al 2004). High-grade astrocytic tumors predominantly express a set of markers characteristic for

glial progenitors and neuronal progenitors and mature astrocytes, whereas mature neurons and oligodendrocytes are extremely rare in high-grade gliomas (Liu et al 2004; Rebetz et al 2008). Tumorspheres from human astrocytic tumors variably differentiate into GFAP positive astrocyte-like cells and rarely into β-III-tubulin-positive immature neuronal cells and GalC-positive oligodendroglial cells *in vitro* (Galli et al 2004; Singh et al 2003). Thus, despite their multipotentiality, tumorspheres preserve the heterogeneous and somewhat restricted and aberrant differentiation potential found in human gliomas. Tumorspheres from a mouse model of high-grade oligodendroglioma, the S100beta-*verbB* p53–/– mice (Weiss et al 2003), primarily give rise to NG2-positive oligodendrocyte progenitor-like cells that fail to further differentiate into mature oligodendrocytes. Although there is variable potential for differentiation among individual high-grade tumors, clonally derived tumorspheres from a given tumor gave rise to similar percentages of glial and neuronal cells. Taken together, these observations suggest that the brain tumor stem cell population within a given tumor is homogeneous. In summary, tumorsphere formation allows for the preservation of the unique malignant features of tumor-inducing cells and the heterogeneity observed between tumor-initiating cells from different tumors. It is therefore an extremely valid assay to isolate and propagate the tumor-initiating population from human, and more recently, from murine brain tumors.

Brain tumor stem cell surface markers

Phenotypic cell isolation strategies that are based on fluorescence-labeled cell surface proteins have been adapted to separate small subpopulations of tumor cells. Human glioma and glioma-derived tumorspheres variably express stem cell-related genes. Of particular interest is the cell surface marker CD133, which is the human homologue of an evolutionary conserved protein prominin-1 (PROM-1). Most PROM-1/CD133 variants are broadly expressed and several splice variants of prominin-1 are differentially expressed in brain cells (Corbeil et al 2009). Expression of a variant of PROM-1/CD133, which is recognized by the AC133 antibody, is more restricted to immature cells and has been used to isolate neuroepithelial progenitors, embryonic neural stem cells from the ventricular zone and the postnatal cerebellum (Corbeil et al 1998; Corbeil et al 2000; Lee et al 2005; Uchida et al 2000) and brain tumor stem cells from adult glioblastoma (Singh et al 2003, 2004a,b). Recent data from one laboratory (Yang et al 2008) showed that tumors from a mouse model of medulloblastoma, the *Patched* mutant mouse, are propagated not by CD133+ neural stem cells but by cells expressing the progenitor markers Math1 and CD15/LeX. CD15/LeX Math1 double positive cells have increased proliferative capacity, but decreased apoptosis and differentiation. CD15/LeX-positive cells are also found in a subset of human medulloblastomas with a poorer prognosis (Read et al 2009). These data suggest that the PROM-1/CD133+ cancer stem cell population and the tumor-propagating cells may be distinct and that some human tumors may be propagated by a progenitor-like tumor cell population. Lastly, not all cancer stem cells are PROM-1/CD133 positive and PROM-1/CD133 expression is downregulated in neural stem cells in the adult sub-ventricular zone (Corti et al 2007; Pfenninger et al 2007). The origin of the PROM-1/CD133 positive cells in human glioblastoma is therefore yet to be determined. One possibility is that they arise from neural stem cells that up-regulate PROM-1/CD133 expression in response to oncogenic mutations.

Brain tumor stem cells and heterogeneous tumor cell populations

Two models have been put forward to explain tumor initiation, cellular heterogeneity and the nature of drug-resistant brain tumor cells. The conventional view of brain tumorigenesis is summarized by the *stochastic model*, which predicts that each cell within the tumor is malignant, and is capable of both initiating and maintaining growth by the generation of neoplastic clones that equally contribute to recurrence following therapeutic intervention (Fig. 2.1A). Tumor cells would have various proliferation potentials and proliferate with stochastic probability. This heterogeneity has been attributed to genomic instability introduced by the initial oncogenic mutation and the selection for cells that can best adapt to the tumor microenvironment. Typically, tumors that recur after an initial response to chemotherapy are resistant to multiple drugs (multi-drug resistance). In the conventional view of tumorigenesis, one or several cells within a tumor acquire genetic changes that confer drug resistance. These cells have a selective advantage, which allows them to overtake the population of tumor cells with fewer mutations.

The second, more recent model is the *hierarchical model* of tumorigenesis or 'cancer stem cell' model (Fig. 2.1B). It hypothesizes that a defined subset of cells, the 'cancer stem cells', has the exclusive ability to initiate and maintain neoplastic growth, and to generate recurrent tumors. The cancer stem cell pool grows tumors in a series of hierarchical cell divisions that generate phenotypically heterogeneous cells similar to the normal brain cell lineages. Prototypic brain tumor stem cells would maintain themselves by dividing relatively slowly in self-renewing divisions

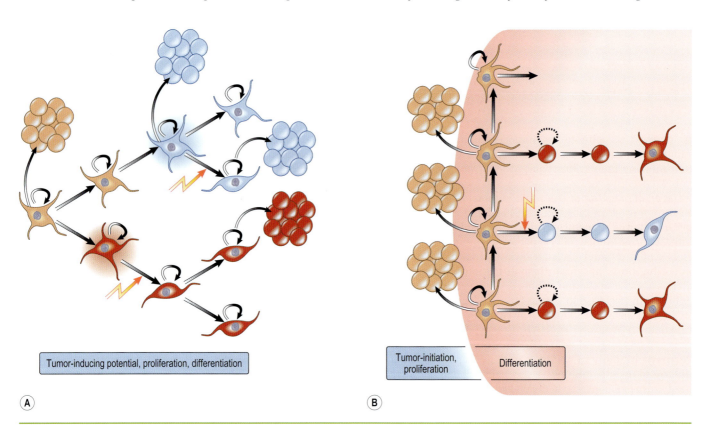

(A)   (B)

Figure 2.1 The stochastic and hierarchical cell model of tumorigenesis. (A) The traditional, stochastic model proposes that all tumor cells are uniformly capable of proliferation (curved arrow) and initiation of neoplastic growth (clones). Not all cells within a tumor divide at the same time but enter proliferation at a stochastic rate. The tumor-initiating cell is a mature brain cell targeted by an oncogenic mutation (red arrow) rather than an immature cell. The cell carrying the mutation is genomically unstable and divides to generate progeny, which is prone to acquire additional mutations (red arrow). These distinct genetic mutations in addition to signals from the microenvironment (shaded circles) select for certain tumor cell types and thereby induce tumor cell heterogeneity. (B) The hierarchical model claims that only a subpopulation of tumor cells due to their stem cell properties can proliferate extensively, induce and sustain tumor growth. Tumor-initiating cells (yellow) are immature cells such as stem cells or progenitors, which have been targeted by an oncogenic mutation, have developed extensive proliferation and self-renewal capacity (curved arrow) and induce and maintain a heterogeneous tumor by dividing along hierarchical lineages. Similar to normal neural stem cells, tumor-initiating stem cells might reside within a niche (pink shaded area), which provides the proper microenvironment to allow for extensive self-renewal and proliferation. First, they self-renew and generate progenitor-like cells with limited proliferative capacity (curved, dashed arrows). These progenitors then generate phenotypically diverse, differentiating cells, which eventually cease to divide. As tumor cells progress and differentiate along this lineage they lose tumor-initiating potential (blue shaded triangle).

but simultaneously giving rise to highly-proliferative progenitor-like cells and phenotypically diverse, non-tumorigenic, cells with limited proliferative potential (Vescovi et al 2006). It is feasible that genomic instability within the cancer stem cell population leads to the accumulation of additional mutations that further increase tumor heterogeneity. In this model, the cancer stem cells are more resistant to treatments that are solely aimed at highly proliferative cell pools, such as radiation and cytotoxic drugs, and survive these conventional treatments to re-establish tumor growth (Bao et al 2006; Sakariassen et al 2007). In addition, brain tumor stem cells, like non-neoplastic neural stem cells, might express high levels of ABC transporters that would confer multi-drug resistance (Vescovi et al 2006).

The cancer stem cell hypothesis

Two experimental observations have especially supported the cancer stem cell hypothesis. First, large numbers of cells (>200 000), either directly harvested from primary tumor tissue or derived from cell lines that have been established by routine adherent, serum supplemented culture techniques are required to produce xenografts in immunosuppressed mice. This biologic behavior is at odds with the traditional, stochastic model (Bruce & Van Der Gaag 1963; Hamburger & Salmon 1977). Second, serum-cultured cell lines derived from high-grade human gliomas, do not represent all phenotypic characteristics and the multitude of genetic aberrations present in the corresponding primary human tumor (Lee et al 2006). One explanation would be that the adherent, serum-containing culture conditions used to establish human tumor cell lines actually select against tumor-initiating cells or irreversibly alter their malignant potential. Alternatively, only sub-populations of tumor cells might have sufficient proliferative capacity to produce tumor xenografts, and culture conditions with the presence of serum might select against these malignant subpopulations. Additional support of the hierarchical model of tumorigenesis is provided by the phenotypic heterogeneity and distinct proliferation capacity of the cancer cells that is reminiscent of normal brain stem cell lineages.

Neural stem cells/progenitors in the developing human brain

During early CNS development in mammals, there is a progressive axial restriction of the neural plate and developing neuroepithelium such that distinct topographic fields give rise to the neuroretina, forebrain, midbrain, and hindbrain (Nowakowski & Hayes 2005). The genetic and epigenetic events which determine this axial map are associated with the expression of a variety of transcriptional factors (TF) from all the major superfamilies, including homeodomain, paired-domain, basic helix–loop–helix (bHLH), winged helix, nuclear orphan receptor, Ets, zinc finger, and T-domain families. These TFs often interact to determine neural stem cell self-renewal and proliferative capacity, and the switch to radial glial cells (secondary neural stem cell) and the ultimate commitment to lineage differentiation of progenitor

cells in a regional and niche-specific manner (Alvarez-Buylla et al 2008; Boncinelli et al 1988; Gilbertson & Gutmann 2007; Hevner 2006; Toth et al 1987; Tropepe et al 2001; Wright et al 1989; Westerman et al 2003). One bHLH factor OLIG2 has documented regulatory activity in both normal and tumor stem cells. OLIG2, plays a major role in the regulation of ventral neuroepithelial cell fate and progenitor oligodendrogenesis, possibly via downregulation of Wnt-signaling, during development and also in the adult CNS (Ahn et al 2008; Dimou et al 2008; Ligon et al 2006). OLIG2 expression is diffusely present in adult gliomas, and also may be a critical lineage-specific determinate of proliferative capacity in both normal and tumorigenic CNS stem cell populations, as demonstrated in a mouse model of malignant glioma (Ligon et al 2007). It is important to note, however, that developmental regulation by transcription factors may differ between primates and non-primate mammals (Mo & Zecevic 2008). A number of the transcription factors, along with other biomolecules, have been used as markers for neural stem cells, progenitor lineages and differentiated neural cells (Table 2.1).

The discovery of neural stem-like cells in both experimental animal and human brain tumors has encouraged researchers to focus on germinal zones within the developing brain and neural stem cell niches in adult brain. The developing fields that are particularly relevant to most primitive/embryonal-like tumors in humans are the retinal neuro-progenitors arising from the retinal neuroepithelium, the cerebellar ventricular zone and the adjacent, more dorsal rhombic lip germinal zone (Wechsler-Reya & Scott 2001) and in the forebrain, a ventricular zone or germinal matrix. Within the forebrain, this matrix ultimately develops into the lateral sub-ventricular zone that has both a temporal and regional heterogeneity with respect to the numbers of neural stem cells and types of progenitor cell populations (Alvarez-Buylla et al 2008), and into a sub-granular layer of the hippocampal dentate gyrus (Li et al 2009).

Tumors arising in the developing brain

Retinal development and retinoblastoma

The retinoblastoma, the most common of the pediatric intraocular tumors, is the only multipotential stem cell tumor of the CNS for which the initiating genetic basis of neoplastic transformation is definitively understood. The transforming event occurs within the immature retina when both alleles of the *Rb* tumor suppressor gene are inactivated within a single cell (Gallie et al 1990; Gennett & Cavenee 1990). Although the tumor commonly exhibits fields of poorly-differentiated small cells with scant, ill-defined cytoplasm, the majority of tumors contain the more typical rosettes associated with either primitive neuroblastic or neurosensory differentiation (Fig. 2.2). Less common are the more highly-differentiated 'fleurettes', which manifest photosensory phenotypic differentiation. Although the presence of these structures with more cytoarchitectural differentiation generally does not have any predictive value for the clinical behavior of these tumors, rare tumors that are entirely composed of rosettes and have an overall reduced cellularity,

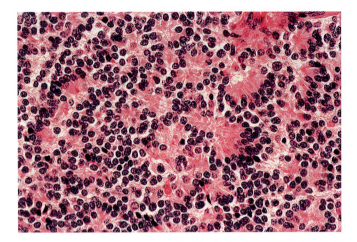

Figure 2.2 Retinoblastoma. The histopathologic appearance of these tumors is often a combination of patternless sheets of primitive cells admixed with the typical rosettes illustrated in this microscopic field. Although the formation of these structures implies an early stage of cellular differentiation, the expression of either photosensory phenotypes or neuronal intermediate filaments is not specifically localized to these structures (H&E).

appear to have a reduced malignant potential. These neoplasms have been designated 'retinocytomas' (Margo et al 1983) to distinguish their different clinical behavior.

The retinoblastoma, as a tumor arising after transformation of an immature progenitor cell in the inner retinal neuroepithelium, clearly gives rise to phenotypes that are associated with the selective regional determination of retinal cell lineages (Gonzalez-Fernandez et al 1992). The normal development of the retina involves multiple topographic considerations. One of the earliest events is the formation of the inner, primitive neuroretinal epithelium and an outer, pigmented epithelium. These two progenitor fields arise when the primitive germinal neuroepithelium of the forebrain forms the inner and outer layers of the optic cup. This appears to be accompanied by the differential, patterned expression of paired box- and homeobox genes in the neuroretinal epithelium (Levine & Green 2004; Martin et al 1992). Within the early developing retina, the primitive neuroretinal cells appear to exert inductive control over the development of the pigmented cells in the outer layer (Buse et al 1993) and the retinal pigmented cells produce factor(s) which affect survival, proliferation and maturation of the retinal progenitor cells (Sheedlo & Turner 1996).

Although *in vitro* culture studies have demonstrated various degrees of plasticity in the formation of both non-neoplastic (Buse & de Groot 1991; Buse et al 1993) and neoplastic (Gonzalez-Fernandez et al 1992) neuroretinal and pigmented epithelial derivatives, examination of retinoblastomas *in situ* strongly suggests that these tumors arise from a loss of normal *Rb* function in a primitive neuroretinal cell rather than from a generally pluripotential neuroepithelial cell. An immature neuroretinal cell, as the putative target for neoplastic transformation, would normally maintain the potential for selective divergent differentiation (Fig. 2.3) (Holt et al 1988; Turner & Cepko 1987; Wetts & Fraser 1988). A study using human retinoblastoma primary tissue

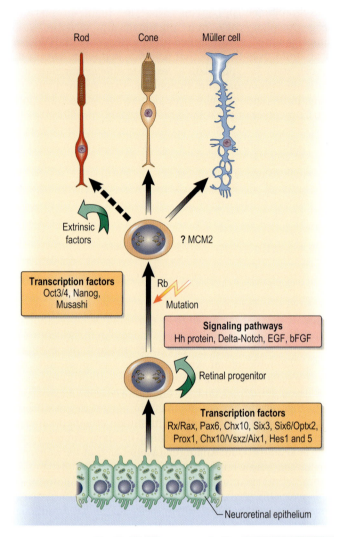

Figure 2.3 Model of retinoblastoma cytogenesis. Divergent phenotypic restriction normally occurs late (following the last mitotic cycle) in the neuroretinal progenitor cell population. The probable target cell in which the *Rb* mutation occurs is a multipotential neuroretinal cell which has not entered its final mitotic cycle. The proliferative retinal progenitor cells are regulated by a number of signaling pathways and transcriptional factors. The retinoblastoma stem cell expresses a number of stem cell transcription factors, including Oct3/4, Nanog, and Musashi. Both groups of intrinsic neuroretinal cells (neurosensory with IRBP/opsin expression and Müller glia with CRA1BP expression) can arise from the transformed progenitor cells. The cone phenotype would be the most probable neurosensory phenotype since it does not appear to be dependent on the extrinsic signals. Alternatively, rod phenotypic expression is dependent on the presence of normal extrinsic signals that would be frequently disrupted in the tumor environment. (Other neuronal phenotypes that would arise from the transformed progenitors are omitted from this scheme for clarity.)

and established cell lines has demonstrated the neural retinal stem cell nature of retinoblastomas by the presence of stem cell markers, including minichromosome maintenance factor 2 (Mcm2), and tumorsphere generation (Seigel et al 2007). The control of cell proliferation in the retinal progenitor cells is highly regulated by a number of signaling pathways, including those receptors activated by Hedgehog,

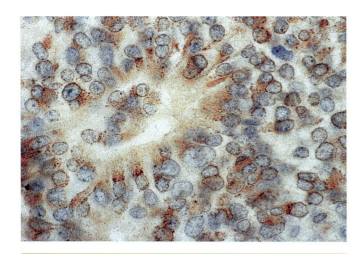

Figure 2.4 Retinoblastoma. Interphotoreceptor retinoid binding protein (IRBP) is the earliest photoreceptor-associated protein demonstrated in retinoblastoma. Its cytoplasmic localization tends to be polarized in the cell. In rosettes and fleurettes, IRBP is particularly present in the apical cell border. (IRBP (RB 504) avidin–biotin immunoperoxidase.)

Delta, EGF, bFGF. The subsequent mechanisms controlling cellular differentiation are tightly orchestrated with the number of cell divisions and the exit from the cell cycle (Giordano et al 2007; Levine & Green 2004; Wallace 2008). Although there is relatively minimal horizontal dispersion of the radially arrayed progenitor cells in primitive neuroretina (Price 1989), there is no divergence of progenitor cells to produce distinct glial and neuronal/neurosensory clones. In contrast to other germinal matrix zones in the forebrain, a diverse array of phenotypes (photoreceptor, neurons, and Müller cells) are generated from retinal progenitor cells following the final mitotic cycle (Turner & Cepko 1987; Holt et al 1988; Wetts & Fraser 1988).

The expression of photoreceptor (Figs 2.4–2.6) and Müller cell (retinal glia) (Figs 2.7, 2.8) associated proteins in retinoblastomas clearly demonstrates the unique regional derivation of these tumors (Gonzalez-Fernandez et al 1992; Holt et al 1988; Turner & Cepko 1987; Wetts & Fraser 1988) and is particularly valuable in the study of specific cell types in retinoblastomas. Inter-photoreceptor retinoid binding protein (IRBP), and cone and rod opsins have strictly defined temporal patterns of expression during normal retinal differentiation. The expression of IRBP occurs very early during neuroretinal development and is normally upregulated before opsin (Gonzalez-Fernandez & Healy 1990; Hauswirth et al 1992; Liou et al 1991). In a series of 22 retinoblastomas (Gonzalez-Fernandez et al 1992), IRBP was detected in over half the tumors (Fig. 2.4), while nearly 70% of the tumors which contained immunoreactive cone (Fig. 2.5) or rod opsin (Fig. 2.6) also demonstrated IRBP. Overall, rod opsin expression was far more restricted in the neoplastic cells than that of either IRBP or cone opsin. This differential expression of cone and rod neoplastic cellular phenotypes corresponds to the normal predominance of cone over rod phenotypes, wherein cone differentiation appears to result from a 'default' mechanism (Adler & Hatlee 1989; Raymond 1991). This suggests that lineage determination by early autonomous commitment of specific cell lineages persists even after

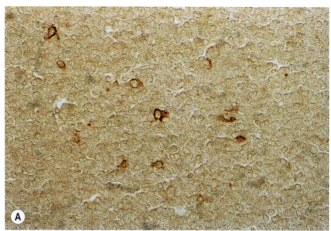

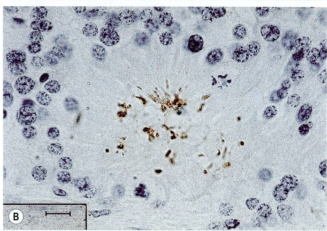

Figure 2.5 Retinoblastoma. (A) Cone opsin can be identified within the more amorphous cellular groups of the retinoblastomas. (B) The most specific localization of cone opsin is in cytoplasmic processes which protrude into the lumen of fleurettes. (Cone opsin (CERN 874) avidin–biotin immunoperoxidase.)

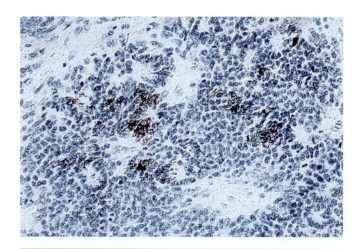

Figure 2.6 Retinoblastoma. Rod opsin is less commonly present in retinoblastomas than cone opsin. Rod opsin is localized both in the cells that form rosettes and in cells within the more amorphous areas of the tumor. (Rod opsin (CERN JS85) avidin–biotin immunoperoxidase.)

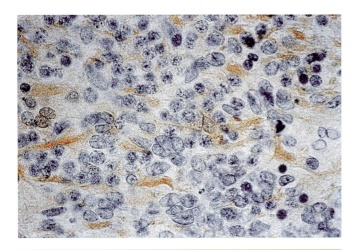

Figure 2.7 Retinoblastoma. Intrinsic glial cell (Müller cell) differentiation within retinoblastomas is accompanied by the presence of cellular retinaldehyde binding protein (CRA1BP) in tumor cells. Unlike the photoreceptor-associated proteins (IRBP, cone and rod opsins), CRA1BP is never localized within neoplastic specialized photosensory structures. (CRA1BP avidin–biotin immunoperoxidase.)

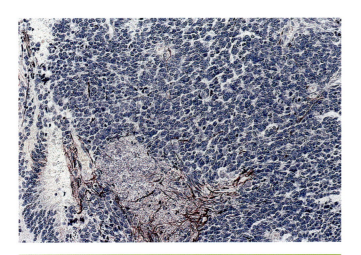

Figure 2.8 Retinoblastoma. Astroglial cells within retinoblastomas are restricted to reactive stromal cells that are frequently located adjacent to blood vessels or in residual, entrapped retina. (GFAP avidin–biotin immunoperoxidase.)

neoplastic transformation (Fig. 2.3). In addition, the magnitude and diversity of microenvironmental effects also appear to be markedly affected by both the cellular position and the stage of differentiation (Reh & Kljavin 1989; Sparrow et al 1990; Watanabe & Raff 1990). Such differences also clearly emphasize the discrepancies and potential caveats arising from the data derived from *in vivo* and *in vitro* studies of cell differentiation in both neoplastic and non-neoplastic cell populations.

Cerebellar development and medulloblastoma

In the early stages of CNS development, the cerebellar progenitor cells arise from two major germinal zones and generate distinct populations of the neural cells that compose the mature cerebellum (see Nowakowski & Hayes 2005, for

review). The first is the peri-ventricular germinal matrix in the cerebellar plate over the fourth ventricle, which forms the typical ventricular, intermediate, and marginal layers during the first 3–8 weeks of development. This fetal cerebellar ventricular zone (VZ) is populated by a band of multipotent stem cells expressing GFAP and OLIG2. They give rise to Purkinje and Golgi II neurons, and the macroglia of the region (Bergmann glia, astrocytes, oligodendrocytes), and the granule neuron precursors (GNP) arising at the rhombic lip (Fig. 2.9A,B).

In addition to these general classes of neural cells, there appears to be parasagittal compartmentalization of the Purkinje cell lineages which arise from these peri-ventricular progenitors during development (Leclerc et al 1992). Although both neuronal and glial differentiation begins relatively early (8–10 weeks gestation) (Yachnis et al 1993), experimental studies in the rodent would suggest that, in contrast to the subdivision of Purkinje cells, the bipotential glial progenitors are diffusely dispersed from the periventricular germinal matrix (not the external granular layer) and appear to persist beyond the neonatal period. Although the major portion of these glial progenitors appeared to progressively undergo oligodendroglial differentiation, *in vitro* studies also demonstrated the potential of these cells to differentiate into type 2 astrocytic lineages (Levine et al 1993). It is tempting to speculate about a relationship between the pool of glial progenitors in the maturing cerebellum and the pilocytic astrocytomas that arise at this site (see below).

The GNP, from the first 10–14 weeks gestation (Rakic & Sidman 1970), migrate over the external surface to populate the second major 'germinal layer' of the cerebellum, the external granular layer (EGL). This 'fetal' layer (Fig. 2.10) is clearly present in the perinatal period, but it does not persist normally beyond the first year (Kadin et al 1970). Neuronal histogenesis from these cells (granular, stellate, and basket neurons) has been clearly documented and experimental studies have also suggested that cells which are putatively derived from the neonatal EGL have the potential for Bergmann gliogenesis (see below). The external granular layer cells divide transiently, then migrate inwards to differentiate into the small neurons of the internal granule cell layer (IGL). The multiple molecular signaling pathways, including Hedgehog, Wnt, and Notch signaling, that have a role in cerebellar development and proliferation of GNPs (Schuller et al 2008; Yang et al 2008) may also play roles in the development and growth of medulloblastomas (Fig. 2.9C–E). Although the EGL, as a putative source of medulloblastomas, may last longer than 12 months (Stevenson & Echlin 1934), it is not clear whether these small numbers of cells would necessarily have the same developmental plasticity as the fetal or neonatal EGL. One key observation with respect to oncogenic targets within the fetal EGL, however, is the report by Kadin and co-workers (1970) of a neonatal midline medulloblastoma with striking continuity with the EGL. In this case, there was multifocal proliferation of the EGL as irregular extensions into the molecular layer which linked regions of normal EGL to definitive tumor.

Other groups of primitive cells, whose histogenetic potential is completely unknown, have also been described in the human cerebellum during the first postnatal year. The

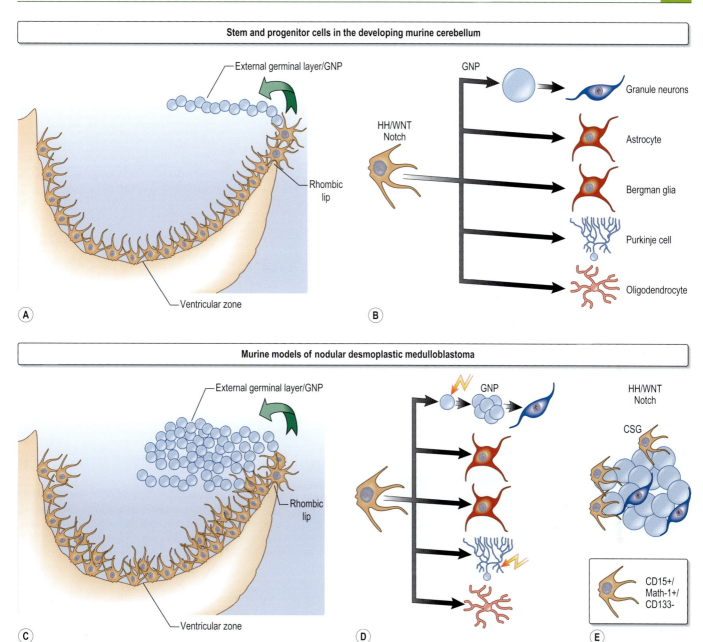

Stem and progenitor cells in the developing murine cerebellum

Murine models of nodular desmoplastic medulloblastoma

Figure 2.9 Stem and progenitor cells in the developing murine cerebellum as initiating cells of medulloblastoma. (A,B) Stem and progenitor cell lineages in the developing murine cerebellum. (A) The ventricular zone and the external germinal layer are the two major germinal zones in the developing cerebellum in rodents and human. In rodents, multipotent stem cells (yellow) with expression of GFAP or Olig2 reside within the fetal cerebellar ventricular zone. They give rise to granule neuron precursors (GNP; blue circles) in the rhombic lip that migrate along the cerebellar surface to form the external germinal layer. (B) Multipotent cerebellar stem cells give rise to GNP, which differentiate solely into granule neurons, and astrocytes, Bergmann glia, Purkinje neurons and oligodendrocytes. Recent studies showed that the Wingless/WNT pathway, the Hedgehog (HH) pathway and the NOTCH pathway, respectively regulate different aspects of murine cerebellar development. HH for example, stimulates proliferation of GNP in the external granule layer. WNT and NOTCH both regulate growth of stem cells in the ventricular zone. Very little is known about the role of HH, WNT and NOTCH in human cerebellar development. (C–E) Stem and progenitor cells as cellular origin of murine nodular/desmoplastic medulloblastoma. (C) Mutation in HH signaling lead to nodular/desmoplastic medulloblastoma in mouse models. Ectopic HH signaling targeted to multipotent stem cells (yellow) in the ventricular zone or GNP in the external germinal layer (blue circle) give rise to medulloblastoma in mouse models. In spite of increased numbers of stem cells, tumor formation due to ectopic HH signaling occurs only due to increased proliferation of GNP. These data suggest that the cellular origin of this tumor, which in some instances might be multipotent stem cells, is distinct from the tumor-propagation population. (D) Ectopic HH signaling either in the multipotent stem cell or the GNP leads to strongly increased proliferation in the GNP but not in other lineages. (E) In medulloblastoma mouse models with ectopic HH signaling, the tumor-propagation population is negative for the CD133 but positive for progenitor markers Math1 and CD15.

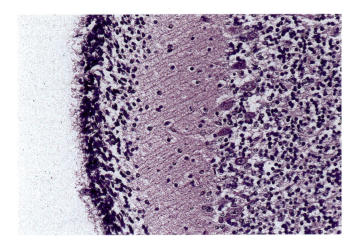

Figure 2.10 Human cerebellum in late gestation. Human cerebellar cortex at 35 weeks gestation readily demonstrates a prominent superficial external granular layer, Purkinje cell layer, and internal granular layer. The external granular layer persists into the first postnatal year as a thin rim of subpial cells (H&E).

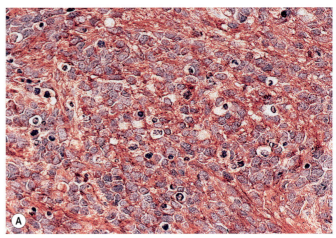

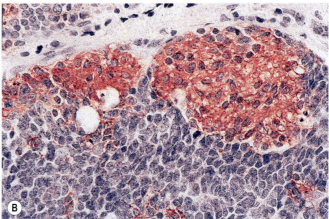

Figure 2.11 Medulloblastoma. Immunohistochemistry for neuron-associated protein, such as the β-III tubulin, can document neuroblastic cell populations within medulloblastomas. This type of differentiation with the primitive cell populations can be extensive (A) or highly focal (B). (TUJ1 avidin–biotin immunoperoxidase.)

first group is composed of small foci of embryonal cells that are situated in proximity to the germinal zone of the posterior medullary velum (Raaf & Kernohan 1944). The second group is the nests of primitive 'matrix cells', located within the deep cerebellar nuclei, that appear to persist during the first 4 months (Jellinger 1972). Given these locations, which were documented in carefully studied post-mortem cases, these cellular rests would appear to be derived from the peri-ventricular germinal matrix rather than the external granular layer. It is therefore tempting to speculate that these cells, as oncogenic targets, may have a distinctive potential for divergent differentiation (both neuronal and glial) similar to the periventricular matrix cells that contribute to the cerebellum.

In the cerebellum, there is a regional predilection for the most common primitive tumor in the central nervous system, the medulloblastoma. It comprises approximately one-quarter of all intracranial tumors in children, with a peak incidence near the end of the 1st decade (for review, see Lopes & VandenBerg 2007; Giangaspero et al 2007). Four histopathologic variants are defined in the current WHO classification: (1) classic medulloblastoma comprised of primitive cells populations arranged in amorphous sheets or ribbons of undifferentiated cells that may be variably interspersed with neuroblastic type (Homer Wright) rosettes; (2) desmoplastic/nodular medulloblastomas that comprise about 10–12% of cases and are distinctive for a biphasic architecture with a follicular arrangement of tumor cells; (3) medulloblastomas with extensive nodularity marked by more extensive neuronal differentiation; (4) anaplastic medulloblastomas that are populated by increased numbers of tumor cells with nuclei that have an increased size and pleomorphism, often accompanied by more conspicuous apoptosis; and (5) large cell medulloblastomas that are essentially more monomorphic than anaplastic medulloblastomas and that contain predominant populations of poorly-differentiated tumor cells with large, vesiculated nuclei and conspicuous apoptosis. In addition, rarer examples of cell

populations within medulloblastomas that exhibit variable muscle cell and melanotic differentiation may be found. Although immunohistochemical evidence for variable neuronal differentiation is present in all tumors (Fig. 2.11), the desmoplastic/nodular and extensively nodular medulloblastomas have the most conspicuous neuronal differentiation within the nodules. Highly cellular sheets and trabeculae of typical tumor cells with conspicuous mitoses encompass the nodules or islands characterized by lower cellularity and cells with finely fibrillated processes (Figs 2.12, 2.13). This architecture is particularly well highlighted by reticulin deposition only in the peripheral cellular areas. The reticulin-free islands prominently demonstrate neuronal class III β-tubulin and neurofilament immunoreactivity. This characteristic nodular architectural pattern of the desmoplastic variant may not be present in the recurrent tumor specimens following treatment, suggesting that treatment may have altered or eliminated the tumor cell or stromal component necessary for this distinctive pattern.

Current experimental models suggest that a multipotent stem cell or a lineage-restricted progenitor is the cellular origin of medulloblastoma. Proliferation of GNPs is indeed

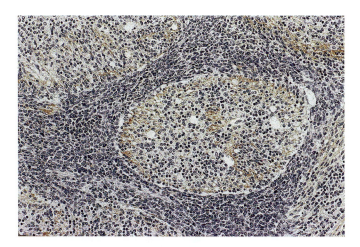

Figure 2.12 Desmoplastic medulloblastoma. Desmoplastic medulloblastomas exhibit a more stereotyped form of focal cellular differentiation with the biphasic formation of central nodules with increased differentiation which are surrounded by more primitive cells. The islands of more differentiated cells usually demonstrate neuronal differentiation with the presence of neurofilament (NF-M/H) epitopes. (SM133 avidin–biotin immunoperoxidase.)

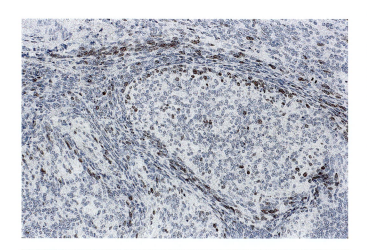

Figure 2.13 Desmoplastic medulloblastoma. The highly cellular trabeculae of tumor cells which demarcate the islands of cellular differentiation show higher labeling indices of Ki-67 in comparison with the more differentiated areas which correspond to neuronal differentiated zones. (MIB1 avidin–biotin immunoperoxidase.)

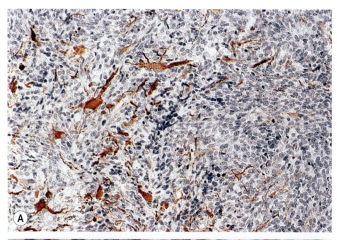

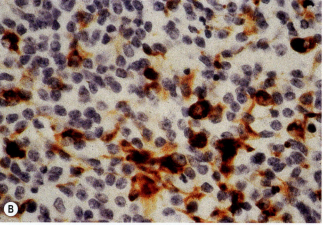

Figure 2.14 Medulloblastoma. (A) Reactive stromal astrocytes are commonly identified in these medulloblastomas by the typical cytoarchitecture. (B) GFAP immunoreactivity in a leptomeningeal metastatic implant of a medulloblastoma is definitive evidence for GFAP immunoreactivity in neoplastic cells and not reactive stromal astrocytes. (GFAP avidin–biotin immunoperoxidase.)

increased in transgenic mice lacking one copy of the inhibitory receptor, *Patched*, which develop medulloblastoma, suggesting that tumors arise from lineage-committed progenitors. However, medulloblastomas may also appear to be multipotential such that tumor cell populations expressing glial markers and neuronal markers may be present, pointing to a stem cell origin. However, it must be noted that the glial phenotypes that are attributed to GFAP expression, are typically far less conspicuous and may represent GFAP-expressing multipotent progenitors rather than differentiated astrocytes (Fig. 2.14A,B). Recently, Yang and Wechsler-Reya (2007) and Ligon and colleagues (2008) have addressed this controversial topic quite elegantly by generating mouse models that carry mutations in the sonic hedgehog pathway in either cerebellar neural stem cells or granule cell progenitors (Schuller et al 2008; Yang et al 2008). By using the Cre-Lox system to delete *Patched*, a negative regulator of sonic hedgehog signaling specifically in granule cell progenitors (with Math-Cre) or in multipotent stem cells (with GFAP-Cre), one group of researchers demonstrated that both cells can give rise to medulloblastoma when devoid of *Patched*. Tumor formation however, occurs due to increased proliferation of granule cell progenitors and not stem cells, independent of the cellular origin of the patched mutation. A second group introduced an oncogenic mutant of *Smoothened*, a positive regulator of sonic hedgehog signaling, using different progenitor-specific Cre-lines to reach a similar conclusion (Schuller 2008). Taken together, these data introduce the novel concept that tumor-initiating cells and tumor-propagating cells represent distinct differentiation stages of a hierarchical population (Fig. 2.9C–E). It will be important to analyze whether these two populations are present in human medulloblastoma, whether they show a distinct therapeutic response and whether other oncogenic mutations in medulloblastoma target multipotent stem cells and progenitors. Noteworthy is that the desmoplastic/nodular and extensive nodular variants are associated with alterations in the hedgehog signaling pathway, including a loss of PTCH. Amplification of the MYC gene in animal models (MYCC or MYCN) may be more associated with the acquisition of anaplastic cellular features and, in humans, it is associated with the large cell variant (Fan & Eberhart 2008).

Forebrain development and pediatric tumors with a primitive cell component

The germinal zone in the wall of the early human neural tube is the pseudo-stratified ventricular layer that is bounded by an outer cell-free marginal zone. All ventricular layer cells span from the adluminal surface to the pial surface (Fig. 2.15). Cellular proliferation in this primitive neuroepithelium occurs by polarized symmetric cell divisions, during which the mitoses occur only at the ventricular (apical) surface with intracellular nuclear movements occurring (interkinetic nuclear migration) from apical to basal zones according to the cell cycle. As brain development proceeds to early neurogenesis, two germinal zones begin to form around the lumen of the lateral ventricle: the ventricular and the sub-ventricular zones. The neuroepithelial cells in the ventricular zone initiate expression of radial glial cell markers (Table 2.1), while initially retaining the apical-basal polarity and elongating as the neural tube thickens during neurogenesis. These radial glial cells (RG) may therefore be considered as secondary neural stem cells. During this period, most proliferating ventricular zone cells are labeled with radial glial (RG) markers such as vimentin, glial fibrillary acidic protein (GFAP), and glutamate astrocyte-specific transporter (GLAST). The intermediate filament proteins, glial fibrillary acidic protein (GFAP) and vimentin, are expressed concomitantly in RG from the initiation of neurogenesis in humans (Cameron & Rakic 1991; Howard et al 2006; Zecevic 2004). A sub-population of these RG cells also express the neuronal markers β-III tubulin, MAP-2, and phosphorylated neurofilament peptides (Fig. 2.16A–C). A small population of cells in the ventricular zone are immunoreactive with only neuronal markers suggesting the early emergence of restricted neuronal progenitors. Basal progenitors are generated by asymmetric divisions of the neural stem cells, both late ventricular neuroepithelial cells and the ventricular radial glia, to initially populate the basal ventricular zone and then to accumulate in the sub-ventricular zone.

The sub-ventricular zone increases in cellularity by both symmetric and asymmetric divisions of these detached cells to constitute different progenitor cell lineages. These lineages may be bipotential to manifest both glial and neuroblastic phenotypes or multiple glial phenotypes (oligodendroglial and astrocytic) or unipotential for neuroblastic or glial phenotypes. Many of the progenitor cell populations appear to be committed at early stages to either neuronal or glial lineages. The number of multipotential progenitors in the ventricular zone gradually decreases, whereas the number of more restricted progenitors increases systematically during the 3-month course of human corticogenesis. Multipotential progenitors appear to co-exist with restricted

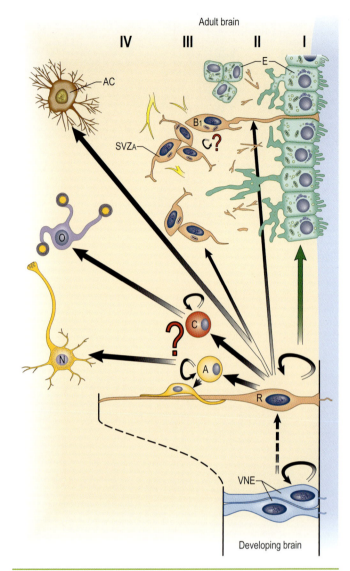

Figure 2.15 Schematic of the developing and adult human sub-ventricular zone in the forebrain. At the bottom, the germinal zone in the wall of the early human neural tube is the pseudo-stratified ventricular layer (VNE) in which all cells span from the adluminal surface to pial surface. As brain development proceeds to early neurogenesis, the neuroepithelial cells in the ventricular zone initiate expression of radial glial cell markers (R) while initially retaining the apical-basal polarity and elongating as the neural tube thickens during neurogenesis. These radial glial (RG) cells are considered to be secondary neural stem cells. These cells at later stages may serve as migratory guides for neuroblasts (yellow). During this period, most proliferating ventricular zone cells are labeled with RG. The sub-ventricular zone increases in cellularity by both symmetric and asymmetric divisions of these detached cells to constitute different progenitor cell lineages. The adult human sub-ventricular zone (SVZ$_A$) located in the lateral wall of the lateral ventricles differs from the murine SVZ by a conspicuous hypocellular gap (Layer II) and an arrangement into more distinct layers that are populated by different cellular phenotypes. (Adapted from Quinones-Hinojosa, A., Sanai, N., Soriano-Navarro, M., et al. Cellular composition and cytoarchitecture of the adult human subventricular zone: a niche of neural stem cells. J Comp Neurol 2006; 494, 415-434; 2. Chaichana, K. L., Capilla-Gonzalez, V., Gonzalez-Perez, O., et al. Preservation of glial cytoarchitecture from ex vivo human tumor and non-tumor cerebral cortical explants: A human model to study neurological diseases. J Neurosci Methods 2007; 164, 261–270.)

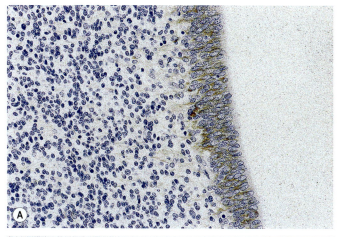

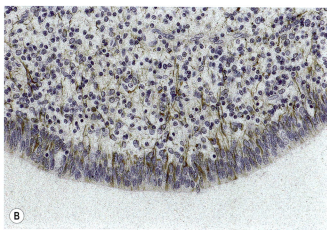

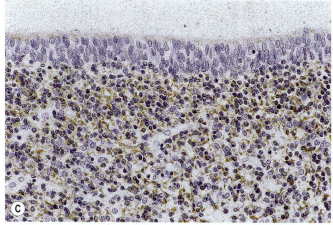

Figure 2.16 Human ventricular matrix and sub-ventricular zone at 26 weeks gestation. (A) The primitive pseudostratified cell layer is strongly immunoreactive for the intermediate filament protein vimentin. A similar pattern of immunoreactivity is present in the epithelial formations of medulloepitheliomas (see Fig. 2.17). Vimentin avidin–biotin immunoperoxidase. (B) GFAP immunohistochemistry highlights the radial glia within the pseudostratified neuroepithelium and thick processes of progenitors within the subependymal zone. GFAP avidin–biotin immunoperoxidase. (C) Abundant immunoreactivity for class β-III tubulin is localized in primitive neuroblast-progenitors within the sub-ventricular zone. Note that the pseudostratified cell layer does not contain cells that are immunoreactive for β-III tubulin. (TUJ1 avidin–biotin immunoperoxidase.)

neuronal progenitors and ventricular radial glia during initial corticogenesis in the human telencephalon and diversification of cells in the ventricular and sub-ventricular zones appears to begin at an earlier point and is more conspicuous than in rodents (Howard et al 2006; Zecevic 2004). It is important to note that different sub-types of radial glial cells co-exist at a given stage of development and that there is regional heterogeneity in the radial glial cell populations (Howard et al 2008). During neurogenesis, radial glial cells have extensive proliferative capacities and are therefore a potential target to acquire and amplify oncogenic mutations. Their role in the formation of human pediatric tumors remains to be fully defined.

Medulloepithelioma

Experimental data for the hypothetical distinction between pluripotential neuroepithelial stem cells (ventricular layer) and multipotential neural progenitors (basal ventricular zone and SVZ) were provided by *in vivo* studies of an experimental mouse teratocarcinoma (OTT-6050), from which two distinctive types of primitive, transplantable neural stem cell populations were derived (VandenBerg et al 1981a; VandenBerg et al 1981b). In the first type, the neural stem cells produced a primitive neuroepithelium resembling ventricular germinal matrix from which the migrating cells displayed either neuronal or glial differentiation. Ependymal

differentiation occurred in the more mature neoplastic neuroepithelium. In contrast, the second type of neural stem cell lost the ability to constitute a polarized neuroepithelium and formed only amorphous groups of cells without neuroepithelial structures. Although the developmental potential for either astrocytic or neuronal differentiation was retained, no ependymal differentiation occurred *in vivo*.

The first group of human tumors, that is predominantly composed of primitive cell populations, is relatively uncommon in the forebrain region. Within this group are neoplasms, which putatively arise from transformation of pluripotential neuroepithelial progenitors, as well as progenitors with more restricted potential for either neuronal or glial lineage formation. These include medulloepithelioma, cerebral neuroblastomas and ganglio-neuroblastomas, and ependymoblastomas. While the medulloepithelioma commonly displays multipotential cellular lineages, the ependymoblastomas appear to be significantly more restricted to ependymal lineages, respectively. In addition, tumors with extremely primitive phenotypes that may have variable evidence for neuronal and/or glial differentiation, analogous to the cerebellar medulloblastoma, have been described under the designation of supratentorial PNET (McLendon et al 2007). These tumors manifest the biologic potential of the primitive neural progenitors of the forebrain that give rise to both glial and neuronal lineages. Therefore, forebrain neoplasms generally appear to manifest similar

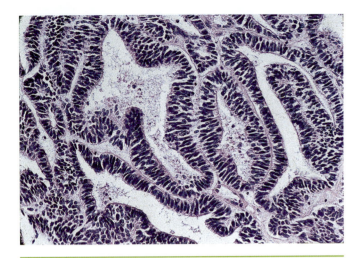

Figure 2.17 Medulloepithelioma. Medulloepithelioma recalls the structure of the primitive neuroepithelium due to the tubular and ribbon-like formations lined by mitotically active, pseudostratified cells. Other areas of the tumors typically display more amorphous collections of differentiating primitive neural cells (H&E).

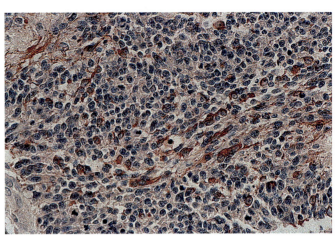

Figure 2.19 Medulloepithelioma. Immunoreactivity β-III tubulin demonstrates progenitors that are intermixed within the amorphous zones separating the tubular neuroepithelial arrangements. In contrast to vimentin and GFAP, this epitope is rarely present within the neuroepithelial structures. (TUJ1 avidin–biotin immunoperoxidase.)

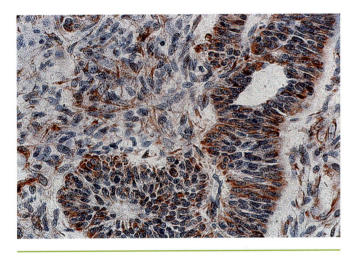

Figure 2.18 Medulloepithelioma. The great majority of tumor cells composing the neuroepithelium and the adjacent regions demonstrate strong immunoreactivity for vimentin. (Vimentin avidin–biotin immunoperoxidase.)

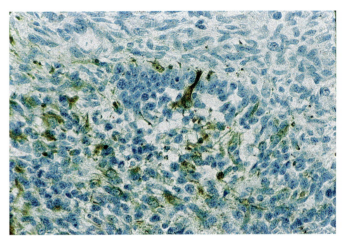

Figure 2.20 Medulloepithelioma. GFAP immunoreactivity is conspicuous in numerous primitive cells adjacent to the more neuroepithelial structures that contain occasional elongated GFAP immunoreactive cells. (GFAP avidin–biotin immunoperoxidase.)

spectra of biologic potentials to those of the various types of progenitor cells and derivative lineages which arise in the developing brain.

The medulloepithelioma appears to display a somewhat analogous histogenetic potential to the ventricular neuro-epithelial stem cell. This very rare tumor occurs early in the pediatric period, usually within the cerebral hemispheres. The hallmark histopathologic feature of these neoplasms is the mitotically active, pseudostratified columnar epithelium, often arranged in ribbons of tubules or papillary rosettes with variable interposition of delicate stromal elements and more amorphous groups of primitive cells. The epithelial structures recall the primitive neuroepithelium of the ventricular germinal matrix (Fig. 2.17). Analogous to this normal developing neuroepithelium, many cells are vimentin

immunoreactive (Fig. 2.18). Neuroblastic/neuronal (Fig. 2.19), radial glial/astrocytic (Fig. 2.20), and/or ependymal cell populations are either intimately admixed with the tubules or present in more well-demarcated fields in about half of the tumors (Russell & Rubinstein 1989). Early ependymal differentiation occurs within the neuroepithelium to form rosettes with abundant proliferative cells that resemble the analogous structures in ependymoblastomas. Similar to the neuroregulators in the primitive neuroepithelial component of the experimental mouse ovarian teratomas (Caccamo et al 1989), immunoreactivity for growth factors that are known to have biologic activity on CNS progenitor cell populations (insulin-like growth factor I and basic fibroblastic growth factor) is abundant in this primitive epithelium (Shiurba et al 1991).

Desmoplastic infantile astrocytoma/ganglioglioma

The second group of tumors, those with a significant but not preponderant primitive cell population, is the desmoplastic infantile astrocytoma/ganglioglioma (Fig. 2.21A) (Vanden-Berg 1993). These are rare neoplasms arising in the cerebral hemispheres within the first 2 years of life. The histogenetic potential of the former reflects bipotential neuroblastic (Figs 2.21B, 2.22) and glial (Figs 2.23, 2.24) progenitor cells as putative oncogenic targets while the latter, appearing quite similar in its histopathologic features, is restricted along an astroglial lineage. One distinctive feature of the neoplastic astroglial lineage in both neoplasms is the production of a basal lamina, often associated with normal subpial astrocytes. A second feature is that the neuronal component seldom achieves the cytoarchitectural maturation that is common in the gangliogliomas that are more common in the mature brain. Therefore the progenitor cell populations, as targets for neoplastic transformation in both tumors, most likely share a common lineage with subpial astroglia and may be related to the potential foci of perinatal and early postnatal neurocytogenesis that might persist in the cerebral

sub-pial zones (Brun 1965). The experimental data from immortalized supratentorial progenitor cells in rats certainly suggest that region-specific extrinsic factors may have significant effects on the hierarchical commitment of undifferentiated cells to glial and neuronal lineages and in the expression of specific phenotypes of either a glial or neuronal cell type (Mehler et al 1993; Renfranz et al 1991). Such studies may explain the capacity for unipotential or bipotential differentiation from the same group of transformed progenitor cells and could account for the common features between the two types of infantile desmoplastic tumors, differing primarily in the degree of divergent cytogenesis.

Neural stem cells in the mature forebrain

The largest germinal region in the adult human brain is the sub-ventricular zone of the lateral wall of lateral ventricles (Fig. 2.15). Only a limited number of studies have carefully described this zone (Kukekov et al 1999; Quinones-Hinojosa

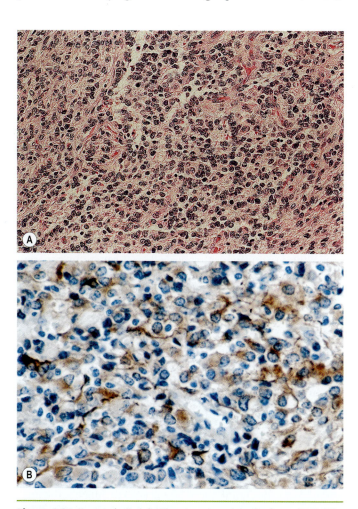

Figure 2.21 Desmoplastic infantile astrocytoma/ganglioglioma (DIG). (A) DIG invariably contain variable populations of primitive neural cells (H&E). (B) These primitive neural cells demonstrate variable MAP2 (a/b/c) immunoreactivity. (AP18 avidin–biotin immunoperoxidase.)

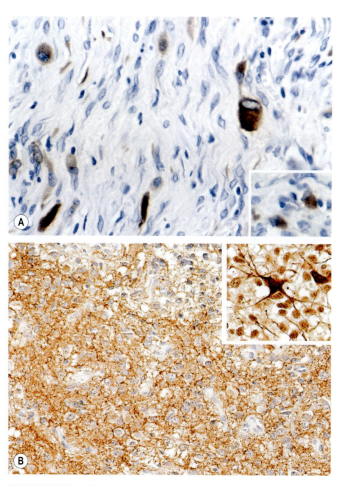

Figure 2.22 Desmoplastic infantile astrocytoma/ganglioglioma (DIG). (A) The neuroblastic cell populations in DIG are immunoreactive for β-III tubulin in both the more primitive and the larger, more polygonal cells. TUJ1 avidin–biotin immunoperoxidase. (B) Synaptophysin immunoreactivity is also present in primitive cellular populations. Inset: Maturing neurons are very infrequent, but may be detected with Bielschowsky silver staining. (SY38 avidin–biotin immunoperoxidase.)

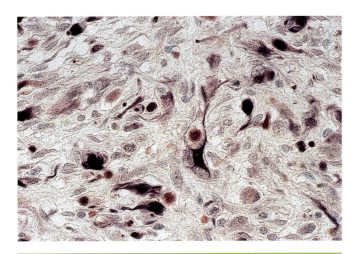

Figure 2.23 Desmoplastic infantile astrocytoma/ganglioglioma (DIG). Double-labeling for GFAP (dark purple) and neurofilament protein (NF-M/H) (red-brown) demonstrates the distinctive populations of neoplastic glial and neuronal cells. Despite the putative bipotential progenitors in the primitive cell population, cells co-expressing both glial and differentiated neuronal markers are not seen in the DIG. (GFAP/NFTP1A3 double immunoperoxidase.)

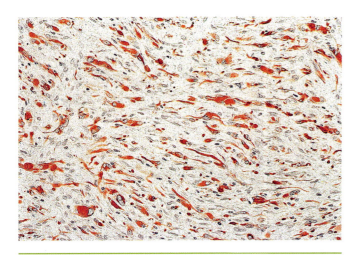

Figure 2.24 Desmoplastic infantile astrocytoma/ganglioglioma (DIG). GFAP immunohistochemistry highlights the neoplastic astrocytes with well-developed processes within the moderately desmoplastic stroma. (GFAP avidin–biotin immunoperoxidase.)

et al 2006; Sanai et al 2005; Bernier et al 2000). The germinal sub-ventricular zone (SVZ) is located in the lateral wall of the lateral ventricles. It differs from the adult murine SVZ by a conspicuous hypocellular gap (Layer II) and an arrangement into more distinct layers that are populated by different cellular phenotypes. In Layer I, the ependymal cells (green) form a simple cuboidal epithelium that has apical microvilli and basal expansions that are closely associated with networks of interconnected astrocytic processes (shown in brown). Layer III is mainly comprised of cell bodies of distinct populations of cells with astrocytic phenotypes. A sub-population of these SVZ astrocytic cells have proliferative potential and have the capacity to form neurospheres in

culture that contain multipotent and self-renewing cells and may correspond to the B1 cells of the murine SVZ. Cells with the ultrastructural features of oligodendrocytes and displaced ependymal cells are also present but less frequent in this layer. These oligodendrocytes do not appear to be myelinating processes and the displaced ependymal cell clusters do not have any definite orientation towards the ventricle. Layer IV, contains myelinated processes and is the transition zone between the SVZ astrocytes and the adjacent brain parenchyma. The bottom of the schematic shows a hypothetical progression from a germinal ventricular zone to an intermediate cellular sub-ventricular zone populated by radial astrocytes that may function as secondary multipotent stem cells and by transit-amplifying cells that give rise to neuroblast (yellow) and glial (red) progenitors. Radial astrocytes may differentiate into various astrocytic phenotypes, including the SVZ cells in Layer III of the adult SVZ and parenchymal astrocytes (Chaichana et al 2007; Quinones-Hinojosa et al 2006). The levels of proliferation in the adult human SVZ are smaller compared with that in other mammals whereas the cellular architecture is distinct. Magnetic resonance imaging (MRI) has revealed that glioblastoma which are associated with the sub-ventricular zone are multifocal and recur at distant sites to the primary tumor (Lim et al 2007). These data indirectly point to a multipotent stem cell-like cell or progenitor cell as the tumor-initiating cell of a glioblastoma sub-group with poor prognosis. The adult human SVZ indeed contains proliferating adult neural stem cells (Quinones-Hinojosa et al 2006). One possible scenario is that multifocal glioblastoma originate in mutated stem cells, which give rise to mutant progenitor cells that migrate away from the germinal areas and proliferate aberrantly once they reach a favorable microenvironment. Further comprehensive analyses of the adult human neural stem cell and its progeny are necessary to determine whether they give rise to glioblastoma by generating brain cancer stem cells.

At postnatal stages in the murine SVZ, radial glial cells turn into parenchymal and germinal zone astrocytes, which are the multipotent neural stem cells or type B cells (Merkle et al 2004). Adult neural stem cells self-renew to generate more stem cells and, depending on their positional and temporal information, give rise to neurons and glia cells. The major germinal region in adult rodents is the subependyma of the rostral lateral ventricle or sub-ventricular zone (SVZ) (Doetsch et al 1999; Gritti et al 1996). Neurogenesis persists also in the sub-granular layer of the dentate gyrus in the hippocampus, which has a cellular hierarchy somewhat similar to that of the SVZ (Vescovi et al 2006).

In the murine adult SVZ, multipotent stem cells are polarized cells (Mirzadeh et al 2008) residing in a stem cell niche directly underlying the ependymal layer which is composed of extracellular matrix including basal lamina and blood vessels (Kokovay et al 2008; Tavazoie et al 2008). Multipotent stem cells are slow-dividing, self-renewing and can be stimulated to give rise to fast-dividing type C transit-amplifying cells. Transit-amplifying cells produce the type A neuroblasts and glial progenitors (Doetsch et al 2002; Jackson et al 2006; Menn et al 2006) (Fig. 2.25).

Multipotential stem cells have a long life span and extensive proliferative capacity, which makes them likely targets

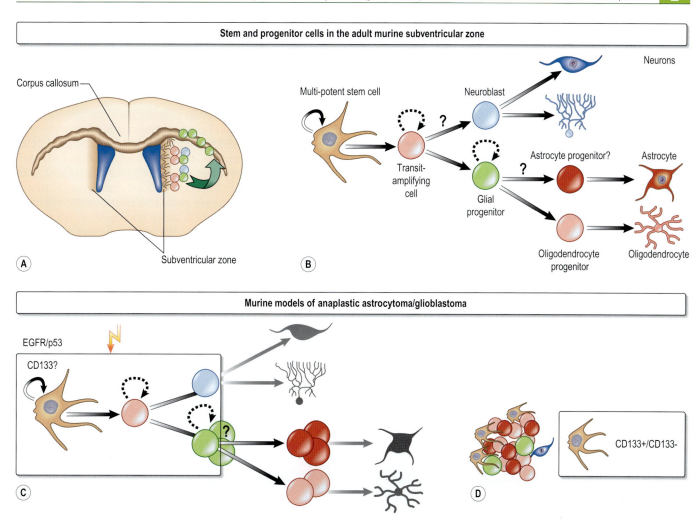

Figure 2.25 The role of stem cells and progenitor cells in the developing murine cerebral hemispheres as origin of astrocytoma. (A,B) Stem and progenitor cells in the adult murine sub-ventricular zone generate differentiated brain cells by dividing along a hierarchical lineage. (A) The sub-ventricular zone is the major germinal area of the mature rodent brain and harbors self-renewing multipotent stem cells (yellow), transit-amplifying cells (pink), neuroblasts (blue) and glial progenitors (green). While stem cells and transit amplifying cells remain in the sub-ventricular zone, progenitors migrate away (arrow) along the rostral migratory stream to generate differentiated cells in other brain areas. (B) Multipotent stem cells divide to generate another stem cell (self-renewal) and a transit-amplifying cell presumably in an asymmetric cell division. Transit-amplifying cells generate neuronal progenitors (neuroblasts) and glial progenitors. Neuroblasts give rise to mature neurons in the olfactory bulbs and glial progenitors give rise to astrocytic and oligodendrocyte progenitors, which in turn generate astrocytes and oligodendrocytes, respectively. (C,D) Murine models of anaplastic astrocytoma/glioblastoma. (C) Oncogenic activation of EGFR signaling, loss of p53 and NF1 tumor suppressors in the immature stem cell lineage generate glial progenitors which proliferate extensively and fail to further differentiate. These aberrantly specified progenitors eventually give rise to tumor cells and are potentially the precursors of cancer stem cells. (D) Brain tumor stem cells in astrocytoma and glioblastoma express the cell surface protein CD133 and generate differentiation-defective glial progenitors, which make up the bulk of tumor cells, and a smaller population of differentiated astrocytes.

for an initial transforming mutation. Their similarities to glioma cancer stem cells suggest that the malignant cell population might arise from transformed neural stem cells (Dirks 2005; Galli et al 2004; Hemmati et al 2003; Singh et al 2003; Singh et al 2004a; Singh et al 2004b). To begin to identify the cellular origin of astrocytoma, Holland and colleagues (2000) have pioneered cell type-specific activation of oncogenes in a mature de-differentiated astrocyte, an immature multipotent stem cell or a glial progenitor cell, respectively. Cell-type specific gene transfer was made possible in mouse models by using the replication-competent ALV splice acceptor RCAS/tva system which consists of the avian leukosis virus (ALV)-based RCAS viral vector and transgenic mice that express the RCAS receptor TVA from either nestin or GFAP promotor. Neural and glial progenitor cells positive for the intermediate filament nestin appear to be more sensitive to the transforming effect of platelet-derived growth factor-B (PDGF-B), epidermal growth factor receptor (EGFR) and the combined activity of Ras and Akt, respectively, than astrocytes expressing GFAP (Dai et al 2001; Holland et al 2000; Holland et al 1998). These data suggest that progenitor cells and perhaps multipotent stem cells, rather then mature astrocytes, are the cellular origin of astrocytoma. This interpretation is complicated by the fact that GFAP is also expressed in multipotent stem cells and not only differentiated astrocytes (Doetsch et al 1999).

Evidence of an immature cell as the origin of brain cancer stem cells has been corroborated by more recent data showing that infusion of PDGF into the lateral ventricle of adult mouse brains was sufficient to induce type B cell proliferation resulting into large hyperplasia with glioma-like features (Jackson et al 2006). In a very elegant study, Alcantara Llaguno and colleagues (2009) deleted a combination of three tumor suppressors, neurofibromin-1, PTEN and p53 specifically in nestin-positive, neural stem/progenitor cells by inducible site-specific recombination. Nestin-positive cells in the SVZ of triple-mutant mice developed precancerous defects including a growth advantage and differentiation changes and developed astrocytoma with complete penetrance. These data convincingly show that immature cells such as neural stem/progenitor cells targeted by oncogenic mutations give rise to astrocytoma (Fig. 2.25).

Forebrain tumors with unique potentials for differentiation

The group of forebrain tumors that display relatively unique developmental potentials are those tumors that usually arise in the late pediatric or young adult periods and are composed of distinctive neuronal or glial phenotypes and develop either near or in the midline of the neuraxis on in subventricular regions of the lateral or third ventricles.

Central neurocytoma

With respect to sub-ventricular zone progenitors, the central neurocytoma is a neoplasm that has several important features. These tumors are uncommon and develop during the first two decades of life; the majority arise in association with the lateral ventricles and, to a lesser extent, the third ventricle (Leenstra et al 2007). Although these tumors are composed of a rather homogeneous population of small cells

with variable, but not significant mitotic activity, they usually behave clinically like a well-differentiated cellular phenotype (Fig. 2.26). Immunohistochemical and ultrastructural studies have unequivocally demonstrated that the majority of cells composing central neurocytomas have neuronal phenotypes (Fig. 2.27) with features that suggest partial cytoarchitectural maturity of interneuron phenotypes in the striatum and thalamus. These include synaptic terminals, often with clear and dense core vesicles, and abundant profiles of cellular processes with parallel arrays of microtubules. GFAP-immunoreactive cells are typically stromal astrocytes with extensive fibrillary processes (Fig. 2.28). Infrequently, tumor cell populations with more primitive neural stem cell (e.g., OLIG2 Musashi 1) (Figs 2.29, 2.30) and GFAP immunoreactivity appear in cases that appear to have a more aggressive

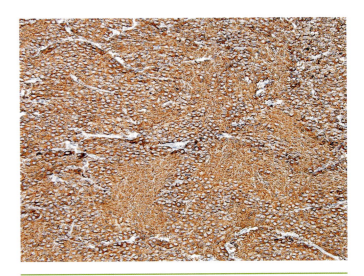

Figure 2.27 Central neurocytoma. The neurocytomas commonly have diffuse immunoreactivity to β-III tubulin in both the cellular and fibrillated zones. (TUJ1 with Ventana Ultraview immunoperoxidase.)

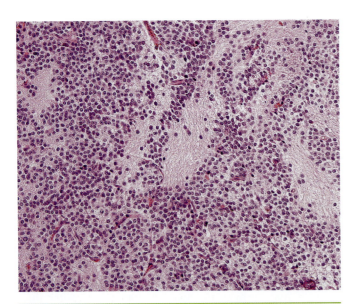

Figure 2.26 Central neurocytoma. Central neurocytomas typically are composed of homogenous cells with round nuclei with stippled chromatin that are arranged in both cellular and fibrillated acellular zones that are interlaced with a delicate microvasculature (H&E).

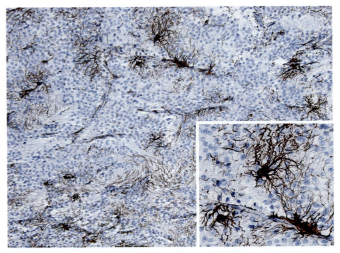

Figure 2.28 Central neurocytoma. GFAP-immunoreactive stromal cells in typical neurocytomas have extensive fibrillary processes and often are intimately associated with the delicate microvascular stroma. (GFAP with Ventana Ultraview immunoperoxidase.)

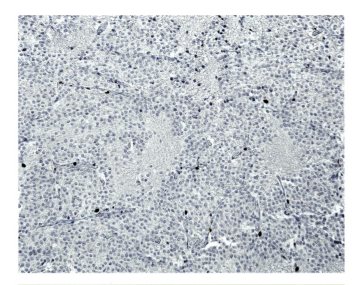

Figure 2.29 Central neurocytoma. The neural stem cell biomarker OLIG2 is present only in small numbers of tumor cells that are often adjacent to the microvasculature. (OLIG2 with Ventana Ultraview immunoperoxidase.)

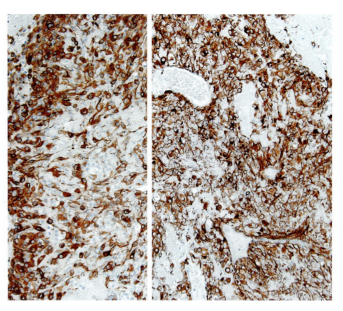

Figure 2.31 Atypical central neurocytoma. (Left) In atypical central neurocytomas, β-III tubulin immunoreactivity is not as diffuse and is present in small cells with delicate processes. (TUJ1 with Ventana Ultraview immunoperoxidase.) (Right) In the same atypical central neurocytoma, there is a marked increased in GFAP immunoreactive cells with similar cytoarchitecture as the cells containing, β-III tubulin. Note the absence of the well-differentiated stromal astrocytes with the extensive fibrillary processes. (GFAP with Ventana Ultraview immunoperoxidase.)

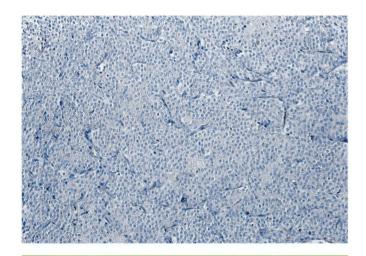

Figure 2.30 Central neurocytoma. Immunohistochemistry for CD133 shows no immunoreactive cells are present in central neurocytomas. (CD133 Abcam #19898 with Ventana Ultraview immunoperoxidase.)

biologic behavior (Fig. 2.31) (von Deimling et al 1990). *In vitro* studies using both non-adherent tumorsphere cultures and adherent monolayers have demonstrated bipotential cytogenetic potentials and GFAP expression is an early event in monolayer culture (Westphal et al 1994). The characteristic phenotype and ventricular location of these tumors suggests that the neurocytoma might arise by the transformation of neuronally biased, transit-amplifying progenitor cells located in the adult sub-ventricular zone (Sim et al 2006).

Pilocytic astrocytoma

The histopathologic and molecular features, preferential locations (Scheithauer et al 2007), and recent experimental data from animal models suggest that pilocytic astrocytomas arise from transformation of a regionally specific radial glial

cell or progenitor cell population in the maturing or mature CNS. Pilocytic astrocytomas are the most common glioma in children, with the highest incidence during the first two decades. In adults, pilocytic astrocytomas tend to develop about one decade earlier than the low-grade diffuse-type astrocytomas and comprise an overall smaller percentage of astrocytic tumors (5% of gliomas) compared to all grades of diffuse type astrocytomas. Although pilocytic astrocytomas most commonly arise in the infratentorial region of children, other preferred sites tend to involve regions near or adjacent to the midline of the neuroaxis, including: optic nerve, optic chiasm/hypothalamus, thalamus and basal ganglia, and brainstem. Tumors involving the optic system are especially associated with NF1 mutations, and in children, the most common supratentorial site involves the optic pathways and hypothalamus followed by the thalamic/basal ganglia region. The tumors typically have a relatively small proliferative cell population and have limited capacity for invasion into adjacent neuropil. In contrast to the limited capacity for brain invasion, these tumors are relatively motile and may readily travel along white matter tracts and into the leptomeningeal surfaces where presumptive proteolytic activity, expressed by the high-grade diffuse-type astrocytomas, may not be required for dispersion.

The tumor cells are typically arranged into a biphasic pattern with bipolar, fibrillated and elongated (piloid) cells that recall elongated radial glia admixed with areas of less stellate cells with short processes that resemble protoplasmic astrocytes. The piloid cells tend to be packed in bundles which are often accentuated and dense in perivascular arrangements. The less stellate cells show more lacy patterns, which are often associated with microcystic changes (Figs 2.32A, 2.33A). The diffuse, but heterogeneous immunoreactivity for OLIG2 (Tanaka et al 2008), DBX, GFAP, and vimentin but not β-III tubulin, NeuN (Preusser et al 2006) or NFP H/M implicate an immunophenotype suggestive of a slowly proliferating radial glial cell or bipotential glial progenitor with limited neurogenic potential (Figs 2.32B, 2.34, 2.35). The clinicopathologic features also implicate a cellular target for tumor initiation that is most susceptible or that

occurs in highest numbers during a time that radial glial cells or neuroglial progenitors would be expected to be sufficiently abundant. Dissociation and analysis of pilocytic astrocytomas have also demonstrated non-clonogenic populations of CD133+ cells that can be cultured in tumorspheres (Singh et al 2003) and CD133+ cells can be detected within intact human tumors by immunohistochemistry (Fig. 2.33B).

Comparative analyses of gene expression in sporadic pilocytic astrocytomas demonstrates that these tumors are uniquely delineated from non-neoplastic white matter and other low-grade gliomas, and are more similar to fetal astrocytes and to oligodendroglial lineages (SOX10, PEN5, PLP, PMP-22, MBP, oligodendroglial myelin glycoprotein)

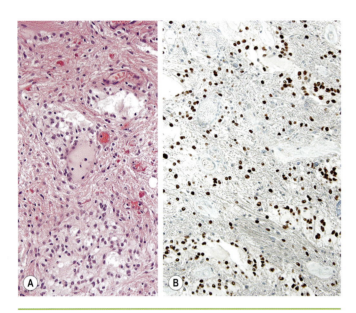

Figure 2.32 Pediatric pilocytic astrocytoma. (A) Pilocytic astrocytoma arising in the posterior fossa showing the typical biphasic pattern of tumor cells (H&E). (B) OLIG2 immunoreactivity in the same tumor is conspicuous and particularly high in the less stellate cells. (OLIG2 with Ventana Ultraview immunoperoxidase.)

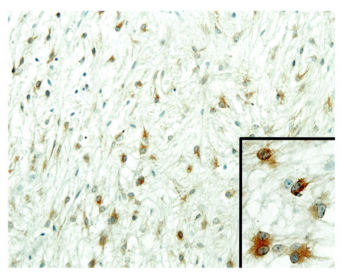

Figure 2.34 Pediatric pilocytic astrocytoma. DCX immunoreactivity is most conspicuous in the cell bodies and delicate processes of the more stellate cells. (DCX (C-18 domain: sc-8066) avidin–biotin immunoperoxidase.)

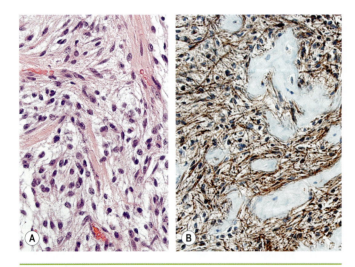

Figure 2.33 Pediatric pilocytic astrocytoma. (A) The elongated tumor cells may be a conspicuous component of the tumors that may form variably sized bundles of processes (H&E). (B) These cells may focal exhibit CD133 immunoreactivity. (CD133 Abcam #19898 with Ventana Ultraview immunoperoxidase.)

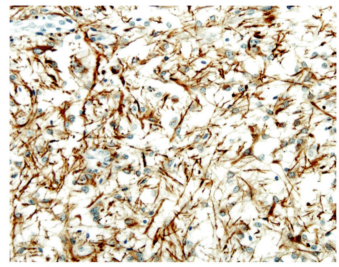

Figure 2.35 Pediatric pilocytic astrocytoma. GFAP immunoreactivity in the same field as Fig. 2.34 is conspicuous and labels many cells with elongated processes. (GFAP avidin–biotin immunoperoxidase.)

(Bannykh et al 2006; Colin et al 2006; Gutmann et al 2002). Consistent with presence of oligodendroglial progenitors, pilocytic astrocytomas, especially optic nerve tumors, contain significant numbers of O4 immunoreactive cells, and the highest numbers of A2B5+ glial progenitor cells are present in pilocytic astrocytomas of the posterior fossa. An expression analysis of 21 juvenile pilocytic astrocytomas presented additional evidence for the relationship of pilocytic astrocytomas to a population of radial glia or early progenitors. Neurogenesis was one of the major biological processes with detection of 18 deregulated genes with the upregulation of four neurogenesis-related genes in these tumors (Wong et al 2005). Recent analyses of both sporadic and NF1-associated tumors indicate cell-lineage specific genetic signatures that correspond to regional progenitor cell populations (Sharma et al 2005). Data from a murine NF1 model indicate that the hyperactivation of the RAS signaling pathway with loss of neurofibromin in BLBP+ cells results in an expansion of the glial progenitors and optic glioma formation (Hegedus et al 2007; Zhu et al 2005). Recent studies showing the presence of a BRAF fusion gene with constitutive BRAF kinase activity in a majority of sporadic pilocytic astrocytomas suggests that the susceptible progenitor cells need only mechanism to activate the mitogen-activated kinase pathway for development of pilocytic astrocytomas (Jones et al 2008; Pfister et al 2008). Thus, the sporadic and NF-1 associated pilocytic astrocytomas, despite the same histologic features, may develop and grow via different genetic alterations that target the same down-stream signaling pathways in region-specific lineage progenitors.

Subependymal giant cell astrocytoma

The subependymal giant cell astrocytomas (SEGA), almost always arise during the first two decades in association with the tuberous sclerosis complex (Lopes et al 2007). The tumors are circumscribed with negligible capacity for invasive spread, frequently nodular, and multicystic with calcifications. They arise in the wall of the lateral ventricles at the level of the basal ganglia or, less commonly, adjacent to the third ventricle. The tumor cells exhibit a wide spectrum of cytoarchitectures: small elongated cells in a variably fibrillated matrix, intermediate size polygonal cells, and variable numbers of giant, ganglion-like cells. The majority of tumor cells demonstrate variable immunoreactivity for GFAP and S-100 protein in addition to neuronal-associated epitopes such as class β-III tubulin, NF-H/M (Figs 2.36, 2.37) and neurotransmitters with variable ultrastructural features suggestive of neuronal differentiation, including microtubules, occasional dense-core granules, and rare synapse formation (Lopes & VandenBerg 2007).

The tuberous sclerosis complex (TSC) is a multi-system genetic disorder with variable phenotypic expression, due to a mutation in one of the two genes, TSC1 and TSC2, and a subsequent hyperactivation of the downstream mTOR pathway, resulting in increased cell growth and proliferation in specific cellular targets (Napolioni et al 2009). In the CNS, the putative cellular target may be a radial glial cell or bipotential progenitor with a limited proliferative capacity that resides in the sub-ventricular zone. A recent study of a congenital subependymal giant cell astrocytoma has

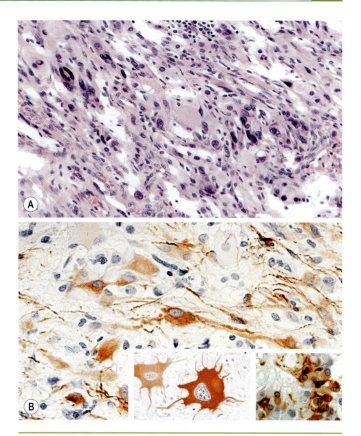

Figure 2.36 Subependymal giant cell astrocytoma. (A) The tumor cell populations in subependymal giant cell astrocytomas exhibit a wide range of cytoarchitectures. The typical appearance consists of cells ranging from polygonal with abundant, glassy cytoplasm to randomly oriented, more elongated and smaller cells in a variably fibrillated matrix. Giant cells are highly variable but always present (H&E). (B) GFAP immunoreactivity is present in the same spectrum of cells as shown above (insets). (GFAP avidin–biotin immunoperoxidase.)

demonstrated the expression of NESTIN, SOX2, GLAST, vimentin, and BLBP in the giant cell sub-populations of tumor cells (Phi et al 2008).

Infiltrating gliomas and brain tumor stem cells

Oligodendroglioma

The molecular pathogenesis of oligodendroglioma is not well understood and it has been debated whether the cellular origin of oligodendroglioma is a multipotent stem cell, a glial progenitor or a differentiated glial cell. PDGFR and epidermal growth factor receptor (EGFR) signaling, respectively, are activated in normal oligodendrogenesis and in oligodendroglioma. PDGF induces de-differentiation of astrocytes, which supports the notion that mature glial cells are the cellular origin of oligodendroglioma (Dai et al 2001). However, similarities between pathways regulating oligodendrogenesis, oligodendrocyte progenitor proliferation and oligodendroglioma suggest that tumors arise from lineage-restricted glial progenitors (Persson et al 2010). For

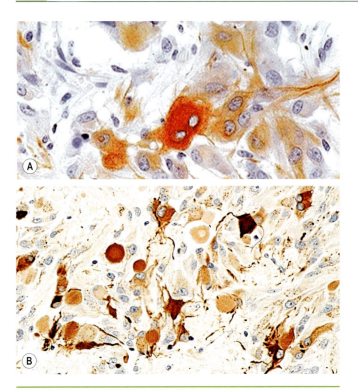

Figure 2.37 Subependymal giant cell astrocytoma. (A) β-III tubulin is detectable in polygonal cells with delicate processes. TUJ1 avidin–biotin immunoperoxidase. (B) Neurofilament epitopes (H/M NFP) are readily detectable in the same polygonal cell populations. (SMI 33 avidin–biotin immunoperoxidase.)

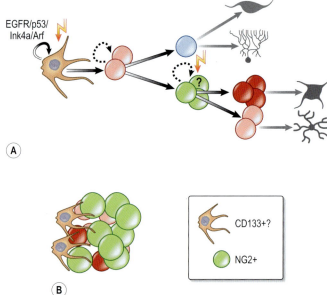

Figure 2.38 A murine model of high-grade oligodendroglioma. (A) Ectopic activation of EGFR signaling by expression of the *verbB* oncogene under control of the S100β promoter in the early oligodendrocytic lineage in combination with loss of p53 or Ink4a/Arf, respectively, induces a shift from asymmetric to symmetric cell division of glial progenitors. Symmetrically dividing cells fail to segregate cell fate markers and differentiation factors properly, which leads to aberrant cell fate specification and proliferation and possibly to genomic instability. Symmetrically dividing cells acquire additional mutations and eventually fail to differentiate and evade normal cell cycle control. (B) Multipotent stem cells (yellow) might be present within oligodendroglioma-derived tumorspheres perhaps as contaminating normal stem cells but do not represent the tumor-initiating population. The symmetrically dividing progenitors (green), which express NG2, rather initiate and propagate oligodendroglioma.

example, ectopic EGFR stimulates the proliferation and inhibits the differentiation of oligodendrocyte progenitors and consequently, oligodendrocyte progenitor-like cells generate hyperplasia in the white matter (Ivkovic et al 2008). In addition, PDGFRα-positive adult neural stem cells in the SVZ generate oligodendrocytes *in vivo*. PDGF infused in the ventricle of adult mice induces massive SVZ stem cell proliferation and large glioma-like hyperplasias with expression of markers for astrocytes but not oligodendrocytes (Jackson et al 2006). Oligodendroglioma in human and mouse models, however, predominantly express markers for immature oligodendrocytes or oligodendrocyte progenitors such as NG2, PDGFRα and OLIG2 and not astrocyte or neuronal markers (Ligon et al 2004). These observations suggest that glial-restricted progenitors progress to a neoplastic state in response to ectopic growth factor receptor signaling and loss of tumor suppressors. Mutated glial-restricted progenitors propagate the tumor by generating an excess of oligodendroglial progenitor-like cells at the expense of mature cells (Fig. 2.38).

A small-scale study has identified CD133+ tumorspheres from high-grade oligodendroglioma (Beier et al 2008). The question remains whether glial-restricted progenitors expression progenitor markers such as NG2 rather than multipotent stem cells might be the cellular origin of CD133+ cells, which can be addressed in mouse models and not in human patients (Figs 2.38, 2.39). A transgenic mouse model of oligodendroglioma expressing the *verbB* oncogene in glial-restricted progenitors and lacking p53 develop high-grade

oligodendroglial tumors (Fig. 2.39) (Weiss et al 2003). In this mouse model, the *verbB* oncogene ectopically activates EGFR signaling in S100β-positive cells in the SVZ and white matter throughout the brain at early postnatal stages. Ectopic EGFR induces premalignant changes such as aberrant self-renewal, impaired differentiation along the glial lineages and hyperproliferation in *verbB*+ neurospheres. Similar but more severe changes were detected in glioma stem cells isolated from oligodendroglial tumors of S100β-*verbB* p53 KO mice, based on their ability to form tumorspheres (Fig. 2.39). Glioma tumorspheres fulfil criteria of brain tumor stem cells, including expression of stem cell markers (Fig. 2.39), aberrant self-renewal and differentiation *in vitro*, and their ability to generate massive high-grade oligodendroglial tumors upon serial orthotopic injections (Harris et al 2008). Orthotopic tumors derived from tumorspheres mimic the features of endogenous high-grade oligodendroglial-like tumors (Galli et al 2004) such as high cellularity, high mitotic index, perineuronal satellitosis, the characteristic 'fried egg' appearance of cells and microvascular hyperplasia (Fig. 2.40). Premalignant changes such as increased self-renewal, impaired differentiation and hyperproliferation

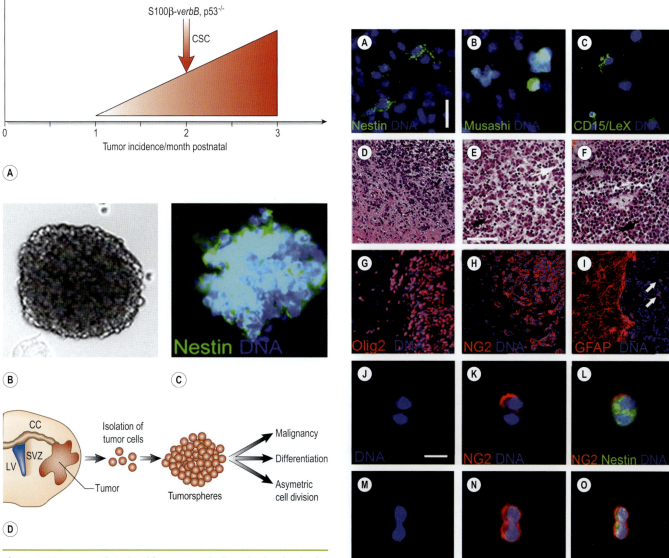

Figure 2.39 Tumor cells isolated from murine high-grade oligodendroglial tumors form self-renewing tumorspheres. (A) S100β-*verbB* transgenic mice lacking p53 develop high-grade oligodendroglial tumors within 2–3 months postnatally after onset of oncogene expression. (B) Tumor cells grow self-renewing tumorspheres. (C) Tumorspheres express high-levels of the stem and progenitor marker nestin. (D) Schematic of tumor cell isolation, culturing of tumorspheres and analyses of malignancy, differentiation and symmetric vs asymmetric cell division mode.

Figure 2.40 Tumorsphere-derived cells express stem and transit amplifying cell markers, generate orthotopic oligodendroglial tumors by dividing symmetrically. (A–C) Tumorspheres express stem and transit amplifying cell markers. (A) Dissociated tumorspheres express markers for nestin (B) the stem cell marker musashi and (C) the stem cell and transit amplifying cell marker CD15/LeX. Scale bar is 20 μM. (D–F) Tumorspheres generate orthotopic high-grade oligodendroglial tumors which mimic the endogenous tumor. (D) Orthotopic tumors are highly infiltrative (E) and similar to endogenous tumors display (F) the typical 'fried egg' appearance of oligodendrocyte progenitor cells with a high-mitotic index. Scale bar is 100 μM. (G,H) Orthotopic tumors consists mainly of oligodendrocyte progenitor-like cells. (G) Similar to endogenous tumors, orthotopic tumors are predominantly expressing Olig2 (H) NG2 (I) but not the astrocyte marker GFAP. (J–O) Asymmetric cell division of NG2 progenitors from wildtype SVZ vs symmetric cell division of NG2 cells from tumorspheres. (J–L) Pair assay depicting a single asymmetric cell division of NG2 cell. NG2 segregates asymmetrically to one of the two daughters only, whereas nestin segregates always symmetrically generating a NG2+ and a NG2- daughter. (M–O) NG2 cells from tumorspheres divide predominantly symmetrically giving rise to two NG2/nestin+ daughters. (J,M) DNA is stained with DAPI in blue. (K,N) NG2 is in red. (L,O) Nestin is in green in the merged image. Scale bar 10 μM.

and malignant progression are accompanied by a shift from asymmetric cell divisions to symmetric cell divisions mode (Fig. 2.40). This opens up the possibility that normal asymmetric cell division prevents premalignant changes and perhaps neoplastic progression. Reminiscent of asymmetric cell division defective invertebrate neuroblasts (Morrison & Kimble 2006), mammalian glial progenitors with defects in asymmetric cell division might be genetically unstable and therefore predisposed to acquire additional mutations and to undergo neoplastic transformation (Fig. 2.41). In support of our hypothesis, several confirmed oncogenes and putative tumor suppressors are known regulators of asymmetric cell

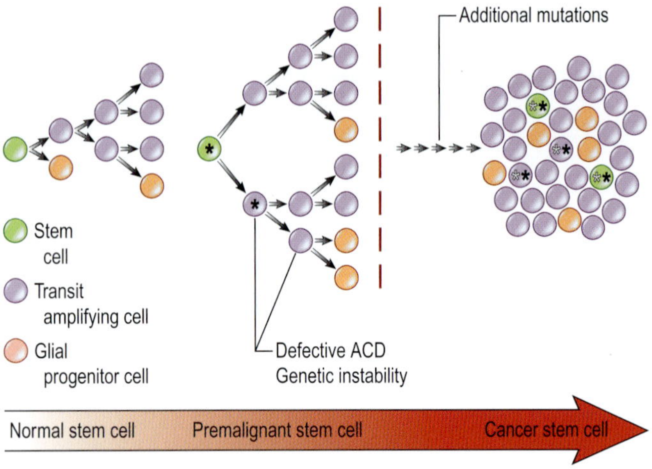

Figure 2.41 Model of the stepwise neoplastic transformation of progenitor cells by a defect in asymmetric cell division. Normal stem and progenitor cells divide asymmetrically to self-renew and generate more committed cells. Oncogenic mutations such as ectopic activation of EGFR signaling (black asterisks) disrupt asymmetric cell division and thereby induce premalignant defects and generate aberrantly self-renewing and differentiating cells. Premalignant progenitors are genetically unstable and are predisposed to acquire additional mutations (white asterisks), which transforms them into malignant, tumor-propagating cells.

division (Morrison & Kimble 2006). The potential link of defects in asymmetric cell division and the development of glioma should be investigated further.

Gliomatosis cerebri

Gliomatosis cerebri is a biologically aggressive, rare glial neoplastic process with the hallmark feature of extensive tumor cell dispersion into a minimum of three cerebral lobes that conspicuously preserves the underlying brain cytoarchitecture, including neuronal cell bodies and axonal structures. The invasive pattern can mimic the subpial spread, neuronal satellitosis, perivascular localization at the infiltrating tumor margins of oligodendrogliomas and glioblastomas (secondary structures of Scherer), or the more amorphous diffuse pattern of dispersion in low-grade astrocytomas. Despite the extensive brain involvement by tumor cells, there is no discrete mass which is detectable by high-resolution neuroimaging. The presence of the infiltrating tumor cells is typically associated with an overall increase in the volume, with variable mass effect, of the involved brain regions with minimally hypodense or isodense changes with T2-weighted MRI and hyperintensity in FLAIR MR imaging. The most commonly affected regions are the cerebral hemispheres followed by the mid-brain, thalamus, and basal ganglia; and, to a lesser extent, the cerebellum and brain stem. The hypothalamus, optic nerves and chiasm, and the spinal cord appear to be involved in less than 10% of reported cases. Although the age varies widely from the neonatal period to the 9th decade, the mean age at diagnosis in children is 12 years and the peak incidence occurs between the 4th and 5th decades of life in adults (Fuller & Kros 2007).

The phenotypic features of the glial tumor cells are typically astrocytic, although a smaller number of cases involve cells with either oligodendroglial features (Balko et al 1992; Pal et al 2008) or a mixture of glial phenotypes. The tumor cells appear typically as small glial cells with elongated fusiform nuclei that have variable pleomorphism and hyperchromasia. Necrosis and microvascular hyperplasia are always absent, consistent with the morphometric features that are more consistent with low-grade gliomas. A vessel quantitative study that demonstrated normal immunohistochemical profiles of the microvasculature in brain areas involved with gliomatosis cerebri also confirmed that angiogenesis is completely absent in these lesions (Bernsen et al 2005). Mitotic indices are highly variable (MIB ≤1–30), but typically low. However, cases may present with tumor cells displaying greater cellular anaplasia (Vates et al 2003) and gliomatosis cerebri may evolve over time, into higher grade phenotypes with or without the appearance of remote, discrete lesions have been reported (Kong et al 2008; Inoue et al 2008).

Immunoreactivity for S100, GFAP, and MAP2 is present but variable in the majority of cases, similar to low-grade infiltrating gliomas (Fuller & Kros 2007; Romeike & Mawrin 2009). Although definitive molecular analyses of gliomatosis cerebri are problematic due to the diffuse, low density dispersion of the tumor cells in small biopsies, these neoplastic cells appear to be clonal and have molecular lesions in common with diffusely infiltrating, low-grade gliomas (Romeike & Mawrin 2008). The neoplastic cells in gliomatosis cerebri express biomarkers that are associated motility in all grades of infiltrating gliomas, CD44 (hyaluronic acid receptor) and matrix metallopeptidases (Kunishio et al 2003; Mawrin et al 2005). However, two studies have highlighted key differences between low-grade infiltrating gliomas and gliomatosis cerebri. One study of gliomatosis cerebri in a 29-year-old male demonstrated the predominant expression of FGFR1 mRNA (β-type) in biopsies with typically low-grade appearing tumor cells (Yamada et al 2001). FGFR1 expression more commonly occurs in malignant gliomas. This aberrant expression in gliomatosis cerebri may reflect a highly migratory neural stem cell/early progenitor cell with an aberrant proliferative phenotype. During development, translocation of midline radial glia and the formation of the corpus callosum require FGFR1 signaling (Smith et al 2006) and FGFR1 signaling increases proliferation and inhibits the spontaneous differentiation of adult neural stem cells via MAPK and Erk1/2 activation (Ma et al 2009). The abundant nestin immunoreactivity in GFAP negative tumor cells of gliomatosis cerebri is also consistent with the hypothesis of a migratory neural stem/early progenitor cell origin (Hilbig et al 2006). A more recent study of four cases of primary gliomatosis cerebri (Kong et al 2008) demonstrated increased, but variable, expression of stem cell-related biomarkers Sox2 and Mushahi-1. In contrast to glioblastoma, there was no significant expression of CD133 in these cell populations.

Glioblastoma

In addition to their similarities with normal neural stem cells, glioblastoma tumorspheres exhibit tumor-specific properties, such as increased self-renewal, aberrant proliferation and differentiation, altered karyotypes and expression of cell fate markers and most importantly malignancy. Brain tumor stem cells derived from human and murine tumorspheres faithfully reproduce the primary tumor, from which they were derived upon xenotransplantation (Galli et al 2004; Harris et al 2008; Lee et al 2006). Injection of human glioblastoma tumorspheres generated tumors with typical features of high-grade glioma such as slow growth, the presence of necrotic areas surrounded by typical pseudopalisading, increased microvascular proliferation and high mitotic figures. Most strikingly, distinctive of high-grade gliomas, implanted tumorspheres are highly migratory and infiltrate the brain parenchyma much more effectively then do serum-cultured cell lines. Analogous to xenograft data, large-scale expression data in combination with karyotypic analyses have showed that serum-free conditions of tumorsphere cultures preserve the global expression profile and the genotypic characteristics of the parental tumor much more robustly than the serum-containing regimen that has been traditionally utilized to establish glioma cell lines (Galli et al 2004; Lee et al 2006; Tunici et al 2004).

In a seminal study, the Dirks lab showed that CD133-positive cells from adult glioblastoma exhibited cancer stem cells properties, whereas CD133-negative cells did not. Strikingly, very few (100–1000) CD133-positive cells sufficiently induced tumor formation in xenografts, and are capable of serial transplantation, whereas much larger numbers (100 000) of CD133-negative cells were unable to do so. Glioblastoma xenografts obtained from CD133-positive cells consist of a minor population of CD133-positive and a majority of CD133-negative cells suggesting that a tumor hierarchy exists in which the CD133-positive tumor stem cell fraction is proliferating to generate CD133-negative non-stem cell tumor cells (Singh et al 2003; Singh et al 2004a; Singh et al 2004b). Although the majority of primary human glioblastomas and tumorspheres variably express CD133 (20–60%) (Fig. 2.42) (Beier et al 2008; Galli et al 2004; Gunther et al 2008), some tumors may have very low fractions (<1%) as determined by flow cytometry and immunohistochemical analysis. This may also be affected by the heterogeneous, faster and slower dividing progenitor cell populations that may also be present (Figs 2.43–2.45). Noteworthy, a subset of primary glioblastoma gave rise to

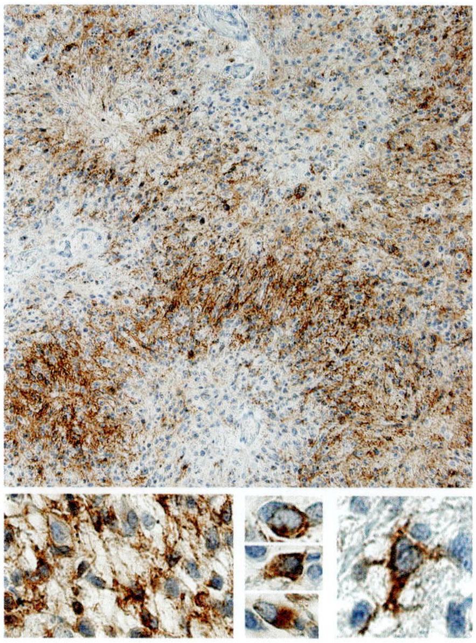

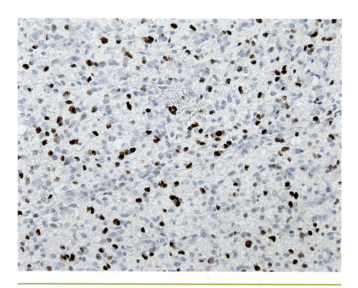

Figure 2.43 Glioblastoma. Glioblastomas typically have conspicuous OLIG2+ cell populations, of which a significant fraction is also MIB-1 positive (not shown). (OLIG2 with Ventana Ultraview immunoperoxidase.)

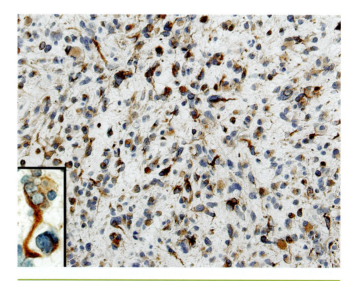

Figure 2.44 Glioblastoma. Glioblastomas have significant heterogeneity of DBX immunoreactive cell populations composed of cells with delicate unipolar or bipolar cytoplasmic processes. (DCX (C-18 domain: sc-8066) avidin–biotin immunoperoxidase.)

Figure 2.42 Glioblastoma. Tumor cell populations within individual tumors show heterogeneous immunoreactivity for CD133 epitope. This tumor showed a very high percentage of CD133+ cells by flow cytometry (56/62% for epitopes 1/2) and most of the immunoreactive cells were distributed in conspicuous zones. Higher magnification shows the CD133+ cells to have cytoplasm without processes or with short fibrillated processes. (CD133 Abcam #19898 with Ventana Ultraview immunoperoxidase.)

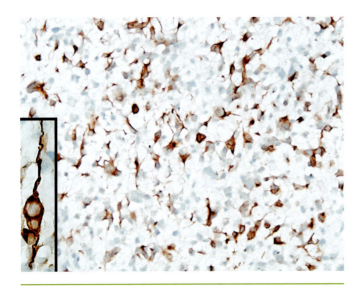

Figure 2.45 Glioblastoma. β-III tubulin immunoreactivity is heterogeneous and present in tumor cells with long, delicate cellular processes in addition to more polygonal cells. (TUJ1 avidin–biotin immunoperoxidase.)

CD133-negative cell clones with stem cell-like properties and somewhat limited *in vivo* tumorigenicity, generating less infiltrative, slower proliferating tumors (Gunther et al 2008). An important question for future research is whether the differential status of CD133-positive cells and distinct capacities for tumorsphere formation in individual gliomas reflect merely experimental differences or are *de facto* related to the distinct cellular origin of tumorigenesis. Since gliomas are initiated by various mutations and carry multiple genetic defects, we anticipate that marker signatures for brain tumor stem cells will vary among glioma patients and will reflect the heterogeneous nature of the tumor-initiating mutation and the cellular evolution of individual tumors. Definitions of specific signatures of brain tumor stem cells for individual brain cancer patients will be the challenge of personalized medicine. We envision that positive and negative selection for a variety of cell surface markers but also specific signaling pathways and metabolic states will be used in the future to regularly isolate brain tumor stem cells from patient tissue.

A critical view of the cancer stem cell hypothesis

Despite recent progress studying tumor-initiating cells in human glioma, we are just beginning to understand their nature. A fundamental question that needs to be addressed is whether brain tumor stem cells in tumorspheres and tested in xenograft transplantations are indeed the tumor-initiating cells in the patient. Lineage tracing experiments to follow the fate of mutated cells along with improved detection of brain tumor stem cells will address the relationship of tumor-initiating cells and brain tumor stem cells in mouse models.

An important open question regarding a therapeutic approach is whether in analogy to the multipotent SVZ stem cells, brain tumor stem cells are slow dividing or are more similar to the fast-proliferating transit-amplifying cells or bi-potent progenitors. Tumorsphere cells are proliferating at a higher rate than normal neurospheres and frequently grow independently of growth factors. Tumorspheres like neurospheres are heterogeneous consisting also of progenitor cells. It is not known whether the brain tumor stem cells or the progenitor cells are contributing to increased proliferation of tumorspheres *in vitro*. We predict that brain tumor stem cells *in vivo* are more similar to transit amplifying cells and lineage-restricted progenitors, which proliferate frequently and generate differentiating progeny.

Adult neural stem cells in the sub-ventricular zone form close contacts with endothelial cells and reside in a vascular niche (Mirzadeh et al 2008; Shen et al 2008; Tavazoie et al 2008). One key question in brain tumor research is about the role of tumor microvascular stroma in affecting an analogous microenvironmental niche that may regulate proliferation and self-renewal of cancer stem cells. Recent data indeed suggest that presumptive tumor stem cells in medulloblastoma crosstalk with endothelial cells of the tumor micro-perivascular niche (Yang & Wechsler-Reya 2007). It will be important to incorporate the effects of bi-directional signals between the microenvironment and the tumor stem cells into any model system in order to elucidate the mechanism of tumor initiation and maintenance.

A fundamental question of cancer biology is the amount of tumorigenic cells within individual tumors. Based on work in leukemia, the hierarchical model of tumorigenesis has initially suggested that cancer stem cells are rare. Current research on melanoma cancer stem cells however, shows that xenotransplantation assay conditions clearly determine the detectable frequency of tumor-initiating cells (Quintana et al 2008). It has been proposed that a single stem cell can give rise to a single neurosphere and that the number of neurospheres in a culture roughly corresponds to the number of stem cells within this culture (Doetsch et al 2002). However, the one-to-one relationship of stem cells to neuro/tumorspheres is difficult to demonstrate experimentally and non-stem cells, such as transit amplifying cells can form spheres *in vitro* (Reynolds & Rietze 2005; Capela 2002). It is therefore likely that tumorsphere assays are underestimating the number of stem cells within the tumor (Reynolds & Rietze 2005). Standardized isolation, tumorsphere and xenotransplantation assay conditions need to be adopted in order to correctly estimate the number of brain tumor stem cells and to compare it between brain tumor patients in order to accurately evaluate the prognostic and predictive value of brain cancer stem cells.

Due to the similarities, it has been suggested that brain tumor stem cells arise from adult neural stem cells or immature progenitors rather than differentiated cells. Recent data from mouse models have been discussed here and show that astrocytoma, oligodendroglioma and medulloblastoma arise from stem and/or progenitor cells. However, currently, we do not fully understand the underlying mechanisms by which stem and progenitor cells in response to oncogenic mutations progress to a neoplastic state.

Therapeutic implications of the tumor stem cells in gliomas

Several small-scale studies suggest that the expression of CD133 and tumorsphere-forming capacity have prognostic value and that glioblastoma with CD133-negative and CD133-positive stem cells have distinct gene expression patterns. In a larger scale expression study, human glioblastoma were grouped in proneural, proliferative and mesenchymal tumors. Neural stem cell markers including CD133 and tumorsphere formation were upregulated in the proliferative molecular subclass, which correlates with poor prognosis (Phillips et al 2006). Thus far, CD133 expression and tumorsphere formation is completely absent in secondary glioblastomas, which are histologically similar, but molecularly different to primary glioblastomas (Kleihues & Ohgaki 1999).

Anaplastic oligodendrogliomas, oligoastrocytomas, and glioblastoma with oligodendroglial components are high-grade oligodendroglial tumors, which are difficult to classify due to intratumoral diversity and the absence of clear histological markers. Since oligodendroglioma and glioblastoma respond differently to treatment, proper diagnosis is essential for outcome. A small-scale study correlates growth frequency of tumorspheres and a distinct CD133-positive population in high-grade oligodendroglial tumors with poor prognosis (Beier et al 2008). In combination, the presence of CD133-positive stem cells or cell populations with other stem cell biomarkers, and frequency of tumorsphere formation might become useful criteria in predicting the therapeutic response and in establishing novel prognostic sub-classes of glioma. Comprehensive, large-scale studies are necessary to evaluate the prognostic and predictive value of CD133-positive stem cells or cell populations with other stem cell biomarkers, which may vary according to the glioma subtype. A recent study showed that brain tumor stem cells are more resistant to conventional treatment than non-stem tumor cells (Bao et al 2006). More evidence is needed to conclude that glioma stem cells survive radiation and perhaps chemotherapy, and give rise to recurring secondary tumors. Successful elimination of brain tumor stem cells by novel stem cell-directed therapies might turn out to be equally important to the cytotoxic therapies directed against non-stem neoplastic cells to prevent tumor growth and recurrence.

Key points

- The biologic properties of neural stem cells and derivative progenitor lineages are highly regulated in both a temporal and spatial fashion throughout the neuraxis.

- CNS neural tumor stem cells share the following traits with neural stem cells: (1) capacity for self-renewal (symmetric cell divisions) and for generation of progenitor cell populations (asymmetric cell divisions) with variable potential(s) to differentiate, depending on the tumor; (2) expression of specific sets of neural biomarkers (CD133, Nestin, etc.); (3) responsiveness to their microenvironment, including the perivascular niche; (4) increased DNA repair mechanisms and ABC transporter-mediated drug efflux that confer decreased sensitivity to radiation and chemo-therapy; and (5) distinct growth requirements, including spheroid formation under non-adherent conditions.

- There may be a clear biologic distinction between the tumor-initiating stem cell, as a slow-dividing, niche-dependent cell and the tumor-propagating stem cells with an increased proliferative potential that can essentially propagate and maintain the tumor.

- A fundamental question is whether cancer stem cells in tumorspheres and tested in xenograft transplantations are indeed the tumor-initiating cells in the patient.

- Germinal zones within the developing brain and neural stem cell niches in adult brain may be the primary sources of cells that may undergo neoplastic transformation and migrate away to initiate tumorigenesis in non-germinal regions.

- The regional properties of neural stem cells and related progenitor lineages in the immature CNS affect their temporal capacity for neoplastic transformation and the resultant tumor histopathology; however, primitive tumors with similar histopathology may not have identical neural stem cell origins.

- The developing fields that are particularly relevant to most primitive/embryonal-like tumors in humans are the retinal neuro-progenitors arising from the retinal neuroepithelium; the cerebellar ventricular zone and the adjacent, more dorsal rhombic lip germinal zone, in the hindbrain; and in the forebrain, a ventricular zone or germinal matrix.

- Adult brain stem cell and derivative progenitor lineage niches are primarily the lateral sub-ventricular zone with (temporal and regional heterogeneity) and the subgranular layer of the hippocampal dentate gyrus.

- The human and murine sub-ventricular zones have distinct cellular architectures but appear to be composed of similar cell types, including ependymal cells, slow-dividing multipotent neural stem cells or type B astrocytes, fast-dividing, growth factor-activated stem cells or transit amplifying cells and glial and neuronal progenitors.

- Forebrain tumors with unique potentials for differentiation in children and young adults arise from radial glial cells, bi-potential progenitors, or transit-amplifying progenitor cells located in region-specific niches.

- Gliomas with similar histopathologic features in pediatric and adult populations may arise from tumor initiating stem cells and may harbor tumor-propagating stem cells at various stages of differentiation.

- The highly proliferative cell populations of malignant gliomas more closely resemble growth factor receptor-activated stem cells or transit amplifying cells and lineage-restricted progenitors, which proliferate frequently and generate differentiating progeny.

- Successful elimination of brain tumor stem cells by novel stem cell-targeted therapies may be equal to, or more efficacious than, the cytotoxic therapies directed against non-stem tumor cells for preventing tumor growth and recurrence.

- An understanding of the underlying mechanisms by which neural stem and progenitor cells respond to oncogenic mutations and progress to a neoplastic state are important for improving therapeutic cellular targeting.

- Standardized conditions for isolation from surgical specimens, tumorsphere production, and xeno-transplantation need to be adopted in order to correctly estimate the number of brain tumor stem cells to accurately evaluate their comparative prognostic and predictive value for therapeutic strategies.

REFERENCES

Adler, R., Hatlee, M., 1989. Plasticity and differentiation of embryonic retinal cells after terminal mitosis. Science 243, 391–393.

Ahn, S.M., Byun, K., Kim, D., et al., 2008. Olig2-induced neural stem cell differentiation involves downregulation of Wnt signaling and induction of Dickkopf-1 expression. PLoS One 3, e3917.

Alcantara Llaguno, S., Chen, J., Kwon, C.H., et al., 2009. Malignant astrocytomas originate from neural stem/progenitor cells in a somatic tumor suppressor mouse model. Cancer Cell 15, 45–56.

Alvarez-Buylla, A., Kohwi, M., Nguyen, T.M., et al., 2008. The heterogeneity of adult neural stem cells and the emerging complexity of their niche. Cold Spring Harb. Symp. Quant. Biol. 73, 357–365.

Bailey, P., Cushing, H.A., 1926. Classification of the tumors of the glioma group on a histogenetic basis with a correlated study of prognosis. Lippincott, Philadelphia, PA.

Bailey, P., 1948. Intracranial tumors, second ed. Thomas, Springfield, IL.

Balko, M.G., Blisard, K.S., Smamha, J., 1992. Oligodendroglial gliomatosis cerebri. Human Pathol. 23, 706–707.

Bannykh, S.I., Stolt, C.C., Kim, J., et al., 2006. Oligodendroglial-specific transcriptional factor SOX10 is ubiquitously expressed in human gliomas. J. Neurooncol. 76, 115–127.

Bao, S., Wu, Q., McLendon, R.E., et al., 2006. Glioma stem cells promote radioresistance by preferential activation of the DNA damage response. Nature 444, 756–760.

Beier, D., Wischhusen, J., Dietmaier, W., et al., 2008. CD133 expression and cancer stem cells predict prognosis in high-grade oligodendroglial tumors. Brain Pathol. 18, 370–377.

Bernier, P.J., Vinet, J., Cossette, M., Parent, A., 2000. Characterization of the subventricular zone of the adult human brain: evidence for the involvement of Bcl-2. Neurosci. Res. 37 (1), 67–78.

Bernsen, H., Van der Laak, J., Küsters, B., et al., 2005. Gliomatosis cerebri: quantitative proof of vessel recruitment by cooptation instead of angiogenesis. J. Neurosurg. 103, 702–706.

Boncinelli, E., Somma, R., Acampora, D., et al., 1988. Organization of human homeobox genes. Hum. Reprod. 3, 880–886.

Bruce, W.R., Van Der Gaag, H.A., 1963. Quantitative assay for the number of murine lymphoma cells capable of proliferation in vivo. Nature 199, 79–80.

Brun, A., 1965. The subpial granular layer of the foetal cerebral cortex in man. Its ontogeny and significance in congenital cortical malformations. Acta Pathol. Microbiol. Scand Suppl. 179, 173–198.

Buse, E., de Groot, H., 1991. Generation of developmental patterns in the neuroepithelium of the developing mammalian eye: the pigment epithelium of the eye. Neurosci. Lett. 126, 63–66.

Buse, E., Eichmann, T., deGroot, H., et al., 1993. Differentiation of the mammalian retinal pigment epithelium in vitro: influence of presumptive retinal neuroepithelium and head mesenchyme. Anat. Embryol. (Berl.) 187, 259–268.

Caccamo, D.V., Herman, M.M., Frankfurter, A., et al., 1989. An immunohistochemical study of neuropeptides and neuronal cytoskeletal proteins in the neuroepithelial component of a spontaneous murine ovarian teratoma. Primitive neuroepithelium displays immunoreactivity for neuropeptides and neuron-associated beta-tubulin isotype. Am. J. Pathol. 135, 801–813.

Cameron, R.S., Rakic, P., 1991. Glial cell lineage in the cerebral cortex: a review and synthesis. Glia 4, 124–137.

Capela, A., Temple, S., 2002. LeX/ssea-1 is expressed by adult mouse CNS stem cells, identifying them as nonependymal. Neuron 35, 865–875.

Chaichana, K.L., Capilla-Gonzalez, V., Gonzalez-Perez, O., et al., 2007. Preservation of glial cytoarchitecture from ex vivo human tumor and non-tumor cerebral cortical explants: A human model to study neurological diseases. J. Neurosci. Methods 164, 261–270.

Colin, C., Baeza, N., Bartoli, C., et al., 2006. Identification of genes differentially expressed in glioblastoma versus pilocytic astrocytoma using suppression subtractive hybridization. Oncogene 25, 2818–2826.

Corbeil, D., Joester, A., Fargeas, C.A., et al., 2009. Expression of distinct splice variants of the stem cell marker prominin-1 (CD133) in glial cells. Glia 57, 860–874.

Corbeil, D., Roper, K., Hellwig, A., et al., 2000 The human AC133 hematopoietic stem cell antigen is also expressed in epithelial cells and targeted to plasma membrane protrusions. J. Biol. Chem. 275, 5512–5520.

Corbeil, D., Roper, K., Weigmann, A., et al., 1998. AC133 hematopoietic stem cell antigen: human homologue of mouse kidney prominin or distinct member of a novel protein family? Blood 91, 2625–2626.

Corbin, J.G., Gaiano, N., Juliano, S.L., et al., 2008. Regulation of neural progenitor cell development in the nervous system. J. Neurochem. 106, 2272–2287.

Corti, S., Nizzardo, M., Nardini, M., et al., 2007. Isolation and characterization of murine neural stem/progenitor cells based on Prominin-1 expression. Exp. Neurol. 205, 547–562.

Dai, C., Celestino, J.C., Okada, Y., et al., 2001. PDGF autocrine stimulation dedifferentiates cultured astrocytes and induces oligodendrogliomas and oligoastrocytomas from neural progenitors and astrocytes in vivo. Genes Dev. 15, 1913–1925.

Dimou, L., Simon, C., Kirchhoff, F., et al., 2008. Progeny of Olig2-expressing progenitors in the gray and white matter of the adult mouse cerebral cortex. J. Neurosci. 28, 10434–10442.

Dirks, P.B., 2005. Brain tumor stem cells. Biol. Blood Marrow. Transplant. 11, 12–13.

Doetsch, F., Caille, I., Lim, D.A., et al., 1999, Subventricular zone astrocytes are neural stem cells in the adult mammalian brain. Cell 97, 703–716.

Doetsch, F., Petreanu, L., Caille, I., et al., 2002. EGF converts transit-amplifying neurogenic precursors in the adult brain into multipotent stem cells. Neuron 36, 1021–1034.

Emmenegger, B.A., Wechsler-Reya, R.J., 2008. Stem cells and the origin and propagation of brain tumors. J. Child Neurol. 23, 1172–1178.

Fan, X., Eberhart, C.G., 2008. Medulloblastoma stem cells. J. Clin. Oncol. 26, 2821–2827.

Fuller, G.N., Kros, J.M., 2007. Gliomatosis cerebri. In: Louis, D.N., Ohgaki, H., Wiestler, O.D., et al. (Eds.), WHO classification of tumours of the central nervous system, fourth ed. IARC, Lyon, pp. 218–221.

Galli, R., Binda, E., Orfanelli, U., et al., 2004. Isolation and characterization of tumorigenic, stem-like neural precursors from human glioblastoma. Cancer Res. 64, 7011–7021.

Gallie, B.L., Squire, J.A., Goddard, A., et al., 1990. Mechanism of oncogenesis in retinoblastoma. Lab. Invest. 62, 394–408.

Giangaspero, F., Eberhart, C.G., Haapasalo, H., et al., 2007. Medulloblastoma. In: Louis, D.N., Ohgaki, H., Wiestler, O.D., et al. (Eds.), WHO classification of tumours of the central nervous system, fourth ed. IARC, Lyon, pp. 131–140.

Gennett, I.N., Cavenee, W.K., 1990. Molecular genetics in the pathology and diagnosis of retinoblastoma. Brain Pathol. 1, 25–32.

Gilbertson, R.J., Gutmann, D.H., 2007. Tumorigenesis in the brain: location, location, location. Cancer Res. 67, 5579–5582.

Giordano, F., De Marzo, A., Vetrini, F., et al., 2007. Fibroblast growth factor and epidermal growth factor differently affect differentiation of murine retinal stem cells in vitro. Mol. Vis. 13, 1842–1850.

Gonzalez-Fernandez, F., Healy, J.I., 1990. Early expression of the gene for interphotoreceptor retinol-binding protein during photoreceptor differentiation suggests a critical role for the interphotoreceptor matrix in retinal development. J. Cell Biol. 111, 2775–2784.

Gonzalez-Fernandez, F., Lopes, M.B., Garcia-Fernandez, J.M., et al., 1992. Expression of developmentally defined retinal phenotypes in the histogenesis of retinoblastoma. Am. J. Pathol. 141, 363–375.

Gritti, A., Parati, E.A., Cova, L., et al., 1996. Multipotential stem cells from the adult mouse brain proliferate and self-renew in response to basic fibroblast growth factor. J. Neurosci. 16, 1091–1100.

Gunther, H.S., Schmidt, N.O., Phillips, H.S., et al., 2008. Glioblastoma-derived stem cell-enriched cultures form distinct subgroups according to molecular and phenotypic criteria. Oncogene 27, 2897–2909.

Gutmann, D.H., Hedrick, N.M., Li, J., et al., 2002. Comparative gene expression profile analysis of neurofibromatosis 1-associated and sporadic pilocytic astrocytomas. Cancer Res. 62, 2085–2091.

Hamburger, A.W., Salmon, S.E., 1977. Primary bioassay of human tumor stem cells. Science 197, 461–463.

Harris, M.A., Yang, H., Low, B.E., et al., 2008. Cancer stem cells are enriched in the side population cells in a mouse model of glioma. Cancer Res. 68, 10051–10059.

Hauswirth, W.W., Langerijt, A.V., Timmers, A.M., et al., 1992. Early expression and localization of rhodopsin and interphotoreceptor retinoid-binding protein (IRBP) in the developing fetal bovine retina. Exp. Eye. Res. 54, 661–670.

Hegedus, B., Dasgupta, B., Shin, J.E., et al., 2007. Neurofibromatosis-1 regulates neuronal and glial cell differentiation from neuroglial progenitors in vivo by both cAMP- and Ras-dependent mechanisms. Cell Stem. Cell 1, 443–457.

Hemmati, H.D., Nakano, I., Lazareff, J.A., et al., 2003. Cancerous stem cells can arise from pediatric brain tumors. Proc. Natl. Acad. Sci. USA 100, 15178–15183.

Hevner, R.F., 2006. From radial glia to pyramidal-projection neuron: transcription factor cascades in cerebral cortex development. Mol. Neurobiol. 33, 33–50.

Hilbig, A., Barbosa-Coutinho, L.M., Toscani, N., et al., 2006. Expression of nestin and vimentin in gliomatosis cerebri. Arq. Neuropsiquiatr. 64, 781–786.

Holland, E.C., Celestino, J., Dai, C., et al., 2000. Combined activation of Ras and Akt in neural progenitors induces glioblastoma formation in mice. Nat. Genet. 25, 55–57.

Holland, E.C., Hively, W.P., DePinho, R.A., et al., 1998. A constitutively active epidermal growth factor receptor cooperates with disruption of G1 cell-cycle arrest pathways to induce glioma-like lesions in mice. Genes Dev. 12, 3675–3685.

Holt, C.E., Bertsch, T.W., Ellis, H.M., et al, 1988. Cellular determination in the Xenopus retina is independent of lineage and birth date. Neuron 1, 15–26.

Howard, B., Chen, Y., Zecevic, N., 2006. Cortical progenitor cells in the developing human telencephalon. Glia 53, 57–66.

Howard, B.M., Zhicheng, M., Filipovic, R., et al., 2008. Radial glia cells in the developing human brain. Neuroscientist 14, 459–473.

Inoue, T., Kanamori, M., Sonoda, Y., et al., 2008. [Glioblastoma multiforme developing separately from the initial lesion 9 years after successful treatment for gliomatosis cerebri: a case report] No Shinkei Geka 36, 709–715.

Ivkovic, S., Canoll, P., Goldman, J.E., 2008. Constitutive EGFR signaling in oligodendrocyte progenitors leads to diffuse hyperplasia in postnatal white matter. J. Neurosci. 28, 914–922.

Jackson, E.L., Garcia-Verdugo, J.M., Gil-Perotin, S., et al., 2006. PDGFR alpha-positive B cells are neural stem cells in the adult SVZ that form glioma-like growths in response to increased PDGF signaling. Neuron 51, 187–199.

Jellinger, K., 1972. Embryonal cell nests in human cerebellar nuclei. Z. Anat. Entwicklungsgesch 138, 145–154.

Jones, D.T., Kocialkowski, S., Liu, L., et al., 2008. Tandem duplication producing a novel oncogenic B R A F fusion gene defines the majority of pilocytic astrocytomas. Cancer Res. 68, 8673–8677.

Kadin, M.E., Rubinstein, L.J., Nelson, J.S., 1970. Neonatal cerebellar medulloblastoma originating from the fetal external granular layer. J. Neuropathol. Exp. Neurol. 29, 583–600.

Kim, C.F., Dirks, P.B., 2008. Cancer and stem cell biology: how tightly intertwined? Cell Stem Cell 3, 147–150.

Kleihues, P., Ohgaki, H., 1999. Primary and secondary glioblastomas: from concept to clinical diagnosis. Neuro. Oncol. 1, 44–51.

Kokovay, E., Shen, Q., Temple, S., 2008. The incredible elastic brain: how neural stem cells expand our minds. Neuron 60, 420–429.

Kong, D.S., Kim, M.H., Park, W.Y., et al., 2008. The progression of gliomas is associated with cancer stem cell phenotype. Oncol. Rep. 19, 639–643.

Kukekov, V.G., Laywell, E.D., Suslov, O., et al., 1999. Multipotent stem/progenitor cells with similar properties arise from two neurogenic regions of adult human brain. Exp. Neurol. 156, 333–344.

Kunishio, K., Okada, M., Matsumoto, Y., Nagao, S., 2003. Matrix metalloproteinase-2 and -9 expression in astrocytic tumors. Brain Tumor Pathol. 20, 39–45.

Leclerc, N., Schwarting, G.A., Herrup, K., et al., 1992. Compartmentation in mammalian cerebellum: Zebrin II and P-path antibodies define three classes of sagittally organized bands of Purkinje cells. Proc. Natl. Acad. Sci. USA 89, 5006–5010.

Lee, A., Kessler, J.D., Read, T.A., et al., 2005. Isolation of neural stem cells from the postnatal cerebellum. Nat. Neurosci. 8, 723–729.

Lee, J., Kotliarova, S., Kotliarov, Y., et al., 2006. Tumor stem cells derived from glioblastomas cultured in bFGF and EGF more closely mirror the phenotype and genotype of primary tumors than do serum-cultured cell lines. Cancer Cell 9, 391–403.

Leenstra, J.L., Rodriguez, F.J., Frechette, C.M., et al., 2007. Central neurocytoma: management recommendations based on a 35-year experience. Int. J. Radiat. Oncol. Biol. Phys. 67, 1145–1154.

Levine, E.M., Green, E.S., 2004. Cell-intrinsic regulators of proliferation in vertebrate retinal progenitors. Semin Cell Dev. Biol. 15, 63–74.

Levine, J.M., Stincone, F., Lee, Y.S., 1993. Development and differentiation of glial precursor cells in the rat cerebellum. Glia 7, 307–321.

Li, G., Kataoka, H., Coughlin, S.R., et al., 2009. Identification of a transient subpial neurogenic zone in the developing dentate gyrus and its regulation by Cxcl12 and reelin signaling. Development 136, 327–335.

Ligon, K.L., Alberta, J.A., Kho, A.T. et al., 2004. The oligodendroglial lineage marker OLIG2 is universally expressed in diffuse gliomas. J. Neuropathol. Exp. Neurol. 63, 499–509.

Ligon, K.L., Fancy, S.P., Franklin, R.J., et al., 2006. Olig gene function in CNS development and disease. Glia 54, 1–10.

Ligon, K.L., Huillard, E., Mehta, S., et al., 2007. Olig2-regulated lineage-restricted pathway controls replication competence in neural stem cells and malignant glioma. Neuron 53, 503–517.

Lim, D.A., Cha, S., Mayo, M.C., et al., 2007. Relationship of glioblastoma multiforme to neural stem cell regions predicts invasive and multifocal tumor phenotype. Neuro. Oncol. 9, 424–429.

Liou, G.I., Geng, L., Baehr, W., 1991. Interphotoreceptor retinoid-binding protein: biochemistry and molecular biology. Prog. Clin. Biol. Res. 362, 115–137.

Liu, Y., Han, S.S., Wu, Y., et al., 2004. CD44 expression identifies astrocyte-restricted precursor cells. Dev. Biol. 276, 31–46.

Lopes, M.B.L., VandenBerg, S.R., 2007. Tumors of the central nervous system. In: Fletcher, C.D.M. (Ed.), Diagnostic histopathology of tumors, third ed. Elsevier, Philadelphia, PA, pp. 1653–1732.

Lopes, M.B.S., Wiestler, O.D., Stemmer-Rachamimov, A.O., et al., 2007. Tuberous sclerosis complex and subependymal giant cell astrocytoma. In: Louis, D.N., Ohgaki, H., Wiestler, O.D., et al. (Eds.), WHO classification of tumours of the central nervous system, fourth ed. IARC, Lyon, pp. 218–221.

McLendon, R.E., Judkins, A.R., Eberhart, C.G., et al., 2007. Central nervous system primitive neuroectodermal tumours. In: Louis, D.N., Ohgaki, H., Wiestler, O.D., et al. (Eds.), WHO classification of tumours of the central nervous system, fourth ed. IARC, Lyon, pp. 141–146.

Ma, D.K., Ponnusamy, K., Song, M.R., et al., 2009. Molecular genetic analysis of FGFR1 signalling reveals distinct roles of MAPK and PLCgamma1 activation for self-renewal of adult neural stem cells. Mol. Brain 2, 16–29.

Margo, C., Hidayat, A., Kopelman, J., et al., 1983. Retinocytoma. A benign variant of retinoblastoma. Arch. Ophthalmol. 101, 1519–1531.

Martin, P., Carriere, C., Dozier, C., et al., 1992. Characterization of a paired box- and homeobox-containing quail gene (Pax-QNR) expressed in the neuroretina. Oncogene 7, 1721–1728.

Mawrin, C., Schneider, T., Firsching, R., et al., 2005. Assessment of tumor cell invasion factors in gliomatosis cerebri. J. Neurooncol. 73, 109–115.

Mehler, M.F., Rozental, R., Dougherty, M., et al., 1993. Cytokine regulation of neuronal differentiation of hippocampal progenitor cells. Nature 362, 62–65.

Menn, B., Garcia-Verdugo, J.M., Yaschine, C., et al., 2006. Origin of oligodendrocytes in the subventricular zone of the adult brain. J. Neurosci. 26, 7907–7918.

Merkle, F.T., Tramontin, A.D., Garcia-Verdugo, J.M., et al., 2004. Radial glia give rise to adult neural stem cells in the subventricular zone. Proc. Natl. Acad. Sci. USA 101, 17528–17532.

Mirzadeh, Z., Merkle, F.T., Soriano-Navarro, M., et al., 2008. Neural stem cells confer unique pinwheel architecture to the ventricular surface in neurogenic regions of the adult brain. Cell Stem Cell 3, 265–278.

Mo, Z., Zecevic, N., 2008. Is Pax6 critical for neurogenesis in the human fetal brain? Cereb. Cortex 18, 1455–1465.

Morrison, S.J., Kimble, J., 2006. Asymmetric and symmetric stem-cell divisions in development and cancer. Nature 441, 1068–1074.

Napolioni, V., Moavero, R., Curatolo, P., 2009. Recent advances in neurobiology of tuberous sclerosis complex. Brain Dev. 31, 104–113.

Nowakowski, R.S., Hayes, N.L., 2005. Cell proliferation in the developing mammalian brain. In: Rao, M.S., Jacobson, M. (Eds.), Developmental biology, fourth ed. Kluwer Academic/Plenum, New York, pp. 21–39.

Pal, L., Behari, S., Kumar, S., et al., 2008. Gliomatosis cerebri – an uncommon neuroepithelial tumor in children with oligodendroglial phenotype. Pediatr. Neurosurg. 44, 212–215.

Persson, A., Petritsch, C., Itsara, M., et al., 2010. Non-stem cell origin of oligodendondrogliomas. Cancer Cell. 18, 669–682.

Pfenninger, C.V., Roschupkina, T., Hertwig, F., et al., 2007. CD133 is not present on neurogenic astrocytes in the adult subventricular zone, but on embryonic neural stem cells, ependymal cells, and glioblastoma cells. Cancer Res. 67, 5727–5736.

Pfister, S., Janzarik, W.G., Remke, M., et al., 2008. BRAF gene duplication constitutes a mechanism of M A P K pathway activation in low-grade astrocytomas. J. Clin. Invest. 118, 1739–1749.

Phi, J.H., Park, S.H., Chae, J.H., et al., 2008. Congenital subependymal giant cell astrocytoma: clinical considerations and expression of radial glial cell markers in giant cells. Childs Nerv. Syst. 24, 1499–1503.

Phillips, H.S., Kharbanda, S., Chen, R., et al., 2006. Molecular subclasses of high-grade glioma predict prognosis, delineate a pattern of disease progression, and resemble stages in neurogenesis. Cancer Cell 9, 157–173.

Preusser, M., Laggner, U., Haberler, C., et al., 2006. Comparative analysis of NeuN immunoreactivity in primary brain tumours: conclusions for rational use in diagnostic histopathology. Histopathology 48, 438–444.

Price, J., 1989. Cell lineage and lineage markers. Curr. Opin. Cell Biol. 1, 1071–1074.

Quinones-Hinojosa, A., Sanai, N., Soriano-Navarro, M., et al., 2006. Cellular composition and cytoarchitecture of the adult human subventricular zone: a niche of neural stem cells. J. Comp. Neurol. 494, 415–434.

Quiñones-Hinojosa, A., Chaichana, K., 2007. The human subventricular zone: A source of new cells and a potential source of brain tumors. Exp. Neurol. 205, 313–324.

Quintana, E., Shackleton, M., Sabel, M.S., et al., 2008. Efficient tumour formation by single human melanoma cells. Nature 456, 593–598.

Raaf, J., Kernohan, J., 1944. Relation of abnormal collections of cells in posterior medullary velum of cerebellum to origin of medulloblastoma. Arch. Neurol. Psychiatry 52, 163–169.

Rakic, P., Sidman, R.L., 1970. Histogenesis of cortical layers in human cerebellum, particularly the lamina dissecans. J. Comp. Neurol. 139, 473–500.

Raymond, P.A., 1991. Retinal regeneration in teleost fish. Ciba. Found Symp. 160, 171–186; discussion 186–191.

Read, T.A., Fogarty, M.P., Markant, S.L., et al., 2009. Identification of CD15 as a marker for tumor-propagating cells in a mouse model of medulloblastoma. Cancer Cell 15, 135–147.

Rebetz, J., Tian, D., Persson, A., et al., 2008. Glial progenitor-like phenotype in low-grade glioma and enhanced CD133-expression and neuronal lineage differentiation potential in high-grade glioma. PLoS one 3, e1936.

Reh, T.A., Kljavin, I.J., 1989. Age of differentiation determines rat retinal germinal cell phenotype: induction of differentiation by dissociation. J. Neurosci. 9, 4179–4189.

Renfranz, P.J., Cunningham, M.G., McKay, R.D., 1991. Region-specific differentiation of the hippocampal stem cell line HiB5 upon implantation into the developing mammalian brain. Cell 66, 713–729.

Reynolds, B.A., Rietze, R.L., 2005. Neural stem cells and neurospheres–re-evaluating the relationship. Nat. Methods 2, 333–336.

Reynolds, B.A., Weiss, S., 1992. Generation of neurons and astrocytes from isolated cells of the adult mammalian central nervous system. Science 255, 1707–1710.

Reynolds, B.A., Weiss, S., 1996. Clonal and population analyses demonstrate that an EGF-responsive mammalian embryonic C N S precursor is a stem cell. Dev. Biol. 175, 1–13.

Romeike, B.F., Mawrin, C., 2008. Gliomatosis cerebri: growing evidence for diffuse gliomas with wide invasion. Expert Rev. Neurother. 8, 587–597.

Romeike, B.F., Mawrin, C., 2009. MAP-2 immunoexpression in gliomatosis cerebri. Histopathology 54, 504–505.

Rubinstein, L.J., 1972. Presidential address. Cytogenesis and differentiation of primitive central neuroepithelial tumors. J. Neuropathol. Exp. Neurol. 31, 7–26.

Rubinstein, L.J., 1985. Embryonal central neuroepithelial tumors and their differentiating potential. A cytogenetic view of a complex neuro-oncological problem. J. Neurosurg. 62, 795–805.

Rubinstein, L.J., 1987. The correlation of neoplastic vulnerability with central neuroepithelial cytogeny and glioma differentiation. J. Neurooncol. 5, 11–27.

Russell, D.S., Rubinstein, L.J., 1989. Pathology of tumours of the nervous system, fifth ed. Edward Arnold, London, pp. 105, 171–172, 247–251.

Sakariassen, P.O., Immervoll, H., Chekenya, M., 2007. Cancer stem cells as mediators of treatment resistance in brain tumors: status and controversies. Neoplasia 9, 882–892.

Sanai, N., Alvarez-Buylla, A., Berger, M.S., 2005. Neural stem cells and the origin of gliomas. N. Engl. J. Med. 353, 811–822.

Scheithauer, B.W., Hawkins, C., Tihan, T., et al., 2007. Pilocytic astrocytoma. In: Louis, D.N., Ohgaki, H., Wiestler, O.D., et al. (Eds.), WHO classification of tumours of the central nervous system, fourth ed. IARC, Lyon, pp. 14–20.

Schuller, U., Heine, V.M., Mao, J., et al., 2008. Acquisition of granule neuron precursor identity is a critical determinant of progenitor cell competence to form Shh-induced medulloblastoma. Cancer Cell 14, 123–134.

Seigel, G.M., Hackam, A.S., Ganguly, A., et al., 2007. Human embryonic and neuronal stem cell markers in retinoblastoma. Mol. Vis. 13, 823–832.

Sharma, M.K., Zehnbauer, B.A., Watson, M.A., et al., 2005. RAS pathway activation and an oncogenic R A S mutation in sporadic pilocytic astrocytoma. Neurology 65, 1335–1336.

Sheedlo, H.J., Turner, J.E., 1996. Influence of a retinal pigment epithelial cell factor(s) on rat retinal progenitor cells. Brain Res. Dev. Brain Res. 93, 88–99.

Shen, Q., Wang, Y., Kokovay, E., et al., 2008. Adult S V Z stem cells lie in a vascular niche: a quantitative analysis of niche cell-cell interactions. Cell Stem Cell 3, 289–300.

Shiurba, R.A., Buffinger, N.S., Spencer, E.M., et al., 1991. Basic fibroblast growth factor and somatomedin C in human medulloepithelioma. Cancer 68, 798–808.

Sim, F.J., Keyoung, H.M., Goldman, J.E., et al., 2006. Neurocytoma is a tumor of adult neuronal progenitor cells. J. Neurosci. 26, 12544–12555.

Singh, S.K., Clarke, I.D., Terasaki, M., et al., 2003. Identification of a cancer stem cell in human brain tumors. Cancer Res. 63, 5821–5828.

Singh, S.K., Clarke, I.D., Hide, T., et al., 2004a. Cancer stem cells in nervous system tumors. Oncogene 23, 7267–7273.

Singh, S.K., Hawkins, C., Clarke, I.D., et al., 2004b. Identification of human brain tumour initiating cells. Nature 432, 396–401.

Smith, K.M., Ohkubo, Y., Maragnoli, M.E., et al., 2006. Midline radial glia translocation and corpus callosum formation require F G F signaling. Nat. Neurosci. 9, 787–797.

Sparrow, J.R., Hicks, D., Barnstable, C.J., 1990. Cell commitment and differentiation in explants of embryonic rat neural retina. Comparison with the developmental potential of dissociated retina. Brain Res. Dev. Brain Res. 51, 69–84.

Stevenson, L., Echlin, R., 1934. The nature and origin of some tumors of the cerebellum (medulloblastoma). Neurol. Psychiatry 31, 93–109.

Tanaka, Y., Sasaki, A., Ishiuchi, S., et al., 2008. Diversity of glial cell components in pilocytic astrocytoma. Neuropathology 28, 399–407.

Tavazoie, M., Van der Veken, L., Silva-Vargas, V., et al., 2008. A specialized vascular niche for adult neural stem cells. Cell Stem Cell 3, 279–288.

Toth, L.E., Slawin, K.L., Pintar, J.E., et al., 1987. Region-specific expression of mouse homeobox genes in the embryonic mesoderm and central nervous system. Proc. Natl. Acad. Sci. USA 84, 6790–6794.

Tropepe, V., Hitoshi, S., Sirard, C., et al., 2001. Direct neural fate specification from embryonic stem cells: a primitive mammalian neural stem cell stage acquired through a default mechanism. Neuron 30, 65–78.

Tunici, P., Bissola, L., Lualdi, E., et al., 2004. Genetic alterations and in vivo tumorigenicity of neurospheres derived from an adult glioblastoma. Mol. Cancer 3, 25.

Turner, D.L., Cepko, C.L., 1987. A common progenitor for neurons and glia persists in rat retina late in development. Nature 328, 131–136.

Uchida, N., Buck, D.W., He, D., et al., 2000. Direct isolation of human central nervous system stem cells. Proc. Natl. Acad. Sci. USA 97, 14720–14725.

VandenBerg, S.R., 1993. Desmoplastic infantile ganglioglioma and desmoplastic cerebral astrocytoma of infancy. Brain Pathol. 3, 275–281.

VandenBerg, S.R., Chatel, M., Griffiths, O.M., et al., 1981a. Neural differentiation in the OTT-6050 mouse teratoma. Production of a tumor fraction restricted to stem cells and neural cells after centrifugal elutriation. Virchows Arch. A Pathol. Anat. Histol. 392, 281–294.

VandenBerg, S.R., Hess, J.R., Herman, M.M., et al., 1981b. Neural differentiation in the OTT-6050 mouse teratoma. Production of a tumor fraction showing melanogenesis in neuroepithelial cells after centrifugal elutriation. Virchows Arch. A Pathol. Anat. Histol. 392, 295–308.

Vates, G.E., Chang, S., Lamborn, K.R., et al., 2003. Gliomatosis cerebri: a review of 22 cases. Neurosurgery 53, 261–271.

Vescovi, A.L., Galli, R., Reynolds, B.A., 2006. Brain tumour stem cells. Nat. Rev. Cancer 6, 425–436.

Vescovi, A.L., Reynolds, B.A., Fraser, D.D., et al., 1993. bFGF regulates the proliferative fate of unipotent (neuronal) and bipotent (neuronal/astroglial) EGF-generated CNS progenitor cells. Neuron 11, 951–966.

von Deimling, A., Janzer, R., Kleihues, P., et al., 1990. Patterns of differentiation in central neurocytoma. An immunohistochemical study of eleven biopsies. Acta Neuropathol. 79, 473–479.

Wallace, V.A., 2008. Proliferative and cell fate effects of Hedgehog signaling in the vertebrate retina. Brain Res. 1192, 61–75.

Watanabe, T., Raff, M.C., 1990. Rod photoreceptor development in vitro: intrinsic properties of proliferating neuroepithelial cells change as development proceeds in the rat retina. Neuron 4, 461–467.

Wechsler-Reya, R., Scott, M.P., 2001. The developmental biology of brain tumors. Annu. Rev. Neurosci. 24, 385–428.

Weiss, W.A., Burns, M.J., Hackett, C., et al., 2003. Genetic determinants of malignancy in a mouse model for oligodendroglioma. Cancer Res. 63, 1589–1595.

Westermann, B.A., Murre, C., Oudejans, C.B.M., 2003. The cellular Pax-Hox-Helix connection. Biochim. Biophys. Acta 1629, 1–7.

Westphal, M., Stavrou, D., Nausch, H., et al., 1994. Human neurocytoma cells in culture show characteristics of astroglial differentiation. J. Neurosci. Res. 38, 698–704.

Wetts, R., Fraser, S.E., 1988. Multipotent precursors can give rise to all major cell types of the frog retina. Science 239, 1142–1145.

Wong, K.K., Chang, Y.M., Tsang, Y.T., et al., 2005. Expression analysis of juvenile pilocytic astrocytomas by oligonucleotide microarray reveals two potential subgroups. Cancer Res. 65, 76–84.

Wright, C.V., Cho, K.W., Oliver, G., et al., 1989. Vertebrate homeodomain proteins: families of region-specific transcription factors. Trends Biochem. Sci. 14, 52–56.

Yachnis, A.T., Rorke, L.B., Lee, V.M., et al., 1993. Expression of neuronal and glial polypeptides during histogenesis of the human cerebellar cortex including observations on the dentate nucleus. J. Comp. Neurol. 334, 356–369.

Yamada, S.M., Hayashi, Y., Takahashi, H., et al., 2001. Histological and genetic diagnosis of gliomatosis cerebri: case report. J. Neurooncol. 52, 237–240.

Yang, Z.J., Ellis, T., Markant, S.L., et al., 2008. Medulloblastoma can be initiated by deletion of Patched in lineage-restricted progenitors or stem cells. Cancer Cell 14, 135–145.

Yang, Z.J., Wechsler-Reya, R.J., 2007. Hit 'em where they live: targeting the cancer stem cell niche. Cancer Cell 11, 3–5.

Zecevic, N., 2004. Specific characteristic of radial glia in the human fetal telencephalon. Glia 48, 27–35.

Zhu, Y., Harada, T., Liu, L., et al., 2005. Inactivation of NF1 in C N S causes increased glial progenitor proliferation and optic glioma formation. Development 132, 5577–5588.

3

Classification and pathogenesis of brain tumors

Michael Gonzales

Introduction

Classification of tumors of the central nervous system (CNS) continues to be based, primarily, on histopathological features with new entities included in upgrades of classification schemes because of novel morphological and biologic features. The decade to the mid-2000s saw fundamental advances in the understanding of how molecular-genetic phenomena contribute to the pathogenesis of brain tumors and influence their behavior. As well as giving important insights into tumor biology, these molecular genetic data supplement morphological classification schemes and, for some tumors, provide an evidence base for adjuvant treatment protocols.

Classification and grading of CNS tumors – historical aspects

The first macroscopic descriptions of brain tumors were published by Cruveilhier in 1829. In 1836, Bressler described a number of brain tumors and categorized them macroscopically as fatty, fleshy and bony tumors, medullary sarcomas, melanoses, cystic tumors and hydatids (cited in Leestma 1980). Then, in 1860, Virchow described the neuroglia (literally 'nerve glue') as the interstitial matrix of the brain in which individual cells are suspended. Most of the subsequent insights into the pathology of brain tumors in the remainder of the nineteenth century can be attributed to Virchow. He was the first to attempt a correlation between macroscopic and microscopic features and the first to use the term 'glioma'. The gliomas were described as slowly growing, poorly circumscribed lesions which diffusely infiltrated but did not destroy the brain parenchyma. In contrast, the sarcomas were clearly demarcated, grew rapidly, exerting what is now recognized as mass effect on adjacent structures, and were frequently hemorrhagic and necrotic. Golgi, in 1884, proposed a narrower definition of gliomas as tumors composed of fibrous cells. He regarded these as benign. Later, in 1890, Virchow reinterpreted tumors of the dura, which are now recognized as meningiomas. He called these 'psammomas' because they contained the concentrically lamellated, calcified structures now known as psammoma bodies, and separated them from dural sarcomas.

Using the heavy metal impregnation techniques perfected by Cajal in 1913 and del Rio-Hortega in 1919 to demonstrate the morphology of the different cells in the brain, Bailey and Cushing (1926), published their scheme for classifying gliomas.

This was based on a hypothesis of CNS histogenesis from primitive medullary epithelium, now called primitive neuroectoderm, via glial and neuronal precursors. Their scheme proposed 14 tumor types (Fig. 3.1), each resulting from developmental arrest at a particular stage in neuronal-glial histogenesis (Ribbert 1918). Tumors could be classified by correlating the morphological features of their component cells with those of normal cells at each defined stage of histogenesis.

Although useful because it directed attention to the process of differentiation, Bailey and Cushing's classification suffered from its essentially hypothetical construction and the realization that cells at each proposed stage of histogenesis are difficult to recognize morphologically. An important contribution was later made by Cox (1933), who suggested that incorporated, non-neoplastic cells take on morphological features similar to those of cells at the different stages of histogenesis proposed by Bailey and Cushing. For these reasons, neuropathologists found this classification difficult to apply with acceptable uniformity.

The Bailey and Cushing scheme, however, dominated thinking about the gliomas until 1949, when James Kernohan (1949) and his colleagues at the Mayo Clinic put forward a much simpler classification. Kernohan had long believed that glial tumors develop from terminally differentiated cells and that different histopathological appearances do not represent different tumor types but rather different degrees of de-differentiation of one tumor type. He dispensed with the confusing histogenetic terminology of Bailey and Cushing and reduced the number of categories of glial tumors to five: astrocytoma, ependymoma, oligodendroglioma, neuroastrocytoma, and medulloblastoma. He also recognized that mixed glial tumors, particularly oligoastrocytomas, could occur, but did not include these as a separate category. Most importantly, however, Kernohan re-introduced the idea, previously advanced by Tooth in 1912, that the biologic behavior of these tumors could be reckoned from their histopathological features and proposed a four-tier grading system for astrocytomas and ependymomas. This was based on increasing anaplasia and decreasing differentiation with increasing grade of tumor, similar to the principles for grading carcinomas previously developed by Broders (1925).

The Kernohan scheme marked the beginning of an era in which attention was directed at formulating an acceptable grading system rather than refining different classifications based on histogenesis. The major reason for this shift in emphasis was an increasing awareness among neuropathologists, neurosurgeons and neurooncologists that a meaningful classification of CNS tumors should provide some indication of biologic behavior as a basis for developing effective treatment protocols.

Several problems were encountered in applying the Kernohan scheme. Some features, particularly assessment of

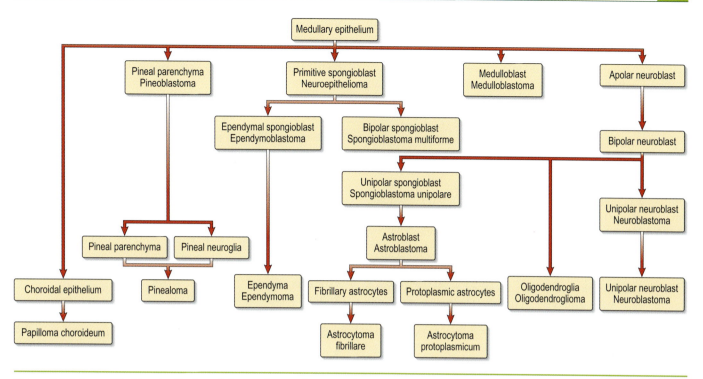

Figure 3.1 Bailey and Cushing classification of gliomas. (From Bailey P & Cushing H (1926) A Classification of Tumours of the Glioma Group on a Histogenetic Basis. Philadelphia: J B Lippincott; pp 146–167.)

anaplasia and degree of cellularity, were found to be subjective and prone to inter-observer variation. This subjectivity engendered meaningless, indeterminate gradings such as I–II and II–III. Another problem was that necrosis was included as a feature of both astrocytoma grade III and grade IV. These two grades were separated by the denser cellularity, more severe anaplasia and higher mitotic figure count in grade IV compared with grade III tumors. A communication accompanying the publication of the scheme reported postoperative survival data for 161 patients (Svien et al 1949). These showed a significantly longer mean survival period and better 3-year survival rate for grade III (14.3%) compared with grade IV (3.8%) tumors. However, there was not a significant difference in the 3-year survival rates for grade II and grade III tumors (15.8% and 14.3%, respectively). These data suggested that a three-tier grading system more accurately reflected the biology of these tumors.

A system proposing three grades: astrocytoma, astrocytoma with anaplastic foci, and glioblastoma multiforme was put forward by Ringertz (1950). In this system, separation between the grades of tumor on histologic criteria was much more precise, with the presence of necrosis of any type defining glioblastoma multiforme. Despite its simplicity, the three-tier system was not widely accepted until the mid-1980s when it was again proposed as a preferable scheme to four-tier systems and promoted for the grading of ependymomas and oligodendrogliomas as well as astrocytic tumors.

The association of necrosis in astrocytomas, graded by the three-tier system, with aggressive biologic behavior and reduced postoperative survival was highlighted in a number of reports in the 1980s (Burger & Vollmer 1980; Nelson et al 1983; Burger et al 1985; Fulling & Garcia 1985; Garcia et al 1985). However, survival statistics indicated a very wide range in postoperative survival periods of patients with tumors graded as anaplastic astrocytoma with anaplastic foci, now known as anaplastic astrocytoma (Fulling & Garcia 1985). This led to closer scrutiny of grading schemes and movement towards a system based on specific histologic features with the aim of determining which features were independent indicators of biologic behavior and survival. These efforts were embodied in the St Anne-Mayo grading scheme, developed by Daumas-Duport & Szikla in 1981, later supported by survival data (Daumas-Duport et al 1988a). In this system, tumors were graded according to the accumulation of four morphological features: nuclear atypia, mitoses, endothelial cell proliferation, and necrosis. Grade I tumors had none of these features; grade II tumors had one feature (usually nuclear atypia); grade III tumors had two features (nuclear atypia, mitoses), and grade IV tumors had three or four features (nuclear atypia, mitoses, endothelial cell proliferation ± necrosis). In their 1988 publication, Daumas-Duport and her colleagues reported the results of applying the St Anne-Mayo system to 287 astrocytic tumors (Daumas-Duport et al 1988a). Their data showed clear distinction between four grades of malignancy with median survival times of 4 years for grade II, 1.6 years for grade III, and 0.7 years for grade IV, respectively. They also reported a 94% concordance between different pathologists.

As with all grading systems, problems emerged in applying the St Anne-Mayo scheme. Doubts arose as to whether grade I lesions should be regarded as tumors given that they contain none of the features assessed for grading. Only two of the 287 astrocytomas (0.7%) analysed were assessed as grade I. In addition, there is no significant difference in the 3-year survival of St Anne-Mayo grade II, III and IV tumors (Daumas-Duport et al 1988a) compared with grade I, II and

III tumors assessed by the Ringertz three-tier system (Burger et al 1985). The conclusion is therefore compelling that, by the criteria of relative frequency and biologic behavior, astrocytic gliomas segregate into three rather than four grades. Limitations of the St Anne-Mayo system in indicating the prognosis of childhood astrocytomas (Brown et al 1998) and some discordance between proliferation indices and grades of tumor (Giannini et al 1999a) have also been noted.

The first World Health Organization (WHO) classification of tumors of the central nervous system was published in 1979 (Zulch 1979). This was a classification of all central nervous system tumors, not just of gliomas. Inclusion of tumor entities was determined by a panel of neuropathology luminaries: Klaus Zulch, Lucien Rubinstein, Kenneth Earle, John Hume Adams, and John Kepes, after a painstaking review of 230 tumors over the previous 10 years. This initial classification was revised in 1988 and 1990 and an updated classification published in 1993 (Kleihues et al 1993). As in the initial 1973 scheme, each tumor was assigned a grade within a 'malignancy' scale from benign (grade I) to malignant (grade IV). This grading scheme was based on a combination of survival data and histopathological features. However, the authors of the updated 1993 scheme cautioned that not all CNS tumors display a range of malignancies from grade I to grade IV. Further revisions of the WHO classification and grading scheme were published in 2000 (Kleihues & Cavenee 2000) and 2007 (Louis et al 2007a). The 2000 revision initiated sections dealing with the molecular genetics of each tumor. This is continued in the 2007 scheme (see Box 3.1).

Several other grading schemes have been formulated in North American and European neurooncology centers, each supported by local survival data (DeArmond et al 1987) and individual institutions continue to adhere to the St Ann-Mayo and Ringertz systems. However, the WHO classification is the most widely followed, particularly by neuropathologists participating in cooperative neurooncology trials.

A comparison of the Ringertz, Kernohan, WHO, and St Anne-Mayo grading schemes is shown in Figure 3.2.

A separate classification scheme for childhood brain tumors was proposed in 1985 (Rorke et al 1985). This alternative scheme has been corroborated by studies that have emphasized the limitations of applying adult classification schemes to pediatric brain tumors and identified histologic features that are important in separating tumor sub-types with differing biologic behaviors (Gilles et al 2000a,b).

The 2007 WHO classification and grading scheme comprises seven major categories based on cell or tissue of origin (Louis et al 2007a; Appendix).

- Tumors of neuroepithelial tissue
- Tumors of cranial and paraspinal nerves
- Tumors of the meninges
- Lymphomas and hemopoietic neoplasms
- Germ cell tumors
- Tumors of the sellar region
- Metastatic tumors.

A number of new entities are included: pilomyxoid astrocytoma, atypical choroid plexus papilloma, angiocentric glioma, papillary glioneuronal tumor, rosette forming glioneuronal tumor of the fourth ventricle, papillary tumor of the pineal region, pituicytoma and spindle cell oncocytoma of the adenohypophysis. The stated rationale for inclusion of these new entities includes evidence of a different age distribution, location, genetic profile or clinical behavior (Louis et al 2007b).

Tumors of neuroepithelial tissue

Tumors arising from neuroepithelium are divided into nine categories: astrocytic, oligodendroglial, oligoastrocytic and ependymal tumors, choroid plexus tumors, other neuroepithelial tumors (for which histogenesis is uncertain), neuronal and mixed neuronal-glial tumors, tumors of the pineal region and embryonal tumors. Neuroepithelial tumors, as a group, have an incidence rate, in the USA, of 7.67/100 000 per year in males and 5.35/100 000 per year in females (CBTRUS 2005).

Astrocytic tumors
- Pilocytic astrocytoma WHO I
  - Pilomyxoid astrocytoma WHO II
- Subependymal giant cell astrocytoma WHO I
- Pleomorphic xanthoastrocytoma WHO II
- Diffuse astrocytoma WHO II
  - Fibrillary astrocytoma
  - Gemistocytic astrocytoma
  - Protoplasmic astrocytoma
- Anaplastic astrocytoma WHO III
- Glioblastoma WHO IV
  - Giant cell glioblastoma
  - Gliosarcoma
- Gliomatosis cerebri WHO III/IV.

Astrocytic tumors are classified as in the 2000 WHO scheme but are listed in order from lowest to highest grade on the WHO 'malignancy scale'. Again, typical pilocytic astrocytoma, pleomorphic xanthoastrocytoma (PXA) and subependymal giant cell astrocytoma (SEGCA) are separated from the more common diffuse astrocytoma, anaplastic astrocytoma and glioblastoma multiforme. Each is histopathologically distinct.

Pilocytic astrocytomas typically occur in children and young adults. They are slowly growing, relatively circumscribed neoplasms with a predilection for midline structures – optic nerve and chiasm, hypothalamus, and dorsal brainstem. They may also arise in cerebellar hemispheres and rarely in cerebral hemispheres in adults (Palma & Guidetti 1985). The majority have a non-aggressive course following either complete or incomplete surgical resection and are accorded a grading of WHO I. However, recurrence and progression of pilocytic astrocytomas in adults has been reported (Stüer et al 2007). Progression free survival for patients with incompletely resected pilocytic astrocytomas has been linked to the level of expression of the oligodendroglial differentiation markers, Olig-1, Olig-2, myelin basic protein (MBP) and platelet derived growth factor receptor-α (PDGFR-α) (Wong et al 2005; Takei et al 2008).

Pilomyxoid astrocytoma is a new entity. This tumor was first recognized in the late 1990s (Tihan et al 1999) as a

Box 3.1 2007 WHO classification of tumors of the central nervous system

TUMORS OF NEUROEPITHELIAL TISSUE

Astrocytic tumors

- Pilocytic astrocytoma
  - Pilomyxoid astrocytoma
- Subependymal giant cell astrocytoma
- Pleomorphic xanthoastrocytoma
- Diffuse astrocytoma
  - Fibrillary astrocytoma
  - Gemistocytic astrocytoma
  - Protoplasmic astrocytoma
- Anaplastic astrocytoma
- Glioblastoma
  - Giant cell glioblastoma
  - Gliosarcoma
- Gliomatosis cerebri

Oligodendroglial tumors

- Oligodendroglioma
- Anaplastic oligodendroglioma

Oligoastrocytic tumors

- Oligoastrocytoma
- Anaplastic oligoastrocytoma

Ependymal tumors

- Subependymoma
- Myxopapillary ependymoma
- Ependymoma
  - Cellular
  - Papillary
  - Clear Cell
  - Tanycytic
- Anaplastic ependymoma

Choroid plexus tumors

- Choroid plexus papilloma
- Atypical choroid plexus papilloma
- Choroid plexus carcinoma

Other neuroepithelial tumors

- Astroblastoma
- Chordoid glioma of the third ventricle
- Angiocentric glioma

Neuronal and mixed neuronal-glial tumors

- Dysplastic gangliocytoma of cerebellum (Lhermitte–Duclos)
- Desmoplastic infantile astrocytoma/ganglioglioma
- Dysembryoplastic neuroepithelial tumor
- Gangliocytoma
- Ganglioglioma
- Anaplastic ganglioglioma
- Central neurocytoma
- Extraventricular neurocytoma
- Cerebellar liponeurocytoma
- Papillary glioneuronal tumor
- Rosette-forming glioneuronal tumor of fourth ventricle
- Paraganglioma

Tumors of the pineal region

- Pineocytoma
- Pineal parenchymal tumor of intermediate differentiation
- Pineoblastoma
- Papillary tumor of the pineal region

Embryonal tumors

- Medulloblastoma
- Desmoplastic/nodular medulloblastoma
  - Medulloblastoma with extensive nodularity
  - Anaplastic medulloblastoma
  - Large cell medulloblastoma

- CNS primitive neuroectodermal tumor
  - CNS neuroblastoma
  - CNS ganglioneuroblastoma
  - Medulloepithelioma
  - Ependymoblastoma
- Atypical teratoid/rhabdoid tumor

TUMORS OF CRANIAL AND PARASPINAL NERVES

- Schwannoma (neurilemoma, neurinoma)
  - Cellular
  - Plexiform
  - Melanotic
- Neurofibroma
  - Plexiform
- Perineurioma
  - Perineurioma, NOS
  - Malignant perineurioma
- Malignant peripheral nerve sheath tumor (MPNST)
  - Epithelioid MPNST
  - MPNST with mesenchymal differentiation
  - Melanotic MPNST
  - MPNST with glandular differentiation

TUMORS OF THE MENINGES

Tumors of meningothelial cells

- Meningioma
  - Meningothelial
  - Fibrous (fibroblastic)
  - Transitional (mixed)
  - Psammomatous
  - Angiomatous
  - Microcystic
  - Secretory
  - Lymphoplasmacyte-rich
  - Metaplastic
  - Chordoid
  - Clear Cell
  - Atypical
  - Papillary
  - Rhabdoid
  - Anaplastic (malignant)

Mesenchymal tumors

- Lipoma
- Angiolipoma
- Hibernoma
- Liposarcoma
- Solitary fibrous tumor
- Fibrosarcoma
- Malignant fibrous histiocytoma
- Leiomyoma
- Leiomyosarcoma
- Rhabdomyoma
- Rhabdomyosarcoma
- Chondroma
- Chondrosarcoma
- Osteoma
- Osteosarcoma
- Osteochondroma
- Hemangioma
- Epithelioid hemangioendothelioma
- Hemangiopericytoma
- Anaplastic hemangiopericytoma
- Angiosarcoma
- Kaposi's sarcoma
- Ewing sarcoma – PNET

Primary melanocytic lesions

- Diffuse melanocytosis
- Melanocytoma

Box 3.1 Continued

- Malignant melanoma
- Meningeal melanomatosis

Other neoplasms related to the meninges

- Hemangioblastoma

LYMPHOMAS AND HEMATOPOIETIC TUMORS

- Malignant lymphomas
- Plasmacytoma
- Granulocytic sarcoma

GERM CELL TUMORS

- Germinoma
- Embryonal carcinoma
- Yolk sac tumor
- Choriocarcinoma

- Teratoma
  - Mature
  - Immature
  - Teratoma with malignant transformation
- Mixed germ cell tumors

TUMORS OF THE SELLAR REGION

- Craniopharyngioma
  - Adamantinomatous
  - Papillary
- Granular cell tumor
- Pituicytoma
- Spindle cell oncocytoma of the adenohypophysis

Metastatic tumors

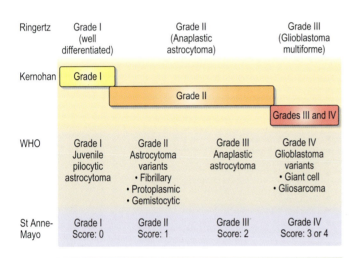

Figure 3.2 Comparison of the four common histopathology-based grading schemes. Boxes indicate the overlap between the Kernohan 4-tier and Ringertz 3-tier systems. Kernohan and St Anne Mayo systems do not grade pilocytic astrocytoma, which, in the WHO system, is regarded as a Grade I tumor. (From Gonzales M F (1997) Grading of gliomas. J Clin Neurosci 4: 16–18.)

variant of pilocytic astrocytoma, occurring predominantly in children. A grading of WHO II reflects relatively aggressive behavior (Chikai et al 2004; Fernandez et al 2003; Komotar et al 2004).

Sub-ependymal giant cell astrocytomas occur almost exclusively in patients with tuberous sclerosis complex (Ahlsén et al 1994; Ess et al 2005). Despite documentation of anaplastic features (mitoses, vascular endothelial cell hyperplasia, necrosis), their behavior is universally benign (Cuccia et al 2003; Kim et al 2001) and they are graded as WHO I.

Pleomorphic xanthoastrocytoma (PXA) occurs predominantly in children and young adults often located superficially, with occasional extension into overlying meninges.

When first reported (Kepes et al 1979), PXAs appeared to behave in a non-aggressive manner. However, progression and shortened postoperative survival, linked to anaplastic features, were noted in subsequent case studies (Weldon-Linne et al 1983; Whittle et al 1989; McLean et al 1998). The term 'pleomorphic xanthoastrocytoma with

anaplastic features' has been proposed for these variants (Giannini et al 1999b) but this specific terminology is not used in the 2007 classification scheme and PXAs are graded as WHO II. The presence of necrosis in PXA has been shown to be associated with a significantly shortened progression free survival (Pahapill et al 1996). Pleomorphic xanthoastrocytoma may rarely form the glial component of a ganglioglioma (Kordek et al 1995) and co-existence of PXA and ganglioglioma as separate composite tumors has also been reported (Perry et al 1997a). The histogenesis of PXA is controversial. In their original series, Kepes and colleagues proposed an origin from sub-ependymal astrocytes, based on ultrastructural similarities between these and PXA tumor cells. However, expression of neuronal markers (Powell et al 1996) and the hemopoietic progenitor cell antigen, CD34 (Reifenberger et al 2003), has also been noted. The rare occurrence in association with cortical dysplasia also raises the possibility that PXA may arise in a pre-existing hamartomatous or maldevelopmental lesion (Lach et al 1996; Im et al 2004).

Diffuse astrocytoma, anaplastic astrocytoma and glioblastoma multiforme represent the great bulk of astrocytic gliomas. Histopathologically, they form an often overlapping morphological and behavioral continuum in contrast to the clear separation between pilocytic, subependymal giant cell and pleomorphic xanthoastrocytomas. Diffuse astrocytoma has three sub-types: fibrillary, gemistocytic, and protoplasmic, separated on the basis of unique histopathological features. Despite gemistocytic astrocytoma having a particular propensity to progress to anaplastic astrocytoma and glioblastoma (Krouwer et al 1991; Schiffer et al 1988), diffuse astrocytomas are accorded a grading of WHO II. Anaplastic astrocytoma (WHO grade III) and glioblastoma multiforme (WHO grade IV) are distinguished from diffuse astrocytoma by their denser hypercellularity, greater nuclear and cellular pleomorphism, greater numbers of mitotic figures, endothelial cell proliferation, and necrosis. Either of these last two features (i.e., endothelial cell proliferation *and/or* necrosis) defines glioblastoma in the WHO scheme. Although not tabulated in the 2007 scheme, so-called 'primary' and 'secondary' glioblastomas are nevertheless recognized on the basis of molecular-genetic alterations in tumor cell DNA. Primary glioblastoma occurs in older individuals (mean age 62 years) and presents with a short clinical history, of the order of 3 months. Secondary glioblastoma is associated with a longer clinical history, over several years, in younger individuals (mean age 45 years), often with documented occurrences of lower grade tumors. Mutations of the TP53 gene, occurring early in tumor evolution, are the hallmark of secondary glioblastoma, while amplification and re-arrangement of the epidermal growth factor receptor (EGFR) gene are characteristic of primary glioblastoma (Ohgaki et al 2004; Ohgaki & Kleihues 2007). Loss of heterozygosity (LOH) at chromosome 10q is common to both forms of glioblastoma (Ohgaki et al 2004).

Giant cell glioblastoma and *gliosarcoma* are histologic sub-types of glioblastoma. The giant cell variant comprises approximately 5% of glioblastomas. The characteristic histopathological feature is the presence of large, bizarrely-shaped tumor cells containing multiple hyperchromatic nuclei. Atypical mitotic figures are often noted. Despite a short clinical history, giant cell glioblastoma has the molecular-genetic footprint of secondary glioblastoma – frequent TP53 mutations, LOH on chromosome 10q and lack of EGFR amplification (Meyer-Puttlitz et al 1997).

Gliosarcomas make up approximately 2% of glioblastomas and are distinguished by the admixture of neoplastic mesenchymal elements with the astrocytic component. Despite the apparent separation of glial and mesenchymal components, cytogenetic and molecular genetic studies, documenting particularly TP53 and *PTEN* mutations, indicate that both components represent neoplastic glial cells (Paulus et al 1994; Biernat et al 1995).

Gliomatosis cerebri describes the phenomenon of diffuse infiltration of at least three lobes of the cerebrum by neoplastic glial cells, usually astrocytes (Nevin 1938). While involvement of the cerebrum is the commonest pattern seen, the process may also involve the optic chiasm and nerves, hypothalamus, mesencephalon, thalamus, basal ganglia, cerebellum and spinal cord (Vates et al 2003). Atypical cells accumulate between fiber tracts in white matter. Rare cases of oligodendroglial gliomatosis cerebri are described (Balko et al 1992). Most examples of gliomatosis cerebri conform to WHO grade III or IV depending on the presence of endothelial cell proliferation and necrosis (Vates et al 2003).

Oligodendroglial and oligoastrocytic tumors
- Oligodendroglial tumors
    - Oligodendroglioma WHO II
    - Anaplastic oligodendroglioma WHO III
- Oligoastrocytic tumors
    - Oligoastrocytoma WHO II
    - Anaplastic oligoastrocytoma WHO III.

The classification and grading of oligodendroglial and oligoastrocytic tumors is identical to the 2000 scheme. Two grades, oligodendroglioma/oligoastrocytoma (WHO II) and anaplastic oligodendroglioma/anaplastic oligoastrocytoma (WHO grade III) are recognized. Both anaplastic variants show increased tumor cell density as well as mitoses and vascular endothelial cell hyperplasia. Small cells with features reminiscent of gemistocytes, but with round nuclei are also noted in anaplastic oligodendrogliomas and anaplastic oligoastrocytomas. These demonstrate GFAP immunoreac-

tivity in their cytoplasm and have been termed, minigemistocytes and gliofibrillary oligodendrocytes (Kros et al 1996; Matyja et al 2001). The astrocytic component of oligoastrocytic tumors varies in amount and may be intimately admixed with oligodendroglial cells (diffuse type) or separate from them (biphasic or compact type) (Hart et al 1974). The latter may not be detected in small biopsies. Interpretation of necrosis in anaplastic variants remains problematic. The presence of necrosis in an otherwise typical anaplastic oligodendroglioma does not indicate shorter survival (Miller et al 2006). Necrosis in anaplastic oligoastrocytoma however, is associated with a significantly reduced survival (Miller et al 2006). The 2007 WHO panel recommendation is that anaplastic oligoastrocytoma with necrosis should be classified as 'glioblastoma with an oligodendroglial component' with the proviso that this will have a better outcome than typical glioblastoma (He et al 2001; Kraus et al 2001), particularly if loss of chromosome 1p can be demonstrated (Kraus et al 2001; Eoli et al 2006).

The two-tier WHO scheme for grading oligodendroglial tumors contrasts with previous schemes proposing four grades (Smith et al 1983; Mörk et al 1986). Daumas-Duport and colleagues proposed a two-tier grading scheme based on histopathological and imaging features: grade A with no endothelial cell hyperplasia and no contrast enhancement; grade B with either endothelial cell hyperplasia or contrast enhancement (Daumas-Duport et al 1997). Follow-up of 79 patients (59 grade A, 20 grade B) showed median survival times of 11 years in grade A and 3.5 years in grade B (Daumas-Duport et al 1997).

Whole of arm deletion of chromosome 1p, either alone or in combination with whole of arm deletion of chromosome 19q is now recognized to be the molecular-genetic signature of oligodendroglial tumors. Co-deletion is seen in up to 80% of oligodendrogliomas (Jeuken et al 2004; Gonzales et al 2006) but is less common in oligoastrocytomas. Co-deletion is predictive of responsiveness to alkylating chemotherapeutic agents (Cairncross et al 1998) as well as prolonged recurrence free survival (Cairncross et al 1998; Ino et al 2000, 2001). At the current stage of evolution of the WHO classification scheme, there is no formal recommendation to use this molecular-genetic signature to confirm an oligodendroglial lineage in CNS tumors.

Ependymal tumors
- Subependymoma WHO I
- Myxopapillary ependymoma WHO I
- Ependymoma WHO II
    - Cellular
    - Papillary
    - Clear cell
    - Tanycytic
- Anaplastic ependymoma WHO III.

As in the 2000 scheme, there are four categories of ependymal tumors: subependymoma, myxopapillary ependymoma, ependymoma (with cellular, papillary, clear cell and tanycytic variants) and anaplastic ependymoma. Myxopapillary ependymoma and sub-ependymoma are graded as WHO I, ependymoma and each of its sub-types as grade II, and anaplastic ependymoma as grade III. As in previous classification schemes, separation of subependymoma and myxopapillary ependymoma from ependymoma, is based on their characteristic histopathological features and specific anatomical locations. The histopathological diagnosis of anaplastic ependymoma is appropriate where there are appreciable numbers of mitotic figures, vascular endothelial cell hyperplasia and/or necrosis. However, tumors with areas of necrosis, not accompanied by brisk mitotic activity or endothelial cell proliferation should not be interpreted as anaplastic ependymoma (Kurt et al 2006). Ependymomas with these features are more common in the posterior cranial fossa and usually have low proliferation indices (Korshunov et al 2000).

Choroid plexus tumors
- Choroid plexus papilloma WHO I
- Atypical choroid plexus papilloma WHO II
- Choroid plexus papilloma WHO III.

The three entities in the choroid plexus tumor category represent a spectrum from benign to malignant. *Atypical choroid plexus papilloma* has been added since the 2000 classification and is distinguished from choroid plexus papilloma by increased mitotic activity. Inclusion of atypical papilloma in the 2007 classification is formulated on a single study of 164 choroid plexus tumors (Jeibmann et al 2006). The recommendation of this study was that a tumor with two or more mitotic figures in 10 high-power fields be regarded as atypical. The histopathological diagnosis of *choroid plexus carcinoma* is appropriate for a tumor with at least four of five anaplastic features: greater than 5 mitoses per 10 high-power fields; increased cellular density; nuclear pleomorphism; blurring of the papillary pattern with invasion of the fibrovascular cores of the papillary structures, and necrosis (Paulus & Brandner 2007). Invasion of adjacent brain parenchyma may also be seen. Immunoreactivity of choroid epithelium for transthyretin (Paulus & Janisch 1990) and synaptophysin (Kepes & Collins 1999) is helpful in separating these choroid plexus tumors from other papillary neoplasms, in particular metastatic papillary carcinoma.

Other neuroepithelial tumors
- Astroblastoma
  - Chordoid glioma of the third ventricle WHO II
  - Angiocentric glioma WHO I.

This category has replaced 'Glial tumors of uncertain origin' in the 2000 scheme.

The term *astroblastoma* was first proposed by Bailey and Bucy in 1930 for a tumor with exaggerated gliovascular structuring in the form of prominent perivascular pseudorosettes formed by astrocytic rather than ependymal cells. There has been considerable disagreement among neuropathologists as to whether this neoplasm is a true entity, separate from astrocytoma, or a sub-type of astrocytoma, particularly as areas with features described in astroblastoma can be found in anaplastic astrocytoma and glioblastoma. Because of a lack of sufficient clinicopathological data, astroblastoma is not accorded a grading in the 2007 scheme. However, astroblastomas tend to be circumscribed, a char-acteristic which facilitates gross total resection and achievement of a favorable outcome (Bonnin & Rubinstein 1989; Brat et al 1999a).

With less than 50 examples reported, the histogenesis of chordoid glioma of the third ventricle remains enigmatic. The first case report proposed an unusual variant of meningioma, expressing glial fibrillary acidic protein (GFAP) (Wanschitz et al 1995). More recently, an origin from ependyma has been formulated on the basis of ultrastructural features (Leeds et al 2006; Jain et al 2008). Because of locally aggressive behavior (Kurian et al 2005), chordoid gliomas are graded as WHO II.

Angiocentric glioma is a low-grade (WHO I), non-aggressive tumor of probable but uncertain glial histogenesis, which occurs most frequently in the cerebral hemispheres. Less than 30 examples have been reported, most commonly in children and young adults (Lellouch-Tubiana et al 2005; Wang et al 2005; Preusser et al 2006). The majority of patients have a history of complex partial seizures.

Neuronal and mixed neuronal-glial tumors
- Dysplastic gangliocytoma of cerebellum (Lhermitte–Duclos) WHO I
- Desmoplastic infantile astrocytoma/ganglioglioma WHO I
- Dysembryoplastic neuroepithelial tumor WHO I
- Gangliocytoma WHO I
- Ganglioglioma WHO I
- Anaplastic ganglioglioma WHO III
- Central neurocytoma WHO II
- Extraventricular neurocytoma WHO II
- Cerebellar liponeurocytoma WHO II
- Papillary glioneuronal tumor WHO I
- Rosette-forming glioneuronal tumor of the fourth ventricle WHO I
- Paraganglioma (spinal) WHO I.

With the exceptions of anaplastic ganglioglioma and a minority of neurocytomas, neuronal and mixed neuronal-glial tumors behave non-aggressively. Many are epilepsy-associated. Two new entities are included: papillary glioneuronal tumor and rosette-forming glioneuronal tumor of the fourth ventricle.

Whether *dysplastic gangliocytoma of the cerebellum* is a tumor or a hamartoma remains unresolved. The lesion was first described in 1920 (Lhermitte & Duclos 1920). An association with Cowden's syndrome has been documented (Padberg et al 1991).

Superficially located astrocytic tumors with pronounced desmoplastic stroma were described as 'meningocerebral astrocytomas' by Taratuto and colleagues in 1984. Then, VandenBerg and colleagues (1987) documented a group of desmoplastic supratentorial neuroepithelial tumors with divergent differentiation and called these 'desmoplastic infantile ganglioma' (DIG). This entity was incorporated into the 1993 WHO classification. The term 'desmoplastic infantile astrocytoma/ganglioma', used in the 2000 and 2007 classifications, evolves from the recognition that these tumors display a histologic spectrum from predominantly astrocytic to mixed astrocytic/ganglion cell. These tumors invariably behave non-aggressively and are graded as WHO I.

Dysembryoplastic neuroepithelial tumor (DNET) was first reported by Daumas-Duport and her colleagues in 1998 (Daumas-Duport et al 1988b). Despite some initial consideration that DNETs were maldevelopmental hamartomatous lesions, they are regarded as neoplasms. They have a stereotyped clinical presentation of early onset complex partial seizures in young individuals that often become refractory to medical treatment. Macroscopically, DNETs are multinodular lesions, either confined to an expanded cortex or involving both cortex and white matter. Most are located in the temporal lobe and frequently involve mesial structures (Daumas-Duport 1993). They have also been described in the caudate nucleus (Cervera-Pierot et al 1997), cerebellum (Daumas-Duport et al 1988b; Kuchelmeister et al 1995) and pons (Leung et al 1994). The characteristic histopathological feature is the glioneuronal element composed of small neuronal cells arranged in columns that are frequently oriented at right angles to the cortical surface. These may enclose small cyst-like spaces filled with myxoid/mucinous material and containing mature neurons. The small cells were initially described as having oligodendroglial features but their processes are immunoreactive for synaptophysin and neuron-specific enolase (Leung et al 1994), suggesting a neuronal lineage. By electron microscopy, they are seen to contain dense core neurosecretory granules and microtubules and where their processes make contact with other cells, electron dense membrane thickenings, typical of synapses, can be identified (Leung et al 1994).

Three histologic sub-types of DNET have been described: simple, complex and non-specific (Daumas-Duport 1993). The simple form consists only of the glioneuronal element, while the complex form contains one or more nodules of glial cells, either astrocytes or oligodendrocytes, in addition to the glioneuronal element, and the adjacent cerebral cortex shows dysplastic features in the form of dyslamination and maloriented neuronal cell bodies. The non-specific form is controversial, since it lacks the glioneuronal element and multinodular architecture. Clinically and radiologically, this overlaps with other low-grade glial tumors, in particular pilocytic astrocytoma and oligodendroglioma. Follow-up studies have confirmed the benign nature of the majority of DNETs (Daumas-Duport et al 1988b; Daumas-Duport 1993; Taratuto et al 1995). However, the possibility that a minority of DNETs may evolve into or co-exist with oligodendrogliomas has been raised (Gonzales et al 2007).

Gangliocytoma and *ganglioglioma* represent a histologic spectrum of neuroepithelial tumors varying from predominantly or exclusively mature ganglion cells in gangliocytoma to a mixture of ganglion cells and glia, usually astrocytes, in ganglioglioma. These tumors occur at any site within the CNS. However, most gangliogliomas occur in the temporal lobe and are commonly associated with temporal lobe epilepsy (Wolf & Wiestler 1995; Luyken et al 2003). Both gangliocytoma and ganglioglioma are graded as WHO I.

Anaplasia in *anaplastic ganglioglioma* (WHO III), refers to features in the glial component that are commonly seen in anaplastic astrocytoma and glioblastoma multiforme, i.e., increased mitoses, vascular endothelial proliferation, necrosis and elevated proliferation indices. Malignant

transformation, i.e., the development of anaplastic features in recurrences of a previous benign ganglioma has been noted (Mittelbronn et al 2007). In one study, expression of the anti-apoptotic protein, survivin, in >5% of glial cells was associated with recurrence and development of anaplastic features (Rousseau et al 2006).

Central neurocytoma is a histologically distinct tumor composed of small cells with immunohistochemical and ultrastructural features of neurons (Hassoun et al 1982; Townsend & Seaman 1986). The tumor arises most commonly in the lateral ventricle near the foramen of Monro. Before the first descriptions of neuronal cell lineage, these tumors were regarded as ependymomas or intraventricular oligodendrogliomas. Examples in which tumor cells express both neuronal and astrocytic lineage markers have been described (Tsuchida et al 1996). Some of these have been designated *glioneurocytomas* (Min et al 1995), while others with mature ganglion cells admixed with neurocytic cells have been called *ganglioneurocytomas* (Funato et al 1997). Tumors with histopathological, immunohistochemical and ultrastructural features similar to central neurocytoma, but occurring in cerebral hemispheric white matter are designated cerebral or *extraventricular neurocytomas* (Nishio et al 1992). Neurocytomas involving the spinal cord have also been described (Coca et al 1994; Tatter et al 1994). The majority of central neurocytomas behave non-aggressively and are graded as WHO II. However, rare cases of craniospinal dissemination have been reported (Yamamoto et al 1996; Eng et al 1997). Likelihood of local recurrence was linked to the Ki-67/MIB-1 proliferation index in one study (Soylemezoglu et al 1997). Some neurocytic tumors occurring in the cerebellum may show a prominent component of mature adipocytes. These are classified as *cerebellar liponeurocytoma* and are graded as WHO II as local recurrence has been documented (Jenkinson et al 2003). Before the 2000 WHO classification, these were regarded as a variant of medulloblastoma (Bechtel et al 1978; Budka & Chimelli 1994; Soylemezoglu et al 1996). However, molecular-genetic studies have indicated clear differences between cerebellar liponeurocytoma and medulloblastoma (Horstmann et al 2004).

Papillary glioneuronal tumor is one of two new entities included in the neuronal and mixed neuronal-glial tumor category. Originally described in 1996 as pseudo-papillary ganglioneurocytoma (Komori et al 1996) but later as papillary glioneuronal tumor (Komori et al 1998), this is a low-grade (WHO I), non-aggressive tumor occurring most commonly in the temporal lobe (Komori et al 1998). The distinctive histopathological feature is the presence of vascularized papillary structures covered by one or more layers of small glial cells, which may include Olig2 immunoreactive oligodendroglia (Tanaka et al 2005). A mixture of small and intermediate neuronal cells as well as large mature ganglion cells is present between the papillae. These are immunoreactive for a number of neuronal antigens: synaptophysin, neuron-specific enolase (NSE), class III tubulin, and neuronal nuclear antigen (NeuN) (Komori et al 1998; Chen et al 2006).

Rosette-forming glioneuronal tumor of the fourth ventricle is the second new entity in the neuronal and mixed neuronal-glial tumor category with a grading of WHO I. When first reported, this neoplasm was regarded as a dysembryoplastic neuroepithelial tumor involving the cerebellum (Kuchelmeister et al 1995). A larger case series subsequently established the distinctive nature of this neoplasm (Komori et al 2002). The most common location is the region of the fourth ventricle, with limited involvement of the vermis, brainstem and cerebral aqueduct (Komori et al 2002). The characteristic histopathological features are Homer Wright rosettes and perivascular pseudo-rosettes composed of small neurocytic cells. The delicate processes of these neurocytic cells are strongly immunoreactive for synaptophysin (Komori et al 2002). The rosettes and pseudo-rosettes are dispersed among a population of astrocytes that often have spindled morphology. Small oligodendroglial-like cells may also be present.

Rosette-forming glioneuronal tumor of the fourth ventricle should not be confused with *glioneuronal tumor with neuropil-like islands*. The latter is an aggressive neoplasm in which discrete islands of neuropil-like material, staining strongly for synaptophysin are present within an otherwise typical anaplastic astrocytoma or glioblastoma (Teo et al 1999). These neuropil islands have a peripheral corona of small oligodendroglial-like cells and, occasionally, larger cells expressing neuronal antigens (NeuN; Hu) (Teo et al 1999; Prayson & Abramovich 2000). These tumors behave aggressively, in-keeping with their high-grade glial component (Teo et al 1999; Varlet et al 2004). Glioneuronal tumor with neuropil-like islands is not included as a separate entity in the 2007 classification. Rather, it is referred to in the discussion of variations in the histopathological appearances of anaplastic astrocytoma and glioblastoma multiforme (Kleihues et al 2007).

Paraganglioma is a tumor of neural crest origin, occurring in the intradural extramedullary compartment, usually in the region of the cauda equina (Gelabert-Gonzalez 2005). These are graded as WHO I and have the same histopathological features as paragangliomas occurring outside the CNS.

Tumors of the pineal region
- Pineocytoma WHO I
- Pineal parenchyma tumor of intermediate differentiation WHO II/III
- Pineoblastoma WHO IV
- Papillary tumor of the pineal region WHO II/III.

Tumors of the pineal region are classified as in the 2000 scheme. *Papillary tumor of the pineal region* is a new entity in this category. *Pineocytomas* are low-grade (WHO I), slowly growing tumors that do not extend beyond the pineal and do not seed the craniospinal axis (Fauchon et al 2000). Tumor cells have morphological features similar to pinocytes and are arranged in rosettes as well as diffuse sheets. Delicate tumor cell processes invariably show immunoreactivity for synaptophysin. Reactivity for a range of neuronal lineage markers: neuron specific enolase (NSE); neurofilament protein (NFP); tau protein; class III β tubulin, may be seen (Yamane et al 2002), as well as expression of photosensory proteins such as retinal S antigen and rhodopsin (Perentes et al 1986; Illum et al 1992).

Pineal parenchymal tumor of intermediate differentiation is composed of small neurocytic cells arranged in diffuse

sheets and showing synaptophysin immunoreactivity. Well-formed Homer Wright rosettes are less prominent compared with typical pineocytoma. These tumors are graded as WHO II or III depending on the presence of mitotic figures, presence or absence of necrosis and degree of expression of neurofilament protein (NFP) (Jouvet et al 2000; Fauchon et al 2000).

Pineoblastoma is an aggressive (WHO IV) pineal parenchymal tumor that may seed the craniospinal axis and metastasize outside the CNS, particularly to bone (Constantine et al 2005). Peritoneal seeding following ventriculoperitoneal shunting has also been reported (Gururangan et al 1994), as well as implantation following stereotactic biopsy (Rosenfeld et al 1990). Histologically, pineoblastomas resemble primitive neuroectodermal tumors with undifferentiated small tumor cells containing hyperchromatic nuclei arranged in diffuse sheets. Scattered Homer Wright and Flexner–Wintersteiner rosettes may be seen. Mitotic figures and necrosis are common. Pineoblastoma may be a component of the trilateral retinoblastoma syndrome (bilateral retinoblastoma and pineoblastoma) (De Potter et al 1994).

Papillary tumor of the pineal region was first described as a distinct neoplasm by Jouvet and colleagues in 2003. The cell lineage of this tumor remains uncertain. Jouvet and colleagues suggested an origin from specialized ependymal cells in the sub-commissural organ based on immunohistochemical and ultrastructural features. These cells come to reside in the definitive pineal gland. The essential features differentiating this tumor from pineal parenchymal tumors are expression of a range of cytokeratins (Fèvre-Montange et al 2006) and only focal weak immunostaining for synaptophysin (Jouvet et al 2003). Less than 50 cases of papillary tumor of the pineal region have been reported and biologic behavior appears to be variable, corresponding to WHO grades II and III (Fèvre-Montange et al 2006).

Embryonal tumors
- Medulloblastoma WHO III
  - Desmoplastic/nodular medulloblastoma
  - Medulloblastoma with extensive nodularity
  - Anaplastic medulloblastoma
  - Large cell medulloblastoma
- CNS primitive neuroectodermal tumor WHO III
  - CNS neuroblastoma
  - CNS ganglioneuroblastoma
  - Medulloepithelioma
  - Ependymoblastoma
- Atypical teratoid/rhabdoid tumor WHO III.

Embryonal tumors comprise medulloblastoma, primitive neuroectodermal tumor (PNET) and atypical teratoid/rhabdoid tumor (ATRT). All three are associated with aggressive behavior and are graded as WHO III.

Medulloblastoma was classified as an entity separate from CNS primitive neuroectodermal tumor (cPNET) in the 2000 WHO scheme. Previously, all embryonal tumors of the CNS, irrespective of location were regarded as PNETs (Rorke 1983). The 2000 refinement of the classification arose from the recognition that medulloblastomas develop from the external granular layer of the cerebellar cortex rather than primitive neuroectoderm and have a different genetic fingerprint to supratentorial PNETs (Russo et al 1999; Cenacchi & Giangaspero 2004). Medulloblastoma is also more responsive to chemotherapy and radiotherapy than PNET (McNeill et al 2002).

Several histologic sub-types of *medulloblastoma* are recognized. In the *desmoplastic/nodular* variant, circumscribed reticulin free zones, termed 'pale islands' and composed of cells with neurocytic features, are dispersed among densely packed cells with small, angulated, hyperchromatic, often overlapping nuclei, with scant cytoplasm, as seen in the usual form of medulloblastoma (McManamy et al 2007). These pale islands may be present only in regions of the tumor. The term *medulloblastoma with extensive nodularity* indicates a tumor in which the pale islands are large and prominent throughout. Desmoplasia and nodules appear not to influence survival (Verma et al 2008). *Anaplastic medulloblastoma* displays a greater degree of nuclear atypia and higher mitotic and apoptotic activity compared to conventional medulloblastoma. Progression from conventional to anaplastic medulloblastoma has been documented. Mixed patterns of conventional and anaplastic medulloblastoma can also be seen in the one tumor. Anaplastic medulloblastoma also overlaps with large cell medulloblastoma. The latter is composed of large epithelioid cells with prominent nucleoli and exhibits abundant mitotic figures and apoptotic debris as well as areas of necrosis (Giangaspero et al 1992; Verma et al 2008).

Central nervous system (CNS) primitive neuroectodermal tumor (cPNET) is retained in the 2007 classification. This is a complex group of embryonal tumors, occurring in the supra-tentorial compartment and composed of cells resembling primitive neuroectoderm of the developing nervous system. Remnants of these cells are recognized as the periventricular germinal matrix in the neonatal brain. These tumors predominate in young children with few cPNETs having been described in adults (Ohba et al 2008). The rare development of cPNET several years after cranial irradiation for glial tumors has been described (Barasch et al 1988; Baborie et al 2007). Evidence of differentiation along neuronal or glial lineages may be detected by immunohistochemistry. Where there is predominant or exclusive neuronal differentiation without formation of mature ganglion cells, the term *CNS neuroblastoma* is appropriate, whereas *CNS ganglioneuroblastoma* contains mature ganglion cells in addition to features of neuroblastoma. While there is histologic overlap with medulloblastoma, cPNET can be distinguished by promoter methylation of the *RAS* association family 1 (RASSF1A) gene (Chang et al 2005) and the p14/ARF gene (Inda et al 2006).

Medulloepithelioma and *ependymoblastoma* are categorized as variants of cPNET and are not listed as separate embryonal tumors, as in the 2000 and previous WHO classification schemes. Both are uncommon embryonal tumors occurring in neonates and young children.

Atypical teratoid/rhabdoid tumor (ATRT) is another uncommon, aggressive, complex embryonal tumor composed of rhabdoid (i.e., resembling rhabdomyoma or rhabdomyosarcoma), primitive neuroectodermal, mesenchymal and epithelial elements (Rorke et al 1996). These tumors occur almost exclusively in children under 3 years of age. A small number of adult ATRTs have been reported (Makuria et al 2008). The commonest sites are cerebral hemispheric white matter, cerebellum, cerebellopontine angle and brainstem. Spinal seeding via cerebrospinal fluid is a common complication of ATRT (Hilden et al 2004). Diagnosis of ATRT is facilitated by demonstrating either deletion/mutation or reduced expression of the INI-1 gene located at 22q11.2 (Biegel 2006). Molecular analysis can now be supplemented by immunohistochemical staining for BAF47, the protein product of the INI-1 gene (Haberler et al 2006).

Tumors of cranial and paraspinal nerves

- Schwannoma WHO I
  - Cellular
  - Plexiform
  - Melanotic
- Neurofibroma WHO I
  - Plexiform
- Perineurioma
  - Perineurioma NOS WHO I/II
  - Malignant perineurioma WHO III
- Malignant peripheral nerve sheath tumor (MPNST) WHO II/III/IV
  - Epithelioid MPNST
  - MPNST with mesenchymal differentiation
  - Melanotic MPNST
  - MPNST with glandular differentiation.

Except for the inclusion of malignant perineurioma, the classification of tumors of cranial and paraspinal nerves is unchanged from the 2000 classification.

Conventional *schwannoma* (syn: neurilemmoma; neurinoma) has a biphasic histologic appearance with compact Antoni A tissue mixed with the more loosely arranged cells of Antoni B tissue. Variably formed Verocay bodies, with a prominent palisaded arrangement of nuclei, may be noted in Antoni A areas. A meningothelial cell component may be seen in NF-2 associated schwannomas (Ludeman et al 2000). Intracranial schwannomas preferentially involve the eighth cranial nerve in the cerebellopontine angle and internal auditory meatus. They may also involve the trigeminal and facial nerves (Akimoto et al 2000; Ugokwe et al 2005). Very rarely, schwannomas develop within brain parenchyma, unassociated with cranial nerves (Casadei et al 1993).

Cellular schwannomas lack well-formed Verocay bodies and are composed predominantly of Antoni A tissue. Scattered mitoses may also be noted in this variant, as well as high proliferation indices and a propensity for local recurrence (Casadei et al 1995).

The *plexiform* variant of schwannoma invariably involves nerves in skin and subcutaneous tissue. The entity has a loose association with NF-2 and schwannomatosis (Reith & Goldblum 1996).

Melanotic schwannoma most commonly involves spinal nerves and has to be distinguished from melanocytic tumors (Er et al 2007). This is best achieved by electron microscopy demonstrating basal lamina material surrounding individual tumor cells. Melanosomes will be seen in melanotic schwannoma and psammoma bodies may also be present, particularly in tumors occurring as part of the Carney complex (Kurtkaya-Yapicier et al 2003).

Neurofibromas exhibit a mixture of Schwann cells and fibroblasts. Small axonal structures, with immunostaining for neurofilament protein (NFP), are noted and there may be small numbers of perineurial cells, demonstrating immunostaining for epithelial membrane antigen (EMA). The plexiform variant is characteristic of NF-1.

Perineurioma was first described in 1978 as a soft tissue tumor in which perineurial cells were recognized on the basis of their ultrastructural features (Lazarus et al 1978). The entity was first included in the WHO classification of tumors of the nervous system in 2000. Virtually all reported examples of perineurioma have involved peripheral nerves, particularly those in the fingers and palms (Fetsch & Miettinen 1997). The particular immunohistochemical characteristics of perineurioma are expression of epithelial membrane antigen (EMA) and the glucose transporter protein, Glut-1 (Hirose et al 2003). Deletion of part or all of chromosome 22q is also characteristic of perineurioma (Giannini et al 1997). While the vast majority of perineuriomas are benign (WHO grade I), local recurrence and distant spread have been reported (Fukunaga 2001).

Malignant peripheral nerve sheath tumor (MPNST) has a spectrum of histopathological appearances. This includes *epithelioid* and *glandular* variants and a variant with *mesenchymal differentiation (malignant Triton tumor)* in addition to the common spindle cell variant. Fundamentally, MPNSTs display features of anaplasia or malignancy not seen in benign nerve sheath tumors. These include diffuse or regional dense hypercellularity, an interdigitating, fascicular arrangement of pleomorphic spindle cells, nuclear enlargement and atypia, frequent mitotic figures (>4 per 10 ×400 high-power fields) and invasion of adjacent soft tissue. MPNSTs with these features are graded as WHO III. The presence of necrosis indicates WHO grade IV. The majority of MPNSTs are associated with NF-1 and most commonly involve paraspinal soft tissue, soft tissue of the buttock and thigh and the brachial plexus. Very rare involvement of cranial nerves by MPNST has been reported (Kudo et al 1983; McLean et al 1990).

Tumors of the meninges

Tumors of meningothelial cells
- Meningioma
  - Meningothelial WHO I
  - Fibrous (fibroblastic) WHO I
  - Transitional (mixed) WHO I
  - Psammomatous WHO I
  - Angiomatous WHO I
  - Microcystic WHO I
  - Secretory WHO I
  - Lymphoplasmacyte-rich WHO I
  - Metaplastic WHO I
  - Chordoid WHO II

- Clear cell WHO II
- Atypical WHO II
- Papillary WHO III
- Rhabdoid WHO III
- Anaplastic (malignant) WHO III.

Meningiomas remain an enigmatic group of tumors that continue to pose challenges in grading and correlation between histopathological features and biologic behavior. In the 2007 classification and grading scheme, grade I meningiomas are regarded as having a low potential for local recurrence and aggressive behavior, whereas grade II and III tumors have a higher potential.

As in the 2000 WHO classification scheme, there are nine histologic sub-types of WHO grade I meningiomas.

Chordoid and *clear cell* sub-types are associated with a higher rate of local recurrence and are graded as WHO II (Couce et al 2000; Zorludemir et al 1995).

Criteria for the histopathological diagnosis of *atypical* and *anaplastic (malignant) meningioma* incorporated into the 2000 and 2007 WHO classification schemes, derive from two large studies undertaken by Perry and colleagues at the Mayo Clinic (Perry et al 1997b, 1999). In those studies, atypical meningioma was defined by 'a mitotic figure count of 4 or more per 10×40 high-power fields (i.e., an area of 0.16 mm^2) *OR* three or more of the following features: increased cellularity; small cells with a high nuclear: cytoplasmic ratio; prominent nucleoli; uninterrupted patternless or sheet-like growth, and foci of spontaneous or geographic necrosis'. The likelihood of recurrence of meningiomas with these features was found to be eight times that of conventional grade I meningiomas. Another earlier study emphasized the importance of necrosis as a predictor of the likelihood of local recurrence (McLean et al 1993).

In the Mayo Clinic studies, *anaplastic (malignant) meningiomas* (WHO grade III) exhibited 'features of frank malignancy far in excess of the abnormalities present in atypical meningioma', e.g., 'clear cytological malignancy similar to that seen in carcinoma, melanoma or sarcoma and/or a very high mitotic index (20 or more mitotic figures per 10 high-power fields)'.

Despite the apparent histopathological differences between WHO grade I, atypical (WHO grade II) and anaplastic (malignant; WHO grade III) meningiomas, up to 12% of grade I tumors recur within 5 years (Perry et al 1997b). Histopathological features indicating the recurrence potential of a grade I meningioma, have yet to be defined. The 1997 study by Perry and colleagues found that brain invasion was a very strong indicator of recurrence. However, the median survival of patients with invasive grade I meningiomas was not significantly different from that for patients with invasive atypical (grade II) tumors. The 2007 WHO classification scheme does not include brain invasion as a criterion for either atypical or malignant meningioma.

Several molecular-genetic studies have linked deletions of chromosomes 1p and 14q in WHO grade I meningiomas, with and without brain invasion, to a higher likelihood of local recurrence (Cai et al 2001; Maillo et al 2007; Pfisterer et al 2008). In one of these studies, deletions were closely linked to high MIB-1 labeling indices (Pfisterer et al 2008).

Deletion of the p16 locus at chromosome 9p.21 or mono-somy of chromosome 9 appear to be associated with a high likelihood of progression of atypical to anaplastic meningioma and shorter survival (Perry et al 2002; Lopez-Gines et al 2004).

Papillary and rhabdoid meningiomas are aggressive variants that are graded as WHO III. *Papillary meningioma* is composed of areas that are recognizable architecturally as meningioma, mixed with papillary or pseudo-papillary structures. These have variably formed fibrovascular cores, covered by a stratified arrangement of atypical tumor cells. Solid papillary structures, resulting from invasion of the fibrovascular cores, may be present. The majority of papillary meningiomas invade brain parenchyma (Ludwin et al 1975). Sporadic examples of metastasis outside the craniospinal compartment, particularly to lung, have also been reported (Ludwin et al 1975; Pasquier et al 1986; Kros et al 2000).

As in other 'rhabdoid' tumors, *rhabdoid meningioma* has a component of large cells with eccentric nuclei and abundant eosinophilic cytoplasm often containing hyaline perinuclear inclusions, spread among cells that are more easily recognizable as meningothelial. The rhabdoid cells do not display features of skeletal muscle differentiation; rather they show immunostaining for epithelial membrane antigen and vimentin, characteristic of meningothelial cells. By electron microscopy, there is a spectrum, from cells with filamentous paranuclear inclusions, typical of rhabdoid cells to cells with meningothelial features – cell membrane invagination and interdigitation with intercellular tight junctions (Perry et al 1998).

Mesenchymal, non-meningothelial cell tumors
- Lipoma
- Angiolipoma
- Hibernoma
- Liposarcoma
- Solitary fibrous tumor
- Fibrosarcoma
- Malignant fibrous histiocytoma
- Leiomyoma
- Leiomyosarcoma
- Rhabdomyoma
- Rhabdomyosarcoma
- Chondroma
- Chondrosarcoma
- Osteoma
- Osteosarcoma
- Osteochondroma
- Hemangioma
- Epithelioid hemangioendothelioma
- Hemangiopericytoma WHO II
- Anaplastic hemangiopericytoma WHO III
- Angiosarcoma
- Kaposi sarcoma
- Ewing sarcoma – peripheral PNET.

This category was significantly expanded in the 2000 classification scheme in recognition of the broad range of mesenchymal tumors that can involve the meninges. As in the 2000 scheme, benign and malignant forms are listed together with grading ranging from WHO I for benign forms to WHO grade IV for the highly malignant sarcomatous forms. Most, if not all tumors in this category, have histopathological features and biologic behaviors that are identical to their counterparts in soft tissue and bone outside the CNS. Entities that are of particular nosological interest include: solitary fibrous tumor, hemangiopericytoma and Ewing's sarcoma/peripheral primitive neuroectodermal tumor (EWS-pPNET).

Solitary fibrous tumor (SFT) is most commonly seen in the pleural cavity and thorax (Klemperer & Rabin 1931; Suster et al 1995) but has been reported at numerous sites in soft tissues, solid organs and gastrointestinal and genitourinary tracts. There is no consensus regarding the cell of origin of SFTs, although ultrastructural features of fibroblastic and myofibroblastic differentiation have been described (El-Naggar et al 1989; Hasegawa et al 1996). Primary meningeal SFT was first described in 1996 (Caniero et al 1996). At all sites, SFT is composed of spindle cells arranged in intersecting fasciculi reminiscent of fibrosarcoma. These show immunostaining for CD34, vimentin and bcl-2. Immunostaining for epithelial membrane antigen (EMA) is not seen in meningeal SFTs and there is usually no reactivity for S-100 protein, cytokeratins or melanocytic markers (Caniero et al 1996). While the majority of intracranial SFTs behave non-aggressively, rare examples with malignant behavior have been recorded (Ogawa et al 2004). Solitary fibrous tumors show a range of chromosomal abnormalities that differ from meningiomas and deletions of chromosome 3p21-p26 in intracranial SFTs differentiate them from extracranial examples (Martin et al 2002).

Despite the merging of hemangiopericytoma with solitary fibrous tumor in the WHO Classification of Soft Tissue Tumors (Gillou et al 2002), meningeal hemangiopericytoma is classified separate from solitary fibrous tumor in the 2007 CNS tumor scheme. Two grades are recognized: (1) *hemangiopericytoma* (WHO grade II), and (2) *anaplastic hemangiopericytoma* (WHO grade III). Difficulties in classifying hemangiopericytoma arise because of histologic overlap with solitary fibrous tumor and fibrous meningioma with low expression of epithelial membrane antigen (Perry et al 1997c). The histogenesis of meningeal hemangiopericytoma remains controversial. However, like solitary fibrous tumors, a fibroblastic rather than pericytic origin has been suggested (Fletcher 2006).

Confusion arises between CNS primitive neuroectodermal tumor (cPNET) and *peripheral primitive neuroectodermal tumor* (pPNET; Ewing's sarcoma/pPNET)). The latter most often occurs outside the CNS, involving soft tissue, peripheral nerves and solid organs such as adrenal, uterus, ovary, and kidney. Bone involvement overlaps histopathologically with the *Ewing's sarcoma* family of tumors (ESft). pPNETs can be separated from cPNETs by their expression of the MIC2 glycoprotein (CD99) reflecting the presence of a unique chimeric gene designated EWS-FLI1 (Ishii et al 2001; Cenacchi & Giangaspero 2004). Despite the majority of pPNETs occurring outside the CNS, rare examples arising within the craniospinal compartment have been reported (Kampan et al 2006).

Primary melanocytic lesions
- Diffuse melanocytosis
- Melanocytoma
- Malignant melanoma
- Meningeal melanomatosis.

Leptomeningeal melanocytes are of neural crest origin and give rise to a spectrum of primary tumors varying from benign through intermediate grade to highly malignant. These tumors are extremely uncommon and account for <1% of primary CNS neoplasms. Diffuse melanocytosis and melanomatosis usually form part of the neurocutaneous melanosis and nevus of Ota syndromes (Kadonaga & Frieden 1991; Balmaceda et al 1993; Piercecchi-Marti et al 2002). Malignant melanoma is differentiated from melanocytoma by the presence of anaplastic features: increased tumor cell density; nuclear and cellular pleomorphism; frequent mitotic figures with atypical forms, and a higher MIB-1 labeling index (≥8%) (Brat et al 1999b). Malignant melanoma may also invade underlying brain or spinal cord parenchyma. Meningeal melanomatosis describes multiple foci of malignant melanoma, each arising *de novo* or resulting from seeding through the sub-arachnoid space. However, occasional melanocytomas have displayed leptomeningeal spread (Bydon et al 2003). Primary melanocytic tumors of the meninges need to be differentiated from other tumors that may undergo melanization, in particular, melanotic schwannoma and the rare melanotic neuroectodermal tumor of infancy (retinal anlage tumor) (Pierre-Kahn et al 1992).

Other neoplasms related to the meninges
- Hemangioblastoma.

Hemangioblastoma (syn: capillary hemangioblastoma) accounts for approximately 2% of primary intracranial tumors and occurs either sporadically or as a component of von Hippel Lindau (VHL) syndrome (Hussein 2007). Up to 40% are VHL-related and display the characteristic mutation at 3p25–26 (Catapano et al 2005). Sporadic tumors are usually solitary and are located most commonly in the cerebellum. VHL-associated tumors frequently involve spinal cord and brainstem in addition to cerebellum. Leptomeningeal dissemination of VHL-associated hemangioblastoma has been documented (Reyns et al 2003), as has sporadic hemangioblastoma involving cerebrum (Sherman et al 2007). The characteristic histopathological features are variably-sized lobules of stromal cells surrounded by capillary vascular channels and scattered prominent large calibre thin-walled sinusoidal vessels. Cellular and reticular variants are recognized, the former with a more prominent stromal cell component and a higher propensity for local recurrence. A variety of chromosomal alterations also distinguish the two variants (Rickert et al 2006). The histogenesis of stromal cells is contentious. Initial immunohistochemical studies indicated an origin from neuroepithelium (Theunissen et al 1990). Later studies have suggested an origin from hemangioblastic progenitor cells (Gläsker et al 2006). Differentia-

tion from metastatic renal cell carcinoma is facilitated by immunoreactivity for inhibin A in stromal cells of hemangioblastoma and CD10 staining in renal cell carcinoma (Jung & Kuo 2005). Hemangioblastomas, both sporadic and VHL-associated, are graded as WHO I.

Lymphomas and hemopoietic neoplasms
- Malignant lymphoma
- Plasmacytoma
- Granulocytic sarcoma.

Primary central nervous system lymphoma (PCNSL) is an uncommon form of extranodal non-Hodgkin's lymphoma involving, brain parenchyma, meninges and eyes (Commins et al 2006). Approximately 90% are CD20+ diffuse large B cell lymphomas. Burkitt's and Burkitt-like lymphomas, lymphoblastic B cell lymphoma and T cell lymphomas make up the remaining 10% (Kadoch et al 2006). PCNSLs occurring in immunocompromised individuals are usually related to latent Epstein-Barr virus (EBV) infection (Forsyth & DeAngelis 1996). Elevated expression as well as mutations of the proto-oncogenes, *MYC* and *PIM*, ectopic expression of the B lymphocyte growth factor, interleukin-4 (IL4), and deletions and promoter methylation affecting the p14ARF/p53/MDM2 pathway are the commonest among a very large number of molecular-genetic alterations seen in PCNSLs (Montesinos-Rongen et al 2004; Rubenstein et al 2006; Kadoch et al 2006). Unusual forms of lymphoma involving the CNS include anaplastic large cell lymphoma, lymphomatosis cerebri and intravascular lymphoma (Gonzales 2003; Rollins et al 2005; Ponzoni & Ferreri 2006). Intravascular lymphoma may represent the earliest stage of PCNSL as examples accompanied by mass lesions have been documented (Imai et al 2004).

The frequency of PCNSL fluctuated from 2.5 cases per 10 million (>1% of all primary CNS tumors) in 1973 to 30 cases per 10 million (7% of all primary CNS tumors) in 1992 (Corn et al 1997). The peak reached in the late 1980s to early 1990s reflected the high incidence of PCNSL in acquired immunodeficiency syndrome (AIDS) (Camilleri-Broet et al 1997). The development of highly effective antiretroviral therapy (HAART) in the 1990s brought about a dramatic reduction in the incidence of HIV-related central nervous system diseases, including PCNSL (Sacktor et al 2001). PCNSL is an aggressive neoplasm. However, advances in chemotherapeutic regimens and radiotherapy have improved median survival from <12 months to 50–60 months (Abrey et al 2000; Pels et al 2003).

The majority of cranial *plasmacytomas* involve skull bones. Rare parenchymal lesions have been reported in meninges, cavernous sinus and pituitary fossa. Exceptional cases of intracerebral plasmacytoma as an early manifestation of multiple myeloma are recorded (Wavre et al 2007).

Granulocytic sarcoma (previously chloroma) is the designation applied to collections of leukemic cells, usually of myeloid lineage, in a variety of organs. A handful of cases involving brain and spinal cord parenchyma have been reported (Yoon et al 1987; Fujii et al 2002; Colovi et al 2004). These lesions may precede, coincide with or follow the leukemic phase of the disease.

A number of *histiocytic tumors* are not tabulated in the 2007 WHO classification. These include Langerhans cell histiocytosis, Rosai–Dorfman disease, Erdheim–Chester disease, hemophagocytic lymphohistiocytosis and juvenile xanthogranuloma.

These entities however, are outlined in detail in the text of the 2007 WHO Classification of Tumors of the Central Nervous System blue book (Paulus & Perry 2007).

Germ cell tumors

- Germinoma
- Embryonal carcinoma
- Yolk sac tumor
- Choriocarcinoma
- Teratoma
  - Mature
  - Immature
  - Teratoma with malignant transformation
- Mixed germ cell tumor.

CNS germ cell tumors have similar, if not identical, histopathological features to germ cell tumors involving the genitourinary tract and mediastinum and are classified in the same way as their non-CNS counterparts. The most common intracranial germ cell tumor is the pineal germinoma. Other locations include the sellar region and anterior third ventricle (germinoma) (Matsutani et al 1997), choroid plexus (embryonal carcinoma and yolk sac tumor) (Burger & Scheithauer 1994) and basal ganglia (germinoma and teratoma) (Kobayashi et al 1989; Ng et al 1992). Nuclear immunostaining for the OCT4 protein is gradually superseding placental alkaline phosphatase (PLAP) staining for confirming the diagnosis of germinoma and is also seen in CNS embryonal carcinomas (Hattab et al 2005). The majority of CNS germinomas also exhibit strong immunostaining for c-kit (CD117) (Hattab et al 2004). This is useful in distinguishing germinoma from atypical teratoid/rhabdoid tumor (Edgar & Rosenblum 2008).

Tumors of the sellar region

- Craniopharyngioma WHO I
  - Adamantinomatous
  - Papillary
- Granular cell tumor WHO I
- Pituicytoma WHO I
- Spindle cell oncocytoma of the adenohypophysis WHO I.

Craniopharyngioma and granular cell tumor are retained in the sellar region tumor category. Pituicytoma and spindle cell oncocytoma of the adenohypophysis are new entities.

Craniopharyngiomas are proposed to arise either from epithelial rests located along the craniopharyngeal tract (Goldberg & Eshbaught 1960) or by metaplastic transformation of adenohypophyseal cells (Hunter 1955; Asa et al 1983). Some also arise from epithelial cell remnants of Rathke's pouch (Prabhu & Brown 2005). The first description of a tumor arising from craniopharyngeal tract cell rests was published in 1902 (Saxer 1902, cited in Karavitaki & Wass 2008). The term craniopharyngioma was proposed by Cushing in 1932.

The *adamantinomatous* sub-type displays the classical histopathological features of basaloid epithelium at the periphery of cellular islands, maturing centrally to keratinizing squamous epithelium through an intermediate zone of loosely cohesive stellate reticulum cells. Calcification and degeneration of keratin to form 'wet' keratin, recognized macroscopically as oily viscous fluid, are common in this variant (Petito et al 1976). The *papillary* variant, which is seen almost exclusively in adults, consists only of well-differentiated squamous epithelium, rarely undergoes cyst formation or calcification and does not form wet keratin (Crotty et al 1995).

Craniopharyngiomas are regarded as benign tumors and are graded as WHO I. Rare cases of purported malignant transformation are on record (Nelson et al 1988; Kristopaitis et al 2000). The exceedingly uncommon occurrence of intracranial dissemination after surgery, with short survival, has also been reported (Nomura et al 2002).

A variety of terms have been applied to *granular cell tumor* in previous WHO and other classifications of CNS tumors. These have included choristoma, granular cell myoblastoma, granular cell neuroma, pituicytoma, and Abrikossoff tumor. As indicated below, pituicytoma is now recognized as a glial tumor involving neurohypophysis or infundibulum. However, both granular cell tumor and pituicytoma arise from glial elements located in the neurohypophysis and infundibulum, with different sub-populations giving rise to each tumor type (Takei et al 1980). The histopathological features of granular cell tumor involving the sellar region are identical to tumors occurring at sites outside the CNS – diffuse sheets of polygonal shaped cells with abundant, finely granular eosinophilic cytoplasm, immunoreactive for S-100 protein, CD68, α-1-antitrypsin and α-1-antichymotrypsin.

Sellar region granular cell tumors are regarded as benign with a grading of WHO I. So-called 'atypical' granular cell tumors, with a mitotic index of ≥5/10HPF and a Ki-67/MIB-1 labeling index of 7% or higher, have been reported (Kasashima et al 2000).

Pituicytoma has been recognized for many years as a distinctive tumor of the neurohypophysis and infundibulum, having been first described in the early 1960s (Jenevein 1964). Histopathologically, there is a loose fascicular or storiform arrangement of spindle cells with positive immunostaining for S-100 protein and vimentin and variable staining for GFAP (Brat et al 2000). Pituicytomas are regarded essentially as low-grade gliomas (WHO I) and need to be distinguished from other low-grade glial tumors, in particular, pilocytic astrocytoma.

Spindle cell oncocytoma of the adenohypophysis is proposed to arise from folliculo-stellate cells of the anterior pituitary (Roncaroli et al 2002). Normal folliculo-stellate cells are thought to regulate the secretory activity of functioning adenohypophyseal cells and to act as antigen presenting cells (Allaerts & Vankelecom 2005). Spindle cell oncocytomas mimic pituitary adenomas both in their macroscopic and radiological appearances. Histologically, they are composed of both spindle and epithelioid cells and show positive immunostaining for S-100 protein, epithelial membrane antigen (EMA) and galactin 3. Immunostaining for pituitary hormones is negative. Negative staining for synaptophysin in spindle cell oncocytomas assists in distinguishing them from non-functioning pituitary adenomas. The majority of the small number of spindle cell oncocytomas that have been reported have behaved non-aggressively and they are graded as WHO I in the 2007 scheme. Local recurrence of two tumors has been reported, each with initially high Ki-67/MIB-1 labeling indices (Kloub et al 2005).

Metastatic tumors

Metastatic brain tumors occur at a rate 10 times that of primary tumors (Arnold & Patchell 2001). These tumors become established in brain parenchyma and meninges as a result of hematogenous spread. Sites of primary tumors metastasizing to brain, in order of decreasing frequency, are lung, breast, colorectum, skin (melanoma), kidney (renal cell), and thyroid (Nussbaum et al 1996). A primary site is not identified in up to 10% of patients at first presentation (Khan & DeAngelis 2003). Metastatic melanoma more commonly involves frontal and temporal lobes, metastatic carcinoma from the breast preferentially involves the cerebellum and basal ganglia and non-small cell carcinoma arising from the lung most commonly metastasizes to the occipital lobes (Graf et al 1988). Metastatic tumors affecting the spinal cord usually develop in the epidural spaces or extend from involved vertebrae. These most commonly arise from primary tumors in the breast, prostate, lung, and kidney (Mut et al 2005).

Immunohistochemistry is vital in determining the lineage of metastatic tumor cells and probable site of the primary tumor. The immunohistochemistry panel should include antibodies against a range of cytokeratins, melanocyte markers, thyroid transcription factor (TTF-1), neuroendocrine markers, and hormone receptors (reviewed by Becher et al 2006). Pathologists also need to be aware of the not uncommon phenomenon of metastasis to meningiomas. The most common primary site in this situation is the breast (Aghi et al 2005).

Classification of childhood brain tumors

Despite the consensus on terminology achieved in the 1993, 2000, and 2007 WHO classifications, brain tumors of childhood pose special problems. Pediatric neuropathologists routinely deal with complex CNS tumors for which no particular category seems appropriate. Furthermore, the association between individual histopathological features and biologic behavior is less clear for childhood gliomas compared with those in adults (Gilles et al 2000a). Grading schemes based on histopathological features derive from studies of adult tumors and are difficult to apply to childhood tumors (Brown et al 1998). Anatomic location appears to be a significant factor in the biologic behavior of childhood

gliomas. Astrocytomas of the cerebellum, for example, have a much more favorable prognosis than histologically similar tumors in the cerebral hemispheres. The scheme for classifying childhood brain tumors proposed by Rorke and colleagues (1985) emphasizes the mixed nature of glial and neuronal-glial tumors and the influence of anatomic location on tumor behavior. The nosologic problems inherent in the designation 'primitive neuroectodermal tumor (PNET)' are addressed by dividing these tumors into sub-categories: primitive neuroectodermal tumor not otherwise specified (PNET-NOS), PNET with astrocytes, ependymal cells, oligodendroglia, neuronal cells, melanocytes, mesenchymal cells or mixed cellular elements, and medulloepithelioma. Medulloblastoma of the cerebellum and pineoblastoma are regarded as the prototypes of PNET-NOS. Medulloepithelioma is further subdivided into medulloepithelioma NOS, which has a distinctive histologic appearance resembling primitive neural tube, and medulloepithelioma with astrocytes, oligodendrocytes, neuronal cells, melanocytes or mesenchymal cells as well as mixed cellular elements.

Pathogenesis of central nervous system tumors

The pathogenesis of central nervous system tumors, particularly gliomas, fundamentally involves alterations in genes mediating initiation, differentiation, and proliferation of tumor cells. These genes encode growth factors and their receptors, second messenger proteins, which influence cell cycle control, apoptosis and necrosis, transcription factors and proteins mediating angiogenesis and interaction between tumor cells and the extracellular matrix. Alterations involving oncogenes (increase in gene copy number, overexpression) result in gain of function, while inactivation of tumor suppressor genes (deletion, translocation) results in loss of function. In addition, epigenetic phenomena, in particular promoter methylation, affect protein expression. Genetic alterations in progenitor cells and putative glioma stem cells establish a population of cells which may be resistant to adjuvant therapies and responsible for tumor recurrence and progression (Singh et al 2004). Familial tumor syndromes are linked to germline mutations. Environmental factors associated with tumor pathogenesis exert their influence by inducing somatic mutations. Apart from their role in pathogenesis, some gene alterations influence the response to adjuvant treatments and biologic behavior of tumors.

Historically, chemicals and viruses have been emphasized as the major environmental factors contributing to the pathogenesis of CNS tumors. More recently there has been vigorous debate over the potential pathogenetic role of radiofrequency electromagnetic radiation associated with the use of mobile telephones. This debate has resulted from conflicting clinical and epidemiological studies.

Although a link between industrial chemicals and CNS tumors was suggested by a number of early epidemiologic studies (Selikoff & Hammond 1982), this was not confirmed in later investigations and the only evidence for direct tumor induction by chemicals has come from animal studies. Evidence for viral induction of CNS tumors in humans is more compelling and experimental studies in laboratory animals have convincingly demonstrated a causative link between some viruses and CNS tumors in susceptible species.

Chemically induced CNS tumors

Epidemiologic studies

In the late 1970s and early 1980s, epidemiologic studies, in particular in North America and Sweden, reported a higher than expected frequency of CNS tumors among workers in the petrochemical and rubber industries (Selikoff & Hammond 1982). Chemicals to which workers in these industries were exposed, and which have been shown to induce CNS tumors in laboratory animals, include aromatic hydrocarbons, hydrazines, bis(chloromethyl)ether, vinyl chloride, and acrylonitrile. Workers in some of these industries were also concurrently exposed to ionizing radiation. Follow-up studies in Sweden, however, did not confirm an increased risk with industrial exposure to these agents (McLaughlin et al 1987).

Chemical induction of CNS tumors in animals

Chemical induction of CNS tumors in small laboratory animals was first reported by Seligman & Shear (1939) and, since that time, this has been a useful paradigm for studying the biology of high-grade neuroglial tumors. The commonly utilized compounds include the *N*-nitrosoureas, the triazenes, the hydrazines, and the aromatic hydrocarbons and their derivatives. These agents have been administered by a variety of routes including direct injection into the brain or ventricles. Transplacental induction of tumors has also been achieved with the nitrosoureas. These have been found to be particularly effective inducers of CNS tumors because of their tropism for neural tissue. Following transplacental induction by ethyl-nitrosourea, high-grade glial tumors appear in offspring at 300 days. The mechanism of action of the nitrosoureas and other alkylating agents is thought to be the induction of unrepaired damage to DNA leading to point mutations. Further molecular-genetic investigations of gene alterations in CNS tumors induced by nitrosourea compounds led to the identification of the *c-erbB2* oncogene (Schechter et al 1984), supporting induction of point mutations as the likely mechanism of action. However, despite a large body of epidemiologic and animal experimental data it is questionable whether any of these compounds is causally related to human brain tumors.

Oncogenic viruses and brain tumors

The evidence for induction of human CNS tumors by oncogenic viruses is stronger than for chemical induction. There have been several reports of high-grade astrocytomas in patients with progressive multifocal leukoencephalopathy, a demyelinating disorder which follows infection of oligodendrocytes and astrocytes by the JC subtype of human papovavirus (Sima et al 1983). Epstein–Barr virus has also been identified in tumor cells in primary CNS lymphoma in patients with, as well as those without, human immunodeficiency virus infection (Geddes et al 1992). Data regarding direct induction of CNS tumors by oncogenic viruses have come exclusively from animal studies. Both DNA and RNA viruses have been shown to be capable of inducing tumors after intracerebral inoculation into susceptible species of laboratory animals. Of the DNA viruses, adenovirus and SV40, another of the papovaviruses, are particularly effective inducers of neoplasia. Human adenovirus type 12 has a particular affinity for primitive neuroectoderm and induces tumors resembling neuroblastoma, medulloblastoma and medulloepithelioma in the brain, and retinoblastoma after intraocular inoculation. SV40 induces highly malignant sarcomatous tumors, while development of multiple cerebellar medulloblastomas has followed inoculation of JC virus. In recent years, these techniques have been refined and tumors have been induced in mice by the introduction of early sequences of SV40 and adenovirus into the genome by transgenic technology (Kelly et al 1986; Danks et al 1995).

Several avian and murine retroviruses have been known for some time to be capable of inducing CNS tumors (for review, see Bigner & Pegram 1976). The mechanism by which these viruses induce tumors was clarified with the identification of oncogenes. The majority of oncogenes that have been identified to date show sequence homology with retroviruses isolated from animal tumors (Varmus 1984), suggesting that activation of oncogenes may occur by insertion of retroviral sequences. To date, however, this has not been confirmed in transgenic experiments.

Other factors

Hormones have been implicated in the growth and progression of some CNS tumors, in particular meningioma. The overall higher incidence of meningiomas in females and enlargement and rapid growth of meningiomas in the region of the tuberculum sellae and sphenoidal ridge during pregnancy have been recognized for some time (Bickerstaff et al 1958). The demonstration of estrogen, progesterone and androgen receptors in biopsy material from meningiomas (Donnell et al 1979; Schnegg et al 1981) supported the hypothesis that hormones promote tumor growth and raised hopes that hormone treatment might control the growth of aggressive meningiomas. However, such treatment has not been proven to significantly alter the biologic behavior of receptor-positive meningiomas.

There has been considerable debate centered on the contribution of radiofrequency/microwave radiation, particularly through the use of mobile telephones, to the pathogenesis of some brain tumors. Most of the studies have been small and have employed short latency periods. One meta-analysis found an association between the use of mobile telephones and an increased incidence of ipsilateral gliomas and acoustic neuromas in 10 case controlled studies that utilized a >10-year latency period (Hardell et al 2008). Another meta-analysis found an association between mobile phone use and all brain tumors, again in studies with a >10-year latency period (Kan et al 2008).

A variety of other factors: alcohol, tobacco, ionizing radiation, and trauma, have, at different times, been suggested to contribute to the development of CNS tumors. Most data come from epidemiologic studies.

REFERENCES

Abrey, L.E., Yahalom, J., DeAngelis, L.M., 2000. Treatment of primary CNS lymphoma: the next step. J. Clin. Oncol. 18, 3144–3150.

Aghi, M., Kiehl, T.-R., Brisman, J.L., 2005. Breast carcinoma metastatic to epidural cervical spine meningioma: case report and review of the literature. J. Neurooncol. 75, 149–155.

Ahlsén, G., Gillberg, I.C., Lindblom, R., et al., 1994. Tuberous sclerosis in Western Sweden. A population study of cases with early childhood onset. Arch. Neurol. 51, 76–81.

Akimoto, J., Ito H., Kudo M., 2000. Primary intracranial malignant schwannoma of trigeminal nerve. A case report with review of the literature. Acta Neurochir. (Wien) 142, 591–595.

Allaerts, W., Vankelecom, H., 2005. History and perspective of pituitary folliculo-stellate cell research. Eur. J. Endocrinol. 153, 1–12.

Arnold, S.M., Patchell, R.A., 2001. Diagnosis and management of brain metastases. Hematol. Oncol. Clin. North Am. 15, 1085–1107.

Asa, S.L., Kovacs, K., Bilbao, J.M., 1983. The pars tuberalis of the human pituitary: a histologic, immunohistochemical, ultrastructural and immunoelectron microscopic analysis. Virchows Arch. Anat. Histopathol. 399, 49–59.

Bailey, P., Cushing, H., 1926. A Classification of Tumors of the Glioma Group on a Histogenetic Basis. Lippincott, Philadelphia, PA, pp. 146–167.

Bailey, P., Bucy, P.C., 1930. Astroblastomas of the brain. Acta. Psychiat. et. Neurol. 5, 439–461.

Balko, M.G., Blisard, K.S., Samaha, F.J., 1992. Oligodendroglial gliomatosis cerebri. Hum. Pathol. 23, 706–707.

Balmaceda, C.M., Fetell, M.R., Powers, J., et al., 1993. Nevus of Ota and leptomeningeal melanocytic lesions. Neurology 43, 381–386.

Barasch, E.S., Altieri, D., Decker, R.E., et al., 1988. Primitive neuroectodermal tumor presenting as delayed sequela to cranial irradiation and intrathecal methotrexate. Pediatr. Neurol. 4, 375–378.

Baborie, A., Chakrabarty, A., Kuruvath, S., et al., 2007. 40 year old male with history of brain tumor 10 years ago. Brain Pathol. 17, 337–338.

Becher, M.W., Abel, T.W., Thompson, R.C., et al., 2006. Immunohistochemical analysis of metastatic neoplasms of the central nervous system. J. Neuropathol. Exp. Neurol. 65, 935–944.

Bechtel, J.T., Patton, J.M., Takei, Y., 1978. Mixed mesenchymal and neuroectodermal tumor of the cerebellum. Acta. Neuropathol. 41, 261–263.

Bickerstaff, E.R., Small, J.M., Guest, I.A., 1958. The relapsing course of certain meningiomas in relation to pregnancy and menstruation. J. Neurol. Neurosurg. Psychiatry 21, 89–91.

Biegel, J.A., 2006. Molecular genetics of atypical teratoid/rhabdoid tumor. Neurosurg. Focus 20, E11.

Biernat, W., Aguzzi, A., Sure, U., et al., 1995. Identical mutations of the p53 tumor suppressor gene in the gliomatous and sarcomatous components of gliosarcomas suggest a common origin from glial cells. J. Neuropathol. Exp. Neurol. 54, 651–656.

Bigner, D.D., Pegram, C.N., 1976. Virus-induced experimental brain tumors and putative associations of viruses with human brain tumors: a review. Adv. Neurol. 15, 57–83.

Bonnin, J.M., Rubinstein, L.J., 1989. Astroblastomas: a pathological study of 23 tumors with post-operative follow up in 13 patients. Neurosurgery 25, 6–13.

Brat, D.J., Cohen, K.J., Sanders, J.M., et al., 1999a. Clinicopathologic features of astroblastoma. J. Neuropathol. Exp. Neurol. 58, 509.

Brat, D.J., Giannini, C., Scheithauer, B.W., et al., 1999b. Primary melanocytic neoplasms of the central nervous system. Am. J. Surg. Pathol. 23, 745–758.

Brat, D.J., Scheithauer, B.W., Staugaitis, S.M., et al., 2000. Pituicytoma: a distinctive low grade glioma of the neurohypophysis. Am. J. Surg. Pathol. 24, 362–368.

Broders, A.C., 1925. The grading of carcinoma. Minn. Medicine 8, 726–730.

Brown, W.D., Gilles, F.H., Tavare, C.J., et al., 1998. Prognostic limitations of the Daumas-Duport grading scheme in childhood supratentorial astroglial tumors. J. Neuropathol. Exp. Neurol. 57, 1035–1040.

Budka, H., Chimelli, L., 1994. Lipomatous medulloblastoma in adults: a new tumor type with possible favorable prognosis. Hum. Pathol. 25, 730–731.

Burger, P.C., Vollmer, R.T., 1980. Histologic factors of prognostic significance in glioblastoma multiforme. Cancer 46, 1179–1186.

Burger, P.C., Vogel, F.S., Green, S.B., et al., 1985. Glioblastoma multiforme and anaplastic astrocytoma. Pathologic criteria and prognostic implications. Cancer 56, 1106–1111.

Burger, P.C., Scheithauer, B.W., 1994. Tumors of the Central Nervous System. Atlas of Tumor Pathology. Fascicle 10. Armed Forces Institute of Pathology, Washington DC, p. 142.

Bydon, A., Guitierrez, J.A., Mahmood, A., 2003. Meningeal melanocytoma: an aggressive course for a benign tumor. J. Neurooncol. 64, 259–263.

Cai, D.X., Banerjee, R., Scheithauer, B.W., et al., 2001. Chromosome 1p and 14q FISH analysis in clinicopathologic subsets of meningioma: diagnostic and prognostic implications. J. Neuropathol. Exp. Neurol. 60, 628–636.

Camilleri-Broet, S., Davi, F., Feuillard, J., et al., 1997. AIDS-related primary brain lymphomas: histopathologic and immunohistochemical study of 51 cases: The French Study Group for HIV-Associated Tumors. Hum. Pathol. 28, 367–374.

Caniero, S.S., Scheithauer, B.W., Nascimento, A.G., et al., 1996. Solitary fibrous tumor of the meninges. A lesion distinct from fibrous meningioma. A clinicopathological and immunohistochemical study. Am. J. Clin. Pathol. 106, 217–224.

Casadei, G.P., Komori, T., Scheithauer, B.W., et al., 1993. Intracranial parenchymal schwannoma. A clinicopathological and neuroimaging study of nine cases. J. Neurosurg. 79, 217–222.

Casadei, G.P., Scheithauer, B.W., Hirose, T., et al., 1995. Cellular schwannoma. A clinicopathological, DNA flow cytometric, and proliferation marker study of 70 patients. Cancer 75, 1109–1119.

Catapano, D., Muscarella, L.A., Guarnieri, V., et al., 2005. Hemangioblastomas of central nervous system: molecular genetic analysis and clinical management. Neurosurg. 56, 1215–1221.

• Cairncross, G., Ueki, K., Zlatescu, M.C., et al., 1998. Specific chromosomal losses predict chemotherapeutic response and survival in patients with anaplastic oligodendrogliomas. J. Natl. Cancer Inst. 90, 1473–1479.

CBTRUS, 2005. Statistical report: Primary Brain Tumors in the United States, 1998–2002. CBTRUS, Chicago, IL.

• Cenacchi, G., Giangaspero, F., 2004. Emerging tumor entities and variants of CNS neoplasms. J. Neuropathol. Exp. Neurol. 63, 185–192.

Cervera-Pierot, P., Varlet, P., Chodkiewicz, J.-P., et al., 1997. Dysembryoplastic neuroepithelial tumors located in the caudate nucleus area; report of four cases. Neurosurgery 40, 1065–1070.

Chang, Q., Pang, J.C., Li, K.K., et al., 2005. Promoter hypermethylation profile of RASSF1A, FHIT and sFRP1 in intracranial primitive neuroectodermal tumors. Hum. Pathol. 36, 1265–1272.

Chen, L., Piao, Y.S., Xu, Q.Z., et al., 2006. Papillary glioneuronal tumor: a clinicopathological and immunohistochemical study of two cases. Neuropathology 26, 243–248.

• Chikai, K., Ohnishi, A., Kato, T., et al., 2004. Clinico-pathological features of pilomyxoid astrocytoma of the optic pathway. Acta. Neuropathol. (Berl.) 108, 109–114.

Coca, S., Moreno, M., Martos, J.A., 1994. Neurocytoma of the spinal cord. Acta Neuropathol. 87, 537–540.

Colovi, N., Colovi, M., Cemerikie, V., et al., 2004. Granulocytic sarcoma of the brain in a patient with acute myeloid leukemia. Acta Chir. Iugosl. 51, 129–131.

Commins, D.L., 2006. Pathology of primary central nervous system lymphoma. Neurosurg. Focus 21, E2.

Constantine, C., Miller, D.C., Gardner, S., et al., 2005. Osseous metastasis of pineoblastoma: a case report and review of the literature. J. Neurooncol. 74, 53–57.

Corn, B.W., Marcus, S.M., Topham, A., et al., 1997. Will primary central nervous system lymphoma be the most frequent brain tumor diagnosed in the year 2000. Cancer 79, 2409–2413.

Couce, M.E., Aker, F.V., Scheithauer, B.W., et al., 2000. Chordoid meningioma: a clinicopathological study of 42 cases. Am. J. Surg. Pathol. 24, 899–905.

Cox, L.B., 1933. The cytology of the glioma group; with special reference to the inclusion of cells derived from the invaded tissue. Am. J. Pathol. 9, 839–898.

Crotty, T.B., Scheithauer, B.W., Young, W.F. Jr., et al., 1995. Papillary craniopharyngioma: a clinicopathological study of 48 cases. J. Neurosurg. 83, 206–214.

Cuccia, V., Zuccaro, G., Sosa, F., et al., 2003. Subependymal giant cell astrocytoma in children with tuberous sclerosis. Childs Nerv. Syst. 19, 232–243.

Cushing, H., 1932. The craniopharyngioma. In: Intracranial tumors. Bailliere, Tindall & Cox, London, pp. 93–98.

• Danks, R.A., Orian, J.M., Gonzales, M.F., et al., 1995. Transformation of astrocytes in transgenic mice expressing SV40 T antigen under the transcriptional control of the glial fibrillary acidic protein promoter. Cancer Res. 55, 4302–4310.

Daumas-Duport, C., Szikla, G., 1981. Delimitation et configuration spatiale des gliomas cerebraux: Donnees histologiques, incidences therapeutiques. Neurochirurgie 27, 273–284.

• Daumas-Duport, C., Scheithauer, B.W., O'Fallon, J., et al., 1988a. Grading of astrocytomas. A simple and reproducible method. Cancer 62, 2152–2165.

• Daumas-Duport, C., 1993. Dysembryoplastic neuroepithelial tumors. Brain Pathol. 3, 283–295.

• Daumas-Duport, C., Scheithauer, B.W., Chodkiewicz, J.-P., et al., 1988b. Dysembryoplastic neuroepithelial tumor (DNET): A surgically curable tumor of young subjects with intractable partial seizures. Report of 39 cases. Neurosurgery 23, 545–556.

• Daumas-Duport, C., Tucker, M.L., Kolles, H., et al., 1997. Oligodendrogliomas. Part II: A new grading system based on morphological and imaging criteria. J. Neurooncol. 34, 61–78.

DeArmond, S.J., Nagashima, T., Cho, K.G., et al., 1987. Correlation of cell kinetics and degree of anaplasia in human brain tumors. In: Chatel, M., Darcel, M., Pecker, J. (Eds.), Brain oncology. Martinus Nijhof, Dordrecht, pp. 67–74.

De Potter, P., Shields, C.L., Shields, J.A., et al., 1994. Clinical variations of trilateral retinoblastoma: a report of 13 cases. J. Pediatr. Ophthalmol. Strabismus 31, 26–31.

Donnell, M.S., Meyer, G.A., Donegan, W.L., 1979. Estrogen-receptor protein in intracranial meningiomas. J. Neurosurg. 50, 499–502.

• Edgar, M., Rosenblum, M.K., 2008. The differential diagnosis of central nervous system tumors. A critical examination of some recent immunohistochemical applications. Arch. Pathol. Lab. Med. 132, 500–509.

El-Naggar, A.K., Ro, J.Y., Ayala, A.G., et al., 1989. Localized fibrous tumor of the serosal cavities. Immunohistochemical, electron-microscopic, and flow-cytometric DNA study. Am. J. Clin. Pathol. 92, 561–565.

Eng, D.Y., DeMonte, F., Ginsberg, L., et al., 1997. Craniospinal dissemination of central neurocytoma – report of two cases. J. Neurosurg. 86, 547–552.

• Eoli, M., Bissola, L., Bruzzone, M.G., et al., 2006. Reclassification of oligoastrocytomas by loss of heterozygosity studies. Int. J. Cancer 119, 84–90.

Er, U., Kazanci, A., Eyiparmak, T., et al., 2007. Melanotic Schwannonma. J. Clin. Neurosci. 4, 676–678.

Ess, K.C., Kamp, C.A., Tu, B.P., et al., 2005. Developmental origin of subependymal giant cell astrocytoma in tuberous sclerosis complex. Neurology 64, 1446–1449.

Fauchon, F., Jouvet, A., Paquis, P., et al., 2000. Parenchymal pineal tumors: a clinicopathological study of 76 cases. Int. J. Radiat. Oncol. Biol. Phys. 46, 959–968.

Fetsch, J.F., Miettinen, M., 1997. Sclerosing perineurioma: a clinicopathological study of 19 cases of a distinctive soft tissue lesion with a predilection for the fingers and palms of young adults. Am. J. Surg. Pathol. 21, 1433–1442.

Fèvre-Montange, M., Hasselblatt, M., Figarella-Branger, D., et al., 2006. Prognosis and histopathologic features in papillary tumors of the pineal region: a retrospective multi-center study of 31 cases. J. Neuropathol. Exp. Neurol. 65, 1004–1011.

Fernandez, Z., Figarella-Branger, D., Girard, N., et al., 2003. Pilocytic astrocytomas in children: prognostic factors – a retrospective study of 80 cases. Neurosurgery 53, 544–553.

Fletcher, C.D., 2006. The evolving classification of soft tissue tumors: an update based on the new WHO classification. Histopathology 48, 3–12.

Forsyth, P.A., DeAngelis, L.M., 1996. Biology and management of AIDS-associated primary CNS lymphoma. Hematol. Oncol. Clin. North Am. 10, 1125–1134.

Fujii, N., Ikeda, K., Takahashi, N., et al., 2002. Multilineage involvement in hypereosinophilic syndrome terminating in granulocytic sarcoma and leukaemic transformation with trisomy 8. Br. J. Haematol. 119, 716–719.

Fukunaga, M., 2001. Unusual malignant perineurioma of soft tissue. Virchows Arch. 439, 212–214.

Fulling, K.H., Garcia, D.M., 1985. Anaplastic astrocytomas of the adult cerebrum. Prognostic value of histologic features. Cancer 55, 928–931.

Funato, H., Inoshita, N., Okeda, R., et al., 1997. Cystic ganglioneurocytoma outside the ventricular region. Acta. Neuropathol. 94, 95–98.

Garcia, D.M., Fulling, K.H., Marks, J.E., 1985. The value of radiation therapy in addition to surgery for astrocytomas of the adult cerebrum. Cancer 55, 919–927.

Geddes, J.F., Bhattacharjee, M.B., Savage, F., et al., 1992. Primary cerebral lymphoma: a study of 47 cases probed for Epstein–Barr virus genome. J. Clin. Pathol. 45, 587–590.

Gelabert-Gonzalez, M., 2005. Paragangliomas of the lumbar region. Report of two cases and review of the literature. J. Neurosurg. Spine 2, 354–365.

Giangaspero, F., Rigobello, L., Badiali, M., et al., 1992. Large-cell medulloblastomas. A distinct variant with highly aggressive behavior. Am. J. Surg. Pathol. 16, 687–693.

Giannini, C., Scheithauer, B.W., Jenkins, R.B., et al., 1997. Soft tissue perineurioma: Evidence of abnormality of chromosome 22, criteria for diagnosis, and review of the literature. Am. J. Surg. Pathol. 21, 164–173.

Giannini, C., Scheithauer, B.W., Burger, P.C., et al., 1999a. Cellular proliferation in pilocytic and diffuse astrocytomas. J. Neuropathol. Exp. Neurol. 58, 46–53.

Giannini, C., Scheithauer, B.W., Burger, P.C., et al., 1999b. Pleomorphic xanthoastrocytoma: what do we really know about it? Cancer 85, 2033–2045.

Gilles, F.H., Brown, W.D., Leviton, A., et al., 2000a. Limitations of the World Health Organization classification of childhood supratentorial astrocytic tumors. Children Brain Tumor Consortium. Cancer 88 (6), 1477–1483.

Gilles, F.H., Leviton, A., Tavare, C.J., et al., 2000b. Definitive classes of childhood supratentorial neuroglial tumors. The Childhood Brain Tumor Consortium. Cancer 3 (2), 126–139.

Gillou, L., Fletcher, J.A., Fletcher, C.D.M., et al., 2002. Extrapleural solitary fibrous tumor and hemangiopericytoma. In: Fletcher, C.D., Unni, K.K., Mertens, F. (Eds.) World Health Organization Classification of Tumors. Pathology and genetics of tumors of soft tissue and bone. IARC Press, Lyon, pp. 86–90.

Gläsker, S., Li, J., Xia, J.B., et al., 2006. Hemangioblastomas share protein expression with embryonal hemangioblast progenitor cell. Cancer Res. 66, 4167–4172.

Goldberg, G.M., Eshbaught, D.E., 1960. Squamous cell nests of the pituitary gland as related to the origin of craniopharyngiomas: a study of their presence in the newborn and infants up to age four. Arch. Pathol. 70, 293–299.

Golgi, C., 1884. Uber die glioma des gehirns (Untersuchungen uber den feineren bau des nervensustems). Fisscher, Jena.

Gonzales, M.F., 1997. Grading of gliomas. J. Clin. Neurosci. 4, 16–18.

Gonzales, M.F., 2003. Primary meningeal anaplastic large cell lymphoma. Pathology 35, 451–452.

Gonzales, M.F., Dale, S., Susman, M., et al., 2006. Quantitation of chromosome 1p and 19q deletions in glial tumors by interphase FISH on formalin-fixed paraffin-embedded tissue. J. Clin. Neurosci. 13, 96–101.

Gonzales, M.F., Dale, S., Susman, M., et al., 2007. DNT-like oligodendrogliomas or DNTs evolving into oligodendrogliomas: two illustrative cases. Neuropathology 27, 324–330.

Graf, A.H., Buchberger, W., Langmayr, H., et al., 1988. Site preference of metastatic tumors of the brain. Virchows Arch. A Pathol. Anat. Histopathol. 412, 493–498.

Gururangan, S., Heidemann, R.L., Kovnar, E.H., et al., 1994. Peritoneal metastases in two patients with pineoblastoma and ventriculo-peritoneal shunts. Med. Pediatr. Oncol. 22, 417–420.

Haberler, C., Laggner, U., Slavc, I., et al., 2006. Immunohistochemical analysis of INI1 protein in malignant pediatric CNS tumors: lack of INI1 in atypical teratoid/rhabdoid tumors and in a fraction of primitive neuroectodermal tumors without rhabdoid phenotype. Am. J. Surg. Pathol. 30, 1462–1468.

Hart, M.N., Petito, C.K., Earle, K.M., 1974. Mixed gliomas. Cancer 33, 134–140.

Hardell, L., Carlberg, M., Söderqvist, F., et al., 2008. Meta-analysis of long-term mobile phone use and the association with brain tumors. Int. J. Oncol. 32, 1097–1103.

Hasegawa, T., Hirose, T., Seki, K., et al., 1996. Solitary fibrous tumor of the soft tissue. An immunohistochemical and ultrastructural study. Am. J. Clin. Pathol. 106, 325–331.

Hassoun, J., Gambarelli, D., Grisoli, F., et al., 1982. Central neurocytoma: An electron microscopic study of two cases. Acta. Neuropathol. 56, 151–156.

Hattab, E.M., Tu, P., Wilson, J.D., et al., 2004. C-kit and HER2/NEU expression in primary intracranial germinoma. J. Neuropathol. Exp. Neurol. 63, 547.

Hattab, E.M., Tu, P., Wilson, J.D., et al., 2005. OCT4 immunohistochemistry is superior to placental alkaline phosphatase (PLAP) in the diagnosis of central nervous system germinoma. Am. J. Surg. Pathol. 29, 368–371.

He, J., Mokhtari, K., Sanson, M., et al., 2001. Glioblastomas with an oligodendroglial component: a pathological and molecular study. J. Neuropathol. Exp. Neurol. 60, 863–871.

Hilden, J.M., Meerbaum, S., Burger, P., et al., 2004. Central nervous system atypical teratoid/rhabdoid tumor: results of therapy in children enrolled in a registry. J. Clin. Oncol. 22, 2877–2884.

Hirose, T., Tani, T., Shimada, T., et al., 2003. Immunohistochemical demonstration of EMA/Glut1-positive perineurial cells and CD-34 positive fibroblastic cells in peripheral nerve sheath tumors. Mod. Pathol. 16, 293–298.

Horstmann, S., Perry, A., Reifenberger, G., et al., 2004. Genetic and expression profiles of cerebellar liponeurocytomas. Brain Pathol. 14, 281–289.

Hunter, I.J., 1955. Squamous metaplasia of cells of the anterior pituitary gland. J. Pathol. Bacteriol. 69, 141–145.

Hussein, M.R., 2007. Central nervous system capillary hemangioblastoma: the pathologist's viewpoint. Int. J. Exp. Pathol. 88, 311–324.

Illum, N., Korf, H.W., Julian, K., et al., 1992. Concurrent uveoretinitis and pineocytoma in a child suggests a causal relationship. Br. J. Ophthalmol. 76, 574–576.

Im, S.H., Chung, C.K., Kim, S.K., et al., 2004. Pleomorphic xanthoastrocytoma: a developmental glioneuronal tumor with prominent glioproliferative changes. J. Neurooncol. 66, 17–27.

Imai, H., Kajimoto, K., Taniwaki, M., et al., 2004. Intravascular large B cell lymphoma presenting with mass lesions in the central nervous system: a report of five cases. Pathol. Int. 54, 231–236.

Inda, M.M., Minoz, J., Coullin, P., et al., 2006. High promoter hypermethylation frequency of p14/ARF in supratentorial PNET but not medulloblastoma. Histopathology 48, 579–587.

Ino, Y., Zlatescu, M.C., Sasaki, H., et al., 2000. Long patient survival and therapeutic responses in histologically disparate high grade gliomas with chromosome 1p loss. J. Neurosurg. 92, 983–990.

Ino, Y., Betensky, R.A., Zlatescu, M.C., et al., 2001. Molecular subtypes of anaplastic oligodendroglioma: implications for patient management at diagnosis. Clin. Cancer Res. 7, 839–845.

Jain, D., Sharma, M.C., Sarkar, C., et al., 2008. Chordoid glioma: report of two rare examples with unusual features. Acta. Neurochir. (Wien) 150 (3), 295–300.

Jeibmann, A., Haselblatt, M., Gerss, J., et al., 2006. Prognostic implications of atypical histologic features in choroid plexus papilloma. J. Neuropathol. Exp. Neurol. 65, 1069–1073.

Jenevein, E.P., 1964. A neurohypophyseal tumor originating from pituicytes. Am. J. Clin. Pathol. 41, 522–526.

Jenkinson, M.D., Bosma, J.J., Du, P.D., et al., 2003. Cerebellar liponeurocytoma with an unusually aggressive clinical course; case report. Neurosurgery 53, 1425–1427.

Jouvet, A., Saint-Pierre, G., Fauchon, F., et al., 2000. Pineal parenchymal tumors: a correlation of histologic features with prognosis in 66 cases. Brain Pathol. 10, 49–60.

Jouvet, A., Fauchon, K., Liberski, P., et al., 2003. Papillary tumor of the pineal region. Am. J. Surg. Pathol. 27, 505–512.

Jeuken, J.W., von Deimling, A., Wesseling, P., 2004. Molecular pathogenesis of oligodendroglial tumors. J. Neurooncol. 70, 161–181.

Jung, S.H., Kuo, T.T., 2005. Immunoreactivity of CD10 and inhibin alpha in differentiating hemangioblastoma of the central nervous system from metastatic clear cell renal cell carcinoma. Mod. Pathol. 2005, 788–794.

Kadoch, C., Treseler, P., Rubenstein, J.L., 2006. Molecular pathogenesis of primary central nervous system lymphoma. Neurosurg. Focus 21, E1.

Kadonaga, J.N., Frieden, I.J., 1991. Neurocutaneous melanosis. Definition and review of the literature. J. Am. Acad. Dermatol. 24, 747–755.

Kampan, W.A., Kros, J.M., De Jong, T.H.R., et al., 2006. Primitive neuroectodermal tumors (PNETs) located in the spinal canal; relevance of classification as central or peripheral PNET. J. Neurooncol. 77, 65–72.

Kan, P., Simonsen, S.E., Lyon, J.L., et al., 2008. Cellular phone use and brain tumor: a meta-analysis. J. Neurooncol. 86, 71–78.

Karavitaki, N., Wass, J., 2008. Craniopharyngiomas. Endocrinol. Metab. Clin. North Am. 37, 173–193.

Kasashima, S., Oda, Y., Nozaki, J., et al., 2000. A case of atypical granular cell tumor of the neurohypophysis. Pathol. Int. 50, 568–573.

Kelly, F., Kellerman, O., Mechali, F., et al., 1986. Expression of SV40 oncogenes in F9 embryonal carcinoma cells, in transgenic mice and transgenic embryos. In: Botchan, M., Grodicker, T.C., Sharp, P.A. (Eds.), DNA tumor viruses. Control of gene expression and replication. Cold Spring Harbor Laboratory, New York, pp. 363–372.

● Kepes, J.J., Rubinstein, L.J., Eng, L.F., 1979. Pleomorphic xanthoastrocytoma: A distinctive meningocerebral glioma in young subjects with a relatively favorable prognosis. A study of 12 cases. Cancer 44, 1839–1852.

Kepes, J.J., Collins, J., 1999. Choroid plexus epithelium (normal and neoplastic) express synaptophysin. A potentially useful aid in differentiating carcinoma of the choroid plexus from metastatic papillary carcinoma. J. Neuropathol. Exp. Neurol. 58, 398–401.

● Kernohan, J.W., Mabon, R.F., Svien, H.J., et al., 1949. A simple classification of gliomas. Proc. Staff Meetings Mayo Clinic 24, 71–74.

Khan, R.B., DeAngelis, L.M., 2003. Brain metastases. In: Schiff, D., Wen, P.Y. (Eds.), Cancer neurology in clinical practice. Humana Press, Totowa, NJ.

Kim, S.K., Wang. K.C., Cho, B.K., et al., 2001. Biologic behavior and tumorigenesis of subependymal giant cell astrocytomas. J. Neurooncol. 52, 217–225.

● Kleihues, P., Burger, P.C., Scheithauer, B.W., et al., 1993. Histologic typing of tumors of the central nervous system, 2nd edn. WHO International Classification of Tumors. Springer-Verlag, New York.

● Kleihues, P., Cavenee, W., 2000. World Health Organization Classification of Tumors. Pathology and genetics of tumors of the nervous system. IARC Press, Lyon.

● Kleihues, P., Burger, P.C., Rosenblum, M., et al., 2007. Anaplastic astrocytoma. In: Louis, D.N., Ohgaki, H., Cavenee, W.K. (Eds.), WHO Classification of Tumors of the Central Nervous System. IARC Press, Lyon, p. 31.

Klemperer, P., Rabin, C.B., 1931. Primary neoplasms of the pleura. A report of five cases. Arch. Pathol. 11, 385–412.

Kloub, O., Perry, A., Tu, P.H., et al., 2005. Spindle cell oncocytoma of the adenohypophysis: report of two recurrent cases. Am. J. Surg. Pathol. 29, 247–253.

Kobayashi, T., Yoshida, J., Kida, Y., 1989. Bilateral germ cell tumors involving the basal ganglia and thalamus. Neurosurgery 24, 579–583.

Komotar, R.J., Burger, P.C., Carson, B.S., et al., 2004. Pilocytic and pilomyxoid hypothalamic/chiasmatic astrocytomas. Neurosurgery 54, 72–79.

Komori, T., Scheithauer, B.W., Anthony, D.C., et al. 1996. Pseudo-papillary ganglioneurocytoma. J. Neuropathol Exp. Neurol. 55, 654.

Komori, T., Scheithauer, B.W., Anthony, D.C., 1998. Papillary glioneuronal tumor; a new variant of mixed neuronal-glial neoplasm. Am. J. Surg. Pathol. 22, 1171–1183.

● Komori, T., Scheithauer, B.W., Hirose, T., 2002. A rosette-forming glioneuronal tumor of the fourth ventricle: infratentorial form of dysembryoplastic neuroepithelial tumor? Am. J. Surg. Pathol. 26, 582–591.

Kordek, R., Biernat, W., Sapieja, W., et al., 1995. Pleomorphic xanthoastrocytoma with a gangliogliomatous component; an immunocytochemical and ultrastructural study. Acta Neuropathol. 89, 194–197.

Korshunov, A., Golanov, A., Timirgaz, V., 2000. Immunohistochemical markers for intracranial ependymoma recurrence. An analysis of 88 cases. J. Neurol. Sci. 177, 72–82.

● Kraus, J.A., Lanszus, K., Glesmann, N., et al., 2001. Molecular genetic alterations in glioblastomas with oligodendroglial component. Acta Neuropathol. 101, 311–320.

Kristopaitis, T., Thomas, C., Petruzelli, G.J., et al., 2000. Malignant craniopharyngioma. Arch. Pathol. Lab. Med. 124, 1356–1360.

Kros, J.M., Schouten, W.C., Janssen, P.J., et al., 1996. Proliferation of gemistocytic cells and glial fibrillary acidic protein (GFAP)-positive oligodendroglial cells in gliomas: a MIB-1/GFAP double labelling study. Acta Neuropathol. 91, 99–103.

Kros, J.M., Cella, F., Bakker, S.L., et al., 2000. Papillary meningioma with pleural metastasis: case report and literature review. Acta Neurol. Scand 102, 200–202.

Krouwer, H.G., Davis, R.L., Silver, P., et al., 1991. Gemistocytic astrocytomas; a reappraisal. J. Neurosurg. 74, 399–406.

Kuchelmeister, K., Demirel, T., Schlorer, E., et al., 1995. Dysembryoplastic neuroepithelial tumor of the cerebellum. Acta Neuropathol. (Berl.) 89, 385–390.

Kudo, M., Matsumoto, M., Terao, H., 1983. Malignant peripheral nerve sheath tumor of acoustic nerve. Arch. Pathol. Lab. Med. 107, 293–297.

Kurian, K.M., Summers, D.M., Statham, P.F., et al., 2005. Third ventricular chordoid glioma: clinicopathological study of two cases with evidence of poor clinical outcome despite low grade histologic features. Neuropathol. Appl. Neurobiol. 31, 354–361.

Kurt, E., Zheng, P.P., Hop, W.C., et al., 2006. Identification of relevant prognostic histopathological features in 69 intracranial ependymomas, excluding myxopapillary ependymomas and subependymomas. Cancer 106, 388–395.

Kurtkaya-Yapicier, O., Scheithauer, B., Woodruff, J.M., 2003. The pathobiologic spectrum of schwannomas. Histol. Histopathol. 18, 925–934.

Lach, B., Duggal, N., DaSilva, V.F., et al., 1996. Association of pleomorphic xanthoastrocytoma with cortical dysplasia and neuronal tumors. A report of three cases. Cancer 78, 2551–2563.

Lazarus, S.S., Med, S.M., Trombetta, L.D., 1978. Ultrastructural identification of a benign perineurial cell tumor. Cancer 41, 1823–1829.

● Leeds, N.E., Lang, F.F., Ribalta, T., et al., 2006. Origin of chordoid glioma of the third ventricle. Arch. Pathol. Lab. Med. 130, 460–464.

Leestma, J.E., 1980. Brain tumors. American Journal of Pathology Teaching Monograph Series. American Association of Pathologists, Maryland, p. 243.

● Lellouch-Tubiana, A., Boddaert, N., Bourgeois, M., et al., 2005. Angiocentric neuroepithelial tumor (ANET): a new epilepsy-related clinicopathological entity within distinctive MRI. Brain Pathol. 15, 281–286.

Leung, S.Y., Gwi, E., Ng, H.K., et al., 1994. Dysembryoplastic neuroepithelial tumor. A tumor with small neuronal cells resembling oligodendroglioma. Am. J. Surg. Pathol. 18, 604–614.

Lhermitte, J., Duclos, P., 1920. Sur un ganglioneurome diffuse du coertex du cervelet. Bull Assoc. Fran. Etude Cancer 9, 99–107.

Lopez-Gines, C., Cerda-Nicolas, M., Gil-Benso, et al., 2004. Association of loss of chromosome 14 in meningioma progression. Cancer Genet. Cytogenet. 15, 123–128.

● Louis, D.N., Ohgaki, H., Wiestler, O.D., et al., 2007a. WHO Classification of Tumors of the Central Nervous System. IARC, Lyon.

● Louis, D.N., Ohgaki, H., Wiestler, O.D., et al., 2007b. The 2007 WHO Classification of Tumors of the Central Nervous System. Acta Neuropathol. 114, 97–110.

Ludeman, W., Stan, A.C., Tatagiba, M., et al., 2000. Sporadic unilateral vestibular schwannoma with islets of meningioma: case report. Neurosurgery 47, 451–452.

Ludwin, S.K., Rubinstein, L.J., Russell, D.S., 1975. Papillary meningioma: a malignant variant of meningioma. Cancer 36, 1363–1373.

● Maillo, A., Orfao, A., Espinosa, A.B., et al., 2007. Early recurrences in histologically benign/grade I meningiomas are associated with large tumors and coexistence of monosomy 14 and del(1p36) in the ancestral tumor cell clone. Neuro. Oncol. 9, 438–446.

Makuria, A.T., Rushing, E.J., McGrail, K.M., et al., 2008. Atypical teratoid rhabdoid tumor (AT/RT) in adults: review of four cases. J. Neurooncol. 88, 321–330.

Matsutani, M., Sano, K., Takakura, K., et al., 1997. Primary intracranial germ cell tumors: a clinical analysis of 153 histologically verified cases. J. Neurosurg. 86, 446–455.

● Martin, A.J., Summersgill, B.M., Fisher, C., et al., 2002. Chromosomal imbalances in meningeal solitary fibrous tumors. Cancer Genet. Cytogenet. 135, 160–164.

Matyja, E., Taraszewska, A., Zabek, M., 2001. Phenotypic characteristics of GFAP-immunopositive oligodendroglial tumors Part I: Immunohistochemical study. Folia Neuropathol. 39, 19–26.

● McLaughlin, J.K., Malker, H.S., Blot, W.J., et al., 1987. Occupational risks of intracranial gliomas in Sweden. J. Natl. Cancer Inst. 78, 253–257.

McLean, C.A., Laidlaw, J.D., Brownbill, D.S., et al., 1990. Recurrence of acoustic neurilemmoma as a malignant spindle-cell neoplasm. Case report. J. Neurosurg. 73, 946–950.

- McLean, C.A., Jolley, D., Cukier, E., et al., 1993. Atypical and malignant meningiomas: importance of micronecrosis as a prognostic indicator. Histopathology 23, 349–353.

McLean, C.A., Jellinek, D.A., Gonzales, M.F., 1998. Diffuse leptomeningeal spread of pleomorphic xanthoastrocytoma. J. Clin. Neurosci. 5, 230–233.

McManamy, C.S., Pears, J., Weston, C.L., et al., 2007. Nodule formation and desmoplasia in medulloblastomas – defining the nodular/desmoplastic variant and its biologic behavior. Brain Pathol. 17, 151–164.

- McNeill, D.E., Cote, T.R., Clegg, L., et al., 2002. Incidence and trends in pediatric malignancies medulloblastoma/primitive neuroectodermal tumor: a SEER update. Surveillance epidemiology and end results. Med. Pediatr. Oncol. 39, 190–194.

Meyer-Puttlitz, B., Hayashi, Y., Waha, A., et al., 1997. Molecular genetic analysis of giant cell glioblastomas. Am. J. Pathol. 151, 853–857.

- Miller, C.R., Dunham, C.P., Scheithauer, B.W., et al., 2006. Significance of necrosis in grading of oligodendroglial neoplasm. A clinicopathological and genetic study of 1093 newly-diagnosed high-grade gliomas. J. Clin. Oncol. 24, 5419–5426.

Min, K.W., Cashman, R.E., Brumback, R.A., 1995. Glioneurocytoma: tumor with glial and neuronal differentiation. J. Child Neurol. 10 (3), 219–226.

Mittelbronn, M., Schittenhelm, J., Lemke, D., et al., 2007. Low grade ganglioglioma rapidly progressing to a WHO IV tumor showing malignant transformation in both astroglial and neuronal cell components. Neuropathology 27, 463–467.

Montesinos-Rongen, M., Van Roost, D., Schaller, C., et al., 2004. Primary diffuse large B cell lymphomas of the central nervous system are targeted by aberrant somatic hypermutation. Blood 103, 1869–1875.

Mörk, S.J., Halvorsen, T.B., Lindegaard, K.-F., et al., 1986. Oligodendrogliomas. Histologic evaluation and prognosis. J. Neuropathol. Exp. Neurol. 45, 65–78.

Mut, M., Schiff, D., Shaffrey, M.E., 2005. Metastasis to nervous system: spinal epidural and intramedullary metastases. J. Neurooncol. 75, 43–56.

Nelson, J.S., Tsukada, Y., Schoenfeld, D., 1983. Necrosis as a prognosis criteria in malignant supratentorial astrocytic gliomas. Cancer 52, 550–554.

Nelson, G.A., Bastian, F.O., Schlitt, M., et al., 1988. Malignant transformation of craniopharyngioma. Neurosurgery 22, 427–429.

Nevin, S., 1938., Gliomatosis cerebri. Brain 61, 170–191.

Ng, H.K., Poon, W.S., Chan, Y.L., 1992. Basal ganglia teratomas: report of three cases. Aust. NZ J. Surg. 62, 436–440.

Nishio, S., Takeshita, I., Kaneko, Y., et al., 1992. Cerebral neurocytoma. A new subset of benign neuronal tumors of the cerebrum. Cancer 70, 529–537.

Nomura, A., Kurimoto, M., Nagi, S., et al., 2002. Multiple intracranial seeding of craniopharyngioma after repeated surgery: case report. Neurol. Med. Chir. (Tokyo) 42, 268–271.

Nussbaum, E.S., Djalilian, H.R., Cho, K.H., et al., 1996. Brain metastases. Histology, multiplicity, surgery, and survival. Cancer 78, 1781–1788.

Ogawa, K., Tada, T., Takahashi, S., et al., 2004. Malignant solitary fibrous tumor of the meninges. Virchows Arch. 444, 459–464.

Ohba, S., Yoshida, K., Hirose, Y., et al., 2008. A supratentorial primitive neuroectodermal tumor in an adult: a case report and review of the literature. J. Neurooncol. 86, 217–224.

- Ohgaki, H., Dessen, P., Jourde, B., et al., 2004. Genetic pathways to glioblastoma: a population-based study. Cancer Res. 64, 6892–6899.

- Ohgaki, H., Kleihues, P., 2007. Genetic pathways to primary and secondary glioblastoma. Am. J. Pathol. 170, 1445–1453.

Padberg, G.W., Schot, J.D., Vielvoye, G.J., et al., 1991. Lhermitte-Duclos disease and Cowden disease: a single phakomatosis. Ann. Neurol. 29, 517–523.

- Pahapill, P.A., Ramsay, D.A., Del Maestro, R.F., 1996. Pleomorphic xanthoastrocytoma: Case report and analysis of the literature concerning the efficacy of resection and the significance of necrosis. Neurosurgery 38, 822–829.

Palma, L., Guidetti, B., 1985. Cystic pilocytic astrocytomas of the cerebral hemispheres. Surgical experience with 51 cases and long-term results. J. Neurosurg. 62, 811–815.

Pasquier, B., Gasnier, F., Pasquier, D., et al., 1986. Papillary meningioma. Clinicopathologic study of seven cases and review of literature. Cancer 58, 299–305.

Paulus, W., Janisch, W., 1990. Clinicopathological correlations in epithelial choroid plexus neoplasms; a study of 52 cases. Acta. Neuropathol. (Berl.) 80, 635–641.

Paulus, W., Batas, A., Ott, G., et al., 1994. Interphase cytogenetics of glioblastoma and gliosarcoma. Acta Neuropathol. 88, 420–425.

Paulus, W., Brandner, S., 2007. Choroid plexus tumors. In: Louis, D.N., Ohgaki, H., Wiestler, O.D., et al. (Eds.), WHO Classification of Tumors of the Central Nervous System. IARC, Lyon, pp. 82–85.

- Paulus, W., Perry, A., 2007. Histiocytic tumors. In: Louis, D.N., Ohgaki, H., Wiestler, O.D., et al. (Eds.), WHO Classification of Tumors of the Central Nervous System. IARC, Lyon, pp. 193–196.

Pels, H., Schmidt-Wolf, I.G., Glasmacher, A., et al., 2003. Primary central nervous system lymphoma: results of a pilot and phase II study of systemic and intraventricular chemotherapy with deferred radiotherapy. J. Clin. Oncol. 21, 4489–4495.

Perentes, E., Rubinstein, L.J., Hermann, M.M., et al., 1986. S-antigen immunoreactivity in human pineal glands and pineal parenchymal tumors. A monoclonal antibody study. Acta Neuropathol. (Berl.) 71, 224–227.

Perry, A., Giannini, C., Scheithauer, B.W., et al., 1997a. Composite pleomorphic xanthoastrocytoma and ganglioglioma. Report of four cases and review of the literature. Am. J. Surg. Pathol. 21, 763–771.

- Perry, A., Stafford, S.L., Scheithauer, B.W., et al., 1997b. Meningioma grading: an analysis of histologic parameters. Am. J. Surg. Pathol. 21, 1455–1465.

- Perry, A., Scheithauer, B.W., Nascimento, A.G., 1997c. The immunophenotypic spectrum of meningeal hemangiopericytoma: a comparison with fibrous meningioma and solitary fibrous tumor of meninges. Am. J. Surg. Pathol. 21, 1354–1360.

Perry, A., Scheithauer, B.W., Stafford, S.L., et al., 1998. 'Rhabdoid' meningioma: An aggressive variant. Am. J. Surg. Pathol. 22, 1482–1490.

- Perry, A., Scheithauer, B.W., Stafford, S.L., et al., 1999. 'Malignancy' in meningiomas: a clinicopathologic study of 116 patients, with grading implications. Cancer 85, 2046–2056.

- Perry, A., Banerjee, R., Lohse, C.M., et al., 2002. A role for chromosome 9p21 deletions in the malignant progression of meningiomas and the prognosis of anaplastic meningiomas. Brain Pathol. 12, 183–190.

Petito, C.K., De Girolami, U., Earle, K., 1976. Craniopharyngiomas. A clinical and pathological review. Cancer 37, 1944–1952.

- Pfisterer, W.K., Coons, S.W., Aboul-Enein, F., et al., 2008. Implicating chromosomal aberrations with meningioma growth and recurrence: results from FISH and MIB-1 analysis of grades I and II meningiomas. J. Neurooncol. 87, 43–50.

Piercecchi-Marti, M.D., Mohamed, H., Liprandi, A., et al., 2002. Intracranial meningeal melanocytoma associated with ipsilateral nevus of Ota. Case report. J. Neurosurg. 96, 619–623.

Pierre-Kahn, A., Cinalli, G., Lellouch-Tubiana, A., et al. 1992. Melanotic neuroectodermal tumor of skull and meninges in infancy. Pediatr. Neurosurg. 18, 6–15.

Ponzoni, M., Ferreri, A.J., 2006. Intravascular lymphoma: a neoplasm of 'homeless' lymphocytes? Hematol. Oncol. 24, 105–112.

- Powell, S.J., Yachnis, A.T., Rorke, L.B., et al., 1996. Divergent differentiation in pleomorphic xanthoastrocytoma. Evidence for neuronal differentiation and possible relationship to ganglion cell tumors. Am. J. Surg. Pathol. 20, 80–85.

- Prayson, R.A., Abramovich, C.M., 2000. Glioneuronal tumor with neuropil-like islands. Human Pathol. 31, 1435–1438.

- Preusser, M., Novak, K., Czech, T., et al., 2006. Angiocentric glioma: report of eight cases (Abstract P1064). Acta Neuropathol. 112, 382–383.

• Reifenberger, G., Kaulich, K., Wiestler, O.D., et al., 2003. Expression of the CD34 antigen in pleomorphic xanthoastrocytomas. Acta Neuropathol. 105, 358–364.

Reith, J.D., Goldblum, J.R., 1996. Multiple cutaneous plexiform schwannomas. Report of a case and review of the literature with particular reference to the association with types 1 and 2 neurofibromatosis and schwannomatosis. Arch. Pathol. Lab. Med. 120, 399–401.

Reyns, N., Assaker, R., Louis, E., et al., 2003. Leptomeningeal hemangioblastomatosis in a case of von Hippel-Lindau disease: case report. Neurosurgery 52, 1212–1215.

Ribbert, H., 1918. Uber das spongioblastoma und das gliom. Virchows Arch. 225, 195–213.

Rickert, C.H., Hasselblatt, M., Jeibmann, A., et al., 2006. Cellular and reticular variants of hemangioblastoma differ in their cytogenetic profiles. Hum. Pathol. 37, 1452–1457.

• Ringertz, N., 1950. Grading of gliomas. Acta. Pathol. Microbiol. Scand 27, 51–65.

Rollins, K.E., Kleinschmidt-DeMasters, B.K., Corboy, J.R., et al., 2005. Lymphomatosis cerebri as a cause of white matter dementia. Hum. Pathol. 36, 282–290.

Roncaroli, F., Scheithauer, B.W., Cenacchi, G., et al., 2002. Spindle cell oncocytoma of the adenohypophysis: a tumor of folliculostellate cells? Am. J. Surg. Pathol. 26, 1048–1055.

Rorke, L.B., 1983. The cerebellar medulloblastoma and its relationship to primitive neuroectodermal tumors. J. Neuropathol. Exp. Neurol. 42, 1–15.

• Rorke, L.B., Gilles, F.H., Davis, R.L., et al., 1985. Revision of the World Health Organization classification of brain tumors for childhood brain tumors. Cancer 56, 1869–1886.

Rorke, L.B., Packer, R.J., Biegel, J.A., 1996. Central nervous system atypical teratoid/rhabdoid tumors of infancy and childhood: definition of an entity. J. Neurosurg. 85, 56–65.

Rosenfeld, J.V., Murphy, M.A., Chow, C.W., 1990. Implantation metastasis of pineoblastoma after stereotactic biopsy. A case report. J. Neurosurg. 73, 287–290.

Rousseau, A., Kujas, M., Bergemer-Fouquet, A.M., et al., 2006. Survivin expression in ganglioglioma. J. Neurooncol. 77, 153–159.

Rubenstein, J.L., Fridlyand, J., Shen, A., et al., 2006. Gene expression and angiotropism in primary CNS lymphoma. Blood 107, 3716–3723.

Russo, C., Pellarin, M., Tingby, O., et al., 1999. Comparative genomic hybridization in patients with supratentorial and infratentorial primitive neuroectodermal tumors. Cancer 86, 331–339.

Sacktor, N., Lyles, R.H., Skolasky, R., et al., 2001. HIV-associated neurological disease incidence changes: Multicenter AIDS Cohort Study 1990–1998. Neurology 56, 257–260.

Schechter, A.L., Stern, D.F., Vaidyanathan, L., et al., 1984. The neu oncogene: an erb-B-related gene encoding a 185,000-Mr, tumour antigen. Nature 312, 513–516.

Schiffer, D., Chio, A., Giordana, M.T., et al., 1988. Prognostic value of histologic factors in adult cerebral astrocytoma. Cancer 61, 1386–1393.

Schnegg, J.F., Gomez, F., LeMarchand-Beraud, T., et al., 1981. Presence of sex steroid hormone receptors in meningioma tissue. Surg. Neurol. 15, 415–418.

Seligman, A.M., Shear, M.J., 1939. Studies in carcinogenesis. VIII. Experimental production of brain tumors in mice with methylcholanthrene. Am. J. Cancer 37, 364–399.

Selikoff, I.J., Hammond, E.C., 1982. Brain tumors in the chemical industry. Ann. N. Acad. Sci. 381, 1–363.

Sherman, J.H., Le, B.H., Okonkwo, D.O., et al., 2007. Supratentorial dural-based hemangioblastoma not associated with von Hippel Lindau complex. Acta Neurochir. (Wien) 149, 969–972.

Sima, A.A.F., Finklestein, S.D., McLachlan, D.R., 1983. Multiple malignant astrocytomas in a patient with spontaneous progressive multifocal leukoencephalopathy. Ann. Neurol. 14, 183–188.

• Singh, S.K., Hawkins, C., Clark, I.D., et al., 2004. Identification of human brain tumor initiating cells. Nature 432, 396–401.

Smith, M.T., Ludwig, C.L., Godfrey, A.D., et al., 1983. Grading of oligodendrogliomas. Cancer 52, 2107–2114.

Soylemezoglu, F., Soffer, D., Onol, B., et al., 1996. Lipomatous medulloblastoma in adults: a distinctive clinicopathological entity. Am. J. Surg. Pathol. 20, 413–418.

Soylemezoglu, F., Scheithauer, B.W., Esteve, J., et al., 1997. Atypical central neurocytoma. J. Neuropathol. Exp. Neurol. 56, 551–556.

Stüer, C., Vilz, B., Majores, M., et al. 2007. Frequent recurrence and progression in pilocytic astrocytoma in adults. Cancer 110, 2799–2808.

Suster, S., Nascimento, A.G., Miettinen, M., et al., 1995. Solitary fibrous tumors of soft tissue. A clinicopathological and immunohistochemical study of 12 cases. Am. J. Surg. Pathol. 19, 1257–1266.

Svien, H.J., Mabon, R.F., Kernohan, J.W., et al., 1949. Astrocytomas. Proc. Staff Mayo Clin. 24, 54–63.

• Takei, H., Yogeswaren, S.T., Wong, K.-K., et al., 2008. Expression of oligodendroglial differentiation markers in pilocytic astrocytomas identifies two clinical subsets and shows a significant correlation with proliferation index and progression free survival. J. Neurooncol. 86, 183–190.

Takei, Y., Seyama, S., Pearl, G.S., et al., 1980. Ultrastructural study of human neurohypophysis. II. Cellular elements of neural parenchyma, the pituicytes. Cell Tissue Res. 205, 273–287.

Tanaka, Y., Yokoo, H., Komori, T., et al., 2005. A distinct pattern of Olig2-positive cellular distribution in papillary glioneuronal tumors: a manifestation of oligodendroglial phenotype? Acta Neuropathol. (Berl.) 110, 39–47.

Taratuto, A.L., Monges, J., Lylyk, P., et al., 1984. Superficial cerebral astrocytoma attached to dura. Report of six cases. Cancer 54, 2505–2512.

Taratuto, A.L., Pomata, H., Seviever, G., et al., 1995. Dysembryoplastic neuroepithelial tumor: morphological, immunocytochemical, and deoxyribonucleic acid analysis in a pediatric series. Neurosurgery 36, 474–481.

Tatter, S.B., Borges, L.F., Louis, S.N., 1994. Central neurocytomas of the cervical spinal cord. Report of two cases. J. Neurosurg. 81, 288–293.

Teo, J.G., Gultekin, S.H., Bilsky, M., et al., 1999. A distinctive glioneuronal tumor of the adult cerebrum with neuropil-like (including 'rosetted') islands: report of 4 cases. Am. J. Surg. Pathol. 23, 501–510.

Theunissen, P.H., Debets-Te Baerts, M., Blaauw, G., 1990. Histogenesis of intracranial hemangiopericytoma and hemangioblastoma. An immunohistochemical study. Acta. Neuropathol. 80, 68–71.

Tihan, T., Fisher, P.G., Kepner, J.L., et al., 1999. Pediatric astrocytomas with monomorphous pilomyxoid features and a less favorable outcome. J. Neuropathol. Exp. Neurol. 58, 1061–1068.

Townsend, J.J., Seaman, J.P., 1986. Central neurocytoma – a rare benign intraventricular tumor. Acta Neuropathol. 71, 167–170.

Tsuchida, T., Matsumoto, M., Shirayama, Y., et al., 1996. Neuronal and glial characteristics of central neurocytoma: an electron microscopical analysis of two cases. Acta Neuropathol. (Berl.) 91, 573–577.

Ugokwe, K., Nathoo, N., Prayson, R., et al., 2005. Trigeminal nerve schwannoma with ancient change. Case report and review of the literature. J. Neurosurg. 102, 1163–1165.

• VandenBerg, S.R., May, E.E., Rubinstein, L.J., et al., 1987. Desmoplastic supratentorial neuroepithelial tumors of infancy with divergent differentiation potential ('desmoplastic infantile gangliogliomas'). Report of 11 cases of a distinctive embryonal tumor with favorable prognosis. J. Neurosurg. 66, 58–71.

• Varlet, P., Soni, D., Miquel, C., et al., 2004. New variants of malignant glioneuronal tumors: a clinicopathological study of 40 cases. Neurosurgery 55, 1377–1391.

• Varmus, H.E., 1984. The molecular genetics of cellular oncogenes. Annu. Rev. Genet. 18, 553–612.

• Vates, G.E., Chang, S., Lamborn, K.R., 2003. Gliomatosis cerebri: a review of 22 cases. Neurosurgery 53, 261–271.

Verma, S., Tavare, C., Gilles, F., 2008. Histologic features and prognosis in pediatric medulloblastoma. Pediatr. Dev. Pathol. 11 (5), 337–343.

Virchow, R., 1860. Cellular pathology. Translated from the second German edition. A. Hirschwald (trans). Chance, London.

Virchow, R., 1890. Das Psamom. Virchow Arch. Anat. Pathol. 160, 32.

● **Wang**, **M.**, **Tihan**, **T.**, **Rojiani**, **A.M.**, **et al.**, 2005. Monomorphous angiocentric glioma: a distinctive epileptogenic neoplasm with features of infiltrating astrocytoma and ependymoma. J. Neuropathol. Exp. Neurol. 64, 875–881.

Wanschitz, **J.**, **Schmidbauer**, **M.**, **Maier**, **H.**, **et al.**, 1995. Suprasellar meningioma with expression of glial fibrillary acidic protein: a peculiar variant. Acta Neuropathol. 90, 539–544.

Wavre, **A.**, **Baur**, **A.**, **Betz**, **M.**, **et al.**, 2007. Case study of intracerebral plasmacytoma as initial presentation of multiple myeloma. Neuro. Oncol. 9, 370–372.

Weldon-Linne, **G.M.**, **Victor**, **T.A.**, **Groothuis**, **D.R.**, **et al.**, 1983. Pleomorphic xanthoastrocytoma: ultrastructural and immunohistochemical study of a case with a rapidly fatal outcome following surgery. Cancer 52, 2055–2063.

Whittle, **I.R.**, **Gordon**, **A.**, **Misra**, **B.K.**, **et al.**, 1989. Pleomorphic xanthoastrocytoma: report of four cases. J. Neurosurg. 70, 463–468.

● **Wong**, **K.K.**, **Chang**, **Y.M.**, **Tsang**, **Y.T.**, **et al.**, 2005. Expression analysis of juvenile pilocytic astrocytomas by oligonucleotide microarray reveals two potential subgroups. Cancer Res. 65, 76–84.

Yamamoto, **T.**, **Komori**, **T.**, **Shibata**, **N.**, **et al.**, 1996. Multifocal neurocytoma/ganglioneurocytoma with extensive leptomeningeal dissemination in the brain and spinal cord. Am. J. Surg. Pathol. 20, 363–370.

● **Yamane**, **Y.**, **Mena**, **H.**, **Nakazato**, **Y.**, 2002. Immunohistochemical characterization of pineal parenchymal tumors using novel monoclonal antibodies to the pineal body. Neuropathology 22, 66–76.

Yoon, **D.H.**, **Cho**, **K.J.**, **Suh**, **Y.L.**, 1987. Intracranial granulocytic sarcoma (chloroma) in a nonleukemic patient. J. Korean Med. Sci. 2, 173–178.

Zorludemir, **S.**, **Scheithauer**, **B.W.**, **Hirose**, **T.**, **et al.**, 1995. Clear cell meningioma. A clinicopathologic study of a potentially aggressive variant of meningioma. Am. J. Surg. Pathol. 19, 493–505.

Zulch, **K.J.**, 1979. Histologic typing of tumors of the central nervous system. International Histologic Classification of Tumors, No. 21. World Health Organization, Geneva.

Epidemiology of brain tumors

Graham G. Giles

Introduction

The epidemiologic study of primary tumors of the brain and spinal cord (CNS tumors) is complex. From the point of view of monitoring trends, there are difficulties with ascertainment and with the taxonomy of incident cases. The estimation of incidence is influenced by the availability of medical services and the rules that govern cancer registration. Populations that are well served by modern imaging modalities tend to have increased levels of detection that lead to higher reported incidence. Cancer registries that include diagnoses without histologic examination of the primary tumor and/or that include tumors of uncertain behavior also tend to report elevated incidence. Thus, apparent differences in incidence between registries can be difficult to interpret.

From an etiologic perspective, historically, a lack of histologic specificity in case selection for research has probably masked the ability of epidemiologic studies to detect causal factors which, in themselves, are likely to vary by histologic type. The heterogeneity of histologic diagnoses within CNS tumors suggests that multiple etiologies are likely to be involved, and points to the need for increased diagnostic specificity in future epidemiologic investigations (Armstrong et al 1990; Davis et al 2008). Table 4.1 shows incidence rates for the major histologic types of CNS tumors classified according to the rubrics of the International Classification of Diseases for Oncology, 3rd Edition (Fritz et al 2000).

Although age and sex specific rates are published for many of these subtypes from several series, they must be viewed in the context of the caveats discussed above. Hospital series benefit from pathology slide review, but suffer from selection bias while population series might be complete, but are not usually subject to centralized pathologic review of diagnosis. It is important to obtain details of histologic verification and review when assessing such data. Epidemiologic studies of specific histologic subtypes have been uncommon. CNS tumors are usually investigated either as one entity or at best, being grouped broadly into gliomas or meningiomas.

There are also difficulties with the accuracy of information on exposures. Three research designs have been used to explore risk factors for CNS tumors. The weakest design compares the number of new cases or deaths from CNS tumors for a sub-group of the population with the number that would be expected based on the application of general population rates to that sub-population. The measure obtained is called a standardized mortality ratio (SMR) or standardized incidence ratio (SIR), a SMR of 1 indicates that the risk does not differ from that of the general population. The second, and most frequently used research design for exploration of risk factors for CNS tumors, is the case–control study. These studies are retrospective in nature and in essence compare the recall of a sample of CNS tumor cases with the recall of a sample of unaffected controls in regard to the exposures of interest, e.g., diet, smoking, X-rays, occupational exposures, etc. Case–control studies estimate risk by calculating an odds ratio (OR) which is commonly reported with a 95% confidence interval (CI) in parenthesis. One problem with this design is that there is some doubt about the accuracy of recall by people suffering from CNS tumors. The concern is about possible effects of the disease process and treatment on recall accuracy and the rapidly failing state of health of patients has required researchers to often resort to collecting surrogate information from proxies. The information biases introduced by differential recall and surrogate data can easily result in modestly elevated estimates of risk (e.g., ORs from 1.1 to 2.0). The relative rarity of CNS tumors has resulted in the accumulation of a large series of small case–control studies that lack statistical power. The combination of information bias and low statistical power has inevitably led to a number of spurious 'findings' that it has not been possible to replicate. The third, and strongest, design is the prospective cohort study. Cohort studies are less prone to bias and study a group of people over time, collecting information about individuals and their patterns of exposure and relating this to the incidence of disease. Cohort studies provide an estimate of relative risk (RR). However, their effectiveness is compromised when only small numbers of the cohort members develop the disease of interest. The rarity of CNS cancers has meant that few prospective cohort studies have reported any substantive findings. As a consequence of the limitations associated with research into the etiology of CNS tumors, there is continuing uncertainty and only a small amount of established knowledge about their causes.

The following discussion attempts to synthesize salient information and evidence from a large number of studies and reports that are highly variable in their quality. In this process, some judgments have had to be made in regard to which studies to include. (The interested reader is pointed to other recent reviews of the literature: see Baldwin & Preston-Martin 2004; Connelly & Malkin 2007; Fisher et al 2007; Ohgaki 2009, for additional materials and views.) The consensus of the Brain Tumor Epidemiology Consortium echoes much of this chapter (Bondy et al 2008).

Descriptive epidemiology

CNS tumors account for only 1.5% of malignancies diagnosed in Australia (AIHW et al 2008a), but are the 12th ranking cause of cancer mortality with 2.8% deaths, and are

Table 4.1 The incidence of CNS tumors by histologic type and behavior; a comparison of rates from CBTRUS with Victoria, Australia*

Histology groupings	All tumors						Malignant tumors only				
	Victoria incidence counts			Rates per 100000			Victoria incidence counts			Rates	
	All ages	0–19 years	>20 years	CBTRUS[US]	Vic[WS]	Vic[US]	All ages	0–19 years	>20 years	Vic[WS]	Vic[US]
Tumors of neuroepithelial tissue	3451	271	3180	6.45	5.86	6.95	3088	146	2942	4.87	6.10
Astrocytoma, pilocytic	148	78	70	0.34	0.41	0.32	0	0	0	0.00	0.00
Astrocytoma, protoplasmic and fibrillary	34	2	32	0.09	0.06	0.07	34	2	32	0.06	0.07
Astrocytoma, anaplastic	379	10	369	0.44	0.62	0.76	379	10	369	0.62	0.76
Astrocytoma, unique variants	44	11	33	0.09	0.10	0.09	10	3	7	0.02	0.02
Astrocytoma, NOS	142	17	125	0.43	0.26	0.29	142	17	125	0.26	0.29
Glioblastoma	1927	22	1905	3.09	2.83	3.83	1927	22	1905	2.83	3.83
Oligodendroglioma	51	0	51	0.32	0.09	0.11	51	0	51	0.09	0.11
Oligodendroglioma, anaplastic	41	0	41	0.17	0.06	0.08	41	0	41	0.06	0.08
Ependymoma, incl. anaplastic	121	31	90	0.26	0.27	0.25	121	31	90	0.27	0.25
Ependymoma, variants	33	1	32	0.08	0.06	0.07	0	0	0	0.00	0.00
Glioma, mixed	210	6	204	0.18	0.36	0.42	210	6	204	0.36	0.42
Glioma, malignant NOS	50	13	37	0.41	0.10	0.10	50	13	37	0.10	0.10
Choroid plexus	15	5	10	0.04	0.03	0.03	4	2	2	0.01	0.01
Neuroepithelial	8	0	8	0.02	0.01	0.02	8	0	8	0.01	0.02
Non-malignant and malignant neuronal/glial, neuronal and mixed	130	31	99	0.22	0.27	0.27	18	0	18	0.03	0.04
Pineal parenchymal	15	2	13	0.03	0.03	0.03	7	1	6	0.00	0.00
Embryonal/primitive/medulloblastoma	103	42	61	0.23	0.29	0.22	86	39	47	0.14	0.12
Tumors of cranial and spinal nerves	577	8	569	1.46	0.95	1.16	6	1	5	0.13	0.09
Nerve sheath, non-malignant and malignant	577	8	569	1.46	0.95	1.16	6	1	5	0.13	0.09
Tumors of meninges	1922	24	1898	5.55	2.93	3.85	51	3	48	0.09	0.11
Meningioma	1838	16	1822	5.35	2.78	3.68	42	2	40	0.03	0.04
Other mesenchymal, non-malignant and malignant	17	4	13	0.06	0.04	0.04	9	1	8	0.05	0.06
Hemangioblastoma	67	4	63	0.14	0.12	0.14	0	0	0	0.00	0.00
Lymphomas and hematopoietic neoplasms	194	1	193	0.47	0.27	0.39	194	1	193	0.16	0.22
Lymphoma	194	1	193	0.47	0.27	0.39	194	1	193	0.16	0.22
Germ cell tumors and cysts	35	19	16	0.08	0.09	0.07	28	15	13	0.17	0.22
Germ cell tumors, cysts and heterotopias	35	19	16	0.08	0.09	0.07	28	15	13	0.17	0.22
Tumors of the sellar region	97	19	78	1.49	0.18	0.20	17	1	16	0.04	0.05
Pituitary	17	1	16	1.37	0.02	0.03	12	0	12	0.02	0.03
Craniopharyngioma	80	18	62	0.12	0.17	0.17	5	1	4	0.01	0.02
Local extensions from regional tumors	1	0	1	0.02	0.00	0.00	1	0	1	0.00	0.00
Chordoma/chondrosarcoma	1	0	1	0.02	0.00	0.00	1	0	1	0.00	0.00
Unclassified tumors	15	0	15	1.00	0.03	0.03	6	0	6	0.01	0.01
Hemangioma	6	0	6	0.11	0.01	0.01	0	0	0	0.00	0.00
Neoplasm, unspecified	6	0	6	0.88	0.01	0.01	3	0	3	0.01	0.01
All other	3	0	3	0.01	0.01	0.01	3	0	3	0.01	0.01
No histological confirmation	1152	66	1086	–	1.50	2.38	584	48	536	0.76	1.21
Total (C70–C72 only)	7094	376	6718	–	11.20	14.30	3715	202	3513	5.70	7.50
Total (including C751–C753 and C300)	7444	408	7036	16.52	11.80	15.00	3975	215	3760	6.23	8.01

Additional group – no histological confirmation added to CBTRUS groups (probably included in 'Neoplasm, unspecified' group in US figures.
Incident cases in 10 years 1997–2006. CBTRUS[US], CBTRUS (Central Brain Tumor Registry of the USA) 2000–2004 rates standardized to US 2000 Standard population; Vic[US], Victoria 1997–2006 rates standardized to US 2000 Standard population; Vic[WS], Victoria rates standardized to World Standard (Segi) population.
*Includes all malignant, uncertain behavior tumors of primary sites C70–C72, C751–C753 and C300 (with morphology 9522, 9523) grouped according to ICDO-3 morphology.

responsible for 6.1% of the years of life lost from cancer before age 75 years. They are of particular importance in childhood, accounting for up to 25% of malignant tumors diagnosed before the age of 15 (Parkin et al 1998). CNS tumors vary in incidence by age, sex, ethnic group, country, and also over time. How much of this variation is due to either artifactual influences or to etiologic differences has been the subject of continual debate. CNS tumor diagnosis has been facilitated by advances in imaging technology made over the course of this century. Access to medical technology might, therefore, explain some of the observed variations between and within populations. One difficulty lies in the proportion of inoperable, image-detected tumors that are seldom verified histologically. The inclusion of these tumors can significantly affect apparent incidence and reduce comparability between populations.

Trends by age and sex

Population-based incidence statistics are routinely obtained from cancer registries. Some registries intentionally include tumors of benign or uncertain behavior in their incidence and there is growing support for this approach, championed by the Central Brain Tumor Registry of the USA, CBTRUS (McCarthy et al 2005). Most registries, however, continue to restrict data collection to malignant primary tumors but the extent to which they are successful probably varies depending on the degree of histologic verification and the specificity of pathologists reports. The international variation in CNS invasive tumor incidence is about 10-fold, with male rates age-adjusted to the world population, ranging from 0.6/100 000 in Algeria to 10.2 in Croatia; rates for Asian countries generally tend to be lower than those for the

USA and Europe, and rates for women lower than those for men (Curado et al 2007).

Examples of age-standardized incidence rates for total malignant CNS tumors are given in Figure 4.1, which illustrates rates up to age 85 years and beyond. Table 4.1 gives age-standardized incidence rates for the principal histologic types of CNS tumor comparing data from CBTRUS (2008) with those from the Victorian Cancer Registry (Australia) for all CNS tumors, including those of benign and uncertain behavior. The rates for the state of Victoria have been standardized to both the US 2000 census and to the World Standard

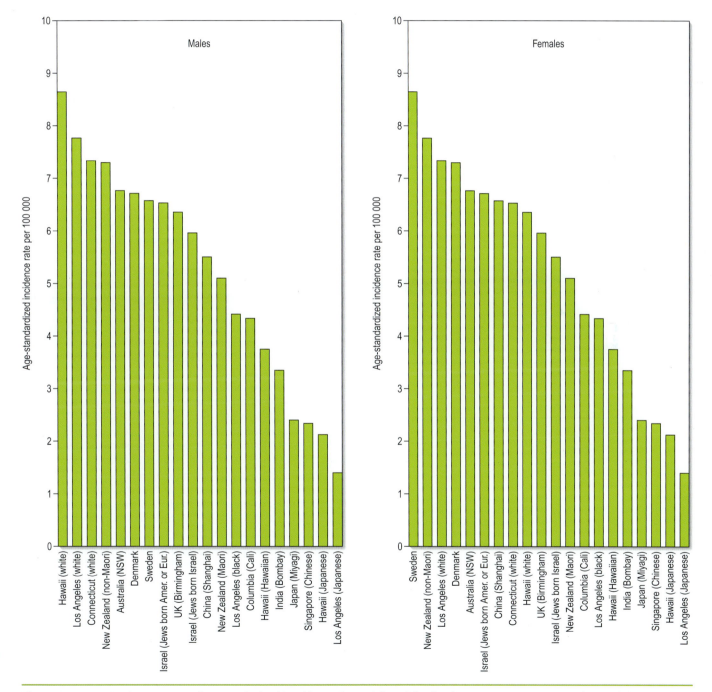

Figure 4.1 International comparisons of age standardized (World) rates by sex (all ages) for all malignant CNS tumors. (From Parkin D, Whelan S, Ferlay J et al. (eds) (1997) Cancer Incidence in Five Continents. Lyon: International Agency for Research on Cancer; vol. VII. IARC Scientific Publication No. 143.)

Population (Segi). Victoria rates, excluding non-malignant tumors, and standardized to the world population are also included for comparison with other international series. Table 4.1 illustrates some problems met when comparing data from different sources and the impact of including non-malignant tumors in CNS tumor totals. For example, Victoria seems to have a low incidence of oligodendrogliomas, but this is because oligoastrocytomas in Victoria are coded to the rubric 'glioma, mixed' and, when this group is added to the two oligodendroglioma groupings, the summed rates become comparable. Further, although Victoria accepts all morphology behavior codes for CNS tumors, it does not do this for endocrine tumors and this is the reason for the low rate in Victoria for pituitary tumors, which are largely benign.

The distribution of CNS tumor incidence with age is characterized by a peak in childhood, an exponential rise from the early 20s until age 70 years, and then a decline with increasing age thereafter; rates for men being higher than those for women at all ages.

Age incidence curves are illustrated in Figure 4.2 for CNS tumors for males and females from selected populations

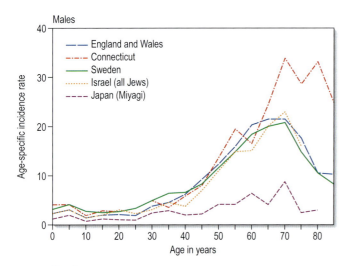

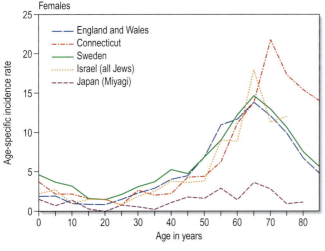

Figure 4.2 Age and sex specific incidence rates for all malignant CNS tumors from selected cancer registries. (From Parkin D, Whelan S, Ferlay J et al. (eds) (1997) Cancer Incidence in Five Continents. Lyon: International Agency for Research on Cancer; vol. VII. IARC Scientific Publication No. 143.)

taken from *Cancer Incidence in Five Continents*, Vol. IX (Curado et al 2007). Given the potential for artifactual influences, the age-specific incidence of CNS tumors is remarkably consistent between populations. Artifactual variation in rates is likely to be strongest for elderly populations and for this reason, the cumulative rates chosen to illustrate trends over time have been restricted to age 65 years (Table 4.2). Velema & Walker (1987) examined age and sex specific incidence rates for the age range 35–65 years for 51 populations. The modeled slope of the age incidence curve on a log–log scale was reported to be 2.6 for both sexes. There were no significant deviations from this model. Although the age curves had the same slope, they were at different levels for different populations (highest for Israel and lowest for Asia), and were thought to reflect differences in exposure or susceptibility to etiologic factors. The slope was the same for registries that included only malignant tumors as for registries that included tumors of benign and uncertain behavior, their inclusion merely increasing the level of incidence. The slope of 2.6 was somewhat less than slopes of 4–5 commonly observed for epithelial tumors, and close to a slope of 2.7 observed for soft tissue sarcomas (Cook et al 1969). According to the multistage theory of carcinogenesis (Armitage & Doll 1954), this implies that fewer events are required for the malignant transformation of glial cells compared with epithelial cells. In Moolgavkar's two-stage model (Moolgavkar et al 1980), the slope of the curve is dependent on the growth characteristics of the cells, and the level of the curve is related to the probability of cell transformation. This model suggests that differences in the slope reflect differences in growth characteristics between glial and epithelial tissues.

Histologic types also vary in their incidence by age and sex (Fig. 4.3). Rates for males are usually higher than for females. CNS tumors in childhood (0–14 years) differ from those of adults, particularly in regard to the distribution of histologic types and intracranial location (Lacayo & Farmer 1991). In children, medulloblastomas and astrocytomas are more common than other types, whereas gliomas and meningiomas are more common in adults. In children, the majority (70%) of tumors are located below the tentorium, compared with only 30% for adults (Rubinstein 1972). Table 4.3 contains rates for the principal histologic types of CNS tumors in childhood from selected cancer registries (Parkin et al 1998). There are some clear differences between the distributions across populations, the most striking being the increased rate of primitive neuroectodermal tumors for male Maoris and Hawaiians; this might indicate a particular predisposition to this tumor. Historical differences between white and black children in the USA, however, were found to have been influenced by differential trends in histologic confirmation and in the proportion of unspecified tumors (Bunin 1987).

The age curves of malignant CNS tumors by histologic type for adults have been examined (Velema & Percy 1987) in similar fashion to the analysis of all CNS tumors by geographic location (Velema & Walker 1987). Velema & Percy discovered that the slopes of the incidence curves for the 35–65 year age range differed significantly by histologic type. The slope increased from 0.4 for ependymomas to 1.0 for oligodendrogliomas, 1.7 for astrocytomas, 2.8 for meningiomas, and 3.9 for glioblastomas. These data point to a

Table 4.2 CNS tumors: cumulative rates per cent to age 65 from the nine volumes of *Cancer Incidence in Five Continents*

	Vol I	Vol II	Vol III	Vol IV	Vol V	Vol VI	Vol VII	Vol VIII	Vol IX
Males									
Australia (NSW)	n/a	n/a	n/a	0.40	0.46	0.43	0.44	0.42	0.42
China (Shanghai)	n/a	n/a	n/a	0.30	0.27	0.31	0.36	0.35	0.35
Colombia (Cali)	0.32	0.34	0.33	0.20	0.28	0.25	0.31	0.32	0.34
Connecticut (white)	0.40	0.43	0.42	0.50	0.46	0.45	0.47	0.44	0.43
Denmark	0.53	0.60	0.54	0.50	0.60	0.37	0.47	0.48	0.41
Hawaii (Hawaiian)	0.21	0.19	0.30	0.20	0.24	0.24	0.25	0.23	0.33
Hawaii (Japanese)	0.18	0.24	0.24	0.10	0.17	0.24	0.12	0.20	0.22
Hawaii (white)	0.28	0.40	0.37	0.50	0.43	0.54	0.51	0.41	0.44
India (Mumbai)	n/a	0.08	0.10	0.10	0.14	0.15	0.21	0.23	0.24
Japan (Miyagi)	0.02	0.20	0.09	0.10	0.15	0.15	0.17	0.18	0.17
Los Angeles (black)	n/a	n/a	n/a	0.30	0.42	0.31	0.30	0.29	0.24
Los Angeles (white)	n/a	n/a	n/a	0.40	0.62	0.39	0.50	0.45	0.47
Singapore (Chinese)	0.10	0.15	0.10	0.10	0.12	0.15	0.14	0.15	0.12
Sweden	0.54	0.62	0.64	0.60	0.63	0.72	0.46	0.45	0.40
UK (Birmingham)	0.44	0.45	0.46	0.50	0.44	0.38	0.44	0.39	0.38
Females									
Australia (NSW)	n/a	n/a	n/a	0.30	0.30	0.30	0.32	0.30	0.29
China (Shanghi)	n/a	n/a	n/a	0.20	0.21	0.31	0.34	0.39	0.41
Colombia (Cali)	0.12	0.15	0.13	0.20	0.14	0.19	0.24	0.26	0.27
Connecticut (white)	0.28	0.34	0.27	0.30	0.32	0.32	0.28	0.32	0.29
Denmark	0.44	0.50	0.50	0.40	0.56	0.64	0.33	0.32	0.32
Hawaii (Hawaiian)	0.34	0.32	0.16	0.30	0.32	0.14	0.17	0.25	0.35
Hawaii (Japanese)	0.06	0.07	0.11	0.10	0.11	0.12	0.09	0.15	0.21
Hawaii (white)	0.18	0.20	0.46	0.20	0.23	0.34	0.29	0.28	0.33
India (Bombay)	n/a	0.07	0.10	0.10	0.10	0.11	0.15	0.16	0.19
Japan (Miyagi)	0.03	0.18	0.05	0.1	0.12	0.11	0.12	0.13	0.12
Los Angeles (black)	n/a	n/a	n/a	0.20	0.40	0.21	0.30	0.20	0.22
Los Angeles (white)	n/a	n/a	n/a	.030	0.55	0.28	0.31	0.34	0.32
Singapore (Chinese)	0.07	0.12	0.10	0.10	0.06	0.12	0.10	0.10	0.10
Sweden	0.52	0.61	0.62	0.60	0.63	0.71	0.36	0.32	0.28
UK (Birmingham)	0.31	0.34	0.33	0.40	0.36	0.24	0.31	0.28	0.31

From 1. Muir C, Waterhouse J, Mack T et al. (1987) Cancer Incidence in Five Continents, vol V No. 88. Lyon: IARC Scientific Publications, and 2. Stukonis, M. Cancer incidence cumulative rates – international comparison. Lyon: IARC, Internal technical report, 1978.

different carcinogenic mechanism for glioblastoma compared with other CNS tumors. The steeper slope suggests that it might take more cellular events to transform a glial cell to a glioblastoma than is required for transformation to a lower grade tumor.

Socioeconomic status (SES) might explain some of the variation in CNS tumor incidence and mortality between populations. People of higher SES generally have better access to healthcare and are medically investigated more often than people of lower SES. In England and Wales the SMRs for males and females aged between 15 and 64 years in social class I were 1.08 and 1.37, respectively, compared with SMRs of 0.92 and 1.0 for males and females of social class V (Logan 1982). Proportionally more deaths occurred after age 55 for persons from social class I compared with social class V. Before the age of 55 years, the proportions of deaths by social class were very similar. Positive associations with SES have also been reported from the USA (Demers et al 1991; Inskip et al 2003; Chakrabarti et al 2005). It appears that SES is more strongly linked with tumors of more indolent course than those that are quickly fatal (Inskip et al 2003).

Time trends

There has been a continuing debate concerning the validity of increasing trends in CNS tumors (Desmeules et al 1992). Long-term trends in mortality are subject to all the known shortcomings of death certificates (Garfinkel & Sarokhan 1982; Bahemuka et al 1988). Some of the older population-based cancer registries, such as Connecticut, have been able to model age–period–cohort trends in incidence (Rousch et al 1987). There have been reports that incidence might have been increasing for the elderly (Greig et al 1990), but these have been explained as a diagnostic artifact related to the advent of CT scanning, given the low levels of histologic verification in the elderly (Boyle et al 1990; Modan et al 1992). Similar increases have not been observed for other countries with long-established cancer registries such as Denmark and Sweden (Ahlbom & Rodvall 1989). The comparatively modest increases seen for younger age groups also suggest that increased detection might be the cause of growing incidence in the elderly. Such detection effects have been shown previously in comparisons of US incidence series (Walker et al 1985). An increase of 35% in childhood CNS tumors between 1973 and 1994 in the USA was explained by the increased use of CT and MRI (Smith et al 1998), but it was suggested that an environmental cause, though unlikely, could not be excluded (Black 1998). More recent analyses of US data noted the contribution of CNS lymphoma to the increase in incidence and, after its exclusion, an overall decreasing trend for other CNS tumors (Hoffman et al 2006). Apparently increasing trends for CNS tumor sub-types were observed to be influenced by better classification of CNS tumors, some sub-types increasing as the numbers

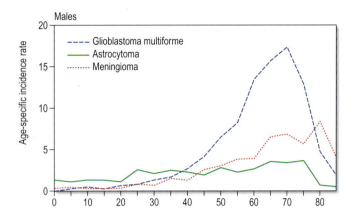

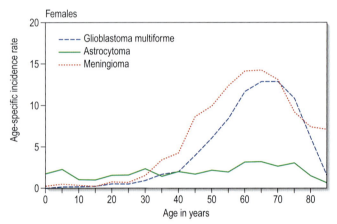

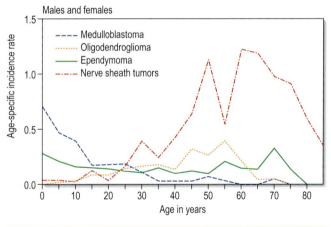

Figure 4.3 Age and sex specific incidence rates for main histologic groups of CNS tumors. (From Victorian Cancer Registry, Unpublished data, 2009.)

of non-specified gliomas decreased over time, but increases for meningiomas and nerve sheath tumors remain unexplained (Hoffman et al 2006; McCarthy et al 2008).

Table 4.2 contains cumulative risks (incidence rates %) from 35 to 65 years of age for CNS tumors from selected cancer registries in Vols I–IX of *Cancer Incidence in Five Continents* (Stukonis 1978; Curado et al 2007), which together cover the period from the 1950s to 2004. The cumulative risk is a directly age-standardized rate that closely approximates actuarial estimates of risk (Day 1987). The rates have been

Table 4.3 CNS tumor incidence for children aged 0–14 years by histologic type

	Astrocytoma	Ependymoma	PNET	Total
US SEER White	16.0	3.2	6.5	31.8
US SEER Black	13.5	3.6	3.9	27.4
US SEER Hawaiian	10.7	3.2	11.8	28.5
Costa Rica	8.3	1.8	3.9	17.4
Israel (Jews)	9.5	2.3	7.9	29.9
China (Tianjin)	6.9	1.5	3.2	17.3
Singapore (Chinese)	6.8	2.3	6.1	19.1
Thailand	2.7	0.9	2.4	10.1
India (Bombay)	3.3	0.6	3.0	11.2
Denmark	15.1	2.3	7.0	38.8
Sweden	22.2	4.3	7.1	41.0
England & Wales	10.3	3.0	5.8	27.0
Australia (Vic)	13.0	2.8	5.5	29.6
New Zealand (Maori)	9.1	2.0	12.0	31.6
New Zealand (Non-Maori)	15.8	1.9	6.6	32.0

Age standardized rates per million child years. From Parkin, D, Kramarova, E, Draper, G, et al. International Incidence of Childhood Cancer., Vol. II. Lyon, France: International Agency for Research on Cancer, 1998 IARC Scientific Publication.

truncated to age 65 to discount the effect of over-zealous investigation of the elderly (Peto 1981). All risks included in the table are observed to be less than 1%, and although some variation is present, e.g., some decline in Scandinavia, and rises in Japanese and Indian populations, there is little evidence of a substantive change in trends over time.

Trends by place and ethnicity

CNS tumor incidence varies from population to population and such variation is sometimes taken as ecological evidence of the importance of environmental risk factors. Incidence rates standardized to the world population are illustrated in Figure 4.1 for males and females separately. Some of the variation in rates shown in the figure is due to varying levels of detection linked with the availability of, and access to, medical technology. It is interesting that Japan, which has comparable technological development to western industrialized countries, has rates of CNS cancer that are one-third or less of those observed for the USA. Incidence for other Asian countries is also low. As already noted in Table 4.2, the exclusion of cases older than 65 years does not remove all of the variation between populations. Historically, geographic variation for CNS tumors in childhood has been greater than that for other childhood malignancies (Breslow & Langholz 1983), suggesting that real differences might exist between populations, due to genetic or environmental factors. Childhood CNS tumor rates (per million) for selected cancer registries, taken from the *International Incidence of Childhood Cancer*, Vol. II (Parkin et al 1998), are given in Table 4.3. These estimates do not provide strong evidence of international variation in total CNS tumor rates, but some support for differences in subtypes, especially astrocytoma.

Similarly, variation in CNS tumor rates between ethnic groups can give clues to possible genetic influences. Cumulative rates per cent to age 65 years for some ethnic subpopulations reported by *Cancer Incidence in Five Continents*, Vols I–IX are given in Table 4.2 (Curado et al 2007). Historically, Jews living in Israel and Jewish populations in the USA have had elevated rates (MacMahon 1960; Newill 1961; Muir et al 1987; Steinitz et al 1989). Asians tend to have low rates.

Jewish migrants to Israel from Europe, America, Africa, and Asia have higher incidence rates than Jews born in Israel (Steinitz et al 1989), but much of this excess occurred in the elderly and might have been a consequence of increased screening.

Changes in cancer incidence and mortality for migrants who move from low to high incidence countries are also used broadly to support causal links with environmental factors. Early analysis of Australian mortality data from 1961 to 1972 showed elevated rates of CNS tumors for adult males from Poland and Africa, and for adult females from Austria and Yugoslavia, but there were no clear patterns with duration of residence, and childhood mortality rates were not statistically different from those for the Australian born (Armstrong et al 1983). McCredie et al (1990) reviewed CNS tumor incidence by ethnic group in New South Wales and reported no statistically significant differences for males, but a significantly lower rate for female migrants from Asia. An analysis of Canadian mortality data for 1970–1973 showed excess mortality risk for immigrants from Britain, Germany, Italy, and Holland (Neutel et al 1989). The increased risk was higher for males than for females and was not apparent for the second generation. Unlike other cancers for which strong environmental links have been established, the ethnic and migrant data give little support for such links with CNS tumors.

Rural residence has been reported to be associated with increased risk of gliomas by some studies (Choi et al 1970a; Musicco et al 1982; Mills et al 1989b), but not all (Burch et al 1987). This association has been hypothesized to be related to agricultural exposures, e.g., zoonotic viruses and pesticides (Sanderson et al 1997). Childhood CNS tumors have also been associated with farm residence (Gold et al 1979; Cordier et al 1994). A review of case–control studies, published between 1979 and 1998, that considered a possible relationship between fetal or childhood exposure to farm residence (Yeni-Komshian & Holly 2000) reported ORs ranging from 0.9 to 2.5 for maternal exposures and from 0.6 to 6.7 for childrens' exposures. Of those studies large enough to analyze by histological type, increased risk associated with farm residence was reported only for primitive neuroectodermal tumors prenatally, OR 3.7 (0.8, 24) or in childhood, OR 5.0 (1.1, 4.7). The low statistical power and case–control design provide little confidence in these estimates.

Trends in survival

Historically, survival statistics for specific histologic types of CNS tumor have been limited to patients from specialist centers or from clinical trials, but this is now changing and more population-based estimates are being produced. Population-based survival estimates are usually adjusted using life tables and are reported as relative survival. Relative survival proportions have the advantage of being more comparable between populations than crude proportions, especially when deaths tend to occur at older ages when competing causes are common.

Overall survival from CNS tumors is comparatively poor with only small gains being made in recent decades. The EUROCARE weighted analysis of all brain tumors for the 1983–1985 period gave 5-year relative survival estimates of 15% for adult males and 18% for adult females (Berrino

et al 1995). Relative 5-year survival proportions for all gliomas diagnosed at all ages in Finland improved over time: 1953–1968 (21%); 1969–1978 (31%), and 1979–1988 (36%) (Kallio et al 1991). In the USA, overall 5-year survival proportions for CNS tumors improved from 18% in 1960–1963 to 24% in 1981–1986 (Boring et al 1991). USA-based national surveys of patterns of care in 1980 and 1985 gave actuarial 5-year survival proportions by age and by Karnofsky ratings (Mahaley et al 1989). For patients in the 1980 survey, the 5-year survival proportions averaged 5.7% for glioblastoma; 33.5% for astrocytoma; 91.6% for meningioma, and 60.9% for medulloblastoma. The estimate of 5-year survival from CNS tumors by (Davis et al 1998), using US SEER data, was 20% for the period 1986–1991 (this analysis excluded benign forms). Estimates were 1% for glioblastoma multiforme (GBM); 34% for astrocytoma; 60% for medulloblastoma; 65% for oligodendroglioma, and 60% for ependymoma. Distinct from the poor estimates for GBM, people with low-grade gliomas can have reasonable survival expectations and quality of life (Claus & Black 2006). Using SEER data for 1973–2001, 5-, 10-, 15- and 20-year survival estimates for those with supratentorial, low-grade gliomas were 60%, 43%, 32% and 26%, respectively. Ohgaki (2009) compares survival estimates from CBTRUS 1992–1997 with that from Zurich for several sub-groups of glioma; reporting Swiss 5-year survival for pilocytic astrocytoma 100%; low-grade diffuse astrocytoma 58%; anaplastic astrocytoma 11%; glioblastomas 1%; oligodendroglioma 78%, and anaplastic oligodendroglioma 30%. Recent survival statistics from CBTRUS (2008) for the period 1973–2004 are given in Table 4.4 by histologic type and by age <15 years and for all ages. The 1-, 5- and 10-year relative survival estimates for all malignant CNS tumors are 52%, 30%, and 26%, respectively. In comparison the 1-, 5- and 10-year relative survival proportions for malignant brain tumors in Australia

Table 4.4 Relative survival estimates (%) for malignant CNS tumors by histologic type and age group (<15 years and all ages) 1973–2004 (CBTRUS 2008)

Survival (relative)	1-year		5-year		10-year	
Age (years)	<15	All ages	<15	All ages	<15	All ages
Histology group						
Pilocytic astrocytoma	98	96	95	92	94	90
Protoplasmic and fibrillary astrocytoma	92	74	80	47	79	38
Anaplastic astrocytoma	71	60	49	33	46	22
Astrocytoma NOS	87	60	78	38	74	31
Glioblastoma	48	30	18	3	15	2
Oligodendroglioma	95	91	89	72	83	56
Anaplastic oligodendroglioma		77		45		34
Ependymoma	86	89	53	73	47	65
Mixed glioma	89	86	72	58	65	45
Glioma malignant NOS	70	51	46	32	43	29
Neuroepithelial	85	59	60	40	57	33
Malignant neuronal/glial, neuronal/mixed	76	84	56	63	53	56
Embryonal primitive medulloblastoma	79	80	56	57	49	48
Lymphoma	n/a	38	n/a	18	n/a	11
Total CNS malignant tumors	n/a	52	n/a	30	n/a	26

From CBTRUS. Primary Brain Tumors in the United States, 2000–2004. Hinsdale, Illinois: Central Brain Tumor Registry of the United States, 2008.

diagnosed between 1982 and 2004 are 41%, 19%, and 15%, respectively, with little evidence of change over time (AIHW et al 2008b). Using data for malignancies diagnosed in Australia during 2000–2004 taken from AIHW et al 2004, the 5-year relative survival estimates for glioma sub-groups are as follows: astrocytoma grade I 93%; astrocytoma grade II 40%; astrocytoma grade III 27%; astrocytoma grade IV (glioblastoma) 3%; oligodendroglioma grade II 71%; oligodendroglioma grade III 33%; and mixed glioma 48% (AIHW and AACR, unpublished data).

Survival differs by age group, children generally having a better prognosis than adults. The Eurocare study gave weighted estimates of 5-year survival as 51% for boys and 58% for girls diagnosed between 1983 and 1985 (Berrino et al 1995). In Australia between 1978 and 1982, the 5-year survival proportions for children aged <15 years were as follows: astrocytoma 73%; medulloblastoma 43%, and ependymoma 44% (Australian Paediatric Cancer Registry 1989). Survival proportions for childhood CNS tumors in Victoria improved between 1970 and 1979 and between 1980 and 1989 (Giles et al 1993). Although the 5-year survival from astrocytoma (70% to 80%) and medulloblastoma (50% to 53%) both increased within these two time periods, only survival from ependymoma increased significantly (37% to 59%). Children in England and Wales diagnosed during 1971–1974 obtained 5-year survival proportions of 56% for astrocytoma; 24% for medulloblastoma, and 36% for ependymoma (Office of Population Censuses and Surveys 1981). Astrocytomas in childhood are commonly of lower grade than those in adults and this improves prognosis. A review of astrocytomas from the Manchester Children's Tumour Registry (Kibirige et al 1989) observed higher 5-year survival proportions for children with juvenile astrocytomas (75%) compared with children having higher grade, adult astrocytomas (15%). The EUROCARE study examined variation in survival from childhood CNS malignancies across Europe between 1978 and 1992 and found it to be substantial; the 5-year survival estimates for all CNS tumors were >60% for Northern Europe, Italy and Poland; 50–60% for the UK, Germany, Switzerland and Slovakia, and <50% for France and Estonia (Magnani et al 2001). The EUROCARE study also made comparisons of its estimates with those from SEER, Canada and Victoria for childhood CNS tumors diagnosed in the 1980s and reported some similarities in outcome with 5-year survival estimates for ependymoma ranging from 55–64%, for astrocytoma from 71–80% and PNET from 48–55% (Magnani et al 2001). In comparison, the 1-, 5- and 10-year relative survival proportions for malignant brain tumors in Australians aged <15 years when diagnosed between 1998 and 2004 were 73%, 56%, and 53%, respectively, with little evidence of change since 1982 (AIHW et al 2008b). The latest CBTRUS survival statistics (2008) for children aged <15 years can be found in Table 4.4 for each histologic group.

Host factors

Personal characteristics, medical history including immunologic status, family history, and genetic factors have been reported to be associated with CNS tumor risk. In most instances these associations are weak and inconsistent, a result of too many small studies trying to cover multiple factors. The strongest associations seen with respect to host factors are rare genetic syndromes, a family history of CNS tumors, and congenital malformations.

Associations with maternal and reproductive factors tend to be isolated reports from small studies that require corroboration. Positive associations have been reported with a prior history of abortion (Choi et al 1970a) and increased maternal age (Selvin & Garfinkel 1972). The occurrence of CNS tumors during pregnancy has been reviewed by Roelvink et al (1987), who concluded that some CNS tumors are hormone sensitive and might respond to the changing hormonal milieu during pregnancy. Many CNS tumors have been shown to possess hormone receptors (Romić Stojković et al 1990). The relationships are not established and might prove to be provocative rather than causal. It is interesting that meningiomas, which occur more often for women than men, have been associated with a prior history of breast cancer (Schoenberg et al 1975; Smith et al 1978), a hormone-dependent malignancy. Schlehofer and colleagues (1992b) reported that menopausal women had a much reduced risk of meningioma, which decreased further for women who had had a bilateral oophorectomy prior to menopause. Menopausal women were at increased risk of gliomas and acoustic neuromas unless the menopause had been surgically induced. These findings support a role for female hormones in CNS tumor development. A large population-based study of reproductive history in Swedish women showed very little by way of association (Lambe et al 1997). Their main finding was a 24% reduction in the risk of glioma, but not meningioma, for ever-parous women, compared with nulliparous.

Older age (≥14 vs <12 years of age) at menarche has been associated with increased risk of glioma, OR 1.90 (1.09, 3.32) (Hatch et al 2005). Huang et al (2004) also reported that glioma risk increased with older age at menarche (p for trend = 0.009), but only for postmenopausal women, while another study reported no association (Lee et al 2006). On the other hand, menopausal status and age at menopause are reported not to be associated with meningioma or glioma risk (Wigertz et al 2008). Having a first birth before age 20 compared with none has been reported to be associated with reduced risk of glioma, OR 0.43 (0.23, 0.83), but with little effect of number of births (Hatch et al 2005). This is supported by a report of decreased glioma risk associated with ever-parous compared with never-parous, OR 0.8 (0.6, 1.0) (Wigertz et al 2008). A protective effect for meningioma has been observed for pregnancy that increased with number and age at first pregnancy; for three or more pregnancies compared with none, the OR was 0.3 (0.2, 0.6) (Lee et al 2006). In another study, meningioma risk for women aged <50 years (but not for older women) increased with number of pregnancies leading to a live birth, the OR was 1.8 (1.1, 2.8) for women giving birth to three children compared with nulliparous women (Wigertz et al 2008).

Breast-feeding has been associated with glioma risk, OR 2.2 (1.3, 3.9) for breast-feeding 36 months or more compared with breast-feeding 3 months or less (Wigertz et al 2008). Another study that compared women who never breast-fed with women who breast-fed >18 months over their lifetime, reported an OR 1.8 (1.1, 2.9) (Huang et al 2004). There is inconsistent evidence of an association between the use of the oral contraceptive pill or hormone replacement therapy and meningioma risk (Lee et al 2006; Claus et el. 2007; Wigertz et al 2006), and the use of exogenous hormones has been associated with both a reduced risk (Hatch et al 2005; Huang et al 2004) and no risk (Wigertz et al 2006) of glioma.

In regard to characteristics at birth, associations have been described with first birth and greater birth weight (Gold et al 1979; Emerson et al 1991; Kuijten & Bunin 1993). Being a first-born was the only significant risk factor to emerge from a large case–control study in Melbourne, Australia; OR 2.0 (1.4, 2.9) (Cicuttini et al 1997). In a prospective study of occurrence of childhood CNS tumors in Norway, associations have been shown with season of birth (higher in winter), birth weight and medulloblastoma (positive), and paternal age (negative) (Heuch et al 1998). A US case–control study has also reported season of birth to be associated with glioma and meningioma risk, with peaks in January–February and troughs in July–August, suggesting the importance of seasonally varying exposures during the pre- or postnatal period in the development of adult brain tumors (Brenner et al 2004).

The risk of astrocytoma in childhood has been associated with older maternal age and a history of prior fetal deaths (Emerson et al 1991). A record linkage study in Australia reported strong associations between congenital malformations and CNS tumor risk, especially malformations of the nervous system, OR 27.8 (6.1, 127) and those of the eye, face, and neck, OR 16.8 (2.7, 103) (Altmann et al 1998). A similar study of 5.2 million children in Norway and Sweden also reported malformations of the nervous system to be associated with increased risk of CNS cancers (Norway SIR, 58 (41, 80); Sweden SIR 8.3 (4.0, 15) (Bjørge et al 2008).

Several intercurrent diseases and chronic conditions including hypertension, stroke, diabetes, epilepsy, and cranial trauma, have also been investigated in regard to their potential influence on CNS tumor risk. Hypertension was not associated with either glioma or meningioma risk for Seventh-Day Adventists (Mills et al 1989b). Stroke has been reported to be associated with risk (OR 6.26) of meningioma for women (Mills et al 1989b), and with glioblastoma (Dobkin 1985), and with both (Schwartzbaum et al 2005). Diabetes has been associated with both increased risk (Mills et al 1989b; Schwartzbaum et al 2005) and decreased risk of glioma (Aronson & Aronson 1965), and with increased risk of glioma and meningioma (Schwartzbaum et al 2005). Epilepsy (or its treatment) has been associated with excess risk of CNS tumors (Clemmesen et al 1974; Schwartzbaum et al 2005), but the two are confounded. A recent review concluded that epilepsy did not cause brain tumors, but that the tumors caused epilepsy (Singh et al 2005). The role of trauma has been a contentious issue, but is now considered not to be causal in relation to glioma (Hochberg et al 1990; Schlehofer et al 1992a). Some reports suggest an increased risk of meningioma associated with a history of head injury (Schoenberg 1991; Phillips et al 2002) and follow-up of 228 055 hospitalizations for head injury in Danish residents has shown a non-significant 15% increase for CNS tumors, SIR 1.15 (0.9, 1.3); and the (statistically insignificant) SIRs for glioma were

1.0, meningioma 1.2, and neurilemmoma 0.8. Based on only 15 cases, an SIR of 2.6 (1.4, 4.2) was reported for hemangiomas (Inskip et al 1998). A recent consensus stated head injury is probably not a risk factor for CNS tumors (Bondy et al 2008). Tonsillectomy has been positively associated with glioma in one study (Mills et al 1989b), and either not or negatively associated with glioma in two others (Gold et al 1979; Preston-Martin et al 1982). A pooled analysis of case–control studies reported no associations between previous medical conditions and risk of meningioma, but identified for glioma increased risks associated with epilepsy and decreased risks associated with infectious diseases and allergic and atopic conditions (Schlehofer et al 1999).

An association between allergy and CNS tumor risk has long been recognized (Vena et al 1985; McWhorter 1988) and has been associated with decreased risk of CNS tumor in some studies (Hochberg et al 1990; Ryan et al 1992; Schlehofer et al 1992a, 1999), especially for glioma, but not in all (Cicuttini et al 1997). An early review of evidence from cohort studies, which are less prone to bias than case–control studies, but which had small numbers of CNS cancers, concluded there was no strong evidence against, and some for, the hypothesis that allergies reduce glioma risk (Schwartzbaum et al 2003). Because it has offered one of the few leads regarding etiology, the association has sparked further research that has confirmed reduced risks (ORs 0.60–0.70) for glioma (Brenner et al 2002; Wigertz et al 2007; Linos et al 2007) and weaker evidence for meningioma (Linos et al 2007; Schoemaker et al 2007) associated with various markers of allergy. Both increased (Hagströmer et al 2005) and decreased risk of brain tumors associated with atopic disease (Wang & Diepgen 2006; Linos et al 2007) has also been reported. Immunoglobulin E serum concentration (a marker of allergy/atopy status) has also been reported to be associated with reduced risk of adult glioma (Wiemels et al 2004). Asthma and eczema have been associated with reduced risk of childhood brain tumors, especially PNET (Harding et al 2008). Others have examined the use of antihistamines and have reported an increased risk for glioma for adults (Scheurer et al 2008) and for childhood brain tumors (Cordier et al 1994); the medications for allergies seemingly abnegating any protective effect. As allergies and atopy promote immune and inflammatory responses, others have examined the use of aspirin and other non-steroidal anti-inflammatory drugs (NSAIDS) and report a 33–50% protective effect against glioma for adults (Scheurer et al 2008; Sivak-Sears et al 2004). Examining genetic variants for key molecules in the immune/inflammatory response pathway, certain cytokine (IL4R and IL13) polymorphisms associated with asthma have been reported to be inversely related with risk of GBM (Schwartzbaum et al 2005). However, further research produced null associations with individual polymorphisms, but suggestive associations with certain IL4R and IL13 haplotypes (Wiemels et al 2007). Using a pooled analysis of cytokine SNPs measured in two large independent case–control studies (overall 756 cases and 1190 controls), the IL4 (rs2243248, 21098T>G) and IL6 (rs1800795, 2174G>C) polymorphisms were shown to be significantly associated with risk of glioma, although even with these numbers, statistical power remained an issue (Brenner et al 2007).

Multiple primary tumors following primary brain tumors have been investigated by the Connecticut and Denmark cancer registries. For Connecticut residents diagnosed with CNS tumors between 1935 and 1982, significant excesses of melanoma and acute non-lymphocytic leukemia were observed (Tucker et al 1985). In Denmark between 1943 and 1984, the RRs for second primaries were kidney 3.2; bone 6.9; connective tissue 4.9; melanoma (females only) 2.5; secondary brain tumors 2.0, and CLL (males only) 3.2 (Osterlind et al 1985). The association between breast cancer and subsequent meningioma has already been referred to (Schoenberg et al 1975). Second cancers after medulloblastoma have been reported for the USA and Sweden (Goldstein et al 1997), and excesses of cancers of the salivary glands, cervix uteri, CNS, and thyroid and acute lymphoblastic leukemia were observed. About half of these were considered to be a consequence of radiation treatment. An association between meningioma and developing breast cancer as a second primary has been reported (Helseth et al 1989; Custer et al 2002). Second primary brain tumors are reported to be increased following bladder cancer, sarcoma, leukemia, colorectal cancer, and endometrial cancer (Ahsan et al 1995). Primary brain tumors are associated with an increased risk of both CNS second tumors and non-CNS second cancers, especially non-Hodgkin lymphoma and melanoma (Salminen et al 1999). A significantly increased risk for developing meningioma after colorectal cancer and after breast cancer has been reported (Malmer et al 2000). Among patients who were diagnosed first with cancer of the brain or CNS, statistically significant excesses are reported for cancers of bone, SIR 14.4; soft tissue, SIR 4.6; brain and CNS, SIR 5.9; salivary gland, SIR 5.1; thyroid gland, SIR 2.7; acute myelocytic leukemia, SIR 4.1, and melanoma of the skin, SIR 1.7 (Inskip 2003). Following childhood CNS tumors, about 1 in 180 will develop a second non-CNS primary cancer in the 15 years following diagnosis; the SIRs being 10.6 for thyroid cancer, 2.75 for leukemia, and 2.47 for lymphoma (Maule et al 2008).

Familial clustering and genetics

As for many other malignancies, familial clustering has been observed, ORs of 2–3 being associated with a family history of CNS tumors (Wrensch et al 1997a). The literature is based largely on case reports and it is difficult to determine whether such instances are related to genetic or environmental factors shared by family members. In his review, Tijssen (1985) pointed to the concordance of histology and age at diagnosis in eight pairs of monozygotic twins; the occurrence of similar neuroglial tumors in (often consecutive) siblings; the decreased age at onset for the children of families in which both parents and children were affected with neuroglial tumors; the dominance of glioblastoma and medulloblastoma in familial CNS tumors; and the occurrence of familial meningioma in several generations, probably associated with neurofibromatosis (Sorensen et al 1985). Case–control studies have also addressed the issue of familial aggregation of CNS and other malignancies, but either identify no risk (Cicuttini et al 1997), or those that they do (ORs 1.6 to 3.0) are based on small numbers and generally lack statistical significance (Hill et al 2003; Hill et al 2004). Population-based and hospital-based family studies have

also examined this issue and have also reported mixed results ranging from no association (O'Neill et al 2002) to increased risks varying by glioma grade and age at onset with the highest SIR (9.0) being for low-grade disease and for younger siblings (Malmer et al 2002). Other family studies not only demonstrate increased risk for CNS tumors, but also increased risk for melanoma, sarcoma, and pancreatic cancers (Scheurer et al 2007b). Analysis of the Utah Population Database, which contains 1401 CNS tumors (astrocytoma/glioblastoma) with at least three generations of genealogy data, identified significantly increased risks of astrocytoma (RR 3.2) and GBM (RR 2.3) for first-degree relatives and of astrocytoma for second-degree relatives (RR 1.9) (Blumenthal & Cannon-Albright 2008). Risk estimates increased when analysis was restricted to index cases with early age at onset (<20 years of age), especially for astrocytoma, RR 9.7, $p = 0.004$ (Blumenthal & Cannon-Albright 2008).

Hirayama reported that of 168 Japanese children with CNS tumors, eight had a family history of CNS tumors compared with the 3.6 expected (Hirayama 1989). Mahaley and colleagues (1989) reported a family history of 16% in the patterns of care survey. Farwell and Flannery (1984) reported increased RRs for CNS tumors in the families of children with CNS neoplasms. The RR for CNS tumors for siblings was 8 and for parents, 5. When the analysis was limited to children with medulloblastomas, the RR for CNS tumors risk to siblings increased to 30.

Certain hereditary and congenital diseases are known to carry an increased risk of CNS tumors (Farrell & Plotkin 2007). They include neurofibromatosis (Blatt et al 1986); Bourneville's disease; Li–Fraumeni tumor syndrome (also known as the SBLA syndrome) (Lynch et al 1989); ataxia telangiectasia (Swift et al 1986); Gorlin syndrome, and Turcot syndrome (Bolande 1989). An excess risk of CNS tumors for persons with blood group A has not been substantiated (Yates & Pearce 1960; Choi et al 1970b). Several cytogenetic studies of CNS tumors have shown abnormalities, especially the loss or translocation of parts of chromosome 22 in familial meningioma and acoustic neuroma, and gains on chromosome 7, or losses on 9 or 10, in gliomas, and disturbances involving chromosomes 1, 6, 17, and 19 in other CNS tumors (Zang & Singer 1967; Bigner et al 1984; Bolger et al 1985; Seizinger et al 1986; Black 1991a, 1991b; Sehgal 1998; Ohgaki & Kleihues 2007; Ney & Lassman 2009). The loss of tumor suppressor genes seems to be a fundamental mechanism in the development of several types of CNS tumors (Bansal et al 2006; Tomkova et al 2008). In recent decades, understanding of the molecular biology of these tumors has grown, examples of which include the determination of elevated epidermal growth factor receptor, as well as platelet-derived growth factor receptor signaling, and the inactivation of p53, p16, and PTEN tumor-suppressor genes that negatively regulate specific enzymatic activities in normal glial cells (Rao & James 2004; Koul 2008). The role of other growth factors and related pathways in CNS tumorigenesis and progression continues to be elucidated (Ohgaki & Kleihues 2007; Hlobilkova et al 2007; Luwor et al 2008; Trojan et al 2007).

Epidemiologic studies have an important and growing role in identifying which individual attributes and environmental exposures increase susceptibility to, and the probability of, adverse genetic mutations (Li et al 1998; Ohgaki & Kleihues 2007). Perhaps even more important, is the strength brought by epidemiologic designs to the study of interaction between environmental exposures and common variants in genes involved in biological pathways relevant to etiologic hypotheses such as nitrosamine exposure. Epidemiologic studies of genetic association, comparing cases with controls, are limited only by statistical power and possible selection bias by ethnic status. There have been a large number of reports from genetic association studies of candidate genes for various malignancies, including CNS tumors, based largely on small case–control studies. Invariably, this research activity has produced a number of false positive associations. A meta-analysis restricted to studies published up to March 15, 2008 with at least 500 cases has reported 31 genetic associations with glioma (18 of which were statistically significant) and one with meningioma which was also statistically significant (Dong et al 2008). The meningioma association was with an SNP in *BRIP1*, OR 1.61 (1.26, 2.06). The 18 statistically significant gene-variant associations with glioma were in 11 genes: one in *ATR*, OR 1.4; four in *CHAF1*, ORs 1.25–1.47; two in *DCLRE1B*, ORs 0.36; two in *ERCC1*, ORs 0.76 and 0.79; one in *IL4*, OR 1.44; one in *IL6*, OR 0.70: one in *NEIL3*, OR 1.29; one in *MSH5*, OR 0.67; one in *POLD1*, OR 0.53; three in *RPA3*, ORs 1.43–1.47 and one in *TP53*, OR 1.34 (Dong et al 2008). Although many other smaller studies of gene-variant associations have been published, these are generally unreliable. The increasing accuracy and throughput speed and decreasing cost of genotyping herald a new era of gene-variant association studies that will measure many thousands of SNPs rather than a few (Dong et al 2008). This will require large collaborations to pool the DNAs from thousands of cases and controls and such efforts are already underway in association with genome-wide association studies (Malmer et al 2007; Bondy et al 2008). While this move is laudable, progress will be confounded if the heterogeneity within CNS tumors is not taken into account, and strong arguments remain for continuing a candidate gene approach to gene-variant associations-specific histology groups, albeit measuring many more SNPs (Bondy et al 2008).

Because of the small effect sizes (ORs of 1.1–1.6) associated with common gene-variants, the study of gene–environment interaction requires much larger sample sizes than previously considered. Although statistical power can be increased by pooling data from several studies, what is difficult to achieve with respect to studying gene–environment interaction, is the standard measurement of relevant environmental exposures across individual studies. This is even more difficult when pooling case–control studies that measure exposures retrospectively and are subject to recall bias. One way forward would be to pool data for cases and controls from prospective cohort studies, but this approach also has limitations, including small numbers of incident cases and lack of commonality of exposure assessment.

Environmental factors

The literature contains many reports of associations between environmental agents and increased risk of CNS tumors. Given the large number of studies, their low statistical power,

and the number of multiple comparisons made, it is to be expected that many of these will have been chance associations (Ahlbom 1990). Isolated reports and contradictory findings, therefore, have to be viewed with a degree of skepticism. There are also methodological problems with a number of the published studies. Consistent reports from different studies are few. Taken together, the established risk factors for CNS tumors explain only a small proportion of their incidence. The strongest established risk factor for CNS tumors is ionizing radiation, especially early in life. The amount of text devoted to certain risk factors in this section essentially reflects the amount of literature on the topic, rather than its tangible importance to CNS tumor risk.

Radiation

The relationship between ionizing radiation and CNS tumors is one of the best established. However, this relationship has not been investigated as extensively as it has for leukemia and certain other cancers because the brain was for some time considered to be relatively resistant to radiation carcinogenesis (National Research Council 1980). Evidence has grown that exposures *in utero* (Bithell & Stewart 1975; Monson & MacMahon 1984) and high-dose irradiation in childhood (Ron et al 1988) and in adult life (Preston-Martin et al 1983) increase CNS tumor risk with some histology groups more than others. The association between low-dose radiological exposures *in utero* and CNS tumor risk being more difficult to establish with certainty (Bunin 2000; Gurney & van Wijngaarden 1999; Linet et al 2003), any association possibly being tumor type specific. For example a national birth cohort study in Sweden, where X-ray exposures were captured by antenatal records, reported no overall increased risk for childhood brain tumor after prenatal abdominal X-ray exposure, adjusted OR 1.02 (0.64, 1.62); but primitive neuroectodermal tumors had the highest risk estimate, OR 1.88 (0.92, 3.83) (Stalberg et al 2007). The combination of rare outcomes, such as individual histology groups of CNS tumor, and a low-dose exposure impose severe limitations on epidemiologic capacity to characterize risks with any precision.

Children irradiated for tinea capitis have been shown to have increased incidence of CNS tumors, especially meningiomas (RR 9.5), gliomas (RR 2.6), and nerve sheath tumors (RR 18.8) (Ron et al 1988). The study of almost 11 000 irradiated children after a median follow-up of 40 years, recently reported an ERR per Gy of 4.63 (2.43, 9.12) and 1.98 (0.73, 4.69) for benign meningiomas and malignant brain tumors, respectively. The estimated ERR per Gy for malignant brain tumors decreased with increasing age at irradiation from 3.56 to 0.4, while no trend with age was seen for meningiomas. The ERR for both types of tumor remains elevated at 30-plus years after exposure (Sadetzki et al 2005). The increased risk after exposures of between 1 and 2 Gy indicates the possibility of late effects from low dose radiotherapy in childhood. A follow-up of a cohort of over 28 000 Swedish children irradiated for skin hemangioma has shown a relative risk of 2.7 (1.0, 5.6) per Gy, and an increased risk with early age, the RR being 4.5 if irradiated in the first 5 months of life (Karlsson et al 1998).

Early data from atomic bomb survivors were inconsistent (Darby et al 1985), but with additional follow-up, to

1995, a statistically significant dose-related excess of CNS tumors has been observed for the survivor cohort with an excess relative risk (ERR) per sievert (ERRSv) of 1.2 (0.6, 2.1). The highest ERRSv was for schwannoma, 4.5 (1.9, 9.2). Non-statistically significant ERRSv were reported for meningiomas, 0.6 (–0.01, 1.8), gliomas, 0.6 (–0.2, 2.0) and other CNS tumors, 0.5 (–0.2, 2.2). For nervous system tumors other than schwannoma, ERRSv were higher for men than for women and for those exposed during childhood than for those exposed during adulthood (Preston et al 2002, 2007, 2008). A follow-up study of the Chernobyl clean-up workers has reported a SIR for brain cancer of 2.14 (1.07, 3.83) based on 11 cases (Rahu et al 2006), but there was no evidence of a dose response and the relationship to radiation exposure remains to be established.

GBM and ependymomas have been induced in primates given high-dose radiation (Kent & Pickering 1958; Traynor & Casey 1971; Haymaker et al 1972; Krupp 1976). Case reports for humans have been reviewed by Salvati et al (1991). For adults, high-dose irradiation of the head has been shown to increase the risk of meningioma (Munk et al 1969). The role of low-dose ionizing radiation is less clear. Dental X-rays have been shown to increase the risk of meningioma, especially for women (Preston-Martin et al 1980, 1983; Preston-Martin 1985; Ryan et al 1992), but not glioma where an OR estimate was 0.42 (Ryan et al 1992). Increased risks for dentists and dental nurses have been reported (Ahlbom et al 1986). Others have examined dental X-rays and report a marginal OR estimate of 2.1 (1.0, 4.3) for meningioma, but risks close to unity for other CNS tumors (Rodvall et al 1998). Longstreth et al (2004) reported an association between ≥6 full-mouth series of dental X-rays 15–40 years before diagnosis and risk of meningioma, OR 2.06 (1.03, 4.17), but no association with modern X-ray dose regimes. Studies of occupational exposure to ionizing radiation have not reported increased risks for brain tumors (Sont et al 2001; Mohan et al 2003; Cardis et al 2005). A recent case–control study of meningioma and ionizing radiation reported no significant associations with diagnostic or occupational exposures (Phillips et al 2005). Blettner et al (2007), in the German component of the INTERPHONE study, reported no statistically significant increased risk between any exposure to medical ionizing radiation and CNS tumors, OR 0.63 (0.48, 0.83) for glioma, 1.08 (0.80, 1.45) for meningioma and 0.97 (0.54, 1.75) for acoustic neuroma. In the same study, radiotherapy to the head and neck regions was associated with non-significant ORs of 2.32 (0.90, 5.96) for meningioma and 6.45 (0.62, 67.16) for and acoustic neuroma, the wide confidence intervals reflecting the small sample size (Blettner et al 2007).

A role for non-ionizing radiation in the etiology of human CNS tumors has been controversial. This form of radiation does not have tumor initiating properties, but has been considered possibly to have promoting effects, if any (Poole & Trichopoulos 1991). It has been suggested that residential magnetic fields may relate to the development of CNS tumors in children (Wertheimer & Leeper 1979). Several studies of residential and occupational magnetic field exposures followed (Easterly 1981; Ahlbom 1988; Coleman & Beral 1988; Savitz et al 1988). The National Radiation Protection Board's review gave pooled estimates of the ORs for CNS tumors

from studies of measured fields as 1.85 (0.91, 3.77); from distance studies as 1.09 (0.50, 2.37); and for wire coding studies as 2.04 (1.11, 3.76) (National Radiation Protection Board 1992). Feychting & Ahlbom (1993) failed to find any significant associations between electromagnetic field (EMF) exposures and childhood CNS tumors. Most studies of magnetic fields and childhood tumors have suffered from problems of selection and recall bias, lack of control of confounders, and poor statistical power. The study by Feychting & Ahlbom (1993) made some progress in that it was free of bias and was able to examine some potential confounders (SES and traffic pollution showed no effect). Subsequent studies also failed to find further support for an effect on brain tumors (Preston-Martin et al 1996; Miller et al 1997; Dockerty et al 1998). Reviews of childhood CNS tumors in relation to EMF have concluded that there is little or no evidence in support of a link between EMF exposure and childhood brain cancer development (Kheifets 2001; IARC 2002; Ahlbom et al 2001; NIEHS 1999). A recent meta-analysis on this topic gave a summary OR of 0.88 (0.57, 1.37) for distance <50 m and 1.14 (0.78, 1.67) for calculated or measured magnetic fields above 0.2 μT. For measured or calculated exposures above 0.3 or 0.4 μT, the summary OR was 1.68 (0.83, 3.43), which did not vary by exposure assessment method, so the possibility of a moderate risk increase at high exposures could not be excluded (Mezei et al 2008). The occupational literature between 1993 and 2007 on EMF and CNS tumors has also been re-examined in a meta-analysis; although there was an overall pooled estimate of a 10% increase in risk for brain cancer, the lack of a clear pattern of EMF exposure and risk did not support a hypothesis that these exposures are responsible for the observed excess risk (Kheifets et al 2008). This was also the finding of a recent case–control study of glioma and meningioma (Coble et al 2009).

A possible association between mobile (cellular) telephone use and CNS tumor risk remains highly topical, having aroused considerable debate over the last decade. Several authorities have reviewed the extensive literature on possible health effects, including CNS tumors, and have generally not recognized a substantially increased risk but, because of the limited amount of follow-up currently available, could not exclude a long-term risk associated with high levels of use (Krewski 2001; Boice & McLaughlin 2006). The various published studies report inconsistent findings and those that accept the positive reports call for adherence to the precautionary principle, especially in face of the possibility of long-term risks and the increasing prevalence of mobile phone use by children (Hardell 2007; Krewski et al 2007; Carpenter & Sage 2008). A recent meta-analysis of studies having users with 10 or more years of exposure produced combined ORs of 1.5 (1.2, 1.8) for glioma, 1.3 (0.95, 1.9) for acoustic neuroma, and 1.1 (0.8, 1.4), for meningioma (Kundi 2009). Research on this topic is challenging, for the reasons that have been given earlier in this chapter. Added to the usual challenges of studying CNS tumors is the considerable problem of measuring exposure to mobile phone use and how to translate this into valid estimates of intracranial exposure to radio-frequency radiation (Cardis et al 2007). The research design that has most commonly been adopted to address this question is the case–control study, which is notoriously prone to bias. This design has been chosen because of the relative rarity of CNS tumors and because of the small numbers of cases and lack of appropriate exposure assessment in existing cohort studies. The best approach to the problem so far, is an international consortium of case–control studies called INTERPHONE, coordinated by the International Agency for Research on Cancer (Cardis et al 2007). To facilitate data pooling, INTERPHONE centers in different countries have adopted similar research protocols. These arrangements do not detract from the fact that INTER-PHONE is a case–control study and, although it has paid considerable attention to addressing potential problems with exposure assessment and bias, any modest risk estimates it produces will be received with some skepticism (Berg et al 2005; Vrijheid et al 2006a,b). Although often limited in statistical power, many of the individual INTERPHONE centers have already published their analyses (Lonn et al 2005; Schoemaker et al 2005; Schüz et al 2006; Hours et al 2007). The main study findings remain to be published, but considering the individual center publications already available, the main findings are likely to be either close to unity or reflect modest risks obtained from sub-group analysis, especially of long-term (>10 years) users and ipsilateral CNS tumor location (Kundi 2009). In regard to the latter, it has been shown that 97–99% of the total electromagnetic energy deposited in the brain is absorbed at the side of the head the phone is held during calls (Cardis et al 2008). Whatever the outcome, it is unlikely to sway the opinion of one reviewer:

> *Based on the epidemiological evidence available now, the main public health concern is clearly motor vehicle collisions, a behavioral effect rather than an effect of radiofrequency exposure as such. Even if the studies in progress were to find large relative effects for brain cancer, the absolute increase in risk would probably be much smaller than the risk stemming from motor vehicle collisions.*

(Rothman 2000)

Infection

The role of infection in CNS tumor etiology is not fully understood. Isolated reports have usually been countered by lack of associations in other studies. Associations between tuberculosis (TB) and glioma have been reported (Ward et al 1973; MacPherson 1976). It has been suggested that the development of both TB and glioma might be related to an impaired immune system. A positive reaction to a TB test was associated with an increased, but statistically insignificant OR of 1.46 for glioma, and an OR of 1.49 for meningioma for Seventh-Day Adventists (Mills et al 1989b). *Toxoplasma gondii* infection has a predilection for neural tissue, which has been related to astrocytoma in one study (Schuman et al 1967); however, no association between *T. gondii* antibodies and glioma was reported by a recent Australian study that, on the contrary, showed an association (OR 2.06) with meningioma (Ryan et al 1993). Bithell et al (1973) reported an association between maternal chickenpox infection and medulloblastoma, but this finding has not been replicated (Adelstein & Donovan 1972; Gold 1980). There have also been reports of astrocytoma in patients with

multiple sclerosis (Reagan & Freiman 1973). Associations with sick pets and with farm residence have also been reported (Bunin et al 1994a).

Exposures in early life have been investigated in regard to maternal factors such as infections, but the evidence is often indirect and/or weak and inconsistent (Baldwin & Preston-Martin 2004; Shaw et al 2006). Similarly, ecological analyses of seasonal patterns of birth have been interpreted as suggestive of an infectious etiology (Brenner et al 2004; Koch et al 2006). Varicella zoster infection has continued to be of interest since earlier reports of maternal chickenpox infection during pregnancy (Bithell et al 1973), and in San Francisco, it has been shown to be protective against adult glioma, OR 0.4 (0.3, 0.6) (Wrensch et al 1997b), an observation repeated in further analyses, but not for other viruses, EBV, HCMV, VSV, HSV simplex (Wrensch et al 2001, 2005; Polterman et al 2006; Scheurer et al 2007a). C-type viruses resembling animal leukemia/sarcoma viruses have been detected in human CNS tumors (Yohn 1972). DNA from BK virus, a human papovavirus, has also been detected in human CNS tumors (Corallini et al 1987), and there has been a single report of multifocal high-grade astrocytoma in a patient with progressive multifocal leukoencephalopathy related to JC virus infection (Sima et al 1983). Footprints of simian virus 40 (a contaminant of polio vaccine given to millions of people between 1955 and 1962) have been detected in human CNS tumors, but follow-up studies have suggested no effect (Strickler et al 1998; Brenner et al 2003; Engels 2002).

CNS tumors, particularly sarcomas, have been induced in animals by several oncogenic viruses including Rous sarcoma virus, adenovirus type 12, chicken-embryo-lethal-orphan virus, simian virus 40, JC papillovirus, and both murine and avian sarcoma viruses (Pitts et al 1983; Tracy et al 1985; Kornbluth et al 1986). Evidence is accumulating that viruses may play a role in CNS carcinogenesis by gene rearrangement and amplification of normal proto-oncogenes (Charman et al 1988; Del Valle et al 2008).

Occupation

The male excess of glioma suggests that occupational exposures might be related to its occurrence (Moss 1985; Kessler & Brandt-Rauf 1987). As with other tumors, the study of occupation and CNS tumors has not been without its problems. In their review of brain tumors and occupational risk factors, Thomas & Waxweiler (1986) complained of diagnostic non-specificity, the paucity of case–control studies, the reliance on mortality studies, and the statistical inevitability of finding associations in studies which involve multiple comparisons. Little has changed. There have been more case–control studies since the mid-1980s, but these studies are not particularly suited to assessing occupational exposures, as they depend on recall, and have invariably been too small to contribute useful information. A recent comparatively large case–control study of 879 cases was inadequate for other than the detection of already identified job titles and exposures (Krishnan et al 2003). The authors commented that the large sample size enabled them to stratify results by gender and histology, but that some findings were still based on very small numbers and, due to the large number of occupations examined, some significant results may have been produced by chance (Krishnan et al 2003). Disease associations with occupational exposures are best approached by following prospectively large numbers of people known to be exposed to the agent(s) of interest, especially where the exposures have been measured with some precision.

Nevertheless, studies relating CNS tumors to occupation have continued to be published in the same tradition, tending to be based largely on job title rather than exposure to specific agents. Occupations in the electrical and electronics, oil refining, rubber, airplane manufacture, machining, farming, and pharmaceutical and chemical industries have been associated with increased CNS tumor risk (Waxweiler et al 1976). Suspect exposures include: benzene and other organic solvents; lubricating oils; acrylonitrile; vinyl chloride; formaldehyde; polycyclic aromatic hydrocarbons; phenol and phenolic compounds, and both ionizing and non-ionizing radiation (Thomas et al 1987a). A possible carcinogenic role for formaldehyde has been postulated following increased mortality from CNS tumors in embalmers (Walrath & Fraumeni 1983), subsequently supported by increased incidence for anatomists and pathologists (Harrington & Oakes 1984; Stroup et al 1986). A recent review of occupational causes of cancer highlighted non-ionizing radiation as a possible cause of brain cancer (Clapp et al 2008). Some publications report increased risk estimates, which are statistically non-significant (Buffler et al 2007; Wesseling et al 2002; Krishnan et al 2003; De Roos et al 2003). Others report significantly increased risks for a range of occupations including firefighters (Kang et al 2008), workers in the semiconductor industry (Beall et al 2005), asphalters (Pan et al 2005), and dentists (Simning & van Wijngaarden 2007). Research has also focused on lead exposure as a possible risk factor, particularly for meningioma, but risk may be limited to persons with a particular genetic susceptibility (Cocco et al 1998; van Wijngaarden & Dosemeci 2006; Rajaraman et al 2006).

There has been a sustained interest in electrical workers and their exposure to electromagnetic fields (EMF) (Lin et al 1985; Thomas et al 1987b; Speers et al 1988; Loomis & Savitz 1990; Schlehofer et al 1990). In their review of EMF and CNS tumor risk, Poole & Trichopoulos (1991) point out similar deficiencies to those reported by Thomas & Waxweiler (1986); of the 17 case–control studies that examined occupational exposures to EMF, only five were sufficiently large and well-designed to ascertain exposure to EMF more completely than using routine data from tumor registration or death certification. The available cohort studies tended not to suggest an appreciable association between occupational EMF exposure and CNS system tumors. EMF exposures in an occupational setting have already been discussed in terms of a comprehensive review. This concluded that the lack of a clear pattern of EMF exposure and risk did not support a hypothesis that these exposures are responsible for the observed excess risk (Kheifets et al 2008).

There are inconsistent reports concerning employment in oil refining. In a review of 10 refinery cohort studies from the USA, the International Agency for Research on Cancer (1989) concluded that of the elevated risks reported, only one was statistically significant, and it was limited to workers of short duration of employment. A recent nested case–control study of 15 cases of CNS neoplasms and 150 controls at a petroleum exploration and extraction research facility reported a range of non-statistically significant ORs near or below 1.0 for every exposure and factor analyzed (Buffler et al 2007).

Farming and farm residence have been associated with increased risk of CNS tumor. Farmers can come into contact with a variety of chemical agents and zoonotic viruses, but there is no firm evidence inculpating any specific exposure (Blair et al 1985). In New Zealand (Reif et al 1989), the farming risk was reported to be strongest for livestock farmers (OR 2.59). A meta-analysis of studies of farming and CNS cancer estimated a RR of 1.3 (1.09, 1.56) (Khuder et al 1998). A large international case–control study reported no associations with animals for either glioma or meningioma and an OR of 0.66 (0.5, 0.9) for general farm workers (Menegoz et al 2002). A French case–control study has reported non-statistically significant risks for glioma and meningioma and pesticide exposure (Provost et al 2007). In a case–control study from Nebraska, significant associations were reported between some specific agricultural pesticide exposures and the risk of glioma for male, but not female, farmers. However, most of the positive associations were limited to proxy respondents (Lee et al 2005). A case–control study from the USA failed to identify any association between glioma or meningioma and pesticides, but women who reported using herbicides had an OR of 2.4 (1.4, 4.3) for meningioma (Samanic et al 2008)

One report of higher levels of organochlorine compounds in the adipose tissue of glioblastoma cases compared with controls, indicates a possible carcinogenic role for pesticide exposure (Unger & Olsen 1980). Organochlorine exposure has been observed to be higher for woodworkers with glioma compared with woodworker controls (Cordier et al 1988). In a follow-up of men in the American Cancer Society Prevention Study II, an RR of 2 (1.25, 3.27) was observed for fatal CNS cancer for men who worked in a wood-related occupation (Stellman et al 1998). Men employed in agricultural crop production in Missouri had an OR of 1.5 for CNS tumors of several cell types (Brownson et al 1990), and French farmers are reported to have an SIR of 1.25 for CNS cancer; ecologic analysis ascribing this to pesticide use in vineyards (Viel et al 1998).

A variety of chemical carcinogens, including N-nitroso compounds, polycyclic aromatic hydrocarbons, acrylonitrile, and vinyl chloride, have been shown to cause brain tumors in experimental animals (Maltoni et al 1977, 1982; Swenburg 1982; Ward & Rice 1982; Zeller et al 1982; Zimmerman 1982). Rice & Ward (1982) indicated that the age dependence of chemically induced CNS tumors in experimental animals was greatest during prenatal life. Transplacental CNS carcinogenesis has been observed to occur, particularly in regard to exposure to nitrosoureas (Druckrey 1973). These observations have prompted studies of parental (usually paternal) occupational exposures in regard to the risk of tumors in children (Arundel & Kinnier-Wilson 1986; Savitz & Chen 1990). Some studies have specifically examined CNS tumors (Peters et al 1981; Olshan et al 1986; Johnson et al 1987; Nasca et al 1988; Wilkins & Koutras 1988; Johnson & Spitz 1989), but some studies have included neuroblastomas with CNS tumors (Wilkins & Hundley 1990).

Savitz & Chen (1990) summarized the findings of studies of CNS tumors as follows: inconsistent associations with motor vehicle related occupations; an unreplicated OR of 4.4 for machine repairmen; elevated risks for painters in three of four studies; and consistently elevated ORs associated with occupations in chemical and petroleum industries and electrical-related occupations. Occupational and industrial exposures to ionizing radiation were consistent with ORs of 2.0. They noted isolated reports of associations with metal-related occupations, farming, construction, aircraft industry, and printing. A case–control study in the USA detected an OR for CNS cancer of 2.3 (1.3, 4.0) for paternal occupation as an electrical worker, and an OR for astroglial tumors of 2.1 (1.1, 3.9) for paternal occupation in the chemical industry (McKean-Cowdin et al 1998). Maternal occupation in the chemical industry was associated with OR 3.3 (1.4, 7.7) for astroglial tumors. A European case–control study that focused on parental exposure to solvents and polycyclic aromatic hydrocarbons (PAH) during the 5-year period before birth reported elevated ORs for paternal employment in agriculture and in motor vehicle occupations. Paternal exposure to PAH was associated with an increased risk of PNET (OR 2), and maternal exposure to 'high' levels of solvents gave ORs of 2.3 (0.9, 5.8) with astroglial tumors and 3.2 (1.0, 10.3) with PNET (Cordier et al 1997). A review of parental occupation concluded that there was evidence of an association between childhood CNS tumors and paternal exposure to paint, but that better research was needed before definitive statements or actions could be made (Colt & Blair 1998). An international case–control study of childhood brain cancer reported several maternal and child farm exposures associated with increased risk, including various animals and agricultural chemicals (Efird et al 2003). No associations with parental occupation were reported by a study from Taiwan (Mazumdar et al 2008).

Diet

Associations between diet and CNS tumors in humans remain weak and inconsistent. International correlations have been reported between CNS tumors and *per capita* consumption of total fat, animal protein, and fats and oils (Armstrong & Doll 1975), but these correlations could easily be due to international differences in technological development and ethnic differences in susceptibility. Most dietary epidemiologic studies of CNS tumors have been retrospective case–control studies, have used poor measures of dietary intake, and have been too small to detect modest risks. The question of diet and CNS tumors is best explored by prospective cohort studies and there are plans to do this by pooling data from several large international cohorts (Smith-Warner et al 2006).

A long-standing dietary hypothesis is that the consumption, and endogenous production, of N-nitroso compounds and their precursors, might increase brain tumor risk (Preston-Martin & Correa 1989), but the reports from case–control studies have been inconsistent and a prospective study of Seventh-Day Adventists (Mills et al 1989a) reported discrepant and non-significant associations with dietary items. Nothing has stopped a steady stream of case–control studies providing additional low quality information on CNS

tumor risk. Burch et al (1987) reported a protective effect of fruit, but not vegetables. Preston-Martin (1989) reported a non-significant protective association between citrus fruit and meningioma. A case–control study from Germany (Boeing et al 1993) reported an increased glioma risk associated with the consumption of ham, processed pork, and fried bacon, but no association with endogenous N-nitrosation, or with the intake of vitamin C, or fruit and vegetables. An Australian case–control study reported no increased risk for glioma or meningioma with the regular consumption of foods rich in N-nitroso precursors, nor were there any decreases in risk associated with the regular use of foods and supplements containing endogenous nitrosation inhibitors (Ryan et al 1992). A case–control study from Israel also failed to find any direct association with nitrosamine intake (Kaplan et al 1997) and neither did a case–control study from Nebraska, showing instead protective effects of fruit and vegetables and related nutrients (Chen et al 2002). The latter report is supported by a case–control study from San Francisco that observed inverse associations between antioxidant and phytoestrogen intakes and glioma risk (Tedeschi-Blok et al 2006). A meta-analysis of cured meat consumption and glioma risk concluded that the available data did not provide clear support for an association (Huncharek et al 2003). Further, a pooled analysis of gliomas from three US prospective cohort studies reported no associations with fruit or vegetables or carotenoid consumption (Holick et al 2007b).

Some have approached the N-nitroso dietary hypothesis in regard to childhood CNS tumors. The consumption of orange juice and vitamin supplements (which contain antioxidant substances such as ascorbic acid that inhibit endogenous nitrosation activity) have been associated with reduced risk of childhood CNS tumors (Preston-Martin & Henderson 1983; Howe et al 1989). In a study of PNET in children aged <6 years, vegetable and fruit juice consumption, and the maternal use of vitamin supplements during pregnancy were reported to be protective, but no significant effect was observed in regard to nitrosamines from food (Bunin et al 1993). A pooled analysis of an international collaborative study of childhood CNS tumors also provided supportive evidence of a non-specific protective effect of maternal vitamin supplementation during pregnancy, OR 0.5 (0.3, 0.8) (Preston-Martin et al 1998). A review of childhood cancer in relation to cured meat considered that, at this time, it cannot be concluded that eating cured meat has increased the risk of childhood brain cancer and that unbiased evaluation of the hypothesis may derive from the conduct of cohort studies (Blot et al 1999). The review's concern was based on the studies potential for bias, especially recall bias, and/or confounding, the relatively weak magnitude of the associations reported, and the inconsistency between study findings. The hypothesis continues to attract support, particularly in regard to maternal consumption of relevant dietary constituents (Pogoda et al 2001; Dietrich et al 2005). An international case–control study of maternal diet and childhood brain cancer risk has reported histology-specific risks and the cured meat association was limited to astrocytomas, with ORs comparing extreme quartiles of consumption ranging from 1.8 to 2.5 across astrocytoma subtypes (Pogoda et al 2009).

Alcohol

The evidence linking alcoholic beverages with CNS tumors is sparse and inconsistent, and largely negative. Choi (1970b) reported that fewer CNS tumor patients had ever drunk alcohol compared with controls. Brain tumor risk has been associated in one study with increased consumption of wine (Burch et al 1987). This finding was not supported by Preston-Martin et al (1989a), who reported no association with alcohol intake. Ryan reported decreased risks for glioma and meningioma, with all forms of alcohol consumption, a significant reduction in risk (OR 0.58) being observed for glioma and wine consumption (Ryan et al 1992). Boeing and colleagues (1993) reported no associations between lifetime alcoholic beverage consumption, either for total alcohol or for single beverages. A significant positive association between childhood CNS tumors and the mother drinking beer in pregnancy was observed by Howe et al (1989). This finding was also seen in a study of childhood astrocytic glioma and PNET, where maternal beer drinking yielded an OR of 4.0 (1.1–22.1) for either tumor (Bunin et al 1994b). A prospective analysis within a large managed-care cohort reported no association between glioma risk and alcohol (Efird et al 2004).

Tobacco

Associations have been shown between passive smoking and childhood CNS tumors (Gold et al 1979; Preston-Martin et al 1982). In a cohort study in Japan, non-smoking wives of men who smoked more than 20 cigarettes a day were shown to have a rate of brain tumor almost five times (95% CI, 1.72–14.11) that of women married to non-smokers (Hirayama 1985). Ryan et al (1992) reported no associations with glioma, but direct and passive smoking increases risk for meningioma, especially for women. Increasing risk of CNS tumors was associated with increasing consumption of 'plain cigarettes' (Burch et al 1987). No association was reported in a cohort of Seventh-Day Adventists (Mills et al 1989a). Choi and colleagues (1970b) did not find any increased risk of CNS tumors associated with smoking, and neither did Brownson et al (1990). The passive smoking findings are difficult to interpret given the lack of direct association between smoking and CNS tumors (Hirayama 1985). A pooled analysis of prospective cohort studies reported no association with glioma risk between baseline or updated smoking status, intensity, duration, or age at smoking initiation for men or women (Holick et al 2007). A prospective analysis within a large managed-care cohort reported individuals who smoked marijuana at least once a month, after adjusting for cigarette smoking and other confounders, had a 2.8-fold (1.3, 6.2) increased risk for glioma (Efird et al 2004).

Drugs

Clemmesen first raised the question of anticonvulsants causing brain tumor among epileptics who were long-term users (Clemmesen et al 1974). An increased risk of childhood brain tumor was shown in mothers who had used barbiturates during pregnancy (Gold et al 1979), but this was not supported by a later study (Preston-Martin et al 1982). A

review of the evidence (MacMahon 1985) concluded that there was no effect on CNS tumors in humans. A recent study of Danish epileptics confirmed an excess risk of CNS tumors after diagnosis of epilepsy, which then declined with further follow-up, indicating that epilepsy, rather than the phenobarbital used to treat it, was associated with the CNS tumor (Olsen et al 1989). A review concludes that the evidence for human carcinogenicity of older antiepileptic drugs is not consistent, they are considered only possibly carcinogenic, and the review suggests that modern drugs used to treat epilepsy are unlikely to be related to risk (Singh et al 2005).

Mills reported increased, but statistically non-significant risks for meningioma associated with the regular use of analgesics and tranquilizers and increased risk of glioma associated with the regular use of tranquilizers (Mills et al 1989b). Preston-Martin & Henderson (1983) reported increased risk of childhood CNS tumors for children whose mothers took antihistamines or diuretics during pregnancy. These findings were not confirmed in a later study of adult CNS tumors (Ryan et al 1992). The regular long-term use of antihistamines by those reporting a history of asthma or allergies is significantly associated with a 3.5-fold increase in the risk for glioma, while the regular use of NSAIDs is reported to reduce glioma risk by 33% (Scheurer et al 2008).

Other associations

Some studies have reported a relationship between serum cholesterol and increased risk of CNS tumors (Smith & Shipley 1989). This has been refuted by a large cohort study in Finland (Knekt et al 1991). Extremely loud noise is reported to be a risk factor for acoustic neuroma (Preston-Martin et al 1989b). A relative risk of 1.7 for childhood brain tumors has been reported with residential proximity to traffic densities of more than 500 vehicles a day (Savitz & Feingold 1989), a suspected agent being benzene from car exhaust. A suggested role for pesticide exposure and childhood CNS tumor risk was reviewed (Zahm & Ward 1998), but at that time, there was insufficient evidence to inculpate pesticides as a cause of childhood CNS tumors, most of the data were from case reports and small case–control studies that had poorly measured exposures. An updated review included an additional 21 studies, 15 of which reported statistically significant increased risks between either childhood pesticide exposure or parental occupational exposure and childhood cancer (Infante-Rivard & Weichenthal 2007). Although the evidence for an association between pesticide exposure and CNS tumors is growing, the studies have several problems that have already been alluded to above, including exposure assessment and poor control of confounders (Infante-Rivard & Weichenthal 2007).

Non-neuroepithelial tumors

Renal transplant patients have long been known to be at increased risk of CNS (Hoover & Fraumeni 1973). The incidence of CNS lymphomas has increased since the HIV/AIDS epidemic produced large numbers of immune compromised people. There is evidence, however, that CNS lymphoma was increasing prior to this time, and that the increase was unrelated to trends in organ transplantation (Eby et al 1988). Since the HIV epidemic, cases of cerebral Kaposi's sarcoma have been reported (Charman et al 1988), as have increases in cerebral lymphomas (Biggar et al 1987). Since the introduction of combination antiretroviral therapy, the incidence of cerebral lymphoma has decreased in parallel with AIDS-defining infections (Bonnet & Chêne 2008).

The annual incidence of pituitary tumors is said to be approximately 1/100 000 population (Schoenberg 1991). Little is known of the epidemiology of pituitary tumors. They appear to occur more often in black Americans than in whites (Heshmat et al 1976). Different histologic types of tumor occur in the pineal region, pinealomas being very rare. The incidence of pineal tumors in Japan is up to nine times higher than elsewhere, and the regional variation of pineal tumors within Japan is very marked (Hirayama 1985). Such strong geographic variation suggests that an environmental factor is involved in etiology, or that genetic factors are specific to a geographically discrete population.

Metastatic tumors

Most epidemiologic studies of CNS tumors have concentrated on primary tumors, and data regarding metastatic disease are limited. An annual incidence rate of 8.3/100 000 was reported in one North American study between 1973 and 1974 (Walker et al 1985). Rates of 11/100 000 and 5.4/100 000 were previously reported in another North American study (Percy et al 1972) and a British study (Brewis et al 1966), respectively. In the study of Walker et al (1985), metastases were more common for men than women (9.7 vs 7.1/100 000). The rate was <1/100 000 before the age of 35 years and increased to >30/100 000 after the age of 60 years. The most common primary site was the lung. For women, metastases from the breast were equal in frequency to metastases from the lung. Metastases from cutaneous malignant melanoma were the third commonest secondary neoplasm. The true extent of metastasis to the brain is unknown, but likely to be far greater than previously estimated (Sul & Posner 2007).

Future prospects for epidemiology

Although the epidemiology of CNS tumors remains poorly understood, there is little need for any more studies, particularly case–control studies, similar to those that have been conducted over recent decades. The pooled results of multi-centered case–control studies coordinated by the SEARCH program of the International Agency for Research on Cancer have largely been published, but their net contribution to our understanding of the epidemiology of CNS tumors is not extensive; the individual studies tend to be small, the measurement of exposures is poor, and the strengths of association are weak. Their combined analysis probably represents what is maximally achievable using conventional case–control designs.

The future for epidemiologic studies of CNS tumors is in research that embraces molecular biology in the search for accurate and specific markers of genetic susceptibility, and accurate assessment of temporally relevant environmental exposures to carcinogenic agents, for specific histologic subtypes of CNS tumor (Bondy et al 2008). Such studies would best be couched within large prospective cohort studies,

several of which are currently in progress around the world, that will be able to pool data to test hypotheses and gene-environment interactions with rigor.

REFERENCES

Adelstein, **A.M.**, **Donovan**, **J.W.**, 1972. Malignant disease in children whose mothers had chickenpox, mumps, or rubella in pregnancy. BMJ 4 (5841), 629–631.

Ahlbom, **A.**, 1988. A review of the epidemiologic literature on magnetic fields and cancer. Scand. J. Work Environ. Health 14 (6), 337–343.

Ahlbom, **A.**, 1990. Some notes on brain tumor epidemiology. Ann. N. Y. Acad. Sci. 609, 179–190.

Ahlbom, **A.**, **Norell**, **S.**, **Rodvall**, **Y.**, **et al.**, 1986. Dentists, dental nurses, and brain tumours. BMJ. (Clin. Res. Ed.) 292 (6521), 662.

Ahlbom, **A.**, **Rodvall**, **Y.**, 1989. Brain tumour trends. Lancet. (letter) ii, 1272.

Ahlbom, **I.C.**, **Cardis**, **E.**, **Green**, **A.**, **et al.**, 2001. Review of the epidemiologic literature on EMF and Health. Environ. Health Perspect 109 (Suppl. 6), 911–933.

Ahsan, **H.**, **Neugut**, **A.I.**, **Bruce**, **J.N.**, 1995. Association of malignant brain tumors and cancers of other sites. J. Clin. Oncol. 13 (12), 2931–2935.

AIHW (Australian Institute of Health and Welfare) and AACR (Australasian Association of Cancer Registries), 2008a. Cancer in Australia: an overview, Vol. CAN 46. AIHW, Canberra.

AIHW (Australian Institute of Health and Welfare) and AACR (Australasian Association of Cancer Registries), 2008b. Cancer survival and prevalence in Australia: cancers diagnosed from 1982 to 2004, Vol. 42. AIHW, Canberra.

Altmann, **A.E.**, **Halliday**, **J.L.**, **Giles**, **G.G.**, 1998. Associations between congenital malformations and childhood cancer. A register-based case–control study. Br. J. Cancer 78 (9), 1244–1249.

Armitage, **P.**, **Doll**, **R.**, 1954. The age distribution of cancer and a multi-stage theory of carcinogenesis. Br. J. Cancer 8 (1), 1–12.

Armstrong, **B.**, **Almes**, **M.**, **Buffler**, **P.**, **et al.**, 1990. A cluster classification for histologic diagnoses on CNS tumors in an epidemiological study. Neuroepidemiology 9, 2–16.

Armstrong, **B.**, **Doll**, **R.**, 1975. Environmental factors and cancer incidence and mortality in different countries, with special reference to dietary practices. Int. J. Cancer 15 (4), 617–631.

Armstrong, **B.K.**, **Woodings**, **T.L.**, **Stenhouse**, **N.S.**, **et al.**, 1983. Mortality from cancer in migrants to Australia 1962–1971. University of Western Australia, Perth.

Aronson, **S.M.**, **Aronson**, **B.E.**, 1965. Central nervous system in diabetes mellitus: lowered frequency of certain intracranial neoplasms. Arch. Neurol. 12, 390–398.

Arundel, **S.E.**, **Kinnier-Wilson**, **L.M.**, 1986. Parental occupations and cancer: a review of the literature. J. Epidemiol. Community Health 40 (1), 30–36.

Australian Paediatric Cancer Registry, 1989. Childhood cancer incidence and survival, Australia 1978 to 1984. Australian Paediatric Cancer Registry, Brisbane.

Bahemuka, **M.**, **Massey**, **E.W.**, **Schoenberg**, **B.S.**, 1988. International mortality from primary nervous system neoplasms: distribution and trends. Int. J. Epidemiol. 17 (1), 33–38.

Baldwin, **R.T.**, **Preston-Martin**, **S.**, 2004. Epidemiology of brain tumors in childhood – a review. Toxicol. Appl. Pharmacol. 199 (2), 118–131.

Bansal, **K.**, **Liang**, **M.L.**, **Rutka**, **J.T.**, 2006. Molecular biology of human gliomas. Technol. Cancer Res. Treat. 5 (3), 185–194.

Beall, **C.**, **Bender**, **T.**, **Cheng**, **H.**, **et al.**, 2005. Mortality among semiconductor and storage device-manufacturing workers. J. Occup. Environ. Med. 47 (10), 996–1014.

Berg, **G.**, **Schuz**, **J.**, **Samkange-Zeeb**, **F.**, **et al.**, 2005. Assessment of radiofrequency exposure from cellular telephone daily use in an epidemiological study: German Validation study of the international case–control study of cancers of the brain – INTERPHONE-Study. J. Expo. Anal. Environ. Epidemiol. 15 (3), 217–224.

Berrino, **F.**, **Esteve**, **J.**, **Coleman**, **M.P.**, 1995. Basic issues in the estimation and comparison of cancer patient survival. In: **Berrino**,

F., Sant, M., Verdecchia, A., et al., (Eds.), IARC Sci. Lyon, No. 132. pp. 1–14.

Biggar, R.J., Horm, J., Goedert, J.J., et al., 1987. Cancer in a group at risk of acquired immunodeficiency syndrome (AIDS) through 1984. Am. J. Epidemiol. 126 (4), 578–586.

Bigner, S.H., Mark, J., Mahaley, M.S., et al., 1984. Patterns of the early, gross chromosomal changes in malignant human gliomas. Hereditas. 101 (1), 103–113.

Bithell, J.F., Draper, G.J., Gorbach, P.D., 1973. Association between malignant disease in children and maternal virus infections. BMJ 1 (5855), 706–708.

Bithell, J.F., Stewart, A.M., 1975. Pre-natal irradiation and childhood malignancy: a review of British data from the Oxford Survey. Br. J. Cancer 31 (3), 271–287.

Bjørge, T., Cnattingius, S., Lie, R.T., et al., 2008. Cancer risk in children with birth defects and in their families: a population based cohort study of 5.2 million children from Norway and Sweden. Cancer Epidemiol. Biomarkers Prev. 17 (3), 500–506.

Black, P.M., 1991a. Brain tumors. Part 1. N. Engl. J. Med. 324 (21), 1471–1476.

Black, P.M., 1991b. Brain tumors. Part 2. N. Engl. J. Med. 324 (22), 1555–1564.

Black, W.C., 1998. Increasing incidence of childhood primary malignant brain tumors – enigma or no-brainer? J. Natl. Cancer Inst. 90 (17), 1249–1251.

Blair, A., Malker, H., Cantor, K.P., et al., 1985. Cancer among farmers. A review. Scand. J. Work. Environ. Health 11 (6), 397–407.

Blatt, J., Jaffe, R., Deutsch, M., et al., 1986. Neurofibromatosis and childhood tumors. Cancer 57 (6), 1225–1229.

Blettner, M., Schlehofer, B., Samkange-Zeeb, F., et al., 2007. Medical exposure to ionising radiation and the risk of brain tumours: INTERPHONE study group, Germany. Eur. J. Cancer 43 (13), 1990–1998.

Blot, W.J., Henderson, B.E., Boice, J.D. Jr, 1999. Childhood cancer in relation to cured meat intake: review of the epidemiological evidence. Nutr. Cancer 34 (1), 111–118.

Blumenthal, D.T., Cannon-Albright, L.A., 2008. Familiality in brain tumors. Neurology. 71 (13), 1015–1020.

Boeing, H., Schlehofer, B., Blettner, M., et al., 1993. Dietary carcinogens and the risk for glioma and meningioma in Germany. Int. J. Cancer 53 (4), 561–565.

Boice, J.D., McLaughlin, J.K., 2006. Concerning mobile phone use and risk of acousticneuroma. Br. J. Cancer 95 (1), 130.

Bolande, R., 1989. Teratogenesis and oncogenesis: a developmental spectrum. In: Lynch, H.T. (Ed.), Genetic epidemiology of cancer. CRC Press, Boca Raton, FL, pp. 58–68.

Bolger, G.B., Stamberg, J., Kirsch, I.R., et al., 1985. Chromosome translocation t(14:22) and oncogene (c-sis) variant in a pedigree with familial meningioma. N. Engl. J. Med. 312 (9), 564–567.

Bondy, M.L., Scheurer, M.E., Malmer, B., et al., 2008. Brain tumor epidemiology: consensus from the Brain Tumor Epidemiology Consortium. Cancer 113 (Suppl. 7), 1953–1968.

Bonnet, F., Chêne, G., 2008. Evolving epidemiology of malignancies in HIV. Curr. Opin. Oncol. 20 (5), 534–540.

Boring, C.C., Squires, T.S., Tong, T., 1991. Cancer statistics, 1991. CA. Cancer J. Clin. 41 (1), 19–36.

Boyle, P., Maisonneuve, P., Saracci, R., et al., 1990. Is the increased incidence of primary malignant brain tumors in the elderly real? J. Natl. Cancer Inst. 82 (20), 1594–1596.

Brenner, A., Linet, M., Fine, H., et al., 2002. History of allergies and autoimmune diseases and risk of brain tumors in adults. Int. J. Cancer 99 (2), 252–259.

Brenner, A.V., Butler, M.A., Wang, S.S., et al., 2007. Single-nucleotide polymorphisms in selected cytokine genes and risk of adult glioma. Carcinogenesis 28 (12), 2543–2547.

Brenner, A.V., Linet, M.S., Selker, R.G., et al., 2003. Polio vaccination and risk of brain tumors in adults: no apparent association. Cancer Epidemiol. Biomarkers Prev. 12 (2), 177–178.

Brenner, A.V., Linet, M.S., Shapiro, W.R., et al., 2004. Season of birth and risk of brain tumors in adults. Neurology 63 (2), 276–281.

Breslow, N.E., Langholz, B., 1983. Childhood cancer incidence: geographical and temporal variations. Int. J. Cancer 32 (6), 703–716.

Brewis, M., Poskanzer, D.C., Rolland, C., et al., 1966. Neurological disease in an English city. Acta. Neurol. Scand. 42 (Suppl. 24), 1–89.

Brownson, R.C., Reif, J.S., Chang, J.C., et al., 1990. An analysis of occupational risks for brain cancer. Am. J. Public Health 80 (2), 169–172.

Buffler, P., Kelsh, M., Kalmes, R., et al., 2007. A nested case–control study of brain tumors among employees at a petroleum exploration and extraction research facility. J. Occup. Environ. Med. 49 (7), 791–802.

Bunin, G., 1987. Racial patterns of childhood brain cancer by histologic type. J. Natl. Cancer Inst. 78 (5), 875–880.

Bunin, G., 2000. What causes childhood brain tumors? Limited knowledge, many clues. Pediatr. Neurosurg. 32 (6), 321–326.

Bunin, G.R., Buckley, J.D., Boesel, C.P., et al., 1994a. Risk factors for astrocytic glioma and primitive neuroectodermal tumor of the brain in young children: a report from the Children's Cancer Group. Cancer Epidemiol. Biomarkers Prev. 3 (3), 197–204.

Bunin, G.R., Kuijten, R.R., Boesel, C.P., et al., 1994b. Maternal diet and risk of astrocytic glioma in children: a report from the Children's Cancer Group (United States and Canada). Cancer Causes Control 5 (2), 177–187.

Bunin, G.R., Kuijten, R.R., Buckley, J.D., et al., 1993. Relation between maternal diet and subsequent primitive neuroectodermal brain tumors in young children. N. Engl. J. Med. 329 (8), 536–541.

Burch, J.D., Craib, K.J., Choi, B.C., et al., 1987. An exploratory case–control study of brain tumors in adults. J. Natl. Cancer Inst. 78 (4), 601–609.

Cardis, E., 2007. Commentary: Low dose-rate exposures to ionizing radiation. Int. J. Epidemiol. 36 (5), 1046–1047.

Cardis, E., Deltour, I., Mann, S., et al., 2008. Distribution of RF energy emitted by mobile phones in anatomical structures of the brain. Phys. Med. Biol. 53 (11), 2771–2783.

Cardis, E., Vrijheid, M., Blettner, M., et al., 2005. Risk of cancer after low doses of ionising radiation: retrospective cohort study in 15 countries. BMJ 331 (7508), 77.

Carpenter, D.O., Sage, C., 2008. Setting prudent public health policy for electromagnetic field exposures. Rev. Environ. Health 23 (2), 91–117.

CBTRUS, 2008. Primary brain tumors in the United States, 2000–2004. Central Brain Tumor Registry of the United States, Hinsdale, IL.

Chakrabarti, I., Cockburn, M., Cozen, W., et al., 2005. A population-based description of glioblastoma multiforme in Los Angeles County, 1974–1999. Cancer 104 (12), 2798–2806.

Charman, H.P., Lowenstein, D.H., Cho, K.G., et al., 1988. Primary cerebral angiosarcoma. Case report. J. Neurosurg. 68 (5), 806–810.

Chen, H., Ward, M.H., Tucker, K.L., et al., 2002. Diet and risk of adult glioma in eastern Nebraska, United States. Cancer Causes Control 13 (7), 647–655.

Choi, N.W., Schuman, L.M., Gullen, W.H., 1970a. Epidemiology of primary central nervous system neoplasms. I. Mortality from primary central nervous system neoplasms in Minnesota. Am. J. Epidemiol. 91 (3), 238–259.

Choi, N.W., Schuman, L.M., Gullen, W.H., 1970b. Epidemiology of primary central nervous system neoplasms. II. Case–control study. Am. J. Epidemiol. 91 (5), 467–485.

Cicuttini, F.M., Hurley, S.F., Forbes, A., et al., 1997. Association of adult glioma with medical conditions, family and reproductive history. Int. J. Cancer 71 (2), 203–207.

Clapp, R.W., Jacobs, M.M., Loechler, E.L., 2008. Environmental and occupational causes of cancer: new evidence 2005–2007. Rev. Environ. Health 23 (1), 1–37.

Claus, E.B., Black, P.M., 2006. Survival rates and patterns of care for patients diagnosed with supratentorial low-grade gliomas: data from the SEER program, 1973–2001. Cancer 106 (6), 1358–1363.

Claus, E.B., Black, P.M., Bondy, M.L., et al., 2007. Exogenous hormone use and meningioma risk: what do we tell our patients? Cancer 110 (3), 471–476.

Clemmesen, J., Fuglsang-Frederiksen, V., Plum, C.M., 1974. Are anticonvulsants oncogenic? Lancet 1 (7860), 705–707.

Coble, J.B., Dosemeci, M., Stewart, P.A., et al., 2009. Occupational exposure to magnetic fields and the risk of brain tumors. Neuro. Oncol. 11 (3), 242–249.

Cocco, P., Dosemeci, M., Heineman, E.F., 1998. Brain cancer and occupational exposure to lead. J. Occup. Environ. Med. 40 (11), 937–942.

Coleman, M., Beral, V., 1988. A review of epidemiological studies of the health effects of living near or working with electricity generation and transmission equipment. Int. J. Epidemiol. 17 (1), 1–13.

Colt, J.S., Blair, A., 1998. Parental occupational exposures and risk of childhood cancer. Environ. Health Perspect 106 (Suppl. 3), 909–925.

Connelly, J.M., Malkin, M.G., 2007. Environmental risk factors for brain tumors. Curr. Neurol. Neurosci. Rep. 7 (3), 208–214.

Cook, P.J., Doll, R., Fellingham, S.A., 1969. A mathematical model for the age distribution of cancer in man. Int. J. Cancer 4 (1), 93–112.

Corallini, A., Pagnani, M., Viadana, P., et al., 1987. Association of BK virus with human brain tumors and tumors of pancreatic islets. Int. J. Cancer 39 (1), 60–67.

Cordier, S., Iglesias, M.J., Le Goaster, C., et al., 1994. Incidence and risk factors for childhood brain tumors in the Ile de France. Int. J. Cancer 59 (6), 776–782.

Cordier, S., Lefeuvre, B., Filippini, G., et al., 1997. Parental occupation, occupational exposure to solvents and polycyclic aromatic hydrocarbons and risk of childhood brain tumors (Italy, France, Spain). Cancer Causes Control 8 (5), 688–697.

Cordier, S., Poisson, M., Gerin, M., et al., 1988. Gliomas and exposure to wood preservatives. Br. J. Ind. Med. 45 (10), 705–709.

Curado, M.P., Edwards, B.S.H., et al., 2007. Cancer incidence in five continents, Vol. 9. IARC, Lyon.

Custer, B.S., Koepsell, T.D., Mueller, B.A., 2002. The association between breast carcinoma and meningioma in women. Cancer 94 (6), 1626–1635.

Darby, S.C., Nakashima, E., Kato, H., 1985. A parallel analysis of cancer mortality among atomic bomb survivors and patients with ankylosing spondylitis given X-ray therapy. J. Natl. Cancer Inst. 75 (1), 1–21.

Davis, F.G., Freels, S., Grutsch, J., et al., 1998. Survival rates in patients with primary malignant brain tumors stratified by patient age and tumor histological type: an analysis based on Surveillance, Epidemiology, and End Results (SEER) data, 1973–1991. J. Neurosurg. 88 (1), 1–10.

Davis, F.G., Malmer, B.S., Aldape, K., et al., 2008. Issues of diagnostic review in brain tumor studies: From the Brain Tumor Epidemiology Consortium. Cancer Epidemiol. Biomarkers Prev. 17 (3), 484–489.

Day, N., 1987. Cumulative rate and cumulative risk. In: Muir, C., Mack, T., Powell, J., et al. (Eds.), Cancer incidence in five continents, Vol 5. IARC, Lyon, pp. 787–789.

De Roos, A.J., Stewart, P.A., Linet, M.S., et al., 2003. Occupation and the risk of adult glioma in the United States. Cancer Causes Control 14 (2), 139–150.

Del Valle, L., White, M.K., Khalili, K., 2008. Potential mechanisms of the human polyomavirus JC in neural oncogenesis. J. Neuropathol Exp. Neurol. 67 (8), 729–740.

Demers, P.A., Vaughan, T.L., Schommer, R.R., 1991. Occupation, socioeconomic status, and brain tumor mortality: a death certificate-based case–control study. J. Occup. Med. 33 (9), 1001–1006.

Desmeules, M., Mikkelsen, T., Mao, Y., 1992. Increasing incidence of primary malignant brain tumors: influence of diagnostic methods. J. Natl. Cancer Inst. 84 (6), 442–445.

Dietrich, M., Block, G., Pogoda, J.M., et al., 2005. A review: dietary and endogenously formed N-nitroso compounds and risk of childhood brain tumors. Cancer Causes Control 16 (6), 619–635.

Dobkin, B.H., 1985. Stroke associated with glioblastoma. Bull. Clin. Neurosci. 50, 111–118.

Dockerty, J.D., Elwood, J.M., Skegg, D.C., et al., 1998. Electromagnetic field exposures and childhood cancers in New Zealand. Cancer Causes Control 9 (3), 299–309.

Dong, L.M., Potter, J.D., White, E., et al., 2008. Genetic susceptibility to cancer: the role of polymorphisms in candidate genes. JAMA 299 (20), 2423–2436.

Druckrey, H., 1973. Chemical structure and action in transplacental carcinogenesis and teratogenesis. In: Tomatis, L.M. (Ed.), Transplacental carcinogenesis, Vol 4. IARC, Lyon, pp. 29–44.

Easterly, C.E., 1981. Cancer link to magnetic field exposure: a hypothesis. Am. J. Epidemiol. 114 (2), 169–174.

Eby, N.L., Grufferman, S., Flannelly, C.M., et al., 1988. Increasing incidence of primary brain lymphoma in the US. Cancer 62 (11), 2461–2465.

Efird, J.T., Friedman, G.D., Sidney, S., et al., 2004. The risk for malignant primary adult-onset glioma in a large, multiethnic, managedcare cohort: cigarette smoking and other lifestyle behaviors. J. Neurooncol. 68 (1), 57–69.

Efird, J.T., Holly, E.A., Preston-Martin, S., et al., 2003. Farm-related exposures and childhood brain tumours in seven countries: results from the SEARCH International Brain Tumour Study. Paediatr. Perinat. Epidemiol. 17 (2), 201–211.

Emerson, J.C., Malone, K.E., Daling, J.R., et al., 1991. Childhood brain tumor risk in relation to birth characteristics. J. Clin. Epidemiol. 44 (11), 1159–1166.

Engels, E.A., Sarkar, C., Daniel, R.W., et al., 2002. Absence of simian virus 40 in human brain tumors from northern India. Int. J. Cancer 101 (4), 348–352.

Farrell, C.J., Plotkin, S.R., 2007. Genetic causes of brain tumors: neurofibromatosis, tuberous sclerosis, von Hippel-Lindau, and other syndromes. Neurol. Clin. 25 (4), 925–946, viii.

Farwell, J., Flannery, J.T., 1984. Cancer in relatives of children with central-nervous-system neoplasms. N. Engl. J. Med. 311 (12), 749–753.

Feychting, M., Ahlbom, A., 1993. Magnetic fields and cancer in children residing near Swedish high-voltage power lines. Am. J. Epidemiol. 138 (7), 467–481.

Fisher, J., Schwartzbaum, J., Wrensch, M., et al., 2007. Epidemiology of brain tumors. Neurologic clinics 25 (4), 867–890.

Fritz, A., Percy, C., Jack, A., et al., 2000. International classification of diseases for oncology, third ed. WHO, Geneva.

Garfinkel, L., Sarokhan, B., 1982. Trends in brain cancer tumor mortality and morbidity in the United States. Ann. N. Y. Acad. Sci. 381, 1–5.

Giles, G., Thursfield, V., Staples, M., et al., 1993. Incidence and survival from childhood cancers in Victoria 1970–1979 and 1980–1989. Anti-Cancer Council Victoria, Melbourne.

Gold, E., Gordis, L., Tonascia, J., et al., 1979. Risk factors for brain tumors in children. Am. J. Epidemiol. 109 (3), 309–319.

Gold, E.B., 1980. Epidemiology of brain tumors. In: Lilienfeld, A.M. (Ed.), Reviews in Cancer epidemiology, Vol 1. Elsevier, North Holland, New York, pp. 245–292.

Goldstein, A.M., Yuen, J., Tucker, M.A., 1997. Second cancers after medulloblastoma: population-based results from the United States and Sweden. Cancer Causes Control 8 (6), 865–871.

Greig, N.H., Ries, L.G., Yancik, R., et al., 1990. Increasing annual incidence of primary malignant brain tumors in the elderly. J. Natl. Cancer Inst. 82 (20), 1621–1624.

Gurney, J.G., van Wijngaarden, E., 1999. Extremely low frequency electromagnetic fields (EMF) and brain cancer in adults and children: review and comment. Neuro. Oncol. 1 (3), 212–220.

Hagströmer, L., Ye, W., Nyren, O., et al., 2005. Incidence of cancer among patients with atopic dermatitis. Arch. Dermatol. 141 (9), 1123–1127.

Hardell, L., Carlberg, M., Soderqvist, F., et al., 2007. Long-term use of cellular phones and brain tumors: increased risk associated with use for > or = 10 years. Occup. Environ. Med. 64 (9), 626–632.

Harding, N.J., Birch, J.M., Hepworth, S.J., et al., 2008. Atopic dysfunction and risk of central nervous system tumours in children. Eur. J. Cancer 44 (1), 92–99.

Harrington, J.M., Oakes, D., 1984. Mortality study of British pathologists 1974–1980. Br. J. Ind. Med. 41 (2), 188–191.

Hatch, E.E., Linet, M.S., Zhang, J., et al., 2005. Reproductive and hormonal factors and risk of brain tumors in adult females. Int. J. Cancer 114 (5), 797–805.

Haymaker, W., Rubinstein, L.J., Miquel, J., 1972. Brain tumors in irradiated monkeys. Acta. Neuropathol. 20 (4), 267–277.

Helseth, A., Mørk, S.J., Glattre, E., 1989. Neoplasms of the central nervous system in Norway. V. Meningioma and cancer of other sites. An analysis of the occurrence of multiple primary neoplasms in meningioma patients in Norway from 1955 through 1986. APMIS 97 (8), 738–744.

Heshmat, M.Y., Kovi, J., Simpson, C., et al., 1976. Neoplasms of the central nervous system. incidence and population selectivity in the Washington D C, metropolitan area. Cancer 38 (5), 2135–2142.

Heuch, J.M., Heuch, I., Akslen, L.A., et al., 1998. Risk of primary childhood brain tumors related to birth characteristics: a Norwegian prospective study. Int. J. Cancer 77 (4), 498–503.

Hill, D.A., Inskip, P.D., Shapiro, W.R., et al., 2003. Cancer in first-degree relatives and risk of glioma in adults. Cancer Epidemiol. Biomarkers Prev. 12 (12), 1443–1448.

Hill, D.A., Linet, M.S., Black, P.M., et al., 2004. Meningioma and schwannoma risk in adults in relation to family history of cancer. Neuro. Oncol. 6 (4), 274–280.

Hirayama, T., 1985. Passive smoking–a new target of epidemiology. Tokai J. Exp. Clin. Med. 10 (4), 287–293.

Hirayama, T., 1989. Family history and childhood malignancies with special reference to genetic environmental interaction. In: Lynch, H.T. (Ed.), Genetic epidemiology and cancer. CRC Press, Boca Raton, FL, pp. 111–118.

Hlobilkova, A., Ehrmann, J., Sedlakova, E., et al., 2007. Could changes in the regulation of the PI3K/PKB/Akt signaling pathway and cell cycle be involved in astrocytic tumor pathogenesis and progression? Neoplasma 54 (4), 334–341.

Hochberg, F., Toniolo, P., Cole, P., et al., 1990. Nonoccupational risk indicators of glioblastoma in adults. J. Neurooncol. 8 (1), 55–60.

Hoffman, S., Propp, J.M., McCarthy, B.J., 2006. Temporal trends in incidence of primary brain tumors in the United States, 1985–1999. Neuro. Oncol. 8 (1), 27–37.

Holick, C.N., Giovannucci, E.L., Rosner, B., et al., 2007a. Prospective study of intake of fruit, vegetables, and carotenoids and the risk of adult glioma. Am. J. Clin. Nutr. 85 (3), 877–886.

Holick, C.N., Giovannucci, E.L., Rosner, B., et al., 2007b. Prospective study of cigarette smoking and adult glioma: dosage, duration, and latency. Neuro. Oncol. 9 (3), 326–334.

Hoover, R., Fraumeni, J.F. Jr, 1973. Risk of cancer in renal-transplant recipients. Lancet 2 (7820), 55–57.

Hours, M., Bernard, M., Montestrucq, L., et al., 2007. [Cell phones and risk of brain and acoustic nerve tumours: the French INTERPHONE case–control study]. Rev. Epidemiol. Sante Publique 55 (5), 321–332.

Howe, G.R., Burch, J.D., Chiarelli, A.M., et al., 1989. An exploratory case–control study of brain tumors in children. Cancer Res. 49 (15), 4349–4352.

Huang, K., Whelan, E.A., Ruder, A.M., et al., 2004. Reproductive factors and risk of glioma in women. Cancer Epidemiol. Biomarkers Prev. 13 (10), 1583–1588.

Huncharek, M., Kupelnick, B., Wheeler, L., 2003. Dietary cured meat and the risk of adult glioma: a meta-analysis of nine observational studies. J. Environ. Pathol. Toxicol. Oncol. 22 (2), 129–137.

IARC Working Group on Evaluation of Carcinogenic Risks to Humans, 2002. Non-ionizing radiation. Part 1, Static and extremely low frequency (ELF) electric and magnetic fields, Vol. 80. IARC, Lyon. [IARC monographs on the evaluation of carcinogenic risks to humans.]

Infante-Rivard, C., Weichenthal, S., 2007. Pesticides and childhood cancer: an update of Zahm and Ward's 1998 review. J. Toxicol. Environ. Health B. Crit. Rev. 10 (1–2), 81–99.

Inskip, P.D., 2003. Multiple primary tumors involving cancer of the brain and central nervous system as the first or subsequent cancer. Cancer 98 (3), 562–570.

Inskip, P.D., Mellemkjaer, L., Gridley, G., et al., 1998. Incidence of intracranial tumors following hospitalization for head injuries (Denmark). Cancer Causes Control 9 (1), 109–116.

Inskip, P.D., Tarone, R.E., Hatch, E.E., et al., 2003. Sociodemographic indicators and risk of brain tumors. Int. J. Epidemiol. 32 (2), 225–233.

International Agency for Research on Cancer, 1989. Occupational exposures in petroleum refining: crude oil and major petroleum fuels. IARC, Lyon. [IARC Monographs Evaluation Carcinogenic Risks Humans, IARC Working Group on the Evaluation of Carcinogenic Risks to Humans.]

Johnson, C.C., Annegers, J.F., Frankowski, R.F., et al., 1987. Childhood nervous system tumors – an evaluation of the association with paternal occupational exposure to hydrocarbons. Am. J. Epidemiol. 126 (4), 605–613.

Johnson, C.C., Spitz, M.R., 1989. Childhood nervous system tumors: an assessment of risk associated with paternal occupations involving use, repair or manufacture of electrical and electronic equipment. Int. J. Epidemiol. 18 (4), 756–762.

Kallio, M., Sankila, R., Jaaskelainen, J., et al., 1991. A population-based study on the incidence and survival rates of 3857 glioma patients diagnosed from 1953 to 1984. Cancer 68 (6), 1394–1400.

Kang, D., Davis, L.K., Hunt, P., et al., 2008. Cancer incidence among male Massachusetts firefighters, 1987–2003. Am. J. Ind. Med. 51 (5), 329–335.

Kaplan, S., Novikov, I., Modan, B., 1997. Nutritional factors in the etiology of brain tumors: potential role of nitrosamines, fat, and cholesterol. Am. J. Epidemiol. 146 (10), 832–841.

Karlsson, P., Holmberg, E., Lundell, M., et al., 1998. Intracranial tumors after exposure to ionizing radiation during infancy: a pooled analysis of two Swedish cohorts of 28,008 infants with skin hemangioma. Radiat. Res. 150 (3), 357–364.

Kent, S.P., Pickering, J.E., 1958. Neoplasms in monkeys (Macaca mulatta): spontaneous and irradiation induced. Cancer 11 (1), 138–147.

Kessler, E., Brandt-Rauf, P.W., 1987. Occupational cancers of the brain and bone. Occup. Med. 2 (1), 155–163.

Kheifets, L., Monroe, J., Vergara, X., et al., 2008. Occupational electromagnetic fields and leukemia and brain cancer: an update to two meta-analyses. J. Occup. Environ. Med. 50 (6), 677–688.

Kheifets, L.I., 2001. Electric and magnetic field exposure and brain cancer: a review. Bioelectromagnetics 5, S120–S131.

Khuder, S.A., Mutgi, A.B., Schaub, E.A., 1998. Meta-analyses of brain cancer and farming. Am. J. Ind. Med. 34 (3), 252–260.

Kibirige, M.S., Birch, J.M., Campbell, R.H., et al., 1989. A review of astrocytoma in childhood. Pediatr. Hematol. Oncol. 6 (4), 319–329.

Knekt, P., Reunanen, A., Teppo, L., 1991. Serum cholesterol concentration and risk of primary brain tumours. BMJ 302 (6768), 90.

Koch, H.J., Klinkhammer-Schalke, M., Hofstadter, F., et al., 2006. Seasonal patterns of birth in patients with glioblastoma. Chronobiol. Int. 23 (5), 1047–1052.

Kornbluth, S., Cross, F.R., Harbison, M., et al., 1986. Transformation of chicken embryo fibroblasts and tumor induction by the middle T antigen of polyomavirus carried in an avian retroviral vector. Mol. Cell. Biol. 6 (5), 1545–1551.

Koul, D., 2008. PTEN signaling pathways in glioblastoma. Cancer Biol. Ther. 7 (9), 1321–1325.

Krewski, D., Byus, C.V., Glickman, B.W., et al., 2001. Recent advances in research on radiofrequency fields and health. J. Toxicol. Environ. Health B. Crit. Rev. 4 (1), 145–159.

Krewski, D., Yokel, R.A., Nieboer, E., et al., 2007. Human health risk assessment for aluminium, aluminium oxide, and aluminium hydroxide. J. Toxicol. Environ. Health B. Crit. Rev. 10 (Suppl. 1), 1–269.

Krishnan, G., Felini, M., Carozza, S.E., et al., 2003. Occupation and adult gliomas in the San Francisco Bay Area. J. Occup. Environ. Med. 45 (6), 639–647.

Krupp, J.H., 1976. Nine-year mortality experience in proton-exposed Macaca mulatta. Radiat. Res. 67 (2), 244–251.

Kuijten, R.R., Bunin, G.R., 1993. Risk factors for childhood brain tumors. Cancer Epidemiol. Biomarkers Prev. 2 (3), 277–288.

Kundi, M., 2009. The controversy about a possible relationship between mobile phone use and cancer. Environ. Health Perspect 117 (3), 316–324.

Lacayo, A., Farmer, P.M., 1991. Brain tumors in children: a review. Ann. Clin. Lab. Sci. 21 (1), 26–35.

Lambe, M., Coogan, P., Baron, J., 1997. Reproductive factors and the risk of brain tumors: a population-based study in Sweden. Int. J. Cancer 72 (3), 389–393.

Lee, E., Grutsch, J., Persky, V., et al., 2006. Association of meningioma with reproductive factors. Int. J. Cancer 119 (5), 1152–1157.

Lee, W.J., Colt, J.S., Heineman, E.F., et al., 2005. Agricultural pesticide use and risk of glioma in Nebraska, United States. Occup. Environ. Med. 62 (11), 786–792.

Li, Y., Millikan, R.C., Carozza, S., et al., 1998. p53 mutations in malignant gliomas. Cancer Epidemiol. Biomarkers Prev. 7 (4), 303–308.

Lin, R.S., Dischinger, P.C., Conde, J., et al., 1985. Occupational exposure to electromagnetic fields and the occurrence of brain tumors. An analysis of possible associations. J. Occup. Med. 27 (6), 413–419.

Linet, M.S., Wacholder, S., Zahm, S.H., 2003. Interpreting epidemiologic research: lessons from studies of childhood cancer. Pediatrics 112 (1 Pt 2), 218–232.

Linos, E., Raine, T., Alonso, A., et al., 2007. Atopy and risk of brain tumors: a meta-analysis. J. Natl. Cancer Inst. 99 (20), 1544–1550.

Logan, W., 1982. Cancer mortality by occupation and social class 1851–1971. IARC, Lyon.

Longstreth, W.T. Jr, Phillips, L.E., Drangsholt, M., et al., 2004. Dental X-rays and the risk of intracranial meningioma: a population-based case–control study. Cancer 100 (5), 1026–1034.

Lonn, S., Ahlbom, A., Hall, P., et al., 2005. Long-term mobile phone use and brain tumor risk. Am. J. Epidemiol. 161 (6), 526–535.

Loomis, D.P., Savitz, D.A., 1990. Mortality from brain cancer and leukaemia among electrical workers. Br. J. Ind. Med. 47 (9), 633–638.

Luwor, R.B., Kaye, A.H., Zhu, H.J., 2008. Transforming growth factor-beta (TGF-beta) and brain tumors. J. Clin. Neurosci. 15 (8), 845–855.

Lynch, H.T., Marcus, J.M., Watson, P., 1989. Genetic epidemiology of breast cancer. In: Lynch, H.T., Hirayama, T. (Eds.), Genetic epidemiology of cancer. CRC Press, Boca Raton, pp. 289–332.

MacMahon, B., 1960. The ethnic distribution of cancer mortality in New York City, 1955. Acta. Unio. Int. Contra. Cancrum. 16, 53–57.

MacMahon, B., 1985. Phenobarbital: epidemiological evidence. In: Wald, N.J., Doll, R. (Eds.), Interpretation of negative epidemiological evidence for carcinogenicity, Vol 65. IARC, Lyon, pp. 153–158.

Macpherson, P., 1976. Association between previous tuberculous infection and glioma. BMJ 2 (6044), 1112.

Magnani, C., Aareleid, T., Viscomi, S., et al., 2001. Variation in survival of children with central nervous system (CNS) malignancies diagnosed in Europe between 1978 and 1992: the EURO-CARE study. Eur. J. Cancer 37 (6), 711–721.

Mahaley, M.S. Jr, Mettlin, C., Natarajan, N., et al., 1989. National survey of patterns of care for brain-tumor patients. J. Neurosurg. 71 (6), 826–836.

Malmer, B., Henriksson, R., Gronberg, H., 2002. Different aetiology of familial low-grade and high-grade glioma? A nationwide cohort study of familial glioma. Neuroepidemiology 21 (6), 279–286.

Malmer, B., Tavelin, B., Henriksson, R., et al., 2000. Primary brain tumors as second primary: a novel association between meningioma and colorectal cancer. Int. J. Cancer 85 (1), 78–81.

Malmer, B.S., Feychting, M., Lonn, S., et al., 2007. Genetic variation in p53 and ATM haplotypes and risk of glioma and meningioma. J. Neurooncol. 82 (3), 229–237.

Maltoni, C., Ciliberti, A., Carretti, D., 1982. Experimental contributions in identifying brain potential carcinogens in the petrochemical industry. Ann. N. Y. Acad. Sci. 381, 216–249.

Maltoni, C., Ciliberti, A., Di Maio, V., 1977. Carcinogenicity bioassays on rats of acrylonitrile administered by inhalation and by ingestion. Med. Lav. 68 (6), 401–411.

Maule, M., Scélo, G., Pastore, G., et al., 2008. Risk of second malignant neoplasms after childhood central nervous system malignant tumours: An international study. Eur. J. Cancer 44 (6), 830–839.

Mazumdar, M., Liu, C.Y., Wang, S.F., et al., 2008. No association between parental or subject occupation and brain tumor risk. Cancer Epidemiol. Biomarkers Prev. 17 (7), 1835–1837.

McCarthy, B.J., Kruchko, C., 2005. Consensus conference on cancer registration of brain and central nervous system tumors. Neuro. Oncol. 7 (2), 196–201.

McCarthy, B.J., Propp, J.M., Davis, F.G., et al., 2008. Time trends in oligodendroglial and astrocytic tumor incidence. Neuroepidemiology 30 (1), 34–44.

McCredie, M., Coates, M.S., Ford, J.M., 1990. Cancer incidence in European migrants to New South Wales. Ann. Oncol. 1 (3), 219–225.

McKean-Cowdin, R., Preston-Martin, S., Pogoda, J.M., et al., 1998. Parental occupation and childhood brain tumors: astroglial and primitive neuroectodermal tumors. J. Occup. Environ. Med. 40 (4), 332–340.

McWhorter, W.P., 1988. Allergy and risk of cancer. A prospective study using NHANESI followup data. Cancer 62 (2), 451–455.

Menegoz, F., Little, J., Colonna, M., et al., 2002. Contacts with animals and humans as risk factors for adult brain tumours. An international case–control study. Eur. J. Cancer 38 (5), 696–704.

Mezei, G., Gadallah, M., Kheifets, L., 2008. Residential magnetic field exposure and childhood brain cancer: a meta-analysis. Epidemiology 19 (3), 424–430.

Miller, R.D., Neuberger, J.S., Gerald, K.B., 1997. Brain cancer and leukemia and exposure to power-frequency (50- to 60-Hz) electric and magnetic fields. Epidemiol. Rev. 19 (2), 273–293.

Mills, P.K., Beeson, W.L., Phillips, R.L., et al., 1989a. Dietary habits and breast cancer incidence among Seventh-Day Adventists. Cancer 64 (3), 582–590.

Mills, P.K., Preston-Martin, S., Annegers, J.F., et al., 1989b. Risk factors for tumors of the brain and cranial meninges in Seventh-Day Adventists. Neuroepidemiology 8 (5), 266–275.

Modan, B., Wagener, D.K., Feldman, J.J., et al., 1992. Increased mortality from brain tumors: a combined outcome of diagnostic technology and change of attitude toward the elderly. Am. J. Epidemiol. 135 (12), 1349–1357.

Mohan, A.K., Hauptmann, M., Freedman, D.M., et al., 2003. Cancer and other causes of mortality among radiologic technologists in the United States. Int. J. Cancer 103 (2), 259–267.

Monson, R.R., MacMahon, B., 1984. Pre-natal X-ray exposure and cancer in children. In: Boice, J.D., Fraumeni, J.F. (Eds.), Radiation carcinogenesis: epidemiology and biological significance. Raven Press, New York, pp. 97–105.

Moolgavkar, S.H., Day, N.E., Stevens, R.G., 1980. Two-stage model for carcinogenesis: Epidemiology of breast cancer in females. J. Natl. Cancer Inst. 65 (3), 559–569.

Moss, A.R., 1985. Occupational exposure and brain tumors. J. Toxicol. Environ. Health 16 (5), 703–711.

Muir, C., Waterhouse, J., Mack, T., et al., 1987. Cancer incidence in five continents, Vol. 5. IARC, Lyon.

Munk, J., Peyser, E., Gruszkiewicz, J., 1969. Radiation induced intracranial meningiomas. Clin. Radiol. 20 (1), 90–94.

Musicco, M., Filippini, G., Bordo, B.M., et al., 1982. Gliomas and occupational exposure to carcinogens: case–control study. Am. J. Epidemiol. 116 (5), 782–790.

Nasca, P.C., Baptiste, M.S., MacCubbin, P.A., et al., 1988. An epidemiologic case–control study of central nervous system tumors in children and parental occupational exposures. Am. J. Epidemiol. 128 (6), 1256–1265.

NIEHS (National Institute of Environmental Health Sciences), 1999. Report on health effects from exposure to power line frequency electric and magnetic fields. Report No. 99–4493. NIEHS, Research Triangle Park, NC.

National Radiation Protection Board, 1992. Electromagnetic fields and the risk of cancer. National Radiological Protection Board. Report of an advisory group on non-ionising radiation, pp. 1–138.

National Research Council, 1980. The effects on populations of exposure to low levels of ionizing radiation. National Academy of Sciences, Washington DC.

Neutel, C.I., Quinn, A., Brancker, A., 1989. Brain tumor mortality in immigrants. Int. J. Epidemiol. 18 (1), 60–66.

Newill, V.A., 1961. Distribution of cancer mortality among etimic subgroups of the white population of New York City, 1953–1958. J. Natl. Cancer Inst. 26, 405–417.

Ney, D.E., Lassman, A.B., 2009. Molecular profiling of oligodendrogliomas: impact on prognosis, treatment, and future directions. Curr. Oncol. Rep. 11 (1), 62–67.

Office of Population Censuses and Surveys, 1981. Cancer statistics: Incidence, survival and mortality in England and Wales. Studies on medical and population subjects. HMSO, London.

Ohgaki, H., 2009. Epidemiology of brain tumors. Methods. Mol. Biol. 472, 323–342.

Ohgaki, H., Kleihues, P., 2007. Genetic pathways to primary and secondary glioblastoma. Am. J. Pathol. 170 (5), 1445–1453.

Olsen, J.H., Boice, J.D. Jr, Jensen, J.P., et al., 1989. Cancer among epileptic patients exposed to anticonvulsant drugs. J. Natl. Cancer Inst. 81 (10), 803–808.

Olshan, A.F., Breslow, N.E., Daling, J.R., et al., 1986. Childhood brain tumors and paternal occupation in the aerospace industry. J. Natl. Cancer Inst. 77 (1), 17–19.

O'Neill, B.P., Blondal, H., Yang, P., et al., 2002. Risk of cancer among relatives of patients with glioma. Cancer Epidemiol. Biomarkers Prev. 11 (9), 921–924.

Osterlind, A., Olsen, J.H., Lynge, E., et al., 1985. Second cancer following cutaneous melanoma and cancers of the brain, thyroid, connective tissue, bone, and eye in Denmark, 1943–1980. Natl. Cancer Inst. Monogr. 68, 361–388.

Pan, S.Y., Ugnat, A.M., Mao, Y., 2005. Occupational risk factors for brain cancer in Canada. J. Occup. Environ. Med. 47 (7), 704–717.

Parkin, D., Kramarova, E., Draper, G., et al., 1998. International incidence of childhood cancer, Vol. 2. IARC, Lyon.

Percy, A.K., Elveback, L.R., Okazaki, H., et al., 1972. Neoplasms of the central nervous system. Epidemiologic considerations. Neurology 22 (1), 40–48.

Peters, F.M., Preston-Martin, S., Yu, M.C., 1981. Brain tumors in children and occupational exposure of parents. Science 213 (4504), 235–237.

Peto, R., 1981. Trends in U.S. cancer. In: Peto, R., Schneiderman, M. (Eds.), Quantification of occupational cancer. Banbury Report 9. Cold Spring Harbor, NY, pp. 269–284.

Phillips, L.E., Frankenfeld, C.L., Drangsholt, M., et al., 2005. Intracranial meningioma and ionizing radiation in medical and occupational settings. Neurology 64 (2), 350–352.

Phillips, L.E., Koepsell, T.D., van Belle, G., et al., 2002. History of head trauma and risk of intracranial meningioma: population-based case–control study. Neurology 58, 1849–1852.

Pitts, O.M., Powers, J.M., Hoffman, P.M., 1983. Vascular neoplasms induced in rodent central nervous system by murine sarcoma viruses. Lab. Invest. 49 (2), 171–182.

Pogoda, J.M., Preston-Martin, S., 2001. Maternal cured meat consumption during pregnancy and risk of pediatric brain tumor in offspring: potentially harmful levels of intake. Public Health Nutr. 4 (2), 183–189.

Pogoda, J.M., Preston-Martin, S., Howe, G., et al., 2009. An international case–control study of maternal diet during pregnancy and childhood brain tumor risk: a histology-specific analysis by food group. Ann. Epidemiol. 19 (3), 148–160.

Poltermann, S., Schlehofer, B., Steindorf, K., et al., 2006. Lack of association of herpes viruses with brain tumors. J. Neurovirol. 12 (2), 90–99.

Poole, C., Trichopoulos, D., 1991. Extremely low-frequency electric and magnetic fields and cancer. Cancer Causes Control 2 (4), 267–276.

Preston, D.L., Cullings, H., Suyama, A., et al., 2008. Solid cancer incidence in atomic bomb survivors exposed in utero or as young children. J. Natl. Cancer Inst. 100 (6), 428–436.

Preston, D.L., Ron, E., Tokuoka, S., et al., 2007. Solid cancer incidence in atomic bomb survivors: 1958–1998. Radiat. Res. 168 (1), 1–64.

Preston, D.L., Ron, E., Yonehara, S., et al., 2002. Tumors of the nervous system and pituitary gland associated with atomic bomb radiation exposure. J. Natl. Cancer Inst. 94 (20), 1555–1563.

Preston-Martin, S., 1985. The epidemiology of primary nervous system tumors in children. Ital. J. Neurol. Sci. 6 (4), 403–409.

Preston-Martin, S., Correa, P., 1989. Epidemiological evidence for the role of nitroso compounds in human cancer. Cancer Surv. 8 (2), 459–473.

Preston-Martin, S., Henderson, B.E., Pike, M.C., 1982. Descriptive epidemiology of cancers of the upper respiratory tract in Los Angeles. Cancer 49 (10), 2201–2207.

Preston-Martin, S., Mack, W., Henderson, B.E., 1989a. Risk factors for gliomas and meningiomas in males in Los Angeles County. Cancer Res. 49 (21), 6137–6143.

Preston-Martin, S., Paganini-Hill, A., Henderson, B.E., et al., 1980. Case–control study of intracranial meningiomas in women in Los Angeles County, California. J. Natl. Cancer Inst. 65 (1), 67–73.

Preston-Martin, S., Pogoda, J.M., Mueller, B.A., et al., 1996. Maternal consumption of cured meats and vitamins in relation to pediatric brain tumors. Cancer Epidemiol. Biomarkers Prev. 5 (8), 599–605.

Preston-Martin, S., Pogoda, J.M., Mueller, B.A., et al., 1998. Results from an international case–control study of childhood brain tumors: the role of prenatal vitamin supplementation. Environ. Health Perspect 106 (Suppl. 3), 887–892.

Preston-Martin, S., Thomas, D.C., Wright, W.E., et al., 1989b. Noise trauma in the aetiology of acoustic neuromas in men in Los Angeles County, 1978–1985. Br. J. Cancer 59 (5), 783–786.

Preston-Martin, S., Yu, M.C., Henderson, B.E., et al., 1983. Risk factors for meningiomas in men in Los Angeles County. J. Natl. Cancer Inst. 70 (5), 863–866.

Provost, D., Cantagrel, A., Lebailly, P., et al., 2007. Brain tumors and exposure to pesticides: a case–control study in south western France. Occup. Environ. Med. 64 (8), 509–514.

Rahu, M., Rahu, K., Auvinen, A., et al., 2006. Cancer risk among Chernobyl cleanup workers in Estonia and Latvia, 1986–1998. Int. J. Cancer 119 (1), 162–168.

Rajaraman, P., Stewart, P.A., Samet, J.M., et al., 2006. Lead, genetic susceptibility, and risk of adult brain tumors. Cancer Epidemiol. Biomarkers Prev. 15 (12), 2514–2520.

Rao, R.D., James, C.D., 2004. Altered molecular pathways in gliomas: an overview of clinically relevant issues. Semin. Oncol. 31 (5), 595–604.

Reagan, T.J., Freiman, I.S., 1973. Multiple cerebral gliomas in multiple sclerosis. J. Neurol. Neurosurg Psychiatry 36 (4), 523–528.

Reif, J.S., Pearce, N., Fraser, J., 1989. Occupational risks for brain cancer: a New Zealand Cancer Registry-based study. J. Occup. Med. 31 (10), 863–867.

Rice, J.M., Ward, J.M., 1982. Age dependence of susceptibility to carcinogenesis in the nervous system. Ann. N. Y. Acad. Sci. 381, 274–289.

Rodvall, Y., Ahlbom, A., Pershagen, G., et al., 1998. Dental radiography after age 25 years, amalgam fillings and tumors of the central nervous system. Oral. Oncol. 34 (4), 265–269.

Roelvink, N.C., Kamphorst, W., van Alphen, H.A., et al., 1987. Pregnancy-related primary brain and spinal tumors. Arch. Neurol. 44 (2), 209–215.

Romić Stojković, R., Jovancević, M., Santel, D.J., et al., 1990. Sex steroid receptors in intracranial tumors. Cancer 65 (9), 1968–1970.

Ron, E., Modan, B., Boice, J.D. Jr, et al., 1988. Tumors of the brain and nervous system after radiotherapy in childhood. N. Engl. J. Med. 319 (16), 1033–1039.

Rothman, K.J., 2000. Epidemiological evidence on health risks of cellular telephones. Lancet 356 (9244), 1837–1840.

Rousch, G., Holford, T., Schymurra, M., et al., 1987. Cancer risk and incidence trends: the Connecticut Perspective. Hemisphere, Washington, pp. 335–359.

Rubinstein, L., 1972. Tumors of the central nervous system, Vol. 2. Atlas of tumor pathology. Armed Forces Institute of Pathology, Washington DC.

Ryan, P., Hurley, S.F., Johnson, A.M., et al., 1993. Tumors of the brain and presence of antibodies to Toxoplasma gondii. Int. J. Epidemiol. 22 (3), 412–419.

Ryan, P., Lee, M.W., North, B., et al., 1992. Risk factors for tumors of the brain and meninges: results from the Adelaide Adult Brain Tumor Study. Int. J. Cancer 51 (1), 20–27.

Sadetzki, S., Chetrit, A., Freedman, L., et al., 2005. Long-term follow-up for brain tumor development after childhood exposure to ionizing radiation for tinea capitis. Radiat. Res. 163 (4), 424–432.

Salminen, E., Pukkala, E., Teppo, L., 1999. Second cancers in patients with brain tumours – impact of treatment. Eur. J. Cancer 35 (1), 102–105.

Salvati, M., Artico, M., Caruso, R., et al., 1991. A report on radiation-induced gliomas. Cancer 67 (2), 392–397.

Samanic, C.M., De Roos, A.J., Stewart, P.A., et al., 2008. Occupational exposure to pesticides and risk of adult brain tumors. Am. J. Epidemiol. 167 (8), 976–985.

Sanderson, W.T., Talaska, G., Zaebst, D., et al., 1997. Pesticide prioritization for a brain cancer case–control study. Environ. Res. 74 (2), 133–144.

Savitz, D.A., Chen, J.H., 1990. Parental occupation and childhood cancer: review of epidemiologic studies. Environ. Health Perspect 88, 325–337.

Savitz, D.A., Feingold, L., 1989. Association of childhood cancer with residential traffic density. Scand. J. Work. Environ. Health 15 (5), 360–363.

Savitz, D.A., Wachtel, H., Barnes, F.A., et al., 1988. Case–control study of childhood cancer and exposure to 60-Hz magnetic fields. Am. J. Epidemiol. 128 (1), 21–38.

Scheurer, M.E., El-Zein, R., Bondy, M.L., et al., 2007a. RE: Lack of association of herpes viruses with brain tumors. J. Neurovirol. 13 (1), 85–87.

Scheurer, M.E., Etzel, C.J., Liu, M., et al., 2007b. Aggregation of cancer in first-degree relatives of patients with glioma. Cancer Epidemiol. Biomarkers Prev. 16 (11), 2491–2495.

Scheurer, M.E., El-Zein, R., Thompson, P.A., et al., 2008. Long-term anti-inflammatory and antihistamine medication use and adult glioma risk. Cancer Epidemiol. Biomarkers Prev. 17 (5), 1277–1281.

Schlehofer, B., Blettner, M., Becker, N., et al., 1992a. Medical risk factors and the development of brain tumors. Cancer 69 (10), 2541–2547.

Schlehofer, B., Blettner, M., Preston-Martin, S., et al., 1999. Role of medical history in brain tumor development. Results from the international adult brain tumor study. Int. J. Cancer 82 (2), 155–160.

Schlehofer, B., Blettner, M., Wahrendorf, J., 1992b. Association between brain tumors and menopausal status. J. Natl. Cancer Inst. 84 (17), 1346–1349.

Schlehofer, B., Kunze, S., Sachsenheimer, W., et al., 1990. Occupational risk factors for brain tumors: results from a population-based case–control study in Germany. Cancer Causes Control 1 (3), 209–215.

Schoemaker, M.J., Swerdlow, A.J., Ahlbom, A., et al., 2005. Mobile phone use and risk of acoustic neuroma: results of the INTER-PHONE case–control study in five North European countries. Br. J. Cancer 93 (7), 842–848.

Schoemaker, M.J., Swerdlow, A.J., Auvinen, A., et al., 2007. Medical history, cigarette smoking and risk of acoustic neuroma: an international case–control study. Int. J. Cancer 120 (1), 103–110.

Schoenberg, B.S., 1991. Epidemiology of primary intracranial neoplasms: disease distribution and risk factors. In: Salcman, M. (Ed.), Neurobiology of brain tumors. Williams & Wilkins, Baltimore, pp. 3–18.

Schoenberg, B.S., Christine, B.W., Whisnant, J.P., 1975. Nervous system neoplasms and primary malignancies of other sites. The unique association between meningiomas and breast cancer. Neurology 25 (8), 705–712.

Schuman, L.M., Choi, N.W., Gullen, W.H., 1967. Relationship of central nervous system neoplasms to Toxoplasma gondii infection. Am. J. Public Health Nations Health 57 (5), 848–856.

Schüz, J., Bohler, E., Berg, G., et al., 2006. Cellular phones, cordless phones, and the risks of glioma and meningioma (INTERPHONE Study Group, Germany). Am. J. Epidemiol. 163 (6), 512–520.

Schwartzbaum, J., Jonsson, F., Ahlbom, A., et al., 2003. Cohort studies of association between self-reported allergic conditions, immune-related diagnoses and glioma and meningioma risk. Int. J. Cancer 106 (3), 423–428.

Schwartzbaum, J., Jonsson, F., Ahlbom, A., et al., 2005. Prior hospitalization for epilepsy, diabetes, and stroke and subsequent glioma and meningioma risk. Cancer Epidemiol. Biomarkers Prev. 14 (3), 643–650.

Sehgal, A., 1998. Molecular changes during the genesis of human gliomas. Semin. Surg. Oncol. 14 (1), 3–12.

Seizinger, B.R., Martuza, R.L., Gusella, J.F., 1986. Loss of genes on chromosome 22 in tumorigenesis of human acoustic neuroma. Nature. 322 (6080), 644–647.

Selvin, S., Garfinkel, J., 1972. The relationship between parental age and birth order with the percentage of low birth-weight infants. Hum. Biol. 44 (3), 501–509.

Shaw, A.K., Li, P., Infante-Rivard, C., 2006. Early infection and risk of childhood brain tumors (Canada). Cancer Causes Control 17 (10), 1267–1274.

Sima, A.A., Finkelstein, S.D., McLachlan, D.R., 1983. Multiple malignant astrocytomas in a patient with spontaneous progressive multifocal leukoencephalopathy. Ann. Neurol. 14 (2), 183–188.

Simning, A., van Wijngaarden, E., 2007. Literature review of cancer mortality and incidence among dentists. Occup. Environ. Med. 64 (7), 432–438.

Singh, G., Driever, P.H., Sander, J.W., 2005. Cancer risk in people with epilepsy: the role of antiepileptic drugs. Brain 128 (Pt 1), 7–17.

Sivak-Sears, N.R., Schwartzbaum, J.A., Miike, R., et al., 2004. Case–control study of use of nonsteroidal antiinflammatory drugs and glioblastoma multiforme. Am. J. Epidemiol. 159 (12), 1131–1139.

Smith, F.P., Slavik, M., MacDonald, J.S., 1978. Association of breast cancer with meningioma: report of two cases and review of the literature. Cancer 42 (4), 1992–1994.

Smith, G.D., Shipley, M.J., 1989. Plasma cholesterol concentration and primary brain tumours. BMJ 299 (6690), 26–27.

Smith, M.A., Freidlin, B., Ries, L.A., et al., 1998. Trends in reported incidence of primary malignant brain tumors in children in the United States. J. Natl. Cancer Inst. 90 (17), 1269–1277.

Smith-Warner, S.A., Spiegelman, D., Ritz, J., et al., 2006. Methods for pooling results of epidemiologic studies: the Pooling Project of Prospective Studies of Diet and Cancer. Am. J. Epidemiol. 163 (11), 1053–1064.

Sont, W.N., Zielinski, J.M., Ashmore, J.P., et al., 2001. First analysis of cancer incidence and occupational radiation exposure based on the National Dose Registry of Canada. Am. J. Epidemiol. 153 (4), 309–318.

Sorensen, S.A., Mulvihill, J.J., Nielsen, A., 1985. Malignancy in neurofibromatosis. In: Muller, H., Weber, W. (Eds.), Familial cancer. Karger, Basel, pp. 119–120.

Speers, M.A., Dobbins, J.G., Miller, V.S., 1988. Occupational exposures and brain cancer mortality: a preliminary study of east Texas residents. Am. J. Ind. Med. 13 (6), 629–638.

Stalberg, K., Haglund, B., Axelsson, O., et al., 2007. Prenatal X-ray exposure and childhood brain tumours: a population-based case–control study on tumour subtypes. Br. J. Cancer 97 (11), 1583–1587.

Steinitz, R., Parkin, D.M., Young, J.L., et al., 1989. Cancer incidence in Jewish migrants to Israel, 1961–1981. IARC Sci. Publ. 98, 1–311.

Stellman, S.D., Demers, P.A., Colin, D., et al., 1998. Cancer mortality and wood dust exposure among participants in the American Cancer Society Cancer Prevention Study-II (CPS-II). Am. J. Ind. Med. 34 (3), 229–237.

Strickler, H.D., Rosenberg, P.S., Devesa, S.S., et al., 1998. Contamination of poliovirus vaccines with simian virus 40 (1955–1963) and subsequent cancer rates. JAMA 279 (4), 292–295.

Stroup, N.E., Blair, A., Erikson, G.E., 1986. Brain cancer and other causes of death in anatomists. J. Natl. Cancer Inst. 77 (6), 1217–1224.

Stukonis, M., 1978. Cancer incidence cumulative rates – international comparison. IARC, Internal technical report, Lyon.

Sul, J., Posner, J.B., 2007. Brain metastases: epidemiology and pathophysiology. Cancer Treat. Res. 136, 1–21.

Swenburg, J.A., 1982. Current approaches to the experimental investigation of chemicals in relation to cancer of the brain. Ann. N. Y. Acad. Sci. 381, 43–49.

Swift, M., Morrell, D., Cromartie, E., et al., 1986. The incidence and gene frequency of ataxia-telangiectasia in the United States. Am. J. Hum. Genet 39 (5), 573–583.

Tedeschi-Blok, N., Lee, M., Sison, J.D., et al., 2006. Inverse association of antioxidant and phytoestrogen nutrient intake with adult glioma in the San Francisco Bay Area: a case–control study. BMC Cancer 6, 148.

Thomas, T.L., Stewart, P.A., Stemhagen, A., et al., 1987a. Risk of astrocytic brain tumors associated with occupational chemical exposures. A case-referent study. Scand. J. Work Environ. Health 13 (5), 417–423.

Thomas, T.L., Stolley, P.D., Stemhagen, A., et al., 1987b. Brain tumor mortality risk among men with electrical and electronics jobs: a case–control study. J. Natl. Cancer Inst. 79 (2), 233–238.

Thomas, T.L., Waxweiler, R.J., 1986. Brain tumors and occupational risk factors. Scand. J. Work. Environ. Health 12, 1–15.

Tijssen, C.C., 1985. Genetic aspects of brain tumours – tumours of neuroepithelial and meningeal tissue. In: Muller, H., Weber, W. (Eds.), Familial cancer. Karger, Basel, pp. 98–102.

Tomkova, K., Tomka, M., Zajac, V., 2008. Contribution of p53, p63, and p73 to the developmental diseases and cancer. Neoplasma 55 (3), 177–181.

Tracy, S.E., Woda, B.A., Robinson, H.L., 1985. Induction of angiosarcoma by a c-erbB transducing virus. J. Virol. 54 (2), 304–310.

Traynor, J.E., Casey, H.W., 1971. Five-year follow-up of primates exposed to 55 MeV protons. Radiat. Res. 47 (1), 143–148.

Trojan, J., Cloix, J.F., Ardourel, M.Y., et al., 2007. Insulin-like growth factor type I biology and targeting in malignant gliomas. Neuroscience 145 (3), 795–811.

Tucker, M.A., Boice, J.D. Jr, Hoffman, D.A., 1985. Second cancer following cutaneous melanoma and cancers of the brain, thyroid, connective tissue, bone, and eye in Connecticut, 1935–1982. Natl. Cancer Inst. Monogr. 68, 161–189.

Unger, M., Olsen, J., 1980. Organochlorine compounds in the adipose tissue of deceased people with and without cancer. Environ. Res. 23 (2), 257–263.

van Wijngaarden, E., Dosemeci, M., 2006. Brain cancer mortality and potential occupational exposure to lead: findings from the National Longitudinal Mortality Study, 1979–1989. Int. J. Cancer 119 (5), 1136–1144.

Velema, J.P., Percy, C.L., 1987. Age curves of central nervous system tumor incidence in adults: variation of shape by histologic type. J. Natl. Cancer Inst. 79 (4), 623–629.

Velema, J.P., Walker, A.M., 1987. The age curve of nervous system tumor incidence in adults: common shape but changing levels by sex, race and geographical location. Int. J. Epidemiol. 16 (2), 177–183.

Vena, J.E., Bona, J.R., Byers, T.E., et al., 1985. Allergy-related diseases and cancer: an inverse association. Am. J. Epidemiol. 122 (1), 66–74.

Viel, J.F., Challier, B., Pitard, A., et al., 1998. Brain cancer mortality among French farmers: the vineyard pesticide hypothesis. Arch. Environ. Health 53 (1), 65–70.

Vrijheid, M., Cardis, E., Armstrong, B.K., et al., 2006a. Validation of short term recall of mobile phone use for the INTERPHONE study. Occup. Environ. Med. 63 (4), 237–243.

Vrijheid, M., Deltour, I., Krewski, D., et al., 2006b. The effects of recall errors and of selection bias in epidemiologic studies of mobile phone use and cancer risk. J. Expo. Sci. Environ. Epidemiol. 16 (4), 371–384.

Walker, A.E., Robins, M., Weinfeld, F.D., 1985. Epidemiology of brain tumors: the national survey of intracranial neoplasms. Neurology 35 (2), 219–226.

Walrath, J., Fraumeni, J.F. Jr, 1983. Mortality patterns among embalmers. Int. J. Cancer 31 (4), 407–411.

Wang, H., Diepgen, T.L., 2006. Atopic dermatitis and cancer risk. Br. J. Dermatol. 154 (2), 205–210.

Ward, D., Mattison, M.L., Finn, R., 1973. Association between previous tuberculosis infection and cerebral glioma. BMJ (1), 83–84.

Ward, D., Rice, J.M., 1982. Review of naturally occurring and chemically induced tumors of the central and peripheral nervous systems in mice and rats in the national Toxicology Program/NCI Carcinogenesis Testing Program. Ann. N. Y. Acad. Sci. 381, 265–273.

Waxweiler, R.G., Stringer, W., Wagner, J.K., 1976. Neoplastic risk among workers exposed to vinyl chloride. Ann. N. Y. Acad. Sci. 271, 40–48.

Wertheimer, N., Leeper, E., 1979. Electrical wiring configurations and childhood cancer. Am. J. Epidemiol. 109 (3), 273–284.

Wesseling, C., Pukkala, E., Neuvonen, K., et al., 2002. Cancer of the brain and nervous system and occupational exposures in Finnish women. J. Occup. Environ. Med. 44 (7), 663–668.

Wiemels, J.L., Wiencke, J.K., Kelsey, K.T., et al., 2007. Allergy-related polymorphisms influence glioma status and serum IgE levels. Cancer Epidemiol. Biomarkers Prev. 16 (6), 1229–1235.

Wiemels, J.L., Wiencke, J.K., Patoka, J., et al., 2004. Reduced immunoglobulin E and allergy among adults with glioma compared with controls. Cancer Res. 64 (22), 8468–8473.

Wigertz, A., Lönn, S., Hall, P., et al., 2008. Reproductive factors and risk of meningioma and glioma. Cancer Epidemiol. Biomarkers Prev. 17 (10), 2663–2670.

Wigertz, A., Lönn, S., Mathiesen, T., et al., 2006. Risk of brain tumors associated with exposure to exogenous female sex hormones. Am. J. Epidemiol. 164 (7), 629–636.

Wigertz, A., Lönn, S., Schwartzbaum, J., et al., 2007. Allergic conditions and brain tumor risk. Am. J. Epidemiol. 166 (8), 941–950.

Wilkins, J.R. 3rd, Hundley, V.D., 1990. Paternal occupational exposure to electromagnetic fields and neuroblastoma in offspring. Am. J. Epidemiol. 131 (6), 995–1008.

Wilkins, J.R. 3rd, Koutras, R.A., 1988. Paternal occupation and brain cancer in offspring: a mortality-based case–control study. Am. J. Ind. Med. 14 (3), 299–318.

Wrensch, M., Fisher, J.L., Schwartzbaum, J.A., et al., 2005. The molecular epidemiology of gliomas in adults. Neurosurg. Focus 19 (5):E5.

Wrensch, M., Lee, M., Miike, R., et al., 1997a. Familial and personal medical history of cancer and nervous system conditions among adults with glioma and controls. Am. J. Epidemiol. 145 (7), 581–593.

Wrensch, M., Weinberg, A., Wiencke, J., et al., 1997b. Does prior infection with varicella-zoster virus influence risk of adult glioma? Am. J. Epidemiol. 145 (7), 594–597.

Wrensch, M., Weinberg, A., Wiencke, J., et al., 2001. Prevalence of antibodies to four herpesviruses among adults with glioma and controls. Am. J. Epidemiol. 154 (2), 161–165.

Yates, P.O., Pearce, K.M., 1960. Recent change in blood-group distribution of astrocytomas. Lancet 1 (7117), 194–195.

Yeni-Komshian, H., Holly, E.A., 2000. Childhood brain tumours and exposure to animals and farm life: a review. Paediatr. Perinat. Epidemiol. 14 (3), 248–256.

Yohn, D.S., 1972. Oncogenic viruses: expectations and applications in neuropathology. Prog. Exp. Tumor. Res. 17, 74–92.

Zahm, S.H., Ward, M.H., 1998. Pesticides and childhood cancer. Environ. Health Perspect 106 (Suppl. 3), 893–908.

Zang, K.D., Singer, H., 1967. Chromosomal constitution of meningiomas. Nature 216 (5110), 84–85.

Zeller, W.J., Ivankovic, S., Habs, M., et al., 1982. Experimental chemical production of brain tumors. Ann. N. Y. Acad. Sci. 381, 250–263.

Zimmerman, H.M., 1982. Production of brain tumors with aromatic hydrocarbons. Ann. N. Y. Acad. Sci. 381, 320–324.

Neurogenetics and the molecular biology of human brain tumors

Ivan Radovanovic and Abhijit Guha

General principles of cancer biology

The majority of human brain tumors arise sporadically, with only a few that are clearly linked with cancer pre-disposing environmental factors or genetic syndromes. Among cancer pre-disposing environmental factors are clearly established ones, such as radiation, while others such as excessive use of cell phones remain the subject of on-going debate (Bondy et al 2008; Croft et al 2008). Cancer pre-disposing genetic syndromes, which present earlier in the pediatric population, are associated with both benign and malignant brain tumors and will be discussed later in the chapter. What is common among sporadic and pre-disposed brain tumors, similar to other cancers, is the fundamental fact that *cancer is a genetic disease* (Fig. 5.1). Alterations in regulation/activity of several normal genes which regulate proliferation, apoptosis, migration and other fundamental cellular processes, often in a cumulative manner, are involved in the genesis and subsequent progression of the brain tumor. Broadly speaking, these genetic alterations include gain-of-function mutations or amplification (oncogenes – the so-called 'accelerators' of cellular growth) and loss-of-function mutations or deletions (tumor suppressor genes, TSGs – the so-called 'brakes' of cellular growth) (Fig. 5.1). Another general point of importance is that the overall growth and therapeutic response of a cancer is not just the result of primary genetic alterations in the tumor cells, but also how these alterations affect and can be effected by stromal endothelial cells, immune cells and further influenced by environmental epigenetic regulation, as depicted in (Fig. 5.2). Collectively, this complex genetic interplay leads to molecular heterogeneity and subsequent pathological heterogeneity, within the same tumor. When a reproducible repertoire of these key growth regulatory genes becomes aberrant in their function and also bypasses the normal cellular death machinery (apoptosis) which destroys aberrant cells, cancer arises. It is the goal of molecular oncology to understand these genetic alterations at the level of the gene, the transcripts and ultimately the proteins, the final workhorse of genetic function. The complexity of understanding the genome, transcriptome and ultimately the proteome, increases exponentially, as depicted in Figure 5.2. However, this slow, thorough and collaborative effort between clinicians and basic scientists is required if we are to develop novel biological targeted therapies (Fig. 5.1, and see Table 5.5), which we believe is the hope for improving the prognosis of currently incurable cancers such as GBMs.

Clonal or field effect and cancer stem cell hypothesis

Debate exists as to whether these genetic alterations that induce cancer such as astrocytomas occur in one astrocyte-clone or a field of astrocytes, both of which then expand to acquire additional alterations leading to tumor progression and heterogeneity, as depicted in Figure 5.3. Multifocal astrocytomas and the entity of gliomatosis cerebri (Romeike & Mawrin 2008), do suggest that in certain cases, there exists a field induction. However, this is not definitive proof since due to the well-recognized invasive capability of astrocytoma cells, one cannot exclude migration from one region to another.

In addition, recent evidence suggests that transformation likely occurs in a 'cancer stem cell' rather than a fully differentiated one, as demonstrated quite elegantly many years ago in leukemias. These cancer stem cells have unlimited capacity to self-replicate (which is a pre-requisite for all transformed cells) and are able to differentiate into several lineages (Fig. 5.4) (Singh et al 2004; Sanai et al 2004). Indeed many of the growth and antigenic characteristics of normal neural stem cells have similarities to transformed cancer cells such as gliomas, making the hypothesis that it is these neural stem cells, or their subsequent immediate progeny, that become transformed to glioma cancer stem cells, with additional molecular alterations giving rise to different grades of gliomas (Cavenee & Kleihues 2000). The therapeutic implication of this hypothesis is that one needs to target the molecular alterations in the rarer cancer stem cells, rather than against their more abundant differentiated off-springs, to completely eradicate the tumor by preventing re-population. Indeed, putative GBM stem cells which may harbor different molecular signatures and hence response to radiation and anti-angiogenesis therapies have been identified (Singh et al 2004). However, lack of ability to strictly characterize a normal glial stem cell, let alone a glioma stem cell, plus the recognized phenomenon of de-differentiation as a result of transformation, leaves much research to be undertaken in this very important area of work centered on cancer stem cells.

Astrocytomas are classified into four WHO (Cavenee & Kleihues 2000) grades, with the most malignant grade-4 or glioblastoma multiforme (GBM) being the most lethal, with a mean survival of less than 16 months, despite current treatment of radical surgical de-bulking, external beam radiotherapy and concomitant chemotherapy. GBMs may develop de-novo and are termed 'Primary GBMs', or they may progress from lower-grade astrocytomas and are termed 'Secondary GBMs', as depicted in Figure 5.5. Whether the 'Primary GBMs' also arise from progression, perhaps with the lower-grade astrocytoma remaining clinically silent, is of debate. However, molecular characterization suggests that these pathologically heterogeneous tumors

are also molecularly heterogeneous, with at least two if not more molecular pathways leading to development of a GBM (Fig. 5.5). This molecular heterogeneity has recently been highlighted by the National Cancer Institute-sponsored Cancer Genome Atlas (TCGA) project, where early results on screening GBMs already show a large number of primary genetic alterations (Cancer Genome Atlas Research Network 2008). In addition to these primary genetic alterations, there exist many secondary epigenetic alterations leading to alterations in the transcripts and ultimately proteins that will add to the molecular heterogeneity. Although this enormity of genetic alterations may lead one to give up on a singular

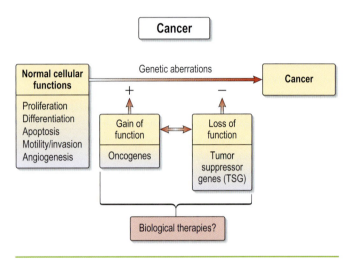

Figure 5.1 Schematic description of general molecular oncogenesis, involving aberrations in normal cell regulatory genes which become aberrant by either loss- or gain-of-function, leading to cancer. Molecular oncology attempts to elucidate these aberrations, their interactions and functional role, with the hope of translating that knowledge to biological therapies.

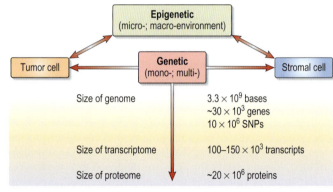

Figure 5.2 Schematic representation showing sizes and distribution of epigenetic and genetic involvement with tumor and stromal cells.

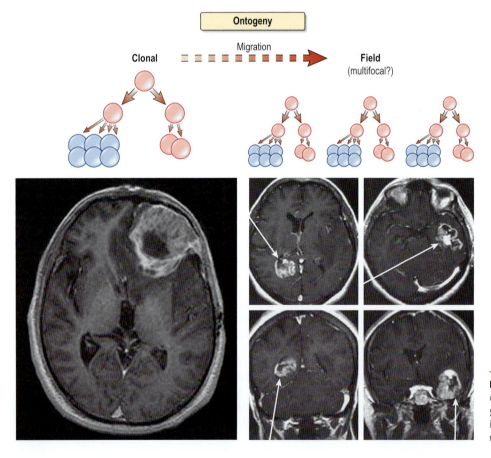

Figure 5.3 'Clonal' and 'Field' for induction of astrocytomas (red circle). Multifocal gliomas suggest the existence of 'field' induction in some astrocytomas, but this may be the result of astrocytoma migration.

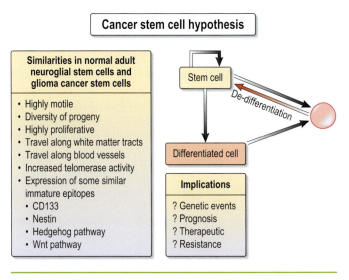

Figure 5.4 Cancer stem cells hypothesis is where the tumor is induced in a self-replicating multi-potent cell vs a well-differentiated cell. The implications of this hypothesis on therapy may be critical in terms of targeting the cancer stem cells, rather than a differentiated offspring. However, this hypothesis remains to be proven, since differentiated transformed GBM cells do replicate and can express many epitopes suggestive of several neural-glial lineage cells as a result of de-differentiation. Much research is required on this very important hypothesis in oncogenesis. (Adapted from Singh et al 2004; Sanai et al 2005).

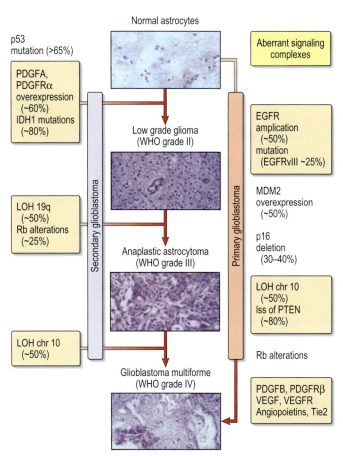

Figure 5.5 Schematic description of molecular pathogenetic pathways in astrocytomas, which leads to the same pathological entity known as a GBM. At least two pathways have been described: 'Primary GBMs' arise de-novo, more in older individuals, and are characterized by aberrations and mutations in EGFR; 'Secondary GBMs' occur through a step-wise progression from lower-grade astrocytomas, which are characterized by mutations in p53, mutations in IDH and aberrant activation of PDGFRa. Like many cancers, there are multiple genetic alterations, composed of loss-of-function (tumor suppressor genes) and gain-of-function (oncogenes), which may play a role in induction of the astrocytoma and/or progression to increased malignancy.

cure for GBMs, it does open up a large number of genetic targets and signaling pathways which may be targeted by current, and still to be discovered, biological therapies, with the hope of slowing down tumor growth in a multi-therapy strategy.

As in other cancers, most gliomas occur spontaneously, without any clear genetic or environmental risk factors. A small subset of gliomas (<5%) occur in the context of germ-line predisposing syndromes such as neurofibromatosis-1, -2 (NF-1, NF-2), Li–Fraumeni, Turcot, and tuberous sclerosis, detailed below. Gliomas from these well-defined cohorts of patients, although small in number, serve an extremely important function in increasing our knowledge of the molecular pathogenesis of the larger sporadic group, as the tumors share many similar genetic alterations.

Aberrations in cell cycle regulatory pathway

Like the majority of human cancers, perturbations in both the p53 and Rb-regulated cell cycle regulatory pathways, are present in human brain tumors including gliomas (Fig. 5.6). p53 protein is a transcription factor that can inhibit cell cycle progression or induce apoptosis in response to stress or DNA damage. Inactivation of p53 function, either by mutations in conjunction with loss of heterozygosity (LOH) of the p53 loci on chromosome #17p (found in 30–40% of all astrocytomas grades (el-Azouzi et al 1989), or aberrant regulation by over-expression of MDM2 or loss of p19, leads to alteration of these critical cell regulatory process (Fig. 5.5). Approximately one-third of all astrocytomas with chromosome #17p loss have p53 mutations with 25% in GBMs, 34% in AA and 30% in LGAs (Fulci et al 1998). Most mutations are missense

mutations found on the conserved domains of Exon 5–8, with no clear studies reporting brain specific mutations, except one study that identified a preponderance of Exon 4 mutations in GBMs (Li et al 1998). Of interest, LOH of *17p* or p53 mutations are rarely found in GBMs with EGFR amplification, which is more closely associated with 'Primary' GBMs as discussed above and in Figure 5.5. However, in these 'Primary' GBMs alterations in p53 function exist, although their may be secondary to aberrant regulation of p53 by proteins such as MDM2 (Figs 5.5, 5.6). MDM2 acts in a feedback loop to limit the action of p53, both by inhibiting its transactivating activity and by catalyzing its destruction (Haupt et al 1997). Less than 5% of astrocytomas demonstrate MDM2 amplification (none of these has primary p53 mutations (Rasheed et al 1999), although 50% of GBMs overexpress MDM2 without gene amplification. Normally, p19 keeps in check this negative regulation of p53 by inhibiting MDM2 expression, with loss of p19 which occurs in

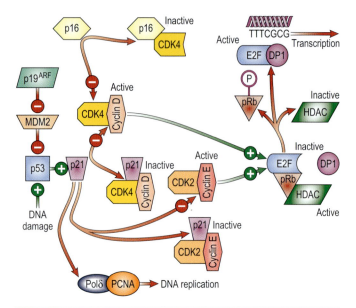

Figure 5.6 Schemata of the critical p53 and pRB mediated cell cycle regulatory pathway, with direct and indirect regulatory proteins, all or some of which may be involved in causing aberrant regulation of these two pathways in majority of human cancers, including astrocytomas. Specifically in astrocytomas, alterations in p53 function may be by direct mutation or loss, or secondary through overexpression of MDM2 or loss of p19. Similarly, there may be direct mutation/loss of pRb or indirect via overexpression of CDK4 or loss of CDK inhibitors such as p16.

occurs in ~30% of GBMs (Rasheed et al 1999), resulting in aberrant activation of MDM2 and thereby providing another mechanism leading to aberrant p53 regulation in astrocytomas (Fig. 5.6).

Similar to the p53 pathway, aberrant loss of p16/cdk4/cyclinD/pRb cell-cycle regulation, integral in G1 to S phase transition, is also prevalent in majority of astrocytomas (Fig. 5.6). Primary LOH of Rb or point mutations occur in 30–40% of GBMs, while amplification or over-expression of *cdk4* is found in 10–20% of GBMs (Reifenberger et al 1994). Inactivation of p16, through homozygous deletion of *CDKN2A* gene, occurs in 24% of AA and 33% of GBMs (Rasheed et al 1999). Rare point mutations of *CDKN2A* or more commonly transcriptional silencing due to *CDKN2A* promoter methylation, also inactivates or downregulates p16 function in many GBMs, resulting in a high proliferative index as demonstrated by Ki67 staining (Ono et al 1996). Of interest, 'Primary GBMs' demonstrate a higher rate of p16 deletion compared to 'Secondary GBMs', whereas *p*Rb LOH and *CDK4* amplification occurs with similar frequency.

Alterations of these critical cell-cycle regulatory proteins alone, although common in GBMs, are probably not sufficient to induce gliomas by themselves, as demonstrated in mouse models (Holland 2001). For example, mice null for p16^{Ink4a} and p19^{ARF} or p53 do not readily form gliomas (Holland 2001), unless bred to other mice harboring additional cell signaling or apoptosis genetic alterations. These include mice with mutations in *NF-1* (neurofibromatosis-1) resulting in aberrant activation of p21-Ras mediated signaling, or activated EGFR mutations (EGFRvIII), both prevalent in human GBMs.

Aberrant growth factors and growth factor receptors

Receptor protein tyrosine kinases (RPTK) and associated downstream aberrant signaling pathways have been clearly linked to the progression of astrocytomas, as schematized in Figure 5.5. Among the many RPTKs, platelet-derived growth factor receptor (PDGFR) and epidermal growth factor receptor (EGFR), have garnered the most interest in astrocytomas.

PDGFR

Two isoforms of PDGFR have been described, PDGFR-α and PDGFR-β, each isoform being encoded by a separate gene (PDGFR-α: chromosome 4; PDGFR-β: chromosome 5) (Hart et al 1988). PDGF is a dimeric growth factor composed of homo- or heterodimers of PDGF-A (chromosome 7), which binds only PDGFR-α, and PDGF-β (chromosome 22), which can bind to both PDGFRs, although at higher affinity to PDGFR-β (Hart et al 1988). The importance of PDGF and PDGFR was noted by astrocytomas developing in primates infected with the simian sarcoma virus (SSV) carrying the *v-sis* oncogene, which is an oncogenic form of PDGF-B (Deinhardt 1980). Human astrocytomas have been shown to overexpress both PDGF ligands and their cognate receptors (Nister et al 1988), resulting in paracrine or autocrine growth stimulatory loops. Unlike EGFRs, rearrangements and amplification of PDGFs or PDGFRs are rare, with amplification in PDGFR-α in ~8% of GBMs and none yet detected for PDGFR-β (Fleming et al 1992). However, overexpression of PDGFR-α receptor is found in ~24% of human astrocytomas, and is likely an early induction factor as it is found in all grades (Fig. 5.5). However, only higher-grade astrocytomas also overexpress the ligands, suggestive of autocrine stimulatory loops contributing to tumor progression. PDGFR-β overexpression is usually found in higher astrocytoma grades, where it may contribute with other angiogenesis-specific cytokines such as VEGF and angiopoietins to the florid GBM vasculature. The functional relevance of these PDGF stimulatory loops in astrocytomas has been tested with neutralizing antibodies, small molecule inhibitors and dominant-negative mutants (Shamah et al 1993). These encouraging pre-clinical data have led to clinical trials targeting PDGF mediated stimulation in astrocytomas (Rao & James 2004).

EGFR

In contrast to PDGFR-α, overexpression of EGFR or ErbB1 (chromosome 7p11-p12) is a late event promoting malignant progression to a GBM, with amplification and often accompanying activating mutations. Amplification of EGFR is detected in only ~3% of low-grade astrocytomas, ~7% of anaplastic astrocytomas but in 40–50% of GBMs (Collins 1995). The normal 170 kDa EGFR binds to EGF, transforming growth factor-α (TGF-α), vaccinia virus growth factor and amphiregulin, resulting in receptor dimerization and activation of downstream signaling pathways (Heldin 1995). This dimerization can form homodimers, or heterodimers with other members of the EGFR family, including ErbB2, ErbB3 and ErbB4 (Heldin 1995). Recently, polymorphisms in the 5′-untranslated region of EGF have been implicated to play a role in gliomagenesis (Bhowmick et al 2004), with

GBM patients with the –GA or –GG genotype having higher tumoral levels of EGF, irrespective of EGFR status. These GBM patients had a significantly shorter overall progression-free survival, compared with the common –AA genotype.

Oncogenic mutant forms of EGFR, notably v-erb-B, have been reported in a variety of human cancers, as has the oncogenic form of ErbB2 (v-neu), especially in breast cancer. In a large number of GBMs with EGFR gene amplification, mutant forms of EGFR are detected, the most common of which is the truncated 140 kDa EGFRvIII or ΔEGFR. EGFRvIII results from intragenic deletions in exons 2–7 (801 bases encoding amino acid #6–273) of the extracellular domain of normal EGFR, resulting in a constitutively phosphorylated (activated) mutant EGFRvIII (Ekstrand et al 1994). In addition to constitutive activation, aberrations in EGFRvIII turnover and persistent signaling in subcellular locations may be another mechanism how it is more transforming than normal EGFR (Moscatello et al 1996).

GBMs which express EGFRvIII have increased in vitro and in vivo growth advantage in experimental conditions, with some ambiguity as to whether it is a negative survival prognosticator in patients. Our recent studies demonstrate that the cohort of GBMs, especially those patients younger than 50 years of age, expressing EGFRvIII have a worse prognosis (Feldkamp et al 1999b). Of interest, the prevalence of EGFRvIII in GBMs may be higher than initially predicted by the number of GBMs with amplifications, as it may also arise not just from intragenic deletion but also aberrant splicing at the RNA level. This second mechanism seems to occur in other human cancers where EGFRvIII has been detected (breast, ovarian, and non-small cell lung), while intragenic deletion is only found in GBMs (Moscatello et al 1995). Due to the prevalence and importance of aberrations in EGF and EGFRs in human GBMs, it has become a highly sought after biological therapeutic target in GBMs, with a variety of potential approaches including neutralizing antibodies, small molecule inhibitors and immunotoxins.

The above discussion is intentionally focused on PDGFR and EGFR, however, a large number of other relevant RPTKs in astrocytomas exist. These include insulin-like growth factors (IGFs) or somatomedins, which along with their receptors (IGFR) are elevated in GBMs, associated tumor cyst fluid and CSF, compared with normal adult brains (Prisell et al 1987). Hepatocyte growth factor/scatter factor (HGF/SCF) and its receptor c-Met have also been noted in glioma pathogenesis, with co-expression more frequently in GBMs than in low-grade astrocytomas (Koochekpour et al 1997; Laterra et al 1997).

Aberrant signal transduction pathways

A variety of aberrant signaling pathways, resulting from primary mutations or secondary to upstream activation of receptors as described above, contribute to alterations in proliferation, angiogenesis, invasion and apoptosis of astrocytomas, resulting in overall growth. The more known relevant pathways are discussed in greater detail below.

p21-Ras
The three human p21-Ras genes encode for four proteins (Ha, N, K4A, K4B) and belong to the important small-G protein-mediated signaling family. Activating mutations (residue 12, 13, 61) of p21-Ras are prevalent in greater than 30% of all human cancers, making this the most common human oncogene (Bos 1989). Much is known of how activation of p21-Ras is regulated by activated RPTKs and its downstream effectors, leading to alterations in cell behavior. p21-Ras activation requires post-translational modification to bind to the inner cell membrane, where exchange of GDP for GTP can occur by nucleotide exchange factors, such as mSos (mammalian homolog of the Son of sevenless) gene (James et al 1993; Pelicci et al 1992). Normal inactivation of p21-Ras:GTP to p21-Ras:GDP requires binding of a family of enzymes called Ras-GAPs (GTPase activating protein, among which are p120GAP and neurofibromin (lost in NF-1 tumors). Hence, in addition to primary activating mutations of p21-Ras, decreased levels of these Ras:GAPs in theory, would also lead to elevated levels of active p21-Ras:GTP. This has been documented in NF-1-associated peripheral nerve tumors and astrocytomas by our group (Feldkamp et al 1999a).

Activated p21-Ras leads to activation of several downstream signals, which ultimately converge into the nucleus to alter transcription and thereby the cell response. One of these is activation of Raf and subsequent activation of MAP-Kinase (ERK1,2), leading to its translocation to the nucleus and resultant proliferative signals. Others include activation of PI3-kinase signaling (discussed in greater detail below), PLCγ and PKC.

Unlike 30% of all human cancers, primary oncogenic p21-Ras mutations are not prevalent in GBMs. However, data initially from our laboratory and subsequently confirmed by others, demonstrate that levels of activated p21-Ras are elevated in GBMs likely from aberrant upstream signals generated by overexpressed and mutated receptors such as PDGFR and EGFR. We and others went on to demonstrate that activated p21-Ras is of functional importance in GBM proliferation, angiogenesis and overall growth using a variety of in vitro and in vivo models, including transgenic mouse glioma models. These experiments were undertaken by genetic modulation of activated p21-Ras, but of more therapeutic relevance using small molecule inhibitors of activated p21-Ras (Feldkamp et al 1999c), which are under current clinical investigations.

PI3K-PTEN-AKT
The PI3-kinase pathway is another major signaling pathway implicated in gliomagenesis. PI3-K can be activated either through p21-Ras-dependent or -independent mechanisms, with activation of AKT/PKB and mTOR (mammalian target of rapamycin), which in turn activates a multitude of downstream effecter pathways leading to cell survival, proliferation, and cytoskeletal organization (Stambolic et al 1998). PI3-K pathway activation in GBMs is not only from upstream activated RPTKs, but also from loss of its major negative regulator PTEN/MMAC located on chromosome 10q23 (Fig. 5.5). Loss of PTEN expression, either through mutation, deletion, or gene inactivation, is one of the most common genetic aberrations of GBMs, and is not found in lower-grade astrocytomas (Stambolic et al 1998; Steck et al 1997). PTEN mutations in 'Primary GBMs' are somewhat more common (~32%) and are associated with amplifications/mutations of

EGFR, compared with mutations in 'Secondary GBMs' (~4%) (Stambolic et al 1998). The prevalence of loss of PTEN protein expression is higher than the mutational rate and approaches ~70–95% of GBMs, suggesting other mechanisms of PTEN loss such as gene inactivation (Maher et al 2001).

Aberrations in PI3-kinase signaling have been demonstrated to be of high functional relevance in GBMs, as restoration of normal PTEN activity in human GBM cells leads to G1 cell cycle arrest. Mouse glioma models based on deletion of PTEN also attest to this importance in astrocytoma progression, as demonstrated by our lab and others. Activation of AKT/PKB leads to activation of several downstream signaling molecules and pro-survival pathways (Maher et al 2001). Among these is mTOR and its downstream target S6, involved in mRNA translation. Since the PI3-K:AKT:mTOR pathway is commonly activated in GBMs, there is considerable interest in designing specific drugs against these molecules. Clinical interest is somewhat limited by bioavailability and toxicity issues, an area of active research. Pharmacologic inhibitors of AKT/PKB are still at the preclinical stage, while mTOR inhibitors based on rapamycin and its analogs CCI-779 and RAD001 are being evaluated in early clinical trials in recurrent GBMs (Huang & Houghton 2003).

JAK-STAT

Activation of the JAK (Janus tyrosine kinases)/STAT (signal transducers and activators of transcription) signaling pathway by various cytokine receptors is important in cellular regulation (Schaefer et al 2002). The JAK family of proteins consists of cytoplasmic proteins with four members, JAK1 JAK2, JAK3, and TYK2, which share seven regions of high homology between them known as JAK homology regions (JH1–JH7). The C-terminal JH-1 domain encodes the catalytic kinase, with the N-terminal JH3–JH7 implicated in receptor association. Seven STAT proteins, have been identified in mammals (STAT1–4, STAT5a, STAT5b, and STAT6) (Kisseleva et al 2002). JAK is recruited to the intracellular domains of certain types of activated receptors, notably the interferon receptors (IFNRs), where it itself is phosphorylated and activated. Activated JAKs in turn phosphorylates downstream substrates, notably STATs, which are latent cytoplasmic transcription factors that on phosphorylation become activated and form homo- or heterodimers. These dimers then translocate to the nucleus to regulate gene transcription. In addition to the STATs, JAKs can also recruit other molecules to the receptor, to activate the MAPK or PI3-K pathways.

Studies in brain tumors on JAK-STATs are not entirely clear. One group found Jak1 and STAT3 to be more elevated in low-grade vs high-grade gliomas, while another group found STAT3 was constitutively activated in glioma and medulloblastoma tumors (Schaefer et al 2002). Analysis of these gliomas found activated STAT3 to be mainly localized to endothelial cells, perhaps resulting in inducing transcription of VEGF and thereby playing a role in glioma angiogenesis. Preclinical studies with emerging agents that inhibit this pathway suggest that targeting the JAK-STAT pathway may be of potential therapeutic benefit in gliomas.

PKC

Protein kinase C (PKC) is a large family of phospholipid-dependent serine/threonine kinases, which are involved in a variety of signal transduction pathways (Blumberg 1991). There are many isozymes of PKC, which differ in their enzymatic properties, tissue expression and intracellular localization. All consist of an N-terminal regulatory domain and a C-terminal kinase domain. The inhibitory effect of the regulatory domain can be inhibited by calcium, anionic phospholipid, diacylglycerol (DAG), or tumor promoting phorbol esters (TPA), depending on the isozyme, hence activating the protein. Three classes of PKC isozymes have been described based on their activation by calcium and DAG (Nishizuka 1992). Conventional PKC isozymes (α, $\beta1$, $\beta2$, γ) are dependent on calcium for their activation, while the novel isozymes (δ, ε, η, θ, μ) do not require calcium for their activation. Both classes are activated by DAG, while atypical isozymes (ζ, λ) are neither calcium-dependent, nor activated by DAG. The set of isozymes expressed in a cell varies during development, transformation, differentiation and senescence (Nishizuka 1992).

PKC is expressed at high levels in the normal developing brain, where it is an important glial mitogen and maturation factor (Clark et al 1991; Honegger 1986). The demonstration that TPA application and activation of PKC could induce tumors, along with the high fetal and neonatal CNS expression, sparked interest to investigate the role of PKC in the pathogenesis of astrocytomas. Malignant astrocytoma cell lines and specimens were found to have increased expression of PKC similar to fetal astrocytes, perhaps as a result of de-differentiation (Couldwell & Antel 1992). In addition, stimulation of aberrant receptors such as EGFR in GBM cells, resulted not only in activation of p21-Ras and PI3-kinase, but also PKC mediated signaling (Couldwell & Antel 1992). However, which PKC isoform(s) are elevated and in which grades of astrocytomas, remains a topic of debate. Several groups have implicated increased PKCα levels in GBMs, with genetic or pharmacological inhibition resulting in growth inhibition (Couldwell & Antel 1992). Current pharmacologic inhibitors of PKC have had some promise in preclinical studies in GBMs, however, clinical trials with tamoxifen, a non-specific PKC inhibitor with acceptable toxicity as per extensive use in breast cancer patients, did not show efficacy (Couldwell & Antel 1992). Development of more specific and potent PKC inhibitors holds some future promise.

Regulators of astrocytoma tumor angiogenesis

Malignant astrocytomas are one of the most vascularized of all human cancers. The tumor-induced vessels in addition to being numerous are also abnormal, in that they do not maintain the blood–brain barrier (BBB), leading to peritumoral edema. In addition, they often lack a normal capillary bed leading to shunting and often to intra-tumoral hemorrhage. Like other solid cancers, anti-angiogenic therapy, either alone or often in conjunction with radiation or chemotherapy, is an area of intense interest in astrocytomas. Several angiogenic cytokines have been implicated in the tumor-induced neo-angiogenesis, but most factors such as PDGF, FGFs, TGFβ have pleiotropic effects, in addition to their contribution to angiogenesis. However, VEGF and angiopoietins are two angiogenic specific growth factor families, with aberrant expression in astrocytomas. VEGF is highly expressed by GBM cells and is principally induced by tumor hypoxia and aberrant cytokine expression by astrocytoma cells such as PDGF, EGF, etc. Expression of VEGFRs is also upregulated secondary to the hypoxia, making VEGF or VEGFR a therapeutic target, which is currently under clinical trial with compounds such as Avastin.

Similar to VEGF, angiopoietins are specific for angiogenesis by virtue of their receptor (Tie2) almost specifically being expressed in endothelial cells. We have demonstrated Tie2 to be over-expressed and phosphorylated in GBMs. The functional role of activated Tie2 in GBM vasculature is under current study, with preliminary evidence from our lab that it may be a second therapeutic anti-angiogenesis specific target. In addition to VEGF, angiopoietins and their receptors, other genes are known to regulate astrocytoma angiogenesis either directly or indirectly. The differential expression of these angiogenesis-related transcripts was recently shown to generate a molecular signature of astrocytomas, which could segregate varying grades and subtypes (Godard et al 2003).

Regulators of astrocytoma metabolism

It is recognized that tumor cells develop aberrant metabolic pathways, such as those involved in glucose metabolism, as it provides macromolecular building blocks such as lipids, nucleic acids and proteins to promote cellular proliferation, as well as resistance to apoptosis (Vander Heiden et al 2009). In essence, tumor and rapidly proliferating cells shift from normal oxidative glycolysis to aerobic glycolysis even in the presence of oxygen. Specifically in malignant gliomas, we have recently shown this switch to aerobic glycolysis is dependent to a great extent from a switch of normal Hexosekinase 1 isoform to Hexosekinase 2 isoform, involved in the first entrance of glucose within the tumor cell (Wolf et al 2011). In addition, the TCGA data (Parsons et al 2008; Wolf et al 2011) has led to identification of mutation of isocitrate dehydrogenase 1(IDH1) in a large percentage of low grade gliomas and secondary gliomas that develop from them (see Fig. 5.5). IDH1 is involved in cellular metabolism, but how it specifically contributes to gliomagenesis is under study.

Regulators of astrocytoma invasion and cytoskeleton

The main obstacle for curing gliomas with local therapies such as surgery or radiation is their inherent invasiveness, which is present even in low-grade tumors. Invasion requires degradation of the extra-cellular matrix (ECM) by proteolytic enzymes expressed by tumor cells. Matrix metalloproteases (MMPs, including collagenases, stromelysins and gelatinases), and serine proteases (including urokinase-type plasminogen activator, uPA, and its receptor, uPAR) play a fundamental role in this process. An imbalance between expression and/or activity of MMPs and their endogenous tissue inhibitors (TIMPs), is in-part responsible for tumor cell invasion. This is similar to the balance of pro-angiogenic factors and endogenous anti-angiogenic factors that regulate

the 'angiogenic switch' (Folkman 1992). In fact, the factors that regulate invasion are an integral and vital part of the angiogenesis cascade.

There is a positive correlation between grade and level of MMP-2, -9 and -12 expression in astrocytomas (Kachra et al 1999). MMP-2 and -9 have additional interest due to their co-localization around proliferating blood vessels, suggesting a role in both angiogenesis and tumor invasion (Kachra et al 1999). Angiogenic factors directly regulate MMP expression, such as VEGF-mediated induction of MMP-1, -3, and -9 in vascular smooth muscle cells (Webb et al 1997). This would be required to break down the ECM allowing not only tumor cell invasion, but also sprouting of new blood vessels. Endogenous negative tissue regulators of MMPs or TIMPs are also important regulators of astrocytoma invasion and angiogenesis. The reports on TIMP-1 and TIMP-2 expression in astrocytomas remains inconclusive, with most of the earlier studies demonstrating decreased levels with increasing glioma grade, whereas recent studies have shown an increase in TIMP-1 in GBMs compared with low-grade astrocytomas and normal brain (Kachra et al 1999). Pre-clinical investigations with over- or underexpression of TIMPs using cell culture and transgenic models may be of use in helping decipher which of the TIMPs are of functional relevance in astrocytoma invasion. Therapeutic trials with metalloprotease inhibitors have not mirrored the promising pre-clinical studies, attributing to the complexity of the various molecular regulators of invasion and angiogenesis.

Aberrant regulation of apoptosis

Transformation not only requires aberrant proliferative and differentiation signals, but also altered cell-death machinery or apoptosis. In astrocytomas, the most common perturbation of apoptosis is activation of anti-apoptotic or pro-survival pathways mediated by aberrant activation of the PI3-K:Akt:mTOR pathway, as discussed above. Other altered apoptotic regulators in astrocytomas include members of the death receptor family, such as Fas. Human gliomas overexpress Fas ligand (FasL), Bcl-2 and TGF-β2, all considered to regulate the apoptotic and immune process, though their expression was not prognostic (Choi et al 2004). Resistance to Fas mediated apoptosis is known to contribute to tumor growth by evading the host immune system. The molecular mechanism(s) of resistance to Fas-mediated apoptosis and sensitization to Fas-induced cell death by IFNγ interferon in human astrocytoma cells was investigated by studying expression of 33 genes linked to Fas signaling (Choi et al 2004). IFNγ increase mRNA expression of caspase-1, 4, and 7, in addition to those of Fas and TRAIL in a time and dose-dependant manner. Studies using specific caspase inhibitors showed that Fas induced cell death were mediated by caspase-1, 3, and 8 in the Fas-sensitive human GBM lines. Interestingly, caspase-1 but not caspase-3 or 8 were upregulated by IFNγ in Fas-sensitive CRT-J cell but not in Fas-resistant U373-MG cells (Song et al 2003). Resistance to induction of cell death by apoptosis in response to radiation or chemotherapy is one of the therapeutic hurdles of GBMs. It has been shown that GBMs overexpress or carry genetic amplifications of members of the inhibitors of apoptosis

(IAP) family such as Survivin, XIAP, cIAP1 or cIAP2, whereas IAP levels are rather low or absent in non-neoplastic cells. The underlying mechanism of the anti-apoptotic activity of IAP has been proposed to be by direct/indirect caspase inhibition, or through their transcriptional activity mediated by the stimulation of NF-κB. Recently it has been reported that the infection of malignant glioma cells with adeno-viruses encoding antisense RNA to X-linked IAP depletes endogenous XIAP levels and promotes global caspase activation and apoptosis. In addition, this Ad-XIAP as gene therapy induce cell death in intracranial glioma xenografts, prolongs survival in nude mice and reduces tumorigenicity, reinforcing their potential as therapeutic target for human gliomas.

Cancer pre-disposition syndromes linked with brain tumors

Less than 5% of all brain tumors are linked with a distinct pre-disposition syndrome, where there is a congregation of brain tumors in a family. This congregation may be a result of familial transmission of a genetic aberration, which pre-disposes to brain and peripheral nerve tumors, or may result from a de-novo germline mutation with subsequent familial transmission in future generations. A direct family member of a sporadic patient with a glioma has a slightly elevated risk of also having a glioma, however, this risk does not increase to significant levels such as in breast cancer. Although relatively small in number, these pre-disposition syndromes are important to study and dissect at a clinical-epidemiological, pathological and molecular level, as they add much to our knowledge and hence potential treatment of the larger sporadic tumor bearing population. They allow us to study cohorts, influence of epigenetic factors on the disease pattern, often share molecular alterations with spo-radic counterparts, develop small animal pre-clinical models based on modulating the pre-disposition gene to study emerging drugs and biological therapies, etc. The following will serve to highlight some of these pre-disposition syn-dromes, and their link with brain tumors.

Neurofibromatosis type I (NF-1)

NF-1 is a relatively frequent autosomal dominant genetic disorder with an incidence of about 1 per 3000–4000 persons (Friedman 1999). In terms of a new NF-1 patient, inheritance of the defective gene from one of the parents in an autosomal dominant manner occurs in 50%, while the other 50% is a new germline (usually sperm) mutation in the *NF-1* gene of the patient itself (Thomson et al 2002). NF-1 (Von Recklinghausen disease) was first recognized as a clinical entity at the end of the nineteenth century by Von Recklinghausen and is characterized by a large array of tumoral and non-tumoral manifestations with very variable severity and occurrence (McClatchey 2007). One of the hall-marks of NF-1 is the development of neurofibromas, which are benign tumors of peripheral nerves of mixed cellular composition. Neurofibromas can grow as superficial subcu-taneous and dermal tumors that remain benign and do not cause significant clinical morbidity but can be disfiguring.

In about 30% of NF-1 patients, these tumors grow as plexi-form neurofibromas that typically originate from larger peripheral nerves or nerve roots (McClatchey 2007). Plexi-form neurofibromas can cause nerve dysfunction, pain and tend to undergo transformation in malignant peripheral nerve sheath tumors (MPNSTs) in approximately 10% of the cases (McClatchey 2007). Other tumor types, including gliomas, mainly in the form of low-grade optic pathways gliomas (mainly WHO grade I pilocytic astrocytomas) in children (Gutmann 2008), myeloid leukemias and pheo-chromocytomas also belong to the spectrum of NF-1. Non-tumoral manifestations of NF-1 comprise skin pigmentation abnormalities such as café-au-lait macules, cognitive diffi-culties, hamartomas of the iris (Lisch nodules), fibrous dys-plasia, typical bone lesions of the sphenoid wing, vertebrae, and tibia. The severity and the onset of NF-1 manifesta-tions, although age-dependent, are unpredictable and highly variable between patients, even within a single affected family. Due to the plethora of sometimes varying and over-lapping clinical features, NIH set the criteria for clinical diagnosis of NF-1 (Cawthon et al 1990a; Viskochil et al 1990) (Table 5.1), which, if required, can be supplemented with molecular testing.

The *Nf-1* gene was identified by positional cloning in 1990 as very large gene (about 350 kb) on chromosome 17q11.21 encoding for an equally large protein named neu-rofibromin (220–280 kDa) (Viskochil et al 1990; Cawthon et al 1990b; Wallace et al 1990). The *Nf-1* gene is evolution-ary highly conserved and has homologues in most eukaryo-tes such as the fruit fly and yeast. Genetically, the NF-1 gene can be classified as a TSG and affected patients harbor either

Table 5.1 Diagnostic criteria for NF-1 and NF-2

Neurofibromatosis type 1 Two or more of the following:	Neurofibromatosis type 2 Any of the following:
Six or more café-au-lait macules >5 mm diameter in prepubertal and >15 mm in post-pubertal individuals	Bilateral vestibular Schwannoma (vS), seen on CT or MRI
Two or more neurofibromas of any type or one plexiform neurofibroma	A family history of NF-2 (1st-degree relative) and either:
Freckling in the axillary or inguinal region	(a) unilateral vS diagnosed at <30 years of age *OR*
Optic glioma	(b) two of the following: meningioma, glioma, Schwannoma, juvenile posterior subcapsular lenticular opacities/juvenile cortical cataracts
Two or more Lisch nodules (iris hamartomas)	Individuals with the following clinical features should be evaluated for NF-2:
A distinct osseous lesion such as a sphenoid dysplasia or thinning of the long bone cortex with or without pseudoarthrosis	Unilateral vS at <30 years of age *PLUS* one of the following: meningioma, glioma, Schwannoma, juvenile posterior subcapsular lenticular opacities/juvenile cortical cataracts
A 1st-degree relative (parent, sibling or offspring) with NF-1 by the above criteria	Multiple meningiomas plus unilateral vS diagnosed at <30 years of age *OR* one of the following: meningioma, glioma, Schwannoma, juvenile posterior subcapsular lenticular opacities/juvenile cortical cataracts

Based on Stumpf et al (1988).

inherited or new germline constitutional heterozygous inactivation of *Nf-1*. Loss of heterozygosity by somatic mutation of the wildtype allele then results in tumor initiation. The fact that *NF-1* mutation is also found in sporadic tumors that are part of the NF-1 spectrum such as MPNST, myeloid leukemias and recently from the TCGA in GBMs (Cancer Genome Atlas Research Network 2008) supports the tumor suppression function of NF-1 with some tissue specificity.

The high number of sporadic NF-1 cases with new mutations is likely due to the very large size of the NF-1 gene together with an especially high mutation rate of the NF-1 locus. This occurs by small deletions or truncating mutations but also alternative mechanisms such as gene conversion with NF-1 pseudogenes on other chromosomes as well as intragenic recombination between repeated sequences within the NF-1 gene (Thomson et al 2002; Dorschner et al 2000). The relatively variable NF-1 expressivity does not translate in a strong genotype-phenotype correlation, although genetic modifiers seem to influence the phenotypic variability seen in NF-1 patients (Szudek et al 2002, 2003). Sporadic NF-1 cases can either occur by transmission from an unaffected parent with germline mosaicism for NF-1 mutation, by a de novo mutation in one parent germ cell subsequently involved in fertilization, or occur post-zygotically at early stages of egg development and therefore result in somatic mosaicism in the patient (Kehrer-Sawatzki & Cooper 2008). The latter scenario would also account for the very variable phenotype seen in NF-1 patients.

The tumor suppressor and physiological functions of NF-1 were extensively studied in mouse models. In *NF-1⁻/⁻* homozygous mouse mutants, constitutional inactivation of the *NF-1* gene results in embryonic lethality at embryonic day 13.5 from cardiac defects reflecting a key role of NF-1 in endothelial cells of the developing heart (Gitler et al 2003; Jacks et al 1994). Although *NF-1⁺/⁻* heterozygous mice have a predisposition to tumors seen in NF-1 patients such as myeloid leukemia and pheochromocytoma, they do not recapitulate the full clinical spectrum of NF-1 disease. Further refinement of *NF-1* mouse models allowed studying the role of NF-1 in specific tissues as well as NF-1 specific tumor development. For example, tissue specific ablation of *NF-1* in neurons results in abnormal development of the cerebral cortex, a phenotype consistent with cognitive abnormalities found in human patients (Zhu et al 2001) and chimeric mice partially composed of *NF-1⁻/⁻* cells develop true neurofibromas showing that loss of heterozygosity of the wildtype *NF-1* allele is necessary for neurofibroma development (Cichowski et al 1999). Crossing *NF-1⁺/⁻* mice with other tumor suppressor deficient mice revealed genetic cooperation of NF-1 in tumorigenesis. *NF-1⁺/⁻; p53⁺/⁻* mice develop MPNSTs and malignant gliomas. Most tumors seen in those mice have lost the wildtype allele of both *p53* and *NF-1* (Reilly et al 2000). As *NF-1* and *p53* alleles are both located on the same chromosome in humans (chromosome 17) but also in mice (chromosome 11) this likely occurs by the loss of the wild type chromosome 11 (Cichowski et al 1999; Reilly et al 2000; Vogel et al 1999). Interestingly, the penetrance and severity of the phenotype is dependent on the genetic background and an imprinted locus on chromosome 11, which is consistent with the variable expressivity of the human disease and the implication of genetic modifiers (Reilly et al 2000;

Richards et al 1995). Furthermore, there is evidence to suggest that that early inactivation of *p53* inactivation relative to *NF-1* is important for malignant astrocytoma formation (Zhu et al 2005).

NF-1⁺/⁻ p53⁺/⁻ mouse models mainly develop malignant gliomas that are only occasionally seen in NF-1 patients and not low-grade optic gliomas, which are a hallmark of NF-1 disease seen in about 15% of NF-1 patients. This is consistent with the prominent role played by p53 in the pathogenesis of secondary GBMs (McClatchey 2007). Mice with specific inactivation of *NF-1* only in astrocytes (*NF-1*lox/lox; *GFAP-Cre* mice) do not result in tumor formation when the surrounding cells have a NF-1⁺/⁺ background (Bajenaru et al 2002). However NF-1⁻/⁻ astrocytes in a heterozygous background where surrounding central nervous system cells, especially neurons, are *NF-1⁺/⁻*, develop optic nerve glioma. Likewise, recent studies showed that neurofibroma formation requires not only *NF-1* deficient Schwann cells but also NF-1 heterozygous bone marrow cells (Yang et al 2008), demonstrating the importance of microenvironment in the pathogenesis of NF-1. These results demonstrate the critical role of the microenvironment in the pathogenesis of NF-1 related tumors.

On the cellular level, neurofibromin functions as a negative regulator of Ras signaling. It has a domain homologous to GTPase activating proteins for Ras (Ras-GAPs), which act by dephosphorylating Ras-GTP resulting in inhibition of Ras activity (Bernards & Settleman 2004) (Fig. 5.7). Increased Ras activity by loss of NF-1 seems to be critical in NF-1 tumor pathogenesis (Basu et al 1992), and activation of well studied Ras dependent pathways such as Raf/MEK, PI3-K/ AKT and Rac are elevated in *NF-1⁻/⁻* cells and tumors (Cichowski & Jacks 2001; Basu et al 1992; Guha et al 1996; Lau et al 2000; Woods et al 2002). Moreover, NF-1 has been

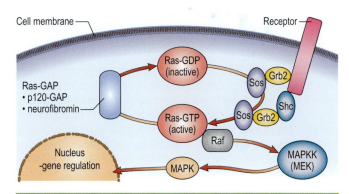

Figure 5.7 Schematic drawing of activation of the Ras/Raf/MAPK pathway. The activated receptor provides phosphotyrosine residues for intracellular signaling adapter proteins such as Grb2, which itself is linked with guanine exchange factor enzymes such as Sos, which can convert inactive Ras-GDP to activated Ras-GTP. Activated Ras-GTP can activate a variety of subsequent signaling molecules or effectors such as Raf to transmit signals and subsequently regulate transcription at the nuclear level. The above signaling cascade is negatively regulated at many levels, including the Ras-GAPs, which converts active Ras-GTP back to inactive Ras-GDP. One of the more prominent Ras-GAPs in humans is neurofibromin, the gene product lost in NF-1, leading to continued growth promoting signaling through active Ras-GTP. Mutations which abrogate the function of Ras-GAPs are the most common oncogenic alterations in human cancers.

shown to regulate adenylyl-cyclase (AC) activity and cAMP levels in *Drosophila*, leading to learning disabilities in NF-1 deficient flies (Guo et al 1997; Guo et al 2000) but also in mammalian cells such as astrocytes and Schwann cells (Dasgupta et al 2003; Kim et al 2001; Tong et al 2002). Recently, mTOR has emerged as a key factor upregulated in NF-1 deficient cells (Dasgupta et al 2005; Johannessen et al 2005) and dependent on Ras mediated signaling. The effect of mTOR on tumor formation seems to be mediated by CyclinD1 and less by the classical mTOR target HIF1 (Johannessen et al 2008). Rapamycin and others related inhibitors of mTOR are therefore believed to be promising agents to treat NF-1 related tumors.

Neurofibromatosis type 2 (NF-2)

NF-2 is about 1/10th as frequent as NF-1, with a live birth incidence of 1/40 000. It too is autosomal dominant in transmission with 50% of the new cases inherited from one of the parents, while the other 50% is a new germline mutation (McClatchey 2007; Evans et al 1992; Rouleau et al 1993; Trofatter et al 1993). Like NF-1, loss of heterozygosity of the second normal *NF-2* allele is the initiator step of schwannoma formation. Although 95% of peripheral and intracranial schwannomas occur in sporadic patients, sporadic somatic mutations of both *NF-2* genes with loss of expression of the gene product Merlin, are found in nearly all non-NF-2 schwannomas (Stemmer-Rachamimov et al 1997). Similar to the clinical diagnosis of NF-1, the NIH clinical criteria stand well to make the diagnosis (Table 5.1) in most cases, although since cloning of the *NF-2* gene, molecular diagnosis on normal cells from the patient can confirm if required.

The TSG function of NF-2 has well been documented in animal models. In mice, biallelic disruption of the *NF-2* gene results in embryogenic lethality and heterozygous mice develop a variety of malignant and metastatic tumors. Transgenic mice with targeted *NF-2* inactivation in Schwann cells develop schwannomas resembling human tumors (Giovannini et al 2000). During mouse embryogenesis, *NF-2* promoter activity studies have found prominent expression in embryonic ectoderm and later in the developing brain. The *NF-2* promoter is mainly active at sites of cell migration during neural tube closure and in anatomical areas prone to tumor development in NF-2 patients, such as the acoustic and trigeminal ganglion (Akhmametyeva et al 2006). Further studies showed a role for Merlin in tissue fusion and cell migration during embryogenesis as well as in critical interactions between normal Schwann cells and axons in adult peripheral nerves, suggesting a role of Merlin in cell–cell and cell–matrix adhesion (McLaughlin et al 2007; Nakai et al 2006). This is consistent with the structure of Merlin (moesin-ezrin-radixin-like-protein), which is strongly related to ERM proteins (ezrin, radixin, and moesins) and its localization at the membrane-cytoskeleton interface (Trofatter et al 1993). The role of Merlin in adhesion is supported by its interactions with focal adhesion complexes proteins such as paxillin and focal adhesion kinase (Fernandez-Valle et al 2002), as well as other adhesion molecules such as β1-integrin and lyillin (Bono et al 2005). In addition, Merlin is involved in cytoskeletal organization by regulating actin polymerization

(Muranen et al 2007; Manchanda et al 2005) and by being a phosphorylation target of p21-activated kinase (PAK) downstream of Rac and Cdc42, small GTPase molecules involved in cell migration, adhesion and cytoskeleton organization (Hirokawa et al 2004; Kaempchen et al 2003; Kissil et al 2003; Shaw et al 2001). Therefore, the TSG function of Merlin, which is capable of inducing cell cycle arrest and blocking cell proliferation after being activated by de-phosphorylation at serine 518, is most likely indirect via contact inhibition of growth (Morrison et al 2001) and interaction with different signaling pathways. For example de-phosphorylated Merlin binds to CD44 which is a hyaluronan receptor resulting in growth inhibition. Besides its contact and adhesion functions, Merlin has also directs interactions with members of several pathways involved in cell proliferation including Raf/Ras/MABK/MEK/Erk and PI3-kinase-Akt (Tikoo et al 1994), which are major signaling funnels of growth factor tyrosine kinase receptors (RPTKs). Another example suggesting participation in RPTK signaling is that Merlin forms tertiary complexes with Magicin and Grb2, an adaptor protein coordinating RPTK and Ras signaling (Wiederhold et al 2004) (Fig. 5.7). Furthermore, Merlin can suppress the action of Ras and Rac that, again, are both major components of RPTK downstream signaling (Nakai et al 2006; Morrison et al 2007). Other studies have suggested a role for Merlin in regulating RPTK activity by controlling and coordinating their availability at the cell membrane (McClatchey & Giovannini 2005). Finally, irrespective of their direct interactions with Merlin, RPTKs such as PDGF-R as well as members of the EGFR and TGFR-β families, have been found at elevated levels in schwannomas (Cole et al 2008; Curto et al 2007; Doherty et al 2008; Fraenzer et al 2003). Consequently, even if the large array of Merlin interactions does not at present allow a fully unified view of Merlin signaling organization, several drug targets rationally amenable to investigational therapies can be recognized. In Phase 1 trials, these include EGFR (Herceptin), Ras/Raf/Mek (Sorafenib), PI3-K-Akt (OSU3013, Rapamycin), PDGFR (Sorafenib) and promising pre-clinical studies with Gleevec from our group (Mukherjee et al 2009).

Tuberous sclerosis

Tuberous sclerosis is a multi-system familial autosomal dominant or sporadic genetic disorder caused by mutations in the TSC1 and TSC2 genes. The clinical spectrum of the disease includes hamartomas and benign tumors in various organs, predominantly in the brain, heart, skin, eyes, kidney, lungs, and liver. The various findings in tuberous sclerosis are grouped in major or minor diagnostic criteria, Table 5.2. The diagnosis of tuberous sclerosis is made when two major criteria or one major and two minor criteria are found (Curatolo et al 2008).

Brain abnormalities are found in nearly 90% of affected subjects and include cortical tubers (the term 'tuber' designates the potato-like appearance of hypertrophic and sclerotic cortical gyri) and subependymal nodules which can both be considered as hamartomas as well as subependymal giant cell astrocytomas (SEGA), which are benign but true neoplasms resulting from the transformation of subependymal nodules. Most of brain structural abnormalities appear

Table 5.2 Diagnostic criteria for tuberous sclerosis (TSC)

TSC: Major diagnostic criteria	TSC: Minor diagnostic criteria
• Facial angiofibromas or forehead plaque pits in dental enamel	• Hamartomatous rectal polyps
• Non-traumatic ungula or periungual fibroma	• Bone cysts
• Hypomelanotic macules (three or more)	• Cerebral white matter dysplasia
• Shagreen patch (connective tissue nevus) migration lines	• Gingival fibromas
• Multiple retinal nodular hamartomas	• Non-renal hamartoma
• Cortical tuber	• Retinal achromic patch
• Subependymal nodule	• Confetti-like skin lesions
• Subependymal giant-cell astrocytoma	• Multiple renal cysts
• Cardiac Rhabdomyoma	
• Lymphangiomyomatosis, renal angiomyolipoma	

Table 5.3 Diagnostic criteria for Von Hippel–Lindau disease (VHL)

Tumors in Von Hippel-Lindau Disease
Retinal hemangioma
Cerebellar hemangioblastoma
Spinal cord hemangioblastoma
Clear cell renal carcinoma
Endolymphatic sac tumors
Pancreatic islet cell tumors
Pheochromocytoma
Cystadenomas of the broad ligament and epididymis

in fetal life and can be diagnosed antenatal with fetal ultrasound or MRI (Curatolo & Brinchi 1993). Clinically, the neurological manifestations of tuberous sclerosis are epileptic seizures, various degrees of mental impairment, behavioral problems and autism (Curatolo et al 1991).

On the histological level, tubers are characterized by dysplastic cortical foci showing a disorganized neuronal and glial architecture associated with cellular abnormalities such as giant neuronal cells and dysmorphic astrocytes. Subependymal nodules are hamartomas mainly in generally located in the subependymal wall of the lateral ventricle. Subependymal nodules may progress into SEGA (Nabbout et al 1999), which are usually benign and slow growing tumors of mixed neuroglial lineage. Most often SEGA become symptomatic by CSF pathway obstruction at the Foramen of Monroe and subsequent hydrocephalus.

The genetics of tuberous sclerosis is related to mutations in TCS1 and TCS2 genes, as initially identified by linkage analysis (Fryer et al 1987; Kandt et al 1992). TCS1 is located on chromosome 9q34 (van Slegtenhorst et al 1997) and TCS2 on chromosome 16p13.3 (European Chromosome 16 Tuberous Sclerosis Consortium 1993). In the majority (70–85%) of sporadic and familial cases, mutations in TCS2 are found and are associated with a more severe phenotype. Mutations include large deletions or small truncations (nonsense mutations and small deletion) with no identified hotspots on TCS1 or TCS2. Interestingly the TSC2 gene is adjacent to the polycystic kidney disease type 1 gene (PKD1) and larger deletion in TCS2 can involve PKD1 as well, resulting in a mixed TSC and polycystic kidney phenotype in less than 3% of TS cases. In TSC, inactivation of only one allele (haploinsufficiency) of TSC1 or TSC2 is enough to induce tuber formation and a significant proportion of SEGA, however, formation of renal angiomyolipoma is more often associated with loss of heterozygosity by a second hit somatic mutation (Chan et al 2004; Henske et al 1997).

The gene products of TCS1, a protein called hamartin (1164aa and 130 kDa), and TCS2 (1807aa and 180 kDa), a protein called tuberin, interact within the same signaling pathway by forming an intracellular complex (Tee et al 2002). Although many proteins have been found to interact with hamartin and tuberin, the principal function of the hamartin/tuberin complex in TSC is considered to be the antagonization of mTOR (mammalian target of rapamycin)

mediated downstream signaling (Tee et al 2002; Gao et al 2002; Inoki et al 2002). The hamartin/tuberin stimulates a GTPase that removes GTP from ras homologue enriched in the brain (RHEB), resulting in inhibition of mTOR (Astrinidis & Henske 2005; Kwiatkowski & Manning 2005). As Akt is the main upstream inhibitor of hamartin/tuberin, saying that Akt stimulates mTOR by inhibiting the hamartin/tuberin complex can summarize the signaling pathway. mTOR, a member of phosphoinositide-3-kinase-related kinase family, is a major actor in several cellular processes such as growth regulation, proliferation control and cancer cell metabolism. Aberrant mTOR signaling is primarily or secondarily involved in other genetic syndromes such as Peutz–Jeghers syndrome (mutation in LKB1), PTEN mutation syndromes such as the Lhermitte–Duclos and Cowden syndrome, Von Hippel–Lindau disease or NF-1. In the pathway considered relevant for TSC development, mTOR controls cap-dependent RNA translation by phosphorylation and inactivation of 4E-BPs, which suppresses the activity of the translation initiation factor eIF4E (Jozwiak et al 2005). Another way for mTOR to regulate translation is by phosphorylation of S6K1, a kinase that activates ribosomal subunit protein S6, leading to ribosome recruitment for protein translation (Jozwiak et al 2005). In addition to mTOR regulation, the hamartin and tuberin complex appears to play a role in cell adhesion and migration via an interaction with ezrin-radixin-moesin proteins and the small GTP-binding protein Rho (Carbonara et al 1996). Some studies have shown the potential metastatic potential of benign TSC-related lesions, such as renal angiomyolipomas (Karbowniczek et al 2003; Marcotte & Crino 2006).

Von Hippel–Lindau disease

Von Hippel–Lindau disease (VHL) is an autosomal dominant multisystem genetic disorder characterized by vascular tumors (angiomas) in different organs (Table 5.3). The disease is caused by mutations in the VHL gene, a TSG coding for a protein which is part of a multi-protein complex involved in the ubiquitination and degradation of the transcription factor HIF (hypoxia inducible factor). Clinically, Von Hippel–Lindau manifests by the growth of angiomas in the retina and in the central nervous system, as well as by renal clear cell carcinomas, pheochromocytomas, pancreatic islet cell tumors, cystadenomas of the broad ligament in females and epididymis in males. In the central nervous system, VHL leads to the growth of hemangioblastomas mainly in the cerebellum and the spinal cord. Hemangioblastomas are highly vascular benign tumors consisting of stromal cells that are known recognized as primitive hemangioblasts that express erythropoietin receptor and have lost heterozygosity of the *VHL* allele intermingled with non tumoral blood vessels (Chan et al 2005; Chan et al 1999; Vortmeyer et al 2003; Vortmeyer et al 1997).

The *VHL* gene was first positioned by linkage studies on chromosome 3p25, a region involved in sporadic renal cancer (Seizinger et al 1988; Seizinger et al 1991) and identified as a 6 kilobase (kb) transcript (Latif et al 1993). The *VHL* gene contains 3 exons and leads to the synthesis of a 4.5 kb mRNA. The *VHL* promoter contains binding sites for PAX, nuclear respiratory factor 1 (Kuzmin et al 1995) and TCF4 (Giles et al 2006) and can be silenced by hypermethylation (Herman et al 1994). The VHL protein (pVHL) has two functionally similar isoforms that both have tumor suppressor activity, a 28–30 kDa protein containing 213 amino acids and a shorter form of 18 kDa lacking the first 53 amino acids of the 28–30 kDa coding for N-terminal acidic repeat domain. pVHL forms a multi-protein ubiquitin-ligase complex by binding elongin C, elongin B, Cul2 and Rbx1. The complex can then target proteins to the proteasome for degradation. The principal substrates of pVHL ubiquitin-ligase complex are the three α-units of HIF. In normoxic conditions HIF is readily targeted by the pVHL complex and degraded in the proteasome. However, when oxygen concentrations drop or pVHL is not functional, HIF-α gets stabilized and heterodimerized with HIF-β (also known as ARNT1-aryl hydrocarbon receptor nuclear translocator 1). This complex then translocates to the nucleus and activates the transcription of genes involved in cellular adaptation to hypoxia that contain hypoxia-response-elements (HRE) in their promoters. These genes include angiogenesis-inducing factors such vascular endothelial growth factor (VEGF), platelet derived growth factor (PDGF) as well as genes involved in anaerobic glycolysis and erythropoiesis (erythropoietin EPO). The HIF-α susceptibility to oxygen concentration is mediated by EglN (egg laying defective nine) proteins which hydroxylate HIF-α on a conserved proline residues in normoxic conditions. This allows HIF to bind to pVHL and eventually initiate the ubiquitination process. Hypoxia, but also other factors such as reactive oxygen species (ROS) generated in mitochondria under low O_2 conditions and nitric oxide (NO) inhibit EglN function and therefore prevent HIF-α degradation. In summary, mutations in VHL associated with hemangioblastoma results in altered HIF regulation and excessive production of HIF dependent growth factors such as VEGF, PDGF, TGF-α and erythropoietin, which all induce proliferation of vascular tumor cells.

Von Hippel–Lindau disease is an autosomal dominant condition with germline heterozygosity of the VHL locus (Stolle et al 1998), however, the actual mutation of VHL is recessive as most hereditary cancer syndromes and requires the somatic inactivation of the wildtype allele of VHL (Pack et al 1999). Most individuals with VHL have a family history of VHL, although sporadic cases with de novo mutation of VHL have been described (Richards et al 1995). In about 20% of cases, the entire VHL locus has been deleted (Pack et al 1999). There is emerging evidence to suggest a strong correlation between the genetic mutation type of VHL and the clinical phenotype, as well as the biochemical spectrum of the disease (Chen et al 1995; Crossey et al 1994). For example, Type 1 VHL disease is related to no *VHL* allele resulting from deletion, nonsense or missense mutation and is associated with a low incidence of pheochromocytoma and a very high expression of HIF as well as of EglN3. Type 2-VHL results from missense mutations and is found in the vast majority of patients with pheochromocytomas. Type 2 can be further subdivided in 2A (low risk of renal carcinoma, moderate HIF expression, low EglN3), 2B (high risk of renal carcinoma, relatively low HIF expression, low EglN3), and 2C disease (pheochromocytoma only without CNS and retinal hemangioblastomas, very low HIF expression, low EglN3).

Gorlin–Goltz syndrome (basal cell nevus syndrome), medulloblastomas, and the Hedgehog-Gli pathway

This syndrome named after Robert Gorlin and Robert Goltz who described it in 1960 (Gorlin & Goltz 1960) is an autosomal dominant genetic disorder with an estimated prevalence of 1 in 50 000–150 000 (Gorlin 1999). The basal cell nevus syndrome (BCNS) or Gorlin–Gotz syndrome (GS) has a high penetrance but very variable expressivity (Lo Muzio 2008). The first report of the syndrome described the association of basal cell tumors, jaw cysts and bifid ribs (Gorlin & Goltz 1960). Since then many different clinical features have expanded the constellation of findings associated with GS. Currently, the diagnosis of GS is made with the help of defined major and minor criteria (Kimonis et al 1997). The majority of the clinical features are related to osteosqueletal malformations affecting ribs, extremities, the spine and the skull (Epstein 2008; High & Zedan 2005). Other system abnormalities, such as ocular, cardiovascular, genitourinary and gastroenteric disorders, may also be associated with Gorlin syndrome. Tumors found in Gorlin syndrome are basal cell carcinomas, which are the hallmark of the disease, desmoplastic medulloblastoma, which represent a distinct group of medulloblastomas (Lo Muzio 2008; Amlashi et al 2003; Herzberg & Wiskemann 1963), and ovarian fibromas. Meningiomas, craniopharyngiomas, glioblastomas, rhabdomyosarcomas have also been described in patients with BCNS. The different phenotypic manifestations of the BNCs affect patients with very variable severity and there is also a significant ethnic difference in BCC incidence between white or African-American patients affected with BCNS (Goldstein et al 1994).

The gene responsible for the syndrome was localized on chromosome 9q22 by linkage analysis in the early 1990s (Gailani et al 1992). A few years later, the gene was identified as the human homologue of the *Drosophila* 'Patched' gene by positional cloning (Hahn et al 1996; Johnson et al 1996). The *PTCH1* gene has 23 exons encompassing 34 kb and coding for a 1447 amino acids transmembrane protein with 12 transmembrane domains. In BCNS patients, more than 50 mutations of PTCH have been described and include deletions, nonsense or missense mutations and insertions (Boutet et al 2003; Chidambaram & Dean 1996; Lench et al 1997; Unden et al 1996). PTHC1 mutations seem to be mainly clustered in two large extracellular loops of the protein (Wicking et al 1997) and rearrangements of PTCH1 resulting in a truncated protein are frequent (Epstein 2008). Although many different mutations of the PTCH1 gene have been described, there is no clear genotype-phenotype correlation in BCNS (Lindstrom et al 2006).

PTCH has been extensively characterized as a regulator of polarity segmentation in *Drosophila* and has also a prominent role in patterning during mammalian development, including in the central nervous system. PTCH is a key component of the canonical Hedgehog-Gli developmental pathway (HH-Gli). In a physiological context, the HH pathway is involved in a multitude of embryological and adult events regulating cellular and tissue homeostasis. Among other processes, HH-Gli controls the regulation of cell fate and cell numbers, as well as the patterning of organs. The pathway activator HH is a secreted extracellular ligand that acts mainly as a morphogenetic factor, which diffuses in gradients to modulate tissue organization. In the developing neural tube, HH acts as a mitogen and promotes cell proliferation but also neural progenitor survival and patterning specification of the ventral spinal cord (Jiang & Hui 2008; Ruiz i Altaba et al 2003). The HH-Gli pathway plays an important role in regeneration and integrity of adult tissue, including of epithelial organs such as lung, prostate, pancreas but also central nervous system, where HH-Gli regulates the maintenance of progenitor and stem cells (Beachy et al 2004b; Fendrich et al 2008; Karhadkar et al 2004; Watkins et al 2003). The biological effects of activated SHH-GLI pathway are thus context-dependent and can result in different biological responses in different tissues and cell types. This context dependence seems to rely on differential transcriptional responses regulated by the combinatorial balance of activator and repressor GLI transcription factors specifically associated with the HH-Gli pathway (Ruiz i Altaba et al 2007). On a mechanistic level, the transduction cascade of the HH-Gli pathway involves essentially the Hedgehog ligand, two transmembrane membrane proteins, PTCH, which is the HH receptor and Smoothened (SMO), as well as downstream transcription factors GLIs. Suppressor of fused (SUFU) is another important member of the pathway and acts in the signal transduction cascade as a suppressor of Gli. In humans, three members of the Hedgehog family are described: *Sonic Hedgehog*, which is the most widely expressed gene, *Indian Hedgehog*, and *Desert Hedgehog*. Hedgehog proteins are secreted extracellular protein ligands that cleave into a substrate binding cholesterol and palmitate molecules to become active. In the absence of the secreted extracellular ligand HH, the pathway is switched off. In this situation, PTCH inhibits 'Smoothened' (SMO), a seven transmembrane domain protein, and prevents it to activate the downstream GLI transcription factors. When HH is present, the binding of active HH to the second large extracellular loop of PTCH1 results in the removal of PTCH mediated inhibition of SMO. This initiates an intracellular information cascade that ultimately results in activation of GLI family of zinc transcription factors. There are three different Gli proteins: Gli1 and Gli2 that are activators of the pathway (GLIA) and Gli3 that mainly has a repressor function (GLIR) (Jiang & Hui 2008; Ruiz i Altaba et al 2007). The activation of the pathway is a balance between GLIA and GLIR, which results in the expression of a broad variety of genes involved among other functions in cell proliferation, survival, self-renewal, differentiation, developmental patterning, and vasculogenesis. Therefore, the main consequence of *PTCH1* loss of

function is over activation of the HH-Gli pathway resulting in developmental anomalies and neoplastic growths constituting the BCNS spectrum (Lindstrom et al 2006). Mutations of PTCH can result in ligand independent constitutive activation of the pathway and promotes tumorigenesis as seen in BNCs (Lindstrom et al 2006).

Medulloblastomas are the most frequent malignant brain tumor in children. They supposedly arise from granule cell precursors in the developing child cerebellum and have a poor survival prognosis of 40–70% at 5 years. Only a minority of medulloblastomas is part of the BNCs, but this association nevertheless suggests that a defined genetic defect in the HH-pathway is sufficient to induce tumorigenesis in the brain (Guessous et al 2008). In that respect, the study of Gorlin syndrome and the related HH-pathway has significantly advanced our understanding of Medulloblastoma pathogenesis. Once again, the evidence of a direct link between a genetic mutation and tumor formation comes from transgenic mouse models. While homozygous null PTCH mice die during embryogenesis, mouse models harboring a heterozygous mutation of PTCH (Ptch1+/−) develop medulloblastomas with a penetrance of a little more than 10% and exhibit several features found in BCNS (Wetmore et al 2001). When in addition to PTCH heterozygosity, p53 in non-functional (Ptch1+/−; Trp53−/− mice), medulloblastoma form in almost 100% of the mice (Taylor et al 2002) illustrating how a second genetic hit can cooperate to dramatically accelerate tumorigenesis. Even if BCNS related medulloblastomas are only a minority of all cases of medulloblastoma, there is evidence that the HH-Gli pathway also plays a prominent role in sporadic medulloblastomas. Mutations in several components of the HH-Gli pathway such as PTCH, SUFU, SMO have been repeatedly reported in subsets of medulloblastomas but seem to be predominant in the desmoplastic type, a sub-group accounting for about 25% of medulloblastomas with distinct histological features affecting older patient and with a more favorable prognosis (Guessous et al 2008). Likewise, a germline mutation of the suppressor of fused gene (SUFU) was found in a sub-set of children with medulloblastoma without BNCs (Taylor et al 2002). Recent studies have provided a molecular classification of medulloblastoma that has some prognostic value. Signature genes and pathways that seem to influence outcome, clinical behavior such as the development of metastasis as well as the patient population characteristics include HH-Gli, NOTCH, PDGF and WNT signaling, genes that are consistently involved in the development and maintenance of granule cell precursors in the cerebellum. Other genes involved in neuronal differentiation, cell cycle, biosynthesis and interestingly photoreceptor differentiation are determinant in the sub-classification of medulloblastomas (Kool et al 2008; Thompson et al 2006). Finally, there is accumulating evidence that the HH pathway, even in the absence of specific mutations, plays a critical role in many other human tumors including gastrointestinal cancers, prostate cancer, melanomas, hematological malignancies, and gliomas (Karhadkar et al 2004; Watkins et al 2003; Stecca et al 2007; Lindemann 2008; Clement et al 2007; Berman et al 2003; Beachy et al 2004a). Because these tumors are dependent on the ligand, they are amenable to chemical inhibitors such as cyclonamine, a natural inhibitor of the pathway blocking activation of SMO, or related synthetic compounds (Ruiz i Altaba 2008).

Li–Fraumeni syndrome

Li–Fraumeni syndrome is an autosomal dominant cancer predisposition syndrome characterized by a variety of early onset tumors. The syndrome, described in 1969 by Li and Fraumeni (initially including families with children developing early onset rhabdomyosarcomas) was characterized by the presence of five cancers: sarcoma, adrenocortical carcinoma (ACC), breast cancer, leukemia, and brain tumors, mainly gliomas and choroid plexus carcinomas (Garber et al 1991; Li & Fraumeni 1969a,b). LFS is highly penetrant, has a heterogenous clinical spectrum, is more frequently found in women than in men (mainly due to the occurrence of breast carcinoma in female patients) and is associated with germline mutations in the Tp53 gene or in genes functionally associated with p53 (Bell et al 1999; Malkin et al 1990). Several criteria have been developed to identify families at risk for a germline Tp53 mutation. Inclusion criteria have evolved over time with the contribution of Birch and colleagues (1994) and Eeles (1995) and, more recently, by Chompret and colleagues (2000, 2001, 2002) (Table 5.4). Diagnosis criteria discriminate between classic LFS, LFS-like or incomplete LFS variants. Importantly, diagnostic criteria defined by Chompret have increased the sensitivity of germline p53 mutation detection by including patients with typical LFS tumors (sarcomas, brain tumors, adrenocortical carcinoma and breast cancers at an early age) but no family history (Chompret et al 2000, 2001; Chompret 2002; Gonzalez et al 2009). The underlying molecular biology of all LFS forms is related to the deficiency of p53 pathway function. This is either by direct mutation in the p53 gene, as found in about 80% of families with classic LFS; 40% in

LF-like and 6% in incomplete LFS (Birch et al 1994; Eeles 1995; Chompret 2002), or in related p53 pathway genes such as checkpoint kinase 2 (CHEK2, 22q12.2) (Bell et al 1999; Bachinski et al 2005) or a locus identified on chromosome 1q23 (Bell et al 1999). CHEK2 is a factor involved in DNA damage response and replication checkpoints. CHEK2 phosphorylates p53, resulting in mitosis discontinuation and initiation of DNA repair. Germline mutations of TP53 are most commonly missense mutations in the DNA binding domain of p53 similar to somatic mutations, however with a different frequency distribution of hotspots (Varley et al 2001). Splicing mutations are also found in a significant number of cases and appear to be more frequent in germline cases than sporadic cases (Olivier et al 2003).

The clinical guidelines for the management of patients affected by the Li–Fraumeni syndrome include thorough familial genetic counseling (including prenatal or preimplantation diagnosis for couples affected with the syndrome), early screening for tumor development (i.e., female patients should have regular bilateral mammograms and can be considered for prophylactic mastectomy) and instructions on avoiding ionizing radiation and DNA-damaging products in everyday life (Varley et al 1997).

Turcot syndrome

In 1959, Turcot and co-workers described a familial association of brain tumors with colon adenocarcinoma and new cases have been subsequently regularly reported. The molecular basis of Turcot syndrome was elucidated in 1995 by demonstrating mutation in the classic colon carcinoma associated gene – adenomatous polyposis coli (APC, on chromosome 5q21–22) in the majority of the families analyzed but a few families had mutation in the non-polyposis coli associated mismatch repair genes hMLH1 (on chromosome 3p21.3) and hPMS2 (on chromosome 7p22), genes responsible for hereditary non-polyposis colorectal cancer syndrome (HNPCC or Lynch syndrome) (Hamilton et al 1995). The reported brain tumors in Turcot syndrome patients are mainly gliomas and medulloblastomas, however sporadic reports have described other tumors associated with the syndrome, including ependymomas, lymphomas, meningiomas, craniopharyngiomas, and pituitary adenomas (Paraf et al 1997).

Turcot syndrome patients with documented *APC* mutations also have findings consistent with familial adenomatous polyposis syndrome (FAP), such as ocular fundus lesions and jaw lesions but usually have a less pronounced colonic polyposis. Paraf and colleagues (1997) proposed to divide the syndrome into two types: brain tumor polyposis type 1 (individuals without FAP syndrome) with higher risk of glioblastomas, and brain tumor polyposis type 2 (individuals with FAP syndrome) with higher risk of medulloblastoma.

Clinical translation and future directions

Our knowledge of the molecular biology of astrocytoma pathogenesis has advanced considerably in the last two decades. The clinical consequences of these discoveries are the plethora of novel, rationally-targeted therapies which are

Table 5.4 Diagnostic criteria of Li–Fraumeni syndrome

Classic Li-Fraumeni syndrome (Li & Fraumeni 1969)	Li-Fraumeni like syndrome (Birch et al 1994)
• A proband with a sarcoma diagnosed before 45 years of age AND • A first-degree relative with any cancer under 45 years of age AND • A first-degree relative or a second-degree relative with any cancer under 45 years of age or a sarcoma at any age	• A proband with any childhood cancer or sarcoma, brain tumor, or adrenal cortical tumor diagnosed before 45 years of age AND • A first- or second-degree relative with a typical LFS cancer (sarcoma, breast cancer, brain tumor, adrenal cortical tumor, or leukemia) at any age AND • A first- or second-degree relative with any cancer under the age of 60 years

Incomplete Li-Fraumeni syndrome (Chompret et al 2000)

• A proband with sarcoma, brain tumor, breast cancer, or adrenocortical carcinoma before 36 years of age, and at least one first- or second-degree relative with cancer (other than breast cancer if the proband has breast cancer) under the age of 46 years or a relative with multiple primaries at any age,
• A proband with multiple primary tumors, two of which are sarcoma, brain tumor, breast cancer, and/or adrenocortical carcinoma, with the initial cancer occuring before the age of 36 years, regardless of the family history
• A proband with adrenocortical carcinoma at any age of onset, regardless of the family history

Modified from: www.genetests.com and Gonzalez et al (2009).

Table 5.5 Biological targeted agents being investigated in glioma

Product	Developer	Status	1st line+TMZ / 2nd line SA	Approval/ Launch
Enzastaurin	Eli Lilly	Phase I/II	– / +	2008
Tarceva	Genentech	Phase II	?	2008
PTK/ZK	Novartis	Phase II	+ / –	2009
SARASAR	SP	Phase I	+ / +	2008
Cilengitide	MerckKGaA	Phase II	+ / +	2008
109881	Sanofi-Aventis	Phase II	?	NA
247550	BMS	Phase II	– / +	NA

being developed (Table 5.5). Although many are of promise in preclinical *in-vitro* and *in-vivo* studies, only a few, if any, have shown efficacy on clinical testing. The reasons for this are many and include our yet incomplete understanding of the molecular biology of astrocytomas; the limitations of the preclinical models we test our agents in; delivery of the biological agents to the target; molecular tumor heterogeneity; dose-limiting toxicity, and most importantly, cross-talk and redundancy of many of these biological pathways.

These obstacles need to be better examined and can be hurdled, but likely will not result in single agent 'magic bullet' therapy. In the future, we will need to not only 'molecularly profile' each individual tumor, but do this repeatedly, as the molecular genetics of the tumor change as it grows and interacts with stromal elements and the microenvironment (Fig. 5.2). Of course, repeated sampling is not usually possible in brain tumors, so emerging non-invasive biological-based imaging modalities will be critical. The issue of delivery will remain, as, although the blood–brain barrier (BBB) is broken in the center of GBMs, it is quite intact in the periphery full of invading tumor cells which leads to recurrence. To circumvent this hurdle, novel delivery modalities such as convection enhanced delivery (CED) holds promise, and are currently being tested in the clinic. Despite these measures, we will need a changing 'cocktail' of biological targeted therapies in addition to the current standard of surgery/radiation/chemotherapy. We have to be vigilant of the toxicity of these multi-modal therapies as we strive to make incremental improvements in the quantity and quality of life of our patients afflicted with gliomas.

REFERENCES

Akhmametyeva, E.M., Mihaylova, M.M., Luo, H., et al., 2006. Regulation of the neurofibromatosis 2 gene promoter expression during embryonic development. Dev. Dyn. 235, 2771–2785.

Amlashi, S.F., Riffaud, L., Brassier, G., et al., 2003. Nevoid basal cell carcinoma syndrome: relation with desmoplastic medulloblastoma in infancy. A population-based study and review of the literature. Cancer 98, 618–624.

Astrinidis, A., Henske, E.P., 2005. Tuberous sclerosis complex: linking growth and energy signaling pathways with human disease. Oncogene. 24, 7475–7481.

Bachinski, L.L., Olufemi, S.E., Zhou, X., et al., 2005. Genetic mapping of a third Li–Fraumeni syndrome predisposition locus to human chromosome 1q23. Cancer Res. 65, 427–431.

Bajenaru, M.L., Zhu, Y., Hedrick, N.M., et al., 2002. Astrocyte-specific inactivation of the neurofibromatosis 1 gene (NF-1) is insufficient for astrocytoma formation. Mol. Cell. Biol. 22, 5100–5113.

Basu, T.N., Gutmann, D.H., Fletcher, J.A., et al., 1992. Aberrant regulation of ras proteins in malignant tumor cells from type 1 neurofibromatosis patients. Nature 356, 713–715.

Beachy, P.A., Karhadkar, S.S., Berman, D.M., 2004a. Mending and malignancy. Nature 431, 402.

Beachy, P.A., Karhadkar, S.S., Berman, D.M., 2004b. Tissue repair and stem cell renewal in carcinogenesis. Nature 432, 324–331.

Bell, D.W., Varley, J.M., Szydlo, T.E., et al., 1999. Heterozygous germ line hCHK2 mutations in Li–Fraumeni syndrome. Science 286, 2528–2531.

Berman, D.M., Karhadkar, S.S., Maitra, A., et al., 2003. Widespread requirement for Hedgehog ligand stimulation in growth of digestive tract tumors. Nature 425, 846–851.

Bernards, A., Settleman, J., 2004. GAP control: regulating the regulators of small GTPases. Trends Cell Biol. 14, 377–385.

Bhowmick, D.A., Zhuang, Z., Wait, S.D., et al., 2004. A functional polymorphism in the EGF gene is found with increased frequency in glioblastoma multiforme patients and is associated with more aggressive disease. Cancer Res. 64, 1220–1223.

Birch, J.M., Hartley, A.L., Tricker, K.J., et al., 1994. Prevalence and diversity of constitutional mutations in the p53 gene among 21 Li–Fraumeni families. Cancer Res. 54, 1298–1304.

Blumberg, P.M., 1991. Complexities of the protein kinase C pathway. Mol. Carcinog. 4, 339–344.

Bondy, M.L., Scheurer, M.E., Malmer, B., et al., 2008. Brain tumor epidemiology: consensus from the Brain Tumor Epidemiology Consortium. Cancer 113 (7 Suppl), 1953–1968.

Bono, P., Cordero, E., Johnson, K., et al., 2005. Layilin, a cell surface hyaluronan receptor, interacts with merlin and radixin. Exp. Cell Res. 308, 177–187.

Bos, J.L., 1989. ras oncogenes in human cancer: a review. Cancer Res. 49, 4682–4689.

Boutet, N., Bignon, Y.J., Drouin-Garraud, V., et al., 2003. Spectrum of PTCH1 mutations in French patients with Gorlin syndrome. J. Invest. Dermatol. 121, 478–481.

Cancer Genome Atlas Research Network, 2008. Comprehensive genomic characterization defines human glioblastoma genes and core pathways. Nature 455, 1061–1068.

Carbonara, C., Longa, L., Grosso, E., et al., 1996. Apparent preferential loss of heterozygosity at TSC2 over TSC1 chromosomal region in tuberous sclerosis hamartomas. Genes Chromosomes Cancer 15, 18–25.

Cavenee, W., Kleihues, P., 2000. Pathology and genetics of tumors of the nervous system, first ed. IARC Press, Lyon.

Cawthon, R.M., O'Connell, P., Buchberg, A.M., et al., 1990a. Identification and characterization of transcripts from the neurofibromatosis 1 region: the sequence and genomic structure of EVI2 and mapping of other transcripts. Genomics 7, 555–565.

Cawthon, R.M., Weiss, R., Xu, G.F., et al., 1990b. A major segment of the neurofibromatosis type 1 gene: cDNA sequence, genomic structure, and point mutations. Cell 62, 193–201.

Chan, C.C., Chew, E.Y., Shen, D., et al., 2005. Expression of stem cells markers in ocular hemangioblastoma associated with von Hippel-Lindau (VHL) disease. Mol. Vis. 11, 697–704.

Chan, C.C., Vortmeyer, A.O., Chew, E.Y., et al., 1999. VHL gene deletion and enhanced V E G F gene expression detected in the stromal cells of retinal angioma. Arch. Ophthalmol. 117, 625–630.

Chan, J.A., Zhang, H., Roberts, P.S., et al., 2004. Pathogenesis of tuberous sclerosis subependymal giant cell astrocytomas: biallelic inactivation of TSC1 or TSC2 leads to mTOR activation. J Neuropathol. Exp. Neurol. 63, 1236–1242.

Chen, F., Kishida, T., Yao, M., et al., 1995. Germline mutations in the von Hippel-Lindau disease tumor suppressor gene: correlations with phenotype. Hum. Mutat. 5, 66–75.

Chidambaram, A., Dean, M., 1996. Genetics of the nevoid basal cell carcinoma syndrome. Adv. Cancer Res. 70, 49–61.

Choi, C., Jeong, E., Benveniste, E.N., 2004. Caspase-1 mediates Fas-induced apoptosis and is up-regulated by interferon-gamma in human astrocytoma cells. J. Neurooncol. 67, 167–176.

Chompret, A., Abel, A., Stoppa-Lyonnet, D., et al., 2001. Sensitivity and predictive value of criteria for p53 germline mutation screening. J. Med. Genet. 38, 43–47.

Chompret, A., Brugieres, L., Ronsin, M., et al., 2000. P53 germline mutations in childhood cancers and cancer risk for carrier individuals. Br. J. Cancer 82, 1932–1937.

Chompret, A., 2002. The Li–Fraumeni syndrome. Biochimie 84, 75–82.

Cichowski, K., Jacks, T., 2001. NF-1 tumor suppressor gene function: narrowing the G A P. Cell 104, 593–604.

Cichowski, K., Shih, T.S., Schmitt, E., et al., 1999. Mouse models of tumor development in neurofibromatosis type 1. Science 286, 2172–2176.

Clark, E.A., Leach, K.L., Trojanowski, J.Q., et al., 1991. Characterization and differential distribution of the three major human protein kinase C isozymes (PKC alpha, P K C beta, and P K C gamma) of the central nervous system in normal and Alzheimer's disease brains. Lab. Invest. 64, 35–44.

Clement, V., Sanchez, P., de Tribolet, N., et al., 2007. HEDGEHOG-GLI1 signaling regulates human glioma growth, cancer stem cell self-renewal, and tumorigenicity. Curr. Biol. 17, 165–172.

Cole, B.K., Curto, M., Chan, A.W., et al., 2008. Localization to the cortical cytoskeleton is necessary for NF-2/merlin-dependent epidermal growth factor receptor silencing. Mol. Cell Biol. 28, 1274–1284.

Collins, V.P., 1995. Gene amplification in human gliomas. Glia. 15, 289–296.

Couldwell, W.T., Antel, J.P., Yong, V.W., 1992. Protein kinase C activity correlates with the growth rate of malignant gliomas: Part II. Effects of glioma mitogens and modulators of protein kinase C. Neurosurgery 31, 717–724; discussion 724.

Croft, R.J., McKenzie, R.J., Inyang, I., et al., 2008. Mobile phones and brain tumors: a review of epidemiological research. Australasia Phys. Eng. Sci. Med. 31 (4), 255–267.

Crossey, P.A., Richards, F.M., Foster, K., et al., 1994. Identification of intragenic mutations in the von Hippel-Lindau disease tumor suppressor gene and correlation with disease phenotype. Hum. Mol. Genet. 3, 1303–1308.

Curatolo, P., Bombardieri, R., Jozwiak, S., 2008. Tuberous sclerosis. Lancet 372, 657–668.

Curatolo, P., Brinchi, V., 1993. Antenatal diagnosis of tuberous sclerosis. Lancet 341, 176–177.

Curatolo, P., Cusmai, R., Cortesi, F., et al., 1991. Neuropsychiatric aspects of tuberous sclerosis. Ann. NY Acad. Sci. 615, 8–16.

Curto, M., Cole, B.K., Lallemand, D., et al., 2007. Contact-dependent inhibition of EGFR signaling by NF-2/Merlin. J. Cell Biol. 177, 893–903.

Dasgupta, B., Dugan, L.L., Gutmann, D.H., 2003. The neurofibromatosis 1 gene product neurofibromin regulates pituitary adenylate cyclase-activating polypeptide-mediated signaling in astrocytes. J. Neurosci. 23, 8949–8954.

Dasgupta, B., Yi, Y., Chen, D.Y., et al., 2005. Proteomic analysis reveals hyperactivation of the mammalian target of rapamycin pathway in neurofibromatosis 1-associated human and mouse brain tumors. Cancer Res. 65, 2755–2760.

Deinhardt, F., 1980. Viral oncology. In: Klein, G. (Ed.), Biology of primate retroviruses. Raven Press, New York, pp. 357–398.

Doherty, J.K., Ongkeko, W., Crawley, B., et al., 2008. ErbB and Nrg: potential molecular targets for vestibular schwannoma pharmacotherapy. Otol. Neurotol. 29, 50–57.

Dorschner, M.O., Sybert, V.P., Weaver, M., et al., 2000. NF-1 microdeletion breakpoints are clustered at flanking repetitive sequences. Hum. Mol. Genet. 9, 35–46.

Eeles, R.A., 1995. Germline mutations in the TP53 gene. Cancer Surv. 25, 101–124.

Ekstrand, A.J., Longo, N., Hamid, M.L., et al., 1994. Functional characterization of an EGF receptor with a truncated extracellular domain expressed in glioblastomas with EGFR gene amplification. Oncogene. 9, 2313–2320.

el-Azouzi, M., Chung, R.Y., Farmer, G.E., et al., 1989. Loss of distinct regions on the short arm of chromosome 17 associated with tumorigenesis of human astrocytomas. Proc. Natl. Acad. Sci. USA 86, 7186–7190.

Epstein, E.H., 2008. Basal cell carcinomas: attack of the hedgehog. Nat. Rev. Cancer 8, 743–754.

European Chromosome 16 Tuberous Sclerosis Consortium., 1993. Identification and characterization of the tuberous sclerosis gene on chromosome 16. Cell 75, 1305–1315.

Evans, D.G., Huson, S.M., Donnai, D., et al., 1992. A genetic study of type 2 neurofibromatosis in the United Kingdom. II. Guidelines for genetic counselling. J. Med. Genet. 29, 847–852.

Feldkamp, M.M., Angelov, L., Guha, A., 1999a. Neurofibromatosis type 1 peripheral nerve tumors: aberrant activation of the Ras pathway. Surg. Neurol. 51, 211–218.

Feldkamp, M.M., Lala, P., Lau, N., et al., 1999b. Expression of activated epidermal growth factor receptors, Ras-guanosine triphosphate, and mitogen-activated protein kinase in human glioblastoma multiforme specimens. Neurosurgery 45, 1442–1453.

Feldkamp, M.M., Lau, N., Guha, A., 1999c. Growth inhibition of astrocytoma cells by farnesyl transferase inhibitors is mediated by a combination of anti-proliferative, pro-apoptotic and anti-angiogenic effects. Oncogene. 18, 7514–7526.

Fendrich, V., Esni, F., Garay, M.V., et al., 2008. Hedgehog signaling is required for effective regeneration of exocrine pancreas. Gastroenterology 135, 621–631.

Fernandez-Valle, C., Tang, Y., Ricard, J., et al., 2002. Paxillin binds schwannomin and regulates its density-dependent localization and effect on cell morphology. Nat. Genet. 31, 354–362.

Fleming, T.P., Saxena, A., Clark, W.C., et al., 1992. Amplification and/or overexpression of platelet-derived growth factor receptors and epidermal growth factor receptor in human glial tumors. Cancer Res. 52, 4550–4553.

Folkman, J., 1992. The role of angiogenesis in tumor growth. Semin. Cancer Biol. 3, 65–71.

Fraenzer, J.T., Pan, H., Minimo, L. Jr., et al., 2003. Overexpression of the NF-2 gene inhibits schwannoma cell proliferation through promoting PDGFR degradation. Int. J. Oncol. 23, 1493–1500.

Friedman, J.M., 1999. Epidemiology of neurofibromatosis type 1. Am. J. Med. Genet. 89, 1–6.

Fryer, A.E., Chalmers, A., Connor, J.M., et al., 1987. Evidence that the gene for tuberous sclerosis is on chromosome 9. Lancet 1, 659–661.

Fulci, G., Ishii, N., Van Meir, E.G., 1998. p53 and brain tumors: from gene mutations to gene therapy. Brain Pathol. 8, 599–613.

Gailani, M.R., Bale, S.J., Leffell, D.J., et al., 1992. Developmental defects in Gorlin syndrome related to a putative tumor suppressor gene on chromosome 9. Cell 69, 111–117.

Gao, X., Zhang, Y., Arrazola, P., et al., 2002. Tsc tumor suppressor proteins antagonize amino-acid-TOR signaling. Nat. Cell Biol. 4, 699–704.

Garber, J.E., Goldstein, A.M., Kantor, A.F., et al., 1991. Follow-up study of twenty-four families with Li–Fraumeni syndrome. Cancer Res. 51, 6094–6097.

Giles, R.H., Lolkema, M.P., Snijckers, C.M., et al., 2006. Interplay between VHL/HIF1alpha and Wnt/beta-catenin pathways during colorectal tumorigenesis. Oncogene. 25, 3065–3070.

Giovannini, M., Robanus-Maandag, E., van der Valk, M., et al., 2000. Conditional biallelic NF-2 mutation in the mouse promotes manifestations of human neurofibromatosis type 2. Genes Dev. 14, 1617–1630.

Gitler, A.D., Zhu, Y., Ismat, F.A., et al., 2003. NF-1 has an essential role in endothelial cells. Nat. Genet. 33, 75–79.

Godard, S., Getz, G., Delorenzi, M., et al., 2003. Classification of human astrocytic gliomas on the basis of gene expression: a correlated group of genes with angiogenic activity emerges as a strong predictor of subtypes. Cancer Res. 63, 6613–6625.

Goldstein, A.M., Pastakia, B., DiGiovanna, J.J., et al., 1994. Clinical findings in two African-American families with the nevoid basal cell carcinoma syndrome (NBCC). Am. J. Med. Genet. 50, 272–281.

Gonzalez, K.D., Noltner, K.A., Buzin, C.H., et al., 2009. Beyond Li–Fraumeni syndrome: clinical characteristics of families with p53 germline mutations. J. Clin. Oncol. 27, 1250–1256.

Gorlin, R.J., Goltz, R.W., 1960. Multiple nevoid basal-cell epithelioma, jaw cysts and bifid rib. A syndrome. N. Engl. J. Med. 262, 908–912.

Gorlin, R.J., 1999. Nevoid basal cell carcinoma (Gorlin) syndrome: unanswered issues. J. Lab. Clin. Med. 134, 551–552.

Guessous, F., Li, Y., Abounader, R., 2008. Signaling pathways in medulloblastoma. J. Cell Physiol. 217, 577–583.

Guha, A., Lau, N., Huvar, I., et al., 1996. Ras-GTP levels are elevated in human NF-1 peripheral nerve tumors. Oncogene. 12, 507–513.

Guo, H.F., The, I., Hannan, F., et al., 1997. Requirement of Drosophila NF-1 for activation of adenylyl cyclase by PACAP38-like neuropeptides. Science 276, 795–798.

Guo, H.F., Tong, J., Hannan, F., et al., 2000. A neurofibromatosis-1-regulated pathway is required for learning in Drosophila. Nature 403, 895–898.

Gutmann, D.H., 2008. Using neurofibromatosis-1 to better understand and treat pediatric low-grade glioma. J. Child Neurol. 23, 1186–1194.

Hahn, H., Wicking, C., Zaphiropoulous, P.G., et al., 1996. Mutations of the human homolog of Drosophila patched in the nevoid basal cell carcinoma syndrome. Cell 85, 841–851.

Hamilton, S.R., Liu, B., Parsons, R.E., et al., 1995. The molecular basis of Turcot's syndrome. N. Engl. J. Med. 332, 839–847.

Hart, C.E., Forstrom, J.W., Kelly, J.D., et al., 1988. Two classes of P D G F receptor recognize different isoforms of PDGF. Science 240, 1529–1531.

Haupt, Y., Maya, R., Kazaz, A., et al., 1997. Mdm2 promotes the rapid degradation of p53. Nature 387, 296–299.

Heldin, C.H., 1995. Dimerization of cell surface receptors in signal transduction. Cell 80, 213–223.

Henske, E.P., Wessner, L.L., Golden, J., et al., 1997. Loss of tuberin in both subependymal giant cell astrocytomas and angiomyolipomas supports a two-hit model for the pathogenesis of tuberous sclerosis tumors. Am. J. Pathol. 151, 1639–1647.

Herman, J.G., Latif, F., Weng, Y., et al., 1994. Silencing of the V H L tumor-suppressor gene by DNA methylation in renal carcinoma. Proc. Natl. Acad. Sci. USA 91, 9700–9704.

Herzberg, J.J., Wiskemann, A., 1963. [The fifth phakomatosis. Basal cell nevus with hereditary malformation and medulloblastoma.]. Dermatologica 126, 106–123.

High, A., Zedan, W., 2005. Basal cell nevus syndrome. Curr. Opin. Oncol. 17, 160–166.

Hirokawa, Y., Tikoo, A., Huynh, J., et al., 2004. A clue to the therapy of neurofibromatosis type 2: NF-2/Merlin is a PAK1 inhibitor. Cancer J. 10, 20–26.

Holland, E.C., 2001. Gliomagenesis: genetic alterations and mouse models. Nat. Rev. Genet. 2, 120–129.

Honegger, P., 1986. Protein kinase C-activating tumor promoters enhance the differentiation of astrocytes in aggregating fetal brain cell cultures. J. Neurochem. 46, 1561–1566.

Huang, S., Houghton, P.J., 2003. Targeting mTOR signaling for cancer therapy. Curr. Opin. Pharmacol. 3, 371–377.

Inoki, K., Li, Y., Zhu, T., et al., 2002. TSC2 is phosphorylated and inhibited by Akt and suppresses mTOR signaling. Nat. Cell Biol. 4, 648–657.

Jacks, T., Shih, T.S., Schmitt, E.M., et al., 1994. Tumor predisposition in mice heterozygous for a targeted mutation in NF-1. Nat. Genet. 7, 353–361.

James, G.L., Goldstein, J.L., Brown, M.S., et al., 1993. Benzodiazepine peptidomimetics: potent inhibitors of Ras farnesylation in animal cells. Science 260, 1937–1942.

Jiang, J., Hui, C.C., 2008. Hedgehog signaling in development and cancer. Dev. Cell 15, 801–812.

Johannessen, C.M., Johnson, B.W., Williams, S.M., et al., 2008. TORC1 is essential for NF-1-associated malignancies. Curr. Biol. 18, 56–62.

Johannessen, C.M., Reczek, E.E., James, M.F., et al., 2005. The NF-1 tumor suppressor critically regulates TSC2 and mTOR. Proc. Natl. Acad. Sci. USA 102, 8573–8578.

Johnson, R.L., Rothman, A.L., Xie, J., et al., 1996. Human homolog of patched, a candidate gene for the basal cell nevus syndrome. Science 272, 1668–1671.

Jozwiak, J., Jozwiak, S., Grzela, T., et al., 2005. Positive and negative regulation of TSC2 activity and its effects on downstream effectors of the mTOR pathway. Neuromolecular Med. 7, 287–296.

Kachra, Z., Beaulieu, E., Delbecchi, L., et al., 1999. Expression of matrix metalloproteinases and their inhibitors in human brain tumors. Clin. Exp. Metastasis 17, 555–566.

Kaempchen, K., Mielke, K., Utermark, T., et al., 2003. Upregulation of the Rac1/JNK signaling pathway in primary human schwannoma cells. Hum. Mol. Genet. 12, 1211–1221.

Kandt, R.S., Haines, J.L., Smith, M., et al., 1992. Linkage of an important gene locus for tuberous sclerosis to a chromosome 16 marker for polycystic kidney disease. Nat. Genet. 2, 37–41.

Karbowniczek, M., Yu, J., Henske, E.P., 2003. Renal angiomyolipomas from patients with sporadic lymphangiomyomatosis contain both neoplastic and non-neoplastic vascular structures. Am. J. Pathol. 162, 491–500.

Karhadkar, S.S., Bova, G.S., Abdallah, N., et al., 2004. Hedgehog signaling in prostate regeneration, neoplasia and metastasis. Nature 431, 707–712.

Kehrer-Sawatzki, H., Cooper, D.N., 2008. Mosaicism in sporadic neurofibromatosis type 1: variations on a theme common to other hereditary cancer syndromes? J. Med. Genet. 45, 622–631.

Kim, H.A., Ratner, N., Roberts, T.M., et al., 2001. Schwann cell proliferative responses to cAMP and NF-1 are mediated by cyclin D1. J. Neurosci. 21, 1110–1116.

Kimonis, V.E., Goldstein, A.M., Pastakia, B., et al., 1997. Clinical manifestations in 105 persons with nevoid basal cell carcinoma syndrome. Am. J. Med. Genet. 69, 299–308.

Kisseleva, T., Bhattacharya, S., Braunstein, J., et al., 2002. Signaling through the JAK/STAT pathway, recent advances and future challenges. Gene. 285, 1–24.

Kissil, J.L., Wilker, E.W., Johnson, K.C., et al., 2003. Merlin, the product of the NF-2 tumor suppressor gene, is an inhibitor of the p21-activated kinase, Pak1. Mol. Cell. 12, 841–849.

Koochekpour, S., Jeffers, M., Rulong, S., et al., 1997. Met and hepatocyte growth factor/scatter factor expression in human gliomas. Cancer Res. 57, 5391–5398.

Kool, M., Koster, J., Bunt, J., et al., 2008. Integrated genomics identifies five medulloblastoma subtypes with distinct genetic profiles, pathway signatures and clinicopathological features. PLoS One 3, e3088.

Kuzmin, I., Duh, F.M., Latif, F., et al., 1995. Identification of the promoter of the human von Hippel–Lindau disease tumor suppressor gene. Oncogene. 10, 2185–2194.

Kwiatkowski, D.J., Manning, B.D., 2005. Tuberous sclerosis: a G A P at the crossroads of multiple signaling pathways. Hum. Mol. Genet. 14 (Spec No. 2), R251–R258.

Laterra, J., Nam, M., Rosen, E., et al., 1997. Scatter factor/hepatocyte growth factor gene transfer enhances glioma growth and angiogenesis in vivo. Lab. Invest. 76, 565–577.

Latif, F., Tory, K., Gnarra, J., et al., 1993. Identification of the von Hippel-Lindau disease tumor suppressor gene. Science 260, 1317–1320.

Lau, N., Feldkamp, M.M., Roncari, L., et al., 2000. Loss of neurofibromin is associated with activation of RAS/MAPK and PI3-K/AKT signaling in a neurofibromatosis 1 astrocytoma. J. Neuropathol. Exp. Neurol. 59, 759–767.

Lench, N.J., Telford, E.A., High, A.S., et al., 1997. Characterisation of human patched germ line mutations in naevoid basal cell carcinoma syndrome. Hum. Genet. 100, 497–502.

Li, F.P., Fraumeni, J.F. Jr., 1969a. Rhabdomyosarcoma in children: epidemiologic study and identification of a familial cancer syndrome. J. Natl. Cancer Inst. 43, 1365–1373.

Li, F.P., Fraumeni, J.F. Jr., 1969b. Soft-tissue sarcomas, breast cancer, and other neoplasms. A familial syndrome? Ann. Intern. Med. 71, 747–752.

Li, Y., Millikan, R.C., Carozza, S., et al., 1998. p53 mutations in malignant gliomas. Cancer Epidemiol. Biomarkers Prev. 7, 303–308.

Lindemann, R.K., 2008. Stroma-initiated hedgehog signaling takes center stage in B-cell lymphoma. Cancer Res. 68, 961–964.

Lindstrom, E., Shimokawa, T., Toftgard, R., et al., 2006. PTCH mutations: distribution and analyses. Hum. Mutat. 27, 215–219.

Lo Muzio, L., 2008. Nevoid basal cell carcinoma syndrome (Gorlin syndrome). Orphanet J. Rare Dis. 3, 32.

Maher, E.A., Furnari, F.B., Bachoo, R.M., et al., 2001. Malignant glioma: genetics and biology of a grave matter. Genes Dev. 15, 1311–1333.

Malkin, D., Li, F.P., Strong, L.C., et al., 1990. Germ line p53 mutations in a familial syndrome of breast cancer, sarcomas, and other neoplasms. Science 250, 1233–1238.

Manchanda, N., Lyubimova, A., Ho, H.Y., et al., 2005. The NF-2 tumor suppressor Merlin and the ERM proteins interact with N-WASP and regulate its actin polymerization function. J. Biol. Chem. 280, 12517–12522.

Marcotte, L., Crino, P.B., 2006. The neurobiology of the tuberous sclerosis complex. Neuromolecular Med. 8, 531–546.

McClatchey, A.I., Giovannini, M., 2005. Membrane organization and tumorigenesis–the NF-2 tumor suppressor, Merlin. Genes Dev. 19, 2265–2277.

McClatchey, A.I., 2007. Neurofibromatosis. Annu. Rev. Pathol. 2, 191–216.

McLaughlin, M.E., Kruger, G.M., Slocum, K.L., et al., 2007. The NF-2 tumor suppressor regulates cell-cell adhesion during tissue fusion. Proc. Natl. Acad. Sci. USA 104, 3261–3266.

Morrison, H., Sherman, L.S., Legg, J., et al., 2001. The NF-2 tumor suppressor gene product, merlin, mediates contact inhibition of growth through interactions with CD44. Genes Dev. 15, 968–980.

Morrison, H., Sperka, T., Manent, J., et al., 2007. Merlin/neurofibromatosis type 2 suppresses growth by inhibiting the activation of Ras and Rac. Cancer Res. 67, 520–527.

Moscatello, D.K., Holgado-Madruga, M., Godwin, A.K., et al., 1995. Frequent expression of a mutant epidermal growth factor receptor in multiple human tumors. Cancer Res. 55, 5536–5539.

Moscatello, D.K., Montgomery, R.B., Sundareshan, P., et al., 1996. Transformational and altered signal transduction by a naturally occurring mutant EGF receptor. Oncogene. 13, 85–96.

Mukherjee, J., Kamnasaran, D., Balasubramaniam, A., et al., 2009. Human schwannomas express activated platelet-derived growth factor receptors and c-kit and are growth inhibited by Gleevec (Imatinib Mesylate). Cancer Res. 69, 5099–5107.

Muranen, T., Gronholm, M., Lampin, A., et al., 2007. The tumor suppressor merlin interacts with microtubules and modulates Schwann cell microtubule cytoskeleton. Hum. Mol. Genet. 16, 1742–1751.

Nabbout, R., Santos, M., Rolland, Y., et al., 1999. Early diagnosis of subependymal giant cell astrocytoma in children with tuberous sclerosis. J. Neurol. Neurosurg. Psychiatry 66, 370–375.

Nakai, Y., Zheng, Y., MacCollin, M., et al., 2006. Temporal control of Rac in Schwann cell-axon interaction is disrupted in NF-2-mutant schwannoma cells. J. Neurosci. 26, 3390–3395.

Nishizuka, Y., 1992. Intracellular signaling by hydrolysis of phospholipids and activation of protein kinase C. Science 258, 607–614.

Nister, M., Libermann, T.A., Betsholtz, C., et al., 1988. Expression of messenger RNAs for platelet-derived growth factor and transforming growth factor-alpha and their receptors in human malignant glioma cell lines. Cancer Res. 48, 3910–3918.

Olivier, M., Goldgar, D.E., Sodha, N., et al., 2003. Li–Fraumeni and related syndromes: correlation between tumor type, family structure, and TP53 genotype. Cancer Res. 63, 6643–6650.

Ono, Y., Tamiya, T., Ichikawa, T., et al., 1996. Malignant astrocytomas with homozygous CDKN2/p16 gene deletions have higher Ki-67 proliferation indices. J. Neuropathol. Exp. Neurol. 55, 1026–1031.

Pack, S.D., Zbar, B., Pak, E., et al., 1999. Constitutional von Hippel-Lindau (VHL) gene deletions detected in VHL families by fluorescence in situ hybridization. Cancer Res. 59, 5560–5564.

Paraf, F., Jothy, S., Van Meir, E.G., 1997. Brain tumor-polyposis syndrome: two genetic diseases? J. Clin. Oncol. 15, 2744–2758.

Parsons, D.W., Jones, S., Zhang, X., et al., 2008. An integrated genomic analysis of human glioblastoma multiforme. Science 321, 1807–1812.

Pelicci, G., Lanfrancone, L., Grignani, F., et al., 1992. A novel transforming protein (SHC) with an SH2 domain is implicated in mitogenic signal transduction. Cell 70, 93–104.

Prisell, P., Persson, L., Boethius, J., et al., 1987. Somatomedins in tumor cyst fluid, cerebrospinal fluid, and tumor cytosol in patients with glial tumors. Acta Neurochir. (Wien) 89, 48–52.

Rao, R.D., James, C.D., 2004. Altered molecular pathways in gliomas: an overview of clinically relevant issues. Semin. Oncol. 31 (5), 595–604.

Rasheed, B.K., Wiltshire, R.N., Bigner, S.H., et al., 1999. Molecular pathogenesis of malignant gliomas. Curr. Opin. Oncol. 11, 162–167.

Reifenberger, G., Reifenberger, J., Ichimura, K., et al., 1994. Amplification of multiple genes from chromosomal region 12q13–12q14 in human malignant gliomas: preliminary mapping of the amplicons shows preferential involvement of CDK4, SAS, and MDM2. Cancer Res. 54, 4299–4303.

Reilly, K.M., Loisel, D.A., Bronson, R.T., et al., 2000. NF-1; Trp53 mutant mice develop glioblastoma with evidence of strain-specific effects. Nat. Genet. 26, 109–113.

Richards, F.M., Payne, S.J., Zbar, B., et al., 1995. Molecular analysis of de novo germline mutations in the von Hippel-Lindau disease gene. Hum. Mol. Genet. 4, 2139–2143.

Romeike, B.F., Mawrin, C., 2008. Gliomatosis cerebri: growing evidence for diffuse gliomas with wide invasion. Expert Rev. Neurother. 8 (4), 587–597.

Rouleau, G.A., Merel, P., Lutchman, M., et al., 1993. Alteration in a new gene encoding a putative membrane-organizing protein causes neuro-fibromatosis type 2. Nature 363, 515–521.

Ruiz i Altaba, A., Mas, C., Stecca, B., 2007. The Gli code: an information nexus regulating cell fate, stemness and cancer. Trends Cell Biol. 17, 438–447.

Ruiz i Altaba, A., Nguyen, V., Palma, V., 2003. The emergent design of the neural tube: prepattern, SHH morphogen and GLI code. Curr. Opin. Genet. Dev. 13, 513–521.

Ruiz i Altaba, A., 2008. Therapeutic inhibition of Hedgehog-GLI signaling in cancer: epithelial, stromal, or stem cell targets? Cancer Cell. 14, 281–283.

Sanai, N., Alvarez-Buylla, A., Berger, M.S., 2005. Neural stem cells and the origin of gliomas. N. Engl. J. Med. 358 (8), 811–822.

Sanai, N., Tramontin, A.D., Quiñones-Hinojosa, A., et al., 2004. Unique astrocyte ribbon in adult human brain contains neural stem cells but lacks chain migration. Nature 427 (6976), 740–744.

Schaefer, L.K., Ren, Z., Fuller, G.N., et al., 2002. Constitutive activation of Stat3alpha in brain tumors: localization to tumor endothelial cells and activation by the endothelial tyrosine kinase receptor (VEGFR-2). Oncogene. 21, 2058–2065.

Seizinger, B.R., Rouleau, G.A., Ozelius, L.J., et al., 1988. Von Hippel-Lindau disease maps to the region of chromosome 3 associated with renal cell carcinoma. Nature 332, 268–269.

Seizinger, B.R., Smith, D.I., Filling-Katz, M.R., et al., 1991. Genetic flanking markers refine diagnostic criteria and provide insights into the genetics of Von Hippel Lindau disease. Proc. Natl. Acad. Sci. USA 88, 2864–2868.

Shamah, S.M., Stiles, C.D., Guha, A., 1993. Dominant-negative mutants of platelet-derived growth factor revert the transformed phenotype of human astrocytoma cells. Mol. Cell Biol. 13, 7203–7212.

Shaw, R.J., Paez, J.G., Curto, M., et al., 2001. The NF-2 tumor suppressor, merlin, functions in Rac-dependent signaling. Dev. Cell 1, 63–72.

Singh, S.K., Hawkins, C., Clarke, I.D., et al., 2004. Identification of human brain tumor initiating cells. Nature 432 (7015), 396–401.

Song, J.H., Song, D.K., Pyrzynska, B., et al., 2003. TRAIL triggers apoptosis in human malignant glioma cells through extrinsic and intrinsic pathways. Brain Pathol. 13, 539–553.

Stambolic, V., Suzuki, A., de la Pompa, J.L., et al., 1998. Negative regulation of PKB/Akt-dependent cell survival by the tumor suppressor PTEN. Cell 95, 29–39.

Stecca, B., Mas, C., Clement, V., et al., 2007. Melanomas require HEDGEHOG-GLI signaling regulated by interactions between GLI1 and the RAS-MEK/AKT pathways. Proc. Natl. Acad. Sci. USA 104, 5895–5900.

Steck, P.A., Pershouse, M.A., Jasser, S.A., et al., 1997. Identification of a candidate tumor suppressor gene, MMAC1, at chromosome 10q23. 3 that is mutated in multiple advanced cancers. Nat. Genet. 15, 356–362.

Stemmer-Rachamimov, A.O., Xu, L., Gonzalez-Agosti, C., et al., 1997. Universal absence of merlin, but not other E R M family members, in schwannomas. Am. J. Pathol. 151, 1649–1654.

Stolle, C., Glenn, G., Zbar, B., et al., 1998. Improved detection of germline mutations in the von Hippel-Lindau disease tumor suppressor gene. Hum. Mutat. 12, 417–423.

Stumpf, S., Alksne, J.F., Annegers, J.F., et al., 1988. Neurofibromatosis. Conference statement. National Institutes of Health Consensus Development Conference. Arch. Neurol. 45, 575–578.

Szudek, J., Evans, D.G., Friedman, J.M., 2003. Patterns of associations of clinical features in neurofibromatosis 1 (NF-1). Hum. Genet. 112, 289–297.

Szudek, J., Joe, H., Friedman, J.M., 2002. Analysis of intrafamilial phenotypic variation in neurofibromatosis 1 (NF-1). Genet. Epidemiol. 23, 150–164.

Taylor, M.D., Liu, L., Raffel, C., et al., 2002. Mutations in SUFU predispose to medulloblastoma. Nat. Genet. 31, 306–310.

Tee, A.R., Fingar, D.C., Manning, B.D., et al., 2002. Tuberous sclerosis complex-1 and -2 gene products function together to inhibit mammalian target of rapamycin (mTOR)-mediated downstream signaling. Proc. Natl. Acad. Sci. USA 99, 13571–13576.

Thompson, M.C., Fuller, C., Hogg, T.L., et al., 2006. Genomics identifies medulloblastoma subgroups that are enriched for specific genetic alterations. J. Clin. Oncol. 24, 1924–1931.

Thomson, S.A., Fishbein, L., Wallace, M.R., 2002. NF-1 mutations and molecular testing. J. Child Neurol. 17, 555–561; discussion 571–552, 646–551.

Tikoo, A., Varga, M., Ramesh, V., et al., 1994. An anti-Ras function of neurofibromatosis type 2 gene product (NF-2/Merlin). J. Biol. Chem. 269, 23387–23390.

Tong, J., Hannan, F., Zhu, Y., et al., 2002. Neurofibromin regulates G protein-stimulated adenylyl cyclase activity. Nat. Neurosci. 5, 95–96.

Trofatter, J.A., MacCollin, M.M., Rutter, J.L., et al., 1993. A novel moesin-, ezrin-, radixin-like gene is a candidate for the neurofibromatosis 2 tumor suppressor. Cell 72, 791–800.

Turcot, J., Despres, J.P., St Pierre, F., 1959. Malignant tumors of the central nervous system associated with familial polyposis of the colon: report of two cases. Dis. Colon Rectum 2, 465–468.

Unden, A.B., Holmberg, E., Lundh-Rozell, B., et al., 1996. Mutations in the human homologue of Drosophila patched (PTCH) in basal cell carcinomas and the Gorlin syndrome: different in vivo mechanisms of PTCH inactivation. Cancer Res. 56, 4562–4565.

Vander Heiden, M.G., Cantley, L.C., Thompson, C.B., 2009. Understanding the Warburg effect: the metabolic requirements of cell proliferation. Science 324, 1029–1033.

van Slegtenhorst, M., de Hoogt, R., Hermans, C., et al., 1997. Identification of the tuberous sclerosis gene TSC1 on chromosome 9q34. Science 277, 805–808.

Varley, J.M., Evans, D.G., Birch, J.M., 1997. Li–Fraumeni syndrome – a molecular and clinical review. Br. J. Cancer 76, 1–14.

Varley, J.M., McGown, G., Thorncroft, M., et al., 2001. Significance of intron 6 sequence variations in the TP53 gene in Li–Fraumeni syndrome. Cancer Genet. Cytogenet. 129, 85–87.

Viskochil, D., Buchberg, A.M., Xu, G., et al., 1990. Deletions and a translocation interrupt a cloned gene at the neurofibromatosis type 1 locus. Cell 62, 187–192.

Vogel, K.S., Klesse, L.J., Velasco-Miguel, S., et al., 1999. Mouse tumor model for neurofibromatosis type 1. Science 286, 2176–2179.

Vortmeyer, A.O., Frank, S., Jeong, S.Y., et al., 2003. Developmental arrest of angioblastic lineage initiates tumorigenesis in von Hippel-Lindau disease. Cancer Res. 63, 7051–7055.

Vortmeyer, A.O., Gnarra, J.R., Emmert-Buck, M.R., et al., 1997. von Hippel-Lindau gene deletion detected in the stromal cell component of a cerebellar hemangioblastoma associated with von Hippel-Lindau disease. Hum. Pathol. 28, 540–543.

Wallace, M.R., Marchuk, D.A., Andersen, L.B., et al., 1990. Type 1 neurofibromatosis gene: identification of a large transcript disrupted in three NF-1 patients. Science 249, 181–186.

Watkins, D.N., Berman, D.M., Burkholder, S.G., et al., 2003. Hedgehog signaling within airway epithelial progenitors and in small-cell lung cancer. Nature 422, 313–317.

Webb, K.E., Henney, A.M., Anglin, S., et al., 1997. Expression of matrix metalloproteinases and their inhibitor TIMP-1 in the rat carotid artery after balloon injury. Arterioscler Thromb. Vasc. Biol. 17, 1837–1844.

Wetmore, C., Eberhart, D.E., Curran, T., 2001. Loss of p53 but not A R F accelerates medulloblastoma in mice heterozygous for patched. Cancer Res. 61, 513–516.

Wicking, C., Gillies, S., Smyth, I., et al., 1997. De novo mutations of the Patched gene in nevoid basal cell carcinoma syndrome help to define the clinical phenotype. Am. J. Med. Genet. 73, 304–307.

Wiederhold, T., Lee, M.F., James, M., et al., 2004. Magicin, a novel cytoskeletal protein associates with the NF-2 tumor suppressor merlin and Grb2. Oncogene. 23, 8815–8825.

Wolf, A., Agnihotri, S., Micallef, J., et al., 2011. Hexokinase 2 is a key mediator of aerobic glycolysis and promotes tumor growth in human glioblastoma multiforme. J. Exp. Med. 208, 313–326.

Woods, S.A., Marmor, E., Feldkamp, M., et al., 2002. Aberrant G protein signaling in nervous system tumors. J. Neurosurg. 97, 627–642.

Yang, F.C., Ingram, D.A., Chen, S., et al., 2008. NF-1-dependent tumors require a microenvironment containing NF-1+/− and c-kit-dependent bone marrow. Cell 135, 437–448.

Zhu, Y., Guignard, F., Zhao, D., et al., 2005. Early inactivation of p53 tumor suppressor gene cooperating with NF-1 loss induces malignant astrocytoma. Cancer Cell 8, 119–130.

Zhu, Y., Romero, M.I., Ghosh, P., et al., 2001. Ablation of NF-1 function in neurons induces abnormal development of cerebral cortex and reactive gliosis in the brain. Genes Dev. 15, 859–876.

6 Biologic therapy for malignant glioma

Susan M. Chang and Derek R. Johnson

Introduction

High-grade gliomas have traditionally been treated with a combination of surgical resection, radiation therapy, and cytotoxic chemotherapy. The current standard-of-care regimen for initial treatment of glioblastoma multiforme employs temozolomide, an orally administered methylating agent with excellent bioavailability, both concomitantly with radiation therapy and as a monthly adjuvant therapy following completion of radiation (Stupp et al 2005). Other traditional chemotherapeutic approaches such as combination therapy with lomustine (CCNU), procarbazine, and vincristine are still commonly employed for treatment of oligodendroglioma and recurrent high-grade glioma (Tatter 2002). Despite new approaches to cytotoxic chemotherapy administration, such as implantation of carmustine wafers into the tumor resection cavity (Westphal et al 2003) and delivery of chemotherapy more directly and efficiently with techniques such as blood–brain barrier disruption (Fortin et al 2005) and convection-enhanced delivery (Lidar et al 2004), the utility of traditional chemotherapeutic agents continues to be limited by poor efficacy, toxicity, and cellular resistance.

In recent years, improved understanding of the molecular biology of brain tumors has led to a new approach to therapy. The identification of a number of the pathways used by tumors to proliferate, avoid apoptosis, and trigger angiogenesis has allowed the development of low molecular weight kinase inhibitors and monoclonal antibodies that disrupt these abilities. This approach is typified by the success of the tyrosine kinase inhibitor imatinib mesylate (Gleevec) in the treatment of chronic myelogenous leukemia (Druker 2004). Within each pathway, potential targets include ligands, ligand receptors, and the multiple downstream signaling cascades initiated by receptor activation. Relevant pathways in glioma include platelet-derived growth factor (PDGF); epidermal growth factor (EGF); hepatocyte growth factor/scatter factor (HGF/SF); insulin-like growth factor (IGF); vascular endothelial growth factor (VEGF); placental growth factor (PlGF), and others. There is great optimism that the use of molecularly targeted agents will lead to significantly improved survival for patients with malignant gliomas.

Most molecularly targeted therapies currently available fall into one of two general categories: monoclonal antibodies against either growth factors or the extracellular ligand-binding domains of growth factor receptors or the growth factor ligands, and small molecule inhibitors of the intracellular kinases and their downstream effectors. Each of these approaches to therapy has theoretical advantages. Antibodies trigger the host immune response, and can lead to down-regulation of cellular surface receptors. A major limitation of antibody-based therapy is poor blood–brain barrier penetration. Bevacizumab, an antibody against VEGF, which will be reviewed in detail later, binds to VEGF on the abluminal side of blood vessels, thereby avoiding this problem. Most other targeted antibody therapies, such as cetuximab, which binds to EGFR, need to enter the brain parenchyma in order to reach their targets. Some clinical trials have examined the administration of antibody therapy directly into the tumor resection cavity (Reardon et al 2002), but systemic administration is far more common. Small molecule kinase inhibitors have the advantage of being better able to penetrate the blood–brain barrier. While more than 500 kinases are encoded in the human genome, to date only approximately 30 have been targeted as anti-cancer therapies in clinical trials (Zhang et al 2009). Most known kinase inhibitors act competitively at the ATP binding site, which is highly conserved across kinase genes (Table 6.1).

Tumor growth factor pathways

Uncontrolled cellular growth, proliferation, and survival are hallmarks of malignancy. Each of these characteristics represents a breakdown of the normal processes involved in cell maturation and death. Mutations and epigenetic changes allow tumor cells to enhance the activity of promoters of growth and escape the influence of inhibitory signaling. Growth factor receptor kinases and their intracellular signal transduction pathways are key to this process, and present a rational target for pharmaceutical intervention (Table 6.2).

Epidermal growth factor

Epidermal growth factor (EGF) and the epidermal growth factor receptor (EGFR) have long been recognized for their role in tumor growth (Cohen 1983). There are four transmembrane epidermal growth factor receptors: EGFR (also known as human EGF receptor 1 or HER1), HER2, HER3, and HER4. When EGF or one of its related ligands binds to the extracellular receptor domain of an EGFR, it leads to the dimer formation and activation of the intracellular tyrosine kinase domain followed by trans-autophosphorylation, allowing the initiation of a large number of signaling cascades. The two EGF-triggered signaling cascades with the greatest relevance for glioma are the RAS-RAF-MEK-MAPK pathway and the PI3K-Akt-mTOR pathway (Scaltriti & Baselga 2006). While many tumors co-express EGF and EGFR, forming an autocrine signaling loop, the role of excessive EGF ligand appears less clinically relevant than that of EGFR (McLendon et al 2007). There are multiple means by

Table 6.1 Selected trials of agents targeting angiogenesis

Target	Agent	Clinical trials	Results
VEGF	Bevacizumab	Phase II: Bevacizumab for recurrent MG	Ongoing
		Phase II: Bevacizumab + irinotecan for recurrent GBM	PFS6 43%, OS6 77% (Vredenburgh et al 2007)
		Phase II: Bevacizumab vs bevacizumab + irinotecan for recurrent GBM	BV PFS6 35%, median OS 9.7m BV+CPT PFS6 50.2%, median OS 8.9m (Cloughesy et al 2008)
		Phase II: Bevacizumab for recurrent GBM followed by bevacizumab + irinotecan after progression	PFS6 29%, OS6 57% for bevacizumab arm No additional response after addition of irinotecan (Kreisl et al 2009)
		Phase II: Bevacizumab + cetuximab + irinotecan for recurrent GBM	Not superior to bevacizumab + irinotecan alone (Lassen et al 2008)
		Phase II: TMZ + XRT followed by bevacizumab + TMZ for newly diagnosed GBM	Ongoing
		Phase II: TMZ + XRT followed by bevacizumab + erlotinib for newly diagnosed GBM	Ongoing
		Phase II: Bevacizumab + TMZ + XRT followed by bevacizumab + everolimus for newly diagnosed GBM	Ongoing
		Phase II: Bevacizumab + TMZ + XRT followed by bevacizumab + TMZ + irinotecan for newly diagnosed GBM	Ongoing
		Phase II: Bevacizumab + TMZ + erlotinib for non-progressive GBM after TMZ/XRT	Ongoing
		Phase II: Bevacizumab + etoposide for recurrent GBM	Ongoing
		Phase II: Bevacizumab + metronomic TMZ for recurrent GBM	Ongoing
		Phase II: Bevacizumab + carmustine for recurrent MG	Ongoing
		Phase II: Bevacizumab + erlotinib for recurrent GBM	Ongoing
		Phase II: Bevacizumab + sorafenib for recurrent GBM	Ongoing
		Phase II: Bevacizumab + bortezomib for recurrent GBM	Ongoing
		Phase II: Bevacizumab + enzastaurin for recurrent MG	Ongoing
		Phase II: Bevacizumab + tandutinib for recurrent MG	Ongoing
		Phase II: Bevacizumab + temsirolimus for recurrent GBM	Ongoing
		Phase II: Bevacizumab + TMZ + XRT vs bevacizumab + irinotecan + XRT for recurrent GBM	Ongoing
		Phase I: Vorinostat + bevacizumab + irinotecan for recurrent GBM	Ongoing
		Phase II: Gliadel followed by bevacizumab/irinotecan for recurrent GBM	Ongoing
		Phase II: Bevacizumab + TMZ vs bevacizumab + etoposide for patients who have failed bevacizumab + irinotecan	Ongoing
	Aflibercept	Phase I: Aflibercept + TMZ + XRT for newly diagnosed or recurrent GBM	Ongoing
		Phase II: Aflibercept for recurrent malignant glioma	Ongoing
VEGFR	Cediranib	Phase III: Cediranib vs lomustine vs cediranib + lomustine for recurrent GBM	Ongoing
		Phase I/II: Cediranib + TMZ + XRT for newly diagnosed GBM	Ongoing
		Phase II: Cediranib for recurrent GBM	Median OS 211d (Batchelor et al 2007)
		Phase I: Cediranib + lomustine for primary recurrent malignant brain tumor	Ongoing
	CT-322	Phase I: CT-322 + TMZ + XRT for newly diagnosed GBM	Ongoing
		Phase II: CT-322 ± irinotecan for recurrent GBM	Ongoing
Notch	MK0752	Phase I: MK0752 for pediatric patients with recurrent CNS cancer	Ongoing

which the EGFR can become overactive in glioma; normal EGFR can be over-expressed due to genetic mutations leading to polysomy or amplification of the EGFR locus (Ekstrand et al 1991), or EGFR itself can be subject to mutation. The most common EGFR mutation in glioma, EGFRvIII, is an in-frame deletion of the extracellular ligand binding domain, which results in activity of the intracellular tyrosine kinase in the absence of EGF binding (Pelloski et al 2007). Amplification and overexpression of the EGFR gene are seen in approximately half of all glioblastomas (Brandes et al 2008). Among tumors with EGFR amplification, approximately half express the constitutively active EGFRvIII mutation. EGFRvIII preferentially activates the PI3K-Akt-mTOR pathway as well as other second-messenger pathways not responsive to unmutated EGFR (McLendon et al 2007).

Several EGFR-targeted therapies are being investigated as treatments for malignant glioma. Antibodies, such as cetuximab (Erbitux) and panitumumab (Vectibix), bind to EGFR and trigger the host immune response, leading to downregulation of EGFR. While cetuximab has been shown to be effective against malignant glioma cells in culture and animal models (Eller et al 2002), no clinical trials examining efficacy of anti-EGFR antibodies in malignant glioma have yet been published. Small molecules, by virtue of their action on the constitutively active intracellular tyrosine kinase domain of EGFR rather than the extracellular receptor domain, are better able to modulate the activity of the important EGFR-vIII mutation of EGFR. One phase II trial of erlotinib, a EGFR tyrosine kinase inhibitor, in combination with temozolomide and radiation therapy in patients with newly diagnosed glioblastoma or gliosarcoma recently demonstrated improved survival relative to historical controls (Prados et al 2009), while a similar study did not suggest benefit (Brown et al 2008). Further studies are ongoing to define treatment effect and identify subpopulations likely to receive maximum benefit. Previous studies of erlotinib and gefitinib suggested that they are of greatest benefit to patients with tumors that coexpress EGFRvIII and PTEN (Mellinghoff et al 2005). These data remain controversial and await prospective confirmation.

Table 6.2 Selected trials of agents targeting tumor growth factors

Target	Agent	Clinical trials	Results
EGFR	Cetuximab	Phase II: Bevacizumab + cetuximab + irinotecan for recurrent GBM	Not superior to bevacizumab + irinotecan alone (Lassen et al 2008)
		Phase I/II: Cetuximab + TMZ + XRT for newly diagnosed GBM	Ongoing
	Nimotuzumab	Phase III: Nimotuzumab + TMZ + XRT vs standard therapy for newly diagnosed GBM	Ongoing
		Phase II: Nimotuzumab for recurrent pontine glioma in pediatric patients	Ongoing
	Erlotinib	Phase I: Erlotinib or erlotinib + TMZ for malignant glioma	PFS6 11% (Prados et al 2006)
		Phase II: Erlotinib + TMZ + XRT for newly diagnosed GBM	Median PFS 8.2m, Median survival 19.3m MGMT status predicts outcome (Prados et al 2009)
		Phase II: Erlotinib for recurrent GBM	Median PFS 12 weeks (Raizer et al 2004)
		Phase I/II: Erlotinib + XRT for young patients with newly diagnosed glioma	Ongoing
		Phase II: TMZ + XRT followed by bevacizumab + erlotinib for newly diagnosed GBM	Ongoing
		Phase II: Bevacizumab + TMZ + erlotinib for non-progressive GBM after initial TMZ + XRT	Ongoing
		Phase II: Erlotinib + sirolimus for recurrent GBM	Ongoing
		Phase II: Erlotinib + temsirolimus for patient with recurrent MG	Ongoing
		Phase II: Erlotinib + bevacizumab for recurrent MG	Ongoing
		Phase I: Erlotinib + dasatinib for recurrent MG	Ongoing
		Phase II: Erlotinib + sorafenib for recurrent GBM	Ongoing
	Gefitinib	Phase II: Gefitinib for first recurrence of GBM	PFS-6 13% (Rich et al 2004)
		Phase I: Everolimus + gefitinib for recurrent GBM	PFS-6 5% (Kreisl et al 2009)
HGF/SF	AMG-102	Phase II: AMG-102 for recurrent malignant glioma	Ongoing

The most common side-effect of anti-EGFR therapy is a papulopustular rash related to the role of EGFR in keratinocyte maturation. The rash is typically self-limited, even with continuation of anti-EGFR therapy, although post-inflammatory hyperpigmentation is often seen. Development of the characteristic rash has been linked to tumor response to anti-EGFR therapy, and may be a useful surrogate marker of response (Perez-Soler 2003). Gastrointestinal side-effects including diarrhea, nausea, and vomiting are also common following anti-EGFR therapy. These symptoms are related to impairment of EGFR's role in maintaining mucosal integrity, and represent a major dose-limiting toxicity for the EGFR tyrosine kinase inhibitor class of therapies. Interstitial lung disease (ILD), which can be fatal, represents a rare but severe toxicity of the EGFR tyrosine kinase inhibitors (Tsuboi & Le Chevalier 2006) (Table 6.3).

Platelet derived growth factor

The platelet derived growth factor (PDGF) pathway shares much in common with the EGFR pathway. The family consists of four ligands, PDGF-A through PDGF-D, and two tyrosine kinase receptors, PDGFR-α and PDGFR-β. Both PDGF and PDGFR are frequently over-expressed in malignant gliomas. As in EGF, receptor activation leads to dimerization, trans-autophosphorylation, and the initiation of multiple downstream signaling cascades including the PI3K-Akt-mTOR and RAS-RAF-MEK-MAPK systems.

The prototypical anti-PDGFR therapy is imatinib (Gleevec), a PDGF receptor tyrosine kinase inhibitor that also has action against Bcl-Abl and c-kit. Imatinib has been evaluated as a therapy for glioma in phase II clinical trials both as monotherapy (Wen et al 2006) and in combination with

hydroxyurea (Reardon et al 2005). While both approaches have favorable side-effect profiles, neither was shown effective as a therapy for unselected patients with recurrent glioblastoma. Further studies investigating imatinib in combination with other agents, such as temozolomide, are ongoing (Table 6.4).

Hepatocyte growth factor/scatter factor

Hepatocyte growth factor (HGF), also known as scatter factor (SF), acts upon the receptor tyrosine kinase c-Met to trigger many cellular processes including proliferation, survival, migration, and invasion. As with EGFR and PDGFR, c-Met mediates both the PI3K-Akt-mTOR and RAS-RAF-MEK-MAPK second messenger systems. The diverse actions of c-Met are collectively known as the invasive growth program. C-Met activity is crucial to embryogenesis, as demonstrated by early intrauterine death of HGF or c-Met knockout mice. In mature animals, HGF and c-Met play a much more limited role, primarily in tissue healing after injury. Abnormal c-Met signaling is seen a variety of tumors, including glial tumors, where its promotion of invasive growth is associated with a poor prognosis (Abounader & Laterra 2005). As with other receptor tyrosine kinases, c-Met over-expression appears to be the primary process leading to aberrant activation of the pathway (Migliore & Giordano 2008). The HGF/c-Met system also interacts with other pathways implicated in tumorigenesis. HGF stimulation produces EGFR activation (Reznik et al 2008) and VEGF production in tumor cells (Abounader & Laterra 2005).

Clinical trials are ongoing to evaluate the role of HGF/c-Met inhibitors in the treatment of malignancy. AMG102 is a fully human monoclonal antibody against HGF that

Table 6.3 Selected trials of agents targeting growth factor effectors

Target	Agent	Clinical trials	Results
RAS	Tipifarnib	Phase I/II: Tipifarnib for recurrent MG in patients receiving or not receiving enzyme-inducing antiepileptic drugs (EIAEDs)	No-EIAED: GBM PFS6 16.7% EIAED: GBM PFS6 6.5% (Cloughesy et al 2006)
		Phase I: Tipifarnib + TMZ + XRT for newly diagnosed GBM	Ongoing
		Phase II: Tipifarnib + XRT for newly diagnosed GBM	Ongoing
	Lonafarnib	Phase I: Lonafarnib + TMZ for recurrent GBM	Ongoing
RAF	Sorafenib	Phase I/II: Sorafenib + TMZ + XRT for newly diagnosed GBM	Ongoing
		Phase II: Sorafenib + TMZ following TMZ + XRT for newly diagnosed GBM	Ongoing
		Phase II: Sorafenib + protracted TMZ in recurrent GBM	Ongoing
		Phase II: Sorafenib + erlotinib for recurrent GBM	Ongoing
		Phase I/II: Sorafenib + erlotinib, tipifarnib, or temsirolimus for recurrent GBM	Ongoing
		Phase I/II: Sorafenib + temsirolimus for recurrent GBM	Ongoing
		Phase II: Sorafenib + bevacizumab for recurrent GBM	Ongoing
AKT	Perifosine	Phase II: Perifosine for recurrent MG	Suspended
mTOR	Sirolimus	Phase I: Sirolimus + vandetanib for recurrent GBM	Ongoing
		Phase II: Sirolimus + erlotinib for recurrent GBM	Ongoing
	Temsirolimus	Phase II: Temsirolimus for recurrent GBM	PFS6 7.8% (Galanis et al 2005)
		Phase I/II: Temsirolimus for recurrent GBM	PFS6 2.5% (Chang et al 2005)
		Phase I: Temsirolimus + TMZ + XRT for newly diagnosed GBM	Ongoing
		Phase II: Temsirolimus + bevacizumab in recurrent GBM	Ongoing
		Phase I/II: Temsirolimus + erlotinib for recurrent GBM	Ongoing
		Phase I/II: Sorafenib + temsirolimus for recurrent GBM	Ongoing
	Everolimus	Phase II: Everolimus for recurrent MG	Ongoing
		Phase I: Everolimus + TMZ for GBM	Ongoing
		Phase I: Everolimus + imatinib + hydroxyurea for recurrent GBM	Ongoing
		Phase I/II: Everolimus + AEE788 for recurrent GBM	Ongoing
		Phase I: Everolimus + gefitinib for recurrent GBM	PFS6 5% (Kreisl et al 2009)
PKC-Beta	Enzastaurin	Phase III: Enzastaurin vs lomustine for recurrent GBM	Terminated for futility (Fine et al 2008)
		Phase II: Enzastaurin + XRT for newly diagnosed GBM	Ongoing
		Phase I/II: Enzastaurin + TMZ + XRT for newly diagnosed GBM	Ongoing
		Phase II: Enzastaurin + bevacizumab for recurrent MG	Ongoing
		Phase I: Enzastaurin + carboplatin for recurrent brain tumors	Ongoing
		Phase I: Enzastaurin + TMZ for recurrent MG	Ongoing

prevents interaction between HGF and c-Met. A multicenter phase II study of AMG102 for treatment of advance malignant glioma is ongoing. Several small molecule inhibitors of c-Met receptor tyrosine kinase activity are in various stages of development and testing. XL184, which inhibits VEGFR-2 and KDR in addition to c-Met, is being evaluated as a treatment for recurrent glioblastoma in a phase II trial. Several other agents including XL880 and ARQ197 are currently being tested in tumors outside of the nervous system.

Insulin-like growth factor

The insulin-like growth factor system consists of three ligands, two receptors, and six insulin-like growth factor binding proteins (IGFBPs). Insulin-like growth factor 1 (IGF-I) and insulin-like growth factor 1 receptor (IGF-I-R) are the components of the system with the greatest relevance to brain tumor formation. The IGF-I pathway is active during fetal brain development and relatively quiescent in normal mature neural tissue, but emerges again to drive growth of malignant brain tumors (Trojan 2007). The role of IGFBPs in glioma formation is less clear; they bind with IGF-I and increase its half-life, while also competing with IGF-I-R for IGF-I binding. Elevated plasma levels of IGFBPs have been demonstrated in patients with several types of solid tumors, and elevated plasma IGFBP-2 has been shown to correlate with increased tumor recurrence and decreased disease-free survival in patients with glioblastoma multiforme (Lin et al 2009). As with previously discussed growth factor systems, both the PI3K-Akt-mTOR and RAS-RAF-MEK-MAPK pathways are involved in IGF-I-R pathway signal transduction (Trojan 2007).

No selective inhibitors of the IGF pathway have yet been evaluated in clinical trials for treatment of central nervous system tumors. SCH 717454, a fully human antibody directed against the IGF-1-R is currently being examined in phase II studies for the treatment of colorectal cancer and osteosarcoma or Ewing's sarcoma. Multiple IGF-I-R tyrosine kinase inhibitor small molecules are in development. Agents such as BMS-754807 and OSI-906 are being evaluated in phase I trials of non-CNS malignancies, and still more options are in pre-clinical testing.

Table 6.4 Selected trials of agents targeting multiple signaling pathways

Target	Agent	Clinical trials	Results
PDGFR, c-kit, Abl	Imatinib	Phase I/II: Imatinib for recurrent glioma	GBM PFS6 3% AA PFS6 10% (Wen et al 2006)
		Phase II: Imatinib for recurrent glioma	GBM PFS6 16% AA PFS6 9% (Raymond et al 2008)
		Phase III: Hydroxyurea ± imatinib for recurrent GBM	Completed
		Phase II/III: Imatinib + hydroxyurea for recurrent GBM	Completed
		Phase II: Imatinib + everolimus + hydroxyurea for recurrent MG	Ongoing
		Phase I: Imatinib + hydroxyurea + vatalanib for recurrent MG	Ongoing
		Phase I: Imatinib + TMZ for MG	Ongoing
EGFR, VEGFR	AEE788	Phase I/II: AEE788 for recurrent GBM	Completed
		Phase I/II: AEE788 + everolimus for recurrent GBM	Ongoing
	Vandetanib	Phase I: Vandetanib + sirolimus for recurrent GBM	Ongoing
		Phase I/II: Vandetanib + TMZ/XRT for newly diagnosed GBM	Ongoing
		Phase I: Vandetanib + etoposide for recurrent MG	Ongoing
		Phase I: Vandetanib + Imatinib + hydroxyurea for recurrent MG	Ongoing
		Phase I/II: Vandetanib for recurrent MG	Ongoing
EGFR, HER2	Lapatinib	Phase I/II: Lapatinib for recurrent GBM	Ongoing
		Phase II: Lapatinib + pazopanib for recurrent MG	Ongoing
PDGFR, VEGFR, c-kit, Flt-3	Sunitinib	Phase II: Sunitinib for recurrent GBM	Ongoing
		Phase I: Sunitinib + irinotecan for recurrent MG	Ongoing
Flt-3, PDGFR, c-kit	Tandutinib	Phase II: Tandutinib + bevacizumab for recurrent MG	Ongoing
		Phase I/II: Tandutinib for recurrent MG	Ongoing
Raf, VEGFR, PDGFR, c-kit, Flt-3	Sorafenib	Phase I/II: Sorafenib + TMZ/XRT for newly diagnosed GBM	Ongoing
		Phase II: Sorafenib + TMZ following TMZ/XRT for newly diagnosed GBM	Ongoing
		Phase II: Sorafenib + protracted TMZ in recurrent GBM	Ongoing
		Phase II: Sorafenib + erlotinib for recurrent GBM	Ongoing
		Phase I/II: Sorafenib + erlotinib, tipifarnib, or temsirolimus for recurrent GBM	Ongoing
		Phase I/II: Sorafenib + temsirolimus for recurrent GBM	Ongoing
		Phase II: Sorafenib + bevacizumab for recurrent GBM	Ongoing
VEGFR, c-Met, RET	XL184	Phase II: XL84 for recurrent GBM	Ongoing
VEGFR, PDGFR	Vatalanib	Phase I: Vatalanib + Imatinib + Hydroxyurea for recurrent malignant glioma	Ongoing
		Phase I/II: XRT + TMZ ± vatalanib for newly diagnosed GBM	Ongoing
VEGFR, PDGFR, c-kit	Pazopanib	Phase I: Vatalanib + TMZ + XRT for newly diagnosed GBM in patients taking EIAEDs	Ongoing
		Phase II: Pazopanib for recurrent GBM	Ongoing
Src family, many others	Dasatinib	Phase I: Dasatinib + erlotinib for recurrent MG	Ongoing
		Phase II: Dasatinib for recurrent GBM	Ongoing

PI3K-Akt-mTOR second messenger system

The phosphoinositide-3-kinase (PI3K) second messenger cascade is a downstream mediator of several growth factor receptors such as EGF. Through activation of this system, EGF is able to inhibit apoptosis and promote cellular survival. PI3K converts phosphatidylinositol (3,4)-bisphosphate (PIP2) into phosphatidylinositol (3,4,5)-trisphosphate (PIP3), leading to the translocation of Akt (also known as protein kinase B) to the cellular surface where it is activated. Once activated by phosphorylation, Akt both increases transcription of pro-survival genes and inactivates pro-apoptotic proteins. Akt has several targets, including mammalian target of rapamycin (mTOR). Akt activation also increases vascular endothelial growth factor (VEGF) production, thereby serving as a link between these two important systems (Jiang & Liu 2008). The major negative regulator of the PI3K-Akt-mTOR pathway is PTEN (phosphatase and tensin homolog), which converts PIP3 to PIP2, thereby deactivating Akt. Overactivation of the PI3K-Akt-mTOR pathway in glioblastoma occurs in two primary ways: by excessive EGFR input and through decreased PTEN inhibitory feedback. The previously mentioned EGFR-vIII mutation of EGFR preferentially activates the PI3K-Akt-mTOR pathway (McLendon et al 2007). The PTEN gene, located on chromosome 10q, is a commonly mutated tumor suppressor gene in a variety of cancers. In glioblastoma, loss of heterozygosity at 10q is found in approximately 70% of tumors, and PTEN mutations are seen in 25% of tumors (Ohgaki & Kleihues 2007). PTEN mutations are far more common in primary glioblastomas than in secondary glioblastomas. In low-grade gliomas and secondary glioblastomas, PTEN promoter methylation is more often seen, representing an alternative pathway to PTEN inactivation (Wiencke et al 2007). Loss of PTEN function is associated with an aggressive tumor phenotype due to unopposed stimulation of Akt activation.

The best studied therapeutic target within the PI3K-Akt-mTOR pathway is mTOR. Temsirolimus (Torisel) and everolimus (Certican) are analogs of sirolimus (Rapamycin) with more favorable pharmacokinetic properties. Phase II trials of temsirolimus in patients with recurrent glioblastoma showed minimal efficacy as a monotherapy in unselected patients, but little treatment-related toxicity (Galanis et al 2005). Follow-up studies to examine temsirolimus in combination with other agents or as a monotherapy in pathologically defined subsets of glioblastoma are ongoing. Akt itself is the target of the small molecule inhibitor perifosine (Momota et al 2005), which is currently being evaluated in a phase II trial as a therapy for recurrent malignant glioma.

Ras-Raf-MEK-MAPK second messenger system

Ras is a signal transduction protein that lies downstream of EGFR and PDGFR. Ras is activated by farnesylation, also known as prenylation, a process in which an isoprenoid is attached to the C-terminal cysteine residue by the enzyme farnesyltransferase. Ras activates a number of signaling cascades, but its action on the mitogen-activated protein (MAP) kinases is especially important for tumor formation. The MAP kinases are a family of serine/threonine-specific protein kinases that regulate a number of processes key to tumor propagation and survival including mitosis, differentiation, apoptosis, and release of angiogenic growth factors. While mutations in the Ras-Raf-MEK-MAPK pathway itself are rare in glioblastoma (Knobbe et al 2004), pathway activity is frequently increased due to previously discussed mutation and over-expression of upstream receptor kinases.

The activation of Ras by farnesylation presents an opportunity for intervention to inhibit the Ras-Raf-MEK-MAPK pathway before it branches to exert its diverse downstream effects. Farnesyltransferase inhibitors (FTIs) are small molecule inhibitors of enzyme action that indirectly inhibit Ras. Tipifarnib (Zarnestra, previously known as R115777) and lonafarnib (Sarsa, previously known as SCH66336) have been evaluated in humans with recurrent glioblastoma multiforme or anaplastic glioma. In phase II trials in patients with recurrent high-grade glioma tipifarnib demonstrate modest activity but was well tolerated (Cloughesy et al 2006). Ongoing trials are examining FTIs in combination with radiation therapy, temozolomide, and other molecularly targeted therapies. While the FTIs represent approach to Ras-Raf-MEK-MAPK pathway modification that is farthest along in development, other classes of compounds are being investigated. Raf is one of several targets of the small molecule sorafenib (Hahn & Stadler 2006), and several clinical trials of sorafenib for malignant glioma are underway. AAL881 is a small molecule inhibitor of Raf and VEGFR that extended survival in mice with glioblastoma xenografts (Sathornsumetee et al 2006).

Angiogenesis pathway inhibitors

The pivotal role of angiogenesis in tumor survival and growth, and the logical consequence that inhibition of angiogenesis may be useful in anticancer therapy, has been recognized since the early 1970s (Folkman 1971). Since that time, a number of angiogenesis pathways have been identified, but it was not until 2004 that bevacizumab (Avastin) became the first targeted anti-angiogenesis therapy to be approved by the Food and Drug Administration (FDA) for the treatment of solid tumors.

Vascular endothelial growth factor

Tumors utilize many different pro-angiogenic factors and pathways to produce their blood supply. The prototypical example, and the pathway that has been the target of the most therapeutic manipulation to date, is the vascular endothelial growth factor (VEGF) system. The VEGF family includes a number of growth factors and receptors. The term VEGF is commonly used to refer to VEGF-A, but VEGF-B, VEGF-C, VEGF-D, VEGF-E, VEGF-F, and placental growth factor (PlGF) also act upon VEGF receptors. Likewise, the term vascular endothelial growth factor receptor (VEGFR) is commonly applied to VEGFR-2, the primary receptor of the VEGF pathway, while VEGFR-1 and VEGFR-3 play less direct roles in neoangiogenesis and tumor growth (Kerbel 2008). Most human solid tumors, including primary brain tumors, express VEGF at elevated levels. VEGF expression is triggered by a number of factors, notably hypoxia and acidosis. In high-grade tumors, the hypoxia that results when the tumor outgrows its blood supply stabilizes hypoxia-inducible transcription factors 1α and 2α, which then lead to increased VEGF gene transcription and improved stability of the VEGF ligand (Semenza 2003). After tumor cells create VEGF, it then acts on endothelial cells to trigger increased vessel formation. When the VEGFR-2 of a vascular endothelial cell is triggered by VEGF-A, it triggers a variety of downstream effects. First, VEGFR-2, a transmembrane tyrosine kinase, dimerizes. It can then begin to activate the PLCγ-PKC-Raf kinase-MEK-MAPK pathway, which leads to cellular proliferation. Additionally, activated VEGFR-2 triggers the phosphatidylinositol 3 kinase (PI3K)-Akt pathway which facilitates cellular survival (Kerbel 2008). VEGF is also a trigger of vascular endothelial cellular migration, allowing the growth of vascular networks (Jain et al 2007a). Blood vessels produced by aberrant VEGF signaling have increased leakiness, leading to elevated interstitial fluid pressure within tumors and the formation of peritumoral edema (Jain et al 2007b).

The first anti-angiogenesis agent shown to have efficacy against malignant glioma was bevacizumab (Avastin), a monoclonal antibody against vascular endothelial growth factor. Prior to its use in glioma, bevacizumab had been demonstrated to improve outcome in non-CNS malignancies, such as colon cancer, when given in combination with cytotoxic chemotherapy (Hurwitz et al 2004). Bevacizumab-induced VEGF blockade is postulated to lead to improved chemotherapy response by allowing normalization of blood vessels, increasing their ability to deliver anti-cancer therapies. Given this background, initial trials of bevacizumab in glioma patients combined the therapy with irinotecan, a conventional chemotherapeutic agent. In a phase II trial, the combination of bevacizumab and irinotecan led to increased 6-month progression-free survival (PFS6) relative to historical controls (Vredenburgh et al 2007). It remains unclear whether the therapeutic benefit was the result of Avastin alone, or whether the addition of irinotecan confers additive anti-tumor effect. A company-sponsored phase II trial of bevacizumab alone vs in combination with irinotecan showed a trend towards improved outcome with combination therapy but this difference was not statistically significant (Cloughesy et al 2008). In another phase II trial, patients with recurrent glioblastoma were first treated with bevacizumab monotherapy, then bevacizumab in combination with irinotecan after tumor progression. This trial showed increased PFS6 with bevacizumab, but no additional response when irinotecan was added after progression (Kreisl et al 2009). A phase III trial will be needed to more fully determine the risks and benefits of the addition of irinotecan to bevacizumab therapy. Further studies of bevacizumab are ongoing including combination therapy trials with other targeted agents such as erlotinib. While bevacizumab is the best-studied of the VEGF pathway modifiers, several other agents are currently being evaluated. Aflibercept (VEGF Trap) is a soluble receptor that binds to circulating VEFG and PlGF and has been shown to be effective against human gliomas in mouse models (Gomez-Manzano et al 2008). A clinical trial of aflibercept in patients with recurrent malignant glioma is ongoing. Small molecule therapies aimed at inhibiting the action of VEGFR include vatalanib (PTK787/ZK22584), pazopanib, cediranib (AZD2171 or Recentin), and CT-322 (Angiocept). While none of these therapies has shown unequivocal survival benefit in patients with glioma, cediranib therapy did lead to a rapid and dramatic radiographic response due to reversible vascular normalization (Batchelor et al 2007). In addition to the therapies above, which are targeted solely at the VEGF pathway, several agents currently under investigation act on VEGF as well as other targets of glioma growth. Examples include sunitinib (Sutent), vandetanib (Zactima), sorafenib (Nexavar), and axitinib (AG 013736).

Anti-VEGF therapy is generally well tolerated. In a study of 55 patients with recurrent glioblastoma treated with bevacizumab and chemotherapy, side-effects attributable to Avastin included venous thromboembolism, hypertension, gastrointestinal perforation, bleeding, and impaired wound healing (Norden et al 2008). Fatigue is also a commonly noted. Small molecule inhibitors of VEGFR, such as sorafenib and sunitinib, cause mucositis, diarrhea, hand-foot reaction and skin rash in addition to bevacizumab-like side-effects. Sunitinib has also been associated with reversible loss of hair pigmentation as a consequence of suppression of c-kit signaling (Robert et al 2005).

Placental growth factor

Placental growth factor (PlGF) is a ligand of vascular endothelial growth factor receptor 1 (VEGFR-1). Four human forms of PlGF have been described, PlGF-1 through PlGF-4. PlGF binding to VEGFR-1 induces expression of a set of proteins distinct from that seen after VEGF binding to VEGFR-1 (Fischer et al 2007). Increased PlGF expression has been noted in several conditions characterized by pathologic angiogenesis. With respect to tumor angiogenesis, PlGF expression was found to correlate with disease progression and decreased patient survival in colorectal cancer (Wei et al 2005). Normal mature tissue exhibits minimal PlGF expression, and pre-clinical animal testing of PlGF blocking agents has shown little toxicity. Aflibercept (VEGF Trap), a soluble decoy receptor with the ability to bind both VEGF and PlGF, is currently being evaluated for malignant glioma in clinical trials.

Neuropilin (NRP)

Neuropilin-1 (NRP1) and neuropilin-2 (NRP2) are transmembrane glycoproteins that serve as cell surface receptors for semaphorins and various ligands involved in angiogenesis. As class III semaphorin receptors, NRP1 and NRP2 help guide axonal growth during the development of the nervous system (Pan et al 2007). In mature organisms, neuropilins are primarily employed as proangiogenic co-receptors. NRP1 binds VEGF-A, VEGF-B, VEGF-E, PlGF, and HGF/SF while NRP2 binds VEGF-A, VEGF-C, PlGF, and HGF/SF. After binding and activation, neuropilins influence angiogenesis by stabilizing VEGF/VEGFR binding (Sulpice et al 2008). Neuropilins are also thought to exert an effect on vascular endothelial cell motility that is independent of their action on the VEGF/VEGFR complex. In pre-clinical testing, monoclonal antibodies targeted against the extracellular ligand binding domains of NRP1 reduced angiogenesis and vascular remodeling. Significantly, co-treatment with anti-VEGF and anti-NRP antibodies showed greater antiangiogenic power than either antibody alone (Pan et al 2007). To date, no specific inhibitors of neuropilin function have been evaluated in clinical trials.

Notch/delta-like ligand 4

The Notch intracellular signaling pathway regulates a variety of processes related to cell growth, differentiation, and death, by mediating gene transcription. Notch and its ligands are expressed in the vascular endothelium during blood vessel formation, and have been shown to play an essential role in normal vascular development and tumor angiogenesis (Kerbel 2008). In humans, there are four notch receptors and five ligands, the most pertinent for glioma formation being Notch1 and delta-like ligand 4 (DLL4), respectively. DLL4 is upregulated in glioblastoma tumor cells and tumor endothelial cells, and an in-vitro study of mouse xenografts has shown that Notch activation by DLL4 leads to decreased angiogenesis, but improved vessel structure and function. This, in turn, was associated with reduced apoptosis and intratumoral hypoxia, leading to growth of glioblastoma xenografts (Li et al 2007). Notch1/DLL4 signaling is functionally tied to both the VEGF and EGFR pathways. In tumors, VEGF acts through VEGFR-1 and VEGFR-2 to activate the phosphatidylinositol 3-kinase/Akt pathway and induce the expression of Notch1 and DLL4 in arterial endothelial cells (Liu et al 2003). Notch1 activity then upregulates EGFR expression, amongst many other functions (Purow et al 2008).

Preclinical data have generated optimism about the potential utility of Notch pathway therapies for treatment of cancer (Noguera-Troise et al 2006). MK0752 is a gamma secretase inhibitor, which inhibits the Notch signaling pathway by preventing the cleavage of the Notch receptor and release of the intracellular domain (Deangelo et al 2006). Several phase I trials of MK0752 in patients with different types of tumors, including recurrent or refractory CNS malignances in young patients, are ongoing. Notch1 and DLL4 may also be indirectly inhibited by VEGF Trap, which is able to block VEGF-induced expression of Notch1 and DLL4.

Protein kinase C-β

The protein kinase C family is a group of serine/threonine kinases that phosphorylate a variety of targets involved in cellular signaling. Many members of the PKC family also function as receptors for phorbol esters, a class of tumor promoters that mimic diacylglycerol. Increased PKCβ activity has been demonstrated in a variety of tumor types, including malignant glioma, and has been shown to stimulate angiogenesis through interplay with the VEGF system (Xia et al 1996). PKCβ activation in endothelial cells is one of the downstream effects of activation of VEGFR by VEGF. PKCβ has also been shown to activate the phosphoinositide 3-kinase (PI3K) second messenger cascade which, as previously discussed, plays an important role in cellular survival and regulation of apoptosis.

The potent small-molecule PKCβ inhibitor enzastaurin is the anti-PKC agent farthest along in development and testing. In preclinical evaluation, enzastaurin is able to inhibit VEGF-stimulated angiogenesis and suppress growth of human glioblastoma xenografts (Graff et al 2005). Phase I testing in non-CNS tumors demonstrated that enzastaurin was very well tolerated (Carducci et al 2006), and an initial phase II trial of enzastaurin monotherapy for recurrent glioma showed an encouraging radiographic response rate (Fine et al 2005), but a phase III trial of enzastaurin versus lomustine (CCNU) was terminated early for futility (Fine et al 2008). Clinical trials evaluating enzastaurin in combination with other therapies such as radiation, temozolomide, and bevacizumab are ongoing.

Thalidomide and analogs

Thalidomide was one of the first anti-angiogenesis agents evaluated for use in the treatment of cancer. Hepatic metabolism of thalidomide produces a metabolite that inhibits basic fibroblast growth factor (bFGF) induced angiogenesis (Bauer et al 1998). Thalidomide also inhibits tumor necrosis factor alpha (TNF-α) (Sampaio et al 1991), which has been shown to upregulate production of bFGF and VEGF. Further, thalidomide is thought to have anti-tumor properties unrelated to its anti-angiogenic actions, through means such as causing oxidative DNA damage and interfering with cell surface adhesion molecules (Adlard 2000). Clinical trials of thalidomide as monotherapy for recurrent malignant gliomas showed transient cytostatic activity, but no significant sustained response (Fine et al 2000). The more potent thalidomide analog lenalidomide has also been evaluated in patients with recurrent glioblastoma and it showed minimal antitumor efficacy (Fine et al 2007). Given the negative results of monotherapy trials in malignant glioma, ongoing trials are examining thalidomide and analogs in combination with other agents.

Integrin therapies

Integrins are transmembrane glycoproteins that interact with the extracellular matrix and serve as receptors for multiple extracellular ligands. The integrin itself is an

Table 6.5 Selected trials of agents targeting integrins

Target	Agent	Clinical trials	Results
Integrins	Cilengitide	Phase I/II: Cilengitide + TMZ + XRT, followed by cilengitide + TMZ for newly diagnosed GBM	PFS6 65% MGMT status predicts outcome (Stupp et al 2007)
		Phase II: Cilengitide for recurrent GBM	PFS6 15%, median OS 9.9m (Reardon et al 2008)
		Phase III: Cilengitide + TMZ + XRT in patients with newly diagnosed GBM and methylated MGMT	Ongoing
		Phase II: Cilengitide + TMZ + XRT in patients with newly diagnosed GBM and unmethylated MGMT	Ongoing

obligate heterodimer composed of an α and a β domain. There are a large number of integrins, each identified by its component α and β domains, but αvβ3 and αvβ5 are the forms that have been most investigated in glial tumors (Nabors et al 2007). Through ligand binding, integrins play a role in the regulation of many cellular processes including proliferation, migration, angiogenesis, and survival (Parise et al 2000). Integrin signaling has been shown to play a role in a wide variety of tumors, and integrin expression is increased in glioblastoma cells (Gingras et al 1995) and in tumor-associated vasculature (Gladson 1996) (Table 6.5).

Cilengitide (EMD 121974) is a peptide that competitively binds to integrins αvβ3 and αvβ5, disrupting normal signaling (Nabors et al 2007). In a phase II study of two different doses of cilengitide monotherapy in patients with newly diagnosed glioblastoma, the therapy was well-tolerated and anti-tumor activity was suggested by radiographic response in 9% of patients, with a trend towards prolonged progression free survival (PFS) and overall survival (OS) in the high-dose (2000 mg twice weekly) group relative to the low-dose (500 mg twice weekly) group (Reardon et al 2008). A phase I/IIa trial of cilengitide 500 mg twice weekly in combination with radiation and temozolomide showed prolonged PFS and OS in comparison with a previous cohort of patients that had been treated with radiation and temozolomide alone. Tumor MGMT status correlated with outcome; patients whose tumors did not express MGMT were more likely to reach the 6-month PFS endpoint (Stupp et al 2007). Further trials of cilengitide in combination with radiation and temozolomide with and without cilengitide are ongoing.

Tumor imaging in anti-angiogenic therapy

Assessing response to therapy in malignant gliomas treated with anti-angiogenic agents presents a unique challenge. Change in the gadolinium enhancement pattern of a malignant glioma is a widely accepted marker of treatment response or tumor progression (Macdonald et al 1990). By preventing the formation of new blood vessels and promoting normalization of existing vessels, anti-angiogenesis agents can create a disassociation between tumor growth and visible enhancement, possibly leading to overestimation of tumor response or unrecognized disease progression. In addition to changing the contrast enhancement pattern of gliomas, anti-angiogenic therapy can alleviate edema and markedly reduce the volume of T2 signal abnormality (Batchelor et al 2007). Further, anti-angiogenic therapy may change glioma growth patterns by forcing the tumor to grow along pre-existing blood vessels, where it can go unnoticed until presenting as a distant recurrence (Norden et al 2008). Given these challenges, the need for imaging methods and markers that better reflect tumor response and progression is clear. Several MRI and PET techniques have been developed which provide physiologic and metabolic information about brain tumors in addition to the standard anatomical data, but these techniques are not yet ready to supplant contrast enhanced MRI for routine clinical use (Gerstner et al 2008).

Apoptosis control pathways

Avoidance of apoptosis, a physiological process of programmed cell death, is critical for cancer development and growth. Conventional chemotherapy and radiation act largely by causing intracellular damage which leads to apoptosis through what is known as the 'intrinsic pathway'. In the intrinsic pathway, cellular damage leads to the accumulation of the p53 tumor suppressor protein which then induces transcription of several pro-apoptotic genes and inhibits expression of anti-apoptotic genes (notably BCL-2). These genes lead to the activation of caspases, or cysteine-aspartic acid proteases, a family of cysteine proteases which ultimately serve as the 'executioner' proteins of apoptosis. In addition to leading to a growth advantage by allowing avoidance of cellular growth checkpoints, p53 inactivation is also thought to confer resistance to ionizing radiation, although this idea remains controversial (Cuddihy & Bristow 2004). Tumors may avoid the intrinsic apoptosis pathway in several ways, including mutation of the TP53 gene or functional inhibition of p53 signaling by negative regulators. Inactivating mutations of p53 are common in malignant glioma, particularly in anaplastic astrocytoma, anaplastic oligodendroglioma, and secondary glioblastoma (Nozaki et al 1999). In primary glioblastoma, mutation of the p53 is less common, but functional inhibition of p53 may play a similar role. The primary negative regulator of p53 is murine double minute 2 (MDM2), called HDM2 in humans. Overexpression of MDM2 due to amplification of the MDM2 gene has been described in a variety of human cancers (Shangary & Wang 2008). MDM2 amplification is more common in primary than in secondary glioblastomas, and early data suggests that some MDM2 genotypes are associated with favorable outcome in certain patient groups (Zawlik et al 2008).

Apoptosis can also be triggered by the 'extrinsic pathway', a system that does not rely on p53 signaling. In the extrinsic pathway, a pro-apoptotic ligand triggers receptors on the cell surface, leading to the down-stream activation of caspases and subsequent apoptosis. In the best studied example of this pathway, apoptosis ligand2/tumor necrosis factor-related apoptosis-inducing ligand (Apo2L/TRAIL) binds to the receptors death receptor 4 (DR4) or death receptor 5 (DR5) triggering the apoptosis program. Apo2L/TRAIL binding to DR4 or DR5 leads to receptor oligomerization, followed by formation of the death-inducing signaling complex (DISC) which includes the protein Fas-associated death domain (FADD). It is FADD which activates the caspases in the extrinsic pathway. For reasons that are not yet clear, extrinsic pathway activation by Apo2L/TRAIL selectively leads to apoptosis in malignant cells, while sparing most other normal cells (Ashkenazi et al 2008).

The apoptosis pathway program has been exploited in several ways for the treatment of malignant glioma. With regard to the intrinsic pathway, ABT-737, a small molecule inhibitor of BCL-2, has been shown to increase survival in intracranial xenograft models of glioblastoma (Tagscherer et al 2008). Recently, several small-molecule inhibitors of MDM2 have shown anti-tumor activity in pre-clinical testing, and clinical trials of MDM2 inhibitors for systemic malignancies are expected in the near future. Approaches to the extrinsic pathway have included intravenous rhApo2L/TRAIL therapy, monoclonal antibodies directed against the death receptors, TRAIL-expressing stem cell transplants, and gene therapy. Currently, trials of intravenous rhApo2L/TRAIL and anti-DR antibodies are ongoing for a variety of systemic malignancies, and trials of these therapies for glioma are likely to occur soon (Ashkenazi et al 2008).

Future direction of targeted therapies

A wide variety of monoclonal antibodies and small molecule inhibitors have been evaluated in the ongoing search for a therapy capable of significantly extending the lifespan of patients with malignant glioma. To date, these molecularly targeted therapies have yielded disappointing results in clinical trials, leading to a re-examination of many aspects of drug development and clinical trial design. The North American Brain Tumor Consortium (NABTC), a large multi-institutional consortium with a focus on evaluating novel brain tumor therapies through clinical trials, recently reviewed these issues and proposed new clinical trial paradigms to guide future research (Chang et al 2008).

A major issue identified by the NABTC is insufficient data from early studies regarding dose selection, drug penetration into the CNS, and extent of biological activity within the CNS. With traditional chemotherapy, aimed at causing apoptosis of neoplastic cells via cellular damage, the optimum dose is thought to be the maximum tolerated dose (MTD) that the patient can tolerate without significant side-effects. This is not necessarily the case when targeting signaling pathways; the optimum biological dose (OBD) may be less than the MTD, or conversely the MTD may be too low to show significant biological activity. Further, direct testing of drug concentrations within fresh glial tumor tissue is rarely performed; data about drug penetration into brain tissue come from indirect methods. In the future, early stage clinical trials may include an arm in which the agent in question is given preoperatively to small groups of patients undergoing resection of their brain tumors for therapeutic reasons. The resected tissue could then be used to directly assess drug distribution and pharmacokinetics, including quantifying the level of inhibition of the pathway being studied.

Another barrier to the evaluation of novel agents is limited ability to identify subsets of patients that benefit from therapy. In future trials, a much greater emphasis will be placed on prospective analysis of tumor markers and signaling pathway activity in pre-treatment tumor tissue samples. Ideally, tumor tissue from the diagnostic biopsy, as well as tissue from each subsequent resection, would be banked in culture and/or used in xenografts to provide a self-renewing reference sample. When the patient is later enrolled in a clinical trial of a novel therapeutic agent, the tissue sample can be analyzed and its molecular profile correlated with individual response to therapy. Further, once a tentative correlation between a molecular marker and response to therapy is made, the tissue bank can be reviewed to construct an enriched population for a follow-up phase II efficacy study.

Finally, the disappointing results of recent targeted therapy trials have called into question the treatment paradigm of modulating a single target within highly complex and redundant system. While this was the logical way to begin, future work is likely to focus more on pairing targeted therapies with traditional treatments such as radiation and chemotherapy, and simultaneously targeting multiple signaling targets. As previously discussed, there is reason to think that angiogenesis inhibitors may increase the efficacy of traditional chemotherapy, and modification of p53 or EGFR signaling may sensitize tumors to radiation. The judicious addition of these therapies, at the right time and in the right dose, to the standard-of-care radiation and temozolomide regimen may have a much more powerful therapeutic effect than use of the targeted therapies alone. In addition to evaluating targeted therapies in combination with traditional therapies, the simultaneous use of multiple targeted therapies, or the use of single therapies with multiple targets, is likely to improve results. Given the multiple parallel, diverging, and converging signaling pathways exploited by gliomas, it is little surprise that response to single targeted therapies is typically transitory. Given the number of targeted agents currently available and in development, the possibilities for designing rational combinations of therapies are practically endless. It is possible to target multiple targets within a single pathway, for example by combining the VEGF antibody bevacizumab with the VEGF receptor tyrosine kinase cediranib. Alternatively, two parallel pathways that promote the same process, such as VEGF and PlGF in angiogenesis, could be targeted simultaneously. If upregulation of one pathway leads the ability to overcome modification of the other when the agents are used as monotherapies, this approach may lead to more durable responses. Finally, less directly related processes can be chosen, for example by combining a VEGF inhibitor with an EGFR inhibitor. While the number of possible combinations is daunting, and toxicity issues pose a challenge, work in this area is underway. While the examples above imply the use of multiple different therapies, the same principle holds true when considering single therapies with multiple targets. Small molecule receptor tyrosine kinases, by virtue on their action on the highly conserved kinase ATP binding site, often have the ability to modulate several kinase pathways simultaneously. One example is sunitinib (Sutent), which acts on VEGFR, PDGFR, and c-kit.

Conclusion

Despite the limited success of the first wave of targeted therapy, there is ample reason to be optimistic about the prospect of truly effective therapy for malignant gliomas in the future. Specific inhibitors have been developed for only a small portion of the currently recognized potential targets, and additional targets are constantly being identified. Further, the interdependence of the various tumor growth and angiogenesis signaling pathways suggests that rational combinations of therapeutic agents may have effects greater than the sum of their parts. Many ongoing trials are examining simultaneous treatment with multiple targeted agents, targeted agents and cytotoxic chemotherapy, and newer agents with inhibitory effects on multiple glioma pathways. Finally, the pathological heterogeneity of glioblastoma may mask efficacy of targeted therapy in selected subsets of patients. Large multicenter databases correlating pathological tumor characteristics and information about response to novel therapeutics combined with more routine evaluation of somatic mutations and gene expression patterns within individual tumors will lead to a truly personalized approach to therapy choice.

REFERENCES

Abounader, R., Laterra, J., 2005. Scatter factor/hepatocyte growth factor in brain tumor growth and angiogenesis. Neuro. Oncol. 7 (4), 436–451.

Adlard, J.W., 2000. Thalidomide in the treatment of cancer. Anticancer Drugs 11 (10), 787–791.

Ashkenazi, A., Holland, P., Eckhardt, S.G., 2008. Ligand-based targeting of apoptosis in cancer: The potential of recombinant human apoptosis ligand 2/Tumor necrosis factor-related apoptosis-inducing ligand (rhApo2L/TRAIL). J. Clin. Oncol. 26 (21), 3621–3630.

Batchelor, T.T., Sorensen, A.G., di Tomaso E., et al., 2007. AZD2171, a pan-VEGF receptor tyrosine kinase inhibitor, normalizes tumor vasculature and alleviates edema in glioblastoma patients. Cancer Cell 11 (1), 83–95.

Bauer, K.S., Dixon, S.C., Figg, W.D., 1998. Inhibition of angiogenesis by thalidomide requires metabolic activation, which is species-dependent. Biochem. Pharmacol. 55 (11), 1827–1834.

Brandes, A.A., Franceschi, E., Tosoni, A., et al., 2008. Epidermal growth factor receptor inhibitors in neuro-oncology: Hopes and disappointments. Clin. Cancer Res. 14 (4), 957–960.

Brown, P.D., Krishnan, S., Sarkaria, J.N., et al., North Central Cancer Treatment Group Study N0177, 2008. Phase I/II trial of erlotinib and temozolomide with radiation therapy in the treatment of newly diagnosed glioblastoma multiforme: North central cancer treatment group study N0177. J. Clin. Oncol. 26 (34), 5603–5609.

Carducci, M.A., Musib, L., Kies, M.S., et al., 2006. Phase I dose escalation and pharmacokinetic study of enzastaurin, an oral protein kinase C beta inhibitor, in patients with advanced cancer. J. Clin. Oncol. 24 (25), 4092–4099.

Chang, S.M., Lamborn, K.R., Kuhn, J.G., et al., North American Brain Tumor Consortium, 2008. Neurooncology clinical trial design for targeted therapies: Lessons learned from the North American Brain Tumor Consortium. Neuro. Oncol. 10 (4), 631–642.

Chang, S.M., Wen, P., Cloughesy, T., et al., 2005. North American Brain Tumor Consortium and the National Cancer Institute 2005 Phase II study of CCI-779 in patients with recurrent glioblastoma multiforme. Invest. New Drugs 23 (4), 357–361.

Cloughesy, T.F., Prados, M.D., Wen, P.Y., et al., 2008. A phase II, randomized, non-comparative clinical trial of the effect of bevacizumab (BV) alone or in combination with irinotecan (CPT) on 6-month progression free survival (PFS6) in recurrent, treatment-refractory glioblastoma (GBM) [abstract]. J. Clin. Oncol. 26 (Suppl), Abstract 2010b.

Cloughesy, T.F., Wen, P.Y., Robins, H.I., et al., 2006. Phase II trial of tipifarnib in patients with recurrent malignant glioma either receiving or not receiving enzyme-inducing antiepileptic drugs: A North American Brain Tumor Consortium Study. J. Clin. Oncol. 24 (22), 3651–3656.

Cohen, S., 1983. The epidermal growth factor (EGF). Cancer 51 (10), 1787–1791.

Cuddihy, A.R., Bristow, R.G., 2004. The p53 protein family and radiation sensitivity: Yes or no? Cancer Metastasis Rev. 23 (3–4), 237–257.

Deangelo, D.J., Stone, R.M., Silverman, L.B., et al., 2006. A phase I clinical trial of the notch inhibitor MK-0752 in patients with T-cell acute lymphoblastic leukemia/lymphoma (T-ALL) and other leukemias [abstract]. J. Clin. Oncol. 24 (Suppl), Abstract 6585.

Druker, B.J., 2004. Imatinib as a paradigm of targeted therapies. Adv. Cancer Res. 91, 1–30.

Ekstrand, A.J., James, C.D., Cavenee, W.K., et al., 1991. Genes for epidermal growth factor receptor, transforming growth factor alpha, and epidermal growth factor and their expression in human gliomas in vivo. Cancer Res. 51 (8), 2164–2172.

Eller, J.L., Longo, S.L., Hicklin, D.J., et al., 2002. Activity of anti-epidermal growth factor receptor monoclonal antibody C225 against glioblastoma multiforme. Neurosurgery 51 (4), 1005–1014.

Fine, H.A., Figg, W.D., Jaeckle, K., et al., 2000. Phase II trial of the antiangiogenic agent thalidomide in patients with recurrent high-grade gliomas. J. Clin. Oncol. 18 (4), 708–715.

Fine, H.A., Kim, L., Albert, P.S., et al., 2007. A phase I trial of lenalidomide in patients with recurrent primary central nervous system tumors. Clin. Cancer Res. 13 (23), 7101–7106.

Fine, H.A., Kim, L., Royce, C., et al., 2005. Results from phase II trial of enzastaurin (LY317615) in patients with recurrent high grade gliomas [abstract]. J. Clin. Oncol. 23 (Suppl), Abstract 1504.

Fine, H.A., Puduvalli, V.K., Chamberlain, M.C., et al., 2008. Enzastaurin (ENZ) versus lomustine (CCNU) in the treatment of recurrent, intracranial glioblastoma multiforme (GBM): A phase III study [abstract]. J. Clin. Oncol. 26 (Suppl), Abstract 2005.

Fischer, C., Jonckx, B., Mazzone, M., et al., 2007. Anti-PlGF inhibits growth of VEGF(R)-inhibitor-resistant tumors without affecting healthy vessels. Cell 131 (3), 463–475.

Folkman, J., 1971. Tumor angiogenesis: Therapeutic implications. N. Engl. J. Med. 285 (21), 1182–1186.

Fortin, D., Desjardins, A., Benko, A., et al., 2005. Enhanced chemotherapy delivery by intraarterial infusion and blood–brain barrier disruption in malignant brain tumors: The Sherbrooke experience. Cancer 103 (12), 2606–2615.

Galanis, E., Buckner, J.C., Maurer, M.J., et al., North Central Cancer Treatment Group, 2005. Phase II trial of temsirolimus (CCI-779) in recurrent glioblastoma multiforme: A North Central Cancer Treatment Group Study. J. Clin. Oncol. 23 (23), 5294–5304.

Gerstner, E.R., Sorensen, A.G., Jain, R.K., et al., 2008. Advances in neuroimaging techniques for the evaluation of tumor growth, vascular permeability, and angiogenesis in gliomas. Curr. Opin. Neurol. 21 (6), 728–735.

Gingras, M.C., Roussel, E., Bruner, J.M., et al., 1995. Comparison of cell adhesion molecule expression between glioblastoma multiforme and autologous normal brain tissue. J. Neuroimmunol. 57 (1–2), 143–153.

Gladson, C.L., 1996. Expression of integrin alpha v beta 3 in small blood vessels of glioblastoma tumors. J. Neuropathol. Exp. Neurol. 55 (11), 1143–1149.

Gomez-Manzano, C., Holash, J., Fueyo, J., et al., 2008. VEGF trap induces antiglioma effect at different stages of disease. Neuro. Oncol. 10 (6), 940–945.

Graff, J.R., McNulty, A.M., Hanna, K.R., et al., 2005. The protein kinase Cbeta-selective inhibitor, Enzastaurin (LY317615.HCl), suppresses signaling through the AKT pathway, induces apoptosis, and suppresses growth of human colon cancer and glioblastoma xenografts. Cancer Res. 65 (16), 7462–7469.

Hahn, O., Stadler, W., 2006. Sorafenib. Curr. Opin. Oncol. 18 (6), 615–621.

Hurwitz, H., Fehrenbacher, L., Novotny, W., et al., 2004. Bevacizumab plus irinotecan, fluorouracil, and leucovorin for metastatic colorectal cancer. N. Engl. J. Med. 350 (23), 2335–2342.

Jain, R.K., di Tomaso, E., Duda, D.G., et al., 2007a. Angiogenesis in brain tumours. Nat. Rev. Neurosci. 8 (8), 610–622.

Jain, R.K., Tong, R.T., Munn, L.L., 2007b. Effect of vascular normalization by antiangiogenic therapy on interstitial hypertension, peritumor edema, and lymphatic metastasis: Insights from a mathematical model. Cancer Res. 67 (6), 2729–2735.

Jiang, B.H., Liu, L.Z., 2008. AKT signaling in regulating angiogenesis. Curr. Cancer Drug Targets 8 (1), 19–26.

Kerbel, R.S., 2008. Tumor angiogenesis. N. Engl. J. Med. 358 (19), 2039–2049.

Knobbe, C.B., Reifenberger, J., Reifenberger, G., 2004. Mutation analysis of the ras pathway genes NRAS, HRAS, KRAS and BRAF in glioblastomas. Acta. Neuropathol. 108 (6), 467–470.

Kreisl, T.N., Kim, L., Moore, K., et al., 2009. Phase II trial of single-agent bevacizumab followed by bevacizumab plus irinotecan at tumor progression in recurrent glioblastoma. J. Clin. Oncol. 27 (5), 740–745.

Lassen, U., Hasselbalch, B., Sørensen, M., et al., 2008. A phase II trial with cetuximab, bevacizumab, and irinotecan for patients with primary glioblastomas and progression after radiation therapy and temozolomide [abstract]. J. Clin. Oncol. 26 (Suppl), Abstract 2056.

Li, J.L., Sainson, R.C., Shi, W., et al., 2007. Delta-like 4 notch ligand regulates tumor angiogenesis, improves tumor vascular function, and promotes tumor growth in vivo. Cancer Res. 67 (23), 11244–11253.

Lidar, Z., Mardor, Y., Jonas, T., et al., 2004. Convection-enhanced delivery of paclitaxel for the treatment of recurrent malignant glioma: A phase I/II clinical study. J. Neurosurg. 100 (3), 472–479.

Lin, Y., Jiang, T., Zhou, K., et al., 2009. Plasma IGFBP-2 levels predict clinical outcomes of patients with high-grade gliomas. Neuro. Oncol. 11 (5), 468–476.

Liu, Z.J., Shirakawa, T., Li, Y., et al., 2003. Regulation of Notch1 and Dll4 by vascular endothelial growth factor in arterial endothelial cells: Implications for modulating arteriogenesis and angiogenesis. Mol. Cell Biol. 23 (1), 14–25.

Macdonald, D.R., Cascino, T.L., Schold, S.C., et al., 1990. Response criteria for phase II studies of supratentorial malignant glioma. J. Clin. Oncol. 8 (7), 1277–1280.

McLendon, R.E., Turner, K., Perkinson, K., et al., 2007. Second messenger systems in human gliomas. Arch. Pathol. Lab. Med. 131 (10), 1585–1590.

Mellinghoff, I.K., Wang, M.Y., Vivanco, I., et al., 2005. Molecular determinants of the response of glioblastomas to EGFR kinase inhibitors. N. Engl. J. Med. 353 (19), 2012–2024.

Migliore, C., Giordano, S., 2008. Molecular cancer therapy: Can our expectation be MET? Eur. J. Cancer 44 (5), 641–651.

Momota, H., Nerio, E., Holland, E.C., 2005. Perifosine inhibits multiple signaling pathways in glial progenitors and cooperates with temozolomide to arrest cell proliferation in gliomas in vivo. Cancer Res. 65 (16), 7429–7435.

Nabors, L.B., Mikkelsen, T., Rosenfeld, S.S., et al., 2007. Phase I and correlative biology study of cilengitide in patients with recurrent malignant glioma. J. Clin. Oncol. 25 (13), 1651–1657.

Noguera-Troise, I., Daly, C., Papadopoulos, N.J., et al., 2006. Blockade of Dll4 inhibits tumour growth by promoting non-productive angiogenesis. Nature 444 (7122), 1032–1037.

Norden, A.D., Young, G.S., Setayesh, K., et al., 2008. Bevacizumab for recurrent malignant gliomas: Efficacy, toxicity, and patterns of recurrence. Neurology 70 (10), 779–787.

Nozaki, M., Tada, M., Kobayashi, H., et al., 1999. Roles of the functional loss of p53 and other genes in astrocytoma tumorigenesis and progression. Neuro. Oncol. 1 (2), 124–137.

Ohgaki, H., Kleihues, P., 2007. Genetic pathways to primary and secondary glioblastoma. Am. J. Pathol. 170 (5), 1445–1453.

Pan, Q., Chanthery, Y., Liang, W.C., et al., 2007. Blocking neuropilin-1 function has an additive effect with anti-VEGF to inhibit tumor growth. Cancer Cell 11 (1), 53–67.

Parise, L.V., Lee, J., Juliano, R.L., 2000. New aspects of integrin signaling in cancer. Semin Cancer Biol. 10 (6), 407–414.

Pelloski, C.E., Ballman, K.V., Furth, A.F., et al., 2007. Epidermal growth factor receptor variant III status defines clinically distinct subtypes of glioblastoma. J. Clin. Oncol. 25 (16), 2288–2294.

Perez-Soler, R., 2003. Can rash associated with HER1/EGFR inhibition be used as a marker of treatment outcome? Oncology (Williston Park) 17 (Suppl), 23–28.

Prados, M.D., Chang, S.M., Butowski, N., et al., 2009. Phase II study of erlotinib plus temozolomide during and after radiation therapy in patients with newly diagnosed glioblastoma multiforme or gliosarcoma. J. Clin. Oncol. 27 (4), 579–584.

Prados, M.D., Lamborn, K.R., Chang, S., et al., 2006. Phase 1 study of erlotinib HCl alone and combined with temozolomide in patients with stable or recurrent malignant glioma. Neuro. Oncol. 8 (1), 67–78.

Purow, B.W., Sundaresan, T.K., Burdick, M.J., et al., 2008. Notch-1 regulates transcription of the epidermal growth factor receptor through p53. Carcinogenesis 29 (5), 918–925.

Raizer, J.J., Abrey, L.E., Wen, P., et al., 2004 A phase II trial of erlotinib (OSI-774) in patients (pts) with recurrent malignant gliomas (MG) not on EIAEDs [abstract]. J. Clin. Oncol. 22 (Suppl), Abstract 1502.

Raymond, E., Brandes, A.A., Dittrich, C., et al., 2008. European Organisation for Research and Treatment of Cancer Brain Tumor Group Study 2008 Phase II study of imatinib in patients with recurrent gliomas of various histologies: A European Organisation for Research and Treatment of Cancer Brain Tumor Group Study. J. Clin. Oncol. 26 (28), 4659–4665.

Reardon, D.A., Akabani, G., Coleman, R.E., et al., 2002. Phase II trial of murine (131)I-labeled antitenascin monoclonal antibody 81C6 administered into surgically created resection cavities of patients with newly diagnosed malignant gliomas. J. Clin. Oncol. 20 (5), 1389–1397.

Reardon, D.A., Egorin, M.J., Quinn, J.A., et al., 2005. Phase II study of imatinib mesylate plus hydroxyurea in adults with recurrent glioblastoma multiforme. J. Clin. Oncol. 23 (36), 9359–9368.

Reardon, D.A., Fink, K.L., Mikkelsen, T., et al., 2008. Randomized phase II study of cilengitide, an integrin-targeting arginine-glycine-aspartic acid peptide, in recurrent glioblastoma multiforme. J. Clin. Oncol. 26 (34), 5610–5617.

Reznik, T.E., Sang, Y., Ma, Y., et al., 2008. Transcription-dependent epidermal growth factor receptor activation by hepatocyte growth factor. Mol. Cancer Res. 6 (1), 139–150.

Rich J.N., Reardon D.A., Peery T., et al., 2004. Phase II trial of gefitinib in recurrent glioblastoma. J. Clin. Oncol. 22 (1), 133–142.

Robert, C., Soria, J.C., Spatz, A., et al., 2005. Cutaneous side-effects of kinase inhibitors and blocking antibodies. Lancet Oncol. 6 (7), 491–500.

Sampaio, E.P., Sarno, E.N., Galilly, R., et al., 1991. Thalidomide selectively inhibits tumor necrosis factor alpha production by stimulated human monocytes. J. Exp. Med. 173 (3), 699–703.

Sathornsumetee, S., Hjelmeland, A.B., Keir, S.T., et al., 2006 AAL881, a novel small molecule inhibitor of RAF and vascular endothelial growth factor receptor activities, blocks the growth of malignant glioma. Cancer Res. 66 (17), 8722–8730.

Scaltriti, M., Baselga, J., 2006. The epidermal growth factor receptor pathway: A model for targeted therapy. Clin. Cancer Res. 12 (18), 5268–5272.

Semenza, G.L., 2003. Targeting, HIF-1 for cancer therapy. Nat. Rev. Cancer 3 (10), 721–732.

Shangary, S., Wang, S., 2008. Targeting the MDM2-p53 interaction for cancer therapy. Clin. Cancer Res. 14 (17), 5318–5324.

Stupp, R., Goldbrunner, R., Neyns, B., et al., 2007. Phase I/IIa trial of cilengitide (EMD121974) and temozolomide with concomitant radiotherapy, followed by temozolomide and cilengitide maintenance therapy in patients (pts) with newly diagnosed glioblastoma (GBM) [abstract]. J. Clin. Oncol. 25 (Suppl), Abstract 2000.

Stupp, R., Mason, W.P., van den Bent, M.J., et al., 2005. European Organisation for Research and Treatment of Cancer Brain Tumor and Radiotherapy Groups, National Cancer Institute of Canada Clinical Trials Group 2005 Radiotherapy plus concomitant and adjuvant temozolomide for glioblastoma. N. Engl. J. Med. 352 (10), 987–996.

Sulpice, E., Plouet, J., Berge, M., et al., 2008. Neuropilin-1 and neuropilin-2 act as coreceptors, potentiating proangiogenic activity. Blood 111 (4), 2036–2045.

Tagscherer, K.E., Fassl, A., Campos, B., et al., 2008. Apoptosis-based treatment of glioblastomas with ABT-737, a novel small molecule inhibitor of bcl-2 family proteins. Oncogene. 27 (52), 6646–6656.

Tatter, S.B., 2002. Recurrent malignant glioma in adults. Curr. Treat Options Oncol. 3 (6), 509–524.

Trojan, J., Cloix, J.F., Ardourel, M.Y. et al., 2007. Insulin-like growth factor type I biology and targeting in malignant gliomas. Neuroscience 145 (3), 795–811.

Tsuboi, M., Le Chevalier, T., 2006. Interstitial lung disease in patients with non-small-cell lung cancer treated with epidermal growth factor receptor inhibitors. Med. Oncol. 23 (2), 161–170.

Vredenburgh, J.J., Desjardins, A., Herndon, J.E., et al., 2007. Bevacizumab plus irinotecan in recurrent glioblastoma multiforme. J. Clin. Oncol. 25 (30), 4722–4729.

Wei, S.C., Tsao, P.N., Yu, S.C., et al., 2005. Placenta growth factor expression is correlated with survival of patients with colorectal cancer. Gut. 54 (5), 666–672.

Wen, P.Y., Yung, W.K., Lamborn, K.R., et al., 2006. Phase I/II study of imatinib mesylate for recurrent malignant gliomas: North American Brain Tumor Consortium Study 99–08. Clin. Cancer Res. 12 (16), 4899–4907.

Westphal, M., Hilt, D.C., Bortey, E., et al., 2003. A phase 3 trial of local chemotherapy with biodegradable carmustine (BCNU) wafers (Gliadel wafers) in patients with primary malignant glioma. Neuro. Oncol. 5 (2), 79–88.

Wiencke, J.K., Zheng, S., Jelluma, N., et al., 2007. Methylation of the PTEN promoter defines low-grade gliomas and secondary glioblastoma. Neuro. Oncol. 9 (3), 271–279.

Xia, P., Aiello, L.P., Ishii, H., et al., 1996. Characterization of vascular endothelial growth factor's effect on the activation of protein kinase C, its isoforms, and endothelial cell growth. J. Clin. Invest 98 (9), 2018–2026.

Zawlik, I., Kita, D., Vaccarella, S., et al., 2008 Common polymorphisms in the MDM2 and TP53 genes and the relationship between TP53 mutations and patient outcomes in glioblastomas. Brain Pathol. 19 (2), 188–194.

Zhang, J., Yang, P.L., Gray, N.S., 2009. Targeting cancer with small molecule kinase inhibitors. Nat. Rev. Cancer 9 (1):28–39.

7 Gene therapy for human brain tumors

Kathryn Howe, Douglas J. Cook, and James T. Rutka

Introduction

Cancers are defined in part by unrestricted cell growth resulting from altered gene function. The classic hypotheses of tumor initiation invoke an inductive gain of oncogenes or a loss of function of tumor suppressor genes resulting in an uncontrolled cell cycle, unrestricted cellular divisions and accumulation of cells comprising the tumor mass. Gene therapy strategies have been proposed to treat cancers through 'direct' interference with oncogenes or by replacing lost tumor suppressor genes or through 'indirect' means by inducing endogenous mechanisms of cell death (Fig. 7.1). Technically, gene therapy is defined as the use of nucleic acid transfer, either RNA or DNA, to treat or prevent disease (Miller 1992; Mulligan 1993; Crystal 1995). One of the first applications of gene transfer emerged from identification of the defective gene in cystic fibrosis; a chloride channel termed the cystic fibrosis transmembrane conductance regulator that has since been proven in principle in animal models and clinical trials (Engelhardt et al 1994). The concept of gene therapy now also extends to strategies aimed at transfection of tumors with oncolytic viruses, administration of proenzyme-regulated cytotoxic therapy, targeted modulation of tumor suppressors or oncogenes, and stimulating local tumor-directed immune responses, each of which can be combined with one of the most promising therapeutic tools to date, stem cell therapy.

Considerations for gene therapy application

Beyond understanding disease pathogenesis to target specific treatment approaches, successful gene therapy strategies require elucidation of an effective therapeutic gene(s), the ability to specifically target a tissue of interest, and appropriate animal models for *in-vivo* experimentation and pre-clinical studies (reviewed in Robbins & Ghivizzani 1998). To date, the efficiency of gene transfer to target tissues remains the rate-limiting step for successful gene therapy as a result of impeding vector and host factors. Development of new delivery vehicles and optimization of earlier vector-based therapies are currently underway in various animal models of disease with several having progressed to human clinical trials, with modest results despite initial promise (Box 7.1).

As a target tissue, the brain is considered a key organ in which to study gene therapy since it is physiologically and immunologically isolated from the rest of the body by the blood–brain barrier. Delivering potential systemic tumor therapies across blood–brain and blood–tumor barriers is both a challenge and an advantage, and more targeted approaches have been developed to reach tumor sites, preserve surrounding normal neural tissue, and leave systemic tissues unaltered. Within the brain tumor subtypes (reviewed in Sanai et al 2005), high-grade gliomas are an obvious target for cancer gene therapy given their diffuse nature, rapid cellular proliferation, and broad cellular migration amidst a background of normal, post-mitotic neural tissue (DeAngelis 2001). Many of the targeted approaches in gene therapy are specific for actively dividing cells, providing a specific, innate targeting system for tumor cells spreading through the brain. Delivery is generally based on direct injection of the gene vector into the tumor mass or into the resection margin following surgical debulking. Clinical trials using therapeutic genes have included prodrug activating genes (suicide genes), cytokine genes, and tumor suppressor genes. The results of key trials will be reviewed at the end of this chapter.

Delivery systems: gene therapy vehicles

Viral vectors

Generation of viral vectors

Viruses have evolved to become highly efficient at nucleic acid delivery to specific cell types while avoiding host immunosurveillance, making them suitable vectors for transfer of genetic material. One of the earliest laboratory modifications was to minimize viral pathogenicity in order to ensure cell viability long enough to retain and express sufficient copies of gene transfer materials within the target tissue. Examples of viruses currently in use in the laboratory and clinical trials include retrovirus, adenovirus, and herpes simplex virus. There follows a brief outline of each vector in the context of its utility in gene therapy strategies.

Retroviruses

Retroviruses (RVs) belong to a family of enveloped RNA viruses called *Retroviridae* that must first reverse transcribe their RNA genomes into DNA before integration into host cell DNA and subsequent replication using host cell machinery. Entry into host cells depends on appropriate viral vector receptor expression at the cell surface and specific interaction between the viral envelope protein and cell surface receptor (Coffin 1990). Following infection, the RV is uncoated and its RNA genome is reverse transcribed into proviral double stranded DNA by means of the RV *pol* gene. The resulting double stranded DNA is translocated to the nucleus, where it is stably integrated into the host genome via a virally encoded integrase. Integrated provirus is then transcribed and produces RNAs encoding the gag, pol, and env proteins, which allow for packaging of the full-length

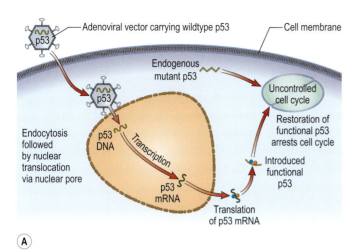

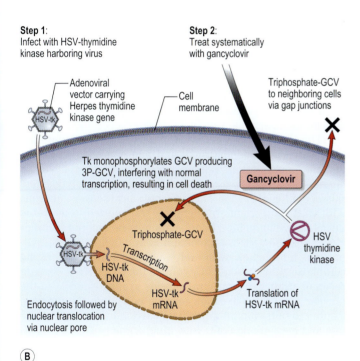

Box 7.1 Current impediments to successful gene therapy in brain tumors

DISTRIBUTION

- Delivering vector, DNA or RNA to the tumor mass and all malignant cells migrating in the nervous system.

EFFICIENCY

- Upon reaching the tumor cell the ability of the vector to infiltrate and kill the malignant cell.

SPECIFICITY

- The ability of the vector to selectively kill or arrest tumor cells while leaving normal cells unaffected.

DURABILITY

- The longevity of the treatment to continuously arrest cell growth or continue to kill malignant cells after initial treatment.

Figure 7.1 Direct vs indirect methods of gene therapy. In the direct method (A) a normal copy of a defective gene is introduced to replace a loss of function contributing to tumor formation. In this case, an adenoviral vector is used to replace mutated p53 in a glioma cell to arrest the cell cycle. In indirect gene therapy (B) an additional gene is introduced that results in cell death. In this case, the herpes simplex virus thymidine kinase gene is introduced via an adenoviral vector to make the cell susceptible to ganciclovir treatment. Upon administering ganciclovir, thymidine kinase phosphorylates the drug to produce triphosphate-ganciclovir, which is integrated into tumor cell DNA and is lethal. The toxic metabolite diffuses to adjacent cells via gap junctions and has the same effect on neighboring tumor cells.

unspliced viral RNA containing the *psi* sequence. Fully infectious viral particles are then budded from the cellular surface.

Most RV vectors currently in use are designed to be replication-incompetent, a safety feature to prevent viral spread after initial infection. Vectors are rendered replication-incompetent through deletion of critical genes for the viral particle (gag), reverse transcriptase activity (pol), and envelope protein (env) synthesis, freeing space for the insertion of the transgene of interest. RV vectors retain the 5′ and 3′ long terminal repeats (LTRs), sequences containing promoter, polyadenylation, reverse transcription and integration signals, and the *psi* packaging signal, each of which is required in *cis* for virus production. The optimization of gene therapy has relied on the development of packaging cell lines and plasmid transfection to produce large quantities of replication-defective virus (Pear et al 1993). The gag, pol, and env polypeptides necessary for viral replication and packaging are provided in the packaging cell lines. RV vector plasmid transfection into packaging cell lines is followed by transcription driven by the viral LTR promoter included in the plasmid. The RNA viral genome is then encapsulated by the viral structural proteins (encoded by *env*) and infectious particles are produced by budding at the cell surface. Bacterial plasmid can either be transiently transcribed (for a few days post-transfection) from unintegrated plasmid molecules or stably transcribed from integrated ones. As infected cells stably produce virus without altering the growth characteristics of the cells, these stable producer lines are suitable for continued recombinant virus production that can be harvested for use in gene therapy.

The prototype RV vector used for gene therapy is the Moloney murine leukemia virus (MMLV), which can accommodate up to 8 kb of foreign DNA through recombinant strategies similar to those previously described. One significant advantage of RV vectors is their stable integration into the DNA of mitotically active cells, enabling the therapeutic gene to be expressed for the life of the cell. In the brain, selective targets include rapidly growing glial tumor cells, activated endothelial cells in neoplastic capillaries, and reactive astrocytes (Shapiro & Shapiro 1998). Ongoing limitations continue to be the low number of infectious particles and transduction rate of tumor cells, despite the use of packaging cell lines to overcome these issues. Animal models suggest 10% transduction rates are necessary for survival benefit, rates which far exceed those reported in human specimens of below 0.002 or 0.03% in two separate clinical studies (Long et al 1999; Puumalainen et al 1998). Inefficient gene transduction has been postulated to result from rapid inactivation by host complement factors as well as poor infiltration of tumor away from the injection sites (Barzon et al 2006). Indeed, application of RVs in clinical trials have yet to show a significant survival benefit or effect on tumor progression.

Adenoviruses

Adenoviruses (AdVs) have been investigated extensively as gene delivery vehicles in clinical trials for cystic fibrosis, and more recently emphasized in malignant glioma clinical trials. In contrast to RVs, AdVs infect a wide variety of cell types, both dividing and non-dividing, and do so efficiently after direct administration of significantly higher viral titers (Wilson 1996). Safety concerns occur, with high systemic doses causing viral toxicity, and have driven the search for means of evading anti-viral immune responses to optimize delivery (Bangari & Mittal 2006).

AdVs consist of a double-stranded linear DNA genome approximately 30–35 kb in length (Graham & Prevec 1995). Gene transfer strategies have traditionally required replication-defective virus, achieved through deletion of early genes 1, 2, 3, and 4 (*E1, E2, E3, E4*), which regulate not only critical viral genes but also inhibit host cell apoptosis (Horwitz 1990). Commonly, it is deletion of the *E1* gene that generates replication deficient virus, as this prevents induction of the *E2*, *E3*, and *E4* promoters necessary for key viral gene products (Graham & Prevec 1995). Infection is initiated by formation of a high-affinity complex between the C-terminal component of the viral fiber protein (knob) and the Coxsackie and adenovirus receptor (CAR) on the cell surface, with internalization mediated by host cell integrins and the Arg-Gly-Asp (RGD) sequence in the viral penton base (Leissner et al 2001). Despite widespread tissue expression of CAR, the low expression on glioma cells presents a challenge for adequate AdV infection. Current research has been directed at improving tropism for glioma cells through a range of modifications, including altering viral knob proteins, improving integrin-penton base interactions through the RGD, and more recently, by developing CAR-independent infection strategies (Van Houdt et al 2007; Kurachi et al 2007). One promising strategy may be the fiber-modified AdV vectors carrying the HIV-1 TAT protein, which bypasses the CAR and has been shown to work in a variety of cell types, including glioma cells (Han et al 2007). Variations of these strategies are currently being applied to overcome low infection rates in neural stem cells (NSC) posing similar challenges (Schmidt et al 2005) that if successful, can improve upon the already promising concept of using NSC glial tumor cell tropism to deliver targeted therapies (Colleoni & Torrente 2008).

Additional challenges include the immunogenicity of AdV infection and loss of therapeutic gene expression 1–2 weeks post-infection, resulting from anti-viral immune responses (Yang et al 1996). Both cellular and humoral immune pathways respond to novel viral capsid epitopes generated from the initial antigen load or leaky viral protein expression (Yang et al 1996). Although less immunogenic,

AdV vectors have been designed containing *E4* and/or *E2* gene deletion, these vectors also have reduced duration of gene expression (Krougliak & Graham 1995; Gao et al 1996; Wang & Finer 1996). Further modifications to AdVs are the 'gutted' or 'helper-dependent' vectors devoid of most viral coding sequences in an attempt reduce viral immunogenicity (Fisher et al 1996; Kochanek et al 1996). While these constructs can accommodate significantly larger DNA sequences, and provide longer high-level transgene expression, purification of isolated gutted virus remains a challenge (reviewed in Segura et al 2008). Despite the obstacles associated with AdV strategies, their high transduction rate of 95–100% and relative safety profile at low titers (Lang et al 2003), are features that continue to drive research into optimizing this delivery tool.

Suicide gene therapy

Suicide gene therapy using Herpes Simplex Virus-1

The herpes simplex virus (HSV)-1 is a large, linear, double-stranded DNA virus 152 kb in length encoding 84 genes (Frampton et al 2005). The genome is well-characterized with reliable HSV-sensitive animal models available to investigate vector strategies and safety profiles (Varghese & Rabkin 2002). The latter is particularly important in the setting of a neurotropic virus such as HSV-1 specific for both neurons and glia that is capable of causing necrotizing encephalitis. Features of HSV-1 that render it attractive for tumor therapy are its broad tissue tropism, large gene transfer capacity through replacement of several nonessential genes (including many coding for neurovirulence), sensitivity to anti-viral drugs, and stability as an intracellular episome that limits insertional mutagenesis (Markert 2000a).

The HSV life cycle is complex, reflecting a set of interactions between virus, neuronal and non-neuronal host cells, and the host immune system, which yield either a lytic or latent infection. *In vivo*, viral progeny released via lytic infection of epithelial or mucosal cells enter local sensory neurons with viral components retrogradely transported to neuronal nuclei, at which point a latent state may be entered (Frampton et al 2005). Virus attachment is initiated by viral glycoprotein interaction with cell surface proteins, forming complexes that subsequently contact the HveA/HveC cognate receptor prior to entry. Viral capsids are transported to the nuclear pore complexes for genome entry into the nucleus, leading to initiation of 'immediate early' (IE) gene transcription and upregulation of DNA synthesis and replication. Activation of late genes is required for structural protein synthesis with the majority of virus assembly occurring within the nucleus, prior to final modifications before budding from the cell surface. While generation of HSV vectors is based on principles universal to viral vectors, such as optimizing tissue tropism, infection, and efficient gene transduction, limiting virulence to ensure host safety and contain the host immune response is a key component of any HSV vector system. Accordingly, IE gene deletion (e.g., *ICP0, ICP4, ICP22, ICP27, ICP47*) not only render viruses replication-deficient, but also less toxic and immunogeneic (Krisky et al 1998).

One of the earliest and most thoroughly studied applications of HSV has been an indirect gene therapy approach involving introduction of a 'suicide' gene, HSV-derived thymidine kinase (HSV-tk), to enhance the effectiveness of a known antiviral therapy such as ganciclovir (GCV), to induce tumor cell death. Transfection of HSV-tk into tumor cells leads to altered phosphorylation of the systemically administered pro-drug ganciclovir, a nucleoside analog, blocking DNA synthesis and ultimately cell division (reviewed in Hamel & Westphal 2003). This strategy was first proposed by Moolten (1986) to target malignant cells using a retrovirus, with subsequent preclinical studies showing complete disappearance of experimental brain tumors in animal models (Culver et al 1992). A significant advantage of this system is that tumor lysis occurs in cells that have not been transfected through a 'bystander effect', with enhanced susceptibility of non-HSV-tk transfected cells to GCV thought to occur through uptake of activated GCV dispersed through leaky gap junctions within the tumor (Hamel et al 1996; Dilber et al 1997). Unfortunately, retrovirus delivery of the HSV-tk/GCV suicide gene has not borne out in a major randomized phase III clinical trial (RCT), as there was no difference in median survival between patients treated with surgical resection and radiotherapy vs those additionally treated with HSV-tk/GCV gene therapy (Rainov 2000). As RV infection is limited to dividing cells and bystander lysis is likely limited by tissue diffusion distances, it is perhaps not surprising that tumor responses have been limited to the site of RV application (either intratumoral injection or surgical resection cavity) (Ram et al 1997). Consequently, studies have been redirected towards AdV delivery in an attempt to improve tumor cell penetration and gene transduction efficiency, with one RCT demonstrating a significant longer median survival time in patients treated with standard therapy plus AdV HSV-tk/GCV gene therapy compared to standard therapy alone (62.4 vs 37.7 weeks, respectively) (Immonen et al 2004). Despite moderate success, AdV infection remains hampered by the scarce CAR expression in gliomas and its inherent inadequacy as a neuropathogen.

Oncolytic virotherapy

Oncolytic virotherapy is based on the development of replication-competent viruses that have the ability to selectively replicate within and kill tumor cells. By permitting replication and viral-induced cell lysis, multiple successions of viral particle release, infection, and cytolysis can occur. Tumor selectivity is based on regulation of viral replication by genes uniquely expressed in malignant cells or by placing expression under the control of tumor-specific promoters (Chiocca 2002). With appropriate attention to the issue of neurovirulence, both HSV and AdV have been developed for this type of virotherapy.

G207 is a conditionally replicating HSV with mutations in both copies of the neurovirulence gene $\gamma_l 34.5$ plus disruption of ribonucleotide reductase *in lieu* of the thymidine kinase used in the suicide gene model. This is the first replication-competent HSV mutant to be used in a clinical trial, with phase I data indicating no dose-limiting toxicities and preliminary results suggestive of decreased tumor volumes (Markert 2000b). Similarly, the HSV1716 mutant with deleted $\gamma_l 34.5$ genes was used in a phase I trial with similar results and progressed to a phase II trial where

intratumoral delivery has shown promising results (Papanastassiou et al 2002). To date, the only other oncolytic virus that has been tested in a clinical trial is a conditionally-replicative AdV, ONYX-015. Through deletion of the E1B-55K gene normally responsible for inactivating host cell p53 tumor suppressor activity, viral replication is restricted to tumor cells harboring non-functional p53. Data from a phase I clinical trial in patients with recurrent gliomas was dismal, with 96% resulting in disease progression following intratumoral delivery (Chiocca et al 2004). While in principle oncolytic viral therapy has unique design advantages and it is encouraging that dose toxicities are not being reached in early clinical trials, limitations to this approach clearly exist and indicate the need to consider alternate anti-tumor strategies.

Tight control: targeting gene expression

As understanding of tumor biology advances, so does the number of possible therapeutic targets available for tumor-specific treatment strategies. An important overarching aim of selective transgene delivery to tumor cells is the preservation of surrounding normal tissue. As alluded to earlier in the discussion of viral vector development, molecular targets have moved beyond the initial selection for relatively non-specific features such as actively dividing cells towards more specific intracellular processes. In particular, knowledge of tumor-specific promoters and the ability to manipulate them according to cell type, cell cycle status, and external stimuli, have enabled more tightly controlled regulation of gene expression and ultimately, cellular control.

Regulation of the cell cycle

Tumor suppressor gene therapy targeting p53
The tumor suppressor gene p53 is one of the most common genetic alterations described with 30–50% of malignant gliomas affected (Hilton et al 2004). Replacement of this 'lost function' has been shown to induce growth arrest or apoptosis in early malignant glioma models, with adenoviral vector gene transfer of wild-type p53 conferring improved survival in nude mice with glioma intracranial xenografts (Kock et al 1996). The concept has been extended to a phase I clinical trial for patients with recurrent glioma, which demonstrated safety but highlighted the challenge of adequate tumor penetration as expression was not found beyond 5 mm from the injection site (Lang et al 2003).

Oncogene therapy targeting the epidermal growth factor receptor (EGFR)
EGFR is a tyrosine kinase receptor found on many cell types that is involved in control of cellular growth but frequently mutated in malignancy. In many tumor cells, EGFR activity is constitutively active and leads to uncontrolled cellular growth. The common glioma EFGR mutant, EGFRvIII, has been targeted for gene therapy in multiple strategies. One method has been delivery of antisense oligonucleotides against EGFR to decrease the overactive tyrosine kinase receptor, an approach that has proven effective in the laboratory setting (Zhang et al 2002). Similarly, overexpression of dominant-negative EGFR using a replication-deficient

adenoviral vector has improved tumor cell responses to radiotherapy in malignant glioma tumor cell lines and animal models (Lammering et al 2001). This has yet to be applied in the clinical setting.

Pro-apoptotic strategies

The apoptotic pathway is frequently altered in tumor cells. As a regulator of cell death, it is an attractive target for gene therapy strategies. Studies to date have included using adenoviral delivery of the pro-apoptotic Fas ligand or tumor necrosis factor-related apoptosis-inducing ligand (TRAIL) to induce apoptosis in multiple glioma cell lines, some of which respond synergistically with co-transfection (Rubinchik et al 2003). An extension of this concept using adenoviral delivery of pro-apoptotic BAX plus radiotherapy has been shown to reduce tumor size in a nude mouse glioma model (Arafat et al 2003). A more targeted approach is the one taken by Komata et al (2001a,b, 2002) who used a telomerase reverse transcriptase promoter specific to malignant glioma cells to induce expression of the pro-apoptotic proteins FADD, caspase-6, and caspase-8, which led to not only to apoptosis but also tumor growth suppression. Clinical application of pro-apoptotic strategies will clearly be limited by the ability to specifically target tumor cells and avoid normal brain tissue. While this probably accounts for studies remaining in preclinical phases, the advent of neural stem cell applications may push new boundaries for this approach (see discussion below).

Therapeutic genes: immunotherapy

By virtue of their location in an immune-privileged site, brain tumor cells easily remain undetected. Immune therapies are therefore designed to enhance and/or promote anti-tumor immune responses through a variety of mechanisms including local cytokine-based upregulation of host immunity, active anti-tumor immunization (vaccination) strategies, or passive immune-based augmentation of chemotherapy or radiation through anti-tumor antibody-mediated approaches.

Cytokine therapy

Cytokines are key mediators of host immune responses, released from various types of immune cells in response to local or systemic stimuli. In simple terms, the system possesses balancing mediators that can be considered either pro-inflammatory or anti-inflammatory/immunosuppressive in nature. Tumor cells evade host immune responses in part through appearing as 'self' by retaining expression of major histocompatibility complex (MHC) molecules (a feature of all normal tissue), and in part because malignant gliomas possess strong immunosuppressive properties, likely through release of the immunosuppressive cytokines transforming growth factor-β (TGFβ) and interleukin (IL)-10 (Thomas & Massague 2005; Filaci et al 2007). Cytokine-specific strategies are based on boosting anti-tumor responses, frequently through IL-2-induced activation of T helper cells, B cells and natural killer cells or inhibiting tumor-driven immunosuppression (Selznick et al 2008). TGFβ in particular has long been noted for its anti-tumor effects, as documented by

in-vitro studies showing significant cytotoxicity and inhibition of proliferation of tumor-infiltrating lymphocytes (TIL) (Kuppner et al 1989). Blocking TGFβ activity with antisense nucleotides or silencing RNA technology has been shown to confer enhanced survival and impair glioma invasiveness and tumorigenicity in in-vivo rodent models, respectively (Fakhrai et al 1996; Friese et al 2004). Whether or not this is also due to inhibition of the pro-angiogenic properties of TGFβ, through regulation of VEGF, was not addressed. For many cytokines, systemic delivery is toxic to the host. As a result, local delivery of cytokine or anti-cytokine therapy remains a challenge outside of direct application to the surgical resection cavity or through tumor injection. Nevertheless, this is a viable method with one example provided by a recent phase I trial investigating adenoviral delivery of the anti-viral cytokine, interferon-β, which showed consistently increased tumor cell apoptosis in postoperative biopsies compared to preoperative controls (Chiocca et al 2008). Alternatively, attempts to amplify the anti-tumor immune response by combining transgenic human IL-2 with the HSV-tk/GCV delivery system has shown some degree of success with tumor regression observed in 50% of malignant glioma patients receiving the therapy (Palu et al 1999; Colombo et al 2005).

Systemic vaccine immunotherapy

Dendritic cell vaccines

While brain tissue may be localized within an immune-privileged site, it is not completely sequestered from the host immune system. Evidence exists suggesting that activated T cells from the periphery can cross the blood–brain barrier and function within the nervous system (Owens et al 1994). Consequently, vaccination with tumor peptides, peptides, or antigen-presenting cells presenting tumor peptides, may drive systemic T-cell responses capable of malignant glial tumor destruction. In contrast, T cells can be harvested from patients, selected for anti-tumor activity, expanded ex vivo and transferred adoptively back to patients.

One of the most promising anti-tumor strategies being researched to date involves priming professional antigen presenting cells, dendritic cells (DCs) with tumor antigen ex vivo. Briefly, ingested tumor antigens are presented on either MHC class I or class II molecules, priming naïve CD8+ve cytotoxic T lymphocytes (CTLs) and CD4+ve helper cells, to elicit targeted tumor cell destruction. Glioma antigens can be fused with MHC-matched glioma cells, pulsed with apoptotic tumor cells, total tumor RNA, tumor lysates, or tumor specific peptides (Parajuli et al 2004). Animal models of intracranial malignant gliomas have established tumor-specific CTL responses can generate protective immunity in animals treated with sensitized DCs (Liau et al 1999; Ni et al 2001). To date, phase I and II clinical trials have further supported the concept, showing strong anti-tumor CTL responses with improved median survival times in patients with resistant malignant gliomas after treatment with autologous DCs pulsed with tumor cell lysates (Yamanaka et al 2005; Yu et al 2004).

While there are clearly multiple variations of strategies that can be approached for DC immunotherapy, one risk of the tumor lysate model described above is generation of an immune response against self-antigens with resultant attack on normal brain tissue. An alternate approach has been to target tumor-specific antigens such as the EGFRvIII, known to be specific to malignant gliomas and expressed in 20–25% of these tumors (Bigner et al 1990). Following successful cell and animal models, early data from a phase II clinical trial has demonstrated a significant increase in time to progression from 7.1–12 months in treated glioma patients compared to a historically matched control cohort (Heimberger et al 2003). At this time, Sampson and colleagues are coordinating ACT III, a phase II/III randomized trial comparing EGFRvIII vaccine plus standard treatment against standard treatment alone in patients with newly diagnosed EGFRvIII-positive malignant gliomas (Celldex Therapeutics, at: www.clinicaltrials.gov). While there remains an ongoing search for tumor-specific targets, a recent study looking at the most promising candidates (EGFRvIII, IL-13Ralpha, gp100, TRP-2) only identified IL-13Rα as a marker with comparable prevalence in malignant gliomas (Saikali et al 2007). One of the newest directions at this time is personalized peptide vaccination using nine amino acid peptide sequences with unique MHC class I binding and CTL activation potential, although it remains to be seen whether this strategy will progress beyond a phase I clinical study (Yamanaka 2008).

Adoptive transfer

Adoptive transfer is an approach based on harvesting tumor-invading lymphocytes (TILs), expansion *ex vivo*, activation by IL-2 stimulation and subsequent re-implantation. The pretense of this design is that TILs may be relatively tumor-specific and will thus mount a localized tumoricidal response upon return as an activated population. While studies to date have been relatively unsuccessful in gliomas (Barzon et al 2006), success achieved using adoptive transfer of TILs in melanoma patients may provide new insights and applications for tumors of the same embryonic origin (Dudley et al 2002).

Adjuvant strategies in radiation and chemotherapy

Antibody-mediated drug delivery is aimed at minimizing systemic drug or radiation administration and toxicity, while targeting and/or improving delivery of the agent within the tumor through inherent alteration of pharmacokinetic properties. Tumor-specific antigens that have been targeted for antibody generation to date include the EGFRvIII mutant, IL-4 receptor, and tenascin (Dunn & Black 2003). Both anti-tenascin and anti-EGFR antibodies have been shown to be effective carriers for iodine radiolabels, with a phase II trial of radiolabeled anti-tenascin suggesting a survival benefit in patients where treatment was administered to the surgical cavity (Reardon et al 2002). Other antibody conjugates serve to deliver immunotoxic compounds typically derived from plant or fungal proteins to improve tumor cytotoxicity. Here again, tumor-specific expression of EGFRvIII provides an ideal target that has been applied in the design of anti-EGFR-*pseudomonas* exotoxin A conjugate therapy – a therapy that has high affinity and cytotoxicity in malignant gliomas *in vitro* (Lorimer et al 1996). Extension of this design is ongoing

with alternate delivery models of EGFR-targeted toxins in malignant glioma patients (Sampson et al 2008). Compounds that are farther along in patient application are the IL-4 and IL-13-pseudomonas exotoxins (PE), with IL-13PE having recently completed a phase I safety trial (Vogelbaum et al 2007). Despite inherent benefits to determining an isolated targeted tumor-specific therapy for malignant gliomas, obstacles to their development as a therapeutic option remain, perhaps indicating that a more realistic goal lies in the design of multi-modal approaches.

Combined immunotherapies

Together, gene therapy, oncolytic virotherapy, and immunotherapy can be combined for multi-modal anti-tumor approaches (Fig. 7.2). Given the relatively new development of immunotherapeutic approaches, combination strategies are only just being explored at this time. An example of these applications is shown by Schneider et al (2008) who down-regulated TGFβ through nanoparticle delivery of antisense oligonucleotides with combined anti-tumor vaccination to improve survival in an animal model of malignant gliomas. Additional concepts involve an adjuvant-like approach with combined viral vector and radiotherapy, the effectiveness of which is being examined in patients with recurrent or progressive glioma using HSV G207 or the oncolytic virus ONYX-015 receiving standard radiotherapy regimens (Selznick et al 2008). Perhaps one of the most exciting new developments involves the delivery of a conditionally-replicating adenoviral oncolytic virus via neural stem cells (NSC), a concept that capitalizes on the unique tumor-targeting features of NSCs to improve penetration of an

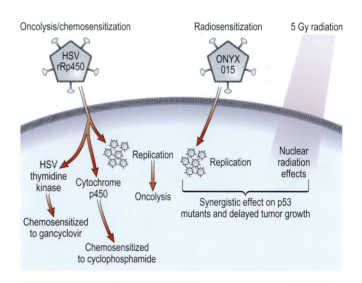

Figure 7.2 Combined strategies in gene therapy are emerging as a means to enhance conventional therapies. To the left the concept of chemosensitization is demonstrated by the use of rRp450 herpes simplex virus that has oncolytic effects, but also introduces herpes-simplex thymidine kinase and cytochrome p450 into tumor cells, sensitizing them to ganciclovir and cyclophosphamide chemotherapy, respectively. To the right radiosensitization is demonstrated as per *in-vitro* experiments that have demonstrated a synergism between the adenoviral oncolytic ONYX-015 virus and low dose (5 Gy) radiation in glioma cell lines. This effect is enhanced in p53 mutant glioma cells.

oncolytic virus within tumor sites (Tyler et al 2008). With extensive possible therapeutic combinations, a key issue now and in the future will be to determine which combination strategies have the greatest potential for success in order to focus efforts on realizable goals.

Neural stem cells: future promise?

One of the key dilemmas of current malignant glioma treatment is the ability of these tumors to disseminate throughout brain parenchyma and thus recur at sites distant from the original location. Adjuvant therapies such as chemotherapy and radiation have provided modest benefits to date and have the additional drawback of side-effects that significantly impact patient quality of life. Both viral and non-viral gene therapy strategies have demonstrated limited tumor penetration with local application, without the additional consideration of distant tumor satellites. And while active immunotherapy may have the potential to target disseminated tumor cells, it faces the limitation of endogenous tumor-driven immunosuppression and heterogeneity of antigenic targets (Ehtesham et al 2005). As a result, the discovery of neural stem cells with potent tumor tropism and the ability to track migratory cells that can be engineered to deliver cytotoxic therapies to tumor satellite regions has been met with much enthusiasm (Fig. 7.3).

Neural stem cells as a targeted delivery system

NSC migratory ability and therapeutic potential was first determined by Aboody et al (2000) who showed cells tracked to tumor sites independent of mode of administration (intracerebral vs intravenous), could be engineered to participate in pro-drug cytotoxic therapy, and that this led to significant tumor shrinkage in a murine glioma model. Adaptations of

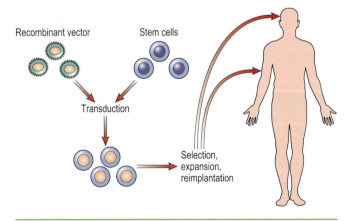

Figure 7.3 Schematic diagram showing application of neural stem cells (NSCs) to deliver gene therapy using vectors. A purified stem cell population from embryonic, umbilical cord-blood derived, or skin cells may be harvested for *ex vivo* gene transfer using vector-based gene transduction techniques. Cells containing the therapeutic gene of interest are isolated, expanded, and reimplanted at various sites, depending on physiological barriers (e.g., blood–brain barrier).

NSC application has included delivery of cytokine-expressing NSC, with particular focus on those known to induce tumoricidal T-cell responses, such as IL-12. Indeed, adenoviral IL-12 gene transfection in NSCs and subsequent administration of IL-12-NSC not only localizes to disseminated tumor sites, but is also associated with increased survival when compared to IL-12-secreting nonmigratory fibroblast controls (Liu et al 2002). Alternatively, induction of tumor cell apoptosis by overexpression of the tumor necrosis factor-related apoptosis-inducing ligand (TRAIL) gene is currently being applied in the development of NSC-driven anti-tumor therapies. Beyond use as a monotherapy, new research suggests TRAIL overexpression via NSCs or adeno-associated virus renders tumor cells more susceptible to the widely-used anti-glioma chemotherapeutic agent, temozolomide (Hingtgen et al 2008). Finally, given the ongoing ethical concerns over the origin of stem cell therapies, it is promising that stem cells of non-embryonic origin such as umbilical cord blood-derived mesenchymal or human skin-derived stem cells are showing therapeutic potential through TRAIL-delivery and direct anti-tumor effects, respectively (Kim et al 2008; Pisati et al 2007).

Clinical trials: one step at a time

Suicide gene delivery

The first gene therapy technique to progress to clinical trials in malignant glioma was based on the indirect HCV-tk/GCV 'suicide' gene model in which tumor cells were selectively targeted by a retroviral (RV) vector and transfected with HCV-tk, making them susceptible to ganciclovir (Moolten 1986). The initial phase I trial of this technique utilized RV producer cells injected directly into the tumor bed following glioma resection (Ram et al 1997). Of 15 patients treated, there were five with anti-tumor effects based on volumetric measurement of enhancing regions of tumor on MRI. These were limited to the smallest tumors by volume suggesting high concentrations of RV are required to achieve an effect. Five more phase I and I/II trials have followed with similar results (Packer et al 2000; Harsh et al 2000; Klatzman et al 1998; Prados et al 2003; Shand et al 1999; see Table 7.1). This therapy was taken into a phase III trial in which 248 patients were randomized to surgical resection and radiation (standard therapy) or standard therapy plus implantation of RV producing cells at the time of surgery (Rainov 2000). There were no differences in time to progression or survival between the two groups, although the safety profile and tolerability of the treatment were confirmed.

Overall, the RV HSK-tk method is hampered by a limited capacity for gene transfer in addition to limited delivery of GCV to transduced cells, suggesting that other strategies are required to complement the system. Moreover, dexamethasone, a steroid routinely utilized in treating edema associated with brain tumors has been shown to inhibit the HSV-tk bystander effect (Robe et al 2005). Early data indicated RV delivery of IL-2 in addition to HSV-tk induced a more potent anti-tumor effect (Palu et al 1999). A subsequent phase I clinical trial enrolled 12 patients and showed safety with no significant toxicities following treatment with RV-producing cells delivering IL-2 in combination with HSV-tk (Colombo

Table 7.1 Published and ongoing clinical trials in gene therapy for brain tumors

Type	Technique	Phase	References
Direct gene therapy	Adenoviral-p53	I	Lang et al 2003
Indirect gene therapy	RV HSV-TK/GCV	I	Germano et al 2003
	RV HSV-TK/GCV	I	Harsh et al 2000
	RV HSV-TK/GCV	I	Packer et al 2000
	RV HSV-TK/GCV	II	Klatzmann et al 1998
	RV HSV-TK/GCV	II	Prados et al 2003
	RV HSV-TK/GCV	II	Shand et al 1999
	RV HSV-TK/GCV	III	Rainov 2000
	Adenoviral HSV-TK/GCV	I	Judy & Eck 2002
	Adenoviral HSV-TK/GCV	I	Germano et al 2003
	Adenoviral HSV-TK/GCV	I	Trask et al 2000
	Adenoviral HSV-TK/GCV	I	Smitt et al 2003
	Adenoviral HSV-TK/GCV	I	Lang et al 2003
	Adenoviral HSV-TK/GCV	III	Immonen et al 2004
	RV HSV-TK/GCV vs Adenoviral HSV-TK/GCV	I/II	Sandmair et al 2000
Oncolytic	HSV G207	I	Markert et al 2000
	HSV 1716	I	Rampling et al 2000
	HSV 1716	I	Papanastassiou et al 2002
	HSV 1716	II	Harrow et al 2004
	ONYX-015	I	Chiocca et al 2004
Immunotherapy	DC-tumor lysate	I	Rutkowski et al 2004
	DC-tumor lysate	I	Yu et al 2004
	DC-tumor lysate	II	Yamanaka et al 2005
Immunogenetherapy	RV HSV-TK/GCV + IL-2	I	Colombo et al 2005

et al 2005). Additionally, in five cases, there was a radiographical decrease in tumor mass at the 12-month follow-up, with one case exhibiting disappearance of a distant non-injected tumor mass.

Similar to the RV methodology, adenovirus has been used as a vector to deliver HSV-tk to tumor cells and has progressed to clinical trials (Judy & Eck 2002; Germano et al 2003). In phase I/II trials there has been promising results with a good safety profile and evidence of tumor effect on serial imaging (Trask et al 2000; Smitt et al 2003; Lang et al 2003). A phase III clinical trial using an adenoviral HSK-tk therapy was conducted in 36 patients, 17 of whom received adenoviral therapy in the tumor bed following resection and 19 of which received standard care (Immonen et al 2004). While the study showed a statistically significant increase in mean survival from 39 to 71 weeks post-treatment, this promising result remains under further investigation.

Both RV and adenoviral techniques have been compared in a combined phase I/II trial where seven patients received AdV-based HSV-tk gene therapy and seven received RV-based HSV-tk (Sandmair et al 2000). There were no serious adverse events for either therapy. Mean survival for RV vs adenovirus based HSV-tk therapy were 7.4 vs 15 months, respectively (a statistically significant difference), suggesting that adenovirus may be a more effective vector for suicide gene delivery.

Direct gene therapy using an adenoviral vector to replace dysfunctional or absent p53 in tumor cells has been taken to a phase I clinical trial (Lang et al 2003). However, there was limited adenoviral penetration of the tumor mass and the method was not pursued further.

Oncolytic virotherapy

Gene therapy using replicating viral vectors for malignant glioma originated from experiments in which a thymidine kinase negative, conditionally replicating, mutant HSV (dlstk) was shown to have oncolytic effects on both immortalized and short-term human malignant glioma cell lines *in vitro* (Martuza et al 1991). *In vivo*, the virus was associated with prolonged survival in mice bearing U87 gliomas. Although this vector was selective for actively replicating cells, concerns over potential virulence in the normal brain and an insensitivity to typical antivirals (owing to the deletion of thymidine kinase), prevented this therapy from moving into clinical trials. However, this pioneering work served as the basis for G207 HSV, a conditionally replicating virus selective to replicating cells through a *lacZ* insertion of the UL39 gene encoding ribonucleotide reductase, thus retaining thymidine kinase and antiviral susceptibility. G207 has limited virulence and decreased concerns of inducing HSV encephalitis secondary to mutations of both copies of the $\gamma_1 34.5$ neurovirulence gene. Markert et al (2000b) published a phase I trial of G207 in which 21 patients with recurrent malignant gliomas received escalating doses of G207 inoculated stereotactically into enhancing components of tumor recurrences. This trial demonstrated safety with no cases of HSV encephalitis, no serious adverse events, and no dose-related toxicities in escalating doses of inoculum. Eight patients had decreased volume of enhancement and there were two long-term survivors at the time of publication. Pathological analysis for LacZ expression demonstrated G207 viral activity in two patients at 56 and 157 days post-inoculation.

A second oncolytic virus, HSV 1716, has also reached clinical trials. This HSV mutant has deletions of both $\gamma_1 34.5$ genes, limiting neurovirulence. In phase I trials there were no serious adverse events noted and virus was recovered from pathologic specimens (Rampling et al 2000; Papanastassiou et al 2002). In phase II testing, the safety profile was confirmed after injection of HSV 1716 adjacent to resection cavities. Two of 12 patients had tumor responses on imaging with three of 12 patients surviving past 15 months (Harrow et al 2004). This promising result awaits further clinical trials.

The third and final oncolytic virus that has proceeded to clinical trials in malignant glioma is ONYX-015 (Bischoff et al 1996). This adenovirus has a deletion in the viral protein E1B-55K that normally inactivates host p53. As a result, p53-negative malignant cells support the replication of this virus despite the loss of this protein. A phase I dose escalation trial of ONYX-015 demonstrated no adverse side-effects, but had limited effect on tumor progression.

Immunotherapy

Immunotherapy for malignant glioma using dendritic cells pulsed with tumor lysate has been evaluated in clinical trials (Yu et al 2004; Rutkowski et al 2004; Yamanaka et al 2005). A phase II trial of peripherally harvested dendritic cells were

using replication-deficient retroviruses and adenoviruses. Hum. Gene Ther. 9, 1769–1774.

Ram, Z., Culver, K.W., Oshiro, E.M., et al., 1997. Therapy of malignant brain tumors by intratumoral implantation of retroviral vector-producing cells. Nat. Med. 3, 1354–1361.

Rainov, N.G., 2000. A phase III clinical evaluation of herpes simplex virus type I thymidine kinase and ganciclovir gene therapy as an adjuvant to surgical resection and radiation in adults with previously untreated glioblastoma multiforme. Hum. Gene Ther. 11, 2389–2401.

Rampling, R., Cruickshank, G., Papanastassiou, V., et al., 2000. Toxicity evaluation of replication-competent herpes simplex virus (ICP 34.5 null mutant 1716) in patients with recurrent malignant glioma. Gene Ther. 7, 859–866.

Reardon, D.A., Akabani, G., Coleman, R.E., et al., 2002. Phase II trial of murine (131)I-labeled antitenascin monoclonal antibody 81C6 administered into surgically created resection cavities of patients with newly diagnosed malignant gliomas. J. Clin. Oncol. 20, 1389–1397.

Robbins, P.D., Ghivizzani, S.C., 1998. Viral vectors for gene therapy. Pharmacol. Ther. 80, 35–47.

Robe, P.A., Nguyen-Khac, M., Jolois, O., et al., 2005. Dexamethasone inhibits the HSV-tk/ganciclovir bystander effect in malignant glioma cells. BMC. Cancer 5, 32.

Rubinchik, S., Yu, H., Woraratanadharm, J., et al., 2003. Enhanced apoptosis of glioma cell lines is achieved by co-delivering FasL-GFP and TRAIL with a complex Ad5 vector. Cancer Gene Ther. 10, 814–822.

Rutkowski, S., De Vleeschouwer, S., Kaempgen, E., et al., 2004. Surgery and adjuvant dendritic cell-based tumor vaccination for patients with relapsed malignant glioma, a feasibility study. Br. J. Cancer 91, 1656–1662.

Saikali, S., Avril, T., Collet, B., et al., 2007. Expression of nine tumor antigens in a series of human glioblastoma multiforme: interest of EGFRvIII, IL-13Ralpha, gp100, and TRP-2 for immunotherapy. J. Neurooncol. 81, 139–148.

Sampson, J.H., Archer, G.E., Mitchell, D.A., et al., 2008. Tumor-specific immunotherapy targeting the EGFRvIII mutation in patients with malignant glioma. Semin. Immunol. 20, 267–275.

Sanai, N., Alverez-Buylla, A., Berger, M.S., 2005. Neural stem cells and the origin of gliomas. NEJM. 353, 811–822.

Sandmair, A.M., Loimas, S., Puranen, P., et al., 2000. Thymidine kinase gene therapy for human malignant glioma, using replication-deficient retroviruses or adenoviruses. Hum. Gene Ther. 11, 2197–2205.

Schmidt, A., Bockmann, M., Stoll, A., et al., 2005. Analysis of adenoviral gene transfer into adult neural stem cells. Virus. Res. 114, 45–53.

Schneider, T., Becker, A., Ringe, K., et al., 2008. Brain tumor therapy by combined vaccination and antisense oligonucleotide delivery with nanoparticles. J. Neuroimmunol. 195, 21–27.

Segura, M.M., Alba, R., Bosch, A., 2008. Advances in helper-dependent adenoviral vector research. Curr. Gene Ther. 8, 222–235.

Selznick, L.A., Mohammed, F.S., Fecci, P., et al., 2008. Molecular strategies for the treatment of malignant glioma – genes, viruses, and vaccines. Neurosurg. Rev. 31, 141–155.

Shand, N., Weber, F., Mariani, L., et al., 1999. A phase 1–2 clinical trial of gene therapy for recurrent glioblastoma multiforme by tumor transduction with the herpes simplex thymidine kinase gene followed by ganciclovir. GLI328 European–Canadian Study Group. Hum. Gene Ther. 10, 2325–2335.

Shapiro, W.R., Shapiro, J.R., 1998. Biology and treatment of malignant glioma. Oncology. (Williston Park) 12, 233–240.

Smitt, P.S., Driesse, M., Wolbers, J., et al., 2003. Treatment of relapsed malignant glioma with an adenoviral vector containing the herpes simplex thymidine kinase gene followed by ganciclovir. Mol. Ther. 7, 851–858.

Thomas, D.A., Massague, J., 2005. TGF-beta directly targets cytotoxic T cell functions during tumor evasion of immune surveillance. Cancer Cell 8, 369–380.

Trask, T.W., Trask, R.P., Aguilar-Cordova, E., et al., 2000. Phase I study of adenoviral delivery of the HSV-tk gene and ganciclovir administration in patients with current malignant brain tumors. Mol. Ther. 1, 195–203.

Tyler, M.A., Ulasov, I.V., Sonabend, A.M., et al., 2008. Neural stem cells target intracranial glioma to deliver an oncolytic adenovirus in vivo. Gene Ther. 16, 262–278.

Van Houdt, W.J., Wu, H., Glasgow, J.N., et al., 2007. Gene delivery into malignant glioma by infectivity-enhanced adenovirus: in vivo versus in vitro models. Neuro. Oncol. 9, 280–290.

Varghese, S., Rabkin, S.D., 2002. Oncolytic herpes simplex virus vectors for cancer virotherapy. Cancer Gene Ther. 9, 967–978.

Vogelbaum, M.A., Sampson, J.H., Kunwar, S., et al., 2007. Convection-enhanced delivery of cintredekin besudotox (interleukin-13-PE38QQR) followed by radiation therapy with and without temozolomide in newly diagnosed malignant gliomas: phase I study of final safety results. Neurosurgery 61, 1031–1037.

Wang, Q., Finer, M.H., 1996. Second-generation adenovirus vectors. Nat. Med. 2, 714–716.

Wilson, J.M., 1996. Adenoviruses as gene-delivery vehicles. N. Engl. J. Med. 334, 1185–1187.

Yamanaka, R., 2008. Cell- and peptide-based immunotherapeutic approaches for glioma. Trends. Mol. Med. 14, 228–235.

Yamanaka, R., Homma, J., Yajima, N., et al., 2005. Clinical evaluation of dendritic cell vaccination for patients with recurrent glioma: results of a clinical phase I/II trial. Clin. Cancer Res. 11, 4160–4167.

Yang, Y., Su, Q., Wilson, J.M., 1996. Role of viral antigens in destructive cellular immune responses to adenovirus vector-transduced cells in mouse lungs. J. Virol. 70, 7209–7212.

Yu, J.S., Liu, G., Ying, H., et al., 2004. Vaccination with tumor lysate-pulsed dendritic cells elicits antigen-specific, cytotoxic T-cells in patients with malignant glioma. Cancer Res. 64, 4973–4979.

Zhang, Y., Zhu, C., Pardridge, W.M., 2002. Antisense gene therapy of brain cancer with an artificial virus gene delivery system. Mol. Ther. 6, 67–72.

Immunology of brain tumors and implications for immunotherapy

David G. Walker

8

Introduction

The prognosis for the commonest primary malignant brain tumor, glioblastoma multiforme, continues to be poor. Because of this, the discussion in this chapter will be restricted to these tumors. Logically, effective treatment strategies and possible cures are more likely to follow from a more profound understanding of the biology of malignant glioma, including their interaction with the immune system.

An interaction between the immune system and the development and response to brain tumors is suggested by three broad observations:

1. Brain tumors are more common in the immunocompromised (Schiff et al 2001).
2. Conversely, a history of autoimmunity and allergy is related to a decreased risk for the development of brain tumors (Linos et al 2007; Wigertz et al 2007).
3. A surprisingly good prognosis is seen in patients who develop local infections following surgery for malignant brain tumors (Bowles & Perkins 1999; Walker and Pamphlett 1999).

Furthermore, three principles have emerged from recent advances in the understanding of the immune response to cancer:

1. The immune system is able to recognize cancer.
2. Antitumor immunity is often suppressed.
3. The potential exists to manipulate the immune response as a tool in the treatment of cancer.

One of the reasons that the goal of cure for malignant glioma has remained elusive is the propensity of glial tumor cells to infiltrate normal brain, thus significantly restricting the effectiveness of traditional therapies. The hope therefore is that the immune system can be manipulated to achieve this goal by seeking out and targeting tumor cells while sparing normal cells. Enthusiasm for an immunotherapeutic approach has at times waned, but more recent experience has provided encouraging evidence for efficacy.

Introduction to immunology and immune responses

The immune system is designed to detect and eliminate foreign biological and non-biological material, as well as restrict unregulated cell growth. All of these may threaten the integrity of the host. These foreign molecules represent antigens, that is, the molecular targets of the immune system. A response to antigens involves multiple interacting levels, including innate immunity, and adoptive immunity, which broadly includes B cells and antibodies, T cells and cell mediated immunity, antigen presenting cells (APCs) and the production of immune memory. Adaptive immunity depends on antigen presentation and activation signals from the innate system to generate a full response. In turn, the innate system effector cells, such as macrophages, require stimulation by the adaptive system to become fully activated. An overview of the immune system is represented in Figure 8.1.

Innate immunity consists of first-line barrier defenses such as skin and mucosal membranes, and an intermediate response that is generated within hours of the detection of a threat. This intermediate reaction is mediated by non-specific immune cells, inflammatory cytokines, and blood-borne proteins such as complement. The innate immune response involves microglia/macrophages, neutrophils and natural killer cells. Neutrophils and macrophages phagocytose microbes and other foreign substances. Natural killer (NK) cells destroy aberrant cells by recognizing characteristic cell surface changes. Common to these responses is the recognition of dangerous cells and substances via recognition of molecules that signal potential danger, such as unmethylated CpG oligonucleotides (characteristic of bacterial DNA), lipopolysaccharide (components of bacterial cell walls) and double stranded RNA. Typically, the innate response will act against bacteria and parasitic invasion, as well as the presence of tumor molecules. During the innate response, inflammatory molecules (cytokines) are released, which have a significant effect on a subsequent adaptive immune response.

An adaptive response (i.e., one that is specifically directed to a known antigen or antigens) is humoral and cellular in its nature. It is based on the concept that self can be distinguished from non-self, and is highly specific. A pool of B and T lymphocytes, each with a unique non-self receptor, continuously circulates through the blood and lymph systems, awaiting exposure to the appropriate antigen. Activation of the adaptive immune response is primarily mediated through T cells and requires T cell receptor binding to the antigen presented on major histocompatibility complex (MHC) molecules and a co-stimulatory second signal. There are two classes of MHC molecules. MHC I molecules are present on the surface of all nucleated cells and present peptides derived from the products of degradation of intracellular proteins to CD8+ (cytotoxic) T cells. MHC II molecules are expressed on the surface of antigen presenting cells (APCs), which process and present antigens originating from outside the APC to CD4+ (helper) T cells. APCs also provide for the activation of T cells, which then enter a phase of clonal expansion that is further amplified by the autocrine and paracrine effects of cytokines such as interleukin-2 and interferon. During proliferation, T cell effector cells emerge and mediate the response of adaptive immunity.

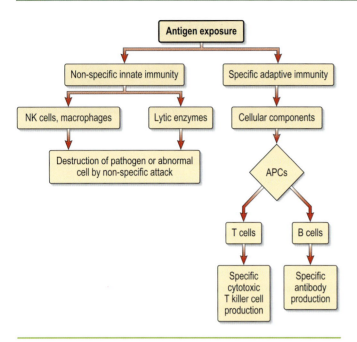

Figure 8.1 Simplified diagram of immune response.

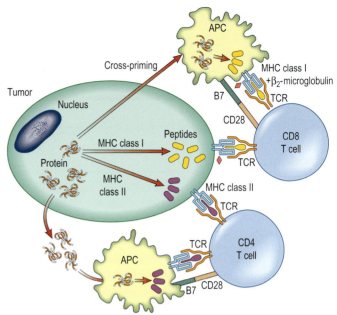

Figure 8.2 Tumor antigen presentation to APCs (From Dietrich PY, Walker, P.R., Calzascia, T., de Tribolet, N., Immunology of brain tumors and implications for immuotherapy. In: Kaye, AH and Laws, ER, eds. Brain Tumors: An Encyclopedic Approach (2nd edition). London: Churchill Livingstone; 2001. 135–150. With permission of Elsevier).

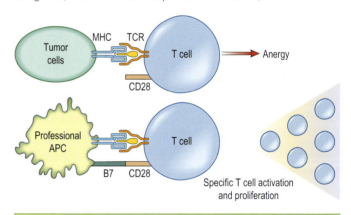

Figure 8.3 The key role of co-stimulatory molecules in T cell activation (From Dietrich PY, Walker, P.R., Calzascia, T., de Tribolet, N., Immunology of brain tumors and implications for immuotherapy. In: Kaye, AH and Laws, ER, eds. Brain Tumors: An Encyclopedic Approach (2nd edition). London: Churchill Livingstone; 2001. 135–150. With permission of Elsevier).

A humoral response involves the production of specific antibodies by plasma cells (which are derived from B cells), although this is likely to have only a minor role against CNS tumors. A cellular response involves helper T cells (CD4+) cells and cytotoxic T cells (CD8+), as well as NKT cells. Much of this cellular response is orchestrated by APCs, the most productive being dendritic cells, which phagocytose antigens and present them to effector cells on their surface in conjunction with surface markers. Integral to this process is the involvement of MHC molecules, present on the surface of cells. This co-stimulation is required for an effective T cell response. Antigen-specific T cell clonal activation requires two signals, first the interaction between the antigen-MHC complex with the T cell receptor, and second, T cell activation, which is provided by the co-stimulatory molecules, allowing for an effective response including further cytokine production, cellular proliferation and cytotoxicity.

Dendritic cells (DCs), which comprise less than 1% of the circulating white blood cell population, are potent antigen presenting cells (APCs) (Parajuli et al 2007) and are central to the regulation, maturation and maintenance of the cellular and humoral immune response. DCs acquire antigens by a variety of mechanisms, which are then processed and presented on the cell surface together with MHC I and II molecules, leading to activation of CD8+ and CD4+ T cells, as well as natural killer (NK) and NKT cells. NK and NKT cells are important in that they can eliminate cellular targets that have reduced MHC expression, which otherwise allows such cells (including glioma cells) to normally escape T cell recognition. The central role of APCs in the processing of tumor antigens and the subsequent stimulation of an effective T cell response are well illustrated in Figures 8.2 and 8.3 (from Dietrich et al 2001).

Once the non-self antigen has been cleared, the adaptive response self-limits with effector cells undergoing programmed cell death, while leaving behind long-term memory cells to ensure the ability to rapidly react should the antigen be encountered subsequently.

Although the CNS is thought not to be strictly 'immune privileged', others have used the term 'immune quiescent' to describe the brain (Yang et al 2006). There is a relative inability within the CNS to initiate an immune response due to the presence of the blood brain barrier which limits the transport of antibodies and cells into the brain parenchyma, the presence of a high concentration of immunoregulatory factors, the absence of lymphoid tissue and drainage and the lack of cellular MHC expression on normal parenchymal cells within the CNS, although the CNS immune environment is available to immune surveillance and the generation of appropriate responses (Hickey 2001).

Immune responses to malignant glioma

The emergence of a tumor may be considered a failure of the immune system. In this context, it is clear that effective antitumor cell-mediated immune responses are not generated in patients with glioma. Multiple factors are likely to play a role in preventing an effective antitumor immune response (Box 8.1).

A range of immunological defects have been reported in astrocytoma patients, including abnormal delayed type hypersensitivity responses and impaired T cell cytotoxicity (Brooks et al 1977; Brooks et al 1976; Dix et al 1999; Elliott et al 1987; Roszman et al 1982; Roszman et al 1985; Young et al 1976). This situation normalizes after tumor resection and then declines again with recurrence of the tumor (Dix et al 1999). Despite the obvious immune defects seen in patients with these tumors, gliomas are infiltrated with lymphocytosis in situ to varying degrees (Palma et al 1978; von Hanwehr et al 1984). There is evidence of an immune response to malignant gliomas, given the presence of T cell clones with antitumor activity, the presence of oligoclonal T cells infiltrating tumors, and the identification of glioma antigens that elicit specific immune responses. However, the immune response is largely ineffective. One of the reasons is that it appears that glioma-infiltrating cytotoxic T cells are inactivated (Black et al 1992).

Cancer cells are masters of disguise and deceit, and achieve this by a number of mechanisms, including downregulation of MHC expression, downregulation of tumor antigens, lack of co-stimulatory molecules on the surface of tumor cells, production of immunosuppressive cytokines, induction of lymphocyte apoptosis and altered dendritic cell function. Specifically for glioma patients, T cell and dendritic cell function is abnormal, and the presence of immunoregulatory cells also hinders an effective response. Glioma cells also have a tendency to actively avoid immune detection (Wiendl et al 2003; Wischhusen et al 2005). In addition, immunosenescence may play a role, in that effective immune responses are less likely in elderly people. This may be one of the factors that explains the increased incidence of these tumors with age (Derhovanessian et al 2008; Wheeler et al 2003).

As mentioned above, immune reactions do occur within the CNS and gliomas also express tumor-associated antigens (Parney et al 2000). These antigens provide a potential stimulus for antiglioma immunity. Although gliomas express tumor-associated antigens, their ability to present these antigens to T cells is controversial. This may relate to their MHC expression. Gliomas are likely to express low levels of class I MHC markers (Miyagi et al 1990; Saito et al 1988). Although MHC I expression can elicit killer cytotoxic T cell stimulation, a far more effective immune response requires the helper T cells. Unlike cytotoxic (CD8+) T cells, helper (CD4+) T cells require class II MHC expression for antigen presentation. Class II molecules are generally expressed by professional antigen presenting cells (Ni & O'Neill 1997). Within the CNS, microglia are the usual class II MHC positive cells (Gehrmann et al 1995; Theele and Streit 1993). Microglia and macrophages are present in increased numbers within human gliomas in situ (Fischer & Reichmann 2001; Leung et al 1997; Roggendorf et al 1996; Rossi et al 1987). However, the absence of antiglioma immunity suggests that these microglia are not functioning as effective immunostimulating cells. Indeed, it is possible that they may be subverted by the tumor into secreting factors that support glioma growth (Mantovani et al 1992).

Glioma cells themselves are poor antigen presenting cells (APCs), since they downregulate the co-stimulatory molecules that are required for activating the immune system (Wintterle et al 2003), and secrete immunosuppressive proteins such as TGF-beta, VEGF and IL-10 (De Vleeschouwer et al 2007; McVicar et al 1992; Naumov et al 2006; Schneider et al 2006). Gliomas have also been shown to secrete IL-6 and IL-8 which can stimulate microglia/macrophages. This may explain the increased numbers of these cells within gliomas. IL-10, secreted by microglia, however, can induce glioma proliferation and migration (Huettner et al 1997). Hence, gliomas may act to subvert inflammatory cells into proglioma functions, perhaps explaining why patients with increased inflammatory cell infiltrates appear to have a worse prognosis (Black et al 1992).

In glioma patients, defects in T cell function include peripheral T cell apoptosis and lymphopenia, impaired T cell responses, inactivation of tumor infiltrating lymphocytes (TILs), probably secondary to glioma derived immunoinhibitory factors including TGF-beta and prostaglandin E, and apoptosis of TILs (Walker et al 2006). Myeloid suppressor cells are also known to infiltrate tumors, and via their secretion of nitric oxide and arginase, induce T cell anergy (Carpentier & Meng 2006). Secretion of prostaglandin E2 (PGE2) appears to induce arginase production by macrophages (Rodriguez et al 2005). It has also been demonstrated that there are changes in the subpopulations of dendritic cells in glioma patients with accumulation of a population of immature cells with poor immunologic function, which may be associated with increased immunodeficiency observed in cancer patients, including those with malignant glioma (Pinzon-Charry et al 2005).

There appears to be an increased population of immunoregulatory T cells (CD4+/CD25+) in cancer patients including those with malignant glioma (Fecci et al 2006; Grauer et al 2007; Sakaguchi 2005). These cells have an important role normally to suppress the immune response and hence avoid autoimmune reactions. However, in excess, they also suppress anti-tumor immunity and their depletion may enhance natural tumor immunosurveillance (El Andaloussi and Lesniak 2006; Waziri et al 2008).

Recent evidence has also identified expression of lectin-like transcript-1 by glioma cells, a molecule which acts to inhibit NK cell function and which also appears to be upregulated by TGF-beta (Roth et al 2007). In addition, several studies such as those by Mitchell et al (2008b), have shown that human cytomegalovirus (HCMV) can be detected in most if not all malignant gliomas. Since HMCV is known to downregulate the immunogenicity of infected cells through inhibition of antigen presentation, downregulation of surface MHC expression, elaboration of TGF-beta from infected cells, and secretion of a viral interleukin 10 homologue (Hengel et al 1998; Kossmann et al 2003; Reddehase 2000), HCMV may contribute to immune evasion of malignant glioma cells (Mitchell et al 2008b).

Tumor antigens (Box 8.2)

The existence of surface antigens on tumor cells that can be recognized by the immune system is central to the idea that the immune system can be manipulated to differentiate tumor cells from their normal counterparts and ultimately help eliminate these tumor cells. Since their original description, numerous tumor antigens have been characterized including those in astrocytomas. They may be potential targets for immunotherapies. Inevitably, the immune responses generated have been ineffective, probably for a combination of reasons, including the fact that tumor antigens are often similar to antigens present on normal cells.

Tumor specific responses have been confirmed by the identification of immunogenic tumor associated antigens (TAAs) across a broad range of cancers. TAAs can arise from any protein expressed in the tumor cell and have their origin in the mutations and aberrant expression that accompany cell transformation. TAAs may represent unique tumor antigens that are specific to a single tumor type (e.g., point mutations, translocations), shared tumor antigens that appear on a number of tumor types but not normal tissue (e.g., ras and p53 mutations, MAGE genes) and antigens that exist in normal tissues but are overexpressed in tumor cells. Tumor antigens are usually classified as one of either: (1) differentiation antigens, (2) the products of viral, mutated, differentially spliced or overexpressed genes, or (3) metabolic pathway proteins.

Previously identified glioma antigens include epidermal growth factor receptor family, in particular the mutated form commonly identified in malignant glioma EGFRvIII, tenascin-C, squamous cell carcinoma antigen recognized by T cells 1 (SART-1), survivin, gp240 glycoprotein (Kurpad et al 1995) and members of the melanoma associated antigens (reviewed in Skog 2006). Among differentiation antigens in glioma, the melanoma-antigen-encoding genes such as MAGE-1, have been shown to be expressed in glioma (Sasaki et al 2001).

Recent evidence has shown that there is a strong association between human cytomegalovirus (HCMV) and glioma (Mitchell et al 2008b). Regardless of the potential role of HMCV in the pathogenesis of glioma, the expression of HMCV proteins may provide an opportunity to target these virally-encoded antigens as a target for cell immunotherapy, especially given the relative ease of eliciting an immune response against viral antigens in contrast to the difficulty of immunization against 'self' tumor antigens.

Despite the theoretical attraction of identifying specific antigen targets, the heterogeneous nature of gliomas may make targeting a single antigen problematic. Indeed, within tumors, non-neoplastic cells have important roles in glioma progression (Zhang et al 2005) and may need to be considered when planning and rationale approach to immunological treatments.

Approaches to immunotherapy (Box 8.3)

Until recently, immunotherapy has provided only modest improvements in outcomes for many cancers. However, the hope remains that immunotherapy can specifically seek out and remove tumor cells, while sparing normal cells. Indeed, the results of recent trials have been far more promising than earlier attempts at immunotherapy for cancer, including malignant glioma.

Passive immunotherapy involves the transfer of immune effectors to seek an immediate impact. Most involve the transfer of tumor-specific antibodies or T cells activated against the tumor. Passive measures may be short-lived however. Active immunotherapy attempts to upregulate a potential immune response to tumor. Active measures theoretically confer long-term immunity against future recurrences.

Passive immunotherapy

Monoclonal antibodies have been used to target specific tumor antigens to cause glioma cell destruction (reviewed in

---

Box 8.2 Tumor antigens in malignant glioma

DIFFERENTIATION ANTIGENS

- MAGE family
- Survivin

ABNORMAL PROTEIN EXPRESSION

- EGFRvIII
- HCMV
- Tenascin
- Gp240 glycoprotein

OVEREXPRESSION OF PROTEINS OF METABOLIC PATHWAY

- Ras
- P53

Box 8.3 Approaches to immunotherapy for malignant glioma

PASSIVE IMMUNOTHERAPY

- Monoclonal antibody delivery
  - Toxin- or radiolabeled monoclonal antibody
- Adoptive T cell transfer

ACTIVE IMMUNOTHERAPY

- Non-specific
  - Systemic and local cytokine delivery
  - Mimicry-induced 'autoimmunity', e.g., CpG oligonucleotides
- Specific
  - Peptide vaccines
  - Dendritic cell vaccines

Gerber & Laterra 2007). Binding of the antibody can lead to cell death through lysis (antibody dependent cellular cytotoxicity) or they may serve as the delivery system for a tumoricidal compound conjugated to the antibody. For example, locally injected 131-I labeled antitenascin antibodies have shown potential in preliminary studies (Reardon et al 2002). This approach may be more effective when used in combination with standard external beam radiotherapy and temozolomide chemotherapy (Bartolomei et al 2004; Reardon et al 2008).

Monoclonal antibodies have also been conjugated with diphtheria and *Pseudomonas* toxins, and these conjoint proteins have been delivered locally by convection enhanced delivery (reviewed in Yang et al 2006). Although phase III trials have been conducted (PRECISE and TRANSMID trials), no survival benefit has been demonstrated at this point. A recent study has also explored the use of immunonanoshells for targeted photothermal therapy (Bernardi et al 2008). In brief, 'nanoshells' are small particles with a silica core of approximately 100 nm and a gold shell of 10 nm that absorb light at a wavelength of 800 nm, which can be delivered externally, thereby creating heat and destroying any nearby cells. The nanoshells can be coated with antibodies designed to target glioma cells. Although an interesting concept, this theoretical approach is likely to be limited practically when applied to clinical scenarios by several factors including which molecular target might be appropriate and also how the immunonanoshells can be delivered to the tumor itself.

Adoptive cell transfer

Another form of passive immunotherapy is adoptive cell transfer (ACT), which is based on the idea that immune cells can be isolated from patients with a tumor, expanded *in vitro* and readministered to mediate a tumor-specific response. There is a good rationale for adoptive cell therapy, since it aims to deliver a large number of highly specific cells with high avidity for tumor cells which can be programmed and activated *in vitro* to have anti-tumor functions (Schumacher & Restifo 2009). T cell infusion can also be preceded by 'conditioning' of the patient by lymphodepletion via chemotherapy or total body irradiation, thus enabling the diminution of immunosuppressive factors and cells prior to infusion of tumor-specific T cells (Dudley et al 2002).

Although ACT has been successful in the treatment of some patients with metastatic melanoma (Rosenberg & Dudley 2009), this has not been the case for malignant glioma thus far. ACT has been used to administer autologous immune cells from the tumor site (Young et al 1977) and lymphokine activated killer cells stimulated with IL-2 (Sankhla et al 1996). Both approaches showed no clear benefit. More recently, irradiated tumor cells exposed to GM-CSF have been administered subcutaneously and T cells harvested from draining lymph nodes. These cells were then expanded *in vitro* and activated with bacterial superantigen, anti-CD3 and IL-2, and then re-administered peripherally with promising early results (Plautz et al 2000). More recent evidence in an animal model from this group suggests that host lymphodepletion increases T cell responses and that CD4+ as well as CD8+ cells have important roles in this approach (Wang et al 2007; Wang et al 2005). The recent identification of human cytomegalovirus (HCMV) in malignant glioma (Mitchell et al 2008b) may imply that HCMV antigens could be appropriate targets in ACT therapy.

Non-specific active immunotherapy

Early attempts at non-specific active immunotherapy were aimed at generating a generalized stimulation of the immune system that might lead to an increased immune response against tumor. In this context, BCG and toxoplasma have been used but have not been shown to be effective (Conley 1980; Mahaley et al 1983). Systemic and local administration of cytokines such as IL-2 have been used without benefit but with toxicity from cerebral edema (Merchant et al 1990; Merchant et al 1992). A recent preclinical study has suggested that IL-21 may be more effective than IL-2 or IL-12 (Daga et al 2007). Other methods for non-specific active immunotherapy have included cytidine-phosphate-guanosine (CpG) oligonucleotides (Carpentier et al 2006), without great success, although a recent preclinical study showed promising results when CpG oligonucleotides were used together with tumor cell lysate as a vaccine (Wu et al 2007). Chiocca et al (Chiocca et al 2008) have described a phase I trial in which an adenoviral vector was used to provide local delivery of interferon-β, and although apoptosis could be demonstrated within the tumor in a dose-dependent fashion, clinical outcome did not appear to be improved.

As described earlier, an association between the immune system and malignant glioma is strongly suggested by the observations of a decreased incidence of these tumors in patients with a history of allergy or autoimmune disease (Linos et al 2007) and also a surprisingly good outcome in patients with these tumors after intracranial infection (Bowles & Perkins 1999; Walker and Pamphlett 1999). These results raise the possibility that molecular mimicry-induced 'autoimmunity' can be employed to treat tumors, and that self-tolerance to tumors may be broken by cross-reactivity against a foreign antigen (Stathopoulos et al 2008). A recent study in an animal model has used the principle of immune-based allorecognition and administration of syngeneic tumor antigen for treatment of malignant glioma (Stathopoulos et al 2008).

An interesting approach may also be to use neural stem cells to provide antitumor stimulation of the immune system (reviewed in Yu et al 2006). Neural stem cells have a strong tendency to migrate to areas of pathology within the CNS, including brain tumors, and in a preclinical study neural stem cells were engineered to secrete IL-12, and then injected into brains of mice with gliomas. Increased infiltration of the tumors with lymphocytes and improved outcomes were demonstrated (Ehtesham et al 2002). In addition, cancer stem cells, which are thought to be a likely source of tumor cells themselves (Singh et al 2003), may themselves be a target for immune therapies (Skog 2006).

Specific active immunotherapy: tumor vaccines

This approach is based on the idea that tumor antigens presented in the context of an adjuvant or other stimulant may induce the immune system to generate an effective immune response against the tumor. A variety of strategies have been employed, including vaccination with an identified tumor associated antigen, and those that use either whole cells or components of whole cells. Tumor antigens include purified peptides, whole proteins and naked DNA encoding for the protein, all administered with an immune adjuvant or immunostimulatory cytokine such as GM-CSF. Whole cell strategies seek to increase the innate immunogenicity of tumor cells through a variety of mechanisms (Waldron & Parsa 2005). Immunogene strategies have also been utilized (Glick 2001; Okada et al 2001).

Several trials of peptide-based immunotherapy for cancer have been conducted in the past decade, but early results were disappointing (Rosenberg et al 2004). More personalized peptide vaccination strategies may be more effective (Yajima et al 2005), particularly when combined with chemotherapy (Sampson et al 2008).

Dendritic cell vaccination

As detailed above, DCs are blood-derived leukocytes that are involved in immune surveillance, antigen capture and antigen presentation. In brief, to create a DC vaccine, DCs are generated *in vitro* from autologous blood monocytes, and are then pulsed with tumor antigens, exposed to maturation stimuli, and then administered to the patient. Typically 1–10 million DCs are given via intradermal injection with the aim of stimulating T cells directed toward the tumor itself. Various sites of injection have been employed and typically the vaccine is given every 1–2 weeks over a variable length of time. DCs have also been injected intratumorally (Yamanaka et al 2005). Dendritic cell (DC) vaccines directly manipulate the presentation of antigens to immune cells.

Advances in recent years have allowed for the efficient isolation, maturation and expansion of dendritic cells *in vitro*. A variety of strategies have been used to generate DC vaccines, including use of peptides eluted from tumor cultures, tumor cell lysates, fusion of irradiated tumor cells with DCs, and transfection of DCs with tumor DNA, RNA or peptide, as well as transfection of the DCs with stimulatory cytokines along with antigenic loading (Nestle et al 1998; Rutkowski et al 2004; Yamanaka et al 2003; Yu et al 2004). Most investigators now believe that tumor lysate is the most effective source of antigens for exposure to DCs in making DC vaccines.

One factor that may limit the effectiveness of DC vaccines, which otherwise may be systemically effective, is the intrinsic immunosuppressive factors in the tumor microenvironment (Parajuli et al 2007). One way of overcoming this is to use immunotherapy in conjunction with other treatments and when the tumor burden is at a minimum. Studies have employed techniques to eliminate regulatory T cells by inhibiting TGF-beta (Friese et al 2004; Jachimczak et al 1993; Liu et al 2007), including in clinical studies (Fakhrai et al 2006). A recent preclinical study demonstrated that elimination of regulatory T cells was essential for effective DC vaccination (Grauer et al 2008).

It has been suggested that effector 'exhaustion' is a significant mechanism underlying the ineffectiveness of current immunotherapy strategies and that mechanisms to counteract tumor-induced tolerance may be important (Overwijk et al 2003; Staveley-O'Carroll et al 1998). In-keeping with this, counteracting the production of PGE2 by glioma cells (which induces arginase production by MSCs and therefore T cell anergy), using cyclooxygenase-2 inhibi-

tors has potential relevance (Rodriguez et al 2005). Others have suggested that small molecule inhibitors of STAT3 may result in immune stimulation in glioma (Hussain et al 2007).

Early results

In glioma studies, dendritic cell vaccines have proven safe and efficacious in animal studies (Heimberger et al 2000; Liau et al 1999; Yamanaka et al 2001; Zhu et al 2005). In a preliminary clinical study using a dendritic cell vaccine generated by exposure to tumor peptides, the safety and bioactivity of the approach was demonstrated (Yu et al 2001). Several groups have published their early results of dendritic cell vaccine (Kikuchi et al 2004; Kikuchi et al 2001; Liau et al 2005; Okada et al 2001; Rutkowski et al 2004; Wheeler et al 2008; Yamanaka et al 2003; Yu et al 2001). In brief, this treatment was shown to be safe with a low incidence of adverse effects.

We have recently published the results of our own experience with DC vaccination (Walker et al 2008). During the study period, 13 patients were enrolled. Nine of these completed the priming phase of six vaccinations. Of the four that failed to complete priming (receiving 2, 4, 4 and 5 vaccinations, respectively), three were withdrawn due to early tumor progression, and one withdrew for personal reasons. Nine patients tumors were graded as glioblastoma multiforme (WHO grade IV) (2/9 recurrent) and four had anaplastic astrocytoma (WHO grade III) (3/4 recurrent). Eight patients were male, and the age of the patient group ranged from 25 to 71 years (mean 51 years). A total of 90 vaccinations were given throughout the study, ranging from 2 to 13 vaccinations in individual patients. There were no adverse events related to the vaccination process.

Of the nine patients that completed the priming phase of vaccination, eight survived beyond 9 months post-surgery; five survived 12 months, and two survived 18 months or longer. Overall, 9 of 13 patients survived for 9 months, 6 of 13 for 12 months, and 3 of 13 for 18 months or longer.

Tumor responses to subsequent adjuvant chemotherapy

Among the group of patients that completed priming vaccination, eight were subsequently treated with temozolomide chemotherapy. Of these, three had progressive disease but five showed an objective radiological response to treatment. One patient (DG12) showed a complete response, which persisted for 3 months. Among these eight patients, four had pre-vaccination temozolomide and two of these showed a response (one complete) to re-introduction of temozolomide post-vaccination. Three of four patients who had no pre-vaccination chemotherapy showed a radiological response to post-vaccination temozolomide.

Case studies

DG03 (Fig. 8.4)

This female patient was the first to be enrolled in the study. At presentation, she was 66 years old, and her initial presentation was of headache and left-sided weakness. She underwent a stereotactic craniotomy and macroscopic resection of a right parietal tumor (Fig. 8.4A). She made an uneventful recovery from surgery and her symptoms were resolved. The histology was consistent with glioblastoma multiforme (WHO grade IV). The patient elected not to undertake postoperative radiotherapy or chemotherapy.

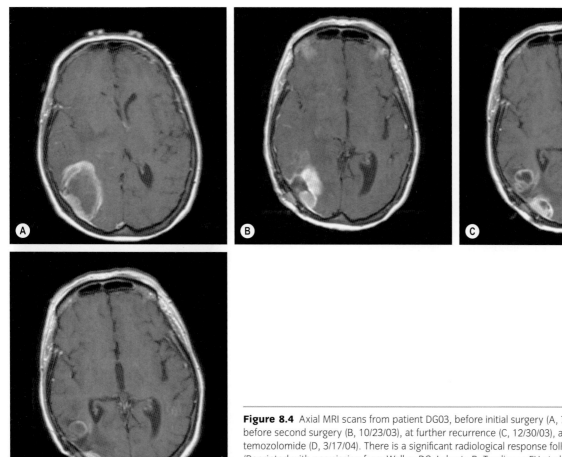

Figure 8.4 Axial MRI scans from patient DG03, before initial surgery (A, 7/29/03), at first recurrence before second surgery (B, 10/23/03), at further recurrence (C, 12/30/03), and after two cycles of temozolomide (D, 3/17/04). There is a significant radiological response following temozolomide. (Reprinted with permission from Walker DG, Laherty R, Tomlinson FH et al. Results of a phase I dendritic cell vaccine trial for malignant astrocytoma: potential interaction with adjuvant chemotherapy. J Clin Neurosci 2008;15:114–121).

Vaccinations commenced 3 weeks postoperatively and she completed the priming phase 12 weeks from that time. After the fourth vaccination, venepuncture was repeated for additional vaccine manufacture. A routine MRI scan after the sixth vaccination showed locally recurrent tumor (Fig. 8.4B), and this was resected. The patient resisted the suggestion of adjuvant therapy and elected not to undertake further vaccination. Two months later, a repeat MRI scan showed further local recurrence (Fig. 8.4C). Adjuvant temozolomide was given. Two 5-day courses at standard adjuvant dosage were given and this resulted in significant shrinkage of the residual tumor (Fig. 8.4D). The patient did not wish to have any further treatment. She eventually died secondary to progressive tumor 12 months after the original surgery.

DG12 (Fig. 8.5)
This 51-year-old female presented with focal neurological deficit 4 years prior to enrolment in our study. At the time, a left occipital lesion was resected macroscopically and histologically this was consistent with an anaplastic astrocytoma (WHO grade III/IV). Surgery was followed by postoperative radiotherapy (60 Gy) and 12 months of monthly adjuvant temozolomide. Prior to re-presentation, the patient experienced worsening visual field loss and an MRI scan showed local tumor recurrence. Further macroscopic resection was performed and the patient entered into the vaccine trial. Nine vaccinations were given in total.

Routine follow-up MRI scans showed local and regional tumor recurrence with diffuse enhancement extending into the ipsilateral temporal lobe, associated with T2-signal change 9 months after her second operation (Fig. 8.5A). Monthly temozolomide was re-introduced (Fig. 8.5B). After four treatments, a complete radiological response was seen, which persisted for 3 months (Fig. 8.5C). Extensive tumor recurrence occurred several months later and the patient died 25 months after entering the trial, and 16 months after the second recurrence.

Effectiveness of dendritic cell vaccination
De Vleeschouwer et al (2006) reviewed the results regarding DC vaccination for patients with malignant glioma. In 11 trials or case reports, over 120 patients had been treated with DC vaccination, using a variety of techniques of DC vaccine manufacture and delivery. Our series of 13 patients added to that growing literature (Walker et al 2008).

Overall, the safety of the treatment has been established (de Vleeschouwer et al 2006). Adverse events have been uncommon and those resulting in death or permanent neurological deficit have not been reported. In addition, immunological responses have consistently been documented (de Vleeschouwer et al 2006; Kikuchi et al 2001; Liau et al 2005). However, as discussed by de Vleeschouwer (2006), there has been criticism of cancer vaccination studies due to the perceived low rate of objective tumor responses (Rosenberg et al

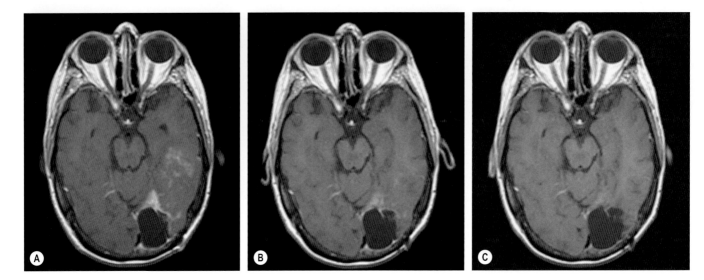

Figure 8.5 Axial MRI scans of patient DG12 after surgery and vaccination showing tumor recurrence (A, 10/5/05). Temozolomide chemotherapy was commenced and subsequent MRI scans showed regression (B, 11/29/05), and complete response (C, 1/30/06). (Reprinted with permission from Walker DG, Laherty R, Tomlinson FH et al. Results of a phase I dendritic cell vaccine trial for malignant astrocytoma: potential interaction with adjuvant chemotherapy. J Clin Neurosci 2008;15:114–121).

2004), yet traditional response criteria are unlikely to measure a beneficial effect of DC vaccination. Hence, overall survival benefit is likely to be of greatest use. Significantly improved survival has been demonstrated in renal cell carcinoma (Jocham et al 2004) and prostate carcinoma (Brower 2005) after treatment with DC vaccines. Early results of a phase III trial for melanoma performed at the Queensland Institute of Medical Research has also strongly suggested a beneficial effect (C. Schmidt, pers comm).

Wheeler et al (2008) have recently published a large trial of patients with GBM who were treated with a DC vaccine. Overall, this phase II trial confirmed the safety of this immunotherapy, and strongly suggested efficacy compared with standard therapy. There was also a strong correlation between documented immunological response to vaccination and survival. De Vleeschouwer et al (2008) have described the results of 56 patients with recurrent GBM treated with DC vaccination after repeat surgery with promising results. Extended survival in some patients was seen, especially those that were young and there was a strong correlation with extent of tumor resection.

DC vaccination has also been used in the context of priming of DCs with specific antigens. The recent confirmation that HCMV is present in most if not all malignant gliomas has led to one group targeting HCMV antigens by loading DCs with pp65-RNA (which codes for a HCMV protein) and delivering this DC vaccine to GBM patients (Mitchell et al 2008a). Early results have been promising, with a progression free survival in a small trial of greater than 12 months, and an overall survival of greater than 20 months.

Timing of vaccination and radiotherapy
In our original trial, consideration was given as to the possible negative interaction between DC vaccination and postoperative radiotherapy. It was decided that postoperative radiotherapy, may be deferred. This decision was made in consultation with the patient's wishes after discussing the pros and cons of postoperative radiotherapy.

Initially we believed there were theoretical reasons that might support delaying postoperative radiotherapy until after vaccination treatment, since ionizing radiation is lethal to T cells. Hence, any T cell response induced by vaccination occurring locally within the brain tumor might be nullified by external beam radiotherapy. Second, at the tissue level, radiotherapy results in obliteration of small blood vessels and hence we believed that this may have been counter-productive to the aims of the vaccine, i.e., since the effectiveness of the vaccine relies on blood–borne T cells invading the tumor and attacking tumor cells. By delaying radiotherapy, our belief was that the potential side-effects of radiotherapy would be deferred, the chances of the vaccine being efficacious would increase, and it was unlikely there would be any adverse effect on survival. We were unable to firmly support this concept, but our first patient did have a surprisingly good overall outcome, and response to subsequent temozolomide, despite not having postoperative radiotherapy. On balance however, radiotherapy is likely to be of benefit in conjunction with glioma vaccines, by ensuring minimal residual disease and increasing tumor cell death and therefore exposure of the immune system to tumor antigens.

Combination of chemotherapy and vaccination
The results of recent multicenter, randomized trials have strongly indicated that temozolomide, when given at a low dose throughout postoperative radiotherapy, followed by monthly temozolomide at a higher dose, leads to an improved outcome when compared with postoperative radiotherapy alone (Stupp et al 2005). Chemotherapy and immunotherapy have often been regarded as antagonistic forms of therapy, based primarily on two assumptions (Lake & Robinson 2005): first, that apoptosis produced by chemotherapy is nonstimulatory to the immune system, and second, that lymphopenia, a common side-effect of chemotherapy, has been assumed to be detrimental to an anti-tumor immune response. However, these assumptions are not likely to be valid, and in fact a large amount of recent data support the concept that

chemotherapy and immunotherapy combine effectively in cancer treatment (reviewed in Lake & Robinson 2005).

The advantages of chemotherapy in patients with malignant glioma who have already received DC vaccination have been noted by others. Wheeler et al (2004) retrospectively compared the survival and progression times of 25 vaccinated and 13 non-vaccinated *de novo* glioblastoma patients receiving chemotherapy. Vaccinated patients receiving subsequent chemotherapy exhibited significantly longer survival (42% 2-year survival) relative to patients receiving isolated vaccination or chemotherapy (8% 2-year survival for both groups). This group has suggested that a mechanism may be that vaccination targets TRP-2 tumor cells, making the remaining tumor cells more chemosensitive (Liu et al 2005). Another case of a child with recurrent malignant glioma has been described and had a surprisingly good outcome when temozolomide was combined with DC vaccination (De Vleeschouwer et al 2004). Recent results have also shown improved responses when DC vaccination is combined with temozolomide in a mouse model (Kim et al 2007).

The combination of vaccination and adjuvant chemotherapy appears attractive in the treatment of cancer in general. In other systems, chemotherapy and vaccination have been shown to combine effectively for the adjuvant treatment of cancers (Casati et al 2005; Dauer et al 2005). The combination of vaccination and traditional therapies has several theoretical advantages (Emens & Jaffee 2005; Lake & Robinson 2005):

1. Chemotherapy can combine with surgery and radiation to achieve a state of minimal residual disease, thus altering the balance of the disease burden and vaccine-induced T cell response in favor of the T cell. Patients with minimal residual disease are most appropriate for combining therapeutic cancer vaccines with traditional treatment modalities.

2. Chemotherapy can be used to groom the local tumor microenvironment to support a productive immune response.

3. Chemotherapy can globally alter immunoregulation within the host.

4. Chemotherapy produces a broader range of tumor antigens available.

5. Chemotherapy improves antigen presentation, by increased antigen cross-presentation (Nowak et al 2003a); partial activation of dendritic cells; priming of APCs for CD40 signal (Nowak et al 2003b), and killing subsets of APC (Nowak et al 2002).

6. Improved T cell response by lack of induction of tolerance by apoptotic tumor cells (Nowak et al 2003a), and lymphopenia-related proliferation increases tumor specific T cell response (Kaech et al 2003).

7. Partial sensitization of tumor cells to CTL lysis (Bergmann-Leitner and Abrams 2001; Yang and Haluska 2004).

8. Promotion of long-term antigen-independent memory (Wherry et al 2004).

9. Improved regulation including increased delivery of exogenous antigen (Nowak et al 2003a); increased CD4+ help (Nowak et al 2003b); reduction in function of negative regulatory cells (Ghiringhelli et al 2004; Polak and Turk 1974), and induction of homeostatic proliferation (Dudley et al 2002).

Timing of vaccination with respect to adjuvant chemotherapy

Post-chemotherapy delivery of vaccination may be more effective compared with pre-treatment (Lake & Robinson 2005), although in the series of Wheeler et al (2004), as well as in our previous patients (Walker et al 2008), chemotherapy followed vaccination. In addition, if immunotherapy is delayed following chemotherapy, all the benefits disappear. Hence in theory, a protocol in which immunotherapy immediately follows chemotherapy, probably in repeating cycles, might be most effective (Lake & Robinson 2005). The optimal timing of the therapies is not known, but as discussed by others (Lake & Robinson 2005) the important factors that may influence timing of vaccination for patients with malignant glioma:

1. It is clear that vaccination is most likely to be effective with minimal tumor burden, which is likely to be towards the end of radiotherapy. In an animal model, research from Lake's group in Perth, Australia, has suggested that partial rather than complete surgical removal of solid tumors leads to an improved response to DC vaccination (Broomfield et al 2005). Residual tumor presumably provides antigenic stimulation and in the case of malignant glioma may be relevant given that complete surgical removal is impossible.

2. Theoretically, T cells should be stimulated when tumor cells are being killed by adjuvant therapy, i.e., when tumor antigens are available subsequent to cell death. This is during the period of radiochemotherapy.

3. DC vaccination should probably be performed when intake of oral steroids is minimal. In the normal course of events, it is expected that steroid requirements would be minimal after completion of radiotherapy.

4. It has been assumed that chemotherapy-induced lymphopenia would inhibit the effectiveness of DC vaccination in cancer patients, but this has not been proven. Indeed, there are reasons to believe that vaccination during a period of recovery from lymphopenia is ideal, since the T cell population will be repopulated with those specific to tumor antigens in this context (Emens & Jaffee 2005).

A recent case report of a patient with malignant glioma treated with a peptide vaccine together with temozolomide has shown that the two therapies can be combined safely and that when vaccination is given during the nadir of temozolomide induced lymphopenia, there may be an enhanced cytotoxic T cell response and a lag in the recovery of regulatory T cells (Heimberger et al 2008). Sampson et al (2008) have recently published results of an EGFRvIII-specific peptide vaccine in patients with newly diagnosed, EGFRvIII+ GBM in combination with temozolomide chemotherapy with a median progression free survival of over 16 months. A phase III randomized study is currently underway. Thus chemotherapy can enhance subsequent responses to a variety of glioma vaccinations.

Key points

- The immune system recognizes and reacts to malignant glioma

- The immune response to malignant glioma is not effective

- A variety of tumor antigens represent potential targets to be used for immunotherapy, including EGFRvIII and HCMV

- Passive and active immunotherapy has been trialled against malignant glioma

- Immunization using tumor vaccines, including dendritic cell vaccines, has proven to be safe although efficacy is not yet proven

- Tumor vaccines are likely to be effective when used in combination with adjuvant chemotherapy.

REFERENCES

Bartolomei, M., Mazzetta, C., Handkiewicz-Junak, D., et al., 2004. Combined treatment of glioblastoma patients with locoregional pre-targeted 90Y-biotin radioimmunotherapy and temozolomide. Q. J. Nucl. Med. Mol. Imaging 48, 220–228.

Bergmann-Leitner, E.S., Abrams, S.I., 2001. Treatment of human colon carcinoma cell lines with anti-neoplastic agents enhances their lytic sensitivity to antigen-specific CD8+ cytotoxic T lymphocytes. Cancer Immunol. Immunother 50, 445–455.

Bernardi, R.J., Lowery, A.R., Thompson, P.A., et al., 2008. Immuno-nanoshells for targeted photothermal ablation in medulloblastoma and glioma: an in vitro evaluation using human cell lines. J. Neurooncol. 86, 165–172.

Black, K.L., Chen, K., Becker, D.P., et al., 1992. Inflammatory leukocytes associated with increased immunosuppression by glioblastoma. J. Neurosurg. 77, 120–126.

Bowles, A.P. Jr., Perkins, E., 1999. Long-term remission of malignant brain tumors after intracranial infection: a report of four cases. Neurosurgery 44, 636–642; discussion 642–633.

Brooks, W.H., Roszman, T.L., Mahaley, M.S., et al., 1977. Immunobiology of primary intracranial tumors. II. Analysis of lymphocyte subpopulations in patients with primary brain tumors. Clin. Exp. Immunol. 29, 61–66.

Brooks, W.H., Roszman, T.L., Rogers, A.S., 1976. Impairment of rosette-forming T lymphocytes in patients with primary intracranial tumors. Cancer 37, 1869–1873.

Broomfield, S., Currie, A., van der Most, R.G., et al., 2005. Partial, but not complete, tumor-debulking surgery promotes protective antitumor memory when combined with chemotherapy and adjuvant immunotherapy. Cancer Res. 65, 7580–7584.

Brower, V., 2005. Cancer vaccine field gets shot of optimism from positive results. Nat. Med. 11, 360.

Carpentier, A., Laigle-Donadey, F., Zohar, S., et al., 2006. Phase 1 trial of a CpG oligodeoxynucleotide for patients with recurrent glioblastoma. Neuro. Oncol. 8, 60–66.

Carpentier, A.F., Meng, Y., 2006. Recent advances in immunotherapy for human glioma. Curr. Opin. Oncol. 18, 631–636.

Casati, A., Zimmermann, V.S., Benigni, F., et al., 2005. The immunogenicity of dendritic cell-based vaccines is not hampered by doxorubicin and melphalan administration. J. Immunol. 174, 3317–3325.

Chiocca, E.A., Smith, K.M., McKinney, B., et al., 2008. A phase I trial of Ad.hIFN-beta gene therapy for glioma. Mol. Ther. 16, 618–626.

Conley, F.K., 1980. Influence of chronic Toxoplasma infection on ethylnitrosourea-induced central nervous system tumors in rats. Cancer Res. 40, 1240–1244.

Daga, A., Orengo, A.M., Gangemi, R.M., et al., 2007. Glioma immunotherapy by IL-21 gene-modified cells or by recombinant IL-21 involves antibody responses. Int. J. Cancer 121, 1756–1763.

Dauer, M., Herten, J., Bauer, C., et al., 2005. Chemosensitization of pancreatic carcinoma cells to enhance T cell-mediated cytotoxicity induced by tumor lysate-pulsed dendritic cells. J. Immunother 28, 332–342.

De Vleeschouwer, S., Fieuws, S., Rutkowski, S., et al., 2008. Postoperative adjuvant dendritic cell-based immunotherapy in patients with relapsed glioblastoma multiforme. Clin. Cancer Res. 14, 3098–3104.

de Vleeschouwer, S., Rapp, M., Sorg, R.V., et al., 2006. Dendritic cell vaccination in patients with malignant gliomas: current status and future directions. Neurosurgery 59, 988–999; discussion 999–1000.

De Vleeschouwer, S., Spencer Lopes, I., Ceuppens, J.L., et al., 2007. Persistent IL-10 production is required for glioma growth suppressive activity by Th1-directed effector cells after stimulation with tumor lysate-loaded dendritic cells. J. Neurooncol. 84, 131–140.

De Vleeschouwer, S., Van Calenbergh, F., Demaerel, P., et al., 2004. Transient local response and persistent tumor control in a child with recurrent malignant glioma: treatment with combination therapy including dendritic cell therapy. Case report. J. Neurosurg. 100, 492–497.

Derhovanessian, E., Solana, R., Larbi, A., et al., 2008. Immunity, ageing and cancer. Immun. Ageing 5, 11.

Dietrich, P.-Y., Walker, P.R., Calzascia, T., et al., 2001. Immunology of brain tumors and implications for immunotherapy. In: Kaye, A.H., Laws, E.R. Jr. (Eds.), Brain tumors: an encyclopedic approach, second ed. Churchill Livingstone, Edinburgh, pp. 135–150.

Dix, A.R., Brooks, W.H., Roszman, T.L., et al., 1999. Immune defects observed in patients with primary malignant brain tumors. J. Neuroimmunol 100, 216–232.

Dudley, M.E., Wunderlich, J.R., Robbins, P.F., et al., 2002. Cancer regression and autoimmunity in patients after clonal repopulation with antitumor lymphocytes. Science 298, 850–854.

Ehtesham, M., Kabos, P., Kabosova, A., et al., 2002. The use of interleukin 12-secreting neural stem cells for the treatment of intracranial glioma. Cancer Res. 62, 5657–5663.

El Andaloussi, A., Lesniak, M.S., 2006. An increase in CD4+CD25+FOXP3+ regulatory T cells in tumor-infiltrating lymphocytes of human glioblastoma multiforme. Neuro. Oncol. 8, 234–243.

Elliott, L.H., Brooks, W.H., Roszman, T.L., 1987. Activation of immunoregulatory lymphocytes obtained from patients with malignant gliomas. J. Neurosurg. 67, 231–236.

Emens, L.A., Jaffee, E.M., 2005. Leveraging the activity of tumor vaccines with cytotoxic chemotherapy. Cancer Res. 65, 8059–8064.

Fakhrai, H., Mantil, J.C., Liu, L., et al., 2006. Phase I clinical trial of a TGF-beta antisense-modified tumor cell vaccine in patients with advanced glioma. Cancer Gene Ther. 13, 1052–1060.

Fecci, P.E., Mitchell, D.A., Whitesides, J.F., et al., 2006. Increased regulatory T-cell fraction amidst a diminished CD4 compartment explains cellular immune defects in patients with malignant glioma. Cancer Res. 66, 3294–3302.

Fischer, H.G., Reichmann, G., 2001. Brain dendritic cells and macrophages/microglia in central nervous system inflammation. J. Immunol. 166, 2717–2726.

Friese, M.A., Wischhusen, J., Wick, W., et al., 2004. RNA interference targeting transforming growth factor-beta enhances NKG2D-mediated antiglioma immune response, inhibits glioma cell migration and invasiveness, and abrogates tumorigenicity in vivo. Cancer Res. 64, 7596–7603.

Gehrmann, J., Matsumoto, Y., Kreutzberg, G.W., 1995. Microglia: intrinsic immuneffector cell of the brain. Brain. Res. Brain Res. Rev. 20, 269–287.

Gerber, D.E., Laterra, J., 2007. Emerging monoclonal antibody therapies for malignant gliomas. Expert Opin. Investig. Drugs 16, 477–494.

Ghiringhelli, F., Larmonier, N., Schmitt, E., et al., 2004. CD4+CD25+ regulatory T cells suppress tumor immunity but are sensitive to cyclophosphamide which allows immunotherapy of established tumors to be curative. Eur. J. Immunol. 34, 336–344.

Glick, R.P., Lichtor, T., Cohen, E.P., 2001. Cytokine-based immunogene therapy for brain tumors. In: Liau, L.M., Becker, D.P., Cloughesy, T.F., et al. (eds). Brain tumor immunotherapy. Human Press, New Jersey, pp. 273–288.

Grauer, O.M., Nierkens, S., Bennink, E., et al., 2007. CD4+FoxP3+ regulatory T cells gradually accumulate in gliomas during tumor growth and efficiently suppress antiglioma immune responses in vivo. Int. J. Cancer 121, 95–105.

Grauer, O.M., Sutmuller, R.P., van Maren, W., et al., 2008. Elimination of regulatory T cells is essential for an effective vaccination with tumor lysate-pulsed dendritic cells in a murine glioma model. Int. J. Cancer 122, 1794–1802.

Heimberger, A.B., Crotty, L.E., Archer, G.E., et al., 2000. Bone marrow-derived dendritic cells pulsed with tumor homogenate induce immunity against syngeneic intracerebral glioma. J. Neuroimmunol 103, 16–25.

Heimberger, A.B., Sun, W., Hussain, S.F., et al., 2008. Immunological responses in a patient with glioblastoma multiforme treated with sequential courses of temozolomide and immunotherapy: case study. Neuro. Oncol. 10, 98–103.

Hengel, H., Brune, W., Koszinowski, U.H., 1998. Immune evasion by cytomegalovirus–survival strategies of a highly adapted opportunist. Trends Microbiol 6, 190–197.

Hickey, W.F., 2001. Basic principles of immunological surveillance of the normal central nervous system. Glia 36, 118–124.

Huettner, C., Czub, S., Kerkau, S., et al., 1997. Interleukin 10 is expressed in human gliomas in vivo and increases glioma cell proliferation and motility in vitro. AntiCancer Res. 17, 3217–3224.

Hussain, S.F., Kong, L.Y., Jordan, J., et al., 2007. A novel small molecule inhibitor of signal transducers and activators of transcription 3 reverses immune tolerance in malignant glioma patients. Cancer Res. 67, 9630–9636.

Jachimczak, P., Bogdahn, U., Schneider, J., et al., 1993. The effect of transforming growth factor-beta 2-specific phosphorothioate-anti-sense oligodeoxynucleotides in reversing cellular immunosuppression in malignant glioma. J. Neurosurg. 78, 944–951.

Jocham, D., Richter, A., Hoffmann, L., et al., 2004. Adjuvant autologous renal tumor cell vaccine and risk of tumor progression in patients with renal-cell carcinoma after radical nephrectomy: phase III, randomised controlled trial. Lancet 363, 594–599.

Kaech, S.M., Tan, J.T., Wherry, E.J., et al., 2003. Selective expression of the interleukin 7 receptor identifies effector CD8 T cells that give rise to long-lived memory cells. Nat. Immunol. 4, 1191–1198.

Kikuchi, T., Akasaki, Y., Abe, T., et al., 2004. Vaccination of glioma patients with fusions of dendritic and glioma cells and recombinant human interleukin 12. J. Immunother 27, 452–459.

Kikuchi, T., Akasaki, Y., Irie, M., et al., 2001. Results of a phase I clinical trial of vaccination of glioma patients with fusions of dendritic and glioma cells. Cancer Immunol. Immunother 50, 337–344.

Kim, C.H., Woo, S.J., Park, J.S., et al., 2007. Enhanced antitumor immunity by combined use of temozolomide and TAT-survivin pulsed dendritic cells in a murine glioma. Immunology 122, 615–622.

Kossmann, T., Morganti-Kossmann, M.C., Orenstein, J.M., et al., 2003. Cytomegalovirus production by infected astrocytes correlates with transforming growth factor-beta release. J. Infect. Dis. 187, 534–541.

Kurpad, S.N., Zhao, X.G., Wikstrand, C.J., et al., 1995. Tumor antigens in astrocytic gliomas. Glia 15, 244–256.

Lake, R.A., Robinson, B.W., 2005. Immunotherapy and chemotherapy – a practical partnership. Nat. Rev. Cancer 5, 397–405.

Leung, S.Y., Wong, M.P., Chung, L.P., et al., 1997. Monocyte chemoattractant protein-1 expression and macrophage infiltration in gliomas. Acta. Neuropathol. (Berl.) 93, 518–527.

Liau, L.M., Black, K.L., Prins, R.M., et al., 1999. Treatment of intracranial gliomas with bone marrow-derived dendritic cells pulsed with tumor antigens. J. Neurosurg. 90, 1115–1124.

Liau, L.M., Prins, R.M., Kiertscher, S.M., et al., 2005. Dendritic cell vaccination in glioblastoma patients induces systemic and intracranial T-cell responses modulated by the local central nervous system tumor microenvironment. Clin. Cancer Res. 11, 5515–5525.

Linos, E., Raine, T., Alonso, A., et al., 2007. Atopy and risk of brain tumors: a meta-analysis. J. Natl. Cancer Inst. 99, 1544–1550.

Liu, G., Akasaki, Y., Khong, H.T., et al., 2005. Cytotoxic T cell targeting of TRP-2 sensitizes human malignant glioma to chemotherapy. Oncogene 24, 5226–5234.

Liu, Y., Wang, Q., Kleinschmidt-DeMasters, B.K., et al., 2007. TGF-beta2 inhibition augments the effect of tumor vaccine and improves the survival of animals with pre-established brain tumors. J. Neurooncol. 81, 149–162.

Mahaley, M.S. Jr., Bigner, D.D., Dudka, L.F., et al., 1983. Immunobiology of primary intracranial tumors. Part 7: Active immunization of patients with anaplastic human glioma cells: a pilot study. J. Neurosurg. 59, 201–207.

Mantovani, A., Bottazzi, B., Colotta, F., et al., 1992. The origin and function of tumor-associated macrophages. Immunol. Today 13, 265–270.

McVicar, D.W., Davis, D.F., Merchant, R.E., 1992. In vitro analysis of the proliferative potential of T cells from patients with brain tumor: glioma-associated immunosuppression unrelated to intrinsic cellular defect. J. Neurosurg. 76, 251–260.

Merchant, R.E., Ellison, M.D., Young, H.F., 1990. Immunotherapy for malignant glioma using human recombinant interleukin-2 and activated autologous lymphocytes. A review of pre-clinical and clinical investigations. J. Neurooncol. 8, 173–188.

Merchant, R.E., McVicar, D.W., Merchant, L.H., et al., 1992. Treatment of recurrent malignant glioma by repeated intracerebral injections of human recombinant interleukin-2 alone or in combination with systemic interferon-alpha. Results of a phase I clinical trial. J. Neurooncol. 12, 75–83.

Mitchell, D.A., Archer, G.E., Bigner, D.D., et al., 2008a. Efficacy of a phase II vaccine targeting Cytomegalovirus antigens in newly diagnosed GBM. J. Clin. Oncol. 26, abstract 2042.

Mitchell, D.A., Xie, W., Schmittling, R., et al., 2008b. Sensitive detection of human cytomegalovirus in tumors and peripheral blood of patients diagnosed with glioblastoma. Neuro. Oncol. 10, 10–18.

Miyagi, K., Ingram, M., Techy, G.B., et al., 1990. Immunohistochemical detection and correlation between MHC antigen and cell-mediated immune system in recurrent glioma by APAAP method. Neurol. Med. Chir. (Tokyo) 30, 649–655.

Naumov, G.N., Bender, E., Zurakowski, D., et al., 2006. A model of human tumor dormancy: an angiogenic switch from the nonangiogenic phenotype. J. Natl. Cancer Inst. 98, 316–325.

Nestle, F.O., Alijagic, S., Gilliet, M., et al., 1998. Vaccination of melanoma patients with peptide- or tumor lysate-pulsed dendritic cells. Nat. Med. 4, 328–332.

Ni, K., O'Neill, H.C., 1997. The role of dendritic cells in T cell activation. Immunol. Cell. Biol. 75, 223–230.

Nowak, A.K., Lake, R.A., Marzo, A.L., et al., 2003a. Induction of tumor cell apoptosis in vivo increases tumor antigen cross-presentation, cross-priming rather than cross-tolerizing host tumor-specific CD8 T cells. J. Immunol. 170, 4905–4913.

Nowak, A.K., Robinson, B.W., Lake, R.A., 2002. Gemcitabine exerts a selective effect on the humoral immune response: implications for combination chemo-immunotherapy. Cancer Res. 62, 2353–2358.

Nowak, A.K., Robinson, B.W., Lake, R.A., 2003b. Synergy between chemotherapy and immunotherapy in the treatment of established murine solid tumors. Cancer Res. 63, 4490–4496.

Okada, H., Pollack, I.F., Lieberman, F., et al., 2001. Gene therapy of malignant gliomas: a pilot study of vaccination with irradiated autologous glioma and dendritic cells admixed with IL-4 transduced fibroblasts to elicit an immune response. Hum. Gene Ther. 12, 575–595.

Overwijk, W.W., Theoret, M.R., Finkelstein, S.E., et al., 2003. Tumor regression and autoimmunity after reversal of a functionally tolerant state of self-reactive CD8+ T cells. J. Exp. Med. 198, 569–580.

Palma, L., Di Lorenzo, N., Guidetti, B., 1978. Lymphocytic infiltrates in primary glioblastomas and recidivous gliomas. Incidence, fate, and relevance to prognosis in 228 operated cases. J. Neurosurg. 49, 854–861.

Parajuli, P., Mathupala, S., Mittal, S., et al., 2007. Dendritic cell-based active specific immunotherapy for malignant glioma. Expert. Opin. Biol. Ther. 7, 439–448.

Parney, I.F., Hao, C., Petruk, K.C., 2000. Glioma immunology and immunotherapy. Neurosurgery 46, 778–791.

Pinzon-Charry, A., Ho, C.S., Laherty, R., et al., 2005. A population of HLA-DR+ immature cells accumulates in the blood dendritic cell compartment of patients with different types of cancer. Neoplasia 7, 1112–1122.

Plautz, G.E., Miller, D.W., Barnett, G.H., et al., 2000. T cell adoptive immunotherapy of newly diagnosed gliomas. Clin. Cancer Res. 6, 2209–2218.

Polak, L., Turk, J.L., 1974. Reversal of immunological tolerance by cyclophosphamide through inhibition of suppressor cell activity. Nature 249, 654–656.

Reardon, D.A., Akabani, G., Coleman, R.E., et al., 2002. Phase II trial of murine (131)I-labeled antitenascin monoclonal antibody 81C6 administered into surgically created resection cavities of patients with newly diagnosed malignant gliomas. J. Clin. Oncol. 20, 1389–1397.

Reardon, D.A., Zalutsky, M.R., Akabani, G., et al., 2008. A pilot study: 131I-antitenascin monoclonal antibody 81c6 to deliver a 44-Gy resection cavity boost. Neuro. Oncol. 10, 182–189.

Reddehase, M.J., 2000. The immunogenicity of human and murine cytomegaloviruses. Curr. Opin. Immunol. 12, 390–396.

Rodriguez, P.C., Hernandez, C.P., Quiceno, D., et al., 2005. Arginase I in myeloid suppressor cells is induced by COX-2 in lung carcinoma. J. Exp. Med. 202, 931–939.

Roggendorf, W., Strupp, S., Paulus, W., 1996. Distribution and characterization of microglia/macrophages in human brain tumors. Acta. Neuropathol. (Berl.) 92, 288–293.

Rosenberg, S.A., Dudley, M.E., 2009. Adoptive cell therapy for the treatment of patients with metastatic melanoma. Curr. Opin. Immunol. 21, 233–240.

Rosenberg, S.A., Yang, J.C., Restifo, N.P., 2004. Cancer immunotherapy: moving beyond current vaccines. Nat. Med. 10, 909–915.

Rossi, M.L., Hughes, J.T., Esiri, M.M., et al., 1987. Immunohistological study of mononuclear cell infiltrate in malignant gliomas. Acta. Neuropathol. (Berl.) 74, 269–277.

Roszman, T.L., Brooks, W.H., Elliott, L.H., 1982. Immunobiology of primary intracranial tumors. VI. Suppressor cell function and lectin-binding lymphocyte subpopulations in patients with cerebral tumors. Cancer 50, 1273–1279.

Roszman, T.L., Brooks, W.H., Steele, C., et al., 1985. Pokeweed mitogen-induced immunoglobulin secretion by peripheral blood lymphocytes from patients with primary intracranial tumors. Characterization of T helper and B cell function. J. Immunol. 134, 1545–1550.

Roth, P., Mittelbronn, M., Wick, W., et al., 2007. Malignant glioma cells counteract antitumor immune responses through expression of lectin-like transcript-1. Cancer Res. 67, 3540–3544.

Rutkowski, S., De Vleeschouwer, S., Kaempgen, E., et al., 2004. Surgery and adjuvant dendritic cell-based tumor vaccination for patients with relapsed malignant glioma, a feasibility study. Br. J. Cancer 91, 1656–1662.

Saito, T., Tanaka, R., Yoshida, S., et al., 1988. Immunohistochemical analysis of tumor-infiltrating lymphocytes and major histocompatibility antigens in human gliomas and metastatic brain tumors. Surg. Neurol. 29, 435–442.

Sakaguchi, S., 2005. Naturally arising Foxp3-expressing CD25+CD4+ regulatory T cells in immunological tolerance to self and non-self. Nat. Immunol. 6, 345–352.

Sampson, J.H., Archer, G.E., Bigner, D.D., et al., 2008. Effect of EGFRvIII-targeted vaccine (CDX-110) on immune response and TTP when given with simultaneous standard and continuous temozolomide in patients with GBM. J. Clin. Oncol. 26, abstract 2011.

Sankhla, S.K., Nadkarni, J.S., Bhagwati, S.N., 1996. Adoptive immunotherapy using lymphokine-activated killer (LAK) cells and interleukin-2 for recurrent malignant primary brain tumors. J. Neurooncol. 27, 133–140.

Sasaki, M., Nakahira, K., Kawano, Y., et al., 2001. MAGE-E1, a new member of the melanoma-associated antigen gene family and its expression in human glioma. Cancer Res. 61, 4809–4814.

Schiff, D., O'Neill, B., Wijdicks, E., et al., 2001. Gliomas arising in organ transplant recipients: an unrecognized complication of transplantation? Neurology 57, 1486–1488.

Schneider, T., Sailer, M., Ansorge, S., et al., 2006. Increased concentrations of transforming growth factor beta1 and beta2 in the plasma of patients with glioblastoma. J. Neurooncol. 79, 61–65.

Schumacher, T.N., Restifo, N.P., 2009. Adoptive T cell therapy of cancer. Curr. Opin. Immunol. 21, 187–189.

Singh, S.K., Clarke, I.D., Terasaki, M., et al., 2003. Identification of a cancer stem cell in human brain tumors. Cancer Res. 63, 5821–5828.

Skog, J., 2006. Glioma-specific antigens for immune tumor therapy. Expert Rev. Vaccines 5, 793–802.

Stathopoulos, A., Samuelson, C., Milbouw, G., et al., 2008. Therapeutic vaccination against malignant gliomas based on allorecognition and syngeneic tumor antigens: proof of principle in two strains of rat. Vaccine 26, 1764–1772.

Staveley-O'Carroll, K., Sotomayor, E., Montgomery, J., et al., 1998. Induction of antigen-specific T cell anergy: An early event in the course of tumor progression. Proc. Natl. Acad. Sci. USA 95, 1178–1183.

Stupp, R., Mason, W.P., van den Bent, M.J., et al., 2005. Radiotherapy plus concomitant and adjuvant temozolomide for glioblastoma. National Cancer Institute of Canada Clinical Trials Group. N. Engl. J. Med. 352 (10), 987–996.

Theele, D.P., Streit, W.J., 1993. A chronicle of microglial ontogeny. Glia 7, 5–8.

von Hanwehr, R.I., Hofman, F.M., Taylor, C.R., et al., 1984. Mononuclear lymphoid populations infiltrating the microenvironment of primary CNS tumors. Characterization of cell subsets with monoclonal antibodies. J. Neurosurg. 60, 1138–1147.

Waldron, J., Parsa, A.T., 2005. Immunotherapy. In: Berger, M.S., Prados, M. (Eds.), Textbook of neuro-oncology. Elsevier Saunders, Philadelphia, pp. 87–92.

Walker, D.G., Chuah, T., Rist, M.J., et al., 2006. T-cell apoptosis in human glioblastoma multiforme: implications for immunotherapy. J. Neuroimmunol. 175, 59–68.

Walker, D.G., Laherty, R., Tomlinson, F.H., et al., 2008. Results of a phase I dendritic cell vaccine trial for malignant astrocytoma: potential interaction with adjuvant chemotherapy. J. Clin. Neurosci. 15, 114–121.

Walker, D.G., Pamphlett, R., 1999. Prolonged survival and pulmonary metastasis after local cure of glioblastoma multiforme. J. Clin. Neurosci. 6, 67–68.

Wang, L.X., Shu, S., Disis, M.L., et al., 2007. Adoptive transfer of tumor-primed, in vitro-activated, CD4+ T effector cells (TEs) combined with CD8+ TEs provides intratumoral TE proliferation and synergistic antitumor response. Blood 109, 4865–4876.

Wang, L.X., Shu, S., Plautz, G.E., 2005. Host lymphodepletion augments T cell adoptive immunotherapy through enhanced intratumoral proliferation of effector cells. Cancer Res. 65, 9547–9554.

Waziri, A., Killory, B., Ogden, A.T., 3rd, et al., 2008. Preferential in situ CD4+CD56+ T cell activation and expansion within human glioblastoma. J. Immunol. 180, 7673–7680.

Wheeler, C.J., Black, K.L., Liu, G., et al., 2008. Vaccination elicits correlated immune and clinical responses in glioblastoma multiforme patients. Cancer Res. 68, 5955–5964.

Wheeler, C.J., Black, K.L., Liu, G., et al., 2003. Thymic CD8+ T cell production strongly influences tumor antigen recognition and age-dependent glioma mortality. J. Immunol. 171, 4927–4933.

Wheeler, C.J., Das, A., Liu, G., et al., 2004. Clinical responsiveness of glioblastoma multiforme to chemotherapy after vaccination. Clin. Cancer Res. 10, 5316–5326.

Wherry, E.J., Barber, D.L., Kaech, S.M., et al., 2004. Antigen-independent memory CD8 T cells do not develop during chronic viral infection. Proc. Natl. Acad. Sci. USA 101, 16004–16009.

Wiendl, H., Mitsdoerffer, M., Weller, M., 2003. Hide-and-seek in the brain: a role for HLA-G mediating immune privilege for glioma cells. Semin. Cancer Biol. 13, 343–351.

Wigertz, A., Lonn, S., Schwartzbaum, J., et al., 2007. Allergic conditions and brain tumor risk. Am. J. Epidemiol. 166, 941–950.

Wintterle, S., Schreiner, B., Mitsdoerffer, M., et al., 2003. Expression of the B7-related molecule B7-H1 by glioma cells: a potential mechanism of immune paralysis. Cancer Res. 63, 7462–7467.

Wischhusen, J., Schneider, D., Mittelbronn, M., et al., 2005. Death receptor-mediated apoptosis in human malignant glioma cells: modulation by the CD40/CD40L system. J. Neuroimmunol. 162, 28–42.

Wu, A., Oh, S., Gharagozlou, S., et al., 2007. In vivo vaccination with tumor cell lysate plus CpG oligodeoxynucleotides eradicates murine glioblastoma. J. Immunother. 30, 789–797.

Yajima, N., Yamanaka, R., Mine, T., et al., 2005. Immunologic evaluation of personalized peptide vaccination for patients with advanced malignant glioma. Clin. Cancer Res. 11, 5900–5911.

Yamanaka, R., Abe, T., Yajima, N., et al., 2003. Vaccination of recurrent glioma patients with tumor lysate-pulsed dendritic cells elicits immune responses: results of a clinical phase I/II trial. Br. J. Cancer 89, 1172–1179.

Yamanaka, R., Homma, J., Yajima, N., et al., 2005. Clinical evaluation of dendritic cell vaccination for patients with recurrent glioma: results of a clinical phase I/II trial. Clin. Cancer Res. 11, 4160–4167.

Yamanaka, R., Zullo, S.A., Tanaka, R., et al., 2001. Enhancement of antitumor immune response in glioma models in mice by genetically modified dendritic cells pulsed with Semliki forest virus-mediated complementary DNA. J. Neurosurg. 94, 474–481.

Yang, M.Y., Zetler, P.M., Prins, R.M., et al., 2006. Immunotherapy for patients with malignant glioma: from theoretical principles to clinical applications. Expert Rev. Neurother. 6, 1481–1494.

Yang, S., Haluska, F.G., 2004. Treatment of melanoma with 5-fluorouracil or dacarbazine in vitro sensitizes cells to antigen-specific CTL lysis through perforin/granzyme- and Fas-mediated pathways. J. Immunol. 172, 4599–4608.

Young, H., Kaplan, A., Regelson, W., 1977. Immunotherapy with autologous white cell infusions ('lymphocytes') in the treatment of recurrent glioblastoma multiforme: a preliminary report. Cancer 40, 1037–1044.

Young, H.F., Sakalas, R., Kaplan, A.M., 1976. Inhibition of cell-mediated immunity in patients with brain tumors. Surg. Neurol. 5, 19–23.

Yu, J.J., Sun, X., Yuan, X., et al., 2006. Immunomodulatory neural stem cells for brain tumor therapy. Expert Opin. Biol. Ther. 6, 1255–1262.

Yu, J.S., Liu, G., Ying, H., et al., 2004. Vaccination with tumor lysate-pulsed dendritic cells elicits antigen-specific, cytotoxic T-cells in patients with malignant glioma. Cancer Res. 64, 4973–4979.

Yu, J.S., Wheeler, C.J., Zeltzer, P.M., et al., 2001. Vaccination of malignant glioma patients with peptide-pulsed dendritic cells elicits systemic cytotoxicity and intracranial T-cell infiltration. Cancer Res. 61, 842–847.

Zhang, J., Sarkar, S., Yong, V.W., 2005. The chemokine stromal cell derived factor-1 (CXCL12) promotes glioma invasiveness through MT2-matrix metalloproteinase. Carcinogenesis 26, 2069–2077.

Zhu, X., Lu, C., Xiao, B., et al., 2005. An experimental study of dendritic cells-mediated immunotherapy against intracranial gliomas in rats. J. Neurooncol. 74, 9–17.

9 Histopathology of brain tumors

M. Beatriz S. Lopes and Bernd W. Scheithauer

Introduction

Over the last two decades, the histologic evaluation of tumors of the nervous system has been dramatically affected by novel technical methods expanding upon immunohistochemical and ultrastructural study. These include not only molecular genetic methods, but the demonstration of specific cytoskeletal and membrane proteins, growth factors, and oncogene detection. In addition, growth kinetics in brain tumors have provided the neurooncologist with a greater understanding of brain tumor biology. Molecular genetic information, in particular, has enhanced our understanding of the various pathways involved in tumor pathogenesis. The identification of specific signaling pathways that may aid in predicting tumor behavior has possible therapeutic implications, serving as treatment targets.

The recent 2007 World Health Organization (WHO) Classification of Tumors of the Central Nervous System (Louis et al 2007) takes into consideration this new body of knowledge. Both neuropathology and oncology has greatly benefitted from the introduction of the novel findings introduced into the clinical arena.

Both histologic sub-types and the distribution of CNS tumors in children vs adults differ markedly, no doubt reflecting the complex histogenesis of the nervous system and the distinctive cells serving as targets of neoplastic transformation. The majority of childhood brain tumors arise in the posterior fossa, whereas the adult tumors affect primarily the supratentorial compartment. This age-related distinction is most dramatically illustrated by medulloblastoma and glioblastoma, the most frequently occurring malignant tumors in these two populations. Another age-related dissimilarity is the prevalence of the more circumscribed, relatively benign, astrocytic tumors in adolescents and young adults. These age- and site-related distinctions serve as important reminders that histologic diagnosis of brain tumors cannot be satisfactorily assessed in the absence of clinical, radiologic and neurosurgical data.

This chapter will focus upon a review of the tumors of the central nervous system in terms of the 2007 World Health Organization (WHO) Classification. Special mention will be given to the categories of neuroepithelial tumors, including gliomas and glioneuronal tumors, meningiomas and other tumors of the meninges, as well as new entities. Our review will stress the distinctive cytologic and histopathologic properties of these tumors, their salient clinical features and molecular genetic profile.

Tumors of neuroepithelial tissue

Astrocytic tumors

Astrocytomas are tumors in which neoplastic cells show distinctive, albeit variable, features of astrocytes. The WHO classification (Table 9.1) recognizes seven sub-types grouped into two major categories. These include diffusely invasive astrocytomas (diffuse astrocytoma, anaplastic astrocytoma, glioblastoma) and the relatively more circumscribed tumors (pilocytic and pilomyxoid astrocytoma, pleomorphic xanthoastrocytoma, subependymal giant cell astrocytoma). The so-called 'gliomatosis cerebri', a clinicopathologic and radiologic entity, is also a diffuse glioma, usually of the astrocytic type.

Aside from the capacity to diffusely invade gray or white matter, diffuse astrocytic tumors have a distinct tendency to undergo anaplastic transformation over time. They also tend to feature morphologic heterogeneity. Glioblastomas, as the highest grade of diffuse astrocytomas, demonstrate the most invasive growth and extensive migratory capacities. On the other hand, the more circumscribed variants feature more limited infiltration of surrounding brain and only very infrequently undergo anaplastic transformation.

Grading diffuse astrocytomas

Diffuse astrocytomas are graded on the basis of increasing anaplasia, and are designated WHO grade II (diffuse astrocytoma), WHO grade III (anaplastic astrocytoma), and WHO grade IV (glioblastoma). Although a number of histopathologic grading systems have been employed in the past (see Kleihues et al 2007a, for review), the WHO classification is now widely used and recommended to achieve uniformity of diagnoses (Kleihues et al 2007a). As regards specific criteria of histologic grading according to the WHO scheme, astrocytic tumors with nuclear atypia alone are considered grade II; those which in addition demonstrate mitotic activity are grade III; and tumors showing not only atypia and mitoses, but either 'microvascular proliferation' or necrosis, are considered grade IV. The non-specific term 'microvascular proliferation' refers to both multilayer 'endothelial' (actually pericytic proliferation), or glomeruloid appearance of the microvasculature. This simplified system is quite adequate for assessment of tumor grades when a tumor is optimally sampled. Tumor grading can, however, become challenging when sampling of a tumor is limited, in particular in stereotactic biopsies. In these cases, the presence of atypia

Table 9.1 Astrocytic tumors

Tumor	WHO grade
Circumscribed variants	
Pilocytic astrocytoma	I
Pilomyxoid astrocytoma	II
Subependymal giant cell astrocytoma	I
Pleomorphic xanthoastrocytoma	II
Diffuse variants	
Diffuse astrocytoma	II
Fibrillary astrocytoma	II
Gemistocytic astrocytoma	II
Protoplasmic astrocytoma	II
Anaplastic astrocytoma	III
Glioblastoma	IV
Giant cell glioblastoma	IV
Gliosarcoma	IV
Gliomatosis cerebri	III

combined with microvascular proliferation but without observed mitoses or necrosis would suggest glioblastoma, particularly when MIB-1 labeling indices are high. Multiple tissue targets and correlation with neuroimaging parameters are essential to overcome morphologic heterogeneity and limitation of sampling.

The presence of mitotic activity is a key feature for distinguishing low-grade (WHO grade II) from high-grade (WHO grades III and IV) astrocytomas. Immunohistochemical techniques have been used to more accurately assess proliferative activity, particular immunostaining for the Ki-67 protein, as defined by reactivity using the monoclonal antibody MIB-1 on formalin-fixed and paraffin tissue. Although MIB-1 labeling index alone is, according to current criteria, insufficient to definitively grade gliomas, there is a good overall correlation between labeling indices and WHO grade in diffuse astrocytomas (Giannini et al 1999a).

It is of note that histologic grading is not the only determinator of patient survival. Patient survival depends upon the combination of several clinical features, including patient's age and neurological status, tumor location, surgical extension and adjuvant therapeutic treatments like radiotherapy and chemotherapy.

Diffuse astrocytoma (WHO grade II)

Three cytologic variants of diffuse astrocytoma are histopathologically recognized. These include *fibrillary*, *gemistocytic*, and *protoplasmic astrocytoma*. This subclassification of astrocytomas roughly equates the morphology of neoplastic astrocytes to that of astrocytes in normal and reactive brain. Generally, this cytologic subdivision of astrocytoma variants is predicated upon predominant 'cell type' present in a given tumor, various cells often being admixed in the same neoplasm. Among these variants, *fibrillary astrocytomas* are the most common. *Gemistocytic astrocytoma* is the second most frequent. Representing no more than 20% of astrocytomas, they are defined as tumors with >60% of gemistocyte content (Krouwer et al 1991). In actuality, gemistocytic cells are commonly observed in astrocytomas of all grades (see Fig. 9.1A). Representing less than 1% of diffuse astrocytomas (Russell & Rubinstein 1989), *protoplasmic astrocytomas* are the least frequently occurring astrocytoma variant.

On gross examination, the consistency of diffuse astrocytomas depends upon the predominant component of the tumor. Protoplasmic astrocytomas appear as gelatinous masses given their frequent presence of mucin-containing microcystics. In contrast, the high proportion of fibrillary astrocytes in fibrillary astrocytomas confers firmness. Intraoperative smears of astrocytomas usually demonstrate a fibrillary matrix background of tumoral cytoplasmic processes. Given their marked variation in cytology, the cytoplasm of tumor cells may range from ones with barely discernible cytoplasm to cells fusiform or elongated (Fig. 9.1A,B). Gemistocytic astrocytomas are composed of round to slightly angulated cells with abundant, well defined, eosinophilic cytoplasm and eccentric nuclei (Fig. 9.1C). The tumor cells often have eccentric, shorter, less conspicuous processes than the long circumferentially radiating processes of reactive astrocytes. The stellate cells of protoplasmic astrocytomas possess a meshwork of poorly fibrillated, short, delicate processes.

Diffuse astrocytomas are generally diffusely immunoreactive for glial fibrillary acidic protein (GFAP). An exception is the protoplasmic astrocytoma, which demonstrates only minor GFAP immunoreactivity (Perentes & Rubinstein 1987; Russell & Rubinstein 1989). The relative expression of GFAP appears to be related to differentiation and proliferative potential (Rutka & Smith 1993). Vimentin, an intermediate filament protein with a relatively wide cellular distribution, particularly abundant in normal and neoplastic mesenchymal tissues, is regularly expressed in astrocytomas, its distribution being similar to that of GFAP, albeit with less prominence (Schiffer et al 1986). A number of other proteins are also expressed in astrocytic tumors, including S-100 protein and neuron-specific enolase (NSE) (Perentes & Rubinstein 1987). It is of note that these protein markers are of restricted diagnostic utility, particularly in distinguishing astrocytomas from other neuroepithelial tumors.

Regardless of the predominant cell type, diffuse astrocytomas (WHO grade II) exhibit mild to moderate cytologic atypia and cellularity. Mitotic activity is lacking in small specimens and MIB-1 labeling indices are usually <4% (von Deimling et al 2007). By definition, microvascular proliferation of the 'endothelial proliferation' type and necrosis are lacking. Collected evidence has shown that the presence of gemistocytes signifies a poor prognosis, even in low-grade diffuse astrocytomas (Krouwer et al 1991; Watanabe et al 1997). Certainly, gemistocytic astrocytomas are particularly prone to progress to anaplastic astrocytoma and glioblastoma (Krouwer et al 1991; Russell & Rubinstein 1989). Nonetheless, the WHO does not recommend the classification of these tumors as anaplastic astrocytoma based solely on predominance of gemistocytic pattern.

Anaplastic astrocytoma (WHO grade III)

All types of diffuse astrocytomas have a variable capacity for progression to anaplastic astrocytomas. Although anaplastic progression is anticipated in 50–70% of tumors (Russell & Rubinstein 1989), the latent period to progression is quite variable with a mean time interval of 4–5 years (Ohgaki et al 2004; Ohgaki et al 2005). Anaplastic astrocytomas may also arise *de novo*, without an intermediate phase of anaplastic progression from lower-grade tumor.

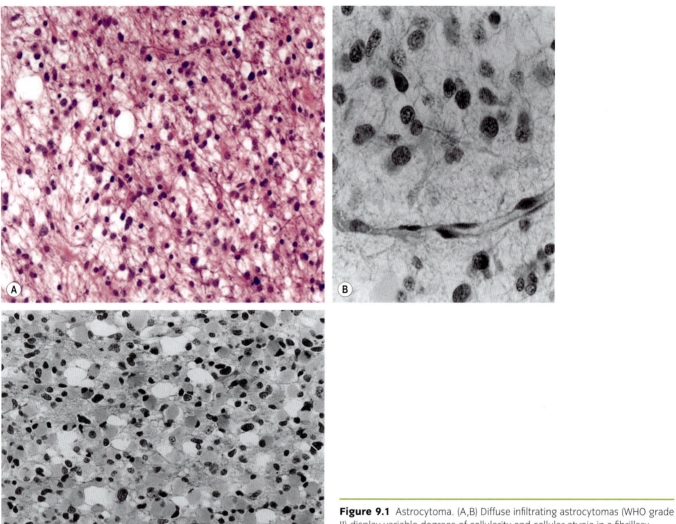

Figure 9.1 Astrocytoma. (A,B) Diffuse infiltrating astrocytomas (WHO grade II) display variable degrees of cellularity and cellular atypia in a fibrillary matrix. The majority of the tumors demonstrate mixed populations of fibrillary and gemistocytic astrocytes. Delicate vessels are present (B). (C) Gemistocytic astrocytomas are composed of a majority of cells with abundant, round cytoplasm and commonly eccentric nuclei. (A–C, H&E).

As a rule, anaplastic astrocytomas show a higher degree of cytologic atypia and nuclear pleomorphism than grade II astrocytomas. Although cellularity is a subjective parameter, anaplastic astrocytomas generally show higher cellularity (Fig. 9.2). In general, grade III astrocytomas have a less dense fibrillary matrix than do diffuse, grade II astrocytomas. Mitotic activity is present, but tends to vary in different portions of the tumor. Ki-67 labeling indices are usually elevated, ranging from 5% to 10% (Kleihues et al 2007b). Microvascular proliferation, again of the 'endothelial proliferation' type, and necrosis should not be present.

Glioblastoma (WHO grade IV)

Glioblastomas represent the most malignant neoplasm of the diffuse astrocytic tumors, representing 15–20% of all intracranial tumors and approximately 50% of gliomas in adults (Burger et al 1991). On the basis of clinical data in combination with molecular genetic alterations, two subtypes of glioblastoma have been described (Kleihues & Ohgaki 1999).

These are termed *primary glioblastoma* and *secondary glioblastoma* (Kleihues & Ohgaki 1999; Watanabe et al 1996). *Primary glioblastomas* arise in older patients (mean 62 years) over a relative short duration (usually less than 3 months) without an antecedent lower-grade lesion, whereas *secondary glioblastomas* develop in younger patients (mean 45 years) with a prior history of lower-grade astrocytoma. *Secondary glioblastomas* have a far lower incidence rate comprising as few as 5% of all glioblastomas in some estimates. This suggests that a significant proportion of patients with the lower-grade astrocytomas do not survive to develop glioblastomas (Ohgaki & Kleihues 2005). As sub-types, the primary and secondary glioblastomas have similar histopathologic features, but appear to develop via different molecular genetic mechanisms (see below). Glioblastomas may also occur in the pediatric group (Dohrmann et al 1975) or, even rarely, congenitally (Itoh et al 1987); in these populations they must be differentiated from embryonal tumors (see below).

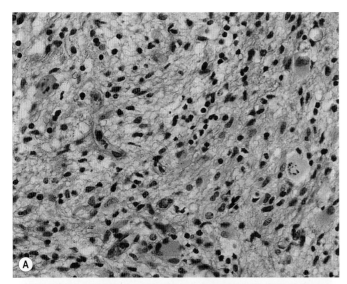

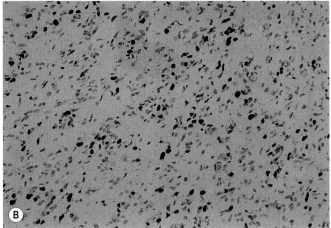

Figure 9.2 Anaplastic astrocytoma. (A) Hypercellularity, cellular atypia and high mitotic activity are features of anaplastic astrocytomas (WHO grade III) (H&E). (B) Ki-67 immunohistochemistry shows moderate elevated labeling indices. (Ki-67 (MIB-1) avidin biotin–immunoperoxidase).

Glioblastomas have neuroimaging and macroscopic features that reflect the aggressive nature of the lesion. Salient features include an expansive lesion on CT or MRI, with features of contrast enhancement and variable, often central, lack of enhancement. Whereas the latter represents necrosis, the zone of enhancement corresponds to hypercellular, often solid tumor with neovascularization (Earnest et al 1988). The heterogeneous signal frequently noted on T_2-weighted MR images correlates a combination of hypocellular tumor and edema. Despite the rather circumscribed neuroimaging and gross appearance of the glioblastomas, diffuse infiltration of the surrounding brain parenchyma by isolated, single cells or small clusters of neoplastic cells is an almost invariable finding. The extent of parenchymal infiltration is highly variable, as has been demonstrated by detailed tumor mapping studies (Burger & Kleihues 1989). Spreading of the tumor cells along fiber tracts may be particularly extensive, the most common example being their extension across the corpus callosum to the opposite hemisphere ('butterfly' pattern).

Histologically, glioblastomas exhibit marked cellular heterogeneity. Cytoplasmic and nuclear pleomorphism may be minimal or striking. Such tumors range from closely packed lesions consisting largely of small cells with scant cytoplasm and oval to nearly round, variably hyperchromatic nuclei, to tumors consisting largely of bizarre, multinucleated giant cells (Fig. 9.3A–D). Most tumors exhibit a mixed pattern of cytologic abnormalities. Mitotic figures, including atypical forms, are often readily identified, but their numbers vary considerably within different portions of the tumor. Similarly, MIB-1 labeling indices, although mostly high in the majority of the tumors (mean = 15–20%), show great regional variation (Burger et al 1986; Ellison et al 1995; Wakimoto et al 1996).

Glioblastomas are distinguished from grade III astrocytomas by the presence of either microvascular (endothelial) proliferation or of necrosis (Kleihues et al 2007c). Micronecrosis or broad geographic zones of necrosis, when surrounded by dense palisades of tumor cells, are attributable to true tumoral necrosis in that palisading is generally lacking in radiation necrosis. In recurrent tumors, the presence of intrinsic tumoral necrosis often cannot be distinguished from the effects of prior treatment, particularly radiation therapy. Other histopathologic features that may be present in glioblastomas are cytoplasmic lipidization, stromal mucin accumulation, myxoid change, and desmoplasia in areas of meningeal, particularly dural, invasion (Kepes et al 1984; Russell & Rubinstein 1989).

As in low-grade astrocytomas, glioblastomas show immunoreactivity for GFAP to a variable degree. Gemistocytic-like and giant cells are strongly GFAP positive while small, less differentiated cells may show only weak staining. Other glial markers including S-100 protein and vimentin are also reliably positive in the majority of glioblastomas.

Glioblastoma variants

Two distinct histopathologic sub-variants of glioblastomas are recognized in the 2007 WHO classification (Kleihues et al 2007c).

The first of these, *giant cell glioblastoma*, has distinctive neuroradiologic and, to a lesser extent, clinical features. They show a slight predilection for the temporal lobe (Margetts & Kalyan-Raman 1989) and, on both neuroimaging and gross examination, appear remarkably circumscribed. Affected patients may exceed the median survival time of those with more ordinary glioblastomas, which are clearly more infiltrative in nature (Margetts & Kalyan-Raman 1989; Russell & Rubinstein 1989). Histologically, giant cell glioblastomas are in large part composed of large, bizarre, multinucleated giant cells with abundant eosinophilic cytoplasm and large, bizarre nuclei (Fig. 9.3D). The frequent presence of more ordinary fibrillary cells or small astrocytes confirms the astrocytic nature of these tumors. Mitotic activity is elevated and atypical mitoses are commonly seen. One histologic feature, admittedly variable, is an increase in reticulin fibers, most conspicuous in relation to blood vessels and areas of necrosis. The giant cells are positive for S-100 protein but vary greatly in GFAP immunoreactivity, the latter being a more prominent feature of the fusiform cells. Molecular genetics of giant cell glioblastomas resemble those of secondary glioblastomas, with frequent *TP53* and *PTEN* gene

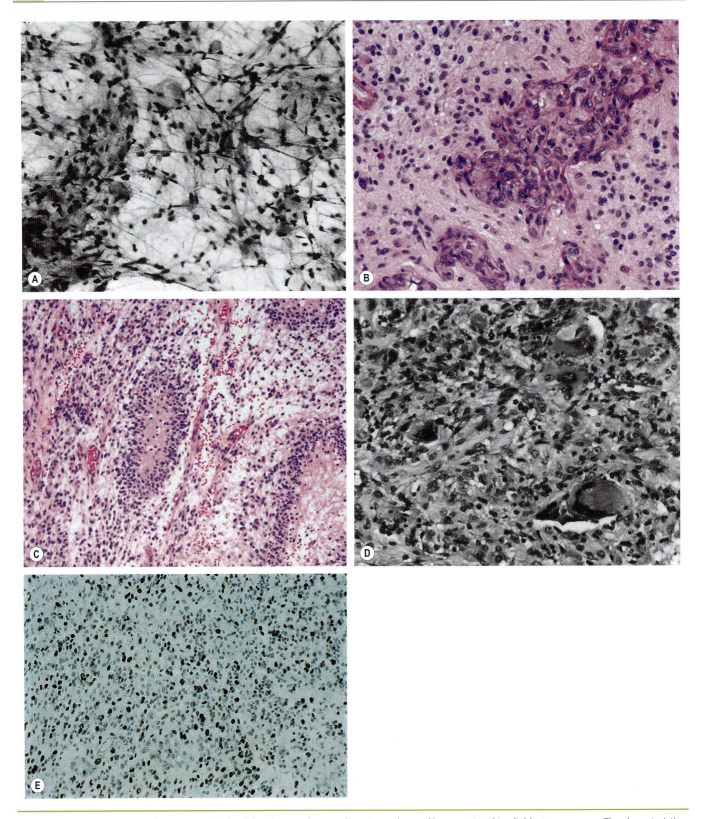

Figure 9.3 Glioblastoma multiforme. (A) Marked cellular pleomorphism and atypia can be readily appreciated in glioblastoma smears. The characteristic fibrillary matrix of astrocytomas is highlighted in smears. (B,C) Cellular atypia, high mitotic activity, exuberant microvascular proliferation, and necrosis constitute the histopathologic features of glioblastomas. (D) Multinucleated giant cells with abundant cytoplasm and bizarre nuclei are the predominant feature of giant cell glioblastomas (A–D, H&E). (E) The Ki-67 labeling index is remarkably high in glioblastomas. Compare this picture with anaplastic astrocytoma (Fig. 9.2). (Ki-67 (MIB-1) avidin biotin–immunoperoxidase).

mutations and rare *EGFR* gene amplification or *p16* deletion (Meyer-Puttlitz et al 1997; Peraud et al 1997; Peraud et al 1999). Thus, it appears that the majority of giant cell glioblastomas develop *de novo* with a short preoperative history (Peraud et al 1997).

The second principal variant of glioblastoma is *gliosarcoma*. Defined as a glioblastoma with a sarcomatous component, its frequency ranges from 2% to 8% of all glioblastomas. (Morantz et al 1976; Albrecht et al 1993; Meis et al 1991; Kleihues et al 2007c). Clinical features are similar to those of ordinary glioblastoma. Histologically, the proportions of glial and sarcomatous components is highly variable, both within individual tumors and in the group as a whole. The relative proportions of the two cell populations are such that the glial component tends over time to become overshadowed. As a result, the lesion may eventuate in what appears to be a primarily sarcomatous process. As a rule, the two components are readily distinguishable on the basis of histologic features alone, particularly with the application of reticulin and collagen stains to highlight the sarcomatous component. Immunohistochemistry for GFAP delineates the neoplastic glial component. In most cases, the sarcomatous component resembles either fibrosarcoma or pleomorphic undifferentiated sarcoma ('malignant fibrous histiocytoma'). Osteocartilaginous and particularly rhabdomyoblastic elements are rarely observed (Barnard et al 1986; Hayashi et al 1993). Immunohistochemical and ultrastructural studies have suggested that the sarcomatous elements might be derived from undifferentiated mesenchymal cells within the adventitia of tumoral vessels (Grant et al 1989; Ho 1990; Ng & Poon 1990; Haddad et al 1992). However, given the capacity of neoplastic glia to produce basal lamina and to elaborate extracellular matrix of a kind associated with mesenchymal differentiation, it may be an oversimplification to assume that the 'sarcomatous' element is invariably nonglial in origin (Paulus et al 1994a). Molecular genetic analyses have shown that the glial and mesenchymal elements of gliosarcomas share similar genetic aberrations (Albrecht et al 1993; Paulus et al 1994a; Biernat et al 1995; Boerman et al 1996), including identical *TP53* and *PTEN* gene mutations in both components. This suggests a monoclonal origin of gliosarcoma, the sarcomatous element representing a phenotypic shift or metaplasia of the glial cells (Biernat et al 1995; Reis et al 2000).

Small cell glioblastoma is a less well-defined variant of glioblastoma and at present has no official place in the 2007 WHO classification. Nevertheless, its recognition is important in the differential diagnosis of high-grade gliomas composed of small cells, particularly anaplastic oligodendrogliomas in adults and supratentorial primitive neuroectodermal tumor (PNET) in children. Small cell glioblastomas are characterized by a predominance of small, anaplastic cells with oval to bean-shaped nuclei and relatively scant cytoplasm. Although they may resemble primitive cells of supratentorial PNET, they exhibit immunoreactivity for glial markers and, as a rule, lack staining for neuronal markers. The histopathologic features similar to oligodendroglial neoplasms include nuclear monotony, micro-calcifications, clear perinuclear haloes, and perineuronal satellitosis. Remarkable for this category of glioblastoma is the presence of *EGFR* gene amplification and 10q deletions in the majority of the cases studied (Burger et al 2001; Perry et al 2004). To further complicate classification, glioblastomas with *bona fide* PNET elements have recently been described (Perry et al 2009).

Molecular cytogenetics of astrocytic tumors

In the last two decades, molecular biology has provided considerable insight into the mechanisms of diffuse astrocytoma tumorigenesis. The intent of this chapter is to highlight key events that may play a role in astrocytic in the process; the reader may obtain more extensive discussion of this topic in several outstanding reviews. The process of tumorigenesis and of anaplastic progression is reflected in several genetic events. Indeed, a number of specific genetic alterations correlate with different tumor grades, from WHO grade II diffuse astrocytoma to tumors of grade IV (glioblastoma) (Kleihues et al 2007c). Key steps include progressive loss of cell cycle regulation in the setting of stimulated growth signaling pathways.

The tumor suppressor gene *TP53* plays a major rôle in several processes, including cell cycle arrest, DNA damage repair, apoptosis and cellular differentiation. Loss of heterozygosity (LOH) on chromosome 17p and *TP53* mutation(s) occur in approximately 30% of astrocytomas, independent of histologic grade (Frankel et al 1992; Fults et al 1992; von Deimling et al 1992a). Inactivating mutations of the *TP53* gene seem to represent one of the earliest genetic alterations, being seen in approximately 50% of diffuse astrocytomas (WHO grade II) (Sidranski et al 1992; von Deimling et al 1992a; Louis et al 1993). Anaplastic progression from grade II to grade III (anaplastic astrocytomas) is usually accompanied by genetic losses on chromosome 19q, *CDK4* overexpression/amplification, *RB* gene pathway alterations, LOH on chromosome 13q, and chromosome 11p loss (Kitange et al 2003). The recent Cancer Genome Atlas report has confirmed that deregulation of *RB*, *TP53* and *PI3K/PTEN* pathways are obligatory events in almost all glioblastomas (The Cancer Genome Atlas Research Network 2008).

Mutations on the isocitrate dehydrogenase (IDH) genes have been recently associated to potential mechanisms of glioma pathogenesis (Parsons et al 2008). IDH1 and IDH2 are NADP-dependent enzymes that catalyze the production of α-ketoglutarate from isocitrate in the cellular metabolism. Mutations of *IDH1*, and less frequently *IDH2*, have recently been identified glioblastomas, in particular in secondary glioblastomas (Parsons et al 2008). Several subsequent studies showed that diffuse astrocytoma (WHO grade II), anaplastic astrocytoma (WHO grade III), in addition to low- and high-grade oligodendroglial tumors (WHO grades II and III) carry an *IDH1* mutation (Balss et al 2008; Ichimura et al 2009; Watanabe et al 2009; Yan et al 2009). In the great majority of gliomas, the mutation results in an amino acid substitution at residue 123 (Arg132His) of the *IDH1* gene (Parsons et al 2008). In contrast, *IDH1* mutations are rarely seen or absent in primary glioblastomas, in the more circumscribed astrocytomas including pilocytic astrocytomas and pleomorphic xanthoastrocytoma, and in ependymomas (Watanabe et al 2009; Yan et al 2009; Ichimura et al 2009). The majority of *IDH1* mutations are seen in combination with either *TP53* mutations or co-deletion of 1p/19q chromosomes, indicating that *IDH* mutations are one of the earliest events in the pathogenesis of infiltrating gliomas (Yan et al 2009).

Approximately 10–17% of anaplastic astrocytomas show *EGFR* gene amplification (Smith et al 2001; Liu et al 2005). Of these, approximately 20–75% express the EGFR vIII mutant (Liu et al 2005; Aldape et al 2004). Approximately 18% of anaplastic astrocytomas have *PTEN* point mutations, which appear to correlate with a significantly worse prognosis (Smith et al 2001). With respect to the role of growth factors in early stages of tumorigenesis and cell proliferation, a number of different factors, including cytokines may play a role in astrocytic tumorigenesis (Van Meir 1995). Altered growth factor activity, either by changes in ligand or receptor expression, occurs in the astrocytic tumors. These include PDGF, bFGF, TGFα, TGFβ, and IGF-1 (Hirano et al 1999; Hu et al 2004).

As previousy commented upon, glioblastomas has been subdivided into molecularly distinct entities on the basis of their clinical and mutually exclusive genetic pathways alterations. Besides *IDH1* mutations, the most prevalent genetic alteration (about 65%) in secondary glioblastomas is *TP53* gene mutation and chromosome 17p loss. In contrast, primary glioblastomas exhibit a 40–60% frequency of amplification of the *EGFR* gene located on chromosome 7p12 (Collins 1995; Smith et al 2001). Clinical and epidemiologic data concerning these two sets of glioblastomas have been described in detail elsewhere (von Deimling et al 1993a; Watanabe et al 1996). However, these two seemingly exclusive pathways do not account for all glioblastomas. Not all primary glioblastomas show *EGFR* amplification; indeed, *TP53* mutations (or overexpression) may be seen instead (Kleihues et al 2007c).

Several other cell cycle regulatory pathways in which genetic lesions progressively develop during anaplastic progression are seen in diffuse astrocytomas. For example: (1) deletions of the *p16* (*CDKN2a*) gene occur in about 30% of primary glioblastomas, often in association with *EGFR* gene amplification (Ohgaki et al 2004), and (2) *PTEN* mutations are observed in about 45% of primary glioblastomas, its inactivation being involved in both primary and secondary glioblastomas (Tohma et al 1998; Zhou et al 1999). In contrast to adult primary glioblastomas, *EGFR* amplification is very uncommon in the pediatric glioblastomas wherein *TP53* alterations are the most common genetic event (Sure et al 1997; Sung et al 2000).

Pilocytic astrocytoma (WHO grade I)

Pilocytic astrocytomas occur most frequently in children and young adults, their peak incidence being during the first two decades but without gender predilection. In adult patients, such tumors tend to appear one decade earlier (mean, 22 years) than do diffuse or infiltrative astrocytomas (Garcia & Fulling 1985). Pilocytic astrocytomas occur both sporadically and in association with neurofibromatosis type 1 (NF-1), wherein it particularly affects the optic pathways. Although they affect all levels of the neuraxis, they characteristically involve midline structures, such as cerebellum, third ventricular region, optic nerve and chiasma, brain stem, and spinal cord. Although supratentorial pilocytic astrocytomas show a tendency to involve the temporo-parietal region, thalamus, hypothalamus, or third ventricle, some examples

also affect the frontoparietal lobes (Forsyth et al 1993). Pilocytic astrocytomas comprise a large proportion (58%) of spinal astrocytomas, a site at which they tend to occur in an older age population (Minehan et al 1995). Compared with the diffuse astrocytomas previously discussed, pilocytic astrocytomas are: (a) biologically less aggressive, (b) have a more favorable prognosis (Clark et al 1985; Forsyth et al 1993), (c) are relatively circumscribed, displacing rather than widely infiltrating the surrounding brain, and (d) only rarely undergo malignant transformation. Nonetheless, infiltration into adjacent leptomeninges or white matter tracts, especially of the brain stem, optic nerves and optic chiasm is a relatively common feature of pilocytic astrocytoma (Tomlinson et al 1994). Leptomeningeal infiltration may play a role in the rare disseminated forms that do not manifest anaplastic features (Mishima et al 1992). Despite their rather indolent behavior and low proliferative activity, pilocytic astrocytomas may recur. This is particularly true of tumors found at unfavorable sites, and thus are only subtotally resected (Brown et al 1992).

Macroscopic features common to pilocytic astrocytomas include the formation of a cyst associated with a solid, mural nodule. This is particularly the case in cerebellar and hypothalamic-third ventricle region. Microscopically, pilocytic astrocytomas typically show a biphasic pattern of growth consisting of: (a) bipolar or 'piloid' highly fibrillated cells accompanied by Rosenthal fibers (Fig. 9.4B), and (b) a loose-knit, microcystic component made up of stellate cells resembling protoplasmic astrocytes, often associated with granular bodies or hyaline protein droplets (Fig. 9.4A). Immunoreactivity for GFAP typically highlights the densely fibrillated elements and is highly variable in microcystic areas. Vimentin is mostly demonstrable in both components (Schiffer et al 1986); the same is true of S-100 protein. The biphasic pattern is not invariably present in tumors affecting the optic pathways and spinal cord. Cellular atypia and multinucleation is common and considered degenerative in nature. Glomeruloid microvascular proliferation is a relatively common feature of pilocytic astrocytoma, however does not imply malignant transformation like microvascular 'endothelial' proliferation in diffuse astrocytomas. Mitotic activity is relatively low, the reported range being 0–4 mitoses per 10HPF, and MIB-1 labeling indices range from 0 to 4% (mean, 1.1%) (Giannini et al 1999a).

Histologic malignancy is rare in pilocytic astrocytomas. Brisk mitotic activity may be the most useful indicator of anaplastic progression, a rare manifestation in these tumors (Schwartz & Ghatak 1990). In a series of 107 pilocytic astrocytomas of the cerebellum (Tomlinson et al 1994), anaplastic progression occurred in only 0.9% of cases; these tumors had relatively high fractions of S-phase cells on DNA flow cytometry. As a rule, the prognosis of such tumors is more favorable than that for patients with diffuse astrocytomas having similar features of malignancy (Tomlinson et al 1994). Not surprisingly, no clinically meaningful definition of 'atypical pilocytic astrocytoma' has been formulated.

In contrast to diffuse astrocytomas, *IDH1* mutations and inactivation of the *TP53* gene does not seem to play a role in the pathogenesis of pilocytic astrocytomas (Ohgaki et al 1993; Patt et al 1996; Louis 1997; Ishii et al 1998; Watanabe et al 2009). Overexpression of p53 protein by immunohisto-

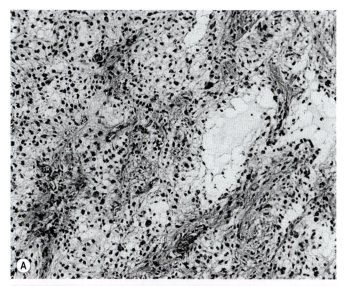

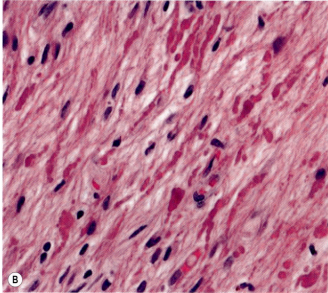

Figure 9.4 Pilocytic astrocytoma. (A,B) A characteristic biphasic pattern is present in pilocytic astrocytomas. (A) Stellate cells compose a loose-textured tissue often associated with microcystic changes. (B) Bipolar, piloid cells arranged in bundles are often associated with Rosenthal fibers. (A,B, H&E).

chemistry may be seen but without associated *TP53* mutations (Lang et al 1994). Allelic losses on chromosome 17q have been described in sporadic pilocytic astrocytomas, including the region encoding the *NF-1* gene (von Deimling et al 1993b). However, a role for *NF-1* as a tumor suppressor gene in the genesis of pilocytic astrocytomas has not yet been confirmed (von Deimling et al 1993b; Platten et al 1996; Gutmann et al 1996). The most significant finding distinguishing between pilocytic and diffuse astrocytomas appears to be alterations in the BRAF fusion gene (Jones et al 2008). A tandem duplication producing a novel oncogenic BRAF fusion gene has been demonstrated in about 66% of pilocytic astrocytomas, whereas this alteration has not been seen in high-grade, diffuse astrocytomas. Different molecular

profiles among tumors appear to occur in accordance with their location. Recent studies of pilocytic tumors arising sporadically as well as in patients with NF-1 showed different gene expression profiles in tumors in supratentorial vs infratentorial lesions (Sharma et al 2008).

Pilomyxoid astrocytoma (WHO grade II)

A rare, distinctive lesion, the *pilomyxoid astrocytoma*, has been considered a variant of pilocytic astrocytoma (Tihan et al 1999; Scheithauer et al 2007a) affecting mainly the supra-sellar/ hypothalamic region of infants and young children (<3 years of age). Its precise pathogenetic relationship to conventional pilocytic astrocytomas remains to be clarified.

Unlike the latter, pilomyxoid astrocytomas are more monomorphous in histologic pattern, feature vague perivascular pseudorosettes composed of elongated cells, exhibit a prominent myxoid stroma, and inconspicuous Rosenthal fibers or eosinophilic granular bodies. They also have a significantly higher recurrence rate, and may undergo CSF dissemination with far greater frequency (Scheithauer et al 2007a).

Pleomorphic xanthoastrocytoma (WHO grade II)

This uncommon, superficially situated glioma occurs most often in children or young adults and shows no gender predilection (Kepes et al 1979; Pasquier et al 1985; Kawano 1991; Giannini et al 1999b). The vast majority are supratentorial with a predilection for the temporal lobe, the basis for associated seizures in up to 78% of cases (Kawano 1991).

Pleomorphic xanthoastrocytomas are somewhat circumscribed masses, presenting as a cyst with a superficially situated mural nodule. Leptomeningeal involvement is common but, as a rule, the dura is uninvolved (Kepes et al 1979; Strom & Skullerud 1983; Kawano 1991). Although a well-defined macroscopic border with the subjacent brain is generally present, limited infiltration of brain parenchyma is apparent upon careful examination. Infiltration of Virchow–Robin spaces may be conspicuous but is not of prognostic significance (VandenBerg 1992).

The histopathologic appearance of PXA is stereotypic. Most tumors exhibit moderate cellularity and considerable pleomorphism, their cells ranging from spindle cells through plump and/or polygonal cells to multinucleated giant cells (Fig. 9.5A). Nuclei are pleomorphic, exhibit great variety of shape and size, and are commonly hyperchromatic. Nuclear cytoplasmic inclusions are a common finding. Cytoplasmic lipidization, especially of scattered giant cells, may be seen but is highly variable. Mitotic figures are scant and MIB-1 labeling indices are low (Giannini et al 1999a). Glomeruloid vasculature may be seen, but endothelial proliferation and necrosis are absent. Focal chronic inflammation is a frequent feature. The astroglial character of the cells is readily apparent and confirmed by GFAP immunoreactivity, albeit not uniform, often lacking particularly giant cells (Fig. 9.5C). Ganglion-like cells may be found in otherwise typical PXA and even neuronal differentiation has been reported at the immunohistochemical level (Furuta et al 1992; Lindboe et al 1992; Kordek et al 1995; Perry et al 1997a; Giannini et al 2002). PXA has also been reported as the glial component of ganglioglioma (Perry et al 1997a).

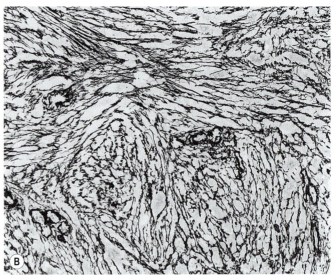

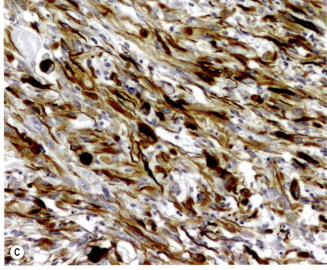

Figure 9.5 Pleomorphic xanthoastrocytoma. (A) Marked cellular heterogeneity, moderate cellular pleomorphism, and xanthomatous changes are present in the PXA (H&E). (B) The characteristic intercellular reticulin stroma defines fascicles of cells and surrounds individual tumor cells. (Gordon and Sweet's reticulin). (C) The astroglial nature of PXA is demonstrated by GFAP immunohistochemistry, although GFAP can be rather irregular in tumor cells. (GFAP avidin biotin–immunoperoxidase).

A characteristic feature of PXA is its variable texture, ranging from firm to indistinguishable from the adjacent brain. This contributes to the gross impression of tumoral demarcation. The increased firmness of many tumors is due in part to the presence of an extracellular matrix, visualized on reticulin (Fig. 9.5B) or collagen stains, which often delineate clusters or even individual tumor cells. Although stroma may be present in various portions of the tumor, it is most conspicuous in areas of leptomeningeal involvement. Although ultrastructural studies demonstrate some degree of pericellular basal lamina (Weldon-Linne et al 1983; Kepes et al 1989), a feature of subpial astrocytes (Russell & Rubinstein 1989; Whittle et al 1989), it is a common finding in astrocytes abutting stroma. Nonetheless, a histogenetic relationship between PXA and specialized subpial astrocytes has been suggested (Kepes et al 1979; Russell & Rubinstein 1989; Whittle et al 1989).

Pleomorphic xanthoastrocytomas are designated WHO grade II tumors. However, the biologic behavior of PXA varies and its potential for anaplastic progression is real. Although the initial description of the entity suggested that PXA should be considered a low-grade neoplasm (Kepes

et al 1979), a significant number recur and a small minority exhibit anaplastic progression (Weldon-Linne et al 1983; Kepes et al 1989; Daita et al 1991; Giannini et al 2002). The latter is far less frequent than in diffuse astrocytomas. Nonetheless, when compared with the other prognostically favorable variants of astrocytomas, i.e., pilocytic and subependymal giant cell astrocytomas, PXA are significantly more prone to aggressive behavior. The histopathologic features of their infiltrating margin may provide an important clue to the potential of PXA to recur and undergo anaplastic transformation (Weldon-Linne et al 1983; Kepes et al 1989; Daita et al 1991). Tumors exhibiting significant mitotic activity, i.e., >5 mitoses per 10-high-power (×40) field and/or necrosis are considered 'pleomorphic xanthoastrocytoma with anaplastic features' (Giannini et al 2007a). The designation has not, however, been fully accepted by the WHO, and no histologic grade has been designated.

Little is known of the molecular genetic events underlying the pathogenesis of PXA. The genetic mutations seen in diffuse infiltrating astrocytomas, mainly *IDH1* and *TP53* mutations and *EGFR* gene amplification, do not appear to play a significant role (Giannini et al 2007a; Watanabe et al 2009). *TP53* mutations have been found in isolated cases and p53 protein overexpression is seen in a minority. On the other hand, anaplastic transformation of PXA may be related to both increased proliferation and genetic mutations. *TP53* mutations have been described in recurrent PXA and in examples having progressed to anaplastic (Muñoz et al 1996; Paulus et al 1996). Amplification of the *EGFR* gene has also been described in an example of recurrent PXA with anaplasia (Paulus et al 1996).

Subependymal giant cell astrocytoma (WHO grade I)

Subependymal giant cell astrocytoma (SEGA) is a benign, slowly growing tumor typically occurring in the first two decades. Nearly all arise in the setting of the tuberous sclerosis complex (TSC). Indeed, despite opinion to the contrary (Shepherd et al 1991), a rare number of histologically similar tumors are unassociated with this phakomatosis. Classic tumors arise in the wall of the anterior lateral ventricles, either at the level of the foramen of Monro or simply overlying the basal ganglia. Extension into the third ventricle is uncommonly seen. Symptoms generally are related to obstructive hydrocephalus. Grossly, SEGAs are typically circumscribed, solid nodules sharply demarcated from underlying parenchyma. Calcifications are often present. Hemorrhage is rarely the presenting event.

Histologically, SEGAs are composed of heterogeneous cells exhibiting a broad range of astroglial phenotypes (Fig. 9.6A). Three principal cell types may be seen enmeshed in a variably fibrillated matrix: small spindle cells, intermediate size polygonal or 'gemistocytic' cells, and giant cells, some ganglionic in appearance. In all cell types, their nuclei feature delicate, granular chromatin and distinct nucleoli. The majority of tumor cells demonstrate immunoreactive for glial markers, but GFAP staining (Fig. 9.6B) and S-100 protein varies considerably. The reactions confirm the essentially astroglial nature of SEGA. It is of note, however, that numerous SEGA exhibit both glial and neuronal markers, including class III β-tubulin, neurofilament proteins, and neurotransmitter substances (Lopes et al 1996). Class III β-tubulin appears to be encountered showing wider distribution than other neuronal epitopes. More rarely, ganglion cells are immunoreactive for a broad spectrum of neuronal markers (Lopes et al 1996; Sharma et al 2004). Ultrastructurally, individual cells of SEGA show a combination of astrocytic and neuronal features, the latter including microtubules, occasional dense core granules and/or secretory vesicles, and even synapses. These features are similar to those seen in tubers, the hamartomatous cortical lesions of tuberous sclerosis.

Unlike diffuse astrocytomas, the biologic behavior of SEGA is relatively unrelated to histology. Mitotic activity and MIB-1 labeling indices are generally low, confirming their benign nature (Lopes et al 2007). Nonetheless, recurrence (Halmagyi et al 1979) and craniospinal dissemination (Telfeian et al 2004) have been reported in examples with increased MIB-1 labeling indices, despite a lack of obviously malignant features. On rare occasions, clinically benign SEGA appear malignant, featuring monomorphous spindle or epithelioid cytology, brisk mitotic activity and necrosis (Shepherd et al 1991).

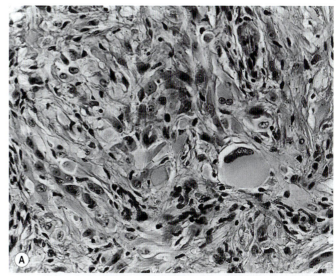
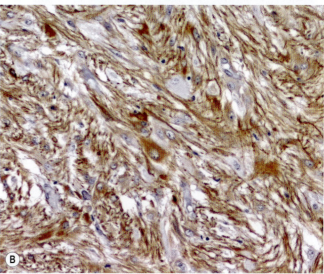

Figure 9.6 Subependymal giant cell astrocytoma. (A) Cellular heterogeneity is typical for SEGA, with spindle, polygonal, and ganglion-like cells (H&E). (B) The majority of tumor cells display variable immunoreactivity for GFAP. (GFAP avidin biotin–immunoperoxidase).

The two major genetic bases of TSC have their origin in abnormalities of chromosomes 9q (*TSC1*) and 16p (*TSC2*). Both have been implicated in tumorigenesis TSC (Lopes et al 2007). Although allelic loss of these genes has infrequently been demonstrated in cerebral lesions, loss of heterozygosity of either the *TSC1* or *TSC2* gene reportedly occurs in occasional SEGAs (Henske et al 1996; Nilda et al 2001; Chan et al 2004; Ess et al 2005). Additional studies have demonstrated loss of immunoreactivity for tuberin, the *TSC2* gene product, in a number of SEGAs, thus confirming the tumor suppressor function of this gene (Henske et al 1997; Mizuguchi et al 1997).

Oligodendroglial tumors

Oligodendroglioma (WHO grade II)

This distinctive glioma accounts for approximately 3% of all primary brain tumors and 9% of adult gliomas (Ohgaki &

Kleihues 2005; CBTRUS 2008). Their adjusted overall incidence rates range from 0.31 to 0.34/100 000 person-years in a large American series (CBTRUS 2008). Although they occur at any age, the majority affect adults with a peak incidence between 35–44 years. Whereas in young adults (20–34 years), oligodendrogliomas represent nearly 10% of all primary brain tumors, in the pediatric age group, the figure is about 2%. As in most glial tumors, there is a slight male gender preference with a male:female ratio of 1.16:1 (CBTRUS 2008).

Oligodendrogliomas most often affect the frontotemporal region, but may arise in any part of the neuraxis in relative proportion to its volume of white matter. Involvement of more than one lobe is not unusual, and bilateral hemispheric spread is common. Oligodendrogliomas are rarely seen in the cerebral deep gray matter, brain stem, cerebellum and spinal cord. Primary leptomeningeal oligodendrogliomas have been reported (Bourne et al 2006).

Macroscopically, oligodendrogliomas are soft and perhaps somewhat translucent. Foci of microcalcification may be present but only on occasion are large areas of coarse calcification encountered. Due to the extensive vascularity of the tumors, evidence of recent or remote tumoral hemorrhage may be seen.

Histologically, the cells of most tumors have ill-defined cytoplasm and are loosely cohesive, either in a poorly fibrillated matrix or in aggregates between nerve fiber tracts. The nuclei are typically round with chromatin more delicate than that of astrocytes (Fig. 9.7A–C). Cytoplasmic processes are usually scant. Thus, intercellular spaces are less fibrillary than those of typical astrocytomas. The tumor cells may be arranged in a broad spectrum of histologic patterns. Most tumors are diffuse, involve cerebral cortex, and have a somewhat defined edge within involved subcortical white matter. Circumscribed hypercellular lobules are occasionally conspicuous. Delicate, acutely branching vessels result in a pattern loosely termed 'chicken wire'. Parallel rows of cells forming palisades simulating polar spongioblastoma are a rare finding. Microcyst formation due to stromal mucin accumulation is a common feature, particularly in low-grade tumors. Reactive astrocytes are frequently encountered throughout the tumor. In low-grade (WHO II) tumors, cell proliferation is low. Mitotic figures may be present in small numbers (<5/10 hpf). MIB-1 labeling indices (LI) are also generally low (mean <2; tumors with MIB-1 LI >5% appear to be associated with shorter survival (Coons et al 1997). Capillaries may be prominent but microvascular endothelial proliferation is generally limited to anaplastic oligodendroglioma.

The majority of proteins and antigenic markers that characterize mature oligodendrocytes and oligodendrocytic cells during brain development are unreliably expressed in neoplastic oligodendrocytes. Their variable expression is further complicated by frequent loss of the markers during tissue processing. Thus, no specific immunocytochemical markers of neoplastic oligodendrocytes are found in fixed, routinely processed and paraffin-embedded tissue. Although the bHLH transcription factors, OLIG1 and OLIG2 are associated with oligodendroglial differentiation in development, neither appears to be expressed in oligodendrogliomas alone (Bouvier et al 2003; Ohnishi et al 2003; Ligon et al 2004). Likewise, markers of developing or mature oligodendrocytes

have yielded mixed results. These include myelin basic protein (MBP) (Figols et al 1985; Nakagawa et al 1986), myelin-associated glycoprotein (MAG) (Perentes & Rubinstein 1987), and proteolipid protein (PLP). Like all glial tumors, oligodendrogliomas show strong immunoreactivity for S-100 protein. Similarly, Leu-7 (CD57) (Perentes & Rubinstein 1986), galactocerebroside (de la Monte 1989), and MAP-2 (Blümcke et al 2001) may be seen, but these markers are not particularly useful for discriminating between oligodendrogliomas and other gliomas. The majority of low-grade oligodendrogliomas do not express vimentin (Jagadha et al 1986), but anaplastic (WHO grade III) oligodendrogliomas are more likely to do so (Cruz-Sanchez et al 1991). We exploit this property for diagnostic purposes. Neoplastic oligodendrocytes with a more prominent, demarcated cell borders and short cellular processes, so-called gliofibrillary oligodendrocytes (Herpers & Budka 1984; Wondrusch et al 1991; Kros et al 1992), often exhibit GFAP immunoreactivity (Fig. 9.7D) (Kros et al 1990). Such cells are occasionally a significant proportion of oligodendrogliomas (Herpers & Budka 1984; Nakagawa et al 1986). The GFAP immunoreactivity of these lesions, as well as that seen in oligodendrogliomas rich in 'minigemistocytes' with their even more sizeable globoid cell bodies, must not be misinterpreted as differentiation indicative of mixed oligoastrocytoma. The latter exhibit obvious fibrillary astrocytes and/or full-size, ordinary gemistocytes. Nonetheless, GFAP immunoreactive cells do tend to increase in number with anaplastic progression of oligodendrogliomas (Herpers & Budka 1984; Kros et al 1990). Low-grade oligodendrogliomas (WHO grade II) lack immunoexpression of nuclear p53 protein, an observation in keeping with their low incidence of *TP53* mutation.

Anaplastic oligodendroglioma (WHO grade III)

Anaplastic oligodendrogliomas represent about 20–35% of oligodendroglial tumors and account for <5% of newly diagnosed malignant gliomas (Cairncross et al 1992). Anaplastic oligodendrogliomas either evolve from progression of a low-grade oligodendroglioma or appear *de novo*. The majority of these tumors arise in older patients. Their peak incidence is between 45 and 50 years of age (Reifenberger et al 2007).

Anaplastic oligodendrogliomas are characterized by the presence of histopathologic features similar to those of anaplastic astrocytomas. These include hypercellularity, significant and often widespread nuclear atypia, brisk mitotic activity, microvascular endothelial proliferation, and necrosis (Fig. 9.8) (Reifenberger et al 2007). No general agreement has been reached on what constitute the most important criteria for 'anaplastic oligodendroglioma'. Some investigators have found mitotic activity and necrosis to be the most important prognostic indicators (Burger 1989). Yet others have found MIB-1 labeling to be the most significant feature relevant to survival (Coons et al 1997; Schiffer et al 1997). Tumors exhibiting cytological features of oligodendroglioma but with endothelial proliferation and necrosis typical of that seen in glioblastoma are regarded as anaplastic oligodendrogliomas, not glioblastomas.

Molecular cytogenetics of oligodendroglial tumors

Oligodendroglial tumors have a distinct molecular genetic profile different from that of diffuse astrocytomas. The

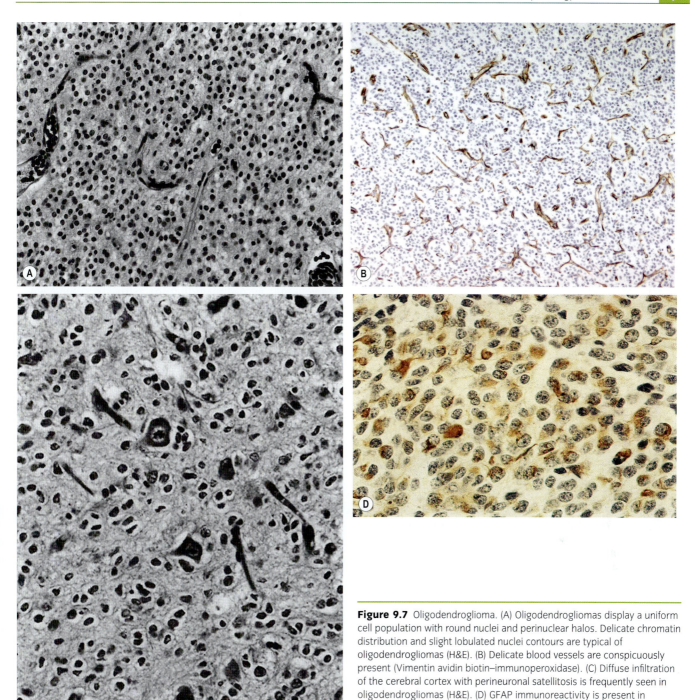

Figure 9.7 Oligodendroglioma. (A) Oligodendrogliomas display a uniform cell population with round nuclei and perinuclear halos. Delicate chromatin distribution and slight lobulated nuclei contours are typical of oligodendrogliomas (H&E). (B) Delicate blood vessels are conspicuously present (Vimentin avidin biotin–immunoperoxidase). (C) Diffuse infiltration of the cerebral cortex with perineuronal satellitosis is frequently seen in oligodendrogliomas (H&E). (D) GFAP immunoreactivity is present in 'gliofibrillary' oligodendrocytes. These GFAP-positive cells should be differentiated from reactive, stromal astrocytes. (GFAP avidin biotin–immunoperoxidase).

majority (60–92%) of oligodendrogliomas in adults have genetic losses on chromosomes 1p (1p34.2-p36.1; 1p36.22-p36.31, 1p36.3-pter) and 19q (19q13.3) (Reifenberger & Louis 2003; Jeuken et al 2004). Inversely, the presence of 1p/19q co-deletion in a glioma is significantly associated with an oligodendroglial phenotype (Felsberg et al 2004). It is of note that oligodendrogliomas in the pediatric group only rarely demonstrate these deletions (Kim et al 2005; Kreiger et al 2005). Combined 1p/19q deletions have been associated with longer survival and a better response to therapy in both low-grade and anaplastic oligodendrogliomas as well as in anaplastic oligoastrocytomas (Felsberg et al 2004; Smith et al 2000; Kanner et al 2006; Kujas et al 2005; McLendon et al 2005).

Certain clinical and radiographic features of oligodendroglial tumors with 1p/19q co-deletions appear to be distinctive. Neuroimaging aspects of tumors with 1p deletion include indistinct borders on T1-weighted images and mixed signal intensities on both T1-weighted and T2-weighted studies (van den Bent 2004; Megyesi et al 2004). Whether

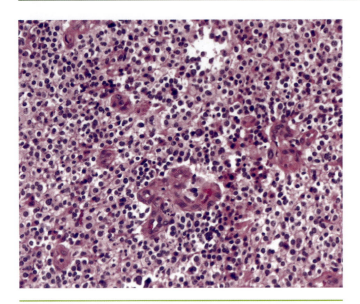

Figure 9.8 Anaplastic oligodendroglioma. Hypercellularity, cellular pleomorphism, mitotic figures, and microvascular endothelial proliferation are characteristics of anaplastic oligodendrogliomas. The characteristic round nuclei of the cells are retained by the anaplastic tumors (H&E).

tumors with this genetic signature show a predilection for specific brain locations remains unsettled (Zlatescu et al 2001). Nonetheless, it has been suggested that oligodendrogliomas arising in the temporal lobes are less likely to have 1p/19q co-deletions than those of the frontal, parietal and occipital lobes (Mueller et al 2002).

High frequency of *IDH1* mutations have been found in oligodendrogliomas (WHO grade II), oligoastrocytomas (WHO grade II), and their anaplastic (WHO grade III) counterparts (Ichimura et al 2009; Watanabe et al 2009). The majority of *IDH1* mutations are seen in association with co-deletion of 1p/19q chromosomes (Ichimura et al 2009).

Malignant progression of oligodendroglial tumors is associated with the accumulation of other genetic abnormalities. Increasing alterations in cell-cycle regulatory genes, notably deletional mutations in addition to methylation at 9p21 loci which affect CDKN2A/B/p14ARF, have been described (Engelhard et al 2002; Reifenberger & Louis 2003). Other important progression-associated alterations include 10q loss and *PTEN* mutation, but these occur in only a minority of tumors (Reifenberger et al 2007).

Mixed oligoastrocytomas

Oligoastrocytoma (WHO grade II)

Oligoastrocytomas are tumors composed of oligodendrocytes and a significant population of neoplastic astrocytes. The predominant component is often oligodendroglial (Rubinstein 1972), but relative proportions vary considerably. The two neoplastic cell populations may be diffusely distributed or, less often, in geographically distinct zones. Oligoastrocytomas arise primarily in the cerebral hemispheres, the frontal lobes being most frequently affected, followed by the temporal lobes (von Deimling et al 2007). As in low-grade oligodendrogliomas, patients with oligoastrocytomas usually

present in the 4th and 5th decade and exhibit a slight male predilection (von Deimling et al 2007).

Histologically, oligoastrocytomas are diffusely infiltrating tumors. Although containing two distinct neoplastic cellular components, neoplastic oligodendroglia and astrocytes, cells with indeterminate or transitional features often abound. Oligoastrocytomas must be distinguished from oligodendrogliomas containing varying numbers of reactive astrocytes. The latter are a regular feature of all infiltrative gliomas. As previously stated, the simple detection of GFAP immunoreactivity in 'gliofibrillary' or 'minigemistocytic' oligodendrocytes should not be overinterpreted as indicative of an astrocytic component.

Anaplastic oligoastrocytoma (WHO grade III)

The frequency with which oligoastrocytomas undergo anaplastic transformation is unknown. Although the alterations often affect both oligodendroglial and astrocytic components, it is generally agreed upon that the astrocytic component is more susceptible to anaplastic change (Muller et al 1997; Russell & Rubinstein 1989). Anaplastic oligoastrocytomas (WHO grade III) are mixed gliomas with the usual histologic features of anaplasia, including increased cellularity, nuclear atypia, brisk mitotic activity, microvascular proliferation and foci of necrosis. As in anaplastic oligodendrogliomas, patients with anaplastic oligoastrocytomas exhibiting allelic deletions on 1p or combined 1p/19q deletions have significant longer survival (Felsberg et al 2004).

The presence of necrosis in anaplastic oligoastrocytomas is rightly seen as evidence of yet further progression of such tumors, in essence a transition to grade IV oligoastrocytoma. However, the finding has prompted some to apply the designation '*glioblastoma with oligodendroglioma component*' (von Deimling et al 2007). For others and in-keeping with long-held WHO policy, the term glioblastoma should be restricted to high-grade tumors of solely astrocytic type (Scheithauer et al 2008). The distinction between anaplastic oligoastrocytoma of WHO grade III and these higher-grade mixed tumors is of clinical relevance given their potential chemosensitivity. Indeed, a minority exhibit 1p/19q co-deletion. Moreover, their survival is intermediate between that of astrocytoma of grades III and IV (Miller et al 2006). This being the case and in an effort to avoid terminologic confusion on the part of clinicians, some of us apply the designation 'grade IV oligoastrocytoma' (Scheithauer et al 2008).

Molecular cytogenetics of mixed oligoastrocytomas

Molecular genetic studies have shown that oligoastrocytomas are genetically heterogeneous (von Deimling et al 2007). One subset of tumors appears genetically related to oligodendrogliomas, whereas another is related to diffuse infiltrating astrocytomas. About 30–70% of oligoastrocytomas are characterized by chromosomes 1p and 19q deletions in both oligodendroglial and astrocytic components (Reifenberger et al 1994; Kraus et al 1995; Maintz et al 1997). Another 30% of tumors have genetic alterations frequently seen in diffuse astrocytomas, including *TP53* gene mutations and/or 17p loss (Reifenberger et al 1994; Maintz et al 1997). It appears that the subsets of oligoastrocytomas with 1p/19q co-deletions are often oligodendroglial-dominant, while those with *TP53* mutations and/or 17p loss are more often astrocytic-dominant

(Maintz et al 1997). As previously mentioned, large percentage of oligoastrocytomas (grades II and III) carry *IDH1* mutations (Ichimura et al 2009; Watanabe et al 2009).

The histogenesis of mixed oligoastrocytomas remains unclear. Molecular data showing similar genetic alterations in both oligodendroglial and astrocytic components favored the notion that oligoastrocytomas arise from a glial precursor cell able to undergo bipotential differentiation. Recent stem cell research has provided evidence supporting the existence of bi- and multipotential glial progenitors in the adult brain, ones analogous to the murine O-2A progenitor cells (Nishiyama et al 1999; Rakic 2003; Tramontin et al 2003). The existence of progenitor cell populations as targets for neoplastic transformation in the adult nervous system may provide a key to understanding the histogenesis of oligodendrogliomas and the morphologic diversity of mixed oligoastrocytomas.

Ependymal tumors

Ependymoma (WHO grade II)

According to the Central Brain Tumor Registry of the United States (CBTRUS 2008), ependymomas account for about 2.1% of all primary CNS tumors and 5.8% of gliomas, but these figures vary greatly by patient age group. The tumors show a distinctly bimodal age distribution, the first peak being in early childhood and the second during the 4th to 5th decades. During the first 4 years of life, ependymal tumors comprise approximately 11% of neuroepithelial tumors. The overall mean age in the adult population is 41 years (CBTRUS 2008). In all age groups, ependymal tumors exhibit an equal gender distribution (McLendon et al 2007b).

Ependymomas arise at any level along the ventricular system and spinal canal, but their anatomic distribution varies according to patient age. Most pediatric ependymomas arise in the posterior fossa, specifically the fourth ventricle (Horn et al 1999). A large proportion of adult ependymomas arise in the spinal cord, wherein they represent about 60% of gliomas (Salazar et al 1983). Spinal cord ependymomas most often affect the cervical region, but approximately 40% of spinal tumors arise in the filum terminale (McCormick & Stein 1990). Supratentorial tumors are more common in adults than children. At least half of such tumors are hemispheric, showing no association with the ventricular system (Guyotat et al 2002; Korshunov et al 2004; Roncaroli et al 2005). Multiple spinal cord ependymomas typically occur in association with NF-2.

Macroscopically, ependymomas are well demarcated, macroscopically pushing aside surrounding brain parenchyma. Despite a sharp parenchymal interface, a small proportion of tumors actually gain access to the ventricular system or undergoes subarachnoid spread. This is particularly true of fourth ventricular ependymomas which, via the foramina, come to involve surrounding cisterns, occasionally encasing the brainstem. Cystic degeneration and calcifications are common features of ependymomas.

Histologically, most ependymomas are composed of uniform cells often oval or round nuclei, chromatin distributed in a 'salt-and-pepper' pattern, and well-defined cytoplasm, often disposed in tapering processes. A characteristic feature of the latter is radially disposed around vessels (perivascular pseudorosettes) (Fig. 9.9A). Although diagnostic of ependymoma, 'true' rosettes with epithelial-like lumens are much less common. Ependymomas vary in histologic pattern from distinctly glial appearing tumors rich in cellular processes (Fig. 9.9B) to ones more epithelial-appearing. Both exhibit vimentin and variable GFAP immunostaining (Fig. 9.9D). More importantly, ependymoma also exhibits EMA reactivity often in a characteristic paranuclear, dot-like pattern or in a ring-like or linear pattern highlight lumina of true rosettes or cell membranes, respectively. Cytokeratins are infrequently or only weakly expressed (Vege et al 2000). Occasional mitotic figures (<5/10 hpf), nuclear atypia, and even non-palisading necrosis may be present without indicating anaplastic change.

The WHO classification recognizes four variants of ependymoma: *cellular, papillary, clear cell,* and *tanycytic* (McLendon et al 2007b). These tumors have basically the same clinical outcome, but their recognition as variants of ependymoma is important in distinguishing them from other gliomas, including anaplastic gliomas, choroid plexus tumors, and even oligodendrogliomas. All are circumscribed and architecturally solid. *Cellular ependymomas* are rather patternless tumors, exhibit little in the way of rosetting and when process-rich, may resemble diffuse astrocytomas. The *papillary ependymomas* tend to show conspicuous papilla formation; as a result, such tumors may mimic choroid plexus tumors or, far less often, metastatic carcinomas. The ependymal nature of such tumors is most easily confirmed by their immunoreactivity for GFAP and lack of cytokeratin staining (Takeuchi et al 2002). The *clear cell ependymomas* (Fig. 9.9C) feature a distinctive honeycomb appearance due to cytoplasmic clearing of their often polygonal, crowded cells. Pseudorosettes may occur, but are inconspicuous. The clear cell variant most commonly affects children and young adults (Katoh et al 2004). At least half of clear cell ependymomas arise at supratentorial sites; most infratentorial tumors affect the cerebellum rather than the fourth ventricle. This ependymoma variant poses a problem in differential diagnosis from oligodendroglioma. The proper diagnosis is suggested by other ependymoma features such as sharp demarcation, contrast enhancement and/or cyst formation on CT and MRI. Histologically, clear cell ependymoma is distinguishable by its GFAP and vimentin-reactivity. The ultrastructural finding of lumens containing intercellular microvilli and cilia as well as junctional complexes is diagnostic of ependymoma (Kawano et al 1989). *Tanycytic ependymomas* are rare and typically affect the spinal cord, although several supratentorial examples have been reported in association with the lateral and third ventricles (Ragel et al 2005). These monomorphous tumors are composed of relatively well-differentiated cells, remarkably elongated cells, the delicate tapering processes of which are GFAP reactive and show only minor EMA immunoreactivity. Most tanycytic ependymomas feature only vague, large perivascular pseudorosettes, true ependymal rosettes being exquisitely rare.

Ependymoma and its variants correspond histologically to WHO grade II. There is no consensus as to what features precisely define anaplastic progression in ependymomas and, in many hands, conventional histopathologic assessment grade in both pediatric and adult patients is poorly correlated with prognosis. This is, in large part, due to the

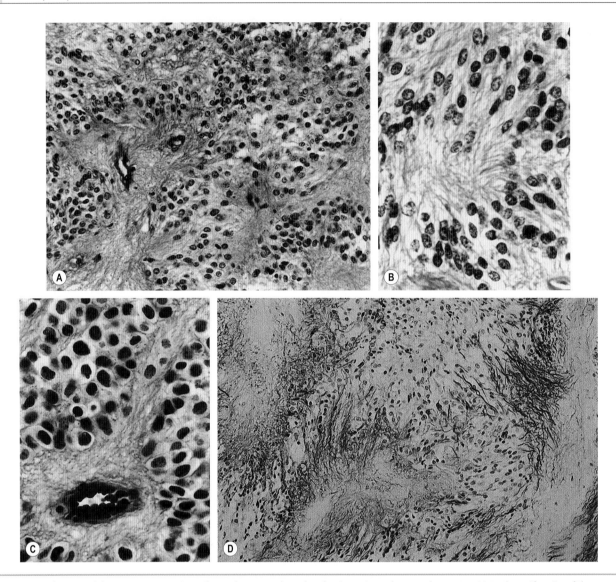

Figure 9.9 Ependymoma. (A) Low-power overview of ependymomas show the classic perivascular pseudorosettes. Note the uniformity of the round nuclei. (B) Perivascular pseudo-rosettes and ependymal rosettes are hallmarks of ependymomas. (C) Ependymomas with clear cell areas can resemble oligodendrogliomas because of the perinuclear halos and nuclear uniformity. (A–C, H&E). (D) Fibrillary processes of neoplastic ependymal cells are strongly immunoreactive for GFAP. (GFAP avidin biotin–immunoperoxidase).

overriding importance of extent of resection and of tumor location and patient age, infratentorial location and age <4 years being negative prognostic factors (Figarella-Branger et al 2000). One morphologic factor of prognostic significance, particularly in supratentorial ependymomas, appears to be proliferative activity, both mitotic index (Schiffer et al 1991) and MIB-1 labeling indices, regardless of other aspects of histologic grade (Schröder et al 1993; Rushing et al 1998; Bennetto et al 1998; Prayson 1999). These studies have shown that high proliferative indices have a positive correlation with the histologic grade and early recurrence. Additionally, other studies have found the combinations of low expression of p27/Kip1, high p53 immunoreactivity, low p14[ARF] immunoreactivity, and elevated survivin immunohistochemistry to define tumors with shorter progression free survivals (Korshunov et al 2001; Korshunov et al 2000; Preusser et al 2005). A recent study in pediatric intracranial

ependymomas identified low expression of nucleolin, a retinoblastoma susceptibility gene-related nucleolar phosphoprotein, to be the single most important biological predictor of outcome in ependymomas, one independent of histological grade (Ridley et al 2008).

Anaplastic ependymoma (WHO grade III)

Anaplastic progression may affect ependymomas occurring at most sites but is a very uncommon occurrence in spinal cord examples (Russell & Rubinstein 1989). The overall frequency of anaplastic transformation of low-grade tumors over time is less than that of diffuse astrocytic tumors (Carter et al 2002).

Anaplastic ependymomas are histologically characterized by increased cellularity, brisk mitotic activity, and the presence of microvascular endothelial proliferation. Microscopic or even geographic necrosis may be present, but in itself is not a robust indicator of anaplasia, being seen in otherwise unremarkable, low-grade ependymomas. On the other hand, pseudo-palisading necrosis is a feature associated with anaplasia.

Anaplastic ependymoma must be distinguished from ependymoblastoma, highly malignant, embryonal tumors affecting primarily infants and children under the age of 5 years. In contrast to anaplastic ependymomas, ependymoblastomas tend to diffusely infiltrate adjacent structures and show a distinct tendency to undergo craniospinal seeding.

Myxopapillary ependymoma (WHO grade I)

The myxopapillary ependymoma is a slow-growing variant of ependymoma that commonly affects the cauda equina region of young adults (mean age, 36.4 years) (Morantz et al 1979; Sonneland et al 1985; Pulitzer et al 1988). There is a significant male predilection (M:F = 1.7 : 1) (Sonneland et al 1985). The tumors are discrete, sausage-shaped, arise from the filum terminale, and compress spinal nerve roots of the cauda equina. Only infrequently do myxopapillary ependymomas present as extradural lesions in the presacral space or in retrosacral soft tissue. Such 'ectopic tumors' presumably arise from ependymal rests (Morantz et al 1979; Pulitzer et al 1988). Although the majority of the tumors are biologically benign and slow-growing, local recurrences are common and CSF dissemination may occur (Patterson et al 1961; Rubinstein & Logan 1970; Sonneland et al 1985). The prognosis of this unique ependymoma variant is related to resectability. Only a minority are found to be intact, bag-like lesions at the time of surgery. Every effort should be made to resect the tumor intact. Needle puncture or intraoperative rupture of the tumor capsule facilitates recurrence and diminishes the likelihood of cure (Sonneland et al 1985).

Histologically, myxopapillary ependymomas are composed of papillary arrangements of elongated fibrillary cells surrounding a cuff of mucinous or hyalinized perivascular stroma. Mucin may also accompany neoplastic cells not in contact with vessels and may therefore be a product of the tumor as well as a stromal response. Electron microscopy has confirmed the ependymal nature of these lesions, revealing cytoplasmic intermediate filaments, pockets of microvilli and cilia often associated with numerous surface membrane interdigitations, and abundant basal lamina (Rawlinson et al 1973; Specht et al 1986). The presence of GFAP immunoreactivity distinguishes this tumor from schwannomas, although the latter may be focally GFAP-positive. Paragangliomas, characterized by limited S-100 protein and strong chromogranin staining, also occur in this region (Sonneland et al 1986).

Subependymoma (WHO grade I)

Subependymomas are well circumscribed, generally asymptomatic nodules located in the walls of the fourth (66–70% of cases) and lateral ventricles (Scheithauer 1978; Lombardi et al 1991). The septum pellucidum, foramen of Monro and, less commonly, spinal cord parenchyma may also be affected (Pagni et al 1992). The majority are incidental post-mortem findings, but symptomatic examples occur with some frequency, usually in older adults, and present either with obstructive hydrocephalus and increased intracranial pressure. Less frequent is spontaneous tumoral hemorrhage.

Histologically, subependymomas exhibit features of both ependymal and astrocytic differentiation. Hypocellular, and composed in large part of densely packed, fibrillated processes, the tumor's low-power architecture is characterized by clusters of cells surrounded by skeins of such processes. Ependymal features such as pseudo-rosettes are inconspicuous and true rosettes are rare. Astrocytic-appearing cells, elongated to plump, occasionally somewhat gemistocytic in appearance, are an usually focal feature. The association of astrocytic and ependymal features has also been confirmed on ultrastructural and tissue culture studies (Fu et al 1974; Azzarelli et al 1977). Microcystic degeneration and microcalcification are commonly encountered, as are vascular hyalinization and hemosiderin deposition, the basis and result of prior subclinical hemorrhage. Nuclear atypia and limited mitotic activity may be present, but are of no prognostic significance. The same is true of typically low-level MIB-1 labeling. Like other ependymal tumors, subependymomas are immunoreactive for vimentin, GFAP, S-100 protein, for vimentin, GFAP, and S-100 protein. Membrane or paranuclear dot-like EMA positivity corresponding to microlumena may be focally seen.

Tumor location and surgical factors, such as extent and attempted resection of tumors of the floor of the fourth ventricle, are the most important of prognostic factors (Lombardi et al 1991).

Molecular cytogenetics of ependymal tumors

In comparison with either astrocytic or oligodendroglial tumors, the molecular pathology of ependymal tumors is less understood. Nonetheless, ependymal tumors do differ in terms of their specific molecular biologic abnormalities (Carter et al 2002; Goussia et al 2001). In contrast to the diffuse astrocytomas, mutations or deletions of TP53, IDH1 Rb, p16, and PTEN are rare in ependymomas, as are genetic losses on chromosome 10q. Similarly, losses on 1p and 19q, changes characteristic of oligodendrogliomas, are also uncommon. Genetic losses on chromosome 22q are the most common abnormality exhibited by ependymoma, monosomy 22 occurring in about one-third of tumors (Ebert et al 1999). Losses on chromosome 6q and gains of 1q are also seen, especially in anaplastic examples. Polysomy of chromosome 7 on CISH has been reported to occur in about two-thirds of adult ependymomas (Santi et al 2005), but amplification of EGFR and CDK4 is uncommon.

In addition, there is some evidence that different patterns of genetic abnormality are seen relative to the tumor location and patient age. With respect to the former, NF2 gene mutations on chromosome 22 are more commonly seen in spinal than intracranial ependymomas (Ebert et al 1999). Myxopapillary ependymomas have losses of chromosome 13 and 14q/14 and gains in chromosomes 9 and 18 (Carter et al 2002; Mahler-Araujo et al 2003). In contrast, ependymomas arising in the posterior fossa often exhibit gains of 1q and 9, and losses of 6q are particular features (Carter et al 2002; Mahler-Araujo et al 2003).

Pediatric ependymomas have different molecular genetic signatures than adult ependymomas. Genetic losses on chromosome 22q are less frequently seen in pediatric tumors (von Haken et al 1996); one contributing factor for this disparity may be the tendency of tumors with 22q losses to arise in the spinal cord (see above), a rare location of pediatric ependymomas. Losses on chromosome 17p are common in sporadic pediatric tumors (von Haken et al 1996), while polysomy 7 is more common in pediatric tumors (66% vs 25%) (Santi et al 2005). By comparative genomic hybridization, pediatric ependymomas more frequently showed balanced profiles (Carter et al 2002). Pediatric ependymomas express *ERBB2* and *ERBB4* (Gilbertson et al 2002). Promoter sites of *CDKN2A*, *CDKN2B*, and *p14*ARF are less methylated in pediatric than adult tumors (Rousseau et al 2003). In contrast, methylation of the tumor suppressor gene *HIC-1* (chromosome 17p13.3) is commonly encountered in ependymomas of the first decade (Waha et al 2004).

Choroid plexus tumors

Choroid plexus papilloma (WHO grade I)

Choroid plexus tumors are rare, comprising only 2.0% of intracranial gliomas and about 0.5% of all brain tumors (Paulus & Brandner 2007). The majority are benign papillomas arising in the lateral ventricles of children (Laurence 1979; Russell & Rubinstein 1989). In adults, the fourth ventricle is the most commonly affected site (Russell & Rubinstein 1989). Third ventricular tumors are rare. Occasional examples arise from choroid plexus in the cerebellopontine angle. Clinical symptoms are usually due to increased intracranial pressure, either secondary to CSF obstruction or to increased production of CSF. A slight male prevalence is noted.

Choroid plexus papillomas are grossly demarcated tumors that resemble a cauliflower. Calcification is common and varies considerably. Their histopathologic appearance is one of a benign, papillary neoplasm composed of a single, often pseudostratified layer of columnar epithelium surrounding a delicate fibrovascular core (Fig. 9.10A). In contrast to normal choroid plexus epithelium, papillomas are hypercellular, exhibit some degree of cellular pleomorphism and consist of cells lacking a hobnail surface contour. Oncocytic and xanthomatous changes may be present (Kepes 1983; Bonnin et al 1987). In terms of signs of atypia, mitotic figures are generally inconspicuous, architectural complexity is usually minor, and necrosis as well as parenchymal invasion are minimal. When prominent, combinations of these features, particularly two or more mitotic figures per 10 hpf, indicate malignant transformation and an increased likelihood of recurrence and cerebrospinal spread (Paulus & Brandner 2007). The mean MIB-1 labeling index reported for ordinary choroid plexus papillomas is 1.9% (Vajtai et al

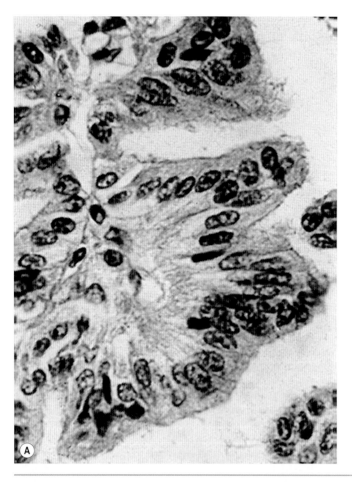
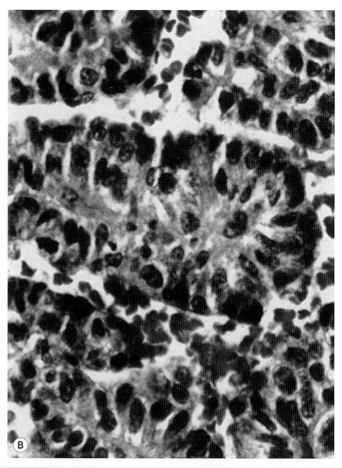

Figure 9.10 Choroid plexus tumors. (A) Papillomas demonstrate papillary structures composed of single or multiple layers of columnar epithelium surrounding a delicate fibrovascular core. (B) Although the papillary structures may still be present, carcinomas exhibit a high degree of cellular pleomorphism and mitotic figures (H&E).

1996). Atypical choroid plexus adenoma is defined as adenomas with increased mitotic activity (Paulus & Brandner 2007). In general, these tumors have other atypical features including increased cellularity, nuclear pleomorphism and solid growth but are more differentiated than carcinomas (Paulus & Brandner 2007).

Choroid plexus papillomas express markers consistent with their origin from ventricular neuroepithelium. These include S-100 protein and often GFAP. Cytokeratin is also a common feature (Miettinen et al 1986; Lopes et al 1989). Transthyretin (pre-albumin) is consistently expressed in choroid plexus tumors (Herbert et al 1990), though this marker is not tissue specific and may be seen in metastatic carcinoma (Albrecht et al 1991). Several potentially specific markers of choroid plexus tumors have been recently described, including: (a) stanniocalcin-1, a glycoprotein normally expressed in human choroid plexus that might participate in the regulation of CSF calcium levels, and (b) Kir7.1, a potassium inwardly-rectifying channel family member that may play a role in the transepithelial transport of potassium (Hasselblatt et al 2006b). Expression of the latter has been observed in the apical cell membrane of choroid plexus epithelial cells.

Choroid plexus carcinoma (WHO grade III)

Most choroid plexus carcinomas arise *de novo*. Malignant transformation of choroid plexus papillomas accounts for <20% of cases of papillomas (Vajtai et al 1996). About 80% of carcinomas arise in children, the majority <2 years of age. The median age of carcinoma patients lies between 26 and 32 months (Packer et al 1992; Pierga et al 1993).

Most carcinomas arise within the lateral ventricles, where, unlike papillomas, they are more often frankly invasive of parenchyma. In addition, subarachnoid spread and CSF dissemination are far more common in carcinomas (Meyers et al 2004). Metastases outside the neuraxis are rare (Vraa-Jensen 1950). Many carcinomas have obvious papillarity, but in many their cells are arranged in patternless sheets (Fig. 9.10B). Marked cellularity and cytologic atypia, brisk mitotic activity, and extensive necrosis are usually present. MIB-1 labeling indices are elevated (mean 13.8%) (Vajtai et al 1996).

In that the majority of choroid plexus carcinomas arise in children, distinction from other malignant pediatric tumors such as germ cell tumors (malignant teratoma, embryonal carcinoma) and atypical teratoid/rhabdoid tumor (AT/RT) are of importance. The differential diagnosis with AT/RT may be difficult, since rare examples of choroid plexus carcinoma show inactivating mutations of the *hSNF5/INI-1* gene on chromosome 22q11.2, the alteration typical of AT/RT (Gessi et al 2003). In the rare adult cases, the principle differential diagnosis is metastatic adenocarcinoma. The presence of vimentin, S-100 protein, and GFAP in the absence of more specific epithelial markers may facilitate the diagnosis.

Other neuroepithelial tumors

The 2007 WHO classification recognizes three tumors in this category. While exhibiting distinctly glial phenotypes, they differ from the gliomas described above. The three tumors are: *astroblastoma*, *chordoid glioma of the third ventricle*, and *angiocentric glioma*. Given the astrocytic phenotype seen in most examples of *gliomatosis cerebri*, the 2007 WHO classification moved this lesion to the category of Astrocytic tumors. Nonetheless, we will mention gliomatosis in the present section, since its clinico-radiological features differ from those of diffuse astrocytomas.

Astroblastomas

Astroblastomas are rare supratentorial gliomas of young patients. In the two largest series published to date, ages range from 3 to 58 years with a predilection for females (Bonnin & Rubinstein 1989; Brat et al 2000). Two congenital astroblastomas have been described (Pizer et al 1995).

Astroblastomas are typically supratentorial tumors but may develop at deep hemispheric sites. An intraventricular location or a spatial relationship to the ventricular system is rare. Neuroimaging studies demonstrate a similarity to ependymoma, including the appearance of lobulation, solid and cystic components, and minimal vasogenic edema. Postgadolinium T1-weighted images typically demonstrate heterogeneous enhancement of the solid portion with rim enhancement of the cyst wall (Port et al 2003).

Histologically, key features of astroblastoma include distinctive perivascular arrangements of variably cohesive, polygonal cells, some with broad, tapering processes forming perivascular rosettes. On phosphotungstic acid-hematoxylin stain, the processes are negative for glial fibrils, a feature often seen in ependymomas. Extensive vascular sclerosis and perivascular collagen deposition are typical features. Microcalcification may also be seen. In contrast to diffuse astrocytomas which only occasionally form vague perivascular arrangements, astroblastomas are well-circumscribed gliomas that lack diffuse infiltration. Unlike ependymoma, astroblastomas tend to be superficially situated in the cerebral hemispheres rather than proximate to the ventricular system.

Astroblastomas demonstrate vimentin, S-100 protein, and GFAP immunoreactivity, but the latter may vary among individual tumor cells, being particularly evident in cells forming perivascular rosettes. As in ependymoma, EMA immunoreactivity may be seen (Brat et al 2000).

Although the WHO classification does not apply specific grades to astroblastomas, the tumors are subdivided in low- and high-grade forms, based upon the presence or absence of histologic features generally associated with glial anaplasia. These include mitotic activity, microvascular hyperplasia, and palisading necrosis (Aldape & Rosenblum 2007). As expected, high-grade tumors tend to have elevated MIB-1 labeling indices than do low-grade tumors (15.5% vs 3.2%) (Brat et al 2000), and are more frequently associated with recurrence and progression (Bonnin & Rubinstein 1989; Thiessen et al 1998). Molecular genetic studies on these tumors are very scarce, due to their rarity. Gains on chromosomes 19 and 20q have been described in a small number of cases; changes not seen in either ependymomas or diffuse astrocytomas (Brat et al 2000).

Chordoid glioma of the third ventricle (WHO grade II)

The chordoid glioma of the third ventricle is a rare, slow-growing glioma forming a well-defined, predominantly solid mass in the third ventricular region of adults. Mean patient age is 46 years with a slight female predominance (1.5:1) (Brat et al 1998; Vajtai et al 1999; Pasquier et al 2002; Raizer et al 2003). Only one pediatric example occurring in a 12-year-old male, has been described (Castellano-Sanchez et al 2001). Neuroimaging features are characteristic and include a well-demarcated, predominantly solid to somewhat cystic tumor, which is isointense to gray matter on T1, T2 and FLAIR sequences and shows homogeneous enhancement on post-gadolinium T1-weighted images (Grand et al 2002).

Histologically, chordoid gliomas are composed of cohesive, epithelioid tumor cells arranged in cords, clusters or lobules delimited by a delicate reticulin-positive network. A vacuolated, mucin-rich, PAS-positive matrix is present between single and clustered tumor cells, thus yielding the 'chordoid' appearance. The tumors are well-demarcated from the adjacent brain but may invoke impressive chronic astrocytosis replete with Rosenthal fibers and often prominent lymphoplasmacytic infiltration. The tumor cells are strongly and diffusely immunopositive for vimentin, GFAP, and CD34 (Reifenberger et al 1999). The majority of tumors exhibit variable, often focal immunoreactivity for cytokeratins, EMA, and S-100 protein (Brat & Scheithauer 2007). Anaplastic features, including microvascular proliferation and necrosis are absent. Mitotic figures are sparse or absent and the MIB-1 labeling index low (0.5% to <5%) (Brat et al 1998; Reifenberger et al 1999).

Ultrastructural features strongly indicate glial, specifically ependymal, differentiation. These include the presence of abundant intermediate filaments as well as microvilli, intermediate junctions (zonulae adherentes) and focal surface basal lamina formation. Cilia are not evident, but rare abnormal intracytoplasmic cilia may be seen (Pasquier et al 2002; Raizer et al 2003).

Limited data is available regarding the molecular genetics of chordoid glioma. A comparative genomic hybridization analysis of four tumors revealed no chromosomal imbalances (Reifenberger et al 1999). Detailed genetic analyses of five cases revealed no aberrations of the kind implicated in astrocytic tumors, including ones affecting *TP53*, *CDKN2A*, *EGFR*, *CDK4* and *MDM2* (Reifenberger et al 1999).

The majority of the chordoid gliomas have an indolent growth pattern and total surgical resection appears curative (Raizer et al 2003). Nonetheless, their relatively high morbidity and mortality appears to be related to tumor size at presentation, and the frequent inability to safely achieve a total resection.

Angiocentric glioma (WHO grade I)

Angiocentric gliomas are epilepsy-associated supratentorial tumors affecting primarily children and young adults. Only about 30 cases have been described (Burger et al 2007). Mean patient age at surgery is 17 years (range, 2.3–70 years) with no gender predilection.

The tumors, typically superficial in location and supratentorial, show a preference for the frontoparietal, followed by temporal and hippocampal areas. Neuroimaging shows a rather demarcated, solid lesion without enhancement. Calcifications are rarely seen (Lellouch-Tubiana et al 2005).

Histologically, angiocentric gliomas consist of uniform elongate, fibrillated cells. Cytologically, nuclei are also fusiform and feature rather coarse chromatin. The cells are

either disposed in distinctive angiocentric patterns or lie isolated in intact parenchyma. The former consist of longitudinal and/or circumferential orientation (Wang et al 2005). Perpendicular orientation of tumor cells beneath the pia is also a characteristic. Occasionally, the cells are compacted in a manner resembling schwannomas, albeit without Verocay body-like arrangement. The tumors show strong immunopositivity for vimentin, S-100 protein, and GFAP. In addition, EMA positivity may be seen in a 'dot-like' pattern and in conjunction with ultrastructural findings indicative of ependymal differentiation (Wang et al 2005).

Angiocentric gliomas are largely indolent tumors that may be cured by gross total resection (Burger et al 2007).

Gliomatosis cerebri

Gliomatosis cerebri is a rare glioma characterized by geographically widespread infiltration of sizable portions of the neuraxis in the absence of a discrete tumor. The process affects patients over a wide age range (neonatal to elderly), the peak incidence being in the 5th to 6th decade (Taillibert et al 2006). It often may involve: (1) multiple, at least three, cerebral lobes, (2) an entire hemisphere or large portions of both, and (3) contiguous infratentorial structures and/or the spinal cord. MR imaging shows areas of high signal on T2-weighted images (Kandler et al 1991). Grossly, the only macroscopic evidence of the tumor is diffuse enlargement of the involved structures and loss of distinction between gray and white matter.

The microscopic hallmark of gliomatosis cerebri is variably non-destructive, diffuse infiltration of brain parenchyma by pleomorphic glial cells, typically astrocytes. Cytologically, they feature barely discernible cytoplasm and fusiform to oval nuclei showing a range of chromasia. As mentioned, gliomatosis usually exhibits an astrocytic phenotype with variable GFAP immunoreactivity. Far less frequently, the tumors with an oligodendroglial or mixed oligoastrocytic cytology are encountered (Vates et al 2003). Some investigators consider gliomatosis cerebri with oligodendroglial features to represent not a pattern of tumor growth, but a specific tumor entity (Fuller & Kros 2007).

Gliomatosis cerebri is usually an aggressive glioma with an overall behavior corresponding to a WHO grade III neoplasm (Fuller & Kros 2007). However, given the small biopsies available in most cases, the association between the histological grade and behavior may show poor correlation. Proliferation indices vary with degree of anaplasia and reported. MIB-1 labeling indices show marked variation (<1–30%) (Fuller & Kros 2007).

There is no evidence for a unique pattern of molecular profile in gliomatosis cerebri. The few studies done so far have shown that changes seen in diffuse astrocytomas, such as *TP53* mutation, are present in gliomatosis cerebri but in lower frequency (Fuller & Kros 2007).

Neuronal and mixed neuronal-glial tumors

Neuronal tumors

Gangliocytomas (WHO grade I)

Gangliocytomas are rare, slow-growing lesions which generally arise in children and young adults. They are relatively well circumscribed lesions generally involving the temporal lobes or cervicothoracic spinal cord (Becker et al 2007; Russo et al 1995). By definition, they consist of mature neurons in a paucicellular, non-neoplastic glial stroma. Less common than gangliogliomas, cerebral examples of gangliocytoma also occur in the setting of chronic seizure disorders. Other locations include the hypothalamic-pituitary region and, rarely, the pineal gland (Towfighi et al 1996). Tumors arising in the sellar pituitary region have been associated with endocrine disorders (Towfighi et al 1996; Becker et al 2007). Hypothalamic gangliocytomas may present with precocious puberty (Boyko et al 1991).

The differential diagnosis of gangliocytoma includes cerebral cortical dysplasia and hypothalamic neuronal hamartoma. Unlike cortical dysplasia, the ganglion cells of gangliocytomas show greater pleomorphism, including the presence of bizarre and multinucleate forms. Gangliocytomas possess no potential for anaplastic progression.

Dysplastic gangliocytoma of the cerebellum (WHO grade I)

Dysplastic gangliocytoma of the cerebellum, also termed Lhermitte–Duclos disease, may be considered a special variant of gangliocytoma. Affecting the cerebellum, it shows combined features of a hamartoma and neoplasia. The lesion usually becomes clinically apparent during the fourth decade (mean age at presentation, 34.8) (Abel et al 2005). Occasionally, patients present earlier in life, mainly as a result of megalencephaly and intracranial hypertension (Tuli et al 1997). MR imaging shows a distinctive T2-weighted image having a striped or laminated appearance wherein narrow, high signal bands alternate with isointense stripes (Abel et al 2005).

Dysplastic gangliocytomas consist of abnormal hypertrophic neurons superficially resembling Purkinje cells in association with large myelinated fibers lying parallel beneath the pia. When present, the granular layer is often reduced in thickness; underlying white matter typically shows decreased myelination. Studies of the abnormal neurons differ in their findings. Some report the expression of synaptic and surface membrane proteins related to Purkinje cells (Shiruba et al 1988; Faillot et al 1990), whereas others suggest a relation to granular cell neurons (Reznik & Schoenen 1983; Yachnis et al 1988). It is likely that dysplastic gangliocytomas arise from cytogenetically heterogeneous cells.

Dysplastic gangliocytomas of the cerebellum are linked to Cowden disease, an autosomal dominant disorder characterized by multiple hamartomas and neoplasms (Eberhart et al 2007, for review). Both conditions relate to germline mutations in the *PTEN* gene on chromosome 10 (Padberg et al 1991; Nelen et al 1996; Liaw et al 1997; Zhou et al 2003). Although the association of the two disorders is well documented, the precise relationships between them and germline *PTEN* mutations are not fully understood. Recently, adult-onset of dysplastic gangliocytoma has been revised from a major diagnostic feature to a pathognomonic criterion of Cowden disease (Zhou et al 2003). Childhood-onset dysplastic gangliocytoma may be distinguished from those of adult-onset by lack of germline *PTEN* mutations and absence of the Cowden disease phenotype (Zhou et al 2003).

The recent studies by Abel et al (2005) have suggested that the pathogenesis of dysplastic gangliocytoma is related to loss of the inhibitory influence of *PTEN* upon its downstream phosphatidylinositol 3-kinase (PI3K) pathway, with resultant deleterious effects upon neuronal migration and regulation of cell size. These authors believe that the lesion may be considered a process of hypertrophy superimposed upon a developmental malformation.

Like other gangliocytomas, this progressive cerebellar lesion ultimately requires resection. Postoperative recurrence is common following a subtotal resection (Banerjee & Gleathil 1979; Marano et al 1988). In a recent series, 31% of patients with long-term follow-up underwent at least one additional resection for recurrent disease (Abel et al 2005).

Central neurocytoma and extraventricular neurocytoma (WHO grade II)

Central neurocytomas are supratentorial, intraventricular tumors of small neurons. They typically affect young adults and are associated with a favorable prognosis following resection alone (von Deimling et al 1990). Central neurocytomas are rare, their incidence ranging from 0.25 to 0.5% of all intracranial tumors in large surgical series (Hassoun et al 1993). Most present as well demarcated, often calcified masses arising in the septum pellucidum and projecting into the lateral ventricles, often in the region of the foramen of Monro. Large tumors may show extension into the third ventricle (Hessler et al 1992). Tumors resemble neurocytomas but occurring at other sites within brain parenchyma are termed extraventricular neurocytomas (Figarella-Branger et al 2007).

The histopathologic features of central neurocytoma are stereotypic (Fig. 9.11). The cellular tumors consist of monotonous small neurons with ill-defined cytoplasm and round nuclei, all set in a background of diffuse or rosetted neuropil. Delicate blood vessels form a branching network somewhat resembling that of oligodendroglioma. Mature ganglion cells are rarely seen in central neurocytomas (von Deimling et al 1990). Mitotic activity is low and the MIB-1

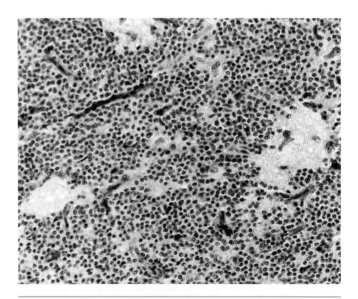

Figure 9.11 Central neurocytoma. Central neurocytomas characteristically consist of homogeneous cell populations with ill-defined borders and a fine fibrillary matrix, especially recognizable in the anuclear areas (H&E).

labeling index is generally low (Robbins et al 1995). In most instances, microvascular proliferation and necrosis are not present.

The neuronal nature of central neurocytomas is confirmed by their immunoreactivity for synaptophysin and other neuronal proteins, including neurofilament proteins and NeuN (von Deimling et al 1990; Hessler et al 1992; Figarella-Branger et al 2007). GFAP is largely restricted to reactive stromal astrocytes (Hessler et al 1992), although some authors have suggested that GFAP staining of tumor cells is associated with more aggressive behavior (Söylemezoglu et al 1997). Ultrastructural features of neurocytoma emphasize their high degree of neuronal maturation, including clear and dense-core vesicles, processes containing parallel microtubules, and the formation of synapses (Hassoun et al 1984; Townsend & Seaman 1986; Nishio et al 1988; von Deimling et al 1990; Kubota et al 1991; Hessler et al 1992).

Central neurocytomas are benign lesions, most behaving in a WHO grade II manner. Only a small number of neurocytomas show mitotic activity, nuclear atypia, endothelial proliferation, or microfoci of necrosis. Although these features tend to be associated with a less favorable outcome, particularly recurrence, they are less well correlated with prognosis than in glial neoplasms (Louis et al 1990; von Deimling et al 1990; Hessler et al 1992, Yasargil et al 1992; Kim et al 1996; Söylemezoglu et al 1997). It has been suggested that tumors exhibiting an increased MIB-1 labeling index (>2%) and vascular endothelial proliferation should be termed 'atypical central neurocytoma' (Söylemezoglu et al 1997). Tumor recurrence is also linked to subtotal resection (Robbins et al 1995; Yasargil et al 1992; Kim et al 1996; Eng et al 1997).

Extraventricular neurocytomas are histologically similar to central neurocytomas. The tumors show an isomorphous population of small cells with perinuclear halos arranged in a finely fibrillary stroma. Ganglion-like cells may be seen intermixed with the neurocytic elements. The main differential diagnosis of these tumors is oligodendrogliomas. Similar to central neurocytomas, extraventricular tumors show neuronal differentiation by immunohistochemical stains. The majority of extraventricular neurocytomas have a benign clinical behavior. However, subtotal resection, atypical histologic features, and high cell proliferation rates appear to correlate with recurrence (Brat et al 2001).

Cerebellar liponeurocytoma (WHO grade II)
Cerebellar liponeurocytomas – neuronal tumors arising in the cerebellum of adults – are very rare. Histologically, they are characterized by neuronal/neurocytic differentiation and focal lipidization (Kleihues et al 2007d). They arise in an older population than patients with central neurocytoma. Most occur in the fifth and sixth decades of life, the mean age at presentation being 50 years (Kleihues et al 2007d).

Liponeurocytomas are well-demarcated masses involving either or both cerebellar hemispheres and the vermis. On neuroimaging studies, CT scans display hypo- to isodensity compared with normal brain parenchyma and moderate, heterogeneous contrast enhancement (Alkadhi et al 2001). T1-weighted MRI sequences show areas of high signal intensity within an overall hypointense tumor, a pattern consistent with focal lipidization (Alkadhi et al 2001; Shin et al 2002).

The tumors are histopathologically characterized by a biphasic pattern of relatively uniform round cells resembling that of neurocytoma, albeit intermingled with a varying proportion of lipidized cells. Mitoses are infrequent and microvascular proliferation and/or necrosis are inconspicuous or absent. The overall proliferative activity of cerebellar liponeurocytomas is comparatively low, with MIB-1 LIs ranging from 1–6% (mean, 3%) (Kleihues et al 2007d).

Immunoreactivity for neuronal markers including synaptophysin and other neuronal proteins is readily detected in both the neurocytic and lipidized cells. Cells immunoreactive for GFAP, S-100, and vimentin may be seen but are more variable in number and distribution (Kleihues et al 2007d). Predictably, ultrastructural studies show evidence of neuronal differentiation, including processes containing parallel microtubules, dense core-vesicles and rare synaptic junctions. Such neuronal cells may also contain cytoplasmic lipid, which appears to coalesce to form large macrodroplets (Taddei et al 2001).

The histogenesis of cerebellar liponeurocytoma and its relationship to other neuronal and neuronal-glial tumors is not well understood. Molecular genetics studies have shown them to have a genetic profile distinct from that of medulloblastomas (Horstmann et al 2004). Unlike medulloblastomas, the tumors lack the frequent finding of isochromosome 17q and show *TP53* missense mutations in about 20% of the cases, a percentage much higher than that observed in either medulloblastoma or central neurocytoma.

Although cerebellar liponeurocytomas appear to have a favorable prognosis, recurrence is seen in nearly two-thirds of cases (Kleihues et al 2007d). Anaplastic progression has not been described, even in recurrent tumors.

Mixed neuronal-glial tumors
Mixed neuronal-glial tumors are more common than the purely neuronal tumors discussed above. Many of these tumors are associated with seizure disorders, particularly gangliogliomas. In the last few years, several reports have described mixed neuronal-glial neoplasms that have distinctive morphological appearance. The 2007 WHO classification incorporated two of these, *papillary glioneuronal tumor* and *rosette-forming glioneuronal tumor of the fourth ventricle*. Both tumors are low-grade and their recognition is important in order to avoid their misidentification as ordinary gliomas and to prevent unnecessary adjuvant treatment.

Gangliogliomas (WHO grade I)
Representing approximately 1% of all brain tumors (Kalyan-Raman & Olivero 1987) and 4–5% of pediatric CNS neoplasms (Sutton et al 1983), gangliogliomas are the most common of the mixed neuronal-glial tumors. The great majority arise in the temporal lobe, although any part of the neuraxis may be affected (Becker et al 2007). The majority are associated with seizures. Indeed, gangliogliomas may represent up to 20% of lesions subject to temporal lobectomy for refractory seizure disorders (Berger et al 1993; Jay et al 1993).

Grossly, gangliogliomas are relatively well-demarcated and characteristically exhibit a cyst-mural nodule architecture. Focal calcification may be seen. Histologically, they exhibit a variable admixture of neoplastic neuronal and glial cells (Fig. 9.12A,B). The neuronal cell elements are

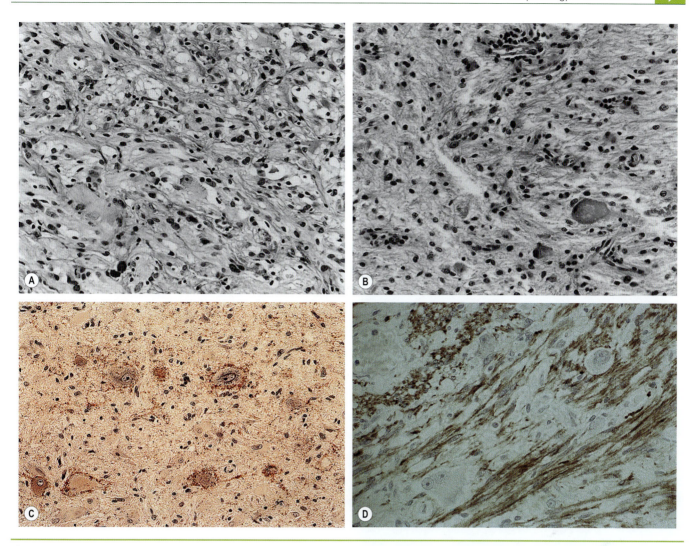

Figure 9.12 Ganglioglioma. (A,B) Mixed population of abnormal ganglionic cells and neoplastic astrocytes, often enmeshed in a fibrillary matrix. Lymphocytic infiltrate and prominent vasculature are common features of gangliogliomas (B) (H&E). (C) Synaptophysin immunohistochemistry highlights the ganglionic elements within the fibrillary glial matrix (Synaptophysin avidin biotin–immunoperoxidase). (D) The glial component of these tumors is readily identified by GFAP immunohistochemistry. (GFAP avidin biotin–immunoperoxidase).

dysmorphic, and vary in size, shape, and distribution. Bizarre forms are present, but binucleation may be rare. The glial component is typically astrocytic, but in rare instances, oligodendrocytes may be present (Allegranza et al 1990). Immunohistochemistry for GFAP and for neuron-associated cytoskeletal proteins, such as neurofilament protein and MAP2, as well as synaptophysin, chromogranin and NeuN (Fig. 9.12C,D) aids in the distinction between glial and neuronal cells. The relative proportions of neoplastic and neurons vary. The stroma of gangliogliomas often includes fibrovascular tissue as well as lymphocytic infiltrates. On occasion, glomeruloid capillaries and/or hyalinized vessels are sufficiently abundant as to mimic a vascular malformation.

It is the glial component, usually astrocytic in nature and more often pilocytic than fibrillary in appearance that possesses the potential for recurrence and anaplastic transformation. Nonetheless, the latter is rare (Russell & Rubinstein 1989). It may be clinically suspected in patients with a recent exacerbation of chronic seizure activity and radiologic features suggestive of progression. The histologic appearance

of the glial element of anaplastic ganglioma (WHO grade III) may be similar to that of anaplastic astrocytomas and may ultimately come to resemble glioblastoma.

Desmoplastic infantile ganglioglioma (WHO grade I)
Desmoplastic infantile ganglioglioma (DIG), a rare variant of the mixed neuronal-glial neoplasms occurs almost exclusively during infancy. It typically presents as a very large supratentorial tumor, with solid and cystic components. Most manifest clinical symptoms between 2 and 24 months of age (mean, 6 months; median, 4 months) with a slight male predominance (VandenBerg 1993; Brat et al 2007). Approximately 10 cases of tumors with the clinical, radiologic, and histopathologic features of DIG have been described in older patients, their ages ranging from 5 to 25 years (Onguru et al 2005; Pommepuy et al 2006).

Most DIGs arise in the frontal and/or parietal lobes and are grossly well demarcated. Nonetheless, on microscopic examination, the interface between the tumor and surrounding brain may be infiltrative to a minor extent. The most

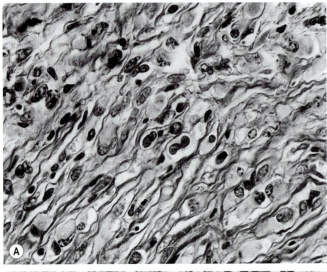

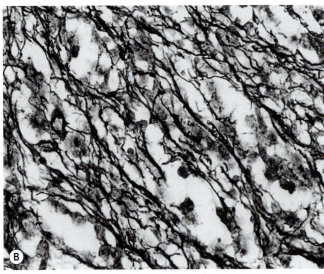

Figure 9.13 Desmoplastic infantile ganglioglioma. (A) Heterogeneous populations of neuroepithelial cells arranged in small clusters or single cells intermixed within a prominent stroma are the hallmark of these tumors (H&E). (B) Reticulin stain accentuates the desmoplastic stroma of these tumors (Gordon and Sweet's reticulin).

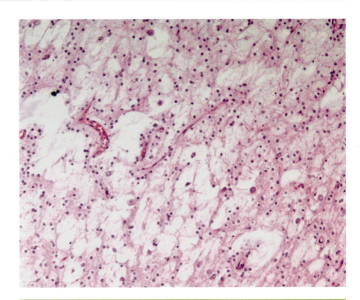

Figure 9.14 Dysembryoplastic neuroepithelial tumor. Multiple intracortical nodules are a principal diagnostic component of DNT. The nodules are basically composed of olilgodendrocyte-like cells, with a few astrocytes and neurons intermixed in an abundant extracellular mucoid matrix (H&E).

conspicuous feature of DIG is its remarkably desmoplastic stroma, which may confer a woody firmness. The latter is most apparent in the leptomeningeal component and/or the interface with involved dura.

Histologically, DIGs exhibit an admixture of neoplastic astrocytes and eosinophilic globoid cells, some of which, despite their superficial resemblance to astrocytes, represent neurons within a desmoplastic stroma (Fig. 9.13). In addition, a minority of DIGs exhibit primitive neuroectodermal tumor-like elements (VandenBerg 1991, 1993). Mitoses and limited foci of necrosis occur mainly in association with such primitive elements, which are not indicative of anaplastic progression or innately malignant in behavior.

Tumors with similar clinical and radiologic features, but limited to astrocytic differentiation, have been termed 'desmoplastic cerebral astrocytomas of infancy' (Taratuto et al 1984; De Chadarévian et al 1990). The histogenetic

relationship between these two desmoplastic tumors of infancy remains unclear (Brat et al 2007).

The most important clinical feature of DIG and desmoplastic infantile astrocytoma (DIA) is their association with a favorable clinical outcome following complete or even subtotal resection (Gambarelli et al 1982; VandenBerg et al 1987; Ng et al 1990; VandenBerg 1991, 1993). Only a few have exhibited aggressive behavior with tumor progression following subtotal resection or cerebrospinal dissemination (Brat et al 2007).

Dysembryoplastic neuroepithelial tumor (WHO grade I)
The now well characterized dysembryoplastic neuroepithelial tumor (DNT) is a rare lesion usually arising in children and young adults with longstanding complex partial seizures. DNTs may represent <1% of all brain tumors (Daumas-Duport 1993); but, in specialized centers for epilepsy surgery, their frequency is considerably higher.

DNTs are intracortical, typically multinodular lesions affecting the medial temporal lobe (Daumas-Duport 1993). They may also arise in other cerebral lobes (Nolan et al 2004). Only a small minority of DNTs involve non-cortical areas, such as the caudate nucleus, cerebellum, and brainstem (Nolan et al 2004; Kuchelmeister et al 1995; Fijumoto et al 2000).

Microscopically, the hallmark of DNT is their multiple nodule architecture. The nodules, often 'patterned', are composed of 'oligodendrocyte-like cells' an occasionally pilocytic or fibrillary-appearing astrocytes. Between the nodules is a typical 'specific component' wherein neurons lie embedded in a mucoid matrix. Thus, some of the neurons appear to float in mucin (Fig. 9.14). Often, cerebral cortex surrounding DNTs displays cortical dysplasia. Cellular atypia is an unusual feature of DNT, but scant mitotic activity may be seen. MIB-1 proliferative indexes are generally very low (<1%) (Taratuto et al 1995; Prayson et al 1996). Immunohistochemical studies for neuronal and glial markers have confirmed the glioneuronal nature of these lesions (Hirose et al 1994). Ultrastructural studies suggest that their constituent 'oligodendrocyte-like cells' are capable of divergent glioneuronal differentiation (Hirose et al 1994).

Considering the varied morphology of these lesions, and that the revealing features are best appreciated at lower power magnification, adequate sampling of intact specimens is diagnostically important. Indeed, non-representative or minute specimens often prompt erroneous diagnoses of oligodendroglioma or oligoastrocytomas. The distinction of DNT from diffuse gliomas is extremely important, since they are associated with a favorable prognosis, even following subtotal resection (Daumas-Duport et al 1988). Radiation and chemotherapy play no role in their treatment. Tumor recurrence has rarely been observed and then only in cases of incomplete resection (Prayson et al 1996).

DNT-like lesions have been reported to occur in locations other than the cerebral cortex. These include examples arising in the area of the septum pellucidum and caudate nucleus (Cervera-Pierot et al 1997; Baisden et al 2001). Like cortical DNTs, these lesions are characterized by an often-nodular proliferation of oligodendrocyte-like cells in a mucin-rich matrix, mucin-entrapped 'floating neurons' within the intervening cortical 'specific component'. The nodules do vary in cellular make-up, occasionally consisting almost entirely of astrocytes. As previously noted, cortical dysplasia may surround the lesion.

Papillary glioneuronal tumor (WHO grade I)
This uncommon tumor is characterized by its pseudopapillary architecture consisting of hyalinized vessels surrounded by a single layer of pseudostratified, small, cuboidal glial cells, as well as interpapillary focal collections or sheets of neurons ranging from neurocytes to small ganglion cells (Nakazato et al 2007a).

The tumors most commonly arise in the white matter and radiographically are rather well-circumscribed, consisting of a contrast-enhancing mass accompanied by a cyst. The tumors occur over a wide range of ages and show no gender predilection (Komori et al 1998; Bouvier-Labit et al 2000; Tsukayama & Arakawa 2002).

Like gangliogliomas, the papillary glioneuronal tumors exhibit little or no mitotic activity and a low MIB-1 labeling index. Although only a few cases have been reported to date, follow-up indicates they are benign in behavior. Only one case of tumor has undergone recurrence (Nakazato et al 2007a).

Rosette-forming glioneuronal tumor of the fourth ventricle (WHO grade I)
This rare lesion of the fourth ventricle is characterized by its biphasic architecture, consisting of small, neurocytic cells arranged in small, Home Wright-like rosettes or perivascular pseudo-rosettes associated with an astrocytic element with pilocytic features (Komori et al 2002; Preusser et al 2003). Ganglion cells may be present. The glial component features occasional Rosenthal fibers, granular bodies or hyaline droplets and microcalcifications.

On neuroimaging, the tumors are located midline, occupy the fourth ventricle and involve the cerebellar vermis. Multicentric lesions with involvement of the cerebellar vermis, midbrain, pons and thalamus have been described (Komori et al 2002; Preusser et al 2003). As in the case of other mixed neuronal-glial tumors, these rare tumors appears to have an indolent course (Hainfellner et al 2007), although postoperative deficits reflective of the tumor's location may be seen.

Pineal parenchymal tumors

Pineal parenchymal tumors (PPT) are rare but do comprise approximately 15–30% of the pineal region tumors (Bruce & Stein 1990; Schild et al 1993; Hoffman et al 1994; Jouvet et al 2000; Fauchon et al 2000). Defined as tumors of pineocytes, the WHO classification recognizes three sub-types including pineocytoma, PPT of intermediate differentiation, and pineoblastoma, representing a spectrum of tumoral features ranging from well-differentiated to primitive. Between the two extremes, are tumors of intermediate differentiation.

The three PPTs are also distinctive from a clinical point of view. Pineocytomas occur most often in older adults, tend to be circumscribed and show no propensity to cerebrospinal (CSF) seeding. Pineocytomas have protracted survival times, the 5-year figure being 67% in one series (Schild et al 1993). Thus, they are considered grade I tumors in the WHO classification (Nakazato et al 2007a). The intermediate PPT of intermediate differentiation lack pineocytomatous rosettes and behavior, somewhat in accord with the relative presence of proliferative activity and neurofilament protein staining (Nakazato et al 2007b; Fèvre-Montange et al 2008). These tumors are designated as either grade II or III by the WHO classification (Nakazato et al 2007b). Their potential for local infiltration and CSF dissemination is significant, and their clinical behavior appears to be more aggressive than pineocytomas (Schild et al 1993). The primitive pineoblastoma has a clinical behavior similar to other primitive neuroectodermal tumors of the CNS (see below), in that they generally arise in children and young adults, are highly infiltrative tumors, have the potential for dissemination by the CSF pathways, and behave as a grade IV malignancy. Patients with pineoblastomas have a short survival time (16 months in a large cohort study) (Fauchon et al 2000), and low 5-year progression free survival (38% in another series) (Reddy et al 2000).

Pineocytomas (WHO grade I)
Pineocytomas account for about 7–30% of the PPTs, most occurring in adults. Early series with less stringent morphologic criteria reported a wider range of patient age at diagnosis, including young patients (range, 11–78 years) (Herrick & Rubinstein 1979; Vaquero et al 1992).

Pineocytomas are typically well-demarcated masses which compress adjacent parenchyma and show little tendency to infiltration. Microscopically, they are moderately cellular neoplasms that typically exhibit the formation of diagnostic 'pineocytomatous rosettes', consisting of a circular arrangement of cytologically uniform cells, the processes of which form large, often circular, delicately fibrillated zone (Borit et al 1980) (Fig. 9.15A). The rosettes far exceed the size of Homer Wright rosettes. Silver impregnation studies for pineocytic processes demonstrates delicate, argyrophilic processes within the centers of the rosettes (De Girolami and

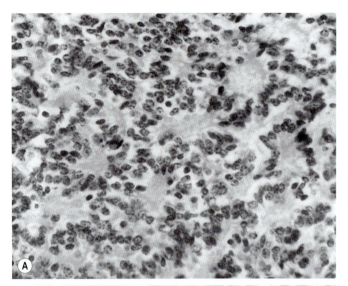

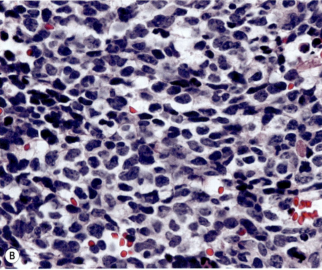

Figure 9.15 Pineal parenchymal tumors. (A) Pineocytomas typically show groups of uniform cells surrounding delicate anuclear areas, forming the so-called pineocytomatous rosettes. (B) In contrast, pineoblastomas are composed of small, primitive cells arranged in sheet-like arrangements and with high mitotic activity (H&E).

processes, neurosensory cilia with a 9+0 microtubule arrangement, intermediate filament bundles, centrioles, dense-core and clear vesicles, as well as annulate lamellae (Kline et al 1979; Markesbery et al 1981; Hassoun et al 1983, 1984; Hassoun & Gambarelli 1989) – all features of normal pineocytic/neurosensory cells.

Pineal parenchymal tumor of intermediate differentiation (WHO grade II or III)

A significant proportion of PPTs do not morphologically fit into the categories of pineocytoma or pineoblastoma and exhibit behavior intermediately between these two distinct tumors. This has led to the introduction of the category of PPT of intermediate differentiation which, in one reported series, accounted for 56% of all PPTs (Jouvet et al 2000). The tumors exhibit a spectrum of differentiation characterized by increased cellularity, and Homer Wright-like rather than pineocytomatous rosettes. In addition, they lack the small cell, primitive appearance of pineoblastoma. Some exhibit minor atypia and low mitotic activity, whereas others show moderate mitotic activity and areas of necrosis (Nakazato et al 2007b; Fèvre-Montange et al 2008). Definite grading criteria have not been established relative to this category but it is likely that a low and higher grade will be established (Scheithauer et al 2008). One study has suggested that proliferative activity and immunoreactivity for neurofilament protein may be the essential criteria dividing PPTs of intermediate differentiation into two separate grades (Fèvre-Montange et al 2008). Although criteria have not been adopted by the WHO, they are loosely considered as encompassing grades II and III.

Pineoblastoma (WHO grade IV)

Pineoblastomas are the most primitive of PPTs. More common than pineocytomas, they account for up to 18% of the pineal region tumors (Bruce & Stein 1990; Hoffman et al 1994) and for 50–75% of the PPTs (D'Andrea et al 1987; Edwards et al 1988; Schild et al 1993; Hoffman et al 1994; Nakazato et al 2007b). Unlike pineocytomas and PPT of intermediate differentiation, they preferentially occur in the first two decades of life (Nakazato et al 2007b).

Pineoblastomas are poorly demarcated masses, showing a high tendency to invade adjacent brain and to disseminate through the neuraxis. Postoperative systemic metastases have been described, in one case to a thoracic vertebra and in another to the sacrum (Charafe-Jauffret et al 2001). Microscopically, they are highly cellular neoplasms composed of small, poorly-differentiated cells with round to oval, hyperchromatic nuclei containing coarse chromatin. The cells are arranged in patternless sheets, but Homer Wright rosettes may be present. Silver carbonate impregnation may demonstrate small cell processes. The ultrastructural features are those of a poorly-differentiated neuroepithelial neoplasm, only occasionally with distinctive photosensory features (Kline et al 1979; Markesbery et al 1981; Min et al 1994). This is evidenced by the presence of Flexner–Wintersteiner rosettes and fleurettes (Stefanko & Manschot 1979; Sobel et al 1981; Russell & Rubinstein 1989). Photosensory-associated protein retinal S-antigen (S-Ag), has been reported across the spectrum of PPTs including pineoblastomas (Perentes et al 1986), pineocytomas (Per-

Zvaigzne 1973). Similar albeit shorter processes with terminal expansions are also noted in more diffuse portions of the tumors. Occasional bizarre giant cells may be seen, a feature upon which some diagnose 'pleomorphic pineocytoma' (Jouvet et al 2000). Such pleomorphic cells are of no prognostic significance (Jouvet et al 2000). Mitotic figures are rare. Focal infarct-like necrosis may occasionally be seen. Calcification may be prominent.

Pineocytomas express neuronal-associated proteins; neurofilament protein and synaptophysin are present in virtually all specimens. Retinal S-antigen (S-Ag) has also been demonstrated in pineocytomas (Korf et al 1986; Perentes et al 1986; Mena et al 1995), a feature no doubt related to the transient photosensory differentiation occurring in pineocytes during development (Reiter 1981). Ultrastructural features of pineocytomas include tangled microtubule-containing entes et al 1986; Jouvet et al 2000) and intermediate PPTs (Jouvet et al 2000). Interphotoreceptor retinoid-binding protein (IRBP), an interphotoreceptor matrix protein that functions in retinoid transport between the photoreceptor cells and the retinal pigment epithelium, is yet another photosensory marker that has been demonstrated in a PPT of intermediate differentiation (Lopes et al 1993).

The presence of photosensory proteins in pineoblastomas not only reflects a biochemical relationship between the retina and the pineal, but also suggests a link between the two embryonal tumors – retinoblastoma and pineoblastoma. It also explains the occurrence of so-called trilateral retinoblastoma (Johnson et al 1985), the concurrence of bilateral retinoblastoma and pineoblastoma. More rarely, the tumors may also exhibit differentiation to mesenchymal tissues (striated muscle, cartilage) and melanotic pigmentation (Schmidbauer et al 1989; McGrogan et al 1992).

Papillary tumor of the pineal region (WHO grade II or III)

This category of pineal region tumor is new to the 2007 WHO classification (Jouvet et al 2007). Its descriptive designation, papillary tumor of the pineal region (PTPR), indicates our lack of histogenetic insight. PTPR appears to be a rare neuroepithelial tumor. First described in 2003 by Jouvet and colleagues, approximately 50 cases have been reported to date (Jouvet et al 2003; Shibahara et al 2004; Fèvre-Montange et al 2006b; Hasselblatt et al 2006a; Kern et al 2006; Kuchelmeister et al 2006; Kawahara et al 2007; Roncaroli & Scheithauer 2007; Dagnew et al 2007). The tumor affects mainly adults with a median age of 29 (range 5–66 years) and shows a slight female predilection (Fèvre-Montange et al 2006b). Patients often present with headache due to hydrocephalus. On imaging, PTPR form well-defined masses, often having a cystic component. MRI shows them to be isointense on T1-weighted images, hyperintense on T2-weighted images, and contrast enhancing (Kawahara et al 2007).

Microscopically, PTPR consist of a solid to papillary proliferation of epithelial-appearing cells within fibrovascular cores. The cells are generally large, cuboidal to somewhat columnar, with well-defined cell membranes and round to oval nuclei with stippled chromatin. Some cells are vacuolated and contain amylase-resistant, PAS positive material. Perivascular pseudo-rosettes, true rosettes and tubules are present to varying degrees. The vessels are often hyalinized, but vascular proliferation is not a feature. Some degree of necrosis is almost always present. Mitotic activity may be moderate (Jouvet et al 2007).

Immunohistochemical stains reveal both neuroepithelial and neuroendocrine differentiation of the tumors. The tumors are uniformly positive for broad spectrum cytokeratin, particularly in the papillae. Staining for GFAP is only focally seen in perivascular cells, but S100, MAP-2, NCAM, NSE, and vimentin (Jouvet et al 2007) reactivity may be evident. In addition, synaptophysin and chromogranin A may be weakly positive. As in ependymomas, EMA positivity in ring- and dot-like patterns can be seen (Jouvet et al 2003; Fèvre-Montange et al 2006b; Shibahara et al 2004). It is of note that PTRTs are also negative for the choroid plexus

tumor markers Kir7.1 and stanniocalcin-1 (Hasselblatt et al 2006b). The MIB-1 labeling index varies, roughly even distributions of cases with indices <5%, 5–10%, and >10% being noted (Fèvre-Montange et al 2006b).

Electron microscopy demonstrates both ependymal and neurosecretory differentiation, based upon the presence of microvilli, zipper-like junctions, dense core granules, numerous mitochondria, and rough endoplasmic reticulum filled with secretory material and ependymal-like processes terminating on vessel (Jouvet et al 2003; Dagnew et al 2007). Based on the immunohistochemical and ultrastructure, an origin from specialized ependymal cells of the subcommissural organ has been postulated (Jouvet et al 2003). A recent microarray analysis of gene expression in two PTPRs lends support to this theory (Fèvre-Montange et al 2006a). Other genetic data is limited, but one study of five PTPRs using comparative genomic hybridization demonstrated a variety of chromosomal imbalances, the most common being losses on chromosomes 10 and 22q and gains on chromosomes 4, 8, 9, and 12 (Hasselblatt et al 2006b).

Due to the rarity of PTPR, the issue of prognosis remains to be clarified. One study analyzing the follow-up of 29 cases (Fèvre-Montange et al 2006b) calculated a 5-year overall survival of 73% and a 5-year progression-free survival of 27%. Tumors recurred locally but spinal metastases were rare. Gross total resection was the only factor associated with survival and recurrence, but it failed to reach statistical significance. Increased mitotic activity did not appear to affect recurrence or survival.

Embryonal tumors

This group of clinically aggressive neoplasms that usually occur in early life, many in the first decade of life, is distinct from the spectrum of anaplastic neuroepithelial tumors occurring in adults, e.g., astrocytic, oligodendroglial, and ependymal tumors. All embryonal tumors, regardless of type, share the common histologic features of high cellularity, brisk mitotic activity, and a tendency to at least focal necrosis. Most show a distinct propensity to leptomeningeal spread by way of cerebrospinal pathways. All deserve their WHO grade IV designation (Louis et al 2007).

Despite the common properties noted above, the various embryonal tumors fall into categories on the basis of their distinct histopathological features and presumed histogeneses. Most common is the *medulloblastoma* which arises in the cerebellum. Embryonal tumors indistinguishable from medulloblastomas, but situated at other sites along the neuraxis are designated *CNS/supratentorial primitive neuroectodermal tumor* (CNS-PNET).

The designation CNS-PNET reflects the concept that embryonal tumors are derived from primitive neuroepithelial progenitor or perhaps stem cells distributed throughout the neuraxis and displaying similar histopathologic features as well as biologic behavior. Implicit in this concept is the notion that the potential for divergent phenotypic differentiation in a PNET is the result of transformation of stem or undifferentiated neuroepithelial cells (Gould et al 1990; Fan & Eberhart 2008). Pluripotential differentiation may take place if neoplastic transformation occurs in a true stem cell, in a lineage committed but not fully differentiated cell, or

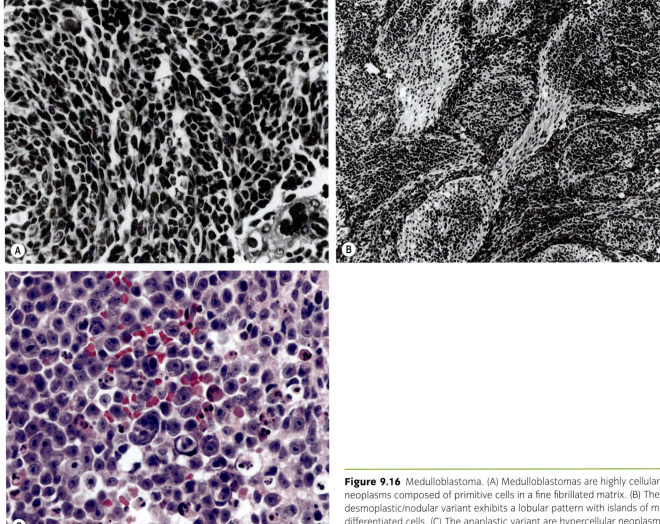

Figure 9.16 Medulloblastoma. (A) Medulloblastomas are highly cellular neoplasms composed of primitive cells in a fine fibrillated matrix. (B) The desmoplastic/nodular variant exhibits a lobular pattern with islands of more differentiated cells. (C) The anaplastic variant are hypercellular neoplasms displaying areas of cellular wrapping and nuclear molding (A–C, H&E).

even in a fully differentiated cell (Fan & Eberhart 2008). Recent data has substantiated previous observations (Russell & Rubinstein 1989) that CNS-PNET is a heterogeneous group of tumors that may show distinct genetic abnormalities and, therefore, have treatment and prognostic implications.

Specific sub-types of embryonal tumors include the *cerebral neuroblastoma/ganglioneuroblastoma* and *ependymoblastoma*, embryonal tumors of neuronal and ependymal lineages, respectively. The *medulloepithelioma*, a very rare embryonal neoplasm having a characteristic, but non-small cell morphology, is also an entity in the 2007 WHO classification. Lastly, a*typical teratoid/rhabdoid tumors* also fall into the embryonal tumor category, but as a category distinct from medulloblastomas and PNETs.

Medulloblastoma (WHO grade IV)

Medulloblastoma is the most common of embryonal tumors, representing about 90% of them (Ellison 2002). Most present during the first decade of life with a peak incidence at age 7 years and a slight male predilection (Giangaspero et al 2007). In adults, the majority of medulloblastomas occur in

the 3rd decade. Only rare examples are encountered beyond the 5th decade of life.

The majority of medulloblastomas, about 75%, are situated in the cerebellar vermis. This is particularly the case in children. Hemispheric tumors are most common in adults, and are frequently of the desmoplastic/nodular subtype (Giangaspero et al 2007). Macroscopically, the tumors are soft and appear rather demarcated from the adjacent cerebellum. Necrosis may be microfocal, sometimes confluent but only rarely massive. The desmoplastic variant of medulloblastoma may be remarkably firm in consistency.

Classic medulloblastoma is the most common variant and shows typical features of an embryonal or primitive neoplasm. The tumors are highly cellular neoplasms, composed of relatively small cells with scant cytoplasm and ill-defined cell borders (Fig. 9.16A). The nuclei vary in both shape and chromatin pattern. In most cases, they are hyperchromatic and ovoid to angular shaped. As a rule, the cells are arrayed in sheets. Only occasionally are rhythmic nuclear palisades encountered. The tumor cells diffusely infiltrate the cerebellar cortex, obliterating the distinction between granular and molecular layers. Mitoses vary in number as does cellular apoptosis. Microvascular proliferation is rarely observed, but small foci of necrosis are seen in the majority of the tumors.

Obvious neuroblastic differentiation, in the form of Homer Wright (neuroblastic) rosettes, is seen in approximately 40% of classic medulloblastomas (Kleihues et al 1989). Neoplastic ganglion cells are present in only about 7% of tumors with such neuroblastic differentiation. Immunoreactivity for neuronal-associated proteins, such as neurofilament proteins, synaptophysin, and class III β-tubulin, is generally present throughout. In contrast, astroglial differentiation is far less frequent, being seen in approximately 10% of cases as scattered or microclustered cells immunoreactive for GFAP (Kleihues et al 1989; Giangaspero et al 2007).

Desmoplastic/nodular medulloblastoma. This medulloblastoma variant represents about 10–12% of all cases (Burger et al 1987; Kleihues et al 1989) and is distinguished by its characteristic biphasic architecture (Fig. 9.16B), which consists of highly cellular sheets and trabeculae of tumor cells interpreted by hypocellular round to oblong islands of cells exhibiting a more differentiated appearance. The so-called 'pale islands' imparting a follicular or nodular architecture, are highlighted on reticulin stains. The intervening densely cellular element consists of often smaller cells enmeshed in reticulin, whereas the cells comprising the nodules are not. The nodular areas contain cells with more advanced differentiation, as evidenced by more open chromatin and the formation of delicate processes. Immunoreactivity for neuronal-associated markers and for the neurotrophin receptors TrkA and TrkC (Eberhart et al 2001) are well seen within the nodules thus underscoring their more advanced neuronal differentiation. Indirect evidence of differentiation within the reticulin-free nodules is their lower Ki-67 labeling index, a finding suggesting the emergence of postmitotic neuronal cells.

A rare variant of desmoplastic medulloblastoma, termed *medulloblastoma with extensive nodularity*, is often commonly seen in infants. Once referred to as 'cerebellar neuroblastoma' (Katsetos et al 1989), such tumors feature markedly expanded nodules as well as streaming of small, maturing round cells resembling those of central neurocytoma.

A less frequent variant of medulloblastoma, *large cell medulloblastoma*, represent about 2–4% of medulloblastomas and have exceptionally aggressive biologic behavior (Giangaspero et al 1992; Giangaspero et al 2007). Histologically, they are characterized by large, round cells with prominent round nuclei and nucleoli, as well as relatively abundant cytoplasm. These tumors also show high level mitotic and apoptotic activity, as well as conspicuous necrosis. This variant of medulloblastoma frequently contains areas of the cellular wrapping and nuclear molding that characterizes *anaplastic medulloblastomas* (Fig. 9.16C), another uncommon variant of medulloblastomas with which the large cell variant is often grouped (Giangaspero et al 2007).

Other rare variants of medulloblastoma include the *medullomyoblastoma*, tumors showing striated muscle cell differentiation with populations of more primitive cells that resemble rhabdomyosarcoma (Rao et al 1990), and

the *melanotic medulloblastoma* with pigmented papillary arrangements. (Kubota et al 2009).

Identifying the histological variants of medulloblastomas has significant clinical implications. Recent studies have shown that they are associated with a different clinical outcome and therapeutic response. This relates not only to their histologic features but to their molecular profiles as well (Eberhart et al 2002a; Eberhart & Burger 2003; Giangaspero et al 2007). The desmoplastic/nodular variant has been associated with a better prognosis than classic medulloblastomas. On the other hand, the large cell and anaplastic medulloblastomas have a far poorer prognosis. Although an official grading system is not widely accepted for medulloblastomas, stratification of tumors according to their degree of differentiation or anaplasia is recommended (Eberhart et al 2002a; Eberhart & Burger 2003; Giangaspero et al 2007). Furthermore, recent studies suggest that a combination of histological classification and molecular profiling of medulloblastomas will be the basis of a more precise grading system (Pomeroy et al 2002; Eberhart et al 2002a,b; Crawford et al 2007; Rossi et al 2008).

Central nervous system primitive neuroectodermal tumors (WHO grade IV)

Central nervous system primitive neuroectodermal tumors (CNS PNET) are the second most common category of embryonal tumors. Histologically, they are indistinguishable from cerebellar medulloblastoma, but are located in other parts of the CNS. Most affect the cerebrum, thus justifying the designation of supratentorial PNETs, but may also arise in the spinal cord and in the suprasellar region.

CNS PNET are very uncommon tumors, thus their precise incidence is unknown. In a survey undertaken by the National Cancer Institute's Surveillance, Epidemiology and End Results program (SEER), of the 768 patients diagnosed either as medulloblastoma or PNET, only 7% were supratentorial (McNeil et al 2002). Most CNS PNET present during the first decade of life (mean, 5.5 years) and have a slight male predilection (McLendon et al 2007a).

The histopathologic features of CNS PNETs are similar to those of medulloblastoma, i.e. hypercellular, patternless and composed of primitive, undifferentiated cells. Intercellular processes form a somewhat fibrillary background in some but not all instances. Specialized cell arrangements such as Homer Wright rosettes and palisades resembling polar spongioblastoma may be seen. Mitotic activity is high and apoptotic figures are commonly seen. The same is true of individual cell and extensive necrosis. Like medulloblastoma, CNS PNET may show evidence of divergent differentiation, as evidenced by immunohistochemical expression of neuronal, glial, epithelial and mesenchymal markers.

A clear distinction should be made between the CNS and peripheral PNETs (pPNETs). In addition to the obviously different sites at which they occur, the pathophysiology and molecular biology of these two forms of embryonal tumor are entirely different. PNETs originating in peripheral nerves and soft tissue are closely related to extraskeletal Ewing's sarcoma. Tumors of the Ewing's sarcoma family are characterized by the t(11;22)(q24;q12) chromosomal translocation and the EWS/FLI-1 fusion transcript (Ushigome et al 2002). Immunoreactivity for CD99, which recognizes the

MIC2 gene product, is typical of the pPNET neoplasms (Ushigome et al 2002). CNS-PNETs do not share this genetic profile and thus lack CD99 expression. Nonetheless, primary intradural pPNETs arising from peripheral nerves residing within the intracranial and intraspinal dura, have been described (Katayama et al 1999; Isatalo et al 2000).

Ependymoblastoma (WHO grade IV)

This rare form of ependymal tumor, usually presents in infants and young children, their median age in one series being 2 years (Mørk & Rubinstein 1985). Nearly all reported examples have been massive, supratentorial tumors in which a relationship to the ventricular system may be hard to assess. They tend to be macroscopically discrete, but microscopic infiltration of surrounding brain and leptomeninges may be seen.

Microscopically, ependymoblastomas are highly cellular and composed of small, poorly-differentiated cells arranged in patternless sheets punctuated by remarkably well-formed ependymoblastic rosettes and tubules. In contrast to the ordinary ependymal rosettes, the ependymoblastic rosettes consist of a thick pseudostratified layer of ependymal cell exhibiting frequent juxtaluminal mitoses. Well-developed perivascular pseudo-rosettes and ependymal rosettes of the type seen in ependymomas are rare. The ultrastructural finding of luminal cytoplasmic specialization, including microvilli, 9+2 cilia, and complex zonulae adherens-type junctions, is clear evidence of ependymal differentiation (Langford 1986). Immunohistochemistry reactivity for GFAP confirms the glial character of these tumors, highlighting groups of primitive cells and occasional cells of the rosettes and tubules. As expected, S-100 protein and vimentin immunoreactivity may also be observed.

For therapeutic and prognostic purposes, ependymoblastomas should be distinguished from anaplastic ependymomas. Ependymoblastomas occur in early childhood, whereas anaplastic ependymomas are tumors often encountered in adults. Their histologic distinction is based upon the overall PNET-like appearance of ependymoblastomas and the multilayered true rosettes and the absence of cytoplasmic and/or nuclear pleomorphism characteristic of anaplastic ependymoma. Furthermore, microvascular endothelial proliferation, an often conspicuous feature of anaplastic ependymomas, is generally absent in ependymoblastomas. Although necrosis may be seen in both tumors, palisading necrosis is primarily a feature of anaplastic ependymomas.

Cerebral neuroblastoma (WHO grade IV)

Cerebral neuroblastomas are rare embryonal tumors. They affect mainly children, often early in the first decade, usually arise in the frontotemporal region, but may arise in any part of the neuraxis, including the brainstem and spinal cord (Horten & Rubinstein 1976; Bennett & Rubinstein 1984). Most are massive, multicystic tumors with a discrete border relative to adjacent brain. In some instances, desmoplasia confers a firm texture and somewhat lobulated appearance.

Histologically, central neuroblastomas are highly cellular, the constituent small cells having poorly defined cytoplasm, round to ovoid nuclei, and hyperchromatic nuclei (Fig. 9.17A). Varying stages of neuronal differentiation may be evident in most cases, evidenced by cells with more

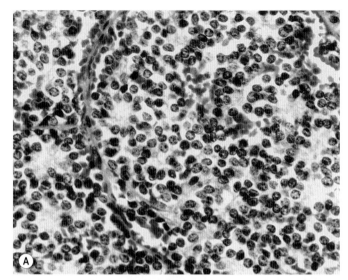
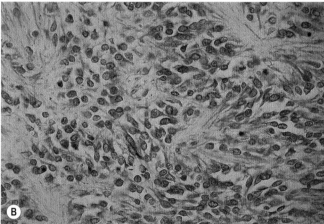

Figure 9.17 Neuroblastoma. (A) Monotonous sheets of poorly-differentiated small cells are intermixed with the characteristic Homer Wright (neuroblastic) rosettes (H&E). (B) Delicate cellular processes (neurites), here highlighted by the neuronal-associated class III β-tubulin, form the fibrillated matrix of these tumors. (TUJ1 avidin biotin–immunoperoxidase).

abundant cytoplasm, conspicuous process formation, and vesicular nuclei. Emerging nucleoli may be seen. The cells tend to be arranged in monotonous sheets, the intercellular spaces containing varying numbers of neuritic processes. Characteristic Homer Wright (neuroblastic) rosettes are present in varying number. Parallel arrangements of compactly aligned cellular groups with rhythmic nuclear palisading, similar to those of medulloblastomas, may be seen. Neurites are detectable by either silver impregnation (Bodian, Bielschowski methods) or by immunohistochemistry for neuronal markers such class III β-tubulin, neurofilaments and synaptophysin (Fig. 9.17B). Ultrastructural features of neuroblastic differentiation include microtubule-containing cell processes, neurosecretory granules or vesicles, and occasional synapses (Russell & Rubinstein 1989). Unlike CNS-PNETs (see below), cerebral neuroblastomas and ganglioneuroblastomas do not demonstrate divergent glial and neuronal differentiation. Therefore, GFAP preparations are negative except in stromal astrocytes.

Scant ganglionic differentiation, either as isolated cells or as clusters, may occur in moderate proportion of the cases. In such instances, the designation *cerebral gangli-oneuroblastoma* is applied (McLendon et al 2007a).

Medulloepithelioma (WHO grade IV)

Medulloepithelioma is the rarest of embryonal tumors, usually affecting children in the first 5 years of life (mean age, 29 months) and exhibiting no gender predilection (Caccamo et al 1989; Molloy et al 1996; McLendon et al 2007a). Intracranial examples produce symptoms and signs of increased intracranial pressure. Most patients die within 1 year of diagnosis, but rare long-term survivors have been noted (Scheithauer & Rubinstein 1979; Molloy et al 1996; Norris et al 2005).

The majority of the medulloepitheliomas are located in the cerebral hemispheres (Caccamo et al 1989), but other sites including the sella/suprasellar region and spinal cord may be affected (McLendon et al 2007a).

The hallmark histologic feature of medulloepithelioma is the formation of primitive epithelium resembling embryonic neural tube. It consists of mitotically active, pseudo-stratified columnar epithelium, often arranged in ribbons, tubules or even papillae. These are delimited by a PAS-positive, external limiting membrane. Immunohistochemically, strong nestin and vimentin immunoreactivity is seen in the epithelial structures, but only occasionally are neuroblastic or glial cytoskeletal proteins, such as class III β-tubulin and GFAP, expressed (Caccamo et al 1989; Tohyama et al 1992; Khoddami & Becker 1997). In contrast, glial and neuronal differentiation can readily be demonstrated in the differentiating components present in many tumors (Caccamo et al 1989). On balance, the morphologic spectrum of this rare embryonal tumor is remarkably similar to those noted during the formation and differentiation of the embryonic neural tube (Cameron & Rakic 1991). Not only can medulloepitheliomas show the full spectrum of glioneuronal differentiation, but some feature specialized mesenchymal elements as well.

Atypical teratoid/rhabdoid tumor (WHO grade IV)

The designation 'atypical teratoid/rhabdoid tumor' (AT/RT) refers to a group of childhood brain tumors that share one common feature – 'rhabdoid' cells. Other tissue elements include primitive neuroectodermal, mesenchymal and rarely mature epithelial cells (Rorke et al 1996; Burger et al 1998). Most AT/RT arise in the posterior fossa, although supratentorial tumors are often seen involving multiple other CNS sites (Judkins et al 2007). The great majority of patients are <3 years of age. Males are more commonly affected than females. AT/RTs are extremely aggressive and are associated with a median and mean survivals of 11 and 24 months, respectively (Judkins et al 2007) (Fig. 9.18).

Grossly, AT/RTs are large, soft and feature often extensive necrosis and hemorrhage. Dissemination in CSF pathways is present at diagnosis in one-third of cases; cranial nerves are also commonly involved (Judkins et al 2007). The very poor prognosis of the tumor is probably due in part to its proclivity for craniospinal seeding (Burger et al 1998).

As previously noted, the tumors are distinguished by the presence of rhabdoid cells. These large, polygonal cells

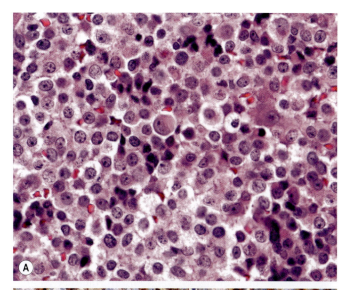

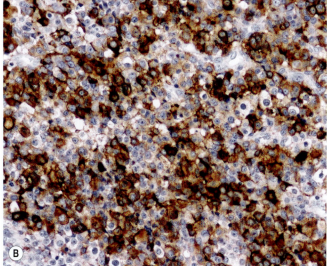

Figure 9.18 Atypical teratoid/rhabdoid tumor. (A) Typical appearance of rhabdoid cells with eosinophilic globoid cytoplasm and eccentric nuclei (H&E). (B) Strong expression of EMA is seen in the great majority of AT/RT (EMA avidin biotin–immunoperoxidase).

feature ample eosinophilic cytoplasm containing a spherical fibrillary paranuclear inclusion, and vesicular nuclei with prominent nucleoli. Similar large cells lacking an inclusion ('pale cells') may also be seen. Both cell types may be abundant or accompanied by a complex mixture of primitive neuroepithelial tumor resembling medulloblastoma, mesenchymal spindle cells, clear cells and rarely true epithelial elements. Both rhabdoid and so-called pale cells are EMA- and vimentin positive. Although they lack true myoid differentiation, both these and accompanying spindle cells may be immunoreactive for smooth muscle actin and desmin. Occasionally, they also show reactivity for cytokeratins, GFAP, synaptophysin and neurofilament protein. Only on rare occasions is reactivity for germ cell markers, including PLAP, AFP and β-HCG, seen in AT/RT (Wharton et al 2003).

The most significant immunohistochemical characteristic of AT/RT is lack of expression of the INI1 protein. The negative reaction is a sensitive marker of AT/RT (Judkins et al 2004; Haberler et al 2006). In normal tissues and most neoplasms, INI1 is constitutively expressed as a nuclear protein; but in AT/RTs, some schwannomas, and epithelioid sarcoma, there is loss of nuclear expression in all but normal stroma endothelial cells. This is due to abnormalities on chromosome 22q11.2, the region containing the *INI1/hSNF5* gene (see below).

Molecular cytogenetics of embryonal tumors

The majority of the data available on molecular genetic studies in these tumors are relevant to medulloblastomas, the most common of the embryonal tumors. Extensive discussion of this topic is available in several outstanding reviews, particularly the 2007 WHO publication of the Classification of Tumors of the Central Nervous System (Giangaspero et al 2007).

Cytogenetic studies have shown isochromosome 17q [i (17q)] to be the most frequent abnormality in medulloblastomas, occurring in about one-third of all tumors (Giangaspero et al 2007). Molecular studies have confirmed this finding, showing frequent loss of heterozygosity (LOH) for chromosome 17p (Steichen-Gersdorf et al 1997). Although this is region contains the *TP53* gene locus, mutations of this gene are rarely seen in medulloblastomas (Raffel et al 1993; Steichen-Gersdorf et al 1997; Kraus et al 2002). Loss of 17p appears to be a negative prognostic indicator in medulloblastomas (Nicholson et al 1999; Lamont et al 2004). A variety of other cytogenetic alterations have been documented, including deletions on chromosomes 1q, 10q, 11p/11q, 16q and 9q. In the latter, the locus of the basal cell nevus syndrome (Gorlin syndrome) at 9q22 (*PTCH*) is located. Germline mutations of the *PTCH* gene predisposes to the development of medulloblastomas, particularly the desmoplastic/nodular variant (Schofield et al 1995). Mutations of this gene have also been found in sporadic medulloblastomas (Raffel et al 1997; Zurawel et al 2000). Mutations in the adenomatous polyposis coli gene (*APC*) and its corresponding Wnt signaling pathway are associated with Turcot Syndrome (germline mutation in *APC*) and with medulloblastomas; however, only a minority of sporadic medulloblastomas have somatic mutations in the *APC*/Wnt pathway (Huang et al 2000). In several studies, amplification of *myc* oncogenes has been associated with aggressive tumor behavior (Eberhart & Burger 2003). Increased *c-myc* mRNA expression is a negative prognostic marker (Aldosari et al 2002; Eberhart et al 2004), being highly associated with the large cell/anaplastic medulloblastoma variant (Eberhart & Burger 2003; Giangaspero et al 2007). Alternatively, down-regulation of *N-myc* and high expression of the neurotrophin receptor TrkC have been associated with protracted survival (Segal et al 1994; Ellison 2002). Several neural transcription factors implicated in the development of the brain have been shown to be deregulated in medulloblastomas. These include PAX5, PAX6, ZIC, NEUROD, SOX4, OTX1 and OTX2. Generally, altered expression of these proteins is unassociated with genetic mutations or copy number changes (see Giangaspero et al 2007 for review).

In contrast to medulloblastomas, relatively little is known regarding genetic abnormalities in CNS-PNETs. Nonetheless, data indicates that chromosomal and genetic aberrations in these tumors differ from those seen in medulloblastomas. Specifically, isochromosome 17q is exceptional in CNS-PNETs and LOH 17p is not encountered (Thomas & Raffel 1991; Russo et al 1999; Kraus et al 2002; McCabe et al 2006). Gene expression profiling of CNS-PNETs has shown a molecular heterogeneity and a lack of clustering, possibly a reflection the diverse spectrum of tumors included this category (Russo et al 1999; McCabe et al 2006).

Cytogenetic analyses of AT/RT were essential to their characterization and distinction from medulloblastoma. These studies revealed specific abnormalities of chromosome 22, either monosomy or partial deletion of 22q11.2 (Rorke et al 1996; Biegel 1999). This region contains the *hSNF5/INI1* gene (recently renamed *SMARCB1/INI* gene), which encodes BAF47, a component of the SWI/SNF chromatin remodeling complex (Biegel et al 2002). Rhabdoid tumors in all anatomical locations have a similar molecular genetic phenotype. Mutation or deletion of both copies of the *SMARCB1/INI* gene is seen in approximately 70% of the tumors (Roberts & Biegel 2009). An additional 20–25% of tumors have reduced expression at the RNA or protein level, indicating a loss-of-function event.

Tumors of the cranial and spinal nerves

The three principal lesions in this group are: *schwannoma, neurofibroma, and perineurioma*. The latter is infrequently encountered in neurosurgical practice. Schwann cells are the exclusive constituent of schwannomas. Neurofibromas consist of Schwann perineurial-like cells and fibroblasts. Both types of tumors exhibit distinct histopathologic patterns and clinical associations. Schwannomas usually present as solitary masses involving cranial and spinal nerve. In contrast, neurofibromas are more often solitary than multiple and involve both small or large peripheral nerves.

Schwannomas and neurofibromas may occur either sporadically or as part of the spectrum of neurofibromatosis (NF). Both NF-1 (von Recklinghausen's disease or peripheral neurofibromatosis) and NF-2 (central neurofibromatosis) are associated with the development of nerve sheath tumors. Schwannomas are characteristic of NF-2, in which they are often multifocal and involve both vestibular nerves. Multiple schwannomas, albeit without vestibular tumors, characterize schwannomatosis as well. In contrast, neurofibromas are the characteristic tumor in NF-1, particularly dermal and plexiform examples. Perineuriomas have no syndrome association.

Deletion or mutation of the *NF2* gene, a tumor suppressor gene located at chromosome 22q12 is implicated in the formation of schwannomas. The mutation is genomic in NF-2 and somatic in sporadic schwannoma (Stemmer-Rachamimov et al 2007). Germline mutations of the *NF1* gene located on the chromosome 17q11.2 is associated with neurofibromas occurring in the setting of NF-1. The role of *NF1* in sporadic neurofibromas is still uncertain but is seems to be implicated in sporadic neurofibromas as well (Scheithauer et al 2007b).

Schwannoma (WHO grade I)

Intracranial and intraspinal schwannomas are usually slow-growing tumors of adults. A female predominance is noted in intracranial examples (Russell & Rubinstein 1989; Scheithauer et al 2007). Schwannomas characteristically involve sensory nerves, particularly posterior spinal roots. Motor and autonomic nerves are rarely affected. Intracranial tumors most often involve the vestibular nerve, followed infrequently by the trigeminal and vagus. Intracranial parenchymal schwannomas, unrelated to a major cranial nerve, are rare and presumably arise from minute fascicles accompanying vessels (Casadei et al 1993).

Macroscopically, schwannomas are well circumscribed, perineurium-encapsulated lesions which displace the remainder of the parent nerve. Unlike small neurofibromas, their nerve of origin is often identifiable. Vestibular schwannomas involve the cerebellopontine angle and expand the internal auditory meatus in a nipple-like fashion, whereas spinal examples tend to grow through intervertebral foramina to assume a 'dumbbell' configuration readily evident on neuroimaging. The cut surface of schwannomas is often solid and variably yellow due to lipid accumulation. Cystic and hemorrhagic degeneration is primarily encountered in large tumors.

Histopathologically, most schwannomas exhibit two patterns: *Antoni A and Antoni B* (Fig. 9.19A). The former consists of compact zones of fusiform cells with elongated nuclei occasionally arrayed in a regimented pattern of alternating nuclei and processes (Verocay bodies). The latter is a common feature of spinal schwannomas. Rich pericellular reticulin staining is particularly characteristic of Antoni A tissue. At the ultrastructural level, it corresponds to the presence of pericellular basement membrane and intercellular basement membrane-like material (Erlandson 1985), which, on immunohistochemistry, are strongly reactive for laminin and collagen IV (Miettinen et al 1983; Leivo et al 1989). Antoni B tissue is loose-textured, less cellular and consists of multipolar cells with round nuclei. Cytoplasmic vacuolation and variable nuclear pleomorphism typify such tissue. Reticulin staining is less dense and irregularly distributed. Intercellular collagen fibrils are commonly encountered on histochemistry and ultrastructure (Erlandson 1985). Lipofuscin pigment may also be seen within tumor cells.

Hyalinized blood vessels are usually a prominent feature in schwannomas, some showing sinusoidal dilatations assuming cavernous proportions (Fig. 9.19B). Thrombosis, spontaneous hemorrhages with necrosis, perivascular macrophages and hemosiderin deposition are also frequent. Other degenerative changes, such as marked enlargement and hyperchromasia of the nuclei are common and of no prognostic significance. They are considered degenerative in nature ('ancient schwannoma').

Several clinically significant schwannoma variants have been described. *Cellular schwannoma* is characterized by high cellularity, exclusive or predominance of Antoni A tissue, absence of Verocay bodies, and the presence of variable mitotic activity (Woodruff et al 1981). Such tumors often involve paravertebral regions in the pelvis, retroperitoneum and mediastinum (Woodruff et al 1981). They must not be mistaken for malignant peripheral nerve sheath tumor

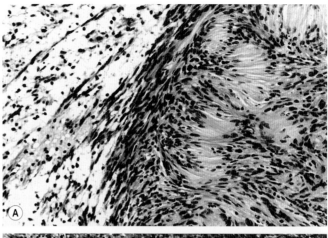

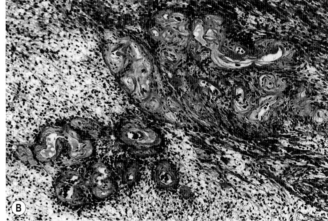

Figure 9.19 Schwannoma. (A) Spindle cells arranged in fascicles and Verocay bodies are features of the Antoni A type of tissue (right), whereas Antoni B (left) displays a loose texture in the tumor. (B) Numerous blood vessels with hyalinized walls are usually present in schwannomas (H&E).

(MPNST) since most cellular schwannomas are associated with an excellent prognosis (Woodruff et al 1981; Casadei et al 1995). Nonetheless, sacral, or intracranial examples show a significant frequency (30–40%) of recurrence as compared with peripherally situated tumors (Casadei et al 1993). *Plexiform schwannomas* are characterized by a plexiform or multinodular growth, presumably involving a nerve plexus or multiple fascicles of a nerve. The majority occur in the dermis and subcutis and resemble microscopically conventional schwannomas. Cranial and large spinal nerves are relatively spared (Iwashita & Enjoji 1987; Kao et al 1989). The association with NF-2 and schwannomatosis is low (5% each) (Berg et al 2008). *Melanotic schwannoma* is a rare variant in which the Schwann cells contain true melanin pigment within ultrastructurally typical melanosomes. Melanotic schwannomas may occur in two varieties – psammomatous and non-psammomatous. The distinction is of importance, since half of psammomatous melanotic schwannomas are associated with Carney complex (Carney 1990).

Nerve sheath tumors share a number of common immunohistochemical features. These will be discussed in combination. All schwannomas are diffusely immunoreactive for S-100 protein and collagen IV/laminin. In contrast, neurofibromas show more variable, less pronounced staining, a not unexpected finding given the mixed composition of these tumors (see below). Leu-7 (HNK-1; CD57) is present in about half of the nerve sheath tumors (Perentes & Rubinstein 1986). Since calretinin is detected in almost all schwannomas but in only a small proportion of neurofibromas, it is a potential marker useful in distinguishing differentiating schwannoma from neurofibroma (Fine et al 2004). Myelin basic protein (MBP) has also been reported in both schwannomas and neurofibromas, albeit in a small proportion of cases (Mogollon et al 1984; Penneys et al 1984). Epithelial membrane antigen (EMA), a marker for perineurial cells (Pinkus & Kurtin 1985), is occasionally detected in neurofibromas (Perentes et al 1987) and is a key feature of so-called 'hybrid' nerve sheath tumors (Hornick et al 2009).

Neurofibroma (WHO grade I)

Neurofibromas are divided into two major groups, the intraneural and the diffusely infiltrative. The latter are more often dermal and/or subcutaneous than massive soft tissue tumors. While the nerve of origin is often inapparent in diffuse tumors, short of an accompanying minor plexiform component in large examples, intraneural neurofibromas typically affect larger, readily recognized nerves and are either solitary and fusiform tumors or, less frequently, plexiform. The latter, particularly when sizeable, are pathognomonic of NF-1. Intraneural neurofibromas tend to involve cervical, brachial, and lumbosacral spinal nerves, but hardly ever affect cranial nerves (Scheithauer et al 2007). Intraspinal neurofibromas are rather frequently associated with NF-1.

Compared with schwannomas, neurofibromas tend to be soft, almost gelatinous in consistency. Solitary and plexiform intraneural tumors demonstrate somewhat similar histopathologic features, being composed in large part of small, spindle-shaped, wavy Schwann cells arranged loosely arrayed within a mucinous to increasingly collagenous matrix, rendering them translucent to opaque and tan, respectively. Varying proportions of perineurial-like cells and fibroblasts are also present. Myelinated and non-myelinated nerve fibers are typically present. Their frequency, especially when still aggregated at the centers of fascicles facilitate the distinction of neurofibromas from schwannomas, wherein nerve fibers tend to be more peripherally displaced within the lesion. Silver stains for axons, myelin preparations, and immunohistochemistry for neurofilament proteins are of utility in demonstrating nerve fibers. Ultrastructural studies indicate that Schwann cells are the principal component of neurofibromas, followed in frequency by perineurial-like cells and fibroblasts (Erlandson & Woodruff 1982). As previously commented, neurofibromas show dominant but not complete immunoreactivity for S-100 protein. Stains for EMA demonstrate the presence of perineurial cells (Perentes et al 1987).

In contrast to schwannomas, intraneural neurofibromas of the plexiform type in particular show a tendency to undergo malignant transformation. Its frequency in plexiform neurofibromas is roughly 5–10% (von Deimling & Perry 2007). Malignant transformation should be clinically suspected on the basis of rapid enlargement of pre-existing neurofibroma, pain, or a change in neurologic symptoms (Ducatman et al 1986). From the histopathologic standpoint, tumors showing hypercellularity, hyperchromasia and nuclear enlargement (3× that of neurofibroma cells) are considered to be undergoing anaplastic transformation (Scheithauer et al 2007). Mitotic figures are not required for the diagnosis, but are often present. The process may be focal or extensive; thus, thorough examination of the specimen is required.

Malignant peripheral nerve sheath tumors (MPNST) (WHO grade II–IV)

MPNSTs are neuroectodermal rather than sarcomatous in nature, fully half represent instances of transformed neurofibromas. In contrast, anaplastic transformation of schwannomas is extremely rare. MPNSTs correspond to about 5% of malignant tumors of the soft tissues with an overall incidence of MPNSTs of 0.001% in the general population and 4.6% among patients with NF-1 (Ducatman et al 1986). Most MPNSTs affect adults in the 3rd to the 6th decades of life. In the setting of NF-1, a somewhat higher incidence of pediatric examples may be encountered (Ducatman et al 1986; Matsui et al 1993; Wanebo et al 1993). Although MPNST may occur *de novo*, approximately 60% of well-sampled MPNST in the Mayo Clinic exhibit a co-existent neurofibroma component (Ducatman et al 1986). The association is even more evident in patients with NF-1 than in sporadic MPNST (81% vs 60%, respectively) (Ducatman et al 1986). Radiation-induced tumors represent about 10% of all cases occurring in both sporadic and syndromic tumors (Ducatman et al 1986; Wanebo et al 1993). MPNST are highly aggressive tumors with overall 5- and 10-year survival rates of 34% and 23%, respectively (Scheithauer et al 2007b).

The distribution of the MPNST is similar to that of solitary intraneural and plexiform neurofibromas, favored sites being the head and neck, trunk, and proximal limbs. Tumors in NF-1 are more often centrally situated (Ducatman et al 1986). A series of 17 intracranial MPNSTs has been recently published; the majority involved the vestibular nerves, followed by the vagal and facial (Scheithauer et al 2009). Examples in primary brain parenchyma are extremely rare (Stefanko et al 1986; Sharma et al 1998; Scheithauer et al 2009).

Grossly, the configuration of many MPNST resembles that of large, often fusiform neurofibromas. Yet others are globular and unassociated with a nerve. The 'capsules' of such tumors consist of infiltrated soft tissue. It is for this reason that wide or *en bloc* excision is required to insure a tumor-free margin. The texture of tumor often varies, depending upon the presence or absence of necrosis. Histologically, MPNSTs show a wide range of cytologic and histologic appearances. The majority consist of fascicles of spindle cells, sometimes arranged in a fascicular, 'herringbone' or storiform pattern. Cytoarchitectural features suggestive of schwannian differentiation may be seen and include cells with a wavy configuration. Most tumors are highly cellular and display nuclear/cellular pleomorphism, as well as brisk mitotic activity. Microvascular proliferation may be seen and necrosis is frequent. The latter may be of the geographic type, accompanied by peripheral palisading. MPNST may correspond to WHO histologic grades II, III or IV, according to the degrees of cellularity, anaplasia, mitotic activity, and necrosis. No generally agreed-upon grading system is in place, but the approach tends to be similar to that applied to soft tissue sarcomas (Fletcher et al 2002).

Heterologous differentiation is seen in approximately 10–15% of MPNSTs and includes mesenchymal (skeletal muscle, bone, cartilage) as well as epithelial (glandular, squamous, neuroendocrine) elements (Scheithauer et al 2007). Plurimorphous MPNST show both. A small number of MPNST (<5%) may be basically composed of lobules or groups of plump cells with round vesicular nuclei and prominent nucleoli and relatively abundant cytoplasm. Such *epithelioid MPNSTs* superficially resemble carcinoma or amelanotic melanoma. Areas of more typical MPNSTs are usually also present. Tumors presenting divergent differentiation are not dramatically different in behavior from ordinary MPNSTs (Ducatman et al 1986).

Overexpression of p53 protein has been described in approximately one half of MPNSTs. Its presence appears to be associated with the malignant progression of neurofibromas to MPNSTs and a poorer prognosis (Halling et al 1996).

Tumor of the meninges

Tumors of meningothelial cells

Meningioma

Meningiomas are common tumors presumably derived from arachnoidal cells as seen in abundance in arachnoidal granulations, and in the stroma of choroid plexus. This distinctive group of tumors account for approximately 35% of all primary CNS neoplasms (CBTRUS 2008); 15% of intracranial tumors, and about 25% of intraspinal tumors (Perry et al 2007). Meningiomas present in mid-life, being rare in childhood. A marked female predominance (3 : 1) is seen in adults, particularly in spinal examples. In contrast, no gender predilection is evident in elderly patients (Perry et al 2007). In children, gender distribution varies, but male predominance has been reported in infants and pre-adolescents (Al-Habib and Rutka 2008). An association between hormones and the risk of meningioma development has been long reported based on a number of findings, including an increased incidence of these tumors in women, growth during pregnancy and the presence of progesterone, and to a lesser extent, estrogen receptors. Multiple meningiomas occur in up to 8% of cases (Nakasu et al 1987), being particularly frequent in the setting of NF-2 and in rare familial predisposition syndromes (Smidt et al 1990; Perry et al 2007) (Fig. 9.20).

Most meningiomas are well demarcated, dura-based, globular masses with little or no capsule. An exception, the flat, carpet-like or '*en plaque*' meningioma, typically occurs at the skull base overlying the sphenoid ridge. Meningiomas grow slowly, compress the brain, and erode adjacent structures. Invasion of the dura and bone occurs with regularity, the latter prompting variable degrees of hyperostosis; neither invasion pattern affects tumor grading. The same is not true of brain invasion (see below).

Meningiomas exhibit a remarkably wide range of histologic appearances (Table 9.2); thus numerous variants are described (Perry et al 2007). These reflect the capacity of

Table 9.2 Meningiomas

Meningioma variant	WHO grade
Meningothelial	I
Fibrous (fibroblastic)	
Transitional (mixed)	
Psammomatous	
Angiomatous	
Microcystic	
Secretory	
Lymphoplasmacyte-rich	
Metaplastic	
Chordoid	II
Clear cell	
Atypical[a]	
Rhabdoid	III
Papillary	
Anaplastic (malignant)[a]	

[a]Meningiomas of any sub-type may be classified as atypical or anaplastic.

meningothelium to undergo a mesenchymal metaplasia. Although the majority of variants show similar behavior, some are associated with systemic diseases (*chordoid* meningioma and Castleman's disease, *lymphoplasmacyte-rich* meningioma and anemia as well as polyclonal gammopathy). Most significantly, four variants of meningiomas (*clear cell, chordoid, papillary, rhabdoid*) exhibit particularly aggressive behavior, e.g., recurrence and rarely metastases.

Histological variants
The *meningothelial*, the *fibrous*, and the *transitional* variants of meningioma are most frequent in occurrence. *Meningothelial* meningiomas are characterized by plump epithelioid cells with poorly-defined cell borders forming lobules and occasional whorls about vessels and stromal collagen. The cells contain nuclei with finely distributed chromatin and inconspicuous nucleoli. Nuclear cytoplasmic invaginations are frequent ('intranuclear pseudoinclusions') (Fig. 9.20B). The *transitional* meningioma possesses not only syncytial-appearing but spindle-shaped cells with a greater tendency to whorl formation. Psammoma bodies are a particularly common feature of this variant. The *fibrous* meningioma consists of spindle cells forming bundles and fascicles embedded in a rich collagenous matrix. Whorls and psammoma bodies are less frequent in this variant.

The *fibrous*, *metaplastic*, and perhaps *angiomatous* (Fig. 9.20C) variants comprise the 'mesenchymal' end of the meningioma spectrum. They all possess a variable degree of reticulin and are rich in collagen, extracellular matrix proteins, such as fibronectin, laminin, and collagens IV and V (Bellon et al 1985).

The somewhat epithelial phenotype of meningiomas is best exemplified by the *microcystic, secretory, clear cell, chordoid*, and *papillary* variants. PAS-positive inclusions are commonly found in the *secretory* variant, its intracytoplasmic lumina being lined by microvilli (Radley et al 1989). *Clear cell* meningiomas, which tend to occur in the posterior fossa (cerebello-pontine angle) or spine cord, are typically composed of patternless, large, glycogen-rich cells with only vague whorl formations (Fig. 9.21D). The *chordoid*

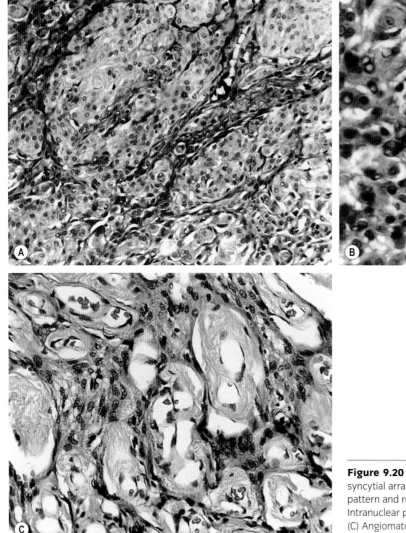

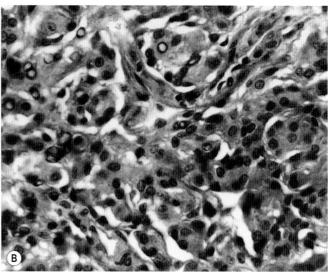

Figure 9.20 Meningioma. (A,B) Meningothelial meningiomas exhibit the syncytial arrangement of cells and whorl formations. The delicate chromatin pattern and regular nuclei are characteristic of meningiomas (B). Intranuclear pseudoinclusions are commonly seen in these tumors. (C) Angiomatous meningiomas display numerous blood vessels intermixed with nests of meningothelial cells (A–C, H&E).

meningioma is characterized by cords and trabecula of eosinophilic, vacuolated cells within a mucin-rich matrix, the result being a mimic of chordoma. Both *clear cell* and *chordoid* meningiomas frequently recur, behaving in a manner analogous to that of atypical meningiomas. Thus, they are considered grade II in the WHO classification (Perry et al 2007). *Clear cell* meningiomas are particularly prone to local recurrence and occasionally undergo spinal seeding (Zorludemir et al 1995).

Papillary meningiomas are characterized by their perivascular pseudopapillary arrangement of tumor cells. Most occur in adolescents and young adults. The *rhabdoid* meningioma consists of rhabdoid cells with open chromatin, some nucleolar prominence and occasionally features of anaplasia, including high mitotic index and necrosis. Both *papillary* and *rhabdoid* meningiomas exhibit aggressive clinical behavior with frequent local recurrences and metastatic potential. Each is considered a grade III neoplasm in the WHO classification (Perry et al 2007).

Meningiomas show immunohistochemical properties of both a mesenchymal and somewhat epithelial nature. Present in virtually 100% of tumors, the principle intermedi-

ate filament is vimentin (Schnitt & Vogel 1986; Russell & Rubinstein 1989). S-100 protein is variably demonstrated in 20–50%, particularly the fibroblastic variant (Schnitt & Vogel 1986; Artlich & Schmidt 1990). Epithelial membrane antigen and cytokeratin are present to a varying degree in the majority of meningiomas, but staining intensity is maximal in epithelial-appearing variants (Schnitt & Vogel 1986; Meis et al 1986; Theaker et al 1987). Claudin-1, tight junction-associated protein, has been also demonstrated in a majority of meningiomas and may, as part of a panel of immunostains, aid in distinguishing meningiomas from histologic mimics (Hahn et al 2006). Meningiomas may also express steroid hormone receptors, more so for progesterone than estrogen (Hsu et al 1997). Lack of PR has been correlated with a less favorable clinical outcome (Hsu et al 1997; Pravdenkova et al 2006; Claus et al 2008).

Grading of meningiomas

Meningiomas occur in three histologic grades: typical (WHO grade I), atypical (WHO grade II), and anaplastic (WHO grade III), according to the histologic features expressed. They reflect the tendency towards aggressiveness, mainly recur-

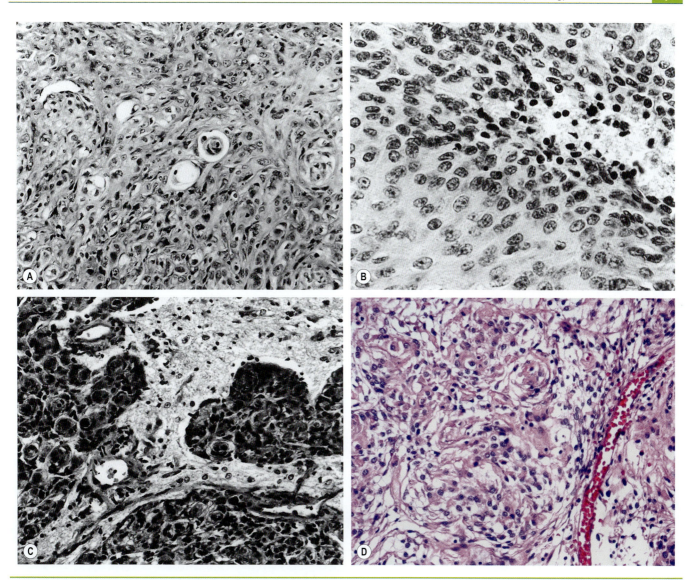

Figure 9.21 Atypical meningioma. (A) Hypercellularity, cellular atypia, and loss of growth pattern are features of atypical meningiomas. (B) Nuclear pleomorphism and prominent nucleoli, associated with areas of necrosis, are present in these tumors. (C) Brain invasion is definitive evidence for the aggressive biologic behavior of meningiomas. (D) Clear cell meningioma are characterized by clear and glycogen-rich cytoplasm. Clear cell meningiomas show aggressive behavior and classified as grade II tumors (A–D, H&E).

rence and malignant behavior (Perry et al 2007). In addition, the special meningioma variants previously described are prone to similar behaviors, these being *clear cell* and *chordoid* (WHO grade II) as well as *papillary* and *rhabdoid* meningiomas (WHO grade III). WHO grade I tumors are benign tumors exhibiting low proliferation, reporting mean MIB-1 labeling indices of around 4% (Perry et al 1998).

Atypical meningioma (WHO grade II)
The WHO classification recognizes a form of meningioma with biologic behavior intermediate between the typical and anaplastic forms. They are associated with a distinct tendency to recur and to be locally aggressive (Perry et al 1997b, 1998). Diagnostic criteria of atypical meningioma include either increased mitotic activity (four or more mitoses per 10 high-power field) or three or more of the following features: hypercellularity, small cells with a

high nuclear:cytoplasmic ratio, diffuse or sheet-like growth, nucleolar prominence, and the presence of necrosis (Fig. 9.21A–B). These features may be seen in any histologic variant of meningioma and may be focal in any given tumor. Thus, careful examination of multiple microsections is necessary in evaluating meningiomas.

Determination of cellular proliferation is of value in identifying tumors likely to recur. Meningiomas with moderate to high MIB-1, mean labeling index 7.2% ± 5.8 in one study, are known to have a greater likelihood of recurrence when compared with grade I meningiomas (Chen & Liu 1990; Perry et al 1998).

Anaplastic (malignant) meningioma (WHO grade III)
In this category are included meningiomas with frankly anaplastic features, often but not invariably including marked nuclear and cellular pleomorphism. These include abundant

mitotic activity and obvious necrosis. Many tumors show cytologic features resembling carcinomas and sarcomas. Otherwise, high mitotic activity, defined as 20 or more mitoses per 10 high-power field, are the key feature of grade III tumors.

Brain invasion

Brain invasion (Fig. 9.21C), defined as infiltration of parenchyma, is considered a strong indicator of aggressive clinical behavior (Perry et al 2007). Tumors with this feature, regardless of their degree of atypia, are prone to recur and should be considered as at least WHO grade II (Perry et al 2007). Careful examination of the tumor–brain interface, aided in some cases by GFAP immunohistochemistry, is necessary to identify brain invasion. This criterion is most meaningful upon evaluation of the first resection specimen, since the brain–tumor interface is markedly affected by prior surgical manipulation.

Molecular cytogenetics of meningiomas

The most common cytogenetic abnormality of meningiomas is allelic loss of 22q, a finding in 40–80% of sporadic tumors. The key genetic abnormality affects 22q12, the location of the *NF2* gene (see Perry et al 2007, for review). This explains the high incidence of meningiomas in this disorder. It is of note that mutations of the *NF2* gene are not restricted to tumors arising in syndromic NF-2. The frequency of *NF2* mutation in sporadic meningiomas is as high as 60% (Perry et al 2007). After chromosome 22, the genes most frequently reported to be altered in sporadic meningiomas are situated on chromosomes 1p, 9p, and 14q. This is particularly the case in tumors of grades II and III. Several other genes appear to be implicated in the tumorigenesis of meningiomas. The reader is referred to several excellent reviews for further information (Riemenschneider et al 2006; Perry et al 2007; Claus et al 2008).

Mesenchymal, non-meningothelial tumors

A variety of mesenchymal tumors arise in the meninges. Although very uncommon, benign tumors in this category include chondroma, osteochondroma, osteoma, and lipoma. Among sarcomas, the most frequent are hemangiopericytoma, chondrosarcoma, and rhabdomyosarcoma. Although these tumors display features similar to their counterparts outside the CNS, it is worthwhile to further discuss hemangiopericytoma given its histologic, immunophenotypic, and ultrastructural peculiarities. The histogenesis of hemangiopericytomas has been the subject of longstanding controversy among general and neuropathologists. It is of note that hemangiopericytoma is considered a non-meningothelial tumor and is unrelated to the angiomatous variant meningioma. Although most hemangiopericytomas are distinct from solitary fibrous tumor, a morphologic spectrum exists between these tumors in their soft tissues counterparts (Guillou et al 2002).

Hemangiopericytoma (WHO grade II–III)

Hemangiopericytomas (HPC) of the meninges account for roughly 1–7% of all meningeal tumors. They are malignant by definition, exhibiting a high rate of recurrence and of late metastasis (Jellinger & Paulus 1991; Mena et al 1991). The majority of the tumors affect adults, males somewhat more often, and occur at a slightly younger age (range, 30–50 years) than meningiomas (Giannini et al 2007b).

Hemangiopericytomas arise from the dura, often in or about the tentorium, and may compress or invade underlying brain tissue. They produce a lytic lesion when involving overlying bone and, unlike meningiomas, do not induce hyperostosis. Grossly, HPC are usually spherical, firm and highly vascular, a feature complicating their resection.

Histologically, HPC are quite cellular and composed of short, plump to spindle cells with ill-defined cytoplasmic borders, and oval to somewhat elongate nuclei (Fig. 9.22A). A delicate cleft-like vascular network dubbed a 'staghorn' pattern is typically present but is not diagnostic. Reticulin deposition (Fig. 9.22B) is often but not invariably present around individual tumor cells. Mitotic activity is quite variable. Necrosis with or without hemorrhage is seen

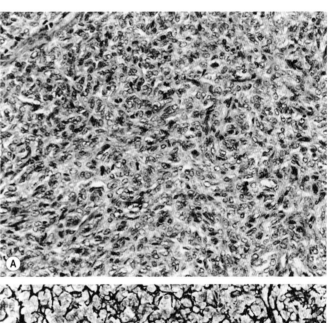

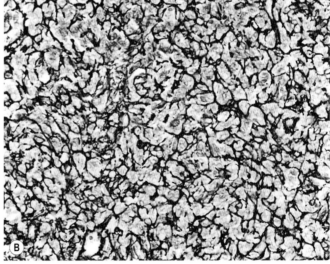

Figure 9.22 Hemangiopericytoma. (A) Hemangiopericytomas are highly cellular neoplasms composed of short, plump spindle cells with moderate pleomorphism (H&E). (B) A branching vascular network is easily demonstrated by reticulin stains (Gordon and Sweet's reticulin).

in high-grade tumors. Immunohistochemical studies show vimentin and variable CD34 immunoreactivity but, unlike meningiomas, S-100 protein and cytokeratin are mostly negative (Nakamura et al 1987; Winek et al 1989; D'Amore et al 1990; Theunissen et al 1990). Focal and weak EMA and claudin-1 may be seen in HPC (Rajaram et al 2004), particularly in patchy, loose-textured areas. Like solitary fibrous tumor, HPCs often express CD99 and bcl-2 (Rajaram et al 2004).

High mitotic rate ($\geq$5–6/10 HPF) in addition to evidence of nuclear pleomorphism and tumor necrosis have been associated with decreased survival (Mena et al 1991). The MIB-1 LI is variable but averages 5–10% (Giannini et al 2007b).

Hemangiopericytoma of the meninges correspond histologically to WHO grade II and is considered a low-grade sarcoma given its high recurrence rate, despite apparently complete excision, and its tendency to metastasize outside the CNS, late in the course, typically after multiple resections. Risk of recurrence is as high as 90% at 15 years (Vuorinen et al 1996). Anaplastic HPC (WHO grade III) shows anaplastic features, which include brisk mitotic activity (at least 5 mit/10 HPF), moderate to marked nuclear atypia, and necrosis often with hemorrhage. Grade III tumors have a shorter time to recurrence than grade II tumors (Ecker et al 2003).

Unlike meningioma, chromosome 22 abnormalities and *NF2* deletions are rarely seen in HPC (Rajaram et al 2004). Rearrangement of chromosome 12q13 is a frequent finding (Herath et al 1994), as are abnormalities of chromosome 3 (Giannini et al 2007b). Other genetic abnormalities seen in meningiomas, such as deletions of 1p, 14q and 4.1B *(DAL-1)* are not found in hemangiopericytomas (Rajaram et al 2004).

Other neoplasms related to leptomeninges

Hemangioblastoma (WHO grade I)

Hemangioblastomas represent less than 2.5% of all intracranial tumors, and can be either sporadic or associated with von Hippel–Lindau (VHL) disease (Plate et al 2007). Their classical location is the cerebellum, but tumors involving the medulla and spinal cord are not uncommon, particularly in patients with VHL (Conway et al 2001). Multiple lesions are diagnostic of this condition (Plate et al 2007). Supratentorial tumors are rare and occur only in association with VHL (Neumann et al 1995; Conway et al 2001; Aldape et al 2007). Retinal hemangioblastomas may be present in almost 60% of patients with VHL. Hemangioblastoma rarely affects peripheral nerve (Plate et al 2007). Patients with the disorder tend to present at a younger age than those with sporadic hemangioblastomas (Aldape et al 2007). Grossly, the tumors are well-circumscribed, mostly cystic lesions associated with one or occasionally more mural nodules. Virtually all tumors abut the leptomeninges. Histologically, they are characterized by an anastomosing network of delicate vessels that separates groups of large polygonal, so-called 'stromal cells', with lipid-laden cytoplasm and hyperchromatic, occasionally large and atypical nuclei. The tumors tend to push aside adjacent brain or spinal cord parenchyma. Frank invasion is very uncommon, but exuberant astrogliosis with Rosenthal fiber formation is a frequent finding. The latter may result

in an erroneous diagnosis of pilocytic astrocytomas in small biopsies or at intraoperative frozen section.

The origin of the stromal cells is not fully understood. They exhibit a wide range of immunohistochemical markers, including intense immunoreactivity for vimentin, inhibin, and neuron-specific enolase (Hoang et al 2003). They may also show variable reactivity for S-100 protein, Leu 7 (CD57) and GFAP. The presence of these glioneuronal markers does not indicate a neuroepithelial histogenesis. The endothelial cells show typical immunoreactivity for endothelial cell markers CD31 and CD34, while stromal cells lack their expression. Expression of VEGF in stromal cells and its receptors in endothelial cells has also been demonstrated (Krieg et al 1998; Zagzag et al 2000), and is the basis of antiangiogenic treatment targeting VEGF signaling (Madhusudan et al 2004).

Hemangioblastomas mimic clear cell tumors, particularly metastatic renal cell carcinoma (RCC). The distinction of these two tumors is of particular importance in the setting of VHL syndrome, since RCC occurs commonly in this setting. Lack of EMA immunoreactivity in hemangioblastoma is, therefore, of diagnostic utility (Mills et al 1990). Expression of inhibin in sporadic and VHL-associated hemangioblastomas is seen in proportions significantly higher than in RCC (Hoang & Amirkhan 2003; Jung & Kuo 2005), and is, therefore, of diagnostic utility in combination with EMA.

Tumors of the hematopoietic system

Primary central nervous system lymphoma

Primary CNS lymphomas (PCNSL) are extranodal, non-Hodgkin's lymphomas unassociated with lymphoma outside the nervous system. Once considered a rare tumor involving the CNS (around 1% of all CNS tumors), its incidence has increased steadily in recent decades, approaching nearly 7% of all primary CNS tumors in some series (Miller et al 1994). Although much of this increase is attributed to increase in the immunocompromised patients, especially in association with AIDS and organ transplantation (Miller et al 1994), there is evidence that PCNSL are increasing in all age groups and in both genders regardless of their immunological status (Eby et al 1988; Hao et al 1999; Olson et al 2002). In the last CBTRUS survey collating data from 2000–2004, PCNSL represents 2.8% of all primary CNS tumors; the slight decrease in incidence being attributed to a decrease in AIDS after the introduction of highly effective antiviral therapy (HAART) (CBTRUS 2008).

In the general population, PCNSL occurs most commonly in the 6th and 7th decade of life. In the immunocompromised population, the age at presentation is lower, with a median in the 30s (Deckert & Paulus 2007). Males are more often affected in both populations. Nearly all PCNSL are high-grade tumors with a median overall patient survival of 50 months (Gavrilovic et al 2006). Patients with AIDS have even shorter survivals, with a median around 36 months (Hoffman et al 2001). Survival continues to improve due to the combination of HAART and standard lymphoma treatment (Hoffman et al 2001; Skiest & Crosby 2003).

PCNSL are usually supratentorial, arising deep within the cerebrum, often involving the basal ganglia and peri-

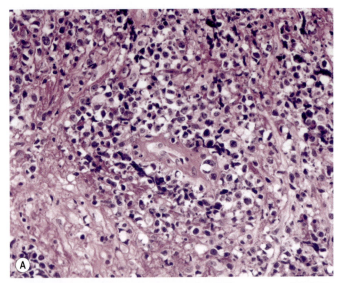

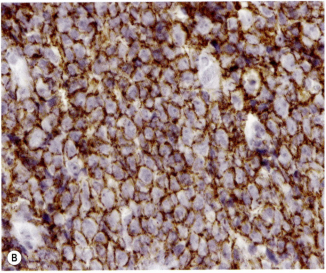

Figure 9.23 Primary CNS lymphoma. (A) Highly anaplastic large cells with numerous mitotic figures and extensive apoptosis are typical of diffuse large B-cell lymphomas. Typically, perivascular arrangements of the tumor cells are seen (H&E). (B) Tumor cells express CD20, a B-cell marker. (CD20 avidin biotin–immunoperoxidase).

ventricular regions. Unlike most primary CNS tumors, they are often multifocal, simulating metastatic tumor. Multiple lesions are particularly common in AIDS and in the post-transplant setting. Since PCNSL diffusely infiltrates brain parenchyma, they may be ill-defined and simulate inflammatory disease (Brecher et al 1998). Intraocular involvement of PCNSL occurs in 15–25% of patients. A cohort of 221 patients with intraocular involvement has recently been reported by the International PCNSL Collaborative Group (Grimm et al 2008).

Grossly, PCNSL are often pale–white, soft lesions with ill-defined borders. Following therapy, or in the setting of AIDS, they may be necrotic and hemorrhagic. Histologically, the vast majority are diffuse B-cell lymphomas (Deckert & Paulus 2007) composed of large cells with round or lobulated nuclei with vesicular chromatin and prominent, coarse nucle-

oli, typically admixed with variable numbers of reactive small, T-lymphocytes and histiocytes (Fig. 9.23A). The tumoral infiltrates are poorly delineated, often patchy in distribution and exhibit an accentuated angiocentric pattern with frequent angioinvasion. Large, reactive astrocytes are typically present and may be a conspicuous cellular element. Immunohistochemical expression of B-cell markers, such as CD20 and CD79a is conspicuous (Fig. 9.23B). Variable numbers of reactive CD3- and CD5-positive T-cells are also seen. In addition to B-cell markers, the majority of PCNSL also express germinal center-associated markers, such as BCL-6, BCL-2, and MUM-1 (Montesinos-Rongen et al 1999; Montesinos-Rongen et al 2008 for review).

Primary T-cell CNS lymphomas are rare and usually affect immunocompetent individuals (Da Silva et al 2006). In Western countries, T-cell PCNSL comprise 2–5% of PCNSL, while in Japan, their incidence is slightly higher (1.7–8.5%) (Da Silva et al 2006; Shibamoto et al 2008). Unlike B-cell PCNSL, the T-cell variety tends to be superficially situated, often involving the leptomeninges (Da Silva et al 2006).

Much more rare are anaplastic lymphomas (Ki-1, often T-cell subtype) and Hodgkin's disease (Paulus et al 1994b; Gerstner et al 2008) The CNS may, however, be involved in the setting of disseminated Hodgkin's disease (Gerstner et al 2008).

Molecular cytogenetics of PCNSL

Molecular studies of PCNSL indicate a germinal center, B cell-derived lineage in the great majority of tumors, recurrent translocations typically involving the immunoglobulin H (*IgH*) and the *BCL6* gene loci (Deckert & Paulus 2007; Montesinos-Rongen et al 2008). The Epstein–Barr virus (EBV) has been identified the great majority of B-cell PCNSL arising in AIDS and in the post-transplantation setting but not in lymphomas occurring in the immunocompetent patients (Morgello 1995).

Key points

- Neuropathologic advances continue to shed light on brain tumor biology

- Further studies based on exciting advances in molecular biology will be even more helpful in guiding diagnosis and therapy.

REFERENCES

Abel, T.W., Baker, S.J., Fraser, M.M., et al., 2005. Lhermitte–Duclos disease: a report of 31 cases with immunohistochemical analysis of the PTEN/AKT/mTOR pathway. J. Neuropath. Exp. Neurol. 64, 341–349.

Albrecht, S., Connelly, J.H., Bruner, J.M., 1993. Distribution of p53 protein expression in gliosarcomas: an immunohistochemical study. Acta. Neuropathol. 85, 222–226.

Albrecht, S., Rouah, E., Becker, L.E., et al., 1991. Transthyretin immunoreactivity in choroid plexus neoplasms and brain metastases. Mod. Pathol. 4, 610–614.

Aldape, K.D., Ballman, K., Furth, A., et al., 2004. Immunohistochemical detection of EGFRvIII in high malignancy grade astrocytomas and evaluation of prognostic significance. J. Neuropathol. Exp. Neurol. 63, 700–707.

Aldape, K.D., Plate, K.H., Vortmeyer, A.O., et al., 2007. Haemangioblastoma. In: Louis, D.N., Ohgaki, H., Wiestler, O.D., et al. (Eds.), WHO classification of tumours of the central nervous system. IARC, Lyon, pp. 184–186.

Aldape, K.D., Rosenblum, M.K., 2007. Astroblastoma. In: Louis, D.N., Ohgaki, H., Wiestler, O.D., et al. (Eds.), WHO classification of tumours of the central nervous system. IARC, Lyon, pp. 88–89.

Aldosari, N., Bigner, S.H., Burger, P.C., et al., 2002. MYCC and MUCN oncogene amplification in medulloblastoma. A fluorescence in situ hybridization study on paraffin sections from the Children's Oncology Group. Arch. Pathol. Lab. Med. 126, 540–544.

Al-Habib, A., Rutka, J.T., 2008. Pediatric meningiomas. In: Lee, J.H. (Ed.), Meningiomas: diagnosis, treatment, and outcome. Springer-Verlag, London, pp. 543–553.

Alkadhi, H., Keller, M., Brandner, S., et al., 2001. Neuroimaging of cerebellar liponeurocytoma. J. Neurosurg 95, 324–331.

Allegranza, A., Pileri, S., Frank, G., et al., 1990. Cerebral ganglioglioma with anaplastic oligodendroglial component. Histopathology 17, 439–441.

Artlich, A., Schmidt, D., 1990. Immunohistochemical profile of meningiomas and their histological subtypes. Hum. Pathol. 21, 843–849.

Azzarelli, B., Rekate, H.L., Roessman, U., 1977. Subependymoma: a case report with ultrastructural study. Acta. Neuropathol. 40, 279–282.

Baisden, B.L., Brat, D.J., Melhem, E.R., et al., 2001. Dysembryoplastic neuroepithelial tumor-lke neoplasm of the septum pellucidum: a lesion often misdiagnosed as glioma. Report of 10 cases. Am. J. Surg. Pathol. 25, 494–499.

Balss, J., Meyer, J., Mueller, W., et al., 2008. Analysis of the IDH1 codon 132 mutation in brain tumors. Acta Neuropathol. 116, 597–602.

Banerjee, A.K., Gleathill, C.A., 1979. Lhermitte–Duclos disease (diffuse cerebellar hypertrophy): prolonged post-operative survival. Ir. J. Med. Sci. 148, 97–99.

Barnard, R.O., Bradford, R., Scott, T., et al., 1986. Gliomyosarcoma. Report of a case of rhabdomyosarcoma arising in a malignant glioma. Acta. Neuropathol. 69, 23–27.

Becker, A.J., Wiestler, O.D., Figarella-Branger, D., et al., 2007. Ganglioglioma and gangliocytoma. In: Louis, D.N., Ohgaki, H., Wiestler, O.D., et al. (Eds.), WHO classification of tumours of the central nervous system. IARC, Lyon, pp. 103–105.

Bellon, G., Caulet, T., Cam, T., et al., 1985. Immunohistochemical localisation of macromolecules of the basement membrane and extracellular matrix of human gliomas and meningiomas. Acta. Neuropathol. 66, 245–252.

Bennett, J.P. Jr, Rubinstein, L.J., 1984. The biologic behavior of primary cerebral neuroblastoma: a reappraisal of the clinical course in a series of 70 cases. Ann. Neurol. 16, 21–27.

Bennetto, L., Foreman, N., Harding, B., et al., 1998. Ki-67 immunolabelling index is a prognostic indicator in childhood posterior fossa ependymomas. Neuropathol. Appl. Neurobiol. 24, 434–440.

Berg, J.C., Scheithauer, B.W., Spinner, R.J., et al., 2008. Plexiform schwannoma: a clinicopathologic overview with emphasis on the head and neck region. Hum. Pathol. 39, 633–640.

Berger, M.S., Ghatan, S., Haglund, M.M., et al., 1993. Low-grade gliomas associated with intractable epilepsy: seizure outcome utilizing electrocorticography during tumor resection. J. Neurosurg 79, 62–69.

Biegel, J.A., 1999. Cytogenetics and molecular genetics of childhood brain tumors. Neuro. Oncol. 1 (2), 139–151.

Biegel, J.A., Kalpana, G., Knudsen, E.S., et al., 2002. The role of INI1 and the SWI/SNF complex in the development of rhabdoid tumors: meeting summary from the workshop on childhood atypical teratoid/rhabdoid tumors. Cancer Res. 62, 323–328.

Biernat, W., Aguzzi, A., Sure, U., et al., 1995. Identical mutations of the p53 tumor suppressor gene in the glial and sarcomatous part of gliosarcomas suggest a common origin from glial cells. J. Neuropathol. Exp. Neurol. 54, 651–656.

Blümcke, I., Becker, A.J., Normann, S., et al., 2001. Distinct expression pattern of microtubule-associated protein-2 in human oligodendrogliomas and glial precursor cells. J. Neuropath. Exp. Neurol. 60, 984–993.

Boerman, R.H., Anderl, K., Herath, J., et al., 1996. The glial and mesenchymal elements of gliosarcoma share similar genetic alterations. J. Neuropathol. Exp. Neurol. 55, 973–981.

Bonnin, J.M., Colon, L.E., Morawetz, R.B., 1987. Focal glial differentiation and oncocytic transformation in choroid plexus papilloma. Acta. Neuropathol. 72, 277–280.

Bonnin, J.M., Rubinstein, L.J., 1989. Astroblastomas: a pathological study of 23 tumors, with a postoperative follow-up in 13 patients. Neurosurgery 25, 6–13.

Borit, A., Blackwood, W., Mair, W.G.P., 1980. The separation of pineocytoma from pineoblastoma. Cancer 45, 1408–1418.

Bourne, T.D., Mandell, J.W., Matsumoto, J.A., et al., 2006. Primary disseminated leptomeningeal oligodendroglioma with 1p deletion. Case report. J. Neurosurg 105 (Suppl.), 465–469.

Bouvier, C., Bartoli, C., Aguirre-Cruz, L., et al., 2003. Shared oligodendrocyte lineage gene expression in gliomas and oligodendrocyte progenitor cells. J. Neurosurg 99, 344–350.

Bouvier-Labit, C., Daniel, L., Dufour, H., et al., 2000. Papillary glioneuronal tumor: clinicopathological and biochemical study of one case with 7-year follow-up. Acta. Neuropathol. 99, 321–326.

Boyko, O.B., Curnes, J.T., Oakes, W.J., et al., 1991. Hamartomas of the tuber cinereum. CT, MR, and pathologic findings. AJNR. Am. J. Neuroradiol. 12, 309–314.

Brat, D.J., Hirose, Y., Cohen, K.J., et al., 2000. Astroblastoma: clinicopathologic features and chromosomal abnormalities defined by comparative genomic hybridization. Brain Pathol. 10, 342–352.

Brat, D.J., Scheithauer, B.W., Eberhart, C.G., et al., 2001. Extraventricular neurocytomas: pathologic features and clinical outcome. Am. J. Surg. Pathol. 25, 1252–1260.

Brat, D.J., Scheithauer, B.W., Staugaitis, S.M., et al., 1998. Third ventricular chordoid glioma: a distinct clinicopathologic entity. J. Neuropathol. Exp. Neurol. 57, 283–290.

Brat, D.J., Scheithauer, B.W., 2007. Chordoid glioma of the third ventricle. In: Louis, D.N., Ohgaki, H., Wiestler, O.D., et al. (Eds.), WHO classification of tumours of the central nervous system. IARC, Lyon, pp. 90–91.

Brat, D.J., VandenBerg, S.R., Figarella-Branger, D., et al., 2007. Desmoplastic infantile astrocytoma and ganglioglioma. In: Louis, D.N., Ohgaki, H., Wiestler, O.D., et al. (Eds.), WHO classification of tumours of the central nervous system. IARC, Lyon, pp. 96–98.

Brecher, K., Hochberg, F.H., Louis, D.N., et al., 1998. Case report of unusual leukoencephalopathy preceding primary CNS lymphoma. J. Neurol. Neurosurg Psychiatry 65, 917–920.

Brown, M.T., Friedman, H.S., Oakes, J., et al., 1992. Chemotherapy for pilocytic astrocytoma. Cancer 71, 3165–3172.

Bruce, J.N., Stein, B.M., 1990. Pineal tumors. Neurosurg Clin. North Am. 1, 123–138.

Burger, P.C., Scheithauer, B.W., Vogel, F.S., 1991. Surgical pathology of the nervous system and its coverings, third ed. Churchill Livingstone, New York.

Burger, P.C., 1989. The grading of astrocytomas and oligodendrogliomas. In: Field, W.S. (Ed.), Primary brain tumors. A review of histologic classification. Springer Verlag, New York, pp. 171–180.

Burger, P.C., Grahmann, F.C., Bliestle, A., et al., 1987. Differentiation in the medulloblastoma. A histological and immunohistochemical study. Acta. Neuropathol. 73, 115–123.

Burger, P.C., Jouvet, A., Preusser, M., et al., 2007. Angiocentric glioma. In: Louis, D.N., Ohgaki, H., Wiestler, O.D., et al. (Eds.), WHO classification of tumours of the central nervous system. IARC, Lyon, pp. 92–93.

Burger, P.C., Kleihues, P., 1989. Cytologic composition of the untreated glioblastoma with implications for evaluation of needle biopsies. Cancer 63, 2014–2023.

Burger, P.C., Pearl, D.K., Aldape, K.D., et al., 2001. Small cell architecture – a histological equivalent of EGFR amplification in glioblastoma multiforme? J. Neuropathol. Exp. Neurol. 60, 1099–1104.

Burger, P.C., Shibata, T., Kleihues, P., 1986. The use of the monoclonal antibody Ki-67 in the identification of proliferating cells: application to surgical neuropathology. Am. J. Surg. Pathol. 10, 611–617.

Burger, P.C., Yu, I.T., Tihan, T., et al., 1998. Atypical teratoid/rhabdoid tumor of the central nervous system: a highly malignant tumor of infancy and childhood frequently mistaken for medulloblastoma: a Pediatric Oncology Group study. Am. J. Surg. Pathol. 22, 1083–1092.

Caccamo, D.V., Herman, M.M., Rubinstein, L.J., 1989. An immunohistochemical study of the primitive and maturing elements of human cerebral medulloepitheliomas. Acta. Neuropathol. 79, 248–254.

Cairncross, J.G., Macdonald, D.R., Ramsay, D.A., 1992. Aggressive oligodendroglioma. A chemosensitive tumor. Neurosurgery 31, 78–82.

Cameron, R.S., Rakic, P., 1991. Glial cell lineage in the cerebral cortex: a review and synthesis. Glia 4, 124–137.

Carney, J.A., 1990. Psammomatous melanotic schwannoma. A distinctive, heritable tumor with special associations, including cardiac myxoma and the Cushing syndrome. Am. J. Surg. Pathol. 14, 206–222.

Carter, M., Nicholson, J., Ross, F., et al., 2002. Genetic abnormalities detected in ependymomas by comparative genomic hybridization. Br. J. Cancer 86, 929–939.

Carter, M., Nicholson, J., Ross, F., et al., 2002. Genetic abnormalities detected in ependymomas by comparative genomic hybridization. Br. J. Cancer 86, 929–939.

Casadei, G.P., Komori, T., Scheithauer, B.W., et al., 1993. Intracranial parenchymal schwannoma. A clinicopathological and neuroimaging study of nine cases. J. Neurosurg 79, 217–222.

Casadei, G.P., Scheithauer, B.W., Hirose, T., et al., 1995. Cellular schwannoma. A clinicopathologic, DNA flow cytometric, and proliferation marker study of 70 patients. Cancer 75, 1109–1119.

Castellano-Sanchez, A.A., Schemankewitz, E., Mazewski, C., et al., 2001. Pediatric chordoid glioma with chondroid metaplasia. Pediatr. Dev. Pathol. 4, 564–567.

CBTRUS, 2008. Statistical Report: Primary brain tumors in the United States, 2000–2004. Central Brain Tumor Registry of the United States, Hinsdale, IL.

Cervera-Pierot, P., Varlet, P., Chodkiewicz, J.P., et al., 1997. Dysembryoplastic neuroepithelial tumors located in the caudate nucleus are: report of four cases. Neurosurgery 40, 1065–1070.

Chan, J.A., Zhang, H., Roberts, P.S., et al., 2004. Pathogenesis of tuberous sclerosis subependymal giant cell astrocytomas: biallelic inactivation of TSC1 or TSC2 leads to mTOR activation. J. Neuropathol. Exp. Neurol. 63, 1236–1242.

Charafe-Jauffret, E., Lehmann, G., Fauchon, F., et al., 2001. Vertebral metastases from pineoblastoma. Arch. Pathol. Lab. Med. 125, 939–943.

Chen, W.Y., Liu, H.C., 1990. Atypical (anaplastic) meningioma: relationship between histologic features and recurrence – a clinicopathologic study. Clin. Neuropathol. 9, 74–81.

Clark, G.B., Henry, J.M., McKeever, P.E., 1985. Cerebral pylocytic astrocytoma. Cancer 56, 1128–1133.

Claus, E.B., Park, P.J., Carroll, R., et al., 2008. Specific genes expressed in association with progesterone receptors in meningioma. Cancer Res. 68, 314–322.

Collins, V.P., 1995. Gene amplification in human gliomas. Glia 15, 289–296.

Conway, J.E., Chou, D., Clatterbuck, R.E., et al., 2001. Hemangioblastomas of the central nervous system in von Hippel-Lindau Syndrome and sporadic disease. Neurosurgery 48, 55–63.

Coons, S.W., Johnson, P.C., Pearl, D.K., 1997. The prognostic significance of Ki-67 labeling indices for oligodendrogliomas. Neurosurgery 41, 878–884.

Crawford, J.R., Tobey, M.D., Packer, R.J., 2007. Medulloblastoma in childhood: new biological advances. Lancet Neurol. 6, 1073–1085.

Cruz-Sanchez, F.F., Rossi, M.L., Buller, J.R., et al., 1991. Oligodendrogliomas: a clinical, histological, immunocytochemical and lectin-binding study. Histopathology 19, 361–367.

D'Amore, E.S.G., Manivel, J.C., Sung, J.H., 1990. Soft-tissue and meningeal hemangiopericytomas: An immunohistochemical and ultrastructural study. Hum. Pathol. 21, 414–423.

D'Andrea, A.D., Packer, R.J., Rorke, L.B., et al., 1987. Pineocytomas of childhood: a reappraisal of natural history and response to therapy. Cancer 59, 1353–1357.

Da Silva, A.N., Lopes, M.B., Schiff, D., 2006. Rare pathological variants and presentations of primary central nervous system lymphomas. Neurosurg Focus 21, E7.

Dagnew, E., Langford, L., Lang, F., et al., 2007. Papillary tumors of the pineal region: case report. Neurosurgery 60, E953–E955.

Daita, G., Yonemasu, Y., Muraoka, S., et al., 1991. A case of anaplastic astrocytoma transformed from pleomorphic xanthoastrocytoma. Brain Tumor. Pathol. 8, 63–66.

Daumas-Duport, C., Scheithauer, B.W., Chodkiewicz, J.-P., et al., 1988. Dysembryoplastic neuroepithelial tumor: A surgically curable tumor of young patients with intractable partial seizures: Report of thirty-nine cases. Neurosurgery 23, 545–556.

Daumas-Duport, C., 1993. Dysembryoplastic neuroepithelial tumors. Brain Pathol. 3, 283–295.

De Chadarévian, J.-P., Pattisapu, J.V., Faerber, E.N., 1990. Desmoplastic cerebral astrocytoma of infancy. Light microscopy, immunocytochemistry, and ultrastructure. Cancer 66, 173–179.

De Girolami, U., Zvaigzne, O., 1973. Modification of the Ach'ucarro-Hortega pineal stain for paraffin-embedded formalin-fixed tissue. Stain Technol. 48, 48–50.

de la Monte, S.M., 1989. Uniform lineage of oligodendrogliomas. Am. J. Pathol. 153, 529–540.

Deckert, M., Paulus, W., 2007. Malignant lymphomas. In: Louis, D.N., Ohgaki, H., Wiestler, O.D., et al. (Eds.), WHO classification of tumours of the central nervous system. IARC, Lyon, pp. 188–192.

Dohrmann, G.J., Farwell, J.R., Flannery, J.T., 1975. Glioblastoma in children. J. Neurosurg 44, 442–448.

Ducatman, B.S., Scheithauer, B.W., Piepgras, D.G., et al., 1986. Malignant peripheral nerve sheath tumors. A clinicopathological study of 120 cases. Cancer 57, 2006–2021.

Earnest, F.I.V., Kelly, P.J., Scheithauer, B.W., et al., 1988. Cerebral astrocytomas: histopathologic correlation of MR and CT contrast enhancement with stereotactic biopsy. Radiology 166, 823–827.

Eberhart, C.G., Burger, P.C., 2003. Anaplasia and grading in medulloblastomas. Brain Pathol. 13, 376–385.

Eberhart, C.G., Kaufman, W.E., Tihan, T., et al., 2001. Apoptosis, neuronal maturation, and neurotrophin expression within medulloblastoma nodules. J. Neuropathol. Exp. Neurol. 60, 462–469.

Eberhart, C.G., Kepner, J.L., Goldthwaite, P.T., et al., 2002a. Histopathologic grading of medulloblastomas: a Pediatric Oncology Group study. Cancer 94, 552–560.

Eberhart, C.G., Kratz, J., Wang, Y., et al., 2004. Histopathological and molecular prognostic markers in medulloblastoma: c-myc, N-myc, TrkC, and anaplasia. J. Neuropathol. Exp. Neurol. 63, 441–449.

Eberhart, C.G., Kratz, J.E., Schuster, A., et al., 2002b. Comparative genomic hybridization detects an increased number of chromosomal alterations in large cell/anaplastic medulloblastomas. Brain Pathol. 12, 36–44.

Eberhart, C.G., Wiestler, O.D., Eng, C., 2007. Cowden disease and dysplastic gangliocytoma of the cerebellum/Lhermitte-Duclos disease. In: Louis, D.N., Ohgaki, H., Wiestler, O.D., et al. (Eds.), WHO classification of tumours of the central nervous system. IARC, Lyon, pp. 226–228.

Ebert, C., von Haken, M., Meyer-Puttlitz, B., et al., 1999. Molecular genetic analysis of ependymal tumors. NF-2 mutations and chromosome 22q loss occur preferentially in intramedullary spinal ependymomas. Am. J. Pathol. 155, 627–632.

Eby, N.L., Grufferman, S., Flannelly, C.M., et al., 1988. Increasing incidence of primary brain lymphomas in the U.S. Cancer 62, 2461–2465.

Ecker, R.D., Marsh, W.R., Pollock, B.E., et al., 2003. Hemangiopericytoma in the central nervous system: treatment, pathological features, and long-term follow up in 38 patients. J. Neurosurg 98, 1182–1187.

Edwards, M.S.B., Hudgins, R.J., Wilson, C.B., et al., 1988. Pineal region tumors in children. J. Neurosurg 68, 689–697.

Ellison, D., 2002. Classifying the medulloblastoma: insights from morphology and molecular genetics. Neuropathol. Appl. Neurobiol. 28, 257–282.

Ellison, D.W., Steart, P.V., Bateman, A.C., 1995. Prognostic indicators in a range of astrocytic tumors: an immunohistochemical study with Ki-67 and p53 antibodies. J. Neurol. Neurosurg Psychiatry. 59, 413–419.

Eng, D.Y., DeMonte, F., Ginsberg, L., et al., 1997. Craniospinal dissemination of central neurocytoma. J. Neurosurg 86, 547–552.

Engelhard, H.H., Stelea, A., Cochran, E.J., 2002. Oligodendroglioma: pathology and molecular biology. Surg. Neurol. 58, 111–117.

Erlandson, R.A., Woodruff, J.M., 1982. Peripheral nerve sheath tumors: an electron microscopic study of 43 cases. Cancer 49, 273–287.

Erlandson, R.A., 1985. Peripheral nerve sheath tumors. Ultrastruct. Pathol. 9, 113–122.

Ess, K.C., Kamp, C.A., Tu, B.P., et al., 2005. Developmental origin of subependymal giant cell astrocytoma in tuberous sclerosis complex. Neurology 64, 1446–1449.

Faillot, T., Sichez, J.-P., Brault, J.-L., et al., 1990. Lhermitte–Duclos disease (dysplastic gangliocytoma of the cerebellum). Report of a case and review of the literature. Acta. Neurochir. 105, 44–49.

Fan, X., Eberhart, C.G., 2008. Medulloblastoma stem cells. J. Clin. Oncol. 26, 2821–2827.

Fauchon, F., Jouvet, A., Paquis, P., et al., 2000. Parenchymal pineal tumors: a clinicopathological study of 76 cases. Int. J. Radiat. Oncol. Biol. Phys. 46, 959–968.

Felsberg, J., Erkwoh, A., Sabel, M.C., et al., 2004. Oligodenroglial tumors: refinement of candidate regions on chromosome arm 1p and correlation of 1p/19q status with survival. Brain Pathol. 14, 121–130.

Fèvre-Montange, M., Champier, J., Szathmari, A., et al., 2006a. Microarray analysis reveals differential gene expression patterns in tumors of the pineal region. J. Neuropathol. Exp. Neurol. 65, 675–684.

Fèvre-Montange, M., Hasselblatt, M., Figarella-Branger, D., et al., 2006b. Prognosis and histopathologic features in papillary tumors of the pineal region: a retrospective multicenter study of 31 cases. J. Neuropathol. Exp. Neurol. 65, 1004–1011.

Fèvre-Montange, M., Szathmari, A., Champier, J., et al., 2008. Pineocytoma and pineal parenchymal tumors of intermediate differentiation presenting cytologic pleomorphism: a multicenter study. Brain Pathol. 18, 354–359.

Figarella-Branger, D., Civatte, M., Bouvier-Labit, C., et al., 2000. Prognostic factors in intracranial ependymomas in children. J. Neurosurg 93, 605–613.

Figarella-Branger, D., Söylemezogly, F., Burger, P.C., 2007. Central neurocytoma and extraventricular neurocytoma. In: Louis, D.N., Ohgaki, H., Wiestler, O.D., et al. (Eds.), WHO classification of tumours of the central nervous system. IARC, Lyon, pp. 106–109.

Figols, J., Iglesias-Rozas, J.R., Kazner, E., 1985. Myelin basic protein (MBP) in human gliomas: a study of twenty-five cases. Clin. Neuropathol. 4, 116–120.

Fijumoto, K., Ohnishi, H., Tsujimoto, M., et al., 2000. Dysembryoplastic neuroepithelial tumor of the cerebellum and brainstem. Case report. J. Neurosurg 93, 487–489.

Fine, S.W., McClain, S.A., Li, M., 2004. Immunohistochemical staining for calretinin is useful for differentiating schwannomas from neurofibromas. Am. J. Clin. Pathol. 122, 552–559.

Fletcher, C.D., Rydholm, A., Singer, S., et al., 2002. Soft tissue tymours: Epidemiology, clinical features, histopathological typing and grading. In: Fletcher, C.D., Unni, K.K., Mertens, F. (Eds.), World Health Organization Classification of Tumors. Pathology and genetics of tumours of soft tissue and bone. IARC, Lyon, pp. 12–18.

Forsyth, P.A., Shaw, E.G., Scheithauer, B.W., et al., 1993. Supratentorial pilocytic astrocytomas. A clinicopathologic, prognostic and flow cytometric study of 51 patients. Cancer 72, 1335–1342.

Frankel, R.H., Bayonna, W., Koslow, M., et al., 1992. p53 mutations in human malignant gliomas: comparison of loss of heterozygosity with mutation frequency. Cancer Res. 52, 1427–1433.

Fu, Y.-S., Chen, A.T.L., Kay, S., et al., 1974. Is subependymoma (subependymal glomerate astrocytoma) an astrocytoma or ependymoma? A comparative ultrastructural and tissue culture study. Cancer 34, 1992–2008.

Fuller, G.N., Kros, J.M., 2007. Gliomatosis cerebri. In: Louis, D.N., Ohgaki, H., Wiestler, O.D., et al. (Eds.), WHO classification of tumours of the central nervous system. IARC, Lyon, pp. 50–52.

Fults, D., Brockmeyer, D., Tullous, M.W., et al., 1992. p53 mutation and loss of heterozygosity on chromosome 17 and 10 during human astrocytoma progression. Cancer Res. 52, 674–679.

Furuta, A., Takahashi, H., Ikuta, F., et al., 1992. Temporal lobe tumor demonstrating ganglioglioma and pleomorphic xanthoastrocytoma components. Case report. J. Neurosurg 77, 143–147.

Gambarelli, D., Hassoun, J., Choux, M., et al., 1982. Complex cerebral tumor with evidence of neuronal, glial and Schwann cell differentiation: A histologic immunocytochemical and ultrastructural study. Cancer 49, 1420–1428.

Garcia, D.M., Fulling, K.H., 1985. Juvenile pilocytic astrocytoma of the cerebrum in adults. A distinctive neoplasm with favorable prognosis. J. Neurosurg 63, 382–386.

Gavrilovic, I.T., Hormigo, A., Yahalom, J., et al., 2006. Long-term follow-up of high-dose methotrexate-based therapy with and without whole brain irradiation for newly diagnosed primary CNS lymphoma. J. Clin. Oncol. 24, 4570–4574.

Gerstner, E.R., Abrey, L.E., Schiff, D., et al., 2008. CNS Hodgkin lymphoma. Blood 112, 1658–1661.

Gessi, M., Giangaspero, F., Pietsch, T., 2003. Atypical teratoid/rhabdoid tumors and choroid plexus tumors: when genetics 'surprise' pathology. Brain Pathol. 13, 409–414.

Giangaspero, F., Eberhart, C.G., Haapasalo, H., et al., 2007. Medulloblastoma. In: Louis, D.N., Ohgaki, H., Wiestler, O.D., et al. (Eds.), WHO classification of tumours of the central nervous system. IARC, Lyon, pp. 132–140.

Giangaspero, F., Rigobello, L., Badiali, M., et al., 1992. Large cell medulloblastomas. A distinct variant with highly aggressive behavior. Am. J. Surg. Pathol. 16, 687–693.

Giannini, C., Paulus, W., Louis, D.N., et al., 2007a. Pleomorphic xanthoastrocytoma. In: Louis, D.N., Ohgaki, H., Wiestler, O.D., et al. (Eds.), WHO classification of tumours of the central nervous system. IARC, Lyon, pp. 22–24.

Giannini, C., Rushing, E.J., Hainfellner, J.A., 2007b. Hemangiopericytoma. In: Louis, D.N., Ohgaki, H., Wiestler, O.D., et al. (Eds.), WHO classification of tumours of the central nervous system. IARC, Lyon, pp. 178–180.

Giannini, C., Scheithauer, B.W., Burger, P.C., et al., 1999a. Cellular proliferation in pilocytic and diffuse astrocytomas. J. Neuropathol. Exp. Neurol. 58, 46–53.

Giannini, C., Scheithauer, B.W., Burger, P.C., et al., 1999b. Pleomorphic xanthoastrocytoma. What do we really know about it? Cancer 85, 2033–2045.

Giannini, C., Scheithauer, B.W., Lopes, M.B., et al., 2002. Immunophenotype of pleomorphic xanthoastrocytoma. Am. J. Surg. Pathol. 26, 479–485.

Gilbertson, R.J., Bentley, L., Hernan, R., et al., 2002. ERBB receptor signaling promotes ependymoma cell proliferation and represents a potential novel therapeutic target for this disease. Clin. Cancer Res. 8, 3054–3064.

Gould, V.E., Rorke, L.B., Jansson, D.S., et al., 1990. Primitive neuroectodermal tumors of the central nervous system express neuroendocrine markers and may express all classes of intermediate filaments. Hum. Pathol. 21, 245–252.

Goussia, A.C., Kyritsis, A.P., Mitlianga, P., et al., 2001. Genetic abnormalities in oligodendroglial and ependymal tumors. J. Neurol. 248, 1030–1035.

Grand, S., Pasquier, B., Gay, E., et al., 2002. Chordoid glioma of the third ventricle: CT and MRI, including perfusion data. Neuroradiology 44, 842–846.

Grant, J.W., Steart, P.V., Aguzzi, A., et al., 1989. Gliosarcoma: An immunohistochemical study. Acta Neuropathol 79, 305–309.

Grimm, S.A., McCannel, C.A., Omuro, A.M., et al., 2008. Primary CNS lymphoma with intraocular involvement: International PCNSL Collaborative Group Report. Neurology 71, 1355–1360.

Guillou, L., Fletcher, J.A., Fletcher, C.D.M., et al., 2002. Extrapleural solitary fibrous tumor and haemangiopericytoma. In: Fletcher, C.D.M., Unni, K.K., Mertens, F. (Eds.), World Health Organization Classification of Tumors. Pathology and genetics of tumours of soft tissue and bone. IARC, Lyon, pp. 86–90.

Gutmann, D.H., Giordano, M.J., Mahadeo, D.K., et al., 1996. Increased neurofibromatosis 1 gene expression in astrocytic tumors: positive regulation by p21-ras. Oncogene 12, 2121–2127.

Guyotat, J., Signorelli, F., Desme, S., et al., 2002. Intracranial ependymomas in adult patients: analyses of prognostic factors. J. Neurooncol. 60, 255–268.

Haberler, C., Laggner, U., Slavc, I., et al., 2006. Immunohistochemical analysis of INI1 protein in malignant pediatric CNS tumors: Lack of INI1 in atypical teratoid/rhabdoid tumors and in a fraction of primitive neuroectodermal tumors without rhabdoid phenotype. Am. J. Surg. Pathol. 30, 1462–1468.

Haddad, S.F., Moore, S.A., Schelper, R.L., et al., 1992. Smooth muscle cells can comprise the sarcomatous component of gliosarcomas. J. Neuropathol. Exp. Neurol. 51, 493–498.

Hahn, H.P., Bundock, E.A., Hornick, J.L., 2006. Immunohistochemical staining for claudin-1 can help distinguish meningiomas from histologic mimics. Am. J. Clin. Pathol. 125, 203–208.

Hainfellner, J.A., Scheithauer, B.W., Giangaspero, F., et al., 2007. Rosette-forming glioneuronal tumor of the fourth ventricle. In: Louis, D.N., Ohgaki, H., Wiestler, O.D., et al. (Eds.), WHO classification of tumours of the central nervous system. IARC, Lyon, pp. 115–116.

Halling, K.C., Scheithauer, B.W., Halling, A.C., et al., 1996. p53 expression in neurofibroma and malignant peripheral nerve sheath tumor. An immunohistochemical study of sporadic and NF-1-associated tumors. Am. J. Clin. Pathol. 106, 282–288.

Halmagyi, G.M., Bignold, L.P., Allsop, J.L., 1979. Recurrent subependymal giant-cell astrocytoma in the absence of tuberous sclerosis. J. Neurosurg 50, 106–109.

Hao, D., DiFrancesco, L.M., Brasher, P.M., et al., 1999. Is primary CNS lymphoma really becoming more common? A population-based study of incidence, clinicopathological features and outcome in Alberta from 1975 to 1996. Ann. Oncol. 10, 65–70.

Hasselblatt, M., Blumcke, I., Jeibmann, A., et al., 2006a. Immunohistochemical profile and chromosomal imbalances in papillary tumors of the pineal region. Neuropathol. Appl. Neurobiol. 32, 278–283.

Hasselblatt, M., Bohm, C., Tatenhorst, L., et al., 2006b. Identification of novel diagnostic markers for choroid plexus tumors: a microarray-based approach. Am. J. Surg. Pathol. 30, 66–74.

Hassoun, J., Devictor, B., Gambarelli, D., et al., 1984. Paired twisted filaments: a new ultrastructural marker of human pinealomas? Acta. Neuropathol. 65, 163–165.

Hassoun, J., Gambarelli, D., Peragut, J.C., et al., 1983. Specific ultrastructural markers of human pinealomas: a study of four cases. Acta. Neuropathol. 62, 31–40.

Hassoun, J., Gambarelli, D., 1989. Pinealomas: need for an ultrastructural diagnosis. In: Fields, W.S. (Ed.), Primary brain tumors. A review of histologic classification. Springer Verlag, New York, pp. 82–85.

Hassoun, J., Söylemezoglu, F., Gambarelli, D., et al., 1993. Central neurocytoma: a synopsis of clinical and histological features. Brain Pathol. 3, 297–306.

Hayashi, H., Ohara, N., Jeon, H.J., et al., 1993. Gliosarcoma with features of chondroblastic osteosarcoma. Cancer 72, 850–855.

Henske, E.P., Scheithauer, B.W., Short, M.P., et al., 1996. Allelic loss is frequent in tuberous sclerosis kidney lesions but rare in brain lesions. Am. J. Hum. Genet. 59, 400–406.

Henske, E.P., Wessner, L.L., Golden, J., et al., 1997. Loss of tuberin in both subependymal giant cell astrocytomas and angiomyolipomas supports a two-hit model for the pathogenesis of tuberous sclerosis tumors. Am. J. Pathol. 151, 1639–1647.

Herath, S.E., Stalboerger, P.G., Dahl, R.J., et al., 1994. Cytogenetic studies of four hemangiopericytomas. Cancer Genet. Cytogenet. 72, 137–140.

Herbert, J., Cavallaro, T., Dwork, A.J., 1990. A marker for primary choroid plexus neoplasms. Am. J. Pathol. 136, 1317–1325.

Herpers, M.J., Budka, H., 1984. Glial fibrillary acidic protein (GFAP) in oligodendroglial tumors: gliofibrillary oligodendroglioma and transitional oligoastrocytoma as subtypes of oligodendroglioma. Acta. Neuropathol. 64, 265–272.

Herrick, M.K., Rubinstein, L.J., 1979. The cytological differentiating potential of pineal parenchymal neoplasms (true pinealomas): a clinicopathologic study of 28 tumors. Brain 102, 289–320.

Hessler, R.B., Lopes, M.B., Frankfurter, A., et al., 1992. Cytoskeletal immunohistochemistry of central neurocytomas. Am. J. Surg. Pathol. 16, 1031–1038.

Hirano, H., Lopes, M.B., Carpenter, J., et al., 1999. The IGF-1 content and pattern of expression correlates with histopathologic grade in diffusely infiltrating astrocytomas. Neuro. Oncol. 1, 109–119.

Hirose, T., Scheithauer, B.W., Lopes, M.B., et al., 1994. Dysembryoplastic neuroepithelial tumor (DNT): an immunohistochemical and ultrastructural study. J. Neuropathol. Exp. Neurol. 53, 184–195.

Ho, K.-L., 1990. Histogenesis of sarcomatous component of the gliosarcoma: an ultrastructural study. Acta. Neuropathol. 81, 178–188.

Hoang, M.P., Amirkhan, R.H., 2003. Inhibin alpha distinguishes hemangioblastoma from clear cell renal cell carcinoma. Am. J. Surg. Pathol. 27, 1152–1156.

Hoffman, H.J., Yoshida, M., Becker, L.E., et al., 1994. Pineal region tumors in childhood. Pediatr. Neurosurg 21, 91–104.

Hoffmann, C., Tabrizian, S., Wolf, E., et al., 2001. Survival of AIDS patients with primary central nervous system lymphoma is dramatically improved by HAART-induced immune recovery. AIDS 15, 2119–2127.

Horn, B., Heideman, R., Geyer, R., et al., 1999. A multi-institutional retrospective study of intracranial ependymoma in children: Identification of risk factors. J. Pediatr. Hematol./Oncol. 21, 203–211.

Hornick, J.L., Bundock, E.A., Fletcher, C.D., 2009. Hybrid schwannoma/serineurioma: clinicopathologic analysis of 42 distinctive benign nerve sheath tumors. Am. J. Surg. Pathol. 33, 1554–1561.

Horstmann, S., Perry, A., Reifenberger, G., et al., 2004. Genetic and expression profiles of cerebelar liponeurocytomas. Brain Pathol. 14, 281–289.

Horten, B.C., Rubinstein, L.J., 1976. Primary cerebral neuroblastoma: a clinicopathologic study of 35 cases. Brain 99, 735–756.

Hsu, D.W., Efird, J.T., Hedley-Whyte, E.T., 1997. Progesterone and estrogen receptors in meningiomas: prognostic considerations. J. Neurosurg 86, 113–120.

Hu, Q.D., Cui, X.Y., Ng, Y.K., et al., 2004. Axoglial interaction via the notch receptor in oligodendrocyte differentiation. Ann. Acad. Med. Singapore 33, 581–588.

Huang, H., Mahler-Araujo, B.M., Sankila, A., et al., 2000. APC mutations in sporadic medulloblastomas. Am. J. Pathol. 156, 433–437.

Ichimura, K., Pearson, D.M., Kocialkowski, S., et al., 2009. *IDH1* mutations are present in the majority of common adult gliomas but rare in primary glioblastomas. Neuro. Oncol. 11, 341–347.

Isatalo, P.A., Agbi, C., Davidson, B., et al., 2000. Primary primitive neuroectodermal tumor of the cauda equina. Hum. Pathol. 31, 999–1001.

Ishii, N., Sawamura, Y., Tada, M., 1998. Absence of p53 gene mutations in a tumor panel representative of pilocytic astrocytoma diversity using a p53 functional assay. Int. J. Cancer 76, 797–800.

Itoh, Y., Kowada, M., Mineura, K., et al., 1987. Congenital glioblastoma of the cerebellum with cytofluorometric deoxyribonucleic acid analysis. Surg. Neurol. 27, 163–167.

Iwashita, T., Enjoji, M., 1987. Plexiform neurilemmoma: a clinicopathological and immunohistochemical analysis of 23 tumors from 20 patients. Virchows Arch. A. Pathol. Anat. Histopathol 411, 305–309.

Jagadha, V., Halliday, W.C., Becker, L.E., 1986. Glial fibrillary acidic protein (GFAP) in oligodendrogliomas: a reflection of transient GFAP expression by immature oligodendroglia. Can. J. Neurol. Sci. 13, 307–311.

Jay, V., Becker, L.E., Otsubo, H., et al., 1993. Pathology of temporal lobectomy for refractory seizures in children. Review of 20 cases including some unique malformative lesions. J. Neurosurg 79, 53–61.

Jellinger, K., Paulus, W., 1991. Mesenchymal, non-meningothelial tumors of the central nervous system. Brain Pathol. 1, 79–87.

Jeuken, J.W., von Deimling, A., Wesseling, P., 2004. Molecular pathogenesis of oligodendroglial tumors. J. Neurooncol. 70, 161–181.

Johnson, D.L., Chandra, R., Fisher, W.S., et al., 1985. Trilateral retinoblastoma: ocular and pineal retinoblastomas. J. Neurosurg 63, 367–370.

Jones, D.T., Kocailkowski, S., Liu, L., et al., 2008. Tandem duplication producing a novel oncogenic BRAF fusion gene defines the majority of pilocytic astrocytomas. Cancer Res. 68, 8673–8677.

Jouvet, A., Fauchon, F., Liberski, P., et al., 2003. Papillary tumor of the pineal region. Am. J. Surg. Pathol. 27, 505–512.

Jouvet, A., Nakazato, Y., Scheithauer, B.W., et al., 2007. Papillary tumor of the pineal region. In: Louis, D.N., Ohgaki, H., Wiestler, O.D., et al. (Eds.), WHO classification of tumours of the central nervous system. IARC, Lyon, pp. 128–129.

Jouvet, A., Saint-Pierre, G., Fauchon, F., et al., 2000. Pineal parenchymal tumors: a correlation of histological features with prognosis in 66 cases. Brain Pathol. 10, 49–60.

Judkins, A.R., Eberhart, C.G., Wesseling, P., 2007. Atypical teratoid/rhabdoid tumor. In: Louis, D.N., Ohgaki, H., Wiestler, O.D., et al. (Eds.), WHO classification of tumours of the central nervous system. IARC, Lyon, pp. 147–149.

Judkins, A.R., Mauger, J., Ht, A., et al., 2004. Immunohistochemical analysis of hSNF5/INI1 in pediatric CNS neoplasms. Am. J. Surg. Pathol. 28, 644–650.

Jung, S.M., Kuo, T.T., 2005. Immunoreactivity of CD10 and inhibin alpha in differentiating hemangioblastoma of central nervous system from metastatic clear cell renal cell carcinoma. Mod. Pathol. 18, 788–794.

Kalyan-Raman, U.P., Olivero, W.C., 1987. Ganglioglioma: A correlative clinicopathological and radiological study of ten surgically treated cases with follow-up. Neurosurgery 20, 428–433.

Kandler, R.H., Smith, C.M., Broome, J.C., et al., 1991. Gliomatosis cerebri: a clinical, radiological and pathological report of four cases. Br. J. Neurosurg 5, 187–193.

Kanner, A.A., Staugatis, S.M., Castilla, E.A., et al., 2006. The impact of genotype on outcome in oligodendroglioma: validation of the loss of chromosome arm 1p as an important factor in clinical decision making. J. Neurosurg 104, 542–550.

Kao, G.F., Laskin, W.B., Olsen, T.G., 1989. Solitary cutaneous plexiform neurilemmoma (schwannoma): a clinicopathologic, immunohistochemical, and ultrastructural study of 11 cases. Mod. Pathol. 2, 20–26.

Katayama, Y., Kimura, S., Watanabe, T., et al., 1999. Peripheral-type primitive neuroectodermal tumor arising in the tentorium. Case report. J. Neurosurg 90, 141–144.

Katoh, M., Satoh, T., Nishiya, M., et al., 2004. Clear cell ependymoma of the fourth ventricle. Neuropathology 24, 330–335.

Katsetos, C.D., Herman, M.M., Frankfurter, A., et al., 1989. Cerebellar desmoplastic medulloblastomas. A further immunohistochemical characterization of the reticulin-free pale islands. Arch. Pathol. Lab. Med. 113, 1019–1029.

Kawahara, I., Tokunaga, Y., Yagi, N., et al., 2007. Papillary tumor of the pineal region: case report. Neurol. Med. Chir. (Tokyo) 47, 568–571.

Kawano, N., Yada, K., Yagishita, S., 1989. Clear cell ependymoma. A histological variant with diagnostic implications. Virchows Arch. [A] 415, 467–472.

Kawano, N., 1991. Pleomorphic xanthoastrocytoma (PXA) in Japan: its clinico-pathologic features and diagnostic clues. Brain Tumor. Pathol. 8, 5–10.

Kepes, J.J., Rubinstein, L.J., Chiang, H., 1984. The role of astrocytes in the formation of cartilage in gliomas. An immunohistochemical study of four cases. Am. J. Pathol. 117, 471–483.

Kepes, J.J., Rubinstein, L.J., Ansbacher, L., et al., 1989. Histopathological features of recurrent pleomorphic xanthoastrocytomas: Further corroboration of the glial nature of this neoplasm. Acta. Neuropathol. 78, 585–593.

Kepes, J.J., Rubinstein, L.J., Eng, L.F., 1979. Pleomorphic xanthoastrocytoma: A distinctive meningocerebral glioma of young subjects with relatively favorable prognosis; a study of 12 cases. Cancer 44, 1839–1852.

Kepes, J.J., 1983. Oncocytic transformation of choroid plexus epithelium. Acta. Neuropathol. 62, 145–148.

Kern, M., Robbins, P., Lee, G., Watson, P., 2006. Papillary tumor of the pineal region: a new pathological entity. Clin. Neuropathol. 25, 185–192.

Khoddami, M., Becker, L.E., 1997. Immunohistochemistry of medulloepithelioma and neural tube. Pediatr. Pathol. Lab. Med. 17, 913–925.

Kim, D.G., Kim, J.S., Chi, J.G., et al., 1996. Central neurocytoma: proliferative potential and biological behavior. J. Neurosurg 84, 742–747.

Kim, S.H., Kim, H., Kim, T.S., 2005. Clinical, histological, and immunohistochemical features predicting 1p/19q loss of heterozygosity in oligodendroglial tumors. Acta. Neuropathol. 110, 27–38.

Kitange, G.J., Templeton, K.L., Jenkins, R.B., 2003. Recent advances in the molecular genetics of primary gliomas. Curr. Opin. Oncol. 15, 197–203.

Kleihues, P., Aguzzi, A., Shibata, T., et al., 1989. Immunohistochemical assessment of differentiation and DNA replication in human brain tumors. In: Fields, W.S. (Ed.), Primary brain tumors. A review of histologic classification. Springer-Verlag, New York, pp. 123–132.

Kleihues, P., Burger, P.C., Aldape, K.D., et al., 2007c. Glioblastoma. In: Louis, D.N., Ohgaki, H., Wiestler, O.D., et al. (Eds.), WHO classification of tumours of the central nervous system. IARC, Lyon, pp. 33–49.

Kleihues, P., Burger, P.C., Rosenblum, M.K., et al., 2007b. Anaplastic astrocytoma. In: Louis, D.N., Ohgaki, H., Wiestler, O.D., et al. (Eds.), WHO classification of tumours of the central nervous system. IARC, Lyon, pp. 30–32.

Kleihues, P., Chimelli, L., Giangaspero, F., et al., 2007d. Cerebellar liponeurocytoma. In: Louis, D.N., Ohgaki, H., Wiestler, O.D., et al. (Eds.), WHO classification of tumours of the central nervous system. IARC, Lyon, pp. 110–112.

Kleihues, P., Louis, D.N., Weistler, O.D., et al., 2007a. WHO grading of tumors of the central nervous system. In: Louis, D.N., Ohgaki, H., Wiestler, O.D., et al. (Eds.), WHO classification of tumours of the central nervous system. IARC, Lyon, pp. 10–11.

Kleihues, P., Ohgaki, H., 1999. Primary and secondary glioblastoma: from concept to clinical diagnosis. Neuro. Oncol. 1, 45–51.

Kline, K.T., Damjanov, I., Katz, S.M., et al., 1979. Pineoblastoma: an electron microscopic study. Cancer 44, 1692–1699.

Komori, T., Scheithauer, B.W., Anthony, D.C., et al., 1998. Papillary glioneuronal tumor: a new variant of mixed neuronal-glial neoplasm. Am. J. Surg. Pathol. 22, 1171–1183.

Komori, T., Scheithauer, B.W., Hirose, T., 2002. A rosette-forming glioneuronal tumor of the fourth ventricle. Infratentorial form of dysembryoplastic neuroepithelial tumor? Am. J. Surg. Pathol. 26, 582–591.

Kordek, R., Biernat, W., Sapieja, W., et al., 1995. Pleomorphic xanthoastrocytoma with gangliomatous component: an immunohistochemical and ultrastructural study. Acta. Neuropathol. 89, 194–197.

Korf, H.W., Klein, D.C., Zigler, J.S., et al., 1986. S-antigen-like immunoreactivity in a human pineocytoma. Acta. Neuropathol. 69, 165–167.

Korshunov, A., Golanov, A., Sycheva, R., 2004. The histologic grade is a main prognostic factor for patients with intracranial ependymomas treated in the microneurosurgical era: an analysis of 258 patients. Cancer 100, 1230–1237.

Korshunov, A., Golanov, A., Timirgaz, V., 2000. Immunohistochemical markers for intracranial ependymoma recurrence. An analysis of 88 cases. J. Neuro. Sci. 177, 72–82.

Korshunov, A., Golanov, A., Timirgaz, V., 2001. p14ARF protein (FL-132) immunoreactivity in intracranial ependymomas and its prognostic significance: an analysis of 103 cases. Acta. Neuropathol. (Berl.) 102, 271–277.

Kraus, J.A., Koopmann, J., Kaskel, P., et al., 1995. Shared allelic losses on chromosomes 1p and 19q suggest a common origin of oligodendroglioma and oligo-astrocytoma. J. Neuropathol. Exp. Neurol. 54, 91–95.

Kraus, J.A., Felsberg, J., Tonn, J.C., et al., 2002. Molecular genetic analysis of the TP53, PTEN, CDKN2A, EGFR, CDK4 and MDM2 tumor-associated genes in supratentorial primitive neuroectodermal tumors and glioblastomas of childhood. Neuropathol. Appl. Neurobiol. 28, 325–333.

Kreiger, P.A., Okada, Y., Simon, S., et al., 2005. Losses of chromosomes 1p and 19q are rare in pediatric oligodendrogliomas. Acta. Neuropathol. (Berl.) 109, 387–392.

Krieg, M., Marti, H.H., Plate, K.H., 1998. Coexpression of erythropoietin and vascular endothelial growth factor in nervous system tumors associated with von Hippel-Lindau tumor suppressor gene loss of function. Blood 92, 3388–3393.

Kros, J.M., Van Eden, C.G., Stefanko, S.Z., et al., 1992. Prognostic implications of glial fibrillary acidic protein containing cell types in oligodendrogliomas. Cancer 66, 1204–1212.

Kros, J.M., de Jong, A.A., van der Kwast, Th.H., 1990. Ultrastructural characterization of transitional cells in oligodendrogliomas. J. Neuropathol. Exp. Neurol. 51, 186–193.

Krouwer, H.G., Davis, R.L., Silver, R., et al., 1991. Gemistocytic astrocytomas: a reappraisal. J. Neurosurg 74, 399–406.

Kubota, K.C., Itoh, T., Yamada, Y., et al., 2009. Melanocytic medulloblastoma with ganglioneurocytomatous differentiation: a case report. Neuropathology. 29, 72–77.

Kubota, T., Hayashi, M., Kawano, H., et al., 1991. Central neurocytoma: immunohistochemical and ultrastructural study. Acta. Neuropathol. 81, 418–427.

Kuchelmeister, K., Demirel, T., Schlorer, E., et al., 1995. Dysembryoplastic neuroepithelial tumor of the cerebellum. Acta. Neuropathol. 89, 385–390.

Kuchelmeister, K., Hugens-Penzel, M., Jodicke, A., Schachenmayr, W., 2006. Papillary tumor of the pineal region: histodiagnostic considerations. Neuropathol. Appl. Neurobiol. 32, 203–208.

Kujas, M., Lejeune, J., Benouaich-Amiel, A., et al., 2005. Chromosome 1p loss: a favorable prognostic factor in low-grade gliomas. Ann. Neurol. 58, 322–326.

Lamont, J.M., McManamy, C.S., Pearson, A.D., et al., 2004. Combined histopahtological and molecular cytogenetic stratification of medulloblastoma patients. Clin. Cancer Res. 10, 5482–5493.

Lang, F.F., Miller, D.C., Pisharody, S., et al., 1994. High frequency of p53 protein accumulation without p53 gene mutation in human juvenile pilocytic, low grade and anaplastic astrocytomas. Oncogene 9, 949–954.

Langford, L.A., 1986. The ultrastructure of the ependymoblastoma. Acta. Neuropathol. 71, 136–141.

Laurence, K.M., 1979. The biology of choroid plexus papilloma in infancy and childhood. Acta. Neurochir. 50, 79–90.

Leivo, I., Engvall, E., Laurila, P., et al., 1989. Distribution of merosin, a laminin-related tissue-specific basement membrane protein, in human Schwann cell neoplasms. Lab. Invest. 61, 426–432.

Lellouch-Tubiana, A., Boddaert, N., Bourgeois, M., et al., 2005. Angiocentric neuroepithelial tumor (ANET): a new epilepsy-realted clinicopathological entity with distinct MRI. Brain Pathol. 15, 281–286.

Liaw, D., Marsh, D.J., Li, J., et al., 1997. Germline mutations of the PTEN gene in Cowden disease, an inherited breast and thyroid cancer syndrome. Nat. Genet. 16, 64–67.

Ligon, K.L., Alberta, J.A., Kho, A.T., et al., 2004. The oligodendroglial lineage marker OLIG2 is universally expressed in diffuse gliomas. J. Neuropathol. Exp. Neurol. 63, 499–509.

Lindboe, C., Cappelen, J., Kepes, J., 1992. Pleomorphic xanthoastrocytoma as a component of a cerebellar ganglioglioma: case report. Neurosurgery 31, 353–355.

Liu, L., Backlund, L.M., Nilsson, B.R., et al., 2005. Clinical significance of EGFR amplification and the aberrant EGFR vIII transcript in conventionally treated astrocytic gliomas. J. Mol. Med. 83, 917–926.

Lombardi, D., Scheithauer, B.W., Meyer, F.B., et al., 1991. Symptomatic subependymoma: a clinicopathological and flow cytometric study. J. Neurosurg 75, 583–588.

Lopes, M.B.S., Altermatt, H.J., Scheithauer, B.W., et al., 1996. Immunohistochemical characterization of subependymal giant cell astrocytomas. Acta. Neuropathol. 91, 368–375.

Lopes, M.B.S., Gonzalez-Fernandez, F., Scheithauer, B.W., et al., 1993. Differential expression of retinal proteins in a pineal parenchymal tumor. J. Neuropathol. Exp. Neurol. 52, 516–524.

Lopes, M.B.S., Rosemberg, S., Cardoso de Almeida, P.C., et al., 1989. Glial fibrillary acidic protein and cytokeratin in choroid plexus tumors: an immunohistochemical study. Pathol. Res. Pract. 185, 339–341.

Lopes, M.B., Wiestler, O.D., Stemmet-Rachamimov, A.O., et al., 2007. Tuberous sclerosis complex and subependymal giant cell astrocytoma. In: Louis, D.N., Ohgaki, H., Wiestler, O.D., et al. (Eds.), WHO classification of tumours of the central nervous system. IARC, Lyon, pp. 218–221.

Louis, D.N., Ohgaki, H., Wiestler, O.D., et al. (Eds.), 2007. WHO classification of tumours of the central nervous system. IARC, Lyon.

Louis, D.N., Swearingen, B., Linggood, R.M., et al., 1990. Central nervous system neurocytoma and neuroblastoma in adults – report of eight cases. J. Neurooncol. 9, 231–238.

Louis, D.N., von Deimling, A., Chung, R.Y., et al., 1993. Comparative study of p53 gene and protein alterations in human astrocytic tumors. J. Neuropathol. Exp. Neurol. 52, 31–38.

Louis, D.N., 1997. A molecular genetic model of astrocytoma histopathology. Brain Pathol. 7, 755–764.

Madhusudan, S., Deplanque, G., Braybrooke, J.P., et al., 2004. Antiangiogenic therapy for von Hippel-Lindau disease. JAMA 291, 943–944.

Mahler-Araujo, M.B., Sanoudou, D., Tingby, O., et al., 2003. Structural Genomic Abnormalities of Chromosomes 9 and 18 in Myxopapillary Ependymomas. J. Neuropathol. Exp. Neurol. 62, 927–935.

Maintz, D., Fiedler, K., Koopmann, J., et al., 1997. Molecular genetic evidence for subtypes of oligoastrocytomas. J. Neuropathol. Exp. Neurol. 56, 1098–1104.

Marano, S.R., Johnson, P.C., Spetzler, R.F., 1988. Recurrent Lhermitte–Duclos disease in a child. J. Neurosurg 69, 599–603.

Margetts, J.C., Kalyan-Raman, U.P., 1989. Giant-celled glioblastoma of brain: a clinico-pathological and radiological study of ten cases (including immunohistochemistry and ultrastructure). Cancer 63, 524–531.

Markesbery, W.R., Haugh, R.M., Young, A.B., 1981. Ultrastructure of pineal parenchymal neoplasms. Acta. Neuropathol. 55, 143–149.

Matsui, I., Tanimura, M., Kobayashi, N., et al., 1993. Neurofibromatosis type 1 and childhood cancer. Cancer 72, 2746–2754.

McCabe, M.G., Ichimura, K., Liu, L., et al., 2006. High-resolution array-based comparative genomic hybridization of medulloblastomas and supratentorial primitive neuroectodermal tumors. J. Neuropathol. Exp. Neurol. 65, 549–561.

McCormick, P.C., Stein, B.M., 1990. Intramedullary tumors in adults. Neurosurg Clin. N. Am. 1, 609–630.

McGrogan, G., Rivel, J., Vital, C., et al., 1992. A pineal tumor with features of 'pineal anlage tumor'. Acta. Neurochir. 117, 73–77.

McLendon, R.E., Herndon, J.E. 2nd, West, B., et al., 2005. Survival analysis of presumptive prognostic markers among oligodendrogliomas. Cancer 104, 1693–1699.

McLendon, R.E., Judkins, A.R., Eberhart, C.G., et al., 2007a. Central nervous system primitive neuroectodermal tumors. In: Louis, D.N., Ohgaki, H., Wiestler, O.D., et al. (Eds.), WHO classification of tumours of the central nervous system. IARC, Lyon, pp. 141–146.

McLendon, R.E., Wiestler, O.D., Kros, J.M., et al., 2007b. Ependymoma and anaplastic ependymoma. In: Louis, D.N., Ohgaki, H., Wiestler, O.D., et al. (Eds.), WHO classification of tumours of the central nervous system. IARC, Lyon, pp. 74–80.

McNeil, D.E., Coté, T.R., Clegg, L., et al., 2002. Incidence and trends in pediatric malignancies medulloblastoma/primitive neuroectodermal tumor: a SEER update. Med. Pediatr. Oncol. 39, 190–194.

Megyesi, J.F., Kachur, E., Lee, D.H., et al., 2004. Imaging correlates of molecular signatures in oligodendrogliomas. Clin. Cancer Res. 10, 4303–4306.

Meis, J.M., Martz, K.L., Nelson, J.S., 1991. Mixed glioblastoma multiforme and sarcoma. A clinicopathologic study of 26 radiation therapy oncology group cases. Cancer 67, 2342–2349.

Meis, J.M., Ordóñez, N.G., Bruner, J.M., 1986. Meningiomas: An immunohistochemical study of 50 cases. Arch. Pathol. Lab. Med. 110, 934–937.

Mena, H., Ribas, J.L., Pezeshkpur, G.H., et al., 1991. Hemangiopericytoma of the central nervous system: a review of 94 cases. Hum. Pathol. 22, 84–91.

Mena, H., Rushing, E.J., Ribas, J.L., et al., 1995. Tumors of pineal parenchymal cells: a correlation of histological features, including nucleolar organizer regions, with survival in 35 cases. Hum. Pathol. 26, 20–30.

Meyer-Puttlitz, B., Hayashi, Y., Waha, A., et al., 1997. Molecular genetic analysis of giant cell glioblastomas. Am. J. Pathol. 151, 853–857.

Meyers, S.P., Khademian, Z.P., Chaung, S.H., et al., 2004. Choroid plexus carcinomas in children: MRI features and patient outcomes. Neuroradiology 9, 770–780.

Miettinen, M., Clark, Virtanen, I., 1986. Intermediate filament proteins in choroid plexus and ependyma and their tumors. Am. J. Pathol. 123, 231–240.

Miettinen, M., Foidart, J.M., Ekblom, P., 1983. Immunohistochemical demonstration of laminin, the major glycoprotein of basement membranes, as an aid in the diagnosis of soft tissue tumors. Am. J. Clin. Pathol. 79, 306–311.

Miller, C.R., Dunham, C.P., Scheithauer, B.W., et al., 2006. Significance of necrosis in grading of oligodendroglial neoplasms: a clinicopathologic and genetic study of newly diagnosed high-grade gliomas. J. Clin. Oncol. 24, 5419–5426.

Miller, D.C., Hochberg, F.H., Harris, N.L., et al., 1994. Pathology with clinical correlations of primary central nervous system non-Hodgkin's lymphoma. Cancer 74, 1383–1397.

Mills, S.E., Ross, G.W., Perentes, E., et al., 1990. Cerebellar hemangioblastoma: immunohistochemical distinction from metastatic renal cell carcinoma. Surg. Pathol. 3, 121–132.

Min, K.W., Scheithauer, B.W., Bauserman, S.C., 1994. Pineal parenchymal tumors: an ultrastructural study with prognostic implications. Ultrastruct. Pathol. 18, 69–85.

Minehan, K.J., Shaw, E.G., Scheithauer, B.W., et al., 1995. Spinal cord astrocytoma: pathological and treatment considerations. J. Neurosurg 83, 590–595.

Mishima, K., Nakamura, M., Nakamura, H., et al., 1992. Leptomeningeal dissemination of cerebellar pilocytic astrocytoma. J. Neurosurg 77, 788–791.

Mizuguchi, M., Kato, M., Yamanouchi, H., et al., 1997. Tuberin immunohistochemistry in brain, kidneys and heart with or without tuberous sclerosis. Acta. Neuropathol. 94, 525–531.

Mogollon, R., Penneys, N., Albores-Saavedra, J., et al., 1984. Malignant schwannoma presenting as a skin mass: confirmation by the demonstration of myelin basic protein within tumor cells. Cancer 53, 1190–1193.

Molloy, P.T., Hachinis, A.T., Rorke, L.B., et al., 1996. Central nervous system medulloepithelioma: a series of eight cases including two arising in the pons. J. Neurosurg 84, 430–436.

Montesinos-Rongen, M., Brunn, A., Bentink, S., et al., 2008. Gene expression profiling suggests primary central nervous system lymphomas to be derived from a late germinal center B cell. Leukemia 22, 400–405.

Montesinos-Rongen, M., Küppers, R., Schlüter, D., et al., 1999. Primary central nervous system lymphomas are derived from germinal-center B cells and show a preferential usage of the V4–34 gene segment. Am. J. Pathol. 155, 2077–2086.

Morantz, R.A., Feigin, I., Ransohoff, J.III, 1976. Clinical and pathological study of 24 cases of gliosarcoma. J. Neurosurg 45, 398–408.

Morantz, R.A., Kepes, J.J., Batnitzky, S., et al., 1979. Extraspinal ependymomas: report of three cases. J. Neurosurg 51, 383–391.

Morgello, S., 1995. Pathogenesis and classification of primary central nervous system lymphoma: an update. Brain Pathol. 5, 383–393.

Mørk, S.J., Rubinstein, L.J., 1985. Ependymoblastoma. A reappraisal of a rare embryonal tumor. Cancer 55, 1536–1542.

Mueller, W., Hartmann, C., Hoffmann, A., et al., 2002. Genetic signature of oligoastrocytomas correlates with tumor location and denotes distinct molecular subsets. Am. J. Pathol. 161, 313–319.

Muller, W., Afra, D., Schroder, R., 1997. Supratentorial recurrences of gliomas: morphological studies in relation to time intervals with 544 astrocytomas. Acta. Neurochir. 37, 75–91.

Muñoz, E.L., Eberhard, D.A., Lopes, M.B.S., et al., 1996. Proliferative activity and p53 mutation as prognostic indicators in pleomorphic xanthoastrocytoma [abstract]. J. Neuropathol. Exp. Neurol. 55, 606.

Nakagawa, Y., Perentes, E., Rubinstein, L.J., 1986. Immunohistochemical characterization of oligodendrogliomas: an analysis of multiple markers. Acta. Neuropathol. 72, 15–22.

Nakamura, M., Inoue, H.K., Ono, N., et al., 1987. Analysis of hemangiopericytic meningiomas by immunohistochemistry, electron microscopy and cell culture. J. Neuropathol. Exp. Neurol. 46, 57–71.

Nakasu, S., Hirano, A., Shimura, T., et al., 1987. Incidental meningiomas in autopsy study. Surg. Neurol. 27, 319–322.

Nakazato, K., Figarella-Branger, D., Becker, A.J., et al., 2007a. Papillary glioneuronal tumor. In: Louis, D.N., Ohgaki, H., Wiestler, O.D., et al. (Eds.), WHO classification of tumours of the central nervous system. IARC, Lyon, pp. 113–114.

Nakazato, Y., Jouvet, A., Scheithauer, B.W., 2007b. Pineocytoma; Pineal parenchymal tumor of intermediate differentiation; Pineoblastoma. In: Louis, D.N., Ohgaki, H., Wiestler, O.D., et al. (Eds.), WHO classification of tumours of the central nervous system. IARC, Lyon, pp. 122–127.

Nelen, M.R., Padberg, G.W., Peeters, E.A., et al., 1996. Localization of the gene for Cowden disease to chromosome 10q22–10q23. Nat. Genet. 13, 114–116.

Neumann, H.P., Lips, C.J.M., Hsia, Y.E., et al., 1995. Von Hippel-Lindau Syndrome. Brain Pathol. 5, 181–193.

Ng, T.H.K., Poon, W.S., 1990. Gliosarcoma of the posterior fossa with features of a malignant fibrous histiocytoma. Cancer 65, 1161–1166.

Ng, T.H.K., Furg, C.F., Ma, L.T., 1990. The pathological spectrum of desmoplastic infantile gangliogliomas. Histopathology 16, 235–241.

Nicholson, J.C., Ross, F.M., Kohler, J.A., et al., 1999. Comparative genomic hybrisization and histological variation in primitive neuroectodermal tumors. Br. J. Cancer 80, 1322–1331.

Nilda, Y., Stemmer-Rachamimov, A.O., Logrip, M., et al., 2001. Survey of somatic mutations in tuberous sclerosis complex (TSC) hamartomas suggest different genetic mechanisms for pathogenesis of TSC lesions. Am. J. Hum. Genet. 69, 493–503.

Nishio, S., Tashima, T., Takeshita, I., et al., 1988. Intraventricular neurocytoma – clinicopathological features of six cases. J. Neurosurg 68, 665–670.

Nishiyama, A., Chang, A., Trapp, B.D., 1999. NG2+ glial cells: A novel glial cell population in the adult brain. J. Neuropathol. Exp. Neurol. 58, 1113–1124.

Nolan, M.A., Sakuta, R., Chuang, N., et al., 2004. Dysembryoplastic neuroepithelial tumors in childhood. Long-term outcome and prognostic features. Neurology 62, 2270–2276.

Norris, L.S., Snodgrass, S., Miller, D.C., et al., 2005. Recurrent central nervous system medulloepithelioma. J. Pediatr. Hematol. Oncol. 27, 264–266.

Ohgaki, H., Dessen, P., Jourde, B., et al., 2004. Genetic pathways to glioblastoma: a population-based study. Cancer Res. 6892–6899.

Ohgaki, H., Eibl, R.H., Schwab, M., et al., 1993. Mutations of the p53 tumor suppressor gene in neoplasms of the human nervous system. Mol. Carcinog. 8, 74–80.

Ohgaki, H., Kleihues, P., 2005. Population-based studies on incidence, survival rates, and genetic alterations in astrocytic and oligodendroglial gliomas. J. Neuropathol. Exp. Neurol. 64, 479–489.

Ohnishi, A., Sawa, H., Tsuda, M., et al., 2003. Expression of the oligodendroglial lineage-associated markers Olig1 and Olig2 in different types of human gliomas. J. Neuropathol. Exp. Neurol. 62, 1052–1059.

Olson, J.E., Janney, C.A., Rao, R.D., et al., 2002. The continuing increase in the incidence of primary central nervous system non-Hodgkin lymphoma. Cancer 95, 1504–1510.

Onguru, O., Celasun, B., Gunhan, O., 2005. Desmoplastic non-infantile ganglioglioma. Neuropathology. 25, 150–152.

Packer, R.J., Perilongo, G., Johnson, D., et al., 1992. Choroid plexus carcinoma of childhood. Cancer 69, 580–585.

Padberg, G.W., Schot, J.D., Vielvoye, G.J., et al., 1991. Lhermitte-Duclos disease and Cowden disease: A single phakomatosis. Ann. Neurol. 29, 517–523.

Pagni, C.A., Canavero, S., Giordana, M.T., et al., 1992. Spinal intramedullary subependymomas: case report and review of the literature. Neurosurgery 30, 115–117.

Parsons, D.W., Jones, S., Zhang, X., et al., 2008. An integrated genomic analysis of human glioblastoma multiforme. Science 321, 1807–1812.

Pasquier, B., Kojder, I., Labat, F., et al., 1985. Le xanthoastrocytome du sujet jeune. Ann. Pathol. 5, 29–43.

Pasquier, B., Péoc'h, M., Morrison, A.L., et al., 2002. Chordoid glioma of the third ventricle: a report of two new cases, with further evidence supporting an ependymal differentiation, and review of the literature. Am. J. Surg. Pathol. 26, 1330–1342.

Patt, S., Gries, H., Giraldo, M., et al., 1996. p53 gene mutations in human astrocytic brain tumors including pilocytic astrocytomas. Hum. Pathol. 27, 586–589.

Patterson, R.H. Jr, Campbell, W.G. Jr, Parsons, H., 1961. Ependymoma of the cauda equina with multiple visceral metastases: report of a case. J. Neurosurg 18, 145–150.

Paulus, W., Bayas, A., Ott, G., et al., 1994a. Interphase cytogenetics of glioblastoma and gliosarcoma. Acta. Neuropathol. 88, 420–423.

Paulus, W., Brandner, S., 2007. Choroid plexus tumors. In: Louis, D.N., Ohgaki, H., Wiestler, O.D., et al. (Eds.), WHO classification of tumours of the central nervous system. IARC, Lyon, pp. 82–85.

Paulus, W., Lisle, D.K., Tonn, J.C., et al., 1996. Molecular genetic alterations in pleomorphic xanthoastrocytoma. Acta. Neuropathol. 91, 293–297.

Paulus, W., Ott, M.M., Strik, H., et al., 1994b. Large cell anaplastic (Ki-1) brain lymphoma of T-cell genotype. Hum. Pathol. 25, 1253–1256.

Penneys, N.S., Mogollon, R., Kowalczyk, A., et al., 1984. A survey of cutaneous neural lesions for the presence of myelin basic protein. An immunohistochemical study. Arch. Dermatol. 120 (2), 210–213.

Peraud, A., Watanabe, K., Plate, K.H., et al., 1997. Mutations versus EGF Receptor expression in giant cell glioblastomas. J. Neuropathol. Exp. Neurol. 56, 1236–1241.

Peraud, A., Watanabe, K., Schwechheimer, K., et al., 1999. Genetic profile of the giant cell glioblastoma. Lab. Invest. 79, 123–129.

Perentes, E., Rubinstein, L.J., 1987. Recent applications of immunoperoxidase histochemistry in human neuro-oncology. Arch. Pathol. Lab. Med. 111, 796–812.

Perentes, E., Nakagawa, Y., Ross, G.W., et al., 1987. Expression of epithelial membrane antigen in perineural cells and their derivatives. An immunohistochemical study with multiple markers. Acta. Neuropathol. 75, 160–165.

Perentes, E., Rubinstein, L.J., Herman, M.M., et al., 1986. S-antigen immunoreactivity in human pineal glands and pineal parenchymal tumors. A monoclonal antibody study. Acta. Neuropathol. 71, 224–227.

Perentes, E., Rubinstein, L.J., 1986. Immunohistochemical recognition of human neuro-epithelial tumors by anti-Leu 7 (HNK-1) monoclonal antibody. Acta. Neuropathol. 69, 227–233.

Perry, A., Aldape, K.D., George, D.H., et al., 2004. Small cell astrocytoma: an aggressive variant that is clinicopathologically and genetically distinct form anaplastic oligodendroglioma. Cancer 101, 2318–2326.

Perry, A., Giannini, C., Scheithauer, B.W., et al., 1997a. Composite pleomorphic xanthoastrocytoma and ganglioglioma: report of four cases and review of the literature. Am. J. Surg. Pathol. 21, 763–771.

Perry, A., Louis, D.N., Scheithauer, B.W., et al., 2007. Meningiomas. In: Louis, D.N., Ohgaki, H., Wiestler, O.D., et al. (Eds.), WHO classification of tumours of the central nervous system. IARC, Lyon, pp. 164–172.

Perry, A., Miller, C.R., Gujrati, M., et al., 2009. Malignant gliomas with primitive neuroectodermal tumor-like components: a clinicopathologic and genetic study of 53 cases. Brain Pathol. 19, 81–90.

Perry, A., Stafford, S.L., Scheithauer, B.W., et al., 1998. The prognostic role of MIB-1, p53 and DNA flow cytometry in completely resected primary meningiomas. Cancer 82, 2262–2269.

Perry, A., Stafford, S.L., Scheitheauer, B.W., et al., 1997b. Meningioma grading. An analysis of histologic parameters. Am. J. Surg. Pathol. 21, 1455–1465.

Pierga, J.Y., Kalifa, C., Terrier-Lacombe, M.J., et al., 1993. Carcinoma of the choroid plexus: a pediatric experience. Med. Pediat. Oncol. 21, 480–487.

Pinkus, G.S., Kurtin, P.J., 1985. Epithelial membrane antigen – a diagnostic discriminant in surgical pathology: immunohistochemical profile in epithelial, mesenchymal, and hematopoietic neoplasms using paraffin sections and monoclonal antibodies. Hum. Pathol. 16, 929–940.

Pizer, B.L., Moss, T., Oakhill, A., et al., 1995. Congenital astroblastoma: an immunohistochemical study. Case report. J. Neurosurg 83, 550–555.

Plate, K.H., Vortmeyer, A.O., Zagzag, D., et al., 2007. von Hippel-Lindau disease and haemangioblastoma. In: Louis, D.N., Ohgaki, H., Wiestler, O.D., et al. (Eds.), WHO classification of tumours of the central nervous system. IARC, Lyon, pp. 215–217.

Platten, M., Giordano, M.J., Dirven, C.M., et al., 1996. Up-regulation of specific NF-1 gene transcripts in sporadic pilocytic astrocytomas. Am. J. Pathol. 149, 621–627.

Pomeroy, S.L., Tamayo, P., Gaasenbeck, M., et al., 2002. Prediction of central nervous system embryonal tumor outcome based on gene expression. Nature 415, 436–442.

Pommepuy, I., Delage-Corre, M., Moreau, J.J., et al., 2006. A report of a desmoplastic ganglioglioma in a 12-year-old girl with review of the literature. J. Neurooncol. 76, 271–275.

Port, J.D., Brat, D.J., Burger, P.C., et al., 2003. Astroblastoma: radiologic-pathologic correlation and distinction from ependymoma. AJNR Am. J. Neuroradiol. 23, 243–247.

Pravdenkova, S., Al-Mefty, O., Sawyer, J., et al., 2006. Progesterone and estrogen receptors: opposing prognostic indicators in meningiomas. J. Neurosurg 105, 163–173.

Prayson, R.A., Morris, H.H., Estes, M.L., et al., 1996. Dysembryoplastic neuroepithelial tumor: a clinicopathologic and immunohistochemical study of 11 tumors including MIB-1 immunoreactivity. Clin. Neuropathol. 15, 47–53.

Prayson, R.A., 1999. Clinicopathologic study of 61 patients with ependymoma including MIB-1 immunohistochemistry. Ann. Diagn. Pathol. 3, 11–18.

Preusser, M., Dietrich, W., Czech, T., et al., 2003. Rosette-forming glioneuronal tumor of the fourth ventricle. Acta. Neuropathol. 106, 506–508.

Preusser, M., Wolfsberger, S., Czech, T., et al., 2005. A survivin expression in intracranial ependymomas and its correlation with tumor cell proliferation and patient outcome. Am. J. Clin. Pathol. 124, 543–549.

Pulitzer, D.R., Martin, P.C., Collins, P.C., et al., 1988. Subcutaneous sacrococcygeal ('myxopapillary') ependymal rests. Am. J. Surg. Pathol. 12, 672–677.

Radley, M.G., Di Sant'Agnese, P.A., Eskin, T.A., et al., 1989. Epithelial differentiation in meningiomas. An immunohistochemical, histochemical and ultrastructural study – with review of literature. Am. J. Clin. Pathol. 92, 266–272.

Raffel, C., Jenkins, R.B., Frederick, L., et al., 1997. Sporadic medulloblastomas contain PTCH mutations. Cancer Res. 57, 842–845.

Raffel, C., Thomas, G.A., Tishler, D.M., et al., 1993. Absence of p53 mutations in childhood central nervous system primitive neuroectodermal tumors. Neurosurgery 33, 103–106.

Ragel, B.T., Townsend, J.J., Arthur, A.S., et al., 2005. Intraventricular tanycytic ependymoma: case report and review of the literature. J. Neurooncol. 71, 189–193.

Raizer, J.J., Shetty, T., Gutin, P.H., et al., 2003. Chordoid glioma: report of a case with unusual histologic features, ultrastructural study and review of the literature. J. Neurooncol. 63, 39–47.

Rajaram, V., Brat, D.J., Perry, A., 2004. Anaplastic meningioma versus meningeal hemangiopericytoma: immunohistochemical and genetic markers. Hum. Pathol. 35, 1413–1418.

Rakic, P., 2003. Developmental and evolutionary adaptations of cortical radial glia. Cereb. Cortex. 13, 541–549.

Rao, C., Friedlander, M.E., Klein, E., et al., 1990. Medullomyoblastoma in an adult. Cancer 65, 157–163.

Rawlinson, D.G., Herman, M.M., Rubinstein, L.J., 1973. The fine structure of a myxopapillary ependymoma of the filum terminale. Acta. Neuropathol. 25, 1–13.

Reddy, A., Janss, A., Phillips, P., et al., 2000. Outcome for children with supratentorial primitive neuroectodermal tumors treated with surgery, radiation, and chemotherapy. Cancer 88, 2189–2193.

Reifenberger, G., Louis, D.N., 2003. Oligodendroglioma: toward molecular definitions in diagnostic neuro-oncology. J Neuropath Exp. Neurol. 62, 111–126.

Reifenberger, G., Weber, T., Weber, R.G., et al., 1999. Chordoid glioma of the third ventricle: immunohistochemical and molecular genetic characterization of a novel tumor entity. Brain Pathol. 9, 617–626.

Reifenberger, J., Reifenberger, G., Liu, L., et al., 1994. Molecular genetic analysis of oligodendroglial tumors shows preferential allelic deletions on 19q and 1p. Am. J. Pathol. 145, 1175–1190.

Reifenberger, G., Kros, J.M., Louis, D.N., et al., 2007. Anaplastic oligodendroglioma. In: Louis, D.N., Ohgaki, H., Wiestler, O.D., et al. (Eds.), WHO classification of tumours of the central nervous system. IARC, Lyon, pp. 60–62.

Reis, R.M., Konu-Lebleblicioglu, D., Lopes, J.M., et al., 2000. Genetic profile of gliosarcomas. Am. J. Pathol. 156, 425–432.

Reiter, R.J., 1981. The pineal gland. Vol I – Anatomy and biochemistry. CRC Press, New York, pp. 121–154.

Reznik, M., Schoenen, J., 1983. Lhermitte–Duclos disease. Acta. Neuropathol. 59, 88–94.

Ridley, L., Rahman, R., Brundler, M.-A., et al., 2008. Multifactorial analysis of predictors of outcome in intracranial ependymoma. Neuro. Oncol. 10, 675–689.

Riemenschneider, M.J., Perry, A., Reifenberger, G., 2006. Histological classification and molecular genetics of meningiomas. Lancet. Neurol. 5, 1045–1054.

Robbins, P., Segal, A., Narula, S., et al., 1995. Central neurocytoma. A clinicopathological, immunohistochemical and ultrastructural study of 7 cases. Pathol. Res. Pract. 191, 100–111.

Roberts, C.W., Biegel, J.A., 2009. The role of SMARCB1/INI1 in development of rhabdoid tumor. Cancer Biol. Ther. 8, 412–416.

Roncaroli, F., Consales, A., Fioravanti, A., 2005. Supratentorial cortical ependymoma: Report of three cases. Neurosurgery 57, E192.

Roncaroli, F., Scheithauer, B.W., 2007. Papillary tumor of the pineal region and spindle cell oncocytoma of the pituitary: new tumor entities in the 2007 WHO classification. Brain Pathol. 17, 314–318.

Rorke, L.B., Packer, R., Biegel, J.A., 1996. Central nervous system atypical teratoid/rhabdoid tumors of infancy and childhood: definition of an entity. J. Neurosurg 85, 56–65.

Rossi, A., Caracciolo, V., Russo, G., et al., 2008. Medulloblastoma: from molecular pathology to therapy. Clin. Cancer Res. 14, 971–976.

Rousseau, E., Ruchoux, M.-M., Scaravilli, F., et al., 2003. CDKN2A, CDKN2B and p14 ARF are frequently and differentially methylated in ependymal tumors. Neuropathol. Appl. Neurobiol. 29, 574–583.

Rubinstein, L.J., Logan, W.J., 1970. Extraneural metastases in ependymoma of the cauda equina. J. Neurol. Neurosurg Psych. 33, 763–770.

Rubinstein, L.J., 1972. Tumors of the central nervous system. Atlas of tumor pathology, fascicle 6. Armed Forces Institute of Pathology, Washington D.C.

Rushing, E.J., Brown, D.F., Hladik, C.L., et al., 1998. Correlation of bcl-2, p53, and MIB-1 expression with ependymoma grade and subtype. Mod. Pathol. 11, 464–470.

Russell, D.S., Rubinstein, L.J., 1989. Pathology of tumors of the nervous system, fifth ed. Edward Arnold, London.

Russo, C., Pellarin, M., Tingby, O., et al., 1999. Comparative genomic hybridization in patients with supratentorial and infratentorial primitive neuroectodermal tumors. Cancer 86, 331–339.

Russo, C.P., Katz, D.S., Corona, R.J., et al., 1995. Gangliocytoma of the cervicothoracic spinal cord. AJNR. Am. J. Neuroradiol. 16, 889–891.

Rutka, J.T., Smith, S.L., 1993. Transfection of human astrocytoma cells with glial fibrillary acidic protein complementary DNA: analysis of expression, proliferation and tumorigenicity. Cancer Res. 53, 3624–3631.

Salazar, O.M., Castro-Vita, H., VanHoutte, P., et al., 1983. Improved survival in cases of intracranial ependymoma after radiation therapy: late report and recommendations. J. Neurosurg 59, 652–659.

Santi, M., Quezado, M., Ronchetti, R., et al., 2005. Analysis of chromosome 7 in adult and pediatric ependymomas using chromogenic in situ hybridization. J. Neurooncol. 72, 25–28.

Scheithauer, B.W., Erdogan, S., Rodriguez, F.J., et al., 2009. Malignant peripheral nerve sheath tumors of cranial nerves and intracranial contents: a clinicopathologic study of 17 cases. Am. J. Surg. Pathol. 33, 325–338.

Scheithauer, B.W., Fuller, G.N., VandenBerg, S.R., 2008. The 2007 WHO classification of tumors of the nervous system: controversies in surgical neuropathology. Brain Pathol. 18, 307–316.

Scheithauer, B.W., Hawkins, C., Tihan, T., et al., 2007a. Pilocytic astrocytomas. In: Louis, D.N., Ohgaki, H., Wiestler, O.D., et al. (Eds.), WHO classification of tumours of the central nervous system. IARC, Lyon, pp. 15–21.

Scheithauer, B.W., Louis, D.N., Hunter, S., et al., 2007b. Schwannoma, neurofibroma, and malignant peripheral nervous sheath tumors. In: Louis, D.N., Ohgaki, H., Wiestler, O.D., et al. (Eds.), WHO classification of tumours of the central nervous system. IARC, Lyon, pp 152–157 and 160–162.

Scheithauer, B.W., Rubinstein, L.J., 1979. Cerebral medulloepithelioma. Report of a case with divergent neuroepithelial differentiation. Childs. Brain 5, 62–71.

Scheithauer, B.W., 1978. Symptomatic subependymoma: report of 21 cases with review of the literature. J. Neurosurg 49, 689–696.

Schiffer, D., Chio, A., Giordana, M.T., et al., 1991. Histologic prognostic factors in ependymoma. Childs Nerv. Syst. 7, 177–182.

Schiffer, D., Dutto, A., Cavalla, P., et al., 1997. Prognostic factors in oligodendrogliomas. Can. J. Neurol. Sci. 24, 313–319.

Schiffer, D., Giordana, M.T., Mauro, A., et al., 1986. Immunohistochemical demonstration of vimentin in human cerebral tumors. Acta. Neuropathol. 70, 209–219.

Schild, S.E., Scheithauer, B.W., Schomberg, P.J., et al., 1993. Pineal parenchymal tumors: Clinical, pathological, and therapeutic aspects. Cancer 72, 870–880.

Schmidbauer, M., Budka, H., Pilz, P., 1989. Neuroepithelial and ectomesenchymal differentiation in a primitive pineal tumor ('pineal anlage tumor'). Clin. Neuropathol. 8, 7–10.

Schnitt, S.J., Vogel, H., 1986. Meningiomas: Diagnostic value of immunoperoxidase staining for epithelial membrane antigen. Am. J. Surg. Pathol. 10, 640–649.

Schofield, D., West, D.C., Anthony, D.C., et al., 1995. Correlation of loss of heterozygosity at chromosome 9q with histological subtype in medulloblastomas. Am. J. Pathol. 146, 472–480.

Schröder, R., Ploner, C., Ernestus, R.I., 1993. The growth potential of ependymomas with varying grades of malignancy measured by the Ki-67 labelling index and mitotic index. Neurosurg Rev. 16, 145–150.

Schwartz, A.N., Ghatak, N.R., 1990. Malignant transformation of benign cerebellar astrocytoma. Cancer 56, 333–336.

Segal, R.A., Goumnerova, L.C., Kwon, Y.K., et al., 1994. Expression of the neurotrophin receptor TrkC is linked to a favorable outcome in medulloblastoma. Proc. Natl. Acad. Sci. USA. 91, 12867–12871.

Sharma, M.C., Ralte, A.M., Gaekwad, S., et al., 2004. Subependymal giant cell astrocytoma – a clinicopathological study of 23 cases with special emphasis on histogenesis. Pathol. Oncol. Res. 10, 219–224.

Sharma, M.K., Mansur, D.B., Reifenberger, G., et al., 2008. Distinct genetic signatures among pilocytic astrocytomas relate to their brain region origin. Cancer Res. 67 (3), 890–900.

Sharma, S., Abbott, R.I., Zagzag, D., 1998. Malignant intracerebral nerve sheath tumor: a case report and review of the literature. Cancer 82, 545–552.

Shepherd, C.W., Scheithauer, B.W., Gomez, M.R., et al., 1991. Subependymal giant cell astrocytoma: a clinical, pathological, and flow cytometric study. Neurosurgery 28, 864–868.

Shibahara, J., Todo, T., Morita, A., et al., 2004. Papillary neuroepithelial tumor of the pineal region. A case report. Acta. Neuropathol. 108, 337–340.

Shibamoto, Y., Ogino, H., Suzuki, G., et al., 2008. Primary central nervous system lymphoma in Japan: Changes in clinical features, treatment and prognosis during 1985–2004. Neuro. Oncol. 10, 560–568.

Shin, J.H., Lee, H.K., Khang, S.K., et al., 2002. Neuronal tumors of the central nervous system: radiologic findings and pathologic correlation. Radiographics 22, 1177–1189.

Shiruba, R.A., Gessaga, E.C., Eng, L.F., et al., 1988. Lhermitte–Duclos disease: An immunohistochemical study of the cerebellar cortex. Acta. Neuropathol. 75, 474–480.

Sidranski, D., Mikkelsen, T., Schwechheimer, K., et al., 1992. Clonal expansion of p53 mutant cells is associated with brain tumor progression. Nature 355, 846–847.

Skiest, D.J., Crosby, C., 2003. Survival is prolonged by highly active antiretroviral therapy in AIDS patients with primary central nervous system lymphoma. AIDS 17, 1787–1793.

Smidt, M., Kirsch, I., Ratner, L., 1990. Deletion of Alu sequences in the fifth c-sis intron in individuals with meningiomas. J. Clin. Invest. 86, 1151–1157.

Smith, J.S., Perry, A., Borell, T.J., et al., 2000. Alterations of chromosome arms 1p and 19q as predictors of survival in oligodendrogliomas, astrocytomas, and mixed oligoastrocytomas. J. Clin. Oncol. 18, 636–645.

Smith, J.S., Tachibana, I., Passe, S.M., et al., 2001. PTEN mutation, EGFR amplification, and outcome in patients with anaplastic astrocytoma and glioblastoma multiforme. J. Natl. Cancer Inst. 93, 1246–1256.

Sobel, R.A., Trice, J.E., Nielsen, S.L., et al., 1981. Pineoblastoma with ganglionic and glial differentiation: report of two cases. Acta. Neuropathol. 55, 243–246.

Sonneland, P.R., Scheithauer, B.W., LeChago, J., et al., 1986. Paraganglioma of the cauda equina region. Clinicopathologic study of 31 cases with special reference to immunocytology and ultrastructure. Cancer 58, 1720–1735.

Sonneland, P.R., Scheithauer, B.W., Onofrio, B.M., 1985. Myxopapillary ependymoma: a clinicopathologic and immunocytochemical study of 77 cases. Cancer 56, 883–893.

Söylemezoglu, F., Scheithauer, B.W., Esteve, J., et al., 1997. Atypical central neurocytoma. J. Neuropathol. Exp. Neurol. 56, 551–556.

Specht, C.S., Smith, T.W., DeGirolami, U., et al., 1986. Myxo-papillary ependymoma of the filum terminale: a light and electron microscopic study. Cancer 58, 310–317.

Stefanko, S.Z., Manschot, W.A., 1979. Pinealoblastoma with retinomatous differentiation. Brain 102, 321–332.

Stefanko, S.Z., Vuzevski, V.D., Maas, A.I.R., et al., 1986. Intracerebral malignant schwannoma. Acta. Neuropathol. 71, 321–325.

Steichen-Gersdorf, E., Baumgartner, M., Kreczy, A., et al., 1997. Deletion mapping on chromosome 17p in medulloblastoma. Br. J. of Cancer 76, 1284–1287.

Stemmer-Rachamimov, A.O., Wiestler, O.D., Louis, D.N., 2007. Neurofibromatosis type 2. In: Louis, D.N., Ohgaki, H., Wiestler, O.D., et al. (Eds.), WHO classification of tumours of the central nervous system. IARC, Lyon, pp. 210–214.

Strom, E.H., Skullerud, K., 1983. Pleomorphic xanthoastrocytoma: report of 5 cases. Clin. Neuropathol. 2, 188–191.

Sung, T., Miller, D.C., Hayes, R.L., et al., 2000. Preferential inactivation of the p53 tumor suppressor pathway and lack of EGFR amplification distinguish de novo high grade pediatric astrocytoma from de novo adult astrocytomas. Brain Pathol. 10, 249–259.

Sure, U., Ruedi, D., Tachibana, O., et al., 1997. Determination of p53 mutations, EGFR overexpression, and los of p16 expression in pediatric glioblastomas. J. Neuropathol. Exp. Neurol. 56, 782–789.

Sutton, L.N., Packer, R.J., Rorke, L.B., et al., 1983. Cerebral gangliogliomas during childhood. Neurosurgery 13, 124–128.

Taddei, G.L., Buccoliero, A.M., Caldarella, A., et al., 2001. Cerebellar liponeurocytoma: immunohistochemical and ultrastructural study of a case. Ultrastruct. Pathol. 25, 59–63.

Taillibert, S., Chodkiewicz, C., Laigle-Donadey, F., et al., 2006. Gliomatosis cerebri: a review of 296 cases from the ANOCEF database and the literature. J. Neurooncol. 76, 201–205.

Takeuchi, H., Kubota, T., Sato, K., et al., 2002. Epithelial differentiation and proliferative potential in spinal ependymomas. J. Neurooncol. 58, 13–19.

Taratuto, A.L., Monges, J., Lylyk, P., et al., 1984. Superficial cerebral astrocytoma attached to dura. Report of six cases in infants. Cancer 54, 2505–2512.

Taratuto, A.L., Pomata, H., Sevlever, G., et al., 1995. Dysembryoplastic neuroepithelial tumor: morphological, immunocytochemical, and deoxyribonucleic acid analyses in a pediatric series. Neurosurgery 36, 474–481.

Telfeian, A.E., Judkins, A., Younkin, D., et al., 2004. Crino Subependymal giant cell astrocytoma with cranial and spinal metastases in a patient with tuberous sclerosis. Case report. J. Neurosurg 100 (Suppl.), 498–500.

The Cancer Genome Atlas Research Network, 2008. Comprehensive genomic characterization defines human glioblastoma genes and core pathways. Nature 455, 1061–1068.

Theaker, J.M., Gatter, K.C., Esiri, M.M., et al., 1987. Epithelial membrane antigen and cytokeratin expression by meningiomas: an immunohistological study. J. Clin. Pathol. 39, 435–439.

Theunissen, P.H., Baerts, M.D.-T., Blaauw, G., 1990. Histogenesis of intracranial haemangiopericytoma and haemangioblastoma. An immunohistochemical study. Acta. Neuropathol. 80, 68–71.

Thiessen, B., Finlay, J., Kulkarni, R., et al., 1998. Astroblastoma: does histology predict biologic behavior? J. Neurooncol. 40, 59–65.

Thomas, G.A., Raffel, C., 1991. Loss of heterozygosity on 6q, 16q, and 17p in human central nervous system primitive neuroectodermal tumors. Cancer Res. 51, 639–643.

Tihan, T., Fisher, P.G., Kepner, J.L., et al., 1999. Pediatric astrocytomas with monomorphous pilomyxoid features and a less favorable outcome. J. Neuropathol. Exp. Neurol. 58, 1061–1068.

Tohma, Y., Gratas, C., Biernat, W., et al., 1998. PTEN (MMAC1) mutations are frequent in primary glioblastomas (de novo) but not in secondary glioblastomas. J. Neuropathol. Exp. Neurol. 57, 684–689.

Tohyama, T., Lee, V.M., Rorke, L.B., et al., 1992. Nestin expression in embryonic human neuroepithelium and in human neuroepithelial tumor cells. Lab. Invest. 66, 303–313.

Tomlinson, F.H., Scheithauer, B.W., Hayostek, C., et al., 1994. The significance of atypia and histologic malignancy in pilocytic astrocytoma of the cerebellum: a clinicopathologic and flow cytometric study. J. Child. Neurol. 9, 301–310.

Towfighi, J., Salam, M.M., McLendon, R.E., et al., 1996. Ganglion cell-containing tumors of the pituitary gland. Arch. Pathol. Lab. Med. 120, 369–377.

Townsend, J.J., Seaman, J.P., 1986. Central neurocytoma – a rare benign intraventricular tumor. Acta. Neuropathol. 71, 167–170.

Tramontin, A.D., Garcia-Verdugo, J.M., Lim, D.A., et al., 2003. Postnatal development of radial glia and the ventricular zone (VZ): a continuum of the neural stem cell compartment. Cereb. Cortex 3, 580–587.

Tsukayama, C., Arakawa, Y., 2002. A papillary glioneuronal tumor arising in an elderly woman: a case report. Brain Tumor. Pathol. 19, 35–39.

Tuli, S., Provias, J.P., Bernstein, M., 1997. Lhermitte-Duclos disease. Literature review and novel treatment strategy. Can. J. Neurol. Sci. 24, 155–160.

Ushigome, S., Machinami, R., Sorensen, P.H., 2002. Ewing sarcoma/primitive neuroectodermal tumor (PNET). In: Fletcher, C.D., Unni, K.K., Mertens, F. (Eds.), World Health Organization Classification of Tumors. Pathology and genetics of soft tissue and bone. IARC, Lyon, pp. 298–300.

Vajtai, I., Varga, Z., Aguzzi, A., 1996. MIB-1 immunoreactivity reveals different labelling in low-grade and in malignant epithelial neoplasms of the choroid plexus. Histopathology 29, 147–151.

Vajtai, I., Varga, Z.X., Scheithauer, B.W., et al., 1999. Chordoid glioma of the third ventricle: confirmatory report of a new entity. Hum. Pathol. 30, 723–726.

van den Bent, M.J., 2004. Advances in the biology and treatment of oligodendrogliomas. Curr. Opin. Neurol. 17, 675–680.

Van Meir, E.G., 1995. Cytokines and tumors of the central nervous system. Glia. 5, 264–288.

VandenBerg, S.R., May, E.E., Rubinstein, L.J., et al., 1987. Desmoplastic supratentorial neuroepithelial tumors of infancy with divergent differentiation potential ('desmoplastic infantile gangliogliomas'). Report on 11 cases of a distinctive embryonal tumor with favorable prognosis. J. Neurosurg 66, 58–71.

VandenBerg, S.R., 1992. Current diagnostic concepts of astrocytic tumors. J. Neuropathol. Exp. Neurol. 51, 644–657.

VandenBerg, S.R., 1993. Desmoplastic infantile ganglioglioma and desmoplastic cerebral astrocytoma of infancy. Brain Pathol. 3, 275–281.

VandenBerg, S.R., 1991. Desmoplastic infantile ganglioglioma: A clinicopathologic review of sixteen cases. Brain Tumor. Pathol. 8, 25–31.

Vaquero, J., Ramiro, J., Martinez, R., et al., 1992. Neurosurgical experience with tumors of the pineal region at Cinica Puerta de Hierro. Acta. Neurochir. 116, 23–32.

Vates, G.E., Chang, S., Lamborn, K.R., et al., 2003. Gliomatosis cerebri: a review of 22 cases. Neurosurgery 53, 261–271.

Vege, K.D., Giannini, C., Scheithauer, B.W., 2000. The immunophenotype of ependymomas. Appl. Immunohistochem Mol. Morphol. 8, 25–31.

von Deimling, A., Burger, P.C., Nakazato, Y., et al., 2007. Diffuse astrocytoma. In: Louis, D.N., Ohgaki, H., Wiestler, O.D., et al. (Eds.), WHO classification of tumours of the central nervous system. IARC, Lyon, pp. 25–29.

von Deimling, A., Eibl, R.H., Ohgaki, H., et al., 1992a. p53 mutations are associated with 17p allelic loss in grade II and grade III astrocytoma. Cancer Res. 52, 2987–2990.

von Deimling, A., Janzer, R., Kleihues, P., et al., 1990. Patterns of differentiation in central neurocytoma: an immunohistochemical study of eleven biopsies. Acta. Neuropathol. 79, 473–479.

von Deimling, A., Louis, D.N., Menon, A.G., 1993b. Deletions on the long arm of chromosome 17 in pilocytic astrocytoma. Acta. Neuropathol. 86, 81–85.

von Deimling, A., Perry, A., 2007. Neurofibromatosis type 1. In: Louis, D.N., Ohgaki, H., Wiestler, O.D., et al. (Eds.), WHO classification of tumours of the central nervous system. IARC, Lyon, pp. 206–209.

von Deimling, A., von Ammon, K., Schoenfeld, A., et al., 1993a. Subsets of glioblastoma multiforme defined by molecular genetic analysis. Brain Pathol. 3, 19–26.

von Haken, M.S., White, E.C., Daneshvar-Shyesther, L., et al., 1996. Molecular genetic analysis of chromosome arm 17p and chromosome arm 22q DNA sequences in sporadic pediatric ependymomas. Genes Chromosomes Cancer 17, 37–44.

Vraa-Jensen, G., 1950. Papilloma of the choroid plexus with pulmonary metastases. Acta. Psych. Neurol. 25, 299–306.

Vuorinen, V., Salinen, P., Haapasalo, H., et al., 1996. Outcome of 31 intracranial hemangiopericytomas. Poor predictive value of cell proliferation indices. Acta. Neurochir. 138, 1399–1408.

Waha, A., Koch, A., Hartmann, W., et al., 2004. Analysis of HIC-1 methylation and transcription in human ependymomas. Int. J. Cancer 110, 542–549.

Wakimoto, H., Aoyagi, M., Nakayama, T., et al., 1996. Prognostic significance of Ki-67 labeling indices obtained using MIB-1 monoclonal antibody in patients with supratentorial astrocytomas. Cancer 77, 373–380.

Wanebo, J.E., Malik, J.M., VandenBerg, S.R., et al., 1993. Malignant peripheral nerve sheath tumors. A clinicopathologic study of 28 cases. Cancer 71, 1247–1253.

Wang, M., Tihan, T., Rojiani, A.M., et al., 2005. Monomorphous angiocentric glioma: a distinctive epileptogenic neoplasm with features of infiltrating astrocytoma and ependymoma. J. Neuropathol. Exp. Neurol. 64, 875–881.

Watanabe, T., Nobusawa, S., Kleihues, P., Ohgaki, H., 2009. IDH1 mutations are early events in the development of astrocytomas and oligodendrogliomas. Am. J. Pathol. 174, 1149–1153.

Watanabe, K., Osamu, T., Yonekawa, Y., 1997. Role of gemistocytes in astrocytoma progression. Lab. Invest. 76, 277–284.

Watanabe, K., Tachibana, O., Sato, K., et al., 1996. Overexpression of the EGF Receptor and p53 mutations are mutually exclusive in the evolution of primary and secondary glioblastomas. Brain Pathol. 6, 217–224.

Weldon-Linne, G.M., Victor, T.A., Groothuis, D.R., et al., 1983. Pleomorphic xanthoastrocytoma: ultrastructural and immunohistochemical study of a case with a rapidly fatal outcome following surgery. Cancer 52, 2055–2063.

Wharton, S.B., Wardle, C., Ironside, J.W., et al., 2003. Comparative genomic hybridization and pathological findings in atypical teratoid/rhabdoid tumor of the central nervous system. Neuropathol. Appl. Neurobiol. 29, 254–261.

Whittle, I.R., Gordon, A., Misra, B.K., et al., 1989. Pleomorphic xanthoastrocytoma: report of four cases. J. Neurosurg 70, 463–468.

Winek, R.R., Scheithauer, B.W., Wick, M.R., 1989. Meningioma, meningeal hemangiopericytoma (angioblastic meningioma), peripheral hemangiopericytoma and acoustic schwannoma. A comparative immunohistochemical study. Am. J. Surg. Pathol. 13, 251–261.

Wondrusch, E., Huemer, M., Budka, H., 1991. Production of glial fibrillary acidic protein (GFAP) by neoplastic oligodendrocytes: gliofibrillary oligodendroglioma and transitional oligoastrocytoma revisited. Brain Tumor. Pathol. 8, 11–15.

Woodruff, J.M., Godwin, T.A., Erlandson, R.A., et al., 1981. Cellular schwannoma. A variety of schwannoma sometimes mistaken for a malignant tumor. Am. J. Surg. Pathol. 5, 733–744.

Yachnis, A.T., Trojanowski, J.Q., Memmo, M., et al., 1988. Expression of neurofilament proteins in the hypertrophic granule cells of Lhermitte–Duclos disease: An explanation for the mass effect and the myelination of parallel fibers in the disease state. J. Neuropathol. Exp. Neurol. 47, 206–216.

Yan, H., Parsons, D.W., Jin, G., et al., 2009. IDH1 and IDH2 mutations in gliomas. N. Engl. J. Med. 360, 765–773.

Yasargil, M.G., von Ammon, K., von Deimling, A., et al., 1992. Central neurocytoma: histopathological variants and therapeutic approaches. J. Neurosurg 76, 32–37.

Zagzag, D., Zhong, H., Scalzitti, J.M., et al., 2000. Expression of hypoxia-inducible factor 1 alpha in brain tumors: Association with angiogenesis, invasion, and progression. Cancer 88, 2606–2618.

Zhou, X.P., Li, Y.J., Hoang-Xuan, K., et al., 1999. Mutational analyses of PTEN gene in gliomas: molecular and pathological correlations. Int. J. Cancer 84, 150–154.

Zhou, X.P., Marsh, D.J., Morrison, C.D., et al., 2003. Germline inactivation of PTEN and dysregulation of the phosphoinositol-3-kinase/Akt pathway cause human Lhermitte-Duclos disease in adults. Am. J. Hum. Genet. 73, 1191–1198.

Zlatescu, M.C., TehraniYazdi, A., Sasaki, H., et al., 2001. Tumor location and growth pattern correlate with genetic signature in oligodendroglial neoplasms. Cancer Res. 61, 6713–6715.

Zorludemir, S., Scheithauer, B.W., Hirose, T., et al., 1995. Clear cell meningioma: a clinicopathologic study of a potentially aggressive variant of meningioma. Am. J. Surg. Pathol. 19, 493–505.

Zurawel, R.H., Allen, C., Chiappa, S., et al., 2000. Analysis of PTCH/SMO/SHH pathway genes in medulloblastoma. Genes Chromosomes Cancer 27, 44–51.

10 Advanced imaging of brain tumors

Ronil V. Chandra and James A. J. King

Introduction

Conventional imaging is the mainstay of brain tumor imaging. This includes preoperative diagnostic imaging, serial assessment in conservatively managed tumors, and assessment of therapeutic response. However, conventional CT and MR imaging techniques only yield information about anatomical location and macroscopic tumoral structure, without assessing tumoral physiology. Tumoral metabolic, cellular architectural, and ultrastructural information is increasingly available for clinical use with novel imaging techniques.

The techniques described in this chapter are now routine in many neurooncology centers, and can contribute to overall patient diagnostic, intraoperative, and postoperative clinical management. Appropriate and informed use can lead to better patient outcomes. Nonetheless, as with all new technology, advanced imaging techniques must always be interpreted in light of the patient's clinical history, examination findings and well established conventional imaging algorithms. Moreover, these physiological techniques, although becoming routine, still require further validation before they become indispensable.

Advanced imaging techniques

Diffusion-weighted imaging

Diffusion-weighted imaging (DWI) can obtain information about tissue microstructure without the use of exogenous contrast agents. Diffusion imaging varies from the simple generation of a DWI or ADC (*apparent diffusion coefficient*) map to diffusion tensor imaging and tractography.

When a molecule of water is agitated by energy, it is randomly displaced. This notion is referred to as molecular diffusion. DWI assesses alteration in the diffusibility of water molecules in tissue. An initial fast echoplanar T2* sequence is used, and then two equal magnetic field strength diffusion encoding gradient (Gdiff) pulses are applied to the brain in opposite directions. The first Gdiff pulse dephases the water molecules, and the second will rephase them. However, any motion from their initial location will result in a different field strength being applied by the second pulse.

If water molecules are free and able to move from their initial position, e.g., in CSF, the opposite gradient pulse cannot rephase the water molecules completely, and thus there is reduced signal intensity. If water molecules remain in the same position, there is complete rephasing and consequent higher signal intensity. The farther a water molecule moves, there will be a gradation of signal intensity loss.

Diffusion-weighted imaging (DWI) has great clinical application in stroke imaging. Cytotoxic cellular edema leads to cellular swelling and restriction of intracellular proton motion, and thus high signal on DWI. Similarly, highly cellular tissues also lead to similar reduced proton motion, and thus diffusion restriction and lower ADC (Cha 2006; Mechtler 2009).

However, one of the limitations of the DW image is that the diffusion information is superimposed on the initial T2* image. The practical consequence of this means that brain or tumoral tissues that have higher T2 signal than surrounding tissue are artifactually of higher signal intensity on the DW image. This phenomenon is called 'T2 shine-through'. Moreover, as the initial image is a T2* image, it is sensitive to magnetic susceptibility, thus calcification, blood products, metal, bone or air will cause artifacts on the DWI image (Cha 2009). Thus the diffusion imaging must be interpreted with conventional anatomical imaging (Cha 2009) to avoid spurious pathological findings.

T2 shine-through can be overcome with the use of an *apparent diffusion coefficient* (ADC) map. This time, an image is obtained without Gdiff – this is called the '*b0 image*' by convention, and a second image with Gdiff applied. The ADC map is then calculated by excluding the T2-weighting, with the resultant information representing true diffusion properties. ADC characterizes the rate of diffusional motion in millimeters squared per second (mm^2/s) (Cha 2009).

Thus, while brain or tumoral tissue may appear of higher signal on the DWI map, one must correlate with the ADC map to confirm that this represents true diffusion restriction, and not T2 shine-through. True diffusion restriction is reduced ADC and of reduced signal intensity on an ADC map. High ADC means unrestricted water motion (Cha 2009).

Diffusion tensor imaging

Water molecules in a glass of water will diffuse equally in all directions – this is termed '*isotropic diffusion*'. This approximates diffusion of CSF within the ventricles. However, the brain parenchyma is of complex structure, with multiple white matter tracts. The diffusion of water molecules within white matter tracts is anisotropic, i.e., not equal in three orthogonal directions. Standard DWI acquires information in three orthogonal planes, i.e., x, y, and z-axes, and results in information about the diffusivity of water molecules in an imaging voxel. However, to assess for 3D anisotropy, directional information is required.

The degree of anisotropy of the diffusion process is represented by *fractional anisotropy* (FA). The FA is a scalar value, between 0 and 1. If the FA = 1, diffusion occurs in one axis only, with restriction in all other directions.

Conversely, if FA = 0, diffusion is isotropic. The FA image pixel value represents a FA value number. Isotropic diffusion, with FA of 0, can also be mathematically represented in 3D as a sphere, while an FA of 1 is represented by an infinite cylinder. Anisotropic diffusion with a FA of between 0 and 1 approximates an ellipsoid, with a direction vector parallel to the direction of maximal diffusivity.

The FA information also has practical implication – in children, while the FA of white matter changes increases during the myelination process, anisotropy is still observed prior to myelination – this may relate to the geometric organization of fibers within a white matter tract (Le Bihan et al 2001). Overall, fiber packing density, degree of myelination, fiber diameter and associated neuroglial cellular packing density could all contribute to white matter FA (Pierpaoli et al 1996). Highly organized white matter tracts, particularly the corpus callosum and corticospinal tracts, have high FA values, gray matter has a low FA values (Pierpaoli et al 1996), and changes in FA in white matter corresponds to changes in microstructural integrity of myelinated tracts (Toh et al 2008a).

The mathematical representation of diffusion, the ellipsoid, can be further characterized by the principal axes: $\lambda_1\lambda_2\lambda_3$. Each of these values '$\lambda$' is called the *eigenvalue*, and their direction, the *eigenvector*. However, to describe this motion mathematically, for each imaging voxel, at least six diffusion measurements have to be obtained. Only then can the directional variation of a water molecule to diffuse in a voxel be measured. This is described in the form of a 3×3 matrix – *the diffusion tensor* – which is a mathematical construct of diffusion in 3D, and the technique is called '*diffusion tensor imaging*' (DTI).

From DTI, a trace-weighted image from the geometric sum of the eigenvectors shows overall diffusivity, i.e., comparable with standard DWI, and mean diffusivity, i.e., comparable with the ADC, can be calculated.

Now there is directional information about water diffusivity within a voxel. The principal direction of the ellipsoid is the principal eigenvector, and if one assumes that the greatest diffusivity occurs along a white matter tract and joins principal eigenvectors within adjacent voxels, a white matter tract map can be constructed. This is based on the observation that tissue structure, such as the myelin sheath of axons, reduces diffusivity perpendicular to the direction of the axon (Gupta et al 2005; Bae et al 2009; Le Bihan et al 2001).

By convention, different orientations have been given different color conventions: red for right/left; green for anterior/posterior; blue for superior/inferior. This preoperative identification of the anatomical white matter tracts linking primary motor and sensory areas has the potential to reduce surgical morbidity from resection (Mechtler 2009).

Note that, while at least six diffusion directions are required to calculate the tensor, the greater the number of directions assessed, the more reliable the tensor calculation. However, there is a trade-off between scan acquisition time and diffusion directions.

Functional MRI

Maintenance of postoperative quality of life is paramount in neurooncology surgery. If eloquent areas of the brain can be identified reliably preoperatively, this can help with appropriate patient preoperative selection; definition of surgical margins; selection of patients for awake craniotomy and cortical stimulation, and possibly better surgical outcome.

The majority of fMRI is based on *blood oxygen level dependant* (BOLD) imaging. When the brain is activated by task, there is conversion of oxyhemoglobin to deoxyhemoglobin and utilization of glucose. There is an increase in local blood flow to supply further glucose and oxyhemoglobin, and removal of deoxyhemoglobin. Deoxyhemoglobin is paramagnetic, unlike oxyhemoglobin, and changes in their relative concentrations are detectable by T2* imaging methods.

While this change in signal intensity is only in the magnitude of a few percent, detection is reproducible, and can reasonably reliably detect primary motor and sensory areas. fMRI paradigms typically utilized include finger or foot tapping, as well as lip puckering to identify different components of the motor strip, or silent word-generation or language-comprehension paradigms for speech areas. This information can then be fused onto a volumetric T1 or T2 weighted image that highlights the tumor, to allow delineation of tumoral involvement.

The non-invasive nature compared with cortical stimulation with awake craniotomy, with high anatomical resolution, makes this a useful investigation in tumors that may involve the primary motor or sensory areas.

MR spectroscopy

MR spectroscopy (MRS) attempts to identify and quantify molecular content within an imaging voxel. However, one must remember than the molecular content being assessed is 10 000 times lower in concentration compared with water molecules in the brain, and that current techniques have low spatial resolution. Thus MRS must be interpreted in light of the clinical and conventional imaging findings.

The magnetic field experienced by a proton when placed in an external magnetic field is reduced by shielding from the electron cloud around the proton. Protons in different molecules thus experience slightly different magnetic fields when placed in the same external magnetic field. However, these differences are tiny relative to the overall strength of the magnet. Thus, instead of measuring absolute resonance frequency of molecules, they are compared to a standard, and quoted as parts per million. The reference molecule is tetramethylsilane, which is arbitrarily defined as 0 ppm.

Tissue localization can be via single voxel or via chemical shift techniques. Single voxel MRS is quicker but interrogates only a small region of the brain. *Chemical shift imaging* however, offers larger coverage, and multiple imaging voxels can be analyzed simultaneously, however it takes a longer time and requires more complex data processing. MRS can be performed at multiple echo times (TE). The shorter TE MRS (typically 35 ms) allows greater detection of metabolites, while the longer TE (up to 270 ms) facilitates greater suppression of macromolecules, and thus only certain metabolites remain evident.

Typical metabolites assessed include lipids (0.9–1.4 ppm), which correlate with cell membrane breakdown; lactate (1.33 ppm), a marker of anaerobic metabolism; N acetyl aspartate (NAA 2.02 ppm), a marker of neuronal density and viability; creatine (3.03), a marker of aerobic metabolism; choline (3.22 ppm), a marker of cell turnover, and myo-inositol (3.56 ppm), a cyclic sugar located in astrocytic cells (Smith et al 2003; Cha 2009; Mullins 2006).

The much greater concentration of water in a voxel means water must be suppressed, and inadequate water suppression leads to a sloping baseline that causes artificial elevation of peaks. Moreover, the magnetic field must be homogenous and adequate shimming is essential to ensure accurate traces.

Note that one imaging voxel is derived of many cells, and the MR spectrum is a summary of the cellular population response. Thus in one voxel, there will be tumor cells, normal brain cells and the response of brain cells to the neoplasm. This makes it important to place a MRS voxel on a location where there is tumor only, to sample mainly tumor cells. Thus if only 25% of the voxel are tumor cells, the choline and NAA levels may not be reflective of the underlying pathology. Moreover, if MRS is used to target sites for stereotactic biopsy, it is important to note that the minimum voxel size for MRS is 1 cm^3 compared with biopsy samples that may be <1 mm^3 (Cha 2009).

Perfusion-weighted imaging

Perfusion attempts to characterize the state of the cerebral and tumoral microvasculature. Tumors can induce angiogenesis, these pathological vessels are histologically disorganized, tortuous and more permeable than normal (Hashizume et al 2000; Aronen & Perkiö 2002; Jain et al 2002). These changes lead to altered local hemodynamics, imaged with perfusion imaging. This form of imaging can thus also be an indirect physiological measure of metabolic activity. There are various PWI methods, including with CT and MR, with the three most widely used MR methods including *dynamic susceptibility contrast* (DSC), *dynamic contrast enhancement* (DCE) and *arterial spin labeling*.

DSC MRI maps are acquired by injection of a bolus of magnetic contrast agent with repeated rapid echo planar T2* imaging. As the gadolinium-based compound passes through the cerebral vasculature, it causes a decrease in T2* signal intensity within the imaging voxel. The proportion of signal reduction is proportional to the concentration of the contrast media in that voxel and the underlying tissue vascularity.

Various perfusion maps can be calculated from the time vs signal intensity curve, with the *cerebral blood volume* (CBV) maps being the most widely used and most reliable in representing tumor angiogenesis and microvascular density (Barajas et al 2009; Cha 2009; Mechtler 2009). CBV is defined as the 'total volume of blood traversing a unit volume of brain in unit time', generally measured in mL/100 g/min. Note that these maps do not give absolute measurement, but rather measurements relative to that of a standard tissue, typically normal white matter (Knopp et al 1999). Thus, they denote 'relative CBV' (rCBV); the rCBV of gray matter is normally higher than white matter (Covarrubias et al 2004).

rCBV values correlate well with angiographic vascularity as well as histological measures for angiogenesis – microvascular density and vascular endothelial growth factor expression (Sadeghi et al 2008; Sugahara et al 1998; Maia et al 2005).

In interpreting DSC perfusion maps, one must consider that it is particularly sensitive to susceptibility artifact from blood product, calcium, melanin, metal or location close to a bone-air interface such as the skull base (Lacerda & Law 2009).

DCE is another type of MR perfusion imaging method that relies on repeated imaging with a T1 sequence and can provide information about endothelial permeability (Cha 2009). The advantage of greater spatial resolution and resistance to susceptibility artifact using T1-imaging is attractive, however currently DSC methods are more common and better validated (Lacerda & Law 2009; Mechtler 2009).

Newer methods of MR perfusion with arterial spin labeling are completely non-invasive, and do not require MR contrast media. Radiofrequency pulses in the arteries feeding a region of brain induce alterations in proton spin in that feeding artery. This in turn induces signal change when these protons enter the tissue of interest. These small signal changes are measurable, however, compared with DSC images the changes induced are smaller, and thus lower spatial image resolution results.

Nuclear medicine

Thallium SPECT

Thallium-201 chloride is a potassium analogue with little brain parenchymal uptake in normal subjects because of the intact blood–brain barrier. However, Thallium-201 does localize in some primary and metastatic tumors. Disruption of the blood–brain barrier itself does not necessarily cause uptake, as resolving hematomas and radiation necrosis do not have significant uptake. Thus, the mechanism is likely a combination of local blood flow dynamics, breakdown of the blood–brain barrier and direct cellular transport (Sasaki et al 1998).

Nonetheless, the uptake in tumors relative to other pathologies has led to its use in glioma staging and postoperative follow-up imaging.

PET

The high rate of 18F-FDG uptake in normal brain limits the detectability of brain tumors, unless there is a marked increase in glucose metabolism (Chen 2007; Chen et al 2006). This is because of active transport across the blood–brain barrier and high physiological uptake by normal brain tissue, particularly the cortex and gray matter, with less uptake in normal white matter (Wong et al 2002). Nonetheless, 18F-FDG uptake is particularly avid in high-grade astrocytic tumors because of up-regulation of glucose transport and increased glucose utilization (Wong et al 2002; Spence et al 2003; Chen 2007). However, FDG uptake is not specific for neoplasm, and can also occur in non-neoplastic processes such as an abscess (Floeth et al 2006). If there is increased uptake in a previously diagnosed low-grade glioma, malignant transformation is likely (De Witte et al 1996; Chen 2007). Moreover, it can be helpful in distinguishing recurrent tumor from radiation necrosis (Langleben & Segall 2000; Chen 2007; Spence et al 2003).

However, false positive diagnoses can occur with clinical or sub-clinical seizures that produce hyper-metabolic activity (Wong et al 2002). Other imaging tracers, such as

11C-methionine, are also promising – there is low uptake in normal brain tissue, and 1.2–3.5 times higher uptake in brain tumors, resulting in higher tumor-to-normal tissue contrast (Spence et al 2003; Chen et al 2006; Chen 2007; Wong et al 2002). 18F DOPA PET also offers greater contrast resolution, with lower normal brain uptake compared with 18F-FDG PET, and has been reported as more sensitive and specific than PET for evaluating low-grade and recurrent tumors (Chen et al 2006; Chen 2007).

Advanced imaging in preoperative diagnosis

When one is confronted with a symptomatic patient with a brain parenchymal abnormality, the fundamental concepts of rapidity of symptom onset, symptom duration and progression are critical. Typically, infarction or intracranial hemorrhages have an abrupt onset without progressive symptoms, and brain tumors a relatively gradual onset with progressive symptoms. A history of remote malignancy always makes intracranial metastasis a consideration.

There are well-established conventional CT and MRI imaging concepts upon which advanced imaging techniques can provide supplementary information that can be confirmatory, or help characterize the abnormality further. Cerebral infarction, cerebral abscess or tumefactive demyelination can mimic brain tumors, and diagnostic biopsy would be best avoided.

Distinguishing tumor and non-tumor pathology

Distinguishing infarct and tumor

The clinical history is invaluable in distinguishing these pathologies, and imaging is often confirmatory. Conventional imaging relies on involvement of typical vascular territories or demonstration of vascular occlusion or normal imaging evolution with ischemia. However, the addition of diffusion imaging is usually confirmatory for arterial ischemia. Acute ischemia results in anoxic cell depolarization, failure of the Na/K pumps, passive influx of water and cytotoxic edema (Le Bihan et al 2001). This results in marked diffusion restriction within minutes in the territory affected (Schaefer et al 2000; Stadnik et al 2003). This manifests as high signal on DWI, which must correspond with reduced ADC to exclude T2 shine through. This occurs within minutes; reduced ADC generally persists for at least 7–14 days, but elevated DWI signal can persist for between 72–144 days (Geijer et al 2001; Lansberg et al 2001; Stadnik et al 2003). While venous infarcts may not have diffusion restriction (Stadnik et al 2003), they are often at typical locations, may be hemorrhagic, and generally are accompanied by venous occlusion.

Tumors can also have diffusion restriction. The diffusivity of water is correlated with tumor cellularity, and highly cellular tumors have reduced ADC (Kono et al 2001; Toh et al 2008b; Mechtler 2009; Sadeghi et al 2008). This is particularly evident in lymphoma, where there can be homogenous mild diffusion restriction, as well as in higher-grade gliomas where diffusion restriction is typically focal and patchy, reflecting a heterogeneous tumoral bed composed of focal high-grade tumor, focal hemorrhage and necrosis.

Perfusion imaging is also helpful, in particular CBV maps. Completed infarcts have low CBV corresponding with the conventional imaging abnormality.

In tumors, MRI rCBV measurements correlate with angiographic assessments of tumor vascular density and the histological extent of tumoral angiogenesis (Cha 2009; Sadeghi et al 2008). However, note that increased tumor microvascularity, while typically seen in higher-grade tumors, can also be seen in benign intracranial neoplasms, in particular meningioma or choroid plexus papillomas (Cha 2009). Nonetheless, progressively higher-grade astrocytic tumors have higher rCBV values both in the mass (Sadeghi et al 2008; Cha 2009), and in the peri-tumoral tissues. Low-grade astrocytomas have little or no elevation of rCBV compared with contralateral normal white matter, while anaplastic astrocytomas have higher rCBV, but lower than glioblastomas (Cha 2009). This progressive increase parallels the microvascular density and vascular endothelial proliferation seen in higher-grade astrocytic tumors (Sugahara et al 1998; Cha 2009).

A neoplastic MRS profile is reduction in NAA from neuronal loss, elevation in Cho from increased cellular turnover, an attenuated Cr peak from reduction in aerobic metabolism, and in some cases of higher-grade gliomas, elevated lactate from anaerobic metabolism or lipids from cellular necrosis and release of free lipids (Cianfoni et al 2007; Cha 2009).

Distinguishing infarct and tumor on MRS is difficult, and relies mainly on marked elevation of lipids and lactate, with minimal elevation of choline, in infarcts compared to tumors, that in turn, generally have greater levels of choline elevation; NAA will be decreased in both pathologies (Fig. 10.1).

Distinguishing abscess and tumor

Clinical and conventional imaging parameters must be used to try to distinguish abscess and tumor. The diagnosis is best established as soon as possible, to facilitate appropriate management, frequently urgent surgical drainage. The conventional MRI appearance of a brain abscess varies according to the histopathological stage, with focal edema and possible patchy enhancement in the early cerebritis phase, progression in edema with new irregular or ill-defined capsular enhancement of a well-defined capsule, often with low T2 capsular signal, and thin uniform enhancement (Desprechins et al 1999; Stadnik et al 2003; Gupta et al 2005).

Conventional MRI features favoring an abscess over tumor in a ring enhancing mass include a pencil thin smooth enhancing rim, which may be thinner on the ventricular side and the presence of adjacent daughter masses (Holmes et al 2004; Luthra et al 2007). However, occasionally tumors can appear almost identical on conventional T1/T2 and post-contrast T1 MRI.

Diffusion imaging is often useful, with marked central diffusion restriction typical within a pyogenic abscess (Bükte et al 2005; Gaviani et al 2005; Gupta et al 2005; Schwartz et al 2006; Cha 2009; Mechtler 2009; Desprechins et al 1999; Lai et al 2002). It is thought the high cellularity, low viscosity and presence of macromolecules within pus are responsible for the restricted diffusion (Bükte et al 2005; Luthra et al

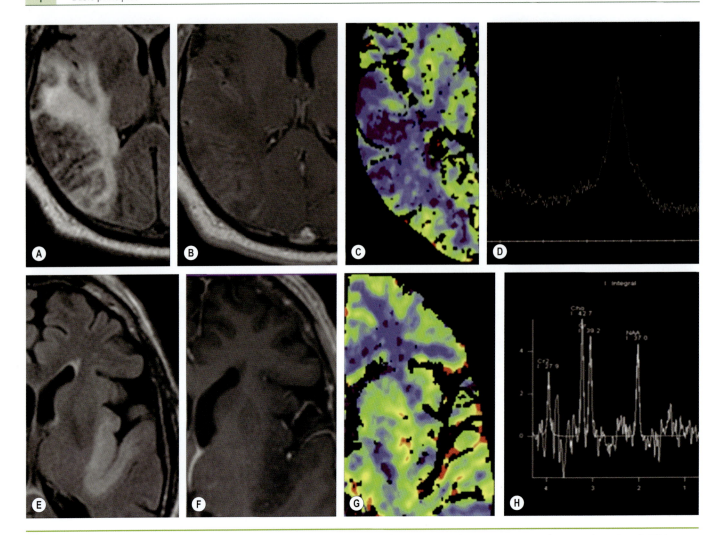

Figure 10.1 Top row: an infarct with mixed FLAIR intensity (A) and faint contrast enhancement (B) that mimics a tumor, however the reduced rCBV (C) and marked lactate peak on MRS (D) help confirm infarction. Bottom row: posterior insular and temporal opercular FLAIR hyperintensity (E) with no contrast enhancement (F) mimicking an infarct. However, no reduction in rCBV (G) and the MRS (H) with mild NAA reduction, elevation of Cho and no significant lactate elevation favor tumor. Biopsy confirmed diffuse astrocytoma (WHO grade II).

2007; Karaarslan & Arslan 2008; Malhotra et al 2009; Desprechins et al 1999; Cha 2009; Gaviani et al 2005). Tumoral cysts or necrotic cores with complex fluid tend not to have reduced diffusivity, with signal closer to CSF signal (Bükte et al 2005; Schwartz et al 2006).

Fungal or tubercular abscesses may occur in specific patient populations, particularly immunocompromised patients, and have features on the conventional imaging that may be helpful – fungal abscesses tend to have non-enhancing intra-cavity extensions or a crenated wall (Luthra et al 2007). Fungal or tubercular abscesses also may have wall and content diffusion restriction, but a fungal abscess core may have elevated ADC (Gaviani et al 2005; Luthra et al 2007).

Perfusion imaging can also be helpful – pyogenic abscesses usually have reduced rCBV while higher-grade gliomas and metastases will have areas of elevated rCBV (Holmes et al 2004; Hakyemez et al 2006a).

MRS can identify certain metabolites that favor an abscess and can help in determining etiology. Pyogenic abscesses tend to have amino acid peaks, with aerobic organisms typically having acetate and succinate peaks; tuberculous abscesses tend to have lipid and lactate peaks without amino acids, and fungal abscesses tend to have trehalose peaks (Luthra et al 2007) (Fig. 10.2).

Distinguishing tumefactive demyelination and tumor

The tumefactive demyelinating lesion (TDL) commonly mimics a brain tumor. There may be clinical, serological or CSF parameters that suggest demyelination, or other typical MRI white matter lesions. However, in their absence, it can be difficult to make a confident diagnosis in the absence of biopsy.

Even with histopathological evaluation, the presence of hypercellular, atypical reactive astrocytes and mitotic figures can also mimic higher-grade tumors and can lead to unnecessary and potentially harmful surgical resection or radiation treatment (Mujic et al 2002; Lucchinetti et al 2008;

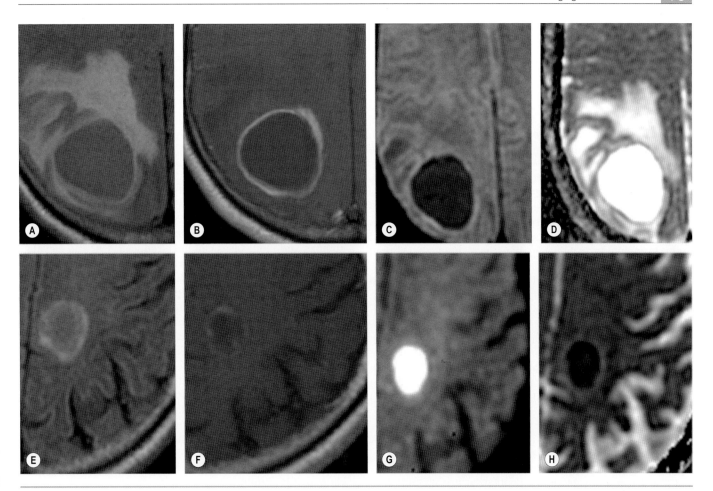

Figure 10.2 Top row: ring enhancing glioblastoma (WHO Grade IV) (A) FLAIR and (B) post-contrast T1 with low central DWI signal (C) and high central ADC signal (D), i.e., no diffusion restriction. Bottom row: ring enhancing abscess (E) FLAIR and (F) post-contrast T1 with central elevated DWI signal (G) and low central ADC signal (H) compatible with diffusion restriction.

Hunter et al 1987; Zagzag et al 1993; Cha et al 2001; Malhotra et al 2009; Tan et al 2004).

Conventional imaging features that favor tumefactive demyelination include a large lesion with little mass effect or edema, ring or arc like enhancement, with the enhancing portion of the ring believed to represent the leading edge and thus typically located on the white matter side (Enzinger et al 2005; Nesbit et al 1991; Given et al 2004; Schwartz et al 2006; Kim et al 2009; Malhotra et al 2009; Tan et al 2004). In addition, one may discern vascular structures passing through the mass in a TDL (Given et al 2004; Cha et al 2001; Malhotra et al 2009; Kim et al 2009) and the cortex is less likely to be involved by a TDL (Kim et al 2009). Furthermore, if the enhancing region on MRI is hypoattenuating to gray matter on unenhanced CT, a TDL is favored (Kim et al 2009).

However, one of the main histopathological differences with a TDL and a high-grade tumor is the lack of neovascularization and angiogenesis within the TDL, which conversely is typical of a high-grade tumor. Thus rCBV values of TDLs are significantly lower than intracranial lymphomas, high grade primary tumors and metastases (Al-Okaili et al 2007; Cha et al 2001; Cha 2006).

Diffusion imaging is typically not helpful in distinguishing tumor and TDL (Kim et al 2009). MRS is typically similar in TDLs and high-grade gliomas – NAA is reduced, choline elevated and mean Cho/Cr ratios are not significantly different (Saindane et al 2002; Malhotra et al 2009). Within TDLs, neuronal loss explains the reduction in NAA, the Cho elevation is thought to result from reactive astrogliosis, demyelination and inflammation (Cianfoni et al 2007). The presence of lactate is variable, and is generally found in plaques with high inflammatory activity (Bitsch et al 1999; Cianfoni et al 2007). MyoI can also be elevated (Bitsch et al 1999).

It has been suggested that there are elevated peaks of glutamine and glutamate, astrocytic neurotransmitters, in TDLs (Cianfoni et al 2007; Malhotra et al 2009). However, elevated glutamine has also been reported in the contralateral normal appearing white matter of glioblastomas, which may relate to neoplastic infiltration (Kallenberg et al 2009) and thus glutamine and glutamate levels may not be distinguishing (Kalis et al 2007).

If there is serial imaging after treatment with corticosteroids, most TDLs show an excellent response and may disappear completely (Given et al 2004; Malhotra et al 2009).

Thus a potential clinical strategy is to proceed with a trial of methylprednisolone and reserve stereotactic biopsy for lesions that are progressive (Malhotra et al 2009).

Distinguishing an arachnoid cyst and epidermoid

Distinguishing an arachnoid cyst from an epidermoid and surrounding normal CSF is important as epidermoids are often resected, with complete resection being the aim. Both appear as CSF attenuating masses on CT scan, and can be difficult to confidently diagnose with conventional imaging. Typically on conventional MRI, they both follow CSF signal, with no enhancement. Often, one can discern subtle alterations in T2 signal in epidermoids compared with the arachnoid cyst, which is a reflection of the pearly macroscopic nature of the epidermoid. Moreover, the epidermoid tends to insinuate in between structures, unlike arachnoid cysts.

However, diffusion imaging is diagnostic, with marked hyperintensity on DWI in the epidermoid (Chen et al 2001; Cha 2009), and reduced ADC compared with normal CSF and similar ADC to brain parenchyma (Schaefer et al 2000; Stadnik et al 2003; Cruz & Sorensen 2006; Chen et al 2001). This may result from the keratinous viscous debris of the epidermoid (Holodny & Ollenschlager 2002; Cha 2009; Mechtler 2009). The appearance of an arachnoid cyst on DWI remains similar to CSF (Holodny & Ollenschlager 2002) (Fig. 10.3).

Histological prediction

Distinguishing metastasis from primary tumor

The most common malignant neoplasms are gliomas and metastases. Although multiplicity favors metastases, multifocal gliomas are not uncommon. Multifocal gliomas are those with gross or microscopic continuity or of CSF dissemination, while multi-centric gliomas do not have any macroscopic or microscopic connection, with no possibility of CSF dissemination (Barnard & Geddes 1987). In a post-mortem autopsy study of 241 patients, 40 patients (16.6%) were found to have multiple tumor foci, in whom 23 (9.5%) were defined as multi-centric. Once those with phakomatosis and demyelination were excluded, 18 patients (7.5%) with multi-centric tumor remained – of these, seven patients (2.9%) had differing histology (Barnard & Geddes 1987).

Nonetheless, the distinction between glioma and metastasis can often be suggested on the clinical history or the detection of extracranial disease. However, there are individuals in whom distinguishing between primary tumor and metastasis can still be difficult, particularly for solitary masses.

In general, as metastases will enhance, the difficulty lies in distinguishing a metastases from a higher-grade primary tumor. Other conventional imaging features favoring metastasis include peripheral location, typically at the gray–white interface and marked edema associated with small tumor burden (Tang et al 2006; Stuckey & Wijedeera 2008). Conventional imaging features favoring a primary glioma include abnormal non-enhancing increased FLAIR cortical signal (Tang et al 2006), marked cortical expansion and extension of nodular abnormal signal across the corpus callosum.

Advanced imaging may be helpful, with patchy diffusion restriction typical of higher-grade gliomas, while enhancing components of most metastases do not have diffusion restriction, and have elevated ADC (Al-Okaili et al 2006; Duygulu et al 2010). Diffusion restriction in metastasis may be seen with particularly hypercellular or mucinous metastasis (Hayashida et al 2006; Karaarslan & Arslan 2008; Stadnik et al 2003). In the necrotic core of a metastasis, elevated ADC is most common, however diffusion restriction has also been reported, particularly in necrotic squamous cell carcinoma and adenocarcinoma metastasis (Stadnik et al 2003; Hartmann et al 2001). In hemorrhagic metastasis, the presence of hemorrhage causes artifact on the diffusion-weighted imaging, thus it is less useful.

While the enhancing components of both higher-grade gliomas and metastases can have reduced ADC and elevated rCBV (Al-Okaili et al 2007), peri-tumoral assessment may be helpful – if there is reduced ADC in peri-tumoral abnormal white matter, an infiltrating glioma is more likely (Chiang et al 2004; Mechtler 2009). Similarly, elevated peri-tumoral choline and CBV are more likely to be seen in high-grade astrocytic tumors compared with metastases (Chiang et al 2004; Cha 2003; Hakyemez et al 2006a; Cha 2009; Mechtler 2009). The reason for these observations is that with metastases, the area of hyperintensity on the T2-weighted images is purely vasogenic edema caused by increased interstitial water content from leaky capillary membranes. However, in high-grade gliomas, the abnormal T2 signal contains a combination of vasogenic edema and infiltrating tumor cells (Cha 2009). Moreover, tumor cells can also be found beyond the outer margins of the T2 signal abnormality in high-grade gliomas (Cha 2009).

Distinguishing lymphoma from primary tumor

Primary CNS lymphomas (PCNL) are mainly high-grade non-Hodgkin's B cell lymphomas (Mechtler 2009). Treatment strategies are vastly different with lymphoma and primary tumors, with chemotherapy the primary treatment modality after biopsy in lymphoma, between surgical resection usual in high-grade primary gliomas (DeAngelis 2001; Horger et al 2009). A history of systemic lymphoma or immune compromise is useful – both congenital and acquired immune compromise increase the incidence of PCNL, particularly the human immunodeficiency virus (Corn et al 1997; DeAngelis 2001). However, PCNL occurring in immunocompromised individuals often has conventional MRI imaging features that mimic a glioblastoma (DeAngelis 2001).

The finding of hyper-attenuation on conventional unenhanced CT in lymphoma compared with astrocytoma may be useful. Moreover on conventional MRI, lymphomas tend to have a peri-ventricular tendency, homogenous isointensity to hypointensity on T1 with most hypointense on T2, with homogenous marked contrast enhancement (Horger et al 2009). Higher-grade gliomas are typically more heterogeneous in their pre- and post-contrast signal intensity, and often with hyperintensity on T2 (Horger et al 2009). Both may involve the corpus callosum (Horger et al 2009).

Overall, lymphomas exhibit lower ADC than both glioblastomas (Guo et al 2002; Cha 2006; Horger et al 2009; Toh

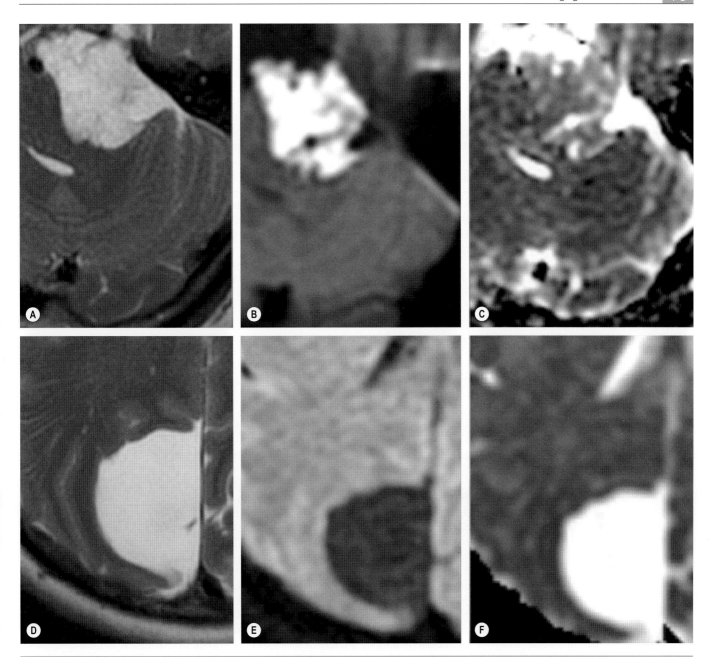

Figure 10.3 Top row: left cerebellopontine angle epidermoid with elevated T2 signal (A), elevated DWI signal (B) and with ADC signal (C) similar to brain parenchyma. Bottom row: arachnoid cyst appears similar in T2 signal intensity (D), but has low DWI signal (E), and ADC signal similar to CSF(F).

et al 2008b) and metastases (Yamasaki et al 2005). Homogenous mild diffusion restriction with ADC reduction is typical of lymphoma (Mechtler 2009), compared with the patchy focal diffusion restriction in higher-grade astrocytomas. While there remains controversy about the relationship between FA and cellularity, lymphomas also have reduced FA compared with glioblastomas (Toh et al 2008b). rCBV may not be helpful, as both have elevated rCBV, but to a higher extent with GBM (Mechtler 2009; Hakyemez et al 2006a). MRS is also similar to astrocytomas (Al-Okaili et al 2006; Smith et al 2003).

Distinguishing pediatric cerebellar tumors

The most common cerebellar tumors in children are *juvenile pilocytic astrocytomas, ependymomas, medulloblastomas,* and *hemangioblastomas*. While they may be distinguishable on the basis of conventional MRI findings, imaging appearances can overlap. Diffusion imaging is useful with lower ADC values reported in medulloblastoma compared with a juvenile pilocytic astrocytoma (Yamasaki et al 2005; Rumboldt et al 2006), with intermediate ADC values for an ependymoma (Rumboldt et al 2006). This probably relates to the densely packed cells and large nuclei seen in medulloblastoma, and thus not surprisingly, the few cases of ADC measurement in atypical teratoid rhabdoid tumor are similar to medulloblastoma (Rumboldt et al 2006). Thus, low ADC values in a pediatric cerebellar tumor should prompt consideration of medulloblastoma or ATRT and thus further spine imaging may be warranted.

MRS may also be helpful, NAA:Cho ratios are lower in cerebellar primitive neuroectodermal tumors compared with astrocytomas and ependymomas (Wang et al 1995).

Distinguishing meningioma from dural metastasis or hemangiopericytoma

Meningiomas account for approximately 20% of all intracranial tumors in hospital-based tumor series (Bondy & Ligon 1996), and for the vast majority of intracranial extra-axial masses. In autopsy series, dural metastases occur in 9% of patients with advanced systemic cancer, most commonly prostate, breast and lung (Laigle-Donadey et al 2005; Nayak et al 2009). In a review of 122 patients with dural metastatic tumor, in 61% involvement was from extension of a skull metastasis, while hematogenous spread accounted for 33%; 56% had a single dural metastasis (Nayak et al 2009). While the majority of cases occurred in those with known systemic malignancy, 11% presented at time of initial cancer diagnosis (Nayak et al 2009). Hemangiopericytomas are also uncommon tumors, accounting for 2–4% of dural tumors, and <1% of intracranial tumors (Akiyama et al 2004). They are more aggressive than meningiomas, with a high rate of local recurrence and propensity for metastases (Mena et al 1991; Akiyama et al 2004).

While preoperatively distinguishing among these pathologies would be useful, the conventional imaging appearances can be identical (Wu et al 2009b; Barba et al 2001; Laigle-Donadey et al 2005). A dural tail, i.e., enhancing thickened dura resembling a tail extending from a mass, has been previously reported as a highly specific sign for meningioma, however, further studies have shown that dural tails can occur with many pathologies, including metastases and hemangiopericytoma (Guermazi et al 2005; Wallace 2004). Hemangiopericytomas have been reported to have: a multi-lobular appearance; narrow base of attachment; irregular margins; strong heterogeneous contrast enhancement; lacking hyperostosis or calcification, and prominent corkscrew arterial feeders (Chiechi et al 1996; Akiyama et al 2004). However, all these features can occur with meningioma, and a dural metastasis could have some similar imaging features. Thus, no conventional imaging sign has been found to be reliable in distinguishing these entities. In one series of 26 patients, 96% of hemangiopericytomas were incorrectly diagnosed preoperatively as meningiomas (Wu et al 2009b).

Advanced imaging is also currently unable to confidently separate these tumors. MRS in meningioma typically reveals absent NAA, markedly elevated choline, and an alanine amino acid peak at 1.45 ppm (Bendszus et al 2001). A spectroscopic study including three patients with hemangiopericytoma found elevated MyoI levels compared with meningioma; both had elevated levels of Ala (Barba et al 2001). It has been suggested that prominent lipid signal on MRS favors a dural metastasis (Bendszus et al 2001), however, this may relate to the relatively large metastasis

examined in that study, as larger studies with smaller metastases have not shown elevated levels of lipid (Sijens & Oudkerk 2002). There has been an attempt at the use of rCBV measurements to distinguish meningioma from dural metastases, however, DSC rCBV methodology is based on an intravascular indicator dilution theory, which assumes the contrast remains intravascular (Wintermark et al 2005). As there is no true blood–brain barrier in meningiomas, uncorrected rCBV measurements are probably artifactually elevated (Zhang et al 2008; Yang et al 2003). In fact, rising intensity above the baseline on the time vs signal intensity T2* MR perfusion curve has been reported for both meningioma and hemangiopericytoma, presumably from contrast exiting the intravascular space, and accumulating in the interstitial compartment (Lim et al 2003).

Prediction of astrocytic tumor grade

Astrocytic tumors are graded according to the World Health Organization (WHO) criteria into categories with increasing biological aggressiveness. With increasing grade, there is increased cellularity, mitotic activity, nuclear polymorphism and vascular epithelial proliferation. The presence of necrosis, characteristically with pseudo-palisading cells, defines a glioblastoma. Glioblastoma accounts for 80% of malignant gliomas (Radhakrishnan et al 1995).

However, for an individual tumor, this can be difficult, as this represents a continuum from well- to poorly-differentiated, and grading is based on the most malignant cell population present.

In general, the presence of contrast enhancement correlates with increasing astrocytic tumor grade, with greater areas of BBB disruption (Cha 2009). However, the circumscribed astrocytomas are an exception to this rule, with contrast enhancement common with pilocytic astrocytoma, pleomorphic xanthoastrocytomas and subependymal giant cell tumors. In addition, meningiomas vividly and homogenously enhance, and thus contrast enhancement does not necessarily correlate with malignant tumor behavior (Cha 2009).

On conventional imaging, the WHO grade II diffuse astrocytomas typically have distinct low T1 and high T2 signal without hemorrhage or contrast enhancement (DeAngelis 2001). The presence of tumoral hemorrhage or contrast enhancement is suggestive of an anaplastic astrocytoma or glioblastoma, however, lower-grade astrocytomas can show contrast enhancement and higher-grade gliomas can have absent or minimal contrast enhancement (Ginsberg et al 1998; Law et al 2003; Knopp et al 1999; Scott et al 2002; Yang et al 2002). Necrosis is the hallmark of a glioblastoma.

The diffusion imaging appearances may be different along the spectrum – some studies report that in general, the higher the astrocytic tumor grade, the lower the mean and minimum ADC (Lee et al 2008; Cha 2006; Kono et al 2001; Yamasaki et al 2005; Yang et al 2002; Cruz & Sorensen 2006). Thus, glioblastomas tend to have lower ADC values than AA, which in turn tend to have lower ADC values than diffuse astrocytomas. However, there is overlap between groups and this should not be used solely to differentiate grades in an individual patient (Stadnik et al 2003; Provenzale et al 2006; Al-Okaili et al 2006) (Fig. 10.4).

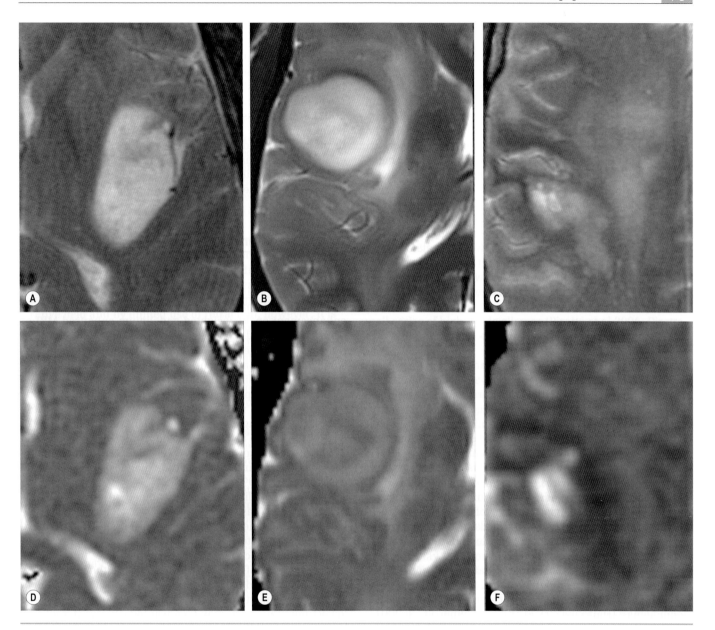

Figure 10.4 T2-weighted images in the top row (A–C), with corresponding ADC maps in the bottom row (D–F). From diffuse astrocytoma (WHO grade II) (A) to anaplastic astrocytoma (WHO grade III) (B) to glioblastoma (WHO grade IV) (C), there is a trend to reduction in ADC values. All cases were operatively confirmed.

The nature of diffusion restriction in high-grade gliomas reflects the histopathological nature – a heterogeneous tumor with mixed areas of viable tumor, necrosis and hemorrhage (Holodny & Ollenschlager 2002). Thus, patchy focal areas of tumoral reduced ADC are typical (Holodny & Ollenschlager 2002). Moreover, as the adjacent abnormal white matter often contains a mixture of infiltrating tumor and vasogenic edema, focal areas of reduced ADC in the peri-tumoral tissues may be found (Lu et al 2003).

While contrast enhancement does depict areas of blood–brain barrier breakdown, it does not provide an assessment of tumoral microvascularity (Lee et al 2008). T1 contrast enhancement represents an alteration in the blood brain barrier that may result from formation of pathological vascular channels or destruction of the normal capillary structure. However, increased cerebral blood volume reflects microvascularity with or without alteration of the blood brain barrier (Knopp et al 1999).

Thus typically, low-grade astrocytic tumors have significantly lower average and maximum rCBV relative to AA or GBM (Aronen & Perkiö 2002; Yang et al 2002; Hakyemez et al 2006a; Jain et al 2008; Mechtler 2009; Law et al 2003; Law et al 2004; Lacerda & Law 2009). The higher rCBV in high-grade primary tumors is thought to relate to increased angiogenesis (Gasparetto et al 2009). However, it is noteworthy that non-astrocytic gliomas are a more heterogeneous group, and low-grade oligodendroglial tumors can also have elevated rCBV (Maia et al 2005; Mechtler 2009; Covarrubias et al 2004). Increased permeability values are also reported in higher-grade glial tumors compared with lower-grade

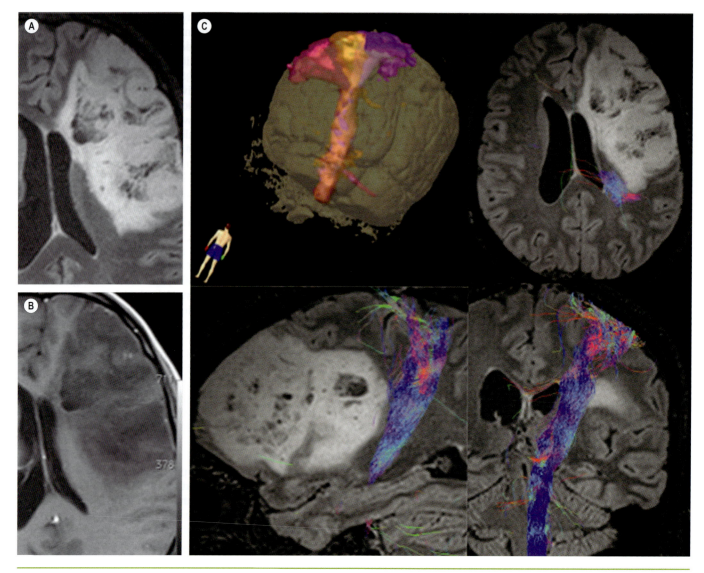

Figure 10.5 Large left frontal protoplasmic astrocytoma (WHO grade II) with FLAIR hyperintensity (A) no contrast enhancement (B) being planned for surgical resection. Images from preoperative planning software incorporating fMRI and motor tractography (C).

for a closed MRI to be brought into the surgical field periodically for intraoperative assessment. Both high-field (1.5T; Sutherland et al 1999; Hall et al 2000; Nimsky et al 2004b) and low-field strength (0.12–0.5T) (Black et al 1997; Nimsky et al 2002; Senft et al 2008) systems have been studied. Higher-field strength magnets generally require movement of the patient or of the scanner but offer improved image quality with shorter acquisition times and a wider spectrum of sequences including diffusion-weighted imaging, MRS and DTI.

A number of studies have documented efficacy and safety of intraoperative MRI systems (Black et al 1997; Tronnier et al 1997; Lewin 1999; Schwartz et al 1999; Hall et al 2000; Bohinski et al 2001a). Despite concerns about infection, deep vein thrombosis and pulmonary embolism with prolongation of anesthesia in the use of iMRI, these complications have not been reported with an increased frequency (Hall et al 2000; Archer et al 2002).

It has been suggested that intraoperative MRI allows more complete resection with lower morbidity (Nimsky et al 2004b). Nimsky in 2004 reported that the percentage of residual tumor volume was significantly reduced between the first intraoperative scan and the final scan (from 21.4% to 6.9%) in resection of glioma (Nimsky et al 2004a). In a recent prospective study of the use of intraoperative MRI in glioma surgery, 47% of patients went on to have further resection after the initial intraoperative scan and the authors claim that extent of resection was optimized by the use of intraoperative MRI, particularly in enhancing tumors (Hatiboglu et al 2009). Immediate surgical morbidity was seen in 28% of patients, with a permanent neurological deficit in 9%, and no mortality.

The use of cortical mapping with bipolar electrical stimulation and frameless stereotactic navigation performed under conscious sedation within the iMRI suite has the potential to further maximize safe resection of brain tumors and has been reported to be safe and effective with a 70% gross total resection rate in a small series (Weingarten et al 2009).

There are only a few studies that have assessed survival in patients undergoing glioma resection in the intraoperative MRI and this is a key issue. In a study of patients undergoing surgery for GBM with iMRI, Schneider et al (2005) reported a significantly longer mean survival for patients undergoing GTR (537d vs 237d) in comparison to those undergoing subtotal resection. This group proposed that intraoperative MRI facilitated a higher percentage of gross total resections in this small cohort of patients with glioblastoma. Perioperative morbidity was considered low at 12.9%. This study is a retrospective review of prospectively collected data and the authors agree that larger randomized studies are needed to address this issue definitively.

Claus et al (2005) found that patients undergoing partial resection of low-grade glioma in the iMRI were at 1.4 times the risk of recurrence and 4.9 times the risk of death of those patients undergoing gross total resection. A retrospective study of costs and benefits of iMRI has documented reduced costs with the use of the intraoperative MRI through a reduced length of stay and reduced rates of repeat resection (Hall et al 2003).

The availability of this resource is limited and the cost is significant, therefore it is critical to determine those patients most likely to benefit from this technology. At present, intraoperative MRI has been shown to be most applicable to resection of benign or low-grade tumors where extent of resection clearly does impact on outcome, such as low-grade glioma, pediatric ependymoma, and possibly high-grade glioma (Schneider et al 2005; Sanai & Berger 2008). This is particularly relevant in children, where the preoperative neuronavigation MRI can be done in the surgical position, resection performed and post-resection scan all performed under the one anesthetic (Lam et al 2001; Nimsky et al 2003; Roth et al 2006; Samdani & Jallo 2007). Further suitable sub-groups include those patients whose tumor is very difficult to distinguish macroscopically from normal brain (again, classically low-grade glioma), patients undergoing reresection where determination of recurrent tumor from gliosis may be difficult, for small tumors to aid localization and confirmation of resection, and where residual may be difficult to visualize (pituitary macroadenoma) (Bohinski et al 2001b; Wu et al 2009a).

Intraoperative ultrasound

Diagnostic cranial ultrasound or echoencephalography has its origins in the 1950s, and has greatest application in the pediatric population. The earliest instruments were limited in image quality and at best, were able to detect shift of the midline as an indication of unilateral intracranial pathology (Leksell 1956). With technologic advances providing improved image quality, diagnostic cranial ultrasound is now ubiquitous in neonatal intensive care units around the world and is a most useful, portable, inexpensive and accurate examination of the neonatal and infantile brain. It frequently plays a role in the diagnosis of infantile brain tumors but is rarely an adequate investigation alone.

Ultrasound imaging is dependent on the pulse echo principle, where a short burst of ultrasound is emitted and the echo of that sound reflected from appropriate surfaces is recorded. A transducer, made from piezoelectric crystal, which can emit and detect ultrasound waves is used in diagnostic ultrasound. Two-dimensional (B mode) imaging and 3D imaging are most relevant to neurosurgery (Rennie et al 2008).

Ultrasound has been applied as an intraoperative tool to aid resection of brain tumors with reports dating from the 1960s (Dyck et al 1966). Its use requires a patent fontanelle, a burrhole or craniotomy site as a window for visualization of the intracranial contents as ultrasound is unable to penetrate the calvarium. The ultrasound probe is covered by a sterile drape with sterile gel before use in the operative field.

The advantages of use of ultrasound intraoperatively include a real-time assessment of anatomic structures, imaging in multiple planes, application of Doppler to identify the vasculature, safety, relatively low infrastructure cost and no requirement for alteration of the operative procedure, instruments, etc. This can be particularly useful to encounter problems with brain shift and inaccuracies of preoperative MRI-based neuronavigation systems. Indeed, several groups have investigated intraoperative 3D ultrasound as a means of updating preoperative MRI-based neuronavigation to account for shift (Gronningsaeter et al 2000a; Gronningsaeter et al 2000b; Unsgaard et al 2002a; Unsgaard et al 2002b; Lindner et al 2006).

The quality of the imaging has been the most significant limitation, although recent technologic advances have made this tool more useful. Ultrasound machines developed specifically for use in the neurosurgical operating room have improved its capacity.

A greater selection of probes (phased, linear, and annular array) has allowed better visualization through a burrhole or craniotomy, of deep-seated lesions (4- to 8-MHz phased array probe optimized at visualizing depths of 3–6 cm and with contact surface area of 13–17 mm) and of superficial lesions (a 10-MHz linear array probe optimized at visualizing depths of 2–4 cm). The use of contrast enhancement (coated microbubbles: sulfur hexafluoride (SF6) and others), has improved differentiation of normal and pathologic tissues (He et al 2008).

Difficulties remain with the differentiation of normal and pathologic tissue at the end of the resection of infiltrating lesions, such as glioma, with blood products in the resection cavity and post-surgical change altering signal characteristics (Rygh et al 2008). The standard B-mode imaging may be enhanced by addition of strain processing by providing greater ability to differentiate normal and pathologic tissue (Selbekk et al 2005). Additionally, the ultrasound requires some degree of operator expertise, which can be readily learnt but does require training in order to maximize usefulness (Lindner et al 2006).

Ultrasound remains a very useful tool for the tumor neurosurgeon and is likely to play an increasing role with further enhancement of image quality.

Fluorescence imaging

5-aminolevulinic acid (5-ALA) is a precursor of hemoglobin that promotes synthesis and accumulation of fluorescent porphyrins in epithelia (skin, gut, etc.) and malignant tissues including glioma (Regula et al 1995; Stummer et al 1998).

Fluorescent porphyrins can be visualized under a specialized operating microscope and hence, may facilitate greater resection of malignant glioma than may be achieved under routine conditions.

This technology has been scrutinized in a randomized multicentre phase III controlled trial comparing fluorescence guided neurosurgery vs routine resection of glioblastoma and shown to improve rates of resection of contrast enhancing tumor (65% vs 36%) and 6-month progression free survival without an increase in adverse events. However, overall, survival did not differ between the two groups (Stummer et al 2006).

Further analysis of the patients in this study, with adjustment for bias, has claimed to provide level 2B evidence that survival depends on complete resection of contrast enhancing tumor in glioblastoma multiforme (Stummer et al 2008b).

This experience has been translated to use of this technology in surgery for cranial metastasis (Morofuji et al 2007; Utsuki et al 2007), ependymoma (Arai et al 2006), and atypical meningioma (Morofuji et al 2008).

It has been proposed that such intraoperative strategies may be combined with photodynamic therapy (ALA-PDT) to improve patient outcomes, with encouraging reports of individual cases (Beck et al 2007; Stummer et al 2008a), although large studies of this treatment have not been reported (Stummer et al 1998; Stepp et al 2007). ALA in combination with Photofrin fluorescence guided resection and repetitive PDT has been investigated in a small single center phase III randomized controlled trial in glioblastoma, with a significant improvement in mean survival in the study group (52.8 weeks vs 24.6 weeks, $p < 0.01$) (Eljamel et al 2008).

Postoperative imaging

Prognostication using ADC

Within the glioma spectrum, minimum tumor ADC value has been shown to inversely correlate with tumor grade (Bulakbasi et al 2004; Kitis et al 2005) and thereby, may be useful to predict outcome. A retrospective study of high-grade glioma patients undergoing diffusion-weighted imaging preoperatively, found a significant negative correlation between minimum ADC and Ki-67 labeling index. The mean minimum ADC was significantly lower in GBM than in anaplastic astrocytoma (although overlap in the absolute values was observed) and the mean minimum ADC of the progressive group was significantly lower than that of the stable group (Higano et al 2006). This was reproduced in a further study of adult high-grade glioma, suggesting tumors with a low minimum ADC tend to have a poorer prognosis (Murakami et al 2007). The same group suggested that the use of minimum ADC and ADC difference values further enhances accurate grading of glial tumors preoperatively (Murakami et al 2009). However, a recent study of patients with low-grade glioma reported that 6-month tumor growth was a better predictor of outcome than perfusion or diffusion-weighted imaging (Caseiras et al 2010).

Early assessment of resection margins

Contrast enhanced MRI within 48–72 hours of surgery has been the traditional method of early assessment of resection margins for glioma surgery following a study demonstrating its superiority over CT published in 1994 (Albert et al 1994). Early imaging avoids confounding post-surgical benign linear contrast enhancement, which can be seen from day 4, up to 3 and 6 months following surgery. MRI was significantly more accurate than surgeon assessment of extent of resection and residual contrast enhancement was the most predictive prognostic factor in patients with glioblastoma (Albert et al 1994). Postoperative assessment of resection of non-enhancing tumors (low-grade glioma, LGG) can be more difficult to quantify, however, FLAIR and T2-weighted imaging performed immediately after surgery is the most useful. DWI is performed routinely in the postoperative setting and, in rare cases, may show evidence of cerebral infarction as a complication of surgery. The entity of diffusion restriction seen adjacent to the resection cavity has also been described, which subsequently in follow-up can demonstrate enhancement in much the same fashion as cerebral infarction would. Thus, early postoperative enhancement has to be assessed in the context of the DWI on the immediate postoperative scan to avoid the incorrect diagnosis of tumor recurrence (Smith et al 2005). Two studies have suggested that transcranial sonography may be more accurate at early detection of residual tumor than CT and MRI and advocate for its complementary use (Becker et al 1999; Mäurer et al 2000).

Early detection of dedifferentiation

Traditional imaging follow-up of LGG has incorporated contrast enhanced MRI with an assessment of size of the lesion, associated mass effect, and the imaging profile in relation to contrast enhancement and diffusion. Tumor volume and evidence of growth has been shown to be an important predictor of outcome in patients with LGG followed with MRI imaging over 6 months (Mandonnet et al 2003; Pallud et al 2006; Brasil Caseiras et al 2010; Rees et al 2009). In a cohort of 21 low-grade gliomas followed prospectively, the mean growth rate was recorded as 3.65 mm/year and a growth rate of higher than 3 mm/year correlated with a greater risk of anaplastic transformation (Hlaihel 2010). While contrast enhancement is a significant predictor of higher tumor grade within series of all gliomas (Asari et al 1994; Pierallini et al 1997), contrast enhancement within documented low-grade gliomas does occur and in a number of studies does not correlate with time to progression (Lev et al 2004; Law et al 2006).

Low-grade glioma follow-up
MRS
The classical MR spectroscopy findings for low-grade glioma are a slightly elevated choline : creatine peak with decreased NAA and no lactate, whereas the classical signature for high-grade glioma is markedly elevated choline : creatine peak, decreased NAA and possible lactate (Smith et al 2003) (Fig. 10.6). Low-grade gliomas have been shown to express higher levels of myoinositol than high-grade gliomas (Castillo et al 2000).

MR spectroscopy has been studied in small series of LGG follow-up. Using a decrease in the NAA/CHO ratio of ≥20%

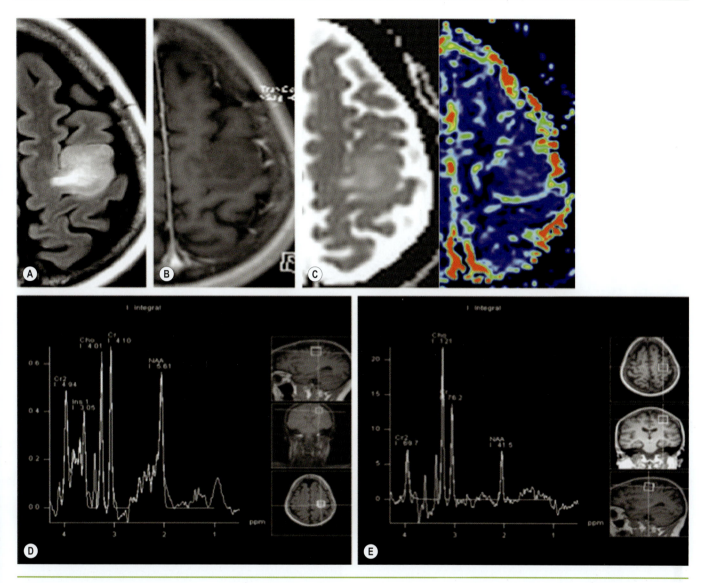

Figure 10.6 A presumed low-grade glioma managed with serial imaging for the previous 5 years. FLAIR hyperintense (A), with no contrast enhancement (B), no reduction in ADC (C), and no elevation of rCBV (D). However, there had been a deterioration in the spectroscopic ratios with further elevation in the level of Cho between D and E over 6 months. This suggested a possible change in tumor biology. Histology revealed an anaplastic oliogoastrocytoma (WHO grade III).

compared with baseline as indicative of progression, this modality was not found to be sufficiently reliable to contribute to the monitoring of LGG (Reijneveld et al 2005). The development of a lipid peak has been suggested to be indicative of dedifferentiation in LGG followed with MRS, although again the studies are very small (Guilloton et al 2008). A further small series of LGG looking at the predictive value of MRS, suggested that a choline to creatine ratio of about 2.4 is associated with an 83% risk of a malignant progression in an average time of 15.4 months (Hlaihel 2010).

MR perfusion
Dynamic susceptibility weighted contrast-material enhanced perfusion MR imaging is a modality of imaging that can provide physiologic information about vascular density, vascular endothelial proliferation and angiogenesis (Shin et al 2002; Law et al 2003; Law et al 2004). Elevations in relative CBV in glioma may be indicative of changes in blood volume

that precede malignant transformation (Fig. 10.7). It has been reported that an assessment of the relative cerebral blood volume within a cerebral glioma, independent of histologic grade (excluding WHO grade 1 pilocytic astrocytoma) can be used to predict a clinical response to treatment, time to progression and survival (Law et al 2008). In a similar study, relative CBV was a better predictor of tumor grade and survival than contrast enhancement (Lev et al 2004). In LGG it has been shown in a retrospective fashion that those patients with a low relative CBV (<1.75) had a significantly longer time to progression than those patients with a relative CBV >1.75 (Law et al 2006) (Fig. 10.8).

PET
18F-FDG PET imaging is dependent on the ability of 18F-FDG to cross the blood–brain barrier and to be phosphorylated in the cell. In diffuse infiltrating glioma, uptake is significantly correlated with the presence of anaplasia, being

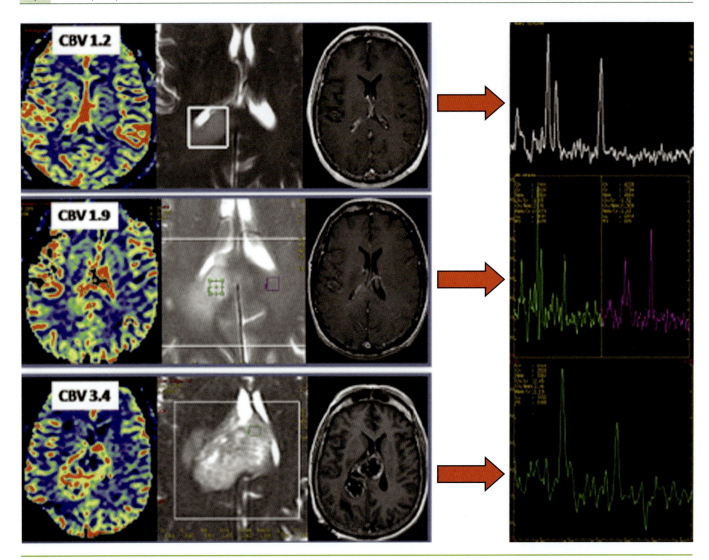

Figure 10.7 Tumor progression 'the angiogenic switch' demonstrated by DSC MR imagining perfusion maps. Top row: Gradient-echo axial DSC MR imaging image with rCBV color overlay map shows low initial perfusion with a rCBV of 1.2 more in-keeping with an LGG than an HGG. Axial FLAIR image shows increased signal within the right splenium of the corpus callosum with some mass effect on the adjacent lateral ventricle. Axial post-contrast T1-weighted image shows no enhancement within the lesion. Spectroscopy of the lesion demonstrates high levels of choline and reduced NAA levels. Middle row: MR imaging at 6 months follow-up. Gradient echo axial DSC MR imaging image with rCBV color overlay map shows an increase in rCBV in comparison to the previous examination (1.2–1.9), more in-keeping with an HGG than an LGG (arrow). However, there is no enhancement, and no change was observed in the spectroscopy. This 'angiogenic switch' may herald early malignant transformation. Bottom row: MR imaging at 8 months follow-up. At this time, there is clear tumor progression, characterised by a marked increase in tumor volume and enhancement as well as mass effect. There is now obvious evidence of rCBV, color overlay shows a further increase in rCBV (3.4), in keeping with tumor progression. It has been demonstrated in the literature that the rCBV increase can precede the contrast enhancement, probably reflecting the angiogenic switch in the tumor biology. (Reproduced from Lacerda & Law 2009.)

highest in high-grade tumors and is a more accurate indicator of tumor grade than MR contrast enhancement (Di Chiro 1987; Law et al 2003). Low-grade lesions generally appear as hypometabolic areas surrounded by normal high activity of the cerebral cortex and exhibit increased uptake in a minority of cases (10%) (Di Chiro 1987). Its utility as a modality of following LGG has been studied. Previously low uptake/low-grade lesions that subsequently develop high uptake have been documented to have undergone malignant transformation (De Witte et al 1996; Padma et al 2003).

18F-FDG PET imaging of brain tumors does have significant limitations (Olivero et al 1995; Ricci et al 1998).

Differentiation of particularly low-grade and recurrent high-grade tumors from normal parenchyma can be difficult on the basis of glucose uptake, due to the inherently high uptake of normal parenchyma. Some tumors do not exhibit high glucose uptake and 18F-FDG uptake and glucose uptake are not always equivalent (Krohn et al 2005). Co-registration with MRI is critical in interpretation of PET by allowing better anatomic localization, thereby differentiating tumors with relatively low uptake in comparison to normal cortex by location (Wong et al 2004). Spatial resolution is improving but remains limited clinically to the detection of lesions >1 cm in diameter.

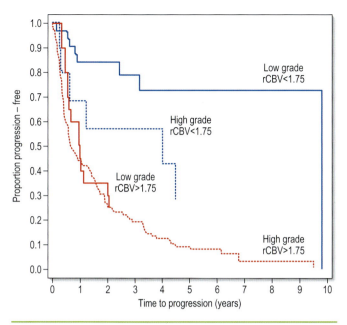

Figure 10.8 Kaplan–Meier survival curves for progression-free survival within the low-grade glioma (LGG) group with (rCBV < 1.75) and (rCBV > 1.75) rCBV groups (*solid lines*) demonstrating a significant difference in time to progression in LGGs stratified by rCBV alone (*p* < 0.0001). When comparing HGGs (*broken lines*), similarly there was a significant difference in progression in HGGs with high (rCBV > 1.75) vs low rCBV (*p* < 0.0001). Among subjects with low rCBV < 1.75), there was a significant difference between high- and low-grade tumors with respect to progression-free survival (*p* = 0.047). However, among subjects with high rCBV (rCBV > 1.75), time to progression was not significantly different (*p* = 0.2666) for low- and high-grade tumors. (From Law et al 2004, with permission.)

Delayed imaging also has been documented to improve diagnostic accuracy (Spence et al 2004).

Assessment of treatment response

Assessment of treatment response is based on clinical and imaging parameters. Imaging is routinely performed at 8–12-weekly intervals for high-grade glioma patients. A number of techniques have been proposed to measure tumor volume on MRI, with computer-assisted volumetric measurement techniques found to be most accurate and reliable (Sorensen et al 2001; Warren et al 2001). In high-grade glioma trials since 1990, the MacDonald criteria have been used, with complete response defined as disappearance of all enhancing tumor on consecutive CT or MRI performed at least 1 month apart, with the patient off steroids and stable or improved. Partial response is defined as >50% reduction in size of the enhancing tumor with steroids stable or reduced and no change in clinical status or improvement. Progressive disease is >25% increase in the size of the tumor, neurological deterioration and a stable or increased corticosteroid requirement. Stable disease is all other situations. By this schema, size is determined as the largest cross-sectional area of tumor (Macdonald et al 1990).

Because of a concern that the above criteria may not identify patients with non-enhancing progressive disease,

especially in the setting of anti-angiogenic therapy, The Neurooncology Working Group of The American Society of Clinical Oncology have proposed a schema to incorporate T2 or FLAIR imaging changes (Chang 2009; van den Bent et al 2009).

Additionally, diffusion-weighted imaging may be used in the assessment of treatment response. In a study of 18 patients with high-grade glioma undergoing conventional treatment with radiation and chemotherapy, higher mean ADC values were documented in patients with stable disease at 1 month post-treatment than those with progressive disease (Mardor et al 2003).

For lower-grade lesions in adults, contrast enhanced MRI has traditionally been used for assessment of treatment response with a schedule of 3-monthly for 1 year; 4-monthly for 1 year; 6-monthly for 1 year, and thereafter yearly. In a study of patients followed after treatment of pediatric cerebellar low-grade astrocytoma based on recurrence patterns, the authors recommended imaging at 6 months, 1, 2, 3.5, and 5 years after complete resection or radiation. For follow-up of patients with residual tumor, 6-monthly for 3 years; yearly for 2 years, and thereafter every 2 years was recommended (Saunders et al 2005).

Assessment for recurrent tumor

Radiation necrosis vs tumor
MR

The MR appearance of radiation necrosis can be diffuse (with abnormal non-enhancing high signal intensity on T2 or FLAIR imaging) or manifest as a focal enhancing mass with central necrosis making it difficult to differentiate from recurrent tumor. The location of the abnormality can be useful in relation to treatment effects occurring within the radiation field but this classically correlates with the site of highest risk for recurrent tumor. Radiation necrosis has a predilection for the periventricular white matter, thought to be due to the less robust blood supply to this area with fewer collateral vessels. Biopsy proven necrosis has been reported to be as high as 24% in a series of 148 patients (Kumar et al 2000) and as low as 4.9% in a series of 426 patients with high-grade glioma, with an actuarial incidence of 13.3% after 3 years in the latter study (Ruben et al 2006). An added difficulty is the presence of mixed necrosis and tumor seen in some patients. Traditional MR methods on which to base clinical management decisions are inadequate.

Newer modalities have shown promise in this area. DWI can provide additional information in this setting, with areas of restricted diffusion found to be consistent with tumor recurrence (Tsui et al 2001). Perfusion MR techniques are under study and do have some value in differentiating tumor from necrosis (Giglio & Gilbert 2003) with increased rCBV (>2.6) shown to be consistent with tumor recurrence (Hazle et al 1997; Sugahara et al 2000). The rCBV in regions of pure necrosis is 0.6 or less. MRS has been studied in a number of series of glioma patients in an attempt to aid differentiation of recurrent tumor from radiation necrosis. An abnormal increase in the choline peak (>50% the contralateral value) or a choline to creatine ratio of >2 was suggestive of recurrent tumor (Träber et al 2002; Ando et al 2004). The sensitivity and specificity of making the diagnosis of recurrent tumor based on a CHO/creatine ratio of 2 was 87% and 89% (Rabinov et al 2002; Lichy et al 2004a; Lichy et al 2004b; Hollingworth et al 2006). It is not felt that such modalities are sufficiently robust to replace biopsy at present.

Nuclear medicine/PET and thallium

The greater availability and lower cost of thallium SPECT makes it an attractive alternative to PET imaging. In a prospective cohort study of patients with low-grade glioma, 201 thallium SPECT was shown to be more sensitive (88%) and specific (76%) than neurostructural imaging (CT/MRI) in differentiating tumor from radiation injury (Gómez-Río et al 2004). In a small retrospective series of patients with high-grade glioma, 201 Tl-SPECT was found to be superior to conventional MR in differentiating necrosis from recurrent tumor with high specificity (100%) (Tie et al 2008). The same modality has been shown with certain caveats to be helpful in differentiating radiation injury from recurrence after gamma knife radiosurgery for metastasis (Serizawa et al 2005).

18F-FDG PET has been reported to be a valuable tool in the discrimination of radiation necrosis from recurrent tumor, with sensitivity of 81–86% and a specificity of 40–94% (Langleben & Segall 2000). FDG uptake is suggestive of viable tumor, whereas absence of uptake suggests necrosis. It has been shown that it is critical to compare PET signal in the area of interest with the expected background activity in that region, facilitated by co-registration with MRI, due to the wide range of activity in regions of treated brain and recurrent tumors. Sensitivity of 96% and specificity of 77% in distinguishing recurrent tumor from radiation necrosis can be achieved when utilizing these criteria (Wang et al 2006).

Pseudo-progression

Pseudo-progression is a clinical and imaging-based diagnosis of a patient immediately at the completion of treatment for glioblastoma who typically remains well with no new symptoms, although up to one-third may be symptomatic (Brandes et al 2008) and have progressive and enhancing lesions seen on MRI, which are a treatment effect and are not related to tumor progression (de Wit et al 2004; Chamberlain et al 2007; Brandsma et al 2008). This phenomenon has been reported in approximately 20% of patients undergoing chemotherapy with temozolomide and radiation for the treatment of glioblastoma (Taal et al 2008) and occurs at an earlier time-frame than radionecrosis would typically be seen (Ruben et al 2006). On subsequent imaging, the contrast enhancement remains stable or is decreased in size (Taal et al 2008). Patients with MGMT methylation were more frequently demonstrating pseudo-progression (Brandes et al 2008).

It is difficult with standard MRI imaging alone to differentiate pseudo-progression from progressive tumor. MR perfusion, ADC measurement, MRS and thallium SPECT can be helpful to try and differentiate true tumor from treatment related chemoradionecrosis, however, they are not definitive, particularly as it is not uncommon to have both components present (Rock et al 2004). Pseudo-progression remains a challenging problem for neurosurgeons and neurooncologists across the world.

Pseudo-response

Bevacizumab is a recently approved humanized monoclonal antibody against vascular endothelial growth factor (VEGF) being used in the treatment of patients with high-grade glioma. The drug has been shown to prolong progression-free survival and control perilesional edema (Stark-Vance 2005; Vredenburgh et al 2007a; Vredenburgh et al 2007b; Guiu et al 2008; Norden et al 2008; Narayana et al 2009; Zuniga et al 2009). It seems to reduce the need for corticosteroids in many patients and the drug has not been found to be associated with unacceptable side-effects or hemorrhage risk.

The use of bevacizumab and other antiangiogenic agents has further complicated the evaluation of response to therapy of high-grade glioma patients. Radiographic response to this therapy has been thought to be indicated by decreased contrast enhancement, and at least partial response has been seen in up to 66% of patients (Stark-Vance 2005). However, several groups have described infiltrative tumor growth occurring in patients on bevacizumab with clinical and radiologic progression (increased areas of T2 and FLAIR signal abnormality) without contrast enhancement, a so-called pseudo-response (Norden et al 2008a; Norden et al 2009b). FLAIR and diffusion-weighted imaging may then become critical tools in the evaluation of high-grade glioma following anti-angiogenic therapy (Norden et al 2009b). In addition to these imaging findings, there is some concern as to whether overall survival is improved by bevacizumab therapy in high-grade glioma (Norden et al 2009a).

Conclusion

Advanced imaging has provided significant gains in the diagnosis and management of brain tumors over the last three decades. Despite this, there remains a paucity of well-designed trials to definitively assess these technologies and their optimal applications. This represents the greatest challenge to those in the neurooncology community over the coming decades.

Key points

- Advanced imaging techniques must be interpreted in light of well established conventional imaging algorithms
- These novel imaging techniques can provide tumoral physiological and cellular architectural information that is not available with conventional CT and MR imaging
- Appropriate use of advanced brain tumor imaging can contribute to better patient management
- However, there remain a paucity of well-designed trials to assess these techniques and their optimal applications.

Acknowledgments

The authors would like to thank Dr Bradford A. Moffat from the Department of Radiology, The Royal Melbourne Hospital, Melbourne, Australia for assistance with illustration preparation.

REFERENCES

Akiyama, M., Sakai, H., Onoue, H., et al., 2004. Imaging intracranial haemangiopericytomas: study of seven cases. Neuroradiology 46 (3), 194–197.

Al-Okaili, R.N., Krejza, J., Wang, S., et al., 2006. Advanced MR imaging techniques in the diagnosis of intraaxial brain tumors in adults. Radiographics 26 (Suppl. 1), S173–S189.

Al-Okaili, R.N., Krejza, J., Woo, J.H., et al., 2007. Intraaxial brain masses: MR imaging-based diagnostic strategy–initial experience. Radiology 243 (2), 539–550.

Albert, F.K., Forsting, M., Sartor, K., et al., 1994. Early postoperative magnetic resonance imaging after resection of malignant glioma: objective evaluation of residual tumor and its influence on regrowth and prognosis. Neurosurgery 34 (1), 45–61.

Anderson, F.A. Jr, 1998. The Glioma Outcomes Project: a resource for measuring and improving glioma outcomes. Neurosurg Focus 4 (6), e8.

Ando, K., Ishikura, R., Nagami, Y., et al., 2004. [Usefulness of Cho/Cr ratio in proton MR spectroscopy for differentiating residual/recurrent glioma from non-neoplastic lesions]. Nippon Igaku Hoshasen Gakkai Zasshi 64 (3), 121–126.

Arai, T., Tani, S., Isoshima, A., et al., 2006. [Intraoperative photodynamic diagnosis for spinal ependymoma using 5-aminolevulinic acid: technical note]. No. Shinkei Geka. 34 (8), 811–817.

Archer, D.P., McTaggart Cowan, R.A., et al., 2002. Intraoperative mobile magnetic resonance imaging for craniotomy lengthens the procedure but does not increase morbidity. Can. J. Anaesth 49 (4), 420–426.

Aronen, H.J., Perkiö, J., 2002. Dynamic susceptibility contrast MRI of gliomas. Neuroimaging Clin. N. Am. 12 (4), 501–523.

Asari, S., Makabe, T., Katayama, S., et al., 1994. Assessment of the pathological grade of astrocytic gliomas using an MRI score. Neuroradiology 36 (4), 308–310.

Bae, M.S., Jahng, G.H., Ryu, C.W., et al., 2009. Effect of intravenous gadolinium-DTPA on diffusion tensor MR imaging for the evaluation of brain tumors. Neuroradiology 51 (12), 793–802.

Barajas, R.F., Chang, J.S., Sneed, P.K., et al., 2009. Distinguishing recurrent intra-axial metastatic tumor from radiation necrosis following gamma knife radiosurgery using dynamic susceptibility-weighted contrast-enhanced perfusion MR imaging. AJNR. Am. J. Neuroradiol 30 (2), 367–372.

Barba, I., Moreno, A., Martinez-Pérez, I., et al., 2001. Magnetic resonance spectroscopy of brain hemangiopericytomas: high myoinositol concentrations and discrimination from meningiomas. J. Neurosurg 94 (1), 55–60.

Barnard, R.O., Geddes, J.F., 1987. The incidence of multifocal cerebral gliomas. A histologic study of large hemisphere sections. Cancer 60 (7), 1519–1531.

Beck, T.J., Kreth, F.W., Beyer, W., et al., 2007. Interstitial photodynamic therapy of nonresectable malignant glioma recurrences using 5-aminolevulinic acid induced protoporphyrin IX. Lasers Surg. Med. 39 (5), 386–393.

Becker, G., Hofmann, E., Woydt, M., et al., 1999. Postoperative neuroimaging of high-grade gliomas: comparison of transcranial sonography, magnetic resonance imaging, and computed tomography. Neurosurgery 44 (3), 469–478.

Bendszus, M., Warmuth-Metz, M., Burger, R., et al., 2001. Diagnosing dural metastases: the value of 1H magnetic resonance spectroscopy. Neuroradiology 43 (4), 285–289.

Berkenstadt, H., Perel, A., Ram, Z., et al., 2001. Anesthesia for magnetic resonance guided neurosurgery: initial experience with a new open magnetic resonance imaging system. J. Neurosurg Anesthesiol 13 (2), 158–162.

Bitsch, A., Bruhn, H., Vougioukas, V., et al., 1999. Inflammatory CNS demyelination: histopathologic correlation with in vivo quantitative proton MR spectroscopy. AJNR. Am. J. Neuroradiol 20 (9), 1619–1627.

Black, P.M., Moriarty, T., Alexander, E. 3rd, et al., 1997. Development and implementation of intraoperative magnetic resonance imaging and its neurosurgical applications. Neurosurgery 41 (4), 831–845.

Bohinski, R.J., Kokkino, A.K., Warnick, R.E., et al., 2001a. Glioma resection in a shared-resource magnetic resonance operating room after optimal image-guided frameless stereotactic resection. Neurosurgery 48 (4), 731–744.

Bohinski, R.J., Warnick, R.E., Gaskill-Shipley, M.F., et al., 2001b. Intraoperative magnetic resonance imaging to determine the extent of resection of pituitary macroadenomas during transsphenoidal microsurgery. Neurosurgery 49 (5), 1133–1144.

Bondy, M., Ligon, B.L., 1996. Epidemiology and etiology of intracranial meningiomas: a review. J. Neurooncol 29 (3), 197–205.

Brandes, A.A., Tosoni, A., Spagnolli, F., et al., 2008. Disease progression or pseudoprogression after concomitant radiochemotherapy treatment: pitfalls in neurooncology. Neuro. Oncol. 10 (3), 361–367.

Brandsma, D., Stalpers, L., Taal, W., et al., 2008. Clinical features, mechanisms, and management of pseudoprogression in malignant gliomas. Lancet Oncol. 9 (5), 453–461.

Brasil Caseiras, G., Ciccarelli, O., Altmann, D.R., et al., 2009. Low-grade gliomas: six-month tumor growth predicts patient outcome better than admission tumor volume, relative cerebral blood volume, and apparent diffusion coefficient. Radiology 253 (2), 505–512.

Braun, V., Albrecht, A., Kretschmer, T., et al., 2006. Brain tumour surgery in the vicinity of short-term memory representation–results of neuronavigation using fMRI images. Acta. Neurochir. (Wien) 148 (7), 733–739.

Broggi, G., Ferroli, P., Franzini, A., et al., 2003. CT-guided neurosurgery: preliminary experience. Acta. Neurochir. 85 (Suppl.), 101–104.

Brucher, J.M., 1993. Neuropathological diagnosis with stereotactic biopsies. Possibilities, difficulties and requirements. Acta. Neurochir. (Wien) 124 (1), 37–39.

Bükte, Y., Paksoy, Y., Genç, E., et al., 2005. Role of diffusion-weighted MR in differential diagnosis of intracranial cystic lesions. Clin. Radiol. 60 (3), 375–383.

Bulakbasi, N., Guvenc, I., Onguru, O., et al., 2004. The added value of the apparent diffusion coefficient calculation to magnetic resonance imaging in the differentiation and grading of malignant brain tumors. J. Comput. Assist. Tomogr. 28 (6), 735–746.

Caseiras, G.B., Chheang, S., Babb, J., et al., 2010. Relative cerebral blood volume measurements of low-grade gliomas predict patient outcome in a multi-institution setting. Eur. J. Radiol. 73 (2), 215–220.

Castillo, M., Smith, J.K., Kwock, L., 2000. Correlation of myo-inositol levels and grading of cerebral astrocytomas. AJNR. Am. J. Neuroradiol 21 (9), 1645–1649.

Ceyssens, S., Van Laere, K., de Groot, T., et al., 2006. [11C]methionine PET, histopathology, and survival in primary brain tumors and recurrence. AJNR. Am. J. Neuroradiol 27 (7), 1432–1437.

Cha, S., 2003. Perfusion MR imaging: basic principles and clinical applications. Magn. Reson. Imaging Clin. N. Am. 11 (3), 403–413.

Cha, S., 2006. Update on brain tumor imaging: from anatomy to physiology. AJNR. Am. J. Neuroradiol 27 (3), 475–487.

Cha, S., 2009. Neuroimaging in neuro-oncology. Neurotherapeutics 6 (3), 465–477.

Cha, S., Pierce, S., Knopp, E.A., et al., 2001. Dynamic contrast-enhanced T2*-weighted MR imaging of tumefactive demyelinating lesions. AJNR. Am. J. Neuroradiol 22 (6), 1109–1116.

Chamberlain, M.C., Glantz, M.J., Chalmers, L., et al., 2007. Early necrosis following concurrent Temodar and radiotherapy in patients with glioblastoma. J. Neurooncol. 82 (1), 81–83.

Chang, S., Clarke, J., Wen, P., 2009. Novel imaging response assessment for drug therapies in recurrent malignant glioma. Educational Book. American Society of Clinical Oncology, Alexandria, VA, pp. 107–111.

Chen, S., Ikawa, F., Kurisu, K., et al., 2001. Quantitative MR evaluation of intracranial epidermoid tumors by fast fluid-attenuated inversion recovery imaging and echo-planar diffusion-weighted imaging. AJNR. Am. J. Neuroradiol 22 (6), 1089–1096.

Chen, W., 2007. Clinical applications of PET in brain tumors. J. Nucl. Med. 48 (9), 1468–1481.

Chen, W., Silverman, D.H., Delaloye, S., et al., 2006. 18F-FDOPA PET imaging of brain tumors: comparison study with 18F-FDG PET and evaluation of diagnostic accuracy. J. Nucl. Med. 47 (6), 904–911.

Chernov, M.F., Muragaki, Y., Ochiai, T., et al., 2009. Spectroscopy-supported frame-based image-guided stereotactic biopsy of parenchymal brain lesions: comparative evaluation of diagnostic yield and diagnostic accuracy. Clin. Neurol. Neurosurg 111 (6), 527–535.

Chiang, I.C., Kuo, Y.T., Lu, C.Y., et al., 2004. Distinction between high-grade gliomas and solitary metastases using peritumoral 3-T magnetic resonance spectroscopy, diffusion, and perfusion imagings. Neuroradiology 46 (8), 619–627.

Chiechi, M.V., Smirniotopoulos, J.G., Mena, H., 1996. Intracranial hemangiopericytomas: MR and CT features. AJNR. Am. J. Neuroradiol 17 (7), 1365–1371.

Cianfoni, A., Niku, S., Imbesi, S.G., 2007. Metabolite findings in tumefactive demyelinating lesions utilizing short echo time proton magnetic resonance spectroscopy. AJNR. Am. J. Neuroradiol 28 (2), 272–277.

Claus, E.B., Horlacher, A., Hsu, L., et al., 2005. Survival rates in patients with low-grade glioma after intraoperative magnetic resonance image guidance. Cancer 103 (6), 1227–1233.

Commins, D.L., Atkinson, R.D., Burnett, M.E., 2007. Review of meningioma histopathology. Neurosurg Focus 23 (4), E3.

Corn, B.W., Marcus, S.M., Topham, A., et al., 1997. Will primary central nervous system lymphoma be the most frequent brain tumor diagnosed in the year 2000? Cancer 79 (12), 2409–2413.

Covarrubias, D.J., Rosen, B.R., Lev, M.H., 2004. Dynamic magnetic resonance perfusion imaging of brain tumors. Oncologist 9 (5), 528–537.

Cruz, L.C. Jr, Sorensen, A.G., 2006. Diffusion tensor magnetic resonance imaging of brain tumors. Magn. Reson. Imaging Clin. N. Am. 14 (2), 183–202.

de Wit, M.C., de Bruin, H.G., Eijkenboom, W., et al., 2004. Immediate post-radiotherapy changes in malignant glioma can mimic tumor progression. Neurology 63 (3), 535–537.

De Witte, O., Levivier, M., Violon, P., et al., 1996. Prognostic value positron emission tomography with [18F]fluoro-2-deoxy-D-glucose in the low-grade glioma. Neurosurgery 39 (3), 470–477.

DeAngelis, L.M., 2001. Brain tumors. N. Engl. J. Med. 344 (2), 114–123.

Demir, M.K., Iplikcioglu, A.C., Dincer, A., et al., 2006. Single voxel proton MR spectroscopy findings of typical and atypical intracranial meningiomas. Eur. J. Radiol. 60 (1), 48–55.

Desprechins, B., Stadnik, T., Koerts, G., et al., 1999. Use of diffusion-weighted MR imaging in differential diagnosis between intracerebral necrotic tumors and cerebral abscesses. AJNR. Am. J. Neuroradiol 20 (7), 1252–1257.

Di Chiro, G., 1987. Positron emission tomography using [18F] fluorodeoxyglucose in brain tumors. A powerful diagnostic and prognostic tool. Invest. Radiol. 22 (5), 360–371.

Duygulu, G., Ovali, G.Y., Calli, C., et al., 2010. Intracerebral metastasis showing restricted diffusion: Correlation with histopathologic findings. Eur. J. Radiol. 74 (1), 117–120.

Dyck, P., Kurze, T., Barrows, H.S., 1966. Intra-operative ultrasonic encephalography of cerebral mass lesions. Bull. Los. Angeles. Neurol. Soc. 31 (3), 114–124.

Eljamel, M.S., Goodman, C., Moseley, H., 2008. ALA and Photofrin fluorescence-guided resection and repetitive PDT in glioblastoma multiforme: a single centre Phase III randomised controlled trial. Lasers. Med. Sci. 23 (4), 361–367.

Enzinger, C., Strasser-Fuchs, S., Ropele, S., et al., 2005. Tumefactive demyelinating lesions: conventional and advanced magnetic resonance imaging. Mult. Scler. 11 (2), 135–139.

Filippi, C.G., Edgar, M.A., Ulu , A.M., et al., 2001. Appearance of meningiomas on diffusion-weighted images: correlating diffusion constants with histopathologic findings. AJNR. Am. J. Neuroradiol 22 (1), 65–72.

Floeth, F.W., Pauleit, D., Sabel, M., et al., 2006. 18F-FET PET differentiation of ring-enhancing brain lesions. J. Nucl. Med. 47 (5), 776–782.

Gasparetto, E.L., Pawlak, M.A., Patel, S.H., et al., 2009. Posttreatment recurrence of malignant brain neoplasm: accuracy of relative cerebral blood volume fraction in discriminating low from high malignant histologic volume fraction. Radiology 250 (3), 887–896.

Gaviani, P., Schwartz, R.B., Hedley-Whyte, E.T., et al., 2005. Diffusion-weighted imaging of fungal cerebral infection. AJNR. Am. J. Neuroradiol 26 (5), 1115–1121.

Geijer, B., Lindgren, A., Brockstedt, S., et al., 2001. Persistent high signal on diffusion-weighted MRI in the late stages of small cortical and lacunar ischaemic lesions. Neuroradiology 43 (2), 115–122.

Giglio, P., Gilbert, M.R., 2003. Cerebral radiation necrosis. Neurologist 9 (4), 180–188.

Ginsberg, L.E., Fuller, G.N., Hashmi, M., et al., 1998. The significance of lack of MR contrast enhancement of supratentorial brain tumors in adults: histopathological evaluation of a series. Surg. Neurol. 49 (4), 436–440.

Giussani, C., Roux, F.E., Ojemann, J., et al., 2010. Is preoperative functional magnetic resonance imaging reliable for language areas mapping in brain tumor surgery? Review of language functional magnetic resonance imaging and direct cortical stimulation correlation studies. Neurosurgery 66 (1), 113–120.

Given, C.A. 2nd, Stevens, B.S., Lee, C., 2004. The MRI appearance of tumefactive demyelinating lesions. AJR. Am. J. Roentgenol. 182 (1), 195–199.

Gómez-Río, M., Martínez Del Valle Torres, D., Rodríguez-Fernández, A., et al., 2004. (201)Tl-SPECT in low-grade gliomas: diagnostic accuracy in differential diagnosis between tumour recurrence and radionecrosis. Eur. J. Nucl. Med. Mol. Imaging 31 (9), 1237–1243.

Greene, G.M., Hitchon, P.W., Schelper, R.L., et al., 1989. Diagnostic yield in CT-guided stereotactic biopsy of gliomas. J. Neurosurg 71 (4), 494–497.

Gronningsaeter, A., Kleven, A., Ommedal, S., et al., 2000a. SonoWand, an ultrasound-based neuronavigation system. Neurosurgery 47 (6), 1373–1380.

Gronningsaeter, A., Lie, T., Kleven, A., et al., 2000b. Initial experience with stereoscopic visualization of three-dimensional ultrasound data in surgery. Surg. Endosc. 14 (11), 1074–1078.

Guermazi, A., Lafitte, F., Miaux, Y., et al., 2005. The dural tail sign – beyond meningioma. Clin. Radiol. 60 (2), 171–188.

Guilloton, L., Cotton, F., Cartalat-Carel, S., et al., 2008. [Supervision of low-grade gliomas with multiparametric MR imaging: research of radiologic indicators of malignancy transformation]. Neurochirurgie 54 (4), 517–528.

Guiu, S., Taillibert, S., Chinot, O., et al., 2008. [Bevacizumab/irinotecan. An active treatment for recurrent high-grade gliomas: preliminary results of an ANOCEF Multicenter Study]. Rev. Neurol. (Paris) 164 (6–7), 588–594.

Gumprecht, H., Lumenta, C.B., 2003. Intraoperative imaging using a mobile computed tomography scanner. Minim Invasive Neurosurg 46 (6), 317–322.

Guo, A.C., Cummings, T.J., Dash, R.C., et al., 2002. Lymphomas and high-grade astrocytomas: comparison of water diffusibility and histologic characteristics. Radiology 224 (1), 177–183.

Gupta, R.K., Hasan, K.M., Mishra, A.M., et al., 2005. High fractional anisotropy in brain abscesses versus other cystic intracranial lesions. AJNR. Am. J. Neuroradiol 26 (5), 1107–1114.

Hakyemez, B., Erdogan, C., Bolca, N., et al., 2006a. Evaluation of different cerebral mass lesions by perfusion-weighted MR imaging. J. Magn. Reson. Imaging 24 (4), 817–824.

Hakyemez, B., Yildirim, N., Gokalp, G., et al., 2006b. The contribution of diffusion-weighted MR imaging to distinguishing typical from atypical meningiomas. Neuroradiology 48 (8), 513–520.

Hall, W.A., Kowalik, K., Liu, H., et al., 2003. Costs and benefits of intraoperative MR-guided brain tumor resection. Acta. Neurochir. 85 (Suppl.), 137–142.

Hall, W.A., Liu, H., Martin, A.J., et al., 2000. Safety, efficacy, and functionality of high-field strength interventional magnetic resonance imaging for neurosurgery. Neurosurgery 46 (3), 632–642.

Hall, W.A., Liu, H., Martin, A.J., et al., 1999a. Comparison of stereotactic brain biopsy to interventional magnetic-resonance-imaging-guided brain biopsy. Stereotact. Funct. Neurosurg 73 (1–4), 148–153.

Hall, W.A., Martin, A., Liu, H., et al., 2001. Improving diagnostic yield in brain biopsy: coupling spectroscopic targeting with real-time needle placement. J. Magn. Reson. Imaging 13 (1), 12–15.

Hall, W.A., Martin, A.J., Liu, H., et al., 1999b. Brain biopsy using high-field strength interventional magnetic resonance imaging. Neurosurgery 44 (4), 807–814.

Hanson, M.W., Glantz, M.J., Hoffman, J.M., et al., 1991. FDG-PET in the selection of brain lesions for biopsy. J. Comput. Assist Tomogr. 15 (5), 796–801.

Hartmann, M., Jansen, O., Heiland, S., et al., 2001. Restricted diffusion within ring enhancement is not pathognomonic for brain abscess. AJNR. Am. J. Neuroradiol 22 (9), 1738–1742.

Hashizume, H., Baluk, P., Morikawa, S., et al., 2000. Openings between defective endothelial cells explain tumor vessel leakiness. Am. J. Pathol. 156 (4), 1363–1380.

Hatiboglu, M.A., Weinberg, J.S., Suki, D., et al., 2009. Impact of intraoperative high-field magnetic resonance imaging guidance on glioma surgery: a prospective volumetric analysis. Neurosurgery 64 (6), 1073–1081; discussion 1081.

Hayashida, Y., Hirai, T., Morishita, S., et al., 2006. Diffusion-weighted imaging of metastatic brain tumors: comparison with histologic type and tumor cellularity. AJNR. Am. J. Neuroradiol 27 (7), 1419–1425.

Hazle, J.D., Jackson, E.F., Schomer, D.F., et al., 1997. Dynamic imaging of intracranial lesions using fast spin-echo imaging: differentiation of brain tumors and treatment effects. J. Magn. Reson. Imaging 7 (6), 1084–1093.

He, W., Jiang, X.Q., Wang, S., et al., 2008. Intraoperative contrast-enhanced ultrasound for brain tumors. Clin. Imaging 32 (6), 419–424.

Hemm, S., Rigau, V., Chevalier, J., et al., 2005. Stereotactic coregistration of 201Tl SPECT and MRI applied to brain tumor biopsies. J. Nucl. Med. 46 (7), 1151–1157.

Hemm, S., Vayssiere, N., Zanca, M., et al., 2004. Thallium SPECT-based stereotactic targeting for brain tumor biopsies. A technical note. Stereotact. Funct. Neurosurg 82 (2–3), 70–76.

Heper, A.O., Erden, E., Savas, A., et al., 2005. An analysis of stereotactic biopsy of brain tumors and nonneoplastic lesions: a prospective clinicopathologic study. Surg. Neurol. 64 (Suppl. 2), S82–S88.

Higano, S., Yun, X., Kumabe, T., et al., 2006. Malignant astrocytic tumors: clinical importance of apparent diffusion coefficient in prediction of grade and prognosis. Radiology 241 (3), 839–846.

Hlaihel, C., 2010. Predictive value of multimodality MRI using conventional, perfusion and spectroscopy MR in anaplastic transformation of low-grade oligodendrogliomas. J. Neurooncol. 97, 73–80.

Hollingworth, W., Medina, L.S., Lenkinski, R.E., et al., 2006. A systematic literature review of magnetic resonance spectroscopy for the characterization of brain tumors. AJNR. Am. J. Neuroradiol 27 (7), 1404–1411.

Holmes, T.M., Petrella, J.R., Provenzale, J.M., et al., 2004. Distinction between cerebral abscesses and high-grade neoplasms by dynamic susceptibility contrast perfusion MRI. AJR. Am. J. Roentgenol. 183 (5), 1247–1252.

Holodny, A.I., Ollenschlager, M., 2002. Diffusion imaging in brain tumors. NeuroImaging Clin. N. Am. 12 (1), 107–124, x.

Horger, M., Fenchel, M., Nägele, T., et al., 2009. Water diffusivity: comparison of primary CNS lymphoma and astrocytic tumor infiltrating the corpus callosum. AJR. Am. J. Roentgenol. 193 (5), 1384–1387.

Hunter, S.B., Ballinger, W.E Jr, Rubin, J.J., 1987. Multiple sclerosis mimicking primary brain tumor. Arch. Pathol. Lab. Med. 111 (5), 464–468.

Jain, R., Ellika, S.K., Scarpace, L., et al., 2008. Quantitative estimation of permeability surface-area product in astroglial brain tumors using perfusion CT and correlation with histopathologic grade. AJNR. Am. J. Neuroradiol 29 (4), 694–700.

Jain, R.K., Munn, L.L., Fukumura, D., 2002. Dissecting tumour pathophysiology using intravital microscopy. Nat. Rev. Cancer 2 (4), 266–276.

Kalis, M., Bowen, B.C., Quencer, R.M., et al., 2007. Metabolite findings in tumefactive demyelinating lesions utilizing short echo time proton magnetic resonance spectroscopy. AJNR. Am. J. Neuroradiol 28 (8), 1427; author reply 1427–1428.

Kallenberg, K., Bock, H.C., Helms, G., et al., 2009. Untreated glioblastoma multiforme: increased myo-inositol and glutamine levels in the contralateral cerebral hemisphere at proton MR spectroscopy. Radiology 253 (3), 805–812.

Kanner, A.A., Vogelbaum, M.A., Mayberg, M.R., et al., 2002. Intracranial navigation by using low-field intraoperative magnetic resonance imaging: preliminary experience. J. Neurosurg 97 (5), 1115–1124.

Karaarslan, E., Arslan, A., 2008. Diffusion weighted MR imaging in non-infarct lesions of the brain. Eur. J. Radiol. 65 (3), 402–416.

Kelly, P.J., Daumas-Duport, C., Kispert, D.B., et al., 1987. Imaging-based stereotaxic serial biopsies in untreated intracranial glial neoplasms. J. Neurosurg 66 (6), 865–874.

Kim, D.S., Na, D.G., Kim, K.H., et al., 2009. Distinguishing tumefactive demyelinating lesions from glioma or central nervous system lymphoma: added value of unenhanced CT compared with conventional contrast-enhanced MR imaging. Radiology 251 (2), 467–475.

Kitis, O., Altay, H., Calli, C., et al., 2005. Minimum apparent diffusion coefficients in the evaluation of brain tumors. Eur. J. Radiol. 55 (3), 393–400.

Knopp, E.A., Cha, S., Johnson, G., et al., 1999. Glial neoplasms: dynamic contrast-enhanced T2*-weighted MR imaging. Radiology 211 (3), 791–798.

Kono, K., Inoue, Y., Nakayama, K., et al., 2001. The role of diffusion-weighted imaging in patients with brain tumors. AJNR. Am. J. Neuroradiol 22 (6), 1081–1088.

Krishnan, R., Raabe, A., Hattingen, E., et al., 2004. Functional magnetic resonance imaging-integrated neuronavigation: correlation between lesion-to-motor cortex distance and outcome. Neurosurgery 55 (4), 904–914; discussion 914–915.

Krohn, K.A., Mankoff, D.A., Muzi, M., et al., 2005. True tracers: comparing FDG with glucose and FLT with thymidine. Nucl. Med. Biol. 32 (7), 663–671.

Kumar, A.J., Leeds, N.E., Fuller, G.N., et al., 2000. Malignant gliomas: MR imaging spectrum of radiation therapy- and chemotherapy-induced necrosis of the brain after treatment. Radiology 217 (2), 377–384.

Lacerda, S., Law, M., 2009. Magnetic resonance perfusion and permeability imaging in brain tumors. NeuroImaging Clin. N. Am. 19 (4), 527–557.

Lai, P.H., Ho, J.T., Chen, W.L., et al., 2002. Brain abscess and necrotic brain tumor: discrimination with proton MR spectroscopy and diffusion-weighted imaging. AJNR. Am. J. Neuroradiol 23 (8), 1369–1377.

Laigle-Donadey, F., Taillibert, S., Mokhtari, K., et al., 2005. Dural metastases. J. Neurooncol. 75 (1), 57–61.

Lam, C.H., Hall, W.A., Truwit, C.L., et al., 2001. Intra-operative MRI-guided approaches to the pediatric posterior fossa tumors. Pediatr. Neurosurg 34 (6), 295–300.

Langleben, D.D., Segall, G.M., 2000. PET in differentiation of recurrent brain tumor from radiation injury. J. Nucl. Med. 41 (11), 1861–1867.

Lansberg, M.G., Thijs, V.N., O'Brien, M.W., et al., 2001. Evolution of apparent diffusion coefficient, diffusion-weighted, and T2-weighted signal intensity of acute stroke. AJNR. Am. J. Neuroradiol 22 (4), 637–644.

Law, M., Oh, S., Babb, J.S., et al., 2006. Low-grade gliomas: dynamic susceptibility-weighted contrast-enhanced perfusion MR imaging – prediction of patient clinical response. Radiology 238 (2), 658–667.

Law, M., Yang, S., Babb, J.S., et al., 2004. Comparison of cerebral blood volume and vascular permeability from dynamic susceptibility contrast-enhanced perfusion MR imaging with glioma grade. AJNR. Am. J. Neuroradiol 25 (5), 746–755.

Law, M., Yang, S., Wang, H., et al., 2003. Glioma grading: sensitivity, specificity, and predictive values of perfusion MR imaging and proton MR spectroscopic imaging compared with conventional MR imaging. AJNR. Am. J. Neuroradiol 24 (10), 1989–1998.

Law, M., Young, R.J., Babb, J.S., et al., 2008. Gliomas: predicting time to progression or survival with cerebral blood volume measurements at dynamic susceptibility-weighted contrast-enhanced perfusion MR imaging. Radiology 247 (2), 490–498.

Le Bihan, D., Mangin, J.F., Poupon, C., et al., 2001. Diffusion tensor imaging: concepts and applications. J. Magn. Reson. Imaging 13 (4), 534–546.

Lee, E.J., Lee, S.K., Agid, R., et al., 2008. Preoperative grading of presumptive low-grade astrocytomas on MR imaging: diagnostic value of minimum apparent diffusion coefficient. AJNR. Am. J. Neuroradiol 29 (10), 1872–1877.

Leksell, L., 1956. Echo-encephalography. I. Detection of intracranial complications following head injury. Acta. Chir. Scand. 110 (4), 301–315.

Lev, M.H., Ozsunar, Y., Henson, J.W., et al., 2004. Glial tumor grading and outcome prediction using dynamic spin-echo MR susceptibility mapping compared with conventional contrast-enhanced MR: confounding effect of elevated rCBV of oligodendrogliomas [corrected]. AJNR. Am. J. Neuroradiol 25 (2), 214–221.

Levivier, M., Goldman, S., Pirotte, B., et al., 1995. Diagnostic yield of stereotactic brain biopsy guided by positron emission tomography with [18F]fluorodeoxyglucose. J. Neurosurg 82 (3), 445–452.

Lewin, J.S., 1999. Interventional MR imaging: concepts, systems, and applications in neuroradiology. AJNR. Am. J. Neuroradiol 20 (5), 735–748.

Lichy, M.P., Bachert, P., Henze, M., et al., 2004a. Monitoring individual response to brain-tumour chemotherapy: proton MR spectroscopy in a patient with recurrent glioma after stereotactic radiotherapy. Neuroradiology 46 (2), 126–129.

Lichy, M.P., Henze, M., Plathow, C., et al., 2004b. [Metabolic imaging to follow stereotactic radiation of gliomas – the role of 1H MR spectroscopy in comparison to FDG-PET and IMT-SPECT]. Rofo. 176 (8), 1114–1121.

Lim, C.C., Roberts, T.P., Sitoh, Y.Y., et al., 2003. Rising signal intensity observed in extra-axial brain tumours – a potential pitfall in perfusion MR imaging. Singapore. Med. J. 44 (10), 526–530.

Lindner, D., Trantakis, C., Renner, C., et al., 2006. Application of intraoperative 3D ultrasound during navigated tumor resection. Minim Invasive Neurosurg 49 (4), 197–202.

Litofsky, N.S., Bauer, A.M., Kasper, R.S., et al., 2006. Image-guided resection of high-grade glioma: patient selection factors and outcome. Neurosurg Focus 20 (4), E16.

Lu, S., Ahn, D., Johnson, G., et al., 2003. Peritumoral diffusion tensor imaging of high-grade gliomas and metastatic brain tumors. AJNR. Am. J. Neuroradiol 24 (5), 937–941.

Lucchinetti, C.F., Gavrilova, R.H., Metz, I., et al., 2008. Clinical and radiographic spectrum of pathologically confirmed tumefactive multiple sclerosis. Brain 131 (Pt 7), 1759–1775.

Luthra, G., Parihar, A., Nath, K., et al., 2007. Comparative evaluation of fungal, tubercular, and pyogenic brain abscesses with conventional and diffusion MR imaging and proton MR spectroscopy. AJNR. Am. J. Neuroradiol 28 (7), 1332–1338.

Macdonald, D.R., Cascino, T.L., Schold, S.C. Jr., et al., 1990. Response criteria for phase II studies of supratentorial malignant glioma. J. Clin. Oncol. 8 (7), 1277–1280.

Maia, A.C. Jr, Malheiros, S.M., da Rocha, A.J., et al., 2005. MR cerebral blood volume maps correlated with vascular endothelial growth factor expression and tumor grade in nonenhancing gliomas. AJNR. Am. J. Neuroradiol 26 (4), 777–783.

Malhotra, H.S., Jain, K.K., Agarwal, A., et al., 2009. Characterization of tumefactive demyelinating lesions using MR imaging and in-vivo proton MR spectroscopy. Mult. Scler. 15 (2), 193–203.

Mandonnet, E., Delattre, J.Y., Tanguy, M.L., et al., 2003. Continuous growth of mean tumor diameter in a subset of grade II gliomas. Ann. Neurol. 53 (4), 524–528.

Mardor, Y., Pfeffer, R., Spiegelmann, R., et al., 2003. Early detection of response to radiation therapy in patients with brain malignancies using conventional and high b-value diffusion-weighted magnetic resonance imaging. J. Clin. Oncol. 21 (6), 1094–1100.

Massager, N., David, P., Goldman, S., et al., 2000. Combined magnetic resonance imaging- and positron emission tomography-guided stereotactic biopsy in brainstem mass lesions: diagnostic yield in a series of 30 patients. J. Neurosurg 93 (6), 951–957.

Mäurer, M., Becker, G., Wagner, R., et al., 2000. Early postoperative transcranial sonography (TCS), C T, and MRI after resection of high-grade glioma: evaluation of residual tumour and its influence on prognosis. Acta. Neurochir. (Wien) 142 (10), 1089–1097.

Mechtler, L., 2009. Neuroimaging in neuro-oncology. Neurol. Clin. 27 (1), 171–201, ix.

Mena, H., Ribas, J.L., Pezeshkpour, G.H., et al., 1991. Hemangiopericytoma of the central nervous system: a review of 94 cases. Hum. Pathol. 22 (1), 84–91.

Morofuji, Y., Matsuo, T., Hayashi, Y., et al., 2008. Usefulness of intraoperative photodynamic diagnosis using 5-aminolevulinic acid for meningiomas with cranial invasion: technical case report. Neurosurgery 62 (Suppl. 1), 102–104.

Morofuji, Y., Matsuo, T., Toyoda, K., et al., 2007. [Skull metastasis of hepatocellular carcinoma successfully treated by intraoperative photodynamic diagnosis using 5-aminolevulinic acid: case report]. No. Shinkei. Geka. 35 (9), 913–918.

Mujic, A., Liddell, J., Hunn, A., et al., 2002. Non-neoplastic demyelinating process mimicking a disseminated malignant brain tumour. J. Clin. Neurosci. 9 (3), 313–317.

Mullins, M.E., 2006. MR spectroscopy: truly molecular imaging; past, present and future. NeuroImaging Clin. N. Am. 16 (4), 605–618, viii.

Murakami, R., Hirai, T., Sugahara, T., et al., 2009. Grading astrocytic tumors by using apparent diffusion coefficient parameters: superiority of a one- versus two-parameter pilot method. Radiology 251 (3), 838–845.

Murakami, R., Sugahara, T., Nakamura, H., et al., 2007. Malignant supratentorial astrocytoma treated with postoperative radiation therapy: prognostic value of pretreatment quantitative diffusion-weighted MR imaging. Radiology 243 (2), 493–499.

Nagar, V.A., Ye, J.R., Ng, W.H., et al., 2008. Diffusion-weighted MR imaging: diagnosing atypical or malignant meningiomas and detecting tumor dedifferentiation. AJNR. Am. J. Neuroradiol 29 (6), 1147–1152.

Nakao, N., Nakai, K., Itakura, T., 2003. Updating of neuronavigation based on images intraoperatively acquired with a mobile computerized tomographic scanner: technical note. Minim Invasive Neurosurg 46 (2), 117–120.

Narayana, A., Kelly, P., Golfinos, J., et al., 2009. Antiangiogenic therapy using bevacizumab in recurrent high-grade glioma: impact on local control and patient survival. J. Neurosurg 110 (1), 173–180.

Nayak, L., Abrey, L.E., Iwamoto, F.M., 2009. Intracranial dural metastases. Cancer 115 (9), 1947–1953.

Nelson, S.J., McKnight, T.R., Henry, R.G., 2002. Characterization of untreated gliomas by magnetic resonance spectroscopic imaging. NeuroImaging Clin. N. Am. 12 (4), 599–613.

Nesbit, G.M., Forbes, G.S., Scheithauer, B.W., et al., 1991. Multiple sclerosis: histopathologic and MR and/or CT correlation in 37 cases at biopsy and three cases at autopsy. Radiology 180 (2), 467–474.

Nimsky, C., Fujita, A., Ganslandt, O., et al., 2004a. Volumetric assessment of glioma removal by intraoperative high-field magnetic resonance imaging. Neurosurgery 55 (2), 358–371.

Nimsky, C., Ganslandt, O., Gralla, J., et al., 2003. Intraoperative low-field magnetic resonance imaging in pediatric neurosurgery. Pediatr. Neurosurg 38 (2), 83–89.

Nimsky, C., Ganslandt, O., Tomandl, B., et al., 2002. Low-field magnetic resonance imaging for intraoperative use in neurosurgery: a 5-year experience. Eur. Radiol. 12 (11), 2690–2703.

Nimsky, C., Ganslandt, O., Von Keller, B., et al., 2004b. Intraoperative high-field-strength MR imaging: implementation and experience in 200 patients. Radiology 233 (1), 67–78.

Norden, A.D., Drappatz, J., Muzikansky, A., et al., 2009a. An exploratory survival analysis of anti-angiogenic therapy for recurrent malignant glioma. J. Neurooncol. 92 (2), 149–155.

Norden, A.D., Drappatz, J., Wen, P.Y., 2009b. Antiangiogenic therapies for high-grade glioma. Nat. Rev. Neurol. 5 (11), 610–620.

Norden, A.D., Young, G.S., Setayesh, K., et al., 2008. Bevacizumab for recurrent malignant gliomas: efficacy, toxicity, and patterns of recurrence. Neurology 70 (10), 779–787.

Olivero, W.C., Dulebohn, S.C., Lister, J.R., 1995. The use of PET in evaluating patients with primary brain tumours: is it useful? J. Neurol. Neurosurg Psychiatry 58 (2), 250–252.

Padma, M.V., Said, S., Jacobs, M., et al., 2003. Prediction of pathology and survival by FDG PET in gliomas. J. Neurooncol. 64 (3), 227–237.

Pallud, J., Mandonnet, E., Duffau, H., et al., 2006. Prognostic value of initial magnetic resonance imaging growth rates for World Health Organization grade II gliomas. Ann. Neurol. 60 (3), 380–383.

Pierallini, A., Bonamini, M., Bozzao, A., et al., 1997. Supratentorial diffuse astrocytic tumours: proposal of an MRI classification. Eur. Radiol. 7 (3), 395–399.

Pierpaoli, C., Jezzard, P., Basser, P.J., et al., 1996. Diffusion tensor MR imaging of the human brain. Radiology 201 (3), 637–648.

Pirotte, B., Acerbi, F., Lubansu, A., et al., 2007a. PET imaging in the surgical management of pediatric brain tumors. Childs. Nerv. Syst. 23 (7), 739–751.

Pirotte, B., Goldman, S., Dewitte, O., et al., 2006. Integrated positron emission tomography and magnetic resonance imaging-guided resection of brain tumors: a report of 103 consecutive procedures. J. Neurosurg 104 (2), 238–253.

Pirotte, B., Goldman, S., Massager, N., et al., 2004a. Combined use of 18F-fluorodeoxyglucose and 11C-methionine in 45 positron emission tomography-guided stereotactic brain biopsies. J. Neurosurg 101 (3), 476–483.

Pirotte, B., Goldman, S., Massager, N., et al., 2004b. Comparison of 18F-FDG and 11C-methionine for PET-guided stereotactic brain biopsy of gliomas. J. Nucl. Med. 45 (8), 1293–1298.

Pirotte, B., Goldman, S., Van Bogaert, P., et al., 2005. Integration of [11C]methionine-positron emission tomographic and magnetic resonance imaging for image-guided surgical resection of infiltrative low-grade brain tumors in children. Neurosurgery 57 (Suppl. 1), 128–139.

Pirotte, B.J., Levivier, M., Goldman, S., et al., 2009. Positron emission tomography-guided volumetric resection of supratentorial high-grade gliomas: a survival analysis in 66 consecutive patients. Neurosurgery 64 (3), 471–481; discussion 481.

Pirotte, B.J., Lubansu, A., Massager, N., et al., 2007b. Results of positron emission tomography guidance and reassessment of the utility of and indications for stereotactic biopsy in children with infiltrative brainstem tumors. J. Neurosurg 107 (Suppl. 5), 392–399.

Provenzale, J.M., Mukundan, S., Barboriak, D.P., 2006. Diffusion-weighted and perfusion MR imaging for brain tumor characterization and assessment of treatment response. Radiology 239 (3), 632–649.

Provenzale, J.M., Wang, G.R., Brenner, T., et al., 2002. Comparison of permeability in high-grade and low-grade brain tumors using dynamic susceptibility contrast MR imaging. AJR. Am. J. Roentgenol. 178 (3), 711–716.

Rabinov, J.D., Lee, P.L., Barker, F.G., et al., 2002. In vivo 3-T MR spectroscopy in the distinction of recurrent glioma versus radiation effects: initial experience. Radiology 225 (3), 871–879.

Radhakrishnan, K., Mokri, B., Parisi, J.E., et al., 1995. The trends in incidence of primary brain tumors in the population of Rochester, Minnesota. Ann. Neurol. 37 (1), 67–73.

Rees, J., Watt, H., Jäger, H.R., et al., 2009. Volumes and growth rates of untreated adult low-grade gliomas indicate risk of early malignant transformation. Eur. J. Radiol. 72 (1), 54–64.

Regula, J., MacRobert, A.J., Gorchein, A., et al., 1995. Photosensitisation and photodynamic therapy of oesophageal, duodenal, and colorectal tumours using 5 aminolaevulinic acid induced protoporphyrin IX – a pilot study. Gut. 36 (1), 67–75.

Reijneveld, J.C., van der Grond, J., Ramos, L.M., et al., 2005. Proton MRS imaging in the follow-up of patients with suspected low-grade gliomas. Neuroradiology 47 (12), 887–891.

Rennie, J.M., Hagmann, C.F., Robertson, N.J., 2008. Neonatal cerebral investigation, second ed. Cambridge University Press, Cambridge.

Ricci, P.E., Karis, J.P., Heiserman, J.E., et al., 1998. Differentiating recurrent tumor from radiation necrosis: time for re-evaluation of positron emission tomography? AJNR. Am. J. Neuroradiol 19 (3), 407–413.

Rock, J.P., Scarpace, L., Hearshen, D., et al., 2004. Associations among magnetic resonance spectroscopy, apparent diffusion coefficients, and image-guided histopathology with special attention to radiation necrosis. Neurosurgery 54 (5), 1111–1119.

Roth, J., Beni Adani, L., Biyani, N., et al., 2006. Intraoperative portable 0.12-tesla MRI in pediatric neurosurgery. Pediatr. Neurosurg 42 (2), 74–80.

Ruben, J.D., Dally, M., Bailey, M., et al., 2006. Cerebral radiation necrosis: incidence, outcomes, and risk factors with emphasis on radiation parameters and chemotherapy. Int. J. Radiat. Oncol. Biol. Phys. 65 (2), 499–508.

Rumboldt, Z., Camacho, D.L., Lake, D., et al., 2006. Apparent diffusion coefficients for differentiation of cerebellar tumors in children. AJNR. Am. J. Neuroradiol 27 (6), 1362–1369.

Rygh, O.M., Selbekk, T., Torp, S.H., et al., 2008. Comparison of navigated 3D ultrasound findings with histopathology in subsequent phases of glioblastoma resection. Acta. Neurochir. (Wien) 150 (10), 1033–1041; discussion 1042.

Sadeghi, N., D'Haene, N., Decaestecker, C., et al., 2008. Apparent diffusion coefficient and cerebral blood volume in brain gliomas: relation to tumor cell density and tumor microvessel density based on stereotactic biopsies. AJNR. Am. J. Neuroradiol 29 (3), 476–482.

Saindane, A.M., Cha, S., Law, M., et al., 2002. Proton MR spectroscopy of tumefactive demyelinating lesions. AJNR. Am. J. Neuroradiol 23 (8), 1378–1386.

Samdani, A., Jallo, G.I., 2007. Intraoperative MRI: technology, systems, and application to pediatric brain tumors. Surg. Technol. Int. 16, 236–243.

Sanai, N., Berger, M.S., 2008. Glioma extent of resection and its impact on patient outcome. Neurosurgery 62 (4), 753–766.

Sasaki, M., Kuwabara, Y., Yoshida, T., et al., 1998. A comparative study of thallium-201 SPET, carbon-11 methionine PET and fluorine-18 fluorodeoxyglucose PET for the differentiation of astrocytic tumours. Eur. J. Nucl. Med. 25 (9), 1261–1269.

Saunders, D.E., Phipps, K.P., Wade, A.M., et al., 2005. Surveillance imaging strategies following surgery and/or radiotherapy for childhood cerebellar low-grade astrocytoma. J. Neurosurg 102 (Suppl. 2), 172–178.

Schaefer, P.W., Grant, P.E., Gonzalez, R.G., 2000. Diffusion-weighted MR imaging of the brain. Radiology 217 (2), 331–345.

Schneider, J.P., Trantakis, C., Rubach, M., et al., 2005. Intraoperative MRI to guide the resection of primary supratentorial glioblastoma multiforme – a quantitative radiological analysis. Neuroradiology 47 (7), 489–500.

Schwartz, K.M., Erickson, B.J., Lucchinetti, C., 2006. Pattern of T2 hypointensity associated with ring-enhancing brain lesions can help to differentiate pathology. Neuroradiology 48 (3), 143–149.

Schwartz, R.B., Hsu, L., Wong, T.Z., et al., 1999. Intraoperative MR imaging guidance for intracranial neurosurgery: experience with the first 200 cases. Radiology 211 (2), 477–488.

Scott, J.N., Brasher, P.M., Sevick, R.J., et al., 2002. How often are nonenhancing supratentorial gliomas malignant? A population study. Neurology 59 (6), 947–949.

Selbekk, T., Bang, J., Unsgaard, G., 2005. Strain processing of intraoperative ultrasound images of brain tumors: initial results. Ultrasound. Med. Biol. 31 (1), 45–51.

Senft, C., Seifert, V., Hermann, E., et al., 2008. Usefulness of intraoperative ultra low-field magnetic resonance imaging in glioma surgery. Neurosurgery 63 (4 Suppl. 2), 257–267.

Serizawa, T., Saeki, N., Higuchi, Y., et al., 2005. Diagnostic value of thallium-201 chloride single-photon emission computerized tomography in differentiating tumor recurrence from radiation injury after gamma knife surgery for metastatic brain tumors. J. Neurosurg 102 (Suppl.), 266–271.

Shin, J.H., Lee, H.K., Kwun, B.D., et al., 2002. Using relative cerebral blood flow and volume to evaluate the histopathologic grade of cerebral gliomas: preliminary results. AJR. Am. J. Roentgenol. 179 (3), 783–789.

Sijens, P.E., Oudkerk, M., 2002. Diagnosing dural metastases. Neuroradiology 44 (3), 275; author reply 276.

Smith, J.K., Castillo, M., Kwock, L., 2003. MR spectroscopy of brain tumors. Magn. Reson. Imaging Clin. N. Am. 11 (3), 415–429, v–vi.

Smith, J.S., Cha, S., Mayo, M.C., et al., 2005. Serial diffusion-weighted magnetic resonance imaging in cases of glioma: distinguishing tumor recurrence from postresection injury. J. Neurosurg 103 (3), 428–438.

Sorensen, A.G., Patel, S., Harmath, C., et al., 2001. Comparison of diameter and perimeter methods for tumor volume calculation. J. Clin. Oncol. 19 (2), 551–557.

Spence, A.M., Mankoff, D.A., Muzi, M., 2003. Positron emission tomography imaging of brain tumors. NeuroImaging Clin. N. Am. 13 (4), 717–739.

Spence, A.M., Muzi, M., Mankoff, D.A., et al., 2004. 18F-FDG PET of gliomas at delayed intervals: improved distinction between tumor and normal gray matter. J. Nucl. Med. 45 (10), 1653–1659.

Stadnik, T.W., Demaerel, P., Luypaert, R.R., et al., 2003. Imaging tutorial: differential diagnosis of bright lesions on diffusion-weighted MR images. Radiographics. 23 (1), e7.

Stark-Vance, V., 2005. Bevacizumab and CPT-11 in the treatment of relapsed malignant glioma. Neuro. Oncol. 7, 369.

Stepp, H., Beck, T., Pongratz, T., et al., 2007. ALA and malignant glioma: fluorescence-guided resection and photodynamic treatment. J. Environ. Pathol. Toxicol. Oncol. 26 (2), 157–164.

Stuckey, S.L., Wijedeera, R., 2008. Multicentric/multifocal cerebral lesions: can fluid-attenuated inversion recovery aid the differentiation between glioma and metastases? J. Med. Imaging Radiat. Oncol. 52 (2), 134–139.

Stummer, W., Beck, T., Beyer, W., et al., 2008a. Long-sustaining response in a patient with non-resectable, distant recurrence of glioblastoma multiforme treated by interstitial photodynamic therapy using 5-ALA: case report. J. Neurooncol. 87 (1), 103–109.

Stummer, W., Pichlmeier, U., Meinel, T., et al., 2006. Fluorescence-guided surgery with 5-aminolevulinic acid for resection of malignant glioma: a randomised controlled multicentre phase III trial. Lancet. Oncol. 7 (5), 392–401.

Stummer, W., Reulen, H.J., Meinel, T., et al., 2008b. Extent of resection and survival in glioblastoma multiforme: identification of and adjustment for bias. Neurosurgery 62 (3), 564–576.

Stummer, W., Stocker, S., Wagner, S., et al., 1998. Intraoperative detection of malignant gliomas by 5-aminolevulinic acid-induced porphyrin fluorescence. Neurosurgery 42 (3), 518–526.

Sugahara, T., Korogi, Y., Kochi, M., et al., 1998. Correlation of MR imaging-determined cerebral blood volume maps with histologic and angiographic determination of vascularity of gliomas. AJR. Am. J. Roentgenol. 171 (6), 1479–1486.

Sugahara, T., Korogi, Y., Tomiguchi, S., et al., 2000. Posttherapeutic intraaxial brain tumor: the value of perfusion-sensitive contrast-enhanced MR imaging for differentiating tumor recurrence from nonneoplastic contrast-enhancing tissue. AJNR. Am. J. Neuroradiol 21 (5), 901–909.

Sutherland, G.R., Kaibara, T., Louw, D., et al., 1999. A mobile high-field magnetic resonance system for neurosurgery. J. Neurosurg 91 (5), 804–813.

Taal, W., Brandsma, D., de Bruin, H.G., et al., 2008. Incidence of pseudo-progression in a cohort of malignant glioma patients treated with chemoirradiation with temozolomide. Cancer 113 (2), 405–410.

Tan, H.M., Chan, L.L., Chuah, K.L., et al., 2004. Monophasic, solitary tumefactive demyelinating lesion: neuroimaging features and neuropathological diagnosis. Br. J. Radiol. 77 (914), 153–156.

Tang, Y.M., Ngai, S., Stuckey, S., 2006. The solitary enhancing cerebral lesion: can FLAIR aid the differentiation between glioma and metastasis? AJNR. Am. J. Neuroradiol 27 (3), 609–611.

Tie, J., Gunawardana, D.H., Rosenthal, M.A., 2008. Differentiation of tumor recurrence from radiation necrosis in high-grade gliomas using 201Tl-SPECT. J. Clin. Neurosci. 15 (12), 1327–1334.

Toh, C.H., Castillo, M., Wong, A.M., et al., 2008a. Differentiation between classic and atypical meningiomas with use of diffusion tensor imaging. AJNR. Am. J. Neuroradiol 29 (9), 1630–1635.

Toh, C.H., Castillo, M., Wong, A.M., et al., 2008b. Primary cerebral lymphoma and glioblastoma multiforme: differences in diffusion characteristics evaluated with diffusion tensor imaging. AJNR. Am. J. Neuroradiol 29 (3), 471–475.

Träber, F., Block, W., Flacke, S., et al., 2002. [1H-MR Spectroscopy of brain tumors in the course of radiation therapy: Use of fast spectroscopic imaging and single-voxel spectroscopy for diagnosing recurrence]. Rofo. 174 (1), 33–42.

Tronnier, V.M., Wirtz, C.R., Knauth, M., et al., 1997. Intraoperative diagnostic and interventional magnetic resonance imaging in neurosurgery. Neurosurgery 40 (5), 891–902.

Tsui, E.Y., Chan, J.H., Ramsey, R.G., et al., 2001. Late temporal lobe necrosis in patients with nasopharyngeal carcinoma: evaluation with combined multi-section diffusion weighted and perfusion weighted MR imaging. Eur. J. Radiol. 39 (3), 133–138.

Unsgaard, G., Gronningsaeter, A., Ommedal, S., et al., 2002a. Brain operations guided by real-time two-dimensional ultrasound: new possibilities as a result of improved image quality. Neurosurgery 51 (2), 402–412.

Unsgaard, G., Ommedal, S., Muller, T., et al., 2002b. Neuronavigation by intraoperative three-dimensional ultrasound: initial experience during brain tumor resection. Neurosurgery 50 (4), 804–812, discussion 812.

Utsuki, S., Miyoshi, N., Oka, H., et al., 2007. Fluorescence-guided resection of metastatic brain tumors using a 5-aminolevulinic acid-induced protoporphyrin IX: pathological study. Brain Tumor. Pathol. 24 (2), 53–55.

van den Bent, M.J., Vogelbaum, M.A., Wen, P.Y., et al., 2009. End point assessment in gliomas: novel treatments limit usefulness of classical Macdonald's Criteria. J. Clin. Oncol. 27 (18), 2905–2908.

Vredenburgh, J.J., Desjardins, A., Herndon, J.E. 2nd, et al., 2007a. Phase II trial of bevacizumab and irinotecan in recurrent malignant glioma. Clin. Cancer Res. 13 (4), 1253–1259.

Vredenburgh, J.J., Desjardins, A., Herndon, J.E. 2nd, et al., 2007b. Bevacizumab plus irinotecan in recurrent glioblastoma multiforme. J. Clin. Oncol. 25 (30), 4722–4729.

Wallace, E.W., 2004. The dural tail sign. Radiology 233 (1), 56–57.

Wang, S.X., Boethius, J., Ericson, K., 2006. FDG-PET on irradiated brain tumor: ten years' summary. Acta. Radiol. 47 (1), 85–90.

Wang, Z., Sutton, L.N., Cnaan, A., et al., 1995. Proton MR spectroscopy of pediatric cerebellar tumors. AJNR. Am. J. Neuroradiol 16 (9), 1821–1833.

Warren, K.E., Patronas, N., Aikin, A.A., et al., 2001. Comparison of one-, two-, and three-dimensional measurements of childhood brain tumors. J. Natl. Cancer Inst. 93 (18), 1401–1405.

Weingarten, D.M., Asthagiri, A.R., Butman, J.A., et al., 2009. Cortical mapping and frameless stereotactic navigation in the high-field intraoperative magnetic resonance imaging suite. J. Neurosurg 111 (6), 1185–1190.

Willems, P.W., Taphoorn, M.J., Burger, H., et al., 2006. Effectiveness of neuronavigation in resecting solitary intracerebral contrast-enhancing tumors: a randomized controlled trial. J. Neurosurg 104 (3), 360–368.

Wintermark, M., Sesay, M., Barbier, E., et al., 2005. Comparative overview of brain perfusion imaging techniques. Stroke 36 (9), e83–e99.

Wong, T.Z., Turkington, T.G., Hawk, T.C., et al., 2004. PET and brain tumor image fusion. Cancer J. 10 (4), 234–242.

Wong, T.Z., van der Westhuizen, G.J., Coleman, R.E., 2002. Positron emission tomography imaging of brain tumors. NeuroImaging Clin. N. Am. 12 (4), 615–626.

Wu, J.S., Shou, X.F., Yao, C.J., et al., 2009a. Transsphenoidal pituitary macroadenomas resection guided by PoleStar N20 low-field intraoperative magnetic resonance imaging: comparison with early postoperative high-field magnetic resonance imaging. Neurosurgery 65 (1), 63–71.

Wu, J.S., Zhou, L.F., Tang, W.J., et al., 2007. Clinical evaluation and follow-up outcome of diffusion tensor imaging-based functional neuronavigation: a prospective, controlled study in patients with gliomas involving pyramidal tracts. Neurosurgery 61 (5), 935–949.

Wu, W., Shi, J.X., Cheng, H.L., et al., 2009b. Hemangiopericytomas in the central nervous system. J. Clin. Neurosci. 16 (4), 519–523.

Yamasaki, F., Kurisu, K., Satoh, K., et al., 2005. Apparent diffusion coefficient of human brain tumors at MR imaging. Radiology 235 (3), 985–991.

Yang, D., Korogi, Y., Sugahara, T., et al., 2002. Cerebral gliomas: prospective comparison of multivoxel 2D chemical-shift imaging proton MR spectroscopy, echoplanar perfusion and diffusion-weighted MRI. Neuroradiology 44 (8), 656–666.

Yang, S., Law, M., Zagzag, D., et al., 2003. Dynamic contrast-enhanced perfusion MR imaging measurements of endothelial permeability: differentiation between atypical and typical meningiomas. AJNR. Am. J. Neuroradiol 24 (8), 1554–1559.

Zagzag, D., Miller, D.C., Kleinman, G.M., et al., 1993. Demyelinating disease versus tumor in surgical neuropathology. Clues to a correct pathological diagnosis. Am. J. Surg. Pathol. 17 (6), 537–545.

Zhang, H., Rödiger, L.A., Shen, T., et al., 2008. Preoperative subtyping of meningiomas by perfusion MR imaging. Neuroradiology 50 (10), 835–840.

Zuniga, R.M., Torcuator, R., Jain, R., et al., 2009. Efficacy, safety and patterns of response and recurrence in patients with recurrent high-grade gliomas treated with bevacizumab plus irinotecan. J. Neurooncol. 91 (3), 329–336.

11 Neuro-ophthalmology of brain tumors

Helen V. Danesh-Meyer

Introduction

The neuro-ophthalmic assessment plays an essential role in the diagnosis and management of brain tumors. The afferent visual pathway includes the retina optic nerve, chiasm, optic tract, lateral geniculate body, optic radiations, and ends in the occipital lobe. Tumors that compress the afferent pathway often present with visual symptoms. Involvement of the efferent visual pathway produces abnormal eye movements, including motility disturbances, gaze palsies, and nystagmus. Examination of the efferent system involves an external orbital assessment for proptosis, and eyelid abnormalities (such as ptosis and lid retraction) as well ocular motility assessment. The pattern of visual function impairment and motility disturbance allows localization of the tumor.

This chapter will present an overview of the relevant anatomy and highlight the key elements of the neuro-ophthalmic history and examination that is necessary to localize the lesion and understand the constellation of clinical features that consequently result from the lesion.

Relevant anatomy of the afferent visual pathway

The pathway for afferent visual information begins in the retina. The optic nerve head is formed from a coalescence of 1 million axons from the retinal ganglion cells which lie in the inner retina. The optic nerve is divided into the intraocular, infraorbital, intracanicular, and intracranial segments. The optic nerve enters the cranium via the optic canals, extending an average of 12 mm at an inclination of 45° to reach the anterior chiasm.

The optic chiasm is comprised of the decussating fibers from the nasal retina (retinal ganglion cells that lie nasal to the macula) that subserve the temporal hemifield. The temporal hemifield includes the blindspot and fibers from the papillomacular bundle. The ratio of crossed to uncrossed fibers within the chiasm is 53:47. Most fibers in the chiasm are projections from the macular region. In the chiasm, the upper nasal quadrant fibers cross dorsally and posteriorly and lower nasal quadrant fibers cross more anteriorly. The uncrossed fibers maintain their position at the lateral aspects of the chiasm and into the optic tracts (Fig. 11.1).

As they enter the optic tract, the crossed (from the contralateral nasal retina) and uncrossed fibers (from the ipsilateral temporal retina) of the chiasm converge. The macular fibers lie dorsolaterally, and the fibers from the upper retinas and lower retinas are situated dorsomedially and ventrolaterally, respectively. The fibers of the optic tract then synapse primarily in the lateral geniculate body by passing posteriorly around the cerebral peduncle and above the posterior cerebral arteries.

However, fibers from the optic tract travel to other locations. The pupillomotor pathways that subserve the pupillary light reflex leave the optic tract within the brachium of the superior colliculus prior to the lateral geniculate nucleus and synapse in the pretectum. The subcortical visual pathway synapses in the superior colliculus.

The lateral geniculate nucleus (LGN) has six layers. Layers 2, 3, and 5 receive visual input from the retinal ganglion cells from the ipsilateral temporal hemiretina (the nasal field). Layers 1, 4, and 6 receive information from the nasal retina (the temporal field).

The optic radiations are formed by the geniculocalcarine fibers leaving the LGN on their way to the calcarine cortex. The temporal radiations travel anteriorly around the lateral ventricle and form Meyer's loop. These fibers contain information from the superior visual fields. The optic radiations terminate in the occipital lobe or the primary visual cortex.

An important retinotopic organization is preserved throughout the course of the afferent visual pathways. Consequently, the visual field and retina have an inverted and reversed relationship. Relative to the point of fixation which is the fovea, the upper visual field falls on the inferior retina, lower visual field on the superior retina, nasal visual field on the temporal retina, and the temporal visual field on the nasal retina. This upside-down and backward information is preserved throughout the afferent pathway.

Because of this unique anatomic configuration of the chiasm, lesions produce typical changes in visual sensory function, particularly visual field defects. For example, if the chiasm is in a normal or a post-fixed position, enlargement of the third ventricle will compress its posterosuperior aspect, causing bitemporal depression of the inferior fields; if the chiasm is pre-fixed, however, the ventricle will compress the posteroinferior aspect, causing bilateral central scotomas, nasal and arcuate defects, or even superior hemianopic defects.

History of visual symptoms

A thorough history of the details of a patient's symptoms is the most important part of the neuro-ophthalmic evaluation. The symptoms a patient may complain of are listed in Table 11.1.

Visual loss

It is essential to establish if the visual loss is monocular or binocular, and if the onset of the visual loss is gradual,

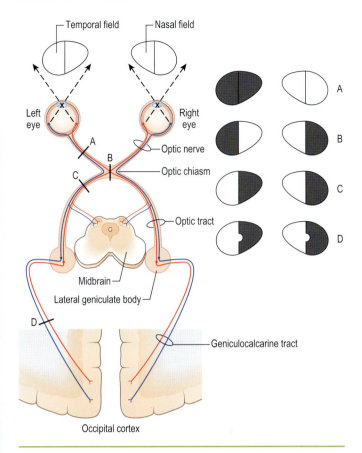

Figure 11.1 The visual pathway showing common patterns of visual field loss. Gray area denotes visual field defects. (A) Monocular visual loss; (B) Bitemporal hemianopia; (C) Right homonymous hemianopia; (D) Right homonymous hemianopia with sparing of central fixation. (From Kaye A H (1991) Essential Neurosurgery. Edinburgh: Churchill Livingstone, 1991. With permission of Elsevier.)

Table 11.1 Symptoms associated with tumors that affect the anterior visual pathway

Symptom	Key feature
Visual loss	Need to distinguish between sudden loss of vision and sudden awareness of visual loss Identify associated features such as pain, diplopia or other symptoms that may suggest an etiology other than optic nerve disease (metamorphopsia, distortion of vision, etc.)
Transient visual obscurations	Feature of raised intracranial pressure Associated with change in posture (supine to upright) Last seconds
Headache	Headaches associated with raised intracranial pressure are worse when lying down, coughing or straining Identify other symptoms of raised intracranial pressure (diplopia, tinnitus, transient visual obscurations)
Diplopia	Need to differentiate between monocular diplopia which is caused by refractive or media opacities and binocular diplopia which is neurologic in origin.

3. Photopsias (positive visual phenomena), such as flashes of lights, shower of sparkles. Photopsia is seen most commonly in retinal disease.

4. A positive scotoma is one that is seen by the patient, such as a purple spot that is often seen after a flash bulb goes off, whereas a negative scotoma refers to a non-seeing area of the visual field. Positive scotomas occur most common with macular disease.

Transient visual obscurations

Transient visual obscurations (TVO) of vision are an important symptom of raised intracranial pressure. Patients usually note unilateral or bilateral 'blacking out' or 'graying out' of vision lasting 10–15 s and recurring many times per day. Classically, it is precipitated by some change in posture or Valsalva manoeuvre (Sadun et al 1984).

Headache

Headache is a common symptom associated with raised intracranial pressure. Such headaches are usually bilateral in the forehead or occiput, and are worse when lying down, on waking, and also when coughing, straining, or bending. The pain is often described as dull, bursting, or throbbing.

Diplopia

Diplopia may be a localizing or a non-localizing symptom. Elevated intracranial pressure may produce unilateral or bilateral abducens palsies. The earliest symptom is often diplopia with horizontal separation of images for distant objects. Later the diplopia may be present on one or both sides.

Examination of afferent visual system

The examination of the afferent visual system involves five key components (Table 11.2):

1. Visual acuity
2. Visual field assessment

sudden, or intermittent. If the visual loss occurs suddenly in one eye, the patient is usually aware of the change, whereas slowly progressive loss may go unnoticed. However, it is necessary to differentiate between sudden loss of vision and the 'sudden awareness of loss of vision'. In the latter, the patient has often incidentally covered the normal seeing eye, and noted poor vision in the other eye, attributing this to an acute event. Details of a previous recording of visual acuity such as a school medical or driver's license examination may be useful in dating a decline in vision. The history taking regarding visual loss should involve ascertainment of any previous known visual loss or relevant past ocular history such as amblyopia, other ocular disorders which may influence vision, and previous eye surgery.

Associated symptoms that should be specifically asked about include:

1. Pain. Pain on eye movement associated with decrease vision occurs in optic neuritis.

2. Metamorphopsia or distortion of vision. Where objects look smaller or straight lines are bent or distorted, a macular rather than an optic nerve abnormality should be suspected.

Table 11.2 Neuro-ophthalmic examination of the afferent visual pathway

Examination	Specific test	Key points
Visual acuity	Snellen VA Near vision	Need to test for best corrected vision with glasses or pinhole Patients over 45 may need reading glasses if testing near vision
Color vision	Ishihara color plates Red desaturation	Optic neuropathies characteristically produce red desaturation Use red target such as top of tropicamide bottle
Pupil	Relative afferent pupillary defect	Assess direct, consensual, anisocoria, convergence and accommodation RAPD Swinging flashlight test for RAPD Brightness sensitivity is excellent surrogate for RAPD
Visual field	Confrontation visual field Amsler grid automated visual field testing	Kinetic red target has highest sensitivity/specificity. But misses significant proportion of mild/moderate defects Amsler measures central 10° Humphrey visual field is Gold Standard
Fundus	Optic nerve swelling or pallor	
Other	Photostress test	

3. Color vision testing
4. Pupil assessment
5. Fundus examination.

Visual acuity

The acuity in each eye should be tested individually. It is helpful to evaluate both distance and near vision. The most widely used tool for measuring distance visual acuity is the Snellen chart, which effectively compares what a patient can see to what a normal person could see at 20 feet (6 meters). The term '20/20' means that the patient sees at 20 feet the line of the Snellen chart that a 'normal' person is expected to see at 20 feet. Most normal people below the age of 40 years can see better than this, and will be able to read the 20/15 (6/5).

The worst numerical value on the chart is 20/200 (or 6/60). If the patient is not able to read the largest letter, visual acuity is then classified as 'counting fingers' (CF), 'hand movements' (HM), 'perception of light' (PL), or 'no perception of light' (NPL).

If a patient is unable to achieve an uncorrected (without help from spectacles) distance acuity of 6/6 or better, the first question which needs to be answered is whether or not this relates to a refractive error in the eye – that is, can the acuity be improved by an appropriate refractive correction? If the patient's glasses are not available then the use of a pin hole eliminates more refractive errors. In practical terms, a pin hole can be expected to improve the acuity by about four lines of the Snellen chart.

Near visual acuity is assessed using pre-printed text sizes, e.g., the Jaeger near vision reading charts will obviously impair near acuity while distance acuity is preserved.

Color vision testing

Methods for testing color vision include:

1. Ishihara pseudo-isochromatic test plates. Each eye should be tested separately. If the patient is not able to see the first plate (Number 12), which is the control plate, then the patient's vision is too poor to perform the remainder of the test and an alternative color vision test should be performed. Visual acuity of approximately 20/400 is required to see these plates. The number of plates correctly identified with each eye is recorded (e.g., 10/14). If only the control plate is identified, then it should be recorded as 'control' only.

2. Color comparison. A comparison of the saturation of colors, between eyes and across the vertical midline may be helpful in identifying subtle optic nerve dysfunction or chiasmal lesions. Use a red pin or the red top of a tropicamide or atropine bottle.

   a. Present the stimulus to each eye separately, approximately 30 cm from the eye being tested.

   b. Place the stimulus in the center of the patient's visual axis and present the stimulus to the two eyes for an equal period of time.

   c. Ask the patient to look directly at the tip of the bottle top.

   d. Ask the patient if 'the bottle top is equally red in both eyes'. An affirmative answer ends the test and the result is recorded as 100% in both eyes.

   e. If the patient indicates that 'redness' of the bottle top differs between the eyes, re-present the stimulus to the eye with normal red perception, and say to the patient, 'if the top of the bottle is 100% red in this eye, then how many percent is the redness of the bottle top in the other eye?'.

The correlation of red comparison by this technique with the presence of a relative afferent pupillary defect when measured with neutral density filters is very high and this test serves as an excellent surrogate for the presence of a relative afferent pupillary defect (Danesh-Meyer et al 2008a).

Pupillary assessment

Pupillary assessment involves identifying any anisocoria, eliciting direct and consensual responses to light on both sides, checking for a relative afferent pupillary defect (RAPD), and examining the response to convergence/accommodation.

The presence of an RAPD is the hallmark of a unilateral or bilateral asymmetric afferent visual abnormality. It is present in optic neuropathies as well as chiasmal and optic tract lesions.

The 'swinging flashlight test' to detect a RAPD defect in effect compares the 'amount of light getting into the brain' through each eye/optic nerve by detecting a change in the size of the pupils as the light source is moved back and forth between the two eyes. The correct way to perform the 'swinging torch test' is to ask the patient to fixate on a distant object (to prevent accommodation and unwanted pupillary constriction). Then shine the light in one eye, then quickly 'flick' it across to the other eye, wait a second or two, then 'flick' it back, and so on.

With the patient fixing in the distance, a bright flashlight is shone from one pupil to the other. With each eye, the light is directed at the pupil long enough to assess the briskness of contraction and the ability to sustain contraction. With an RAPD, the pupil on the side of the optic nerve lesion contracts less briskly or has dilation as its first movement (Thompson et al 1981).

Brightness comparison

There are several circumstances in which it is difficult or not possible to test for an RAPD, such as when the pupils have been pharmacologically dilated, dark irides or a presbyopic examiner. In these circumstances, it is useful to test for brightness comparison. The technique is as follows:

1. Present the same stimulus to each eye separately, approximately 30 cm from the eye being tested.
2. Ensure the eyes are in the primary position.
3. Place the stimulus in the center of the patient's visual axis and ask the patient to fixate on the light.
4. Present the stimulus to the two eyes for an equal period of time.
5. Ask the patient to look directly at the tip of the bottle top.
6. Ask the patient if 'the light is equally bright in both eyes'. An affirmative answer ends the test and the result is recorded as 100% in both eyes.
7. If the patient indicates that the 'brightness' of the bottle top differs between the eyes, re-present the stimuli to the eye with the brighter light perception and say to the patient, 'if the top of the bottle is 100% bright in this eye, then how many percent brightness is the light in the other eye?'.

   The correlation of brightness comparison by this technique with the presence of a relative afferent pupillary defect when measured with neutral density filters is very high and this test serves as an excellent surrogate for the presence of an RAPD (Danesh-Meyer et al 2008a).

Visual field assessment

Assessment of the visual field is one of the fundamental aspects of the afferent visual system examination. The visual field examination helps localize and identify diseases affecting the visual pathways. There are several techniques of visual field testing ranging from confrontation visual field, formal automated perimetry, to Amsler grid testing. The advantage of confrontation visual field testing is that it can be performed by the bedside and does not require specialized equipment. However, it suffers from a relatively low sensitivity and may miss mild to moderate defects. The Gold Standard for visual field testing is automated perimetry with Humphrey visual field testing (Zeiss Meditec, San Diego). This test takes an average of 3–6 min per eye. The Amsler grid can be used to assess the central 10°.

An understanding of the size of the visual field is important prior to visual field testing. The visual fields of each eye overlap centrally. The physiological blindspot corresponds to the optic disc, as it has no overlying photoreceptors and is located 15° temporally in each eye (Table 11.3).

Table 11.3 Size of the visual fields

Direction	Size (degrees)
Superiorly	60
Inferiorly	70–75
Nasally	60
Temporally	100–110
Binocular	120

Confrontation visual fields

Confrontation visual field testing is the most flexible of all techniques. Several different techniques can be used for confrontation fields. The most sensitive technique is the use of a small (5 mm) red target, which is moved inward from beyond the boundary of each quadrant along a line bisecting the horizontal and vertical meridians. The patient is specifically asked to report when the pin is perceived to be red in color. The visual field of each eye should then be checked separately. However, overall confrontation visual field testing has a limited sensitivity (between 25% and 76%). When this test is combined with static finger wiggling in each quadrant, the sensitivity improves to 78% with a specificity of 90%, although the test performance varies with the density of the visual field defect and the underlying etiology. Mild visual field defects are associated with profoundly reduced sensitivities ranging from 0–67%. Red comparison has the best sensitivity for mild defects (<–5 dB), but only a specificity of 28%. To achieve a 50% probability of identifying a visual field defect with a kinetic red target would require a mean deviation of –6 dB loss, which is a moderate visual field loss (Danesh-Meyer et al 2008a).

Important patterns of visual fields (Table 11.3)

In order to understand the pattern of a visual field defect, one must appreciate the topographic relationship between the retina and the visual field.

- The upper visual field falls on the inferior retina (below the fovea)
- The lower nasal field falls on the superior retina (above the fovea)
- The nasal visual field falls on the temporal retina
- The temporal visual field falls on the nasal retina.

Retinal-type field defects

1. Disorders of cones tend to produce a central scotoma as cone density is highest in the center of vision and declines steeply by 3° eccentricity.
2. Disorders of rods tend to produce a ring scotoma, which will affect the mid-periphery first.
3. Macular lesions produce central or paracentral defects (Table 11.4).

Optic nerve-type field defects

Optic neuropathies typically produce nerve fiber bundle defects within the central 30° of the visual field. There are three main types of nerve fiber bundle defects depending on the underlying etiology.

1. Papillomacular bundle: damage to macular fibers that enter the temporal aspect of the disc.

Table 11.4 Patterns of visual field defects

Retinal lesions	Central scotoma (disorder of cones or macula)
	Constriction of periphery or mid-periphery (disorder of rods)
Optic nerve lesions	Central scotoma
	Centro-cecal scotoma
	Paracentral defect
	Arcuate defect
	Altitudinal defect
Chiasmal	Junctional
	Bitemporal visual field loss
Retrochiasmal	Homonymous hemianopic defect
Optic tract	Incomplete homonymous hemianopia
Temporal optic radiations	Superior quadrantanopia
Parietal optic radiations	Inferior quadrantanopia
Superior calcarine fissure	Inferior quadrantanopia
Inferior calcarine fissure	Superior quadrantanopia
Occipital pole	Homonymous paracentral scotoma

a. Central scotoma.

b. Centrocecal scotoma: a central scotoma that is continuous with the blindspot.

c. Paracentral: a defect lying next to, but not involving central fixation.

2. Arcuate defect: damage of fibers from the retina temporal to the disc that enter the superior and inferior poles of the disc.

3. Temporal wedge shape defect: damage of fibers on the nasal side of the disc. These do not necessarily obey the vertical midline.

Chiasmal lesion

1. Junctional scotoma: a lesion of the anterior optic chiasm may produce an optic neuropathy in the ipsilateral eye with a superotemporal field defect in the other eye that respects the vertical meridian. This is thought to be explained by the crossing inferonasal fibers travelling anteriorly towards the contralateral optic nerve before passing into the optic tract. This is known as 'Willebrand's knee', although the anatomical presence of Willebrand's knee is debated.

2. Bitemporal visual field defect: a lesion of the decussating fibers in the optic chiasm causes bitemporal hemifield defects. Compression of the inferior chiasm produces superior and central field defects.

Lesions at or behind the chiasm

These lesions produce characteristic patterns of visual field loss. *Homonymous hemianopic field defects originating from the point of fixation and obeying the vertical meridian.* This occurs contralateral to the side of the lesion. In contrast, optic nerve lesions produce defects that originate from the blindspot and consequently do not respect the vertical meridian. Therefore, it is very helpful to test whether the lesion extends to the midline or to the blindspot.

1. Complete homonymous hemianopias may occur with any lesion of the retrochiasmal visual pathways and do not allow precise localization of the lesions along the retrochiasmal visual pathways. Congruity increases gradually as one proceeds from the chiasm to the striate cortex.

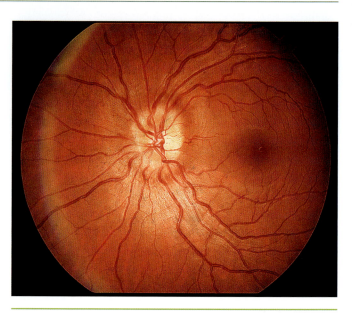

Figure 11.2 Temporal pallor of the right optic nerve head secondary to a clinoidal meningioma compressing the optic nerve.

2. Lesions of the optic tract produce incongruent hemianopias.

3. Damage to Meyer's loop, the temporal optic radiations, produces homonymous superior quadrantanopia.

4. Damage to the parietal optic radiations causes a homonymous inferior quadrantanopia.

5. Lesions of the superior bank of the calcarine fissure produce an inferior quadrantanopia, while a lesion of the inferior calcarine fissure produces a superior quadrantanopia.

6. Macular sparing occurs when the occipital pole is not involved.

7. A lesion of the occipital pole causes a homonymous paracentral scotoma.

Fundus examination

Fundus examination is best performed through a dilated pupil. The optic nerve may appear pale or swollen.

Optic disc pallor (Fig. 11.2)

1. Primary optic atrophy is caused by direct injury of the retinal ganglion cell or its axon and occurs with loss of optic nerve fibers, but minimal damage to optic nerve head anatomy. It occurs as a result of compressive lesions.

2. Secondary optic atrophy is a consequence of severe disc edema. The characteristic appearance is of a grayish disc appearance rather than a white pale disc as seen in primary optic atrophy. The glial proliferation may be sufficient to give a raised appearance to the optic disc margins.

Optic disc swelling

1. Papilledema (Box 11.1). Bilateral optic disc swelling is a sign of raised intracranial pressure. Early papilledema is difficult to detect and requires considerable experience. Features that are helpful in differentiating papilledema from pseudopapilledema:

a. Venous pulsations are absent in papilledema. The presence of venous pulsation of the central retinal vein occurs when the intracranial pressure is <200 mm of water (Walsh et al 1969). The absence of venous pulsation, however, does not mean that intracranial pressure is raised, since about 20% of normal eyes do not show spontaneous pulsation of veins as they enter the optic disc

b. Opacification or burring of the retinal nerve fiber layer adjacent to the superior and inferior disc margins. This is one of the earliest signs of papilledema with the changes being attributed to the swelling of axons from obstructed axoplasmic flow (Hoyt & Knight 1973). The earliest changes are best seen using a red-free light from the ophthalmoscope

c. Nerve fiber layer hemorrhages (splinter hemorrhages)

d. Circumferential retinal folds in peripapillary retina (Bird & Sanders 1973)

e. Cotton wool spots, which are infarcted axons

f. Venous distension and a telangiectatic mesh of small dilated capillaries appears on the disc surface

g. Hard exudates.

2. Unilateral optic disc swelling is most commonly associated with a meningioma located in the anterior orbit.

   a. Optociliary shunt vessel.

Other

1. Photostress test. This test is helpful in differentiating decreased vision from an optic neuropathy from macular disease. In patients with retinal or macular disease, there is a delay in the process of recovery of retinal sensitivity following exposure to bright light. Similarly, severe carotid disease causing global ocular ischemia may cause prolongation of recovery. The test is performed as follows:

   a. Measure the best corrected visual acuity in each eye

   b. The patient should be asked to look at a bright light for 10 s

   c. Record the time it takes for visual acuity to recover to within one line of their best corrected visual acuity

   d. Normal recovery time is <30 s, however, macular or retinal disease may cause prolongation of recovery (Glaser et al 1977).

2. Visually evoked potential measurement is helpful for evaluating optic nerve function.

3. Electroretinogram evaluates retinal function.

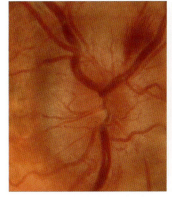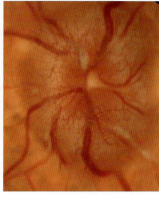

Figure 11.3 Acute papilledema. Note bilateral disc swelling with elevation of the optic nerve head and extensive hemorrhages.

Non-localizing symptoms and signs

Papilledema

Papilledema is the crucial clinical sign of raised intracranial pressure and the term is used synonymously with that disorder. Early papilledema may be difficult to detect with a direct ophthalmoscope.

Intracranial tumors may produce papilledema by several mechanisms:

1. Increase in the total amount of intracranial tissue by the tumor

2. Increase tissue volume by cerebral edema surrounding the tumor

3. The tumor may block the flow of CSF within the ventricular system, producing non-communicating hydrocephalus or within the arachnoid granulations, producing communicating hydrocephalus

4. Compromise cerebral venous outflow

5. The tumor may manufacture CSF.

Features of acute papilledema (Fig. 11.3)
Symptoms
- Often no visual symptoms initially
- Transient visual obscurations:
  - Enlarged blindspot
  - Diplopia
  - Tinnitus or pulsations in ear often worse on lying down.

Signs
- Bilateral swollen optic nerves
- Unilateral or bilateral IVth nerve palsy
- Enlarged blindspot.

Features of chronic papilledema (Fig. 11.4)
Symptoms
- Visual acuity is preserved until very late
- Progressive constriction of visual field loss, usually beginning nasally and leading to generalized constriction. Often undetected until very late
- Visual loss from papilledema can occur with any cause of papilledema.

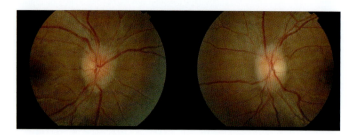

Figure 11.4 Chronic papilledema.

Signs
- Enlarged blindspot
- Pseudo-drusen: small glistening hard exudates become apparent in the superficial disc substance
- Chronic atrophic papilledema may show a pallor of the swollen disc. This is an ominous sign and suggests impending loss of central acuity
- Unilateral or bilateral VIth nerve palsy.

Abducens nerve palsy (VIth nerve palsy)

A unilateral or bilateral abducens nerve paresis may be a false localizing sign. The abducens nerve has a long subarachnoid course, during which it lies between the brainstem and the clivus. With increased intracranial pressure, the nerve may become compressed between the pons and the basilar artery or stretched along the sharp edge of the petrous bone. It resolves within days to weeks once intracranial pressure has normalized.

Hydrocephalus

Hydrocephalus, ventricular enlargement from obstructed flow of CSF, can produce several neuro-ophthalmic symptoms and signs.

1. Disturbances of ocular motility:
   a. Unilateral or bilateral abducens palsy
   b. Divergence paralysis
   c. Trochlear nerve palsy
   d. Oculomotor palsy.
2. Dorsal midbrain syndrome (see below). Obstructive hydrocephalus is a cause of dorsal midbrain syndrome. The earliest sign is light-near dissociation of the pupils. However, often the first recognized feature is vertical gaze paresis and upbeat nystagmus in upgaze. The vertical vestibule-ocular reflex is preserved. Convergence-retraction nystagmus appears next. Finally, there may be tonic downward deviation of both eyes associated with severe lid retraction.

Localizing symptoms and signs

Tumors in the orbit

Tumors in the orbit may present with features of optic nerve compromise because of direct effects on the orbit or its adnexae (Box 11.2).

Clinical features associated with tumors in the orbit are shown in Box 11.3.

Findings on examination
1. Decreased visual acuity.
2. Relative afferent pupillary defect.
3. Decreased color vision.
4. Visual field defect.

Fundus examination
a. Optic nerve pallor. Optic nerve appearance may be normal in the early stages and gradually develops pallor.
b. Optic disc swelling. Mass lesions in the orbit may produce optic nerve swelling by direct compression of the intra-orbital portion of the optic nerve. There may be an associated slowly progressive visual loss and proptosis. Patients with optic nerve meningioma and gliomas often retain good vision. Color vision testing may reveal defects in optic nerve function.
c. Choroidal folds. The presence of choroidal folds and proptosis suggest that a bulky tumor is compressing the posterior globe.
d. Optociliary shunt vessels. Optociliary shunt vessels overlie the optic disc and shunt blood from the retinal to the choroidal circulation. They occur in chronic compression of the intraorbital optic nerve. In this circumstance the triad of ipsilateral visual loss, optic disc swelling that resolves into optic atrophy and optociliary shunt vessels occurs. The triad of optociliary shunt vessels, visual loss and disc pallor is most commonly seen in spheno-orbital meningiomas (Frisen et al 1973; Wright et al 1980).

Abnormal optic nerve function
Patients may complain of sudden loss of vision which may actually represent the sudden awareness of loss of vision that has been inadvertently recognized (by random covering the normal eye). Poor vision may also be an incidental finding when the loss of vision occurs insidiously.

Gaze-evoked amaurosis
Patients with orbital tumors may experience visual loss in the affected eye whenever the eye is placed in a specific eccentric position of gaze. The visual loss disappears when the direction of gaze is changed. The most common lesions responsible for gaze-evoked amaurosis are optic nerve sheath meningiomas or hemangiomas.

Proptosis

Proptosis or protrusion of the globe is the hallmark of orbital disease. It rarely occurs in patients with cavernous sinus disease. Greater than 2 mm of protrusion between the two globes should be considered abnormal. Tumors within the extraocular muscle cone, such as optic nerve meningioma or glioma, produce axial proptosis (protrusion of the eye straight ahead). Masses in other orbital region produce dystopia and the eye is pushed in the opposite direction of the pass (Miller & Newman 2004).

Enophthalmos

Enophthalmos is when the globe is sunken back. Most causes are not due to tumors. However, scirrhous carcinoma of the breast may metastasize to the orbit where it apparently incites a fibrotic reaction that results in progressive enophthalmos.

Limitation of ocular movement

Limitation of ocular motility is not a localizing sign of an orbital tumor. However, if there is associated increased pressure to retropulsion or an increase in intraocular pressure when the patients looks in the field of limitation, it suggests mechanical restriction.

Syndrome of the floor of the orbit

Tumors of the floor of the orbit produce a syndrome with the following features that occur in consecutive stages:

1. Severe pain in the region of the ipsilateral maxilla
2. Anaesthesia of the first two divisions of the trigeminal nerve
3. Growth into the cranial vault
4. Proptosis
5. Diplopia.

Other features

1. Eyelid malposition: retraction or proptosis.
2. Globe displacement.

Common pathology

Optic nerve meningioma

Optic nerve meningiomas (Fig. 11.5) arise from the dural sheath of the intraorbital optic nerve. They occur most commonly in females in the 5th decade, presenting with unilateral painless progressive loss of vision. Patients may experience transient visual loss.

They are often characterized by optic nerve head swelling and the presence of optociliary shunt vessels, which are tortuous dilated veins on the optic disc surface. These drain venous blood from the obstructed central retinal vein, via choroidal veins to the ophthalmic vein (Wright et al 1980; Sibony et al 1984; Sarkies 1987).

Optic nerve meningiomas may extend from the intraorbital, intracanalicular to the intracranial optic nerve. If untreated, they can involve the chiasm and extend into the contralateral optic nerve. Intracanicular optic nerve involvement may also occur in association with a meningioma of the anterior clinoid or tuberculum sellae. Optic nerve meningiomas appear on MRI as a fusiform enlargement of

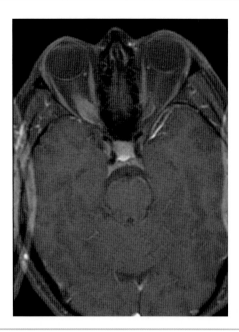

Figure 11.5 Optic nerve meningioma. Magnetic resonance imaging axial image T1 with gadolinium demonstrating right optic nerve meningioma.

the optic nerve/sheath complex. There may also be flattening of the posterior globe due to tumor encroachment. The optic canal may be enlarged. These tumors are hypointense on both T1- and T2-weighted images and typically enhance with gadolinium.

An optic nerve meningioma at the optic canal is rare but should be suspected if there is gradual deterioration of vision with normal neuroimaging (Sanders & Falconer 1964).

Optic nerve glioma

Optic nerve glioma often presents in childhood and can be associated with neurofibromatosis, in which case they are slow growing, presenting with gradual progressive loss of vision and proptosis. Patients with glioma may have quite substantial optic disc swelling and retain good vision. About half are confined to the orbit; the remainder have intracranial extension (Alford & Lofton 1988). MRI will show enlargement of the optic nerve tissue. Lesions on T1-weighted MRI are usually isointense to hypointense and the T2-weighted MRI is hyperintense. The tumor usually enhances but not to the degree typical of meningiomas.

Malignant glioma of adulthood is uncommon. In contrast, these patients present with rapidly progressive unilateral or bilateral visual loss. Significant enhancement of the optic nerve after gadolinium infusion may indicate the presence of optic nerve glioma. Even with aggressive radiation therapy, there is invariable rapid spread of tumor intracranially, and death occurs within months.

Other

- *Carcinomatous or lymphomatous optic neuropathy* is due to meningeal infiltration by neoplastic cells, usually but not always in patients with known metastatic carcinoma or lymphoma.
- *Metastatic.*

Table 11.5 Clinical features of cavernous sinus/orbital apex syndrome

Orbital apex syndrome	Superior orbital fissure syndrome	Cavernous sinus syndrome
Proptosis		
Optic nerve dysfunction	Optic nerve dysfunction	
IIIrd	IIIrd	IIIrd
IVth	IVth	IVth
VIth	VIth	VIth
	V1	V1
	Oculosympathetic pathway	Oculosympathetic pathway
		V2

Tumors involving the cavernous sinus/ superior orbital fissure/orbital apex

Tumors within the orbital apex/superior orbital fissure and cavernous sinus (Table 11.5) primarily produce symptoms and signs related to ocular motor nerve dysfunction. However, there may also be optic nerve dysfunction, oculosympathetic dysfunction, and trigeminal neuropathy. Orbital apex syndrome is usually the term used when multiple ocular motor cranial nerve palsies occur with optic nerve dysfunction. Lesions may be primarily based in the cavernous sinus/superior orbital fissure or may extend laterally from parachiasmal tumors.

Relevant anatomy

Anatomy of superior orbital fissure
The cavernous sinuses, a rich plexuses of veins that surround the internal carotid arteries, lie lateral to the pituitary fossa. Anteriorly, lie the tuberculum sellae and the anterior clinoid processes and posteriorly are the posterior clinoid processes. The lateral wall has two dural layers between which travel cranial nerves III, IV, and the ophthalmic division of the trigeminal nerve (V1). V2 and part of the trigeminal ganglion may lie in the inferolateral wall of the cavernous sinus. Cranial nerve VI lies free in the cavernous sinus. Sympathetic fibers from the superior sympathetic ganglion ascend with the internal carotid artery and join the under surface of cranial nerve VI in the cavernous sinus briefly before fusing with the ophthalmic division of the trigeminal nerve to enter the orbit.

Clinical features
The clinical features may be divided into five categories (Table 11.5):

1. Extraocular muscle palsy. Usually there are simultaneous deficits of two or more ipsilateral ocular motor cranial nerves.

   a. The trochlear nerve is only involved in the cavernous sinus when the other nerves are affected

   b. In the presence of a IIIrd nerve palsy, the eye is turned down and out. If intorsion of the globe, i.e., clockwise rotation of the right eye or anticlockwise rotation of the left eye, can be demonstrated, the trochlear nerve is intact

   c. With intracavernous aneurysms, the abducens nerve may show an isolated palsy, but with meningiomas,

evidence of oculomotor, trochlear, oculosympathetic, and trigeminal nerve damage is usually present (Jefferson 1953).

2. Eyelid and pupil abnormality. Cavernous sinus syndrome can produce sympathetic and/or parasympathetic denervation. Oculosympathetic paralysis (ipsilateral Horner's syndrome) can occur manifesting as mild ptosis miosis and elevation of the lower lid (upside ptosis). Oculomotor nerve dysfunction may lead to ptosis and mydriasis. However, pupillary changes are usually minimal. In cases of combined sympathetic and parasympathetic paralysis, the pupil is midposition and sluggish to both light and near stimuli.

3. Pain. Retro-orbital pain may be the first indication of cavernous sinus disease. An insidious pain, which has a gnawing or burning quality develops when the trigeminal nerve is invaded by a malignant process. The ophthalmic division (and in the cavernous sinus, the maxillary divisions) may be affected most commonly by a meningioma. If all three divisions of the trigeminal nerve are involved, it is more likely to be a neuroma.

4. Proptosis is uncommon with cavernous sinus involvement unless there is extension into the orbital apex/superior orbital fissure. There may be resistance to pressure over the globe and congestion of conjunctival veins.

5. Aberrant regeneration. Primary aberrant regeneration of the IIIrd nerve can occur with cavernous sinus syndrome in the absence of previous IIIrd nerve palsy (Schatz et al 1977).

   a. Pupil-gaze dyskinesis. Dilated pupil will constrict on attempted adduction or depression

   b. Lid-gaze dyskinesis. Ptotic lid may lift on adduction and downgaze.

   Tumors that should be considered include:

1. Meningiomas: these usually arise from the dura near the petrous apex and invade the cavernous sinus from outside. The symptoms and signs associated with meningiomas depend on the location of the tumor and the rate of growth.

   a. Sphenoid wing tumors (Fig. 11.6):
      - Pterional tumors. These usually are large masses before diagnosis and present with features of increased intracranial pressure.
      - En plaque meningiomas are slowly growing and may present with progressive ptosis, proptosis, and downward displacement of the globe due to marked hyperostosis of the greater wing.
      - Tumors of the middle third project back into the temporal lobe and often present with seizures.
      - Tumors affecting the medial and inner sphenoid wing (clinoid) involve the structures in the superior orbital fissure or cavernous sinus.

2. Nasopharyngeal carcinoma.

3. Neuroma.

4. Metastatic carcinoma from lung, breast, and prostate.

5. Perineural spread of squamous cell carcinoma. This may occur from the years after dermatologic excision (ten Hove et al 1997).

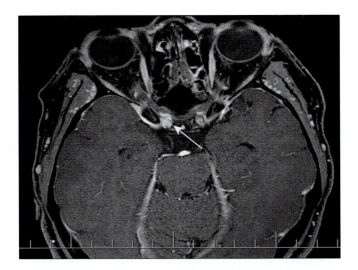

Figure 11.6 Anterior clinoidal meningioma. MRI axial image T1-weighted image with contrast demonstrating an anterior clinoidal meningioma with tail compressing the optic nerve.

Differential diagnosis

1. Aneurysm.
2. Cavernous sinus thrombosis or carotid-cavernous fistula.
3. Lymphoma.
4. Infection.
5. Inflammatory process such as sarcoid.
6. Venous malformations.

Tumors in the suprasellar region

Clinical features of tumors in the suprasellar region are shown in Box 11.4.

Tumors located in the suprasellar region produce specific syndromes from their effects on the intracranial optic nerves, the chiasm, optic tracts, and the hypothalamus. The most common tumors are pituitary adenomas, meningiomas, craniopharyngiomas, and gliomas. Damage to adjacent neurologic and vascular structures such as the cavernous sinus may result in additional symptoms. The arrangement of visual fibers in the chiasm accounts for the characteristic symptoms and signs of visual loss.

Relevant anatomy

The optic chiasm is positioned over the diaphragm sellae in 75–85% of patients. Clinically, the most important anatomical relationship of the chiasm is with the pituitary gland. The chiasm lies approximately 1 cm above the pituitary fossa (Fig. 11.7).

However, in approximately 10% of cases, it can overlie the tuberculum sellae (a 'pre-fixed' chiasm) or in 5–15%, it is located over the dorsum sellae (a 'post-fixed' chiasm). The optic chiasm tilts forward in an angle of about 15–45°. These relationships have a direct bearing on the configuration of the visual field defects resulting from an encroaching pituitary tumor.

Box 11.4 Clinical features of suprasellar lesions

- Progressive visual loss
- Sudden visual loss
- Postfixation blindness
- Hemifield slide phenomenon
- Ocular motor paresis
- See-saw nystagmus
- Hypothalamic involvement
- Features of hydrocephalus
- Visual field abnormality

The chiasm contains decussating axons from both optic nerves. Axons arising from the retinal ganglion cells nasal to the fovea that carry information from the temporal visual fields cross the midline to join the axons from the temporal retinal and form the optic tracts. Hence, each optic tract carries visual information from the contralateral visual fields. Because the vertical midline determined by this decussation passes through the fovea, not the optic disc, the blindspot lies entirely within the temporal visual field.

Symptoms

1. Progressive loss of vision. Most patients do not perceive that peripheral vision is impaired, but complain of an inability to perform various fine motor tasks requiring careful depth perception or binocular vision. Typically, the visual loss is asymmetric, with one eye showing greater involvement than the other. However, patients may complain of slowly dimming vision (Wybar 1977).

2. Sudden loss of vision. Pituitary apoplexy may result in sudden bilateral severe visual loss, even blindness, associated with headache, diplopia, and/or disturbed consciousness. This occurs as a result of hemorrhage or infarction of the pituitary tumor and may extend into the cavernous sinus on one or both sides with the result that there may be external and internal ophthalmoplegia.

3. 'Post-fixation blindness' or disturbance of depth perception (Fig. 11.8). Patients complain of difficulties with tasks such as sewing or using precision tools. The underlying mechanism is that during convergence, there is a crossing of two blind temporal hemifields in patients with bitemporal field defects. The image of an object posterior to fixation falls on blind nasal retinas and consequently disappears. The term 'post-fixation blindness' refers to objects disappearing behind the point of fixation.

4. Diplopia (Fig. 11.9).

    a. Secondary to the *'hemifield slide phenomenon'*. This is a horizontal or vertical diplopia not associated with an ocular motor paresis or ocular misalignment. Such patients have difficulty reading because of doubling or loss of printed letters or words. It occurs because the visual field in patients with complete bitemporal hemianopias have no corresponding retinal points to visually link the hemifield of the two eyes. This loss of physiologic linkage results in a tendency for the hemifields to overlap if there is an underlying tendency for the eyes to be slightly misaligned (Kirkham 1972).

    b. Ocular motor paresis as a result of extension into the subarachnoid space or within the cavernous sinus.

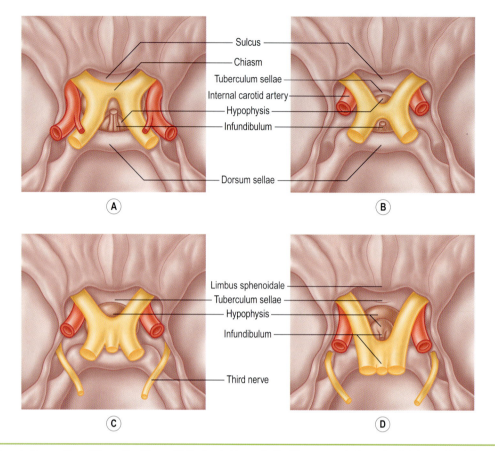

Figure 11.7 Variations in the position of the optic chiasm. (A) Prefixed chiasm; (B, C) chiasm over pituitary gland; (D) post-fixed chiasm. (From Whitnall S E The Anatomy of the Human Orbit, 2nd edn. Oxford: Oxford University Press; p. 385, 1932.)

The diplopia may be painful if the trigeminal nerve is also affected in the cavernous sinus. Ocular motor misalignment combined with a bitemporal field defect suggests the lesion has extended beyond the chiasm or there has been pituitary apoplexy that caused rapid chiasmal expansion.

5. Photophobia (not common) – the mechanism is unknown.

Signs

1. Visual acuity. Classically, patients read down the Snellen chart, missing the letters in their temporal field for each eye, although the visual loss tends to be asymmetric.

2. Color vision. Patients will miss reading the figure that falls in the temporal field if a two digit number is presented or will have temporal red desaturation when tested across the vertical midline.

3. Optic nerve appearance (Fig. 11.10). Patients with chiasmal syndromes may or may not have ophthalmoscopically apparent nerve fiber layer or optic atrophy.

   a. Band or bow-tie atrophy. When optic atrophy is present, it occurs in a distinctive pattern called 'band atrophy', where the pallor extends horizontally in a band across the optic disc. This corresponds to degeneration of the peripheral retinal ganglion cells located nasal to the fovea that course directly into the nasal aspect of the disc and the nasal macula fibers (the papillomacular bundle), which course directly to the temporal disc. There is relative sparing of the superior and inferior portions of the disc, where the majority of spared temporal fibers which subserve the nasal visual field enter (Cushing 1930).

   b. Papilledema. This is more frequently associated with suprachiasmal tumors which may occlude the third ventricle, but rarely with intrasellar lesions.

4. Decompensated phoria. This presents with a manifest comitant strabismus and is a result of loss of normal nasotemporal visual field overlap in patients with complete bitemporal visual field defects.

5. See-saw nystagmus. This is characterized by synchronous alternating elevation and intorsion of one eye and depression and extorsion of the other eye, and occurs in patients with tumors in the diencephalon or chiasmal lesions. It is thought to be caused by damage to the structures near the interstitial nucleus of Cajal.

6. Hypothalamic involvement:

   a. Diabetes insipidus

   b. Hypothalamic hypopituitarism

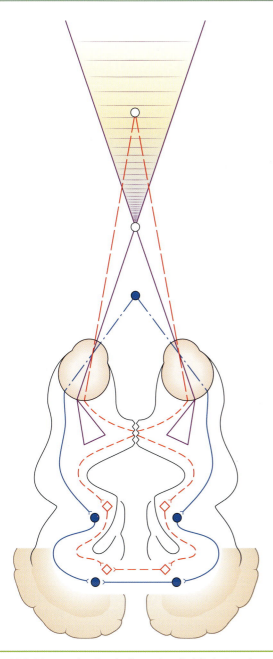

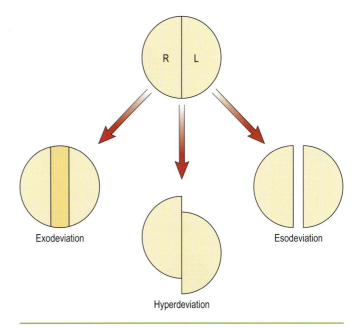

Figure 11.9 A chiasmal lesion interrupts the physiological linkage between the two half fields and allows intermittent overlap or separation of the two nasal fields. L, left temporal projection; R, right temporal projection. (From Kaye A H, Essential Neurosurgery. Edinburgh: Churchill Livingstone, 1991. With permission of Elsevier.)

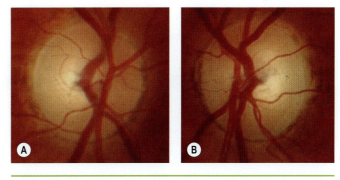

Figure 11.10 (A) Right optic disc showing temporal pallor. (B) Left optic disc demonstrating temporal and nasal pallor and 'bow tie' pattern of atrophy.

Figure 11.8 Diagram showing the formation of a blind triangular area of visual field that occurs just beyond fixation in patients with complete bitemporal hemianopia or dense bitemporal hemianopic scotoma. (From Kirkham T H (1972) The ocular symptomatology of pituitary tumors. Proceedings of Royal Society of Medicine 65: p517–518.)

   c. Growth retardation and delayed sexual development in pre-pubertal children.

7. Features of hydrocephalus from a tumor that has expanded postero-superiorly into the third ventricle and obstructed cerebrospinal fluid flow:

   a. Impairment of upgaze

   b. Pupillary light-near dissociation

   c. Convergence retraction nystagmus

   d. Papilledema.

8. Visual field loss. Two configurations of visual field loss are the 'signatures' of chiasmal involvement.

   a. Bitemporal field defects (Fig. 11.11). The bitemporal hemianopia is seen in lesions that affect the central portion of the chiasm. The classic bitemporal hemianopia may involve only the superior visual fields if the lesion produces extrinsic compression initially from below such as occurs with a pituitary adenoma or any other infrachiasmal lesion (e.g., tuberculum sellae and medial sphenoidal ridge meningiomas). Gradually the defect descends into the lower temporal field and then into the lower nasal quadrant. In general, the upper nasal visual field is often preserved even in advanced chiasmal syndromes.

   Conversely, superior chiasmatic compression may cause only an inferior hemianopic field loss. In most cases of bitemporal hemianopia, the visual

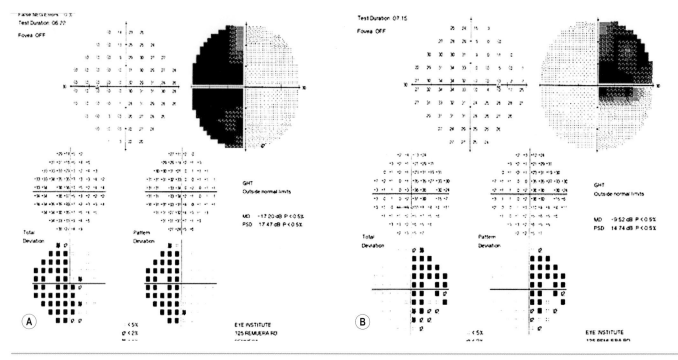

Figure 11.11 Bitemporal hemianopia. (A) Left visual field (Humphrey SITA Standard 24–2) demonstrating temporal field loss. (B) Right visual field showing temporal visual field loss.

acuity is normal. In addition, a suprachiasmal tumor is more likely to produce papilledema because such lesions can extend into and occlude the third ventricle.

Occasionally, a large posterior fossa tumor may cause chiasmal syndrome by compression of the third ventricle through increased intracranial pressure. Most of these cases are also associated with papilledema.

Iatrogenic causes of chiasmal syndrome occur most commonly after removal of a suprasellar meningioma, craniopharyngiomas or clipping of an aneurysm. A chiasmal syndrome can also occur from exuberant packing of the sphenoid sinus with fat following transsphenoidal resection of a pituitary adenoma resulting in inferior compression of the chiasm. The visual field defect usually improves immediately after emergency removal of the fat.

Radiation necrosis of the chiasm may also produce a chiasmal syndrome. This may begin months to several years after high dose radiation therapy.

b. Junctional scotoma or 'anterior chiasmal syndrome'. A lesion that is located more anteriorly compressing the medial aspect of the junction between the chiasm and the optic nerve will affect the ipsilateral optic nerve fibers and the contralateral fibers of Willebrand knee (the crossing of the temporal retinal fibers). This results in an ipsilateral central scotoma and a contralateral superior temporal field cut, and is also called a junctional chiasmal syndrome. When a small lesion damages only the crossing fibers of the ipsilateral eye, the field defect is monocular

and temporal with a midline hemianopic character that extends to the periphery of the visual field. If only the macular crossed fibers from one eye are damaged, the resultant field defect is still monocular and temporal but is scotomatous and located paracentrally.

9. Other visual field defects:

a. Bitemporal hemianopic scotoma

b. Lesions that damage the posterior aspect of the optic chiasm produce typically bitemporal hemianopic scotomas which are often taken for cecocentral scotomas attributed to toxic or hereditary processes rather than a tumor. However, bitemporal hemianopic scotomas will be associated with normal visual acuity and color vision, whereas toxic/nutritional processes are invariably associated with reduced visual acuity and dyschromatopsia

c. Homonymous hemianopic field defects. The homonymous hemianopic field defect is more likely with a pre-fixed chiasm or when the tumor involves the optic tract which is usually incongruous (Kearns & Rucker 1958)

d. Monocular visual field defect. If the posterior portion of the optic nerve is involved the visual field defect may be monocular with a central or cecocentral defect. Compression of the posterior optic nerve against the overlying anterior cerebral artery, the roof of the optic canal, or the falciform ligament may cause an inferior altitudinal defect.

10. Optical coherence tomography. Optical coherence tomography (OCT) is an imaging technique that has been

developed to assess tissue thickness of the optic nerve head retinal nerve fiber layer (RNFL) thickness *in vivo*. It allows high resolution (approximately 10 μm) cross-sectional imaging of the eye. The peripapillary RNFL thickness can be evaluated and quantified using OCT. OCT RNFL has been shown to be able to predict visual recovery following surgery for pituitary tumors. Patients who have thin preoperative RNFL (<85 μm) have less recovery of visual acuity and visual field than patients who have thicker RNFL (Fig. 11.12) (Danesh-Meyer et al 2006, 2008b).

11. Extension into the cavernous sinus (see below):

a. Motility disturbance. Patients will have characteristics of IIIrd, IVth, or VI nerve palsy or a combination of these

b. Trigeminal sensory neuropathy. This is present when the ocular motor nerves are damaged in the cavernous sinus. There is no motor trigeminal nerve involvement

c. Horner's syndrome. If the oculosympathetic fibers are damaged, there will be a post-ganglionic Horner's,

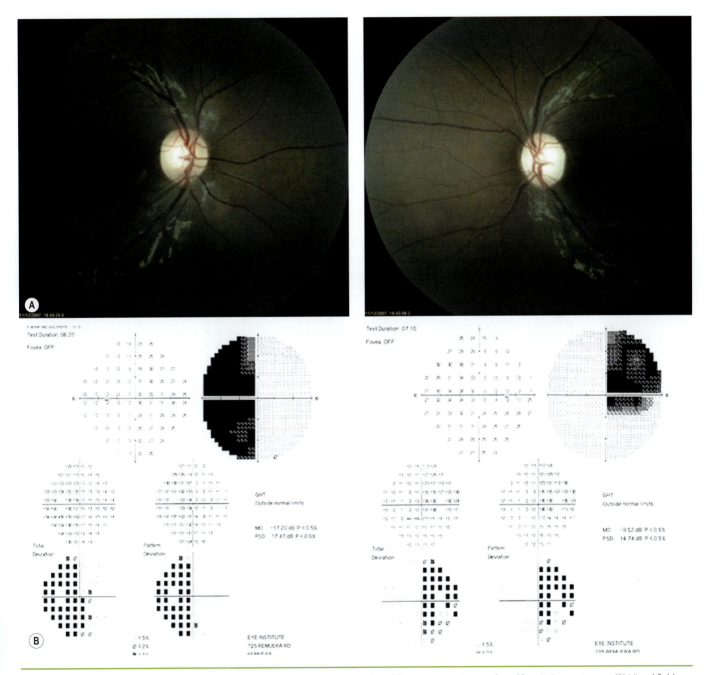

Figure 11.12 OCT predicts recovery of vision. (A) Bilateral pallor of optic nerve head from compression produced by pituitary a tumor. (B) Visual field defect preoperatively. Cont'd

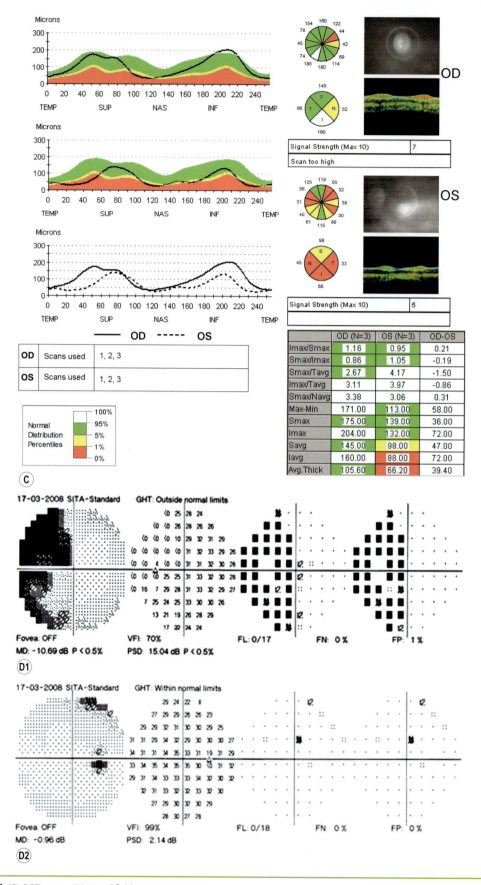

Figure 11.12, cont'd (C) OCT scans. (D) Visual fields postoperatively.

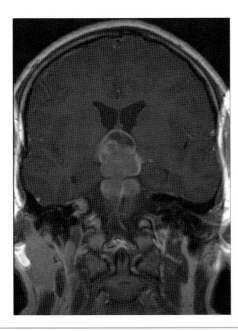

Figure 11.13 Pituitary tumor. Coronal enhanced T1 view with gadolinium enhancement showing pituitary tumor extending into the suprasellar cisterns with compression of the optic chiasm.

usually in combination with VIth involvement. When both the IIIrd and oculosympathetic fibers are damaged, the clinical picture will be one of a IIIrd nerve palsy with a small pupil that will be normally reactive if the paresis is pupil-sparing or poorly or non-reactive if the IIIrd nerve paresis has damaged the pupillomotor fibers.

Features of specific tumors

Pituitary adenomas

Pituitary adenomas (Fig. 11.13) often become symptomatic during pregnancy but regress with delivery. Furthermore, during the 3rd trimester, the pituitary gland may enlarge sufficiently to produce chiasmal compression and visual symptoms. Again, these resolve spontaneously following delivery.

Pituitary apoplexy

Pituitary apoplexy is a term that applies to infarction or hemorrhage of the pituitary occurring in pre-existing pituitary tumors or in a non-tumorous pituitary gland. It is potentially a life-threatening condition.

Pituitary apoplexy has a wide range of clinical presentations. Most patients experience headache with symptoms and signs related to meningeal irritation and ophthalmoplegia due to compression of the ocular motor nerves in the cavernous sinus. The IIIrd nerve is the most commonly affected, followed by the VIth and IVth. Other features associated with it include:

1. Altered consciousness
2. Nausea and vomiting
3. Visual loss due to chiasmal compression
4. Endocrine dysfunction
5. Facial paresthesias
6. Focal hemispheric and cerebellar symptoms.

The presence of nuchal rigidity, photophobia and a reduced level of consciousness may be mistakenly attributed to an aneurismal subarachnoid hemorrhage.

There is no population that seems to have a propensity for pituitary apoplexy. The age range is broad, from the 1st to the 9th decade, with a peak in the 5th decade.

There is no sex predominance or histological sub-type or size of pituitary tumor that confers a higher risk (Rolih & Ober 1993). Most importantly, most cases of pituitary apoplexy (80% in our series) occur in patients who have as of yet undiagnosed pituitary adenomas, with the apoplectic episode often the presenting symptom of the pituitary tumor.

The pathophysiological changes that lead to pituitary apoplexy are still open to speculation. It is well recognized that pituitary adenomas are particularly prone to hemorrhage and necrosis. It has been suggested that a rapidly growing adenoma that outstrips its blood supply may lead to ischemic necrosis and hemorrhage of the gland. Others propose direct compression of the pituitary infundibulum by an expanding mass, thus compromising the blood flow from the portal vessels, resulting in necrosis of the entire gland with hemorrhage as a secondary occurrence. Various other mechanisms have been proposed for hemorrhage and infarction of pituitary adenomas, including inherent fragility of tumor blood vessels and atherosclerotic embolization.

In approximately one-third of patients some sort of precipitating factor is identified. Over the past 20 years, numerous case reports and small series have emphasized the association of pituitary apoplexy with a wide variety of underlying causes. The multiple factors reported as precipitants of pituitary apoplexy can be considered in the following categories:

1. Fluctuations in blood pressure and altered blood flow to pituitary gland.
   a. Hypotension in the setting of cardiac surgery, lumbar laminectomy, or hemodialysis, has been associated with pituitary apoplexy of both normal and adenomatous glands.
   b. Transient increase in intracranial pressure with resultant hypoperfusion of the pituitary gland, as caused by coughing, sneezing, or positive pressure ventilation (Vidal et al 1992; McFadzean 1991).
   c. Minor head trauma, procedures such as angiography, pneumoencephalography, myelography, lumbar puncture, and spinal anaesthesia.
   d. Vascular changes after pituitary irradiation often result in chronic hypoperfusion.
2. Acute increase in blood flow in the pituitary gland is considered a classic triggering factor for pituitary apoplexy.
3. Stimulation of the pituitary gland through increased estrogen states, such as:
   a. Pregnancy
   b. Exogenous estrogen administration
   c. Response to stress
   - Surgical stress: numerous surgical procedures have been implicated in apoplexy through excessive stimulation of the pituitary gland responding to stress by having to produce a larger amount of steroids

• Acute systemic illness such as myocardial infarction or severe infection dynamic testing of the pituitary using gonadotropin releasing hormone (GnRH), thyrotropin releasing hormone (TRH) or other secretogogues.

4. Anticoagulation: whether from administration of anticoagulant drugs, thrombolytic agents, or thrombocytopenia.

Craniopharyngioma

Papilledema in a patient with a chiasmal syndrome should raise the possibility of the tumor being a *craniopharyngioma*. In children with this tumor, half will have papilledema in addition to chiasmal and optic tract field defects, however in adults, disc swelling is uncommon (Stahnke et al 1984). The infiltrative and extensive growth of craniopharyngiomas entails a higher incidence of ocular motor nerve palsies (Baskin & Wilson 1986).

Meningioma

Suprasellar meningiomas (Fig. 11.14) arise from the dura of the tuberculum sellae and rarely from the diaphragma sellae. Cushing's 'syndrome of the chiasm' – consisting of bitemporal visual field defects, bilateral optic atrophy, and a normal sella turcica on plain radiographs – was due to tuberculum sellae meningiomas (Cushing 1930). The major symptoms are painless, progressive visual loss and headache (Symon & Rosenstein 1984).

Primary glioma

Primary gliomas of the chiasm present in childhood with unilateral or bilateral loss of vision, 'amblyopia', strabismus, optic atrophy, or nystagmus (Miller et al 1974).

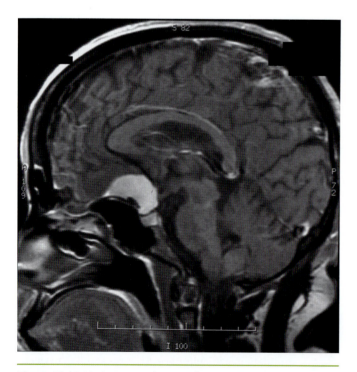

Figure 11.14 Meningioma with suprasellar extension.

Other

Other conditions may mimic a suprasellar tumor such as sarcoid, lymphoma or aneurysms arising from internal carotid artery.

Syndrome of the optic tract

Lesions in the suprasellar region and lesions deep to the temporal lobe may damage the optic tract.

Relevant anatomy

The optic tract fibers travel above and around the infundibulum and below the third ventricle. The blood supply of the optic tract is supplied by thalamic perforators of the posterior cerebral artery and branches of the anterior choroidal artery off the internal carotid artery.

Each optic tract contains fibers from the contralateral hemifield.

Clinical features

1. Optic atrophy. Tumors that compress the optic tract produce optic atrophy as axons die back, but this will not occur with lesions posterior to the lateral geniculate nucleus. The optic atrophy will occur temporally in the eye ipsilateral to the tract lesion, and a bow-tie configuration in the contralateral eye (Savino et al 1978).

2. Incongruous homonymous hemianopia. The field defect associated with an optic tract lesion is typically an incongruous homonymous hemianopia. An incongruous defect is one that asymmetrically involves the two eyes.

3. Relative afferent pupillary defect (RAPD). A RAPD may be present on the side of the greater field loss. If the lesion affects the entire optic tract this will be the side *contralateral* to the lesion as 53% of the fibers cross over. The combination of a homonymous hemianopia and an RAPD is the hallmark of an optic tract lesion.

The clinical features of optic tract lesions are shown in Box 11.5.

A complete tract lesion produces a classic triad:

1. Complete homonymous hemianopia

2. RAPD without any loss of visual acuity or color vision in the eye ipsilateral to the hemianopia (contralateral to the lesion)

3. Hemianopic optic nerve atrophy.

Tumors involving the lateral geniculate body

The more anterior the involvement of the post-chiasmal visual pathway, the more incongruous the homonymous hemianopia.

Box 11.5 Clinical features of optic tract lesions

• Complete homonymous hemianopia
• RAPD
• Preserved VA and color in eye contralateral to lesion
• Band atrophy of optic nerve

Clinical features

1. Congruous or incongruous hemianopic defect:
   a. If the posterior choroidal artery is affected, the result will be a congruous horizontal sectanopia.
   b. Lesions involving the anterior choroidal artery produce a quadruple quadrantanopia (the horizontal sector is spared).

Frontal lobe tumors

Frontal lobe tumors may present with a wide-range of neuro-ophthalmic symptoms and signs. The most common presentation is with papilledema, seizures, and visual loss. The visual loss may be a result of chronic papilledema or direct compression of the optic nerves or chiasm.

The Foster Kennedy syndrome was originally described as the triad of optic atrophy, contralateral papilledema, and anosmia, caused by an olfactory groove meningioma or large frontal lobe tumors. With modern neuroimaging, the diagnosis is often made earlier and anosmia may not be present. The optic atrophy occurs on the side of tumor as a result of direct compression. Because there are few nerve fibers there is no swelling. The contralateral disc swelling is due to papilledema from increased intracranial pressure related to the tumor size.

1. Non-dominant frontal lobe: presents with a personality change toward indifference and apathy and visual loss.
2. Frontal eye fields: head and eyes turning to the opposite side during a seizure. There may be some associated lower face weakness but there is often some weakness of eyelid closure and slower blinking on that side. A failure of voluntary closure of the eyelids bilaterally has been termed 'compulsive eye opening' and 'apraxia of eyelid closure'.

Temporal lobe tumors

Clinical features of temporal lobe lesions are shown in Box 11.6.

Tumors involving the temporal lobes may present late, especially if involving the non-dominant hemisphere. The most common presentation is with features of raised intracranial pressure. If the tumor extends medially or there is herniation of the hippocampus there may be distortion of the brainstem and consequent cranial nerve palsies. There may be involvement of Meyer's loop of the optic radiations.

Clinical features

1. Contralateral superior homonymous quadrantanopia (a 'pie-in-the-sky' defect).

Box 11.6 Clinical features of temporal lobe lesions
- Contralateral superior homonymous quadrantanopia
- Complex visual hallucination
- Papilledema (if large tumor)

2. Complex formed hallucinations lasting seconds and not necessarily confined to the contralateral visual field. The visual hallucinations may be distortions (metamorphosis) with objects smaller (micropsia) or larger (macropsia). However, patients may complain of quite dramatic vivid scenes. The hallucinations are regarded as epileptic phenomena.
3. Papilledema: Temporal lobe tumors may present when they have enlarged causing symptoms of increased intracranial pressure.

Parietal lobe tumors

Clinical features of parietal lobe lesions are shown in Box 11.7.

Clinical features

1. Non-dominant parietal lobe:
   a. Homonymous hemianopia with greater inferior quadrant loss as the parietal radiations carry the information from the inferior visual fields
   b. Visual inattention is commonly seen in parietal tumors and is often associated with sensory inattention and subtle homonymous hemianopia. The patient will fail to see hand movement in the left-half field when hand movements are presented in both right and left fields simultaneously
   c. Defective visual localization: the patient may fail to localize accurately objects in the affected field. For example, there may be an inability to touch the examiner's finger accurately in that field
   d. Tonic deviation of the eyes to the side opposite parietal lesions during attempted Bell's phenomenon
   e. Absent optokinetic nystagmus with rotation of the drum towards the side of the parietal lesion due to a defect of ipsilateral pursuit
   f. Palinopsia or visual perseveration results in the persistence of normal images usually for several minutes but can last for hours within the homonymous hemianopia.
2. Dominant parietal lobe lesions:
   a. Alexia: a tumor of the left angular gyrus of the parietal lobe may cause word blindness. This is potentially reversible (Turgman et al 1979)
   b. Gerstmann syndrome: acalculia, agraphia, finger agnosia, and right-left confusion.

Box 11.7 Clinical features of parietal lobe lesions
- Contralateral inferior homonymous quadrantanopia
- Visual inattention
- Defective visual localization
- Palinopsia
- Tonic deviation of eyes to contralateral side of lesion during attempted Bell's phenomenon
- Alexia
- Gerstmann syndrome (acalculia, agraphia, finger agnosia, left-right confusion)

phenomenon and is reported to occur in close to 20% of patients (Foy et al 1981a; Shaw & Foy 1991).

There is no specific AED that is proven to have particular efficacy for TAE. Monotherapy with phenytoin or carbamazepine is still generally accepted as first-line treatment in patients with partial epilepsy, and both drugs are probably of equal efficacy. Phenytoin has traditionally been the most commonly used AED in the perioperative setting because it is available for intravenous administration. However, intravenous phenytoin poses significant risks of cutaneous, cardiac and systemic side-effects (O'Brien et al 1998; O'Brien et al 2001). Sodium valproate is generally well tolerated and is effective in suppressing the focal seizures that not uncommonly occur in TAE, however, there is evidence that it is not as efficacious as carbamazepine against complex partial seizures (Mattson et al 1992). Adverse effects of sodium valproate such as the dose related thrombocytopenia, and other coagulopathies can be preoperative concerns, although serious bleeding complications are rare (Köse et al 2009). Another concern is the increased risk of sodium valproate treatment for the unborn child of a woman who becomes pregnant while taking the drug, particularly at higher doses (Vajda et al 2004; Meador et al 2009).

Phenobarbital and primidone are also efficacious for seizure control. However, their use frequently results in unacceptable behavioral and cognitive disturbances and therefore they are no longer recommended as first-line therapy for TAE (Mattson et al 1985; Smith et al 1987).

In recent years, there has been a shift in some centers to use newer generation AEDs for TAE. Levetiracetam is one such example and has favorable pharmacokinetic and tolerability profiles, particularly as it is rapidly absorbed orally and is also now available as an intravenous drug. It demonstrates linear kinetics, is minimally hepatically metabolized through a pathway independent of the cytochrome P450 system, has no significant drug–drug interactions and has a wide therapeutic index (Ulloa et al 2009). It is one of the few AEDs that has been specifically studied in TAE and as add-on therapy, it is reported to be effective in reducing seizures in more than half of TAE patients who have had ongoing seizures while being treated with other AEDs (Siddiqui et al 2002; Wagner et al 2003; Newton et al 2006). As monotherapy, it is widely believed to be associated with significantly fewer adverse reactions than older AEDs, and is at least as effective in prophylaxis of early and late postoperative seizures when used for seizure prophylaxis following supratentorial neurosurgery (Milligan et al 2008).

Other new AEDs such as lamotrigine (van Breemen et al 2009), gabapentin (Perry & Sawka 1996), topiramate (Maschio et al 2008), pregabalin (Elger et al 2005) and zonisamide (Maschio et al 2009) have all been demonstrated to be significantly more efficacious than placebo in reducing seizure frequency as 'add on therapy' in patients with partial epilepsy, and a number also as monotherapy. These new AEDs have not yet been evaluated in TAE and there are still relatively few comparative studies of these with the more established drugs. Those few studies have generally found the newer AEDs to be of comparable efficacy, but with an improved patient tolerability profile.

The functional condition of a patient with a high-grade glioma may also influence the likelihood of seizure control.

Chaichana et al (2009) in their study of patients with high-grade gliomas found on multivariate analysis that increased Karnofsky Performance Score (KPS) was significantly associated with the chance of attaining seizure control (RR 0.944, 95% CI 0.914–0.977).

Surgical management

Surgery is currently the only treatment capable of achieving complete seizure control in patients with drug resistant TAE. However, such an outcome is only applicable to a small minority of patients where the tumor is low grade and where it can be safely completely excised along with the surrounding epileptogenic zone. Even then, complete seizure control is far from guaranteed. A consensus has yet to be reached regarding the most appropriate surgery for intractable TAE (Fried & Cascino 1993). As with most neurosurgical treatments, there is at best only Class III evidence for effectiveness of the various surgical approaches for TAE.

Indication for surgery

For most patients with brain tumors, surgery is primarily directed at obtaining a histologic diagnosis, alleviating mass effect and raised intracranial pressure and improving prognosis. If the patient has TAE due to a low-grade tumor that is well controlled with AEDs, surgery for the epilepsy *per se* is generally not recommended. However, in a patient with drug resistant TAE, which is particularly common with low-grade tumors, surgery may be indicated for control of the epilepsy, i.e., 'epilepsy surgery' (Sankhla & Khan 2008). Approximately 38–76% of all supratentorial tumors considered for epilepsy surgery are in the temporal lobe (Rasmussen 1975; Boon et al 1991; Britton et al 1994). Complete seizure control postoperatively is associated with improvement in psychological and intellectual development (of critical importance with children) and general quality of life, and may reduce the incidence of secondary epileptogenesis and prevent the malignant transformation of otherwise benign tumors (Smith et al 1992; Hammond et al 2000; Aronica et al 2001; Kim et al 2001; Blumcke & Wiestler 2002).

Penfield originally observed in 1940 that surgical excision of a tumor could result in good seizure outcome. At that time, the postoperative control rates of TAE were in the order of 0–21% (Penfield et al 1940; White et al 1948). Today, these control rates have vastly improved. Complete seizure control in patients with low-grade gliomas after surgery is reported to be 67% at 12 months (Chang et al 2008), and in patients with high-grade gliomas for the same follow-up period, it was found to be 77% (Chaichana et al 2009). Presumably this improvement in outcome is a result of both the development of more effective AEDs and the more precise surgical resections aided by image guided stereotactic systems. Better selection of patients for epilepsy surgery has been aided by the establishment of comprehensive preoperative evaluation programs, evolution of imaging techniques (particularly high resolution structural MRI), improved electrophysiological techniques and a further understanding of TAE pathogenesis (Ramamurthi et al 1980; Goldring & Gregorie 1984; Deutschman & Haines 1985; Chang et al 1991).

Extent of surgical excision

There remains considerable controversy as to whether surgical resection for TAE associated with low-grade gliomas should just target the lesion, or also include the surrounding ictal onset zone (usually defined by subdural EEG electrode or electrocorticography recordings). As discussed previously, there is considerable evidence that seizures arise predominantly from the peri-tumoral region rather than the tumor itself. However, those advocating lesionectomy alone have reported median seizure free rates of 80% (range 65–94%), which is as good as those achieved by wider resections, including the tumor and the peri-tumoral epileptogenic cortex (Goldring & Gregorie 1984; Spencer et al 1984; Morrell 1985; Hirsch et al 1989; Cascino et al 1990; Awad et al 1991; Boon et al 1991; Cascino et al 1992; Haddad et al 1992; Morris et al 1993; Pilcher et al 1993; Packer et al 1994; Villemure & de Tribolet 1996; Morris et al 1998; Iannelli et al 2000; Luyken et al 2003). Gross total resection of low-grade gliomas has been found to be a strong predictor of seizure control (Chang et al 2008), while macroscopic resection of high-grade glioma has been found to be associated with seizure control that trended toward, but did not reach statistical significance (Chaichana et al 2009).

In contrast, advocates of resection of the lesion and the surrounding ictal onset zone report higher rates of postoperative seizure freedom than with lesionectomy alone (Rasmussen 1975; Goldring & Gregorie 1984; Drake et al 1987; Berger et al 1989; Sperling et al 1989; Berger 1995; Jooma et al 1995a, 1995b; Zentner et al 1997; Rassi-Neto et al 1999; Iannelli et al 2000). Penfield (1940) was among the first to suggest that resection of the surrounding epileptogenic area may improve seizure control. However, for some patients, particularly those with poorly-controlled complex partial seizures, even extensive resections guided by EEG may produce disappointing results (Deutschman & Haines 1985; Whittle & Beaumont 1995). Hwang and colleagues (2001) found no difference in extent of surgical excision with the rate of seizures continuing to occur postoperatively. Kirkpatrick et al (1993) in their retrospective study of 31 patients undergoing temporal lobe tumor resections found seizure control outcome to be independent of both tumor pathology and completeness of tumor resection.

Seizures arising from a brain region remote from the tumor have been reported to occur in up to one-third of patients, and this may explain the failure of epilepsy surgery to control the seizures in some patients with low-grade tumors. This is the phenomenon of 'secondary epileptogenesis', whereby seizures spreading from a focus in one brain region 'kindles' another region to become an independent seizure focus. Early surgical resection of the primary epileptic lesion has been advocated to prevent development of a secondary, potentially irreversible, seizure focus (Morrell & deToledo-Morrell 1999; Hwang et al 2001). Secondary epileptogenesis is reported to occur more frequently with temporal tumors, and commonly involves the mesolimbic structures (Gilmore et al 1994). From a surgical point of view, this raises another controversial issue regarding whether the mesial temporal structures should be resected in addition to a tumor in the temporal neocortex. Whether removal of this additional brain tissue, which has significant risk of inducing postoperative memory loss,

improves the outcome with respect to seizures continues to be a matter of debate.

The role of EEG cortical mapping

Controversy also exists concerning the use of electrocorticography to guide the extent of resection of adjacent or distant seizure foci associated with brain tumors (Fried 1995; Tran et al 1997; Wennberg et al 1999; Duffau et al 2002). Some authors believe that epileptiform discharges recorded on intraoperative electrocorticogram (ECoG) indicate epileptogenic brain and so advocate the use of ECoG to define the boundaries for tailored cortical resections (Berger 1995). These and other investigators (Gonzalez & Elvidge 1962; Drake et al 1987; Awad et al 1991; Berger et al 1993) have reported, especially in children, better long-term seizure control of refractory TAE without the need for ongoing AED therapy using this surgical strategy. Dysembryoplastic neuroepithelial tumors (DNETs), which are particularly epileptogenic, are often associated with a surrounding region of focal cortical dysplasia which must also be removed for optimal seizure control (Takahashi et al 2005). As the site and extent of the associated cortical dysplasia is often difficult to define on MRI, intraoperative electrocorticography can be helpful in guiding the extent of the surgical excision in this case. Others believe that intraoperative ECoG is not reliable enough to determine surgical boundaries, with interictal spikes often being recorded at sites remote to the ictal onset zone. For these authors, the use of chronic video-EEG monitoring with intracranial electrodes or grids to localize the site of the electrographic seizure onset and then 'tailoring' the resection to include the mapped seizure foci is the preferred approach (Murphy et al 2004). Others have reported that chronic intracranial EEG monitoring or intraoperative ECoG did not show a statistically significant relationship with the post-resection seizure control rate for DNETs (Lee et al 2000).

The development of imaging technologies has made available a wide variety of modalities to assist with the non-invasive, pre-surgical evaluation of patients with drug-resistant epilepsy. These include functional magnetic resonance imaging (fMRI) (Chakraborty & McEvoy 2008), positron emission tomography (PET) (Meyer et al 2003), magnetoencephalography (MEG) (Ganslandt et al 1999), single photon emission tomography (SPECT) (Van Paesschen 2004) or subtraction ictal SPECT co-registered to MRI (SISCOM) (Ahnlide et al 2007). Soon after the introduction of these new neuroimaging methods, there was a decrease in the use of invasive intracranial EEG implantations. Recently there has been a resurgence in the use of EEG for preoperative evaluation in TAE, utilizing a more targeted, image guided approach facilitated by the integration or fusion within the stereotactic MRI space of multiple imaging modalities (Liubinas et al 2009). Multimodality image guided (MMIG) surgery combines neuroimaging with invasive ECoG monitoring to maximize the accuracy of a functional cortical map of both the ictal onset zone, and the surrounding eloquent cortex, that is then used to guide the tailored surgical resection. A recent case series of eight patients from our center who underwent tailored cortical resection following MMIG subdural grid implantation with a mean follow-up of 39 months, found seven patients (87.5%) had an Engel Class

I outcome with the other patient having an Engel Class III outcome (Liubinas et al 2009). Another earlier case series of 13 patients who had MMIG bilateral depth electrodes and subdural grids inserted reported similar outcome results (Murphy et al 2002).

The role of awake functional stimulation mapping

In addition to recording epileptiform activity, the other purpose of functional mapping is to locate eloquent cortex (e.g., primary language, motor or visual cortices). This is important when eloquent cortex is involved in, or adjacent to, the proposed surgical resection. This can be carried out preoperatively by stimulating chronic implanted subdural EEG electrodes, usually in the ward setting of the epilepsy monitoring unit. Electrical stimulation functional mapping can also be performed intraoperatively during the craniotomy with the patient awake instead of, or to supplement, the subdural electrode stimulation. The principal advantages of an awake craniotomy over a craniotomy under general anesthetic are the ability to test function, especially speech, as well as the ability to observe any seizure activity during mapping. Other benefits include minimization of drug interferences on the ECoG recordings (if this is used to assist in defining epileptic foci), lower morbidity and decreased required length of postoperative hospital stay when compared with craniotomies performed under general anesthesia (GA). A prospective study of awake craniotomy used routinely and non-selectively for 610 patients with supratentorial lesions, found the technique to be associated with low complication and mortality rates (Serletis & Bernstein 2007). A prospective study comparing outcomes in 26 patients who underwent an awake craniotomy for intrinsic lesions involving eloquent cortex, with those in 27 patients who had the surgery under general anesthesia, found that the mean operative time and blood loss was less, and the tumor cytoreduction volume and short-term neurological improvement to be better in the GA group of patients (Gupta et al 2007). However, none of the results in this study was statistically significant and a larger cohort is required to substantiate such observations. The technique is highly dependent on an experienced surgical and anesthetic team, and requires appropriate patient selection and careful preoperative work-up.

Radiotherapy

Radiotherapy is currently not widely advocated for the principal aim of controlling seizures in patients with TAE. However, in one series of nine patients with malignant brain tumors and medically refractory TAE diagnosed by stereotactic biopsy and treated with radiotherapy, all patients had either significant reduction (>75%) or elimination of seizures (Chalifoux & Elisevich 1996). Moreover, the effect was reported to last beyond the immediate and early post-radiation period. The therapy may thus also lessen the propensity for cerebral tissue to later develop epileptogenicity. Radiosurgery is now being used to control seizures in non-tumoral mesial temporal lobe epilepsy and with the technique reported to provide seizure-free outcome rates comparable with those of resective surgery (Barbaro et al 2009). Radionecrosis, a secondary complication of

radiotherapy, has been reported to also act as a secondary focus for the initiation of seizures. The true epileptogenic effect of brain irradiation is difficult to assess objectively due to several confounding factors specific for the postoperative scenario, such as the concurrent presence of residual or recurrent tumor (Riva et al 2006). Seizure foci arising as a late complication of radiotherapy for leukemia has been documented (Radhakrishnan et al 2008).

REFERENCES

Ahnlide, J.A., Rosén, I., Lindén-Mickelsson Tech, P., et al., 2007. Does SISCOM contribute to favorable seizure outcome after epilepsy surgery? Epilepsia 48 (3), 579–588.

Araque, A., Sanzgiri, R.P., Parpura, V., et al., 1999. Astrocyte-induced modulation of synaptic transmission. Can. J. Physiol. Pharmacol. 77 (9), 699–706.

Aronica, E., Leenstra, S., van Veelen, C.W., et al., 2001. Glioneuronal tumors and medically intractable epilepsy: a clinical study with long-term follow-up of seizure outcome after surgery. Epilepsy Res. 43 (3), 179–191.

Avoli, M., 1987. Mechanisms of generalized epilepsy with spike and wave discharge. Electroencephalogr Clin. Neurophysiol 39 (Suppl), 184–190.

Avoli, M., 1991. Excitatory amino acid receptors in the human epileptogenic neocortex. Epilepsy Res. 10 (1), 33–40.

Avoli, M., Louvel, J., Pumain, R., et al., 2005. Cellular and molecular mechanisms of epilepsy in the human brain. Prog. Neurobiol. 77 (3), 166–200.

Awad, I.A., Rosenfeld, J., Ahl, J., et al., 1991. Intractable epilepsy and structural lesions of the brain: mapping, resection strategies, and seizure outcome. Epilepsia 32 (2), 179–186.

Baker, G.A., Jacoby, A., Buck, D., et al., 1997. Quality of life of people with epilepsy: a European study. Epilepsia 38 (3), 353–362.

Barbaro, N.M., Quigg, M., Broshek, D.K., et al., 2009. A multicenter, prospective pilot study of gamma knife radiosurgery for mesial temporal lobe epilepsy: seizure response, adverse events, and verbal memory. Ann. Neurol. 65 (2), 167–175.

Bateman, D.E., Hardy, J.A., McDermott, J.R., et al., 1988. Amino acid neurotransmitter levels in gliomas and their relationship to the incidence of epilepsy. Neurol. Res. 10 (2), 112–114.

Beaumont, A., Whittle, I.R., 2000. The pathogenesis of tumour associated epilepsy. Acta. Neurochir. (Wien) 142, 1–15.

Begley, C.E., Lairson, D.R., Reynolds, T.F., et al., 2001. Early treatment cost in epilepsy and how it varies with seizure type and frequency. Epilepsy Res. 47 (3), 205–215.

Behrens, P.F., Langemann, H., Strohschein, R., et al., 2000. Extracellular glutamate and other metabolites in and around RG2 rat glioma: an intracerebral microdialysis study. J. Neurooncol. 47, 11–22.

Berdiev, B.K., Xia, J., McLean, L.A., et al., 2003. Acid-sensing ion channels in malignant gliomas. J. Biol. Chem. 278 (17), 15023–15034.

Berger, M.S., 1995. Functional mapping-guided resection of low-grade gliomas. Clin. Neurosurg 42, 437–452.

Berger, M.S., Ghatan, S., Haglund, M.M., et al., 1993. Low-grade gliomas associated with intractable epilepsy: seizure outcome utilizing electrocorticography during tumor resection. J. Neurosurg 79 (1), 62–69.

Berger, M.S., Kincaid, J., Ojemann, G.A., et al., 1989. Brain mapping techniques to maximize resection, safety, and seizure control in children with brain tumors. Neurosurgery 25 (5), 786–792.

Birbeck, G.L., Hays, R.D., Cui, X., et al., 2002. Seizure reduction and quality of life improvements in people with epilepsy. Epilepsia 43 (5), 535–538.

Blumcke, I., Wiestler, O.D., 2002. Gangliogliomas: an intriguing tumor entity associated with focal epilepsies. J. Neuropathol. Exp. Neurol. 61 (7), 575–584.

Boon, P.A., Fried, W.P., Spencer, I., et al., 1991. Intracranial, intraaxial, space occupying lesions in patients with intractable partial seizures: an anatomical, neuropsychological and surgical correlation. Epilepsia 32, 467–476.

Bordey, A., Sontheimer, H., 1998. Electrophysiological properties of human astrocytic tumor cells In situ: enigma of spiking glial cells. J. Neurophysiol 79 (5), 2782–2793.

Brat, D.J., Mapstone, T.B., 2003. Malignant glioma physiology: cellular response to hypoxia and its role in tumor progression. Ann. Intern. Med. 138 (8), 659–668.

Britton, J.W., Cascino, G.D., Sharbrough, F.W., et al., 1994. Low-grade glial neoplasms and intractable partial epilepsy: efficacy of surgical treatment. Epilepsia 35 (6), 1130–1135.

Bromfield, E.B., 2004. Epilepsy in patients with brain tumors and other cancers. Rev. Neurol. Dis. 1 (Suppl 1), S27–S33.

Campbell, K.A., Bank, B., Milgram, N.W., 1984. Epileptogenic effects of electrolytic lesions in the hippocampus: role of iron deposition. Exp. Neurol. 86 (3), 506–514.

Cardone, R.A., Casavola, V., Reshkin, S.J., 2005. The role of disturbed pH dynamics and the Na+/H+ exchanger in metastasis. Nat. Rev. Cancer 5 (10), 786–795.

Carlson, H., Ronne-Engström, E., Ungerstedt, U., et al., 1992. Seizure related elevations of extracellular amino acids in human focal epilepsy. Neurosci. Lett. 140 (1), 30–32.

Cascino, G.D., 1990. Epilepsy and brain tumors: implications for treatment. Epilepsia 31 (Suppl 3), S37–S44.

Cascino, G.D., Kelly, P., Hirschorn, K.A., et al., 1990. Stereotactic resection of intra-axial cerebral lesions in partial epilepsy. Mayo. Clin. Proc. 65, 1053–1060.

Cascino, G.D., Kelly, P., Sharbrough, F.W., et al., 1992. Long-term follow-up of stereotactic lesionectomy in partial epilepsy: predictive factors and electroencephalographic results. Epilepsia 33, 639–644.

Chaichana, K.L., Parker, S.L., Olivi, A., et al., 2009. Long-term seizure outcomes in adult patients undergoing primary resection of malignant brain astrocytomas. J. Neurosurg 111 (2), 282–292.

Chakraborty, A., McEvoy, A.W., 2008. Presurgical functional mapping with functional MRI. Curr. Opin. Neurol. 21 (4), 446–451.

Chalifoux, R., Elisevich, K., 1996. Effect of ionizing radiation on partial seizures attributable to malignant cerebral tumors. Stereotact. Funct. Neurosurg 67 (3–4), 169–182.

Chan, R.C., Thompson, G.B., 1984. Morbidity, mortality, and quality of life following surgery for intracranial meningiomas. A retrospective study in 257 cases. J. Neurosurg 60 (1), 52–60.

Chang, C.N., Ojemann, L.M., Ojemann, G.A., et al., 1991. Seizures of fronto-orbital origin: a proven case. Epilepsia 32 (4), 487–491.

Chang, E.F., Potts, M.B., Keles, G.E., et al., 2008. Seizure characteristics and control following resection in 332 patients with low-grade gliomas. J. Neurosurg 108, 227–235.

Chernov, M.F., Kubo, O., Hayashi, M., et al., 2005. Proton MRS of the peri-tumoral Brain. J. Neuro. Sci. 228, 137–142.

Cirak, B., Inci, S., Palaoglu, S., et al., 2003. Lipid peroxidation in cerebral tumors. Clin. Chim. Acta. 327 (1–2), 103–107.

Coulter, D.A., DeLorenzo, R.J., 1999. Basic mechanisms of status epilepticus. Adv. Neurol. 79, 725–733.

de Bock, F., Dornand, J., Rondouin, G., 1996. Release of TNF alpha in the rat hippocampus following epileptic seizures and excitotoxic neuronal damage. Neuroreport 7 (6), 1125–1129.

De Simoni, M.G., Perego, C., Ravizza, T., et al., 2000. Inflammatory cytokines and related genes are induced in the rat hippocampus by limbic status epilepticus. Eur. J. Neurosci. 7, 2623–2633.

Deutschman, C.S., Haines, S.J., 1985. Anticonvulsant prophylaxis in neurological surgery. Neurosurgery 17 (3), 510–517.

Drake, J., Hoffman, H.J., Kobayashi, J., et al., 1987. Surgical management of children with temporal lobe epilepsy and mass lesions. Neurosurgery 21 (6), 792–797.

Duffau, H., Capelle, L., Lopes, M., et al., 2002. Medically intractable epilepsy from insular low-grade gliomas: improvement after an extended lesionectomy. Acta. Neurochir. (Wien) 144, 563–573.

During, G.R., Mirchandani, P., Leone, A., et al., 1993. Direct hippocampal injection of HSV-1 vector expressing GLUR6 results in spontaneous seizures, hyperexcitability in CA1 cells, and loss of CA1, hilar, and CA3 neurons. J. Soc. Neurosci. 19, 21.

Echlin, F.A., 1959. The supersensitivity of chronically isolated cerebral cortex as a mechanism in focal epilepsy. Electroencephalogr Clin. Neurophysiol 11, 697–722.

Elger, C.E., Brodie, M.J., Anhut, H., et al., 2005. Pregabalin add-on treatment in patients with partial seizures: a novel evaluation of flexible-dose and fixed-dose treatment in a double-blind, placebo-controlled study. Epilepsia 46 (12), 1926–1936.

Engel, J., Pedley, T.A., Aicardi, J., et al., 2007. Epilepsy: A comprehensive textbook, 2nd edn. Lippincott Williams & Wilkins, London.

Ferrier, C.H., Aronica, E., Leijten, F.S., et al., 2006. Electrocorticographic discharge patterns in glioneuronal tumors and focal cortical dysplasia. Epilepsia 47 (9), 1477–1486.

Foy, P.M., Copeland, G.P., Shaw, M.D., 1981a. The incidence of postoperative seizures. Acta. Neurochir. (Wien) 55 (3–4), 253–264.

Foy, P.M., Copeland, G.P., Shaw, M.D., 1981b. The natural history of postoperative seizures. Acta. Neurochir. (Wien) 57 (1–2), 15–22.

Fried, I., 1995. Management of low-grade gliomas: results of resections without electrocorticography. Clin. Neurosurg 42, 453–463.

Fried, I., Cascino, G.D., 1993. Lesional surgery. In: Engel, J. Jr. (Ed.), Surgical treatment of the epilepsies. Raven Press, New York, pp. 501–509.

Gaitatzis, A., Sander, J.W., 2004. The mortality of epilepsy revisited. Epileptic. Disord. 6 (1), 3–13.

Ganslandt, O., Fahlbusch, R., Nimsky, C., et al., 1999. Functional neuronavigation with magnetoencephalography: outcome in 50 patients with lesions around the motor cortex. J. Neurosurg 91 (1), 73–79.

Gardner-Medwin, A.R., 1983. A study of the mechanisms by which potassium moves through brain tissue in the rat. J. Physiol. 335, 353–374.

Gastaut, J.L., Michel, B., Hassan, S.S., et al., 1979. Electroencephalography in brain edema (127 cases of brain tumor investigated by cranial computerized tomography). Electroencephalogr Clin. Neurophysiol 46 (3), 239–255.

Gilles, F.H., Sobel, E., Leviton, A., et al., 1992. Epidemiology of seizures in children with brain tumors. The Childhood Brain Tumor Consortium. J. Neurooncol. 12 (1), 53–68.

Gillies, R.J., Raghunand, N., Karczmar, G.S., et al., 2002. MRI of the tumor microenvironment. J. Magn. Reson. Imaging 16 (4), 430–450.

Gilmore, R., Morris, H. 3rd, Van Ness, P.C., et al., 1994. Mirror focus: function of seizure frequency and influence on outcome after surgery. Epilepsia 35 (2), 258–263.

Glantz, M.J., Cole, B.F., Forsyth, P.A., et al., 2000. Practice parameter: anticonvulsant prophylaxis in patients with newly diagnosed brain tumors. Report of the Quality Standards Subcommittee of the American Academy of Neurology. Neurology 54 (10), 1886–1893.

Goldring, S., Gregorie, E.M., 1984. Surgical management of epilepsy using epidural recordings to localize the seizure focus. Review of 100 cases. J. Neurosurg 60 (3), 457–466.

Goldring, S., Rich, K.M., Picker, S., 1986. Experience with gliomas in patients presenting with a chronic seizure disorder. Clin. Neurosurg 33, 15–42.

Gonzalez, D., Elvidge, A.R., 1962. On the occurrence of epilepsy caused by astrocytoma of the cerebral hemispheres. J. Neurosurg 19, 470–482.

Gowers, W., 1878. On some symptoms of organic brain disease. Brain 1, 48–59.

Gupta, D.K., Chandra, P.S., Ojha, B.K., et al., 2007. Awake craniotomy versus surgery under general anesthesia for resection of intrinsic lesions of eloquent cortex – a prospective randomised study. Clin. Neurol. Neurosurg 109 (4), 335–343.

Haddad, S.F., Moore, S.A., Menezes, A.H., et al., 1992. Ganglioglioma: 13 years of experience. Neurosurgery 31 (2), 171–178.

Haglund, M.M., Berger, M.S., Kunkel, D.D., et al., 1992. Changes in gamma-aminobutyric acid and somatostatin in epileptic cortex associated with low-grade gliomas. J. Neurosurg 77 (2), 209–216.

Hamberger, A., Nyström, B., Larsson, S., et al., 1991. Amino acids in the neuronal microenvironment of focal human epileptic lesions. Epilepsy Res. 9 (1), 32–43.

Hammond, R.R., Duggal, N., Woulfe, J.M., et al., 2000. Malignant transformation of a dysembryoplastic neuroepithelial tumor. Case report. J. Neurosurg 92 (4), 722–725.

Herman, S.T., 2002. Epilepsy after brain insult: targeting epileptogenesis. Neurology 59 (Suppl 5), S21–S26.

Hildebrand, J., 2004. Management of epileptic seizures. Curr. Opin. Oncol. 16 (4), 314–317.

Hirsch, J.F., Sainte Rose, C., Pierre-Khan, A., et al., 1989. Benign astrocytic and oligodendrocytic tumors of the cerebral hemispheres in children. J. Neurosurg 70 (4), 568–572.

Hossmann, K.A., Seo, K., Szymas, J., et al., 1990. Quantitative analysis of experimental peri-tumoral edema in cats. Adv. Neurol. 52, 449–458.

Hwang, S.L., Lieu, A.S., Kuo, T.H., et al., 2001. Preoperative and postoperative seizures in patients with astrocytic tumours: analysis of incidence and influencing factors. J. Clin. Neurosci. 8 (5), 426–429.

Iannelli, A., Guzzetta, F., Battaglia, D., et al., 2000. Surgical treatment of temporal tumors associated with epilepsy in children. Pediatr. Neurosurg 32 (5), 248–254.

Jooma, R., Yeh, H.S., Privitera, M.D., et al., 1995a. Lesionectomy versus electrophysiologically guided resection for temporal lobe tumors manifesting with complex partial seizures. J. Neurosurg 83 (2), 231–236.

Jooma, R., Yeh, H.S., Privitera, M.D., et al., 1995b. Seizure control and extent of mesial temporal resection. Acta. Neurochir. (Wien) 133 (1–2), 44–49.

Kaibara, T., Tyson, R.L., Sutherland, G.R., 1998. Human cerebral neoplasms studied using MR spectroscopy: a review. Biochem. Cell. Biol. 76 (2–3), 477–486.

Kanai, Y., 1997. Family of neutral and acidic amino acid transporters: molecular biology, physiology and medical implications. Curr. Opin. Cell. Biol. 9 (4), 565–572.

Kaplan, P.W., 2004. Neurologic aspects of eclampsia. Neurol. Clin. 22 (4), 841–861.

Kim, S.K., Wang, K.C., Hwang, Y.S., et al., 2001. Intractable epilepsy associated with brain tumors in children: surgical modality and outcome. Childs. Nerv. Syst. 17 (8), 445–452.

Kirkpatrick, P.J., Honavar, M., Janota, I., et al., 1993. Control of temporal lobe epilepsy following en bloc resection of low-grade tumors. J. Neurosurg 78 (1), 19–25.

Kish, S.J., Olivier, A., Dubeau, F., et al., 1988. Increased activity of choline acetyltransferase and acetylcholinesterase in actively epileptic human cerebral cortex. Epilepsy Res. 2 (4), 227–231.

Köhling, R., Senner, V., Paulus, W., et al., 2006. Epileptiform activity preferentially arises outside tumor invasion zone in glioma xenotransplants. Neurobiol. Dis. 22 (1), 64–75.

Kondziolka, D., Bernstein, M., Resch, L., et al., 1987. Significance of hemorrhage into brain tumors: clinicopathological study. J. Neurosurg 67 (6), 852–857.

Köse, G., Arhan, E., Unal, B., et al., 2009. Valproate-associated coagulopathies in children during short-term treatment. J. Child. Neurol. 24 (12), 1493–1498.

Kraft, R., Basrai, D., Benndorf, K., et al., 2001. Serum deprivation and NGF induce and modulate voltage-gated Na(+) currents in human astrocytoma cell lines. Glia. 34 (1), 59–67.

Laake, J.H., Slyngstad, T.A., Haug, F.M., et al., 1995. Glutamine from glial cells is essential for the maintenance of the nerve terminal pool of glutamate: immunogold evidence from hippocampal slice cultures. J. Neurochem. 65 (2), 871–881.

Labrakakis, C., Patt, S., Hartmann, J., et al., 1998. Glutamate receptor activation can trigger electrical activity in human glioma cells. Eur. J. Neurosci. 10 (6), 2153–2162.

Labrakakis, C., Patt, S., Weydt, P., et al., 1997. Action potential-generating cells in human glioblastomas. J. Neuropathol. Exp. Neurol. 56 (3), 243–254.

Lee, D.Y., Chung, C.K., Hwang, Y.S., et al., 2000. Dysembryoplastic neuroepithelial tumor: radiological findings (including PET, SPECT, and MRS) and surgical strategy. J. Neurooncol. 47 (2), 167–174.

Lhatoo, S.D., Johnson, A.L., Goodridge, D.M., et al., 2001. Mortality in epilepsy in the first 11 to 14 years after diagnosis: multivariate analysis of a long-term, prospective, population-based cohort. Ann. Neurol. 49 (3), 336–344.

Lieu, A.S., Howng, S.L., 2000. Intracranial meningiomas and epilepsy: incidence, prognosis and influencing factors. Epilepsy Res. 38 (1), 45–52.

Liigant, A., Haldre, S., Oun, A., et al., 2001. Seizure disorders in patients with brain tumors. Eur. Neurol. 45 (1), 46–51.

Linn, F., Seo, K., Hossmann, K.A., 1989. Experimental transplantation gliomas in the adult cat brain. 3. Regional biochemistry. Acta. Neurochir. (Wien) 99 (1–2), 85–93.

Liubinas, S.V., Cassidy, D., Roten, A., et al., 2009. Tailored cortical resection following image guided subdural grid implantation for medically refractory epilepsy. J. Clin. Neurosci. 16 (11), 1398–1408.

Lo, M., Wang, Y.Z., Gout, P.W., 2008. The x(c)- cystine/glutamate antiporter: a potential target for therapy of cancer and other diseases. J. Cell. Physiol. 215 (3), 593–602.

Logue, V., 1974. Surgery of supratentorial meningiomas: a modern series. J. Neurol. Neurosurg Psychiatr. .37, 1277.

Luyken, C., Blümcke, I., Fimmers, R., et al., 2003. The spectrum of long-term epilepsy-associated tumors: long-term seizure and tumor outcome and neurosurgical aspects. Epilepsia 44 (6), 822–830.

Magistretti, P.J., Pellerin, L., Rothman, D.L., et al., 1999. Energy on demand. Science. 283 (5401), 496–497.

Mahaley, M.S. Jr., Dudka, L., 1981. The role of anticonvulsant medications in the management of patients with anaplastic gliomas. Surg. Neurol. 16 (6), 399–401.

Marco, P., Sola, R.G., Ramón, S., et al., 1997. Loss of inhibitory synapses on the soma and axon initial segment of pyramidal cells in human epileptic peritumoral neocortex: implications for epilepsy. Brain Res. Bull. 44 (1), 47–66.

Maschio, M., Dinapoli, L., Saveriano, F., et al., 2009. Efficacy and tolerability of zonisamide as add-on in brain tumor-related epilepsy: preliminary report. Acta. Neurol. Scand. 120 (3), 210–212.

Maschio, M., Dinapoli, L., Zarabla, A., et al., 2008. Outcome and tolerability of topiramate in brain tumor associated epilepsy. J. Neurooncol. 86 (1), 61–70.

Mathern, G.W., Adelson, P.D., Cahan, L.D., et al., 2002. Hippocampal neuron damage in human epilepsy: Meyer's hypothesis revisited. Prog. Brain Res. 135, 237–251.

Matthew, E., Sherwin, A.L., Welner, S.A., et al., 1980. Seizures following intracranial surgery: incidence in the first post-operative week. Can. J. Neurol. Sci. 7 (4), 285–290.

Mattson, R.H., Cramer, J.A., Collins, J.F., 1992. A comparison of valproate with carbamazepine for the treatment of complex partial seizures and secondarily generalized tonic-clonic seizures in adults. The Department of Veterans Affairs Epilepsy Cooperative Study No. 264 Group. N. Engl. J. Med. 327 (11), 765–771.

Mattson, R.H., Cramer, J.A., Collins, J.F., et al., 1985. Comparison of carbamazepine, phenobarbital, phenytoin, and primidone in partial and secondarily generalized tonic-clonic seizures. N. Engl. J. Med. 313 (3), 145–151.

McNamara, J.O., 1999. Emerging insights into the genesis of epilepsy. Nature. 399 (6738 Suppl), A15–A22.

Meador, K.J., Baker, G.A., Browning, N., et al., 2009. Cognitive function at 3 years of age after fetal exposure to antiepileptic drugs. N. Engl. J. Med. 360 (16), 1597–1605.

Meyer, P.T., Sturz, L., Sabri, O., et al., 2003. Preoperative motor system brain mapping using positron emission tomography and statistical parametric mapping: hints on cortical reorganization. J. Neurol. Neurosurg Psychiatry 74 (4), 471–478.

Miller, L.G., Galpern, W.R., Dunlap, K., et al., 1991. Interleukin-1 augments gamma-aminobutyric acidA receptor function in brain. Mol. Pharmacol. 39 (2), 105–108.

Milligan, T.A., Hurwitz, S., Bromfield, E.B., 2008. Efficacy and tolerability of levetiracetam versus phenytoin after supratentorial neurosurgery. Neurology 71 (9), 665–669.

Moots, P.L., Maciunas, R.J., Eisert, D.R., et al., 1995. The course of seizure disorders in patients with malignant gliomas. Arch. Neurol. 52 (7), 717–724.

Morrell, F., 1985. Secondary epileptogenesis in man. Arch. Neurol. 42 (4), 318–335.

Morrell, F., deToledo-Morrell, L., 1999. From mirror focus to secondary epileptogenesis in man: an historical review. Adv. Neurol. 81, 11–23.

Morris, H.H., Estes, M.L., Gilmore, R., et al., 1993. Chronic intractable epilepsy as the only symptom of primary brain tumor. Epilepsia 34 (6), 1038–1043.

Morris, H.H., Matkovic, Z., Estes, M.L., et al., 1998. Ganglioglioma and intractable epilepsy: clinical and neurophysiologic features and predictors of outcome after surgery. Epilepsia 39 (3), 307–313.

Murphy, M.A., O'Brien, T.J., Cook, M.J., 2002. Insertion of depth electrodes with or without subdural grids using frameless stereotactic guidance systems – technique and outcome. Br. J. Neurosurg 16 (2), 119–125.

Murphy, M.A., O'Brien, T.J., Morris, K., et al., 2004. Multimodality image-guided surgery for the treatment of medically refractory epilepsy. J. Neurosurg 100 (3), 452–462.

Newman, E.A., Zahs, K.R., 1998. Modulation of neuronal activity by glial cells in the retina. J. Neurosci. 18 (11), 4022–4028.

Newton, H.B., Goldlust, S.A., Pearl, D., 2006. Retrospective analysis of the efficacy and tolerability of levetiracetam in brain tumor patients. J. Neurooncol. 78 (1), 99–102.

O'Brien, T.J., Cascino, G.D., So, E.L., et al., 1998. Incidence and clinical consequence of the purple glove syndrome in patients receiving intravenous phenytoin. Neurology 51 (4), 1034–1039.

O'Brien, T.J., Meara, F.M., Matthews, H., et al., 2001. Prospective study of local cutaneous reactions in patients receiving IV phenytoin. Neurology 57 (8), 1508–1510.

Oberndorfer, S., Schmal, T., Lahrmann, H., et al., 2002. [The frequency of seizures in patients with primary brain tumors or cerebral metastases. An evaluation from the Ludwig Boltzmann Institute of Neuro-Oncology and the Department of Neurology, Kaiser Franz Josef Hospital, Vienna]. Wien. Klin. Wochenschr 114 (21–22), 911–916.

Okada, Y., Kloiber, O., Hossmann, K.A., 1992. Regional metabolism in experimental brain tumors in cats: relationship with acid/base, water, and electrolyte homeostasis. J. Neurosurg 77 (6), 917–926.

Pace, A., Bove, L., Innocenti, P., et al., 1998. Epilepsy and gliomas: incidence and treatment in 119 patients. J. Exp. Clin. Cancer Res. 17 (4), 479–482.

Packer, R.J., Sutton, L.N., Patel, K.M., et al., 1994. Seizure control following tumor surgery for childhood cortical low-grade gliomas. J. Neurosurg 80 (6), 998–1003.

Pasquier, B., Péoc'H, M., Fabre-Bocquentin, B., et al., 2002. Surgical pathology of drug-resistant partial epilepsy. A 10-year-experience with a series of 327 consecutive resections. Epileptic. Disord. 4 (2), 99–119.

Pasternack, M., Bountra, C., Voipio, J., et al., 1992. Influence of extracellular and intracellular pH on GABA-gated chloride conductance in crayfish muscle fibres. Neuroscience 47 (4), 921–929.

Pasti, L., Zonta, M., Pozzan, T., et al., 2001. Cytosolic calcium oscillations in astrocytes may regulate exocytotic release of glutamate. J. Neurosci. 21 (2), 477–484.

Patt, S., Labrakakis, C., Bernstein, M., et al., 1996. Neuron-like physiological properties of cells from human oligodendroglial tumors. Neuroscience 71 (2), 601–611.

Patt, S., Steenbeck, J., Hochstetter, A., et al., 2000. Source localization and possible causes of interictal epileptic activity in tumor-associated epilepsy. Neurobiol. Dis. 7 (4), 260–269.

Penfield, W., Erickson, T.C., Tarlov, I., 1940. Relation of intracranial tumours and symptomatic epilepsy Arch. Neurol. Psychiatry 44, 300–316.

Penfield, W., Jasper, H., 1954. Functional localization in the cerebral cortex. Epilepsy and the functional anatomy of the human brain, 2nd edn. Little Brown, Boston, pp. 41–155.

Perry, J.R., Sawka, C., 1996. Add-on gabapentin for refractory seizures in patients with brain tumours. Can. J. Neurol. Sci. 23 (2), 128–131.

Pilcher, W.H., Silbergeld, D.L., Berger, M.S., et al., 1993. Intraoperative electrocorticography during tumor resection: impact on seizure outcome in patients with gangliogliomas. J. Neurosurg 78 (6), 891–902.

Pitkanen, A., Sutula, T.P., 2002. Is epilepsy a progressive disorder? Prospects for new therapeutic approaches in temporal-lobe epilepsy. Lancet. Neurol. 1 (3), 173–181.

Radhakrishnan, A., Sithinamsuwan, P., Harvey, A.S., et al., 2008. Multifocal epilepsy: the role of palliative resection – intractable frontal and occipital lobe epilepsy secondary to radiotherapy for acute lymphoblastic leukaemia. Epileptic. Disord. 10 (4), 362–370.

Ramamurthi, B., Ravi, B., Ramachandran, V., 1980. Convulsions with meningiomas: incidence and significance. Surg. Neurol. 14 (6), 415–416.

Ranson, B., 1992. Glial modulation of neuronal excitability mediated by extracellular pH: a hypothesis. Prog. Brain Res. 94, 37–47.

Rasmussen, T., 1975. Surgery of epilepsy associated with brain tumors. Adv. Neurol. 8, 227–239.

Rassi-Neto, A., Ferraz, F.P., Campos, C.R., et al., 1999. Patients with epileptic seizures and cerebral lesions who underwent lesionectomy restricted to or associated with the adjacent irritative area. Epilepsia 40 (7), 856–864.

Riva, M., Salmaggi, A., Marchioni, E., et al., 2006. Tumour-associated epilepsy: clinical impact and the role of referring centres in a cohort of glioblastoma patients. A multicentre study from the Lombardia Neurooncology Group. Neurol. Sci. 27, 345–351.

Robinson, M.B., Dowd, L.A., 1997. Heterogeneity and functional properties of subtypes of sodium-dependent glutamate transporters in the mammalian central nervous system. Adv. Pharmacol. 37, 69–115.

Rodriguez-Enriquez, S., Moreno-Sanchez, R., 1998. Intermediary metabolism of fast-growth tumor cells. Arch. Med. Res. 29 (1), 1–12.

Roslin, M., Henriksson, R., Bergström, P., et al., 2003. Baseline levels of glucose metabolites, glutamate and glycerol in malignant glioma assessed by stereotactic microdialysis. J. Neurooncol. 61 (2), 151–160.

Rothstein, J.D., Tabakoff, B., 1984. Alteration of striatal glutamate release after glutamine synthetase inhibition. J. Neurochem 43 (5), 1438–1446.

Sankhla, S., Khan, G.M., 2008. Surgical management of epilepsy associated with temporal lobe tumors. J. Pediatr. Neurosci. 3, 121–125.

Sato, H., Tamba, M., Ishii, T., et al., 1999. Cloning and expression of a plasma membrane cystine/glutamate exchange transporter composed of two distinct proteins. J. Biol. Chem. 274 (17), 11455–11458.

Sawada, M., Hara, N., Maeno, T., 1990. Extracellular tumour necrosis factor induces a decreased K. conductance in an identified neuron of Aplysia kurodai. Neurosci. Lett. 115, 219–225.

Sawada, M., Hara, N., Maeno, T., 1991a. Tumour necrosis factor reduces the ACh-induced outward current in identified Aplysia neurons. Neurosci. Lett. 131, 217–220.

Sawada, M., Hara, N., Maeno, T., 1991b. Analysis of a decreased Na. conductance by tumour necrosis factor in identified neurons of Aplysia kurodai. J. Neurosci. Res. 28, 466–473.

Schaller, B., 2005. Influences of brain tumor-associated pH changes and hypoxia on epileptogenesis. Acta. Neurol. Scand. 111 (2), 75–83.

Schuler, V., Lüscher, C., Blanchet, C., et al., 2001. Epilepsy, hyperalgesia, impaired memory, and loss of pre- and postsynaptic GABA(B) responses in mice lacking GABA(B(1)). Neuron. 31 (1), 47–58.

Serletis, D., Bernstein, M., 2007. Prospective study of awake craniotomy used routinely and nonselectively for supratentorial tumors. J. Neurosurg 107 (1), 1–6.

Shaw, M.D., Foy, P.M., 1991. Epilepsy after craniotomy and the place of prophylactic anticonvulsant drugs: discussion paper. J. R. Soc. Med. 84 (4), 221–223.

Sibson, N.R., Dhankhar, A., Mason, G.F., et al., 1997. In vivo 13C NMR measurements of cerebral glutamine synthesis as evidence for glutamate-glutamine cycling. Proc. Natl. Acad. Sci. U. S. A. 94 (6), 2699–2704.

Siddiqui, F., Wen, P., Dworetzky, B., et al., 2002. Use of levetiracetam in patients with brain tumours. Epilepsia 43 (Suppl), 297.

Singh, R., Pathak, D.N., 1990. Lipid peroxidation and glutathione peroxidase, glutathione reductase, superoxide dismutase, catalase, and glucose-6-phosphate dehydrogenase activities in FeCl3-induced epileptogenic foci in the rat brain. Epilepsia 31 (1), 15–26.

Sirven, J.I., Wingerchuk, D.M., Drazkowski, J.F., et al., 2004. Seizure prophylaxis in patients with brain tumors: a meta-analysis. Mayo. Clin. Proc. 79 (12), 1489–1494.

Sloviter, R.S., 1994. The functional organization of the hippocampal dentate gyrus and its relevance to the pathogenesis of temporal lobe epilepsy. Ann. Neurol. 35 (6), 640–654.

Smith, D.B., Mattson, R.H., Cramer, J.A., et al., 1987. Results of a nationwide Veterans Administration Cooperative Study comparing the efficacy and toxicity of carbamazepine, phenobarbital, phenytoin, and primidone. Epilepsia 28 (Suppl), S50–S58.

Smith, N.M., Carli, M.M., Hanieh, A., et al., 1992. Gangliogliomas in childhood. Childs. Nerv. Syst. 8 (5), 258–262.

Soliven, B., Albert, J., 1992. Tumor necrosis factor modulates the inactivation of catecholamine secretion in cultured sympathetic neurons. J. Neurochem 58 (3), 1073–1078.

Spencer, D.D., Spencer, S.S., Mattson, R.H., et al., 1984. Intracerebral masses in patients with intractable partial epilepsy. Neurology 34 (4), 432–436.

Sperling, M.R., Cahan, L.D., Brown, W.J., et al., 1989. Relief of seizures from a predominantly posterior temporal tumor with anterior temporal lobectomy. Epilepsia 30 (5), 559–563.

Strowbridge, B.W., Bean, A.J., Spencer, D.D., et al., 1992. Low levels of somatostatin-like immunoreactivity in neocortex resected from presumed seizure foci in epileptic patients. Brain Res. 587 (1), 164–168.

Taillibert, S., Delattre, J.Y., 2005. Palliative care in patients with brain metastases. Curr. Opin. Oncol. 17 (6), 588–592.

Takahashi, A., Hong, S.C., Seo, D.W., et al., 2005. Frequent association of cortical dysplasia in dysembryoplastic neuroepithelial tumor treated by epilepsy surgery. Surg. Neurol. 64 (5), 419–427.

Tang, C.M., Dichter, M., Morad, M., 1990. Modulation of the N-methyl-D-aspartate channel by extracellular H+. Proc. Natl. Acad. Sci. U. S. A. 87 (16), 6445–6449.

Taphoorn, M.J., 2003. Neurocognitive sequelae in the treatment of low-grade gliomas. Semin. Oncol. 30 (Suppl), 45–48.

Tomson, T., 2000. Mortality in epilepsy. J. Neurol. 247 (1), 15–21.

Tran, T.A., Spencer, S.S., Javidan, M., et al., 1997. Significance of spikes recorded on intraoperative electrocorticography in patients with brain tumor and epilepsy. Epilepsia 38 (10), 1132–1139.

Ulloa, C.M., Towfigh, A., Safdieh, J., 2009. Review of levetiracetam, with a focus on the extended release formulation, as adjuvant therapy in controlling partial-onset seizures. Neuropsychiatr Dis. Treat. 5, 467–476.

Vajda, F.J., O'brien, T.J., Hitchcock, A., et al., 2004. Critical relationship between sodium valproate dose and human teratogenicity: results of the Australian register of anti-epileptic drugs in pregnancy. J. Clin. Neurosci. 11 (8), 854–858.

van Breemen, M.S., Wilms, E.B., Vecht, C.J., 2007. Epilepsy in patients with brain tumours: epidemiology, mechanisms, and management. Lancet. 6, 421–430.

van Breemen, M.S., Rijsman, R.M., Taphoorn, M.J., et al., 2009. Efficacy of anti-epileptic drugs in patients with gliomas and seizures. J. Neurol. 256 (9), 1519–1526.

Van Paesschen, W., 2004. Ictal SPECT. Epilepsia 45 (Suppl), 35–40.

van Veelen, M.L., Avezaat, C.J., Kros, J.M., et al., 1998. Supratentorial low-grade astrocytoma: prognostic factors, dedifferentiation, and the issue of early versus late surgery. J. Neurol. Neurosurg Psychiatry 64 (5), 581–587.

Villemure, J.G., de Tribolet, N., 1996. Epilepsy in patients with central nervous system tumors. Curr. Opin. Neurol. 9 (6), 424–428.

Wagner, G.L., Wilms, E.B., Van Donselaar, C.A., et al., 2003. Levetiracetam: preliminary experience in patients with primary brain tumours. Seizure 12 (8), 585–586.

Waniewski, R.A., Martin, D.L., 1986. Exogenous glutamate is metabolized to glutamine and exported by rat primary astrocyte cultures. J. Neurochem. 47 (1), 304–313.

Wen, P.Y., Marks, P.W., 2002. Medical management of patients with brain tumors. Curr. Opin. Oncol. 14 (3), 299–307.

Wennberg, R., Quesney, L.F., Lozano, A., et al., 1999. Role of electrocorticography at surgery for lesion-related frontal lobe epilepsy. Can. J. Neurol. Sci. 26 (1), 33–39.

White, J.C., Liu, C.T., Mixter, W.J., et al., 1948. Focal epilepsy; a statistical study of its causes and the results of surgical treatment; epilepsy secondary to cerebral trauma and infection. N. Engl. J. Med. 239 (1), 1–10.

Whittle, I.R., Beaumont, A., 1995. Seizures in patients with supratentorial oligodendroglial tumours. Clinicopathological features and management considerations. Acta. Neurochir. (Wien) 135 (1–2), 19–24.

Whittle, I.R., Clarke, M., Gregori, A., et al., 1992. Interstitial white matter brain oedema does not alter the electroencephalogram. Br. J. Neurosurg. 6 (5), 433–437.

Williamson, A., Shepard, G.M., Spencer, D.D., 1991. Evidence for hyperexcitability near neocortical lesions in epileptic patients. Epilepsia 31 (Suppl 3), S67–S73.

Wolf, H.K., Roos, D., Blümcke, I., et al., 1996. Perilesional neurochemical changes in focal epilepsies. Acta. Neuropathol. 91, 376–384.

Ye, Z.C., Rothstein, J.D., Sontheimer, H., 1999. Compromised glutamate transport in human glioma cells: reduction-mislocalization of sodium-dependent glutamate transporters and enhanced activity of cystine-glutamate exchange. J. Neurosci. 19 (24), 10767–10777.

Yuen, T., Bjorksten, A., Finch, S., et al., 2010. Glutamate and its role in tumor associated epilepsy. Manuscipt in preparation.

Zentner, J., Hufnagel, A., Wolf, H.K., et al., 1997. Surgical treatment of neoplasms associated with medically intractable epilepsy. Neurosurgery 41 (2), 378–386, discussion 386–387.

Anesthesia and intensive care management of patients with brain tumors

Jesse Raiten, Robert H. Thiele, and Edward C. Nemergut

13

Introduction

There is no branch of surgery wherein an anesthesiologist can impact the surgical procedure as directly as intracranial neurosurgery. Even subtle changes in anesthetic technique and patient management can directly impact the surgical field and the ease by which the neurosurgeon can complete the intended procedure. Thus, both anesthesiologists and neurosurgeons must have a comprehensive understanding of neurophysiology and neuropathophysiology and the potential impact of various anesthetic agents and techniques. Indeed, Drs Liu and Apuzzo noted in a 2003 editorial that 'as much as any single factor, the development of neuroanesthesia was an essential element in the evolution of the modern neurosurgical operating environment' (Liu et al 2003).

A useful approach to guide the learner in the cogent understanding of neuroanesthesia is to develop goals for the optimal care of all patients presenting for brain tumor resection. Obviously, the first goal is to safely maintain oxygenation and circulation and support the function of vital organs. This goal is not unique to neurosurgical patients and should be the primary goal of any surgical anesthetic. The second goal is to provide the neurosurgeons with an excellent operative field. This requires an understanding of cerebral physiology, especially the effect of anesthetic agents on the cerebral metabolic rate (CMR), the cerebral blood flow (CBF), and intracranial pressure (ICP). The third goal is to conduct the anesthetic such that a rapid emergence from anesthesia is possible. This allows for early neurologic assessment in the operating room and requires an understanding of pharmacokinetics and pharmacodynamics. Secondary goals might include increasing the tolerance to cerebral ischemia, allowing for appropriate neurophysiologic monitoring, and the avoidance of possible toxicity. The above serves as a gross outline to the first half of this chapter. The second half of this chapter will focus on postoperative care of patients with brain tumors, specifically the care of critically ill patients in the intensive care unit (ICU).

Basic neurophysiology and pharmacology

Determinants of the cerebral metabolic rate

All neurons have an electrical potential across their cell membranes (–70 mV at rest) secondary to different intracellular and extracellular ion concentrations. Specific, energy-dependent protein ion channels maintain this potential. Neurons communicate over longer distances through the propagation of action potentials, which is a brief and rapid depolarization of the cell membrane. Neurons communicate with one another via chemical synapse. An action potential causes the release of a neurotransmitter that combines with a post-synaptic receptor on the target neuron. Neurotransmitters function by making the target neuron more or less likely to depolarize (and fire an action potential). Inhibitory neurotransmitters make action potentials less likely by hyperpolarizing the target neuron.

The principal inhibitory neurotransmitter in the central nervous system (CNS) is γ-aminobutyric acid (GABA). The activation of $GABA_A$ receptors opens chloride channels and the activation of $GABA_B$ receptors opens potassium channels. Glycine is another important inhibitory neurotransmitter. The toxin strychnine is an important competitive inhibitor of the glycine receptor. Excitatory neurotransmitters function by making action potentials more likely by depolarizing target neurons. The principal excitatory neurotransmitter in the CNS is glutamate and its metabolites AMPA (α-amino-3-hydroxyl-5-methyl-4-isoxazole-propionate) and NMDA (N-methyl-D-aspartic acid). The activation of specific glutamate receptors results in the activation of sodium and/or calcium channels.

The regulation of all ion channels and electrical potential is energy dependent. The principal substrate for brain metabolism is glucose; however, the brain can also use ketone bodies during a starved state. Regardless, the ultimate utilization of both energy fuels requires entrance into the tricarboxylic acid cycle (TCA), which requires oxygen. As such, the brain requires a continuous supply of oxygen. In the absence of pathology or drugs, the cerebral metabolic requirement for oxygen ($CMRO_2$) is stable between 3.0 and 3.8 (average 3.5) mL O_2/min per 100 g brain tissue. This value can be greater in infants and children. Approximately 50–60% of the brain's energy consumption is used to support electrophysiological function (ions pumps, etc.) leaving about 40–50% for homeostatic functions, such as the maintenance of cellular integrity, etc. The CMR is not constant and may vary widely between specific parts of the brain. CMR is decreased during natural sleep and increased during intense mental or physical activity or arousal of any cause.

Determinants of the cerebral blood flow

Obviously, a continuous supply of oxygen requires uninterrupted blood flow. Important physiologic determinants of the cerebral blood flow (CBF) include blood pressure, CO_2 and O_2, and the CMR. Measurements of the CBF range from 45 to 65 (average 50) mL/min per 100 g brain tissue. White matter requires slightly less blood flow with average values around 20 mL/min per 100 g tissue, whereas gray matter receives more blood flow with average values around 80 mL/min per 100 g tissue. Cerebral perfusion pressure (CPP) can be defined as the difference between mean arterial pressure (MAP) and intracranial pressure (ICP):

$$CPP = MAP - ICP$$

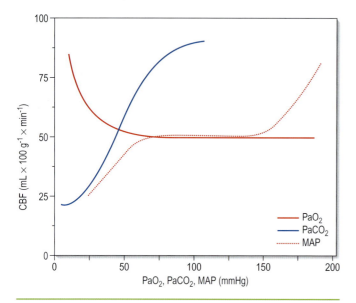

Figure 13.1 Changes in cerebral blood flow (CBF) caused by alterations in $PaCO_2$, PaO_2, and mean arterial pressure (MAP). (From Patel PM, Drummond JC. Cerebral Physiology and the Effects of Anesthetics and Techniques. In Miller's Anesthesia, 6th edition. Philadelphia: Churchill Livingstone; 2005. With permission of Elsevier.)

In the non-pathologic brain, the CBF is maintained across a wide range of cerebral perfusion pressures through the process of myogenic autoregulation. The mechanism is not completely understood (Branston 1995); however, when hypertensive, vascular smooth muscle senses increased pressure and stretch, and responds with contraction and an increase in the cerebrovascular resistance (CBV). During hypotension, vascular smooth muscle senses decreased pressure and responds with dilation and decreases in CBV. This process is not instantaneous and abrupt changes in blood pressure can alter CBF until myogenic regulation can take effect. Regardless, the end result is that CBF is said to be constant between a CPP of 55 and 155 mmHg (Fig. 13.1). At a CPP above 155 mmHg, the cerebral vasculature is maximally constricted and further increases in pressure result in increased CBF and the risks of hypertensive encephalopathy. At a CPP below 55 mmHg, the cerebral vasculature is maximally vasodilated and CBF becomes entirely pressure dependent.

It is important to note that in chronic untreated hypertension, hypertrophy of the cerebral vasculature leads to a 'rightward' shift of the autoregulation curve (Strandgaard 1976). This protects the brain against hypertensive encephalopathy at the risk of limiting the safe level for reducing the CPP. Consequently, patients with chronic untreated hypertension may develop cerebral ischemia at a CPP higher than 55 mmHg. Also, it is important to recognize that even within the range over which autoregulation normally occurs, a rapid change in arterial pressure will result in a transient (3–4 min) alteration in CBF (Greenfield et al 1984).

CO_2 is a potent physiologic determinant of CBF. If one considers the normal $PaCO_2$ to be 40 mmHg, doubling the $PaCO_2$ to 80 mmHg will double the CBF. Further increases in $PaCO_2$ produce little increase in CBF, as the cerebral vasculature is already maximally vasodilated. Conversely, if one considers the normal $PaCO_2$ to be 40 mmHg, halving the $PaCO_2$ to 20 mmHg will halve the CBF. Further decreases in the $PaCO_2$ produce little decrease in CBF, as the cerebral vasculature is already maximally vasoconstricted. Thus, the $PaCO_2$ has a linear relationship with CBF over a four-fold (20–80 mmHg) range (Fig. 13.1).

The $PaCO_2$ is able to exert these powerful effects on the CBF through its ability to impact the pH of the CSF and extracellular fluid. During acute hypocapnia, rapid diffusion of CO_2 out of the CSF leads to a relative excess of HCO_3^- and an increase in CSF pH. The increase in the pH of the CSF and extracellular fluid lead directly to vascular smooth muscle contraction, increases in CVR, and decreases in CBF. During acute hypercapnia, rapid diffusion of CO_2 into the CSF leads to a relative paucity of HCO_3^- and a decrease in CSF pH. The decrease in the pH of the CSF and extracellular fluid lead directly to vascular smooth muscle dilation, decreases in CVR, and increases in CBF. Since CO_2 has no direct effect on CBF (the effect of CO_2 is mediated through a change in the pH of the CSF and the extracellular fluid), the effects of both hypocapnia and hypercapnia on CBF are short-lived and extinguish upon normalization of the extracellular HCO_3^- concentration (Muizelaar et al 1988; Raichle et al 1970). Thus, abrupt restoration of normocapnia after prolonged hyperventilation can result in massive increases in CBF, as rapid diffusion of CO_2 into the CSF leads to a relative paucity of HCO_3^- and a decrease in the pH of the CSF.

It should be noted that most, if not all, pathologic states attenuate or abolish normal CO_2 reactivity. This may occur with both regional and global processes. For example, in traumatic brain injury, the vascular supply to the injured area may be maximally vasodilated and may not respond to CO_2. Thus, deliberate hyperventilation may decrease CBF to normal, uninjured areas.

Oxygen and PaO_2 are less potent determinants of CBF (Fig. 13.1). Nevertheless, hypoxemia (PaO_2 <50 mmHg) can produce striking increases in CBF. This is not directly mediated by PaO_2 but rather by the by-products of anaerobic metabolism (i.e. lactate). This explains the lack of CO_2 reactivity in ischemic areas. Normobaric and hyperbaric hyperoxia (pO_2 >1 atm) may cause small decreases in CBF.

The most important physiologic determinant of CBF is the CMR. In essence, anything that causes a change in CMR will cause a parallel change in CBF. For example, hypothermia decreases the CMR approximately 6–7% for every 1°C decrease in temperature. Thus, at 27°C (a 10°C decrease in temperature), the CMR will have decreased by approximately 60% from baseline, normothermic (37°C) values. This change in CMR would be accompanied by a decrease in CBF by approximately 60%. In contrast, hyperthermia increases CMR by approximately 5–6% for every 1°C increase in temperature up to 42°C. A febrile patient with a fever of 40°C would have an increase in CMR by approximately 15% from baseline, normothermic (37°C) values. This change in CMR would be accompanied by a decrease in CBF by approximately 15%. After 42°C, a dramatic decrease in CMR is observed. This decrease in CMR represents a toxic effect of hyperthermia and protein (electron transport) degradation.

Intracranial pressure (ICP)

Normal ICP in a supine patient ranges from approximately 8–12 mmHg. Pathologic conditions significantly alter ICP. Since CPP is dependent upon the ICP, increases in ICP can significantly limit the CPP and the CBF. The cranium is a rigid structure surrounded by bone that contains three things: the cellular elements of brain, glia, etc. (~80%), blood (~10%), and cerebrospinal fluid (CSF) (~10%). As the volume of the cranium is fixed, an increase in the volume of any element must result in a consequent decrease in the volume of another element or an increase in pressure or both. Intracranial elastance is determined by measuring the change in intracranial pressure in response to a change in intracranial volume (dP/dV). (Many sources will refer to this as intracranial compliance; however, this is incorrect for compliance is dV/dP). Regardless, a slowly growing brain tumor is initially well compensated; however, a point is eventually reached where further increases produce precipitous increases in ICP. Major compensatory mechanisms include the displacement of CSF, and increases in CSF absorption, a decrease in CSF production, and a decrease in the cerebral blood volume (CBV), especially venous blood volume. Since all anesthetic agents have important effects on CBV, CBF, CMR, and ICP and most patients with brain tumors presenting for surgery have reached a point where cerebral elastance is very high, the understanding of these principles is critical to optimal patient care.

Potent inhaled anesthetics

Understanding the complex effects of potent inhaled anesthetic agents is critical to the conduct of optimal perioperative care. There is a tendency among some authors to generalize the effects of potent inhaled agents as being similar; however, that will not be our approach here and we will consider each modern agent individually. To understand the effect of a given potent volatile anesthetic on cerebral hemodynamics, one must understand two basic principles: (1) all potent inhaled anesthetic agents are direct cerebral vasodilators and thereby decrease CVR and tend to increase CBF and ICP in patients with altered intracranial elastance. (2) All potent inhaled anesthetic agents decrease CMR and thereby tend to decrease CBF. It is important to note for all agents, the decrease in CMR stems from a decrease in electrophysiological activity, the maximal decrease in CMR is attained with EEG-silence and represents about 50% of total CMR (as explained above). The net effect for a given agent on CBF and ICP results from the balance of the above two properties. In addition, some potent inhaled anesthetic agents can attenuate normal CO_2 reactivity and autoregulation through their effects on CVR and CBF.

Halothane is the oldest potent inhaled anesthetic still in use. It is the most potent cerebral vasodilator and causes the least decrease in CMR. In addition, it almost completely abolishes normal CO_2 reactivity to the point that even profound hyperventilation can reliably decrease CBF if it is initiated before halothane is administered. At equivalent minimum alveolar concentration (MAC), halothane increases CBF up to 200%. Halothane has been shown to decrease CSF production and decrease CSF absorption; however, these

effects are likely not clinically relevant. The combined sum of these properties have made halothane an unpopular choice for patients with brain tumors and altered intracranial elastance.

Isoflurane is the prototype of all modern inhaled anesthetics in terms of its effects on cerebral physiology. Isoflurane is a weak direct cerebral vasodilator and causes dose-dependent decreases in CMR with the ability to produce an isoelectric EEG at approximately 2 MAC. The effects of isoflurane on CMR are not uniform: isoflurane reduces the CMR predominantly in the neocortex. In addition, isoflurane preserves normal CO_2 reactivity and effectively abolishes autoregulation only at high concentrations. Like halothane, its effects on CSF formation and absorption are likely not clinically relevant. As above, the combined sum of these properties have made isoflurane the proverbial touchstone for all modern anesthetics and the standard to which any new agent is measured. Nevertheless, the net effect of isoflurane administration is a modest, dose-dependent increase in CBF; however, these effects can generally be completely abrogated with judicious hyperventilation. Similarly, isoflurane may increase ICP, especially in patients with altered intracranial elastance; however, hyperventilation can generally attenuate this effect.

Sevoflurane was introduced into anesthetic practice in the 1990s and, in many ways, may be superior to isoflurane. Like isoflurane, sevoflurane can produce an isoelectric EEG at approximately 2 MAC indicative of a 50% reduction in CMR. Also, sevoflurane is only a very weak direct cerebral vasodilator. Indeed, 0.5 MAC sevoflurane produces no significant increase in CBF in a study of healthy volunteers. In fact, increases in CBF with 1.5 MAC sevoflurane are similar to increases in CBF with 0.5 MAC isoflurane (Matta et al 1999). Sevoflurane possesses a low blood:gas partition coefficient (0.68), approximately half that of isoflurane, which allows for a more rapid emergence from general anesthesia. These properties have made sevoflurane a popular choice for neuroanesthesia. That said, some studies have noted the appearance of epileptiform EEG changes in some patients when the concentration of sevoflurane is abruptly increased (Voss et al 2008). The clinical significance of these changes is unknown; however, it is the opinion of the authors that these changes are not likely relevant.

Desflurane was also introduced into anesthetic practice in the 1990s and is structurally similar to isoflurane. Like isoflurane, desflurane can produce an isoelectric EEG at approximately 2 MAC indicative of a 50% reduction in CMR. Also like isoflurane, desflurane has little effect on CO_2 reactivity and effectively abolishes autoregulation only at high concentrations. In addition, desflurane produces the lowest blood:gas partition coefficient (0.42), which allows for rapid emergence from general anesthesia. Unfortunately, desflurane possesses some notable disadvantages. Initiation of desflurane (and abrupt increases in desflurane concentration) cause substantial increases in plasma norepinephrine concentration, which leads to increases in blood pressure (Weiskopf et al 1994). This can translate into abrupt increases in CBF, especially at high desflurane concentrations when autoregulation is already impaired. In addition, several human and animal studies have shown desflurane to produce increases in ICP over both isoflurane and

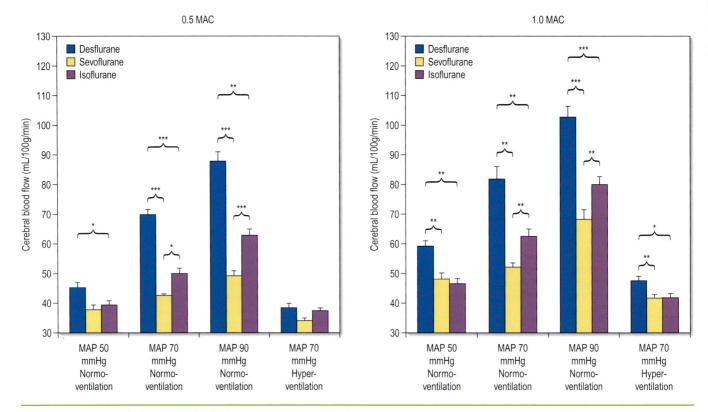

Figure 13.2 Cerebral blood flow (CBF) for desflurane, sevoflurane, and isoflurane at 0.5 and 1.0 minimal alveolar concentrations (MAC) with three different mean arterial pressures (MAP) (50, 70, and 90 mmHg). Note that moderate hypocapnia abrogates most changes. Differences between the agents are indicated (*$p < 0.05$; **$p < 0.01$; ***$p < 0.001$). (From Holmstrom A and Akeson J. Desflurane increases intracranial pressure more and sevoflurane less than isoflurane in pigs subjected to intracranial hypertension. J Neurosurg Anesthesiol 2004;16(2):136–143.)

sevoflurane (Holmstrom & Akeson 2004). Nevertheless, since these effects can almost always be eliminated by even mild hyperventilation, desflurane has become a popular choice for neuroanesthesia.

The effects of the potent volatile agents on CBF and CIP are summarized in Figures 13.2 and 13.3.

Nitrous oxide

Nitrous oxide is a highly insoluble anesthetic agent that allows for rapid emergence from anesthesia. Unfortunately, when used alone, nitrous oxide alters the EEG and causes dramatic increases in both CBF and ICP in patients with supratentorial tumors. When combined with a potent inhaled agent (see above), nitrous oxide increases CBF, ICP and accelerates the blunting of autoregulation. If utilized with an intravenous agent (see below), nitrous oxide has more modest effects on ICP and CBF. Nitrous oxide has also been shown in multiple studies to increase the incidence of postoperative nausea and vomiting (PONV) (Apfel et al 2004; Gan 2006; Myles et al 2007), which may be particularly deleterious to any patient who has just had intracranial surgery.

Finally, it is important to remember that nitrous oxide has a potential to dramatically expand air-filled spaces. Because nitrous oxide is used in high concentrations and is more soluble in blood than nitrogen, it partitions out of the blood into air-filled spaces much faster than nitrogen is reabsorbed out of such spaces. As such, nitrous oxide has been associated with the expansion of intracranial air and the development of a tension pneumocephalus (Artru 1982).

Intravenous anesthetics

The most commonly used intravenous anesthetics are barbiturates (including thiopental and methohexital), propofol, etomidate, and ketamine. All intravenous anesthetics (with the exception of ketamine, see below) produce substantial decreases in CMR, CBF, and ICP. At appropriate doses, propofol, etomidate and thiopental can produce electrical silence on EEG, corresponding to a 50–60% decrease in CMR.

Barbiturates have four main actions in the brain: (1) hypnosis; (2) depression of the CMR; (3) reduction in CBF through increased CVR and flow-metabolism coupling; and (4) anticonvulsant activity. Unlike the potent volatile agents, the barbiturates uniformly reduce the CMR throughout the brain. Unfortunately, all barbiturates possess the capacity to produce significant hypotension, especially in hypovolemic patients, which can result in significant reductions in CPP. If CPP is maintained, barbiturates decrease CMR slightly more than they reduce CBF such that metabolic supply theoretically exceeds the CMR. These factors combine to make the barbiturates, especially, *thiopental,* extremely popular. Unfortunately, thiopental's utility beyond the induction of anesthesia is extremely limited secondary to its long-half life (≈ 12 h) and its potential to produce hypotension.

Methohexital, an oxybarbiturate with a relatively short half-life (3–4 h), would seemingly be a useful agent. Unfortunately, small doses actually lower the seizure threshold, making it useful for electroconvulsive therapy (ECT) but inappropriate for patients undergoing intracranial neurosurgical procedures. Epileptiform patterns are also noted after

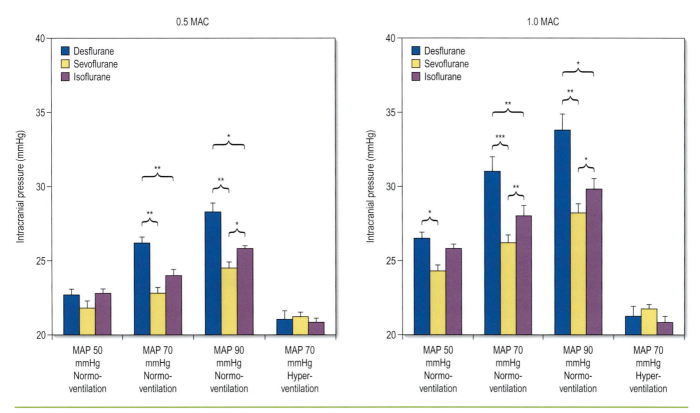

Figure 13.3 Intracranial pressure (ICP) for desflurane, sevoflurane, and isoflurane at 0.5 and 1.0 minimal alveolar concentrations (MAC) with three different mean arterial pressures (MAP) (50, 70, and 90 mmHg). Note that moderate hypocapnia abrogates most changes. Differences between the agents are indicated ($*p < 0.05$; $**p < 0.01$; $***p < 0.001$). (From Holmstrom A and Akeson J. Desflurane increases intracranial pressure more and sevoflurane less than isoflurane in pigs subjected to intracranial hypertension. J Neurosurg Anesthesiol 2004;16(2):136–143.)

high doses and there is a 33% increase in postoperative seizures when a methohexital infusion is utilized. Thus, methohexital is not frequently used in neuroanesthesia.

Etomidate is a carboxylated imidazole and is structurally unrelated to all other intravenous anesthetics. Etomidate is often utilized secondary to its minimal degree of cardiovascular suppression, maintenance of myocardial contractility, and low incidence of hypotension. In patients with high intracranial elastance, etomidate is unique in that it is able to both reduce CMR and CBF without reducing CPP. Unfortunately, etomidate has several undesirable effects. The effects of etomidate on CMR are not uniform, affecting the cortex more than the brainstem. Etomidate is a potent inhibitor of 11-β-hydroxylase in the adrenal glands and can decrease cortisol synthesis. This may be particularly important in patients with Cushing's disease where a low postoperative cortisol can be mistaken for a therapeutic surgical result. In addition, multiple studies suggest that even while reducing CMR, etomidate actually decreases the tolerance to ischemia and results in increased injury compared with control patients. The induction of anesthesia with etomidate is associated with a 70% incidence of myoclonic movement; however, these movements are not associated with seizure activity on the EEG. Nevertheless, etomidate remains an attractive agent for the induction of general anesthesia in patients with significant cardiac compromise.

Ketamine is a phencyclidine derivative that produces 'dissociative anesthesia' where patients appear to be in a

cataleptic state: eyes are open, respiration is maintained, and many reflexes are maintained. Although a direct myocardial suppressant, the cardiovascular effects of ketamine mimic the effects of sympathetic nervous system stimulation with increases in heart rate and blood pressure. Ketamine has been historically unpopular during neurosurgery as administration results in increases in CMR, CBF, and ICP. Ketamine is the only intravenous agent that dilates the cerebral vasculature and increases CBF. The effects on CMR are not uniform as limbic and reticular structures experience increases in CMR, while cortical areas, especially somatosensory and auditory, experience decreases in CMR (and CBF). Seizure activity in the thalamic and limbic areas has been described. These increases in ICP, CMR, and CBF limit ketamine's utility in patients with altered intracranial elastance; however, 'low dose' ketamine produces minimal effects on ICP and may possess neuroprotective qualities secondary to its NMDA receptor antagonism.

Propofol is substituted isopropyl phenol that decreases CMR, CBF, and ICP. Like barbiturates, propofol uniformly reduces the CMR throughout the brain. Propofol possesses the capacity to produce significant hypotension, especially in hypovolemic patients, which can result in significant reductions in CPP. Unlike barbiturates, propofol may independently increase CVR, decreasing CBF to a greater degree than CMR. Propofol has a relatively short half-life ($\approx$1–2 h) and undergoes little prolongation of context-sensitive half time and thus is useful as an infusion in both the intraoperative and postoperative setting.

Opioids

Commonly used opioids in neuroanesthesia include the synthetic opioids *fentanyl, sufentanil, alfentanil, and remifentanil*. Morphine and codeine are rarely used in the intraoperative setting but are occasionally used in the post-operative setting and in the intensive care unit. All opioids have little direct effect on CBF, CMR, or ICP. All opioids attenuate the ventilatory response to hypercarbia and ablate the ventilatory response to hypoxia, thus, if patients are allowed to spontaneously ventilate, all opioids will increase CBF through an increase in $PaCO_2$. In patients with altered intracranial elastance, this may result in a substantial increase in ICP. It is also important to recognize that all opioids, with the exception of meperidine, are vasotonic and their acute administration can result in bradycardia. In patients with a brain tumor, it is important to distinguish the effect from Cushing's reflex. In addition to increasing heart rate, meperidine also has a metabolite, normeperidine, which can induce seizures, especially in patients with renal failure. Finally, like thiopental and propofol, all opioids may reduce blood pressure, CPP, and compensatory cerebrovascular vasodilation with increases in ICP.

Dexmedetomidine

Dexmedetomidine is a highly selective alpha-2 adrenergic receptor agonist. The foremost clinical effects of dexmedetomidine are both a sedative-hypnotic and analgesic effect, which is mediated through the activation of alpha-2 adrenergic receptors in the locus ceruleus and the spinal cord. Unlike all other intravenous agents, dexmedetomidine causes only mild increases in $PaCO_2$, which make it particularly useful for sedation in awake brain tumor patients or in patients undergoing an awake craniotomy. The elimination half-life is approximately 2–3 h; however, a context sensitive half-time ranges from 4 min (after a 10 min infusion) to 2–3 h (after an 8 h infusion). Hypotension and bradycardia can complicate its use, especially if it is given too quickly or if a patient is given too great of a load over too short a period of time.

The effects of various intravenous anesthetics on CBF and CMR are summarized in Figure 13.4.

Muscle relaxants

Neuromuscular blocking agents (NMBAs) are essentially free of any direct effect on CMR, ICP, or CBF. Pancuronium, through its vagolytic activity, can increase heart rate and MAP, potentially increasing CBF and ICP in patients with altered intracranial elastance and autoregulation. Bisbenzylisoquinoliniums (such as mivacurium) may be associated with histamine release and hypotension. Succinylcholine can increase ICP in brain tumor patients secondary to the cerebral activation associated with fasciculations and enhanced muscle spindle activity; however if co-administered with intravenous agent (such as propofol or thiopental), this is likely not clinically relevant.

Succinylcholine has a short duration of action and is useful in the setting of a potential difficult airway or rapid sequence induction, as in the case of a patient with an increased risk of aspiration. Among its side-effects,

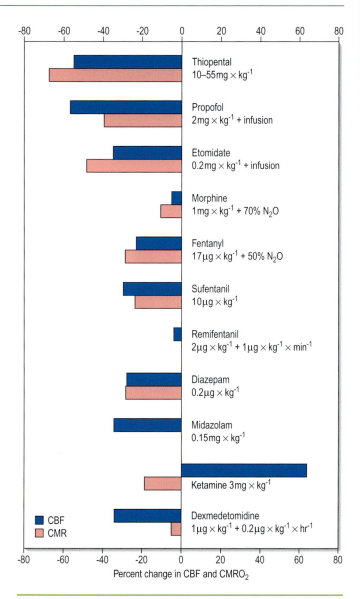

Figure 13.4 Changes in cerebral blood flow (CBF) and cerebral metabolic rate (CMR) caused various intravenous anesthetics. (With permission from Patel PM, Drummond JC. Cerebral Physiology and the Effects of Anesthetics and Techniques. In Miller's Anesthesia, 6th edition. Philadelphia: Churchill Livingstone; 2005. With permission from Elsevier.)

succinylcholine's depolarization of the acetylcholine receptor causes an efflux of potassium, and may increase the serum potassium level. In patients with profound muscle weakness or immobility, the release of potassium may be larger, potentially resulting in dangerous levels of hyperkalemia. This hyperkalemic response may be due to an upregulation of acetylcholine receptors, including new isoforms, which may be observed in the setting of muscle denervation (Martyn et al 2006). Succinylcholine is therefore generally avoided in paraplegic patients, or those enduring long periods of immobility (which may also lead to an up regulation of the acetylcholine receptor). Non-depolarizing neuromuscular blockers may be safely used in patients with weakness or paralysis. Rocuronium is a non-depolarizing agent with rapid onset, and is the muscle relaxant of choice for rapid sequence induction in patients when succinylcholine is contraindicated.

While standard dosing regimens have been established for most muscle relaxants, their administration should be guided by monitoring of muscle twitches. Twitch monitors are readily available and can deliver electrical stimuli at different rates and intensities, allowing the clinician to assess the degree of neuromuscular blockade. This ensures that a patient is not overdosed with paralytics, potentially delaying extubation and contributing to postoperative weakness, or critical illness myopathy. In a patient with hemiplegia, twitch monitoring should occur on the non-affected side, as extra-junctional proliferation of acetylcholine receptors on the plegic side will lead to decreased sensitivity to muscle relaxants. This may lead the clinician to underestimate the degree of muscle relaxation throughout the rest of the body, increasing the risk for excessive drug administration.

Anesthetic management of the patient with a supratentorial brain tumor

A craniotomy for the resection or biopsy of a supratentorial tumor is among the most common neurosurgical procedures. Relevant preoperative considerations include the patient's ICP and intracranial elastance, the location and size of the tumor, and any relevant patient comorbidities. The location and size of the tumor will give the anesthesiologist an indication of the surgical position and the potential for blood loss.

Preoperative assessment

Information regarding each patient's medical comorbidities should be available for review prior to surgery. Generally speaking, patients presenting for the surgical resection of a brain tumor present urgently if not emergently for surgical excision or biopsy. Thus, complete preoperative optimization is not always possible. Nevertheless, if deemed surgical candidates, all patient should be optimized to the greatest degree possible prior to surgery. Patients with significant hepatic disease or cirrhosis require a thorough evaluation of their blood coagulation. Patients with dialysis dependent end stage renal disease (ESRD) should be dialyzed prior to surgery and their serum electrolytes, especially serum potassium, should be checked prior the induction of general anesthesia. While there are no randomized studies to guide management, conventional wisdom dictates that unless resection is deemed emergent, surgery should likely be delayed in patients with acute exacerbations of asthma or chronic obstructive pulmonary disease (COPD), given the diminished pulmonary function after general anesthesia observed in all patients. All patients, especially those with a history of cardiac disease should undergo risk stratification using the American College of Cardiology guidelines (Fleisher et al 2007); however, it should be noted that if significant coronary artery disease or significant valvular disease is discovered, brain tumor patients may not be candidates for preoperative therapy given the fact most therapeutic interventions (coronary artery stents, coronary artery bypass grafting, valve repair or replacement) require varying degrees of systemic anticoagulation, often continuing into the post-procedure period. Nevertheless, knowledge of cardiac function and the presence of significant cardiac disease, even if not presently amenable to therapy, may be useful to the anesthesiologist.

Patients with a significant mass effect, especially if edema is present, should receive preoperative steroids. Dexamethasone is the most commonly used steroid. A regimen such as 10 mg intravenously or orally every 6 h is generally effective. Conventional wisdom has dictated that patients with brain tumors should not be given a preoperative anxiolytic (most commonly midazolam) because of concern about increase $PaCO_2$, CBF, and ICP in a patient whose intracranial elastance is already abnormal. It is also possible that a patient with significant anxiety, may become hypertensive and that may increase $PaCO_2$, CBF, and ICP. Thus, the authors believe that the absolute prohibition of preoperative anxiolytics is not appropriate; however, any patient given a preoperative anxiolytic should be carefully monitored.

In addition to standard monitors, most patients presenting for intracranial neurosurgery require invasive monitoring of blood pressure using an arterial catheter. The preinduction placement of an arterial line may be appropriate in patients with large tumors, significant mass effect, and/or altered intracranial elastance. The induction of anesthesia, laryngoscopy, and endotracheal intubation may be associated with hypertension, with its attendant risks in a patient with impaired elastance and autoregulation. Nevertheless, the placement of an arterial line may be delayed until after the induction of anesthesia in most patients. Procedures with a potential for substantial blood loss (tumors encroaching on the sagittal sinus, large vascular tumors) may also justify the placement of a CVP catheters. Pulmonary artery catheterization is rarely indicated.

Management of anesthesia

Many factors may impact the selection of anesthetic agents. The effects of any agent on ICP, CPP, CBF, $CMRO_2$, and promptness of return to consciousness are major considerations. Other considerations include drug-related protection from ischemia or edema, blood pressure control, and compatibility with neurophysiologic monitoring techniques.

As virtually all of the volatile anesthetics can cause an increase in ICP when accompanied by normocarbia, deep anesthesia with high dose volatile agents is rarely used. Moderate hypocarbia with <1.0 MAC volatile agent represents the most common anesthetic technique. As above, halothane produces the greatest reduction in cerebral vascular resistance and the clearest increase in ICP and is rarely used. If halothane must be used, the decrease in CVR can be blunted or even eliminated if hyperventilation is established before halothane is turned on (Adams et al 1972). As previously noted, isoflurane, sevoflurane, and desflurane produce less of a reduction in CVR and a comparatively diminished elevation of ICP at normocarbia. This response can be blocked by hyperventilation in tumor patients. On balance, isoflurane, sevoflurane, and desflurane may also be considered equally appropriate in patients with brain tumors, so long as the anesthesiologist is aware of each agent's attendant advantages and disadvantages. The authors prefer

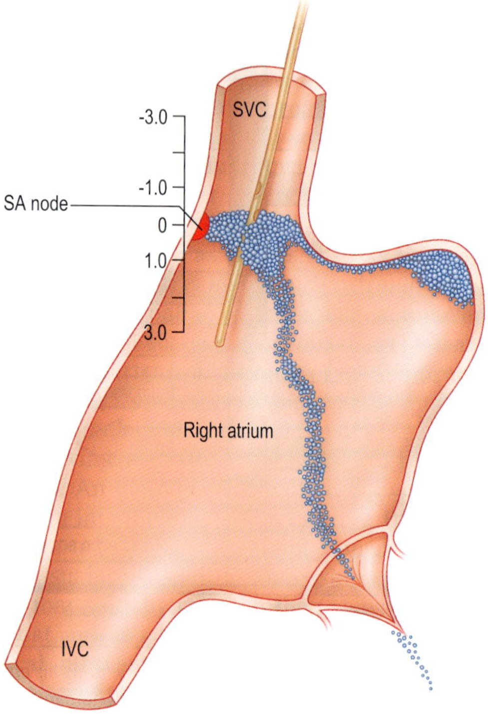

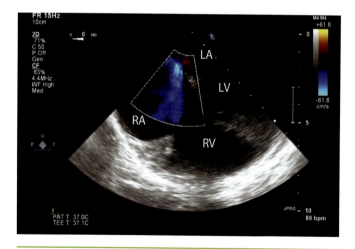

Figure 13.6 Air tends to localize at the atrial-SVC junction, moving through the tricuspid valve or into upright portions of the atrium. The multi orifice catheter placement most likely to aspirate air is shown. IVC, inferior vena cava; SA, sinoatrial; SVC superior vena cava.

Figure 13.7 Color Doppler TEE showing a PFO. LA, left atrium; LV, left ventricle; RA, right atrium; RV, right ventricle. (Image courtesy of Julie Huffmyer, M.D., The University of Virginia.)

contrast-enhanced TEE (Fig. 13.7). If this study reveals the passage of contrast across an incomplete atrial septum without any provocative maneuvers, we believe surgery in the seated position is contraindicated. If contrast crosses the septum only with provocative maneuvers, the surgeon, anesthesiologist, and patient should carefully consider the positioning options available given the size and location of the tumor and the amount of contrast detected in the left atrium. Obviously, if no contrast is visualized in the left

> **Box 13.1** Treatment of venous air embolism
>
> 1. Inform surgical team, flood field with saline. Consider Valsalva or bilateral jugular compression to increase venous pressure to help surgeons to identify entry site
> 2. Discontinue nitrous oxide
> 3. Attempt to aspirate air from right atrial catheter
> 4. Expand intravascular volume with intravenous fluids to increase preload
> 5. If hypotensive, consider vasopressors
> 6. Consider placing patient in the head down position if persistent hypotension develops
> 7. ACLS protocol for cardiovascular collapse.

atrium after provocative maneuvers, the sitting position is not contraindicated. Transcranial Doppler (TCD) may also be used as a screening technique for a PFO and VAE (Stendel et al 2000); however, TCD is less widely available than TEE.

If a VAE occurs, the anesthesiologist and surgeon have three simultaneous goals: (1) stop the entry of air; (2) stabilize the patient, and (3) remove intravascular air, if possible (Box 13.1).

Macroglossia

One of the advantages of the seated position is that it allows for better venous drainage of the head in comparison to the prone position. Nevertheless, there are several reports of patients developing significant edema of the upper airway during posterior fossa surgery (Pivalizza et al 1998). This edema can lead to airway obstruction. It is unclear exactly what puts patients at risk for this complication. Nevertheless, it is reasonable to maintain at least two fingerbreadths' distance between the chin and the sternum to prevent excessive reduction of the anterior-posterior diameter of the oropharynx. In addition, an oral airway should not be left in place during the procedure as it may compress the venous drainage of the tongue. Finally, for anesthesiologists who use TEE to monitor patients during posterior fossa procedures, the use of pediatric probes of smaller diameter may be prudent.

Quadriplegia

The sitting position has been implicated as a cause of rare instances of unexplained postoperative paraplegia. Conventional wisdom suggests (Wilder 1982) that significant neck flexion may result in stretching or compression of the cervical spinal cord. While this has not been firmly established, the authors believe that it is prudent to avoid over flexion of the neck by maintaining at least two fingerbreadths' distance between the chin and the sternum (as noted above). Further, the sitting position may not be optimal for patients with significant reductions in neck mobility secondary to cervical fusion or degenerative joint disease.

Special considerations in transsphenoidal surgery

Patients presenting for transsphenoidal surgery offer many unique challenges to the anesthesiologist. Due to the prominent role of the pituitary gland in the endocrine system, patients require meticulous preoperative assessment, intraoperative management and postoperative care. The successful anesthetic management of patients presenting for transsphenoidal surgery requires a working understanding of the relevant pathophysiology and the possible implications of anesthesia and surgery. While often considered to be relatively uncommon, the transsphenoidal resection of pituitary brain tumors may account for as much as 20% of all intracranial operations performed for primary brain tumors at academic medical centers (Nemergut et al 2005a).

Preoperative concerns

As in the case of any expanding intracranial mass, patients can experience raised intracranial pressure (ICP). Pituitary tumors may increase ICP in two different ways: (1) directly, by mass expansion in the sella with subsequent edema; or (2) indirectly, by obstruction of the third ventricle. Despite the fact that most patients will present with headache, elevated ICP is quite rare. Should ICP be increased, it is critical to avoid any maneuver that might further increase ICP and result in brainstem herniation or impairment of cerebral perfusion.

Optimal anesthetic management necessitates a thorough understanding of the pathophysiology associated with neuroendocrine disease. Advances in laboratory evaluation and radioimaging have allowed for earlier diagnosis and visualization of tumors; however, it is important to note that most tumors have an insidious, non-specific onset. Patients may not seek medical care for years, often not until they have developed severe, multi-organ disease. Special attention in this discussion will be given to acromegaly and Cushing's disease as they present a number of unique challenges to the anesthesiologist (Fig. 13.8).

Acromegaly

Cardiac disease is the most important cause of morbidity and mortality in acromegalic patients (Colao et al 2001; Matta

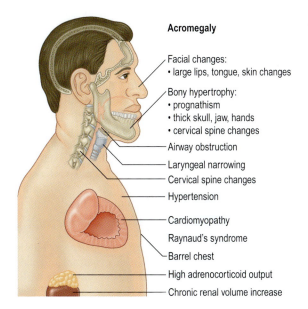
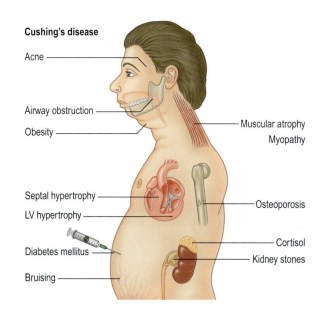
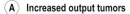
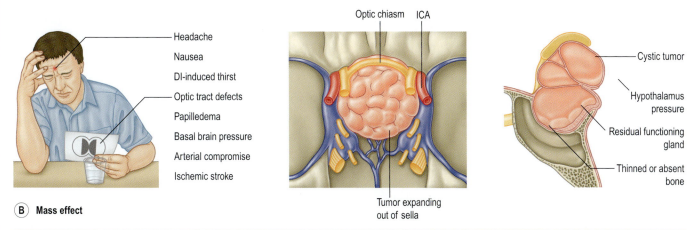

Figure 13.8 (A) Systemic and (B) mass effects of pituitary tumors. A pituitary tumor may present with wide-ranging systemic manifestations secondary to the central role of the pituitary gland in the endocrine system. Also, any expanding intrasellar mass may produce local effects secondary to pressure on adjacent structures within the brain. DI, diabetes insipidus; ICA, internal carotid artery. (With permission from Nemergut EC, Dumont AS, Barry UT, et al. Perioperative management of patients undergoing transsphenoidal pituitary surgery. Anesth Analg 2005;101(4):1170–1181.)

et al 2003). Indeed, the most frequent cause of death in untreated acromegaly is cardiovascular (Rajasoorya et al 1994), with 50% of patients dying before the age of 50. After cardiovascular disease, respiratory disease is the most common cause of death in untreated acromegaly. Sleep apnea secondary to upper airway obstruction (obstructive sleep apnea or OSA) can affect up to 70% of acromegalic patients (Guilleminault et al 1979). It is interesting to note that airway obstruction is three-fold more common among male acromegalics than female acromegalics (Fatti et al 2001). Hypertrophy of the facial bones, especially the mandible, and coarsening of facial features, leads to significant changes in patient appearance. Soft tissues of the nose, mouth, tongue, and lips become thicker and help give acromegalic patients their characteristic facies. In addition to the easily observed external changes, there is thickening of the laryngeal and pharyngeal soft tissues (Kitahata 1971). Hypertrophy of the periepiglottic folds, calcinosis of the larynx (Edge et al 1981), and recurrent laryngeal nerve injury can all contribute to airway obstruction and respiratory disease. Indeed, hypertrophy can cause significant reduction in the size of the glottic opening. Laryngeal stenosis (Williams et al 1994) and abnormal vocal cord function may be present and patients may report hoarseness or changes in vocal tone, quality, or strength. It is interesting to note that vocal cord function is quickly reversed and may return to normal within 10 days of surgery (Wilson 1990).

A high risk of perioperative airway compromise has been well documented in acromegalics with OSA (Piper et al 1995). As such, narcotics and benzodiazepines should be administered with caution to any acromegalic carrying the diagnosis of OSA. Given the high percentage of acromegalic patients with OSA and the fact that OSA is under-diagnosed in most patient populations, the prudent physician should attempt to elicit a history of OSA in all acromegalic patients. Any history of excessive daytime somnolence, snoring, or frank sleep apnea (often noted by the patient's spouse) should alert the physician to the possibility of OSA, especially among male patients.

The combination of these factors has led to the increased incidence of difficulties in airway management in patients presenting with acromegaly (Nemergut et al 2006; Schmitt et al 2000). As might be expected, difficult laryngoscopy and poor laryngeal view has been associated with Mallampati class 3 and 4 airway examinations; however, 20% of acromegalic patients assessed as Mallampati class 1 and 2 have been noted to be difficult to intubate (Nemergut et al 2006; Schmitt et al 2000). As such, the Mallampati classification has poor 'negative predictive value' and difficult endotracheal intubation may be unpredictable in acromegalic patients. Indeed, routine tracheostomy (Southwick et al 1979) had been historically advocated for management of the acromegalic airway; however, this is rarely necessary (Ovassapian et al 1981; Young et al 1993). Flexible fiberoptic laryngoscopy can also be more difficult (Hakala et al 1998).

Cushing's disease

Cushing's disease specifically results from the unregulated hypersecretion of adrenocorticotropic hormone (ACTH) by a pituitary adenoma and consequent hypercortisolism.

Systemic hypertension is among the most common manifestations of Cushing's disease. Indeed, as many as 80% of patients with Cushing's disease have systemic hypertension and 50% of untreated patients have severe hypertension with a diastolic blood pressure >100 mmHg (Ross et al 1966).

As in acromegaly, OSA is also common among patients with Cushing's disease. Polysomnographic studies indicate that as many as 33% of patients with Cushing's disease have mild sleep apnea and 18% of patients have severe sleep apnea (Shipley et al 1992). Complaints of daytime sleepiness are very common (Shipley et al 1992). Weight gain and centripetal obesity are commonly observed in Cushing's disease. As obese patients are more likely to have OSA than nonobese patients, it seems that obesity may play a role in a high prevalence of OSA observed among patients with Cushing's disease. In addition, patients develop fat deposits over the cheeks and temporal regions, giving rise to the rounded 'moon-facies' characteristic of the disease. It does not appear that these changes result in a higher incidence of difficult intubation (Nemergut et al 2006).

Glucose intolerance occurs in at least 60% (Smith et al 2000) of patients with Cushing's disease, with overt diabetes mellitus present in up to one-third of all patients. Indeed, there is evidence that a high prevalence of occult Cushing's disease may exist among patients with diabetes mellitus, type II (Catargi et al 2003). Diffuse osteoporosis may occur in up to 50% of patients presenting with Cushing's disease (Kaltsas et al 2002). Almost 20% of patients may have pathologic fractures and many patients with long-standing Cushing's syndrome have lost height because of osteoporotic vertebral collapse (Ross et al 1982). In addition, aseptic necrosis of the femoral and humeral heads can occur in Cushing's syndrome. Particular care should be taken when positioning patients during surgery.

Many patients with Cushing's disease report generalized weakness and a myopathy of the proximal muscles of the lower limb and the shoulder girdle have been described (Ross et al 1982). Hypercortisolism also results in skin thinning (Ferguson et al 1983). Patients may appear to have senile purpura with many small bruises and a loss of subcutaneous fat. Nevertheless, there are no data to suggest a change in the susceptibility to succinylcholine or nondepolarizing neuromuscular blockers. Cannulation of superficial veins for intravenous access can be extremely difficult and minimal trauma may result in bruising.

Intraoperative considerations

After the induction of anesthesia and tracheal intubation, the patient is positioned for surgery. Transsphenoidal operations are generally performed with the patient supine with some degree of head-up position (Fig. 13.9). The neck is extended and the head is turned slightly to facilitate surgical access to both nares. Any time the operative field is above the right atrium, venous air embolism (VAE) is a theoretical risk. Echocardiography, precordial Doppler, and end-tidal N_2 monitoring may be considered. Although a 10% risk of VAE in the semi-seated position has been reported (Newfield et al 1978), a clinically significant VAE associated with significant morbidity or mortality has not been reported.

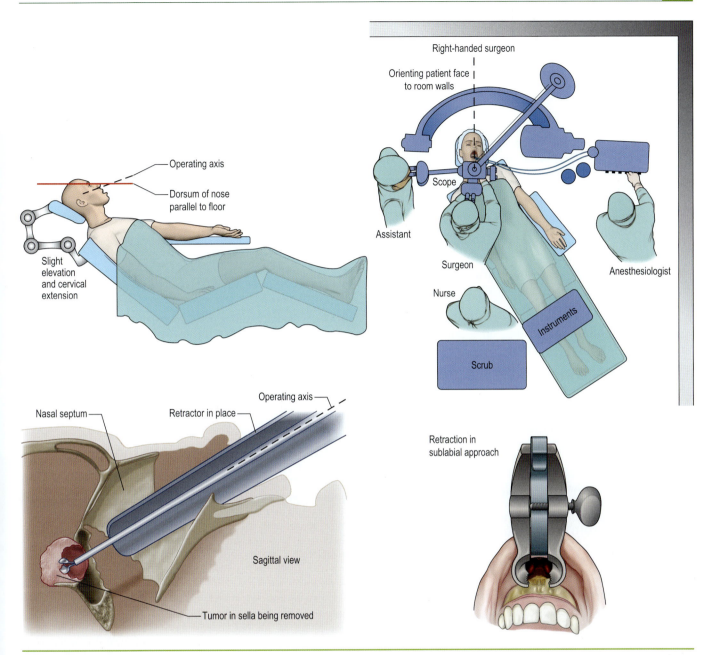

Figure 13.9 Patient position and transsphenoidal surgical approach to the pituitary. (With permission from Nemergut EC, Dumont AS, Barry UT, et al. Perioperative management of patients undergoing transsphenoidal pituitary surgery. Anesth Analg 2005;101(4):1170–1181.)

Topical application or injection of local anesthetic and epinephrine solutions to the mucosal surfaces of the nose are commonly employed during surgical preparation. Cocaine may also be utilized (Fleming et al 1990), but many authors prefer lidocaine-epinephrine mixtures (Kasemsuwan et al 1996). The application of vasoconstrictors serves to shrink mucosa and reduce bleeding. The addition of lidocaine to epinephrine has been shown to increase the arrhythmogenic threshold dose of epinephrine when compared with epinephrine in saline (Horrigan et al 1978). Furthermore, a comparison of 0.5% vs 1% lidocaine used with the same concentration of epinephrine, indicated that mucosal infiltration with the higher dose lidocaine led to more stable hemodynamics (Abou-Madi et al 1980).

Nevertheless, the potential for dysrhythmias or hypertension persists in the presence or absence of inhaled anesthetics (Chelliah et al 2002; Keegan et al 2000; Pasternak et al 2004). Hypertension can be significant and myocardial ischemia with cardiac troponin elevation has been reported in patients without coronary artery disease (Chelliah et al 2002). Hypertension may be successfully treated with intravenous agents such as nitroglycerin, nitroprusside, or phentolamine. Hypertension is normally transient and should be treated with short-acting agents to avoid 'rebound' hypotension after the vasoconstrictive effects of epinephrine have ended.

Many surgeons will place a lumbar intrathecal catheter to assist in visualization of the tumor. The catheter can be used to manipulate cerebrospinal fluid pressure (CSF) pressure by the injection of saline or aspiration of CSF. In patients with large macroadenomas with significant suprasellar extension, some pituitary surgeons will inject intrathecal air. The air serves to increase CSF pressure and may 'push' the suprasellar portion of the tumor into the operative field. The injected air may also serve to outline a tumor, allowing for fluoroscopic visualization. Obviously, strict asepsis should be utilized when anything is injected into the CSF. The anesthesiologist should be cognizant of the fact that nitrous oxide, if used, can rapidly expand this intracranial air.

Transsphenoidal pituitary surgery is normally associated with minimal blood loss; however, there is a potential for significant hemorrhage given the proximity of the pituitary to the carotid arteries. Indeed, carotid artery injury is an infrequent but potentially fatal complication of transsphenoidal surgery (Fukushima et al 1998). Growth hormone-secreting tumors can be associated with impressive dilatation of the intracranial arteries, theoretically increasing the risk for intraoperative hemorrhage. In the case of inadvertent arterial injury, immediate communication among the surgeon, the anesthesiologist, and other members of the operating room team is imperative.

Postoperative considerations and disorders of water balance

Disorders of water balance resulting from perturbations in secretion of anti-diuretic hormone (ADH) are one of the most frequently encountered acute perioperative complications of transsphenoidal surgery (Ciric et al 1997; Hensen et al 1999; Jane et al 2001; Kelly et al 1998; Nemergut et al 2005a; Olson et al 1997; Semple et al 1999; Singer et al 2003). Abnormalities in ADH secretion resulting in postoperative diabetes insipidus (DI) and the syndrome of inappropriate ADH secretion (SIADH) have been reported in 0.5–25% (Ciric et al 1997; Jane et al 2001; Semple et al 1999; Singer et al 2003) of cases, and 9–25% (Jane et al 2001; Kelly et al 1995; Olson et al 1997; Singer et al 2003) of cases, respectively. The treatment of SIADH and DI are discussed below.

Special considerations in malignant hyperthermia

Malignant hyperthermia (MH) is hypermetabolic disease associated with abnormal skeletal muscle metabolism. The incidence is 1:10 000 general anesthetics. Trigger agents for MH include all volatile anesthetics (not including nitrous oxide) and succinylcholine. Predisposing disorders include central core disease and rare myotonias (such as hypokalemic periodic paralysis). MH is inherited in an autosomal dominant fashion, with variable penetrance. In susceptible individuals, exposure to a triggering agent results in a dramatic and uncontrolled increase in skeletal muscle oxidative metabolism. This massive increase in oxygen consumption results in a proportionate rise in CO_2 production and thus an unexpected rise in end-tidal CO_2 is the most sensitive and specific sign of MH. If not treated immediately (see below), the condition leads rapidly to hyperthermia, circulatory collapse, and death.

The halothane-caffeine contracture test is the gold standard for MH testing. The North American test has a

---

Box 13.2 Treatment of malignant hyperthermia

1. Discontinue all triggering agents
2. Hyperventilate with 100% O_2 at 10 L/min
3. Dantrolene 2.5 mg/kg, as needed, for at least 36 h. GET ASSISTANCE WITH MIXING (20 mg vials in 50 cc of sterile distilled water, preferably at 40°C). Note that each 20 mg dantrolene contains 300 mg of mannitol, thus a Foley catheter must also be inserted. Titrate dantrolene (and bicarbonate) to heart rate, temperature, and $PaCO_2$
4. Cool by all routes available (esp. nasogastric lavage, also ice packs)
5. Treat hyperkalemia (calcium chloride, glucose, insulin, bicarbonate, hyperventilation). Do not give potassium if hypokalemia results, however, as it may retrigger MH
6. Beware of dysrhythmias, but do not treat with CCB (lidocaine is safe)
7. Central mixed venous or femoral venous blood gases are superior to ABGs as a guideline for therapy
8. Send creatinine, coags, CK.

Note that as many as 25% of patients may recrudesce. DIC is common, especially if temperature exceeds 41°C. Myoglobinuric renal failure is also common. Severe pain and weakness are sequelae of MH, and muscle recovery can take months.

100% sensitivity and a 78% specificity (requires a positive response in only one of the two tests), while the European test has a 98% sensitivity and a 93% specificity (requires a positive response in both tests). There is also a clinical grading scale that examines muscle rigidity, myonecrosis, respiratory acidosis, temperature, and cardiac involvement to give a likelihood scale (Box 13.2).

Critical care management of the tumor patient following craniotomy

Patients who have undergone a craniotomy for tumor resection should be managed postoperatively in a critical care unit by a team with specialized training in neurocritical care. Data from patients with a variety of neurologic injuries suggests that these patients have better outcomes when cared for in a dedicated neurointensive care unit (NICU) (Rincon et al 2007).

Project Impact, which studied 1038 patients with intracerebral hemorrhage over the course of 3 years, showed that not being in an NICU was associated with an increased in-hospital mortality rate, and having a full-time intensivist was associated with lower mortality (Diringer et al 2001). Varelas and colleagues (2006) demonstrated a 51% reduction in NICU-associated mortality in patients with TBI who were cared for by a neurointensivist. They also found a 12% shorter hospital length of stay, and a 57% greater odds of being discharged to home or rehabilitation (Varelas et al 2006). Given the evidence of improved outcomes in patients with other brain pathologies, it is reasonable to assume that patients having undergone craniotomy for tumor resection will also do better when cared for postoperatively by an intensivist in a NICU setting.

Advances in neurosurgical and anesthetic techniques have helped reduce the morbidity and mortality associated with neurosurgery. However, patients undergoing craniotomy continue to pose numerous challenges for the neurointensivist. While traditional ICP monitors are a staple in the NICU, advances in monitoring techniques may allow for more rapid detection of deleterious conditions before they progress, and allow the clinician to have a more complete, real time understanding of the patient's cerebral metabolic status. Renewed attention is being focused on the deleterious effects of postoperative pain, with novel analgesic techniques including advances in both pharmacologic and regional anesthetic techniques. There is recognition of the negative effects of prolonged postoperative mechanical ventilation, and there is an emphasis on expediting time to extubation for patients in the intensive care unit. In this section we will address diagnosis and management of elevated intracranial pressure (ICP), cerebral monitoring devices, diagnosis and treatment of metabolic and electrolyte derangements, timing of postoperative tracheal extubation, seizure prophylaxis and management, recognition and treatment of altered mental status, and provision of postoperative analgesia.

Increased intracranial pressure

ICP is normally <15 mmHg in an adult and pressures >20 mmHg are considered pathologic. In the healthy brain, homeostatic mechanisms exist to maintain ICP within the normal range. The proper function of these compensatory mechanisms depends on several factors including cerebral autoregulation, an intact blood–brain barrier, and the ability for CSF to be displaced within the ventricular system. In the patient with neurologic injury, a disruption in any of these variables can lead to inability of the body to properly regulate ICP. Such derangements may be seen in patients following craniotomy and tumor resection. While the tumor itself can affect regulatory mechanisms and increase ICP, craniotomy and surgical resection can result in cerebral edema, damage to the blood–brain barrier, and alteration of cerebral blood flow.

Ultimately, the deleterious effects of elevated ICP are related to a reduction in CPP. Optimization of CPP requires knowledge of arterial blood pressure and ICP. While invasive ICP monitors may not be necessary in awake patients who are able to cooperate with mental status exams, many patients in ICU postoperatively are not able to communicate adequately due to tracheal intubation and sedation, residual anesthetics, or neuromuscular blocking drugs. In these patients, other assessment methods are necessary to monitor for increased ICP.

Monitoring intracranial pressure

In 2007, the Brain Trauma Foundation issued guidelines for ICP monitoring (Bratton et al 2007a–d). The Foundation recommended (level 2 evidence) 'intracranial pressure should be monitored in all salvageable patients with a severe traumatic brain injury (GCS score of 3–8 after resuscitation) and an abnormal computed tomography'. With a lower level of recommendation (level 3 evidence) the Foundation stated that 'ICP monitoring is indicated in patients with severe TBI with a normal CT scan if two or more of the following features are noted at admission: age over 40 years, unilateral or bilateral motor posturing, or systolic blood pressure <90 mmHg'.

While ICP monitoring is clearly supported by the Foundation in the aforementioned situations, it is unclear whether or not such techniques improve patient outcome. To our knowledge, all data regarding ICP monitoring and outcome is of the retrospective variety, limiting our ability to establish a causative relationship between monitoring and patient outcome. As ICP monitoring devices are not without risk, we believe that a randomized, prospective, clinical trial would be prudent. In a retrospective study of a database of 9001 TBI patients (546 of whom received ICP monitoring), Lane and colleagues (2000) showed that insertion of an ICP monitor was associated with a significantly decreased rate of death among patients with severe TBI. Lane's group hypothesized that while ICP monitor placement may allow for more informed management decisions, the observed effect may also be due to more aggressive neurosurgical protocols where ICP monitors were placed, or selection bias in patients receiving ICP monitors, rather than the monitors themselves.

In a survey of 628 patients in 28 level 1 trauma centers in the USA, Bulger and colleagues (2002) observed that management of severe brain injury at an aggressive center (defined by placement of an ICP monitor >50% of the time for patients with GCS ≤8 and an abnormal CT scan of the brain), was associated with a significant reduction in mortality. However, among survivors, there was no statistical difference in functional status at discharge. Further differences in care at more aggressive institutions, including higher rates of neurosurgical consultation, intubation on admission, and pharmacologic and surgical techniques to treat increased ICP, likely contributed to the mortality differences (in addition to the placement of an ICP monitor).

Cremer and colleagues (2005), in a retrospective cohort study with prospective assessment of outcome, studied more than 300 patients with severe head injury who were treated at two trauma centers in The Netherlands. One group of patients received supportive intensive care, which included maintaining mean arterial pressure at approximately 90 mmHg and basing therapeutic interventions on clinical and radiographic findings. The second group received care aimed at maintaining ICP <20 mmHg and CPP >70 mmHg. ICP/CPP-targeted management resulted in prolonged requirements for mechanical ventilation and no improvement in outcome as measured by the Glasgow Outcome Scale after ≥12 months.

Regardless of its effect on outcome, the utilization of an ICP monitor is not without associated risk. Complications of ICP monitoring include infection, hemorrhage, malfunction, obstruction and malposition. Hemorrhage requiring hematoma evacuation occurs in 0.5% of patients undergoing ICP monitoring. The infection rate for ICP devices is reported between 1% and 27%, depending on the type of device and the method for determining infection. When comparing monitoring techniques, ventricular devices have an average bacterial colonization rate of 8%, and parenchymal monitors have an infection rate of 14%. May and colleagues (2006) conducted a retrospective study evaluating the use of narrow vs broad-spectrum antibiotic prophylaxis in patients with ICP monitors. They concluded that broad-spectrum antibiotic prophylaxis did not reduce CNS infections, but rather was associated with a shift to resistant Gram-negative organisms in subsequent infectious complications. Routine exchange of ventricular catheters or prophylactic antibiotics is not recommended to reduce the risk of infection associated with ventricular ICP monitors (see Bratton et al 2007a–d).

Management of elevated ICP, secondary

In some cases of elevated ICP to brain tumor, improvement may be seen with craniotomy and tumor resection alone. Patients who require ICP monitoring preoperatively may no longer need invasive monitors postoperatively. However, craniotomy and tumor resection may also result in considerable cerebral edema, damage to the blood–brain barrier, and alteration in cerebral blood flow autoregulation. Any of these factors may contribute to intracranial hypertension postoperatively, which can be managed by a variety of pharmacologic, non-pharmacologic, and surgical techniques.

Sedation and analgesia

Patients in the ICU following craniotomy may experience pain and agitation. Pain is often due to the surgical procedure, and agitation may be secondary to multiple causes including increased ICP, metabolic disturbances, dyssynchrony with the ventilator, and postoperative delirium. It is well known that pain and agitation can increase blood pressure and ICP to dangerous levels in a patient who recently underwent a neurosurgical procedure. Management of sedation and analgesia are fundamental concepts in critical care. The management of postsurgical analgesia in the patient undergoing craniotomy for tumor resection will be discussed in more detail later in this chapter.

A variety of drugs have been used for sedation in the neurocritical care unit to control ICP. Propofol and the benzodiazepines are the most common sedative agents, although newer drugs, such as the alpha-2 agonist dexmedetomidine, may also have a role. Propofol (2,6-diisopropyl phenol) is a water insoluble drug that enhances γ-aminobutyric acid transmission. Propofol decreases ICP in patients with normal or elevated ICP, and anesthetic doses lower the cerebral metabolic rate of oxygen consumption. Importantly, propofol can cause significant hypotension, thus CPP may decrease, particularly in hypovolemic patients. Cerebral autoregulation is preserved in patients without head trauma but may be impaired in patients with head injury. The cerebral electrophysiological effects of propofol vary depending on the dose. At low doses the drug may activate epileptic foci, while at higher doses it has been used to treat seizure activity (Hutchens et al 2006). The systemic effects of propofol are well described, with effects on nearly every organ system. While induction doses (2 mg/kg body weight) frequently cause apnea, infusions of the drug may increase the respiratory rate and diminish the ventilatory response to hypercarbia (Hutchens et al 2006).

In a prospective, multicenter trial of 98 patients comparing propofol with midazolam in the general ICU population, propofol allowed more effective sedation and less patient ventilator dyssynchrony. Sedation with propofol also allowed more predictable and rapid awakening (Chamorro et al 1996). Propofol is a useful sedative in the neurocritical care unit because it allows for rapid awakening of patients, permitting frequent neurologic exams. In general, its neurologic profile is also favorable for patients in the ICU, and it may be a useful agent in patients with increased ICP.

As noted above, dexmedetomidine is a highly selective alpha-2 adrenoreceptor agonist that has anxiolytic and analgesic qualities, without causing respiratory depression. Alpha-2 receptors are found in the brain (pons and medulla), spinal cord (dorsal horn), and in the periphery (vascular smooth muscle). The sedative effects of dexmedetomidine are mediated through activation of receptors in the locus ceruleus (Bekker et al 2005). Although dexmedetomidine may produce a transient hypertensive response due to its activation of the alpha-2B receptor on vascular smooth muscle, the ultimate effect is a reduction in blood pressure and heart rate, related to a reduction in catecholamine levels. In the brain, dexmedetomidine may decrease cerebral blood flow secondary to vasoconstriction mediated by alpha-2 receptor activation on vascular smooth muscle (Bekker et al 2005). The effects of dexmedetomidine on ICP are less clear, with few trials in humans, although some animal trials have demonstrated a decrease in ICP.

While there is a paucity of data on the use of dexmedetomidine in the NICU, it is a promising sedative in this patient population because patients generally remain cooperative and do not develop respiratory depression, thus permitting frequent neurologic checks. Aryan and colleagues (2006) conducted a retrospective study of dexmedetomidine in neurosurgical patients and concluded that it was a safe and effective sedative that could be administered without significant effect on ICP or CPP.

Hyperventilation

Mechanical ventilation to achieve a $PaCO_2$ in the 26–30 mmHg range is a simple maneuver that can transiently reduce ICP through vasoconstriction and decrease intracranial blood flow. This technique can be used in emergent situations when raised ICP poses a life-threatening risk to the patient, and it is commonly used by neuroanesthesiologists in the operating room to manage ICP in patients undergoing craniotomy.

While hyperventilation is an effective technique to lower ICP, the constrictive effect on arterioles is relatively brief, lasting only 11–20 h. As CSF pH equilibrates following hyperventilation induced alkalosis, cerebral arterioles may re-dilate to a larger size than at baseline, which may lead to an increase in ICP (Rangel-Castilla et al 2008). Furthermore, there is concern that hyperventilation, particularly in patients with TBI or stroke, may decrease cerebral blood flow to levels which may increase the risk for cerebral ischemia. That said, multiple sources note that while hyperventilation clearly decreases cerebral blood flow, hyperventilation induced ischemia has not been clearly demonstrated (Rangel-Castilla et al 2008; Stocchetti et al 2005).

A Cochrane Database Review published in 2000 concluded 'The data available are inadequate to assess any potential benefit or harm that might result from hyperventilation in severe head injury. Randomized controlled trials to assess the effectiveness of hyperventilation therapy following severe head injury are needed' (Schierhout et al 2000). Since that time, no randomized, controlled trials of hyperventilation in humans with neurologic injury have been published.

The Brain Trauma Foundation, in its 2007 guidelines (Bratton et al 2007a–d) for the use of hyperventilation in patients with TBI, stated that 'hyperventilation is recommended as a temporizing measure for the reduction of elevated intracranial pressure. Hyperventilation should be avoided during the first 24 h after injury when cerebral blood flow (CBF) is often critically reduced'. They also recommended that 'if hyperventilation is used, jugular venous oxygen saturation (SjO_2) or brain tissue oxygen tension ($PbrO_2$) measurements are recommended to monitor oxygen delivery'. These were level 3 recommendations. With a level 2 recommendation, they advised, 'prophylactic hyperventilation … is not recommended'. It seems clear that there is a temporary role for hyperventilation in the treatment of patients with elevated ICP. Clinicians should be aware that while this is a useful and easy therapy to implement, it is not without its risks and controversies.

Mannitol

Mannitol is an osmotic diuretic that is metabolically inert in humans. It is FDA approved for the treatment of increased intracranial pressure. Mannitol works primarily by increasing plasma osmotic pressure, leading to brain dehydration and a decrease in ICP, with consequent improvement in cerebral perfusion. Serum osmolarity is optimal in the 300–320 mOsm range, above which undesirable side-effects such as hyperosmolarity, hypovolemia, and renal failure may become evident (Rangel-Castilla et al 2008). In patients with intact cerebral autoregulation, mannitol may induce cerebral vasoconstriction, while it may lead to cerebral vasodilation in patients who have lost cerebral pressure autoregulation (Rangel-Castilla et al 2008). Repeat doses of mannitol may lead to a reversal of the osmotic gradient between brain tissue and plasma, thereby causing an exacerbation of vasogenic cerebral edema and paradoxically leading to an increase in ICP (Kaufmann et al 1992).

Limited data suggest that prolonged Osm >320 mOsm/L is associated with a higher mortality (Trost et al 1992). However, a recent retrospective study of 98 patients treated with mannitol in a NICU showed no correlation between serum Osm and the development of renal failure. Elevated APACHE II scores and a history of congestive heart failure were the only factors predictive of impending renal failure in patients treated with mannitol (Gondim et al 2005).

Bell and colleagues (1987) showed, via magnetic resonance imaging, that brain water content could be reduced within 15 min in patients with intrinsic cerebral tumors who were administered an intravenous infusion of 20% mannitol. Bolus administration of mannitol (1 g/kg body weight) can lower the ICP within 1–5 min, with peak action in 20–60 min and an effect lasting 1.5–6 h (Rangel-Castilla et al 2008). Mannitol may be combined with other diuretics to produce a synergistic effect on ICP. Pollay and colleagues (1983) showed in dogs that when mannitol and furosemide were used together, a greater (62.4% vs 56.6%) and more sustained (5 h vs 2 h) fall in ICP was achieved. They observed a significantly increased urine production over controls, as well as a transient, but not significant, fall in serum sodium levels.

Hypertonic therapy

Hypertonic saline (HTS) can be given in concentrations ranging from 3% to 23.4%, and like mannitol, works primarily by increasing intravascular osmotic pressure to draw water out of cerebral parenchyma, thereby reducing intracranial volume and ICP (Rangel-Castilla et al 2008). However, HTS may have additional effects, and likely possesses vasoregulatory, hemodynamic, neurochemical, and immunologic properties (Doyle et al 2001). While mannitol is contraindicated in hypovolemic patients due to its diuretic effects, HTS increases intravascular volume and may raise blood pressure (Rangel-Castilla et al 2008). HTS administration may be associated with osmotic demyelination syndrome, acute renal insufficiency, and hematologic abnormalities. A rebound rise in ICP has also been described with HTS administration, typically occurring after bolus administration or at the end of infusion. This may represent a true rebound rise in ICP, or may reflect the limited half-life of the substrate (Doyle et al 2001).

There have been limited studies comparing HTS with mannitol for management of increased ICP. Vialet and colleagues (2003) compared isovolume infusions of either 7.5% HTS or 20% mannitol in patients with head trauma and elevated ICP refractory to standard therapy. They observed significantly fewer and shorter episodes of elevated ICP in the group receiving hypertonic saline solution. Francony and colleagues (2008) conducted a randomized, controlled trial comparing the effects of equimolar infusions of 20% mannitol with 7.45% HTS in stable patients with a sustained elevation in ICP secondary to TBI or stroke. They demonstrated that a single equimolar infusion of mannitol was as effective as HTS in decreasing ICP in patients with brain injury. However, cerebral perfusion pressure and cerebral blood flow velocities increased in the mannitol group only. As expected, mannitol caused a significantly greater diuresis compared with HTS, while the HTS solution caused a significant elevation in serum sodium and chloride 2 hours after the infusion was initiated.

In another trial comparing 20% mannitol and 7.5% saline/6% dextran solution in patients with elevated ICP, Battison and colleagues (2005) showed a significantly greater and more sustained reduction in ICP with the saline/dextran solution. The use of other, novel hypertonic solutions to control increased ICP has also garnered attention. A recent trial compared 20% mannitol with a hyperosmolar sodium lactate solution in patients with severe TBI and raised ICP (Ichai et al 2009). The authors showed the sodium lactate-based formula to be superior to mannitol in terms of degree of ICP change, length of effect, and frequency of success. Further trials are clearly warranted.

Barbiturate coma

Barbiturates may reduce ICP through reductions in both CBF and cerebral metabolic rate of oxygen consumption. In an uncontrolled study of 10 patients with increased ICP resistant to standard therapy, Chen and colleagues (2008) demonstrated an increase in brain tissue oxygen levels in 70% of patients treated with pentobarbital infusion. While not generally used as an initial agent to treat elevated ICP, barbiturates have been used since 1974 to induce coma in an effort to manage cases of refractory intracranial hypertension. Among 67 patients with severe head injury and refractory intracranial hypertension, 45% had a 'good ICP

Table 13.2 Cerebral salt wasting (CSW) vs syndrome of inappropriate anti-diuretic hormone secretion (SIADH)

	CSW	SIADH
Incidence	More common	Less common
Volume status	Hypovolemic	Normovolemic
Salt balance	Negative	Variable
CVP (cm H_2O)	≤5	6–10

salts, fludrocortisone (Hasan et al 1989). Damaraju and colleagues (1997) were able to attain serum sodium levels >130 mEq/L within 72 h in 76% of CSW patients treated with 50 cc/kg per day normal saline, and 12 g/day oral salts.

Syndrome of inappropriate antidiuretic hormone

SIADH, initially described in patients with lung cancer, commonly occurs in association with intracranial malignancies. Other, less common causes of SIADH include hypothyroidism, glucocorticoid deficiency, vincristine, oxytocin, carbamazepine, clofibrate, chlorpropamide, and NSAIDs (Baylis 2003). Inappropriately high levels of ADH leads to increased water reabsorption from the distal collecting ducts in the kidney. Patients are usually euvolemic, but may be hypervolemic due to retention of excess free water. Symptoms of SIADH are secondary to hyponatremia – headache, nervousness, confusion, lethargy, nausea, vomiting, seizures, coma, and potentially death. They depend on both the rapidity of onset and degree of hyponatremia, with rapid-onset disturbances usually more symptomatic. Sodium levels <120–125 mEq/L are almost always symptomatic. Interestingly, these patients will sometimes exhibit a paradoxical sense of thirst (Baylis 2003).

The treatment of SIADH varies based on the time course. Acute SIADH (<48 h) is generally treated with fluid restriction and, if severe, HTS and/or furosemide. Chronic SIADH (>48 h) is treated with long-term fluid restriction (1200–1800 cc/day), demeclocycline, furosemide, and occasionally phenytoin (which is thought to inhibit ADH release). Care should be taken not to correct hyponatremia too rapidly: there have been reports of profound neurologic deficits following rapid correction of hyponatremia in patients with chronic disease. This phenomena, termed 'osmotic demyelination syndrome' can usually be avoided if the rate and degree of sodium repletion is carefully monitored – do not exceed a correction rate of 1.3 mEq/L per h, limit corrective measures if sodium increases >10 mEq/L in 24 h, and stop corrective measures if sodium increases >125 mEq/L.

Sivakumar and colleagues (1994) investigated the use of central venous pressure (CVP) monitoring to guide therapy in neurosurgical patients with hyponatremia. In a study of 25 patients, CVP was used as the sole distinguishing factor for making the diagnosis of CSW versus SIADH in hyponatremic neurosurgical patients, and therapy was guided accordingly. By basing therapy on CVP (5 cm water or less being hypovolemic, 6–10 cm water being normovolemic), Damaraju's group (1997) was able to achieve serum sodium levels of 130 mEq/L within 72 h in 76% of patients. When CVP data from these studies are pooled, 87% of

patients were hypovolemic, 13% were normovolemic, and none were hypervolemic, suggesting that CSW is the overwhelming cause of volume and electrolyte abnormalities in the neurosurgical setting.

Diabetes insipidus

Unlike CSW and SIADH, which usually are associated with hyponatremia, diabetes insipidus (DI) is generally associated with *hyper*natremia. DI is almost always caused by insufficient release of ADH ('central' DI), although rarely it can be caused by insensitivity to ADH ('nephrogenic' DI). Regardless of the etiology, the result is an inability of the kidneys to retain water. Urine output is increased and patients often experience polydipsia. Patients may also experience altered mental status, weakness, lethargy, coma, seizures, and intracranial bleeding secondary to excessive dehydration and contraction of brain parenchyma.

Central DI may occur secondary to a variety of neurologic insults or procedures, including transsphenoidal surgery (Nemergut et al 2005a), brain tumors (ex. craniopharyngioma), head injury, or following encephalitis or meningitis. Pharmacologic agents including ethanol, phenytoin, and possibly steroids, may also induce DI. DI is relatively common, with an overall incidence of 3.7% (Wong et al 1998). The incidence of DI may be as high as 6.7% in post-craniotomy (tumor) patients (Balestrieri et al 1982). Nephrogenic DI can be caused by drugs (lithium, demeclocycline, colchicine), chronic renal disease, hypercalcemia, hypokalemia, and Sjögren's syndrome. However, central DI is more common than nephrogenic DI in the neurosurgical patient population (Tisdall et al 2006). As noted above, transient DI is fairly common after transsphenoidal surgery (Nemergut et al 2005b).

DI is diagnosed in the presence of a urine osmolality <200 mOsm/L (or urine specific gravity <1.003), a normal or high serum osmolality, in combination with high urine output (>250 cc/h for adults, >3 cc/kg per h in pediatric patients). A supervised water deprivation test can be performed when the diagnosis remains elusive. The patient is made NPO and osmolalities are checked each hour. With fluid restriction, a normal patient's urine output will decrease and urine osmolality will increase (approaching or exceeding 600 mOsm/L). If urine osmolality plateaus (<30 mOsm/L change over 3 h), the patient loses 3% of body weight, or if 6–8 h elapse without urine osmolality approaching 600 mOsm/L, the patient has failed the water deprivation test. A test dose of vasopressin may be administered at this point. It is important to emphasize that this test must be supervised, as the outcome of unchecked water deprivation in a patient with DI may be fatal.

Treatment of DI requires replacing fluid losses, initially with isotonic fluids for resuscitation, and later with hypotonic fluids if increased urine output continues. If DI is diagnosed, most patients will be able to maintain intravascular volume if allowed to drink freely. If patients are unable to match urine losses with oral intake, treatment with desmopressin (DDAVP) should be considered (Robertson et al 1989). If DDAVP is utilized, it is important to follow serum sodium and osmolarity to avoid 'overshoot' hyponatremia. Serum sodium and osmolality should be monitored closely.

Doses are adjusted, titrating to urine output and osmolality (target urine osmolality 150–155 mEq/L within 24 h of initiating treatment). Mild DI (some residual ADH effects are present) can occasionally be treated with carbamazepine (200–600 mg/day), chlorpropamide (100–500 mg/day), or clofibrate (500 mg four times daily). Thiazide diuretics may also be useful (Makaryus et al 2006).

Timing of tracheal extubation

Tracheal extubation may not be possible at the immediate conclusion of surgery, and patients may be taken to the ICU with an endotracheal tube in place. Keeping a patient intubated and on mechanical ventilation is not without risk, and most patients should be extubated as soon as possible. Adverse effects associated with endotracheal intubation and mechanical ventilation include pneumonia, laryngeal injury, hemodynamic changes, the need for sedation, patient discomfort, and difficulty obtaining an accurate neurologic exam. On the other hand, premature extubation can lead to hypoventilation and increases in ICP, aspiration, and the need for reintubation under suboptimal conditions. Numerous criteria have been established to assess whether a patient is ready for extubation (Box 13.3).

When comparing predictors of a successful extubation, the two most likely to be helpful are the 'rapid shallow breathing index' (RSBI, respiratory rate/tidal volume), and negative inspiratory force (NIF). While a NIF >20 cm water does not guarantee a successful extubation, a poor performance in this test usually predicts failure (Yang et al 1991). Other bedside weaning parameters, such as PaO_2/FiO_2 ratio, tidal volume, respiratory rate, vital capacity, and minute ventilation have not consistently proven useful.

Much of the data on ventilator weaning suggests that protocol-driven weaning is superior to physician-directed weaning (Table 13.3). However, none of these large, randomized studies looked specifically at patients following craniotomy and tumor resection. In fact, there is very little data available on extubation criteria in this patient population.

In a randomized, controlled trial of protocol driven spontaneous breathing trials (SBT) and extubation in 100 neurosurgical patients, Namen and colleagues (2001) found no difference in days to first extubation attempt, and no difference in outcomes between the two groups (only the intervention group received an SBT). Extubation was delayed in 82% of patients in the intervention group who passed the SBT, usually due to concerns about the patient's mental status. On multivariate analysis, higher GCS scores, lower RSBI, higher P/F ratios, and higher tidal volumes were all found to be associated with successful extubation in this patient population.

Box 13.3 Traditional (conservative) weaning criteria

NEUROMUSCULAR

- Arousable
- Intact gag reflex
- GCS >12
- Able to hold head off bed for 5 s

CARDIOVASCULAR

- HR <140
- Hemodynamically stable

PULMONARY

- PaO_2 >60 mmHg on FiO_2 ≤40% and PEEP ≤5
- $PaCO_2$ at baseline
- Rapid shallow breathing index (RSBI) <100
- NIF >25 cm water

HEMATOLOGIC/INFLAMMATORY

- Afebrile

METABOLIC/ENDOCRINE

- Electrolytes within normal limits (particularly sodium, calcium, phosphate)
- pH 7.30–7.40

Table 13.3 Protocol vs physician-directed weaning

Patients	n	Study type	Outcome	Reference
Studies in support of protocol directed weaning				
MICU and CCU	300	Randomized, controlled trial	Duration of MV decreased from 6 to 1.5 days ($p = 0.003$)	Ely et al 1996
			Complications (autoextubation, reintubation, tracheostomy, >21 days MV) decreased by 50% ($p = 0.001$)	
			ICU days were similar	
MICU and SICU	357	Randomized, controlled trial	Duration of MV decreased from 44 to 35 h ($p = 0.039$)	Bahrami et al 1997
			Mortality rates were similar	
MICU and SICU	385	Randomized, controlled trial	Duration of MV decreased from 124 h to 68 h ($p = 0.0001$)	Marelich et al 2000
			VAP trended downwards from 7.1% to 3.0% ($p = 0.061$)	
			Mortality and failure rates were similar	
MICU	928	Prospective cohort	Significantly reduced the duration of MV	Grap et al 2003
			Length of stay in the ICU trended downward	
ICU >48 h	104	Retrospective cohort	Duration of MV (22.5–16.6 days, $p = 0.02$) and ICU length (27.6–21.6 days, $p = 0.02$) decreased	Tonnelier et al 2005
			VAP, discontinuation failure rates and ICU mortality were the same	
Studies suggesting protocols make no difference				
MICU	299	Prospective, controlled	No differences in duration of MV, ICU stay or mortality	Krishnan et al 2004
			Similar failure rates	

CCU, cardiac ICU; MICU, medical ICU; MV, mechanical ventilation; SICU, surgical ICU; VAP, ventilation associated pneumonia.

Traditionally, patients must be awake, alert and able to follow commands before being extubated. It is assumed that this level of consciousness and cooperation indicates an intact ability to clear secretions and maintain a patent airway. However, following craniotomy and tumor resection, patients may not be awake and communicative, despite meeting all other criteria for extubation. These patients pose special challenges when assessing for extubation, as aspiration is likely if a patient cannot cough and clear secretions. It is not uncommon for extubation to be delayed based entirely on a depressed mental status, despite normal respiratory mechanics. In a prospective cohort study of brain injured patients, Coplin and colleagues (2000) studied time to extubation and outcomes in 136 intubated patients with brain injuries. They showed that in patients with altered sensorium, extubation is often delayed despite meeting other extubation criteria. Based on their outcome data of reintubation rates and pneumonia, their study did not support delaying extubation in patients with brain injuries who have altered mental status but meet all other extubation criteria.

Without any large, randomized trials of extubation in patients following craniotomy and tumor resection, neurointensivists must extrapolate from the general ICU literature. The usual predictors of a successful extubation seem to apply to post-craniotomy patients, and patients may have better outcomes when weaned to extubation using a protocolized approach incorporating spontaneous breathing trials. While altered mental status and depressed sensorium may be present in patients after craniotomy, these should not necessarily delay extubation.

Seizures

Seizures are common in patients with brain tumors, and are the presenting signs in more than one-third of patients (Michelucci 2006). Low-grade tumors are more likely to present with seizures (Chang et al 2008), and while the presence of preoperative seizures increases the risk of further events postoperatively, the initial seizure may occur following surgery. The seizure rate varies by tumor type, with oligodendrogliomas having the highest overall rate (50%–81%), followed by astrocytomas (40%–66%), ependymomas (33%–50%), glioblastomas (30%–42%), meningiomas (30%–40%), and metastatic lesions (19%–26%).

Seizure activity is associated with negative sequelae. Postoperative seizures can make it difficult to obtain an accurate neurologic exam, cause bodily injury to the patient, and complicate airway management. Seizures result in a burst of metabolic activity in the brain, and can cause structural brain injury that may actually predispose the patient to further seizure activity (Deutschman et al 1985). Status epilepticus, a manifestation of untreated or refractory seizures, has been associated with systemic lactic acidosis, CO_2 narcosis, hyperkalemia, hypoglycemia, shock, cardiac arrhythmias, pulmonary edema, acute renal tubular necrosis and aspiration pneumonia. These findings may be related to changes in cerebral blood flow, increases in cerebral glucose and oxygen consumption, ATP depletion, lactate accumulation, and excitotoxic mechanisms (Wasterlain et al

1993). In patients with low-grade gliomas, the presence of postoperative seizures has been highly correlated with tumor recurrence (Chang et al 2008). This can likely be explained by the strong inverse relationship between achievement of a gross total resection and postoperative seizure activity.

In 1996, more than 50% of physicians caring for patients with brain tumors reported prophylactically prescribing AEDs prior to seizure occurrence (Glantz et al 1996). Despite this practice, a meta-analysis conducted by the American Academy of Neurology showed no significant reduction in the incidence of seizures, or the seizure-free survival rate following prophylactic administration of AEDs in patients with brain tumors. Based on the lack of therapeutic efficacy, and because of the systemic side-effects, inconvenience, and cost associated with AEDs, the subcommittee could not justify the use of AEDs for prevention of seizures (Glantz et al 2000). They also stated that 'in patients with brain tumors who have not had a seizure, tapering and discontinuing anticonvulsants after the first postoperative week is appropriate'. AEDs may be recommended for patients undergoing radiation therapy, which can increase the risk for seizures (Packer et al 2003).

Aside from a history of preoperative seizures, risk factors for postoperative seizures include tumor location (cortical or supratentorial) (Deutschman et al 1985), brain retraction, postoperative metabolic derangements (hypoxia, hyper- and hyponatremia, hyperglycemia, and/or acidosis), and incomplete resection. Whether or not inadequate preoperative AED levels is a risk factor is unclear, as the usefulness of AEDs for preventing postoperative seizures has recently been called into question.

In one study, the administration of phenytoin following craniotomy was associated with a significant reduction in the incidence of epilepsy (North et al 1983). A retrospective review of 23 seizures in patients following craniotomy suggested that inadequate AED levels, found in 83% of patients who seized, were a contributing factor (Kvam et al 1983). On the other hand, in a prospective study comparing carbamazepine, phenytoin and 'no treatment' in post-craniotomy patients, Foy and colleagues (1992) failed to find a significant difference between treatment regimens, or between treatment and 'no treatment' groups, when measuring seizures or death. A high incidence of drug-related side-effects was observed in the treatment group. A meta-analysis by Kuijlen and colleagues (1996) suggested that prophylactically-administered AEDs prevented postoperative convulsions, but this effect was not statistically significant.

AEDs are associated with significant side-effects, their administration is often labor-intensive, and they can be expensive. The most feared complications of AED administration are toxic epidermal necrolysis (TEN) and Steven's–Johnson Syndrome (SJS), both of which can be fatal. There appears to be an increased likelihood of developing TEN–SJS in patients receiving both radiation therapy and AEDs (Ahmed et al 2004). Side-effects from AEDs are seen more frequently in patients with brain tumors (20–40%) than in the general population of patients with epilepsy (Reich et al 1976; Warren et al 1977). A recent study of 195 patients with low-grade gliomas in the Netherlands showed that cognitive deficits were more frequently observed in the setting of AED administration (Taphoorn 2003).

AEDs may interact with other drugs, including chemotherapeutic agents and steroids. Dexamethasone, for instance, has been shown to reduce serum phenytoin levels, thereby increasing the risk of seizures (Lackner 1991). The majority of AEDs (with the exception of valproate) are enzyme-inducers (Vecht et al 2003a,b). At least two studies have reported lower serum concentrations of antineoplastic agents when administered in conjunction with enzyme-inducing AEDs (phenytoin, carbamazepine, phenobarbital) (Chang et al 1998; Fetell et al 1997).

In addition to decreasing serum concentrations, enzyme-inducing AEDs may decrease the efficacy of chemotherapeutic agents. One study in children with ALL showed lower event-free survival rates, and higher hematologic and CNS relapse rates in patients receiving teniposide and methotrexate (Relling et al 2000). A study of adult patients with glioblastoma multiforme showed a significant decrease in survival time in patients taking enzyme-inducing AEDs, when compared to those who were administered non-enzyme-inducing AEDs (10.8 vs 13.9 months) (Oberndorfer et al 2005).

Enzyme-inhibiting AEDs, such as valproate, may increase the toxicity of chemotherapeutic agents. Valproic acid has been shown to increase the incidence of complications (thrombocytopenia, neutropenia) associated with a nitrosourea, cisplatin, and etoposide treatment regimen (Bourg et al 2001; Wen et al 2002).

AEDs are effective at reducing the incidence of seizures in patients who have already experienced an epileptic event. However, the data suggest that the side-effects and costs associated with AED administration do not justify their routine use in patients who have a primary brain tumor, but have not yet experienced a seizure. There is controversy surrounding routine postoperative seizure prophylaxis, thus we cannot recommend routine AED administration in epilepsy free patients following craniotomy. For those who do receive prophylaxis, the treatment duration should be as brief as possible. The physician prescribing AEDs for brain tumor patients requiring chemotherapy should be aware of any potential drug interactions between the anticonvulsants and antineoplastic agents.

Delayed awakening in the ICU

While many patients will awaken from anesthesia immediately upon completion of surgery, some patients may experience unexpected, delayed awakening. When this occurs, the clinician must quickly assess the situation by performing a thorough history and physical exam, and obtaining additional laboratory or radiological studies. Delayed awakening following anesthesia and surgery is not uncommon, and may be due to a variety of etiologies. Residual volatile anesthetic, which may accumulate and be stored in adipose tissue, is common after long operations. The same applies to narcotics and benzodiazepines that may have accumulated in tissues throughout the surgery if administered in large doses, or in a patient with altered metabolism secondary to renal or liver disease. Neuromuscular blocking drugs are often used in neurosurgical procedures to ensure optimal surgical conditions. Excessive dosing, decreased metabolism or clearance, or inadequate drug reversal at the conclusion of surgery may lead to residual paralysis and the appearance of delayed awakening.

Careful review of the anesthetic record, with special attention to when volatile anesthetics were discontinued, narcotic and benzodiazepine use, and amount of neuromuscular blockade reversal agent and recovery of twitches, are important to note. Based on this information, empiric treatment with an appropriate antidote (naloxone for narcotics, flumazenil for benzodiazepines, or a combination of neostigmine and glycopyrrolate for neuromuscular blocking agents) may be indicated. Residual volatile anesthetic may be managed simply by continuing mechanical ventilation until the patient awakens.

When careful review of the history and physical exam does not reveal a cause for the failure to awaken, additional work-up is indicated. In patients following neurosurgery, a head CT scan without contrast is indicated to assess for bleeding, signs of increased ICP, or other acute cerebral pathology. An EEG may be indicated if there is concern for non-convulsive status epilepticus. Laboratory studies, including serum sodium, phosphate, calcium, magnesium, glucose, serum osmolality, and blood urea nitrogen (BUN) are indicated. The patient's body temperature should also be noted, as hypothermia can prolong the effects of drugs or lead to depressed levels of consciousness. Usually, the reason the patient is not awakening will become obvious after careful review of the data.

Postoperative analgesia

While once believed to cause minimal postoperative pain, brain surgery is now recognized to cause significant postoperative discomfort. In a series of 37 patients undergoing elective brain surgery (the majority for tumors), 60% complained of pain postoperatively, and two-thirds of those classified their pain as moderate to severe (De Benedittis et al 1996). Pain was most common in the 48 h following surgery and was described as superficial by 86% of patients. In a series of 187 patients in 2007, Gottschalk and (2007) colleagues observed similar findings. Additionally, these authors observed that infratentorial procedures reported more severe pain and required more opioid and non-opioid analgesics (Gottschalk et al 2007).

Acute pain management in the patient following craniotomy requires diligent attention to ensure proper titration of medication. Inadequate pain control can lead to hypertension, agitation, and vomiting, all of which may contribute to increased ICP. On the other hand, narcotic administration is not without significant side-effects, particularly when high doses are administered. Sedation, respiratory depression, nausea, and constipation are known side-effects. Sedative effects may depress the patient's mental status and complicate neurologic exams, and respiratory depression may lead to increased CO_2 levels and increased cerebral blood flow and pressure.

Codeine phosphate has been used extensively in neurosurgical patients, particularly in the UK, as it is believed to cause less respiratory depression and sedation than other narcotics (Nguyen et al 2001). However, in a study comparing morphine and codeine for postoperative analgesia following intracranial surgery, Goldsack and colleagues (1996) did not observe respiratory depression or sedation from either drug. Both drugs were administered intramuscularly (codeine 60 mg and morphine 10 mg.) They concluded that morphine was a safe alternative, with longer lasting effects than codeine. Sudheer and colleagues (2007) compared the analgesic efficacy and respiratory depressant effects of morphine PCA, tramadol PCA, and codeine 60 mg intramuscularly in 60 craniotomy patients. While arterial CO_2 did rise with all three analgesic regimens, it did so equally between the groups. They concluded that morphine PCA could provide better analgesia without increasing the risk of sedation or ventilatory changes, when compared with codeine.

In an effort to minimize narcotic administration in postoperative neurosurgical patients, a variety of non-opioid based analgesic techniques have been investigated. The simple infiltration of the surgical wound with bupivacaine 0.25% and epinephrine (1:200 000) at the beginning and end of craniotomy was shown to decrease postoperative pain on admission to the PACU (Bloomfield et al 1998). Nguyen and colleagues (2001) studied the effects of ropivacaine scalp block administered after completion of the surgery, but before awakening. They concluded that ropivacaine scalp block decreases the severity of postoperative pain, although the use of codeine postoperatively did not differ between the control and intervention groups. When skull block was performed prior to surgical pinning, Gazoni and colleagues (2008) failed to show superior analgesia postoperatively compared to control, when using a remifentanil-based anesthetic. Different approaches to pain management after craniotomy have been recently reviewed (Nemergut et al 2007).

Key points

- Goals for neuroanesthesia: (1) to safely maintain oxygenation and circulation and support the function of vital organs; (2) to provide the neurosurgeons with an excellent operative field; (3) conduct the anesthetic such that a rapid emergence from anesthesia is possible. Secondary goals might include increasing the tolerance to cerebral ischemia, allowing for appropriate neurophysiologic monitoring, and the avoidance of possible toxicity.

- All potent inhaled anesthetic agents are direct cerebral vasodilators and thereby decrease CVR, tend to increase CBF and ICP in patients with altered intracranial elastance; however, all potent inhaled anesthetic agents decrease CMR and thereby tend to decrease CBF. The net effect for a given agent on CBF and ICP results from the balance of the above two properties.

- Most intravenous agents reduce CBF through a reduction in the CMR.

- Euvolemia, as always, should be the goal of perioperative fluid management.

- Data from patients with a variety of studies suggests that neurosurgical patients have better outcomes when cared for in a dedicated neurointensive care units.

- Craniotomy and tumor resection may result in considerable cerebral edema, damage to the blood–brain barrier, and alteration in cerebral blood flow and autoregulation. Any of these factors may contribute to intracranial hypertension postoperatively, which can be managed by a variety of pharmacologic, non-pharmacologic, and surgical techniques.

- The physiological control of fluid status (via sodium) is different from control of osmolality (via free water balance), although cross-over exists between the systems.

- Both hyperglycemia (>180 mg/dL) and hypoglycemia (<60 mg/dL) are associated with poor outcome in different patient populations. Early enthusiasm for 'intensive insulin therapy' to maintain glucose between 80–110 mg/dL is waning as attempts to do so have highlighted the risks of aggressive glucose control. The most prudent approach may be to maintain glucose within the normal range, minimizing the incidence of hypoglycemia.

- While once believed to cause minimal postoperative pain, brain surgery is now recognized to cause significant postoperative discomfort.

REFERENCES

Abou-Madi, M.N., Trop, D., Barnes, J., 1980. Aetiology and control of cardiovascular reactions during trans-sphenoidal resection of pituitary microadenomas. Can. Anaesth. S. J. 27 (5), 491–495.

Adams, R.W., Gronert, G.A., Sundt, T.M., et al., 1972. Halothane, hypocapnia, and cerebrospinal fluid pressure in neurosurgery. Anesthesiology 37, 510–517.

Ahmed, I., Reichenberg, J., Lucas, A., et al., 2004. Erythema multiforme associated with phenytoin and cranial radiation therapy: a report of three patients and review of the literature. Int. J. Dermatol. 43 (1), 67–73.

Apfel, C.C., Korttila, K., Abdalla, M., et al., 2004. A factorial trial of six interventions for the prevention of postoperative nausea and vomiting. N. Engl. J. Med. 350 (24), 2441–2451.

Artru, A.A., 1982. Nitrous oxide plays a direct role in the development of tension pneumocephalus intraoperatively. Anesthesiology 57 (1), 59–61.

Aryan, H.E., Box, K.W., Ibrahim, D., et al., 2006. Safety and efficacy of dexmedetomidine in neurosurgical patients. Brain Inj. 20 (8), 791–798.

Bahrami, S., Yao, Y.M., Leichtfried, G., et al., 1997. Monoclonal antibody to endotoxin attenuates hemorrhage-induced lung injury and mortality in rats. Crit. Care Med. 25 (6), 1030–1036.

Balakrishnan, G., Raudzens, P., Samra, S.K., 2000. A comparison of remifentanil and fentanyl in patients undergoing surgery for intracranial mass lesions. Anesth. Analg. 91 (1), 163–169.

Balestrieri, F.J., Chernow, B., Rainey, T.G., 1982. Postcraniotomy diabetes insipidus. Who's at risk? Crit. Care Med. 10 (2), 108–110.

Battison, C., Andrews, P.J., Graham, C., et al., 2005. Randomized, controlled trial on the effect of a 20% mannitol solution and a 7.5% saline/6% dextran solution on increased intracranial pressure after brain injury. Crit. Care Med. 33 (1), 196–202; discussion 257–258.

Baylis, P.H., 2003. The syndrome of inappropriate antidiuretic hormone secretion. Int. J. Biochem. Cell Biol. 35 (11), 1495–1499.

Bedell, E.A., Berge, K.H., Losasso, T.J., 1994. Paradoxic air embolism during venous air embolism: transesophageal echocardiographic evidence of transpulmonary air passage. Anesthesiology 80 (4), 947–950.

Bekker, A., Sturaitis, M.K., 2005. Dexmedetomidine for neurological surgery. Neurosurgery 57 (Suppl.), 1–11.

Bell, B.A., Smith, M.A., Kean, D.M., et al., 1987. Brain water measured by magnetic resonance imaging. Correlation with direct estimation and changes after mannitol and dexamethasone. Lancet 1 (8524), 66–69.

Bellander, B.-M., Cantais, E., Enblad, P., et al., 2004. Consensus meeting on microdialysis in neurointensive care. Intensive Care Med. 30 (12), 2166–2169.

Belli, A., Sen, J., Petzold, A., et al., 2008 Metabolic failure precedes intracranial pressure rises in traumatic brain injury: a microdialysis study. Acta Neurochir. (Wien) 150 (5), 461–470.

Bergsneider, M., Hovda D.A., Shalmon E., et al., 1997. Cerebral hyperglycolysis following severe traumatic brain injury in humans: a positron emission tomography study. J. Neurosurg. 86 (2), 241–251.

Bilotta, F., Spinelli, A., Giovannini, F., et al., 2007. The effect of intensive insulin therapy on infection rate, vasospasm, neurologic outcome, and mortality in neurointensive care unit after intracranial aneurysm clipping in patients with acute subarachnoid hemorrhage: a randomized prospective pilot trial. J. Neurosurg. Anesthesiol. 19 (3), 156–160.

Black, S., Ockert, D.B., Oliver, W.C. Jr., et al., 1988. Outcome following posterior fossa craniectomy in patients in the sitting or horizontal positions. Anesthesiology 69 (1), 49–56.

Bloomfield, E.L., Schuber, A., Secic, M., et al., 1998. The influence of scalp infiltration with bupivacaine on hemodynamics and postoperative pain in adult patients undergoing craniotomy. Anesth. Analg. 87 (3), 579–582.

Bourg, V., Lebrun, C., Chichmanian, R.M., et al., 2001. Nitroso-urea-cisplatin-based chemotherapy associated with valproate: increase of haematologic toxicity. Ann. Oncol. 12 (2), 217–219.

Branston, N.M., 1995. Neurogenic control of the cerebral circulation. Cerebrovasc. Brain Metab. Rev. 7 (4), 338–349.

Bratton, S.L., Chestnut, R.M., Ghajar, J., et al., 2007a. Guidelines for the management of severe traumatic brain injury. IV. Infection prophylaxis. J. Neurotrauma. 24 (Suppl.), S26–S31. [Erratum appears in J Neurotrauma 2008, 25 (3), 276–278].

Bratton, S.L., Chestnut, R.M., Ghajar, J., et al., 2007b. Guidelines for the management of severe traumatic brain injury. VI. Indications for intracranial pressure monitoring. J. Neurotrauma. 24 (Suppl.), S37–S44. [Erratum appears in J Neurotrauma 2008, 25 (3), 276–278].

Bratton, S.L., Chestnut, R.M., Ghajar, J., et al., 2007c. Guidelines for the management of severe traumatic brain injury. VII. Intracranial pressure monitoring technology. J. Neurotrauma. 24 (Suppl.), S45–S54. [Erratum appears in J Neurotrauma 2008, 25 (3), 276–278].

Bratton, S.L., Chestnut, R.M., Ghajar, J., et al., 2007d. Guidelines for the management of severe traumatic brain injury. XIV. Hyperventilation. J. Neurotrauma. 24 (Suppl.), S87–S90. [Erratum appears in J Neurotrauma 2008, 25 (3), 276–278.].

Brunkhorst, F.M., Engel, C., Bloos, F., et al., 2008. Intensive insulin therapy and pentastarch resuscitation in severe sepsis. N. Engl. J. Med. 358 (2), 125–139.

Bruno, A., Levine, S.R., Frankel, M.R., et al., 2002. Admission glucose level and clinical outcomes in the NINDS rt-PA Stroke Trial. Neurology 59 (5), 669–674.

Bulger, E.M., Nathens, A.B., Rivara, F.P., et al., 2002. Management of severe head injury: institutional variations in care and effect on outcome. Crit. Care Med. 30 (8), 1870–1876.

Bunegin, L., Albin, M.S., Helsel, P.E. et al., 1981. Positioning the right atrial catheter: a model for reappraisal. Anesthesiology 55 (4), 343–348.

Capes, S.E., Hunt, D., Malmberg, K., et al., 2001. Stress hyperglycemia and prognosis of stroke in nondiabetic and diabetic patients: a systematic overview. Stroke 32 (10), 2426–2432.

Catargi, B., Rigalleau, V., Poussin, A., et al., 2003. Occult Cushing's syndrome in type-2 diabetes. J. Clin. Endocrinol. Metab. 88 (12), 5808–5813.

Chamorro, C., de Latorre, F.J., Montero, A., et al., 1996. Comparative study of propofol versus midazolam in the sedation of critically ill patients: results of a prospective, randomized, multicenter trial. Crit. Care Med. 24 (6), 932–939.

Chang, E.F., Potts, M.B., Keles, G.E., et al., 2008. Seizure characteristics and control following resection in 332 patients with low-grade gliomas. J. Neurosurg. 108 (2), 227–235.

Chang, S.M., Kuhn, J.G., Rizzo, J., et al., 1998. Phase I study of paclitaxel in patients with recurrent malignant glioma: a North American Brain Tumor Consortium report. J. Clin. Oncol. 16 (6), 2188–2194.

Chelliah, Y.R., Manninen, P.H., 2002. Hazards of epinephrine in transsphenoidal pituitary surgery. J. Neurosurg. Anesthesiol. 14 (1), 43–46.

Chen, H.I., Malhotra, N.R., Oddo, M., et al., 2008. Barbiturate infusion for intractable intracranial hypertension and its effect on brain oxygenation. Neurosurgery 63 (5), 880–887.

Ciric, I., Ragin, A., Baumgartner, C., et al., 1997. Complications of transsphenoidal surgery: results of a national survey, review of the literature, and personal experience. Neurosurgery 40 (2), 225–227.

Claassen, J., Carhuapoma, J.R., Kreiter, K.T., et al., 2002. Global cerebral edema after subarachnoid hemorrhage: frequency, predictors, and impact on outcome. Stroke 33 (5), 1225–1232.

Colao, A., Marzullo, P., Di Somma, C., et al., 2001. Growth hormone and the heart. Clinical. Endocrinology 54 (2), 137–154.

Coplin, W.M., Pierson, D.J., Cooley, K.D., et al., 2000. Implications of extubation delay in brain-injured patients meeting standard weaning criteria. Am. J. Respir. Crit. Care Med. 161 (5), 1530–1536.

Cormio, M., Gopinath, S.P., Valadka, A., et al., 1999. Cerebral hemodynamic effects of pentobarbital coma in head-injured patients. J. Neurotrauma. 16 (10), 927–936.

Cremer, O.L., van Dijk, G.W., van Wensen, E., et al., 2005. Effect of intracranial pressure monitoring and targeted intensive care on functional outcome after severe head injury. Crit. Care Med. 33 (10), 2207–2213.

Croughwell, N.D., Newman, M.F., Blumenthal, J.A., et al., 1994. Jugular bulb saturation and cognitive dysfunction after cardiopulmonary bypass. Ann. Thorac. Surg. 58 (6), 1702–1708.

Damaraju, S.C., Rajshekhar, V., Chandy, M.J., 1997. Validation study of a central venous pressure-based protocol for the management of neurosurgical patients with hyponatremia and natriuresis. Neurosurgery 40 (2), 312–317.

De Benedittis, G., Lorenzetti, A., Migliore, M., et al., 1996. Postoperative pain in neurosurgery: a pilot study in brain surgery. Neurosurgery 38 (3), 466–470.

Deutschman, C.S., Haines, S.J., 1985. Anticonvulsant prophylaxis in neurological surgery. Neurosurgery 17 (3), 510–517.

Devos, P., Preiser, J.-C., Melot, C., 2007. Impact of tight glucose control by intensive insulin therapy on ICU mortality and the rate of hypoglycemia: final results of the Glucontrol Study. Intensive Care Med. 33 (S189), 189.

Diringer, M.N., Edwards, D.F., 2001. Admission to a neurologic/neurosurgical intensive care unit is associated with reduced mortality rate after intracerebral hemorrhage. Crit. Care Med. 29 (3), 635–640.

Doyle, J.A., Davis, D.P., Hoyt, D.B., 2001. The use of hypertonic saline in the treatment of traumatic brain injury. J. Trauma. 50 (2), 367–383.

Edge, W.G., Whitwam, J.G., 1981. Chondro-calcinosis and difficult intubation in acromegaly. Anaesthesia 36 (7), 677–680.

Ely, E.W., Baker, A.M., Dunagan, D.P., et al., 1996. Effect on the duration of mechanical ventilation of identifying patients capable of breathing spontaneously. N. Engl. J. Med. 335 (25), 1864–1869.

Enblad, P., Frykholm, P., Valtysson, J., et al., 2001. Middle cerebral artery occlusion and reperfusion in primates monitored by microdialysis and sequential positron emission tomography. Stroke 32 (7), 1574–1580.

Fandino, J., Stocker, R., Prokop, S., et al., 2000. Cerebral oxygenation and systemic trauma related factors determining neurological outcome after brain injury. J. Clin. Neurosci. 7 (3), 226–233.

Fatti, L.M., Scacchi, M., Pincelli, A.I., et al., 2001. Prevalence and pathogenesis of sleep apnea and lung disease in acromegaly. Pituitary 4 (4), 259–262.

Ferguson, J.K., Donald, R.A., Weston, T.S., et al., 1983. Skin thickness in patients with acromegaly and Cushing's syndrome and response to treatment. Clin. Endocrinol. 18 (4), 347–353.

Fetell, M.R., Grossman, S.A., Fisher, J.D., et al., 1997. Preirradiation paclitaxel in glioblastoma multiforme: efficacy, pharmacology, and drug interactions. New Approaches to Brain Tumor Therapy

Central Nervous System Consortium. J. Clin. Oncol. 15 (9), 3121–3128.

Fleisher, L.A., Beckman, J.A., Brown, K.A., et al., 2007. ACC/AHA 2007 Guidelines on Perioperative Cardiovascular Evaluation and Care for Noncardiac Surgery: Executive Summary: A Report of the American College of Cardiology/American Heart Association Task Force on Practice Guidelines (Writing Committee to Revise the 2002 Guidelines on Perioperative Cardiovascular Evaluation for Noncardiac Surgery): Developed in Collaboration With the American Society of Echocardiography, American Society of Nuclear Cardiology, Heart Rhythm Society, Society of Cardiovascular Anesthesiologists, Society for Cardiovascular Angiography and Interventions, Society for Vascular Medicine and Biology, and Society for Vascular Surgery. Circulation 116 (17), 1971–1996. [Erratum appears in Circulation 2008, 118 (9), e141–e142].

Fleming, J.A., Byck, R., Barash, P.G., 1990. Pharmacology and therapeutic applications of cocaine. Anesthesiology 73 (3), 518–531.

Fox, J.L., Falik, J.L., Shalhoub, R.J., 1971. Neurosurgical hyponatremia: the role of inappropriate antidiuresis. J. Neurosurg. 34 (4), 506–514.

Foy, P.M., Chadwick, D.W., Rajgopalan, N., et al., 1992. Do prophylactic anticonvulsant drugs alter the pattern of seizures after craniotomy? J. Neurol. Neurosurg. Psychiatry 55 (9), 753–757.

Francony, G., Fauvage, B., Falcon, D., et al., 2008. Equimolar doses of mannitol and hypertonic saline in the treatment of increased intracranial pressure. Crit. Care Med. 36 (3), 795–800.

Fukushima, T., Maroon, J.C., 1998. Repair of carotid artery perforations during transsphenoidal surgery. Surgical Neurology 50 (2), 174–177.

Gan, T.J., 2006. Risk factors for postoperative nausea and vomiting. Anesth. Analg. 102 (6), 1884–1898.

Gandhi, G.Y., Nuttall, G.A., Abel, M.D., et al., 2005. Intraoperative hyperglycemia and perioperative outcomes in cardiac surgery patients. Mayo Clin. Proc. 80 (7), 862–866.

Gandhi, G.Y., Nuttall, G.A., Abel, M.D., et al., 2007. Intensive intraoperative insulin therapy versus conventional glucose management during cardiac surgery: a randomized trial. Ann. Intern. Med. 146 (4), 233–243.

Gazoni, F.M., Pouratian, N., Nemergut, E.C., 2008. Effect of ropivacaine skull block on perioperative outcomes in patients with supratentorial brain tumors and comparison with remifentanil: a pilot study. J. Neurosurg. 109 (1), 44–49.

Glantz, M.J., Cole, B.F., Forsyth, P.A., et al., 2000. Practice parameter: anticonvulsant prophylaxis in patients with newly diagnosed brain tumors. Report of the Quality Standards Subcommittee of the American Academy of Neurology. Neurology 54 (10), 1886–1893.

Glantz, M.J., Cole, B.F., Friedberg, M.H., et al., 1996. A randomized, blinded, placebo-controlled trial of divalproex sodium prophylaxis in adults with newly diagnosed brain tumors. Neurology 46 (4), 985–991.

Goldsack, C., Scuplak, S.M., Smith, M., 1996. A double-blind comparison of codeine and morphine for postoperative analgesia following intracranial surgery. Anaesthesia 51 (11), 1029–1032.

Gondim Fde, A., Aiyagari, V., Shackleford, A., et al., 2005. Osmolality not predictive of mannitol-induced acute renal insufficiency. J. Neurosurg. 103 (3), 444–447.

Gopinath, S.P., Robertson, C.S., Contant, C.F., et al., 1994. Jugular venous desaturation and outcome after head injury. J. Neurol. Neurosurg. Psychiatry 57 (6), 717–723.

Gopinath, S.P., Valadka, A.B., Uzura, M., et al., 1999. Comparison of jugular venous oxygen saturation and brain tissue PO_2 as monitors of cerebral ischemia after head injury. Crit. Care Med. 27 (11), 2337–2345.

Gottschalk, A., Berkow, L.C., Stevens, R.D., et al., 2007. Prospective evaluation of pain and analgesic use following major elective intracranial surgery. J. Neurosurg. 106 (2), 210–216.

Grap, M.J., Strickland, D., Tormey, L., et al., 2003. Collaborative practice: development, implementation, and evaluation of a weaning protocol for patients receiving mechanical ventilation. Am. J. Crit. Care 12 (5), 454–460.

Greenfield, J.C., Jr., Rembert, J.C., Tindall, G.T., 1984. Transient changes in cerebral vascular resistance during the Valsalva maneuver in man. Stroke 15 (1), 76–79.

Guilleminault, C., van den Hoed, J., 1979. Acromegaly and narcolepsy. Lancet 2 (8145), 750–751.

Gupta, A.K., Hutchinson, P.J., Al-Rawi, P., et al., 1999. Measuring brain tissue oxygenation compared with jugular venous oxygen saturation for monitoring cerebral oxygenation after traumatic brain injury. Anesth. Analg. 88 (3), 549–553.

Guy, J., Hindman, B.J., Baker, K.Z., et al., 1997. Comparison of remifentanil and fentanyl in patients undergoing craniotomy for supratentorial space-occupying lesions. Anesthesiology 86 (3), 514–524.

Hagen, P.T., Scholz, D.G., Edwards, W.D., 1984. Incidence and size of patent foramen ovale during the first 10 decades of life: an autopsy study of 965 normal hearts. Mayo Clin. Proc. 59 (1), 17–20.

Hakala, P., Randell, T., Valli, H., 1998. Laryngoscopy and fibreoptic intubation in acromegalic patients. Br. J. Anaesth. 80 (3), 345–347.

Harrigan, M.R., 1996. Cerebral salt wasting syndrome: a review. Neurosurgery 38 (1), 152–160.

Hasan, D., Lindsay, K.W., Wijdicks, E.F., et al., 1989. Effect of fludrocortisone acetate in patients with subarachnoid hemorrhage. Stroke 20 (9), 1156–1161.

Hensen, J., Henig, A., Fahlbusch, R., et al., 1999. Prevalence, predictors and patterns of postoperative polyuria and hyponatraemia in the immediate course after transsphenoidal surgery for pituitary adenomas. Clin. Endocrinol. (Oxf.) 50 (4), 431–439.

Hillered, L., Persson, L., Nilsson, P., et al., 2006. Continuous monitoring of cerebral metabolism in traumatic brain injury: a focus on cerebral microdialysis. Curr. Opin. Crit. Care 12 (2), 112–118.

Hillered, L., Vespa, P.M., Hovda, D.A., 2005. Translational neurochemical research in acute human brain injury: the current status and potential future for cerebral microdialysis. J. Neurotrauma 22 (1), 3–41.

Holmstrom, A., Akeson, J., 2004. Desflurane increases intracranial pressure more and sevoflurane less than isoflurane in pigs subjected to intracranial hypertension. J. Neurosurg. Anesthesiol. 16 (2), 136–143.

Horrigan, R.W., Eger, E.I., Wilson, C., 1978. Epinephrine-induced arrhythmias during enflurane anesthesia in man: a nonlinear dose-response relationship and dose-dependent protection from lidocaine. Anesth. Analg. 57 (5), 547–550.

Hutchens, M.P., Memtsoudis, S., Sadovnikoff, N., 2006. Propofol for sedation in neuro-intensive care. Neurocrit. Care 4 (1), 54–62.

Ichai, C., Armando, G., Orban, J., et al., 2009. Sodium lactate versus mannitol in the treatment of intracranial hypertensive episodes in severe traumatic brain-injured patients. Intensive Care Med. 35 (3), 471–479.

Jagannathan, J., Okonkwo, D.O., Dumont, A.S., et al., 2007. Outcome following decompressive craniectomy in children with severe traumatic brain injury: a 10-year single-center experience with long-term follow up. J. Neurosurg. 106 (Suppl.), 268–275.

Jane, J.A., Jr., Laws, E.R., Jr., 2001. The surgical management of pituitary adenomas in a series of 3,093 patients. J. Am. Coll. Surg. 193 (6), 651–659.

Jeremitsky, E., Omert, L.A., Dunham, C.M., et al., 2005. The impact of hyperglycemia on patients with severe brain injury. J. Trauma 58 (1), 47–50.

Juvela, S., Siironen, J., Kuhmonen, J., 2005. Hyperglycemia, excess weight, and history of hypertension as risk factors for poor outcome and cerebral infarction after aneurysmal subarachnoid hemorrhage. J. Neurosurg. 102 (6), 998–1003.

Kaal, E.C., Vecht, C.J., 2004. The management of brain edema in brain tumors. Curr. Opin. Oncol. 16 (6), 593–600.

Kagansky, N., Levy, S., Knobler, H., 2001. The role of hyperglycemia in acute stroke. Arch. Neurol. 58 (8), 1209–1212.

Kaltsas, G., Manetti, L., Grossman, A.B., 2002. Osteoporosis in Cushing's syndrome. Front Horm. Res. 30, 60–72.

Kasemsuwan, L., Griffiths, M.V., 1996. Lignocaine with adrenaline: is it as effective as cocaine in rhinological practice? Clin. Otolaryngol. Allied Sci. 21 (2), 127–129.

Kaufmann, A.M., Cardoso, E.R., 1992. Aggravation of vasogenic cerebral edema by multiple-dose mannitol. J. Neurosurg. 77 (4), 584–589.

Keegan, M.T., Atkinson, J.L., Kasperbauer, J.L., et al., 2000. Exaggerated hemodynamic responses to nasal injection and awakening from anesthesia in a Cushingoid patient having transsphenoidal hypophysectomy. J. Neurosurg. Anesthesiol. 12 (3), 225–229.

Kelly, D.F., Laws, E.R. Jr., Fossett, D., 1995. Delayed hyponatremia after transsphenoidal surgery for pituitary adenoma. Report of nine cases. J. Neurosurg. 83 (2), 363–367.

Kelly, J.J., Tam, S.H., Williamson, P.M., et al., 1998. The nitric oxide system and cortisol-induced hypertension in humans. Clin. Exp. Pharmacol. Physiol. 25 (11), 945–946.

Kirkpatrick, P.J., Smielewski, P., Czosnyka, M., et al., 1995. Near-infrared spectroscopy use in patients with head injury. J. Neurosurg. 83 (6), 963–970.

Kitahata, L.M., 1971. Airway difficulties associated with anaesthesia in acromegaly. Three case reports. Br. J. Anaesth. 43 (12), 1187–1190.

Korosue, K., Heros, R.C., Ogilvy, C.S., et al., 1990. Comparison of crystalloids and colloids for hemodilution in a model of focal cerebral ischemia. J. Neurosurg. 73 (4), 576–584.

Kozek-Langenecker, S.A., 2005. Effects of hydroxyethyl starch solutions on hemostasis. Anesthesiology 103 (3), 654–660.

Krinsley, J.S., 2003. Association between hyperglycemia and increased hospital mortality in a heterogeneous population of critically ill patients. Mayo Clin. Proc. 78 (12), 1471–1478.

Krishnan, J.A., Moore, D., Robeson, C., et al., 2004. A prospective, controlled trial of a protocol-based strategy to discontinue mechanical ventilation. Am. J. Respir. Crit. Care Med. 169 (6), 673–678.

Kuijlen, J.M., Teernstra, O.P., Kessels, A.G., et al., 1996. Effectiveness of antiepileptic prophylaxis used with supratentorial craniotomies: a meta-analysis. Seizure 5 (4), 291–298.

Kvam, D.A., Loftus, C.M., Copeland, B., et al., 1983. Seizures during the immediate postoperative period. Neurosurgery 12 (1), 14–17.

Lackner, T.E., 1991. Interaction of dexamethasone with phenytoin. Pharmacotherapy 11 (4), 344–347.

Lane, P.L., Skoretz, T.G., Doig, G., et al., 2000. Intracranial pressure monitoring and outcomes after traumatic brain injury. Can. J. Surg. 43 (6), 442–448.

Lanier, W.L., Stangland, K.J., Scheithauer, B.W., et al., 1987. The effects of dextrose infusion and head position on neurologic outcome after complete cerebral ischemia in primates: examination of a model. Anesthesiology 66 (1), 39–48.

Lanzino, G., Kassell, N.F., Germanson, T., et al., 1993. Plasma glucose levels and outcome after aneurysmal subarachnoid hemorrhage. J. Neurosurg. 79 (6), 885–891.

Liu, C.Y., Apuzzo, M.L.J., 2003. The genesis of neurosurgery and the evolution of the neurosurgical operative environment: part I-prehistory to 2003. Neurosurgery 52 (1), 3–19.

Makaryus, A.N., McFarlane, S.I., 2006. Diabetes insipidus: diagnosis and treatment of a complex disease. Cleve. Clin. J. Med. 73 (1), 65–71.

Mammoto, T., Hayashi, Y., Ohnishi, Y., et al., 1998. Incidence of venous and paradoxical air embolism in neurosurgical patients in the sitting position: detection by transesophageal echocardiography. Acta Anaesthesiol. Scand. 42 (6), 643–647.

Marelich, G.P., Murin, S., Battistella, F., et al., 2000. Protocol weaning of mechanical ventilation in medical and surgical patients by respiratory care practitioners and nurses: effect on weaning time and incidence of ventilator-associated pneumonia. Chest 118 (2), 459–467.

Marion, D.W., Darby, J., Yonas, H., 1991. Acute regional cerebral blood flow changes caused by severe head injuries. J. Neurosurg. 74 (3), 407–414.

Marshall, W.K., Bedford, R.F., Miller, E.D., 1983. Cardiovascular responses in the seated position –impact of four anesthetic techniques. Anesth. Analg. 62 (7), 648–653.

Martyn, J.A.J., Richtsfeld, M., 2006. Succinylcholine-induced hyperkalemia in acquired pathologic states: etiologic factors and molecular mechanisms [see comment]. Anesthesiology 104 (1), 158–169.

Matta, B.F., Heath, K.J., Tipping, K., et al., 1999. Direct cerebral vasodilatory effects of sevoflurane and isoflurane. Anesthesiology 91 (3), 677–680.

Matta, M.P., Caron, P., 2003. Acromegalic cardiomyopathy: a review of the literature. Pituitary 6 (4), 203–207.

May, A.K., Fleming, S.B., Carpenter, R.O., et al., 2006. Influence of broad-spectrum antibiotic prophylaxis on intracranial pressure monitor infections and subsequent infectious complications in head-injured patients. Surg. Infect. 7 (5), 409–417.

McFarlane, C., Lee, A., 1994. A comparison of plasmalyte 148 and 0.9% saline for intra-operative fluid replacement. Anaesthesia 49 (9), 779–781.

McGirt, M.J., Woodworth, G.F., Brooke, B.S., et al., 2006. Hyperglycemia independently increases the risk of perioperative stroke, myocardial infarction, and death after carotid endarterectomy. Neurosurgery 58 (6), 1066–1073.

Michelucci, R., 2006. Optimizing therapy of seizures in neurosurgery. Neurology 67 (Suppl.), S14–S18.

Michenfelder, J.D., Miller, R.H., Gronert, G.A., 1972. Evaluation of an ultrasonic device (Doppler) for the diagnosis of venous air embolism. Anesthesiology 36 (2), 164–167.

Muizelaar, J.P., van der Poel, H.G., Li, Z.C., et al., 1988. Pial arteriolar vessel diameter and CO_2 reactivity during prolonged hyperventilation in the rabbit. J. Neurosurg. 69 (6), 923–927.

Myburgh, J., Cooper, D.J., Finfer, S., et al., 2007. Saline or albumin for fluid resuscitation in patients with traumatic brain injury. N. Engl. J. Med. 357 (9), 874–884.

Myles, P.S., Leslie, K., Chan, M.T.V., et al., 2007. Avoidance of nitrous oxide for patients undergoing major surgery: a randomized controlled trial. Anesthesiology 107 (2), 221–231.

Namen, A.M., Ely, E.W., Tatter, S.B., et al., 2001. Predictors of successful extubation in neurosurgical patients. Am. J. Respir. Crit. Care Med. 163 (3 Pt 1), 658–664.

Nelson, P.B., Seif, S.M., Maroon, J.C. et al., 1981. Hyponatremia in intracranial disease: perhaps not the syndrome of inappropriate secretion of antidiuretic hormone (SIADH). J. Neurosurg. 55 (6), 938–941.

Nemergut, E.C., Dumont, A.S., Barry, U.T., et al., 2005a. Perioperative management of patients undergoing transsphenoidal pituitary surgery. Anesth. Analg. 101 (4), 1170–1181.

Nemergut, E.C., Durieux, M.E., Missaghi, N.B., et al., 2007. Pain management after craniotomy. Best Pract. Res. Clin. Anaesthesiol. 21 (4), 557–573.

Nemergut, E.C., Zuo, Z., 2006. Airway management in patients with pituitary disease: a review of 746 patients. J. Neurosurg. Anesthesiol. 18 (1), 73–77.

Nemergut, E.C., Zuo, Z., Jane, J.A., Jr., et al., 2005b. Predictors of diabetes insipidus after transsphenoidal surgery: a review of 881 patients. J. Neurosurg. 103 (3), 448–454.

Newfield, P., Albin, M.S., Chestnut, J.S., et al., 1978. Air embolism during trans-sphenoidal pituitary operations. Neurosurgery 2 (1), 39–42.

Nguyen, A., Girard, F., Boudreault, D., et al., 2001. Scalp nerve blocks decrease the severity of pain after craniotomy. Anesth. Analg. 93 (5), 1272–1276.

North, J.B., Penhall, R.K., Hanieh, A., et al., 1983. Phenytoin and postoperative epilepsy. A double-blind study. J. Neurosurg. 58 (5), 672–677.

Ober, K.P., 1991. Endocrine crises. Diabetes insipidus. Crit. Care Clin. 7 (1), 109–125.

Oberndorfer, S., Piribauer, M., Marosi, C., et al., 2005. P450 enzyme inducing and non-enzyme inducing antiepileptics in glioblastoma patients treated with standard chemotherapy. J. Neurooncol. 72 (3), 255–260.

Olson, B.R., Gumowski, J., Rubino, D., et al., 1997. Pathophysiology of hyponatremia after transsphenoidal pituitary surgery. J. Neurosurg. 87 (4), 499–507.

Ovassapian, A., Doka, J.C., Romsa, D.E., 1981. Acromegaly – use of fiberoptic laryngoscopy to avoid tracheostomy. Anesthesiology 54 (5), 429–430.

Packer, R.J., Gurney, J.G., Punyko, J.A., et al., 2003. Long-term neurologic and neurosensory sequelae in adult survivors of a childhood brain tumor: childhood cancer survivor study. J. Clin. Oncol. 21 (17), 3255–3261.

Papadopoulos, G., Kuhly, P., Brock, M., et al., 1994. Venous and paradoxical air embolism in the sitting position. A prospective study with transesophageal echocardiography. Acta Neurochir. (Wien) 126 (2–4), 140–143.

Parsons, M.W., Barber, P.A., Desmond, P.M., et al., 2002. Acute hyperglycemia adversely affects stroke outcome: a magnetic resonance imaging and spectroscopy study. Ann. Neurol. 52 (1), 20–28.

Pasternak, J., Atkison, J., Kasperbauer, J., et al., 2004. Hemodynamic responses to epinephrine-containing local anesthetic injection and to emergence from general anesthesia in transsphenoidal hypophysectomy patients. J. Neurosurg. Anesthesiol. 16 (3), 189–195.

Patel, P.M., Drummond, J.C., 2005. Cerebral physiology and the effects of anesthetics and techniques. In: Miller's anesthesia, 6th edn. Churchill Livingstone, Philadelphia, PA.

Perez-Barcena, J., Llompart-Pou, J.A., Homar, J., et al., 2008. Pentobarbital versus thiopental in the treatment of refractory intracranial hypertension in patients with traumatic brain injury: a randomized controlled trial. Crit. Care 12 (4), R112.

Peters, J.P., Welt, L.G., Sims, E.A., et al., 1950. A salt-wasting syndrome associated with cerebral disease. Trans. Assoc. Am. Physicians 63, 57–64.

Piper, J.G., Dirks, B.A., Traynelis, V.C., et al., 1995. Perioperative management and surgical outcome of the acromegalic patient with sleep apnea. Neurosurgery 36 (1), 70–75.

Pivalizza, E.G., Katz, J., Singh, S., et al., 1998. Massive macroglossia after posterior fossa surgery in the prone position. J. Neurosurg. Anesthesiol. 10 (1), 34–36.

Pollay, M., Fullenwider, C., Roberts, P.A., et al., 1983. Effect of mannitol and furosemide on blood-brain osmotic gradient and intracranial pressure. J. Neurosurg. 59 (6), 945–950.

Raichle, M.E., Posner, J.B., Plum, F., 1970. Cerebral blood flow during and after hyperventilation. Arch. Neurol. 23 (5), 394–403.

Rajasoorya, C., Holdaway, I.M., Wrightson, P., et al., 1994. Determinants of clinical outcome and survival in acromegaly. Clin. Endocrinol. 41 (1), 95–102.

Rangel-Castilla, L., Gopinath, S., Robertson, C.S., 2008. Management of intracranial hypertension. Neurol. Clin. 26 (2), 521–541.

Reich, S.D., Bachur, N.R., 1976. Alterations in Adriamycin efficacy by phenobarbital. Cancer Res. 36 (10), 3803–3806.

Relling, M.V., Pui, C.H., Sandlund, J.T., et al., 2000. Adverse effect of anticonvulsants on efficacy of chemotherapy for acute lymphoblastic leukaemia. Lancet 356 (9226), 285–290.

Rincon, F., Mayer, S.A., 2007. Neurocritical care: a distinct discipline? Curr. Opin. Crit. Care 13 (2), 115–121.

Roberts, I., 2000. Barbiturates for acute traumatic brain injury. Cochrane Database of Systematic Reviews (2), CD000033.

Robertson, G.L., 1984. Abnormalities of thirst regulation. Kidney Int. 25 (2), 460–469.

Robertson, G.L., Harris, A., 1989. Clinical use of vasopressin analogues. Hosp. Pract. (Off Ed.) 24 (10), 114–118, 126–118, 133 passim.

Robinson, A.G., 1985. Disorders of antidiuretic hormone secretion. Clin. Endocrinol. Metab. 14 (1), 55–88.

Ross, E.J., Linch, D.C., 1982. Cushing's syndrome – killing disease: discriminatory value of signs and symptoms aiding early diagnosis. Lancet 2 (8299), 646–649.

Ross, E.J., Marshall-Jones, P., Friedman, M., 1966. Cushing's syndrome: diagnostic criteria. Q. J. Med. 35 (138), 149–192.

Sahuquillo, J., Arikan, F., 2006. Decompressive craniectomy for the treatment of refractory high intracranial pressure in traumatic brain injury. Cochrane Database Syst. Rev. (1), CD003983.

Salvant, J.B., Jr., Muizelaar, J.P., 1993. Changes in cerebral blood flow and metabolism related to the presence of subdural hematoma. Neurosurgery 33 (3), 387–393.

Samra, S.K., Dy, E.A., Welch, K., et al., 2000. Evaluation of a cerebral oximeter as a monitor of cerebral ischemia during carotid endarterectomy. Anesthesiology 93 (4), 964–970.

Scheingraber, S., Rehm, M., Sehmisch, C., et al., 1999. Rapid saline infusion produces hyperchloremic acidosis in patients undergoing gynecologic surgery. Anesthesiology 90 (5), 1265–1270.

Schierhout, G., Roberts, I., 2000. Hyperventilation therapy for acute traumatic brain injury. Cochrane Database of Syst. Rev. (2), CD000566.

Schmitt, H., Buchfelder, M., Radespiel-Troger, M., et al., 2000. Difficult intubation in acromegalic patients: incidence and predictability. Anesthesiology 93 (1), 110–114.

Semple, P.L., Laws, E.R., Jr., 1999. Complications in a contemporary series of patients who underwent transsphenoidal surgery for Cushing's disease. J. Neurosurg. 91 (2), 175–179.

Shipley, J.E., Schteingart, D.E., Tandon, R., et al., 1992. Sleep architecture and sleep apnea in patients with Cushing's disease. Sleep 15 (6), 514–518.

Singer, P.A., Sevilla, L.J., 2003. Postoperative endocrine management of pituitary tumors. Neurosurg. Clin. N. Am. 14 (1), 123–138.

Singh, S., Bohn, D., Carlotti, A.P., et al., 2002. Cerebral salt wasting: truths, fallacies, theories, and challenges. Crit. Care Med. 30 (11), 2575–2579.

Sivakumar, V., Rajshekhar, V., Chandy, M.J., 1994. Management of neurosurgical patients with hyponatremia and natriuresis. Neurosurgery 34 (2), 269–274.

Smith, M., Hirsch, N.P., 2000. Pituitary disease and anaesthesia. Br. J. Anaesth. 85 (1), 3–14.

Smythe, P.R., Samra, S.K., 2002. Monitors of cerebral oxygenation. Anesth. Clin. North America 20 (2), 293–313.

Sneyd, J.R., Andrews, C.J., Tsubokawa, T., 2005. Comparison of propofol/remifentanil and sevoflurane/remifentanil for maintenance of anaesthesia for elective intracranial surgery. Br. J. Anaesth. 94 (6), 778–783.

Soriano, S.G., Martyn, J.A., 2004. Antiepileptic-induced resistance to neuromuscular blockers: mechanisms and clinical significance. Clin. Pharmacokinet. 43 (2), 71–81.

Southwick, J.P., Katz, J., 1979. Unusual airway difficulty in the acromegalic patient – indications for tracheostomy. Anesthesiology 51 (1), 72–73.

Stahl, N., Mellergard, P., Hallstrom, A., et al., 2001. Intracerebral microdialysis and bedside biochemical analysis in patients with fatal traumatic brain lesions. Acta Anaesthesiol. Scand. 45 (8), 977–985.

Stendel, R., Gramm, H.J., Schroder, K., et al., 2000. Transcranial Doppler ultrasonography as a screening technique for detection of a patent foramen ovale before surgery in the sitting position. Anesthesiology 93 (4), 971–975.

Stocchetti, N., Maas, A.I., Chieregato, A., et al., 2005. Hyperventilation in head injury: a review. Chest 127 (5), 1812–1827.

Strandgaard, S., 1976. Autoregulation of cerebral blood flow in hypertensive patients. The modifying influence of prolonged antihypertensive treatment on the tolerance to acute, drug-induced hypotension. Circulation 53 (4), 720–727.

Sudheer, P.S., Logan, S.W., Terblanche, C., et al., 2007. Comparison of the analgesic efficacy and respiratory effects of morphine, tramadol and codeine after craniotomy. Anaesthesia 62 (6), 555–560.

Taphoorn M.J., 2003, Neurocognitive sequelae in the treatment of low-grade gliomas. Semin. Oncol. 30 (Suppl.), 45–48.

Thiele, R.H., Pouratain, N., Zuo, Z., et al., 2009. Strict glucose control does not affect mortality after aneurysmal subarachnoid hemorrhage. Anesthesiology 110 (3), 603–610.

Tisdall, M., Crocker, M., Watkiss, J., et al., 2006. Disturbances of sodium in critically ill adult neurologic patients: a clinical review. J. Neurosurg. Anesthesiol. 18 (1), 57–63.

Todd, M.M., Warner, D.S., Sokoll, M.D., et al., 1993. A prospective, comparative trial of three anesthetics for elective supratentorial craniotomy. Propofol/fentanyl, isoflurane/nitrous oxide, and fentanyl/nitrous oxide. Anesthesiology 78 (6), 1005–1020.

Tommasino, C., Moore, S., Todd, M.M., 1988. Cerebral effects of isovolemic hemodilution with crystalloid or colloid solutions. Crit. Care Med. 16 (9), 862–868.

Tonnelier, J.M., Prat, G., Le Gal, G., et al., 2005. Impact of a nurses' protocol-directed weaning procedure on outcomes in patients undergoing mechanical ventilation for longer than 48 hours: a prospective cohort study with a matched historical control group. Crit. Care 9 (2), R83–R89.

Toung, T.J., Rossberg, M.I., Hutchins, G.M., 2001. Volume of air in a lethal venous air embolism. Anesthesiology 94 (2), 360–361. [Erratum appears in Anesthesiology 2001, 94 (4), 723].

Trost, H.A., Gaab, M.R., 1992. Plasma osmolality, osmoregulation and prognosis after head injury. Acta Neurochir. (Wien) 116 (1), 33–37.

Valadka, A.B., Gopinath, S.P., Contant, C.F., et al., 1998. Relationship of brain tissue PO_2 to outcome after severe head injury. Crit. Care Med. 26 (9), 1576–1581.

Van den Berghe, G., Schoonheydt, K., Becx, P., et al., 2005. Insulin therapy protects the central and peripheral nervous system of intensive care patients. Neurology 64 (8), 1348–1353.

Van den Berghe, G., Wilmer, A., Hermans, G., et al., 2006. Intensive insulin therapy in the medical ICU. N. Engl. J. Med. 354 (5), 449–461.

Van den Berghe, G., Wouters, P., Weekers, F., et al., 2001. Intensive insulin therapy in the critically ill patients. N. Engl. J. Med. 345 (19), 1359–1367.

Varelas, P.N., Eastwood, D., Yun, H.J., et al., 2006. Impact of a neurointensivist on outcomes in patients with head trauma treated in a neurosciences intensive care unit. J. Neurosurg. 104 (5), 713–719.

Vecht, C.J., Wagner, G.L., Wilms, E.B., 2003a. Interactions between antiepileptic and chemotherapeutic drugs. Lancet Neurology 2 (7), 404–409.

Vecht, C.J., Wagner, G.L., Wilms, E.B., 2003b. Treating seizures in patients with brain tumors: Drug interactions between antiepileptic and chemotherapeutic agents. Semin. Oncol. 30 (Suppl.), 49–52.

Vialet, R., Albanese, J., Thomachot, L., et al., 2003. Isovolume hypertonic solutes (sodium chloride or mannitol) in the treatment of refractory posttraumatic intracranial hypertension: 2 mL/kg 7.5% saline is more effective than 2 mL/kg 20% mannitol. Crit. Care Med. 31 (6), 1683–1687.

Voss, L.J., Sleigh, J.W., Barnard, J.P., et al., 2008. The howling cortex: seizures and general anesthetic drugs. Anesth. Analg. 107 (5), 1689–1703.

Warren, B.B., Durieux, M.E., 1997. Hydroxyethyl starch: safe or not? Anesth. Analg. 84 (1), 206–212.

Warren, R.D., Bender, R.A., 1977. Drug interactions with antineoplastic agents. Cancer Treat. Rep. 61 (7), 1231–1241.

Wasterlain, C.G., Fujikawa, D.G., Penix, L., et al., 1993. Pathophysiological mechanisms of brain damage from status epilepticus. Epilepsia 34 (Suppl.), S37–S53.

Weiskopf, R.B., Moore, M.A., Eger, E.I., 2nd, et al., 1994. Rapid increase in desflurane concentration is associated with greater transient cardiovascular stimulation than with rapid increase in isoflurane concentration in humans. Anesthesiology 80 (5), 1035–1045.

Wen, P.Y., Marks, P.W., 2002. Medical management of patients with brain tumors. Curr. Opin. Oncol. 14 (3), 299–307.

Wilder, B.L., 1982. Hypothesis: the etiology of midcervical quadriplegia after operation with the patient in the sitting position. Neurosurgery 11 (4), 530–531.

Williams, E.L., Hildebrand, K.L., McCormick, S.A., et al., 1999. The effect of intravenous lactated Ringer's solution versus 0.9% sodium chloride solution on serum osmolality in human volunteers. Anesth. Analg. 88 (5), 999–1003.

Williams, L.S., Rotich, J., Qi, R., et al., 2002. Effects of admission hyperglycemia on mortality and costs in acute ischemic stroke. Neurology 59 (1), 67–71.

Williams, R.G., Richards, S.H., Mills, R.G., et al., 1994. Voice changes in acromegaly. Laryngoscope 104 (4), 484–487.

Wilson, C.B., 1990. Role of surgery in the management of pituitary tumors. Neurosurg. Clin. N. Am. 1 (1), 139–159.

Wong, M.F., Chin, N.M., Lew, T.W., 1998. Diabetes insipidus in neurosurgical patients. Ann. Acad. Med. Singapore 27 (3), 340–343.

Yang, K.L., Tobin, M.J., 1991. A prospective study of indexes predicting the outcome of trials of weaning from mechanical ventilation. N. Engl. J. Med. 324 (21), 1445–1450.

Young, M.L., Hanson, C.W., 3rd, 1993. An alternative to tracheostomy following transsphenoidal hypophysectomy in a patient with acromegaly and sleep apnea. Anesth. Analg. 76 (2), 446–449.

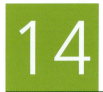

14

Surgical principles in the management of brain tumors

Katharine J. Drummond and Robert G. Ojemann

Preoperative management

General considerations

The decision to remove a brain tumor is based on an evaluation of the clinical history and examination findings, the results of the radiographic studies, an evaluation of the benefits and risks of the management options, and a detailed discussion with the patient. Surgery is recommended only after a thorough consideration of both tumor and patient factors, including the location, size, number, vascularity, type and mass effect of the tumor and the age, performance and neurological status and comorbidities of the patient (Sawaya & Weinberg 2005). When discussing the operation, it is important to assess the patient's hopes, fears and expectations from the procedure. An understanding of lifestyle and occupation to assess the impact of any resulting disability is important. A clear presentation should be made of the impact of tumor removal on presenting symptoms and the immediate and long-term benefits and risks, including the possibility (or otherwise) of cure or prologation of life and the alternative treatments available. The risks discussed should include the general risks of surgery, including death and other catastrophes, the specific risks of removal of the tumor and the risk of declining surgery. The importance of a tissue diagnosis should be discussed. It is prudent to spend adequate time to obtain full, informed consent from the patient, with the family or close friend present, and to keep a written record of these conversations. More than one consultation and a second opinion from another specialist may be necessary (Fearnside & Black 2000).

Once the decision has been made to perform surgery, careful planning is required and several management decisions will need to be made. These include an evaluation of the imaging studies and assessment of the overall medical status. Associated hydrocephalus may need to be managed. The operative approach must be carefully considered and decisions made about special equipment needs, the use of intraoperative monitoring and what form of image-guidance will be used. The surgical plan needs to be considered in the context of the experience of the surgeon and the facilities and expertise locally available. For the majority of malignant and glial tumors, an overall management plan should be devised with a multidisciplinary team.

There should be a clear plan as to the goals of surgery, which may include diagnosis, cure, prolongation of life, relief of symptoms or facilitation of other therapies, depending on the diagnosis. The rationale for extensive resection, particularly in malignant glial tumors, should be clearly discerned and may include cytoreduction, reduction of intracranial pressure, improvement of neurological function, facilitation

of adjuvant therapies and extensive biopsy to avoid sampling error. Overall, maximal safe resection for intra-axial lesions is increasingly the goal of surgery, with evidence accumulating that extent of resection is related to survival (Nikas et al 2000; Salcman 2000; Stummer et al 2008; McGirt et al 2009). In some patients with deep tumors, only a framed stereotactic biopsy may be indicated.

Evaluation of imaging studies

Most brain tumors will be diagnosed by magnetic resonance imaging (MRI) with gadolinium enhancement. The surgeon must decide if this study gives all the information needed to perform the operation. The questions one should consider are:

- Is further imaging required for image-guidance and will fiducial placement be required in advance for registration?
- Does the type of suspected pathology or the surgical approach being considered require angiography (magnetic resonance or conventional) to evaluate abnormal vascularity, the position of normal blood vessels, or the status of the venous sinuses? If there is abnormal vascular supply, should embolization be planned immediately prior to the procedure? If the tumor involves the internal carotid artery, should a test occlusion be done?
- Is computed tomography (CT) needed to evaluate bone anatomy, erosion, calcification, or pathology?
- Would a functional MRI give useful information?
- Would metabolic or biological imaging such as positron emission tomography (PET), single photon emission computed tomography (SPECT) or magnetic resonance spectroscopy (MRS) aid in tumour localization or biopsy planning?
- Will image processing, such as three-dimensional recontruction, fusion of different modalities, fibre-tracking or three dimensional reconstructions, be helpful to plan surgery and increase the usefulness of frameless stereotaxy (Nikas et al 2000; Gumprecht et al 2002; Aquilina et al 2006)?

Medical evaluation and treatment

As part of the initial history the physician must determine if there are any medical problems in the patient's history that require further treatment or evaluation prior to surgery (Rosner 1996; Weintraub et al 1996; Jellinek & Freeman 2000). This assessment should include any adverse response to previous operations, evaluation of current medications, and inquiries about bleeding disorders, diabetes, cardiopulmonary problems, liver or kidney disorders, endocrine deficiency, allergic reactions, and musculoskeletal pathology that might interfere with positioning. Cardiac and antihypertensive medications are usually continued up to the time of surgery. Increasing numbers of patients are now anticoagulated, including newer drugs whose effects and safety profile may be less familiar. A careful medication history is necessary and aspirin, clopidogrel, coumadins and other anticoagulants should be ceased for appropriate periods preoperatively if possible. A single dose of aspirin will impair platelet function for 7–10 days and clopidogrel should be ceased for at least 2 weeks prior to surgery if possible. Advice should be sought from other treating physicians as to the safety of discontinuing or reversing anticoagulants, for instance, in the presence of a cardiac aterial stent or mechanical valve. For urgent procedures, where anticoagulants have not been ceased, haematological advice should be sought.

A full baseline neurological examination is essential in the immediate preoperative period. Increasingly, the preoperative evaluation of the patient will be performed as an outpatient to minimise the costs of inpatient care. This often results in a reduction of opportunities available for examination but it is imperative that this not be negelected. Specialised preoperative assessment is often warranted, particularly to establish the baseline state, including neuropsychological, neuro-ophthalomological or endocrinological examinations.

The usual laboratory preoperative evaluation includes blood count, urinalysis, blood sugar, blood urea nitrogen and creatinine, electrolytes, coagulation studies (prothrombin time, partial thromboplastin time and platelet count), chest X-ray, and electrocardiogram. Abnormalities, particularly hyponatraemia, hypokalemia, hyperglycaemia and coagulation abnormalities, should be corrected. Comprehensive evaluation in the preoperative period will also allow for planning of the postoperative period. Specialist respiratory care (for neuromuscular or lung parenchymal disease), cardiac monitoring or management of diabetes mellitus and electolytes disorders should be planned in advance. Neurological compromise (such as drowsiness) will exacerbate many preoperative medical conditions and this should be anticipated. Patients with acute exacerbations of comorbidities should not undergo elective surgery and patients with chronic disease should have their condition optimized prior to elective surgery.

The initiation of steroids is another decision that needs attention. If there is significant brain edema, it is these authors' practice to prescribe steroids for several days prior to surgery. Depending on the location of the tumor, a decision will also need to be made about commencing anticonvulsant medication. The evidence that anticonvulsant prophylaxis is effective in reducing either preoperative or postoperative seizures is not convincing (Shaw & Foy 1991; Glantz et al 2000; Sirven et al 2004). However, they are often recommended, particularly for high-risk patients, such as those with temporal lobe or motor cortex tumors, because the effects of perioperative seizures can be catastrophic. Management of seizures in the patient who has already had one or more seizures, particularly in relation to choice of anticonvulsant, is increasingly complex and the opinion of an expert neurologist can be helpful.

Management of hydrocephalus

Some patients with brain tumors will have enlarged ventricles on imaging. If there are no symptoms or signs of either normal pressure or high pressure hydrocephalus, nothing needs to be done. If there is a high probability that symptomatic hydrocephalus will be relieved by tumor removal, then the use of perioperative steroids, combined in some patients with cerebrospinal fluid (CSF) drainage at operation, is sufficient treatment. In a few patients, a ventriculostomy will be left for several days postoperatively and a trial occlusion done to determine if a ventriculoperitoneal shunt is needed. A ventriculoperitoneal shunt is inserted if there is symptomatic hydrocephalus and an adequate decompression of the tumor cannot be achieved.

In some elderly patients with symptomatic normal pressure hydrocephalus syndrome associated with cerebellopontine angle or other skull base tumors, a ventriculoperitoneal shunt may be the only operation needed. A small group of elderly patients with symptoms from hydrocephalus and with brain stem compression from a large acoustic neuroma have been managed with insertion of a ventriculoperitoneal shunt and a subtotal removal of the tumor under the same anesthesia, with good results (Ojemann 1993a).

Perioperative management

When the patient arrives in the preoperative area, appropriate intravenous lines are inserted, electrocardiogram leads are placed, and a catheter is inserted into the radial artery for continuous monitoring of blood pressure. Intravenous steroids and prophylactic antibiotics are given (Barker 1994, 2007). Full leg sequential compression devices are placed on each lower extremity for venous thrombosis prophylaxis. Careful induction of anesthesia is done to try to avoid episodes of hypotension, hypertension and raised intracranial pressure. Bispectral index (BIS) monitoring will generally be used to monitor depth of anesthesia and avoid awareness (Punjasawadwong et al 2007). A heating blanket should be used to avoid hypothermia, particularly in long operations. Specialist anesthesia for tumor neurosurgery will allow physiological conditions required for optimal surgery (Kraayenbrink & McAnulty 2006).

After the induction of anesthesia, the eyes are protected with an adhesive, occlusive patch. Eye care must be particularly meticulous if alcoholic scalp preparation solution is used to avoid corneal ulceration. A catheter is placed in the bladder. Diuresis with furosemide or 1–1.5 g/kg mannitol should be considered, particularly for deep lesions, those requiring significant retraction or those associated with significant edema. However, diuresis can also alter brain anatomy and reduce the accuracy of frameless stereotaxy, and should not be used unless necessary (Sloan 2006). During the operation, steroids and antibiotics are continued at 6-h intervals.

A lumbar drain may be inserted for skull base procedures, provided the intracranial pressure is not raised, to reduce brain retraction. In some cerebellopontine angle tumors, the cistern is opened and a catheter placed in the area to drain CSF during the operation (Ojemann 1993a).

bone wax. Small drill holes are made at appropriate intervals and fine hitching sutures are placed to tent the dura to the bone edge to control epidural bleeding. In addition to bipolar coagulation, hemostasis is achieved using topical agents such as absorbable gelatin sponge or oxidized regenerated cellulose (Arand & Sawaya 1996). If one of the paranasal sinuses is intentionally or inadvertently entered, special attention is required to prevent infection and CSF fluid leak. The mucosa should be stripped and the defect filled with antibiotic soaked gelatin sponge, muscle or fat and a vascularised pericranial graft used to cover the defect. Before the dura is opened, the skin margins are covered with antiseptic-soaked sponges and towels are placed around the operative area.

Dural opening

If the intracranial pressure seems raised and the dura 'tight', all measures should be taken to relax the brain before opening, including head elevation, diuresis, hyperventilation and checking the neck position and endotracheal tube. The dura is opened to give adequate visualization, but care is taken to minimize the exposure of normal brain tissue. Normal brain that is exposed or is to be retracted should be protected. The venous anatomy needs to be kept in mind when opening the dura and during the initial exposure. Veins along the anterior third of the superior sagittal sinus, the middle cerebral vein along the sphenoid wing, and the petrosal vein in the cerebellopontine angle can usually be taken if needed to aid the exposure. Cortical veins along the middle and posterior thirds of the sagittal sinus, the internal cerebral veins, vein of Galen, and the vein of Labbe, however, must be preserved to avoid devastating venous infarction. The dural flap should be kept moist and on the stretch with sutures during the procedure. If dura is involved with tumor, such as with a convexity meningioma, it is removed with the tumor.

Surgical approaches

Bifrontal

The patient is placed in the supine position. The elevation and degree of flexion or extension of the head depend on the tumor being treated, but are critical considerations for exposure (Ojemann 1993c). A coronal incision beginning just anterior to the tragus and extending behind the anterior hairline is made through the galea, taking care to preserve the pericranial tissue (Fig. 14.1). If extra pericranial tissue will be needed to cover the floor of the anterior fossa or the frontal sinuses or to patch the convexity dura, the skin along the posterior aspect of the incision is elevated 1–2 cm and the pericranial tissue is incised. The scalp flap is then turned down with or without the pericranial tissue, which may also be turned down as a separate flap. The temporalis muscle is opened just enough to expose the 'key hole'. Burr holes are placed just below the end of the superior temporal line (key hole) and on each side of the superior sagittal sinus anterior to the skin incision. The bone flap is usually cut in one piece, with the bone cut just above the supraorbital ridge being made from each side as far medially as possible. Irregular bone projecting from the inner table of the skull in this location means that it is usually not possible to cut completely across the area. Usually, this leaves a centimeter or less of bone in the midline. The outer table of bone is cut

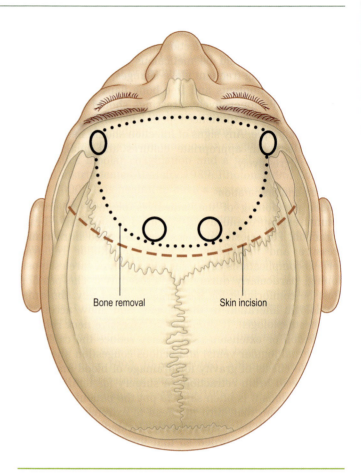

Figure 14.1 Bifrontal approach.

with a small burr on the high-speed drill and then the inner table can be broken as the bone is elevated and the free bone flap removed. The frontal sinuses are almost always entered. It is more important to achieve an exposure low enough for tumor removal with minimal brain retraction than to avoid the frontal sinuses. If the operation is going to be entirely intradural, a small flap of pericranial tissue from the back of the scalp flap can be turned down over the sinus and sewn to the adjacent dura before the dura is opened (Ojemann 1993c, 1996a). If an extradural exposure is also required, pericranium can be secured over the sinus opening at the end of the operation.

Middle frontal

The patient is in the supine position with the ipsilateral shoulder elevated. The head is elevated so that the convexity over the center of the tumor is at the highest point (Ojemann 1993c; Ojemann & Ogilvy 1993). For tumors in the general region of the coronal suture the skin flap is turned forward (Fig. 14.2). The incision starts at the anterior hairline, extends posteriorly along or parallel to the midline (on the opposite side if necessary) as far as needed, and turns inferiorly and then anteriorly to end at about the frontotemporal junction.

Frontotemporal (pterional)

The patient is in the supine position with the ipsilateral shoulder elevated. The degree of head rotation depends on the location of the tumor which is being approached

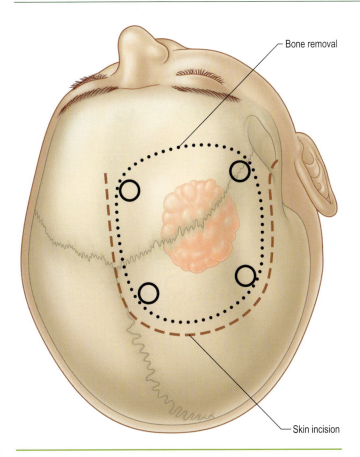

Figure 14.2 Middle frontal approach.

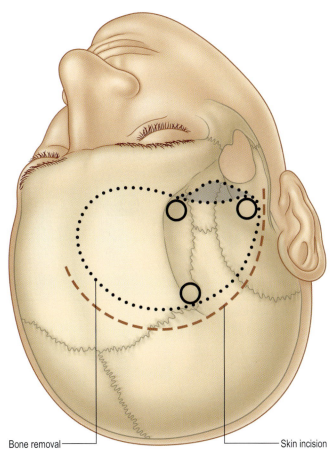

Figure 14.3 Frontotemporal (pterional) approach.

(Ojemann 1993c; Ojemann et al 1995; Ojemann 1996a). The skin incision is made just above the zygomatic process behind the anterior hairline and extends medially to end near the midline at the hairline (Fig. 14.3). If the incision is too far forward, the frontotemporal branch of the facial nerve may be injured. The skin, underlying temporalis muscle, and pericranial tissue are turned down together, exposing the anterior and lateral inferior frontal and anterior temporal bone. The temporalis muscle may be cut to expose the zygomatic process. A burr hole is placed just below the anterior end of the superior temporal line (key hole). A second burr hole is placed over the anterior temporal lobe, and others may be used depending on the surgeon's preference. When cutting across the greater wing of the sphenoid bone, resistance may be felt, and the cut will need to go superiorly around this area with a craniotome or a burr used to cut through this region. After the bone flap is elevated the lateral portion of the sphenoid wing is removed, as is bone over the anterior temporal region, with a combination of bone nibblers and a high speed burr. Access can be extended using the orbitozygomatic approach, which includes removal of the zygoma and orbital rim with the bone flap (Adada & Al-Mefty 2005).

Frontotemporal (extended temporal)
For tumors in the anterior and medial aspects of the temporal lobe and middle fossa, the pterional exposure may be modified by curving the incision around the top of the ear and extending it medially and anteriorly (Fig. 14.4) (Ojemann et al 1995). The bone removal is similar to that described

for the pterional approach but more of the temporal lobe is exposed. This approach allows exposure of the anterior and medial temporal area along the sphenoid wing by providing the ability to retract both the frontal and anterior temporal lobes.

To improve the access to the floor of the middle fossa and sphenoid wing, the skin incision can be carried below the zygoma if it is close to the tragus. The zygomatic arch is transected and the temporalis muscle retracted into the space formerly occupied by the zygomatic arch.

Temporal
The patient may be placed in a semilateral position with the ipsilateral shoulder well elevated, however the full lateral position will avoid excessive head rotation and venous congestion. The head is usually nearly parallel to the floor (Ojemann et al 1995). The degree of head extension depends on the type of tumor being treated. Tumors in the middle and posterior temporal region can be exposed by a horseshoe-shaped scalp flap based along the floor of the middle fossa (Fig. 14.5). The incision starts just behind the anterior hairline, extends medially to the superior temporal line, and goes posteriorly and then inferiorly to end above the mastoid area. If the incision is too far forward or extends below the zygomatic process, the frontotemporal branch of the facial nerve may be injured. After the bone flap is elevated, further bone may be removed to take the exposure to the floor of the middle fossa.

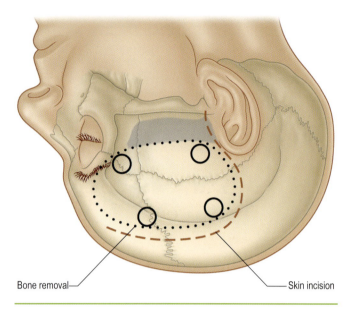

Bone removal—   —Skin incision

Figure 14.4 Frontotemporal (extended temporal) approach.

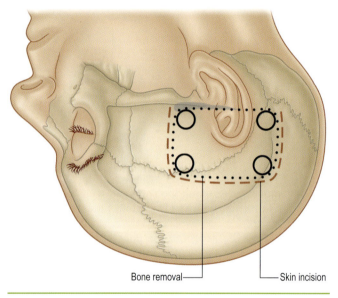

Bone removal—   —Skin incision

Figure 14.5 Temporal approach.

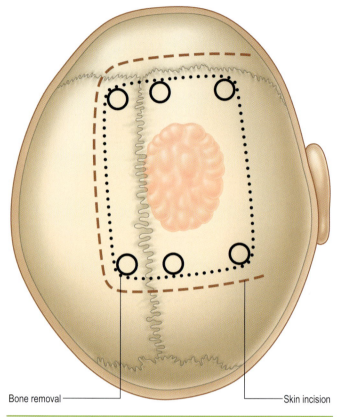

Bone removal—   —Skin incision

Figure 14.6 Posterior frontal-parietal (vertex) approach.

sinus. If the bone is markedly adherent to dura, the bone flap can be elevated in two sections. The first is on the side of the tumor with the medial cut approximately 1 cm from the midline. The second section of bone is then cut and the sagittal sinus exposed under direct vision.

Occipital
The patient is placed in the lateral position using an axillary roll and the head elevated and turned towards the floor to bring the center of the tumor to the highest point (Ojemann 1993c; Ojemann & Ogilvy 1993). Alternatively, the prone or sitting position can be used. The skin incision is horseshoe-shaped, based on the posterior temporal-inferior occipital region, and may be extended across the midline if necessary (Fig. 14.7).

Temporal suboccipital
The patient is positioned with the ipsilateral shoulder well elevated and the head turned to the opposite side, often nearly parallel to the floor (Ojemann et al 1995) or in the full lateral position. The angle of the exposure can be altered by rotating the table from side to side. The incision starts in front of the ear and curves posteriorly no higher than the superior temporal line. About 2 cm posterior to the mastoid area the incision is carried inferiorly (Fig. 14.8). It can stop just below the level of the mastoid process or can be gently curved onto the neck so that the carotid bifurcation and internal jugular vein can be exposed. A bone flap may be removed above and below the transverse sinus in one or two parts. The same precautions noted with the superior sagittal sinus are followed. Further bone is removed as needed to

Posterior frontal parietal (vertex)
The patient is placed in a semisitting or lounging position with the head well elevated so that the scalp over the center of the tumor is uppermost (Ojemann 1993c; Ojemann & Ogilvy 1993; Ojemann et al 1995). A horseshoe-shaped incision is made, extending approximately 2 cm across the midline, with the anterior and posterior branch of the incision placed to give adequate exposure (Fig. 14.6). Often seven or eight burr holes are used, two on each side of the sagittal sinus, one in the midportion of the contralateral side, and two or three across the base. The dural separation and bone cut over the superior sagittal sinus are done last to allow rapid control of bleeding. As the bone flap is elevated, gelatin sponge covered with oxidised regenerated cellulose and a cottonoid are placed directly over the superior sagittal

Skin incision   Bone removal

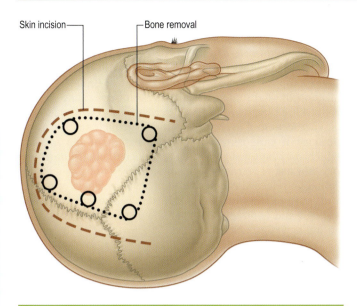

Figure 14.7 Occipital approach.

Skin incision   Bone removal

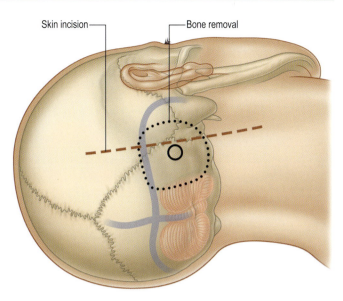

Figure 14.9 Suboccipital (lateral) approach.

Skin incision   Bone removal

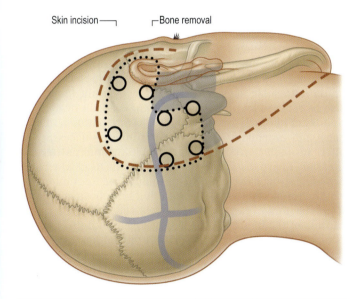

Figure 14.8 Temporal-suboccipital approach.

expose the sigmoid sinus and the dura anterior to the sinus. Modifications of this approach, including the transpetrosal approach (Al-Mefty & Smith 1991), may be used to reach tumors involving the clivus, petrous bone, middle fossa, and cerebellopontine angle.

Suboccipital (lateral)
This approach is used for tumors in the cerebellopontine angle and in the lateral cerebellum. The patient is placed in the full lateral position with the ipsilateral shoulder pulled towards the foot of the bed. Extension, flexion and rotation of the neck depends on the position of the tumour. Alternatively, the patient may be in the sitting position or supine with the ipsilateral shoulder slightly elevated and the head

turned parallel to the floor (Ojemann 1993a, 1996b). The operating table is turned so that the surgeon can sit behind the patient's head with the feet under the table. The line of sight may be altered by rotating the table from side to side. A curvilinear incision is made, centered 2 cm medial to the mastoid process (Fig. 14.9). One or more burr holes are placed in the bone over the lateral posterior fossa and a bone flap is cut over the lateral two-thirds of the cerebellar hemisphere. The supero-inferior position of the bone flap will depend on the position of the lesion. Further bone is removed as needed to expose the transverse and sigmoid sinuses. Mastoid air cells are usually entered and are occluded with bone wax.

Suboccipital (far lateral)
The patient is placed in the lateral position with the head slightly elevated and tilted toward the ipsilateral shoulder (Ojemann et al 1995), or in the prone or sitting position. The skin incision and craniectomy are shown in Figure 14.10. Removal of the rim of the foramen magnum is carried laterally to just behind the occipital condyle. The posterior arch of C1 is removed from the arterial sulcus of the vertebral artery laterally to just beyond the midline medially.

Suboccipital (midline)
The prone, sitting, or lateral oblique position can be used (Tew & Scodary 1993b; Ojemann 1996c). For many tumors of the cerebellar hemispheres the prone position is adequate, but the sitting position is used for tumors in the superior vermis or cerebellum or brainstem (Fig. 14.11). A midline incision is made, staying in the midline plane between the paraspinal-occipital muscles (Fig. 14.12). The muscles are detached to expose the midline bone. A craniotomy is done, with the flap uncovering both medial cerebellar hemispheres including the posterior rim of the foramen magnum. The posterior arch of C1 can be removed if necessary. The dura is opened over each cerebellar hemisphere. The incisions are connected across the lower midline and a dural flap is

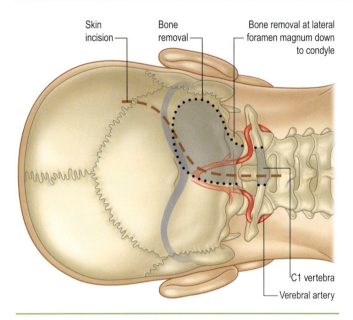

Skin incision — Bone removal — Bone removal at lateral foramen magnum down to condyle

C1 vertebra

Verebral artery

Figure 14.10 Suboccipital (far lateral) approach.

rotated superiorly. Bleeding from the occipital sinus is controlled with metal clips or a running suture. In some patients the dura will also be opened across the foramen magnum, and bleeding from the circular sinus may need to be controlled. When a more lateral exposure is needed for a large tumor of the cerebellar hemisphere, the incision is curved laterally and a scalp flap raised (hockey-stick incision, Fig. 14.12).

Other skull base approaches
The surgeon should be familiar with the different approaches that can be used for tumor removal in the skull base and the principles of skull base surgery (Ojemann 1993b; Sekhar & Janecka 1993; Adada & Al-Mefty 2005). These include craniofacial procedures and approaches to the cavernous sinus. Anterior extradural approaches include transoral, transoral-labimandibular glossotomy, transoral and trans-palatal, transsphenoidal, transethmoidal, transmaxillary, or combinations of these. Lateral extradural-intradural approaches include translabyrinthine, transcochlear, petro-sal, and infratemporal.

Tumor removal
The objective of surgical intervention for benign tumors is usually total removal of the tumor if possible. In some patients, involvement of critical structures may prevent a complete excision. The surgeon must remember that the first priority is to attempt to preserve and/or improve neurologic function. For patients in whom total removal carries significant risk of morbidity, it may be better judgment to leave some tumor and plan to follow the patient or treat the residual tumor with radiation therapy.

For primary intrinsic brain tumors, maximal resection of as much of the tumor tissue as can be safely excised is planned as discussed above. When the tumor is in the speech or motor-sensory areas, the operation may be done under local anesthesia with cortical mapping and clinical monitoring of the awake patient during resection. This is particularly helpful for low-grade gliomas (Nikas et al 2000). Other techniques to maximise extent of resection include early mapping of the resection margins with frameless stereotaxy and intraoperative MRI if available. Enhanced visualization of glial tumors with fluorescent dyes may also be useful (Stummer et al 2008). Microsurgical techniques will allow resection of even large tumors through small cortical incisions if care is taken with placement of the incision (which may be through a gyrus or sulcus), choice of trajectory and use of retractors (Salcman 2000). Retractor blades should be released regularly to improve perfusion of underlying tissue. The ultrasonic aspirator is used to fragment, suspend and aspirate tissue, or the laser can be used as a cutting or vaporizing tool.

Solitary metastatic tumors are completely removed if they present in an operable location and there is a reasonable life expectancy. Occasionally, removal of second or subsequent metastases may also be indicated. Palliative resection of metastases to avoid imminent neurological deficit, even when there are multiple lesions present, may also be warranted.

Brain retraction is minimized by the position of the patient, diuresis, drainage of CSF when indicated, and a well-planned exposure. The brain is protected with cottonoids when retraction is required.

In many patients with benign tumors, safe removal of the tumor is facilitated by an extensive internal decompression using bipolar coagulation and suction, sharp dissection or the ultrasonic aspirator. Retraction of brain tissue can also be reduced by traction on the tumor capsule away from brain and nerve tissue which also allows separation of vascular and arachnoid attachments. It may be necessary to alternate dissection of the tumor capsule and internal decompression. Sharp dissection should always be used when surrounding structures cannot tolerate much traction. Cottonoids are used to protect areas of brain that have been separated from the tumor capsule. Arterial vessels adherent to the capsule of the tumor should be preserved until the surgeon is sure they do not supply important brain tissue. Often, after internal decompression of the tumor, a vessel on the capsule of the tumor can be preserved using microsurgical dissection.

Closure
Careful hemostasis is essential. If not already the case, the patient's blood pressure is raised to close at the anticipated postoperative blood pressure. If a partial removal of tumor has been done, a single layer of Surgicel is left on the area of the resection as well as on any brain tissue that has been incised. The risk of postoperative bleeding from the cut edge of a partially removed high-grade intrinsic tumor is high and meticulous haemostasis is particularly important.

Increasingly, techniques to further improve local tumour control for malignant gliomas that are most likely to recur locally are being employed after tumour resection. At this point in the operation, consideration may be given to interstitial radiotherapy, local chemotherapy or photodynamic therapy.

Usually the retracted, sometimes dried, dura cannot be closed in a watertight fashion. Dura may also have been

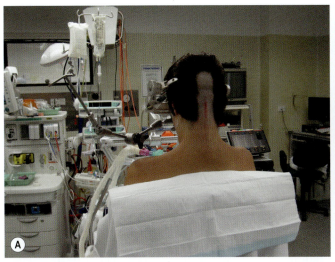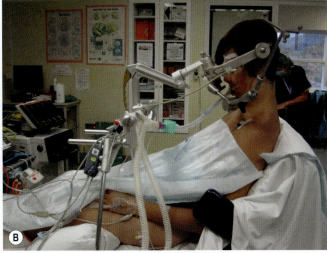

Figure 14.11 The sitting position for approach to the occipital region, posterior fossa and cervicomedullary junction. (**A**) Posterior view. (**B**) Lateral view. The degree of neck flexion required depends on the position of the lesion. The knees should be slightly flexed, arms resting on the thighs and all pressure areas well-padded.

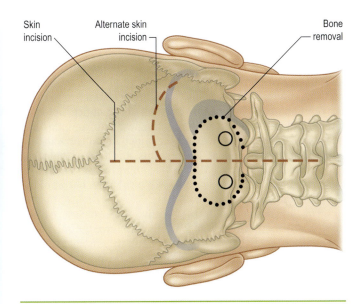

Skin incision Alternate skin incision Bone removal

Figure 14.12 Suboccipital (midline) approach.

removed if attached to the tumor. A graft of pericranial tissue or commercial synthetic dural substitute should be used. The dural closure can be reinforced with a commercial spray sealant. Just prior to completion of the dural closure, the subdural space and area of tumor removal are filled with saline (at body temperature) to displace as much air as possible. Therefore the last part of the dural closure should be at the highest point of the craniotomy. The bone flap is replaced with plates and screws. The bone should be replaced, or a cranioplasty fashioned, even in the posterior fossa, to reduce the incidence of postoperative headache (Harner et al 1995). Burr hole covers can be used, or a commercial filler (hydroxyapatite) used to fill the burr holes and any remaining bony defects. If the air sinuses have been opened, foreign material should be avoided close to the opening as much as possible due to the risk of infection.

Prior to closure of the scalp, the wound is irrigated with an antibiotic solution. The muscle, fascia, and galea are closed in separate layers with absorbable sutures and the skin with nylon or staples.

Image-guided neurosurgery

A neurosurgeon carrying out a craniotomy on an intracranial lesion guides the operation according to several elements, each of which provides some orientation, in combination with training and experience. These include preoperative imaging studies, anatomic landmarks and intra-operative visual and tactile cues, including color and texture. In operations where the anatomy is relatively feature-rich and stereotypic, such as operations on small tumors in the cerebellopontine angle, the surgeon's training and knowledge, the preoperative imaging studies, and the visual and tactile appreciation of normal and lesional anatomy at surgery provide the information necessary to carry out the procedure safely and effectively.

Many operations, however, are marked by a paucity of anatomic visual and tactile cues, with inadequate spatial information for the surgeon to achieve the clinical goal of the operation safely. The anatomic landmarks leading to the lesion may lack the definition necessary to facilitate navigation to a deep intracranial lesion, as is the case with much of the cerebral hemispheres. The lesion may be small, making accurate, adequate craniotomy placement difficult without exposure of additional normal brain. Once exposed, moreover, some lesions may have little tactile and visual distinction from surrounding tissue; impeding safe and effective lesion resection. This might be the case when a lesion resembles the surrounding tissue, or when there is such destruction of anatomy that normal structures of orienting value are not present. Similarly, a surgeon debulking the interior of a tumor may find no landmarks to indicate the proximity of the deep tumor capsule. Therefore, in the majority of tumor cases, the additional spatial information provided by a computer-assisted system for image guidance (frameless stereotaxy) and/or intraoperative imaging (CT, MRI or ultrasound) is necessary (Barnett et al 1993; Germano 1995; Sipos et al 1996; Spicer & Apuzzo 2005; Aquilina et al 2006).

Increasingly, frameless stereotaxy is considered standard and essential for removal of most tumors. It can be of particular value in surgical planning; when planning, however, one does not step through the operation in chronological order. Instead, one envisions the most difficult part of the operation (commonly the final dissection of the lesion), and works from there in reverse order. Thus, the first step in surgical planning is to envision the exposure of the lesion necessary to carry out the final dissection. The required final exposure depends on the size and location of the lesion, and on its consistency and vascular supply. It is wise to broaden the exposure somewhat to compensate for error in the image guidance system and for the expected brain shift that will occur during the craniotomy. After envisioning the exposure needed for the final dissection, one outlines the prerequisite cortical incision to give this final exposure. In sequence, one then determines the dural incision necessary to give that cortical incision, the bony craniotomy necessary to give that dural exposure, and the skin incision necessary to allow that bony craniotomy. Of course, to visualize these steps of the operation, clear surgical goals should have been determined preoperatively, including extent of resection and treatment intent.

Limitations of frameless stereotaxy

The information provided by an image guidance system can be misleading. It may contain random error contributed by imaging, registration and technique (Kaus et al 1997; Butler 1999). Moreover, image-guided surgery hinges on the assumption that the brain behaves as a rigid body: intracranial anatomy is assumed to remain geometrically unchanged at craniotomy as in the preoperative imaging study. However, brain shift at craniotomy results from pressure changes at skull and dural opening, CSF loss, hyperventilation, diuresis, gravity, retraction and resection of tissue. This results in inaccuracies of up to 8 cm in an image guidance system based on pre-operative imaging (Nauta 1993; Dorward et al 1998; Roberts et al 1998; Navabi et al 2001). The information provided by an image guidance system is merely a single source of information that a surgeon must weigh prudently against other sources of information, such as visual and tactile cues, and the surgeon's training and experience. When compared with other lesions, skull base tumors are associated with less brain shift and thus frameless stereotaxy may remain relatively accurate throughout the surgery.

Intraoperative imaging

The pernicious influence of brain shift on the accuracy of image-guided surgery can be countered by intraoperative imaging, which is likely to become the standard of care for removal of many tumors in coming decades. Intraoperative computed imaging antedates frameless stereotaxy (Shalit et al 1982), but the latter found broader use

because of cost and convenience of use. Recently, the appreciation of brain shift has stimulated a resurgence in the popularity of intraoperative imaging. The three chief modalities of intraoperative imaging are MRI (Black et al 1997; Staubert et al 1997; Martin et al 2000; Nimsky et al 2006), CT (Shalit et al 1982; Lunsford et al 1996), and ultrasound (Dempsey 1996; Dohrmann & Rubin 1996; Sawaya & Weinberg 2005). The combination of frameless stereotaxy supplemented by intraoperative MRI updates provides the most advanced neuronavigation to date for the precise and safe removal of brain tumors. The combination of technologies enables the surgeon to see the location of a tool, without needing to re-image with the tool in place. Further imaging can then be performed only when there is significant tissue shift.

Intraoperative MRI is most useful for localization and targeting of lesions, protecting and avoiding eloquent cortex, improving extent of resection (Bohinski et al 2001) and monitoring complications, including hemorrhage.There is no radiation and nuclear magnetic resonance is a particularly powerful criterion for discriminating different tissue types; particularly useful for low-grade glioma which is often not well-differentiated from normal brain. The perceived disadvantages of intraoperative MRI, including the need for customized non-paramagnetic instruments; the longer operating times; the reduction in operating space imposed by the magnets and coils; and the poor image quality have largely now been overcome and there are a number of configurations commercially available. Questions remain regarding the refinement of tissue differentiation, for instance, between tumor and edematous or hemorrhagic brain and the frequency of imaging. However, the most important current limitation is the high cost. Despite this, addition of the capability for intraoperative MRI is becoming commonplace in modern operating rooms and will probably become the standard of care.

The advantages of intraoperative CT are: less capital investment than MRI is required; there is greater geometric fidelity than in MRI; and CT can be built in a mobile version that may be employed elsewhere in the hospital such as at the bedside in the intensive care unit (ICU) when not actually in use in the operating room (Butler et al 1998). The disadvantages of intraoperative CT are: the inconvenience caused by the bulk of the gantry; less contrast between soft tissue types; and the need to remove radiopaque objects such as retractors from the surgical field during scanning.

Intraoperative ultrasound is a convenient, flexible, and cheap tool for intraoperative imaging with real-time, interactive imaging. The role of ultrasound in locating deep tumors and enhancing extent of tumor resection by defining borders and detecting residual tumor has been demonstrated (Hammoud et al 1996; Conrad et al 2002). However, differential echogenicity is not a powerful criterion for discriminating between tissue types, particularly after previous surgery or radiotherapy, and when anatomical resolution is poor, although this may be improved with coregistration with other imaging (Hartov et al 2008).

Image guidance can provide significant navigational aid in many operations. Intraoperative CT and MRI require significant additional personnel and capital resources beyond that required by image guidance systems. It remains to be seen whether the benefit of compensating for brain shift justifies the cost.

Immediate postoperative management

At the conclusion of the operation, careful attention must be paid to the patient's blood pressure and to avoid coughing and straining on extubation. Continuous monitoring should be done during transfer to the recovery room or intensive care unit and appropriate medications should be immediately available to prevent hypertension. The usual precautions to ensure an adequate airway are followed. The patient is positioned with the head elevated.

Throughout the postoperative period, frequent, regular, standardized neurological observation should continue and any change communicated promptly to the neurosurgeon. When a patient does not recover promptly from anesthesia, has an unexpected neurological deficit or is not progressing as anticipated from a neurologic standpoint, an immediate CT scan is done to evaluate the presence of hematoma, hydrocephalus, edema, tension pneumocephalus, and/or infarction. Subsequent treatment depends on the results of that scan. If the patient is deteriorating rapidly, rarely immediate re-exploration without CT scan will be warranted. Other common causes of poor recovery include hypoxia, hypercarbia and seizures, which should also be excluded.

A CT scan should be performed routinely within 24 h to exclude postoperative bleeding and assess cerebral swelling. After resection of intrinsic tumors, a contrast enhanced MRI within 48 h of surgery, to determine the extent of resection before inflammatory enhancement commences is useful (Albert et al 1994).

Should there be a CSF fluid leak, the leak should be stitched where possible, a CT scan done and, if there is no contraindication, a lumbar CSF fluid drain is placed, usually for at least 72 h. Antibiotics, which are usually given for 24 h after surgery, are continued for as long as the drain is in place.

If the operation involves the pituitary stalk or hypothalamus the patient will need to be carefully observed for diabetes insipidus. After removal of a brain tumor, a syndrome of inappropriate antidiuretic hormone secretion may occur. This is generally managed with fluid restriction. If the patient has diabetes mellitus, serum glucose is followed and management is carried out intraoperatively and postoperatively using insulin. Postoperative analgesia requirements should be modest and should be planned in advance of the surgery. Severe or increasing headache should be thoroughly investigated before increasing amounts of analgesia, particularly narcotics, are given. Small doses of morphine (1 mg) given at 20 min intervals and titrated against sedation give safe, adequate analgesia in the early postoperative period.

Depending on the neurologic status and the degree of expected cerebral edema, steroids are tapered as rapidly as possible and peptic ulcer prophylaxis continued until steroids are weaned. An exception is with patients expected to commence radiotherapy in the early postoperative period, who may continue on a low dose of dexamethasone (2–4 mg/day). Thromboembolic complications are common in neurosurgical patients, especially those with malignant tumors. However, there is little evidence to guide the decision to commence postoperative anticoagulation and individual neurosurgeons will decide based on the perceived competing risks of thromboembolism (malignant tumor, hemiparesis, immobility) and of anticoagulation (postoperative hemorrhage). Prophylaxis is not commenced preoperatively for cranial neurosurgery.

In the case of supratentorial tumors anticonvulsants are often continued. How long they should be continued has not been defined (Glantz et al 2000). If there have been no preoperative seizures, this medication is discontinued within 1 week to 3 months, depending on the surgeons preference and perceived epileptogenicity of the lesion and the occurrence of side effects. If the patient has had a preoperative seizure disorder, the anticonvulsant will be continued for at least several months and sometimes indefinitely, and a specialist neurologist should be consulted. Postoperative seizures should be treated aggresively to avoid status epilepticus and the adverse postoperative effects of hypertension with hemorrhage in the resection cavity and hypercarbia with cerebral edema (Drummond et al 1997).

Key points

- The decision to recommend surgery on a brain tumor is based on a comprehensive evaluation of the patient. A surgeon should not hesitate to acquire more information, whether clinical, laboratory, or radiological, if it may clarify the patient's candidacy for surgery.

- The imaging studies are reviewed to determine if there is a safely achievable operation that will improve the patient's quality or length of life and the final decision to operate based on this information and a thorough discussion with the patient and their family.

- Comorbidities must be addressed and managed, including unrelated medical problems that may affect the surgical outcome or related problems such as hydrocephalus.

- In addition to standard neuroanesthesia monitoring, the surgeon must decide if special monitoring such as speech, electrocorticography, or cranial nerve monitoring will be needed.

- Key factors at surgery include careful positioning of the patient, a well-planned exposure, familiarity with microsurgical techniques, avoidance of excessive brain retraction, minimal exposure of normal brain, and meticulous closure.

- Intravenous antibiotics are administered prior to incision and usually continued for 24 h after surgery. Diuretics and corticosteroids may reduce brain edema and avoid excessive brain retraction. Anticonvulsants and thromboembolism prophylaxis should be considered carefully.

- The goals of the operation should be decided in advance and a clear surgical plan determined.

- One plans for early interruption of the tumor blood supply, internal decompression of the tumor, dissection of the tumor capsule into the area of decompression, and possible removal of involved dura and bone. For tumors with an indistinct boundary with normal tissue, there should be removal of as much tumor as possible while preserving normal function.

- The scalp incision is planned to provide optimal exposure while preserving adequate blood supply.

- It is important to understand the venous anatomy. Cortical veins along the middle and posterior thirds of the sagittal sinus, the internal cerebral veins, the vein of Galen and the vein of Labbe must be preserved.

- Careful hemostasis is essential, particularly at closure.

- At surgery, visual and tactile cues are the surgeon's most important sources of information. In operations with a paucity of such cues, additional spatial information may be provided by an image guidance (frameless stereotaxy) system. This information is subject to error including from misregistration and brain shift, and must be cross-checked often against other sources of information.

- The loss of accuracy due to brain shift in image-guided surgery can be countered by the use of intraoperative imaging.

- Upon recovery from anesthesia, a patient is examined neurologically. Unexpected abnormalities may need further investigation such as CT or, in rare cases, immediate re-exploration.

REFERENCES

Adada, B., Al-Mefty, O., 2005. Meningioma: Skull base surgery. In: Black, P.Mc.L., Loeffler, J.S. (Eds.), Cancer of the nervous system, second ed. Lippincott Williams and Wilkins, Philadelphia, PA, pp. 329.

Al-Mefty, O. (Ed.), 1989. 1. Ergonomics and cranial-base surgery 2. Power equipment. In Surgery of the Cranial Base. Kluwer Academic, Boston, MA, pp. 3.

Al-Mefty, O., Smith, R.R., 1991. Clival and petroclival meningiomas. In: Al-Mefty, O. (Ed.), Meningiomas. Raven Press, New York, pp. 517.

Albert, F.K., Forsting, M., Sartor, K., et al., 1994. Early postoperative magnetic resonance imaging after resection of malignant glioma: objective evaluation of residual tumor and its influence on regrowth and prognosis. Neurosurgery 34, 45–61.

Aquilina, K., Edwards, P., Strong, A., 2006. Principles and practice of image-guided neurosurgery. In: Moore, A.J., Newell, D.W. (Eds.), Tumor neurosurgery. Principles and practice. Springer Verlag, London, pp. 123.

Arand, A.G., Sawaya, R., 1996. Intraoperative use of topical hemostatic agents in neurosurgery. In: Wilkins, R.H., Rengachary, S.S. (Eds.), Neurosurgery update I. McGraw-Hill, New York, pp. 615.

Barker, F.G., 1994. Efficacy of prophylactic antibiotics for craniotomy: a meta-analysis. Neurosurgery 35, 484–490.

Barker, F.G., 2007. Efficacy of prophylactic antibiotics against meningitis after craniotomy: a meta-analysis. Neurosurgery 60, 887–894.

Barnett, G.H., Kormos, D.W., Steiner, C.P., et al., 1993. Use of frameless, armless stereotactic wand for brain tumor localization with two-dimensional and three dimensional neuroimaging. Neurosurgery 33, 674–678.

Berger, M.S., Ojemann, G.A., 1992. Intraoperative brain mapping techniques in neuro-oncology. Stereotact. Funct. Neurosurg. 58, 153–161.

Black, P.M., Moriarty, T., Alexander, E. III, et al., 1997. Development and implementation of intraoperative magnetic resonance imaging and its neurosurgical applications. Neurosurgery 41, 831–845.

Boggan, J.E., Powers, S.K., 1996. Use of lasers in neurological surgery. In: Youmans, J.R. (Ed.), Neurological Surgery. WB Saunders, Philadelphia, PA, pp. 795.

Bohinski, R.J., Kokkino, A.K., Warnick, R.E., et al., 2001. Glioma resection in a shared-resource magnetic resonance operating room after optimal image-guided frameless stereotactic resection. Neurosurgery 48, 731–744.

Butler, W.E., 1999. Comparison of three methods of estimating confidence intervals for stereotactic error. Comput. Aided. Surg. 4, 26–36.

Butler, W.E., Piaggio, C.M., Constantinou, C., et al., 1998. A mobile computed tomographic scanner with intraoperative and intensive care unit applications. Neurosurgery 42, 1304–1310.

Cerullo, L.J., 1996. Application of the laser to neurological surgery. In: Wilkins, R.H., Rengachary, S.S. (Eds.), Neurosurgery. McGraw Hill, New York, pp. 609.

Chyatte, D., 1996. Instrumentation and techniques: general, microsurgical and special. In: Tindall, G.T., Cooper, P.R., Barrow, D.L. (Eds.), The practice of neurosurgery. Williams & Wilkins, Baltimore, MD, pp. 428.

Conrad, M., Schonaue, C., Morel, C., 2002. Brain operations guided by real-time two-dimensional ultrasound: new possibilities as a result of improved image quality. Neurosurgery 51, 402–411.

Constantini, S., Epstein, F., 1996. Ultrasound dissection. In: Wilkins, R.H., Rengachary, S.S. (Eds.), Neurosurgery. McGraw-Hill, New York, pp. 607.

Dempsey, R.Z., 1996. Neurosonography. In: Youmans, J.R. (Ed.), Neurological surgery. WB Saunders, Philadelphia, PA, pp. 214.

Dohrmann, G.J., Rubin, J.M., 1996. Intraoperative diagnostic ultrasound. In: Wilkins, R.H., Rengachary, S.S. (Eds.), Neurosurgery. McGraw-Hill, New York, pp. 575.

Dorward, N.L., Alberti, O., Velani, B., et al., 1998. Postimaging brain distortion: magnitude, correlates, and impact on neuronavigation. J. Neurosurg. 88, 656–662.

Drummond, K.J., Fearnside, M.R., Chee, A., 1997. Transcutaneous carbon dioxide measurement after craniotomy in spontaneously breathing patients. Neurosurgery 41, 361–365.

Fearnside, M.R., Black, P.Mc.L., 2000. Informed consent. In: Kaye, A.H., Black, P.Mc.L. (Eds.), Operative neurosurgery. Churchill Livingstone, London, pp. 199.

Germano, I.M., 1995. The NeuroStation system for image-guided frameless stereotaxy. Neurosurgery 37, 348.

Glantz, M.J., Cole, B.F., Forsyth, P.A., et al., 2000. Practice parameter: anticonvulsant prophylaxis in patients with newly diagnosed brain tumors. Report of the Quality Standards Subcommittee of the American Academy of Neurology. Neurology 54, 1886–1893.

Greenberg, I.M., 1996. Self retaining retractors and handrests. In: Wilkins, R.H., Rengachary, S.S. (Eds.), Neurosurgery. McGraw-Hill, New York, pp. 593.

Grossman, R.G., 1993. Preoperative and surgical planning for avoiding complications. In: Apuzzo, M.L. (Ed.), Brain surgery: complication avoidance and management. Churchill Livingstone, New York, pp. 3.

Gugino, L.D., Aglio, L.S., Black, P.Mc.L., 2000. Cortical stimulation techniques. In: Kaye, A.H., Black, P.Mc.L. (Eds.), Operative neurosurgery. Churchill Livingstone, London, pp. 85.

Gumprecht, H., Ebel, G.K., Auer, D.P., et al., 2002. Neuronavigation and functional MRI for surgery in patients with lesion in eloquent brain areas. Minim. Invasive Neurosurg. 45, 151–153.

Hammoud, M.A., Ligon, B.L., El Souki, R., et al., 1996. Use of intraoperative ultrasound for localizing tumors and determining the extent of resection: a comparative study. J. Neurosurg. 84, 737–741.

Harner, S.G., Beatty, C.W., Ebersold, M.J., 1995. Impact of cranioplasty on headache after acoustic neuroma removal. Neurosurgery 36, 1097–1100.

Hartov, A., Roberts, D.W., Paulsen, K.D., 2008. A comparative analysis of coregistered ultrasound and magnetic resonance imaging in neurosurgery. Neurosurgery 62 (Suppl.), 91–99.

Heifetz, M.D., 1993. Use and misuse of instruments. In: Apuzzo, M.L. (Ed.), Brain surgery: complication avoidance and management. Churchill Livingstone, New York, pp. 71.

Jellinek, D.A., Freeman, R., 2000. Perioperative care. In: Kaye, A.H., Black, P.Mc.L. (Eds.), Operative neurosurgery. Churchill Livingstone, London, pp. 15.

Kaus, M., Steinmeier, R., Sporer, T., et al., 1997. Technical accuracy of a neuronavigation system measured with a high-precision mechanical micromanipulator. Neurosurgery 41, 1431–1436.

Kokkino, A.J., Tew, J.M., 2000. Neurosurgical instrumentation, including neuromonitoring. In: Kaye, A.H., Black, P.Mc.L. (Eds.), Operative neurosurgery. Churchill Livingstone, London, pp. 71.

Kraayenbrink, M., McAnulty, G., 2006. Neuroanesthesia. In: Moore, A.J., Newell, D.W. (Eds.), Tumor neurosurgery. Principles and practice. Springer Verlag, London, pp. 71.

Lunsford, L.D., Kondziolka, D., Bissonette, D.J., 1996. Intraoperative imaging of the brain. Stereotact. Funct. Neurosurg. 66, 58–64.

Lustgarten, L., Teddy, P.J., 2000. Patient positioning in neurosurgery. In: Kaye, A.H., Black, P.Mc.L. (Eds.), Operative neurosurgery. Churchill Livingstone, London, pp. 45.

Manwaring, K.H., Hamilton, A.J., 1996. Neurosurgical endoscopy. In: Tindall, G.T., Cooper, P.R., Barrow, D.L. (Eds.), The practice of neurosurgery. Williams & Wilkins, Baltimore, MD, pp. 233.

Martin, C., Alexander 3rd, E., Jolesz, F., et al., 2000. Surgery in the MRI environment. In: Kaye, A.H., Black, P.Mc.L. (Eds.), Operative neurosurgery. Churchill Livingstone, London, pp. 185.

McGirt, M.J., Chaichana, K.L., Gathinji, M., et al., 2009. Independent association of extent of resection with survival in patients with malignant brain astrocytoma. J. Neurosurg. 110, 156–162.

Nauta, H.J.W., 1993. Error assessment during 'image guided' and 'imaging interactive' stereotactic surgery. Comput. Med. Imaging Graphics 18, 279–287.

Navabi, A., Black, P.Mc.L., Gering, D.T., et al., 2001. Serial intraoperative magnetic resonance imaging of brain shift. Neurosurgery 48, 787–798.

Nikas, D.C., Bello, L., Black, P.Mc.L., 2000. Cerebral hemisphere gliomas (adults) – low grade (astrocytomas and oligodendrogliomas). In: Kaye, A.H., Black, P.Mc.L. (Eds.), Operative neurosurgery. Churchill Livingstone, London, pp. 333.

Nimsky, C., Ganslandt, O., Buchfelder, M., et al., 2006. Intraoperative visualization for resection of gliomas: the role of functional neuronavigation and intraoperative 1.5 T MRI. Neurol. Res. 28, 482–487.

Ojemann, R.G., 1993a. The surgical management of cranial and spinal meningiomas. Clin. Neurosurg. 40, 498–535.

Ojemann, R.G., 1993b. Infratentorial procedures – neoplastic disorders – general considerations. In: Apuzzo, M.L. (Ed.), Brain surgery: complication avoidance and management. Churchill Livingstone, New York, pp. 1711.

Ojemann, R.G., 1993c. The surgical management of acoustic neuroma (vestibular schwannoma). Clin. Neurosurg. 40, 321–383.

Ojemann, R.G., 1996a. Meningiomas: Supratentorial meningiomas: Clinical features and surgical management. In: Wilkins, R.H., Rengachary, S.J. (Eds.), Neurosurgery, vol. 1. McGraw-Hill, New York, pp. 873.

Ojemann, R.G., 1996b. Acoustic neuroma (vestibular schwannoma). In: Youmans, J.R. (Ed.), Neurological surgery. WB Saunders, Philadelphia, PA, pp. 2841.

Ojemann, R.G., 1996c. Operative positioning and monitoring for surgery of the fourth ventricle. In: Cohen, A.R. (Ed.), Surgical disorders of the fourth ventricle. Blackwell Science, Cambridge, MA, pp. 161.

Ojemann, R.G., Ogilvy, C.S., 1993. Convexity, parasagittal and parafalcine meningiomas. In: Apuzzo, M.L. (Ed.), Brain surgery: complication avoidance and management. Churchill Livingstone, New York, pp. 187.

Ojemann, R.G., Ogilvy, C.S., Crowell, R.M., et al., 1995. Surgical management of neurovascular disease. Williams & Wilkins, Baltimore, MD.

Punjasawadwong, Y., Boonjeungmonkol, N., Phongchiewboon, A., 2007. Bispectral index for improving anaesthetic delivery and postoperative recovery. Cochrane Database Syst. Rev. (4):CD003843.

Rhoton, A.L. Jr., 1996. General and micro-operative techniques. In: Youmans, J.R. (Ed.), Neurological surgery. WB Saunders, Philadelphia, PA, pp. 724.

Roberts, D.W., Hartov, A., Kennedy, F.E., et al., 1998. Intraoperative brain shift and deformation: a quantitative analysis of cortical displacement in 28 cases. Neurosurgery 43, 749–758.

Rosner, M.J., 1996. Preoperative evaluation: complications, their prevention and treatment. In: Youmans, J.R. (Ed.), Neurological surgery. WB Saunders, Philadelphia, pp. 691.

Salcman, M., 2000. High grade cerebral hemisphere gliomas (adult). In: Kaye, A.H., Black, P.Mc.L. (Eds.), Operative neurosurgery. Churchill Livingstone, London, pp. 317.

Sawaya, R.E., Weinberg, J.S., 2005. Principles of brain tumor surgery in adults. In: Black, P.Mc.L., Loeffler, J.S. (Eds.), Cancer of the nervous system, second ed. Lippincott Williams and Wilkins, Philadelphia, PA, pp. 141.

Sekhar, I.N., Janecka, I.P., 1993. Surgery of cranial base tumors. Raven Press, New York.

Shalit, M.N., Israeli, Y., Matz, S., et al., 1982. Experience with intraoperative CT scanning in brain tumors. Surg. Neurol. 17, 376–382.

Shaw, M.D.M., Foy, P.D., 1991. Epilepsy after craniotomy and the place of prophylactic anticonvulsant drugs: discussion paper. J. Roy. Soc. Med. 84, 221–223.

Sipos, E.P., Tebo, S.A., Zinreich, S.J., et al., 1996. In vivo accuracy testing and clinical experience with the ISG viewing wand. Neurosurgery 39, 194–202.

Sirven, J.I., Wingerchuk, D.M., Drazkowski, J.F., et al., 2004. Seizure prophylaxis in patients with brain tumors: a meta-analysis. Mayo Clin. Proc. 79, 1489–1494.

Sloan, A.E., 2006. Stereotactic resection of malignant brain tumors. In: Badie, B. (Ed.), Neurosurgical operative atlas: Neuro-oncology. Thieme, New York, pp. 115.

Spicer, M.A., Apuzzo, M.L.J., 2005. Image-guided surgery. In: Black, P.Mc.L., Loeffler, J.S. (Eds.), Cancer of the nervous system, second ed. Lippincott Williams and Wilkins, Philadelphia, PA, pp. 155.

Staubert, A., Schlegel, W., Sartor, K., et al., 1997. Intraoperative diagnostic and interventional magnetic resonance imaging in neurosurgery. Neurosurgery 40, 891–900.

Stummer, W., Reulen, H.J., Meinel, T., et al., 2008. Extent of resection and survival in glioblastoma multiforme: identification of and adjustment for bias. Neurosurgery 62, 564–576.

Tew, J.M. Jr., Scodary, D.J., 1993a. Supratentorial procedures – Basic techniques and surgical positioning. In: Apuzzo, M.L. (Ed.), Brain surgery: complication avoidance and management. Churchill Livingstone, New York, pp. 31.

Tew, J.M. Jr., Scodary, D.J., 1993b. Infratentorial procedures – neoplastic disorders – surgical positioning. In: Apuzzo, M.L. (Ed.), Brain surgery: complication avoidance and management. Churchill Livingstone, New York, pp. 1609.

Van Loveren, H., Guthikonda, M., 1996. Guidelines for patient positioning in neurological surgery. In: Tindall, G.T., Cooper, P.R., Barrow, D.L. (Eds.), The practice of neurosurgery. Williams & Wilkins, Baltimore, MD, pp. 413.

Weintraub, H.S., Field, S., Hymos, K., et al., 1996. Perioperative medical evaluation of neurosurgical patients. In: Tindall, G.T., Cooper, P.R., Barrow, D.L. (Eds.), The practice of neurosurgery. Williams & Wilkins, Baltimore, MD, pp. 251.

Wilkins, R.H., 1996. Principles of neurosurgical operative technique. In: Wilkins, R.H., Rengachary, S.S. (Eds.), Neurosurgery. McGraw-Hill, New York, pp. 517.

15 Radiosurgery and radiotherapy for brain tumors

Douglas Kondziolka, Ajay Niranjan, L. Dade Lunsford,
David A. Clump, and John C. Flickinger

Introduction

Radiosurgery and external beam radiotherapy, alone or in combination, are integral components in the management of brain tumors. Stereotactic radiosurgery (SRS) is the process of delivering a precise or conformal, image-guided focus of ionizing radiation to a well-defined target volume in a single procedure. Radiosurgery can halt tumor cell division, cause neoplastic blood vessels to occlude, induce apoptosis or necrosis, and modify the blood–brain barrier around the tumor (Kondziolka et al 1992a, 1992b, 1999b, 2000; Niranjan et al 2004; Witham et al 2005). In contrast, external beam radiation therapy (EBRT) relies upon a distinct radio-biological process from that of SRS, delivering a course of treatment as a fractionated regimen over a period of weeks. In doing so, EBRT exploits the fundamental concepts of radiobiology by optimizing normal tissue repair, promoting reoxygenation and cell-cycle redistribution, as well as allowing for tumor cell repopulation. Bridging the described treatment modalities is fractionated stereotactic radiosurgery (FSR) that employs the advantages of stereotactic guidance to deliver a conformal high-dose of radiation in two to five sessions.

The feasibility of SRS was first realized in 1967 when the first patient was treated with the 179-source cobalt 60 Gamma Knife® delivery system. Although initially designed for functional neurosurgery, the second generation device (1975) opened the door to therapeutic radiosurgery for neoplastic or vascular mass lesions. The third generation increased the number of sources and beam diameters, used greatly improved dose planning systems, and integrated CT and MRI for target definition. Later units facilitated cobalt reloading, and added robotics. In 2006, the Perfexion® model expanded robotics, increased the treated volume of brain to include the head and neck, and eliminated helmet changes (Novotny et al 2008; Niranjan et al 2009). While the vast majority of clinical experience and biological understanding of radiosurgery is the result of the body of work generated by the Gamma Knife delivery system, more recently modified linear accelerators and cyclotrons producing charged particles have been used for radiosurgery, including devices with robotics and image-based target localization (Cyberknife®) (Hakim et al 1998; Friedman et al 2005; Chang et al 2005; Chang & Adler 1997). These later systems allow for accurate, efficient, precise, and reliable delivery of ionizing radiation to the brain, while also facilitating fractionation when necessary.

Applications for brain tumors

Stereotactic radiosurgery

The first two patients treated with the Gamma Knife delivery system had a craniopharyngioma and a pituitary adenoma.

Since that time, SRS for the management of tumors has been enhanced greatly by the introduction of MRI, which facilitated high-resolution brain tissue imaging and precise target delineation. In the 1980s, an increasing number of patients with benign tumors underwent radiosurgery, and in the 1990s, treatment evolved to alter the management of malignant neoplasms. SRS offered an alternative treatment modality with advantages over surgical intervention or conventional EBRT. This is especially evident in the treatment of small or medium-sized lesions, which equates to a target volume <35 mm. While this generalization persists, careful consideration of the clinical scenario including the degree of mass effect, tumor location, and the burden of systemic disease must also be considered.

An advantage of SRS is the ability to efficiently create highly conformal and selective volumetric dose plans for irregular shaped lesions. With the Gamma Knife delivery system, multiple isocenters using narrow radiation beams, or multiple delivery angles, are used to create a three-dimensional radiation volume that matches the imaging-defined tumor margin (Lunsford et al 2006). The steep falloff of radiation into the surrounding normal structures maintains safety, as radiation tolerance within the brain is location and volume dependent.

Because many targets are adjacent to critical brain and cranial nerve structures, conformal radiosurgery is crucial to maintain low morbidity rates with high tumor control. In instances where a large decrease in dose is necessary to limit normal tissue toxicity, consideration of alternative modes of treatment delivery may be necessary. For instance, in proton radiosurgery, dose is delivered with a sharp beam profile and deposited at a determined depth with minimal exit dose; a radiobiologic process termed the *Bragg peak*. Additionally, FSR may be used in this scenario as higher dose per fraction compared with conventional EBRT may be delivered, while maintaining the benefits of normal tissue repair observed with fractionated regimens (Chan et al 2005; Combs et al 2005).

Fractionated radiotherapy

The advantage for fractionating radiotherapy becomes magnified when large volumes of sensitive surrounding normal tissue need to be included in the treatment volume. This is exemplified by the standard 2-cm margin around enhancing tumor and edema routinely used in the treatment of diffusely infiltrative neoplasms such as glioblastoma multiforme. In this instance, a large volume of normal tissue is included in the target volume as infiltrative microscopic disease is intermingled with normal brain tissue.

The effect of fractionating radiotherapy can be represented by various mathematical formulas, most of which have individual limitations. The most commonly used formula is called the linear-quadratic formula which relates the log of surviving cells after a dose fraction of radiation 'd' as being proportional to an alpha-coefficient times the dose per fraction and a beta-coefficient times the dose per fraction squared (Barendsen 1982). By knowing one parameter, the alpha/beta ratio (α/β) for a given tissue or target, one could theoretically change from one radiotherapy course with dose/fractions d_1 and n_1 fractions with a known effect to a second course with dose/fraction d_2 and n_2 fractions with an equivalent effect on that tissue by using the following formula:

$$n_1 \times d_1 \times [1 + d_1/(\alpha/\beta)] = n_2 \times d_2 \times [1 + d_2/(\alpha/\beta)],$$

where n_{1or2} = number of fractions and d_{1or2} = dose per fraction for radiotherapy courses 1 or 2, and α/β = alpha/beta ratio for the tissue of interest.

In order to simplify matters for using and understanding the linear-quadratic formula, some authors have grouped tumors and normal tissue responses into three simple categories (Barendsen 1982). Late responding tissues like brain and spinal cord have low alpha/beta ratios in the range of 1–3 and are preferentially spared injury by the use of low dose fractions compared with most other tissues or tumors. Tumors and acute mucosal reactions are classified as early responding with alpha/beta ratios closer to 10 that are not spared as much by using small dose fractions. Intermediate tissues like small bowel and lung have values close to 5. Because many cell culture dose–response analyses of malignant tumors found alpha/beta values of ≥ 10, fractionated radiotherapy regimens with standard doses (1.8–2.0 Gy) have been utilized. However, not all tumors will respond to this fractionation and dose scheme. For instance, recent studies have determined the alpha/beta ratio for melanoma and a higher dose per fraction is advocated (Dasu 2007; Bentzen et al 1989).

There are significant limitations in using the linear-quadratic formula to calculate equivalent effects for different radiotherapy schedules. First, one needs to know precise alpha/beta ratios for every different type of tumor/target to be treated, and for every normal tissue at risk for complications. And second, the formula must give an accurate prediction within the dose-fractionation range that it is used. While the linear-quadratic formula performs adequately in predicting effects when changing from standard fractionation at 1.8–2 Gy per fraction down to doses of 1.2 Gy or up to 4–5 Gy, it is not accurate for extrapolating from 1.8–2 Gy up to single-fraction doses of 12–25 Gy (McKenna & Ahmad 2009). In addition, alpha/beta ratios are hard to determine for benign tumors. Determining an accurate alpha/beta ratio for a tumor or normal tissue requires a huge body of data correlating effects with different sized dose/fractions with a large number of events (complications or tumor recurrences). Fortunately for benign tumor patients, recurrences and complications are relatively infrequent after radiotherapy or radiosurgery, making alpha/beta ratios difficult to accurately determine. Another limitation is that at doses relevant for radiosurgery, tumor cell culture studies may be inaccurate for determining alpha/beta ratios, since the host endothelial cells may be a more important target than the tumor cells (Garcia-Barros et al 2003).

Fractionated radiotherapy is usually chosen over SRS when large targets >4 cm in average diameter (>32 mL) need to be irradiated in the brain. Acute radiation reactions with large treatment volume appear to be reduced by fractionation. Fractionated radiotherapy seems to be a better choice than radiotherapy for postoperative radiotherapy of large tumors that require a large volume of normal tissue at risk for recurrence to be irradiated. Fractionated radiotherapy with homogeneous dose distributions may be preferred to radiosurgery for treating tumors completely surrounding sensitive structures, such as the optic chiasm, when it is hard to separate tumor from optic nerve on the imaging.

With conventional radiotherapy, tumors/targets are typically treated with a minimum 3–5 mm margin to allow for set-up error for head and neck targets, while a 1.5 cm margin may be needed to account for the movement of lung targets. Thus gross target volumes (GTV) or clinical target volumes (CTV = GTV + any margin needed for microscopic tumor spread) are expanded by 3–5 mm to form planning target volumes (PTV) for conventional radiotherapy. That 3–5 mm margin can be reduced to 0.5–2 mm with the use of relocatable stereotactic frames or by image-guided radiotherapy. This is exemplified by modalities which enable FSR. Image-guided radiotherapy techniques (Cyberknife, Synergy®, Trilogy®, Tomotherapy®, etc.) use either biplanar or 3D imaging obtained on the radiotherapy treatment table immediately prior to each fraction and often mid-fraction to limit treatment set-up errors.

Vestibular schwannomas

The evolution of SRS has impacted the management algorithm of cranial base tumors such as schwannomas, meningiomas, pituitary tumors, craniopharyngiomas, and other lesions. Rather than simply recommending surgical resection (complete or partial), observation (with a variable natural history), or fractionated radiation therapy (with few published outcomes studies), the multidisciplinary team can now offer radiosurgery as primary or in some cases as adjuvant care.

The goals of vestibular schwannoma radiosurgery are to prevent further tumor growth, to preserve cochlear and other cranial nerve function, to maintain or to improve the patient's neurological status, and to avoid the risks associated with open surgical resection. Long-term results have established radiosurgery as an important minimally invasive alternative to microsurgery. Initially, radiosurgery was attractive to patients who were elderly or medically infirm, but was later offered to patients of all ages eligible for stereotactic frame fixation. We have found that the results have been consistent across age groups (Fig. 15.1) (Flickinger et al 2001, 2004).

During the past decade radiosurgery has emerged as an effective alternative to surgical removal of small to moderate-sized vestibular schwannomas. Initially, patients had radiosurgery as an alternative to microsurgical resection due to one or more of the following criteria: advanced patient age, poor medical condition for surgery, recurrent or residual tumor after prior surgery, neurofibromatosis type II, or patient preference (Subach et al 1999; Kondziolka et al 1998b; Flickinger & Kondziolka 1996; Flickinger et al 2001). Currently, most patients select radiosurgery because of

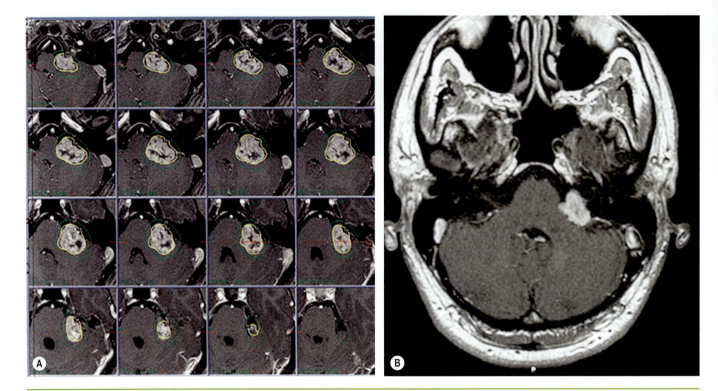

Figure 15.1 Axial MR images showing (A) radiosurgery dose plan for right acoustic tumor with brainstem compression. (B) A follow-up MRI 8 years later showing tumor regression.

published superior clinical outcomes which have established its long term safety and efficacy. To date we have managed 1397 patients with vestibular schwannomas using Gamma Knife stereotactic radiosurgery (see Table 15.1 for further information). The mean patient age in our series was 57 years (range, 12–95). A total of 8% had neurofibromatosis (Kondziolka et al 1998b). Symptoms before radiosurgery included hearing loss (92%), balance symptoms or ataxia (51%), tinnitus (43%), or other neurologic deficit (19.5%). Some 34% of our patients had useful hearing, Gardner–Robertson grade I (speech discrimination score ≥70%; pure tone average ≤30 dB) or grade II (speech discrimination score ≥50%; pure tone average ≤50 dB). Since 1992, the average dose prescribed to the tumor margin was 13 Gy with the 50% isodose line being used in 90% of patients.

Our long-term study documented a 98% clinical tumor control rate (no requirement for surgical intervention) at 5–10 years (Kondziolka et al 1998b). Patients managed from 1992–1997 had a similar success rate (Flickinger et al 2001). Between 1987 and 1992, there were significant modifications in the technique of radiosurgery including a change from CT to MRI-based planning, improved computer workstations and conformal dose planning, the use of more isocenters of radiation, the use of smaller irradiation beams, and a reduction in the average margin dose to 12–13 Gy. Since our modification of these techniques beginning in 1991, there has been a significant reduction in the morbidity of radiosurgery (Niranjan et al 2008; Kano et al 2009a). Currently, the risk for any grade delayed facial nerve dysfunction is below 1% (Niranjan et al 2008; Kano et al 2009a).

Table 15.1 Applications for Gamma Knife radiosurgery for brain tumors at the University of Pittsburgh

Diagnosis	Procedures (n)
Vestibular schwannoma	1397
Trigeminal schwannoma	39
Other schwannoma	62
Meningioma	1302
Pituitary tumor	290
Craniopharyngioma	74
Hemangioblastoma	48
Hemangiopericytoma	39
Glomus tumor	21
Pineocytoma	16
Malignant pineal tumor	13
Chordoma	30
Chondrosarcoma	22
Choroid plexus papilloma	12
Hemangioma	7
Glioblastoma multiforme	327
Anaplastic astrocytoma	128
Fibrillar astrocytoma	42
Mixed glioma	69
Pilocytic astrocytoma	86
Ependymoma	71
Medulloblastoma	24
CNS lymphoma	12
Hypothalamic hamartoma	6
Brain metastasis	3041
Invasive skull base tumor	32
Other tumor	66
Total	**7276**

Total procedures, $n = 9627$; brain tumors, $n = 7276$.

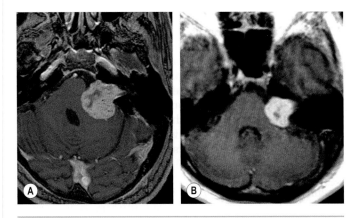

Figure 15.2 Axial MR images before radiosurgery showing (A) right acoustic tumor before radiosurgery. (B) A 2-year follow-up MRI showing tumor regression.

Patients with useful hearing before radiosurgery, continue to report an approximate 75% overall rate for maintenance of useful hearing, depending on tumor size (Lunsford et al 2005). For patients with intracanalicular tumors, the rate of hearing preservation is above 80% (Niranjan et al 2008; Niranjan et al 1999). Radiosurgery has been shown to be a cost-effective, low risk, and an effective alternative to microsurgery for vestibular schwannoma patients (Fig. 15.2).

For smaller tumors, it is likely that more patients now receive radiosurgery as primary management. Although there has not been a randomized trial with level 1 evidence to compare radiosurgery to resection (and one is not likely to be performed), there are now four matched cohort studies, which provide level 2 evidence. These studies reported on patients with similar sized tumors, and evaluated clinical, imaging, and quality of life outcomes. All four reports consistently showed better results after radiosurgery for most clinical measures, similar results for the preoperative symptoms of tinnitus and imbalance, and similar freedom from tumor progression rates (Regis et al 2002; Pollock et al 1995, 2006; Myrseth et al 2005). In some patients, there can be transient expansion of the tumor capsule after irradiation which usually can be observed without further treatment (Pollock 2006; Hasegawa et al 2006). Based on these data, we believe that the only remaining indication for surgical resection in a patient with a small to moderate size tumor is brainstem compression causing disabling imbalance, or patient choice.

Stereotactic radiotherapy

As previously discussed, fractionated delivery of ionizing radiation is likely to result in radiobiological processes that differ from that of radiosurgery specifically as it may relate to repair of normal tissues. FSR may allow for a high-dose of conformal radiation to be delivered to the target, while sparing normal tissues such as the vestibular-cochlear system and time for its interfractional repair. Fractionated regimens have varied from 25.0 Gy provided in 5 fractions, 21.0 Gy in 3 fractions to 18.0 Gy in 3 fractions. The Stanford group has reported their Cyberknife FSR experience with encouraging local control and hearing preservation

(Sakamoto et al 2009). Additionally, the use of FSR may prove to be especially useful in the management of larger, asymptomatic lesions that are in close proximity to the vestibular or trigeminal system. In fact, a LINAC-based FSR and SRS comparison of 25.0 Gy provided in 5 fractions vs 12.5 Gy in 1 fraction demonstrated similar rates of local control, but 5-year trigeminal nerve preservation in favor of the fractionated regimen (Meijer et al 2003). Additional insight into the role of fractionated radiotherapy was established by Andrews et al (2008) who published their outcomes using stereotactic radiotherapy at a total dose of 50.4 or 46.8 Gy. In patients with grades one or two hearing; the median follow-up was 65 weeks. Although no patient had later tumor growth, the hearing preservation rates were better at the lower dose. At 3 years, the hearing preservation rate was 55–60%, and no patient with grade 2 hearing preserved it at the 50.0 Gy dose (Andrews et al 2008). As dose becomes standardized in FSR and long-term results obtained, comparisons between the differing delivery systems will be better appreciated.

Meningiomas

Radiosurgery has proven an effective strategy for patients with meningioma, especially those that are consistent with WHO grade histology. Initially, radiosurgery was only considered for residual or recurrent tumors after prior resection (Kondziolka et al 1991). However, in the early 1990s it became a standard treatment for small basal meningiomas where the risks of resection were excessive. Meningiomas are especially suitable for radiosurgery because these tumors are usually well-demarcated and rarely invade the brain (Flickinger et al 2003). The steep radiation fall-off can directly conform to this well-defined tumor margin while sparing normal tissue (Kondziolka et al 1998a). Delayed tumor recurrence after surgery, surgical morbidity, and surgical mortality (especially in the elderly), has increasingly led to consideration of radiosurgery as the primary management of meningiomas in critical locations. Accordingly, the role of aggressive skull base surgery has waned and small basal tumors have been managed by radiosurgery alone, while larger tumors with mass effect benefit from subtotal resection followed by radiosurgery (for residual tumor) (Kondziolka et al 1999a, 2003).

Our 22-year experience includes 1302 intracranial meningiomas. We evaluated 972 patients with 1045 intracranial meningiomas in detail. The series included 70% who were women, 49% who had undergone a prior resection, and 5% who received prior fractionated radiation therapy. The mean age was 57 years. Tumor locations included middle fossa (351), posterior fossa (307), convexity (126), anterior fossa (88), parasagittal region (113), or other sites (115). The mean tumor volume was 7.4 mL. Follow-up past 5, 7, 10, and 12 years was obtained in 327, 190, 90, and 41 patients, respectively.

The overall control rate for patients who had adjuvant radiosurgery for known WHO grade 1 (benign) meningiomas (prior resection) was 93%. Primary radiosurgery patients (no prior histologic confirmation; $n = 482$), had a tumor control rate of 97%. Adjuvant radiosurgery for patients with WHO grades 2 and 3 tumors had tumor control rates of 50% and 17%, respectively. Delayed resection after radiosurgery was necessary in 51 patients (5%) at a mean of 35 months.

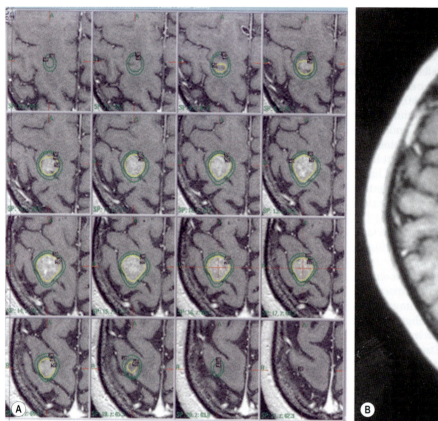
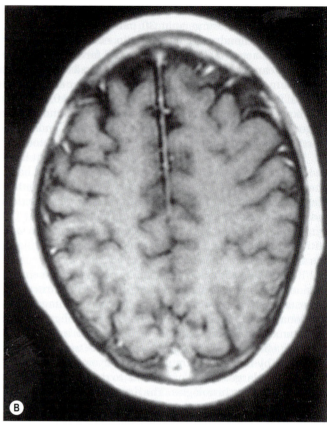

Figure 15.3 Axial MR images during radiosurgery planning for single brain metastasis. (A) A margin dose of 20 Gy was delivered to 50% isodose line. (B) A follow-up MRI 6 months after radiosurgery shows complete resolution.

Glial neoplasms

Malignant gliomas continue to represent one of the most serious challenges in neurooncology. It has been over 30 years since radiation therapy was established as the standard adjuvant treatment following maximal resection in high-grade gliomas including glioblastoma multiforme (GBM). The Brain Tumor Study Group (BTSG) in the 1970s demonstrated in a prospective randomized trial that WBRT to 50–60 Gy resulted in a survival advantage over best supportive care or carmustine alone (Walker et al 1978). Radiation therapy continues to be an essential component in the multidisciplinary management of GBM with the current standard of care consisting of concurrent and adjuvant temozolomide (Stupp et al 2005). Despite improvements, nearly all will require salvage therapy to address recurrent disease within 2 years of diagnosis (Stupp et al 2009). To address this locally progressive disease, therapeutic options have evolved to maximize the current advances in technology and treatment delivery.

While initial treatments consisted of WBRT delivered by opposed lateral fields, more recent evidence suggests that localized therapy is equally effective. Regional therapy is supported by a retrospective analysis of recurrence patterns that suggests 78% of recurrent disease occurs within 2 cm of the tumor bed volume as defined on CT (Hochberg & Pruitt 1980; Oppitz et al 1999; Wallner et al 1989). Imaging advances, including the use of pre- and postoperative gadolinium-enhanced MRI has facilitated in more accurate defining of the tumor volume. Current radiation treatment planning defines the GTV1 as the postoperative T2 or FLAIR enhancement and surgical cavity plus an additional 2 cm to create a CTV1. This CTV1 plus an additional 0.5 cm margin to account for set-up uncertainty is the PTV1 and is typically prescribed to 46.0 Gy in 23 fractions. Following delivery of this prescribed dose to the PTV1, a boost volume, defined by the postoperative T1 enhancement plus a margin is prescribed an additional 14.0 Gy in 7 fractions for a total 60.0 Gy to the tumor bed.

With the majority of recurrences within the previously irradiated volume, there is rationale for dose escalation with the intention to improve primary local control. In order to maximize the benefits of radiation on intrinsic glial tumors of the brain, surgical procedures such as interstitial brachytherapy with temporary or permanent radioactive isotopes, intracavitary irradiation with colloidal isotopes, and balloon placement of radioactive isotopes have been used. Radiosurgery is a minimally invasive method to boost the radiation effect of fractionated radiotherapy for patients with malignant glial tumors (Ulm et al 2005; Mahajan et al 2005; Larson et al 1996).

Radiosurgery has been used mainly for carefully selected patients with residual or deep-seated malignant glial tumors <3.5 cm in diameter as part of a multi-modality approach.

To date, we performed radiosurgery on 327 patients with glioblastomas and 96 patients with anaplastic astrocytomas. Glioblastoma patients had a mean age of 54 years, and a mean tumor volume of 3.4 mL. A total of 65% had a prior resection, and 58% had prior chemotherapy. Anaplastic astrocytoma patients had a mean age of 38 years, and a mean tumor volume of 3.6 mL; 42% had one or more prior resections, and 40% had prior chemotherapy. In comparison to patients who received radiotherapy alone, we found that glioblastoma patients had significant prolongation of survival (Nagai et al 2004). However, no prospective randomized trial has been completed to study the benefit of boost radiosurgery after radiation therapy for glioblastoma multiforme. A randomized trial showed no benefit from up-front radiosurgery plus radiotherapy and carmustine, compared with radiotherapy and carmustine alone (Souhami et al 2004). From our experience, we think that radiosurgery is a useful concept for residual or recurrent smaller-volume malignant gliomas after completion of initial radiation therapy and chemotherapy. It may also provide tumor growth control in the setting of a later recurrence if other treatment options are limited.

Other treatment delivery schemes have been attempted in the re-irradiation of GBM. For instance, fractionated therapy delivered twice-weekly to 36.0 Gy in 6 fractions led to an improved survival of 15.8 months in 12 of 36 responders vs 7.3 months in non-responders (Patel et al 2009). Continuing the multidisciplinary approach to the management of GBM, re-irradiation concurrent with a humanized monoclonal antibody that recognized and blocks the vascular endothelial growth factor (VEGF) receptor, Bevacizumab, have been attempted. Using a FSR regimen consisting of 30.0 Gy delivered in 5 fractions over a 2.5 week period, recurrent GBM was treated with bevacizumab (10 mg/kg) every 14 days on days 1 and 15 of 28-day cycles with radiosurgery being delivered during the second cycle (Gutin et al 2009). This regimen led to a 6-month progression free survival of 65% and a 1-year survival from the time of study enrollment of 54% (Gutin et al 2009). Combining radiation therapy with targeted agents that engage the vascular component of tumors, which is also a proposed target of radiosurgery, future studies will focus on manipulating the signaling pathways that contribute to radioresistance as well as the pathogenesis of GBM.

While the role of radiation therapy in the management of GBM is relatively well-established to improve local control over observation, similar effects are not as clear in low-grade gliomas. As low-grade gliomas are relatively slow-growing tumors, a dose-response with escalation has not been observed. Two randomized controlled trials demonstrated no difference in progression free survival or overall survival between those receiving 45 and 65 in the EORTC trial and those receiving 50.4 and 64.8 Gy in the INTERGROUP study (Karim et al 1996; Shaw et al 2002). Postoperative EBRT has been compared to observation and treatment at the time of progression and while there was no difference in overall survival between the two approaches, immediate EBRT did lead to improved progression-free survival and a decrease in seizure activity (van den Bent et al 2005). In addition to those with uncontrolled seizure activity and neurological deficits, immediate ERBRT is favored in those with adverse risk factors including those >40 years old; those with pure astrocytoma histology; tumor ≥6 cm; tumor crossing the midline, as this sub-group has a median overall survival of only 3.7 years compared with that of 7.8 years in the low-risk sub-group (Pignatti et al 2002).

In addition, radiosurgery also has a smaller role for patients with low-grade astrocytomas of the brain (Hadjipanayis et al 2002; Hadjipanayis et al 2003). To date, we have managed 86 patients with pilocytic astrocytomas and 42 with fibrillary astrocytomas. We have managed 69 patients with mixed gliomas including 19 patients with oligodendrogliomas (Kano et al 2009c). Neurocytomas appear to regress in volume after radiosurgery (Tyler-Kabara et al 2001). Most patients had small volume tumors in critical brain locations, or had residual tumors after prior resection. All had histological confirmation.

Radiosurgery has also been used as the sole radiation modality for the management of patients with small pilocytic astrocytomas in critical brain locations (Kano et al 2009b; Kano et al 2009e). We treated 86 patients whose mean age was 17 years (range, 4–52). Radiosurgery was effective in the management of children with pilocytic tumors, especially those located in the brainstem locations after prior resection. The most common brain location in our patients was the pons. Radiosurgery is also used as an alternative to fractionated radiation therapy in the management of patients with residual or recurrent ependymomas, or as additional treatment after tumor recurrence following radiation therapy. To date, we have treated 71 patients with ependymomas (Kano et al 2009d), and 24 patients with medulloblastomas (Germanwala et al 2008).

REFERENCES

Andrews, D.W., Scott, C.B., Sperduto, P.W., et al., 2004. Whole brain radiation therapy with or without stereotactic radiosurgery boost for patients with one to three brain metastases: phase III results of the RTOG 9508 randomised trial. Lancet 363, 1665–1672.

Andrews, D.W., Werner-Wasik, M., Den, R.B., et al., 2008. Toward dose optimization for fractionated stereotactic radiotherapy for acoustic neuromas: comparison of two dose cohorts. Int. J. Radiat. Oncol. Biol. Phys. 74, 419–426.

Arvold, N.D., Lessell, S., Bussiere, M., et al., 2009. Visual outcome and tumor control after conformal radiotherapy for patients with optic nerve sheath meningioma. Int. J. Radiat. Oncol. Biol. Phys. 75, 1166–1172.

Atteberry, D., Szeifert, G., Kondziolka, D., et al., 2006. Radiosurgical pathology observations on cerebral metastases after gamma knife radiosurgery. Radiosurgery 6, 173–185.

Barendsen, G.W., 1982. Dose fractionation, dose rate and iso-effect relationships for normal tissue responses. Int. J. Radiat. Oncol. Biol. Phys. 8, 1981–1997.

Bentzen, S.M., Overgaard, J., Thames, H.D., et al., 1989. Clinical radiobiology of malignant melanoma. Radiother Oncol. 16, 169–182.

Bhatnagar, A.K., Flickinger, J.C., Kondziolka, D., et al., 2006. Stereotactic radiosurgery for four or more intracranial metastases. Int. J. Radiat. Oncol. Biol. Phys. 64, 898–903.

Chan, A.W., Black, P., Ojemann, R.G., et al., 2005. Stereotactic radiotherapy for vestibular schwannomas: favorable outcome with minimal toxicity. Neurosurgery 57, 60–70.

Chang, E.L., Wefel, J.S., Maor, M.H., et al., 2007. A pilot study of neurocognitive function in patients with one to three new brain metastases initially treated with stereotactic radiosurgery alone. Neurosurgery 60, 277–284.

Chang, E.L., Wefel, J.S., Hess, K.R., et al., 2009. Neurocognition in patients with brain metastases treated with radiosurgery or radiosurgery plus whole-brain irradiation: a randomised controlled trial. Lancet Oncol. 10, 1037–1044.

Chang, S.D., Adler, J.R. Jr., 1997. Treatment of cranial base meningiomas with linear accelerator radiosurgery. Neurosurgery 41, 1019–1027.

Chang, S.D., Gibbs, I.C., Sakamoto, G.T., et al., 2005. Staged stereotactic irradiation for acoustic neuroma. Neurosurgery 56, 1254–1263.

Combs, S.E., Volk, S., Schulz-Ertner, D., et al., 2005. Management of acoustic neuromas with fractionated stereotactic radiotherapy (FSRT): long-term results in 106 patients treated in a single institution. Int. J. Radiat. Oncol. Biol. Phys. 63, 75–81.

Condra, K.S., Buatti, J.M., Mendenhall, W.M., et al., 1997. Benign meningiomas: primary treatment selection affects survival. Int. J. Radiat. Oncol. Biol. Phys. 39, 427–436.

Coke, C.C., Corn, B.W., Werner-Wasik, M., et al., 1998. Atypical and malignant meningiomas: an outcome report of seventeen cases. J. Neurooncol. 39, 65–70.

Dasu, A., 2007. Is the alpha/beta value for prostate tumours low enough to be safely used in clinical trials? Clin. Oncol. (R. Coll. Radiol.) 19, 289–301.

Firlik, K.S., Kondziolka, D., Flickinger, J.C., et al., 2000. Stereotactic radiosurgery for brain metastases from breast cancer. Ann. Surg. Oncol. 7, 333–338.

Flickinger, J.C., Kondziolka, D., 1996. Radiosurgery instead of resection for solitary brain metastasis: the gold standard redefined. Int. J. Radiat. Oncol. Biol. Phys. 35, 185–186.

Flickinger, J.C., Kondziolka, D., Maitz, A.H., et al., 2003. Gamma knife radiosurgery of imaging-diagnosed intracranial meningioma. Int. J. Radiat. Oncol. Biol. Phys. 56, 801–806.

Flickinger, J.C., Kondziolka, D., Niranjan, A., et al., 2001. Results of acoustic neuroma radiosurgery: an analysis of 5 years' experience using current methods. J. Neurosurg. 94, 1–6.

Flickinger, J.C., Kondziolka, D., Niranjan, A., et al., 2004. Acoustic neuroma radiosurgery with marginal tumor doses of 12 to 13 Gy. Int. J. Radiat. Oncol. Biol. Phys. 60, 225–230.

Flickinger, J.C., Kondziolka, D., Pollock, B.E., et al., 1996. Evolution in technique for vestibular schwannoma radiosurgery and effect on outcome. Int. J. Radiat. Oncol. Biol. Phys. 36, 275–280.

Friedman, W.A., Murad, G.J., Bradshaw, P., et al., 2005. Linear accelerator surgery for meningiomas. J. Neurosurg. 103, 206–209.

Garcia-Barros, M., Paris, F., Cordon-Cardo, C., et al., 2003. Tumor response to radiotherapy regulated by endothelial cell apoptosis. Science 300, 1155–1159.

Germanwala, A.V., Mai, J.C., Tomycz, N.D., et al., 2008. Boost Gamma Knife surgery during multimodality management of adult medulloblastoma. J. Neurosurg. 108, 204–209.

Gutin, P.H., Iwamoto, F.M., Beal, K., et al., 2009. Safety and efficacy of bevacizumab with hypofractionated stereotactic irradiation for recurrent malignant gliomas. Int. J. Radiat. Oncol. Biol. Phys. 75, 156–163.

Hadjipanayis, C.G., Kondziolka, D., Flickinger, J.C., et al., 2003. The role of stereotactic radiosurgery for low-grade astrocytomas. Neurosurg. Focus 14, e15.

Hadjipanayis, C.G., Niranjan, A., Tyler-Kabara, E., et al., 2002. Stereotactic radiosurgery for well-circumscribed fibrillary grade II astrocytomas: an initial experience. Stereotact Funct. Neurosurg. 79, 13–24.

Hakim, R., Alexander, E. 3rd, et al., 1998. Results of linear accelerator-based radiosurgery for intracranial meningiomas. Neurosurgery 42, 446–454.

Hasegawa, T., Kida, Y., Yoshimoto, M., et al., 2006. Evaluation of tumor expansion after stereotactic radiosurgery in patients harboring vestibular schwannomas. Neurosurgery 58, 1119–1128.

Hasegawa, T., Kondziolka, D., Flickinger, J.C., et al., 2003a. Brain metastases treated with radiosurgery alone: an alternative to whole brain radiotherapy? Neurosurgery 52, 1318–1326.

Hasegawa, T., Kondziolka, D., Flickinger, J.C., et al., 2003b. Stereotactic radiosurgery for brain metastases from gastrointestinal tract cancer. Surg. Neurol. 60, 506–515.

Hochberg, F.H., Pruitt, A., 1980. Assumptions in the radiotherapy of glioblastoma. Neurology 30, 907–911.

Hug, E.B., Devries, A., Thornton, A.F., et al., 2000. Management of atypical and malignant meningiomas: role of high dose, 3D-conformal radiation therapy. J. Neurooncol 48, 151–160.

Jeremic, B., Pitz, S., 2007. Primary optic nerve sheath meningioma: stereotactic fractionated radiation therapy as an emerging treatment of choice. Cancer 110, 712–722.

Kano, H., Kondziolka, D., Khan, A., et al., 2009a. Predictors of hearing preservation after stereotactic radiosurgery for acoustic neuroma. J. Neurosurg. 111 (4), 863–873.

Kano, H., Kondziolka, D., Niranjan, A., et al., 2009b. Stereotactic radiosurgery for pilocytic astrocytomas part 1: outcomes in adult patients. J. Neurooncol 95 (2), 211–218.

Kano, H., Niranjan, A., Khan, A., et al., 2009c. Does radiosurgery have a role in the management of oligodendrogliomas? J. Neurosurg. 110, 564–571.

Kano, H., Niranjan, A., Kondziolka, D., et al., 2009d. Outcome predictors for intracranial ependymoma radiosurgery. Neurosurgery 64, 279–288.

Kano, H., Niranjan, A., Kondziolka, D., et al., 2009e. Stereotactic radiosurgery for pilocytic astrocytomas part 2: outcomes in pediatric patients. J. Neurooncol. 95 (2), 219–229.

Karim, A.B., Maat, B., Hatlevoll, R., et al., 1996. A randomized trial on dose-response in radiation therapy of low-grade cerebral glioma: European Organization for Research and Treatment of Cancer (EORTC) Study 22844. Int. J. Radiat. Oncol. Biol. Phys. 36, 549–556.

Killory, B.D., Kresel, J.J., Wait, S.D., et al., 2009. Hypofractionated CyberKnife radiosurgery for perichiasmatic pituitary adenomas: early results. Neurosurgery 64, A19–A25.

Kondziolka, D., Flickinger, J.C., Perez, B., 1998a. Judicious resection and/or radiosurgery for parasagittal meningiomas: outcomes from a multicenter review. Gamma Knife Meningioma Study Group. Neurosurgery 43, 405–414.

Kondziolka, D., Levy, E.I., Niranjan, A., et al., 1999a. Long-term outcomes after meningioma radiosurgery: physician and patient perspectives. J. Neurosurg. 91, 44–50.

Kondziolka, D., Lunsford, L.D., Claassen, D., et al., 1992a. Radiobiology of radiosurgery: Part I. The normal rat brain model. Neurosurgery 31, 271–279.

Kondziolka, D., Lunsford, L.D., Claassen, D., et al., 1992b. Radiobiology of radiosurgery: Part II. The rat C6 glioma model. Neurosurgery 31, 280–288.

Kondziolka, D., Lunsford, L.D., Coffey, R.J., et al., 1991. Gamma knife radiosurgery of meningiomas. Stereotact Funct. Neurosurg. 57, 11–21.

Kondziolka, D., Lunsford, L.D., Flickinger, J.C., 1999b. The radiobiology of radiosurgery. Neurosurg. Clin. N. Am. 10, 157–166.

Kondziolka, D., Lunsford, L.D., McLaughlin, M.R., et al., 1998b. Long-term outcomes after radiosurgery for acoustic neuromas. N. Engl. J. Med. 339, 1426–1433.

Kondziolka, D., Lunsford, L.D., Witt, T.C., et al., 2000. The future of radiosurgery: radiobiology, technology, and applications. Surg. Neurol. 54, 406–414.

Kondziolka, D., Martin, J.J., Flickinger, J.C., et al., 2005a. Long-term survivors after gamma knife radiosurgery for brain metastases. Cancer 104, 2784–2791.

Kondziolka, D., Nathoo, N., Flickinger, J.C., et al., 2003. Long-term results after radiosurgery for benign intracranial tumors. Neurosurgery 53, 815–822.

Kondziolka, D., Niranjan, A., Flickinger, J.C., et al., 2005b. Radiosurgery with or without whole-brain radiotherapy for brain metastases: the patients' perspective regarding complications. Am. J. Clin. Oncol. 28, 173–179.

Larson, D.A., Gutin, P.H., McDermott, M., et al., 1996. Gamma knife for glioma: selection factors and survival. Int. J. Radiat. Oncol. Biol. Phys. 36, 1045–1053.

Lee, J.Y., Niranjan, A., McInerney, J., et al., 2002. Stereotactic radiosurgery providing long-term tumor control of cavernous sinus meningiomas. J. Neurosurg. 97, 65–72.

Lunsford, L.D., Kondziolka, D., Niranjan, A., et al., 2006. Concepts of conformality and selectivity in acoustic tumor radiosurgery. Radiosurgery 6, 98–107.

Lunsford, L.D., Niranjan, A., Flickinger, J.C., et al., 2005. Radiosurgery of vestibular schwannomas: summary of experience in 829 cases. J. Neurosurg. 102 (Suppl.), 195–199.

Maesawa, S., Kondziolka, D., Thompson, T.P., et al., 2000. Brain metastases in patients with no known primary tumor. Cancer 89, 1095–1101.

Mahajan, A., McCutcheon, I.E., Suki, D., et al., 2005. Case-control study of stereotactic radiosurgery for recurrent glioblastoma multiforme. J. Neurosurg. 103, 210–217.

Martin, J.J., Niranjan, A., Kondziolka, D., et al., 2007. Radiosurgery for chordomas and chondrosarcomas of the skull base. J. Neurosurg. 107, 758–764.

Mathieu, D., Kondziolka, D., Cooper, P.B., et al., 2007. Gamma knife radiosurgery in the management of malignant melanoma brain metastases. Neurosurgery 60, 471–482.

McKenna, F.W., Ahmad, S, 2009. Fitting techniques of cell survival curves in high-dose region for use in stereotactic body radiation therapy. Phys. Med. Biol. 54, 1593–1608.

Meijer, O.W., Vandertop, W.P., Baayen, J.C., et al., 2003. Single-fraction vs. fractionated LINAC-based stereotactic radiosurgery for vestibular schwannoma: a single institution study. Int. J. Radiat. Oncol. Biol. Phys. 56, 1390–1396.

Mori, Y., Kondziolka, D., Flickinger, J.C., et al., 1998a. Stereotactic radiosurgery for cerebral metastatic melanoma: factors affecting local disease control and survival. Int. J. Radiat. Oncol. Biol. Phys. 42, 581–589.

Mori, Y., Kondziolka, D., Flickinger, J.C., et al., 1998b. Stereotactic radiosurgery for brain metastasis from renal cell carcinoma. Cancer 83, 344–353.

Muthukumar, N., Kondziolka, D., Lunsford, L.D., et al., 1998. Stereotactic radiosurgery for tentorial meningiomas. Acta. Neurochir. (Wien) 140, 315–321.

Muthukumar, N., Kondziolka, D., Lunsford, L.D., et al., 1999. Stereotactic radiosurgery for anterior foramen magnum meningiomas. Surg. Neurol. 51, 268–273.

Myrseth, E., Moller, P., Pedersen, P.H., et al., 2005. Vestibular schwannomas: clinical results and quality of life after microsurgery or gamma knife radiosurgery. Neurosurgery 56, 927–935.

Nagai, H., Kondziolka, D., Niranjan, A., et al., 2004. Results following stereotactic radiosurgery for patients with glioblastoma multiforme. Radiosurgery 5, 91–99.

Niranjan, A., Gobbel, G.T., Kondziolka, D., et al., 2004. Experimental radiobiological investigations into radiosurgery: present understanding and future directions. Neurosurgery 55, 495–505.

Niranjan, A., Lunsford, L.D., Flickinger, J.C., et al., 1999. Dose reduction improves hearing preservation rates after intracanalicular acoustic tumor radiosurgery. Neurosurgery 45, 753–765.

Niranjan, A., Mathieu, D., Flickinger, J.C., et al., 2008. Hearing preservation after intracanalicular vestibular schwannoma radiosurgery. Neurosurgery 63, 1054–1063.

Niranjan, A., Novotny, J. Jr., Bhatnagar, J., et al., 2009. Efficiency and dose planning comparisons between the Perfexion and 4C Leksell Gamma Knife units. Stereotact Funct. Neurosurg. 87, 191–198.

Niranjan, A., Szeifert, G.T., Kondziolka, D., et al., 2002. Gamma Knife radiosurgery for growth hormone-secreting pituitary adenomas. Radiosurgery 4, 93–101.

Novotny, J., Bhatnagar, J.P., Niranjan, A., et al., 2008. Dosimetric comparison of the Leksell Gamma Knife Perfexion and 4C. J. Neurosurg. 109 (Suppl.), 8–14.

Oppitz, U., Maessen, D., Zunterer, H., et al., 1999. 3D-recurrence-patterns of glioblastomas after CT-planned postoperative irradiation. Radiother Oncol. 53, 53–57.

Patel, M., Siddiqui, F., Jin, J.Y., et al., 2009. Salvage reirradiation for recurrent glioblastoma with radiosurgery : radiographic response and improved survival. J. Neurooncol. 92, 185–191.

Perry, A., Scheithauer, B.W., Stafford, S.L., et al., 1999. Malignancy in meningiomas: a clinicopathologic study of 116 patients with grading implications. Cancer 85, 2046–2056.

Peterson, A.M., Meltzer, C.C., Evanson, E.J., et al., 1999. MR imaging response of brain metastases after gamma knife stereotactic radiosurgery. Radiology 211, 807–814.

Pignatti, F., van den Bent, M., Curran, D., et al., European Organization for Research and Treatment of Cancer Radiotherapy Coopera-tive Group., 2002. Prognostic factors for survival in adult patients with cerebral low-grade glioma. J. Clin. Oncol. 20, 2076–2084.

Pollock, B.E., 2006. Management of vestibular schwannomas that enlarge after stereotactic radiosurgery: treatment recommendations based on a 15 year experience. Neurosurgery 58, 241–248.

Pollock, B.E., Driscoll, C.L., Foote, R.L., et al., 2006. Patient outcomes after vestibular schwannoma management: a prospective comparison of microsurgical resection and stereotactic radiosurgery. Neurosurgery 59, 77–85.

Pollock, B.E., Lunsford, L.D., Kondziolka, D., et al., 1995. Outcome analysis of acoustic neuroma management: a comparison of microsurgery and stereotactic radiosurgery. Neurosurgery 36, 215–229.

Regis, J., Pellet, W., Delsanti, C., et al., 2002. Functional outcome after gamma knife surgery or microsurgery for vestibular schwannomas. J. Neurosurg. 97, 1091–1100.

Sakamoto, G.T., Blevins, N., Gibbs, I.C., 2009. Cyberknife radiotherapy for vestibular schwannoma. Otolaryngol. Clin. North. Am. 42, 665–675.

Shaw, E., Arusell, R., Scheithauer, B., et al., 2002. Prospective randomized trial of low- versus high-dose radiation therapy in adults with supratentorial low-grade glioma: initial report of a North Central Cancer Treatment Group/Radiation Therapy Oncology Group/Eastern Cooperative Oncology Group study. J. Clin. Oncol. 20, 2267–2276.

Sheehan, J.P., Niranjan, A., Sheehan, J.M., et al., 2005. Stereotactic radiosurgery for pituitary adenomas: an intermediate review of its safety, efficacy, and role in the neurosurgical treatment armamentarium. J. Neurosurg. 102, 678–691.

Sheehan, J.P., Sun, M.H., Kondziolka, D., et al., 2003. Radiosurgery in patients with renal cell carcinoma metastasis to the brain: long-term outcomes and prognostic factors influencing survival and local tumor control. J. Neurosurg. 98, 342–349.

Souhami, L., Seiferheld, W., Brachman, D., et al., 2004. Randomized comparison of stereotactic radiosurgery followed by conventional radiotherapy with carmustine to conventional radiotherapy with carmustine for patients with glioblastoma multiforme: report of Radiation Therapy Oncology Group 93–05 protocol. Int. J. Radiat. Oncol. Biol. Phys. 60, 853–860.

Stupp, R., Mason, W.P., van den Bent, M.J., et al., 2005. European Organisation for Research and Treatment of Cancer Brain Tumor and Radiotherapy Groups; National Cancer Institute of Canada Clinical Trials Group: N. Engl. J. Med. 352, 987–996.

Stupp, R., Hegi, M.E., Mason, W.P., et al., European Organisation for Research and Treatment of Cancer Brain Tumour and Radiation Oncology Groups; National Cancer Institute of Canada Clinical Trials Group., 2009. Effects of radiotherapy with concomitant and adjuvant temozolomide versus radiotherapy alone on survival in glioblastoma in a randomised phase III study: 5-year analysis of the EORTC-NCIC trial. Lancet Oncol. 10, 459–466.

Subach, B.R., Kondziolka, D., Lunsford, L.D., et al., 1999. Stereotactic radiosurgery in the management of acoustic neuromas associated with neurofibromatosis Type 2. J. Neurosurg. 90, 815–822.

Tyler-Kabara, E., Kondziolka, D., Flickinger, J.C., et al., 2001. Stereotactic radiosurgery for residual neurocytoma. Report of four cases. J. Neurosurg. 95, 879–882.

Ulm, A.J. 3rd, Friedman, W.A., et al., 2005. Radiosurgery in the treatment of malignant gliomas: the University of Florida experience. Neurosurgery 57, 512–517.

van den Bent, M.J., Afra, D., de Witte, O., et al., EORTC Radiotherapy and Brain Tumor Groups and the UK Medical Research Council., 2005. Long-term efficacy of early versus delayed radiotherapy for low-grade astrocytoma and oligodendroglioma in adults: the EORTC 22845 randomised trial. Lancet 366, 985–990.

Walker, M.D., Alexander, E. Jr., Hunt, W.E., et al., 1978. Evaluation of BCNU and/or radiotherapy in the treatment of anaplastic gliomas. A cooperative clinical trial. J. Neurosurg. 49, 333–343.

Wallner, K.E., Galicich, J.H., Krol, G., et al., 1989. Patterns of failure following treatment for glioblastoma multiforme and anaplastic astrocytoma. Int. J. Radiat Oncol. Biol. Phys. 16, 1405–1409.

Witham, T.F., Okada, H., Fellows, W., et al., 2005. The characterization of tumor apoptosis after experimental radiosurgery. Stereotact Funct. Neurosurg. 83, 17–24.

Clinical trials and chemotherapy

Nader Pouratian, Christopher P. Cifarelli,
Mark E. Shaffrey, and David Schiff

Introduction

The armamentarium for treating brain tumors is growing rapidly, including radiation (both fractionated and stereotactic), chemotherapy, immunotherapy, gene therapy, biological therapies, and surgical resection (each addressed individually in separate chapters). Because of the abundance of options and numerous caveats that are specific to brain tumors, defining optimal management is challenging. The challenge is exacerbated by the relatively low incidence of brain tumors compared with tumors in other parts of the body, making it difficult to conduct large-scale clinical trials.

Despite these challenges, clinical trials have been critical for defining the efficacy of the few widely accepted treatment paradigms for brain tumors. For example, Patchell et al (1990) clearly identified a beneficial role for surgical resection of solitary brain metastases in a landmark Phase III clinical trial in 1990. Likewise, Stupp et al (2005) revolutionized the management of glioblastoma when they reported the benefits of combined temozolomide and radiation therapy over radiation therapy alone in a phase III clinical trial. These and other clinical trials discussed in this chapter provide definitive evidence of treatments that should and indeed have changed the management of brain tumors. This is in stark contrast to results of institutional series that must always be interpreted with caution because of their retrospective nature and significant biases (especially selection bias).

In this chapter, we review the critical components of clinical trials including a detailed discussion of the specific challenges and limitations one must be aware of when conducting each phase of clinical trials in patients with brain tumors. Subsequently, we review the specific challenges and considerations of conducting brain tumors clinical trials for chemotherapy and surgical intervention, highlighting the contribution of some of the most significant trials in each of these areas. Finally, we briefly address the increasingly important move towards standardization of reporting of clinical trials and the need for multi-institutional and international collaboration for the successful implementation of brain tumor clinical trials.

Clinical trials design

Clinical trials have traditionally been conducted in three phases (Table 16.1). The primary objective of phase I trials is to determine treatment-related toxicities and the maximally tolerated dose (MTD) or optimal dose. Although not powered or intended to determine efficacy, many often analyze patient outcomes as a secondary outcome measure.

The primary objective of phase II trials is to determine the preliminary efficacy of the treatment in question, usually in a small sample of 40–50 patients using the doses determined in phase I trials. Phase II trials are often open-labeled and single arm in design and are therefore not conclusive for efficacy. The randomized phase II design is also becoming increasingly popular. In either case, identifying a sufficient 'response rate' provides justification to proceed to a larger phase III trial. Because more patients are enrolled in phase II than phase I trials, toxicity is often re-evaluated as a secondary outcome measure. Phase III trials aim to confirm results of phase II trials in a larger series of patients or to modify an established regimen (e.g., a different dosing regimen). These trials are usually blinded and randomize patients to either a 'treatment' or 'control' group. Primary and secondary outcome measures and the proposed statistical analyses must be predefined.

Clinical trials in brain tumor patients, especially chemotherapy clinical trials, require special considerations because of the heterogeneity of the population treated, the relatively small number of brain tumor patients (making sufficient enrollment challenging), potential interactions with regularly prescribed medications that affect hepatic metabolism (e.g., anticonvulsant medications), and limitations imposed by the blood–brain barrier (i.e., question of bioavailability). Methods for controlling for heterogeneity and each phase of clinical trial design are therefore discussed in detail to explore special considerations and limitations for each in patients with brain tumors.

Reducing variability

Controlling for population heterogeneity is a challenge for any clinical trial, which is why well-defined and precise enrollment and exclusion criteria are essential. The heterogeneity of brain tumors, especially that of glioblastoma, is no exception. To minimize the heterogeneity, it is imperative to control for and stratify known prognostic factors (histopathological, chromosomal, and genetic). For example, early studies of 'malignant gliomas' included numerous histopathological entities, including anaplastic astrocytomas, anaplastic oligodendrogliomas, anaplastic oligoastrocytomas, and glioblastoma, which are now well known to have different prognoses based on histopathology alone. Tissue diagnosis and stratification by histopathology is therefore now recognized as critical. Tissue diagnosis is particularly important in trials of tumor recurrence or progression to differentiate tumor progression from radiation-related changes and necrosis that can often masquerade as tumor progression. Moreover, because pathologists can interpret histopathological findings differently, central review of

Table 16.1 Summary of the phases of clinical trials

	Goal	Design	Primary assessment	Secondary assessment	Typical enrollment	Challenges
Phase 0	Demonstrate bioavailability of therapy	Acquire tissue from patients with preoperative exposure to the treatment	Bioavailability and bioactivity of therapeutic agent in resected tumor tissue	–	~10	Necessary prerequisite for novel biological agents who CNS bioavailability is not previously documented
Phase I	Determine treatment-related toxicities and MTD	Non-randomized, open label dose escalation design	Toxicity	Efficacy (OS and PFS)	10–20	Must account for hepatic induction by antiepileptic medications
Phase II	Determine preliminary efficacy	Open label, single-arm design	Preliminary efficacy (e.g., OS, PFS, radiographic response)	Re-evaluation of toxicity; QOL measures	40–50	Selection of appropriate endpoints and surrogate markers of outcome and efficacy
Phase III	Demonstrate unequivocal efficacy or modify an established regimen	Double-blind randomized controlled trial	Efficacy (e.g., OS, PFS, QOL measures)	Other measures of efficacy and QOL	Several hundred	Securing sufficient recruitment, funding, and enrollment for large-scale trial

MTD = maximum tolerated dose; OS = overall survival; PFS = progression-free survival; QOL = quality of life.

histopathology is deemed necessary to avoid introduction of further variability.

Several prognostic classification schemes have been designed to control for heterogeneity. For patients with brain metastases, at least four prognostic indices have been described, including the Radiation Therapy Oncology Group (RTOG) Recursive Partitioning Analysis (RPA) classification, the Score Index for Radiosurgery (SIR), the Brain Score for Brain Mestases (BSBM), and, most recently, the Graded Prognostic Assessment (GPA) (Gaspar et al 1997; Lorenzoni et al 2004; Sperduto et al 2008; Weltman et al 2000). Each predicts prognosis based on various combinations of age, Karnofsky performance status [KPS], primary tumor control, the presence of extracranial metastases, and the number and volume of brain metastases, highlighting the importance of these prognostic factors in stratification and analysis of clinical trials for brain metastases.

For malignant gliomas, the RTOG RPA classification was the first system to systematically control for heterogeneity, providing a classification system that stratifies patients with malignant gliomas with respect to survival (Curran et al 1993; Scott et al 1998). Its power lies in accounting for prognostic factors that are most consistently reported across studies, including tumor grade, age, performance status, and extent of surgical resection. Despite changes in fractionated radiation therapy (XRT) techniques, treatment (including the introduction of temozolomide), and histopathological classification systems since its inception, RPA classification remains a robust predictor of overall survival (Mirimanoff et al 2006). Gorlia et al (2008) described nomograms to predict survival in patients with malignant gliomas that incorporate more recently identified prognostic factors, including XRT with concurrent and adjuvant temozolomide and MGMT promoter methylation status. Likewise, several studies have demonstrated the importance of and impact of chromosomal deletions on patient prognosis, as exemplified by the impact of 1p/19q deletion status on outcomes in patients with anaplastic oligodendrogliomas (Cairncross

et al 1998). It is important therefore to not only stratify patients by historically important prognostic factors but also by emerging molecular, chromosomal, and genetic profiles, such as MGMT promoter methylation status and treatment history.

Phase I trials

Defining toxicity and optimal dosing (which may in fact be distinct from MTD) is fraught with challenges in the brain tumor population because of the difficulty of differentiating between treatment-related and disease-related complications and because the pharmacodynamics, pharmacokinetics, and bioavailability of experimental therapeutics can be influenced by factors (e.g., regularly prescribed medications) that are unique to this population.

In order to facilitate toxicity evaluation, the National Cancer Institute developed the Common Toxicity Criteria (CTC) which outlines the grading of 'adverse' reactions. In the brain tumor population, however, it can be difficult, if not impossible, to determine if an 'adverse' event, particularly a neurological event, truly represents treatment toxicity rather than a disease-related complication. For example, if a patient experiences a seizure while on a chemotherapy trial, this should be considered a grade IV adverse event by CTC criteria, even though the seizure may be due to tumor progression or inadequate anticonvulsant therapy. Other examples of ambiguity may include focal neurological progression or electrolyte abnormalities (e.g., hyponatremia), which are commonly seen as part of the natural history of brain tumor progression. Allocating these events as 'toxicities' may have significant implications for determination of MTD. It is therefore essential that the trial protocol detail in advance how such ambiguous events will be handled.

Determining MTD or optimal dose in brain tumor patients also requires special consideration. Results of phase I trials for other diseases cannot be generalized to the brain tumor population because commonly prescribed enzyme-inducing antiepileptic drugs (EIAEDs) may significantly alter the pharmacokinetics and pharmacodynamics of the investigational therapy and thereby alter the perceived efficacy and toxicity. This was exemplified by a phase II study of paclitaxel in patients with malignant gliomas using doses established for patients with solid tumors; paclitaxel did not result in the expected level or profile of toxicities in brain tumor patients (Prados et al 1996). It was hypothesized that hepatic induction by EIAEDs increased the hepatic clearance and therefore decreased the bioavailability and dose-dependent toxicity of paclitaxel. Chang et al (1998) soon afterwards confirmed the impact of EIAEDs on chemotherapy pharmacokinetics and pharmacodynamics in a phase I trial of paclitaxel for malignant gliomas, stratifying patients by EIAED use. They reported that the dose limiting toxicity of paclitaxel in glioma patients taking EIAEDS was central neurotoxicity rather than myelosuppression, which is the dose-limiting toxicity in patients not on EIAEDs (Chang et al 1998). Since then, several phase I trials have found and confirmed that the toxicity profile of investigational chemotherapeutics can be significantly altered by EIAEDs, including, e.g., tipifarnib (a farnesyl protein transferase inhibitor) and irinotecan (a topoisomerase I inhibitor) (Cloughesy et al 2005; Loghin et al 2007; Prados et al 2004). To account for these potentially significant drug interactions and to preserve resources, the North American Brain Tumor Consortium (NABTC) has modified their clinical trial design template (Chang et al 2008). Before proceeding with phase I pharmacokinetic and toxicity studies in patients receiving EIAEDs, they propose establishing preliminary efficacy in phase II trials in patients not on EIAEDs using established doses from trials in patients with solid tumors.

The design and introduction of molecularly targeted therapies has required even further modifications to the classic design of clinical trials. Scientific advances have made possible the design of therapies targeted to specific aberrant pathways in brain tumor pathogenesis. Bioavailability, biological activity, and efficacy in *in vitro* and xenograft models, however, do not guarantee success in humans with spontaneous tumors. Demonstrating successful entry into the human central nervous system (bioavailability) and biological activity in human brain tumors is therefore considered a necessary prelude to extensive clinical trials. The NABTC therefore introduced the concept of a phase 0 trial. In a phase 0 trial, tissue would be acquired from patients who have had preoperative exposure to the investigational therapy in order to evaluate the agent's bioavailability and biological activity and to determine the optimal biological dose (Chang et al 2008). Ideally, tissue from the same patient could be evaluated with and without exposure to the investigational agent (e.g., in patients undergoing reoperation for recurrent glioma) to demonstrate biological efficacy. The concept of reoperation for the sole purpose of assessing biological activity clearly raises ethical concerns and is not considered standard. Phase 0 trials would not replace the standard phase I dose-escalation trial or toxicity assessment. Clinical trials would only proceed to phase II if the proposed target is successfully modulated and the agent has an acceptable toxicity profile (phase I study) (Chang et al 2008). A similar trend for pretrial investigations has been emerging across multiple oncology disciplines (Booth et al 2008).

Phase II trials

The selection of appropriate and clinically relevant endpoints is vital for phase II trials, because their primary goal is to demonstrate preliminary clinical efficacy and provide justification for phase III trials. Because outcomes are often compared to historical controls, validated and meaningful outcomes measures that can be compared to that of other studies must be used to ensure that potential benefits are not overlooked due to the inevitable introduction of selection bias.

The most frequently reported endpoints are survival (including overall [OS] and progression free [PFS]), radiographic response, and, more recently, quality-of-life measures. Measures of OS and PFS include estimates of median survival (e.g., Kaplan–Meier methods) or determination of survival at a set time (e.g., 1, 2, or 5-year OS; the latter survival estimate allows for more timely completion of studies, especially in the case of some brain tumors like low-grade gliomas (LGG) that can have median survival of >10 years). As one might suspect, however, OS is not necessarily the only or most useful measure of efficacy. For example, in a study comparing the efficacy of postoperative XRT after surgical resection of single brain metastases, Patchell et al (1998) found that while OS was not affected by postoperative XRT, those receiving XRT experienced fewer intracranial recurrences and were less likely to die of neurological causes. There has been an increased awareness that increasing OS without maintaining quality-of-life (QOL) is not desirable. Measuring PFS is therefore likely as important as OS. Conveniently, 6-month PFS has repeatedly been shown to be an important marker (and surrogate measure) of OS (Lamborn et al 2008). Other QOL endpoints are also being considered more commonly for phase II and III trials (Corn et al 2008; Mauer et al 2007; Taphoorn et al 2007). These studies highlight the fact that QOL issues can be significant, including neurocognitive decline and changes in daily function (e.g., nausea, vomiting, somnolence), and may negate the other benefits of intervention. Some of the validated measures of neurocognition and QOL for brain tumor patients include the Mini-Mental Status Examination (MMSE), EORTC Quality of Life Questionnaire C30 (QLQ-C30), EORTC QLQ-Brain Module (QLQ-BN20), Spitzer Quality of Life Index (SQLI), and Functional Assessment of Cancer Therapy-Brain-specific (FACT-Br) testing (Corn et al 2008; Efficace & Bottomley 2002; Li et al 2008; Moinpour et al 2000; Osoba et al 1996).

In many studies, radiographic response is measured as a surrogate marker of outcome and efficacy. Unfortunately, radiographic responses and symptom assessment are often imprecise measures of tumor burden and drug efficacy. In order to standardize the evaluation and reporting of radiographic responses, Macdonald et al (1990) described an explicit scheme for classifying radiographic responses, including complete responses (CR), partial responses (PR), stable disease (SD) and progressive disease (PD). These criteria, which are based on contrast enhancement on CT and MR, standardized the reporting of radiographic responses, making inter-trial comparisons more reliable and meaningful. Despite standardization, it remains unclear what constitutes a 'response', especially when SD may be the expectation rather than CR or PR. In contrast, is SD a response in patients with LGG in whom radiographic progression is not expected in the short term? The Macdonald criteria are also limited by reliance on contrast enhancement, despite it being well known that disease infiltrates beyond the field of enhancement. Moreover, the significance of contrast enhancement is increasingly questionable in an era when adjuvant therapies can masquerade as tumor progression or regression, such as radiation-induced changes and necrosis, temozolomide-induced 'pseudo-progression', and the illusion of glioma regression with VEGF-inhibitors. To address these shortcomings, the Response Assessment in Neuro-Oncology Working Group recently published revised criteria for the measurement of disease burden (both enhancing and non-enhancing components) and the evaluation of radiographic responses, allowing and accounting for multifocal and cystic disease and potential treatment-related radiographic changes (Wen et al 2010). In place of standard imaging, several investigators are focusing on more sophisticated imaging mechanisms including PET, SPECT, and MR spectroscopy and perfusion to assess and predict tumor control and patient survival (Hirai et al 2008; Jenkinson et al 2007; Schlemmer et al 2002; Thompson et al 1999).

The NABTC has modified its clinical trial template to also require tissue availability from all patients included in trials to assess for targets and biomarkers associated with clinical efficacy. After conducting initial phase II trials in a 'general' tumor population, a second phase II study would be conducted in an 'enriched population' based on target presence and biomarkers, in which the activity of targeted biological and molecular agents could be assessed.

Phase III trials

Like phase II trials, selection of appropriate and clinically meaningful endpoints is critical for phase III trials. However, phase III trials face additional challenges, including recruiting sufficient enrollment, proper randomization, and, ideally, double-blinded design, all of which are further complicated in the brain tumor population. Because phase III trials aim to identify a statistically and clinically significant difference between patients randomized to one of at least two arms, power calculations require enrollment of hundreds of patients. Such recruitment is difficult in light of the relatively low incidence of brain tumors and the need to enroll only patients who meet highly stringent selection criteria. Successful and rapid accrual therefore requires multi-institutional and possibly international cooperation, as was seen in the Stupp trial, which established the efficacy of XRT with concurrent and adjuvant temozolomide (Stupp et al 2005). As with other oncology trials, randomization, a critical element for phase III trials, can be difficult in patients with brain tumors, especially when there is a preconceived notion of the superiority of an established therapeutic approach. For example, while a preponderance of retrospective and institutional studies favor surgical resection for low-grade gliomas (LGGs), a prospective randomized trial has not been conducted because of ethical concerns that a beneficial treatment may be withheld from patients. Likewise, blinding patients and caretakers to investigational therapies can be difficult, if not impossible, in clinical trials for brain tumors, especially those that involve radiation therapy (XRT or stereotactic) or surgical interventions. While this unavoidably introduces bias, measures must be taken to reduce this, including use of objective outcome measures and evaluation by blinded reviewers.

Chemotherapy clinical trials

In addition to the general considerations already described for brain tumor clinical trials, chemotherapy clinical trials face additional obstacles. The most important of these are that of ensuring adequate drug delivery while limiting systemic toxicity and overcoming inherent and acquired mechanisms of drug resistance.

Safe and efficacious use of chemotherapeutic agents in the central nervous system (CNS) requires a balance between penetration of the blood–brain barrier (BBB) and avoidance of systemic as well as neurologic toxicity. CNS bioavailability of chemotherapeutic compounds is largely a function of the BBB, with small non-polar lipophilic agents preferentially passing from the vascular space, through endothelial tight junctions, and into target tissues. Clinically, several trials have specifically focused on routes of delivery, directly comparing intravenous (IV), intra-arterial (IA), and intraparenchymal (interstitial) routes.

IV dosing has the advantage of ease of administration with reasonably high doses that avoid first pass hepatic metabolism but is theoretically limited by side-effects of the systemic exposure of cytotoxic agents. Alternatively, the IA route allows for high-dose, vessel-specific administration of chemotherapy via selective angiographic localization. Potential hazards associated with IA treatment include vessel injury, vasospasm and leukoencephalopathy, although some of these effects may be compound specific (Rosenblum et al 1989; Tsuboi et al 1995). Despite theoretical advantages of IA therapy, clinical trials to date have failed to demonstrate a clinical advantage of IA over IV administration. For example, Kochi et al (2000) prospectively compared nimustine (ACNU) dosing via IV vs IA routes for newly diagnosed glioblastoma. The IA dosing was both safe and equally efficacious compared with IV administration, but did not provide a survival advantage (Kochii et al 2000). Additional phase III studies of IA ACNU have confirmed these findings with increased drug delivery but no increase in PFS (Imbesi et al 2006).

Extravascular approaches to chemotherapy delivery attempt to circumnavigate the issue of BBB penetration by directly implanting chemotherapeutic agents at the site of tumor resection (i.e., interstitial or intraparenchymal therapy). In fact, the first successful phase III chemotherapy clinical trial for glioblastoma was with Carmustine (BCNU) wafers (Gliadel®) that were implanted following presumed gross total resection of high-grade gliomas; Valtonen et al (1997) demonstrated a survival advantage over resection alone. Initial follow-up studies reported increased morbidity with Gliadel wafers, but a long-term analysis of 288 patients receiving Gliadel over 10 years at a single institution failed to demonstrate any increased morbidity, including infection, cyst formation, or malignant edema (Attenello et al 2008). This type and duration of follow-up highlights the fact that phase I clinical trials may not capture the entire profile of toxicities and that long-term toxicity (and efficacy) should continue to be evaluated even after conclusion of phase I trials.

Convection enhanced delivery (CED) has also emerged as a viable means of direct implantation of therapeutic agents, taking advantage of the ability of bulk flow via continuous infusion under positive pressure to provide a homogenous high concentration of large molecules within the tumor site (Lonser et al 2002). This approach has been undertaken with Cintredekin Besudotox (Interleukin-13-PE38QQR) with promising early results based on low levels of dose-limited toxicities. However, the follow-up phase III trial, called PRECISE for Phase III Randomized Evaluation of Convection Enhanced Delivery of IL13-PE38QQR, failed to show a benefit compared to Gliadel therapy (data not yet published). Further clinical trials will be essential to determine whether CED can provide superior drug delivery, tumor control, and patient outcomes in selected populations or with different therapeutic regimens (Tanner et al 2007; Vogelbaum et al 2007).

To increase CNS bioavailability, some have focused on devising strategies to destabilize the BBB and therefore make it more permeable to chemotherapeutics. Strategies include concurrent administration of intra-arterial mannitol or bradykinin with both intravenous and intra-arterial chemotherapeutic agents; BBB disruption therapy is thought to promote increased drug delivery without a significant increase in morbidity (Hall et al 2006; Macnealy et al 2008). Unfortunately, no study has been able to utilize this approach to directly show increased drug tumor delivery, nor have any of these small trials shown a significant improvement in survival in comparison to control treatment. Larger studies are currently underway. In addition to tight junctions that are well-known to impede drug delivery through the BBB, there are inherent and inducible mechanisms of reducing BBB permeability to chemotherapeutics. For example, ATP-binding cassette (ABC) efflux transporters and cytochrome P-450 enzyme systems have both been shown to be expressed in the endothelial cells of the BBB (Dauchy et al 2008). Among the ABC transporters, P-glycoprotein and the multi-drug resistance-related protein (MRP1) are expressed by gliomas, indicating multiple layers of redundancy for drug metabolism and cellular efflux (de Faria et al 2008).

Besides issues of drug delivery, investigators need to be cognizant of mechanisms of drug- and treatment-resistance. Interestingly, cross-resistance can occur between drugs that do not share a common primary target or bear any structural similarity, thus advancing the notion of upregulation of generalized resistance mechanisms (Gottesman & Pastan 1993). Perhaps the best studied chemoresistance mechanism from a clinical perspective is the role of O^6-methylguanine methyltransferase (MGMT) in resistance of gliomas to alkylating agents, such as temozolomide, that create persistent O^6-methylguanine adducts. The presence of persistent adducts forces the DNA repair machinery into futile cycling until p53-mediated apoptosis induces cell-death. Gene silencing of the MGMT repair protein via promoter methylation has been show to correlate with improved outcome in high-grade glioma patients treated with temozolomide (Hegi et al 2005). This treatment resistance factor has been deemed so important that there has been a call to require stratification by MGMT methylation status in all future clinical trials of glioblastoma (Gorlia et al 2008). Recent development of an anti-MGMT monoclonal antibody has made it possible to assess MGMT status on the basis of immunocytochemistry, although early attempts to correlate this data with clinical outcome have proven to be largely unsuccessful (Preusser et al 2008).

The recent advances in the identification of tumor progenitor cells within glioblastoma tumors add yet another layer of complexity with regard to considerations of chemoresistance. Using microarray analysis of genetic markers in glioblastoma-derived neurosphere cell populations, Murat et al (2008) have identified several upregulated HOX gene clusters, including the cell-cycle checkpoint gene GADD45G, suggesting enhanced DNA repair mechanisms in tumor progenitor cells. Moreover, the DNA damage induced by ionizing radiation in tumor progenitor cells expressing prominin-1 (CD133) is efficiently repaired via cell cycle checkpoint kinases, Chk1 and Chk2, thereby confirming another mechanism of treatment resistance in glioma management (Bao et al 2006).

Examples of significant chemotherapy trials

Gliomas

Prior to the advent of effective chemotherapeutic agents, surgical resection along with palliative radiotherapy was the mainstay of treatment for high-grade gliomas. Since that time, several landmark trials have expanded the current chemotherapeutic armamentarium for gliomas to include alkylating agents, like temozolomide, and nitrosoureas, like carmustine (BCNU).

In a randomized multi-center phase II trial, Yung et al (2000) effectively compared the PFS and safety in patients with recurrent high-grade glioblastomas treated with temozolomide vs procarbazine (PCB). Both PFS and 6-month OS were significantly improved in the temozolomide groups, with the latter metric being 60% with temozolomide vs 44% for PCB (Yung et al 2000). These data prompted further study of temozolomide, especially in management of newly diagnosed glioblastoma and in conjunction with radiotherapy. Stupp et al (2005) reported a statistically significant increase in 2-year OS (26.5%) in the temozolomide plus radiotherapy group compared with conventional radiotherapy alone (10.4%), thus serving as the basis for current glioma management in the majority of patients worldwide.

The use of BCNU-impregnated wafers in glioma treatment has also been the subject of several large multi-center trials to determine both safety and short-term/long-term efficacy. Currently employed as an interstitial agent with delivery via passive diffusion from implanted polymer-based wafers, the first prospective, randomized double-blind study of carmustine vs placebo found that the treatment group had a median survival time of 58 weeks from surgical intervention vs approximately 40 weeks in the control group (Valtonen et al 1997). Retrospective analysis of combination therapy, using carmustine wafers along with radiation and temozolomide has also been performed, with patients receiving the combination therapy demonstrating a median survival of 21 months without increased perioperative morbidity (McGirt et al 2009). Unfortunately, the use of Gliadel in this study was limited to cases where the neurosurgeon determined there to be a gross total resection, making it impossible to compare extent of resection with the afore-mentioned treatment arms and further confounding these results. Moreover, the study does not control for MGMT promoter methylation status, possibly overlooking an important subset of patients in whom combination treatment may be efficacious. Further prospective trials will be needed to adequately assess this multimodal approach.

Primary central nervous system lymphoma (PCNSL)

The incidence of PCNSL and associated deaths has increased over the past 20 years, prompting many groups to reassess treatment paradigms (Panageas et al 2005). Early interventions consisting of whole brain radiotherapy and chemotherapeutic agents were generally palliative, with a median expected survival of 12–18 months and a 2-year survival below 5%, as presented by the Radiation Therapy Oncology Group (RTOG-8315) (Nelson et al 1992). In the first multi-center trial examining the role of combination high-dose intrathecal methotrexate with whole brain radiation, DeAngelis et al (2002) were able to demonstrate a 94% response rate, with a median PFS of 24 months and an overall median survival of 36.9 months. Unfortunately, up to 15% of treatment arm patients experienced severe delayed drug related neurotoxicity. Follow-up studies have incorporated the prospective use of additional agents, including rituximab, procarbazine and vincristine, along with reduced dosing of whole brain radiation and have documented decreased cognitive deficits (Correa et al 2009). This treatment paradigm has evolved as a standard protocol, thereby placing patients on an initial chemotherapeutic regimen in an attempt to limit radiation associated adverse effects. Despite increasing incidence, the rarity of PCNSL has ensured that almost all trials are pilot/phase II, highlighting one of the primary challenges of clinical trials for brain tumors: sufficient enrollment.

Medulloblastoma and primitive neuroectodermal tumors (PNETs)

In the pediatric population, current management of medulloblastoma and PNETs incorporates chemotherapeutic agents along with craniospinal radiation. In the largest clinical trial of pediatric patients with high-stage medulloblastoma, Zeltzer et al (1999) demonstrated an advantage of concurrent vincristine and radiation followed by post-radiation VCP (vincristine, CCNU, and prednisone) compared with traditional '8-in-1' therapy, which was the prior standard of care, with 5-year PFS of $63 \pm 5\%$ and $45 \pm 5\%$, respectively (Zeltzer et al 1999). Subsequent studies from the UK Children's Cancer Study Group (UKCCSG) have confirmed the efficacy of concurrent radiation and several agents, including vincristine, etoposide, carboplatin and cyclophosphamide for PNETs, including refractory and metastatic medulloblastoma (Taylor et al 2005). In an analysis of 68 patients treated between 1992 and 2000, improved PFS was only seen in patients with lesions confined to the infratentorial region and when the radiation and chemotherapy were administered in temporal proximity to each other and surgical resection (at least within 110 days) (Taylor et al 2005). Unfortunately, in lesions with supratentorial or spinal metastases, no significant improvement in survival could be identified compared with the radiation and surgery group, prompting the search for additional biological therapies.

Significant evidence exists for the involvement of the Ras oncogene in several pediatric brain tumors, including recurrent high-grade glioma, medulloblastoma and PNETs (Gerosa et al 1989; MacDonald et al 2001). A key component in the Ras pathway is the post-translational farnesylation of the Ras protein. A prospective study of tipifarnib, a potent inhibitor of farnesyl transferase was found to be well tolerated in pediatric patients with recurrent medulloblastomas and PNETs, but ineffective as a single agent. Further trials using a multimodal approach will be necessary (Fouladi et al 2007).

Surgical clinical trials

As the decades pass since the first operations on brain tumors, one would expect that the role of surgery in the treatment of CNS malignancies would be extraordinarily clear. As technology to assist surgeons has advanced with improvements in imaging, mapping, visualization and guidance, it is a reasonable expectation that proof of surgical efficacy and extent of surgical resection will follow. However, there is still a relative lack of Class I data that justify the morbidity and expense of surgical resection for many CNS tumors. This relative paucity of data often speaks to the difficulties encountered in the design of effective clinical trials that offer clinical equipoise, reasonable accrual timeframes and justification of expense. A few trials that have greatly impacted the way patients are surgically treated will be highlighted in addition to some areas where there are still remains a lack of general consensus and quality data.

Perhaps the highest quality data from a clinical trial that demonstrated surgical efficacy is for the surgical resection of solitary brain metastases. Although nearly 20 years since publication, this trial persists as a landmark for surgical clinical trials of brain tumors. In 1990, Patchell et al randomized 48 patients with solitary brain metastases to treatment with surgery and WBRT (25 patients) and compared this to a cohort of patients treated with WBRT alone (23 patients). Patients were evaluated for local recurrence and survival. This study demonstrated that the addition of surgery to WBRT reduced the local recurrence rate in these patients from 52% to 20% ($p < 0.02$). The length of survival was improved in the surgical group from 15 to 40 weeks ($p < 0.01$). Patients in the surgery and WBRT arm also remained functionally independent for a longer period of time, 38 weeks compared vs 8 weeks ($p < 0.005$). This study demonstrated a clear benefit to adding surgery to WBRT. The patients treated with surgery lived longer, had fewer local recurrences and had a better quality of life as determined by a longer time of functional independence. This was an ideal surgical trial. The endpoint was clear, the number of patients needed to accrue was relatively small, the treatment effect was large and the results were definitive.

Since the time of the publication of Patchell's study in 1990, there have been surprisingly few studies that have added to our knowledge base with respect to the surgical treatment of metastatic brain disease. It is now known through subsequent studies that control of the primary and systemic disease plays a critical role in the determination of survival following surgical treatment. In fact, in the clinical trial setting, the benefit of surgery can be eliminated if the patient population has a high rate of systemic disease progression (Mintz et al 1996; Shaffrey et al 2004). There still remains notable uncertainty with respect to surgical treatment of multiple metastases and recurrent solitary metastases. However, in patients who have symptomatic, surgically accessible solitary metastases (regardless of the primary) and who are RPA Class I (KPS ≥70, age ≤65 years, controlled primary tumor), surgical treatment has been proven a mainstay of therapy.

Although there is little doubt that the surgical treatment of glioblastoma in symptomatic patients can extend survival, the question of the relative impact of the extent of resection on survival is somewhat less clear. Several studies fail to identify a difference in survival based on extent of resection. There have been substantial limitations in the studies to assess the extent of resection of glioblastoma on survival. In general, these studies have not been prospective or randomized. Often, these surgical studies have exhibited significant selection bias by including those patients in surgical cohorts who are most likely to do well with surgical treatment (most favorable location, functional status, and performance status). In the past, there have not been standardized means of assessment of the extent of resection, often using a surgeon's intraoperative assessment of extent of resection.

Simpson et al (1993) published the results of a study on the influence of tumor site, size and the extent of resection on the survival of patients with glioblastoma. The study included 645 patients that were accrued through three consecutive randomized RTOG trials employing surgery and irradiation plus or minus chemotherapy. In each instance, the therapeutic question did not have an impact on survival; thus, the data could be summarized and analyzed independently of the treatment arms. Patients undergoing complete resection had a median survival of 11.3 months as compared with 6.6 months for biopsy only. However, there was also a significant difference in median survival for patients that had subtotal resection vs biopsy only (10.4 vs 6.6 months). Patients with frontal lobe tumors fared the best. In a Cox multivariate model, age <40, high KPS, complete tumor resection and frontal lobe location influenced outcome most favorably. The assessment of the extent of resection was performed by either CT scan or MRI, which is less than ideal. The study is further limited by having analyzed outcomes and factors that were not determined prior to the initiation of the original trials, which is a prerequisite for a properly conducted phase III trial. Despite the retrospective analysis of the endpoints, this study is classified as Class II due to the prospective nature of the data collection.

Perhaps the most highly publicized series on the surgical resection of glioblastoma was that published by Lacroix and colleagues in 2001. This study demonstrated a significant increase in survival when 98% or more of the enhancing disease of a glioblastoma was resected ($p = 0.02$) (Lacroix et al 2001). Fewer than 50% of the patients were able to achieve a 98% or greater resection. The positive attributes of this study included a sizable patient population ($n = 416$) and analysis of pre- and postoperative MRI studies. However, the study still suffered from the limitations of a retrospective study and probable selection bias; <10% of patients had tumors of the posterior fossa or deep gray matter. Despite the enormous influence of this study, ultimately it represents Class III data.

In 2006, Stummer and colleagues published results of a surgical clinical trial, the primary intent of which was to evaluate the extent of resection of glioblastoma using an enhanced fluorescence visualization technique with the injection of 5-ALA and the use of an UV filter on the operating microscope. Randomization of 270 patients occurred between cohorts where glioblastoma resection was performed with or without 5-ALA. Complete resection of the tumor occurred in 65% of the patients using 5-ALA, and only in 29% of the control group ($p < 0.0001$). As a secondary endpoint, survival was analyzed as well. There was a significant improvement in the 6-month progression free survival rate for the 5-ALA group 41% vs 21% ($p = 0.0003$). This study represents Class I data for the use of 5-ALA to improve the complete resection rate of glioblastoma and class II data for the correlation of extent of resection with survival because survival was not a predetermined primary endpoint (Stummer et al 2008).

The tumors that most underscore the struggle to design adequate surgical clinical trials for brain tumors are the low-grade gliomas. Although surgery has been a foundation in the diagnosis and treatment of these neoplasms, there remains no clear consensus regarding the role of extent of resection in overall survival. This quandary is not unique to surgical treatment alone as the efficacy of many interventions, such as fractionated radiotherapy and chemotherapy, struggle for the same validation for this diagnosis. There are many real and potential benefits to surgical resection of low-grade gliomas: cytoreduction, reduction of mass effect, improvement of neurological deficits, improvement of seizure control, and reduction of sampling error as compared to biopsy. A definitive answer with regard to prolongation of survival with tumor resection is still not known, although there is gestalt from a body of Class III evidence which leads one to believe that some evidence favors extensive tumor resection (Sanai & Berger 2008).

Planning a surgical trial to compare conservative to extensive surgical treatment is a complicated problem that is fraught with challenges. First, given the body of known literature, there are ethical concerns with regard to randomization of low-grade glioma patients to a non-surgical treatment arm; such a trial was rejected in concept phase by the American College of Surgeons Oncology Group. Thus, a trial would likely have to be designed with a prospective cohort construction. Such a trial would require enrollment of 1100 patients and would have to be observed for at least 10 years (Pouratian et al 2007). Statistical analysis would have to take into account such variables as patient age, tumor size, tumor location, molecular genetics and a wide range of potential treatment variables, including radiation and chemotherapy. The time for accrual and expense of this trial would be phenomenal, even without considerations for central tumor pathological review and central film review. Such a trial would be feasible, but the resources and commitment are currently being spent on more fertile and less hostile ground.

Reporting of clinical trials

No matter how well a clinical trial is constructed and conducted, and regardless of how exciting the results, proper reporting of the trial results is mandatory for proper interpretation. To permit critical appraisal of trials and to promote the quality of trials, standardized guidelines for the careful reporting of the results of randomized controlled trials (i.e., phase III trials) have been developed and the pitfalls of not adhering to these have been clearly outlined (Altman et al 2001). These guidelines are referred to as the CONSORT (Consolidated Standards of Reporting Trials) criteria. The adoption and endorsement of CONSORT criteria for randomized trials has been shown to improve with quality of reports of RCTs (Moher et al 2001).

The great majority of neurooncology trials represent phase I and II efforts. Neurooncology trials have numerous issues and features that differentiate them from protocols for other malignancies, including issues of anticonvulsant effects on chemotherapy metabolism, corticosteroids confounding radiographic interpretation, and the phenomena of postoperative enhancement and pseudo-progression mimicking tumor, to name a few. A respected group of neurooncologists has therefore recently put together guidelines for optimal reporting of phase I and II medical and surgical clinical trials (Chang et al 2007; Chang et al 2005). These guidelines, given the acronym GNOSIS (Guidelines for Neuro-Oncology: Standards for Investigational Studies), are also extremely useful in assisting an investigator designing a clinical therapeutic protocol. These criteria include a checklist of components necessary for proper reporting of clinical trials, including details of title, abstract, introduction, methods (including eligibility criteria and treatment plans), results (including patient flow, data analysis, and outcomes), discussion, and acknowledgements.

To facilitate the communication and documentation of ongoing clinical trials, the National Institutes of Health provide an online registry of ongoing trials which can be easily searched at http:// www.clinicaltrials.gov.

Benefits of collaboration

Primary brain tumors comprise <1.5% of all cancers, and even relatively common sub-types such as glioblastoma present a challenge to timely accrual to large clinical trials. To identify clinically meaningful treatment effects, studies of >500 patients are often required. Such large studies are often conducted under the auspices of government funded cooperative groups. In North America, these groups include the Radiation Therapy Oncology Group (RTOG), Eastern Cooperative Oncology Group (ECOG), North Central Cancer Treatment Group (NCCTG), and National Cancer Institute of Canada (NCIC). These cooperative groups frequently co-endorse each other's clinical trial protocols in order to avoid wasting valuable resources (both monetary and subjects) and competing for accrual of small patient populations. In Europe, the European Organisation for Research and Treatment of Cancer (EORTC) is the principal cooperative group. Recent years have highlighted the benefits of

multi-institutional and multi-national collaboration. The pivotal phase III trial demonstrating the benefit of adding temozolomide to radiotherapy for glioblastoma was a joint effort between EORTC and NCIC; this trial required only 20 months to enroll 573 patients (Stupp et al 2005). More recently, cooperation among RTOG, EORTC, NCIC and NCCTG enabled RTOG 0525, a phase III trial exploring benefit of dose-dense temozolomide in newly diagnosed glioblastoma, to enroll almost 1200 patients in <2.5 years – a particularly remarkable rate considering patients undergoing stereotactic biopsy for diagnosis were excluded. Similar international collaborations are planned for phase III trials in 1p/19q-co-deleted anaplastic gliomas (NCCTG N0577) and non-co-deleted anaplastic gliomas (EORTC CATNON study).

Conclusion

The framework for multi-institutional and international cooperation to address significant questions with respect to the optimal treatment of brain tumors has now been established. With the significant advances in the genetics and molecular pathogenesis of brain tumors, the neurooncology community has never been better equipped to use clinical trials to more definitively delineate the role of various treatment strategies for all different types of brain tumors. Given this opportunity, we must remain cognizant of the limitations and challenges that are specific to the brain tumor patient population and the needs to conduct and report the results of clinical trials in a meticulous manner. More importantly, we must be aware of ethical considerations that may deem clinical trials as unsuitable for evaluating the efficacy of some treatment strategies. Despite these considerations, given the state of our knowledge, technology, and international cooperation, it seems likely that clinical trials will provide answers for the neurooncology community at an accelerated pace.

REFERENCES
- Altman, D.G., Schulz, K.F., Moher, D., et al., 2001. The revised CONSORT statement for reporting randomized trials: explanation and elaboration. Ann. Intern. Med. 134 (8), 663–694.
Attenello, F.J., Mukherjee, D., Datoo, G., et al., 2008. Use of Gliadel (BCNU) wafer in the surgical treatment of malignant glioma: a 10-year institutional experience. Ann. Surg. Oncol. 15 (10), 2887–2893.
Bao, S., Wu, Q., McLendon, R.E., et al., 2006. Glioma stem cells promote radioresistance by preferential activation of the DNA damage response. Nature 444 (7120), 756–760.
Booth, C.M., Calvert, A.H., Giaccone, G., et al., 2008. Endpoints and other considerations in phase I studies of targeted anticancer therapy: recommendations from the task force on Methodology for the Development of Innovative Cancer Therapies (MDICT). Eur. J. Cancer 44 (1), 19–24.
Cairncross, J.G., Ueki, K., Zlatescu, M.C., et al., 1998. Specific genetic predictors of chemotherapeutic response and survival in patients with anaplastic oligodendrogliomas. J. Natl. Cancer Inst. 90 (19), 1473–1479.
- Chang, S., Vogelbaum, M., Lang, F.F., et al., 2007. GNOSIS: guidelines for neuro-oncology: standards for investigational studies – reporting of surgically based therapeutic clinical trials. J. Neurooncol. 82 (2), 211–220.
- Chang, S.M., Kuhn, J.G., Rizzo, J., et al., 1998. Phase I study of paclitaxel in patients with recurrent malignant glioma: a North American Brain Tumor Consortium report. J. Clin. Oncol. 16 (6), 2188–2194.

• **Chang, S.M., Lamborn, K.R., Kuhn, J.G., et al.**, 2008. Neurooncology clinical trial design for targeted therapies: lessons learned from the North American Brain Tumor Consortium. Neuro. Oncol. 10 (4), 631–642.

• **Chang, S.M., Reynolds, S.L., Butowski, N., et al.**, 2005. GNOSIS: guidelines for neuro-oncology: standards for investigational studies-reporting of phase 1 and phase 2 clinical trials. Neuro. Oncol. 7 (4), 425–434.

Cloughesy, T.F., Kuhn, J., Robins, H.I., et al., 2005. Phase I trial of tipifarnib in patients with recurrent malignant glioma taking enzyme-inducing antiepileptic drugs: a North American Brain Tumor Consortium Study. J. Clin. Oncol. 23 (27), 6647–6656.

Corn, B W, Moughan, J., Knisely, J.P. et al., 2008. Prospective evaluation of quality of life and neurocognitive effects in patients with multiple brain metastases receiving whole-brain radiotherapy with or without thalidomide on Radiation Therapy Oncology Group (RTOG) trial 0118. Int. J. Radiat. Oncol. Biol. Phys. 71 (1), 71–78.

Correa, D.D., Rocco-Donovan, M., Deangelis, L.M., et al., 2009. Prospective cognitive follow-up in primary CNS lymphoma patients treated with chemotherapy and reduced-dose radiotherapy. J. Neurooncol. 91 (3), 315–321.

• **Curran, W.J., Jr., Scott, C.B., Horton, J., et al.**, 1993. Recursive partitioning analysis of prognostic factors in three Radiation Therapy Oncology Group malignant glioma trials. J. Natl. Cancer Inst. 85 (9), 704–710.

Dauchy, S., Dutheil, F., Weaver, R.J., et al., 2008. ABC transporters, cytochromes P450 and their main transcription factors: expression at the human blood-brain barrier. J. Neurochem. 107 (6), 1518–1528.

de Faria, G.P., de Oliveira, J.A., de Oliveira, J.G., et al., 2008. Differences in the expression pattern of P-glycoprotein and MRP1 in low-grade and high-grade gliomas. Cancer Invest 26 (9), 883–889.

DeAngelis, L.M., Seiferheld, W., Schold, S.C., et al., 2002. Combination chemotherapy and radiotherapy for primary central nervous system lymphoma: Radiation Therapy Oncology Group Study 93–10. J. Clin. Oncol. 20 (24), 4643–4648.

Efficace, F., Bottomley, A., 2002. Health related quality of life assessment methodology and reported outcomes in randomised controlled trials of primary brain cancer patients. Eur. J. Cancer 38 (14), 1824–1831.

Fouladi, M., Nicholson, H.S., Zhou, T., et al., 2007. A phase II study of the farnesyl transferase inhibitor, tipifarnib, in children with recurrent or progressive high-grade glioma, medulloblastoma/primitive neuroectodermal tumor, or brainstem glioma: a Children's Oncology Group study. Cancer 110 (11), 2535–2541.

Gaspar, L., Scott, C., Rotman, M., et al., 1997. Recursive partitioning analysis (RPA) of prognostic factors in three Radiation Therapy Oncology Group (RTOG) brain metastases trials. Int. J. Radiat. Oncol. Biol. Phys. 37 (4), 745–751.

Gerosa, M.A., Talarico, D., Fognani, C., et al., 1989. Overexpression of N-ras oncogene and epidermal growth factor receptor gene in human glioblastomas. J. Natl. Cancer Inst. 81 (1), 63–67.

• **Gorlia, T., van den Bent, M.J., Hegi, M.E., et al.**, 2008. Nomograms for predicting survival of patients with newly diagnosed glioblastoma: prognostic factor analysis of EORTC and NCIC trial 26981–22981/CE.3. Lancet Oncol. 9 (1), 29–38.

Gottesman, M.M., Pastan, I., 1993. Biochemistry of multidrug resistance mediated by the multidrug transporter. Annu. Rev. Biochem. 62, 385–427.

Hall, W.A., Doolittle, N.D., Daman, M., et al., 2006. Osmotic blood-brain barrier disruption chemotherapy for diffuse pontine gliomas. J. Neurooncol. 77 (3), 279–284.

Hegi, M.E., Diserens, A.C., Gorlia, T., et al., 2005. MGMT gene silencing and benefit from temozolomide in glioblastoma. N. Engl. J. Med. 352 (10), 997–1003.

Hirai, T., Murakami, R., Nakamura, H., et al., 2008. Prognostic value of perfusion MR imaging of high-grade astrocytomas: long-term follow-up study. AJNR Am. J. Neuroradiol. 29 (8), 1505–1510.

Imbesi, F., Marchioni, E., Benericetti E., et al., 2006. A randomized phase III study: comparison between intravenous and intraarterial ACNU administration in newly diagnosed primary glioblastomas. Anticancer Res. 26 (1B), 553–558.

Jenkinson, M.D., Du Plessis, D.G., Walker, C., et al., 2007. Advanced MRI in the management of adult gliomas. Br. J. Neurosurg. 21 (6), 550–561.

Kochii, M., Kitamura, I., Goto, T., et al., 2000. Randomized comparison of intra-arterial versus intravenous infusion of ACNU for newly diagnosed patients with glioblastoma. J. Neurooncol. 49 (1), 63–70.

• **Lacroix, M., Abi-Said, D., Fourney, D.R., et al.**, 2001. A multivariate analysis of 416 patients with glioblastoma multiforme: prognosis, extent of resection, and survival. J. Neurosurg. 95 (2), 190–198.

Lamborn, K.R., Yung, W.K., Chang, S.M., et al., 2008. Progression-free survival: an important end point in evaluating therapy for recurrent high-grade gliomas. Neuro. Oncol. 10 (2), 162–170.

Li, J., Bentzen, S.M., Renschler, M., et al., 2008. Relationship between neurocognitive function and quality of life after whole-brain radiotherapy in patients with brain metastasis. Int. J. Radiat. Oncol. Biol. Phys. 71 (1), 64–70.

Loghin, M.E., Prados, M.D., Wen, P., et al., 2007. Phase I study of temozolomide and irinotecan for recurrent malignant gliomas in patients receiving enzyme-inducing antiepileptic drugs: a North American brain tumor consortium study. Clin. Cancer Res. 13 (23), 7133–7138.

Lonser, R.R., Walbridge, S., Garmestani, K., et al., 2002. Successful and safe perfusion of the primate brainstem: in vivo magnetic resonance imaging of macromolecular distribution during infusion. J. Neurosurg. 97 (4), 905–913.

Lorenzoni, J., Devriendt, D., Massager, N., et al., 2004. Radiosurgery for treatment of brain metastases: estimation of patient eligibility using three stratification systems. Int. J. Radiat. Oncol. Biol. Phys. 60 (1), 218–224.

• **Macdonald, D.R., Cascino, T.L., Schold, S.C., Jr., et al.**, 1990. Response criteria for phase II studies of supratentorial malignant glioma. J. Clin. Oncol. 8 (7), 1277–1280.

MacDonald, T.J., Brown, K.M., LaFleur, B., et al., 2001. Expression profiling of medulloblastoma: PDGFRA and the RAS/MAPK pathway as therapeutic targets for metastatic disease. Nat. Genet. 29 (2), 143–152.

Macnealy, M.W., Newton, H.B., McGregor, J.M., et al., 2008. Primary meningeal CNS lymphoma treated with intra-arterial chemotherapy and blood-brain barrier disruption. J. Neurooncol. 90 (3), 329–333.

Mauer, M.E., Taphoorn, M.J., Bottomley, A., et al., 2007. Prognostic value of health-related quality-of-life data in predicting survival in patients with anaplastic oligodendrogliomas, from a phase III EORTC brain cancer group study. J. Clin. Oncol. 25 (36), 5731–5737.

McGirt, M.J., Than, K.D., Weingart, J.D., et al., 2009. Gliadel (BCNU) wafer plus concomitant temozolomide therapy after primary resection of glioblastoma multiforme. J. Neurosurg. 110 (3), 583–588.

Mintz, A.H., Kestle, J., Rathbone, M.P., et al., 1996. A randomized trial to assess the efficacy of surgery in addition to radiotherapy in patients with a single cerebral metastasis. Cancer 78 (7), 1470–1476.

Mirimanoff, R.O., Gorlia, T., Mason, W., et al., 2006. Radiotherapy and temozolomide for newly diagnosed glioblastoma: recursive partitioning analysis of the EORTC 26981/22981-NCIC CE3 phase III randomized trial. J. Clin. Oncol. 24 (16), 2563–2569.

Moher, D., Jones, A., Lepage, L., 2001. Use of the CONSORT statement and quality of reports of randomized trials: A comparative before-and-after evaluation. JAMA 285 (15), 1992–1995.

Moinpour, C.M., Lyons, B., Schmidt, S.P., et al., 2000. Substituting proxy ratings for patient ratings in cancer clinical trials: an analysis based on a Southwest Oncology Group trial in patients with brain metastases. Qual. Life Res. 9 (2), 219–231.

Murat, A., Migliavacca, E., Gorlia, T., et al., 2008. Stem cell-related 'self-renewal' signature and high epidermal growth factor receptor expression associated with resistance to concomitant chemoradiotherapy in glioblastoma. J. Clin. Oncol. 26 (18), 3015–3024.

Nelson, D.F., Martz, K.L., Bonner, H., et al., 1992. Non-Hodgkin's lymphoma of the brain: can high dose, large volume radiation therapy improve survival? Report on a prospective trial by the

Radiation Therapy Oncology Group (RTOG), RTOG 8315. Int. J. Radiat. Oncol. Biol. Phys. 23 (1), 9–17.

Osoba, D., Aaronson, N.K., Muller, M., et al., 1996. The development and psychometric validation of a brain cancer quality-of-life questionnaire for use in combination with general cancer-specific questionnaires. Qual. Life Res. 5 (1), 139–150.

Panageas, K.S., Elkin, E.B., DeAngelis, L.M., et al., 2005. Trends in survival from primary central nervous system lymphoma, 1975–1999: a population-based analysis. Cancer 104 (11), 2466–2472.

● **Patchell, R.A., Tibbs, P.A., Regine, W.F., et al.**, 1998. Postoperative radiotherapy in the treatment of single metastases to the brain: a randomized trial. JAMA 280 (17), 1485–1489.

● **Patchell, R.A., Tibbs, P.A., Walsh, J.W., et al.**, 1990. A randomized trial of surgery in the treatment of single metastases to the brain. N. Engl. J. Med. 322 (8), 494–500.

Pouratian, N., Asthagiri, A., Jagannathan, J., et al., 2007. Surgery Insight: the role of surgery in the management of low-grade gliomas. Nat. Clin. Pract. Neurol. 3 (11), 628–639.

Prados, M.D., Schold, S.C., Spence, A.M., et al., 1996. Phase II study of paclitaxel in patients with recurrent malignant glioma. J. Clin. Oncol. 14 (8), 2316–2321.

Prados, M.D., Yung, W.K., Jaeckle, K.A., et al., 2004. Phase 1 trial of irinotecan (CPT-11) in patients with recurrent malignant glioma: a North American Brain Tumor Consortium study. Neuro. Oncol. 6 (1), 44–54.

Preusser, M., Charles Janzer, R., Felsberg, J., et al., 2008. Anti-O6-methylguanine-methyltransferase (MGMT) immunohistochemistry in glioblastoma multiforme: observer variability and lack of association with patient survival impede its use as clinical biomarker. Brain Pathol. 18 (4), 520–532.

Rosenblum, M.K., Delattre, J.Y., Walker, R.W., et al., 1989. Fatal necrotizing encephalopathy complicating treatment of malignant gliomas with intra-arterial BCNU and irradiation: a pathological study. J. Neurooncol. 7 (3), 269–281.

Sanai, N., Berger, M.S., 2008. Glioma extent of resection and its impact on patient outcome. Neurosurgery 62 (4), 753–766.

Schlemmer, H.P., Bachert, P., Henze, M., et al., 2002. Differentiation of radiation necrosis from tumor progression using proton magnetic resonance spectroscopy. Neuroradiology 44 (3), 216–222.

Scott, C.B., Scarantino, C., Urtasun, R., et al., 1998. Validation and predictive power of Radiation Therapy Oncology Group (RTOG) recursive partitioning analysis classes for malignant glioma patients: a report using RTOG 90–06. Int. J. Radiat. Oncol. Biol. Phys. 40 (1), 51–55.

Shaffrey, M.E., Mut, M., Asher, A.L., et al., 2004. Brain metastases. Curr. Probl. Surg. 41 (8), 665–741.

Simpson, J.R., Horton, J., Scott, C., et al., 1993. Influence of location and extent of surgical resection on survival of patients with glioblastoma multiforme: results of three consecutive Radiation Therapy Oncology Group (RTOG) clinical trials. Int. J. Radiat. Oncol. Biol. Phys. 26 (2), 239–244.

Sperduto, P.W., Berkey, B., Gaspar, L.E., et al., 2008. A new prognostic index and comparison to three other indices for patients with brain metastases: an analysis of 1,960 patients in the RTOG database. Int. J. Radiat. Oncol. Biol. Phys. 70 (2), 510–514.

● **Stummer, W., Pichlmeier, U., Meinel, T., et al.**, 2006. Fluorescence-guided surgery with 5-aminolevulinic acid for resection of malignant glioma: a randomised controlled multicentre phase III trial. Lancet Oncol. 7 (5), 392–401.

● **Stummer, W., Reulen, H.J., Meinel, T., et al.**, 2008. Extent of resection and survival in glioblastoma multiforme: identification of and adjustment for bias. Neurosurgery 62 (3), 564–576.

● **Stupp, R., Mason, W.P., van den Bent, M.J., et al.**, 2005. Radiotherapy plus concomitant and adjuvant temozolomide for glioblastoma. N. Engl. J. Med. 352 (10), 987–996.

Tanner, P.G., Holtmannspotter, M., Tonn, J.C., et al., 2007. Effects of drug efflux on convection-enhanced paclitaxel delivery to malignant gliomas: technical note. Neurosurgery 61 (4), E880–E882.

Taphoorn, M.J., van den Bent, M.J., Mauer, M.E., et al., 2007. Health-related quality of life in patients treated for anaplastic oligodendroglioma with adjuvant chemotherapy: results of a European Organisation for Research and Treatment of Cancer randomized clinical trial. J. Clin. Oncol. 25 (36), 5723–5730.

Taylor, R.E., Bailey, C.C., Robinson, K.J., et al., 2005. Outcome for patients with metastatic (M2–M3) medulloblastoma treated with SIOP/UKCCSG PNET-3 chemotherapy. Eur. J. Cancer 41 (5), 727–734.

Thompson, T.P., Lunsford, L.D., Kondziolka, D., 1999. Distinguishing recurrent tumor and radiation necrosis with positron emission tomography versus stereotactic biopsy. Stereotact Funct Neurosurg. 73 (1–4), 9–14.

Tsuboi, K., Yoshii, Y., Hyodo, A., et al., 1995. Leukoencephalopathy associated with intra-arterial ACNU in patients with gliomas. J. Neurooncol. 23 (3), 223–231.

● **Valtonen, S., Timonen, U., Toivanen, P., et al.**, 1997. Interstitial chemotherapy with carmustine-loaded polymers for high-grade gliomas: a randomised double-blind study. Neurosurgery 41 (1), 44–49.

Vogelbaum, M.A., Sampson, J.H., Kunwar, S., et al., 2007. Convection-enhanced delivery of Cintredekin Besudotox (interleukin-13-PE38QQR) followed by radiation therapy with and without temozolomide in newly diagnosed malignant gliomas: phase 1 study of final safety results. Neurosurgery 61 (5), 1031–1038.

Weltman, E., Salvajoli, J.V., Brandt, R.A., et al., 2000. Radiosurgery for brain metastases: a score index for predicting prognosis. Int. J. Radiat. Oncol. Biol. Phys. 46 (5), 1155–1161.

Wen, P.Y., Macdonald, D.R., Reardon, D.A., et al., 2010. Updated response assessment criteria for high-grade gliomas: Response Assessment in neuro-oncology working group. J. Clin. Onc. 28 (11), 1963–1972.

Yung, W.K., Albright, R.E., Olson, J., et al., 2000. A phase II study of temozolomide vs. procarbazine in patients with glioblastoma multiforme at first relapse. Br. J. Cancer 83 (5), 588–593.

● **Zeltzer, P.M., Boyett, J.M., Finlay, J.L., et al.**, 1999. Metastasis stage, adjuvant treatment, and residual tumor are prognostic factors for medulloblastoma in children: conclusions from the Children's Cancer Group 921 randomized phase III study. J. Clin. Oncol. 17 (3), 832–845.

17 Mouse models for brain tumor therapy

Nikki Charles, Andrew B. Lassman, and Eric C. Holland

Introduction

Malignant gliomas and medulloblastomas are the most common brain tumors in adults and children, respectively (CBTRUS 2008). Despite advances in surgical techniques, radiotherapy targeting, and chemotherapy efficacy, gliomas, and a majority of medulloblastomas remain incurable fatal tumors in almost all patients. Animal models that effectively replicate the human diseases both histologically and molecularly provide an important tool for better understanding of glioma and medulloblastoma biology. They also serve as an invaluable resource for the testing of novel therapies. Ultimately, the translation of such therapies to clinical trials in humans leads to further investigation of the reasons for treatment success or failure, and for further evaluation in animal models. Therefore, models provide a key link in the process of moving research from bench to bedside and back. This chapter will focus on *in vivo* models, especially those generated through cell type specific gene transfer using the RCAS/tv-a system, described further below.

Gliomas and medulloblastomas are molecularly complex. Identifying the few molecular abnormalities that contribute to tumor formation or maintenance among the plethora of derangements is critical to improved understanding and treatment. Over 100 years ago, Koch laid out his 'postulates' for the analogous assessment of the cause of infectious disease (Koch 1884). In short, he postulated that an infectious agent causes a disease if: (1) it is always observed whenever a disease occurs; (2) it never occurs in the absence of the disease, and (3) it induces the disease when isolated from one host and implanted into another (translated into English, in Rivers 1937). These postulates are also applicable to tumor modeling, where an oncogenic molecular abnormality (e.g., PDGF pathway activation) is the 'infectious' agent of Koch. PDGF signaling is activated in a sub-set of human glioblastomas (GBMs) and forced activation of PDGFR in glia induces glioma formation (see below). Admittedly, 'always' and 'never' are not valid terms, but this reflects the molecular heterogeneity of tumors rather than negating the concepts of the postulates. In other words, it is reasonable to conclude that tumors modeled with PDGFR activation fulfill Koch's postulates for one molecular tumor sub-type observed in humans.

Medulloblastoma molecular biology

The most extensively modeled signaling pathway best characterized in medulloblastomas is the Sonic Hedgehog cascade. Gorlin syndrome (Gorlin 1987) is a constellation of heritable abnormalities including medulloblastomas, as a consequence of germline inactivation/loss of the 'Patched' (PTCH) tumor suppressor gene (Chidambaram et al 1996; Johnson et al 1996). Evidence that sporadic medulloblastomas, particularly those of desmoplastic histology (Raffel et al 1997) also demonstrate PTCH signaling abnormalities (Zurawel et al 2000) reinforces the contribution of PTCH to medulloblastoma formation.

PTCH is a receptor for Sonic Hedgehog (SHH). Cerebellar Purkinje cells normally secrete SHH in the external granular layer (EGL). The action of SHH on PTCH is inhibitory, reducing the basal inhibition normally exerted by PTCH on another molecule called 'Smoothened' (SMO) (Murone et al 1999). Disinhibited SMO then induces expression of GLI (Murone et al 1999), a transcription factor so named because it is highly amplified in gliomas (Kinzler et al 1987; Wong et al 1987) but it is also now known to be amplified in other cancers (Roberts et al 1989).

Abnormalities at any point in this cascade can induce medulloblastomas. These include enhanced SHH activity (by gene amplification or protein overexpression) (Oro et al 1997), PTCH inactivation (by genomic loss or inactivating mutation), SMO overexpression, or GLI overexpression. Finally, suppressor of fused (SUFU) translocates GLI from nucleus to cytoplasm reducing its oncogenic activity as a transcription factor. Therefore, inactivation of SUFU also predisposes to medulloblastoma formation (Taylor et al 2002). Modeling proves that SHH signaling abnormalities observed in humans are causal. However, it should be noted that desmoplastic histology is uncommon, and that the majority of human medulloblastomas are insufficiently modeled at this time.

Turcot syndrome is another familial tumor condition involving medulloblastomas (Turcot et al 1959). Oncogenic WNT/β-catenin signaling pathway abnormalities predispose to tumor formation in one Turcot syndrome sub-type (Hamilton et al 1995). WNT abnormalities are also observed in a subset of sporadic medulloblastomas, further supporting their biologic importance (Kool et al 2008). However, most *in vivo* medulloblastoma modeling to date has not focused on WNT abnormalities.

MYC is an oncogenic transcription factor overexpressed or amplified in medulloblastomas, where amplification also predicts short survival (Gulino et al 2008). p53 abnormalities are also prevalent. However, neither MYC (Fults et al 2002) nor p53 (Marino et al 2000) abnormalities alone are sufficient to cause medulloblastomas. Rather, they cooperate with other abnormalities (Rao et al 2003; Wetmore et al 2001). In this manner, they are similar to abnormalities of INK4A-ARF that reduce latency and increase frequency of the formation of gliomas, but are generally insufficient to cause gliomas in the absence of other oncogenic abnormalities described below.

Glioma molecular biology

There are many ways to categorize the molecular abnormalities that contribute to glioma biology. A functional scheme easily allows interrogation by modeling and is the classification used here. Abnormalities of normal cell cycle control (proliferation), signal transduction cascades, and receptor tyrosine kinases are common in gliomas and have been modeled extensively.

Cell cycle control

The cell cycle encompasses four phases: G1, S (during which DNA is synthesized), G2, and M (when mitosis occurs). Functionally, two cascades drive proliferation: INK4A/CDK4/RB/E2F and ARF/MDM2/p53 (Sherr 2001a), and both have been modeled extensively. INK4A (Serrano et al 1993), also called p16 in both humans and mice, is a tumor suppressor that inhibits the cyclin dependent kinase (CDK)4/6-Cyclin D complex. Cyclins (lettered A, B, C, etc.) are pro-mitotic molecules that heterodimerize with CDKs (numbered 1, 2, 3, etc.) (Pardee 1989). By inhibiting CDK4/6-Cyclin D, INK4A indirectly reduces the phosphorylation of RB. Hypophosphorylated RB binds and reduces the activity of the pro-mitotic transcription factor E2F. However, in the absence of INK4A, the CDK4/6-Cyclin D complex is disinhibited, phosphorylating RB which releases E2F. The transcriptional activating function of E2F promotes a positive feedback loop leading to its own expression, as well as that of the cyclins and CDKs, leading to cell division. Therefore, inactivation or loss of INK4A, overexpression of CDK4, and inactivation or loss of RB, all effectively have the same functional consequence of increased proliferation.

ARF, also called p19 in mice and p14 in humans, is another tumor suppressor encoded by the INK4A gene, but through the use of an alternative reading frame (ARF) and different promoter (Quelle et al 1995). Normally, ARF binds to MDM2 (Tao & Levine 1999) which then releases p53 and reduces proliferation among numerous other actions (Oren 2001). This induces the expression of several CDK inhibitor proteins (CIPs) such as p21CIP1 (El-Deiry et al 1993; Harper et al 1993), reducing the action of CDK-Cyclin heterodimers and, consequently, mitosis. Therefore, in the absence of ARF, MDM2 forms an inhibitor complex with p53, disinhibiting the expression of p21CIP as well as other pro-mitotic factors promoting proliferation. Inactivation or loss of ARF, overexpression of MDM2, and inactivation or loss of p53, all effectively have the same functional consequence of increased proliferation.

There is molecular cross-talk between the INK4A/CDK4/RB/E2F and ARF/MDM2/p53 pathways. If one is disinhibited, feedback loops from the other can provide an inhibitory signal. For example, E2F induces ARF expression, ARF induces E2F degradation, and p53 increases MDM2 expression (Bates et al 1998; Martelli et al 2001; Wu et al 1993). In addition, these cascades are more complex and not as linear as described here. However, conceptually, these two arms of cell cycle control can both be modeled, either alone or together. Alterations of at least one, if not both, have been described in almost all gliomas (Ichimura et al 2000).

For example, more than two-thirds of GBMs harbor abnormalities of the INK4A pathway, such as *CDK4* amplification, or loss/inactivating mutation of both *INK4* or *RB* loci (Ichimura et al 2000). Epigenetic mechanisms, such as methylation, can also silence wild-type gene expression (Nakamura et al 2001). These abnormalities are also more prevalent in high-grade gliomas than lower-grade tumors (Ichimura et al 2000).

Similarly, functional disruption of *ARF* occurs in the majority of gliomas, although typically in association with loss of exons shared with *INK4A* (Fulci et al 2000). MDM2 amplification is detected in only 10% of GBMs, occasionally in combination with CDK4 amplification (He et al 1994). However, overexpression in the absence of gene amplification can also disrupt proliferation control (Landers et al 1994). p53 loss occurs in approximately one-third of GBMs (Ichimura et al 2000). ARF, p53, and MDM2 alternations are typically mutually exclusive genetic events presumably as a consequence of their redundant functional effect (Fulci et al 2000; He et al 1994; Kleihues & Ohgaki 1999). Taken together, potential disruption of normal proliferation control is detected in almost all GBMs at one of several contributing genetic loci.

Receptor tyrosine kinases (RTKs)

Platelet derived growth factor (PDGF) and epidermal growth factor (EGF) are ligands that transmit their signals to both normal and cancer cells through receptors such as PDGFR and EGFR. Upon ligand binding, receptor dimerization leads through a series of steps to activation of the tyrosine kinase activity of the intracellular domain of the receptor. Through a series of phosphorylations, signal transduction cascade (e.g., AKT and RAS described below) then induce various cellular activities such as proliferation, invasion, or reduced apoptosis. Therefore, abnormal receptor activation contributes to tumorigenesis and maintenance.

EGFR is amplified or duplicated in one-third to one-half of astrocytomas (Kleihues & Ohgaki 1999), although protein overexpression occurs in more than 90% (Schlegel et al 1994). The frequency of these abnormalities is also higher in high-grade than low-grade tumors (Hurtt et al 1992), and is far more common in primary than secondary GBMs that arise from a low-grade tumor (Kleihues & Ohgaki 1999). In addition, constitutively activating EGFR mutations lead to ligand independent activation in approximately one-half of GBMs, depending on the detection technique and series (Kuan et al 2001). The most common of these is variant III (EGFRvIII), although other mutations occur (Kuan et al 2001), including several newly described alterations in the extracellular domain (Lee et al 2006).

PDGFR is overexpressed in approximately one-quarter of gliomas (Fleming et al 1992), with prevalence correlating with grade. Concurrent abnormalities of both PDGF and PDGFR lead to an oncogenic autocrine stimulatory loop (Di Rocco et al 1998; Guha et al 1995; Hermanson et al 1992). PDGF/PDGFR anomalies are particularly prevalent among tumors with oligodendroglial histology (Di Rocco et al 1998; Smith et al 2000). As described below, models generated with PDGF signaling abnormalities also exhibit features of high-grade oligodendrogliomas, with the specific

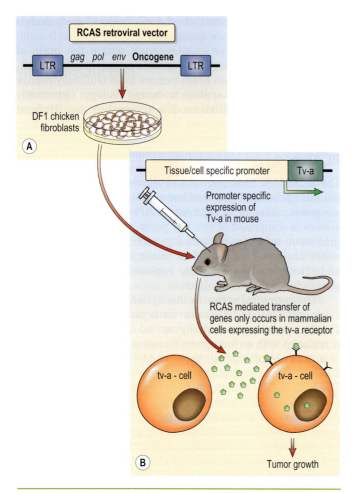

A

B

RCAS mediated transfer of genes only occurs in mammalian cells expressing the tv-a receptor

tv-a - cell

tv-a - cell

Tumor growth

Figure 17.1 The RCAS/tv-a method of postnatal gene transfer for modeling CNS tumors. The RCAS vector (A) has the *gag, pol,* and *env* viral genes required for viral packaging. RCAS is grown in DF1 chicken fibroblast cells which are injected into the brains of new born mice (B) genetically engineered to express tv-a (the RCAS receptor) under control of a specific promoter. These DF1 cells survive temporarily in the brain where they produce RCAS virions that infect tv-a expression cells. Tumor growth is initiated from RCAS-infected cells.

cells in Gtv-a or Ntv-a mice (Fisher et al 1999). The threshold for transformation is high because tumors form only as a consequence of experimentally induced oncogenic abnormalities following RCAS-infection. Moreover, inefficient infection leads to a limited population of infected cells because RCAS virions cannot replicate in murine cells. Therefore, one advantage of RCAS/tv-a modeling is the ability to conclude that the experimentally induced oncogenic abnormalities are highly transforming. However, this is also disadvantageous for detecting mutations that contribute to tumor formation but are otherwise insufficient.

To address this problem, the RCAS/tv-a system can also be combined with additional modeling techniques to allow even more powerful investigation of tumor biology. For example, proliferation control normally exerted by the tumor suppressor inhibitor of CDK4-A (INK4A) or the protein encoded by its alternate reading frame (ARF) is lost or

functionally disrupted in most human gliomas, as discussed further below. Crossing *Ink4a-Arf* knockout mice with Gtv-a or Ntv-a mice yields *Ink4a-Arf* null animals susceptible to RCAS infection. Therefore, oncogenes encoded by one or multiple RCAS vectors are transferrable in a cell type specific manner to Gfap or nestin expressing cells in *Ink4a-Arf* null animals, allowing investigation of the role of *Ink4a-Arf* loss in tumor formation and latency.

However, loss of some tumor suppressor genes is embryonically lethal making it difficult to determine the importance of germline deletions to tumor biology. The RCAS/tv-a modeling system can be adapted to targeted tumor suppressor deletion through combinations with the Cre-*lox* system. Cre recombinase catalyzes the excision of DNA flanked on the 5′ and 3′ end by *lox*P sequences ('floxed'). The loxP sequence is 33 base pairs and is too small for knock-in around a gene of interest to affect gene function or expression spontaneously. Crossing mice transgenic for a floxed sequence with tv-a mice allows cell-type specific gene removal following infection by an RCAS vector engineered to carry Cre recombinase (RCAS-Cre). For example, as above, *PTEN* (Li et al 1997) is lost or otherwise disrupted in most human glioblastomas (Sano et al 1999), but homozygous *Pten* loss is embryonically lethal (Di Cristofano et al 1998; Podsypanina et al 1999; Suzuki et al 1998). RCAS-Cre infection of mice transgenic for both tv-a and floxed *Pten* allows interrogation of the role *Pten* plays in tumor formation and latency. Combination of these techniques is also possible, e.g., by crossing Ntv-a, *Ink4a-Arf* null, and *Pten* floxed mice and infecting them with RACAS-Cre (Hu et al 2005).

Medulloblastoma

Several mouse models of medulloblastoma exist. As noted above, human medulloblastomas are believed to arise in undifferentiated neural progenitor cells (i.e., granule neuron precursor (GNP) cells) of the developing cerebellum (Marino 2005; Wechsler-Reya & Scott 2001). The SHH/Patched signaling pathway normally functions in the brain to promote proliferation in GNPs; therefore, activated SHH/Patched signaling is the major pathway targeted for modeling medulloblastomas in mice.

One approach to elevating Gli signaling in these cells is by suppressing Ptch activity. Approximately 15% of *Ptch* heterozygous mice develop aggressive medulloblastomas (Goodrich et al 1997; Wetmore et al 2000). Loss of *p53, Lig4,* or several other genes encoding proteins involved in DNA repair dramatically enhances medulloblastoma formation in *Ptch* mutant mice (Wetmore et al 2000).

Another approach to modeling the abnormalities of SHH signaling that occur in humans is the forced overexpression of Shh itself. Shh is the ligand for the Ptch receptor downregulating Ptch activity. Two main experimental strategies employ retroviral transfer of SHH to the developing cerebellum. For example, 76% of mice developed medulloblastomas following microinjection of murine leukemia virus overexpressing Shh *in utero* (Weiner et al 2002). RCAS-mediated transfer of SHH to nestin expressing neural precursor cells in newborn pups also induces medulloblastomas (Fig. 17.2). For example, injection of an RCAS vector encoding SHH (RCAS-SHH) into the cerebellum induces medulloblastomas

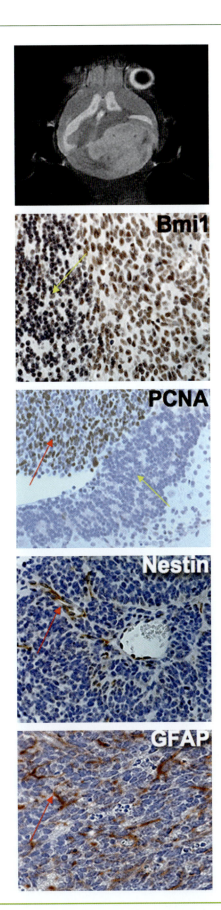

Figure 17.2 Medulloblastoma generated by the RCAS/tv-a system. MRI (top) of a SHH-induced medulloblastoma. Immunohistochemical analysis demonstrates Bmi1, PCNA, nestin and GFAP expression as indicated (red arrow points to positive tumor cells and yellow arrow to adjacent IGL cells).

in approximately 10% of Ntv-a mice (Rao et al 2003). However, the frequency of tumor formation increases to approximately 25% when combined with MYC activation (Rao et al 2003), although MYC alone is insufficient (Fults et al 2002). MYC activation may contribute by maintaining or promoting an undifferentiated stem-like phenotype that is more sensitive to malignant transformation (Lassman et al 2004). MYC also cooperates with other SHH abnormalities such as *Ptch* loss (Fults et al 2002). AKT can also synergize with SHH to induce medulloblastomas, with tumors forming in approximately 50% of Ntv-a mice injected with both RCAS-SHH and RCAS-AKT (Rao et al 2004).

The RCAS system has also been used to overexpress SHH with BCL2 or IGF2 to enhance medulloblastoma tumor incidence. Loss of the tumor suppressor *Pten* by Cre-*lox* targeted deletion in combination with SHH overexpression gives rise to a minor medulloblastoma subtype referred to as 'medulloblastoma with extensive nodularity' (Hambardzumyan et al 2008a). Additionally, mutations leading to constitutive activation of Smoothened in the developing cerebellum is a third approach to model medulloblastomas in mice (Fults 2005; Piedimonte et al 2005). Tumors closely mimicking that observed in humans arise in ~48% of mice (Hallahan et al 2004).

In some models of medulloblastomas, the Shh/Ptch pathway components are not directly targeted. Overexpression of IFNs, a class of cytokines that play a role in host response to viral infection in the brain (Sarciron & Gherardi 2000; Suzuki 1999), lead to highly aggressive medulloblastomas in >80% of mice (Lin et al 2004). Although *p53* is wildtype in most human sporadic medulloblastomas, the loss of p53 function plays an important role in medulloblastoma formation in murine models. In mice, dysfunction of genes controlling cell cycle activity and DNA repair leads to the development of tumors histologically consistent with medulloblastomas (Hambardzumyan et al 2008a). Combined *p53* and *Parp* loss results in medulloblastomas in about 50% of mice (Eberhart 2003), while targeted deletion of both *p53* and *Rb* also result in medulloblastomas (Marino 2005).

Gliomas

The abnormalities of PDGF signaling observed in human gliomas have been extensively modeled in mice. Early studies used a retroviral system employing Maloney murine leukemia virus (MMLV). MMLV differs from RCAS in two major ways: expression of a specific receptor (such as TV-A) is not required for infection, and the splice site can accept inserts larger than those that RCAS can accommodate. Intracranial injection of MMLV-PDGF induces gliomas in almost 50% of newborn mice (Uhrbom et al 1998). However, the histologic sub-types are heterogeneous, likely as a result of the multiple infected cells of origin resulting from the broad infectibility of host cells. RCAS-PDGF, with infection restricted to tv-a expressing cells, induces gliomas in approximately 40% of Gtv-a mice. This frequency increases to approximately 70% when Ntv-a mice are used (Dai et al 2001). In addition, the frequency and grade of induced tumors is dependent on PDGF dose (Shih et al 2004). The lower threshold to tumor formation in Ntv-a mice in comparison to Gtv-a mice is likely explained by the more mature astrocytic vs stem-like character of Gfap expressing vs nestin expressing cells, respectively. Further supporting this explanation, RCAS-PDGF converts astrocytic cells to those with characteristics of glial progenitors *in vitro* (Dai et al 2001), suggesting that a dedifferentiated/undifferentiated state is necessary for tumor formation. Nestin-expressing cells already exhibit undifferentiated character and do not require dedifferentiation from a more mature phenotype. In addition, the histology of tumors that arise in Gtv-a and Ntv-a mice differ. Ntv-a mice form both oligodendrogliomas as well as mixed oligoastrocytomas, but Gtv-a mice form almost exclusively oligodendrogliomas. This suggests that dedifferentiation of Gfap expressing astrocytes leads to a pluripotent stem-like cell that can form tumors of either oligodendroglial or mixed histology (Dai et al 2001).

The threshold and latency to tumor formation are reduced by cell cycle abnormalities which alone are generally insufficient for gliomagenesis. For example, mice null for both *Ink4a* and *Arf* do not develop gliomas without other cooperative abnormalities (Serrano et al 1996). Similarly, disruption of cell cycle control by combined *p53* and *Rb* loss in Gfap-expressing cells does not cause gliomas (Marino et al 2000). When the INK4A and ARF arms of cell cycle control are modeled independently, such as by loss of *Ink4a* with *Arf* retention (Krimpenfort et al 2001; Sharpless et al 2001; Sherr 2001b) or CDK4 overexpression, gliomas do not form (Huang et al 2002). Similarly, *Rb* loss in Gfap-expressing cells does not cause gliomas (Marino et al 2000). Similarly, when functional consequences of ARF abnormalities are specifically modeled by *p53* nullizygosity, gliomas do not form (Marino et al 2000). However, in contrast to these observations, *Arf* null mice do form low-grade oligodendrogliomas at low frequency following prolonged latency (Kamijo et al 1999). The implication of this finding is currently unclear, but may suggest that *Arf* is the more

potent tumor suppressor gene at the *INK4A-ARF* locus. Nonetheless, in general, cell cycle dysregulation is insufficient for glioma formation.

Ink4a-Arf loss increases the frequency of tumor formation from 40% to 70% in Gtv-a mice injected with RCAS-PDGF (Fig. 17.3) (Dai et al 2001). Moreover, higher-grade tumors typically form in *Ink4a-Arf* null mice than in those with wild-type *Ink4a-Arf*. These results demonstrate that *Ink4a-Arf* loss lowers the threshold to tumor formation. *Ink4a-Arf* loss also reduces the threshold to tumor formation with oncogenic changes other than PDGF expression. For example, RAS and AKT are activated in approximately 100% and 70% of GBMs as described above. However, co-injection of RCAS-RAS and RCAS-AKT does not induce tumors in Gtv-a mice. By contrast, 40% of *Ink4a-Arf* null Gtv-a mice develop gliomas following expression of oncogenic forms of RAS + AKT (Uhrbom et al 2002). Ntv-a, *Ink4a-Arf* wildtype mice do develop GBMs following co-injection of RCAS-RAS + RCAS-AKT at a frequency of approximately 25%, although Gtv-a mice do not (Holland et al 2000; Uhrbom et al 2002). This observation further demonstrates the lower threshold to tumor formation from stem-like (nestin-expressing) cells of origin than from more mature (Gfap-expressing) cells demonstrated with RCAS-PDGF above. This point is supported further by the observation that tumor frequency is higher in *Ink4a-Arf* null Ntv-a mice (50%) relative to Gtv-a mice (40%) (Uhrbom et al 2002). Supporting the observation that ARF may be more important to tumor suppression than INK4A, mice nullizygous for *Arf* develop malignant astrocytomas in the setting of forced RAS activation (Uhrbom et al 2005), whereas RAS alone is unable to induce tumors in *Ink4a-Arf* wild type mice (Holland et al 2000).

RAS-driven tumors are histologically distinct from the PDGF-driven tumors that exhibit more oligodendroglial histology. Tumors induced by RCAS-RAS injection of *Ink4a-Arf*

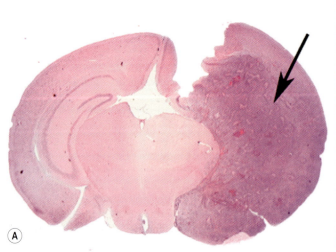
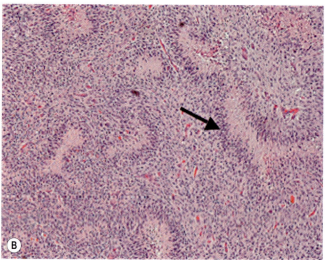

Figure 17.3 RCAS-mediated PDGF gene transfer to nestin-expressing cells in the brain generates high-grade gliomas. (A) Whole mount of a glioma bearing mouse brain stained with hematoxylin and eosin (H&E) at low magnification demonstrates a large infiltrative tumor (arrow). (B) At high magnification, the tumor exhibits histological features of high grade human gliomas including pseudopalisading necrosis (arrow) and microvascular proliferation.

(or *Arf*) null Gtv-a or Ntv-a mice exhibit areas of sarcomatous histology with spindled cells and absent GFAP expression. There is, however, intratumoral heterogeneity, and other areas demonstrate a typical astrocytic histology and GFAP expression. The astrocytic areas also demonstrate spontaneous activation of AKT (Uhrbom et al 2002). The contribution of AKT is mainly to the maintenance of an astrocytic phenotype. Although AKT is activated in the majority of human GBMs (Holland et al 2000; Rajasekhar et al 2003), RCAS-AKT alone is insufficient to induce GBMs in either Ntv-a or Gtv-a mice (Holland et al 2000). AKT is also unable to induce gliomas in the setting of *Ink4a-Arf* loss (Hu et al 2005; Uhrbom et al 2002). However, forced AKT activation induces predominantly astrocytomas in *Ink4a-Arf* null animals co-injected with RCAS-RAS (Uhrbom et al 2002). In addition, RAS + AKT induced astrocytomas convert to oligodendroglial histology when treated with inhibitors of AKT effectors such as mTOR (Hu et al 2005). Finally, as described above, RCAS-PDGF induces high-grade gliomas with oligodendroglial histology. By contrast, concurrent activation of AKT and overexpression of PDGF induces mixed oligoastrocytomas and increased expression of the astrocytic marker GFAP (Dai et al 2005).

GLI signaling in mouse gliomas

Although GLI was first described in the context of gliomas (Collins 1993), its role in tumor formation has been studied in more detail in medulloblastomas. There have been several isolated studies exploring the importance of GLI and the broader SHH/PTCH/SMO/GLI cascade in gliomas. For example, *GLI* amplification occurs in a small sub-set of gliomas (Bigner et al 1988; Hui et al 2001; Mao & Hamoudi 2000) and SMO inhibition by the drug cyclopamine reduces glioma cell proliferation (Bar et al 2007; Clement et al 2007; Dahmane et al 2001; Ehtesham et al 2007). More recently, one report has suggested a potential role of the SHH pathway in gliomagenesis. Using the RCAS/tv-a system in Gli reporter mice, Becher and colleagues (2008) demonstrated that sonic signaling was activated in mouse gliomas induced by PDGF overexpression. Immunohistochemical analysis of gliomas demonstrated elevated Shh protein expression localized to stem cell niches within gliomas (PVN regions) and its expression was strongly correlated with increasing glioma grade.

Therapeutic responses in mouse models of brain tumors

Radio-resistant cells in the perivascular niche of medulloblastomas

Radioresistance caused by Akt activation in brain tumor stem-like cells of the tumor perivascular niche (PVN) is most clearly understood in medulloblastomas. For example, Hambardzumyan and colleagues (2008a) demonstrated that PVN stem-like cells respond to radiation by increasing nestin expression (potentially their 'stem-ness') and activating the Pi3k/Akt proliferation/survival pathway. Several medulloblastoma mouse models were used to show p53 dependent induction of apoptosis in the main tumor population

following irradiation and p53-dependent arrest of the cell cycle in the PNV stem-like cells of tumors. The bulk of the medulloblastoma tumor mass undergoes apoptosis 6 h after radiation, while the stem-like populations residing in the tumor PVN arrest then re-enter the cell cycle 72 h later. These stem-like populations residing in PVN also increase their stem-like character (nestin expression) and activate the Akt signaling pathway 6 h after irradiation. This coincides with a decrease in the expression of Pten. Radiation induced p53-dependent cell cycle arrest in PVN stem-like cells was shown to be Pten dependent (Hambardzumyan et al 2008a).

Pre-treatment of medulloblastoma-bearing mice with perifosine, a small molecule inhibitor of Akt signaling, sensitized PVN stem-like cells to radiation-induced apoptosis (Hambardzumyan et al 2008a). This medulloblastoma model demonstrated that the Pi3k/Akt pathway is activated in response to radiation and mediates the resistance to radiation within these brain tumors. These findings in medulloblastomas could be extrapolated to gliomas to further understand the mechanisms responsible for their infamous radioresistant phenotype. Human gliomas often show less response than medulloblastomas to radiotherapy and chemotherapy, as do modeled tumors (Hambardzumyan et al 2008b). However, parallels exist between the two tumor types including the presence of a stem-like cell niche in the perivascular space of PDGF-induced gliomas (Fig. 17.4).

Cells expressing CD133 and nestin represent the stem-like populations in both medulloblastomas and gliomas (Calabrese et al 2007; Galli et al 2004; Singh et al 2004). In medulloblastomas, these nestin positive, stem-like PVN cells activate the Akt pathway to mediate their radioresistant phenotype (Hambardzumyan et al 2008a). A similar mechanism may contribute to radioresistance in gliomas.

The importance of AKT signaling in PDGF-induced gliomas has been demonstrated in preclinical trials in glioma-bearing mice by blocking the activity of mTOR using the rapamycin analog temsirolimus (Uhrbom et al 2004). These data suggest that PDGF-driven human gliomas may also be dependent on mTOR activity for proliferation as well. Unpublished data indicate that blocking mTOR alone is insufficient to completely inhibit all points in the pathway, and combinations of drugs that target both Akt and mTOR activity may have greater efficacy.

Bioluminescence imaging

Bioluminescence imaging is a sensitive *in vivo* technique based on the detection of light emitted by luciferases from tissues (Momota & Holland 2005; Shah 2005). The luciferase gene, isolated from fireflies (firefly luc) or the sea pansy (renilla luc), cleaves its substrates (D-luciferin or coelenterazine, respectively) in ATP-dependent reactions to produce light.

Reporter mouse lines can be engineered to express luciferase under the control of specific promoters resulting in light output regulated by the activity of that promoter. As mammalian tissues do not normally emit bioluminescence, luciferase expression is limited to cells specifically engineered to express the bioluminescent reporter (Uhrbom et al

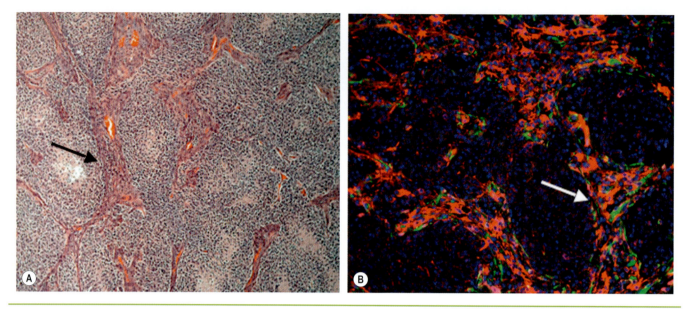

Figure 17.4 Microvascular proliferating structures in PDGF-induced gliomas. H&E stain (A) showing well formed structures that immunofluoresce (B) for nestin in green, pS6 in purple and SHH in red. Arrows show regions of microvascular proliferation.

2004). The amount of luciferase produced *in vivo* can be quantified by photons as a measure of promoter activity. Bioluminescent imaging offers the advantage of identifying mice with tumors and specifically measuring tumor cell response to treatment non-invasively, allowing each mouse to be its own control.

Bioluminescence has been used in mouse models of brain tumors (Becher et al 2008; Parr et al 1997; Uhrbom et al 2004). Depending on the promoter used in the transgene, bioluminescent imaging can be applied to study cell proliferation, pathological activation of signaling pathways and tumor cell response to pharmacological inhibitors for treatment of brain tumors. For example, one study examined Rb disruption (frequently abnormal in human gliomas) in a PDGF-induced mouse glioma model (Uhrbom et al 2004). The human E2F1 promoter was used to drive expression of the firefly luciferase gene (Ef-luc) in a transgenic mouse line. The E2F1 reporter mouse was crossed to RCAS/Ntv-a mouse. This approach allows monitoring of cell proliferation because E2F1 is regulated by Rb, a transcription factor known to promote cell cycle progression (Alonso et al 2008). Elevated Rb pathway activity was tracked over time and the efficacy of drug treatment monitored in real time. This system allowed analysis of the pharmacodynamics and potency of drugs that disrupt tumor cell proliferation.

In another report, bioluminescence was also used to monitor activation of the sonic pathway in PDGF induced gliomas (Becher et al 2008). A mouse transgenic line was used containing an expression cassette where firefly luciferase was expressed under a Gli1-responsive promoter. The Gli1 reporter mouse was crossed to the RCAS/Ntv-a line to generate reporter mice that could be infected with PDGF producing viruses (Dai et al 2001). This model was used to demonstrate both activation of the SHH signaling pathway in SHH-driven medulloblastomas as well as the importance of SHH/Patched pathway in glioma biology. Gli activity was

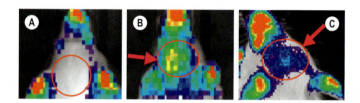

Figure 17.5 Bioluminescence imaging reporter mice can be used for monitoring medulloblastomas and gliomas. Using a transgenic background in which luciferase is driven from a Gli1-responsive promoter, light can be detected over the top of the head in living animals. Control mice (A) show light emitted from the nose and ears only. In medulloblastoma (B) and glioma (C) bearing mice, additional light is visible (arrow). The medulloblastomas are driven by SHH. The gliomas are driven by PDGF but nonetheless demonstrate SHH signaling as visible light.

found to be highly elevated in gliomas and strongly correlated with increasing grade (Fig. 17.5).

Conclusions

Mouse models that accurately replicate human medulloblastomas and gliomas molecularly, by imaging, and histologically provide an opportunity to better understand tumorigenesis and to test new therapies. The RCAS/tv-a system in particular allows cell type specific gene transfer postnatally, generates tumors in the natural host environment, and can be used to distinguish causal molecular aberrations from epiphenomena. Future work will further strengthen our understanding of tumor molecular biology, and lead to new insights into the design of better therapies for brain tumors.

Key points

- Mouse medulloblastomas and gliomas modeled with the RCAS/tv-a system accomplish cell type specific postnatal gene transfer and recapitulate the histology, imaging, and molecular features of a subset of human tumors, distinguishing causal oncogenic abnormalities from epiphenomena.

- Brain tumor stem cells show the capacity for multipotentiality, proliferation, self-renewal, and differentiation, and they are a potential source of chemo- and radiotherapy resistance.

- Pre-clinical experiments with medulloblastoma mouse models driven by sonic hedgehog signaling abnormalities demonstrate that perivascular stem-like cells remain resistant to radiation by activating cell survival pathways and proliferation arrest, then re-enter the cell cycle to proliferate and repopulate the tumor.

- Bioluminescent mouse tumor models allow non-invasive quantitation of biologic pathway activation in tumors *in vivo*, and rapid detection of tumor formation and response to therapy.

REFERENCES

Al-Hajj, M., Wicha, M.S., Benito-Hernandez, A., et al., 2003. Prospective identification of tumorigenic breast cancer cells. Proc. Natl. Acad. Sci. USA 100 (7), 3983.

Alonso, M.M., Alemany, R., Fueyo, J., et al., 2008. E2F1 in gliomas: a paradigm of oncogene addiction. Cancer Lett. 263 (2), 157.

Ayuso-Sacido, A., Roy, N.S., Schwartz, T.H., et al., 2008. Long-term expansion of adult human brain subventricular zone precursors. Neurosurgery 62 (1), 223.

Bar, E.E., Chaudhry, A., Lin, A., et al., 2007. Cyclopamine-mediated hedgehog pathway inhibition depletes stem-like cancer cells in glioblastoma. Stem Cells 25 (10), 2524.

Bates, P., Young, J.A., Varmus, H.E., 1993. A receptor for subgroup A Rous sarcoma virus is related to the low density lipoprotein receptor. Cell 74 (6), 1043.

Bates, S., Phillips, A.C., Clark, P.A., et al., 1998. p14ARF links the tumour suppressors R B and p53. Nature 395 (6698), 124.

Becher, O.J., Hambardzumyan, D., Fomchenko, E.I., et al., 2008. Gli activity correlates with tumor grade in platelet-derived growth factor-induced gliomas. Cancer Res. 68 (7), 2241.

Bigner, S.H., Burger, P.C., Wong, A.J., et al., 1988. Gene amplification in malignant human gliomas: clinical and histopathologic aspects. J. Neuropathol. Exp. Neurol. 47 (3), 191.

Bleau, A.M., Hambardzumyan, D., Ozawa, T., et al., 2009. PTEN/PI3K/Akt pathway regulates the side population phenotype and ABCG2 activity in glioma tumor stem-like cells. Cell Stem Cell 4 (3), 226.

Blume-Jensen, P., Hunter, T., 2001. Oncogenic kinase signalling. Nature 411 (6835), 355.

Bonnet, D., Dick, J.E., 1997. Human acute myeloid leukemia is organized as a hierarchy that originates from a primitive hematopoietic cell. Nat. Med. 3 (7), 730.

Bos, J.L., 1989. Ras oncogenes in human cancer: a review. Cancer Res. 49 (17), 4682.

Cai, J., Cheng, A., Luo, Y., et al., 2004. Membrane properties of rat embryonic multipotent neural stem cells. J. Neurochem. 88 (1), 212.

Calabrese, C., Poppleton, H., Kocak, M., et al., 2007. A perivascular niche for brain tumor stem cells. Cancer Cell 11 (1), 69.

Cavallaro, M., Mariani, J., Lancini, C., et al., 2008. Impaired generation of mature neurons by neural stem cells from hypomorphic Sox2 mutants. Development 135 (3), 541.

CBTRUS, 2008. Central Brain Tumor Registry of the United States 2008. statistical report: primary brain tumors in the United States. CBTRUS, Hinsdale, IL.

Chidambaram, A., Goldstein, A.M., Gailani, M.R., et al., 1996. Mutations in the human homologue of the Drosophila patched gene in Caucasian and African-American nevoid basal cell carcinoma syndrome patients. Cancer Res. 56 (20), 4599.

Choe, G., Horvath, S., Cloughesy, T.F., et al., 2003. Analysis of the phosphatidylinositol 3'-kinase signaling pathway in glioblastoma patients in vivo. Cancer Res. 63 (11), 2742.

Cichowski, K., Jacks, T., 2001. NF1 tumor suppressor gene function: narrowing the GAP. Cell 104 (4), 593.

Clement, V., Sanchez, P., de Tribolet, N., et al., 2007. HEDGEHOG-GLI1 signaling regulates human glioma growth, cancer stem cell self-renewal, and tumorigenicity. Curr. Biol. 17 (2), 165.

Cole, S.P., Bhardwaj, G., Gerlach, J.H., et al., 1992. Overexpression of a transporter gene in a multidrug-resistant human lung cancer cell line. Science 258 (5088), 1650.

Collins, V.P., 1993. Amplified genes in human gliomas. Semin. Cancer Biol. 4 (1), 27.

Dahmane, N., Sanchez, P., Gitton, Y., et al., 2001. The Sonic Hedgehog-Gli pathway regulates dorsal brain growth and tumorigenesis. Development 128 (24), 5201.

Dai, C., Celestino, J.C., Okada, Y., et al., 2001. PDGF autocrine stimulation dedifferentiates cultured astrocytes and induces oligodendrogliomas and oligoastrocytomas from neural progenitors and astrocytes in vivo. Genes Dev. 15 (15), 1913.

Dai, C., Lyustikman, Y., Shih, A., et al., 2005. The characteristics of astrocytomas and oligodendrogliomas are caused by two distinct and interchangeable signaling formats. Neoplasia 7 (4), 397.

Das, S., Srikanth, M., Kessler, J.A., 2008. Cancer stem cells and glioma. Nat. Clin. Pract. Neurol. 4 (8), 427.

Davies, M.P., Gibbs, F.E., Halliwell, N., et al., 1999. Mutation in the PTEN/MMAC1 gene in archival low grade and high grade gliomas. Br. J. Cancer 79 (9-10), 1542.

De Miguel, M.P., Cheng, L., Holland, E.C., et al., 2002. Dissection of the c-Kit signaling pathway in mouse primordial germ cells by retroviral-mediated gene transfer. Proc. Natl. Acad. Sci. USA 99 (16), 10458.

Dean, M., Fojo, T., Bates, S., 2005. Tumour stem cells and drug resistance. Nat. Rev. Cancer 5 (4), 275.

Di Cristofano, A., Pesce, B., Cordon-Cardo, C., et al., 1998. Pten is essential for embryonic development and tumour suppression. Nat. Genet. 19 (4), 348.

Di Rocco, F., Carroll, R.S., Zhang, J., et al., 1998. Platelet-derived growth factor and its receptor expression in human oligodendrogliomas. Neurosurgery 42 (2), 341.

Doetsch, F., Caille, I., Lim, D.A., et al., 1999. Subventricular zone astrocytes are neural stem cells in the adult mammalian brain. Cell 97 (6), 703.

Donnenberg, V.S., Donnenberg, A.D., 2005. Multiple drug resistance in cancer revisited: the cancer stem cell hypothesis. J. Clin. Pharmacol. 45 (8), 872.

Du, J., Bernasconi, P., Clauser, K.R., et al., 2009. Bead-based profiling of tyrosine kinase phosphorylation identifies S R C as a potential target for glioblastoma therapy. Nat. Biotechnol. 27 (1), 77.

Eberhart, C.G., 2003. Medulloblastoma in mice lacking p53 and PARP: all roads lead to Gli. Am. J. Pathol. 162 (1), 7.

Ehtesham, M., Sarangi, A., Valadez, J.G., et al., 2007. Ligand-dependent activation of the hedgehog pathway in glioma progenitor cells. Oncogene 26 (39), 5752.

El-Deiry, W.S., Tokino, T., Velculescu, V.E., et al., 1993. WAF1, a potential mediator of p53 tumor suppression. Cell 75 (4), 817.

Emmenegger, B.A., Wechsler-Reya, R.J., 2008. Stem cells and the origin and propagation of brain tumors. J. Child Neurol. 23 (10), 1172.

Eramo, A., Lotti, F., Sette, G., et al., 2008. Identification and expansion of the tumorigenic lung cancer stem cell population. Cell Death Differ. 15 (3), 504.

Eriksson, P.S., Perfilieva, E., Bjork-Eriksson, T., et al., 1998. Neurogenesis in the adult human hippocampus. Nat. Med. 4 (11), 1313.

Fang, D., Nguyen, T.K., Leishear, K., et al., 2005. A tumorigenic subpopulation with stem cell properties in melanomas. Cancer Res. 65 (20), 9328.

Feldkamp, M.M., Lala, P., Lau, N., et al., 1999. Expression of activated epidermal growth factor receptors, Ras-guanosine triphosphate, and mitogen-activated protein kinase in human glioblastoma multiforme specimens. Neurosurgery 45 (6), 1442.

Ferri, A.L., Cavallaro, M., Braida, D., et al., 2004. Sox2 deficiency causes neurodegeneration and impaired neurogenesis in the adult mouse brain. Development 131 (15), 3805.

Fisher, G.H., Orsulic, S., Holland, E., et al., 1999. Development of a flexible and specific gene delivery system for production of murine tumor models. Oncogene 18 (38), 5253.

Fleming, T.P., Saxena, A., Clark, W.C., et al., 1992. Amplification and/or overexpression of platelet-derived growth factor receptors and epidermal growth factor receptor in human glial tumors. Cancer Res. 52 (16), 4550.

Fulci, G., Labuhn, M., Maier, D., et al., 2000. p53 gene mutation and ink4a-arf deletion appear to be two mutually exclusive events in human glioblastoma. Oncogene 19 (33), 3816.

Fults, D., Pedone, C., Dai, C., et al., 2002. MYC expression promotes the proliferation of neural progenitor cells in culture and in vivo. Neoplasia 4 (1), 32.

Fults, D.W., 2005. Modeling medulloblastoma with genetically engineered mice. Neurosurg. Focus 19 (5), E7.

Gage, F.H., 2000. Mammalian neural stem cells. Science 287 (5457), 1433.

Galli, R., Binda, E., Orfanelli, U., et al., 2004. Isolation and characterization of tumorigenic, stem-like neural precursors from human glioblastoma. Cancer Res. 64 (19), 7011.

Goodrich, L.V., Milenkovic, L., Higgins, K.M., et al., 1997. Altered neural cell fates and medulloblastoma in mouse patched mutants. Science 277 (5329), 1109.

Gorlin, R.J., 1987. Nevoid basal-cell carcinoma syndrome. Medicine (Baltimore) 66 (2), 98.

Guha, A., Dashner, K., Black, P.M., et al., 1995. Expression of P D G F and P D G F receptors in human astrocytoma operation specimens supports the existence of an autocrine loop. Int. J. Cancer 60 (2), 168.

Guha, A., Feldkamp, M.M., Lau, N., et al., 1997. Proliferation of human malignant astrocytomas is dependent on Ras activation. Oncogene 15 (23), 2755.

Gulino, A., Arcella, A., Giangaspero, F., 2008. Pathological and molecular heterogeneity of medulloblastoma. Curr. Opin. Oncol. 20 (6), 668.

Hallahan, A.R., Pritchard, J.I., Hansen, S., et al., 2004. The SmoA1 mouse model reveals that notch signaling is critical for the growth and survival of Sonic Hedgehog-induced medulloblastomas. Cancer Res. 64 (21), 7794.

Hambardzumyan, D., Becher, O.J., Rosenblum, M.K., et al., 2008a. PI3K pathway regulates survival of cancer stem cells residing in the perivascular niche following radiation in medulloblastoma in vivo. Genes Dev. 22 (4), 436.

Hambardzumyan, D., Squatrito, M., Carbajal, E., et al., 2008b. Glioma formation, cancer stem cells, and akt signaling. Stem Cell Rev. 4 (3), 203.

Hamilton, S.R., Liu, B., Parsons, R.E., et al., 1995. The molecular basis of Turcot's syndrome. N. Engl. J. Med. 332 (13), 839.

Harper, J.W., Adami, G.R., Wei, N., et al., 1993. The p21 Cdk-interacting protein Cip1 is a potent inhibitor of G1 cyclin-dependent kinases. Cell 75 (4), 805.

He, J., Reifenberger, G., Liu, L., et al., 1994. Analysis of glioma cell lines for amplification and overexpression of MDM2. Genes Chromosomes Cancer 11 (2), 91.

Hermanson, M., Funa, K., Hartman, M., et al., 1992. Platelet-derived growth factor and its receptors in human glioma tissue: expression of messenger R N A and protein suggests the presence of autocrine and paracrine loops. Cancer Res. 52 (11), 3213.

Holland, E.C., 2004. Mouse models of human cancer. Wiley-Liss, New York.

Holland, E.C., Celestino, J., Dai, C., et al., 2000. Combined activation of Ras and Akt in neural progenitors induces glioblastoma formation in mice. Nat. Genet. 25 (1), 55.

Holland, E.C., Hively, W.P., DePinho, R.A., et al., 1998. A constitutively active epidermal growth factor receptor cooperates with disruption of G1 cell-cycle arrest pathways to induce glioma-like lesions in mice. Genes Dev. 12 (23), 3675.

Holland, E.C., Varmus, H.E., 1998. Basic fibroblast growth factor induces cell migration and proliferation after glia-specific gene transfer in mice. Proc. Natl. Acad. Sci. USA 95 (3), 1218.

Hu, X., Pandolfi, P.P., Li, Y., et al., 2005. mTOR promotes survival and astrocytic characteristics induced by Pten/AKT signaling in glioblastoma. Neoplasia 7 (4), 356.

Huang, Z.Y., Baldwin, R.L., Hedrick, N.M., et al., 2002. Astrocyte-specific expression of CDK4 is not sufficient for tumor formation, but cooperates with p53 heterozygosity to provide a growth advantage for astrocytes in vivo. Oncogene 21 (9), 1325.

Hughes, S.H., Greenhouse, J.J., Petropoulos, C.J., et al., 1987. Adaptor plasmids simplify the insertion of foreign D N A into helper-independent retroviral vectors. J. Virol. 61 (10), 3004.

Hui, A.B., Lo, K.W., Yin, X.L., et al., 2001. Detection of multiple gene amplifications in glioblastoma multiforme using array-based comparative genomic hybridization. Lab. Invest. 81 (5), 717.

Hurtt, M.R., Moossy, J., Donovan-Peluso, M., et al., 1992. Amplification of epidermal growth factor receptor gene in gliomas: histopathology and prognosis. J. Neuropathol. Exp. Neurol. 51 (1), 84.

Ichimura, K., Bolin, M.B., Goike, H.M., et al., 2000. Deregulation of the p14ARF/MDM2/p53 pathway is a prerequisite for human astrocytic gliomas with G1-S transition control gene abnormalities. Cancer Res. 60 (2), 417.

Jiang, B.H., Aoki, M., Zheng, J.Z., et al., 1999. Myogenic signaling of phosphatidylinositol 3-kinase requires the serine-threonine kinase Akt/protein kinase B. Proc. Natl. Acad. Sci. USA 96 (5), 2077.

Johnson, R.L., Rothman, A.L., Xie, J., et al., 1996. Human homolog of patched, a candidate gene for the basal cell nevus syndrome. Science 272 (5268), 1668.

Kamijo, T., Bodner, S., van de Kamp, E., et al., 1999. Tumor spectrum in ARF-deficient mice. Cancer Res. 59 (9), 2217.

Kania, G., Corbeil, D., Fuchs, J., et al., 2005. Somatic stem cell marker prominin-1/CD133 is expressed in embryonic stem cell-derived progenitors. Stem Cells 23 (6), 791.

Kinzler, K.W., Bigner, S.H., Bigner, D.D., et al., 1987. Identification of an amplified, highly expressed gene in a human glioma. Science 236 (4797), 70.

Kleihues, P., Ohgaki, H., 1999. Primary and secondary glioblastomas: from concept to clinical diagnosis. Neuro. Oncol. 1 (1), 44.

Koch, R., 1884. Die atiologie der tuberkulose. In: Loeffler, F., (Ed.), Mitteilungen aus. dem. Kaiserlichen Gesundheitsamt, Vol. 2. pp. 1–88.

Kool, M., Koster, J., Bunt, J., et al., 2008. Integrated genomics identifies five medulloblastoma subtypes with distinct genetic profiles, pathway signatures and clinicopathological features. PLoS One 3 (8), e3088.

Krimpenfort, P., Quon, K.C., Mooi, W.J., et al., 2001. Loss of p16Ink4a confers susceptibility to metastatic melanoma in mice. Nature 413 (6851), 83.

Kuan, C.T., Wikstrand, C.J., Bigner, D.D., 2001. EGF mutant receptor vIII as a molecular target in cancer therapy. Endocr. Relat. Cancer 8 (2), 83.

Landers, J.E., Haines, D.S., Strauss, J.F., 3rd, et al., 1994. Enhanced translation: a novel mechanism of mdm2 oncogene overexpression identified in human tumor cells. Oncogene 9 (9), 2745.

Lassman, A.B., Dai, C., Fuller, G.N., et al., 2004. Overexpression of c-MYC promotes an undifferentiated phenotype in cultured astrocytes and allows elevated Ras and Akt signaling to induce gliomas from GFAP-expressing cells in mice. Neuron. Glia Biol. 1 (2), 157.

Lee, J.C., Vivanco, I., Beroukhim, R., et al., 2006. Epidermal growth factor receptor activation in glioblastoma through novel missense mutations in the extracellular domain. PLoS Med. 3 (12), e485.

Lendahl, U., Zimmerman, L.B., McKay, R.D., 1990. CNS stem cells express a new class of intermediate filament protein. Cell 60 (4), 585.

Li, J., Yen, C., Liaw, D., et al., 1997. PTEN, a putative protein tyrosine phosphatase gene mutated in human brain, breast, and prostate cancer. Science 275 (5308), 1943.

Lin, W., Kemper, A., McCarthy, K.D., et al., 2004. Interferon-gamma induced medulloblastoma in the developing cerebellum. J. Neurosci. 24 (45), 10074.

Lois, C., Alvarez-Buylla, A., 1994. Long-distance neuronal migration in the adult mammalian brain. Science 264 (5162), 1145.

Lois, C., Alvarez-Buylla, A., 1993. Proliferating subventricular zone cells in the adult mammalian forebrain can differentiate into neurons and glia. Proc. Natl. Acad. Sci. USA 90 (5), 2074.

Maehama, T., Dixon, J.E., 1998. The tumor suppressor, PTEN/MMAC1, dephosphorylates the lipid second messenger, phosphatidylinositol 3, 4, 5-trisphosphate. J. Biol. Chem. 273 (22), 13375.

Mao, X., Hamoudi, R.A., 2000. Molecular and cytogenetic analysis of glioblastoma multiforme. Cancer Genet. Cytogenet. 122 (2), 87.

Marino, S., 2005. Medulloblastoma: developmental mechanisms out of control. Trends Mol. Med. 11 (1), 17.

Marino, S., Vooijs, M., van Der Gulden, H., et al., 2000. Induction of medulloblastomas in p53-null mutant mice by somatic inactivation of Rb in the external granular layer cells of the cerebellum. Genes Dev. 14 (8), 994.

Martelli, F., Hamilton, T., Silver, D.P., et al., 2001. p19ARF targets certain E2F species for degradation. Proc. Natl. Acad. Sci. USA 98 (8), 4455.

Momota, H., Holland, E.C., 2005. Bioluminescence technology for imaging cell proliferation. Curr. Opin. Biotechnol. 16 (6), 681.

Munoz, M., Henderson, M., Haber, M., et al., 2007. Role of the MRP1/ABCC1 multidrug transporter protein in cancer. IUBMB Life 59 (12), 752.

Murone, M., Rosenthal, A., de Sauvage, F.J., 1999. Sonic hedgehog signaling by the patched-smoothened receptor complex. Curr. Biol. 9 (2), 76.

Nakamura, M., Watanabe, T., Klangby, U., et al., 2001. p14ARF deletion and methylation in genetic pathways to glioblastomas. Brain Pathol. 11 (2), 159.

O'Brien, C.A., Pollett, A., Gallinger, S., et al., 2007. A human colon cancer cell capable of initiating tumour growth in immunodeficient mice. Nature 445 (7123), 106.

Oren, M., 2001. The p53 saga: the good, the bad, and the dead. Harvey Lecture 97, 57.

Oro, A.E., Higgins, K.M., Hu, Z., et al., 1997. Basal cell carcinomas in mice overexpressing sonic hedgehog. Science 276 (5313), 817.

Pardee, A.B., 1989. G1 events and regulation of cell proliferation. Science 246 (4930), 603.

Parr, M.J., Manome, Y., Tanaka, T., et al., 1997. Tumor-selective transgene expression in vivo mediated by an E2F-responsive adenoviral vector. Nat. Med. 3 (10), 1145.

Piedimonte, L.R., Wailes, I.K., Weiner, H.L., 2005. Medulloblastoma: mouse models and novel targeted therapies based on the Sonic hedgehog pathway. Neurosurg. Focus 19 (5), E8.

Podsypanina, K., Ellenson, L.H., Nemes, A., et al., 1999. Mutation of Pten/Mmac1 in mice causes neoplasia in multiple organ systems. Proc. Natl. Acad. Sci. USA 96 (4), 1563.

Quelle, D.E., Zindy, F., Ashmun, R.A., et al., 1995. Alternative reading frames of the INK4a tumor suppressor gene encode two unrelated proteins capable of inducing cell cycle arrest. Cell 83 (6), 993.

Raffel, C., Jenkins, R.B., Frederick, L., et al., 1997. Sporadic medulloblastomas contain PTCH mutations. Cancer Res. 57 (5), 842.

Rajasekhar, V.K., Viale, A., Socci, N.D., et al., 2003. Oncogenic Ras and Akt signaling contribute to glioblastoma formation by differential recruitment of existing mRNAs to polysomes. Mol. Cell 12 (4), 889.

Rao, G., Pedone, C.A., Coffin, C.M., et al., 2003. c-Myc enhances sonic hedgehog-induced medulloblastoma formation from nestin-expressing neural progenitors in mice. Neoplasia 5 (3), 198.

Rao, G., Pedone, C.A., Valle, L.D., et al., 2004. Sonic hedgehog and insulin-like growth factor signaling synergize to induce medulloblastoma formation from nestin-expressing neural progenitors in mice. Oncogene 23 (36), 6156.

Reynolds, B.A., Weiss, S., 1992. Generation of neurons and astrocytes from isolated cells of the adult mammalian central nervous system. Science 255 (5052), 1707.

Ricci-Vitiani, L., Lombardi, D.G., Pilozzi, E., et al., 2007. Identification and expansion of human colon-cancer-initiating cells. Nature 445 (7123), 111.

Rivers, T.M., 1937. Viruses and Koch's postulates. J. Bacteriol. 33 (1), 1.

Roberts, W.M., Douglass, E.C., Peiper, S.C., et al., 1989. Amplification of the gli gene in childhood sarcomas. Cancer Res. 49 (19), 5407.

Rushing, E.J., Watson, M.L., Schold, S.C., et al., 1998. Glial tumors in the MNU rat model: induction of pure and mixed gliomas that do not require typical missense mutations of p53. J. Neuropathol. Exp. Neurol. 57 (11), 1053.

Sabers, C.J., Martin, M.M., Brunn, G.J., et al., 1995. Isolation of a protein target of the FKBP12-rapamycin complex in mammalian cells. J. Biol. Chem. 270 (2), 815.

Sakakibara, S., Imai, T., Hamaguchi, K., et al., 1996. Mouse-musashi-1, a neural RNA-binding protein highly enriched in the mammalian CNS stem cell. Dev. Biol. 176 (2), 230.

Sano, T., Lin, H., Chen, X., et al., 1999. Differential expression of MMAC/PTEN in glioblastoma multiforme: relationship to localization and prognosis. Cancer Res. 59 (8), 1820.

Sarciron, M.E., Gherardi, A., 2000. Cytokines involved in Toxoplasmic encephalitis. Scand J. Immunol. 52 (6), 534.

Scheid, M.P., Woodgett, J.R., 2003. Unravelling the activation mechanisms of protein kinase B/Akt. FEBS Letters 546 (1), 108.

Schlegel, J., Stumm, G., Brandle, K., et al., 1994. Amplification and differential expression of members of the erbB-gene family in human glioblastoma. J. Neurooncol. 22 (3), 201.

Scott, P.H., Brunn, G.J., Kohn, A.D., et al., 1998. Evidence of insulin-stimulated phosphorylation and activation of the mammalian target of rapamycin mediated by a protein kinase B signaling pathway. PNAS 95 (13), 7772.

Serrano, M., Hannon, G.J., Beach, D., 1993. A new regulatory motif in cell-cycle control causing specific inhibition of cyclin D/CDK4. Nature 366 (6456), 704.

Serrano, M., Lee, H., Chin, L., et al., 1996. Role of the INK4a locus in tumor suppression and cell mortality. Cell 85 (1), 27.

Shah, K., 2005. Current advances in molecular imaging of gene and cell therapy for cancer. Cancer Biol. Ther. 4 (5), 518.

Sharpless, N.E., Bardeesy, N., Lee, K.H., et al., 2001. Loss of p16Ink4a with retention of p19Arf predisposes mice to tumorigenesis. Nature 413 (6851), 86.

Sherr, C.J., 2001a. The INK4a/ARF network in tumour suppression. Nat. Rev. Mol. Cell Biol. 2 (10), 731.

Sherr, C.J., 2001b. Parsing Ink4a/Arf: 'pure' p16-null mice. Cell 106 (5), 531.

Shih, A.H., Dai, C., Hu, X., et al., 2004. Dose-dependent effects of platelet-derived growth factor-B on glial tumorigenesis. Cancer Res. 64 (14), 4783.

Singh, S.K., Hawkins, C., Clarke, I.D., et al., 2004. Identification of human brain tumour initiating cells. Nature 432 (7015), 396.

Smith, J.S., Wang, X.Y., Qian, J., et al., 2000. Amplification of the platelet-derived growth factor receptor-A (PDGFRA) gene occurs in oligodendrogliomas with grade IV anaplastic features. J. Neuropathol. Exp. Neurol. 59 (6), 495.

Suzuki, A., de la Pompa, J.L., Stambolic, V., et al., 1998. High cancer susceptibility and embryonic lethality associated with mutation of the PTEN tumor suppressor gene in mice. Curr. Biol. 8 (21), 1169.

Suzuki, Y., 1999. Genes, cells and cytokines in resistance against development of toxoplasmic encephalitis. Immunobiology 201 (2), 255.

Tao, W., Levine, A.J., 1999. P19 (ARF) stabilizes p53 by blocking nucleo-cytoplasmic shuttling of Mdm2. Proc. Natl. Acad. Sci. USA 96 (12), 6937.

Taylor, M.D., Liu, L., Raffel, C., et al., 2002. Mutations in SUFU predispose to medulloblastoma. Nat. Genet. 31 (3), 306.

Turcot, J., Despres, J.P., St Pierre, F., 1959. Malignant tumors of the central nervous system associated with familial polyposis of the colon: report of two cases. Dis. Colon Rectum 2, 465.

Uhrbom, L., Dai, C., Celestino, J.C., et al., 2002. Ink4a-Arf loss cooperates with KRas activation in astrocytes and neural progenitors to generate glioblastomas of various morphologies depending on activated Akt. Cancer Res. 62 (19), 5551.

Uhrbom, L., Hesselager, G., Nister, M., et al., 1998. Induction of brain tumors in mice using a recombinant platelet-derived growth factor B-chain retrovirus. Cancer Res. 58 (23), 5275.

Uhrbom, L., Kastemar, M., Johansson, F.K., et al., 2005. Cell type-specific tumor suppression by Ink4a and Arf in Kras-induced mouse gliomagenesis. Cancer Res. 65 (6), 2065.

Uhrbom, L., Nerio, E., Holland, E.C., 2004. Dissecting tumor maintenance requirements using bioluminescence imaging of cell proliferation in a mouse glioma model. Nat. Med. 10 (11), 1257.

Wechsler-Reya, R., Scott, M.P., 2001. The developmental biology of brain tumors. Annu. Rev. Neurosci. 24, 385.

Weigmann, A., Corbeil, D., Hellwig, A., et al., 1997. Prominin, a novel microvilli-specific polytopic membrane protein of the apical surface of epithelial cells, is targeted to plasmalemmal protrusions of non-epithelial cells. Proc. Natl. Acad. Sci. USA 94 (23), 12425.

Weiner, H.L., Bakst, R., Hurlbert, M.S., et al., 2002. Induction of medulloblastomas in mice by sonic hedgehog, independent of Gli1. Cancer Res. 62 (22), 6385.

Wetmore, C., Eberhart, D.E., Curran, T., 2001. Loss of p53 but not A R F accelerates medulloblastoma in mice heterozygous for patched. Cancer Res. 61 (2), 513.

Wetmore, C., Eberhart, D.E., Curran, T., 2000. The normal patched allele is expressed in medulloblastomas from mice with heterozygous germ-line mutation of patched. Cancer Res. 60 (8), 2239.

Wong, A.J., Bigner, S.H., Bigner, D.D., et al., 1987. Increased expression of the epidermal growth factor receptor gene in malignant gliomas is invariably associated with gene amplification. Proc. Natl. Acad. Sci. USA 84 (19), 6899.

Wu, X., Bayle, J.H., Olson, D., et al., 1993. The p53-mdm-2 autoregulatory feedback loop. Genes Dev. 7 (7A), 1126.

Xin, L., Lawson, D.A., Witte, O.N., 2005. The Sca-1 cell surface marker enriches for a prostate-regenerating cell subpopulation that can initiate prostate tumorigenesis. Proc. Natl. Acad. Sci. USA 102 (19), 6942.

Young, J.A., Bates, P., Varmus, H.E., 1993. Isolation of a chicken gene that confers susceptibility to infection by subgroup A avian leukosis and sarcoma viruses. J. Virol. 67 (4), 1811.

Zurawel, R.H., Allen, C., Chiappa, S., et al., 2000. Analysis of PTCH/SMO/SHH pathway genes in medulloblastoma. Genes Chromosomes Cancer 27 (1), 44.

Management of brain tumors in the pediatric patient

Jonathan Roth, Shlomi Constantini, and Jeffrey V. Rosenfeld

18

Introduction and epidemiology

Pediatric brain tumors (PBT) are a unique entity in children and in the overall general brain tumor population. Malignant pediatric brain tumors (MPBT) are second only to acute lymphatic leukemia (ALL) in their incidence, and, during recent years, their incidence is continuing to increase. Some 30% of pediatric deaths due to cancer are caused by MPBT, three times that caused by ALL (Bleyer 1999). The incidence of PBT is $4.5/10^5$. This is significantly less than the incidence of adult BT, which is $16.5/10^5$ (CBTRUS 2008). Incidence of PBT is mildly more common in males (M:F ratio 4.5:4). White children have nearly double the incidence rate of black children (CBTRUS 2008). The reason for this discrepancy, which is maintained in other cancers too, is not known. About 50% of PBTs are malignant. Age has a major impact on incidence, histological type, and outcome of PBT. Younger children (especially younger than 5 years old) have an incidence of $3.5–4/10^5$ with a 5-year survival of about 50%. Older children (10–20 years old) have an incidence of $2–2.5/10^5$ with a 5-year survival of about 75% (Bleyer 1999). The 5-year survival for all pediatric patients is about 65%. This rate decreases continuously with age, down to about 23% among patients 45–54 years old.

Tumor location and histological distribution differ in children and adults (Tables 18.1, 18.2). As opposed to adults, where two-thirds of primary brain tumors are located in the cerebrum, only one-quarter of pediatric tumors are located there. However, nearly 30% of PBT are located in the posterior fossa (including the brain stem and cerebellum), as opposed to 7% of primary brain tumors in adults. Children have a higher rate of midline tumors (including the pineal and pituitary regions, and the ventricular system) as opposed to adults (CBTRUS 2008). Certain tumors are considered 'childhood' histologies, such as pilocytic astrocytomas, medulloblastomas, and germ cell tumors. While other subtypes such as glioblastomas and meningiomas, are rare among children (CBTRUS 2008).

Treatment for the pediatric population has a few goals. First, curing, or controlling the disease and increasing long-term survival; second, preventing long-term complications from the various diagnostic and treatment modalities needed to treat the primary disease, and third, minimizing psychosocial impacts of the diagnosis as well as the treatments on the child and the family.

Genetics and environmental risk factors

Over the last two decades there have been tremendous advances in genetic research. This has become the leading frontier for understanding oncogenesis as well as for the development of newer and advanced treatments. Tumor genetic testing enables reclassification of tumor types not only according to histological characteristics, but also by genetic characteristics, enabling matching of specific chemotherapeutics to specific tumor types. In addition, a tumor's genetic profile may serve as a prognostic factor. A review of molecular genetics and diagnostic techniques in pediatric brain tumors was published by Tamber et al (2006). Molecular genetics in PBT is a complex topic that is beyond the scope of this chapter; however, we will briefly review some of the basic data for specific tumor types.

High-grade astrocytomas

High-grade astrocytomas in children are relatively rare lesions. What has been very interesting, and as yet incompletely characterized, is the fact that the genetic alterations that accompany childhood high-grade astrocytic neoplasms are distinct from those that occur in adults (Rickert et al 2001). Genetic alterations that are the hallmark of adult anaplastic astrocytomas – loss of p53, PTEN, p14ARF, and amplification of epidermal growth factor receptor (EGFR) III mutant – are relatively rare in pediatric anaplastic astrocytomas (Tamber et al 2006).

Common chromosomal losses in pediatric high-grade gliomas include those of chromosomes 16p, 17p, 19p, 19q, and 22 (Rickert et al 2001). Within the spectrum of high-grade gliomas, distinct cytogenetic changes are observed in pediatric anaplastic astrocytomas (typified by gains of chromosome 5q and losses of chromosomes 6q, 9q, 12q, and 22q), and in pediatric glioblastoma, (typified by gains in chromosomes 1q and 16p and losses of chromosomes 8q and 17p). The finding of 1q amplification is noteworthy because it may be a marker of poor survival.

In addition to being characterized by their respective patterns of structural chromosomal abnormalities, pediatric high-grade astrocytomas may be distinguished from their adult counterparts on the basis of differential expression of oncogenes and tumor suppressor genes that are involved in signal transduction pathways critical to the process of gliomagenesis. Although amplification of the EGFR gene is observed in up to 40% of adult glioblastomas and 15% of adult anaplastic astrocytomas, this amplification is not a common finding in pediatric high-grade astrocytomas (Cheng et al 1999). Similarly, whereas de novo adult glioblastomas have a high frequency of mutations in the PTEN tumor suppressor gene, pediatric malignant gliomas rarely contain such mutations. When mutations of PTEN are observed, they may herald a poor prognosis for children with high-grade astrocytomas. The majority of adult secondary glioblastomas demonstrate mutations of the p53 tumor

Table 18.1 Distribution of primary brain and CNS tumors by location according to age (%)

	<19 years old	Adults
Cerebellum	16	3
Brain stem	12	4.3
Ventricles	5.6	1.8
Cerebrum	24	65
Pineal	3	
Pituitary	8	7
Cranial nerves	4.6	1
Spinal cord	5.6	4.2

Data from CBTRUS (2008). 2007–2008 CBTRUS Statistical Report: Primary Brain and Central Nervous System Tumors Diagnosed in Eighteen States in 2000–2004. Published by the Central Brain Tumor Registry of the United States, Hinsdale, IL. website: www.cbtrus.org.

Table 18.2 Distribution of primary brain and CNS tumors by histology according to age (%)

Children (years)	0–14	15–19	Adults	
Pilocytic astrocytoma	20.9[a]	14[a]	Meningioma	30.1[a]
Embryonal (including medulloblastoma)	16.8[a]	6.7	Glioblastoma	20.3[a]
Glioblastoma	2.8	3.2	Nerve sheath	8
Other astrocytomas	10.5[a]	10.4[a]	Pituitary	6.3
Ependymoma	7	4.6	Astrocytoma (grades II–III)	9.8
Germ cell tumors	3.9	6.8	Olidodendroglioma	3.7
Craniopharyngioma	3.1	2.7	Lymphoma	3.1
Pituitary	0.8	10.1[a]	Ependymoma	2.3
Others	32	36	Craniopharyngioma	0.7
			Others	14

[a]Most common pathologies.
Data from CBTRUS (2008). 2007–2008 CBTRUS Statistical Report: Primary Brain and Central Nervous System Tumors Diagnosed in Eighteen States in 2000–2004. Published by the Central Brain Tumor Registry of the United States, Hinsdale, IL. website: www.cbtrus.org.

suppressor gene located on chromosome 17p. A relatively small subset of pediatric high-grade gliomas, mostly occurring in older children, also harbor frequent p53 mutations; p53 mutations are seldom seen in malignant gliomas of children younger than 3 years. This finding again suggests that malignant gliomas in very young children may follow a distinct molecular pathway as compared to malignant gliomas in older children and adults (Cheng et al 1999).

Low-grade and pilocytic astrocytomas

Whereas tremendous advances have been made in the understanding of the molecular pathogenesis of pediatric high-grade astrocytomas, there have been comparatively few studies focusing on the low-grade and pilocytic astrocytomas of childhood. Cytogenetic studies have revealed a normal karyotype in the majority of pilocytic astrocytomas examined (Sanoudou et al 2000). Where abnormal profiles have been observed, no consistent karyotype abnormalities have been identified.

Individuals with neurofibromatosis type 1 (NF-1) have an increased propensity to develop pilocytic astrocytomas, especially of the optic/hypothalamic region. As sporadic (non-NF-1) pilocytic astrocytomas occasionally show loss of heterozygosity (LOH) on chromosome 17q (the location of the NF-1 tumor suppressor gene), one would predict that mutations of the NF-1 gene with consequent loss of expression would be found in sporadic pilocytic astrocytomas. In fact, this appears not to be the case. In actuality, the expression of the NF-1 tumor suppressor gene in sporadic pilocytic astrocytomas is often upregulated, perhaps as a reactive response to excessive cellular proliferation. This is in contrast to pilocytic astrocytomas arising in NF-1 patients, where loss of NF-1 expression is an obligatory finding (Wimmer et al 2002). The precise origin of the differing contribution of the NF-1 gene product in the setting of NF-1 vs non-NF-1 pilocytic astrocytomas has yet to be elucidated.

Even with the use of various sensitive p53 mutation detection assays, it appears that p53 mutations are absent or at most infrequently present in the setting of pediatric pilocytic astrocytomas (Cheng et al 1999; Ishii et al 1998). Taken together, these findings indicate that abnormalities of p53 do not contribute in any significant way to the genesis of pilocytic astrocytomas. Most cases of pediatric pilocytic astrocytoma show immunopositivity for p16 and CDK4, indicating that abnormalities in the pRb/cyclinD1/CDK4/p16 pathway likely do not play an important role in the evolution of these tumors (Cheng et al 1999). PTEN mutations are also likely not a significant contributor to the pathogenesis of these lesions, as mutations in this tumor suppressor gene tend to be reserved for higher-grade tumors.

Ependymomas

Chromosome 22 defects are frequently found in ependymomas. Mutation of the NF-2 gene product on chromosome 22 has been documented to predispose to the formation of various tumor types, including ependymomas, especially in patients with NF-2 (Ebert et al 1999). However, the vast majority of sporadic (non-NF-2) cases lack mutations in the NF-2 gene.

Pediatric intracranial ependymomas appear to have a chromosomal signature distinct from their adult counterparts (Hirose et al 2001). This finding suggests that pediatric intracranial ependymomas may progress along substantially different pathways from those giving rise to adult supratentorial or spinal ependymomas. Where chromosomal aberrations are observed in pediatric ependymomas, monosomy 17 appears to be one of the most common lesions, with approximately 50% frequency. Gain of chromosome 1q is also a frequent finding in pediatric ependymomas (Dyer et al 2002). Several studies have demonstrated an association between the presence of 1q gain and a poor clinical course, suggesting that the presence of one or more genes located on 1q may be a factor in tumor progression and/or response to therapy (Dyer et al 2002; Hirose et al 2001).

Our understanding of the origins of ependymomas increased dramatically with the recent Taylor and colleagues (2005) publication, in which histologically identical but genetically distinct ependymomas showed patterns of gene expression that recapitulate those of radial glial cells in corresponding regions of the central nervous system. In that study, supratentorial, infratentorial, and intraspinal ependymomas demonstrated distinct genetic signatures and were shown to arise from restricted populations of radial glial stem cells. For the supratentorial tumors, CDK4 and several notch signaling pathway genes were overexpressed; for the infratentorial tumors, IFG-1 and several HOX homeobox genes were overexpressed; and for the spinal tumors, ID genes and aquaporins were overexpressed. The implications of this study are that ependymomas should be treated with therapies that target the cell signal pathways, maintaining subsets of ependymoma stem cells, rather than the histological or clinical forms of the disease.

Atypical teratoid rhabdoid tumor (AT/RT)

AT/RT frequently demonstrates deletion of the long arm of chromosome 22q11.2 (Reddy 2005). Further molecular studies have led to identification of the INI1/hSNF-5 tumor suppressor gene at this location (Versteege et al 1998). A somatic mutation in this gene predisposes children to develop AT/RT. Some children with AT/RT are born with heterozygous germline mutations of the hSNF-5 gene, suggesting that these children were predisposed to develop AT/RT (Taylor et al 2000); in most cases, however, these germline mutations arise de novo. This suggests that tumors which are histologically diagnosed as primitive neuroectodermal tumors/medulloblastomas but which also harbor hSNF-5 mutations are most likely AT/RT.

Medulloblastoma

Recent gene expression studies have shown that medulloblastomas are molecularly distinct from supratentorial primitive neuroectodermal tumors (sPNETs) (Pomeroy et al 2002).

The ERBB or epidermal growth factor family of receptor tyrosine kinases plays a crucial role in regulating cellular proliferation, apoptosis, migration, and differentiation. Activation of these receptors through ligand binding, dimerization, and autophosphorylation culminates in downstream signaling through mitogen-activated protein kinase (MAPK), AKT, and STAT. Interestingly, one of the four members of the ERBB family, ERBB2, has been shown to be highly expressed in medulloblastoma. A high level of ERBB2 and ERBB4 coexpression signifies an increased risk of metastases and is associated with poor prognosis for medulloblastomas. Compounds such as OSI-774 (erlotinib, also known as gefitinib) inhibit ERBB2 signaling in human medulloblastoma cells and may have therapeutic potential (Hernan et al 2003).

The PDGFR and downstream activation of the RAS/MAPK signaling pathway (including MAP2K1, MAP2K2, and MAPK1/3) have also been revealed as potential mediators of medulloblastoma metastasis (Tamber et al 2006).

Loss of chromosome 17p, often through the formation of an isochromosome 17q i(17)(q10), is the most common chromosome aberration in childhood medulloblastomas, occurring in about 25–35% of cases. Either isolated 17p deletion or i(17)(q10) it has been reported as a significant negative prognostic factor (Gilbertson et al 2001; Pan et al 2005). Recent cytogenetic analysis using matrix comparative genomic hybridization (CGH) suggested that overexpression of CDK6 correlates with a poor prognosis (Mendrzyk et al 2005).

As it is anticipated that genetic tumor markers will increasingly influence the selection of adjuvant therapy for the individual patient, it is crucial to collect tumor tissue samples for genetic analysis. In addition, as it is anticipated that genetic research will continue to evolve, there is a need for multicenter cooperation. Tumor banks are being developed for ongoing and future genetic research.

Environmental hazards

Infectious agents, especially certain viruses, have been associated with increased risk for certain cancers (Martin-Villalba et al 2008; Pagano et al 2004; Reiss & Khalili 2003). Human polyomavirus has been associated with increased brain tumor risk (Reiss & Khalili 2003). Protein transfer from the virus to surrounding cells and secondary deregulation of cell proliferation factors have been suggested. This may be due either to inactivation of tumor suppressor genes or to up-regulating cell proliferation. Weggen et al (2000) have found evidence of several human polyomavirus sequences in human medulloblastomas, meningiomas, and ependymomas. However, currently, there are no clinical implications for these findings.

Radiation has been associated with increased risk of brain tumors. Head irradiation for treatment of children with tinea capitis has been shown to be a major risk factor for future benign and malignant tumors (Sadetzki et al 2005). This increased risk has been shown to be even higher among children with neurofibromatosis (Kleinerman 2009). Recent data suggest that even low dose radiation (such as in CT scans) may induce secondary malignancies, and thus should be reduced whenever possible (Brenner et al 2001; Hall et al 2004). The oncogenic mechanism of radiation is by inducing genetic changes, either down-regulating tumor suppressor genes or upregulating oncogenic genes.

Cell phone exposure has been the focus of various epidemiological studies over the last few years. To date, no clear evidence exists to support, or disprove, the potential risk imposed by cell phones when used by children, but excessive use is discouraged. In adults, the current literature suggests that exposure to the low dose radiation emitted by cell phones does not pose additional risk for developing brain tumors (Kan et al 2008).

An interesting seasonal variation in the incidence of pediatric medulloblastoma has been reported (Hoffman et al 2007). Children born during the Fall (especially during October), had an increased risk for medulloblastomas. Potential causes for this seasonal association may be related to higher levels of community infections during pregnancy and early childhood, or seasonal variation in exposure to various chemicals; however, no clear pathophysiological mechanism has been established.

Diagnosis, investigation, and preoperative considerations

History and examination

The midline location of many pediatric brain tumors results in a paucity of focal neurological signs and delay in diagnosis until the lesion has reached a significant size. Manifestations of pediatric brain tumors may be related to elevated intracranial pressure (secondary to the tumor mass or to secondary hydrocephalus), focal neurological signs, epilepsy,

Table 18.3 Presenting symptoms and signs of pediatric brain tumors

Among 3702 children <18 years old	(%)	Among 232 children <4 years old	(%)
Headache	33	Macrocephaly	41
Nausea and vomiting	32	Nausea and vomiting	30
Abnormal gait or coordination	27	Irritability	24
Papilledema	13	Lethargy	21
Seizures	13	Abnormal gait and coordination	19
Unspecified symptoms of raised intracranial pressure	10	Weight loss	14
Squint	7	Clinically apparent hydrocephalus (bulging fontanelle, splayed sutures)	13
Changes in behavior or school performance	7	Seizures	10
Macrocephaly	7	Headache	10
Cranial nerve palsies	7	Papilledema	10
Lethargy	6	Unspecified focal signs	10
Abnormal eye movements (nystagmus, Parinaud syndrome)	6	Unspecified symptoms of elevated intracranial pressure	9
Hemiplegia	6	Focal motor weakness	7
Weight loss	5	Head tilt	7
Focal motor weakness	5	Decreased level of consciousness	7
Unspecified visual or eye abnormalities	5	Squint	6
Altered level of consciousness	5	Abnormal eye movements	6
		Developmental delay	5
		Hemiplegia	5

From Wilne S, Collier J, Kennedy C, et al. Presentation of childhood CNS tumours: a systematic review and meta-analysis. Lancet Oncol 2007;8(8):685–695.

Table 18.4 Presenting symptoms and signs according to tumor location

	(%)
Supratentorial tumors:	
Unspecified symptoms of raised ICP	47
Seizure	38
Papilledema	21
Posterior fossa tumors:	
Nausea or vomiting	75
Headaches	67
Abnormal gait or coordination	60
Papilledema	34
Brain stem tumors:	
Abnormal gait or coordination	78
Cranial nerve deficits	52
Pyramidal signs	33
Headaches	23
Squint	19
Centrally located tumors (area of third ventricle):	
Headaches	49
Abnormal eye movements	20
Nausea and vomiting	20
Papilledema	20

From Wilne S, Collier J, Kennedy C, et al. Presentation of childhood CNS tumours: a systematic review and meta-analysis. Lancet Oncol 2007;8(8):685–695.

cognitive and behavioral disturbances, and/or endocrine and growth disturbance. A recent meta-analysis reviewed childhood CNS tumor presentation (Wilne et al 2007). Headache, nausea and vomiting were the most common presenting symptoms, however, they appeared only in 30–40% of patients (Table 18.3). Presenting symptoms were strongly correlated to the tumor location (Table 18.4).

A common complaint among children is headache. Among Swedish school children, 40% experienced a headache by the age of 7 years old, and 75% by the age of 15 years old. Approximately 20% of children in the USA have chronic headaches. Although most are due to benign reasons, some may be the presenting symptom of brain tumors. It is important, however, to recognize that not all brain tumors present with headaches, especially in the younger age groups. In one study, 18% of children younger than 5 years old, 52% between 6–10 years old, and 68% between 11 and 20 years old with brain tumors presented with headaches (Flores et al 1986). In another study, 62% of children with brain tumors presented with headaches, and >50% had at least three associated symptoms, such as nausea, vomiting, visual effects, problems with walking, weakness, or changes in personality, school performance or speech (CBTC 1991). In our series of PBT, while 40% presented with headaches, only 3% had headaches alone as the sole presenting symptom.

Symptoms of brain tumors in young children are often nonspecific and easily dismissed by the physician who first encounters the child. Symptoms may include 'cerebellar fits', which may be mistakenly identified as seizures but are actually acute periods of obtundation, representing incipient coning and dangerous levels of brainstem compression due to a tight posterior fossa. Visual obscurations may also indicate high intracranial pressure. Their presence heightens the urgency of surgical intervention. Symptoms may intermittently 'come and go', with the child appearing neurologically intact, giving the impression of a 'functional' cause and thereby delaying diagnosis. Previous studies focusing on delayed diagnosis found that the median period between the first presenting symptom to diagnosis (prediagnostic symptomatic interval or PSI) was about 2 months, and was inversely related to the child's age (Dobrovoljac et al 2002; Kukal et al 2009). PSI also correlated with tumor histology: high-grade tumors associated with a shorter PSI and low-grade tumors associated with a longer PSI. Kukal et al (2009) also showed that PSI is not independently associated with the prognosis, but rather, there is an association with the tumor histology and patient age.

Head circumference is an essential component of the examination, particularly in infants, and should be recorded on a head circumference chart. Visual decline is often missed in young children until the loss is advanced, because the child does not notice or report it. Vision should be formally tested if possible. Visual fields and acuity should be recorded, particularly if there is a possibility that the lesion involves the visual pathways. Sluggish dilated pupils are a sign of severely raised intracranial pressure and are a warning sign of impending neurological deterioration. Only about 20% of children with PBTs will have papilledema and about 50% of them will have a normal neurological exam. Therefore, taking a careful history may be more important than the actual examination (Shai et al 2009). Hearing should be formally tested too, particularly if there is developmental delay or if the lesion is likely to involve hearing pathways.

Pediatric neurologist and pediatrician

It is helpful to involve a pediatric neurologist during the diagnostic phase, particularly if there is a complex neurological picture or epilepsy is a feature. There may be general medical problems, and/or developmental, behavioral, and family issues, which require the expertise of a pediatrician. Preoperative speech pathology and physiotherapy assessments may also be relevant. Pediatric neurologists, as the gatekeepers for MR in many western countries, have to be trained in differentiating between important and unimportant signs of PBTs. To achieve an upward learning curve, an open line of communication must be established between pediatric neurologists, and pediatric neurosurgeons.

Neuropsychology and developmental assessment

A baseline neuropsychology assessment should be completed preoperatively for children over the age of 4 years. Some limited neuropsychological testing can even be done in some 3-year-old children. Formal developmental assessment with the Vineland Adaptive Behavior Scale can also be performed on children <3 years of age. Results of any neuropsychology assessment may be obfuscated by raised intracranial pressure or mood change. Nevertheless, it will be helpful in determining prognosis for recovery of cognitive function postoperatively and also has important medicolegal implications. A complete developmental assessment is essential in the young child for the same reasons.

Endocrinology

Any child with endocrine or growth disturbance identified preoperatively, as well as any child with the possibility of endocrine complications postoperatively, should be assessed preoperatively by endocrinologists. Weight, height, and, when relevant, pubertal status of the child should be documented and their nutritional state and fluid balance assessed.

Endocrinopathy is common among children with craniopharyngiomas, as well as children with optic pathway/ hypothalamic gliomas (Halac & Zimmerman 2005; Janss et al 1995). Endocrinological screening is important preoperatively, as well as postoperatively, as major endocrinopathies may follow treatment.

Epilepsy

Epilepsy should be fully characterized and preferably investigated by an electroencephalogram (EEG) or in cases of more frequent epilepsy by Video-EEG Monitoring. All focal seizure investigation should be followed by MR imaging. An attempt at controlling the epilepsy should be made prior to surgery. Prophylactic anticonvulsants are usually commenced preoperatively for supratentorial pathologies; however, this remains a controversial issue (Kombogiorgas et al 2006).

Neuroimaging

Complete CNS imaging (including spinal imaging) is important in order to define the goals of surgery – total gross resection on one extreme, as opposed to biopsy on the other.

Magnetic resonance (MR) with gadolinium-DTPA contrast is superior to computed tomography (CT), defining the exact location and extent of the tumor and aiding with planning the tumor resection.

MRI should be obtained for all patients preoperatively. The sagittal and coronal images are particularly helpful for midline tumors, showing the tumor relationship to the brainstem, the ventricular system, and other surrounding structures, and thus aiding in the planning of surgery. When dealing with potentially metastatic tumors (such as germ cell tumors, ependymomas, and medulloblastomas), spinal screening MRI should be completed along with cranial MRI in order to detect spinal metastases and leptomeningeal spread before blood enters the canal during surgery and makes it more difficult to distinguish between blood and tumor. Diffusion-weighted and perfusion MR imaging may help characterize the tumor, and assess treatment response (Provenzale et al 2006).

New white matter protocols with diffusion tensor imaging (DTI) have recently become useful in identifying functional pathways and their relation to the tumor. Especially when integrated into navigation workstations, DTI may increase surgical safety (Hendler et al 2003).

It is important to note that some children are diagnosed following an acute event. Thus a CT scan, which is quick to perform and has greater availability than MRI, is often the primary diagnostic tool. CT is superior to MRI in defining skull involvement, and is extremely important when evaluating skull base tumors that may invade the skull. However, these tumors are uncommon in children. An MRI should preferably follow the initial CT, and, when the child is young and may need general anesthesia for the diagnostic MRI, the MRI may be completed immediately prior to surgery. In addition, navigational/stereotactic techniques should be planned, and designated fiducial markers placed on the child's head prior to imaging.

A variety of other imaging tools are available, and useful within the proper context. Brain ultrasound (US), especially in small children with open fontanelles, may serve as a screening tool, but an MRI is absolutely indicated for further evaluation. Magnetic resonance spectroscopy (MRS) has been used in various applications, for diagnosis, differentiation between tumor recurrence and radiation necrosis, tumor follow up, and prognosis (Fayed et al 2006; Schlemmer et al 2002). However, the sensitivity and specificity of MRS is not high, and thus MRS can only be used as a complementary tool to other studies or histological diagnosis. Nuclear medicine has a role in diagnosis and follow-up for children with brain tumors. Bone scans can be useful for showing 'hot areas' for skull-involving tumors, such as Ewing sarcoma and osteosarcoma. FDG PET scans show hypermetabolism related to tumors; however, this technique has a low spatial resolution and is also a complementary investigation (Chen 2007). Similarly, SPECT scans may show increased uptake, especially in astrocytomas, but these too serve as complementary investigations (Benard et al 2003).

Timing of neuroimaging

Neuroimaging is warranted whenever a new neurological deficit occurs; whether motor, cranial nerve related, or an abnormal ophthalmological finding. Torticollis may be suggestive of a craniovertebral or a posterior fossa lesion; thus, when no other cause explains a new-onset torticollis, CNS imaging is indicated. Neuroimaging is also indicated for enlarging head circumferences beyond the baseline growth curve, suggesting hydrocephalus or an intracranial mass.

New onset of a seizure disorder may be the presenting sign of a brain tumor. Yet most seizures among children are not secondary to tumors, but secondary to cortical dysplasias, trauma, and metabolic diseases. The role of MR in the workup of an unprovoked seizure in a child has been discussed in the literature. Shinnar et al (2001) found two tumor cases among 411 children with an unprovoked seizure that had an MRI. Byars et al (2007) found no mass lesions among 249 similar children, and Sharma et al (2003), found two tumors among 475 first seizure children. Currently, based on the available data, MRI following an unprovoked seizure remains a recommendation. MRI should be done emergently if the child remains with a focal deficit that does not resolve within several hours (such as in Todd's paresis), or in a prolonged status epilepticus not resolving within hours. A non-urgent MRI is recommended following an unprovoked focal seizure (with or without generalization), or when the EEG does not suggest a benign epilepsy of childhood, or any other primary seizure syndrome, or in children under the age of 1 year (Hirtz et al 2000).

Other investigations

Other diagnostic investigations include germ cell tumor markers, such as alpha-feto-protein (αFP), beta-human-chorionic-gonadotrophin (β-hCG), and placental alkaline phosphatase in the serum and CSF. The presence of these markers serves in some treatment protocols as a major indicator for decision-making, as well as a baseline marker for tumor follow-up (Echevarria et al 2008).

Dexamethasone

Steroids are often commenced several days before surgery to reduce peritumoral edema. The child's condition often improves noticeably with this medication. Cushingoid effects of prolonged high doses should be avoided.

Operative principles

The goals of surgery are to accurately define the extent of the tumor including the presence of leptomeningeal deposits, to resect as much of the tumor as can be achieved without causing further significant neurological deficit and to correct secondary hydrocephalus and re-establish CSF pathways. Maximizing the extent of resection, while minimizing morbidity is achieved using operative adjuncts such as intraoperative navigation systems, real-time imaging and preoperative as well as real-time functional monitoring. In the following section, we address the various factors that are used to achieve these goals. The goal of resecting maximal tumor is modified for specific tumor types such as germ cell tumors, which are very sensitive to adjuvant therapy. Collection of CSF for cytology and tumor markers has important prognostic implications for those tumors with a propensity to seed into the CSF pathways. Note that lumbar CSF has much better predictive value and higher positively rate than ventricular CSF (Gajjar et al 1999).

Physiology of the child

The child is not a small adult, and the surgeon must be aware of the differences in surgical and anesthetic techniques required for children as compared with adults. This particularly relates to airway considerations, blood volume, thinness of the scalp and skull, delicacy of the tissues, surface area to weight ratio, intravenous fluid requirements, and drug metabolism. The child is easily prone to hypothermia, hypovolemia, and anemia, all of which should be prevented. The young child needs a particularly gentle approach both in general body handling and during surgery, and the surgeon must minimize blood loss with meticulous hemostatic techniques.

In addition, the sulci and sylvian fissure are not well developed in young children, and are not as readily used as planes of dissections or surgical corridors as in the mature brain.

Timing of surgery

The child with a posterior fossa tumor and obstructive hydrocephalus is in a parlous situation and provides a challenge for the neurosurgeon, particularly in relation to the timing and order of surgery. The hydrocephalus is usually controlled following the definitive removal of the tumor, but the conscious state is an important determinant of the timing of surgery. An obtunded patient is an urgent surgical problem requiring prompt action. Steroids may delay the urgency of surgery if the conscious state is only mildly disturbed. The patient should be placed on the next elective list unless obtundation is present, in which case the operation should be done forthwith. Placement of a ventricular drain may be hazardous in the presence of a large posterior fossa tumor, because upward coning and secondary hemorrhage in the brainstem may occur and cause further obtundation and blindness due to the compression of the posterior cerebral arteries at the tentorial edge. The patient usually deteriorates 12–24 h following insertion of a ventriculostomy drain or ventriculoperitoneal shunt. The risk of upward herniation is reported to be 3% (Albright 1983), with a higher risk for large vermian tumors. The treatment is occlusion of the drain, and immediate resective surgery. Third ventriculostomy is an alternative to an external ventricular drain (Ruggiero et al 2004).

It is preferable to proceed immediately with the definitive excision of a posterior fossa tumor rather than initially to treat the hydrocephalus. Even if the patient presents obtunded, immediate placement of an external ventricular drain and resection of the tumor is advised, because the tumor itself may be causing considerable brainstem compression and contributing to the obtundation. In such a case, the ventricular drainage and pressure reduction should be minimal until the posterior fossa has been decompressed, to prevent upward herniation. If the patient has been vomiting for a prolonged period, is dehydrated with electrolyte disturbance, poorly nourished, in poor general condition, and also obtunded, it may be necessary to correct the hydrocephalus first with controlled CSF drainage. This will render the patient in better general condition for major resective surgery. The patient must be observed very closely for any deterioration due to coning or increasing brainstem compression.

Obstructive hydrocephalus due to pineal region tumors is best managed with an endoscopic third ventriculostomy. The tumor can be biopsied at the time of the third ventriculostomy (Al-Tamimi et al 2008). Tumor excision may follow as a secondary procedure if indicated (Cultrera et al 2006).

A controversial issue is a small tumor presenting with a seizure, with no mass effect or secondary hydrocephalus. Despite the lack of literature, it seems that the transformation of low-grade tumors to high-grade ones is extremely rare among children. It may thus be an acceptable treatment to follow intact children with small tumors that appear as low grade on the imaging and present with seizures, as long as the imaging characteristics remain stable, and their seizures are controlled medically.

Positioning

The position of the child depends essentially on the location of the tumor. The surgeon must have a direct line of sight to the tumor and comfortably reach the tumor extremities. The *prone position* is commonly used for posterior fossa tumors and occipital supratentorial lesions.

The surgeon must weigh risks versus benefits when choosing the *sitting position*. There are some high vermis, brain stem, or pineal lesions extending predominantly infratentorially which are better suited to the sitting position compared with the prone position, but each case must be judged individually and depends on the surgeon's experience. The sitting position is not usually chosen in children under 4 years of age. The advantages of the sitting position are that the exposure of the tumor may be excellent, microscope access improved, and hemorrhage and brain swelling minimized. The disadvantages are that the surgeon must sit in an awkward and uncomfortable position, operating with arms elevated and extended for often prolonged periods, and becomes fatigued. In addition, the patient has cardiovascular instability with a tendency to postural hypotension, and the risks of venous air embolism (VAE) and paradoxical air embolism are enhanced. The latter is rare but its effects are disastrous. The risk of air embolism in children, as in adults in the sitting position, is 30–45%, and children are more frequently endangered by this complication than adults (Cucchiara & Bowers 1982; Meyer et al 1994). A discussion of the methods of detection, clinical effects, therapy, and prevention of VAE is beyond the scope of this chapter but is developed further in the literature (Jadik et al 2009; Meyer et al 1994). Pneumocephalus, intracranial hematoma, and cerebral hypoperfusion may also occur in the sitting position. The *lounging position*, with hips flexed and knees flexed up to near shoulder height, maintains the advantages of the full sitting position while significantly lessening the risks of hypotension, reduced cerebral blood flow, and air embolism (von Gosseln et al 1991).

Application of three-point head fixation must be done very carefully between the ages of 18 months and 5 years, and should not be used below the age of 18 months. CSF leaks and depressed skull fractures may easily result if too much pressure is applied. A combined horseshoe and pin system has been suggested for children from 6 months to 14 years of age (Gupta 2006).

Neuroanesthesia

An arterial line, pulse oximeter, and urinary catheter should be placed prior to positioning the patient. Excessive neck flexion should be avoided in the prone position, and the chin should not touch the chest. The eyes need careful protection, particularly when the patient is prone. Towels should be placed and held on either side of the head to prevent any antiseptic preparation entering even fully covered eyes. Careful padding of the face, and especially the eyes, is required for the prone position on the horseshoe ring. The surgeon should check that the patient's eyes are not in close contact with the horseshoe ring itself. The surgeon should also check the peripheral cutaneous pressure points for adequate protection with soft padding. A securing adhesive plaster or silicone bar is placed under the child's buttock, to prevent the child from gliding during tilting of the operative table. Kinking of the endotracheal tube is not usually a problem in either sitting or prone position if nasal intubation is used. Once the patient is in the final position, the anesthetist will need to check the position of the endotracheal tube to ensure that it has not entered the right mainstem bronchus.

Prophylactic broad-spectrum antibiotic cover is given at the time of induction. We currently use Vancomycin and Ceftriaxone, or Cephalothin. Careful attention should be directed to maintenance of body temperature, particularly in the younger child, because hypothermia is a consequence of undue periods of body exposure. Further intravenous steroids are administered at the induction. It is not necessary to administer anti-convulsants for a posterior fossa tumor. If the cranial contents appear tight radiologically, mannitol is administered intravenously in a dose of 0.25–0.5 g/kg at the time of the scalp incision. This helps reduce intracranial pressure and aids operative exposure. The cerebral protective effect may also be helpful. Mannitol can also be delivered later in the course of the operation if swelling is becoming a problem. Precordial Doppler and end-tidal CO_2 monitoring are performed when the patient is in the sitting position.

Surgical approaches

The surgeon must exercise flexibility and versatility of approach to achieve the safest and usually the most direct route to the tumor. For tumors involving the base of the skull or the basal cisterns, the same principles as apply to adult skull base surgery should be applied to the child. The aim is maximal exposure of the lesion with minimization of brain retraction. Skull base approaches are increasingly being used in children to enable resections of tumors such as chordoma, meningioma, and sarcoma (Borba et al 1996; Tuite et al 1996). The transsphenoidal approach may be indicated for some selected sellar and parasellar lesions (Kassam et al 2007). This approach is suitable for intrasellar craniopharyngiomas and those with a globular suprasellar extension (infradiaphragmatic), as well as pituitary tumors (Abe & Ludecke 1999). The transnasal transsphenoidal approach using endoscopy is well suited to the child's small nasal passages (Kassam et al 2007).

Adjuncts to operative neurosurgery

Stereotaxy

Various technical adjuncts to tumor excision are being used to increase the precision of brain tumor surgery and to decrease morbidity (Rosenfeld 1996). Intraoperative *ultrasound* is a simple method for identifying larger subcortical lesions. *Frameless stereotaxy* is becoming an indispensable aid to brain tumor surgery, enabling the surgeon to accurately plan the trajectory, choose the entry point (enabling smaller craniotomies in many cases), and provide useful intraoperative navigation (Roth et al 2006a,b, 2007). Frameless stereotaxy may be used for stereotactic biopsies; however, *framed stereotaxy* is advisable for biopsy of small deep seated lesions.

Neuroendoscopy

Transventricular endoscopic procedures have become commonly used for various pathologies. CSF drainage-related procedures, such as endoscopic third ventriculostomy (ETV) and septum pellucidotomy, are being widely used (Drake 2007; Oertel et al 2009). In addition, endoscopic resection of intraventricular tumors has been described in patients with and without hydrocephalus (Souweidane 2005a,b) (Fig. 18.1). In patients with obstructive hydrocephalus secondary to midline tumors (pineal, tectal, thalamic), the common practice is endoscopic biopsy with or without an ETV (O'Brien et al 2006; Souweidane et al 2000). Use of fine 1–2 mm malleable fiberscopes can provide the surgeon with unparalleled views of the tumor and the tumor bed at close range and from unusual angles. This technique may enable the surgeon to minimize surgical morbidity and to improve the completeness of the excision. The endoscope and frameless stereotactic system can be combined to improve placement and navigation of the endoscope (Souweidane 2005b).

Functional magnetic resonance and diffusion tensor imaging

Preoperative functional MR (fMR) can be used in cooperative children from about the age of 5 years to identify the side of speech dominance with some confidence. Functional MR localization of the sensorimotor cortex can be integrated into frameless stereotactic images, correlating accurately with

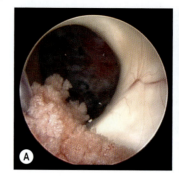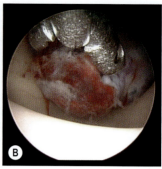

Figure 18.1 An endoscopic view through the right foramen of Monro showing a suprasellar tumor extending into the third ventricle (A). An endoscopic biopsy was performed (B).

electrophysiological localization of the sensorimotor cortex (Schulder et al 1998). Co-registration of the fMR speech cortex localization into the frameless stereotactic system can also be performed. This technique may prove useful to more confidently resect tumors which lie close to or within the language or sensorimotor cortex (Stapleton et al 1997).

DTI has been used for imaging reconstruction of the main white matter tracts, such as the pyramidal tracts (Hendler et al 2003). Combination of preoperative DTI with navigation may additionally aid intraoperative identification of the highly functional white matter tracts, thus assisting the surgeon during removal of intraaxial tumors situated near the pyramidal tract, such as brain stem tumors, or cerebral tumors adjacent to the motor tracts.

Electrophysiological monitoring

Electrophysiological monitoring includes several modalities, such as motor evoked potentials (MEP), somatosensory evoked potentials (SSEP), brain stem auditory evoked responses (BAER), cortical stimulation, and cranial nerve nuclei stimulation. MEP and SSEP provide continuous monitoring during resection of lesions that are adjacent to the pyramidal and sensory tracts. The most common anatomical areas for these lesions are brainstem tumors. Early identification of a decrease in MEP or SSEP response alerts the surgeon to potential damage, and helps to tailor the surgery for maximum resection while also maximizing patient safety. Cortical stimulation (either in an awake patient or with the aid of EMG recording in an anesthetized patient, without muscle relaxants) helps identify the motor strip and plan a non-eloquent corridor for surgery. In young children, while the motor thresholds are too high under general anesthesia to obtain an accurate motor map, SSEP can be used successfully to identify the sensory cortex. SSEP can be measured with electrocorticography, using an electrode strip.

Cranial nerve nuclei stimulation aids in resection of brainstem tumors. Stimulation of the brainstem surface (usually the fourth ventricular floor) maps functional areas, thus again aiding in finding a non-functional corridor to the tumor (Morota et al 1995, 1996).

Cortical mapping versus awake craniotomy

Cortical mapping is useful for resection of lesions close to or within the speech or sensori-motor cortex. It is possible to perform electrical mapping of the cortex in awake patients over the age of 8 years, but this is a very unpleasant experience for the child. Taylor & Bernstein's youngest patient in a series of 200 cases was 12 years of age (Taylor & Bernstein 1999). In the Toronto group, out of 610 patients the youngest was also 12 years old (Serletis & Bernstein 2007). If mapping of the speech or motor cortex is required prior to the definitive resection of a tumor in a child, we would prefer to insert cortical electrode grids, map the cortex extraoperatively, and resect the lesion at a second stage procedure. This two-staged approach is usually used when the child has an epileptic focus and a structural lesion. The standard grids have electrode spacing of 1 cm, which does not permit accurate mapping using extraoperative stimulation. Special grids with an electrode spacing of 0.5 cm are required.

Intraoperative imaging

Real-time intraoperative imaging systems enable navigation based upon images acquired intraoperatively. These imaging systems consist of intraoperative MR (iMR) scanners, CT scanners, or ultrasound (US) systems. By obtaining intraoperative images, the navigation dataset may be updated during the operation, thereby compensating for anatomical changes such as brain, tumor, or cavity shifts (Roth et al 2006a). Using iMR systems for navigational imaging and postoperative imaging alleviates the need for routinely requiring additional preoperative and early postoperative CT or MR scans (Roth et al 2006b). Intraoperative MR systems acquire images in a variety of sequences, such as T1 (with or without contrast), T2, and FLAIR, thereby differentiating pathological tissue from normal brain tissue and maximizing resection control (Figs 18.2–18.4). Contrast-enhanced fast fluid-attenuated inversion-recovery (FLAIR) MR provides marked contrast enhancement clearly showing tumor boundaries and is a sensitive method of detecting residual or recurrent tumor (Essig et al 1999). Note that in the pediatric population, complete resection of low-grade gliomas has been shown to be a good prognostic factor (Black 2000; Cohen et al 2001).

The intraoperative ultrasound (IOUS) SonoWand system enables acquisition of high-resolution IOUS images (Figs 18.5–18.7). Combined with 3D reconstruction used as a basis for navigation, the new, updated images are presented simultaneously with preoperative image reconstructions in the same spatial orientation, to improve anatomic orientation. IOUS such as the SonoWand system have shown similar results to iMR differentiating normal brain tissue from glial tumors (Tronnier et al 2001). In certain cases, the tumor to tissue resolution is even better using the IOUS system, especially when comparing high-end US equipment with low-end iMR machines (Roth et al 2007). The IOUS system maximizes the accuracy and efficiency of neuronavigation, enabling surgeons to fine-tune the resection with optimal effectiveness.

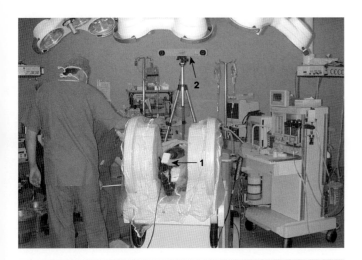

Figure 18.2 The intraoperative MR system (0.12-tesla iMR portable system, PoleStar N-10, Odin Medical Technologies, Yokneam, Israel; distributed by Medtronic, Louisville, CO, USA) in position for imaging acquisition. A coil is placed on the patient's head (1). An infrared camera (2) is placed in front of the system. After imaging acquisition, the magnetic drums are lowered to below the surgical bed and surgery is resumed.

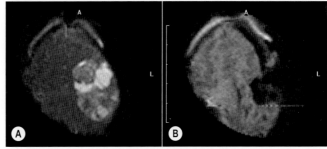

Figure 18.3 (A) Preoperative MR image of left parietal teratoma in a 3-year-old child (e-steady sequence). (B) Intraoperative image after resection was finished (T1-weighted sequence).

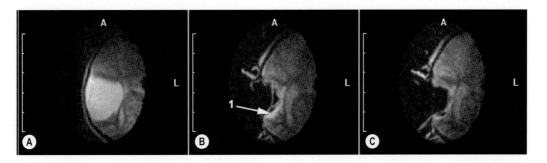

Figure 18.4 (A) Preoperative MR image of a right temporal pilocytic astrocytoma in a 3-year-old child (T2-weighted sequence). (B) Intraoperative image shows a small residual tumor rim (1). (C) Intraoperative image of the tumor cavity shows complete tumor removal.

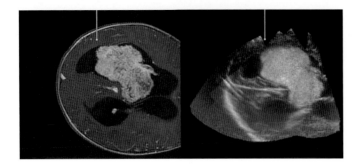

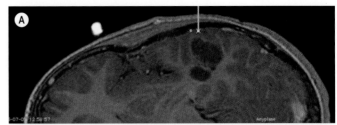

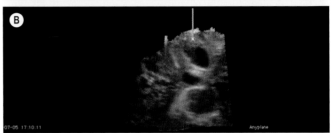

Figure 18.5 Preoperative MR scans and IOUS images before dural opening, showing a choroid plexus papilloma in a 2-year-old child. The images show the lesion from various angles, as determined by the trajectory of the wand. Total removal was achieved. The IOUS images show the falx, ventricular system and the tumor.

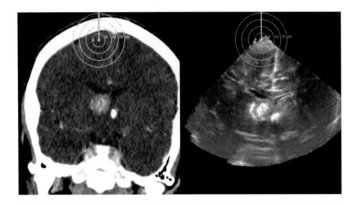

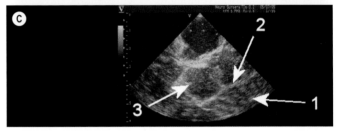

Figure 18.6 Preoperative CT images and IOUS scans before dural opening of a 10-year-old child with tuberous sclerosis. A left subependymal giant cell astrocytoma bulging in to the left ventricle is seen. In addition, some calcifications are seen adjacent to the tumor and contralaterally. The CT and US images are presented in the same angulations as determined by the wand. Total resection was achieved. The IOUS images demonstrate the interhemispheric space, corpus callosum and ventricles.

Figure 18.7 Preoperative MR scans (A) and IOUS images after partial (B) and complete (C) resection of a low-grade astrocytoma in a 15-year-old child. The dual presentation of preoperative MRI and IOUS help to easily interpret the US images. Cerebellum (1) and tentorium (2) are seen, as well as the midbrain (3).

Postoperative care

Intensive nursing is provided in the general ward or the neurointensive therapy unit, depending on the magnitude of the surgery. Any potential or manifest endocrine deficiency or hypothalamic thirst center dysregulation will require close monitoring and management by the pediatric endocrinologist, and ongoing epilepsy may require the ongoing involvement of the neurologist.

Additional aspects that require special emphasis in the postoperative care of children following brain tumor surgery are the requirement for adequate analgesia. This may involve patient controlled analgesia (PCA) for older children, or carefully monitored opiate infusion for younger children. Postoperative neurological deficits such as cerebellar symptoms and mutism after posterior fossa surgeries, cranial neuropathy after brainstem-involving procedures, and/or nausea and vomiting after procedures adjacent to the obex, all cause additional discomfort and stressful impact on the child and the family. Thus, there is often a need for rehabilitation taking place in an environment that includes specialist pediatric providers. Additionally, there is need for family counseling and support.

Timing of postoperative neuroimaging

Identification of residual or recurrent tumor is critical in planning therapy, determining the response to therapy, and the prognosis. Surgically induced MR-detectable contrast enhancement and extracellular methemoglobin formation all occur within 24 h of the completion of surgery, interfering with the detection of small amounts of residual tumor (Oser et al 1997). It is often difficult to perform a scan within this time-frame. It is important to perform a postoperative cranial MR within 72 h of surgery, usually giving a good indication as to the completeness of the excision. If the tumor has a propensity to metastasize, a spinal MR scan should be included if it could not be done preoperatively, but the surgeon should be aware that blood in the spinal canal from posterior fossa surgery will obscure any pathology for several days.

Surveillance neuroimaging protocols should be developed for each tumor type to minimize the number of postoperative scans required to most likely yield a positive result based on the frequency of recurrence. Surveillance imaging is not valuable in identifying recurrence of cerebellar astrocytoma or supratentorial ganglioglioma, but is probably worthwhile for posterior fossa ependymoma, optic/hypothalamic astrocytoma, and medulloblastoma (Steinbok et al 1996).

Reoperation or 'second look' surgery

Reoperation for residual disease may be indicated to obtain a complete clearance of tumor. This particularly applies to ependymomas where complete excision is the most important factor affecting long-term survival. Several operations may be required to achieve this aim if the tumor is accessible (Hukin et al 1998). Intraoperative imaging will verify the total resection of the tumor, and reduce the need for second look surgery.

Interpretation of the pathology

Pediatric neuropathology is a challenging discipline because of the wide range of often uncommon tumor types with often subtle and variegated histological features. Prognostication based on pediatric neuropathology is less predictable than the adult equivalent. This is especially so in the case of gliomas with anaplastic features. Unusual tumor types have been described in children such as the desmoplastic glioblastoma of infancy (Al-Sarraj & Bridges 1996), pleomorphic xanthoastrocytoma, the atypical teratoid/rhabdoid tumor which can be mistaken for glioblastoma and PNET tumors (Parwani et al 2005; Rorke et al 1996). The teratoid/rhabdoid tumor is very aggressive in behavior, with a poor response to chemotherapy, and should be separated from the medulloblastoma group, otherwise any analysis of results and response to chemotherapy is skewed (Squire et al 2007). The increasing emphasis on tumor markers, immunocytochemistry, proliferation indices, and cytogenetics to more accurately classify brain tumors and predict their behavior are discussed elsewhere in this book.

Tumor seeding via shunt systems

The development of extraneural metastasis is uncommon following the placement of a ventriculoperitoneal or ventriculoatrial shunt (Pollack et al 1994). Medulloblastoma confers the greatest risk (Berger et al 1991). Pineal tumors may also metastasize this way (Back et al 1997).

Adjuvant treatments

The role of surgery changes according to the specific tumor type. Tumors that may be treated solely by an aggressive surgical approach include ependymomas, low-grade gliomas (including posterior fossa pilocytic astrocytomas and grade II astrocytomas), choroid plexus papillomas, pituitary adenomas, and most meningiomas.

However, certain tumors may not be amenable to total resection without a significant associated morbidity due to their invasion of critical structures, such as the brain stem, optic tracts, and hypothalamus. Some tumors have a high recurrence rate despite 'total gross resection', this may be secondary to local invasion (such as in high-grade gliomas and medulloblastomas), or to concurrent metastasis (e.g., medulloblastomas, ependymomas, germ cell tumors).

Thus, over the years, various adjuvant treatments have evolved, including radiation-based treatments and chemotherapeutic regimens.

Certain tumors are extremely sensitive to the adjuvant treatments. When weighing the risks and benefits of the various treatments (including surgery, chemotherapy, and radiation), the logical decision for some tumors is to treat mainly by chemotherapy and or radiation, while surgery (if at all) is applied for diagnosis only. A classic example of this approach is in treating germ cell tumors. These typically midline lesions occur either in the suprasellar area or in the pineal region. These tumors are extremely sensitive to chemotherapy and radiation. Over the last few years, their diagnosis and treatment has shifted from surgical resection, to diagnosis based on serum (or CSF) markers – αFP, β-hCG, and placental alkaline phosphatase. Only if all markers are negative is there an indication for a biopsy (Echevarria et al 2008). However, when presenting with obstructive hydrocephalus from aqueductal compression, these patients are treated by an endoscopic third ventriculostomy and endoscopic biopsy (Nishioka et al 2006; Shono et al 2007).

Another example of treatment paradigm shift is in the treatment of craniopharyngiomas. This is a benign tumor, typically situated in the suprasellar region, often rising into the third ventricle. Until a few years ago, the ultimate treatment was a total gross resection. Despite a low recurrence rate, the neurocognitive and hormonal outcomes were dismal, mostly from injury to adjacent structures along the hypothalamic-pituitary axis. While surgery is still the primary treatment, with maximal resection as the goal, additional and effective adjuvant regimens enable a less aggressive surgical approach, with lower surgery-associated morbidity and good tumor control. These treatments include radiation, intralesional chemotherapy (such as Bleomycin or Interferon), and intratumoral radiation (Backlund 1989; Derrey et al 2008; Hukin et al 2007; Ierardi et al 2007; Puget et al 2006; Sainte-Rose et al 2005; Sands et al 2005).

As the focus of this chapter is the surgical aspect of pediatric brain tumors, we will only provide a brief review of the adjuvant treatments, focusing on their essentials and the major relevant tumor subpopulations.

Radiation

For many childhood CNS tumors, radiation therapy plays an essential role in treatment. For most childhood brain tumors, chemotherapy cannot eliminate all the cancer cells, thus radiation is frequently employed. Despite the beneficial oncolytic effect of radiation therapy, there are potential long-term complications. The developing immature brain is vulnerable to radiation, particularly the white matter (Kitahara et al 2005; Kitajima et al 2007).

Neurocognitive decline, neuroendocrinopathy, cranial neuropathy, retinopathy, vasculopathy (including secondary Moyamoya disease), myelopathy, and spinal growth disturbance are all secondary to injury of the developing brain, spine, and adjacent structures (Butler et al 2006; Darzy et al 2007; Duffner 2004; Ishikawa et al 2006; Mihalcea & Arnold 2008; Williams et al 2005).

Secondary cavernous angiomas secondary to microvascular injury may occur (Baumgartner et al 2003; Duhem et al 2005). Secondary tumors (benign, such as meningiomas, and malignant, such as high-grade gliomas and thyroid carcinoma) occur due to various genetic insults, and may occur many years after the radiation treatment (Kleinschmidt-Demasters et al 2006; Mazonakis et al 2003; Nicolardi &

DeAngelis 2006; Umansky et al 2008). The risk of secondary tumors may be higher among syndromatic children, such as NF and nevoid basal cell carcinoma syndrome (Choudry et al 2007; Kleinerman 2009).

We do not advise whole brain radiotherapy in children before the age of 3 years because of the long-lasting and often profound effects on cognitive development, and neuroendocrine function.

Due to all the risks of general radiation, the improved precision of conformal radiation techniques has been increasingly utilized to treat pediatric brain tumors (Habrand & De Crevoisier 2001; Kirsch & Tarbell 2004; Lo et al 2008).

Stereotactic radiosurgery

Stereotactic radiosurgery is a technique in which a high *single* dose of radiation is applied to a defined intracranial volume. The radiation is delivered through multiple low doses from multiple directions, all stereotactically targeted to a predefined volume. The head is fixated in a pin frame during the treatment. The advantage of this technique is the steep target to periphery radiation exposure dose cut off. This enables treatment of an intracranial pathology with less surrounding damage. However, controversy still exists concerning the safety of radiosurgery in children in general, and for pathologies adjacent to crucial structures, such as brain stem, cranial serves, and hypothalamus, in particular. Another limitation of radiosurgery is the size of the lesion that can be treated while maintaining the steep target to periphery dose cut off. Thus, lesions larger than 2.5–3 cm in diameter are not suitable for radiosurgical treatments. In addition, as the patient's head is fixated in a pin frame, this treatment necessitates general anesthesia in order to treat children.

Currently, three stereotactic radiosurgical techniques exist: gamma knife radiosurgery (GKR), linear accelerator (LINAC), and proton beam radiosurgery. Gamma knife radiosurgery (GKR) is based on emission of photon energy from 201 cobalt sources. LINAC uses high X-ray energy produced by collision of accelerated electrons on a heavy metal. Proton beam utilizes the Bragg peak effect of steep energy decay at a constant distance. As opposed to GKR and LINAC systems, proton beam radiosurgery is effective for larger lesions that are superficial to the brain. Classic pathologies for proton beam treatment are clival tumors, thus sparing the brainstem from high radiation doses (Chen et al 2007).

Fractionated stereotactic radiosurgery

Fractionated stereotactic radiosurgery is a technique in which the radiation is given in several doses over a few days, and to a larger target compared to radiosurgery. The head is fixated by a patient-fitted mask. The target to periphery dose exposure cut off is less than in standard single-dose radiosurgery, and the additional radiation induces risk to the surrounding structures.

Intensity modulated radiation treatment

Intensity modulated radiation treatment (IMRT) is another conformal method that delivers high photon energy by a linear accelerator (Kirsch & Tarbell 2004; Teh et al 1999). IMRT treats tumors with multiple fixed photon fields that travel through a collimator made up of mobile leaves of metal. During treatment, individual leaves move in and out of the radiation field to sculpt the radiation dose around particular structures. Although IMRT can be an elegant way to deliver radiation to a target while limiting the radiation dose to normal structures, these structures are still exposed to a high dose of radiation.

Chemotherapy

Adjuvant chemotherapy has become part of the protocol for most adult brain tumors, and in some pediatric tumors too. In fact, since in the very young population radiation therapy is associated with devastating neurocognitive and neuroendocrine sequelae, the need to add adequate chemotherapy is even stronger.

Medulloblastoma

For the average-risk group, a pilot study used reduced-dose craniospinal irradiation (23.4 Gy) with concurrent weekly vincristine during radiotherapy, and 8 cycles of adjuvant chemotherapy (consisting of lomustine, cisplatin, and vincristine) administered after the completion of radiotherapy (Packer et al 1999). A total of 65 children between the ages of 3 and 10 years old were enrolled in the study. Progression-free survival for this group was $86 \pm 4\%$ at 3 years and $79 \pm 7\%$ at 5 years. These study results for the combination of reduced-dose craniospinal irradiation and effective chemotherapy are comparable with or even better than the results typically achieved using standard-dose craniospinal irradiation alone (5-year progression-free survival probability, $67\% \pm 7.4\%$). Companion data from an earlier randomized trial comparing radiation doses conducted by the Pediatric Oncology Group (POG) and the Children's Cancer Group (CCG) suggest a difference in neurocognitive levels measured more than 3 years after irradiation (Mulhern et al 1998). The decline in intelligence quotient (IQ) scores was most significant in children younger than 8.5 years. The full-scale IQ scores of patients after treatment with 36 Gy craniospinal irradiation (70 average) were lower than those of patients after treatment with 23.4 Gy (85 average). The greater toxicity associated with higher dose craniospinal irradiation, together with the comparable disease control achieved using adjuvant chemotherapy and reduced-dose craniospinal irradiation, support the use of reduced-dose craniospinal irradiation together with chemotherapy as the new 'standard' for therapy in children with medulloblastoma. This approach is now widely accepted as the standard in North America. In the concluded POG-CCG trial for average-risk medulloblastoma (A9961), all patients were treated with a reduced dose of craniospinal irradiation (23.4 Gy) combined with a posterior fossa boost (55.8 Gy), and vincristine was administered weekly during radiotherapy (Packer et al 2006). After completion of radiotherapy, patients were randomly assigned to groups that received either the standard regimen of lomustine, cisplatin, and vincristine, or an alternative regimen of cyclophosphamide, cisplatin, and vincristine. The 5-year event-free survival for the 379 eligible patients enrolled was $81\% \pm 2\%$, with no difference in event free survival in either arm of the study. On the basis of this result, the current Children's Oncology Group (COG) is conducting a randomized study that is seeking to further reduce the dose of craniospinal irradiation to 18 Gy, while maintaining the same degree of disease control.

Attempts to improve survival rates for high-risk patients (<3 years old, >1.5 cm² residual disease, or presence of metastatic disease) have also relied on a variety of chemotherapy regimens administered before or after radiotherapy.

The best result for *high-risk medulloblastoma* to date has been published by a consortium of investigators led by St Jude Children's Research Hospital (Gajjar et al 2006). Following maximal surgical resection of the tumor, therapy consisted of craniospinal irradiation (36 Gy M0–M1; 39.6 Gy M2–M3) with an additional radiotherapy boost to the primary tumor bed and a 2 cm margin delivered using 3-dimensional conformal technique. At 6 weeks after completion of radiotherapy, these investigators used four courses of cyclophosphamide-based dose-intensive chemotherapy, with hematopoietic stem cell support, for a 16-week period. The 5-year event-free survival for 48 patients with high-risk medulloblastoma was 70% at 5 years.

High-grade gliomas
As in adults with high-grade gliomas, chemotherapy is part of the basic treatment protocol for children with high-grade gliomas.

The standard of care for adult patients with glioblastoma multiforme consists of radiation therapy followed by 6 months of temozolomide. The DNA repair gene, O6-methylguanine-DNA-methyltransferase (MGMT), removes methylated adducts from the O6-guanine position, which represents the principal mechanism of resistance to temozolomide. In adults, epigenetic silencing of MGMT by promoter methylation has been associated with improved outcome for patients with glioblastoma multiforme receiving temozolomide (Hegi et al 2005). However, whether such a correlation exists for children with high-grade glioma remains to be determined.

A multi-institutional study coordinated by St Jude Children's Research Hospital (St Jude High Grade (SJHG)-98) between 1999 and 2002 tested the efficacy of temozolomide in patients with non-brain stem high-grade glioma (48% glioblastoma multiforme, 32% anaplastic astrocytoma) (Broniscer et al 2006). After surgery, patients received radiotherapy and 6 cycles of temozolomide. The study also included an optional window therapy of irinotecan. A total of 31 eligible patients were enrolled. The 1- and 2-year progression free survival estimates in this study were 43% ± 9% and 11 ± 5%, respectively. The 1- and 2-year overall survival estimates were 63% ± 8% and 21% ± 7%, respectively (Broniscer et al 2006). Patients with anaplastic astrocytoma fared significantly better than those with glioblastoma multiforme; 2-year progression free survival estimate was 0 for 15 patients with glioblastoma multiforme compared with 20% ± 10% for patients with anaplastic astrocytoma. The median time to progression (for the combined AA and GBM group) after the start of radiotherapy was 0.8 years (range 0.2–1.9 years). The marked differences in response to temozolomide between adults and children with high grade glioma highlight the distinct underlying biology between these groups and support the development of therapeutic strategies based on tumor biology rather than similarities in histological appearance.

Low-grade gliomas
The current therapy for the vast majority of LGG remains surgery. Long-term event free survival following total gross resection ranges between 50–95%. Children with less than TGR fair less well, with progression free survival of 33–67% (Laws et al 1984; Siegel et al 2006).

Currently, there is much controversy concerning the place for chemotherapy, and the choice of medication protocol.

As an exception, among younger children with optic pathway/hypothalamic astrocytomas, the Gold Standard of treatment is chemotherapy, with surgery indicated for mass reduction of a large exophytic mass, for relief of hydrocephalus, and for tumors not responsive to adjuvant treatments. A recent randomized phase III study (COG A9952) has compared carboplatin and vincristine versus thioguanine, procarbazine, lomustine, and vincristine in children with progressive low-grade astrocytoma (National Cancer Institute 1997). Results are still pending.

Germ cell tumors
Germinomas are extremely radiosensitive, with a >90% 5-year survival using irradiation alone. However, chemotherapy has been shown to be effective too, with 84% complete resolution with chemotherapy alone. Many agents have been suggested, especially cyclophosphamide, ifosfamide, etoposide, and carboplatin. Chemotherapy has also been shown to be effective and lowers the radiation dose needed when given prior to radiotherapy (Echevarria et al 2008).

Non-germinomatous germ cell tumors (NGGCT) are less radiosensitive than pure germinomas (only 30–50% 5-year survival after radiation alone). However, by adding pre-radiation chemotherapy, the 4–5 year survival increased to 65–75% (Echevarria et al 2008).

Other tumor types
As opposed to the clear role of chemotherapy in treatment protocols for medulloblastoma and high grade glioma, no effective chemotherapy has been found to date to treat ependymomas, diffuse pontine gliomas, and atypical teratoid/rhabdoid tumors.

A new chemotherapeutic treatment is rapamycin and its derivative RAD001. Rapamycin has been suggested for sub-ependymal giant cell astrocytomas (Franz et al 2006). The mechanism of rapamycin is by inhibiting the mTOR function. mTOR is an evolutionarily conserved protein kinase, which is expressed from fungi to humans.

Results over the past 10 years have shown that mTOR serves as a major effector of cell growth as opposed to cell proliferation. Mutations in either hamartin or tuberin drive Rheb into the guanosine triphosphate–bound state, which results in constitutive mTOR signaling.

mTOR appears to mediate many of its effects on cell growth through the phosphorylation of the ribosomal protein S6 kinases (S6Ks) and the repressors of protein synthesis initiation factor eIF4E, the 4EBPs. The S6Ks act to increase cell growth and protein synthesis, whereas the 4EBPs serve to inhibit these processes. mTOR interacts with the S6Ks and 4EBPs through an associated protein, raptor. When mTOR is constitutively activated through mutations in either hamartin or tuberin, this results in hamartomatous lesions of tuberous sclerosis in the brain, kidney, heart, lung, and

341

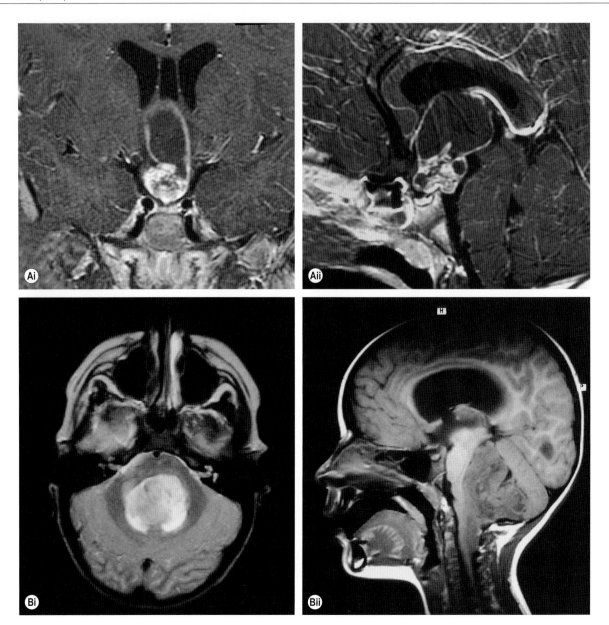

Figure 18.8 MRI scans showing four tumor types which pose a major challenge for the pediatric neurosurgeon. (A) A large craniopharyngioma invading the hypothalamus and extending into the third ventricle. The neurosurgeon must decide whether to adopt an aggressive approach with this tumor and attempt to remove it completely which may effect a cure but with a high risk of major endocrine, fluid balance, growth, and cognitive disability. The alternate approach would be to undertake a partial excision, and accept delayed complications that may follow radiotherapy or re-exploration. (B) A large posterior fossa ependymoma with invasion of the floor of the fourth ventricle, filling and occlusion of the fourth ventricle and extension into the basal cisterns with envelopment of the basal arteries and cranial nerves. How aggressive should the neurosurgeon be? Incomplete removal will have a poor prognosis. Complete removal may result in a cure but risk major morbidity to the brain stem and lower cranial nerve function which may be lifelong or even fatal.

other organs of the body. Interestingly, recentstudies have shown that mTOR signaling is also constitutive in neurofi-bromatosis associated tumors, and that these effects are also mediated by the de-repression of hamartin/tuberin tumor suppressor complex (Johannessen et al 2005, 2008).

Conclusions

The management of PBT is quite different from adult brain tumors. The different pathology, cytogenesis, molecular biology, physiology and sensitivity of the developing brain, are all unique challenges. A multidisciplinary team approach is essential to achieve the best outcomes for PBT. Aggressive high-grade gliomas or medulloblastomas, malignant pineal tumors, diffuse pontine glioma, aggressive skull base tumors, and large craniopharyngiomas, remain a challenge for even the most experienced pediatric neurosurgeon (Fig. 18.8). New knowledge is improving the safety of surgery and the completeness of resection, and advances in radiation therapy and chemotherapy are increasing survival from malignant PBT.

It is the privilege of a pediatric neurosurgeon to develop a special and long-lasting relationship with the child and their parents.

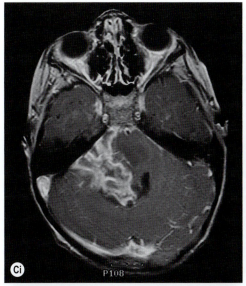

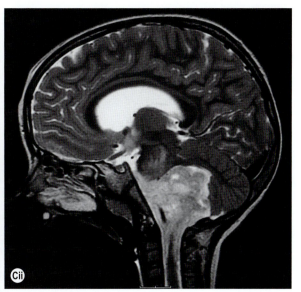

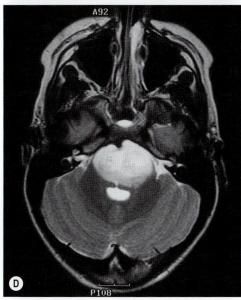

Figure 18.8, cont'd (C) Disseminated primitive neuroectodermal tumor (PNET). The neurosurgeon clearly must rely on adjuvant therapy to effect control of the tumor and this is often only temporary. More effective chemotherapy regimens or biological therapies are needed. (D) Diffuse pontine brain stem glioma. This tumor is a malignant astrocytoma which is inoperable and has a relentless downhill course to death. Short-term remission may be obtained with adjuvant therapy but more effective chemotherapy regimens or biological therapies are needed.

Key points

- The management of brain tumors in children provides tremendous challenges because of the wide range of pathology encountered, the need to preserve the mental and physical development of the child, and the problems created for the parents and family who will require strong support.

- The incidence of brain tumors in children is approximately 4.5 cases per 100 000 population per year.

- Midline tumors such as gliomas of the hypothalamus and pons, posterior fossa tumors, and embryonal tumors are more common in children than adults. Approximately 30% of childhood intracranial tumors arise in the posterior fossa.

- The goals of surgery are to define the extent of the tumor including the presence of leptomeningeal deposits, to resect as much of the tumor as can be achieved without causing further significant neurological deficit, and to correct secondary hydrocephalus and re-establish CSF pathways. If the patient's condition is compromised by the hydrocephalus, this may require initial correction with a delay in the resection of the tumor.

- The precision of the resective surgery is improved by technical adjuncts such as frameless stereotaxy, neuroendoscopy, functional MR, and electrocorticography.

- Postoperative cranial MR is performed within 72 h of surgery and usually gives a good indication as to the completeness of the excision.

- Chemotherapy is the primary adjuvant therapy for young children with malignant brain tumors. Radiotherapy causes serious morbidity when delivered to the immature nervous system and should be delayed. Standard chemotherapy has been disappointing in achieving this goal and high-dose chemotherapy with autologous stem cell rescue is under evaluation. 'Second look' surgery is likely to have a role in clearing residual disease following chemotherapy.

- Chemotherapy is effective in controlling the progression of some low-grade gliomas in children.

- Radiotherapy is a mainstay of treatment for malignant brain tumors in children older than 3–4 years.

- Novel therapies such as immunological and gene therapies are evolving and will be necessary if the prognosis of malignant brain tumors in children is to improve.

- Genetic and molecular analysis of tumors is evolving and will likely play a key role in the reclassification of brain tumors pertaining to selective adjuvant treatments and prognosis.

REFERENCES

Abe, T., Ludecke, D.K., 1999. Transnasal surgery for infradiaphragmatic craniopharyngiomas in pediatric patients. Neurosurgery 44 (5), 957–966.

Albright, A.L., 1983. The value of precraniotomy shunts in children with posterior fossa tumors. Clin. Neurosurg. 30, 278–285.

Al-Sarraj, S.T., Bridges, L.R., 1996. Desmoplastic cerebral glioblastoma of infancy. Br. J. Neurosurg. 10 (2), 215–219.

Al-Tamimi, Y.Z., Bhargava, D., Surash, S., et al., 2008. Endoscopic biopsy during third ventriculostomy in paediatric pineal region tumours. Childs Nerv. Syst. 24 (11), 1323–1326.

Back, M.R., Hu, B., Rutgers, J., et al., 1997. Metastasis of an intracranial germinoma through a ventriculoperitoneal shunt: recurrence as a yolk-sac tumor. Pediatr. Surg. Int. 12 (1), 24–27.

Backlund, E.O., 1989. Colloidal radioisotopes as part of a multimodality treatment of craniopharyngiomas. J. Neurosurg. Sci. 33 (1), 95–97.

Baumgartner, J.E., Ater, J.L., Ha, C.S., et al., 2003. Pathologically proven cavernous angiomas of the brain following radiation therapy for pediatric brain tumors. Pediatr. Neurosurg. 39 (4), 201–207.

Benard, F., Romsa, J., Hustinx, R., 2003. Imaging gliomas with positron emission tomography and single-photon emission computed tomography. Semin. Nucl. Med. 33 (2), 148–162.

Berger, M.S., Baumeister, B., Geyer, J.R., et al., 1991. The risks of metastases from shunting in children with primary central nervous system tumors. J. Neurosurg. 74 (6), 872–877.

Black, P.M., 2000. The present and future of cerebral tumor surgery in children. Childs Nerv. Syst. 16 (10–11), 821–828.

Bleyer, W.A., 1999. Epidemiologic impact of children with brain tumors. Childs Nerv. Syst. 15 (11–12), 758–763.

Borba, L.A., Al-Mefty, O., Mrak, R.E., et al., 1996. Cranial chordomas in children and adolescents. J. Neurosurg. 84 (4), 584–591.

Brenner, D., Elliston, C., Hall, E., et al., 2001. Estimated risks of radiation-induced fatal cancer from pediatric C T. AJR Am. J. Roentgenol. 176 (2), 289–296.

Broniscer, A., Chintagumpala, M., Fouladi, M., et al., 2006. Temozolomide after radiotherapy for newly diagnosed high-grade glioma and unfavorable low-grade glioma in children. J. Neurooncol. 76 (3), 313–319.

Butler, J.M., Rapp, S.R., Shaw, E.G., 2006. Managing the cognitive effects of brain tumor radiation therapy. Curr. Treat. Options Oncol. 7 (6), 517–523.

Byars, A.W., deGrauw, T.J., Johnson, C.S., et al., 2007. The association of M R I findings and neuropsychological functioning after the first recognized seizure. Epilepsia 48 (6), 1067–1074.

CBTC, 1991. The epidemiology of headache among children with brain tumor. Headache in children with brain tumors. The Childhood Brain Tumor Consortium. J. Neurooncol. 10 (1), 31–46.

CBTRUS, 2008. Statistical Report: Primary brain tumors in the United States, 2000–2004. Central Brain Tumor Registry of the United States, Hinsdale, IL.

Chen, C.C., Chapman, P., Petit, J., et al., 2007. Proton radiosurgery in neurosurgery. Neurosurg. Focus 23 (6), E5.

Chen, W., 2007. Clinical applications of P E T in brain tumors. J. Nucl. Med. 48 (9), 1468–1481.

Cheng, Y., Ng, H.K., Zhang, S.F., et al., 1999. Genetic alterations in pediatric high-grade astrocytomas. Hum. Pathol. 30 (11), 1284–1290.

Choudry, Q., Patel, H.C., Gurusinghe, N.T., et al., 2007. Radiation-induced brain tumours in nevoid basal cell carcinoma syndrome: implications for treatment and surveillance. Childs Nerv. Syst. 23 (1), 133–136.

Cohen, K.J., Broniscer, A., Glod, J., 2001. Pediatric glial tumors. Curr. Treat. Options Oncol. 2 (6), 529–536.

Cucchiara, R.F., Bowers, B., 1982. Air embolism in children undergoing suboccipital craniotomy. Anesthesiology 57 (4), 338–339.

Cultrera, F., Guiducci, G., Nasi, M.T., et al., 2006. Two-stage treatment of a tectal ganglioglioma: endoscopic third ventriculostomy followed by surgical resection. J. Clin. Neurosci. 13 (9), 963–965.

Darzy, K.H., Pezzoli, S.S., Thorner, M.O., et al., 2007. Cranial irradiation and growth hormone neurosecretory dysfunction: a critical appraisal. J. Clin. Endocrinol. Metab. 92 (5), 1666–1672.

Derrey, S., Blond, S., Reyns, N., et al., 2008. Management of cystic craniopharyngiomas with stereotactic endocavitary irradiation using colloidal 186Re: a retrospective study of 48 consecutive patients. Neurosurgery 63 (6), 1045–1053.

Dobrovoljac, M., Hengartner, H., Boltshauser, E., et al., 2002. Delay in the diagnosis of paediatric brain tumours. Eur. J. Pediatr. 161 (12), 663–667.

Drake, J.M., 2007. Endoscopic third ventriculostomy in pediatric patients: the Canadian experience. Neurosurgery 60 (5), 881–886.

Duffner, P.K., 2004. Long-term effects of radiation therapy on cognitive and endocrine function in children with leukemia and brain tumors. Neurologist 10 (6), 293–310.

Duhem, R., Vinchon, M., Leblond, P., et al., 2005. Cavernous malformations after cerebral irradiation during childhood: report of nine cases. Childs Nerv. Syst. 21 (10), 922–925.

Dyer, S., Prebble, E., Davison, V., et al., 2002. Genomic imbalances in pediatric intracranial ependymomas define clinically relevant groups. Am. J. Pathol. 161 (6), 2133–2141.

Ebert, C., von Haken, M., Meyer-Puttlitz, B., et al., 1999. Molecular genetic analysis of ependymal tumors. NF-2 mutations and chromosome 22q loss occur preferentially in intramedullary spinal ependymomas. Am. J. Pathol. 155 (2), 627–632.

Echevarria, M.E., Fangusaro, J., Goldman, S., 2008. Pediatric central nervous system germ cell tumors: a review. Oncologist 13 (6), 690–699.

Essig, M., Knopp, M.V., Schoenberg, S.O., et al., 1999. Cerebral gliomas and metastases: assessment with contrast-enhanced fast fluid-attenuated inversion-recovery MR imaging. Radiology 210 (2), 551–557.

Fayed, N., Morales, H., Modrego, P.J., et al., 2006. Contrast/noise ratio on conventional MRI and choline/creatine ratio on proton M R I spectroscopy accurately discriminate low-grade from high-grade cerebral gliomas. Acad. Radiol. 13 (6), 728–737.

Flores, L.E., Williams, D.L., Bell, B.A., et al., 1986. Delay in the diagnosis of pediatric brain tumors. Am. J. Dis. Child 140 (7), 684–686.

Franz, D.N., Leonard, J., Tudor, C., et al., 2006. Rapamycin causes regression of astrocytomas in tuberous sclerosis complex. Ann. Neurol. 59 (3), 490–498.

Gajjar, A., Chintagumpala, M., Ashley, D., et al., 2006. Risk-adapted craniospinal radiotherapy followed by high-dose chemotherapy and stem-cell rescue in children with newly diagnosed medulloblastoma (St Jude Medulloblastoma-96), long-term results from a prospective, multicentre trial. Lancet Oncol. 7 (10), 813–820.

Gajjar, A., Fouladi, M., Walter, A.W., et al., 1999. Comparison of lumbar and shunt cerebrospinal fluid specimens for cytologic detection of leptomeningeal disease in pediatric patients with brain tumors. J. Clin. Oncol. 17 (6), 1825–1828.

Gilbertson, R., Wickramasinghe, C., Hernan, R., et al., 2001. Clinical and molecular stratification of disease risk in medulloblastoma. Br. J. Cancer 85 (5), 705–712.

Gupta, N., 2006. A modification of the Mayfield horseshoe headrest allowing pin fixation and cranial immobilization in infants and young children. Neurosurgery 58 (Suppl.), ONS-E181.

Habrand, J.L., De Crevoisier, R., 2001. Radiation therapy in the management of childhood brain tumors. Childs Nerv. Syst. 17 (3), 121–133.

Halac, I., Zimmerman, D., 2005. Endocrine manifestations of craniopharyngioma. Childs Nerv. Syst. 21 (8–9), 640–648.

Hall, P., Adami, H.O., Trichopoulos, D., et al., 2004. Effect of low doses of ionising radiation in infancy on cognitive function in adulthood: Swedish population based cohort study. BMJ 328 (7430), 19.

Hegi, M.E., Diserens, A.C., Gorlia, T., et al., 2005. MGMT gene silencing and benefit from temozolomide in glioblastoma. N. Engl. J. Med. 352 (10), 997–1003.

Hendler, T., Pianka, P., Sigal, M., et al., 2003. Delineating gray and white matter involvement in brain lesions: three-dimensional alignment of functional magnetic resonance and diffusion-tensor imaging. J. Neurosurg. 99 (6), 1018–1027.

Hernan, R., Fasheh, R., Calabrese, C., et al., 2003. ERBB2 up-regulates S100A4 and several other prometastatic genes in medulloblastoma. Cancer Res. 63 (1), 140–148.

Hirose, Y., Aldape, K., Bollen, A., et al., 2001. Chromosomal abnormalities subdivide ependymal tumors into clinically relevant groups. Am. J. Pathol. 158 (3), 1137–1143.

Hirtz, D., Ashwal, S., Berg, A., et al., 2000. Practice parameter: evaluating a first nonfebrile seizure in children: report of the quality standards subcommittee of the American Academy of Neurology, The Child Neurology Society, and The American Epilepsy Society. Neurology 55 (5), 616–623.

Hoffman, S., Schellinger, K.A., Propp, J.M., et al., 2007. Seasonal variation in incidence of pediatric medulloblastoma in the United States, 1995–2001. Neuroepidemiology 29 (1–2), 89–95.

Hukin, J., Epstein, F., Lefton, D., et al., 1998. Treatment of intracranial ependymoma by surgery alone. Pediatr. Neurosurg. 29 (1), 40–45.

Hukin, J., Steinbok, P., Lafay-Cousin, L., et al., 2007. Intracystic bleomycin therapy for craniopharyngioma in children: the Canadian experience. Cancer 109 (10), 2124–2131.

Ierardi, D.F., Fernandes, M.J., Silva, I.R., et al., 2007. Apoptosis in alpha interferon (IFN-alpha) intratumoral chemotherapy for cystic craniopharyngiomas. Childs Nerv. Syst. 23 (9), 1041–1046.

Ishii, N., Sawamura, Y., Tada, M., et al., 1998. Absence of p53 gene mutations in a tumor panel representative of pilocytic astrocytoma diversity using a p53 functional assay. Int. J. Cancer 76 (6), 797–800.

Ishikawa, N., Tajima, G., Yofune, N., et al., 2006. Moyamoya syndrome after cranial irradiation for bone marrow transplantation in a patient with acute leukemia. Neuropediatrics 37 (6), 364–366.

Jadik, S., Wissing, H., Friedrich, K., et al., 2009. A standardized protocol for the prevention of clinically relevant venous air embolism during neurosurgical interventions in the semisitting position. Neurosurgery 64 (3), 533–539.

Janss, A.J., Grundy, R., Cnaan, A., et al., 1995. Optic pathway and hypothalamic/chiasmatic gliomas in children younger than age 5 years with a 6-year follow-up. Cancer 75 (4), 1051–1059.

Johannessen, C.M., Johnson, B.W., Williams, S.M., et al., 2008. TORC1 is essential for NF1-associated malignancies. Curr. Biol. 18 (1), 56–62.

Johannessen, C.M., Reczek, E.E., James, M.F., et al., 2005. The NF-1 tumor suppressor critically regulates TSC2 and mTOR. Proc. Natl. Acad. Sci. U S A 102 (24), 8573–8578.

Kan, P., Simonsen, S.E., Lyon, J.L., et al., 2008. Cellular phone use and brain tumor: a meta-analysis. J. Neurooncol. 86 (1), 71–78.

Kassam, A., Thomas, A.J., Snyderman, C., et al., 2007. Fully endoscopic expanded endonasal approach treating skull base lesions in pediatric patients. J. Neurosurg. 106 (Suppl.), 75–86.

Kirsch, D.G., Tarbell, N.J., 2004. Conformal radiation therapy for childhood C N S tumors. Oncologist 9 (4), 442–450.

Kitahara, S., Nakasu, S., Murata, K., et al., 2005. Evaluation of treatment-induced cerebral white matter injury by using diffusion-tensor M R imaging: initial experience. AJNR Am. J. Neuroradiol. 26 (9), 2200–2206.

Kitajima, M., Hirai, T., Maruyama, N., et al., 2007. Asymptomatic cystic changes in the brain of children after cranial irradiation: frequency, latency, and relationship to age. Neuroradiology 49 (5), 411–417.

Kleinerman, R.A., 2009. Radiation-sensitive genetically susceptible pediatric sub-populations. Pediatr. Radiol. 39 (Suppl. 1) S27–S31.

Kleinschmidt-Demasters, B.K., Kang, J.S., Lillehei, K.O., 2006. The burden of radiation-induced central nervous system tumors: a single institution s experience. J. Neuropathol. Exp. Neurol. 65 (3), 204–216.

Kombogiorgas, D., Jatavallabhula, N.S., Sgouros, S., et al., 2006. Risk factors for developing epilepsy after craniotomy in children. Childs Nerv. Syst. 22 (11), 1441–1445.

Kukal, K., Dobrovoljac, M., Boltshauser, E., et al., 2009. Does diagnostic delay result in decreased survival in paediatric brain tumours? Eur. J. Pediatr. 168 (3), 303–310.

Laws Jr., E.R., Taylor, W.F., Clifton, M.B., et al., 1984. Neurosurgical management of low-grade astrocytoma of the cerebral hemispheres. J. Neurosurg. 61 (4), 665–673.

Lo, S.S., Fakiris, A.J., Abdulrahman, R., et al., 2008. Role of stereotactic radiosurgery and fractionated stereotactic radiotherapy in pediatric brain tumors. Expert. Rev. Neurother. 8 (1), 121–132.

Martin-Villalba, A., Okuducu, A.F., von Deimling, A., 2008. The evolution of our understanding on glioma. Brain Pathol. 18 (3), 455–463.

Mazonakis, M., Damilakis, J., Varveris, H., et al., 2003. Risk estimation of radiation-induced thyroid cancer from treatment of brain tumors in adults and children. Int. J. Oncol. 22 (1), 221–225.

Mendrzyk, F., Radlwimmer, B., Joos, S., et al., 2005. Genomic and protein expression profiling identifies CDK6 as novel independent prognostic marker in medulloblastoma. J. Clin. Oncol. 23 (34), 8853–8862.

Meyer, P.G., Cuttaree, H., Charron, B., et al., 1994. Prevention of venous air embolism in paediatric neurosurgical procedures performed in the sitting position by combined use of MAST suit and PEEP. Br. J. Anaesth. 73 (6), 795–800.

Mihalcea, O., Arnold, A.C., 2008. Side effect of head and neck radiotherapy: optic neuropathy. Oftalmologia 52 (1), 36–40.

Morota, N., Deletis, V., Epstein, F.J., et al., 1995. Brain stem mapping: neurophysiological localization of motor nuclei on the floor of the fourth ventricle. Neurosurgery 37 (5), 922–930.

Morota, N., Deletis, V., Lee, M., et al., 1996. Functional anatomic relationship between brain-stem tumors and cranial motor nuclei. Neurosurgery 39 (4), 787–794.

Mulhern, R.K., Kepner, J.L., Thomas, P.R., et al., 1998. Neuropsychologic functioning of survivors of childhood medulloblastoma randomized to receive conventional or reduced-dose craniospinal irradiation: a Pediatric Oncology Group study. J. Clin. Oncol. 16 (5), 1723–1728.

National Cancer Institute, 1997. Phase III randomized study of carboplatin and vincristine versus thioguanine, procarbazine, lomustine, and vincristine in children with progressive low grade astrocytoma. Online. Available at: www.cancer.gov/clinicaltrials/COG-A9952. (accessed March 25, 2009).

Nicolardi, L., DeAngelis, L.M., 2006. Response to chemotherapy of a radiation-induced glioblastoma multiforme. J. Neurooncol. 78 (1), 55–57.

Nishioka, H., Haraoka, J., Miki, T., 2006. Management of intracranial germ cell tumors presenting with rapid deterioration of consciousness. Minim. Invasive Neurosurg. 49 (2), 116–119.

O'Brien, D.F., Hayhurst, C., Pizer, B., et al., 2006. Outcomes in patients undergoing single-trajectory endoscopic third ventriculostomy and endoscopic biopsy for midline tumors presenting with obstructive hydrocephalus. J. Neurosurg. 105 (Suppl.), 219–226.

Oertel, J.M., Schroeder, H.W., Gaab, M.R., 2009. Endoscopic stomy of the septum pellucidum: indications, technique, and results. Neurosurgery 64 (3), 482–493.

Oser, A.B., Moran, C.J., Kaufman, B.A., et al., 1997. Intracranial tumor in children: MR imaging findings within 24 hours of craniotomy. Radiology 205 (3), 807–812.

Packer, R.J., Gajjar, A., Vezina, G., et al., 2006. Phase III study of craniospinal radiation therapy followed by adjuvant chemotherapy for newly diagnosed average-risk medulloblastoma. J. Clin. Oncol. 24 (25), 4202–4208.

Packer, R.J., Goldwein, J., Nicholson, H.S., et al., 1999. Treatment of children with medulloblastomas with reduced-dose craniospinal radiation therapy and adjuvant chemotherapy: A Children's Cancer Group Study. J. Clin. Oncol. 17 (7), 2127–2136.

Pagano, J.S., Blaser, M., Buendia, M.A., et al., 2004. Infectious agents and cancer: criteria for a causal relation. Semin. Cancer Biol. 14 (6), 453–471.

Pan, E., Pellarin, M., Holmes, E., et al., 2005. Isochromosome 17q is a negative prognostic factor in poor-risk childhood medulloblastoma patients. Clin. Cancer Res. 11 (13), 4733–4740.

Parwani, A.V., Stelow, E.B., Pambuccian, S.E., et al., 2005. Atypical teratoid/rhabdoid tumor of the brain: cytopathologic characteristics and differential diagnosis. Cancer 105 (2), 65–70.

Pollack, I.F., Hurtt, M., Pang, D., et al., 1994. Dissemination of low grade intracranial astrocytomas in children. Cancer 73 (11), 2869–2878.

Pomeroy, S.L., Tamayo, P., Gaasenbeek, M., et al., 2002. Prediction of central nervous system embryonal tumour outcome based on gene expression. Nature 415 (6870), 436–442.

Provenzale, J.M., Mukundan, S., Barboriak, D.P., 2006. Diffusion-weighted and perfusion MR imaging for brain tumor characterization and assessment of treatment response. Radiology 239 (3), 632–649.

Puget, S., Grill, J., Habrand, J.L., et al., 2006. Multimodal treatment of craniopharyngioma: defining a risk-adapted strategy. J. Pediatr. Endocrinol. Metab. 19 (Suppl.), 367–370.

Reddy, A.T., 2005. Atypical teratoid/rhabdoid tumors of the central nervous system. J. Neurooncol. 75 (3), 309–313.

Reiss, K., Khalili, K., 2003. Viruses and cancer: lessons from the human polyomavirus, JCV. Oncogene 22 (42), 6517–6523.

Rickert, C.H., Strater, R., Kaatsch, P., et al., 2001. Pediatric high-grade astrocytomas show chromosomal imbalances distinct from adult cases. Am. J. Pathol. 158 (4), 1525–1532.

Rorke, L.B., Packer, R.J., Biegel, J.A., 1996. Central nervous system atypical teratoid/rhabdoid tumors of infancy and childhood: definition of an entity. J. Neurosurg. 85 (1), 56–65.

Rosenfeld, J.V., 1996. Minimally invasive neurosurgery. Aust. NZJ Surg. 66 (8), 553–559.

Roth, J., Beni Adani, L., Biyani, N., et al., 2006b. Intraoperative portable 0.12-tesla MRI in pediatric neurosurgery. Pediatr. Neurosurg. 42 (2), 74–80.

Roth, J., Beni-Adani, L., Biyani, N., et al., 2006a. Classical and real-time neuronavigation in pediatric neurosurgery. Childs Nerv. Syst. 22 (9), 1065–1071.

Roth, J., Biyani, N., Beni-Adani, L., et al., 2007. Real-time neuronavigation with high-quality 3D ultrasound SonoWand in pediatric neurosurgery. Pediatr. Neurosurg. 43 (3), 185–191.

Ruggiero, C., Cinalli, G., Spennato, P., et al., 2004. Endoscopic third ventriculostomy in the treatment of hydrocephalus in posterior fossa tumors in children. Childs Nerv. Syst. 20 (11–12), 828–833.

Sadetzki, S., Chetrit, A., Freedman, L., et al., 2005. Long-term follow-up for brain tumor development after childhood exposure to ionizing radiation for tinea capitis. Radiat. Res. 163 (4), 424–432.

Sainte-Rose, C., Puget, S., Wray, A., et al., 2005. Craniopharyngioma: the pendulum of surgical management. Childs Nerv. Syst. 21 (8–9), 691–695.

Sands, S.A., Milner, J.S., Goldberg, J., et al., 2005. Quality of life and behavioral follow-up study of pediatric survivors of craniopharyngioma. J. Neurosurg. 103 (Suppl.), 302–311.

Sanoudou, D., Tingby, O., Ferguson-Smith, M.A., et al., 2000. Analysis of pilocytic astrocytoma by comparative genomic hybridization. Br. J. Cancer 82 (6), 1218–1222.

Schlemmer, H.P., Bachert, P., Henze, M., et al., 2002. Differentiation of radiation necrosis from tumor progression using proton magnetic resonance spectroscopy. Neuroradiology 44 (3), 216–222.

Schulder, M., Maldjian, J.A., Liu, W.C., et al., 1998. Functional image-guided surgery of intracranial tumors located in or near the sensorimotor cortex. J. Neurosurg. 89 (3), 412–418.

Serletis, D., Bernstein, M., 2007. Prospective study of awake craniotomy used routinely and nonselectively for supratentorial tumors. J. Neurosurg. 107 (1), 1–6.

Shai, V., Fatal, V., Constantini, S., 2009. Delay in the diagnosis of pediatric brain tumors in Israel: A survey on 330 children. Submitted for publication.

Sharma, S., Riviello, J.J., Harper, M.B., et al., 2003. The role of emergent neuroimaging in children with new-onset afebrile seizures. Pediatrics 111 (1), 1–5.

Shinnar, S., O'Dell, C., Mitnick, R., et al., 2001. Neuroimaging abnormalities in children with an apparent first unprovoked seizure. Epilepsy. Res. 43 (3), 261–269.

Shono, T., Natori, Y., Morioka, T., et al., 2007. Results of a long-term follow-up after neuroendoscopic biopsy procedure and third ventriculostomy in patients with intracranial germinomas. J. Neurosurg. 107 (Suppl.), 193–198.

Siegel, M.J., Finlay, J.L., Zacharoulis, S., 2006. State of the art chemotherapeutic management of pediatric brain tumors. Expert. Rev. Neurother. 6 (5), 765–779.

Souweidane M.M., 2005a. Endoscopic management of pediatric brain tumors. Neurosurg. Focus 18 (6A), E1.

Souweidane, M.M., 2005b. Endoscopic surgery for intraventricular brain tumors in patients without hydrocephalus. Neurosurgery 57 (Suppl.), 312–318.

Souweidane, M.M., Sandberg, D.I., Bilsky, M.H., et al., 2000. Endoscopic biopsy for tumors of the third ventricle. Pediatr. Neurosurg. 33 (3), 132–137.

Squire, S.E., Chan, M.D., Marcus, K.J., 2007. Atypical teratoid/rhabdoid tumor: the controversy behind radiation therapy. J. Neurooncol. 81 (1), 97–111.

Stapleton, S.R., Kiriakopoulos, E., Mikulis, D., et al., 1997. Combined utility of functional MRI, cortical mapping, and frameless stereotaxy in the resection of lesions in eloquent areas of brain in children. Pediatr. Neurosurg. 26 (2), 68–82.

Steinbok, P., Hentschel, S., Cochrane, D.D., et al., 1996. Value of postoperative surveillance imaging in the management of children with some common brain tumors. J. Neurosurg. 84 (5), 726–732.

Tamber, M.S., Bansal, K., Liang, M.L., et al., 2006. Current concepts in the molecular genetics of pediatric brain tumors: implications for emerging therapies. Childs Nerv. Syst. 22 (11), 1379–1394.

Taylor, M.D., Bernstein, M., 1999. Awake craniotomy with brain mapping as the routine surgical approach to treating patients with supratentorial intraaxial tumors: a prospective trial of 200 cases. J. Neurosurg. 90 (1), 35–41.

Taylor, M.D., Gokgoz, N., Andrulis, I.L., et al., 2000. Familial posterior fossa brain tumors of infancy secondary to germline mutation of the hSNF5 gene. Am. J. Hum. Genet. 66 (4), 1403–1406.

Taylor, M.D., Poppleton, H., Fuller, C., et al., 2005. Radial glia cells are candidate stem cells of ependymoma. Cancer Cell 8 (4), 323–335.

Teh, B.S., Woo, S.Y., Butler, E.B., 1999. Intensity modulated radiation therapy (IMRT), a new promising technology in radiation oncology. Oncologist 4 (6), 433–442.

Tronnier, V.M., Bonsanto, M.M., Staubert, A., et al., 2001. Comparison of intraoperative MR imaging and 3D-navigated ultrasonography in the detection and resection control of lesions. Neurosurg. Focus 10 (2), E3.

Tuite, G.F., Veres, R., Crockard, H.A., et al., 1996. Pediatric transoral surgery: indications, complications, and long-term outcome. J. Neurosurg. 84 (4), 573–583.

Umansky, F., Shoshan, Y., Rosenthal, G., et al., 2008. Radiation-induced meningioma. Neurosurg. Focus 24 (5), E7.

Versteege, I., Sevenet, N., Lange, J., et al., 1998. Truncating mutations of hSNF5/INI1 in aggressive paediatric cancer. Nature 394 (6689), 203–206.

von Gosseln, H.H., Samii, M., Suhr, D., et al., 1991. The lounging position for posterior fossa surgery: anesthesiological considerations regarding air embolism. Childs Nerv. Syst. 7 (7), 368–374.

Weggen, S., Bayer, T.A., von Deimling, A., et al., 2000. Low frequency of SV40, JC and BK polyomavirus sequences in human medulloblastomas, meningiomas and ependymomas. Brain Pathol. 10 (1), 85–92.

Williams, G.B., Kun, L.E., Thompson, J.W., et al., 2005. Hearing loss as a late complication of radiotherapy in children with brain tumors. Ann. Otol. Rhinol. Laryngol. 114 (4), 328–331.

Wilne, S., Collier, J., Kennedy, C., et al., 2007. Presentation of childhood CNS tumours: a systematic review and meta-analysis. Lancet Oncol. 8 (8), 685–695.

Wimmer, K., Eckart, M., Meyer-Puttlitz, B., et al., 2002. Mutational and expression analysis of the NF-1 gene argues against a role as tumor suppressor in sporadic pilocytic astrocytomas. J. Neuropathol. Exp. Neurol. 61 (10), 896–902.

Management of recurrent gliomas and meningiomas

Lewis Hou and Griffith R. Harsh IV

19

Introduction

Renewed growth of a mass at the site of a previously treated brain tumor raises the issues of indications for and choices of treatment. Important considerations include the following:

1. Is the mass a recurrence of the original tumor?
2. Why did the tumor regrow?
3. Does this regrowth pose a threat to the patient's neurologic function and survival?
4. What additional therapy is appropriate?

Confirmation of recurrence

When recurrent growth of a tumor is suspected clinically or radiographically, the full set of imaging studies should be reviewed with careful attention directed toward detecting any change of imaging signals and documenting the size of the lesion. The original pathology specimen should be reviewed.

Differential diagnosis

An enlarging lesion at the site of a previously treated tumor likely represents renewed growth of an incompletely eradicated initial tumor rather than the development of a new pathologic entity. Exceptions are infrequent but those in the following list need to be considered:

- A distinctly new tumor may arise at the site of an irradicated tumor. This is more likely to occur if there is a genetic predisposition to tumor development shared by cells in the area; e.g., multiple neurofibromas can develop along the same nerve root in a patient with neurofibromatosis or multiple gliomas may occur in a patient with tuberous sclerosis.

- A tumor of related histology may supplant the original tumor; e.g., the astrocytic component may replace the oligodendrocytic component as the predominant sub-type of a mixed glioma, or a gliosarcoma may arise from a previously treated glioblastoma.

- The initial therapy may induce a secondary tumor of a different type; e.g., a parasellar sarcoma after irradiation for a pituitary adenoma, or a glioblastoma in the radiation field of a meningioma.

- A metastatic tumor may grow in the original tumor; e.g., a breast metastasis within a pituitary adenoma.

- Non-neoplastic lesions may mimic tumor growth; e.g., an abscess or granuloma at the site of resection of a tumor induced by treatment of the original tumor, or radiation necrosis following focal high dose irradiation (Buckley & Broome 1995; Vogelsang et al 1998).

These alternative diagnoses must be excluded before prognosis is addressed and therapy is chosen. Neurodiagnostic imaging usually permits accurate prediction of the diagnosis. Generally, recurrent tumors have imaging features similar to those of the original lesion. A recurrent meningioma commonly is dural-based and homogeneously enhances, whereas a recurrent malignant glioma will likely have central low intensity, rim enhancement, and hypointense surround on enhanced T1-weighted magnetic resonance imaging (MRI). In some cases, however, attention to subtle differences may be required: a dural tail may differentiate a radiation-induced meningioma from a recurrent pituitary adenoma; a more spherical, sharply demarcated shape may suggest an abscess rather than a recurrent malignant glioma; and a diffuse, irregularly marginated pattern of surrounding edema may indicate radiation necrosis rather than a recurrent tumor.

Two scenarios, malignant progression and radiation effects, often pose particular diagnostic difficulty. In each case, alternative diagnoses are often impossible to distinguish using current imaging modalities alone. Thus, biopsy for histological evaluation and confirmation may be necessary.

Malignant progression

The first scenario is the renewed growth of a low-grade tumor. When low-grade gliomas regrow after therapy, approximately half remain non-anaplastic, but the other 50% have progressed to a more malignant form (McCormack et al 1992). Molecular analyses have delineated genetic correlates of this progression (Ohgaki 2005; Ohgaki et al

2007). Enlarging low-grade tumors will usually resemble the original tumor on imaging studies. When progression in grade has occurred, the new tumor may also resemble the old one, especially if the original tumor enhanced with contrast. Enhancement is highly predictive of likelihood of recurrence; low-grade enhancing tumors are 6–8 times more likely to recur than non-enhancing ones (McCormack et al 1992). Most commonly, new malignant growth in a previously non-enhancing glioma enhances and thus is readily identified. In one study, only 30% (16/42) of low-grade tumors enhanced initially, but 92% (22/24) enhanced at recurrence (McCormack et al 1992). Occasionally, an enlarging malignant focus may not enhance. It might, however, be apparent as a region of hypermetabolism on a 2-deoxyglucose or 11-C methionine PET study, or have an increased rate of enhancement on a dynamic MRI scan, increased activity on a dual isotope single photon emission computerized tomogram (SPECT), or increased choline signal on magnetic resonance spectroscopy (MRS) (Wong et al 2002; Alexiou et al 2008, 2009; Hu et al 2009). The differential specificity of each of these new modalities is approximately 80–90% (Hutter et al 2003). Usually, however, histologic analysis after biopsy or resection is warranted to verify malignant transformation (Hsu et al 1997a,b).

Histologic grade is also a critical determinant of recurrence and outcome in meningiomas. Atypical (approximately 5% of meningiomas) and malignant (approximately 2% of meningiomas) meningiomas contain histologic features that predict more rapid growth, earlier clinical deterioration after treatment of recurrence, and shorter survival (de la Monte et al 1986; Mahmood et al 1993; Kim et al 2006; Bruna et al 2007). The rates of recurrence for benign, atypical, and malignant meningiomas (using previous WHO criteria) in one large series were 7%, 35%, and 73%, respectively (Maier et al 1992).

Progression in grade in typical meningiomas occurs less frequently than in low-grade gliomas. Most recurrent meningiomas retain their original histologic features at recurrence. Rapid regrowth may raise the suspicion of progression, but tissue examination is required to confirm or exclude the development of atypical and malignant histologic features. Benign meningiomas may become atypical or malignant, and atypical tumors may become frankly malignant. In one series utilizing previous WHO criteria, 6 of 23 (26%) originally atypical meningiomas were malignant at recurrence (Palma et al 1997).

Recent reviews of the Mayo Clinic series have prompted revision of the WHO criteria for atypical (grade II) and malignant (anaplastic, grade III) meningioma (Riemenschneider et al 2006). Meningiomas are considered atypical, and thus likely to recur and cause death sooner, if they have either: (1) at least three of five features: sheeting, hypercellularity, small cells, large nuclei, brain invasion or (2) at least four mitoses in 10 high-powered fields. Such atypical tumors recur at 3.5× the frequency (41% vs 12%) of recurrence of tumors of typical histology. Tumors are termed anaplastic (WHO grade III) if meningothelial features are replaced by those of sarcoma, melanoma, or carcinoma or there are at least 20 mitoses per high-powered field. Such anaplastic tumors recur promptly, regrow rapidly, and prove fatal at a median interval of 18 months.

Radiographic characteristics such as multinodularity, central hypodensity, extensive edema, and limited demarcation from cortex and surrounding dura suggest the presence of atypical histology. PET scans can show hypermetabolism and MRI may demonstrate increased tumor blood volume (DiChiro et al 1987).

Radiation effects

The second scenario that causes diagnostic difficulty is renewed enlargement of a tumor mass following radiation. Often, CT and MR imaging inadequately distinguish recurrent tumor from radiation-induced enlargement. Usually only large, very malignant tumors grow sufficiently rapidly to show significant enlargement during, or within 3 months of completing, a course of radiation. When this does occur, the prognosis is particularly poor (Barker et al 1996).

Radiation can cause tumor enlargement in three ways: (1) through an early reaction, occurring during or shortly after irradiation, which is likely to be edema; (2) through an early delayed reaction arising a few weeks to a few months after radiation, which involves edema and demyelination; (3) through a late delayed reaction that occurs 6–24 months after radiation and reflects radiation-induced necrosis (Leibel & Sheline 1987). Regional teletherapy to a dose of 60 Gy is the current standard radiation treatment for most gliomas; most meningiomas receive 50–55 Gy (Walker et al 1978). Although these doses have a low risk of inducing radiation necrosis, regional early and early delayed effects are relatively common. In most cases, tissue swelling represents edema and is transient. Acute symptoms from early and early delayed effects of radiation usually respond quickly to a short course of corticosteroids. The low density, T_1-hypointense, T_2-hyperintense regions of edema correspond to the area irradiated. Chronically, these volumes of brain will demonstrate parenchymal atrophy, enlargement of subarachnoid spaces, and *ex vacuo* ventricular dilatation. Dementia with apathy, inanition, and memory loss and decline in fine motor control are the clinical correlates. In the absence of new tumor growth, enhancement on CT and MRI beyond the initial resection margin is infrequent; when it does occur, it is patchy, irregularly marginated, and it can be distinguished from the more focal appearance of recurrent tumor.

In contrast, the late delayed effect of radiation-induced necrosis appears at about the time malignant tumors might be expected to recur (Scharfen et al 1992). It is thus more likely to be mistaken for recurrent tumor growth. The risk of radiation necrosis increases with the volume of tissue treated, the dose delivered, and the fraction size (Marks et al 1981). Radiation necrosis following fractionated treatment to doses <70 Gy is rare, but it is much more common following brachytherapy or radiosurgery, which deliver high doses of radiation to relatively small volumes over a short time period (Loeffler et al 1990a,b; Scharfen et al 1992). A common protocol for brachytherapy is a 50–60 Gy boost (to 60 Gy of regional external beam radiotherapy) to a 0–5 cm tumor delivered over approximately one week. The radiosurgery equivalent is a 10–20 Gy boost to a 0–3 cm diameter tumor delivered in <1 h (Li et al 1992). Necrosis is radiographically and pathologically evident in almost all cases and symptomatic in about half.

Whether it arises from higher doses of fractionated radiotherapy, brachytherapy, or radiosurgery, radiation necrosis is often difficult to distinguish from recurrent tumor. It forms a ring contrast-enhancing mass that resembles a malignant tumor. It has a CT hypodense, T_1-hypointense, T_2-hyperintense center; an enhancing annular region; and a hypodense, T_1-hypointense, T_2-hyperintense surround. The surround corresponds to edema that strikingly radiates along white matter tracts. The similarity of this appearance to that of recurrent tumors and the time course of its occurrence frequently necessitates additional measures to differentiate radiation-induced necrosis from recurrent tumor. Several functional neurodiagnostic imaging techniques attempt to distinguish between these two possibilities. These include PET scans, SPECT studies, cerebral blood volume mapping, and MRS. Regions of high activity are thought to distinguish recurrent tumor from relatively metabolically inactive and hypovascular radiation necrosis (Alexiou et al 2009). Although specificity in differentiating tumor from radiation necrosis of up to 100% has been claimed, in many cases, these studies are inconclusive and the diagnosis is revealed either by the clinical course or by analysis of a pathology specimen.

When an enlarging mass, which is either recurrent tumor, radiation necrosis, or both, becomes symptomatic, corticosteroid therapy is required (Edwards & Wilson 1980). Up to half the patients receiving brachytherapy and radiosurgery for a malignant glioma develop symptoms that either prove refractory to corticosteroids or require debilitating long-term steroid use (Scharfen et al 1992; Alexander & Loeffler 1998; Combs et al 2005; Biswas et al 2009). Surgery for resection of an enlarging, symptomatic mass is needed in 20–40% of cases following brachytherapy or radiosurgery of a malignant glioma and fewer than 5% of cases of radiosurgery for meningiomas. At reoperation for presumed radiation necrosis following focal radiation treatment of a malignant glioma, necrosis without tumor was found in 5% of cases, tumor alone in 29%, and a mixture of radiation necrosis and tumor in 66% (Scharfen et al 1992). In almost all cases, the tumor that is seen is of reduced viability (Daumas-Duport et al 1984; Rosenblum et al 1985).

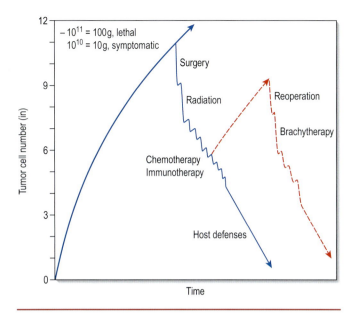

Figure 19.1 Multimodality therapy of malignant gliomas. Various therapeutic methods, including reoperation, are used in the attempt to reduce the number of tumor cells.

Causes of recurrence

Renewed growth of a brain tumor following surgery and possibly radiation and chemotherapy indicates failure of these therapies to reduce the tumor mass to a size and cell number that would permit its eradication by the patient's immune system (Fig. 19.1) (Harsh & Wilson 1990). Failure arises from a number of factors that limit the efficacy of each modality.

Recurrence after surgery

Surgery may fail because of anatomic considerations, pathologic features, or errors in judgment or technique. The involvement of critical structures may limit the initial resection. Investment of the internal carotid artery or its branches by a parasellar meningioma and involvement of the optic pathways, diencephalon, internal capsule, brainstem, or eloquent cortex by a glioma often preclude complete removal. Tumor recurrence, despite removal of all microscopically evident tumor, can occur if there is microscopic infiltration of adjacent structures. Even low-grade cerebral gliomas are usually infiltrative, and microscopic foci of neoplastic cells are frequently found in the dural base of a meningioma (Borovich et al 1986; Sallinen et al 2000; Rokni-Yazdi et al 2009). The dural margin is the likely site of recurrence of completely resected meningiomas (Nakasu et al 1999; Rokni-Yazdi et al 2009). Malignant meningiomas and anaplastic astrocytomas are characteristically widely invasive. Finally, errors in judgment, such as preoperatively underestimating the amount of tumor that can be safely removed or intraoperatively failing to remove tumor that was targeted, result in potentially resectable tumor being left as a nidus of regrowth.

Recurrence after radiation

Radiation therapy may fail because of inadequate targeting, underutilization of the tolerable dose, or radiation resistance of the tumor cells. Proximity to critical anatomical structures can also limit maximal allowable radiation dosage. Furthermore, the correlations between imaging abnormality and tumor extent are incomplete. Pathologic studies have shown that individual tumor cells can be found throughout and even beyond CT hypodense and MRI T_2-hyperintense areas of malignant glioma (Burger et al 1983; Kelly et al 1987; Burger et al 1988). For each individual case, the extent of brain invasion from the contrast-enhancing margin of a malignant glioma or the portion of the dural tail of a meningioma that contains tumor cells is incompletely known (Borovich et al 1986). The choice of field size for irradiation of such lesions is difficult and relies as much on the trade-off between target volume and tolerable dose as on the accurate delineation of tumor boundaries. Failure to include an adequate annulus of tissue around the tumor to accommodate imaging uncertainty and technical error may leave tumor cells incompletely irradiated.

Even if the maximal dose tolerated by infiltrative surrounding brain is delivered, tumor cells may remain viable. Hypoxic, non-proliferating cells and tumor stem cells are particularly radioresistant; with time or change in the physiologic conditions following therapy, re-entry of cells into the cell cycle permits the proliferation that results in clinically apparent tumor recurrence (Hoshino 1984; Dirks 2006). Analysis of patterns of failure demonstrates that, even with maximal tolerable doses of photon radiation of 70–80 Gy, almost all malignant astrocytomas fail centrally (Lee et al 1999). A study of high-dose fractionated proton irradiation following radical resection of glioblastomas showed the following: (1) a dose between 80 and 90 Gy is sufficient to prevent tumor regrowth; (2) outside of this high-dose volume, tumor regrows, usually in areas receiving between 60 and 70 Gy; (3) enlargement of the high-dose volume to include more peripheral areas is likely to induce unacceptably high levels of symptomatic radiation-related necrosis (Fitzek et al 1999).

Recurrence after chemotherapy

Chemotherapy fails as a result of inadequate drug delivery, toxicity, or cell resistance. The blood–brain barrier is deficient in the contrast-enhancing region of the tumor, but surrounding brain usually has an intact blood–brain barrier; lipid-insoluble drugs thus have limited access to tumor cells infiltrating peripheral regions. The margin between drug efficacy and neurotoxicity, bone marrow suppression, pulmonary injury, and gastrointestinal side-effects is often narrow. Non-cycling cells and tumor stem cells are resistant to cell-cycle specific drugs, and potentially vulnerable cells often rapidly develop biochemical means of resistance to chemotherapeutic agents (Hoshino 1984; Kornblith & Walker 1988; Dirks 2006).

Even if these therapies significantly reduce the tumor burden, the patient's immune response may be rendered ineffective by chemotherapy and by the tumor's secretion of factors antagonistic to immune function, such as IL-10, prostaglandin E2, and transforming growth factor (TGF)-β2, and its expression of apoptosis-inducing molecules, such as Fas ligand (FasL) and galectin-1 (Bower et al 2007). Each of these limitations of each component of multimodality therapy may contribute to failure to prevent tumor regrowth. At the time of tumor recurrence, consideration of these reasons for failure is essential to assessment of prognosis and to the choice of subsequent therapy.

Prognostic implications of residual and recurrent tumor

In the management of a recurrent brain tumor, consideration of the prognostic implications of regrowth is essential. The presence of residual tumor and the occurrence of tumor regrowth likely have different prognostic implications.

Residual tumor

Radiologic demonstration of residual tumor after initial treatment may be consistent with preoperative goals and expectations; the prognosis would be that originally formulated. If, however, residual tumor is identified unexpectedly, the prognosis may need to be altered. The prognostic import of residual tumor is best seen in the relationship between extent of resection and likelihood of tumor recurrence.

Residual meningiomas
For meningiomas, the extent of resection dramatically affects patient outcome. The incidence of symptomatic recurrence varies with the amount of tumor remaining after the initial operation: 44% following partial removal; 29% following removal of tumor down to its dural base; 19% after removal of tumor and coagulation of its dural base; and 9% following removal of all tumor and infiltrated dura and bone (Simpson 1957). That resection of the dural base of an otherwise completely removed tumor reduces the recurrence rate by half (10% vs 20%) has been confirmed by subsequent reports (Yamashita et al 1980; Chan & Thompson 1984; Kinjo at al 1993). In one study, total removal produced a much higher chance of freedom from recurrence than did partial removal (93%, 80%, and 68% vs 63%, 45%, and 9% after 5, 10, and 15 years, respectively) (Mirimanoff et al 1985; Kinjo et al 1993). The probabilities of a second operation were 6%, 15%, and 20% at intervals of 5, 10, and 15 years after a total resection but 25%, 44%, and 84% at the same intervals following partial resection. Patients must be followed for decades. Although tumor regression is usually seen within the first 10 years, it has been observed after more than 25 years (Mathiesen et al 1996).

Tumor location is a critical determinant of resectability and, thus, of probability of recurrence. Reported 5–10-year recurrence rates are approximately 5% for intraventricular meningiomas, 20% for parasagittal, falcine, cerebral convexity, parabasal convexity (lateral sphenoid wing and olfactory groove), and cerebellar convexity tumors, and 50% for basal (medial sphenoid, cavernous, orbital, clival, petrous, and tentorial) meningiomas (Phillipon & Cornu 1991; Strassner et al 2009). In one series, 96% of convexity meningiomas were totally removed and only 3% had recurred at 5 years, but for sphenoid ridge meningiomas the total resection rate was 28% and the 5-year recurrence rate was 34% (Mirimanoff et al 1985; Strassner et al 2009). High rates of incomplete removal likely reflect tumor investment of cranial nerves, the brainstem, and the internal carotid, vertebral, or basilar arteries, or invasion of dural sinuses. Widespread invasion of bone, particularly if lytic rather than hyperostotic changes are seen, and infiltration of cortex are also prognostic of frequent and early recurrence. In one series, 40% (12/30) of tumors causing skull lysis recurred, but only 13% (4/31) of hyperostosing tumors recurred, despite the observation that hyperostotic bone almost invariably contains tumor cells (Olmsted & McGee 1977; Bikmaz et al 2007). Similarly, invasion of cortex is ominous; it was noted in 22% of multiply recurrent tumors, 9% of singly recurrent tumors, and only 1% of non-recurrent tumors (Boker et al 1985). Multivariate analysis has identified tumor shape as a significant predictor of risk of recurrence; mushrooming and lobulated tumors are more likely to recur than round ones (Nakasu et al 1999). Meningiomas with radiographically irregular margins are also more likely to invade cortex, to induce edema, to be incompletely resected, and to recur (Suwa et al 1995; Strassner et al 2009).

The tendency to recur is also critically dependent on histology. Based on the WHO classification of 2000, prognostic factors include tumor grade, mitotic index, cellularity, pleomorphism, prominent nucleoli, a small cell population with a high nucleus/cytoplasmic ratio, necrosis, and brain invasion. Furthermore, immunohistologic profiles, including high levels of staining for Ki67 and BCL2, correlate with tumor grade and prognosis (Uzüm & Ataoğlu 2008). The rates of recurrence for benign, atypical, and malignant meningiomas in one large series were 7%, 35%, and 73%, respectively (Maier et al 1992). In another, the median duration of recurrence-free survival, median time to recurrence, and median total survival were 12 years, 5 years, and 19 years for atypical meningiomas and 2 years, 2 years, and 7 years for malignant meningiomas (Palma et al 1997). Shorter interval to recurrence correlates not only with higher tumor grade, but also with higher mitotic index (MI >6: MIB-1 labeling index >3%), dense staining for TGF-β, absence of progesterone receptors, and necrosis (Hsu et al 1997a,b). High proliferation indices – BUdR labeling index >1% and flow cytometric index >19% – separate tumors prone to recurrence from non-recurring ones and correlate with tumor doubling rates of several months rather than years and with time to tumor recurrence of 1–3 years rather than 5–10 years (Jääskeläinen et al 1985; Cho et al 1986; Crone et al 1988). In one study, a high mitotic index occurred in 20% of tumors that eventually recurred but in only 8% of non-recurring tumors. A total of 26% of recurring tumors had necrosis but only 6% of non-recurring tumors did (Boker et al 1985; de la Monte et al 1986). The MIB-1 labeling index of non-recurrent tumors was 1.6%; for tumors that would recur later, it was 3.6% at the first operation, and for recurrent tumors it was 8.8% at the second operation (Matsuno et al 1996). Sequential recurrences of the same tumor usually occur at shorter intervals; tumors show higher labeling indices, sheeting, micronecrosis, and a more complex karyotype (Steudel et al 1996; Cerda-Nicolas et al 1998). Atypical characteristics are prognostic of recurrence almost regardless of the extent of resection (Jääskeläinen et al 1985; de la Monte et al 1986; Jääskeläinen et al 1986; Perry et al 1997; Uzüm & Ataoğlu 2008).

Young age correlates with the likelihood of recurrence of meningiomas because of the longer time at risk and more aggressive tumor behavior. In one series, tumors that eventually recurred initially presented at a mean age of 43 years, as opposed to 53 years for non-recurrent tumors. This relationship holds for the risk of recurrence after reoperation as well; tumors with multiple recurrences initially presented at 36.4 years vs 46.7 years for singly recurrent tumors (Phillipon & Cornu 1991). Gender may also be important. Meningiomas are more likely to be atypical or malignant, and thus recur more frequently and earlier after treatment, in men than in women (Jääskeläinen 1986). These prognostic indicators should influence the decisions regarding the management of both residual and recurrent meningiomas.

When residual tumor is identified by postoperative imaging, the management options include reoperation, irradiation, and observation. Unless a readily correctable technical or medical consideration limited the initial resection, early reoperation will not be warranted. Radiation of residual meningiomas is relatively safe and effective; in one study, radiation following surgery reduced the rate of recurrence of incompletely resected meningiomas from 60% to 32% and increased the interval to recurrence from 66 to 125 months (Carella et al 1982; Barbaro et al 1987; Goldsmith et al 1992). The rates of tumor control following irradiation of incompletely resected benign meningiomas depend on tumor size. The 5-year progression-free survival rate of patients with tumors with maximal diameters >5 cm was 40%, compared with 93% for those with smaller tumors. This difference in tumor control resulted in a difference in 5-year tumor-related mortality: 35% for large tumors and 3% for smaller tumors (Connell et al 1999).

The ability to detect small changes in tumor size radiographically, their relatively slow growth, and the infrequency of malignant transformation argue for delaying reoperation and irradiation of residual benign tumor mass until renewed growth is documented. Follow-up of such cases must be regular (usually annual neurologic and radiographic examinations) and sustained, as the cumulative risk of recurrence continues to increase after 5 and 10 years (Mirimanoff et al 1985). Many atypical and all malignant meningiomas, with their high likelihood of rapid regrowth, however, will warrant adjuvant radiation, even if gross total resection is achieved. For an atypical meningioma, if a Simpson grade I resection is attained and reliable postoperative imaging follow-up is feasible, irradiation can be deferred until regrowth is seen. If the resection is incomplete, renewed regrowth is the rule, and the residual tumor should be irradiated. Confidence that the residual tumor and areas at risk of recurrence are small and focal permits use of stereotactic radiosurgery rather than large field radiotherapy in traditional fractionation. This is better delivered in the early postoperative period rather than delayed until regrowth has occurred (Patil et al 2008; Colombo et al 2009). For malignant meningiomas, which are less likely to be removed completely, early postoperative irradiation of both residual tumor and resection margins is strongly indicated (Harris 2003).

Residual gliomas
Cytoreductive surgery is a fundamental part of the treatment of most systemic malignancies (Devita 1983). In most cases, there is a strong relationship between the extent of resection and outcome. For gliomas, correlation between extent of resection or, more significantly, size of residual tumor, and outcome measures, such as interval to tumor progression and survival, has been strongly suggested by retrospective and prospective series, but not by randomized clinical trials (Rostomily et al 1994). More recently, one study, reported a significant survival advantage when ≥98% resection is achieved (Hentschel 2003).

Correlation of survival with extent of resection for low grade gliomas has been suggested by retrospective uncontrolled reviews and comparisons with historical controls (Ammirati et al 1987b; Vertosick et al 1991; McCormack et al 1992; Chang et al 2009). One study of 461 adult patients with low grade cerebral gliomas found that gross total surgical removal correlated with length of survival (Laws et al 1984). Another reported a median survival duration of 7.4 years following maximal surgical resection. The median survival of a sub-group patients with hemispheric tumors compared favorably (10 years vs 8 years) with that of a comparable series treated with biopsy and radiation alone (Vertosick et al 1991; McCormack et al 1992). Additional studies have demonstrated that extensive resection of low grade gliomas delays tumor recurrence (Berger & Rostomily 1997; Chang et al 2009).

For high-grade gliomas, the correlations between the extent of resection at the initial operation and (1) the time to tumor recurrence and (2) the duration of patient survival have been disputed (Coffey et al 1988). Historical reports and reviews of large series have noted the association of survival and extent of resection for both astrocytomas and oligodendrogliomas (Jelsma & Bucy 1969; Walker et al 1978; Chang et al 1983; Nelson et al 1985; Shaw et al 1992). Extensive reviews of the literature, however, have failed to locate randomized, controlled clinical trials comparing survival after biopsy with that after radical resection of malignant gliomas (Nazzaro & Neuwelt 1990; Quigley & Maroon 1991). Nevertheless, the benefit of surgical cytoreduction has been strongly suggested by the following findings:

1. Reviews of multicentered trials have shown that the more complete the resection, the longer the patient lived (Shapiro 1982; Wood et al 1988, Simpson et al 1993).

2. In a study of 243 patients, multivariate regression analysis identified extent of resection as an important prognostic factor ($p < 0.0001$) for survival (Vecht et al 1990).

3. In a retrospective review of 1215 patients with WHO grade III or IV, increasing extent of surgical resection was associated with improved survival independent of age, degree of disability WHO grade, or subsequent treatment modalities used (McGirt et al 2009).

4. Single center studies have confirmed this relationship: in one study containing 21 glioblastomas and 10 anaplastic astrocytomas, median duration of survival after gross total resection was 90 weeks vs only 43 weeks following subtotal resection, and the 2-year survival rates were 19% and 0%, respectively, even although the two groups were well matched for other prognostically significant variables (Ammirati et al 1987b; Ciric et al 1989); in another study, patients with gross total resection of malignant glioma lived longer (76 vs 19 weeks) than those who underwent only a biopsy, even after correction for tumor accessibility and all other prognostically significant variables (Winger et al 1989) and one large recent series showed that GTR (>98%) significantly increases the duration of survival (Hentschel & Sawaya 2003).

5. In two larger series, patients with resected cortical and subcortical grade IV gliomas lived longer: 50.6 vs 33.0 weeks (Devaux et al 1993) and 39.5 vs 32.0 weeks (Kreth et al 1993) after surgery and radiation than those who underwent biopsy and radiation.

6. Small postoperative tumor volume has been shown to correlate with longer time to tumor progression after

surgery (Levin et al 1980) and longer patient survival (Andreou et al 1983; Rostomily et al 1996).

Although less than ideal, the data that exist for gliomas and experience with tumors outside the central nervous system suggest the benefit of cytoreduction when a near-total removal (2 log reduction of tumor cell number) of a glial tumor can be achieved. Thus, failure to identify and remove readily accessible tumor mass at an initial operation might warrant reoperation before regrowth occurs.

Recurrent tumor

Regrowth of tumors after an initial response (diminution or stability) to surgery and radiation therapy is ominous. This is particularly true if the growth is more rapid or more infiltrative than that of the original tumor. Such growth often exhibits changes in the basic biology of the tumor that make it less responsive to subsequent therapy. A short interval between initial treatment and recurrence of symptoms often indicates rapid regrowth and a poor prognosis. Factors to be considered in estimating prognosis include the biology of the tumor (its pathology, growth rate, and invasiveness), its resectability, its prior response to radiation and chemotherapy, and the age and performance status of the patient (Karnofsky et al 1951). Estimates of the recurrent tumor's size, growth rate, invasiveness, and location must be made in assessing its potential for causing both neurologic deficit and death. Reappearance of a slowly growing, well-demarcated frontal convexity meningioma in a middle-aged patient of good neurologic condition after a 10-year interval of post-surgical quiescence clearly carries a prognosis very different from that of diffuse diencephalic spread of a glioblastoma multiforme in an elderly patient with a poor performance status 3 months after treatment with surgery, radiation, and chemotherapy.

Therapy of recurrent tumors

The choice of therapy of a recurrent tumor is based upon a comparison of the natural history of the regrowing tumor with the risk–benefit calculus of potential therapies.

Therapy of recurrent meningiomas

Meningiomas that recur may warrant reoperation and/or radiation. Recurrent meningiomas can cause neurologic deficit and threaten survival by direct compression of eloquent tissue or by increasing intracranial pressure. An enlarging tumor, even if asymptomatic, should be treated unless anatomic considerations, severe medical problems, or limited life expectancy preclude it. The decision to reoperate must weigh the natural history of the recurrent tumor, its likelihood of causing neurologic injury or death within the patient's expected lifetime, the technical feasibility of achieving a radical resection, the patient's medical condition, and the potential efficacy of alternative treatments.

The pattern of recurrence will influence the choice of therapy. Recurrence is almost always local, although spread of tumor in different directions from the original site and even multifocal recurrence can occur (Fig. 19.2). Regional multifocal tumor deposits result from spread of tumor cells

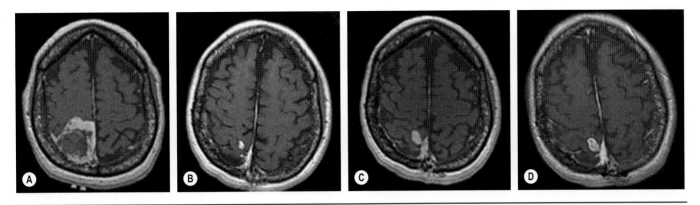

Figure 19.2 Local recurrence of meningioma. This left parasagittal meningioma (axial contrast enhanced T1-weighted MRIs) presented with left leg weakness (A). Postoperative MRI (B) showed thickening of the lateral wall of the superior sagittal sinus and subadjacent falx, as well as a small focus of parenchymal enhancement. In the 4th year of follow-up (C), the plaque of tumor along the sinus thickened and the parenchymal focus enlarged. Both were treated with stereotactic radiosurgery. A scan 6 months later (D) shows loss of central contrast enhancement of the parenchymal nodule, consistent with radiation effect.

through and beneath the dura (Fig. 19.3) (DeVries & Wakhloo 1994). In one pathologic study of dural tails evident radiologically, 15/47 dural tails evident on MRI contained infiltrating tumor cells (Uematsu et al 2005). Regional recurrence was found in 16% (7/45) of cases in one series of recurrent meningiomas; it was associated with younger age, atypical and malignant histologies, and a tendency to recur multiple times (Phillipon & Cornu 1991). This type of recurrence requires more extensive surgical exposure at reoperation and usually mandates postoperative radiation.

Recurrent tumors may recapitulate the pattern of growth of the original tumor or they may behave differently. When the recurrent tumor resembles the initial one, the surgical considerations for reoperation will be similar to those of the original surgery. Many surgeons have found that tumors recurrent after surgery, radiation, or both are more difficult to resect and that reoperation carries an increased risk of complications (Sekhar et al 1996). If the recurrent tumor differs from the original, a different surgical approach may be needed:

1. A convexity meningioma that was initially intradural may regrow extradurally, extend in dumbbell fashion through a trephination, and erode the scalp (Fig. 19.4); excision of such a tumor may necessitate a larger scalp flap, piecemeal removal of bone, and tissue transfer for closure.

2. A falx meningioma may regrow contralaterally and require a bilateral exposure.

3. A parasagittal meningioma may completely occlude a previously patent superior sagittal sinus, such that excision of the sinus and complete removal of the tumor is possible.

4. A globoid clinoidal meningioma may recur as an *en plaque* tumor extending through the optic canal or invading the cavernous sinus, such that a more extensive resection of the skull base is necessary (Fig. 19.5).

If surgery is not feasible, or if tumor remains after reoperation, radiation should be given, particularly if the meningioma's histology is atypical or malignant. The probability of another recurrence after reoperation alone is 42% at 5 years and 56% after 10 years. The mean recurrence-free interval is shorter following each successive surgery: 6 years, 3 years and 10 months, 3 years, and 1 year and 7 months after the first, second, third, and fourth operations, respectively (Mirimanoff et al 1985; Phillipon & Cornu 1991) In one series of sphenoid wing meningiomas, postoperative radiation was delivered to the residua of 31 tumors postoperatively and to 11 recurrent tumors. No tumor recurred during 4 years of follow-up. In a comparable group of patients who did not receive radiation, 16/38 patients with partially resected tumors and 5/6 with recurrent tumors had regrowth (Peele et al 1997).

If a recurrent benign tumor is small (<10 cm^3 in volume), discrete, and difficult to resect, stereotactic radiosurgery is an excellent alternative to microsurgery and fractionated radiotherapy (Fig. 19.6) (Muthukumar et al 1998; Chang & Adler 1997; Shafron et al 1999; Colombo et al 2009). Stereotactic radiosurgery of cavernous sinus meningiomas remaining after radical surgery has provided a 100% control rate at a median follow-up of 2 years (range 6–54 months): 19/34 (56%) tumors regressed; 24% of patients had neurologic improvement; 70% were unchanged, and two patients (6%) developed permanent new neurologic deficits (Duma et al 1993). A subsequent report from the same institution demonstrated a 93.1% control rate for typical meningiomas at both 5- and 10-year follow-up. And for 83 patients who underwent radiosurgery as the sole treatment modality, the 5-year control rate was 96.9% (Lee et al 2002). Similar treatment of 41 tentorial meningiomas, of which 44% were recurrent after 1–4 operations, produced a tumor control rate of 98% at a mean follow-up of 3 years. Nineteen patients improved clinically, 20 remained stable, and two deteriorated, one from tumor growth and one from radiation injury (Muthukumar et al 1998). More recently, staged or fractionated stereotactic radiosurgery has been used to treat recurrent meningiomas of larger size or greater proximity to radiosensitive normal structures than previously thought safe (Pendl et al 2000; Adler et al 2008).

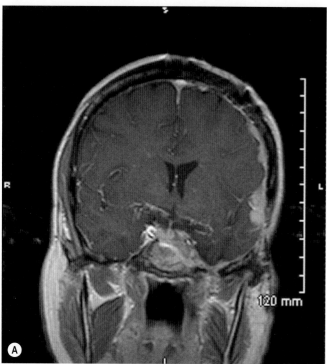

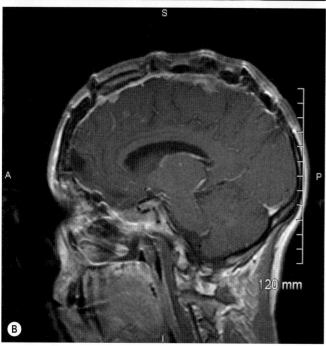

Figure 19.3 Regional multifocal tumor deposits. These may reflect multiple meningiomatosis or result from spread of tumor cells through and beneath the dura. These coronal (A) and sagittal (B) T1 weighted, contrast enhanced MRI scans show numerous left fronto-temporal convexity and superior sagittal sinus meningiomas.

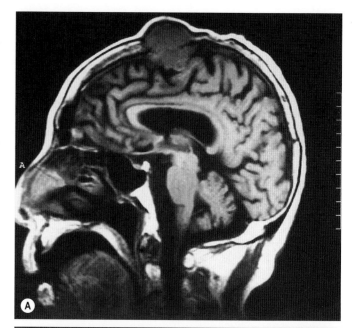

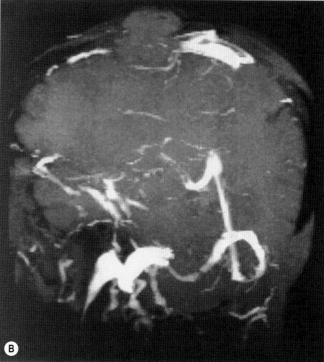

Figure 19.4 Recurrent meningioma. (A) A 78-year-old man developed a convexity skull mass at the site of a falx meningioma that had been resected previously. Extension of the recurrent tumor through the skull and falx was apparent. (B) The superior sagittal sinus was occluded by tumor such that it could be sacrificed and the tumor totally removed.

If the tumor is large, appears more malignant, and grows diffusely, fractionated radiotherapy, which permits treatment of even larger volumes, is appropriate (Carella et al 1982; Barbaro et al 1987; Goldsmith et al 1992; Milosevic et al 1996). In a subset of one series of patients with residual benign meningiomas whose treatments were based on CT or MR imaging, an actuarial progression-free survival rate of 98% at 5 years was achieved (Goldsmith et al 1992). In most cases, atypical or malignant tumors remaining after reoperation should also be irradiated (Hug et al 2000; Modha et al 2005). Depending on the field and dose of the original irradiation and the intervening interval, reir-radiation may be possible (Fig. 19.7) (Milker-Zabel 2009).

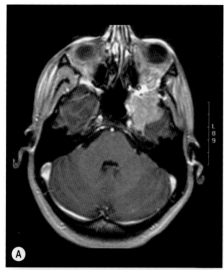

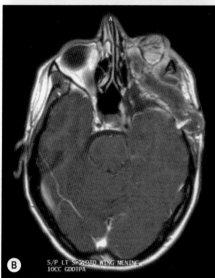

Figure 19.5 Recurrent orbital meningioma. Recurrence of orbital tumor after two craniotomies and proton beam radiosurgery (A: axial T1-weighted MRI with contrast) necessitated orbital exenteration and repair with a graft of rectus abdominis muscle. Ten years later, the tumor had not recurred (B: axial T1-weighted MRI with gadolinium).

Medical therapies considered for recurrent meningiomas include hormonal therapy, chemotherapy and immunotherapy (Sioka & Kyritsis 2009). Detection of receptors for progesterone, estrogen, and somatostatin on meningioma specimens or cells in culture has prompted trials of medical alteration of receptor activity.

Between two-thirds and three-quarters of all meningiomas have progesterone receptors; staining for progesterone receptors is much more common in typical than in atypical or anaplastic types and is thus prognostically favorable (Pravdenkova et al 2006; Roser 2004; Huisman et al 1991). Nonetheless, the antiprogesterone agent, mifepristone (RU486, 200 mg/day) has shown only limited antitumor activity (8/28 (29%) patients with partial response) (Grunberg et al 2006). The antiestrogen, tamoxifen, produced a similarly muted response in a higher proportion of

patients (90%, 9/10) despite the lower proportion of tumors (19%) with estrogen receptors (Huisman et al 1991; Goodwin et al 1993). The potential utility of somatostatin, suggested by the finding of its receptors on most meningiomas, was supported by a tumor control rate of 44% after 6 months of treatment (Chamberlain et al 2007).

Chemotherapy has proven to be of little value for recurrent meningiomas. Initial encouraging reports of activity of hydroxyurea (15–20 mg/kg per day p.o.) against recurrent, non-resectable meningiomas (a cumulative rate of partial response or stability of 78% (26/32 patients in two studies; Mason et al 2002; Newton et al 2004; Newton 2007) prompted Phase II studies which failed to confirm significant efficacy (19/54 or 35% partial response or, more commonly, stability; Fuentes et al 2004; Loven et al 2004; Weston et al 2006). A subset of four atypical or malignant meningiomas showed no response. Similarly, Phase II trials of either temozolomide ($n = 16$) or irinotecan ($n = 16$) have failed to demonstrate significant anti-tumor activity for either agent (Gupta et al 2007; Rockhill et al 2007). Telomerase activity is much more common in anaplastic than in typical meningiomas; even within a group of typical meningiomas, it correlates with a poor prognosis (Langford et al 1997). Telomerase inhibitors may be a reasonable strategy.

Immunotherapy has seen little testing. Treatment of a total of 18 unresectable or recurrent meningiomas, some of which were malignant, with interferon α-2b was followed by disease stability (for up to 8 years) in 14/18 total patients from two studies (Kaba et al 1997; Muhr et al 2001). Given the disappointing results with hormonal and chemotherapeutic strategies, such immunotherapeutic agents should be studied further (Sioka & Kyritsis 2009).

Therapy of recurrent gliomas

The choice of therapy of a recurrent glioma is based on a comparison of the natural history of the regrowing tumor with the risk–benefit ratio of potential therapies. Recurrent gliomas warrant aggressive multimodality therapy if the patient is in good neurologic and general medical condition and therapeutic options offer a realistic chance for significant improvement in neurologic status or extension of survival (Salcman et al 1982).

Patterns of recurrence of gliomas

When gliomas recur, most do so locally. Historically, >80% of recurrent glioblastoma multiforme arose within 2 cm of the original margin of contrast-enhancing tumor (Hochberg & Pruitt 1980; Wallner et al 1989a). In one series, over 90% of glioma cases showed recurrence at the original tumor location, while 5% developed multiple lesions after treatment (Choucair et al 1986). In another study of 36 patients with malignant gliomas receiving 70–80 Gy of fractionated radiation, 32 (89%) had central (at least 95% of the recurrent tumor within the volume receiving at least 95% of the maximum dose) or in-field (at least 80% of tumor within this highest dose volume) recurrence, and three (8%) had marginal recurrence. Only one (3%) fell predominantly outside the high-dose range. Seven patients had multiple sites of recurrence, but only one had a large recurrence outside the high dose volume (Lee et al 1999). This tendency to recur

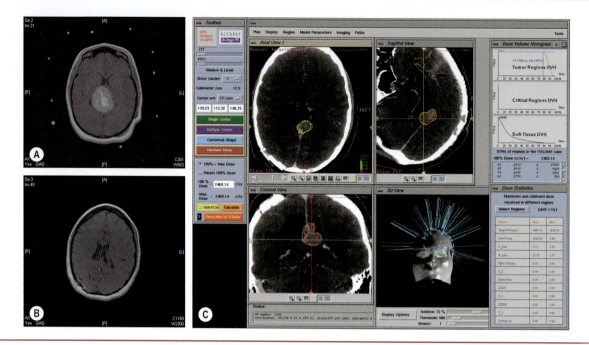

Figure 19.6 Stereotactic radiosurgery of a recurrent meningioma. A large intraventricular WHO grade II meningioma was removed from a young woman (A, preop T1 axial MRI with contrast) with the exception of tumor in the wall of the vein of Galen (B, postop T1 axial MRI with contrast). Subsequent regrowth of tumor was treated with stereotactic radiosurgery (C, CyberKnife treatment plan).

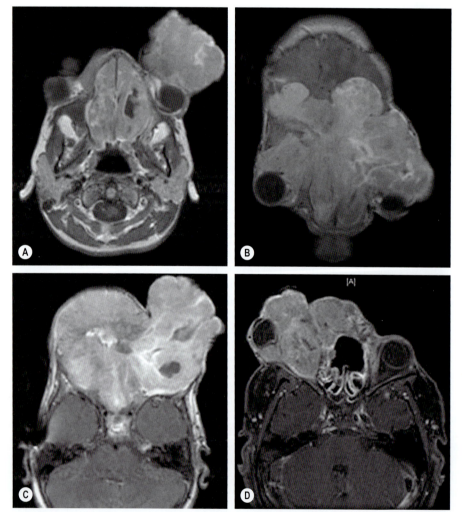

Figure 19.7 Reirradiation of a recurrent meningioma. This WHO grade II meningioma was originally treated with surgery and radiation therapy in 1987. Recurrent tumor (A, axial; B, coronal, and C, axial T1-weighted MRI with contrast) was resected. A subsequent recurrence (D, axial) led to right orbital enucleation in 2002. A subsequent recurrence in the medial left orbit, refractory to somatostatin, warranted enucleation of the blind left eye and reirradiation in 2008.

locally is a function of tumor cell distribution. There is a gradient of tumor cell density in which tumor cell number decreases rapidly at increasing distances from the contrast-enhancing rim of solid tumor. Thus, although individual tumor cells spread through the brain at great distances from the primary site, there are so many more cells locally that the odds favor local reaccumulation of tumor mass (Burger et al 1983; Kelly et al 1987).

Factors contributing to the likelihood of local recurrence include the following:

1. The relative predominance of tumor cell mass in the region
2. The statistical likelihood that a local cell will be the cell that first develops a competitive proliferative advantage
3. The possibility that the physiologic milieu (hypervascularity and increased permeability, disrupted tissue architecture, and paracrine growth factor stimuli) at the site is particularly conducive to regrowth.

As tumor cell proliferation resumes at the initial tumor site, cells again spread rapidly and diffusely. Tumor cell proliferation resumes at distant sites as a result of the influx of these new, mitotically active cells or the renewed growth of cells that spread before the initial treatment (Choucair et al 1986). Biologic therapeutic agents may also affect the pattern of recurrence; recent experience with bevacizumab (Avastin) suggests that tumors treated with this inhibitor of VEGF are more likely to recur as diffusely infiltrative lesions distant from the original site of tumor (Narayana et al 2009). Consequently, treatments targeting local recurrence alone will, at best, be briefly palliative. Treatment of tumor recurrence thus usually involves a combination of modalities aimed at both local and distant disease.

Epidemiology of recurrent glioblastoma

The heterogeneity in defining recurrence and the variability of treatment algorithms employed at different institutions result in a vague profile of recurrent glioblastoma multiforme (Hou et al 2006). In a multi-center trial of reoperation for resection and placement of cavitary biodegradable BCNU-wafer in 222 patients with recurrent glioblastoma and a Karnofsky Performance Score of at least 60, the median interval from initial diagnosis to tumor recurrence was 12 months (Brem et al 1995). Among a cohort of 301 patients with GBM, 223 patients had tumor recurrence at a median interval from initial diagnosis of 4.9 months (Barker et al 1998); 64% of these had a Karnovsky Performance Score >70 at the time of recurrence.

Glioblastoma recurrence is demonstrated on imaging obtained in routine surveillance or in response to new or recurring symptoms. In a questionnaire-based study of patients with recurrent glioblastoma or anaplastic astrocytoma and a KPS >70, self-reported symptoms included fatigue, uncertainty about the future, motor difficulties, drowsiness, communication difficulties, and headache (Osoba et al 2000). While most symptoms likely reflected tumor recurrence, confounding factors such as radiation necrosis and steroid treatment may have contributed to generalized fatigue, and pain and uncertainty about the future may have resulted from the diagnosis alone, independent of current tumor status. Incoordination, weakness, visual loss, and pain were reported more frequently by patients with recurrent glioblastoma than by those with anaplastic astrocytoma, providing evidence that more aggressive disease will cause greater neurological deficit.

Therapy of recurrent malignant glioma

Choice of therapy for a recurrent glioma must consider the tumor's current and previous histology, previous treatment, and location and the patient's age, medical and neurologic conditions, and preferences. An enlarging lesion that was originally a low-grade glioma should undergo biopsy (stereotactically or, if resection is anatomically feasible, by open craniotomy) to confirm histology (Fig. 19.8). If the tumor remains low grade and a large part of the lesion can be resected without inflicting significant neurologic deficit, it should be removed; if previously irradiated to significantly less than maximal tolerable dose, the tumor bed and surrounding area should receive fractionated radiotherapy. The longer the interval since the initial radiotherapy, the higher the dose that can be given safely at recurrence. If the tumor is inaccessible to surgery, radiation alone should be prescribed. If a low-grade tumor previously irradiated to a maximal tolerable dose recurs as a low-grade glioma, it should be resected, if possible. If it is inaccessible, stereotactically delivered focal radiation is an attractive option (Ostertag 1983; Mayer & Sminia 2008).

If the low-grade tumor recurs as a high-grade tumor or if a high-grade tumor recurs, reoperation should be attempted if the patient has a Karnofsky score of at least 70 and removal of all or almost all of the contrast-enhancing tumor is potentially attainable, or if the tumor mass is causing neurologic symptoms that might be palliated by its reduction. Removal of tumor may improve the patient's quality of life by alleviating neurologic deficit or permitting reduction of steroid dose. It may also prolong survival by reducing tumor burden and improving response to radiation, chemotherapy, immunotherapy or biologic therapy (Vick et al 1989; Brem et al 1991).

If the tumor was not irradiated previously, the tumor bed and its annular margin should receive regional radiotherapy. Even when radiotherapy has been used initially, it is an option at recurrence, but doses permitted under standard guidelines for conventional fractionation and volumes are unlikely to be high enough to be effective. Other possibilities include highly conformal conventionally fractionated radiotherapy (e.g., IMRT, intensity modulated radiation therapy), hypofractionated stereotactic radiotherapy, interstitial brachytherapy, and stereotactic radiosurgery (Hucharek & Muscat 1995; Arcicasa et al 1999; Hayat et al 1997; Kim et al 1997; Wiggenraad et al 2009). In one study, the use of highly conformal teletherapy for re-irradiation of recurrent gliomas (mean re-irradiation dose of 38 Gy, range 30.6–59.4 Gy) at a median time of 38 months (range 9–234 months) produced radiographic stability or regression and neurologic improvement in two-thirds of the patients (Kim et al 1997). In another study, 10 patients with recurrent malignant gliomas treated with intensity modulated radiation therapy (daily fractions of 5 Gy to a total median dose of 30 Gy) demonstrated a

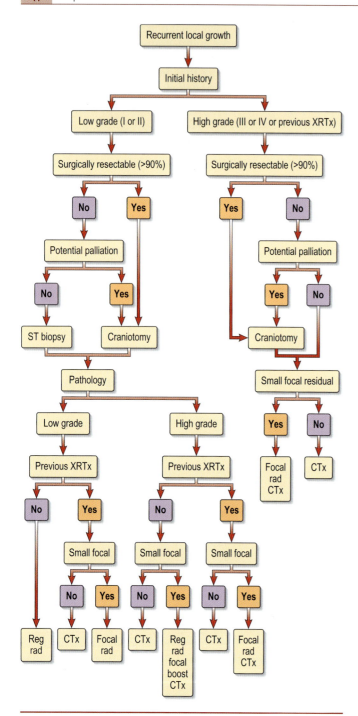

Figure 19.8 Recurrent glioma. Decisions in the management of a recurrent tumor should consider grade, resectability, and prior therapy. CTx, chemotherapy; focal rad/boost, stereotactic radiosurgery, brachytherapy, or radiotherapy; N, neurologic; reg rad, regional fractionated radiation therapy; small focal, less than 10 cm³, radiographically demarcated.

median overall survival duration of 10.1 months from the time of treatment, with 1- and 2-year survival rates of 50% and 33% (Voynov et al 2002).

Hypofractionated stereotactic radiotherapy (SRT) combines high dose per fraction with stereotactic targeting.

Hypofractionated SRT (e.g., 20–30 Gy in 2–5 Gy fractions) of recurrent malignant gliomas resulted in a median duration of subsequent survival of 9.3 months (15.4 months for grade III tumors and 7.9 months for grade IV tumors) in one study (Vordermark et al 2005). Another protocol that delivered 20–50 Gy in 5 Gy fractions to 29 patients with recurrent high-grade astrocytomas resulted in a median duration of survival after retreatment of 11 months (Shepherd et al 1997). Steroid dependent toxicity occurred in 36% of patients; reoperation was required in 6%, and a total dose in excess of 40 Gy predicted radiation damage ($p < 0.005$). Another study used 24 Gy in 3 Gy fractions; 30 Gy in 3 Gy fractions, and 35 Gy in 3.5 Gy fractions to boost previously irradiated residual or recurrent malignant gliomas at a mean of 3.1 months (range 1–46 months) after standard treatment to 60 Gy. A total of 60% of patients required less steroid and 45% improved neurologically. Some 80% of those receiving 30 or 35 Gy responded. The median duration of survival was 10.5 months. No grade III toxicity occurred. Reoperation was not performed (Hudes et al 1999). A fourth protocol combined fractionated stereotactic radiosurgery and Taxol as a radiosensitizer for recurrent malignant gliomas. It resulted in median survival duration of 14.2 months in 14 selected patients (Lederman et al 1998). These four studies suggest that hypofractionated SRT has moderate efficacy and acceptable safety in selected patients.

Although several studies suggested promise for brachytherapy in treating glioblastomas, both initially and at the time of recurrence, tumors in these studies were highly selected for small size and focality – two features that would make them appropriate for stereotactic radiosurgery or radiotherapy, less invasive techniques with equivalent results (Scharfen et al 1992; McDermott et al 1998; Gaspar et al 1999). In a retrospective comparison of interstitial brachytherapy and radiosurgery for recurrent glioblastomas, the median durations of survival in the two groups were similar (11.5 months and 10.2 months, respectively). Patterns of failure were similar. The actuarial risks of reoperation for necrosis at 12 and 24 months were 33% and 48%, respectively, after radiosurgery, and 54% and 65%, respectively, after brachytherapy, with the caveat that the brachytherapy group had larger tumors and longer follow-up (Shrieve et al 1995; Alexander & Loeffler 1998).

Other forms of focal radiation therapy of recurrent gliomas such as photodynamic therapy (PDT), boron neutron capture therapy (BNCT), intraoperative radiation (IORT), and radiolabeled monoclonal antibodies to tumor cells surface receptors have been studied (Hara et al 1995; Muller & Wilson 1995; Popovic et al 1996; Bigner et al 1998; Chanana et al 1999; Reardon et al 2007). A dozen clinical trials have measured the safety and efficacy of irradiation of a tumor's resection cavity by 131I-labeled mAb 81C6 (anti-tenascin C). Promising results for this technique during initial resection suggest its potential utility during reoperation as well (Reardon et al 2007).

Although some of these studies report modest benefit, the diffuse infiltration of malignant tumors at the time of recurrence and the dose-limiting toxicity that occurs after 60–70 Gy of radiation frustrate focal therapies and warrant more systemic approaches such as chemotherapy and biologic and immune therapies.

Chemotherapy

Chemotherapy of infiltrative gliomas at diagnosis and at recurrence is often valuable. Temozolomide (Temodar, TMZ), an oral DNA methylating agent with a benefit-toxicity profile superior to that of antecedent alternative intravenous alkylating agents such as BCNU and CCNU, has become the drug of choice. TMZ is appropriate for those low-grade tumors not treated by chemotherapy at the time of initial presentation; one study reported a response rate of 47% (Pace et al 2003). If the tumor recurs despite TMZ, a protracted schedule of TMZ administration or strategies using CCNU alone, PCV, bevacizumab (Avastin) alone or bevacizumab combined with other drugs (e.g., Irinotecan) can be tried (Triebels et al 2004; Kesari et al 2009; Norden et al 2008; Narayana et al 2009; Taillibert et al 2009).

For grade III tumors, TMZ is also recommended (Chinot 2001). Perhaps reflective of the favorable biology of the tumor, TMZ of anaplastic oligodendrogliomas with deletions of chromosomes 1p and 19q is particularly effective (Cairncross et al 1998; Smith et al 2000). In the initial treatment of patients with GBM, the addition of TMZ to radiotherapy increases the percentage of patients surviving at 2 years to 26.5% from 10.4% for radiotherapy alone and the median duration of survival to 14.6 months from 12.1 months (Stupp et al 2005). At the time of renewed growth of a high-grade tumor, if the tumor has not previously been exposed to TMZ, TMZ should be given. If TMZ has been used but it was discontinued prior to either tumor progression or treatment-limiting toxicity occurring, rechallenge with TMZ or a single nitrosourea agent would be appropriate (Table 19.1) (Brandes et al 2009). Patients treated for recurrent or progressive GBM with TMZ showed an overall response rate of 19% and mean time to progression of 11.7 weeks (Brandes et al 2002). Similarly, treatment of recurrent GBM with a standard TMZ regimen (150–200 mg/m^2 × 5 days in 28-day cycles) produced a progression free survival rate of 6 months (PFS-6) of 21% vs 8% following procarbazine (Yung et al 2000). A more intensive regimen (150 mg/m^2 daily on a week on/week off cycle) yielded a PFS-6 of 48% with an overall PFS-12 of 81% (Wick et al 2004) and combinations of TMZ with the matrix metalloproteinase inhibitor, marimastat, or 13-cis-retinoic acid, produced rates of PFS-6 of 39% and 32%, respectively (Jaeckle et al 2003). If TMZ was used to treat the primary tumor and toxicity occurred, then an agent with a different toxicity risk profile should be used (Taillibert et al 2009).

Limitations of the efficacy of TMZ and related alkylating agents (BCNU, CCNU) reflect cellular drug resistance mechanisms, including the suppression of DNA repair mechanisms. The MGMT cytoprotective repair protein removes TMZ-induced methyl adducts at the O6-guanine in DNA (Zhang et al 2006). Administration of O6-benzlguanine to suppress this DNA repair has increased the cytotoxicity of TMZ in pre-clinical models (Pepponi et al 2003).

Intracavitary implantation of wafers of drug polymers attempts to enhance local drug delivery while avoiding systemic side-effects. The initial randomized, double blinded clinical trial with intracavitary BCNU wafers showed longer median survival (31 vs 23 weeks) and improved survival rates 6 months after treatment of recurrent GBM in the BCNU arm relative to the placebo arm, but the survival curves converged at longer follow-up, and higher rates of symptomatic edema, infection (3.6% vs 0.9%) and seizures (37.3% vs 28.6%) were noted (Brem et al 1995).

Chemotherapy offers little benefit to patients whose tumors recur a second time (Hau et al 2003). Nor is multi-agent chemotherapy more beneficial than single-agent chemotherapy (Nieder et al 2000). And hematological toxicity is worse with more complex combinatorial agents (Poisson et al 1991; Sanson et al 1996).

For cancer patients, quality of life is an important consideration. Patients suffering from recurrent GBM reported greater satisfaction and a higher health-related quality of life (HRQOL) when treated with TMZ than with PCV (Osoba et al 2000) Choice of chemotherapy should consider such findings as well as efficacy, toxicity, and cost.

Biologic and immune therapies

Delineation of the molecular pathways of glial tumorigenesis has fostered development and testing of small molecule inhibitors and monoclonal antibodies targeting their components. Erlotinib and gefitinib, inhibitors of the epidermal growth factor receptor (EGFR), a tyrosine kinase amplified or mutated in a high percentage of glioblastomas, are two examples of such molecular based therapeutic agents However, recent phase II trials have failed to demonstrate convincing effect. Gefitinib provided rates of progression free survival at 8 months (PFS-6) of 14% in a prospective study of 28 patients with recurrent or progressive high-grade glioma and of 13% in 53 patients with recurrent glioblastoma (Franceschi et al 2007; Rich 2004). And, a randomized phase II trial conducted by the European Organization for Research and Treatment of Cancer found a PFS-6 of 12%, for patients with recurrent glioblastomas treated with gefitinib compared to a PFS-6 of 24% for the control group treated with either BCNU or TMZ (Van Den Bent et al 2007). Disappointment over the failure of EGFR inhibitors as single agents has not dimmed optimism that they may be more valuable when used in conjunction with other therapeutic agents.

EGFRvIII, a constitutively active form of the receptor resulting from its most common deletion (found in approx. 30% of GBM), has been targeted by small inhibitory molecules and monoclonal antibodies specific for the mutated receptor. Tyrphostin, an inhibitor of EGFR more active against the mutated than against the wild type receptor, has significantly delayed tumor recurrence in animal models and is entering the clinical phase of trials (Han et al 1996). And

Table 19.1 Recurrent glioblastoma: recommended treatment

Resectable: focal or diffuse (with a resectable symptomatic portion)	Multiple; unresectable focal; or diffuse
Craniotomy for resection ± BCNU wafer, then TMZ, concurrent with and subsequent to radiotherapy (if not already given)[a]	TMZ, concurrent with and subsequent to radiotherapy (if not already given)[b]

From the National Comprehensive Cancer Network (NCCN) Guidelines; Fadul et al 2008.
[a]Level II recommendation.
[b]Level I recommendation for patients 18–70 years old with good health otherwise; Level III recommendation for patients older than 70 having KPS of at least 60.

mAbs raised against the variant receptor have shown anti-tumor effects in cell culture (Aldape et al 2004).

Since EGFR is an initial component of the PI3 kinase (PI3K) pathway, which is crucial to cell survival, proliferation and motility, tumor cells, when chronically activated by the EGFRvIII mutation, become dependent on PI3k and thus potentially sensitized to its disruption (Weinstein 2002; Mellinghoff 2005). Interestingly, the PTEN tumor suppressor protein, an inhibitor of the P13K pathway, is often lost in glioblastoma (Smith 2001). Based on these observations, it has been hypothesized that while possession of the EGFRvIII mutation would sensitize tumors to EGFR kinase inhibitors, loss of PTEN would mitigate this effect by disassociating EGFR inhibition from inhibition of the downstream P13K pathway. Coexpression of EGFRvIII and PTEN at both mRNA and protein levels was significantly associated with a clinical response in glioblastomas treated with EGFR kinase inhibitors (Mellinghoff 2005). Thus, although inhibition of EGFR activity and the PI3K pathway may not be effective against all GBM, it may hold promise against tumors, at diagnosis or at recurrence, selected for having predisposing molecular lesions.

Targeting the tumor's vasculature is another promising strategy (Folkman 1971). Bevacizumab (Avastin), an inhibitor of vascular endothelial growth factor (VEGF) with anti-angiogenic and anti-edema effects, rapidly reduces contrast enhancement at the site of tumor. This response is associated with increased time to tumor progression: bevacizumab and irinotecan produced a PFS-6 rate of 46% in patients with recurrent glioblastoma (Vredenburgh et al 2007). Despite other similarly impressive bevacizumab-induced increases in time to local recurrence of contrast enhancing tumor, lengthened overall survival has not been observed. This suggests that the rapid, often substantial, reduction of contrast enhancement induced by bevacizumab may reflect decreases in vascular permeability rather than true regression of tumor. Furthermore, there is increasing concern both that the suppression of angiogenesis during treatment is transient and that treatment may favor more diffuse, initially hypoangiogenic, growth (Narayana et al 2009). Despite these concerns, an advisory committee to the Food and Drug Administration recently unanimously recommended approval of bevacizumab for treatment of glioblastoma.

Immunotherapy also holds great promise for patients with malignant gliomas (Hall 2004). Efforts to enhance the immune response to tumors include both passive and active strategies (Mitra 2009). Passive approaches include implantation of modified immune cells into a resection cavity. One early study employing lymphokine-activated killer (LAK) cells and IL-2 reported a median duration of survival of 53 weeks after reoperation and implantation compared with 26 weeks following reoperation and chemotherapy (Hayes et al 1995). Another implanting the LAK cells without the IL-2 in 40 patients with recurrent glioblastomas reported a median duration of survival of 9 months and a 1-year survival rate of 34% (Dillman et al 2004). Adoptive immunotherapy, a variety of passive immunotherapy, is receiving great interest. Tissue harvested at surgery is disaggregated and various constituents (simple lysate, DNA, proteins, etc.) are used to prime dendritic cells harvested from the patient's blood or tumor (Yu 2004; Liau 2005). Active immune strategies

employ vaccination. Clinical testing of a vaccine to EGFR vIII has progressed to a Phase III trial based on safety and efficacy against newly diagnosed GBM in Phase I and II trials (Sampson 2008a). Confirmation of the actual clinical benefit of these and other efforts to enhance the immune response awaits completion of Phase III trials.

Monoclonal antibodies to other tumor cell surface receptors have also been used to block other components of growth factor signalling pathways (e.g., PDGF), to deliver toxins specifically to tumor cells (e.g., toxin linked to EGF or IL-13), and, as mentioned above, to selectively irradiate tumor sites (e.g., I131-mAb; Reardon et al 2007; Sampson et al 2008b). For example, *Pseudomonas* exotoxin has been targeted to the IL-13 receptors highly expressed on malignant glioma cells by injecting the toxin conjugated to IL-13 into the resection cavity of recurrent, malignant glioma. *Pseudomonas* exotoxin conjugated to TGFα also has been investigated in a phase I trial, with relative safety but mixed results in terms of efficacy. Overall, toxin delivery by cytokines has demonstrated relative safety and variable efficacy.

Cells carrying therapeutic genes have also been used. Preliminary gene therapy studies using ganciclovir activated by a thymidine kinase gene delivered by a retrovirus produced by a modified mouse fibroblast packaging cell line have proved feasibility and safety but have not yet achieved proof of mechanism or demonstrated efficacy (Ram et al 1995; Harsh et al 2000). In a small study that examined the effects of an intratumoral injection of retroviral vector-producing cells combined with intravenous ganciclovir, the authors obtained a 1-year survival rate of 25% with tumor response in 50% of the cases (Colombo et al 2005).

Numerous such strategies utilize reoperation to harvest tissue for molecular analysis or to guide tumor specific therapies and as a source of agents for vaccination. Reoperation also presents an opportunity to implant drug polymers, immune stimulants, toxins, viruses, radioisotopes, therapeutic cells, and infusion catheters for subsequent delivery of therapeutic agents (Fig. 19.9) (Brem et al 1995; Hayes et al 1995; Ram et al 1995; Colombo et al 2005; Reardon et al 2007; Sampson et al 2008b).

Reoperation for malignant glioma

Rationale for reoperation

Early reoperation, within months of the initial procedure, might be indicated for complications such as intracerebral, subdural, or epidural hematoma, wound dehiscence and infection, or hydrocephalus and CSF leakage. Occasionally, failure to identify and remove readily accessible tumor mass might warrant reoperation. In the Royal Melbourne Hospital experience, 5 of 200 patients underwent early reoperation (Kaye 1992). More frequently, true tumor recurrence after an interval of response to the initial therapy is the reason for considering reoperation. Reoperation is justified if it produces sustained improvement of neurologic condition and quality of life or significant increase of response rates to adjuvant therapy. Palliation of neurologic symptoms by surgery results from reduction of the local mass effect produced by the tumor and tumor-induced edema. Steroid dose may be able to be reduced and steroid side effects diminished.

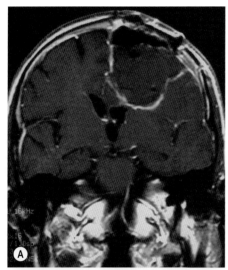
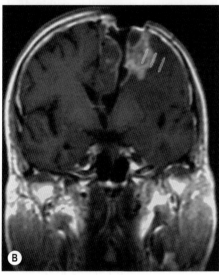

Figure 19.9 Adjuvant therapy. Reoperation provides the opportunity to implant drug polymers, immune stimulants, toxins, viruses, radioisotopes, therapeutic cells, and infusion catheters for subsequent delivery of therapeutic agents. A 39-year-old man developed marginal recurrence about the cystic resection cavity left after removal and irradiation of an anaplastic astrocytoma 3 years previously. As part of a gene therapy trial, three columns of vector producing cells were infused within the tumor, at the tumor margin, and in surrounding tumor-infiltrated brain (A, coronal MRI). Five days later, the tumor and the infused tissue to be analyzed were removed. Care was taken to extend the resection to the margin of eloquent areas and to achieve watertight closure (B, coronal, immediately postoperative MRI).

Multiple studies have shown that initial surgical cytoreduction of a malignant glioma can both improve neurologic deficits and promote maintenance of high performance status. One review of 82 patients examined five categories of neurologic function in each patient. Preoperatively, 191 neurologic deficits were noted. Postoperatively, 151 deficits were improved or stable and 40 were worse (Shapiro et al 1989). Another study showed that patients undergoing gross total resection of their malignant gliomas were likely to have improved neurologic function (97% of 36 patients had either

improved or stable neurologic examinations), higher functional status (mean KPS score improvement of 6.8%), and extended maintenance of good functional status (185 weeks) (Ammirati et al 1987b; Ciric et al 1989). A third study confirmed that more extensive resection was correlated with better immediate postoperative performance, lower 1-month mortality rate, and longer survival: 43% of patients with malignant gliomas improved, 50% remained unchanged, and 7% suffered deterioration in their neurologic condition following resection of at least 75% of their tumor. A more limited resection proved inferior (28% improved, 51% were unchanged, and 21% were worse) (Vecht et al 1990).

Similar results can be achieved by reoperation. In one series, 45% of patients had an improved Karnofsky score following reoperation (Ammirati et al 1987a). In another series focusing on reoperation, when gross tumor resection was achieved, 82% (32/39) of patients had improvement or stability in their Karnofsky score (Wallner et al 1989b). In one-third, patients with Karnofsky scores of ≤50 also underwent reoperation. Two-thirds improved from a dependent to an independent state and the median duration of survival was similar to that for all patients undergoing reoperation (Sipos & Afra 1997).

The doubling rate of malignant gliomas is so high, however, that the benefit from reoperation will be very brief unless adjuvant therapies are able to induce remission of tumor growth. Surgical resection is especially beneficial when reduction of tumor burden improves the response rate to such adjuvant therapies. One early study of multidrug chemotherapy following reoperation for recurrent malignant gliomas used multivariate analysis to identify prognostic factors. During chemotherapy, disease stabilization or partial response occurred in 29 of 51 (57%) patients. Median time to tumor progression was 19 weeks for all pathologies; it was 32 weeks for patients with anaplastic astrocytomas and 13 weeks for those with glioblastoma multiforme. Median survival time was 40 weeks for all pathologies; it was 79 weeks for patients with anaplastic astrocytoma and 33 weeks for those with glioblastoma multiforme. A total of 35% of patients had serious chemotoxicity but none had permanent morbidity or mortality. Factors associated with a longer median time to tumor progression included a higher Karnofsky score, lower grade of initial histology, lack of prior chemotherapy, less myelotoxicity, smaller postoperative tumor volume, greater extent of resection, and a local rather than diffuse pattern of recurrence. Those associated with a longer median survival time were a higher Karnofsky score, anaplastic astrocytoma rather than glioblastoma at recurrence, greater and myelotoxicity, and lobar rather than central location of the tumor (Hucharek & Muscat 1995).

More recent studies from UCSF, Memorial Sloan-Kettering, the University of Washington, and Johns Hopkins University have shown that reoperation followed by chemotherapy leads to stabilization of performance score for significant intervals (Ammirati et al 1987a; Harsh et al 1987; Berger et al 1992; Brem et al 1995). At UCSF, 44% of patients with glioblastomas maintained a performance level of at least 70 (a level consistent with self-care and judged to be survival of high quality (Karnofsky et al 1951) for at least 6 months after reoperation; 18% maintained this level for at least 1 year; and three patients did so for longer than 3

symptoms depends on the location of the tumor and its physical characteristics. Removal is facilitated by a more superficial location in non-eloquent areas; a discrete pseudoencapsulated mass is more easily removed than a less well-marginated diffuse one; drainage of a cystic component will often provide immediate reduction of mass, as well as an avenue for further resection of tumor.

During the interval between initial surgery and tumor recurrence, the patient will usually undergo therapy that might affect tolerance of surgery. The decision to reoperate must consider overall physical condition, tissue viability, blood coagulability, hematologic reserve, and immune function following surgery, radiation, corticosteroids, and chemotherapy. A high risk of multisystem failure, failure to thrive, intracranial hemorrhage, anemia, wound infection, pneumonia, and neurologic damage may exist. This risk should be assessed for each patient by obtaining preoperative chemical, hematologic, and radiographic studies.

In choosing patients for reoperation and subsequent therapy, consideration of the individual patient's profile of these prognostically significant factors permits a reasonable estimate of the likelihood of benefit from the procedure. Quality of life is a very important determinant of benefit as perceived by the patient, family and society. Reoperation and subsequent multimodal therapy should be chosen only if maintenance of a reasonable level of function is anticipated (Fig. 19.10).

Preparation for reoperation

Before surgery, the patient is likely to be receiving corticosteroids; these should be continued. At the time of induction of anesthesia, the patient is fitted with thigh-high intermittent-compression airboots. Additional steroids, prophylactic antibiotics, and osmotic and loop diuretics are given and the patient is hyperventilated. In positioning the patient, the likelihood of elevated intracranial pressure makes attention to elevation of the head above the level of the heart particularly important.

Reoperative exposure

In planning the needed exposure, the tumor can be located by its relationship to the margins of the craniotomy and to the cortical pattern of gyri and sulci on the preoperative MRI scan, by intraoperative frameless stereotaxy, or by intraoperative MRI (Barnett et al 1993; Black et al 1999). The procedure should be planned in advance to ensure adequate skin opening, craniotomy, and durotomy to expose the recurrent mass. All may need enlarging because of the increased extent of the tumor or a desire to perform corticography for mapping of motor or speech function.

The skin incision from the previous operation is usually used. The skin opening can be increased by additional incisions. They should be external to the previous flap, avoid its base and other vascular pedicles, and intersect the previous incision at right angles. The margins of the prior craniotomy flap should be defined. Generally, this is best accomplished with a curette, beginning at the prior trephination. Depending on the interoperative interval, the prior flap may need to be recut. Dissection in the epidural plane can be begun with a curette followed by a No. 3 and then a No. 2 Penfield dissector. The craniotomy plate is further elevated as the

dura is stripped from its inner surface with a dissector. Epidural adhesions fixing dura to the craniotomy margin should be preserved as prophylaxis against postoperative extension of an epidural fluid collection unless the craniotomy needs to be enlarged. In this case, these adhesions are dissected with a curette and trimmed. After the dura is stripped from the undersurface of the cranial plate, an additional segment of bone can be removed with a craniotome.

The durotomy may need to be enlarged, but often it can be limited to part of the dural exposure. It should be planned to minimize traverse of cortical adhesions. For instance, in re-exposing a temporal lesion, the durotomy can be placed over the cyst remaining from the prior resection. Flapping the dura superiorly then allows adhesions to be put on traction such that they may be dissected from cortex, coagulated, and sharply divided. Extending a durotomy along an old incision line should be avoided. The old incision line should be traversed perpendicularly and as infrequently as possible in that it is often the site of the densest adhesions. Microdissection of larger vessels from dural attachments may be necessary. Once the dura is opened and retracted, the exposed cortex is inspected for the surface presentation of the tumor, apparent as abnormal color, consistency, and vascularity.

Localization of the subcortical extent of the tumor is then undertaken. Again, the preoperative imaging studies and stereotactic techniques are of value (Golfinos 1995). Brain shift occurring during dural opening and tumor resection must be considered when using these techniques. Intraoperative MRI or ultrasonography may help correct for this (LeRoux et al 1989; Black et al 1999; Hatiboglu et al 2009). Tumor may also be found by locating a cystic resection cavity or encephalomalacic brain left after the previous operation. In that almost all tumors recur within 2 cm of the original tumor's margin, exposure of the initial tumor's surgical bed will usually reveal at least part of the recurrent mass.

Electrocorticographic mapping of motor, sensory, and speech areas may reduce the chance of inflicting neurologic deficit and may encourage a more extensive resection by revealing the relationship of the site of cortical traverse and of the subsequent subcortical dissection to eloquent brain (Fig. 19.11). This technique is often more difficult at the time of reoperation because of cortical disruption by the tumor and prior surgery (Berger et al 1990). However, long term re-shapings of language, sensory, and motor maps in some patients have allowed gross total resection of recurrent gliomas without neurologic sequelae (Duffau et al 2002; Robles et al 2008).

Generally, the appearance of the tumor itself is the best guide to its extent. Tumor-infiltrated cortex is likely to have increased vascular markings, a pink to gray color, and a firm consistency. Its central core may vary from yellow cystic fluid of low viscosity to high viscosity, soupy, white necrosis which resembles pus, to a yellow-gray, granular, honeycomb-like material. Typically, the center is relatively avascular although it may be traversed by thrombosed blood vessels.

Some advocate incision into the tumor mass and internal debulking with an ultrasonic aspirator or laser as an initial step; however, this often induces significant hemorrhage. Enucleation by circumferential dissection in the pseudoplane about the rim of solid tumor is usually more

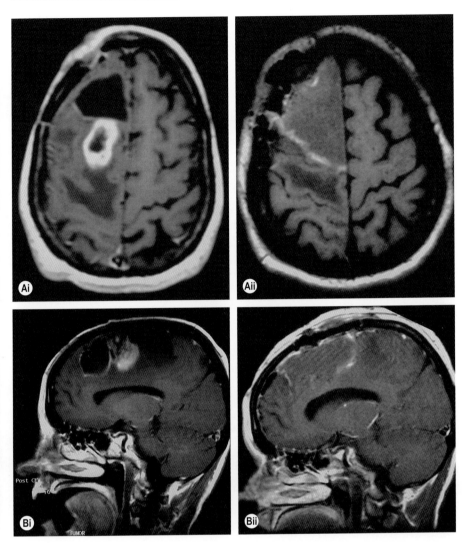

Figure 19.11 Recurrent malignant glioma. A 43-year-old woman developed left arm and leg weakness 11 months following complete resection and irradiation (60 Gy) of a right frontal glioblastoma. Pre-reoperative axial (Ai) and sagittal (Bi) MR scans show ring contrast enhancement just posterior to the resection cavity. Reoperation, guided by intraoperative electrocorticographic mapping of the primary motor area, accomplished gross total removal of the recurrent tumor and surrounding frontal lobe back to the precentral sulcus, as seen on postoperative axial (Aii) and sagittal (Bii) images. After resolution of perioperative edema, full extremity strength returned.

satisfactory. Arteries supplying the tumor and veins draining it can be coagulated and divided as they enter the tumor mass, much as the vascular supply of an arteriovenous malformation is handled. In areas of non-eloquent brain in particular, the softened, necrotic, highly edematous white matter around the tumor provides an excellent plane of dissection. The use of bipolar cautery forceps and suction together accomplishes this dissection while reducing local mass. Beyond the encephalomalacic brain lies more normal brain which, although edematous and possibly injured by prior retraction and radiation therapy, is often functional and should be preserved.

Often, the tumor can be removed as a single specimen without the need for significant retraction of surrounding brain. In general, gentle, transient gentle pressure on a cottonoid paddy lying on the margin of resection provides sufficient exposure of the dissection plane that fixed self-retaining retractors are unnecessary. Retraction of the tumor mass is preferable to retraction of surrounding brain. Often, identification of the appropriate plane for the circumferential dissection is facilitated by this retraction on the tumor; coherence of the tumor mass helps delineate the plane between solid tumor and tumor-infiltrated brain.

Once the tumor mass has been removed, the margins of resection should be inspected to verify completeness of the excision. The margins should be free of tumor that is more firm, glassy, opaque, and hypervascular. Biopsies of the surrounding edematous brain should be sent for frozen-section analysis to verify absence of tumor. If solid tumor or tumor infiltrating into non-eloquent areas remains, it should be removed. In some cases, extension of tumor into eloquent areas or diencephalic structures will preclude resection of the entire mass. In such cases, the tumor should be divided. This often entails coagulation of numerous strands of small, thin-walled blood vessels. This is particularly true if the extension is in the direction of the vascular supply, e.g., medial extension of a temporal lobe tumor toward the posterior aspect of the sylvian fissure. Particular care should be taken to coagulate and sharply divide these vessels. Tearing them without prior coagulation will leave a loose end that will retract and continue to bleed. Such loose ends should be directly coagulated rather than tamponaded with hemostatic packing, which may encourage deeper dissection of a hematoma.

After the resection has been completed, hemostasis should be confirmed by filling the tumor cavity with saline and, during a Valsalva maneuver, observing for wisps of continuing hemorrhage. This should be performed with the patient's blood pressure at least as high as the normal pressure. The cavity is then aspirated, lined with a single layer of oxidized cellulose, and filled again with irrigation fluid. Hyperventilation is then reversed to permit expansion of the brain during closure.

Watertight dural closure is essential. Often, this can be attained by primary suturing, given the decompression from the operation. If the dura is incompetent, it may be supplemented by a pericranial graft or a synthetic dural replacement. Peripheral and central dural tacking sutures are placed. The bone fragments are wired together, and the craniotomy plate is then fixed with titanium miniplates. The wound is irrigated repeatedly with antibiotic solution and then closed in layers with 2–0 absorbable suture in muscle, fascia, and galea. The galeal sutures should be inverted and the knots should be cut short to avoid erosion superficially. They should be placed in sufficient proximity that tension-free closure of the skin is possible. Staples or simple running 4–0 nylon skin sutures usually provide adequate closure except at sites of attenuation, where horizontal mattress sutures may be preferred.

Postoperatively, the patient should be closely monitored for signs of increased intracranial pressure from hematoma or edema. Fluid restriction, dehydration, and corticosteroids should usually be continued. The patient should be mobilized as soon as possible and a gadolinium enhanced MRI scan should be obtained as soon as it is tolerable to assess extent of tumor resection.

Key points

- Extent of initial surgical resection is an important determinant of risk of recurrence for gliomas and meningiomas.

- The high likelihood of recurrence of gliomas and most meningiomas mandates long-term follow-up.

- A recurrent mass on imaging studies may not be tumor; histologic verification is often necessary.

- Treatment of a recurrent tumor must be chosen within the context of the natural history of the disease and the characteristics of the individual patient.

- Reoperation may improve neurologic function and prolong survival in some cases; often, however, radiosurgery or radiation therapy can provide similar benefit to survival in a less invasive manner

REFERENCES

Adler, J.R. Jr., Gibbs, I.C., Puataweepong, P., et al., 2008. Visual field preservation after multisession cyberknife radiosurgery for periopic lesions. Neurosurgery 62 (Suppl. 2), 733–743.

Aldape, K.D., Ballman, K., Furth, A., et al., 2004. Immunohistochemical detection of EGFRVIII in high malignancy grade astrocytoma and evaluation of prognostic significance. J. Neuropathol. Exp. Neurol. 63 (7), 700–707.

Alexander, E., Loeffler, J.S., 1998. Radiosurgery for primary malignant brain tumors. Semin. Surg. Oncol. 14, 43–52.

Alexiou, G., Tsiouris, S., Kyritsis, A., et al., 2009. Glioma recurrence versus radiation necrosis: accuracy of current imaging modalities. J. Neurooncol. 95 (1), 1–11.

Alexiou, G., Tsiouris, S., Polyzoidis, K., et al., 2008. Assessment of recurrent glioma with focus on proliferation. Nucl. Med. Comm. 29 (9), 840–841.

Ammirati, M., Galicich, J.H., Arbit, B., 1987a. Reoperation in the treatment of recurrent intracranial malignant gliomas. Neurosurgery 21, 607–614.

Ammirati, M., Vick, N., Liao, Y., et al., 1987b. Effect of the extent of surgical resection on survival and quality of life in patients with supratentorial glioblastomas and anaplastic astrocytomas. Neurosurgery 21, 201–206.

Androeu, J., George, A.E., Wise, A., et al., 1983. CT prognostic criteria of survival after malignant glioma surgery. AJNR 4, 488–490.

Arcicasa, M., Roncadin, M., Bidoli, E., et al., 1999. Reirradiation and lomustine in patients with relapsed high-grade gliomas. Int. J. Radiat. Oncol. Biol. Phys. 43, 789–793.

Barbaro, N.M., Gutin, P.H., Wilson, C.B., et al., 1987. Radiation therapy in the treatment of partially resected meningiomas. Neurosurgery 20, 525–528.

Barker, F.G., Chang, S.M., Gutin, P.H., et al., 1998. Survival and functional status after resection of recurrent glioblastoma multiforme. Neurosurgery 42, 709–723.

Barker, F.G., Prados, M.D., Chang, S.M., et al., 1996. Radiation response and survival in patients with glioblastoma multiforme. J. Neurosurg. 84, 442–448.

Barnett, G.H., Kormos, D.W., Steiner, C.P., et al., 1993. Use of a frameless armless wand for brain tumor localization with two dimensional and three dimensional imaging. Neurosurgery 33, 674–678.

Berger, M.S., Rostomily, R.C., 1997. Low grade gliomas: Functional mapping, resection strategies, extent of resection, and outcome. J. Neurooncol. 34, 85–101.

Berger, M.S., Ojemann, G.A., Lettich, E., 1990. Neurophysiological monitoring during astrocytoma surgery. Neurosurg. Clin. North Am. 1, 65–80.

Berger, M.S., Tucker, A., Spence, A., et al., 1992. Reoperation for glioma. Clin. Neurosurg. 39, 172–186.

Bigner, D.D., Brown, M.T., Friedman, A.H., et al., 1998. Iodine-131-labeled antitenascin monoclonal antibody 81C6 treatment of patients with recurrent malignant gliomas: phase I trial results. J. Clin. Oncol. 16, 2202–2212.

Bikmaz, K., Mrak, R., Al-Mefty, O., 2007. Management of bone-invasive, hyperostotic sphenoid wing meningiomas. J. Neurosurg. 107 (5), 905–912.

Biswas, T., Okunieff, P., Schell, M., et al., 2009. Stereotactic radiosurgery for glioblastoma: retrospective analysis. Radiat. Oncol. 4, 11.

Black, P.M., Alexander, E., 3rd, Martin, C., et al., 1999. Craniotomy for tumor treatment in an intraoperative magnetic resonance imaging unit. Neurosurgery 45, 423–436.

Boker, D.K., Meurer, H., Gullotta, F., 1985. Recurrent intracranial meningiomas. Evaluation of some factors predisposing for tumor recurrence. J. Neurosurg. Sci. 29, 11–17.

Borovich, B., Doron, Y., Braun, J., et al., 1986. Recurrence of intracranial meningiomas: the role played by regional multicentricity. Part 2: clinical and radiological aspects. J. Neurosurg. 65, 168–171.

Bower, R., Lim, M., Harsh, G.R., 2007. Immunotherapy for gliomas. Part I: Tumor-induced immunosuppression. Contemp. Neurosurg. 29 (14), 1–6.

Brandes, A.A., Ermani, M., Basso, U., et al., 2002. Temozolomide in patients with glioblastoma at second relapse after first line nitrosourea-procarbazine failure: a phase II study. Oncology 63, 38–41.

Brandes, A.A., Tosoni, A., Franceschi, E., et al., 2009. Recurrence pattern after temozolomide concomitant with and adjuvant to radiotherapy in newly diagnosed patients with glioblastoma: correlation with M G M T promote methylation status. J. Clin. Oncol. 27 (8), 1275–1279.

Brem, H., Mahaley, M.S. Jr., Vick, N.A., et al., 1991. Interstitial chemotherapy with drug polymer implants for the treatment of recurrent gliomas. J. Neurosurg. 74 (3), 441–446.

Brem, H., Piantadosi, S., Berger, P.C., et al., 1995. Placebo controlled trial of safety and efficacy of intraoperative controlled delivery by biodegradable polymers of chemotherapy for recurrent gliomas. Lancet 345, 1008–1012.

Bruna, J., Brell, M., Ferrer, I., et al., 2007. Ki-67 proliferative index predicts clinical outcome in patients with atypical or anaplastic meningioma. Neuropathology 27, 114–120.

Buckley, S.C., Broome, J.C., 1995. A foreign body reaction to Surgical(R) mimicking an abscess or tumour recurrence. Br. J. Neurosurg. 9, 561–563.

Burger, P.C., Dubois, P.J., Schold, S.C. Jr., et al., 1983. Computerized tomography and pathologic studies of the untreated, quiescent, and recurrent glioblastoma multiforme. J. Neurosurg. 58, 159–169.

Burger, P.C., Heinz, E.R., Shibata, T., et al., 1988. Topographic anatomy and C T correlations in the untreated glioblastoma multiforme. J. Neurosurg. 68, 698–704.

Cairncross, J.G., Ueki, K., Zlatescu, M.C., et al., 1998. Specific genetic predictors of chemotherapeutic response and survival in patients with anaplastic oligodendrogliomas. J. Natl. Cancer Inst. 90, 1473–1479.

Carella, R.J., Ransohoff, J., Newall, J., 1982. Role of radiation therapy in the management of meningioma. Neurosurgery 10, 332–339.

Cerda-Nicolas, M., Lopez-Gines, C., Barcia-Salorio, J., et al., 1998. Evolution to malignancy in a recurrent meningioma: morphological and cytogenetic findings. Clin. Neuropathol. 17, 210–215.

Chamberlain, M., Glantz, M., Fadul, C., 2007. Recurrent meningioma: salvage therapy with long acting somastatin analogue. Neurology 69, 969–973.

Chan, R.C., Thompson, G.B., 1984. Morbidity, mortality and quality of life following surgery for intracranial meningiomas: a retrospective study in 257 cases. J. Neurosurg. 60, 52–60.

Chanana, A.D., Capala, J., Chadha, M., et al., 1999. Boron neutron capture therapy for glioblastoma multiforme: Interim results from the Phase I/II dose-escalation studies. Neurosurgery 44, 1182–1193.

Chandler, K.L., Prados, M.D., Malec, M., et al., 1993. Long-term survival in patients with glioblastoma multiforme. Neurosurgery 32, 716–720.

Chang, C.H., Horton, J., Schoenfeld, O., et al., 1983. Comparison of postoperative radiotherapy and combined postoperative radiotherapy and chemotherapy in the multidisciplinary management of malignant gliomas. Cancer 52, 997–1007.

Chang, E.F., Clark, A., Jensen, R.L., et al., 2009. Multiinstitutional validation of the University of California at San Francisco Low-Grade Glioma Prognostic Scoring System. J. Neurosurgery 111 (2), 203–210.

Chang, S.D., Adler, J.R. Jr., 1997. Treatment of cranial base meningiomas with linear accelerator radiosurgery. Neurosurgery 41, 1019–1025.

Chinot, O.L., Honoré, S., Dufour, H., et al., 2001. Safety and efficacy of temozolomide in patients with recurrent anaplastic oligodendrogliomas after standard radiotherapy and chemotherapy. J. Clin. Oncol. 19, 2449–2455.

Cho, K.G., Hoshino, T., Nagashima, T., et al., 1986. Prediction of tumor doubling time in recurrent meningiomas: cell kinetics studies with bromodeoxyuridine labelling. J. Neurosurg. 65, 790–794.

Choucair, A.K., Levin, V.A., Gutin, P.H., et al., 1986. Development of multiple lesions during radiation therapy and chemotherapy in patients with gliomas. J. Neurosurg. 65, 654–658.

Ciric, I., Ammirati, M., Vick, N., et al., 1989. Supratentorial gliomas: surgical considerations and immediate postoperative results. Gross total resection versus partial resection. Neurosurgery 21, 21–26.

Coffey, R.J., Lunsford, L.D., Taylor, F.H., 1988. Survival after stereotactic biopsy of malignant gliomas. Neurosurgery 22, 465–473.

Colombo, F., Barzon, L., Franchin, E., et al., 2005. Combined HSV-TK/IL-2 gene therapy in patients with recurrent glioblastoma multiforme: biological and clinical results. Cancer Gene. Ther. 12 (10), 835–848.

Colombo, F., Casentini, L., Cavedon, C., et al., 2009. Cyberknife radiosurgery for benign meningiomas: short-term results in 199 patients. Neurosurgery 64 (Suppl. 2), A7–13.

Combs, S., Widmer, V., Thilmann, C., et al., 2005. Stereotactic radiosurgery (SRS): treatment option for recurrent glioblastoma multiforme (GBM). Cancer 104 (10), 2168–2173.

Connell, P.P., Macdonald, R.L., Mansur, D.B., et al., 1999. Tumor size predicts control of benign meningiomas treated with radiotherapy. Neurosurgery 44, 1194–1200.

Crone, K.R., Challa, V.R., Kute, T.E., et al., 1988. Relationship between flow cytometric features and clinical behaviour of meningiomas. Neurosurgery 23, 720–724.

Daneyemez, M., Gezen, F., Canakçi, Z., et al., 1998. Radical surgery and reoperation in supratentorial malignant glial tumors. Minim. Invasive Neurosurg. 41 (4), 209–213.

Daumas-Duport, C., Blond, S., Vedrenee, C., et al., 1984. Radiolesion versus recurrence: bioptic data in 30 gliomas after interstitial implant or combined interstitial and external radiation treatment. Acta Neurochir. 33 (Suppl.), 291–299.

de la Monte, S., Flickinger, J., Linggood, R.M., 1986. Histopathologic features predicting recurrence of meningiomas following subtotal resection. Am. J. Surg. Pathol. 10, 836–843.

Devaux, B.C., O'Fallon, J.R., Kelly, P.J., 1993. Resection, biopsy, and survival in malignant gliomas. A retrospective study of clinical parameters, therapy, and outcome. J. Neurosurg. 78, 767–775.

Devita, V.T., 1983. The relationship between tumor mass and resistance to chemotherapy. Cancer 51, 1209–1220.

DeVries, J., Wakhloo, A.K., 1994. Repeated multifocal recurrence of grade, I., grade II, and grade III meningiomas: regional multicentricity (primary new growth) or metastases? Surg. Neurol. 41, 299–305.

DiChiro, G., Hatazawa, J., Katz, D.A., et al., 1987. Glucose utilization by intracranial meningiomas as an index of tumor aggressivity and probability of recurrence: an ET study. Radiology 164, 521–526.

Dillman, R.O., Duma, C.M., Schiltz, P.M., et al., 2004. Intracavitary placement of autologous lymphokine-activated killer (LAK) cells after resection of recurrent glioblastoma. J. Immunother. 27 (5), 398–404.

Dirks, P., 2006. Cancer: Stem cells and brain tumours. Nature 444 (7120), 687–688.

Duffau, H., Denvil, D., Capelle, L., 2002. Long term reshaping of language, sensory, and motor maps after glioma resection: A new parameter to integrate in the surgical strategy. J. Neurol. Neurosurg. Psychiatry 72 (4), 511–516.

Duma, C.M., Lunsford, L.D., Kondziolka, D., et al., 1993. Stereotactic radiosurgery of cavernous sinus meningiomas as an addition or alternative to microsurgery. Neurosurgery 32, 699–705.

Edwards, M.S., Wilson, C.B., 1980. Treatment of radiation necrosis. In: Gilbert, H.A., Kagan, A.R. (Eds.), Radiation damage to the nervous system. A delayed therapeutic hazard. Raven Press, New York, pp. 120–143.

Fadul, C.E., Wen, P.Y., Kim, L., et al., 2008. Cytotoxic chemotherapeutic management of newly diagnosed glioblastoma multiforme. J. Neurooncol. 92 (2), 239.

Fitzek, M., Thornton, A., Ley, M., et al., 1999. Accelerated fractionated proton/photon irradiation to 90 cobalt gray equivalent for glioblastoma multiforme: results of a phase II prospective trial. J. Neurosurg. 91, 251–260.

Folkman, J., 1971. Tumor angiogenesis: therapeutic implications. N. Engl. J. Med. 285 (21), 1182–1186.

Franceschi, E., Cavallo, G., Lonardi, S., et al., 2007. Gefitinib in patients with progressive high-grade gliomas: a multicentre phase II study by Gruppo Italiano Cooperativo di Neuro-Oncologia (GICNO). Br. J. Cancer 96 (7), 1047–1051.

Fuentes, S., Chinot, O., Dufour, H., et al., 2004. Hydroxyurea treatment for unresectable meningioma. Neurochirurgi. 50, 461–467.

Gaspar, L.E., Zamarano, L.J., Shamsa, F., et al., 1999. Permanent 125iodine implants for recurrent malignant gliomas. Int. J. Radiat. Oncol. Biol. Phys. 43, 977–982.

Goldsmith, B., Wara, W., Wilson, C.B., et al., 1992. Postoperative external beam irradiation for subtotally resected meningiomas. Int. J. Radiat. Oncol. Biol. Phys. 24 (Suppl. 1), 126–127.

Golfinos, J., Fitzpatrick, B.C., Smith, L.R., et al., 1995. Clinical use of a frameless stereotactic arm: results of 325 cases. J. Neurosurgery 83, 197–205.

Goodwin, J., Crowley, J., Eyre, H., et al., 1993. A phase II evaluation of tamoxifen in unresectable or refractory meningiomas: a Southwest Oncology Group study. J. Neurooncol. 15, 75–77.

Grunberg, S., Weiss, M., Russell, C., et al., 2006. Long term administration of mifepristone (RU486): clinical tolerance during extended treatment of meningioma. Cancer Invest. 24, 727–733.

Gupta, V., Su, Y.S., Samuelson, C.G., et al., 2007. Irinotecan: a potential new chemotherapeutic agent for atypical or malignant meningiomas. Neurosurgery 106, 455–462.

Hall, W.A., 2004. Extending survival in gliomas: surgical resection or immunotherapy? Surg. Neurol. 61 (2), 145–148.

Han, Y., Caday, C., Nanda, A., et al., 1996. Tyrphostin A G 1478 Preferentially inhibits human glioma cells expressing truncated rather than wild-type epidermal growth factor receptors. Cancer Res. 56, 3859–3861.

Hara, A., Nishimura, Y., Sakai, N., et al., 1995. Effectiveness of intra-operative radiation therapy for recurrent supratentorial low grade glioma. J. Neurooncol. 25, 239–243.

Harris, A.E., Lee, J.Y., Omalu, B., et al., 2003. The effect of radiosur-gery during management of aggressive meningiomas. Surg. Neurol. 60 (4), 298–305.

Harsh, G.R., Wilson, C.B., 1990. Neuroepithelial tumors in adults. In: Youmans, J.R. (Ed.), Neurological surgery. WB Saunders, Phila-delphia, PA, pp. 3040–3136.

Harsh, G.R., Levin, V.A., Gutin, P.H., et al., 1987. Reoperation for recurrent glioblastoma and anaplastic astrocytoma. Neurosurgery 21, 615–621.

Harsh, G.R., Deisboeck, T.S., Luis, D.N., et al., 2000. Thymidine kinase activation of ganciclovir in recurrent malignant gliomas: a gene-marking and neuropathological study. J. Neurosurg. 92 (5), 804–811.

Hatiboglu, M.A., Weinberg, J.S., Suki, D., et al., 2009. Impact of intraoperative high-field magnetic resonance imaging guidance on glioma surgery: a prospective volumetric analysis. Neurosur-gery 64 (6), 1073–1081.

Hau, P., Baumgart, U., Pfeifer, K., et al., 2003. Salvage therapy in patients with glioblastoma: is there any benefit? Cancer 98, 2678–2686.

Hayat, K., Jones, B., Bisbrown, G., et al., 1997. Retreatment of patients with intracranial gliomas by external beam radiotherapy and cytotoxic chemotherapy. Clin. Oncol. 9, 158–163.

Hayes, R.L., Koslow, M., Hiesiger, E.M., et al., 1995. Improved long term survival after intracavitary interleukin-2 and lymphokine-activated killer cells for adults with recurrent malignant glioma. Cancer 76, 840–852.

Hentschel, S.J., Sawaya, R., 2003. Optimizing outcomes with maximal surgical resection of malignant gliomas. Cancer Control. 10 (2), 109–114.

Hochberg, F.H., Pruitt, A., 1980. Assumptions in the radiotherapy of glioblastoma. Neurology 30, 407–911.

Hoshino, T.A., 1984. A commentary on the biology and growth kinet-ics of low-grade and high-grade gliomas. J. Neurosurg. 61, 895–900.

Hou, L.C., Veeravagu, A., Hsu, A.R., et al., 2006. Recurrent glioblas-toma multiforme: a review of natural history and management options. Neurosurg. Focus 20, E5.

Hsu, D.W., Efird, J.T., Hedley-Whyte, E.T., 1997a. Progesterone and estrogen receptors in meningiomas: prognostic considerations. J. Neurosurg. 86, 113–120.

Hsu, D.W., Louis, D.N., Efird, J.T., et al., 1997b. Use of MIB-1 (Ki-67) immunoreactivity in differentiating grade II and grade III gliomas. J. Neuropathol. Exp. Neurol 56, 857–865.

Hu, L., Baxters, L., Smith, K., et al., 2009. Relative cerebral blood volume values to differentiate high-grade glioma recurrence from post treatment radiation effect: direct correlation between image-guided tissue histopathology and localized dynamic susceptibility-weighted contrast-enhanced perfusion M R imaging measurements. AJNR Am. J. NeuroRadiology 30 (3), 552–558.

Hucharek, M., Muscat, J., 1995. Treatment of recurrent high grade astrocytoma; results of a systematic review of 1,415 patients. AntiCancer Res. 18, 1303–1311.

Hudes, R.S., Corn, B.W., Werner-Wasik, M., et al., 1999. A phase I dose escalation study of hypofractionated stereotactic radiother-apy as salvage therapy for persistent or recurrent malignant glioma. Int. J. Radiat. Oncol. Biol. Phys. 43, 293–298.

Hug, E.B., Devries, A., Thornton, A.F., et al., 2000. Management of atypical and malignant meningiomas: role of high-dose, 3D-conformal radiation therapy. J. Neurooncol. 48, 151–160.

Huisman, T., Tanghe, H., Koper, J., et al., 1991. Progesterone, oestra-diol, and E G F receptors on human meningiomas and their CT characteristics. Eur. J. Cancer 27, 1453–1457.

Hutter, A., Schwetye, K., Bierhals, A., et al., 2003. Brain neoplasms; epidemiology, diagnosis, and prospects of cost-effective imaging. Neuroimag. Clin. North Am. 13 (2), 237–250.

Jääskeläinen, J., 1986. Seemingly complete removal of histologically benign intracranial meningioma: late recurrence rate and factors predicting recurrence in 657 patients. Surg. Neurol. 26, 461–469.

Jääskeläinen, J., Haltia, M., Laasonen, E., et al., 1985. The growth rate of intracranial meningiomas and its relation to histology: an analysis of 43 patients. Surg. Neurol. 24, 165–172.

Jääskeläinen, J., Haltia, M., Servo, A., et al., 1986. Atypical and anaplastic meningiomas: radiology, surgery, radiotherapy, and outcome. Surg. Neurol. 25, 233–242.

Jaeckle, K.A., Hess, K.R., Yung, W.K., et al., 2003. Phase II evaluation of temozolomide and 13 cis-retinoic acid for the treatment of recurrent and progressive malignant gliomas: a North American Brain Tumor Consortium study. J. Clin. Oncol. 21 (12), 2305–2311.

Jelsma, R., Bucy, P.C., 1969. Glioblastoma multiforme. Its treatment and some factors affecting survival. Arch. Neurol. 20, 161–171.

Kaba, S.E., DeMonte, F., Bruner, J.M., et al., 1997. The treatment of recurrent unresectable and malignant meningiomas with inter-feron alpha-2B. Neurosurgery 40, 271–275.

Karnofsky, D., Burchenal, J.H., Armistead, G.C. Jr., et al., 1951. Tri-ethylene melamine in the treatment of neoplastic disease. AMA Arch. Intern. Med. 87, 477–516.

Kaye, A.H., 1992. Malignant brain tumors. In: Rothenberg, R.E. (Ed.), Reoperative surgery. McGraw-Hill, New York, pp. 51–76.

Kelly, P.J., Daumas-Duport, C., Scheithauer, B., et al., 1987. Stereo-tactic histologic correlation of computed tomography and mag-netic resonance imaging defined abnormalities in patients with glial neoplasms. Mayo Clin. Proc. 62, 450–459.

Kesari, S., Schiff, D., Drappatz, J., et al., 2009. Wen1Phase II study of protracted daily temozolomide for low-grade gliomas in adults. Clin. Cancer Res. 15, 330–336.

Kim, H.K., Thornton, A.F., Greenberg, H.S., et al., 1997. Results of re-irradiation of primary intracranial neoplasms with three-dimensional conformal therapy. Am. J. Clin. Oncol. 20, 358–363.

Kim, Y.J., Ketter, R., Henn, W., et al., 2006. Histopathologic indica-tors of recurrence in meningiomas: correlation with clinical and genetic parameters. Virchows Arch. 449, 529–538.

Kinjo, T., Al-Mefty, O., Kanaan, I., 1993. Grade zero removal of supratentorial convexity meningiomas. Neurosurgery 33 (3), 394–399.

Kornblith, P.L., Walker, M., 1988. Chemotherapy of gliomas. J. Neu-rosurg. 68, 1–17.

Kreth, F.W., Warnke, P.C., Scheremet, R., et al., 1993. Surgical resec-tion and radiation therapy in the treatment of glioblastoma mul-tiforme. J. Neurosurg. 78, 762–766.

Langford, L.A., Piatyszek, M.A., Xu, R., et al., 1997. Telomerase activity in ordinary meningiomas predicts poor outcome. Hum. Pathol. 28, 416–420.

Latif, A.Z., Signorini, D., Gregor, A., et al., 1998. Application of the M R C brain tumor prognostic index to patients with malignant glioma not managed in randomised control trial. J. Neurol. Neu-rosurg. Psychiatry 64, 747–750.

Laws, E.R., Taylor, W.F., Clifton, M.B., et al., 1984. Neurosurgical management of low-grade astrocytoma of the cerebral hemi-spheres. J. Neurosurg. 61, 665–673.

Lederman, G., Arbit, E., Odaimi, M., et al., 1998. Fractionated stere-otactic radiosurgery and concurrent taxol in recurrent glioblast-oma multiforme: a preliminary report. Int. J. Radiat. Oncol. Biol. Phys. 40, 661–666.

Lee, J.Y., Niranjan, A., McInerney, J., et al., 2002. Stereotactic radio-surgery providing long-term tumor control of cavernous sinus meningiomas. J. Neurosurg. 97 (1), 65–72.

Lee, S.W., Fraass, B.A., Marsh, L.H., et al., 1999. Patterns of failure following high-dose 3-D conformal radiotherapy for high-grade astrocytomas: a quantitative dosimetric study. Int. J. Radiat. Oncol. Biol. Phys. 43, 79–88.

Leibel, S.A., Sheline, G.E., 1987. Radiation therapy for neoplasms of the brain. J. Neurosurg. 66, 1–22.

LeRoux, P.D., Berger, M.S., Ojemann, G.A., et al., 1989. Correlation of intraoperative ultrasound tumor volumes and margins with preoperative computerized tomography scans. J. Neurosurg. 71, 691–698.

Levin, V.A., Hoffman, W.F., Heilbron, D.C., et al., 1980. Prognostic significance of the pretreatment C T scan on time to progression for patients with malignant gliomas. J. Neurosurg. 52, 642–647.

Li, A., Shea, W.M., Wyn, C.J., et al., 1992. Radiosurgery as part of the initial management of patients with malignant glioma. J. Clin. Oncol. 10, 1379–1385.

Liau, L., Prins, R.M., Kiertscher, S.M., et al., 2005. Dendritic cell vaccination in glioblastoma patients induces systemic and intracranial T-cell responses modulated by the local central nervous system tumor microenvironment. Clin. Cancer Res. 11, 5515–5525.

Loeffler, J.S., Alexander, I.I., Hochberg, F.H., et al., 1990b. Clinical patterns of failure following stereotactic interstitial irradiation for malignant gliomas. Int. J. Radiat. Oncol. Biol. Phys. 19, 1455–1462.

Loeffler, J.S., Alexander, I.I., Wen, P.Y., et al., 1990a. Results of stereotactic brachytherapy used in the initial management of patients with glioblastoma. J. Natl. Cancer Inst. 82, 1918–1921.

Loven, D., Hardoff, R., Sever, Z.B., et al., 2004. Non-Resectable Slow-Growing Meningiomas Treated by Hydroxyurea. J. Neurooncol. 67, 221–226.

Mahmood, A., Caccamo, D.V., Tomecek, F.J., et al., 1993. Atypical and malignant meningiomas: a clinicopathological review. Neurosurgery 33, 955–963.

Maier, H., Ofner, D., Hittmair, A., et al., 1992. Classic, atypical, and anaplastic meningioma: three histopathological subtypes of clinical relevance. J. Neurosurg. 77, 616–623.

Marks, J.E., Boylan, R.J., Prossal, S.C., et al., 1981. Cerebral radionecrosis; incidence and risk in relation to dose, time, fractionation, and volume. Int. J. Radiat. Oncol. Biol. Phys. 7, 243–252.

Mason, W.P., Gentili, F., Macdonald, D.R., et al., 2002. Stabilization of disease progression by hydroxyurea in patients with recurrent or unresectable meningiomas. J. Neurosurg. 97, 341–346.

Mathiesen, T., Lindquist, C., Kihlstrom, L., 1996. Recurrence of cranial base meningiomas. Neurosurgery 39, 2–7.

Matsuno, A., Fujimaki, T., Sasaki, T., et al., 1996. Clinical and histopathological analysis of proliferative potentials of recurrent and non-recurrent meningiomas. Acta. Neuropathol. 91, 504–510.

Mayer, R., Sminia, P., 2008. Reirradiation tolerance of the human brain. Int. J. Radiat. Oncol. Biol. Phys. 70 (5), 1350–1360.

McCormack, B.M., Miller, D.C., Budzilovich, G.N., et al., 1992. Treatment and survival of low grade astrocytoma in adults 1977–1988. Neurosurgery 31, 636–642.

McDermott, M.W., Sneed, P.K., Gutin, P.H., 1998. Interstitial brachytherapy for malignant brain tumors. Semin. Surg. Oncol. 14, 79–87.

McGirt, M.J., Chaichana, K.L., Gathinji, M., et al., 2009. Independent association of extent of resection with survival in patients with malignant brain astrocytoma. J. Neurosurg. 110 (1), 156–162.

Mellinghoff, I.K., Wang, M.Y., Vivanco, I., et al., 2005. Molecular determinants of the response of glioblastomas to E G F R kinase inhibitors. N. Engl. J. Med. 353 (19), 2012–2024.

Milker-Zabel, S., Zabel-du Bois, A., Huber, P., et al., 2009. Intensity-modulated radiotherapy for complex-shaped meningioma of the skull base: long-term experience of a single institution. Int. J. Radiat. Oncol. Biol. Phys. 68, 858–863.

Milosevic, M.F., Frost, P.J., Laperriere, N.J., et al., 1996. Radiotherapy for atypical or malignant intracranial meningioma. Int. J. Radiat. Oncol. Biol. Phys. 34, 817–822.

Mirimanoff, R.O., Dosoretz, D.E., Linggood, R.M., et al., 1985. Meningioma: analysis of recurrence and progression following neurosurgical resection. J. Neurosurg. 62, 18–24.

Mitra, S., Li, G., Harsh, G. IV., 2009. Passive antibody mediated immunotherapy. In: Yang, I., Lim, M. (Eds.), Brain tumor vaccines and immunotherapy for malignant gliomas. Springer-Verlag, New York, in press.

Modha, A., Gutin, P.H., 2005. Diagnosis and treatment of atypical and anaplastic meningiomas: a review. Neurosurgery 57, 538–550.

Muhr, C., Gudjonsson, O., Lilja, A., et al., 2001. Meningioma treated with interferon alpha 2B evaluated with 11-C L methionine positron emission tomography. Clinical Cancer Res. 7, 2269–2276.

Muller, P.J., Wilson, B.C., 1995. Photodynamic therapy for recurrent supratentorial gliomas. Semin. Surg. Oncol. 11, 346–354.

Muthukumar, N., Kondziolka, D., Lunsford, L.D., et al., 1998. Stereotactic radiosurgery for tentorial meningiomas. Acta Neurochir. 104, 315–320.

Nakasu, S., Nakasu, Y., Nakajima, M., et al., 1999. Preoperative identification of meningiomas that are highly likely to recur. J. Neurosurg. 90, 455–462.

Narayana, A., Kelly, P., Golfinos, J., et al., 2009. Antiangiogenic therapy using bevacizumab in recurrent high-grade glioma: impact on local control and patient survival. J. Neurosurg. 110, 173–180.

Nazzaro, J., Neuwelt, E., 1990. The role of surgery in the management of supratentorial intermediate and high-grade astrocytomas in adults. J. Neurosurg. 73, 331–344.

Nelson, D.F., Nelson, J.S., Davis, D.R., et al., 1985. Survival and prognosis of patients with astrocytoma with atypical or anaplastic features. J. Neurooncol. 3, 99–103.

Newton, H.B., 2007. Hydroxyurea chemotherapy in the treatment of meningiomas. Neurosurg. Focus 23, 4, E11.

Newton, H.B., Slivka, M.A., Stevens, C., 2004. Hydroxyurea chemotherapy for unresectable or residual meningioma. J. Neurooncol. 67, 165–170.

Nieder, C., Grosu, A.L., Molls, M., 2000. A comparison of treatment results for recurrent malignant gliomas. Cancer Treat. Rev. 26, 397–409.

Norden, A., Young, G.S., Setayesh, K., et al., 2008. Bevacizumab for recurrent malignant gliomas: Efficacy, toxicity, and patterns of recurrence. Neurology 70, 779–787.

Ohgaki, H., Kleihues, P., 2007. Genetic pathways to primary and secondary glioblastoma. Am. J. Pathol. 170 (5), 1445–1453.

Ohgaki, H., 2005. Genetic pathways to glioblastomas. Neuropathology 25, 1–7.

Olmsted, W.W., McGee, T.P., 1977. Prognosis in meningiomas through evaluation of skull bone patterns. Radiology 123, 375–377.

Osoba, D., Brada, M., Prados, M.D., et al., 2000. Effect of disease burden on health-related quality of life in patients with malignant gliomas. Neuro. Oncol. 2 (4), 221–228.

Ostertag, C.B., 1983. Biopsy and interstitial radiation therapy of cerebral gliomas. Ital. J. Neurol. Sci. 2 (Suppl.), 121–128.

Pace, A., Vidiri, A., Galiè, E., et al., 2003. Temozolomide chemotherapy for progressive low-grade glioma: clinical benefits and radiological response. Ann. Oncol. 14, 1722–1726.

Palma, L., Celli, P., Franco, C., et al., 1997. Long-term prognosis for atypical and malignant meningiomas: a study of 71 surgical cases. J. Neurosurg. 86, 793–800.

Patil, C.G., Hoang, S., Borchers, D.J. 3rd, et al., 2008. Predictors of peritumoral edema after stereotactic radiosurgery of supratentorial meningiomas. Neurosurgery 63 (3), 435–440.

Peele, K.A., Kennerdell, J.S., Maroon, J.C., et al., 1997. The role of postoperative irradiation in the management of sphenoid wing meningiomas. A preliminary report. Ophthalmology 103, 1761–1766.

Pendl, G., Unger, F., Papaefthymiou, G., et al., 2000. Staged radiosurgical treatment for large benign cerebral lesions. J. Neurosurg. 93 (Suppl. 3), 107–112.

Pepponi, R., Marra, G., Fuggetta, M.P., et al., 2003. The effect of 06-alkylguanine-DNA alkyltransferase and mismatch repair activities on the sensitivity of human melanoma cells to temozolomide, 1,3-bis(2-chloroethyl)1-nitrosourea, and cisplatin. J. Pharmacol. Exp. Ther. 304, 661–668.

Perry, A., Stafford, S.L., Scheithauer, B.W., 1997. Meningioma grading an analysis of histologic parameters. Am. J. Surg. Path. 121, 1455–1465.

Phillipon, J., Cornu, P., 1991. The recurrence of meningiomas. In: Al-Mefty, O. (Ed.), Meningiomas. Raven Press, New York, pp. 87–105.

Pieper, D.R., Al-Mefty, O., 1999a. Management of intracranial meningiomas secondarily involving the infratemporal fossa: radiographic characteristics, pattern of tumor invasion, and surgical implications. Neurosurgery 45, 231–237.

Pieper, D.R., Al-Mefty, O., Hanada, Y., et al., 1999b. Hyperostosis associated with meningioma of the cranial base: secondary changes or tumor invasion. Neurosurgery 44, 742–746.

Poisson, M., Pereon, Y., Chiras, J., et al., 1991. Treatment of recurrent malignant supratentorial gliomas with carboplatin (CBDCA). J. Neurooncol. 10, 139–144.

Popovic, E.A., Kaye, A.H., Hill, J.S., 1996. Photodynamic therapy of brain tumors. J. Clin. Laser. Med. Surg. 14, 251–256.

Pravdenkova, S., Al-Mefty, O., Sawyer, J., et al., 2006. Progesterone and estrogen receptors: opposing prognostic indicators in meningiomas. J. Neurosurg. 105, 163–173.

Quigley, M.R., Maroon, J.C., 1991. The relationship between survival and the extent of the resection in patients with supratentorial malignant gliomas. J Neurosurgery 29, 385–389.

Ram, Z., Culver, K., Oshiro, E., et al., 1995. Summary of results and conclusions of the gene therapy of malignant brain tumors: a clinical study. J. Neurosurg. 82, 343A.

Reardon, D.A., Zalutsky, M.R., Bigner, D.D., 2007. Antitenascin-C monoclonal antibody radioimmunotherapy for malignant glioma patients. Expert Rev. AntiCancer Ther. 7, 675–687.

Rich, J.N., Reardon, D.A., Peery, T., et al., 2004. Phase II trial of gefitinib in recurrent glioblastoma. J. Clin. Oncol. 22 (1), 133–142.

Riemenschneider, M.J., Perry, A., Reifenberger, G., 2006. Histological classification and molecular genetics of meningiomas. Lancet Neurol. 5, 1045–1054.

Robles, S.G., Gatignol, P., Lehéricy, S., et al., 2008. Long-term brain plasticity allowing a multistage surgical approach to world health organization grade II gliomas in eloquent areas. J. Neurosurg. 109 (4), 615–624.

Rockhill, J., Mrugala, M., Chamberlain, M.C., 2007. Intracranial meningiomas: an overview of diagnosis and treatment. Neurosurg. Focus 23:E1.

Rokni-Yazdi, H., Azmoudeh Ardalan, F., Asadzandi, Z., et al., 2009. Pathologic Significance of the 'Dural Tail Sign'. Eur. J. Radiology 70 (1), 10–16.

Rosenblum, M.L., Chiu-Liu, H., Davis, R.L., et al., 1985. Radiation necrosis versus tumor recurrence following interstitial brachytherapy: Utility of tissue culture studies. Mayo Clin. Proc. 621, 527–529.

Roser, F., Nakamura, M., Bellinzona, M., et al., 2004. The prognostic value of progesterone receptor status in meningiomas. J. Clin. Pathol. 57, 1033–1037.

Rostomily, R.C., Spence, A.M., Duong, D., et al., 1994. Multimodality management of recurrent adult malignant gliomas: results of a phase II multiagent chemotherapy study and analysis of cytoreductive surgery. Neurosurgery 35 (3), 378–388.

Rostomily, R.C., Berger, M.S., Keles, G.E., et al., 1996. Radical surgery in the management of low grade and high grade gliomas. In: Yung, W.K. (Ed.), Clinical neurology: International practices and research. Cerebral glioma series. Baillière Tindall, London, pp. 345–369.

Salcman, M., Kaplan, R.S., Durken, T.B., et al., 1982. Effect of age and reoperation on survival in the combined modality treatment of malignant astrocytomas. Neurosurgery 10, 454–463.

Sallinen, P., Sallinen, S., Helen, P., et al., 2000. Grading of diffusely infiltrating astrocytomas by quantitative histopathology, cell proliferation and image cytometric D N A analysis. Comparison of 133 tumours in the context of the W H O 1979 and W H O 1993 grading schemes. Neuropathol. Appl. Neurobiol. 26 (4), 319–331.

Sampson, J.H., Archer, G.E., Mitchella, D.A., et al., 2008A. Tumor-specific immunotherapy targeting the EGFRvIII mutation in patients with malignant glioma. Sem. Immunol. 20, 267–275.

Sampson, J.H., Akabani, G., Archer, G.E., et al., 2008B. Intracerebral infusion of an EGFR-targeted toxin in recurrent malignant brain tumors. Neuro. Oncol. 10 (3), 320–329.

Sanson, M., Ameri, A., Monjour, A., et al., 1996. Treatment of recurrent malignant supratentorial gliomas with ifosfamide, carboplatin and etoposide: a phase II study. Eur. J. Cancer 32A, 2229–2235.

Scharfen, C.D., Sneed, P.K., Wara, W.M., et al., 1992. High activity iodine-125 interstitial implant for gliomas. Int. J. Radiat. Oncol. Biol. Phys. 24, 583–591.

Sekhar, L.N., Patel, S., Cusimano, M., et al., 1996. Surgical treatment of meningiomas involving the cavernous sinus: evolving ideas based on a ten year experience. Acta Neurochir. 65, 58–62.

Shafron, D.H., Friedman, W.A., Buatti, J.M., et al., 1999. Linac radiosurgery for benign meningiomas. Int. J. Radiat. Oncol. Biol. Phys. 43, 321–327.

Shapiro, W.R., 1982. Treatment of neuroectodermal brain tumors. Ann. Neurol. 12, 231–237.

Shapiro, W.R., Green, S.B., Burger, P.C., et al., 1989. Randomized trial of three chemotherapeutic regimens in postoperative treatment of malignant glioma. J. Neurosurg. 71, 1–9.

Shaw, E.G., Scheithauer, B.W., O'Fallon, J.R., et al., 1992. Oligodendrogliomas: the Mayo experience. J. Neurosurg. 76, 428–434.

Shepherd, S.F., Laing, R.W., Cosgrove, V.P., 1997. Hypofractionated stereotactic radiotherapy in the management of recurrent glioma. Int. J. Radiat. Oncol. Biol. Phys. 37, 393–398.

Shrieve, D.C., Alexander, E., Wen, P.C., et al., 1995. Comparison of stereotactic radiosurgery and brachytherapy in the treatment of recurrent glioblastoma multiforme. Neurosurgery 36, 275–284.

Simpson, D., 1957. The recurrence of intracranial meningiomas after surgical treatment. J. Neurol. Neurosurg. Psychiatry 20, 22–39.

Simpson, J.R., Horton, J., Scott, C., et al., 1993. Influence of location and extent of surgical resection on survival of patients with glioblastoma multiforme: results of three consecutive Radiation Therapy Oncology Group (RTOG) clinical trials. Int. J. Radiat. Oncol. Biol. Phys. 26 (2), 239–244.

Sioka, C., Kyritsis, A.P., 2009. Chemotherapy, hormonal therapy, and immunotherapy for recurrent meningiomas. J. NeuroOncology 92, 1–6.

Sipos, L., Afra, D., 1997. Reoperations of supratentorial anaplastic astrocytomas. Acta Neurochir. 39, 99–104.

Smith, J.S., Perry, A., Borell, T.J., et al., 2000. Alterations of chromosome arms 1p and 19q as predictors of survival in oligodendrogliomas, astrocytomas, and mixed oligoastrocytomas. J. Clin. Oncol. 18, 636–645.

Smith, J.S., Tachibana, I., Passe, S.M., et al., 2001. PTEN mutation, EGFR amplification, and outcome in patients with anaplastic astrocytoma and glioblastoma multiforme. J. Natl. Cancer Inst. 93 (16), 1246–1256.

Steudel, W.I., Feld, R., Henn, W., et al., 1996. Correlation between cytogenetic and clinical findings in 215 human meningiomas. Acta Neurochir. 65, 73–76.

Strassner, C., Buhl, R., Mehdorn, M., 2009. Recurrence of intracranial meningiomas: Did better methods of surgical treatment change the outcome in the last 30 years? Neurolog. Res. 31, 478–482.

Stromblad, L.G., Anderson, H., Malmstrom, P., 1993. Reoperation for malignant astrocytomas: personal experience and a review of the literature. Br. J. Neurosurg. 7, 623–633.

Stupp, R., Stupp, O., Mason, P., et al., 2005. Radiotherapy plus Concomitant and Adjuvant Temozolomide for Glioblastoma. N. Engl. J. Med. 352, 987–996.

Suwa, T., Kawano, N., Oka, H., et al., 1995. Invasive meningioma: a tumour with high proliferating and 'recurrence' potential. Acta Neurochir. 136, 127–131.

Taillibert, S., Vincent, L.A., Granger, B., et al., 2009. Bevacizumab and irinotecan for recurrent oligodendroglial tumors. Neurology 72 (18), 1601–1606.

Triebels, V.H., Taphoorn, M.J., Brandes, A.A., et al., 2004. Salvage P C V chemotherapy for temozolomide-resistant oligodendrogliomas. Neurology 63 (5), 904–906.

Uematsu, Y., Owai, Y., Nishibayashi, H., et al., 2005. The dural tail sign of meningiomas. Progr. Comp. Imag. 27 (2), 59–63.

Uzüm, N., Ataoğlu, G.A., 2008. Histopathological parameters with Ki-67 and bcl-2 in the prognosis of meningiomas according to WHO, 2000. classification. Tumori. 94 (3), 389–397.

van den Bent, M.J., Kros, J.M., 2007. Predicative and prognostic markers in neuro-oncology. J. Neuropathol. Exp. Neurol. 66 (12), 1074–1081.

Vecht, C.J., Avezaat, C.J., van Patten, W.L., et al., 1990. The influence of the extent of surgery on the neurologic function and survival in malignant glioma. A retrooperation analysis in 243 patients. J. Neurol. Neurosurg. Psychiatry 53, 466–471.

Vertosick, F.T., Selker, R.G., Arena, V.C., 1991. Survival of patients with well differentiated astrocytomas diagnosed in the era of computed tomography. Neurosurgery 28, 496–501.

Vick, N.A., Ciric, I.S., Eller, T.W., et al., 1989. Reoperation for malignant astrocytoma. Neurology 39 (3), 430–432.

Vogelsang, J.P., Wehe, A., Markais, E., 1998. Postoperative intracranial abscess – clinical aspects in the differential diagnosis to early recurrence of malignant glioma. Clin. Neurol. Neurosurg. 100, 11–14.

Vordermark, D., Kolbl, O., Tuprecht, K., et al., 2005. Hypofractionated stereotactic irradiation: treatment option in recurrent malignant glioma. BMC Cancer 5, 55–60.

Voynov, G., Kaufman, S., Hong, T., et al., 2002. Treatment of recurrent malignant gliomas with stereotactic intensity modulated radiation therapy. Am. J. Clin. Oncol. 25 (6), 606–611.

Vredenburgh, J.J., Desjardins, A., Herndon, J.E., et al., 2007. Bevacizumab plus irinotecan in recurrent glioblastoma multiforme. J. Clin. Oncol. 25 (30), 4722–4729.

Walker, M.D., Alexander, E., Hunt, W.E., et al., 1978. Evaluation of B C N U and/or radiotherapy in the treatment of anaplastic gliomas. J. Neurosurg. 49, 333–343.

Wallner, K.E., Galicich, J.H., Krol, G., et al., 1989a. Patterns of failure following treatment for glioblastoma multiforme and anaplastic astrocytoma. Int. J. Radiat. Oncol. Biol. Phys. 16, 1405–1409.

Wallner, K.E., Galicich, J.H., Malkin, M.G., 1989b. Inability of computed tomography appearance of recurrent malignant astrocytoma to predict survival following reoperation. J. Clin. Oncol. 7, 1492–1496.

Weinstein, I.B., 2002. Cancer. Addiction to oncogenes – the Achilles heal of cancer. Science 297 (5578), 63–64.

Weston, G.J., Martin, A.J., Mufti, G.J., et al., 2006. Hydroxyurea treatment of meningiomas: A pilot study. Skull Base 16, 157–161.

Wick, W., Steinbach, J.P., Kuker, W.M., et al., 2004. One week on/one week off: a novel active regimen of temozolomide for recurrent glioblastoma. Neurology 62 (11), 2113–2115.

Wiggenraad, R.G., Petoukhova, A.L., Versluis, L., et al., 2009. Stereotactic radiotherapy of intracranial tumors: a comparison of intensity-modulated radiotherapy and dynamic conformal arc. Int. J. Radiat. Oncol. Biol. Phys. 74 (4), 1018–1026.

Wilson, C.B., 1980. Reoperation for primary tumors. Semin. Oncol. 2, 19–20.

Winger, M.J., Macdonald, D.R., Cairncross, J.G., 1989. Supratentorial anaplastic gliomas in adults. The prognostic importance of extent of resection and prior low grade glioma. J. Neurosurg. 71, 487–493.

Wong, T., van der Westhuizen, G., Coleman, R., 2002. Positron emission tomography imaging of brain tumors. Neuroimag Clin. North Am. 12 (4), 615–626.

Wood, J.R., Green, S.B., Shapiro, W.R., 1988. The prognostic importance of tumor size in malignant gliomas: a computed tomographic scan study by the Brain Tumor Cooperative Group. J. Clin. Oncol. 6, 338–343.

Yamashita, J., Handa, H., Iwaki, K., et al., 1980. Recurrence of intracranial meningiomas with special reference to radiotherapy. Surg. Neurol. 14, 33–40.

Young, B., Oldfield, E.H., Markesberry, W.R., et al., 1981. Reoperation for glioblastoma. J. Neurosurg. 55, 917–921.

Yu, J., Liu, G., Ying, H., et al., 2004. Vaccination with tumor lysate-pulsed dendritic cells elicits antigen-specific, cytotoxic t-cells in patients with malignant glioma. Cancer Res. 64, 4973–4979.

Yung, W.K., Albright, R.E., Olson, J., et al., 2000. A phase II study of temozolomide vs. procarbazine in patients with glioblastoma multiforme at first relapse. Br. J. Cancer 83 (5), 588–593.

Zhang, M., Chakravarti, A., 2006. Novel radiation-enhancing agents in malignant gliomas. Semin. Radiat. Oncol. 16, 29–37.

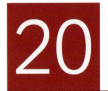

Low-grade astrocytomas

Nader Sanai and Mitchel S. Berger

Epidemiology

Glial tumors constitute approximately 50% of newly-diagnosed primary brain tumors, with low-grade gliomas accounting for approximately 15% of all brain tumors in adults (Guthrie & Laws 1990). Studies conducted in different parts of the world have indicated that the average annual incidence rate of gliomas per 100 000 population is approximately 5.4, equating to an incidence of low-grade astrocytomas in adults of approximately 0.8 per 100 000 population per year. The subset of tumors classified as low-grade gliomas represents a heterogeneous group of tumors with astrocytic, oligodendroglial, ependymal, or mixed cellular histologies. However, our discussion will be limited to the diffuse, infiltrating variety of tumors classified as World Health Organization (WHO) grade II lesions – specifically low-grade astrocytomas (Kleihues & Cavenee 2000). Among low-grade astrocytomas, the most common histologic subtypes are the fibrillary, protoplasmic, and gemistocytic variants. There is no indication in the literature that low-grade astrocytomas are more prevalent in a specific ethnic or national group.

Approximately 1500 new cases of low-grade astrocytoma are diagnosed in North America each year (Davis et al 1996). Age-specific data show that low-grade astrocytomas constitute 15% of brain tumors in adults and 25% of brain tumors in children (Guthrie & Laws 1990). Pediatric low-grade gliomas, which include cerebellar astrocytomas, optic pathway and hypothalamic gliomas, brainstem gliomas, and hemispheric low-grade gliomas, are discussed elsewhere in this volume. These tumors demonstrate a slight male predominance and a biphasic age distribution with the first peak occurring during childhood (ages 6–12 years) and a second peak in adulthood (between the 3rd and 5th decades). The median age of presentation in adults is 35 years.

Family history and genetic factors

There is no evidence in the literature that low-grade astrocytomas are more prevalent along racial or ethnic lineages. Similarly, with the exception of those families afflicted with one of several phakomatoses, hereditary factors have been demonstrated to play a role in the development of these tumors. Hereditary neurologic tumor syndromes involving gliomas include neurofibromatosis (NF-1 and NF-2), tuberous sclerosis (TS), the Li–Fraumeni cancer syndrome, and Turcot syndrome (Chen 1998). For patients with neurofibromatosis, those with type 1 have an increased incidence of optic pathway gliomas. Additionally, nearly 15% of gliomas associated with the NF-1 syndrome are located in the brain

stem, cerebral cortex, or cerebellum. In general, the low-grade gliomas found in patients with neurofibromatosis behave in a more malignant fashion than those found in the general population. Approximately 5% of patients with tuberous sclerosis may have subependymal giant cell astrocytoma. These tumors usually occur during the teenage years, and typically arise in the region of the foramen of Monro. Li–Fraumeni syndrome is a rare autosomal dominant hereditary disorder associated with germline mutations of the p53 tumor suppressor gene. Beyond low-grade astrocytomas, patients with Li–Fraumeni syndrome are at risk for a wide range of malignancies, including breast cancer, acute leukemia, soft tissue sarcoma, bone sarcoma, and adrenal cortical carcinoma. Similarly, Turcot syndrome patients are at risk for low- and high-grade astrocytomas, in addition to hereditary nonpolyposis colorectal cancer and medulloblastomas.

Clinical presentation

Low-grade astrocytomas arise roughly in proportion to the relative mass of the different lobes. Their most common location is within the frontal lobes, followed by temporal and parietal lobe lesions in order of decreasing incidence. Other potential locations include the basal ganglia and thalamus, where the long-term prognosis may be worse than for hemispheric lesions (Franzini et al 1994). Between 50% and 80% of all patients present with seizures as their initial symptom, with the majority remaining otherwise neurologically intact (McCormack et al 1992). Patients may present with or develop other signs and symptoms, which are largely dictated by the tumor's size and location. This includes signs and symptoms of raised intracranial pressure (headache, nausea, vomiting, lethargy, papilledema), focal neurological deficits (weakness, sensory disturbance or neglect, visual neglect, agnosia, aphasia), and impaired executive function (altered personality, disinhibition, apathy).

In some studies, seizures can accompany low-grade astrocytoma presentation in up to 81% of patients (Chang et al 2008a). Of the patients who presented with seizures, ~50% have uncontrolled seizures at the time of resection, despite antiepileptic treatment. Partial seizure type, temporal location, and longer seizure duration also appear to predispose patients to poorer preoperative seizure control (Chang et al 2008a). Careful consideration of a patient's seizure status is of paramount importance for low-grade astrocytoma patients, as seizures significantly impact patients quality of life. Beyond antiepileptic agents, surgical resection is an effective means of reducing seizure burden on patients with low-grade astrocytomas. Postoperatively, the factors associated with freedom from seizures are: gross-total tumor resection, preoperative seizure history of <1 year, and non-simple partial seizure type. However, continued use of antiepileptic drugs can be necessary, and in some patients, an additional operation may be required for persistent seizure activity. In our experience, optimal control of intractable epilepsy without postoperative anticonvulsants is possible when perioperative (i.e., extraoperative or intraoperative) electrocorticographic mapping of separate seizure foci accompanies the tumor resection. With most cases of epilepsy – those with occasional breakthrough seizures – mapping is not needed, but complete tumor resection is. When mapping is not used and radical tumor resection with adjacent brain is carried out, seizures occur less frequently, but most patients must remain on anti-epileptic drugs (Bloom et al 1982).

Conventional neuroimaging studies

The typical computed tomographic (CT) appearance is one of an either discrete or diffuse hypo- to isodense mass lesion, showing minimal or no enhancement with intravenous contrast. In approximately 15–30% of patients, however, tumor enhancement can be appreciated (Piepmeier et al 1996; Magalhaes et al 2005). Calcifications may also occur, particularly among non-astrocytoma lineages, including oligodendrogliomas or mixed oligoastrocytomas. In addition, cystic changes may be seen with any histological subtype.

Magnetic resonance imaging (MRI) is the diagnostic procedure of choice for low-grade astrocytoma, delineating the lesion as hypo- to isointense on T1-weighted images, and hyperintense on T2-weighted images (Fig. 20.1). Similar to CT scans, the majority do not show gadolinium enhancement on MRI. Low-grade astrocytomas are intra-axial lesions, but do not typically exert significant mass effect on surrounding structures. They do, however, display a tendency to reside within and extend along white matter tracts (e.g., corpus callosum, subcortical white matter). Neuroimaging is not diagnostic, but may suggest a particular pathological subtype of low-grade astrocytoma by virtue of the tumor's location and imaging characteristics. Oligodendrogliomas, for example, are frequently located within the frontal lobes, involve the cortex, and display calcifications, in contrast to other low-grade astrocytomas. However, although low-grade astrocytomas share characteristic MRI features, a diagnosis cannot be established based upon imaging alone. In a study of stereotactic biopsies on 20 consecutive adult patients with CT and MR imaging characteristics consistent with low grade astrocytoma, histologic analysis revealed only 50% of these patients to harbor low-grade astrocytoma, whereas 45% had anaplastic astrocytomas (Kondziolka et al 1993). Additionally, T1-weighted MRI with gadolinium often underestimates the extent of a low-grade astrocytoma. The true extent is shown on the T2-weighted sequences, although on these sequences tumor extent and surrounding edema are indistinguishable. More recently, diffusion tensor MR imaging has been used as a surrogate marker of glioma infiltration (Price et al 2004, 2006).

Emerging neuroimaging technologies

Magnetic resonance imaging modalities

Continued improvement in the resolution of anatomic imaging and innovations in functional and physiological imaging modalities have the potential to improve our ability to diagnose, treat, follow, and predict outcome in low-grade astrocytoma patients. The increasing use of 7-Tesla MRIs (as compared to the standard 1.5T magnet) will provide more anatomic detail and exquisite cytoarchitectural data on intracranial lesions (Di Costanzo et al 2006a,b). Proton magnetic resonance spectroscopy (MRS) allows for the non-invasive assessment of metabolite levels within intracranial lesions (Fig. 20.2). Of particular interest are the metabolites N-acetyl aspartate (NAA), choline (Cho), creatine (Cr), and lipids. In contrast to normal brain, astrocytomas typically demonstrate a decrease in NAA and Cr levels and a rise in Cho levels, indicative of their proliferative potential, cellular heterogeneity, and high cell turnover. In general, higher-grade lesions display higher Cho:NAA and Cho:Cr ratios than lower-grade tumors. The utility and reliability of MRS in predicting tumor grade non-invasively is currently being evaluated (Jeun et al 2005; McKnight et al 2007; Shimizu et al 1996), but does not supplant the need for tissue diagnosis. However, MRS may facilitate the identification of targets for surgical biopsy, focusing our attention on regions with elevated Cho peaks, suggestive of increased cellular proliferation and thereby regions of maximal tumor activity. In addition, MRS has proven useful in monitoring low-grade astrocytoma patients following radiotherapy, as it can often distinguish between tumor recurrence and radiation necrosis.

Magnetic resonance techniques have also been developed for assessment of cerebral blood volume (CBV). A 2–3 min dynamic acquisition of T2-weighted images during intravenous injection of a bolus of gadolinium-DTPA allows estimations of CBV. A voxel-by-voxel CBV map can be created by integrating the area under the dynamic contrast uptake curve, and provides a relative measure of CBV with a spatial resolution of approximately $1 \times 2 \times 5$ mm^3 or better. Magnetic resonance perfusion has already demonstrated utility in predicting histopathological diagnosis and tumor grade non-invasively (Cha et al 2005; Hakyemez et al 2005) (Fig. 20.3), and will likely play a role in selecting biopsy locations, evaluating treatment response, and differentiating treatment effects versus recurrent tumor.

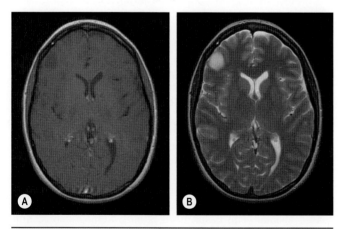

Figure 20.1 T1-weighted, axial (A) and T2-weighted, axial (B) magnetic resonance imaging of a non-contrast-enhancing, low-grade astrocytoma in a 41-year-old female patient. (Adapted from Sanai N, Berger MS: Glioma extent of resection and its impact on patient outcome. Neurosurgery 62:753, 2008.)

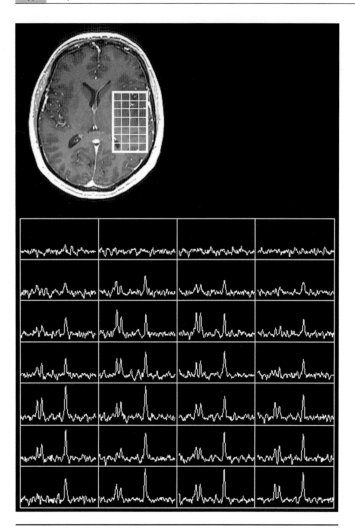

Figure 20.2 A 35-year-old male patient with low-grade insular astrocytoma. Three-dimensional MR spectroscopy demonstrates multiple voxels with elevated choline, reduced NAA, and low creatine, compatible with tumor metabolism. Lipid peaks seen within voxels at the more inferior levels may represent either lipid contamination from the skull base or tumor necrosis products. (Adapted from Sanai N, Berger MS: Glioma extent of resection and its impact on patient outcome. Neurosurgery 62:753, 2008.)

Positron emission tomography

Positron emission tomography (PET) and single-photon emission computed tomography (SPECT) are additional functional/metabolic imaging modalities that contribute to the diagnosis and management of low-grade astrocytoma patients. These modalities supplement the characterization of tumor grade, as low-grade astrocytomas are typically hypometabolic compared with high-grade lesions. Preoperatively, these technologies are also used to identify motor- or language-related regions of cortical function, although with limited specificity. In addition to predicting tumor grade, and preoperative planning, indications for the use of PET or SPECT in low-grade astrocytoma include following patients for evidence of tumor recurrence or dedifferentiation (Minn 2005).

Functional imaging

Functional MRI is based on the increase in blood flow to local vasculature that accompanies neural activity in the brain.

This results in a corresponding local reduction in deoxyhemoglobin, as the increase in blood flow occurs in the absence of a comparable increase in oxygen extraction. Thus, deoxyhemoglobin is used as an endogenous contrast-enhancing agent, and serves as the source of the signal during fMRI. fMRI results can be consistent with electrophysiology, PET, cortical stimulation, and magneto-encephalography and is commonly used to provide preoperative functional and structural information for neurosurgery. Cortical stimulation, which remains the Gold Standard is based upon local circuit disruption or activation and best identifies areas that are essential to language processing. In contrast, fMR imaging is an activation-based method that identifies all regions of the brain demonstrating activity related to a particular task, regardless of whether those areas are essential or supplementary. Consequently, areas that appear negative for language when cortical stimulation is used may still demonstrate fMR imaging activation, producing false-positive results. Decreased specificity may also be expected because fMR imaging is a perfusion-based method and does not directly detect neuronal activity.

Magnetoencephalography

Magnetoencephalography (MEG) has also been increasingly used for preoperative functional mapping. Compared with functional MR (fMR) imaging and positron emission tomography, MEG has the advantage of higher temporal resolution by directly measuring neuronal activation rather than indirect hemodynamic change. Previous studies have also suggested that MEG is more accurate than fMR imaging in identifying functional cortices that have been distorted by a nearby tumor. Overall, MEG is a robust and reliable functional imaging modality that is now used to identify the cortical location of motor and sensory pathways. Integrating MEG data with DTI information into a neuronavigational workstation directs the neurosurgeon towards potential functional sites that can be intraoperatively confirmed using stimulation mapping. Magnetic source imaging (MSI), which is based on the magnetoencephalographic detection of the late neuromagnetic field elicited by simple speech sounds (Szymanski et al 1999), is another adjunct to mapping techniques that can be useful for mapping the somatosensory cortex and determining hemispheric dominance, and may serve as a replacement to the Wada test.

Gross morphologic features

Tumor morphology has traditionally been described in terms of the historical categories of astrocytomas – the protoplasmic and fibrillary histologic subtypes. In general, the protoplasmic astrocytoma of the cerebrum appears grossly as a superficial soft-gray expansion of the cortex, although examination of the cut surface usually reveals involvement of the subjacent white matter. The borders of the tumor are poorly defined and cyst formation is common, especially with deeply seated lesions. The tissue itself is soft, homogeneous, and rather gelatinous in texture. In contrast, the fibrillary astrocytoma is often firmer than the protoplasmic variety and has a rubbery consistency to the touch. The appearance of the cut surface is whiter than that of the protoplasmic variety, and it is therefore more difficult to distinguish tumor from

ten (*PTEN*), which inhibits AKT, and neurofibromin 1 (*NF1*), which inhibits Ras activation. Both of these are frequently genetically altered in GBM (Table 21.1). The net result of these genetic alterations in the RTK/Ras/PI3K pathway in GBMs is a selective growth/proliferation advantage for tumor cells.

Cell cycle aberrations are also present in gliomas. The most frequent genomic aberration in GBM cell-cycle control is the simultaneous deletion of p14^{ARF} and p16^{INK4a}.

p16^{INK4a}, like p21, represses the activity of CDK4 (Fig. 21.5). Deletion of the genomic locus that encodes both gene products as well as other gene products that control cell proliferation (*CDKN2A/B*) occurs in ~50–60% of all GBMs (Parsons et al 2008; McLendon et al 2008). In fact, restoration of this genomic locus in glioma cells significantly inhibits their proliferation (Inoue et al 2004). Inactivation of *CDKN2A/B* or p53 is an important step in gliomagenesis, since nearly all GBMs feature inactivating mutations at either of these two loci (Parsons et al 2008; McLendon et al 2008). In the case of p53, mutations or homozygous deletions occur in ~30–60% of GBMs. Thus, it is clear that loss of cell cycle tumor suppressor genes is a major mechanism for GBM pathogenesis.

An exhaustive description of all the abnormalities and pathways present in gliomas is beyond the scope of this chapter. Suffice it to say that other pathway and signal transduction aberrancies described in gliomagenesis and progression include: (a) apoptosis, where there are abnormalities in p53, Bcl family, Bax, PUMA, p21, to name only a few (Bennett 1999; Fulci et al 2002); (b) vasculogenesis and angiogenesis, where abnormalities of both pro-angiogenic and anti-angiogenic factors have been reported, such as VEGF (Chi et al 2007), basic fibroblast growth factor (bFGF), interleukin-6 and 8 (IL-6 and IL-8), hypoxia inducible factor 1 alpha (HIF1-α), members of the angiopoietin family, thromobospondins, certain interferons, endostatins (Chi et al 2007), vasculostatin (Kaur et al 2003) and stromal-derived factor-1 (SDF1) (Aghi et al 2006), PTEN (where its replacement back by gene transfer diminishes angiogenesis; Abe et al 2003) and (c) invasion, where abnormalities of CD44 (Chi et al 2007), integrins, the zinc-dependent matrix metalloprotease family (MMPs) (Chi et al 2007), brevicans (Viapiano et al 2005; Viapiano & Matthews 2006), glycogen synthase kinase-3 (Nowicki et al 2008) have all been reported. Recent animal models also appear to show that some of the endovascular proliferation in gliomas may derive from the process of vasculogenesis (Aghi & Chiocca 2005), where bone marrow derived cells may be attracted by secretion of stromal derived factor-1 (SDF-1) to the glioma where they contribute to their extensive neovascularity (Aghi et al 2006).

Biomechanics of invasion

In terms of invasion, insufficient attention has been paid to the mechanical and physical properties of the process of invading glioma cells. The histologic features of these tumors reveals extensive infiltration of brain by invading glioma cells (Fig. 21.6). In fact, the invasion process is a mechanically driven one (Ingber 2003a). Malignant astrocytes infiltrate the parenchyma, and in the process, require work and

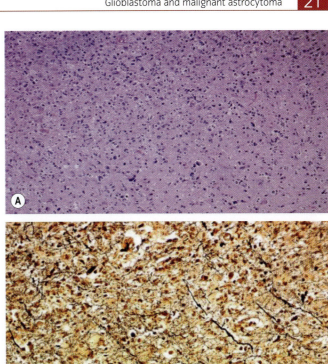

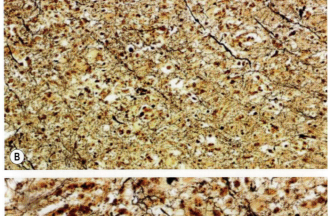

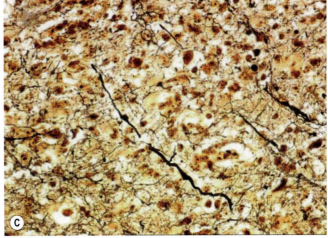

Figure 21.6 Invasion of glioblastoma multiforme into brain. (A) Hematoxylin and eosin histopathology of a GBM reveals extensive cellularity from tumor cell infiltration; note that a distinct tumor-brain boundary does not exist. (B) Silver staining from the same patient sample readily reveals tumor cells entwined among the black staining axons of the white matter. (C) Higher magnification view of panel (B) further illustrates the insidious infiltrative potential of these malignant cells.

mechanical force to do so. At its very premise, the problem at hand can be distilled into a Newtonian mechanical scenario, 'To every action there is an equal and opposite reaction'. Much like when a person walks, he/she imparts a force on the earth, which the earth equally imparts onto the walker; since the mass of the earth is greater than the mass of the walker, it is the person who moves. An analogous system exists in the brain harboring malignant astrocytomas; the tumor cell pushes against the brain, since the brain is more massive than the cell, the malignancy proceeds. At this point in time, we know very little about the mechanobiological events, which define these processes. For instance, does the malignant cell move along the ECM much like a rock-climber would, by gaining firm purchases to move forward; or is the situation analogous to that of an ice-skater, where frictional forces are minimized. Another uncertainty rests within the structure of the cell itself – do the malignant astrocytes traverse the brain as rigid ballistic bodies, 'slicing' its way about, or do these transformed cells assume 'floppy' conformations of their cytoskeletal network, allowing them effectively to diapedese there way throughout the CNS extracellular matrix. Nanotechnological and bioengineering concepts may help elucidate how biomechanics influences invasion.

The dynamic behavior of GBM cells is well illustrated in Figure 21.7. Here it is quite easy to appreciate the highlighted, pink false colored GBM cell, not only migrating extensively, but also undergoing multiple cytoskeletally driven conformations, as it is being tracked over 12 h of con-focal fluorescent video-microscopy. The migratory potential of malignant astrocytes can be even further quantified if their movements are constrained to one dimension polystyrene 'racetracks' (Fig. 21.8). In such a highly stylized assay, actual velocities of cell migration can be tabulated. In this example, for the three cells being tracked, the average migration velocity was ~40 μm/h, with the fastest moving at ~60 μm/h, and the slowest moving at ~20 μm/h. Again it is clear to see that the migrating tumor cell clearly represents a dynamic entity performing work, further highlighting the clearly important, yet poorly delineated role mechanical forces play in this malignant process. While the actuators of this process will inevitably be biological molecules (Bellail et al 2004; Demuth et al 2008; Nakada et al 2007), the 'readout' is clearly mechanical. It has only been through recent developments in nanotechnology that we will begin to uncover some of the fundamental interactions ultimately critical for malignant astrocytic migration (Ingber 2003b,c; Sarkar et al 2004; Sarkar et al 2005, 2007).

Epidemiology and etiologic factors

Epidemiological studies have failed to reveal for the most part, etiologic factors causative of or linked to gliomagenesis. In fact, numerous dietary, experiential and environmental exposures studied in relation to brain tumor risk have shown inconsistent associations; that is, one or more positive studies, but some with no association found. These include: head injury and trauma (Hu et al 1998; Hochberg et al 1984; Preston-Martin et al 1998; Inskip et al 1998; Baldwin & Preston-Martin 2004; Wrensch et al 2002); dietary calcium intake (for glioma) (Tedeschi-Blok et al 2001; Hu et al 1999a); dietary N-nitroso compound intake (for glioma and meningioma) (Chen et al 2002; Lee et al 1997; Schwartzbaum et al 1999a; Preston-Martin & Henderson 1984); dietary antioxidant intake (for Glioma); (Hu et al 1999a;

Chen et al 2002; Lee et al 1997; Schwartzbaum et al 1999a); dietary maternal N-nitroso compound intake (for childhood brain tumors) (Baldwin & Preston-Martin 2004; Wrensch et al 2002); dietary maternal and early life antioxidant intake (for childhood brain tumors); maternal folate supplementation (for primitive neuroectodermal tumors) (Baldwin & Preston-Martin 2004; Bunin et al 1993); tobacco smoking (for glioma and meningioma) (Baldwin & Preston-Martin 2004; Lee et al 1997; Hu et al 1999b); alcohol consumption (for glioma, meningioma and childhood brain tumors) (Preston-Martin 1996; Wrensch et al 1993); and exposure to electromagnetic fields (for childhood and adult brain tumors) (Baldwin & Preston-Martin 2004).

The only exception to a link between a risk factor and a diagnosis of glioma are radiation and some rare genetic syndromes. Radiation exposure with possible links to gliomas may include therapeutic and diagnostic medical procedures, occupation, atmospheric testing of nuclear weapons, and proximity to atomic bomb explosions in Japan (Shintani et al 1999). Survivors of the bombing of Hiroshima have higher incidence rates of glioma as well as other CNS tumors. The historical practice of treatment of children suffering from tinea capitis and skin hemangioma with radiation has also been associated with significantly elevated relative risks for glioma (Preston-Martin 1996; Juven & Sadetzki 2002). Regardless, therapeutic doses of ionizing radiation contribute to the development of only a small proportion of brain tumors; in one study, between 1% and 3% of glioma and meningioma patients, as well as controls, reported a history of at least one therapeutic dose of ionizing radiation prior to diagnosis of their brain tumor (Blettner et al 2007). More recent concern over a source of radiation has been that emanating from cell phones. A number of epidemiologic studies of cell phone use and glioma risk have suggested that short-term cell phone use is likely not associated with glioma risk (Auvinen et al 2002; Christensen et al 2005; Hardell et al 1999; Hardell et al 2002; Hardell et al 2005; Hepworth et al 2006; Inskip et al 2001; Johansen et al 2001; Lahkola et al 2007; Lonn et al 2005; Muscat et al 2000; Schüz et al 2006; Feychting & Anders 2010). There are limited data and inconsistent results pertaining to long-term use and glioma risk (Christensen et al 2005; Hardell et al 1999; Hardell et al 2002; Hardell et al 2005; Hepworth et al 2006; Lahkola et al 2007; Lonn et al 2005; Schüz et al 2006; Feychting & Anders 2010; Ahlbom et al 2004). The largest population-based case-control study reported to date (1522 glioma cases and 3301 controls) conducted in five Nordic Countries and the UK found no consistent evidence for increased risk of glioma related to use of cell phones (Lahkola et al 2007). Therefore, to date, no study has demonstrated good evidence for an association between long-term cell phone use and increased glioma risk.

The relatively rare genetic syndromes associated with gliomas are neurofibromatosis type 1 and 2 (Thiagalingam et al 2004; McKusick 2008; Upadhyaya et al 1997; Narod et al 1992); Turcot syndrome (McKusick 2008; Paraf et al 1997; Turcot et al 1959); tuberous sclerosis (Wrensch et al 2002; Bondy et al 1994); retinoblastoma and Li–Fraumeni syndrome (McKusick 2008; Li et al 1988). Each of these is linked to specific defects in tumor suppressor genes and patients afflicted with these syndromes are also prone to the

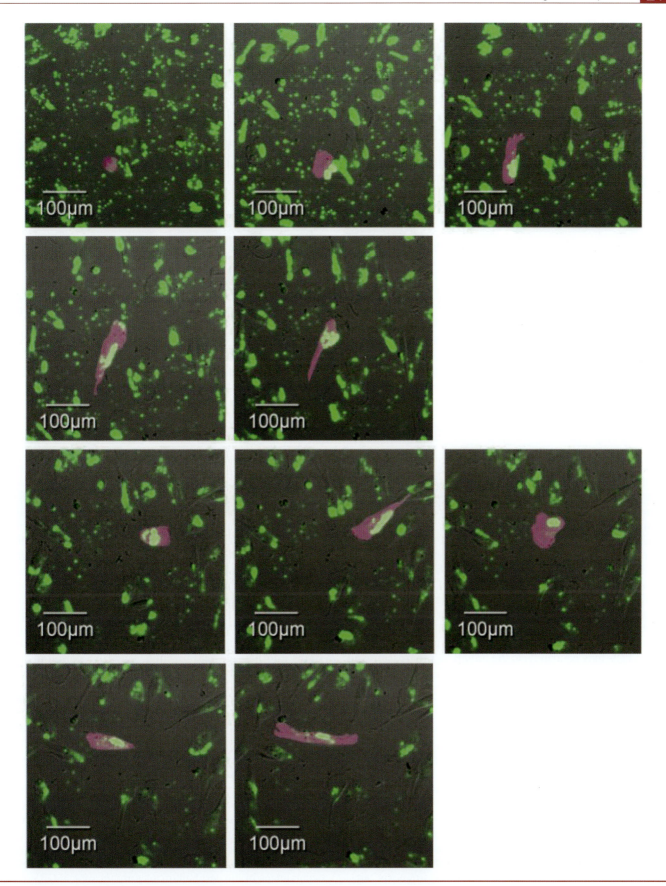

Figure 21.7 Tracking GBM cell migration as well as dynamic cytoskeleton morphologies. Quantum dots (green aggregates) were seeded onto a surface with primary GBM cells. A single cell is tracked (false color image, pink), as it migrates over the substrate, phagocytosing quantum dots and in the process, assuming multiple cytoskeletal morphologies. Each frame represents a 90-min time lapsed interval. (Compiled from unpublished data, Courtesy of A. Sarkar, Ohio State University Medical Center/James Cancer Hospital, Columbus, OH.)

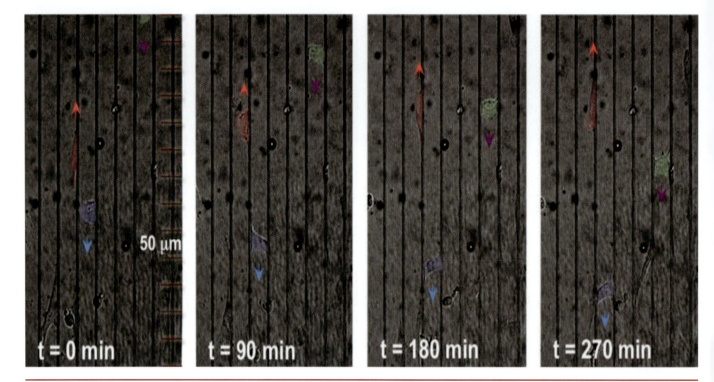

Figure 21.8 Velocity measurements of primary culture GBM cells assayed on tumor 'racetracks'. Polystyrene 'racetracks' with 45 μm troughs were seeded with primary culture GBM cells. Three cells are tracked in false color imagery: a 'red cell' moving from bottom to top, as well as 'blue and green cells' travelling from top to bottom. Time lapsed con-focal video-microscopy was used to obtain these images. (Compiled from unpublished data, Courtesy of A. Sarkar, Ohio State University Medical Center/James Cancer Hospital, Columbus, OH.)

development of other types of cancers. A viral etiology for gliomagenesis or progression has also failed to reveal consistent findings. Data related to varicella-zoster-virus (VZV), JC virus and other papovavirus, SV40 virus, adenoviruses, retroviruses and herpes simplex viruses has generally been inconclusive for a link to glioma risk (Wrensch et al 1997; Wrensch et al 2001; Wrensch et al 2005a; Wrensch et al 2005b; Schwartzbaum et al 2006; Strickler et al 1998). Recently, though, there has been resurgent interest in a possible link between CMV (cytomegalovirus) and gliomas (Cobbs et al 2002; Miller 2009). It is certainly attractive to speculate that expression of viral genes in pre-glioma or glioma cells may contribute to the initiation, progression and maintenance of these tumors.

Prognostic factors

A number of prognostic variables have been studied over the years to determine their influence on overall survival from a diagnosis of malignant glioma. In fact, younger age at diagnosis has been shown to be an independent prognostic variable for survival (Barker et al 1998). In addition, performance score as measured by the Karnofsky scale (KPS) and tumor grade (III vs IV) are also consistently shown to be predictors of outcome. Other variables have been described (Buckner 2003; Chang & Barker 2005). In fact, the following are associated with glioblastoma prognosis: age, Karnofsky Performance Scale (KPS) score, extent of resection, capacity for complete resection, degree of necrosis,

enhancement on preoperative magnetic resonance imaging studies, volume of residual disease, therapeutic approach, pre- and postoperative tumor size, non-central tumor location (defined as infiltration of splenium, basal ganglia, thalamus, or midbrain), patient deterioration, patient condition before radiation therapy, and presurgical serum albumin level (Lacroix et al 2001; Lutterbach et al 2003; Jeremic et al 2003; Schwartzbaum et al 1999b). In order to classify patients into prognostic groups, the Radiation Therapy Oncology Group (RTOG) published a Recursive Partitioning Analysis (RPA) (Curran WJ Jr et al 1993). This scheme uses patient age, functional status (KPS and work ability), mental status and neurological function, length of symptoms, type of surgery, radiation dose delivered, and tumor histology to define 6 patient groups with distinctly different survival prognoses. Stratification may become even more complex, as genetic markers (MGMT promoter methylation) also become included.

Location, presentation, and radiography

Malignant astrocytomas are essentially a supratentorial disease (Ohgaki & Kleihues 2005). While actual percentages may vary from study to study, for the most part, a fronto-temporal location usually predominate in these tumors. The occipital lobe is the least frequent site for predilection and occurrences in the cerebellum account for <1% of GBM cases (Hur et al 2008). In a large series of cases collected from a single institution, the peak incidence in age of those afflicted by this disease was between 45 and 70 years, with a mean age at the time of diagnosis being 53 years (Ohgaki & Kleihues 2005). Men are more frequently diagnosed, often at a ratio of 3 : 2, males : females.

Tumors typically start within the subcortical white matter, but often infiltrate into adjacent nuclear structures such as the cortex, or the deep nuclei. Typical symptoms on presentation may be focal or generalized, and include in order of frequency: headache, neurocognitive symptoms such as personality change or language dysfunction, motor weakness, seizures or decreased level of consciousness (Chang et al 2005). Clinically significant hemorrhages, unlike those, which can occur with metastatic tumors, are relatively infrequent (Kondziolka et al 1987). While the dura typically serves as a boundary halting malignant glioma migration, extracranial disease, while rare, has been reported. When it does occur, the lungs seem to be a potential site, and this has significant implications for transplantation medicine (Armanios et al 2004; Chen et al 2008).

The initial imaging study obtained is typically a CT scan of the head. In AAs, the typical non-contrast enhanced scan reveals a low-density lesion, and calcification if it occurs, is rare. Usually upon contrast admission, there is no enhancement. MRI features are quite variable, with mixed isointense to hypointense signaling on T1-weighted sequences, while T2/FLAIR sequences will produce heterogeneous hyperintensities, and typically little to no enhancement occurs with the administration of contrast (Thoman et al 2006; Mukundan et al 2008). For GBMs, CT findings will often reveal an isointense rim surrounding a hypodense center, with edema seen in the periphery. When contrast is administered, there is often avid, yet irregular enhancement. The MRI findings in GBMs reveal isointense to hypointense signaling on T1-weighted imaging, while T2/FLAIR sequences register a hyperintense signal. Contrast sequences will reveal a ragged lesion, which may or may not have associated cystic structures. Often in comparing the T2/FLAIR image to the T1 contrast enhanced image, the extent of peritumoral edema will extend well beyond the lesion's contrast enhancing boundaries (Thoman et al 2006; Mukundan et al 2008; Earnest F 4th et al 1988; Tovi 1993; Tovi et al 1994).

A variety of MR imaging sequences such as diffusion imaging (Brunberg et al 1995), perfusion imaging (Law et al 2002; Hirai et al 2008), diffusion tensor imaging (Sinha et al 2002; Toh et al 2008; Tropine et al 2004), and spectroscopy (Di Costanzo et al 2008; Fan et al 2004; Yerli et al 2007) are also available and utilized to varying degrees in a reflection of institutional biases. Additionally positron emission tomography (PET) has also been employed to provide radiographically derived metabolic data in the treatment and management of gliomas. By monitoring the accelerated uptake of C-methyl methionine (MET) into brain tumors compared to normal brain parenchyma (Kraus et al 2001), MET-PET proponents believe that it provides more accurate tumor delineation than anatomical based imaging such as MRI (Ogawa et al 1993; Derlon et al 1989; Tovi et al 1990). Regardless of the imaging modality, malignant astrocytoma present in protean radiologic fashion (Fig. 21.9), making the diagnosis ultimately a histopathological entity. Perhaps the only situation in which a malignant astrocytoma, GBM in particular, is radiologically unequivocal, would be in the situation of the imaging entity described as a 'butterfly glioma', although exceptions can be found here as well (Scozzafava et al 2008; Cazenave et al 1986).

Malignant astrocytomas have no real pathognomonic radiographic appearance and it is equally true that other intracranial lesions can often mimic high-grade gliomas (Okamoto et al 2004a,b). The range of lesions can include other neoplastic processes such as lymphoma and a host of non-neoplastic entities (Fig. 21.10), including demyelinating disease, sarcoidosis, Behçet's disease, abscess, toxoplasmosis, tuberculoma, fungal infection, neurocysticercosis, syphilitic gumma, vascular pathologies (stroke, cavernoma, or giant aneurysm), and radiation necrosis.

Approach and management of the patient

Preoperative management

In the patient with a suspected radiologic diagnosis of a cerebral malignant glioma, one of the first management questions relates to the use of corticosteroids and of seizure prophylaxis. In the majority of patients, corticosteroid therapy (with dexamethasone or an equivalent) can control the symptoms of increased intracranial pressure such as headache, nausea, and vomiting in <24 h and remains efficacious for several days. Corticosteroids can also alleviate neurologic symptoms associated with the location of the tumor such as motor weakness, sensory anomalies, speech or visual disturbances, and emotional lability. Steroid use can facilitate the planned surgical resection. Complications of preoperative steroid use are rare, but may involve insomnia, psychological disturbances, agitation, gastric disturbances and bone fractures. We typically begin patients on dexamethasone p.o. at 4 mg every 6 h and will also provide an H2-blocker such as ranitidine. Anticonvulsants are necessary with a history of seizures. Anticonvulsants given prophylactically without a history of seizures have not generally shown benefit. In fact, the American Academy of Neurology has published these guidelines (Glantz et al 2000):

1. In patients with newly diagnosed brain tumors, anticonvulsant medications are not effective in preventing first seizures. Because of their lack of efficacy and their potential side-effects, prophylactic anticonvulsants should not be used routinely in patients with newly diagnosed brain tumors (standard).

2. In patients with brain tumors who have not had a seizure, tapering and discontinuing anticonvulsants after the first postoperative week is appropriate, particularly in those patients who are medically stable and who are experiencing anticonvulsant-related side-effects (guideline).

Decisions on surgical procedure

The neurosurgeon is often confronted with questions regarding the appropriate surgical procedure in a patient with a suspected malignant glioma. The preoperative evaluation of a patient with a suspected malignant glioma should lead the neurosurgeon to a decision related to an attempt to resect the tumor in a gross total fashion or to only perform a stereotactic procedure to obtain tissue for diagnosis and grading.

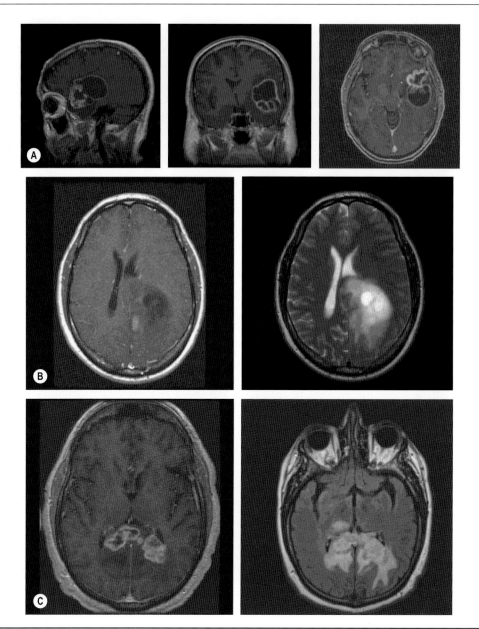

Figure 21.9 MRI imaging reveals multiple radiographic appearances of GBMs. (A) Depicts sagittal, coronal, and axial views of a 'typical' GBM with ragged contrast enhancement and complex multi-cystic structure. (B) Reveals axial views of an intracranial lesion with minimal contrast enhancement; the T2 sequence defines the complex cystic nature of this mass. Operative debulking proved this lesion to be a GBM. (C) Axial imaging with contrast reveals a corpus callosal crossing lesion. Biopsy proved this intracranial pathology to be a 'butterfly' glioma; the FLAIR sequence illustrates how the edema related to the infiltration of tumor cells extend well beyond its contrast enhancing regions.

Occasionally, symptoms related to mass effect and edema from a tumor that may not be amenable to a gross total resection may be ameliorated by generous debulking. Factors that influence the decision for a craniotomy vs a biopsy include tumor location, patient performance status, patient and family preferences and concomitant morbidities. Careful inspection of MRI images can help surgical planning by showing how and where the tumor affects areas of brain, particularly areas where eloquence (sensorimotor, speech, memory, vision, reading) may be affected. At times, additional MR modalities, such as functional MRI to locate memory and speech regions or MEG, can be useful. Diffusion tractography may provide information related to subcortical location of major motor fibers in relation to infiltrating areas of tumor (Fig. 21.11). Software now exists that allows for fusing such images as an aid to intraoperative navigation. On occasion, concerns about vascularity and/or location of major vascular structures necessitate the need for MR angiography or cerebral angiography. If a tumor is to be biopsied, software to track the passage of the needle through brain and into tumor helps alleviate the concern of transgression into a vascular structure located within pial convolutions. For malignant gliomas that appear to have recurred after standard treatment and where there is a question

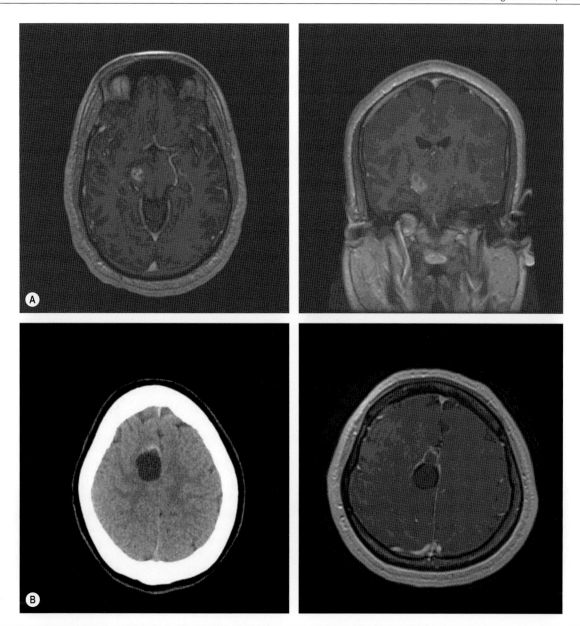

Figure 21.10 Malignant astrocytoma radiographic mimics. (A) depicts in axial and coronal views a raggedly enhancing lesion deep in the right hemisphere. Subsequent biopsy proved this lesion to be demyelinating disease. (B) The bottom set of images includes a non-contrast CT scan as well as a T1-weighted axial MR slice with contrast. Following surgical resection, this 'mass' proved to be neurocysticercosis.

related to recurrence vs necrosis, MR spectroscopy and PET scanning have been sometimes used in an attempt to forestall biopsies. In conclusion, the radiographic evaluation is an integral part of patient management in terms of decision-making for therapy, provision of initial counsel, and follow-up of therapy.

In summary, the decision tree essentially involves no surgical treatment, biopsy alone or an attempt at maximal resection of the enhancing mass and/or its surrounding areas of abnormal signal. Recently, a number of authors have been advocating that gross total resection does correlate with increased survival and quality of life (Buckner 2003; Lacroix et al 2001; Laws et al 2003), thus rendering this surgical decision difficult in patients where circum-

stances may not appear favorable for an aggressive surgical approach. In general and at a minimum, obtaining tissue for histologic diagnosis appears to be a reasonable decision. Cases of demyelinating lesions, abscesses, and/or other types of brain tumors being given a radiologic diagnosis of glioblastoma have occurred with concomitant disastrous results in terms of psychological and treatment impacts on the patients (Fig. 21.10). Except for the brainstem, modern radiologic guidance allows for relatively precise biopsies of brain anomalies with minimal neurologic impact.

Even more difficult is the decision when a certain neurologic deficit will likely be caused by the attempt to remove a lesion completely. For example, is the unilateral sacrifice of occipital visual cortex with a certain homonymous

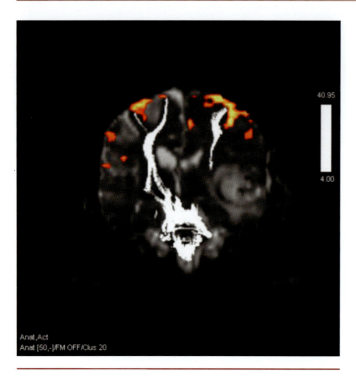
40.95

4.00

Anat,Act
Anat [50,-]/FM OFF/Clus 20

Figure 21.11 Fusion of DTI and fMRI. Coronal section of brain with tumor in left temporal lobe. Motor mapping by fMRI reveals areas of motor activation in cortex. DTI reveals motor tracts. The patient presented with dysphasia and right hemiparesis. DTI shows interruption of left motor tracts by infiltrating tumor and edema.

hemianopsia justified in order to achieve gross total resection of a glioblastoma? Similarly, is sacrifice of cortex and white matter tracts involved in unilateral tongue movement with some temporary dysarthria justified in order to achieve gross total resection of a glioblastoma? The answers to these questions depend largely on the medical condition and willingness of the patient and family to be able to cope with a neurologic deficit in order to maximize the removal of tumor tissue and, possibly, improve survival.

Decisions regarding intraoperative use of Gliadel

Intracavitary chemotherapy with Gliadel is now FDA-approved as an adjunct at first diagnosis since it has been shown to improve average survival by 2 months (Westphal et al 2003). Technical pointers with Gliadel include the need to avoid placement if a large ventricular cavity exists, need for water-tight dural closure and thus avoidance of non-suturable duraplasties such as Duragen, the possibility for wound dehiscence and infection, and the possibility for prolonged steroid use.

Surgical treatment

While surgery remains a hallmark in the treatment of malignant astrocytomas, by definition, such a diffusely infiltrative disease process cannot be cured solely by neurosurgical 'resection'. Surgical resection strategies date back to over

100 years. The goals of surgical interventions are to avoid complications while providing clinical efficacy. Surgery is generally reserved for lesions whose locations tend to be lobar and in non-eloquent brain. Biopsy is generally reserved for patients whose lesions are deep seated, or poor craniotomy candidates. Despite the lack of appropriately designed randomized controlled trials, there is a demonstrable belief that extent of tumor resection in both high-grade and low-grade gliomas leads to better outcomes (Sanai et al 2005; Sanai & Berger 2008a; Ammirati et al 1987; Ciric et al 1987). In fact, the majority of recently published literature appear to show that extent of resection, and even more, a gross total resection of all enhancing areas of tumor as measured by the postoperative MRI obtained within 48–72 h is linked to improved symptomatology and improved outcomes, such as progression-free and overall survivorship (Buckner 2003; Lacroix et al 2001; Laws et al 2003; Sanai & Berger 2008a; McGirt et al 2009). That being said, a Cochrane Database of Systemic Reviews for 'Biopsy versus resection of high grade glioma' concludes, due to a lack of randomized control trials, what most neurosurgeons and neurooncologists take at face value – biopsy is less risky than open surgery, but will not improve symptoms or extend survival, whereas craniotomy can relieve symptoms, but there is uncertainty that it extends survival (Proescholdt et al 2005).

Thus in order to maximize safe, yet aggressive surgical resections, neurosurgeons have come to rely upon preoperative tools such as functional MRI (fMRI), diffusion tensor tractography, as well as magnetoencephalography (MEG) (Alexander et al 2007; Korvenoja et al 2006; Mäkelä et al 2007; Sanai & Berger 2008b) to temper resections when working in and around eloquent brain regions (Fig. 21.11). Several intraoperative mechanisms to maximize tumor resection while sparing neurological function also exist and include awake craniotomy/intraoperative corticography (Gupta et al 2007; Tonn 2007; Taylor & Bernstein 1999; Meyer et al 2001) as well as intraoperative MRI-guided resections (Hirschberg et al 2005; Schneider et al 2005; Hirschl et al 2009), in addition to standard stereotaxy (Kondziolka 2007) (video link). Experimental techniques based on fluorescence guided tumor resections have also been described (Stepp et al 2007; Stummer et al 2003). The proliferation of imaging and intraoperative adjuncts appear to have led to craniotomies that are less invasive than those of the past in terms of skin incision, bony removal and corticectomies and intracerebral surgical pathways. This appears to result in an increased capacity for extended tumor resections with less neurologic morbidity than those performed 15–20 years ago. It is likely that the advent of high-field intraoperative MRIs may provide increased certainty to the neurosurgeon regarding extent of surgical resection and capacity to return to the tumor to complete a resection if needed.

The gross histopathologic features of AAs and GBMs have been well described (Louis et al 2007; Kleihues et al 2000; Kaye & Laws 1995), and as such will only briefly be mentioned here. Typically, AAs encountered at surgery may consist of a poorly-delineated infiltrating mass, often expanding gyri; cysts and hemorrhages are uncommon features. In contrast, GBMs bear significant vascularity, which is often thrombosed, and gross hemorrhagic features occur commonly. Microscopic features of AAs include hypercellularity, nuclear atypia, pleomorphism, and mitotic activity, GFAP positivity, modest proliferation indices (<10%), and an absence of endothelial proliferation or necrosis. Microscopically GBMs appear frankly hypercellular, containing bizarre cells and nuclei, mitosis and proliferation indices are elevated (>10%), GFAP immunoreactivity may or may not be present depending on the extent of cellular dedifferentiation, and must contain necrosis and/or endothelial proliferation. Surgical techniques include subpial dissection, suction, hemostasis, possibly under magnifying loupes or microscopic guidance. When using navigation, preoperative delineation of tumor boundaries may be helpful since as tumor is resected navigation coordinates become less precise. Intraoperative re-registration with iMRI may thus be useful in these cases. Techniques of resection have included 'en bloc' strategies vs piecemeal approaches (from inside the tumor towards outside). Each of these possesses advantages and disadvantages. 'En bloc' strategies when coupled with preoperative delineation of the perimeter of tumor with navigation allow more certainty that gross tumor will be removed in its totality. In addition, by dissection in the gliotic/edematous white matter surrounding the tumor, less bleeding may be encountered. The disadvantages are that relatively normal brain, albeit infiltrated by invading tumor cells, is violated. While some areas (frontal lobes, anterior temporal areas, non-dominant temporal lobes and occipital lobes, cerebellum) allow for this with minimal neurologic morbidity, proximity to eloquent cortex makes 'en bloc' resection techniques difficult (Fig. 21.12). 'Piecemeal' resections possess the opposite advantages and disadvantages. By staying within tumor, the operator remains assured that damage to relatively 'normal' brain structures is minimized. However, the extensive intratumoral vascularity of some tumors may obscure planes of dissection and, when such tumor vascularity is in close proximity to major arterial feeders (such as sylvian vessels), the possibility of straying into and injuring important cerebral arterial supply may lead to devastating neurologic sequelae (Fig. 21.13). Ultimately, most surgeons end up employing either technique based on preference, tumor anatomy, and intraoperative findings.

Radiation therapy

Aggressive care for patients with malignant astrocytomas employs three points of attack: surgery, chemotherapy, and radiation therapy. Once the surgical phase is complete, it is still well understood that viable tumor cells persist within the parenchyma of the brain, hence necessitating chemo and radiation adjuvant therapies to maximize survival. Radiation therapy has been a standard of care in the treatment of malignant gliomas. Excellent studies exist providing Level one evidence for the use of radiation in the treatment of malignant astrocytomas (Buatti et al 2008). Treatment protocols targeting malignant gliomas usually prescribe a radiation dose of 60 Gy in 2 Gy daily fractions provided over a period of 6 weeks (Laperriere et al 2002). In general, hyperfractionation schemes, brachytherapy, or stereotactic radiosurgery have not shown to be as useful in terms of improving

outcome and have been used primarily as salvage treatments upon recurrence (Gabayan et al 2006). There has been one study, conducted as a randomized clinical trial, that compared the provision of standard RT (60 Gy in 30 fractions over 6 weeks) or a shorter course of RT (40 Gy in 15 fractions over 3 weeks) for patients that were 60 years of age or older and were diagnosed with a newly diagnosed malignant glioma (Roa et al 2004). The study concluded that there was no significant difference in survival between patients receiving standard RT or short-course RT and concluded that, in view of the similar KPS scores between the two groups, decreased increment in corticosteroid requirement, and reduced treatment time, the abbreviated course of RT was a reasonable treatment option for older patients with GBM.

Radiation planning which includes a 1–2 cm margin about the lesion is fraught with ambiguity defining the true boundaries of the intracranial lesion. Nevertheless, such a margin ostensibly is targeting the diffusely infiltrative cells which will ultimately lead to recurrence and clinical demise. In this regard, radiation therapy planning schema are becoming more sophisticated in terms of attempting to deliver higher intensity radiation to the tumor and decreasing the amount of radiation to normal tissues (Chang et al 2008). This may be especially useful in children with gliomas, where a few centers have been employing proton beam radiotherapy (Kirsch & Tarbell 2004; DeLaney 2007). As discussed in the next section, the most significant advance in terms of delivery of radiation has been the concomitant use of temozolomide chemotherapy (Stupp et al 2005).

Chemotherapy

Although for a long time the role of chemotherapies in the upfront treatment of malignant gliomas was unclear (Rampling et al 2004), however recent advances have now brought to forefront the role of this modality. Two US Food and Drug Agency (FDA) approved therapies in the treatment of malignant astrocytomas are the oral agent temozolomide, and Gliadel implantable carmustine wafers. Both have changed the prominence of chemotherapy in the aggressive management of patients harboring malignant gliomas. Temozolomide gained FDA approval for use in GBMs in 2005, having already been used in the treatment of AA, whereas Gliadel received FDA approval in the treatment of GBMs a little earlier. Both drugs are alkylating agents. Temozolomide's effectiveness depends on its ability to methylate DNA at the ^{6}O or ^{7}N position on guanine residues; carmustine, a nitrosourea, alkylates and cross-links DNA during all phases of the cell cycle (Garside et al 2007). A Cochrane Review of Gliadel wafers in high-grade gliomas (Westphal et al 2003; Hart et al 2008a; Brem et al 1995; Valtonen et al 1997; Westphal et al 2006) concluded that Gliadel implantation increased survival compared with placebo, as a primary therapy; however it did not confer any survival benefit in therapy for recurrent tumor. A similar Cochrane Review of temozolomide for high-grade gliomas concluded that temozolomide increased survival when employed as concomitant and adjuvant therapy for GBMs, increasing survival by 2 months. It did not increase survival in recurrent disease,

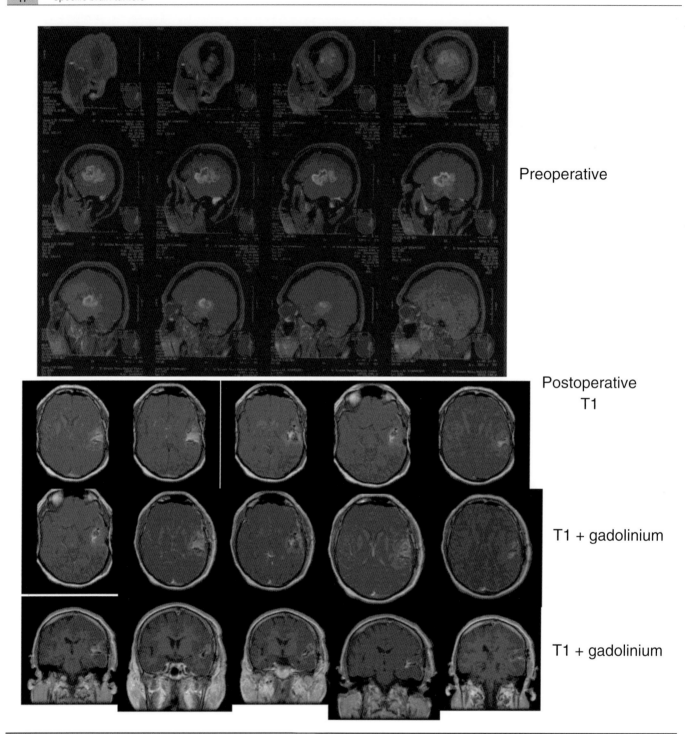

Preoperative

Postoperative
T1

T1 + gadolinium

T1 + gadolinium

Figure 21.12 'En bloc' resection of GBM in left superior temporal gyrus. The patient presented with seizures and temporary aphasia, relieved by dexamethasone. Sagittal T1 with gadolinium images are shown in upper panels. A craniotomy with speech mapping allowed for navigation of tumor circumference and resection in an 'en bloc' fashion. Postoperative images (T1 + gadolinium) reveal the tumor cavity with proteinaceous fluid and Gliadel wafers, but little if any enhancement of rim.

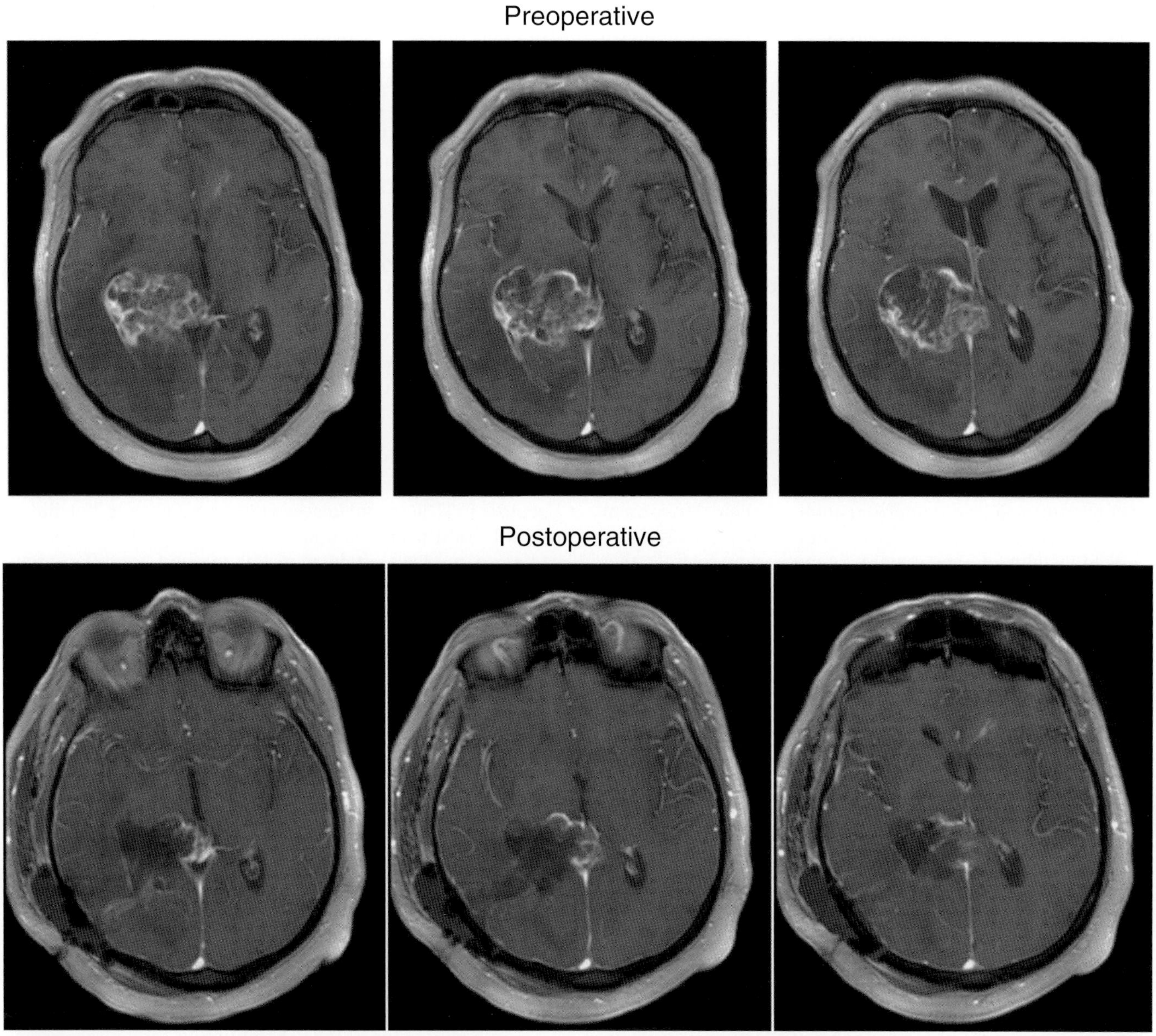

Preoperative

Postoperative

Figure 21.13 Piecemeal resection of GBM in right dominant posterior mesiotemporal lobe. The patient presented with memory loss and aphasia after a seizure. He was left-handed and right hemisphere dominant. His symptoms improved and a craniotomy for debulking of the tumor (shown in upper panels) was performed. At surgery, the lesion was found to be extensively necrotic and piecemeal resection was carried out to avoid straying into dominant mesiotemporal areas. In the midline, tumor was found to be adherent to midline cerebral veins and thus an intraoperative decision to desist from further surgery was made. Postoperative MRIs (lower panel) reveals residual areas of enhancement in the midline.

although it did increase the time to progression (Stupp et al 2005; Hart et al 2008b; Athanassiou et al 2005; Taphoorn et al 2005).

Fine molecular nuances regarding tumor genetics will also play a role in the treatment of patients with malignant gliomas. Elegant work performed by the oncology group in Lausanne, Switzerland, reveals the important interplay between treatment protocol and tumor genetics. ^{6}O-methylguanine-DNA methyltransferase (MGMT) is a DNA-repair enzyme which removes DNA adducts placed by agents such as temozolomide. Patients in their study were randomized to either temozolomide plus radiation therapy vs radiation therapy alone. Median survival was 6 months longer for those with a hypermethylated, epigenetically silenced MGMT gene. The best outcomes occurred in those individuals with downregulated MGMT gene receiving temozolomide and radiation, with the median survival enjoyed by this group at just over 21 months (Hegi et al 2005). This leaves no doubt that rational treatment approaches tailored to individual patient tumor genetics, such as IDH mutation or MGMT methylation status will lead to more customized clinical treatment plans. In fact, knowledge of such molecular pathways also leads to insights on why certain chemotherapy regimes that target expression of signaling factors involved in glioma could fail. A recent trial, e.g., showed that patients in trials using molecular inhibitors of EGFR kinases that had been deemed unsuccessful was able to find a sub-population that, instead, did show evidence of tumor response. The molecular determinants of this response were co-expression of both the EGFRvIII variant and of PTEN (Mellinghoff et al 2005).

Gliadel is currently used both in primary and recurrent tumors where the surgical cavity is lined with the circular polymers/wafers. Its main side-effects have been cerebral edema, CSF leaks/wound breakdowns/infections and seizures (Sabel & Giese 2008). Temozolomide is provided to patients with newly diagnosed malignant gliomas at a dose of 75 mg/m^2 daily during radiation and then at 150–200 mg/m^2 for 5 days of a 28 day cycle, starting 1 month after radiation. Its main side-effect has been myelosuppression.

There has been recent interest in the use of an anti-VEGF (vascular endothelial growth factor) antibody (bevacizumab, Avastin, Genentech) due to its significant effects on regression of gadolinium-enhancing areas (Narayana et al 2009) (Fig. 21.14). A recent phase II clinical trial in patients with recurrent malignant glioma showed a favorable safety and efficacy profile (Vredenburgh et al 2007), prompting initiation of a large phase III clinical trial and, in late 2008, requests to the FDA for accelerated approval of the drug in patients with recurrent malignant glioma (available at: www.gene.com/gene/news/pressreleases/display.do?method=detail&id=11627). It is clear though that an increasing number of neurooncologists are using this agent off-label as treatment in recurrent GBM or even in newly diagnosed GBM concomitantly with standard therapies (Narayana et al 2008).

Tumor recurrence

A common clinical problem that occurs with glioma patients who have undergone surgical and radiation therapy is differentiating the cause of clinical or radiographic evidence of progression, which can be caused by tumor recurrence, radiation necrosis, a combination of both, or a radiation-induced tumor. All of these entities appear as contrast-enhancing, space-occupying mass lesions surrounded by edema, and as a result, CT and MRI cannot differentiate these entities reliably.

Several non-invasive methods exist to aid in differentiating tumor recurrence from radiation necrosis including positron emission tomography (PET), single photon emission computed tomography (SPECT), and magnetic resonance spectroscopy (MRS). PET allows the differentiation of radiation necrosis (which is hypometabolic) from high-grade recurrent tumors with necrosis (which is hypermetabolic) with sensitivities from 80% to 90% and specificities from 50% to 90% (Thompson et al 1999). However, the sensitivities are much lower with low- or intermediate-grade gliomas because of low uptake of fluoro-2-deoxy-D-glucose (FDG).

Thallium-201 SPECT scans measure metabolically active tissues by cell-specific tracer uptake in malignant cells. Because ^{201}Tl accumulates in viable tumor cells but not in normal brain tissue or other non-neoplastic tissue such as radiation necrosis, it is a useful method to differentiate between tumor recurrence and radiation necrosis (Caresia et al 2006; Vos et al 2003).

Unlike PET and SPECT, MR spectroscopy does not use high-energy radiation or require radio-labeled tracers. It provides metabolic information about brain tumors by analyzing spectral patterns of several metabolites. The concentration of N-acetylaspartate (NAA) appears to be related to neuron and axon density, choline (Cho)-containing compounds seem to correlate with alteration in phospholipid membrane turnover, lipid and lactate (Lip-Lac) may be found in areas of abnormal or anaerobic metabolism or necrosis, and creatine (Cr) may be seen in regions rich in energy metabolism. The ratios of these metabolites, based on their spectral patterns, have been shown to be reliable indicators of whether tissues are composed of pure tumor or pure necrosis but less reliable when tissues are composed of varying degrees of mixed tumor and necrosis (Plotkin et al 2004; Rabinov et al 2002; Zeng et al 2007).

The gold standard for differentiating tumor recurrence from radiation necrosis in patients with irradiated gliomas remains tissue biopsy. Because gliomas are histologically heterogeneous, a main concern regarding stereotactic biopsy has been how accurately the biopsy specimens reflect the histological characteristics of the tumor as a whole. Forsyth et al (1995) reported that even when performed by different neurosurgeons at several institutions stereotactic biopsy accuracy rates ranged from 76% to 100% with a median of 95%. In their study, stereotactic biopsy results were predictive of survival outcomes (patients with recurrent tumor had the shortest survival times, all patients with pure radiation necrosis survived, and patients with a mixture of tumor and radiation necrosis had an intermediate survival time), providing indirect evidence for the accuracy of the diagnosis.

The question of attempting a gross total re-resection is also controversial (Tatter 2002). In general, re-resection is appropriate to minimize current symptomatology, to combine with a clinical trial, if the patient is in good medical and

T1 + Gadolinium   FLAIR

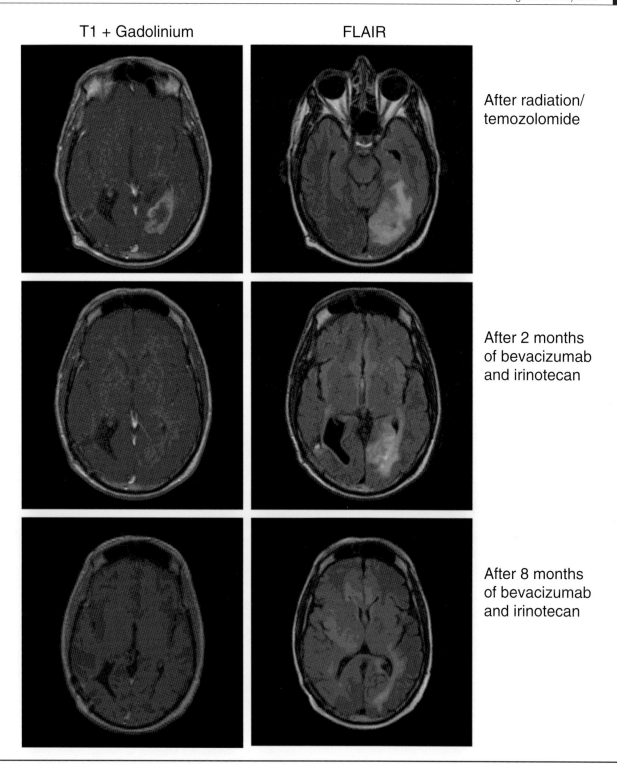

After radiation/
temozolomide

After 2 months
of bevacizumab
and irinotecan

After 8 months
of bevacizumab
and irinotecan

Figure 21.14 Bevacizumab-mediated regression of gadolinium-enhancing area of tumor. Serial MR images show regression (compare top to middle and lower panels) of gadolinium-enhancement and FLAIR abnormality in this patient with a GBM in the left occipital brain, after failure of radiation and temozolomide (top panel). The patient had previously undergone a resection of a cystic GBM in the contralateral occipital lobe. Although the left occipital FLAIR abnormality improved, increased FLAIR signal is visible throughout the hemispheres (lower panel).

neurologic condition and/or if the tumor can be removed without causing unacceptable morbidity. Re-resection can be combined with clinical trials of biologic and/or novel chemotherapy agents. There has also been a recent resurgence of boosting the resection cavity with local radiation either by stereotactic radiosurgery, brachytherapy or the use of an FDA-approved implantable balloon (GliaSite).

Other therapies

The historical perspective of therapies for malignant gliomas is replete with failures in terms of ultimate effectiveness in clinical trials and/or of approval by the FDA. General areas that have met this fate have included immunotherapies, gene therapies, brachytherapies, most chemotherapies, several signal transduction inhibitors and antibody-based cytotoxins to just name a few. Since delivery of drugs and biologics to tumors in the CNS is a major impediment, trials of route of administration have also been attempted, without much success to date. These administration routes have included blood–brain–barrier breakdown with osmotic or drug-based agents, intracavitary administration via Ommaya or other types of reservoirs, intrathecal or intraventricular administration and convection-enhanced delivery (CED). Although promising treatments almost always do not meet expectations in clinical trials, active research in circumventing the reasons that are underlying such lack of clinical efficacy can lead to advances that may ultimately provide success. In fact, there has been recent interest in immunotherapy trials that involve vaccination of patients with an EGFRvIII peptide (Sampson et al 2008) or using dendritic cells pulsed with autologous GBM lysates (Liau et al 2000; Prins et al 2008). Continued interest in CED for delivery of biologics and cytotoxins remains high (Vogelbaum 2007; Kunwar et al 2007), although a recent phase 3 trial did not receive FDA approval for the cytotoxin that was under study. Gene therapy approaches continue to be investigated both at the research and clinical trial level (Chiocca et al 2008; Fulci & Chiocca 2007; Immonen et al 2004). The use of tumor-killing viruses (oncolytic viruses) to selectively target and destroy malignant gliomas is also an active area of research (Martuza et al 1991; Aghi & Chiocca 2009; Markert et al 2009; Chiocca 2008; Chiocca et al 2003; Hardcastle et al 2007). These are only a few examples of areas where research into therapeutics may lead to the next generation of treatments for this dreadful disease.

Key points

- GBMs and AAs are the most common and aggressive primary brain tumors in adults.
- They are histologically characterized by nuclear atypia and mitoses, neovascular proliferation, and invasion. Biomolecular mechanisms relevant for each of these phenotypes are increasingly being elucidated.
- A recent hypothesis characterizes a glioma cell of origin derived from a neural stem cell or glial progenitor in the brain.
- Genetic variations appear to differentiate subsets of GBMs and AAs, with some showing improved response to chemotherapy and outcome. The best characterized of these variations with improved outcome are hypermethylation of the promoter for the MGMT gene and the more recently described mutations of the IDH genes.
- The only established risk factors for gliomas are radiation exposure and certain genetic syndromes (Li–Fraumeni, Turcot, neurofibromatosis type 1, tuberous sclerosis).
- Younger patients (<50 years old), with high Karnofsky performance status, and lower-grade histopathology (WHO grade III astrocytoma), are afforded better outcomes; nevertheless, long-term survival with malignant astrocytomas (WHO grade III and IV) remains elusive.
- Imaging by MRI with and without gadolinium is the diagnostic study of choice. Other MR modalities (functional, diffusion tractography, MRS) can help with surgical planning.
- Steroids are helpful to alleviate symptomatology from tumor edema. Anticonvulsants in the absence of seizures are not recommended, except for a short course in the immediate intraoperative and postoperative period.
- Surgical resection of the entire area of gadolinium enhancement is increasingly being shown to improve outcome, although some controversy remains due to lack of randomized trials. Surgical adjuncts (intraoperative imaging and navigation, functional evaluations, fluorescence-based imaging of tumor residual) can improve the ability for maximum resection with minimal morbidity.
- Intraoperative placement of intracavitary BCNU-loaded polymers (Gliadel) is FDA-approved and has been shown to improve survival.
- Postoperative temozolomide chemotherapy with radiation therapy has been shown to improve survival (Level one evidence).
- Novel therapies with anti-angiogenic agents (Avastin) appear to show promise in relieving edema and diminishing tumor hyperpermeability. Additional novel treatments (gene-based, cell-based, vaccines, small molecules) remain exploratory.
- Tumor recurrence almost always occurs: it is diagnostically and therapeutically dealt with in a similar fashion if the patient displays a suitable clinical status.

REFERENCES

Abe, T., Terada, K., Wakimoto, H., et al., 2003. PTEN decreases in vivo vascularization of experimental gliomas in spite of proangiogenic stimuli. Cancer Res. 63, 2300–2305.

Aghi, M., Chiocca, E.A., 2005. Contribution of bone marrow-derived cells to blood vessels in ischemic tissues and tumors. Mol. Ther. 12, 994–1005.

Aghi, M., Cohen, K.S., Klein, R.J., et al., 2006. Tumor stromal-derived factor-1 recruits vascular progenitors to mitotic neovasculature, where microenvironment influences their differentiated phenotypes. Cancer Res. 66, 9054–9064.

Aghi, M.K., Chiocca, E.A., 2009. Phase ib trial of oncolytic herpes virus G207 shows safety of multiple injections and documents viral replication. Mol. Ther. 17, 8–9.

Ahlbom, A., Green, A., Kheifets, L., et al., 2004. Epidemiology of health effects of radiofrequency exposure. Environ. Health Perspect 112, 1741–1754.

Alcantara Llaguno, S., Chen, J., Kwon, C.H., et al., 2009. Malignant astrocytomas originate from neural stem/progenitor cells in a somatic tumor suppressor mouse model. Cancer Cell 15, 45–56.

Alexander, A.L., Lee, J.E., Lazar, M., et al., 2007. Diffusion tensor imaging of the brain. Neurotherapeutics 4, 316–329.

Alvarez-Buylla, A., Kohwi, M., Nguyen, T.M., et al., 2008. The heterogeneity of adult neural stem cells and the emerging complexity of their niche. Cold Spring Harb. Symp. Quant. Biol. 73, 357–365.

Ammirati, M., Vick, N., Liao, Y.L., et al., 1987. Effect of the extent of surgical resection on survival and quality of life in patients with supratentorial glioblastomas and anaplastic astrocytomas. Neurosurgery 21, 201–206.

Armanios, M.Y., Grossman, S.A., Yang, S.C., et al., 2004. Transmission of glioblastoma multiforme following bilateral lung transplantation from an affected donor: case study and review of the literature. Neuro. Oncol. 6, 259–263.

Athanassiou, H., Synodinou, M., Maragoudakis, E., et al., 2005. Randomized phase II study of temozolomide and radiotherapy compared with radiotherapy alone in newly diagnosed glioblastoma multiforme. J. Clin. Oncol. 23, 2372–2377.

Auvinen, A., Hietanen, M., Luukkonen, R., et al., 2002. Brain tumors and salivary gland cancers among cellular telephone users. Epidemiology (Cambridge MA) 13, 356–359.

Bachoo, R.M., Maher, E.A., Ligon, K.L., et al., 2002. Epidermal growth factor receptor and Ink4a/Arf: convergent mechanisms governing terminal differentiation and transformation along the neural stem cell to astrocyte axis. Cancer Cell 1, 269–277.

Baldwin, R.T., Preston-Martin, S., 2004. Epidemiology of brain tumors in childhood – a review. Toxicol. Appl. Pharmacol. 199, 118–131.

Barker, F.G. II, Huhn, S.L., Prados, M.D., 1998. Clinical characteristics of long-term survivors of glioma. In: Berger, M.S., Wilson, C.B. (Eds.), The gliomas. WB Saunders, Philadelphia, PA, pp. 710–722.

Bellail, A.C., Hunter, S.B., Brat, D.J., et al., 2004. Microregional extracellular matrix heterogeneity in brain modulates glioma cell invasion. Int. J. Biochem. Cell Biol. 36, 1046–1069.

Bennett, M.R., 1999. Mechanisms of p53-induced apoptosis. Biochem. Pharmacol. 58, 1089–1095.

Biernat, W., Kleihues, P., Yonekawa, Y., et al., 1997. Amplification and overexpression of MDM2 in primary (de novo) glioblastomas. J. Neuropathol. Exp. Neurol. 56, 180–185.

Blettner, M., Schlehofer, B., Samkange-Zeeb, F., et al., 2007. Medical exposure to ionising radiation and the risk of brain tumours: Interphone Study Group, Germany. Eur. J. Cancer 43, 1990–1998.

Bondy, M., Wiencke, J., Wrensch, M., et al., 1994. Genetics of primary brain tumors: a review. J. Neurooncol. 18, 69–81.

Brem, H., Piantadosi, S., Burger, P.C., et al., 1995. Placebo-controlled trial of safety and efficacy of intraoperative controlled delivery by biodegradable polymers of chemotherapy for recurrent gliomas. The Polymer-brain Tumor Treatment Group. Lancet 345, 1008–1012.

Brunberg, J.A., Chenevert, T.L., McKeever, P.E., et al., 1995. In vivo MR determination of water diffusion coefficients and diffusion anisotropy: correlation with structural alteration in gliomas of the cerebral hemispheres. Am. J. Neuroradiol. 16, 361–371.

Buatti, J., Ryken, T.C., Smith, M.C., et al., 2008. Radiation therapy of pathologically confirmed newly diagnosed glioblastoma in adults. J. Neurooncol. 89, 313–337.

Buckner, J.C., 2003. Factors influencing survival in high-grade gliomas. Semin. Oncol. 30, 10–14.

Bunin, G.R., Kuijten, R.R., Buckley, J.D., et al., 1993. Relation between maternal diet and subsequent primitive neuroectodermal brain tumors in young children. N. Engl. J. Med. 329, 536–541.

Cairncross, J.G., Ueki, K., Zlatescu, M.C., et al., 1998. Specific genetic predictors of chemotherapeutic response and survival in patients with anaplastic oligodendrogliomas. J. Natl. Cancer Inst. 90, 1473–1479.

Canoll, P., Goldman, J.E., 2008. The interface between glial progenitors and gliomas. Acta. Neuropathol. 116, 465–477.

Caresia, A.P., Castell-Conesa, J., Negre, M., et al., 2006. Thallium-201SPECT assessment in the detection of recurrences of treated gliomas and ependymomas. Clin. Transl. Oncol. 8, 750–754.

Cazenave, C., Reid, S., Virapongse, C., et al., 1986. Reactive gliosis simulating butterfly glioma: a neuroradiological case study. Neurosurgery 19, 816–819.

CBTRUS, 2008. Statistical report: primary brain tumors in the United States, 2000–2004. Central Brain Tumor Registry of the United States, Hinsdale, IL.

Chakravarti, A., Dicker, A., Mehta, M., 2004. The contribution of epidermal growth factor receptor (EGFR) signaling pathway to radioresistance in human gliomas: a review of preclinical and correlative clinical data. Int. J. Radiat. Oncol. Biol. Phys. 58, 927–931.

Chang, J., Thakur, S.B., Huang, W., et al., 2008. Magnetic resonance spectroscopy imaging (MRSI) and brain functional magnetic resonance imaging (fMRI) for radiotherapy treatment planning of glioma. Technol. Cancer Res. Treat. 7, 349–362.

Chang, S.M., Barker, F.G. 2nd, 2005. Marital status, treatment, and survival in patients with glioblastoma multiforme: a population based study. Cancer 104, 1975–1984.

Chang, S.M., Parney, I.F., Huang, W., et al., 2005. Patterns of care for adults with newly diagnosed malignant glioma. JAMA 293, 557–564.

Chen, H., Shah, A.S., Girgis, R.E., et al., 2008. Transmission of glioblastoma multiforme after bilateral lung transplantation. J. Clin. Oncol. 26, 3284–3285.

Chen, H., Ward, M.H., Tucker, K.L., et al., 2002. Diet and risk of adult glioma in eastern Nebraska, United States. Cancer Causes Control 13, 647–655.

Chi, A., Norden, A.D., Wen, P.Y., 2007. Inhibition of angiogenesis and invasion in malignant gliomas. Expert Rev. Anticancer Ther. 7, 1537–1560.

Chiocca, E.A., Aghi, M., Fulci, G., 2003. Viral therapy for glioblastoma. Cancer J. 9, 167–179.

Chiocca, E.A., Smith, K.M., McKinney, B., et al., 2008. A phase I trial of Ad.hIFN-beta gene therapy for glioma. Mol. Ther. 16, 618–626.

Chiocca, E.A., 2008. The host response to cancer virotherapy. Curr. Opin. Mol. Ther. 10, 38–45.

Christensen, H.C., Schüz, J., Kosteljanetz, M., et al., 2005. Cellular telephones and risk for brain tumors: a population-based, incident case-control study. Neurology 64, 1189–1195.

Ciric, I., Ammirati, M., Vick, N., et al., 1987. Supratentorial gliomas: surgical considerations and immediate postoperative results. Gross total resection versus partial resection. Neurosurgery 21, 21–26.

Cobbs, C.S., Harkins, L., Samanta, M., et al., 2002. Human cytomegalovirus infection and expression in human malignant glioma. Cancer Res. 62, 3347–3350.

Curran, W.J. Jr., Scott, C.B., Horton, J., et al., 1993. Recursive partitioning analysis of prognostic factors in three Radiation Therapy Oncology Group malignant glioma trials. J. Natl. Cancer Inst. 85, 704–710.

DeLaney, T.F., 2007. Clinical proton radiation therapy research at the Francis H. Burr Proton Therapy Center. Technol. Cancer Res. Treat. 6, 61–66.

Dell'Albani, P., 2008. Stem cell markers in gliomas. Neurochem. Res. 33, 2407–2415.

Demuth, T., Rennert, J.L., Hoelzinger, D.B., et al., 2008. Glioma cells on the run – the migratory transcriptome of 10 human glioma cell lines. BMC Genomics 9, 54.

Derlon, J.M., Bourdet, C., Bustany, P., et al., 1989. [11C]L-methionine uptake in gliomas. Neurosurgery 25, 720–728.

Di Costanzo, A., Scarabino, T., Trojsi, F., et al., 2008. Proton M R spectroscopy of cerebral gliomas at 3 T: spatial heterogeneity, and tumour grade and extent. Eur. Radiol. 18, 1727–1735.

Doetsch, F., Petreanu, L., Caille, I., et al., 2002. EGF converts transit-amplifying neurogenic precursors in the adult brain into multipotent stem cells. Neuron 36, 1021–1034.

Donahue, B., Scott, C.B., Nelson, J.S., et al., 1997. Influence of an oligodendroglial component on the survival of patients with anaplastic astrocytomas: a report of Radiation Therapy Oncology Group 83–02. Int. J. Radiat. Oncol. Biol. Phys. 38, 911–914.

Earnest, F. 4th, Kelly, P.J., Scheithauer, B.W., et al., 1988. Cerebral astrocytomas: histopathologic correlation of MR and CT contrast enhancement with stereotactic biopsy. Radiology 166, 823–827.

Ekstrand, A.J., Longo, N., Hamid, M.L., et al., 1994. Functional characterization of an EGF receptor with a truncated extracellular domain expressed in glioblastomas with EGFR gene amplification. Oncogene 9, 2313–2320.

Ekstrand, A.J., Sugawa, N., James, C.D., et al., 1992. Amplified and rearranged epidermal growth factor receptor genes in human glioblastomas reveal deletions of sequences encoding portions of the N- and/or C-terminal tails. Proc. Natl. Acad. Sci. USA 89, 4309–4313.

Fan, G., Sun, B., Wu, Z., et al., 2004. In vivo single-voxel proton M R spectroscopy in the differentiation of high-grade gliomas and solitary metastases. Clin. Radiol. 59, 77–85.

Feychting, M., Anders, A., 2010. Radiofrequency fields and glioma. In: Mehta, M., Chang, S., Newton, H., et al., (Eds.), Principles and practices of neuro-oncology: A multidisciplinary approach. Demos Medical, New York.

Forsyth, P.A., Kelly, P.J., Cascino, T.L., et al., 1995. Radiation necrosis or glioma recurrence: is computer-assisted stereotactic biopsy useful? J. Neurosurg. 82, 436–444.

Fulci, G., Chiocca, E.A., 2007. The status of gene therapy for brain tumors. Expert Opin. Biol. Ther. 7, 197–208.

Fulci, G., Ishii, N., Maurici, D., et al., 2002. Initiation of human astrocytoma by clonal evolution of cells with progressive loss of p53 functions in a patient with a 283H TP53 germ-line mutation: evidence for a precursor lesion. Cancer Res. 62, 2897–2905.

Fuller, G.N., Scheithauer, B.W., 2007. The 2007 Revised World Health Organization (WHO) Classification of Tumours of the Central Nervous System: newly codified entities. Brain Pathol. 17, 304–307.

Gabayan, A.J., Green, S.B., Sanan, A., et al., 2006. GliaSite brachytherapy for treatment of recurrent malignant gliomas: a retrospective multi-institutional analysis. Neurosurgery 58, 701–709.

Galli, R., Binda, E., Orfanelli, U., et al., 2004. Isolation and characterization of tumorigenic, stem-like neural precursors from human glioblastoma. Cancer Res. 64, 7011–7021.

Garside, R., Pitt, M., Anderson, R., et al., 2007. The effectiveness and cost-effectiveness of carmustine implants and temozolomide for the treatment of newly diagnosed high-grade glioma: a systematic review and economic evaluation. Health Technol. Assess 11, iii–iv, ix–221.

Glantz, M.J., Cole, B.F., Forsyth, P.A., et al., 2000. Practice parameter: anticonvulsant prophylaxis in patients with newly diagnosed brain tumors. Report of the Quality Standards Subcommittee of the American Academy of Neurology. Neurology 54, 1886–1893.

Godlewski, J., Nowicki, M.O., Bronisz, A., et al., 2008. Targeting of the Bmi-1 oncogene/stem cell renewal factor by microRNA-128 inhibits glioma proliferation and self-renewal. Cancer Res. 68, 9125–9130.

Gupta, D.K., Chandra, P.S., Ojha, B.K., et al., 2007. Awake craniotomy versus surgery under general anesthesia for resection of intrinsic lesions of eloquent cortex – a prospective randomised study. Clin. Neurol. Neurosurg. 109, 335–343.

Hambardzumyan, D., Squatrito, M., Carbajal, E., et al., 2008. Glioma formation, cancer stem cells, and Akt signaling. Stem Cell Rev. 4, 203–210.

Hardcastle, J., Kurozumi, K., Chiocca, E.A., et al., 2007. Oncolytic viruses driven by tumor-specific promoters. Curr. Cancer Drug Targets 7, 181–189.

Hardell, L., Carlberg, M., Mild, K.H., 2005. Case-control study on cellular and cordless telephones and the risk for acoustic neuroma or meningioma in patients diagnosed 2000–2003. NeuroEpidemiology 25, 120–128.

Hardell, L., Mild, K.H., Carlberg, M., 2002. Case-control study on the use of cellular and cordless phones and the risk for malignant brain tumours. Int. J. Radiat. Biol. 78, 931–936.

Hardell, L., Nasman, A., Pahlson, A., et al., 1999. Use of cellular telephones and the risk for brain tumours: A case-control study. Int. J. Oncol. 15, 113–116.

Hart, M.G., Grant, R., Garside, R., et al., 2008a. Chemotherapeutic wafers for high grade glioma. Cochrane Database Syst. Rev. (3), CD007294.

Hart, M.G., Grant, R., Garside, R., et al., 2008b. Temozolomide for high grade glioma. Cochrane Database Syst. Rev. (4), CD007415.

He, J., Mokhtari, K., Sanson, M., et al., 2001. Glioblastomas with an oligodendroglial component: a pathological and molecular study. J. Neuropathol. Exp. Neurol. 60, 863–871.

Hegi, M.E., Diserens, A.C., Gorlia, T., et al., 2005. MGMT gene silencing and benefit from temozolomide in glioblastoma. N. Engl. J. Med. 352, 997–1003.

Hepworth, S.J., Schoemaker, M.J., Muir, K.R., et al., 2006. Mobile phone use and risk of glioma in adults: case-control study. BMJ 332, 883–887.

Hermanson, M., Funa, K., Hartman, M., et al., 1992. Platelet-derived growth factor and its receptors in human glioma tissue: expression of messenger R N A and protein suggests the presence of autocrine and paracrine loops. Cancer Res. 52, 3213–3219.

Hermanson, M., Funa, K., Koopmann, J., et al., 1996. Association of loss of heterozygosity on chromosome 17p with high platelet-derived growth factor alpha receptor expression in human malignant gliomas. Cancer Res. 56, 164–171.

Hirai, T., Murakami, R., Nakamura, H., et al., 2008. Prognostic value of perfusion M R imaging of high-grade astrocytomas: long-term follow-up study. Am. J. Neuroradiol. 29, 1505–1510.

Hirschberg, H., Samset, E., Hol, P.K., et al., 2005. Impact of intraoperative M R I on the surgical results for high-grade gliomas. Min. Invasive Neurosurg. 48, 77–84.

Hirschl, R.A., Wilson, J., Miller, B., et al., 2009. The predictive value of low-field strength magnetic resonance imaging for intraoperative residual tumor detection. J. Neurosurg. 111 (2), 252–257.

Hochberg, F., Toniolo, P., Cole, P., 1984. Head trauma and seizures as risk factors of glioblastoma. Neurology 34, 1511–1514.

Hoelzinger, D.B., Demuth, T., Berens, M.E., 2007. Autocrine factors that sustain glioma invasion and paracrine biology in the brain microenvironment. J. Natl. Cancer Inst. 99, 1583–1593.

Hu, J., Johnson, K.C., Mao, Y., et al., 1998. Risk factors for glioma in adults: a case-control study in northeast China. Cancer Detect Prev. 22, 100–108.

Hu, J., La Vecchia, C., Negri, E., et al., 1999a. Diet and brain cancer in adults: a case-control study in northeast China. Int. J. Cancer 81, 20–23.

Hu, J., Little, J., Xu, T., et al., 1999b. Risk factors for meningioma in adults: a case-control study in northeast China. Int. J. Cancer Journal 83, 299–304.

Hur, H., Jung, S., Jung, T.Y., et al., 2008. Cerebellar glioblastoma multiforme in an adult. J. Korean Neurosurg. Soc. 43, 194–197.

Immonen, A., Vapalahti, M., Tyynelä, K., et al., 2004. AdvHSV-tk gene therapy with intravenous ganciclovir improves survival in human malignant glioma: a randomised, controlled study. Mol. Ther. 10, 967–972.

Ingber, D.E., 2003a. Mechanobiology and diseases of mechanotransduction. Ann. Med. 35, 564–577.

Ingber, D.E., 2003b. Tensegrity I. Cell structure and hierarchical systems biology. J. Cell Sci. 116, 1157–1173.

Ingber, D.E., 2003c. Tensegrity II. How structural networks influence cellular information processing networks. J. Cell Sci. 116, 1397–1408.

Inoue, R., Moghaddam, K.A., Ranasinghe, M., et al., 2004. Infectious delivery of the 132 kb CDKN2A/CDKN2B genomic DNA region results in correctly spliced gene expression and growth suppression in glioma cells. Gene. Ther. 11, 1195–1204.

Inskip, P.D., Mellemkjaer, L., Gridley, G., et al., 1998. Incidence of intracranial tumors following hospitalization for head injuries (Denmark). Cancer Causes Control 9, 109–116.

Inskip, P.D., Tarone, R.E., Hatch, E.E., et al., 2001. Cellular-telephone use and brain tumors. N. Engl. J. Med. 344, 79–86.

Jeremic, B., Milicic, B., Grujicic, D., et al., 2003. Multivariate analysis of clinical prognostic factors in patients with glioblastoma multiforme treated with a combined modality approach. J. Cancer Res. Clin. Oncol. 129, 477–484.

Johansen, C., Boice, J.J., McLaughlin, J., et al., 2001. Cellular telephones and cancer – a nationwide cohort study in Denmark J. National Cancer Institute 93, 203–207.

Juven, Y., Sadetzki, S., 2002. A possible association between ionizing radiation and pituitary adenoma: a descriptive study. Cancer 95, 397–403.

Kaur, B., Brat, D.J., Calkins, C.C., et al., 2003. Brain angiogenesis inhibitor 1 is differentially expressed in normal brain and glioblastoma independently of p53 expression. Am. J. Pathol. 162, 19–27.

Kaye, A.H., Laws, E.R., 1995. Brain tumors: an encyclopedic approach. Churchill Livingstone, Edinburgh, pp. 191–214.

Kefas, B., Godlewski, J., Comeau, L., et al., 2008. microRNA-7 inhibits the epidermal growth factor receptor and the Akt pathway and is down-regulated in glioblastoma. Cancer Res. 68, 3566–3572.

Kernohan, J.W., Mabon, R.F., Svien, H.J., et al., 1949. A simplified classification of the gliomas. Mayo. Clin. Proc. 24, 71–75.

Kirsch, D.G., Tarbell, N.J., 2004. New technologies in radiation therapy for pediatric brain tumors: the rationale for proton radiation therapy. Pediatr. Blood Cancer 42, 461–464.

Kleihues, P., Cavenee, W.K., International Agency for Research on Cancer, 2000. Pathology and genetics of tumours of the nervous system. IARC Press, Lyon.

Kondziolka, D., Bernstein, M., Resch, L., et al., 1987. Significance of hemorrhage into brain tumors: clinicopathological study. J. Neurosurg. 67, 852–857.

Kondziolka, D., 2007. Stereotactic neurosurgery: what's turning people on? Clin. Neurosurg. 54, 23–25.

Korvenoja, A., Kirveskari, E., Aronen, H.J., et al., 2006. Sensorimotor cortex localization: comparison of magnetoencephalography, functional M R imaging, and intraoperative cortical mapping. Radiology 241, 213–222.

Kraus, J.A., Lamszus, K., Glesmann, N., et al., 2001. Molecular genetic alterations in glioblastomas with oligodendroglial component. Acta. Neuropathol. 101, 311–320.

Kunwar, S., Prados, M.D., Chang, S.M., et al., 2007. Direct intracerebral delivery of cintredekin besudotox (IL13-PE38QQR) in recurrent malignant glioma: a report by the Cintredekin Besudotox Intraparenchymal Study Group. J. Clin. Oncol. 25, 837–844.

Kwon, C.H., Zhao, D., Chen, J., et al., 2008. Pten haploinsufficiency accelerates formation of high-grade astrocytomas. Cancer Res. 68, 3286–3294.

Lacroix, M., Abi-Said, D., Fourney, D.R., et al., 2001. A multivariate analysis of 416 patients with glioblastoma multiforme: prognosis, extent of resection, and survival. J. Neurosurg. 95, 190–198.

Lahkola, A., Auvinen, A., Raitanen, J., et al., 2007. Mobile phone use and risk of glioma in 5 North European countries. Int. J. Cancer 120, 1769–1775.

Laperriere, N., Zuraw, L., Cairncross, G., 2002. Radiotherapy for newly diagnosed malignant glioma in adults: a systematic review. Radiother. Oncol. 64, 259–273.

Law, M., Cha, S., Knopp, E.A., et al., 2002. High-grade gliomas and solitary metastases: differentiation by using perfusion and proton spectroscopic MR imaging. Radiology 222, 715–721.

Laws, E.R., Parney, I.F., Huang, W., et al., 2003. Survival following surgery and prognostic factors for recently diagnosed malignant glioma: data from the Glioma Outcomes Project. J. Neurosurg. 99, 467–473.

Lee, M., Wrensch, M., Miike, R., 1997. Dietary and tobacco risk factors for adult onset glioma in the San Francisco Bay Area (California, USA). Cancer Causes Control 8, 13–24.

Li, F.P., Fraumeni J.F. Jr., Mulvihill, J.J., et al., 1988. A cancer family syndrome in twenty-four kindreds. Cancer Res. 48, 5358–5362.

Liau, L.M., Black, K.L., Martin, N.A., et al., 2000. Treatment of a patient by vaccination with autologous dendritic cells pulsed with allogeneic major histocompatibility complex class I-matched tumor peptides. Case Report. Neurosurg. Focus. 9, e8.

Lonn, S., Ahlbom, A., Hall, P., et al., 2005. Long-term mobile phone use and brain tumor risk. Am. J. Epidemiol. 161, 526–535.

Louis, D.N., Ohgaki, H., Wiestler, O.D., et al., 2007. The 2007 WHO classification of tumours of the central nervous system. Acta Neuropathol. 114, 97–109.

Louis, D.N., 2006. Molecular pathology of malignant gliomas. Annu. Rev. Pathol. 1, 97–117.

Lutterbach, J., Sauerbrei, W., Guttenberger, R., 2003. Multivariate analysis of prognostic factors in patients with glioblastoma. Strahlentherapie und. Onkologie: Organ der. Deutschen. Rontgengesellschaft 179, 8–15.

Markert, J.M., Liechty, P.G., Wang, W., et al., 2009. Phase Ib trial of mutant herpes simplex virus G207 inoculated pre-and post-tumor resection for recurrent GBM. Mol. Ther. 17, 199–207.

Martuza, R.L., Malick, A., Markert, J.M., et al., 1991. Experimental therapy of human glioma by means of a genetically engineered virus mutant. Science 252, 854–856.

McGirt, M.J., Chaichana, K.L., Gathinji, M., et al., 2009. Independent association of extent of resection with survival in patients with malignant brain astrocytoma. J. Neurosurg. 110, 156–162.

McKusick, V., (Ed.), 2008. Online Mendelian Inheritance in Man, OMIM (TM). McKusick-Nathans Institute of Genetic Medicine, Johns Hopkins University, and National Center for Biotechnology Information. National Library of Medicine Bethesda, MD.

McLendon, R., Friedman, A., Bigner, D., et al., Cancer Genome Atlas Research Network 2008. Comprehensive genomic characterization defines human glioblastoma genes and core pathways. Nature 455 (7216), 1061–1068.

Mellinghoff, I.K., Wang, M.Y., Vivanco, I., et al., 2005. Molecular determinants of the response of glioblastomas to EGFR kinase inhibitors. N. Engl. J. Med. 353, 2012–2024.

Meyer, F.B., Bates, L.M., Goerss, S.J., et al., 2001. Awake craniotomy for aggressive resection of primary gliomas located in eloquent brain. Mayo. Clin. Proc. 76, 677–687.

Miller, G., 2009. Brain cancer. A viral link to glioblastoma? Science 323, 30–31.

Mukundan, S., Holder, C., Olson, J.J., 2008. Neuroradiological assessment of newly diagnosed glioblastoma. J. Neurooncol. 89, 259–269.

Muscat, J.E., Malkin, M.G., Thompson, S., et al., 2000. Handheld cellular telephone use and risk of brain cancer. JAMA 284, 3001–3007.

Mäkelä, J.P., Forss, N., Jääskeläinen, J., et al., 2007. Magnetoencephalography in neurosurgery. Neurosurgery 61, 147–165.

Nakada, M., Nakada, S., Demuth, T., et al., 2007. Molecular targets of glioma invasion. Cell Mol. Life Sci. 64, 458–478.

Narayana, A., Golfinos, J.G., Fischer, I., et al., 2008. Feasibility of using bevacizumab with radiation therapy and temozolomide in newly diagnosed high-grade glioma. Int. J. Radiat. Oncol. Biol. Phys. 72, 383–389.

Narayana, A., Kelly, P., Golfinos, J., et al., 2009. Antiangiogenic therapy using bevacizumab in recurrent high-grade glioma: impact on local control and patient survival. J. Neurosurg. 110, 173–180.

Narod, S.A., Parry, D.M., Parboosingh, J., et al., 1992. Neurofibromatosis type 2 appears to be a genetically homogeneous disease. Am. J. Hum. Genet. 51, 486–496.

Nowicki, M.O., Dmitrieva, N., Stein, A.M., et al., 2008. Lithium inhibits invasion of glioma cells; possible involvement of glycogen synthase kinase-3. Neuro. Oncol. 10, 690–699.

Nutt, C.L., Mani, D.R., Betensky, R.A., et al., 2003. Gene expression-based classification of malignant gliomas correlates better with survival than histological classification. Cancer Res. 63, 1602–1607.

Ogawa, T., Shishido, F., Kanno, I., et al., 1993. Cerebral glioma: evaluation with methionine PET. Radiology 186, 45–53.

Ogden, A.T., Waziri, A.E., Lochhead, R.A., et al., 2008. Identification of A2B5+CD133- tumor-initiating cells in adult human gliomas. Neurosurgery 62, 505–515.

Ohgaki, H., Kleihues, P., 2005. Population-based studies on incidence, survival rates, and genetic alterations in astrocytic and oligodendroglial gliomas. J. Neuropathol. Exp. Neurol. 64, 479–489.

Ohgaki, H., Kleihues, P., 2007. Genetic pathways to primary and secondary glioblastoma. Am. J. Pathol. 170, 1445–1453.

Okamoto, K., Furusawa, T., Ishikawa, K., et al., 2004a. Mimics of brain tumor on neuroimaging: part I. Radiat. Med. 22, 63–76.

Okamoto, K., Furusawa, T., Ishikawa, K., et al., 2004b. Mimics of brain tumor on neuroimaging: part II. Radiat. Med. 22, 135–142.

Paraf, F., Jothy, S., Van Meir, E.G., 1997. Brain tumor-polyposis syndrome: two genetic diseases? J. Clin. Oncol. 15, 2744–2758.

Parsons, D.W., Jones, S., Zhang, X., et al., 2008. An integrated genomic analysis of human glioblastoma multiforme. Science 321, 1807–1812.

Pelloski, C.E., Ballman, K.V., Furth, A.F., et al., 2007. Epidermal growth factor receptor variant III status defines clinically distinct subtypes of glioblastoma. J. Clin. Oncol. 25, 2288–2294.

Perry, A., Aldape, K.D., George, D.H., et al., 2004. Small cell astrocytoma: an aggressive variant that is clinicopathologically and genetically distinct from anaplastic oligodendroglioma. Cancer 101, 2318–2326.

Phillips, H.S., Kharbanda, S., Chen, R., et al., 2006. Molecular subclasses of high-grade glioma predict prognosis, delineate a pattern of disease progression, and resemble stages in neurogenesis. Cancer Cell 9, 157–173.

Plotkin, M., Eisenacher, J., Bruhn, H., et al., 2004. 123I-IMT SPECT and 1H MR-spectroscopy at 3.0 T in the differential diagnosis of recurrent or residual gliomas: a comparative study. J. Neurooncol. 70, 49–58.

Preston-Martin, S., Henderson, B.E., 1984. N-nitroso compounds and human intracranial tumours. IARC Scientific Publ. 57, 887–894.

Preston-Martin, S., Pogoda, J.M., Schlehofer, B., et al., 1998. An international case-control study of adult glioma and meningioma: the role of head trauma. Int. J. Epidemiol. 27, 579–586.

Preston-Martin, S., 1996. Epidemiology of primary CNS neoplasms. Neurologic Clin. 14, 273–290.

Prins, R.M., Cloughesy, T.F., Liau, L.M., 2008. Cytomegalovirus immunity after vaccination with autologous glioblastoma lysate. N. Engl. J. Med. 359, 539–541.

Proescholdt, M.A., Macher, C., Woertgen, C., et al., 2005. Level of evidence in the literature concerning brain tumor resection. Clin. Neurol. Neurosurg. 107, 95–98.

Rabinov, J.D., Lee, P.L., Barker, F.G., et al., 2002. In vivo 3-T MR spectroscopy in the distinction of recurrent glioma versus radiation effects: initial experience. Radiology 225, 871–879.

Rampling, R., James, A., Papanastassiou, V., 2004. The present and future management of malignant brain tumours: surgery, radiotherapy, chemotherapy. J. Neurol. Neurosurg. Psychiatry 75 (Suppl 2), ii24–ii30.

Roa, W., Brasher, P.M., Bauman, G., et al., 2004. Abbreviated course of radiation therapy in older patients with glioblastoma multiforme: a prospective randomized clinical trial. J. Clin. Oncol. 22, 1583–1588.

Sabel, M., Giese, A., 2008. Safety profile of carmustine wafers in malignant glioma: a review of controlled trials and a decade of clinical experience. Curr. Med. Res. Opin. Online.

Sampson, J.H., Archer, G.E., Mitchell, D.A., et al., 2008. Tumor-specific immunotherapy targeting the EGFRvIII mutation in patients with malignant glioma. Semin. Immunol. 20, 267–275.

Sanai, N., Alvarez-Buylla, A., Berger, M.S., 2005. Neural stem cells and the origin of gliomas. N. Engl. J. Med. 353, 811–822.

Sanai, N., Berger, M.S., 2008a. Glioma extent of resection and its impact on patient outcome. Neurosurgery 62, 753–766.

Sanai, N., Berger, M.S., 2008b. Mapping the horizon: techniques to optimize tumor resection before and during surgery. Clin. Neurosurg. 55, 14–19.

Sarkar, A., Caamano, S., Fernandez, J.M., 2005. The elasticity of individual titin P E V K exons measured by single molecule atomic force microscopy. J. Biol. Chem. 280, 6261–6264.

Sarkar, A., Caamano, S., Fernandez, J.M., 2007. The mechanical fingerprint of a parallel polyprotein dimer. Biophys. J. 92, L36–L38.

Sarkar, A., Robertson, R.B., Fernandez, J.M., 2004. Simultaneous atomic force microscope and fluorescence measurements of protein unfolding using a calibrated evanescent wave. Proc. Natl. Acad. Sci. USA 101, 12882–12886.

Schneider, J.P., Trantakis, C., Rubach, M., et al., 2005. Intraoperative M R I to guide the resection of primary supratentorial glioblastoma multiforme – a quantitative radiological analysis. Neuroradiology 47, 489–500.

Schwartzbaum, J.A., Fisher, J.L., Aldape, K.D., et al., 2006. Epidemiology and molecular pathology of glioma. Nat. Clin. Pract. Neurol. 2, 494–503.

Schwartzbaum, J.A., Fisher, J.L., Goodman, J., et al., 1999a. Hypotheses concerning roles of dietary energy, cured meat, and serum tocopherols in adult glioma development. NeuroEpidemiology 18, 156–166.

Schwartzbaum, J.A., Lal, P., Evanoff, W., et al., 1999b. Presurgical serum albumin levels predict survival time from glioblastoma multiforme. J. Neurooncol. 43, 35–41.

Schüz, J., Böhler, E., Berg, G., et al., 2006. Cellular phones, cordless phones, and the risks of glioma and meningioma (Interphone Study Group, Germany). Am. J. Epidemiol. 163, 512–520.

Scozzafava, J., Johnson, E.S., Blevins, G., 2008. Neurological picture. Demyelinating butterfly pseudo-glioma. J. Neurol. Neurosurg. Psychiatry 79, 12–13.

Shaw, E.G., Scheithauer, B.W., O'Fallon, J.R., et al., 1992. Oligodendrogliomas: the Mayo Clinic experience. J. Neurosurg. 76, 428–434.

Shaw, E.G., Scheithauer, B.W., O'Fallon, J.R., et al., 1994. Mixed oligoastrocytomas: a survival and prognostic factor analysis. Neurosurgery 34, 577–582.

Shintani, T., Hayakawa, N., Hoshi, M., et al., 1999. High incidence of meningioma among Hiroshima atomic bomb survivors. J. Radiat. Res. 40, 49–57.

Singh, S.K., Clarke, I.D., Terasaki, M., et al., 2003. Identification of a cancer stem cell in human brain tumors. Cancer Res. 63, 5821–5828.

Singh, S.K., Hawkins, C., Clarke, I.D., et al., 2004. Identification of human brain tumour initiating cells. Nature 432, 396–401.

Sinha, S., Bastin, M.E., Whittle, I.R., et al., 2002. Diffusion tensor M R imaging of high-grade cerebral gliomas. Am. J. Neuroradiol. 23, 520–527.

Stepp, H., Beck, T., Pongratz, T., et al., 2007. ALA and malignant glioma: fluorescence-guided resection and photodynamic treatment. J. Environ. Pathol. Toxicol. Oncol. 26, 157–164.

Strickler, H.D., Rosenberg, P.S., Devesa, S.S., et al., 1998. Contamination of poliovirus vaccines with simian virus 40 (1955–1963) and subsequent cancer rates. JAMA 279, 292–295.

Stummer, W., Reulen, H.J., Novotny, A., et al., 2003. Fluorescence-guided resections of malignant gliomas – an overview. Acta. Neurochir. Suppl. 88, 9–12.

Stupp, R., Mason, W.P., van den Bent, M.J., et al., 2005. Radiotherapy plus concomitant and adjuvant temozolomide for glioblastoma. N. Engl. J. Med. 352, 987–996.

Taphoorn, M.J., Stupp, R., Coens, C., et al., 2005. Health-related quality of life in patients with glioblastoma: a randomised controlled trial. Lancet Oncol. 6, 937–944.

Tatter, S.B., 2002. Recurrent malignant glioma in adults. Curr. Treat. Options Oncol. 3, 509–524.

Taylor, M.D., Bernstein, M., 1999. Awake craniotomy with brain mapping as the routine surgical approach to treating patients with supratentorial intraaxial tumors: a prospective trial of 200 cases. J. Neurosurg. 90, 35–41.

Tedeschi-Blok, N., Schwartzbaum, J., Lee, M., et al., 2001. Dietary calcium consumption and astrocytic glioma: the San Francisco Bay Area Adult Glioma Study, 1991–1995. Nutr. Cancer 39, 196–203.

Thiagalingam, S., Flaherty, M., Billson, F., et al., 2004. Neurofibromatosis type 1 and optic pathway gliomas: follow-up of 54 patients. Ophthalmology 111, 568–577.

Thoman, W.J., Ammirati, M., Caragine, L.P. Jr., et al., 2006. Brain tumor imaging and surgical management: the neurosurgeon's perspective. Top. Magn. Reson. Imaging 17, 121–126.

Thompson, T.P., Lunsford, L.D., Kondziolka, D., 1999. Distinguishing recurrent tumor and radiation necrosis with positron emission tomography versus stereotactic biopsy. Stereotact. Funct. Neurosurg. 73, 9–14.

Toh, C.H., Castillo, M., Wong, A.M., et al., 2008. Primary cerebral lymphoma and glioblastoma multiforme: differences in diffusion characteristics evaluated with diffusion tensor imaging. Am. J. Neuroradiol. 29, 471–475.

Tonn, J.C., 2007. Awake craniotomy for monitoring of language function: benefits and limits. Acta. Neurochir. (Wien.) 149, 1197–1198.

Tovi, M., Hartman, M., Lilja, A., et al., 1994. MR imaging in cerebral gliomas. Tissue component analysis in correlation with histopathology of whole-brain specimens. Acta. Radiol. 35, 495–505.

Tovi, M., Lilja, A., Bergström, M., et al., 1990. Delineation of gliomas with magnetic resonance imaging using Gd-DTPA in comparison with computed tomography and positron emission tomography. Acta. Radiol. 31, 417–429.

Tovi, M., 1993. MR imaging in cerebral gliomas analysis of tumour tissue components. Acta. Radiol. Suppl. 384, 1–24.

Tropine, A., Vucurevic, G., Delani, P., et al., 2004. Contribution of diffusion tensor imaging to delineation of gliomas and glioblastomas. J. Magn. Reson. Imaging 20, 905–912.

Turcot, J., Despres, J.P., St Pierre, F., 1959. Malignant tumors of the central nervous system associated with familial polyposis of the colon: report of two cases. Dis. Colon. Rectum. 2, 465–468.

Uhrbom, L., Dai, C., Celestino, J.C., et al., 2002. Ink4a-Arf loss cooperates with KRas activation in astrocytes and neural progenitors to generate glioblastomas of various morphologies depending on activated Akt. Cancer Res. 62, 5551–5558.

Uhrbom, L., Nerio, E., Holland, E.C., 2004. Dissecting tumor maintenance requirements using bioluminescence imaging of cell proliferation in a mouse glioma model. Nat. Med. 10, 1257–1260.

Upadhyaya, M., Osborn, M.J., Maynard, J., et al., 1997. Mutational and functional analysis of the neurofibromatosis type 1 (NF1) gene. Hum. Genet 99, 88–92.

Valtonen, S., Timonen, U., Toivanen, P., et al., 1997. Interstitial chemotherapy with carmustine-loaded polymers for high-grade gliomas: a randomized double-blind study. Neurosurg. 41, 44–49.

Vescovi, A.L., Galli, R., Reynolds, B.A., 2006. Brain tumour stem cells. Nat. Rev. Cancer 6, 425–436.

Viapiano, M.S., Bi, W.L., Piepmeier, J., et al., 2005. Novel tumor-specific isoforms of BEHAB/brevican identified in human malignant gliomas. Cancer Res. 65, 6726–6733.

Viapiano, M.S., Matthews, R.T., 2006. From barriers to bridges: chondroitin sulfate proteoglycans in neuropathology. Trends Mol. Med. 12, 488–496.

Vogelbaum, M.A., 2007. Convection enhanced delivery for treating brain tumors and selected neurological disorders: symposium review. J. Neurooncol. 83, 97–109.

Vordermark, D., Ruprecht, K., Rieckmann, P., et al., 2006. Glioblastoma multiforme with oligodendroglial component (GBMO): favorable outcome after post-operative radiotherapy and chemotherapy with nimustine (ACNU) and teniposide (VM26). BMC Cancer 6, 247.

Vos, M.J., Hoekstra, O.S., Barkhof, F., et al., 2003. Thallium-201 single-photon emission computed tomography as an early predictor of outcome in recurrent glioma. J. Clin. Oncol. 21, 3559–3565.

Vredenburgh, J.J., Desjardins, A., Herndon, J.E., 2nd, et al., 2007. Phase II trial of bevacizumab and irinotecan in recurrent malignant glioma. Clin. Cancer Res. 13, 1253–1259.

Watanabe, K., Sato, K., Biernat, W., et al., 1997. Incidence and timing of p53 mutations during astrocytoma progression in patients with multiple biopsies. Clin. Cancer Res. 3, 523–530.

Westphal, M., Hilt, D.C., Bortey, E., et al., 2003. A phase 3 trial of local chemotherapy with biodegradable carmustine (BCNU) wafers (Gliadel wafers) in patients with primary malignant glioma. Neuro. Oncol. 5, 79–88.

Westphal, M., Ram, Z., Riddle, V., et al., 2006. Gliadel wafer in initial surgery for malignant glioma: long-term follow-up of a multicenter controlled trial. Acta. Neurochir. (Wien.) 148, 269–275.

Wrensch, M., Bondy, M.L., Wiencke, J., et al., 1993. Environmental risk factors for primary malignant brain tumors: a review. J. Neurooncol. 17, 47–64.

Wrensch, M., Fisher, J.L., Schwartzbaum, J.A., et al., 2005a. The molecular epidemiology of gliomas in adults. Neurosurg Focus. 19, E5.

Wrensch, M., Minn, Y., Chew, T., et al., 2002. Epidemiology of primary brain tumors: current concepts and review of the literature. Neuro. Oncol. 4, 278–299.

Wrensch, M., Weinberg, A., Wiencke, J., et al., 1997. Does prior infection with varicella-zoster virus influence risk of adult glioma? Am. J. Epidemiol. 145, 594–597.

Wrensch, M., Weinberg, A., Wiencke, J., et al., 2001. Prevalence of antibodies to four herpesviruses among adults with glioma and controls. Am. J. Epidemiol. 154, 161–165.

Wrensch, M., Weinberg, A., Wiencke, J., et al., 2005b. History of Chickenpox and Shingles and Prevalence of Antibodies to Varicella-Zoster Virus and Three Other Herpesviruses among Adults with Glioma and Controls. Am. J. Epidemiol. 161, 929–938.

Yan, H., Parsons, D.W., Jin, G., et al., 2009. IDH1 and IDH2 Mutations in Gliomas. N. Engl. J. Med. 360, 765–773.

Yerli, H., A ildere, A.M., Ozen, O., et al., 2007. Evaluation of cerebral glioma grade by using normal side creatine as an internal reference in multi-voxel 1H-MR spectroscopy. Diagn. Interv. Radiol. 13, 3–9.

Zeng, Q.S., Li, C.F., Zhang, K., et al., 2007. Multivoxel 3D proton M R spectroscopy in the distinction of recurrent glioma from radiation injury. J. Neurooncol. 84, 63–69.

22 Oligodendroglioma

Katharine J. Drummond

Introduction

Oligodendrogliomas are diffusely infiltrating, usually well-differentiated gliomas (WHO grade II) composed of cells morphologically resembling oligodendroglial cells (Reifenberger et al 2007b). They may de-differentiate into more aggressive anaplastic forms. Anaplastic oligodendroglioma (WHO grade III) has a similar appearance but with focal or diffuse features of malignancy (Reifenberger et al 2007a). The oligodendroglial tumor group also includes the oligoastrocytoma (WHO grade II), a tumor consisting of a mixture of two neoplastic cell types morphologically resembling oligodendroglioma and diffuse astrocytoma, which also has a corresponding anaplastic variant (WHO grade III) (von Deimling et al 2007a,b).

The initial description of an oligodendroglioma was published in the classification of gliomas by Bailey and Cushing in 1926. Subsequently, Bailey and Bucy (1929) reported their classic description of 13 oligodendrogliomas. The mixed variant was first described in 1935 (Cooper 1935). These were generally thought to be uncommon intracranial tumors but with the evolution of the histological criteria for diagnosis of oligodendroglioma and oligoastrocytoma, the rate of diagnosis is increasing (Burger 2002; Cairncross et al 2006). Recently published series that have suggested that tumors with oligodendroglial features have a more favorable outcome and response to therapy compared with other gliomas, thus increasing the importance of accurate diagnosis. Controversies in the diagnosis of oligodendroglioma have highlighted the limitations of histopathology and have been early indicators of the importance of biological markers in diagnosis and directing therapy.

Epidemiology

Older series have reported oligodendrogliomas to be uncommon tumors, generally accounting for 4–7% of all primary intracranial gliomas (Rubinstein 1972; Mork et al 1985), and occasionally up to 15% (Burger et al 1991). More recently, with better definition of histopathological diagnostic criteria, some reports suggest that up to 25% of newly diagnosed malignant gliomas have oligodendroglial features (Cairncross et al 2006). Incidence is reported to range between 0.27 and 0.35 per 100000 persons (Ohgaki & Kleihues 2005; CBTRUS 2006). Most series do not report a sex predilection (Rubinstein 1972; Celli et al 1994), although some suggest a slightly higher incidence in males of 1.5–2 : 1, particularly for anaplastic tumors (Russell & Rubinstein 1977; Mork et al 1985; Shaw et al 2004; CBTRUS 2006;

Jaeckle et al 2006). They most frequently occur in the 4th and 5th decades of life with a peak incidence at 26–46 years (Lebrun et al 2004; Shaw et al 2004; Jaeckle et al 2006). There is a biphasic age distribution, with a peak in childhood at 6–12 years, however these remain uncommon tumors in children (Wilkinson et al 1987; Hirsch et al 1989; CBTRUS 2006). Anaplastic tumors present almost a decade later than grade II tumors and comprise 20–35% of oligodendroglial tumors with an incidence of 0.07–0.18 per 100000 (Ohgaki & Kleihues 2005; CBTRUS 2006).

Mixed tumors account for less than 10% of all gliomas (Helseth & Mork 1989; CBTRUS 2006) and between 10% and 19% of supratentorial low-grade glioma (Jaskolsky et al 1987). Only a small percentage of these are anaplastic (Winger et al 1989; Ohgaki & Kleihues 2005). The age and sex distribution is similar to oligodendroglioma (Jaskolsky et al 1987; Beckmann & Prayson 1997; Ohgaki & Kleihues 2005; CBTRUS 2006) as are the clinical and radiological features (Shaw et al 1994; Beckmann & Prayson 1997; Mueller et al 2002).

Clinical presentation

The classic presentation of a patient with an oligodendroglioma is that of epilepsy developing in middle life, as originally described by Bailey and Cushing (1926) (Dam et al 1985), although these tumors may also present in childhood or early adulthood. Until recently, focal or generalized seizures were generally present for many years prior to the diagnosis of a calcified tumor on imaging (Chin et al 1980; Wilkinson et al 1987; Shaw et al 1992; Morris et al 1993). Seizures may have been the only manifestation of a benign intracerebral tumor over many years, and presentation with seizures is generally considered a favorable prognostic factor for oligodendrogliomas, associated with extended survival (Walker et al 1978; Winger et al 1989; Smith et al 1991). Up to two-thirds of patients with oligodendroglioma present with seizures (Lebrun et al 2004), however those who do not have seizures early in the course of their disease do not commonly (14%) develop them later (Hildebrand et al 2005).

With the advent of readily available, high quality imaging for the investigation of seizures, these tumors are increasingly identified early and the classic presentation with a long standing history of seizures is becoming uncommon (Olson et al 2000). Identification of asymptomatic tumors on imaging performed for other reasons (such as a head injury or research) is becoming common. In addition, many patients present with symptoms other than seizures (Olson et al 2000; Lebrun et al 2004), generally associated with the effects of the mass lesion; including focal neurologic deficit related to the position of the lesion, cognitive deficit (Tucha et al 2000; Taphoorn & Klein 2004), headache (Forsyth & Posner 1993) and symptoms of raised intracranial pressure. Presentation with intracerebral cerebral hemorrhage, which may be catastrophic, is more common in oligodendroglioma than other gliomas (Ludwig et al 1986).

Anaplastic oligodendrogliomas also commonly present with seizures. If the tumor has progressed from a grade II oligodendroglioma, a prolonged history may be noted but *de novo* tumors with a short history of seizures, headache or focal neurological deficit also occur (Lebrun et al 2004; Ohgaki & Kleihues 2005).

Imaging features

Oligodendrogliomas are diagnosed on CT or MRI scan performed for the investigation of seizures or other symptoms. CT scan is particularly useful for the identification of calcification, which occurs in greater than 50% of tumors and is often flocculent, but is not diagnostic (Fig. 22.1) (Lee & Van Tassel 1989; Lee et al 1998); thus MRI and CT may be complementary modalities to characterize the tumor and its extent (Margain et al 1991). On CT scan, oligodendrogliomas are hypo- or isodense, well-demarcated and display minimal contrast enhancement. On MRI, they are characteristically amorphous lesions involving the cerebral cortex and subcortical white matter; they are uncommonly cystic and there is usually minimal surrounding white matter edema (Fig. 22.2). They are generally hypointense on T1-weighted images and hyperintense on T2-weighted and fluid attenuated inversion recovery (FLAIR) images. Calcification appears as paramagnetic material (Lee & Van Tassel 1989). Contrast enhancement is generally absent or has a scant wispy, dot-like or lacy appearance in low-grade lesions (Fig. 22.3). High-grade tumors generally, but not invariably, enhance on both CT and MRI and may be associated with hemorrhagic or necrotic

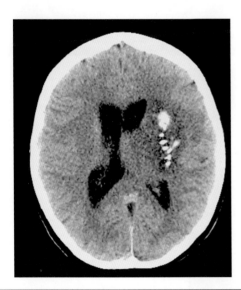

Figure 22.1 Axial CT scan of a slightly hypodense oligodendroglioma extensively involving the left thalamus, basal ganglia and upper brainstem and showing prominent calcification.

areas (Shaw et al 1992; Jenkinson et al 2006). Ring-enhancement is uncommon and is associated with poor prognosis (Cairncross et al 1998). Non-enhancing lesions are generally considered low grade, however a proportion are high grade on histological examination (Fig. 22.3), particularly in older patients, and the diagnosis of a low-grade oligodendroglioma in an older patient should be taken with caution (Recht et al 1992; Barker et al 1997). Pure oligodendrogliomas and mixed tumors cannot be differentiated on imaging (Fig. 22.2C) (Lee et al 1998). Thus, despite quantum advances in imaging, histological diagnosis of all tumors, even those with a typical imaging appearance, remains essential.

More recently, functional, metabolic and other imaging has been used to further characterize these tumors. In particular, identification of imaging characteristics that may predict tumor grade and prognosis have been investigated (Barker et al 1997; Hsu et al 2004; Henson et al 2005). Positron emission tomography (PET) has been used to differentiate low-grade oligodendroglioma and astrocytoma with limited success (Derlon et al 1997; Derlon et al 2005). Given the importance of molecular genetic biological markers such as deletion of 1p and 19q, which are discussed in more detail below, imaging correlates of this molecular signature have been sought. Oligodendrogliomas with the combined deletion have been reported to be more likely located in the frontal, parietal or occipital lobes, crossing the midline, with indistinct margins and calcification (Zlatescu et al 2001; Mueller et al 2002; Megyesi et al 2004), but other reports have not confirmed these findings (Jenkinson et al 2006). They may also have increased activity on thallium-201 single photon emission tomography (SPECT) and FDG ([fluorine-18] fluoro-2-deoxyglucose)-PET compared with other low-grade tumors (Walker et al 2004; Derlon et al 2005). Tumors with intact 1p/19q more often have inhomogeneous signal intensity on MRI (Megyesi et al 2004; Jenkinson et al 2006) and are more likely to be located in the temporal lobe, thalamus and diencephalon (Zlatescu et al 2001; Mueller et al 2002).

Cerebral blood volume (CBV) maps have been used to assess the grade of glioma by measuring vascular density. There is generally a positive correlation of relative CBV with grade. However, for low-grade oligodendrogliomas, CBV may be increased. This may be explained by the dense vascular pattern characteristic of classic oligodendroglial tumors (Sugahara et al 1998; Law et al 2003; Lev et al 2004).

Imaging investigation of oligodendroglioma should include considerations for image-guided surgery, which is now the standard of care (Spicer & Apuzzo 2005; Aquilina et al 2006), and preoperative imaging should include considerations for frameless stereotactic neuronavigation, including if available, adjuncts such as functional MRI (Vlieger et al 2004) and fiber-tracking (Berman et al 2004; Henry et al 2004), to avoid eloquent regions. Metabolic imaging such as PET, SPECT and MR spectroscopy may be useful for targeting biopsy sites (Pirotte et al 2004). Additionally, low-grade gliomas are the indication *par excellence* for intraoperative MRI, as they are poorly-differentiated from surrounding normal brain but well-defined on imaging. Where available, tumor resection using this technology should be considered, as the extent of resection is likely to be improved (Claus et al 2005).

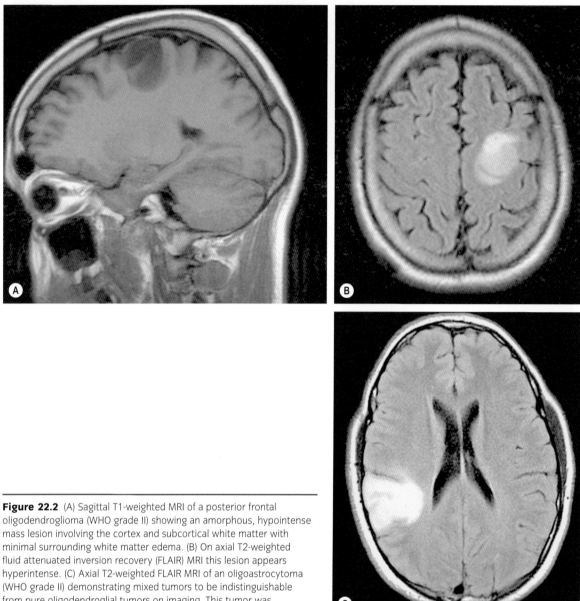

Figure 22.2 (A) Sagittal T1-weighted MRI of a posterior frontal oligodendroglioma (WHO grade II) showing an amorphous, hypointense mass lesion involving the cortex and subcortical white matter with minimal surrounding white matter edema. (B) On axial T2-weighted fluid attenuated inversion recovery (FLAIR) MRI this lesion appears hyperintense. (C) Axial T2-weighted FLAIR MRI of an oligoastrocytoma (WHO grade II) demonstrating mixed tumors to be indistinguishable from pure oligodendroglial tumors on imaging. This tumor was diagnosed incidentally on an MRI performed for research purposes.

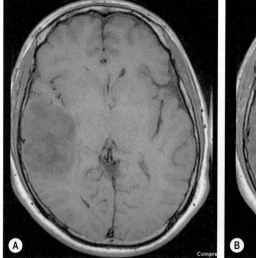
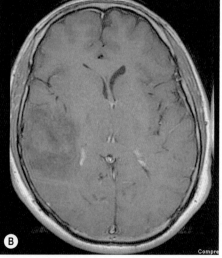

Figure 22.3 Axial T1-weighted MRI of a right temporal oligodendroglioma, without (A) and with (B) contrast administration. There is wispy, poorly-defined enhancement in the otherwise typical tumor. Histopathology revealed anaplastic features. Despite advances in imaging, neither tumor type nor grade can be accurately determined without histopathological examination.

Anatomy and pathology

Oligodendrogliomas occur most frequently in the cerebral hemispheres, in rough proportion to the mass of each lobe (frontal:parietal:temporal:occipital; 3:2:2:1) (Earnest et al 1950; Roberts & German 1966; Chin et al 1980; Burger & Vogel 1982; Shaw et al 1992). They often involve more than one lobe, particularly spanning the frontotemporal-perisylvian-insular region (Fig. 22.4). They are uncommon in the posterior fossa (Packer et al 1985; Wilkinson et al 1987), brainstem (Alvarez et al 1996), and spinal cord (Fortuna et al 1980; Pagni et al 1991). Anaplastic tumors have a similar distribution.

Macroscopic appearance

These tumors are infiltrative, but macroscopically, there is often an abrupt interface between the tumor and the adjacent white matter, the mass appearing solid and well-defined.

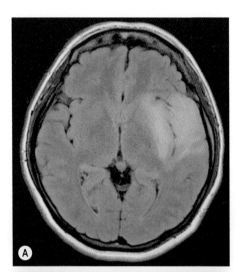

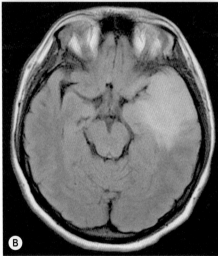

Figure 22.4 Axial T2-weighted fluid attenuated inversion recovery (FLAIR) MRI (A,B) of a WHO grade II oligodendroglioma involving the left temporal lobe, inferior frontal lobe and insula. These tumors commonly involve more than one lobe, particularly spanning the frontotemporal-perisylvian-insular region.

They may also be cystic or mucinous and anaplastic tumors may have areas of necrosis.

They characteristically involve the cortex and subcortical white matter and infiltrate into the leptomeninges and even adhere to the dura. Calcification is frequent. Seeding of the cerebrospinal fluid pathways may occur (Burger 1990) but primary intraventricular oligodendrogliomas are rare (Tekkok et al 1992). Very rarely, tumor cells may be distributed widely through the supra- and infratentorial structures resulting in gliomatosis cerebri (Balko et al 1992). Metastases with multiple intracranial and even systemic lesions have been reported (Macdonald et al 1989; Ogasawara et al 1990; Merrell et al 2006). Hemorrhage within the tumor is not uncommon, and may be related to the structure of the neoplastic capillary bed (Ludwig et al 1986; Reifenberger et al 2007b).

Histopathological diagnosis and grading

There is considerable inter-observer variation in the diagnosis and grading of gliomas. This is most marked for tumors with an oligodendroglial component. Diagnostic criteria and grading systems have evolved over recent decades, and there is no clear marker for neoplastic oligodendroglial cells. Panel review of anaplastic oligodendrogliomas and anaplastic oligoastrocytomas from the EORTC Trial 26951 demonstrated wide discrepancies between the diagnoses provided by the submitting pathologist and those of the expert panel of nine neuropathologists. For anaplastic oligodendrogliomas a consensus diagnosis was reached in 52% of the cases submitted with a diagnosis of anaplastic oligodendroglioma and in only 8% of cases submitted with a diagnosis of anaplastic oligoastrocytoma. There was also considerable inter-observer variation within the panel of experts (Kros et al 2007).

Microscopic appearance

Microscopically, oligodendrogliomas are composed of cells with uniform, round to oval nuclei and a fine chromatin pattern with small nucleoli. The cytoplasm shows minimal process formation, so a fibrillary background appearance is lacking. Perinuclear haloes are characteristic of oligodendrogliomas and are a result of autolysis during fixation for paraffin section; haloes are therefore absent in frozen sections. The tumor cells are present in sheets and lobular groups within a prominent vascular network composed of distinctive short curvilinear capillaries. The perinuclear haloes against the background vascular network is commonly known as the 'fried egg' or 'chicken wire' appearance (Fig. 22.5). Infiltration of the tumor into the cerebral cortex results in perineuronal satellitosis and perivascular and sub-pial tumor cell aggregates. Calcification is common and may be found as microcalcification in the tumor or adjacent brain, or as mineralization of tumor vessels. Oligodendrogliomas have a propensity to include large entrapped reactive astrocytes, as well as small tumor cells with eccentric non-fibrillar glassy cytoplasm strongly positive for glial fibrillary acidic protein (GFAP) and known as mini- or microgemistocytes (Reifenberger et al 2007b). Rare variants include the signet-ring cell oligodendroglioma (Kros et al 1997).

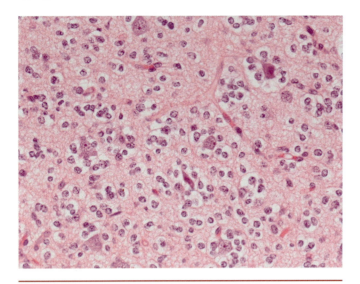

Figure 22.5 The characteristic microscopic appearance of an oligodendroglioma (WHO grade II) made up of lobular groups of cells with uniform, round to oval nuclei and prominent perinuclear haloes. There is a background vascular network composed of distinctive short curvilinear capillaries. The perinuclear halos against the background vascular network is commonly known as the 'fried egg' or 'chicken wire' appearance.

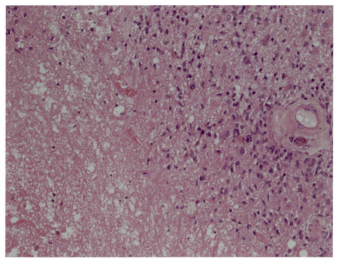

Figure 22.6 The microscopic appearance of a glioblastoma multiforme with oligodendroglial features (WHO grade IV). There is prominent necrosis and endothelial hyperplasia and an astrocytic component but also cells with oligodendroglial features.

Oligodendroglioma (WHO grade II) has the histological appearance described above but can also feature marked nuclear atypia and occasional mitoses. Anaplastic oligodendroglioma (WHO grade III) has typical features of oligodendroglioma but is more cellular, with increased nuclear and cellular pleomorphism and atypia, significant mitotic activity, microvascular proliferation, and areas of focal tumor necrosis (Giannini et al 2001; Reifenberger et al 2007a). Gliofibrillary oligodendrocytes and minigemistocytes are common (Kros et al 1990). It has been suggested that the presence of tumor necrosis alone, even with pseudopallisading, does not upgrade the tumor to glioblastoma multiforme if other typical oligodendroglial features are present, and may not indicate a worse prognosis as compared to other grade III tumors (Miller et al 2006). However, most neuropathologists would consider prominent necrosis within an oligodendroglioma to be indicative of progression of an astrocytic component and these tumors are usually classified as glioblastoma multiforme with an oligodendroglial component (WHO grade IV) (Fig. 22.6). Typical glioblastoma multiforme is uncommonly found as a progressive change in oligodendroglioma but is the most malignant form of this tumor. Histogenesis of these tumor types from oligodendroglial cells is assumed, based on similarities in cellular morphology, however the cell of origin is not clear and origin from glial progenitor cells is also likely (Shih & Holland 2004).

Normal oligodendroglial cells can be identified by several relatively specific marker proteins, including myelin basic protein (MBP), proteolipid protein (PLP), myelin-associated glycoprotein (MAG), galactocerebrosidase, some gangliosides, 2′-3′-cyclic nucleotide-3′-phosphatase (CNP), glycerol-3-phosphate dehydrogenase, lactate dehydrogenase (LDH) and carbonic anhydrase C; however, none of

these proteins is consistently expressed in neoplastic oligodendrocytes, or expression is not restricted to tumor cells (carbonic anhydrase) (Nakagawa et al 1986; 1987; Schwechheimer et al 1992; Sung et al 1996; Reifenberger et al 2007b).

Some oligodendrogliomas show focal immunostaining for S-100 or neuron specific enolase, but this is neither sensitive nor specific. A high percentage of oligodendrogliomas are immunoreactive for the cell surface antigen Leu 7 (CD57) (Nakagawa et al 1986; Reifenberger et al 1987) and the marker of oligodendroglial progenitor cells A2B5 (de la Monte 1990) but the specificity of these markers has not been determined. Other positive markers on immunohistochemistry include vimentin, particularly in anaplastic tumors (Dehghani et al 1998), microtubule-associated protein-2 (MAP-2) (Blumcke et al 2001) and transcription factors OLIG-1 and -2 (Ligon et al 2004; Riemenschneider et al 2004). None of these is specific to oligodendrogliomas, being expressed in other gliomas and neuronal tumors. Positive staining for p53 is rare and *TP53* mutation and deletion of 1p and 19q are mutually exclusive (Ohgaki et al 1991; Reifenberger et al 1994; Reifenberger & Louis 2003; Jeuken et al 2004; Ohgaki & Kleihues 2005).

Most well-differentiated neoplastic oligodendrocytes do not immunostain for GFAP, however entrapped reactive astrocytes, gemistocytes, minigemistocytes and scattered gliofibrillary oligodendrocytes may be found in oligodendrogliomas and are GFAP positive (Reifenberger et al 1987; Kros et al 1990; Kros et al 1991). Large classic gemistocytes have been associated with a poor prognosis (Kros et al 1990). Gliofibrillary oligodendrocytes are GFAP-positive neoplastic cells with morphologic characteristics of oligodendroglial cells. They may represent a transitional or intermediate form between oligodendroglial and astrocytic phenotypes (Kros et al 1990; Kros et al 1991) or may relate to a developmental phenotype of oligodendroglial cells (Choi

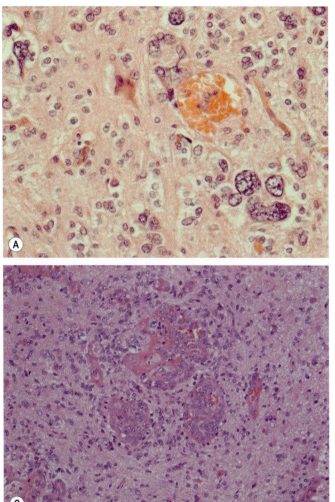

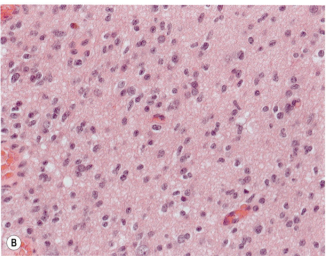

Figure 22.7 The microscopic appearance of an oligoastrocytoma with neoplastic cells expressing both oligodendroglial and astrocytic features. (A) Oligoastrocytoma (WHO grade II) with prominent 'fried egg' oligodendroglial cells and intermingled large pleomorphic neoplastic astrocytes. (B) Oligoastrocytoma (WHO grade II) with a predominant astrocytic component and a few oligodendroglial cells with small round nuclei. (C) Anaplastic oligoastrocytoma with intermingled oligodendroglial and astrocytic cells. The tumor is hypercellular, with cellular and nuclear atypia and prominent endothelial hyperplasia.

& Kim 1984). Synaptophysin, neurofilament or other neuronal marker expression may occur in oligodendrogliomas due to trapped neuropil, particularly at the tumor edge, or due to the presence of neoplastic oligodendroglial cells expressing these markers (Wharton et al 1998a; Perry et al 2002).

Oligoastrocytomas (von Deimling et al 2007a,b) are comprised of neoplastic cells with both astrocytic and oligodendroglial phenotypes (Fig. 22.7). There is a rare biphasic ('compact') variant in which areas of oligodendroglioma and astrocytoma are juxtaposed but more commonly these cells are intimately mixed in the intermingled ('diffuse') variant (Hart et al 1974). True fibrillary, protoplasmic or gemistocytic astrocytic cells should be present and even a prominent component of GFAP positive minigemistocytes or gliofibrillary oligodendrocytes does not warrant a diagnosis of oligoastrocytoma. The minimum astroglial component required for diagnosis is not always well-defined and reliable detection of both cell types is hampered by a lack of specific markers. Thus, inter-observer variability in diagnosis of these tumors is even higher than for pure oligodendroglial tumors (Kim et al 1996; Beckmann & Prayson 1997; Kros et al 2007). Grading is broadly similar to oligodendrogliomas and Ki-67 proliferation index correlates with features of anaplasia.

Genetic features

Oligodendrogliomas are only rarely familial or associated with hereditary cancer syndromes (summarized in Reifenberger et al 2007b). G-banded karyotypes are largely normal or non-clonal (Ransom et al 1992; Thiel et al 1992; Magnani et al 1994).

The hallmark genetic lesion of oligodendroglioma and oligoastrocytoma is allelic loss of the 19q and 1p regions, with loss of heterozygosity (LOH) frequencies ranging from 40% to 86%, and 50% to 83%, respectively (Reifenberger et al 1994; Kraus et al 1995; Reifenberger & Louis 2003; Jeuken et al 2004; Okamoto et al 2004). Co-deletion of 1p and 19q appears to be due to an unbalanced translocation between chromosomes 1 and 19 [t(1;19)(q10;p10)], with loss of one entire copy of 1p and 19q (Griffin et al 2006; Jenkins et al 2006). Partial deletions are uncommon. These regions are likely to encode tumor suppressor genes and mutations in the *p53* tumor suppressor gene and are rarely found in oligodendrogliomas (Ohgaki et al 1991). Candidate genes include the DNA fragmentation factor subunit B gene, myelin-related epithelial membrane protein gene 3, *CDKN2C*, *SHREW1*, *TP73*, *RAD54*, *p190RhoGAP*, *ZNF342* and *PEG3* (Dong et al 2002; Hong et al 2003; Reifenberger & Louis

2003; Wolf et al 2003; Trouillard et al 2004; Alaminos et al 2005; Barbashina et al 2005; McDonald et al 2005; McDonald et al 2006). The 19q and 1p losses are seen in both low-grade and anaplastic oligodendrogliomas and are thus thought to be important early events in oligodendroglial tumorigenesis. Deletion of 1p/19q has generated intense interest, as it has been demonstrated to be associated with prolonged survival and response to chemotherapy (Cairncross et al 1998; Aldape et al 2007; Giannini et al 2008). Other aberrations include gains on chromosome 7 and losses on 4, 6, 11p, 14 and 22q (Reifenberger & Louis 2003; Jeuken et al 2004). Epigenetic silencing by promoter methylation has been found for a number of genes (summarized in (Reifenberger et al 2007b) and includes *MGMT* promoter hypermethylation (Mollemann et al 2005).

Anaplastic oligodendrogliomas (Grade 3) have a slightly lower frequency of 1p/19q deletion than grade II tumors. Progression from grade II to III is associated with an accumulation of genetic abnormalities (Reifenberger & Louis 2003; Jeuken et al 2004). Additional abnormalities include gains on 7 and 15q and losses on 4q, 6, 9p, 10q, 11, 13q, 18 and 22q and these may be related to progression (Thiel et al 1992; Reifenberger et al 1994; Cairncross et al 1998; Jeuken et al 2004; Roerig et al 2005). *CDKN2A* gene deletions, found on 9p, are associated with a poor prognosis and are present in one-third of anaplastic oligodendrogliomas (Cairncross et al 1998; Reifenberger & Louis 2003; Jeuken et al 2004). Losses of 10q are present in approximately 10% of tumors but a normal *PTEN* copy is often retained, suggesting another tumor suppressor gene of importance (Sasaki et al 2001; Reifenberger & Louis 2003; Jeuken et al 2004).

A number of growth factors and their receptors are involved in the tumorigenesis or progression of oligodendroglial tumors. The majority of tumors express both sub-units of the potent mitogen platelet-derived growth factor (PDGF) and their corresponding receptors, likely resulting in autocrine stimulation (Di Rocco et al 1998). Vascular endothelial growth factor (VEGF) and its receptors are also expressed, particularly in anaplastic tumors and may be related to tumor progression (Chan et al 1998; Christov et al 1998). Epithelial growth factor receptor (EGFR) is expressed in approximately half of all oligodendroglial tumors of any grade but without *EGFR* gene amplification (Reifenberger et al 1996). Simultaneous expression of its ligands suggests an autocrine or paracrine loop (Ekstrand et al 1991). Other implicated growth factors include basic fibroblast growth factor (bFGF), transforming growth factor beta (TGF-β), insulin-like growth factor 1 (IGF-1), and nerve growth factor (NGF) (Reifenberger & Louis 2003).

Oligoastrocytoma displays genetic features of both astrocytoma and oligodendroglioma with 1p/19q deletion in 30–50% (Reifenberger et al 1994; Kraus et al 1995; Okamoto et al 2004) and *TP53* mutations in 30% (Reifenberger et al 1994; Mueller et al 2002; Okamoto et al 2004), but usually not in combination, suggesting a similar cellular origin (rather than concurrently developing tumors) and significant genetic heterogeneity. Progression is associated with accumulation of similar genetic abnormalities including loss of 9p, 10p and 11p as well as homozygous deletion of *CDKN2A* (Reifenberger et al 1994; Mueller et al 2002).

Histological grading

There have been a number of grading systems used for oligodendrogliomas and until the last decade, there has been no internationally accepted grading system. Subsequently, the WHO grading system has been widely accepted as standard and this system recognizes oligodendroglial tumors as a continuous spectrum ranging from well-differentiated to frankly malignant tumors. Oligodendrogliomas correspond to WHO grade II and anaplastic oligodendroglioma to WHO grade III (Reifenberger et al 2007a,b). This grading system has been shown to correlate with prognosis (Giannini et al 2001; Felsberg et al 2004; Lebrun et al 2004; Ohgaki & Kleihues 2005) and the features of each tumor are described above.

Grading systems used previously included the three-tiered Ringertz system (Ringertz 1950), the four-tiered Armed Forces Institute of Pathology (AFIP) system (Smith et al 1983) (later updated to divide oligodendroglioma into low grade and anaplastic (Burger & Scheithauer 1994)), and the four-tiered St Anne-Mayo system (Shaw et al 1992). The AFIP classification has also been modified into a three-tiered scheme (Kros et al 1988). Each takes account of similar histological features including cellularity, cellular and nuclear atypia and pleomorphism, mitotic index, endothelial proliferation, and necrosis. A two-tiered system which includes both imaging and histopathological features has also been proposed by Daumas-Duport et al (1997). Despite the differences in these grading systems, they are broadly similar and describe groups of oligodendroglial tumors with prognostic significance.

Assessment of growth fraction in oligodendroglial tumors by means of the proliferation-associated antigen Ki-67, using the MIB-1 antibody may be useful in determining tumor grade and prognosis (Heegaard et al 1995; Coons et al 1997; Dehghani et al 1998). WHO grade II oligodendrogliomas have a Ki-67 index of less than 3–5% (Coons et al 1997; Dehghani et al 1998). Anaplasia is associated with higher labeling indices (Wharton et al 1998b). Minigemistocytes are usually MIB-1 negative but gliofibrillary oligodendrocytes may be positive (Kros et al 1996).

Differential diagnosis

Oligodendrogliomas must be differentiated pathologically from a number of neoplastic and benign lesions (Reifenberger et al 2007b). The availability of only small stereotactic biopsies may make this differentiation more difficult. The distinction between a well-differentiated fibrillary astrocytoma and an oligodendroglioma may be difficult on intraoperative frozen section because of the lack of the 'fried egg' appearance in these preparations. True mixed gliomas show distinct areas of oligodendroglioma along with areas of astrocytoma, however other tumors may have cells that resemble oligodendroglioma. These include juvenile pilocytic astrocytoma, cellular ependymomas (particularly clear cell ependymoma), clear cell meningioma and dysembryoplastic neuroepithelial tumors (DNET). Differentiation can usually be achieved by recognition of areas of typical histology (perivascular pseudorosettes, pilocytic cells) and with electron microscopy (Cenacchi et al 1996). Identification of deletion of 1p/19q may be helpful, as this is rare in non-glial tumors, but not helpful if absent. Intraventricular oligodendrogliomas must be differentiated from central neurocytoma and this is usually possible using neuronal marker staining, however occasionally oligodendrogliomas also express neuronal markers (Wharton et al 1998a; Perry et al 2002). Poorly-differentiated oligodendrogliomas may be confused with malignant astrocytoma or metastatic carcinoma. Oligodendrogliomas may present with intracerebral hemorrhage; fragments of tumor may only be found after careful examination of evacuated blood clot (Hinton et al 1984). Vascular malformations may show areas of oligodendroglial proliferation that imitate an oligodendroglioma and this may also be seen in lobectomy specimens removed for intractable epilepsy. Benign processes such as demyelination and infarction that are rich in macrophages may mimic oligodendroglioma.

Treatment

General principles

The management of low-grade glioma is controversial and this is particularly true of the indolent oligodendroglioma, for which, it has been argued, perhaps no treatment should be offered (Cairncross & Laperriere 1989). Until recently, data on factors associated with prognosis and the efficacy of surgery, radiotherapy and chemotherapy for these lesions have been scant. Despite recent advances in our understanding of the genetic abnormalities that underlie oligodendroglial tumorigenesis and the benefit of adjuvant chemotherapy for anaplastic tumors, management choices are still often not clear. There are few published clinical practice guidelines (Australian Cancer Network Adult Brain Tumour Guidelines Working Party 2008). Treatment options include observation alone, biopsy with subsequent observation, or surgical resection with or without postoperative radiation and/or chemotherapy. Concerns regarding risks of treatment are paramount, particularly in the neurologically intact patient who may be expected to survive a decade or more and especially as the tumor may involve eloquent regions. Whether adjuvant therapy should be 'saved' until malignant progression, should also be considered. The role of surgery in the management of intractable seizures is an additional concern, and variable results have been reported (Lee et al 1989; Smith et al 1991). A recent report suggests that a good seizure outcome after surgery can be achieved in greater than 90% of patients in a selected series (Chang et al 2008).

It is important that biopsy should be performed in all cases of suspected low-grade glioma. The exception is for tumors with a typical appearance in an eloquent or technically challenging area such as the brainstem. However, even patients with tumors with the typical radiological appearance of a low-grade oligodendroglioma may harbor an anaplastic tumor, particularly those aged over 40 years. Thus, biopsy should be performed whenever possible, both to plan treatment and to determine prognosis, particularly in light of the importance of analysis for 1p/19q deletion (Barker et al 1997; Lebrun et al 2004; Nutt 2005).

For anaplastic oligodendroglioma and anaplastic oligoastrocytoma, the issues and recommendations regarding surgery are similar to those for all high-grade gliomas. Gross total surgical resection, where safe, or a maximal de-bulking, followed by postoperative radiotherapy, is considered the standard of care and will not be discussed further here (see Andersen 1978; Walker et al 1978; Walker et al 1980; Sandberg-Wollheim et al 1991; Davies et al 1996; Vuorinen et al 2003; Hart et al 2004; Taylor et al 2004; Australian Cancer Network Adult Brain Tumour Guidelines Working Party 2008).

Surgery

Surgical resection for low-grade glioma has been controversial for decades and there continues to be no good quality evidence for surgical treatment of these tumors. Generally, oligodendroglioma and oligoastrocytoma have been grouped with astrocytoma in retrospective series assessing the effect of extent of resection, and the deficiencies in the data are similar for each type of tumor. Overall, older retrospective studies have supported extent of resection as a prognostic factor in low-grade glioma. However, they generally included a wide range of tumor types and sometimes grades, did not stratify tumors on the basis of genetic or clinical prognostic factors, and were tainted by strong selection bias for good prognosis, surgically accessible tumors in non-eloquent areas in young, well patients. In addition, extent of resection was largely determined according to surgeon estimate or postoperative CT scans, both of which are unreliable, and follow-up was often short. Therefore, some authors have recommended a policy of observation only, as the evidence for a benefit from surgical resection was very poor (Laws et al 1984; Winger et al 1989; Sandeman et al 1990; Soffietti 1990; Smith et al 1991). There are few studies that analyze oligodendroglioma alone. As the prognosis of astrocytoma is not as good as for oligodendroglioma, the relevance to oligodendroglioma of studies analyzing all tumor types together is not clear.

Older studies dealing specifically with oligodendroglioma were marred by the same limitations described above, but generally supported surgical resection (Horrax & Wu 1951; Roberts & German 1966; Reedy et al 1983). The Mayo Clinic experience of 82 patients (Shaw et al 1992) found a median survival time of 12.6 years and 5 and 10 year survival rates of 74% and 59% in patients who had undergone gross total surgical resection, in comparison to 4.9 years, 48% and 26%, respectively, for those patients who underwent a subtotal resection. Other studies which have reported an improvement in survival with more extensive resection include that by Mork and colleagues (1985), who reported an improvement in median survival from 2.7 years to 3.8 years, that by Celli and colleagues (1994) who reported an improvement in 5-year and median survival from 44%, and 4 years to 66% and 9.25 years; and another which reported an improvement in 5-year survival from 41% to 84% (Whitton & Bloom 1990). However, results have varied and although most studies showed a survival advantage of resection over biopsy alone, not all show an advantage of aggressive, extensive resection over more conservative, limited procedures (Sun et al 1988).

The more recent literature is of somewhat better quality, has similar findings and suggests an advantage for tumor resection. The histological definition of the tumors is more rigorous and extent of resection is usually determined by postoperative MRI. However, the studies are still retrospective, often include all types of low-grade glioma and the selection bias for young, well patients with accessible tumors remains (Keles et al 2001; Talos et al 2006). One recent retrospective study of a well-defined population of 216 low-grade gliomas showed that patients in whom at least 90% of the tumor was resected had 5- and 8-year overall survival rates of 97% and 91%, respectively, whereas patients with less than 90% resected had 5- and 8-year overall survival rates of 76% and 60%, respectively. When adjusted for age, Karnofsky performance score, tumor location, and tumor sub-type, extent of resection was an independent predictor of overall survival and malignant progression-free survival (Smith et al 2008). Others have found similar results (McGirt et al 2008) but one study looking specifically at oligodendrogliomas did not agree (El-Hateer et al 2009).

Thus, in the absence of a randomized prospective study, which is unlikely to be performed due to the lack of equipoise and probably also patient acceptance, the weight of evidence favors a surgical resection of as much of the tumor as can be safely excised for oligodendroglioma and oligoastrocytoma. We would advocate aggressive surgical resection for accessible lesions that are unlikely to produce a permanent neurological deficit. However, a neurological deficit in a young patient who is likely to survive years or decades is a disaster, and thus, all measures to reduce the likelihood of this outcome should be employed, including awake surgery with intraoperative electrophysiologic mapping and intraoperative neurological testing (Berger & Ojemann 1992; Gugino et al 2000) and image-guided surgery.

Radiotherapy

After tumor resection and confirmation of the histopathological diagnosis, in most patients with an oligodendroglioma, adjuvant therapy will not be immediately indicated. An EORTC study comparing initial radiotherapy at diagnosis vs delayed therapy at progression showed no difference in overall survival (median 7.4 vs 7.2 years) between the two groups, however, progression-free survival was shorter in the group in whom radiotherapy was delayed (median 5.3 vs 3.4 years) (van den Bent et al 2005). Unfortunately, a number of high-grade tumors were included in the analysis, but these were balanced between the two groups. During observation, the majority of patients displayed slow continued growth of the residual tumor, on average 4 mm diameter per year, with eventual progression to anaplasia (Mandonnet et al 2003). Therefore, it is acceptable to observe patients with an extensively resected oligodendroglioma and otherwise good prognostic factors, including age less than 40 years and favorable cytogenetic features (1p/19q deletion) (Nutt 2005; Kaloshi et al 2007), to avoid the risk of long-term radiotherapy toxicity until disease progression.

To date, there have been no studies addressing when to initiate radiation therapy in patients with oligodendroglioma, with or without an initial period of observation. Indications have included generally recognized poor prognostic factors; age over 40 years, progressive growth, progressive neurological deficit, normal 1p/19q status and signs of progression on imaging. Early seizure control was somewhat better in the early treatment arm in the EORTC study described above (van den Bent et al 2005), therefore uncontrolled seizures may also be an indication. The argument against early radiotherapy is the concern regarding delayed treatment-induced neurocognitive dysfunction (Laack & Brown 2004), which is well documented and related particularly to whole brain radiotherapy and fraction size greater than 2 Gy (Postma et al 2002; Taphoorn 2003; Taphoorn & Klein 2004). Therefore, radiotherapy should be delayed in patients whose prognosis is for prolonged survival and should be considered only for the above-mentioned clear indications. Significant residual tumor after resection has been suggested as an indication for radiotherapy, but has not been validated.

There have been no phase III studies of radiotherapy where accrual has been restricted to oligodendroglial tumors alone. Consequently, results are extrapolated from two prospective randomized studies that have evaluated the effect of radiotherapy dose in all low-grade gliomas. Prior to these two studies, the older literature was unhelpful in determining whether adjuvant therapy should be used for these tumors and was fraught with the same difficulties as that regarding surgical resection (Sheline et al 1964; Chin et al 1980; Lindegaard et al 1987; Cairncross & Laperriere 1989). Many studies showed no benefit from radiotherapy (Muller et al 1977; Afra et al 1978; Dohrmann et al 1978; Reedy et al 1983; Sun et al 1988; Wallner et al 1988; Nijjar et al 1993). However, there was a suggestion in these retrospective studies that radiotherapy may be useful, particularly in patients who had subtotally resected tumors. One showed a difference in survival in 63 patients who underwent a subtotal resection and radiotherapy at a dose of less than 50 Gy, vs a dose of greater than 50 Gy. The median survival, and 5- and 10-year survival rates in the 26 patients who received surgery plus lower dose radiotherapy was 4.5 years, 39% and 20%, but for higher dose radiotherapy was 7.9 years, 62% and 31% (Shaw et al 1992). Another study demonstrated an increase in median and 5- and 10-year survival rates in 41 patients. The 27 patients treated with surgery and radiation had an increased median survival of 84 vs 47 months, and increased 5- and 10-year survival of 83% vs 51%, and 46% vs 36%, respectively. Median time to tumor recurrence was also longer in those treated with surgery and radiation (Gannett et al 1994). Another study of 41 patients treated with surgery plus radiotherapy found the outcome of treatment was not significantly improved with postoperative radiotherapy; however, when these patients were stratified for subtotal vs total resection, there was a significant difference in 5-year survival time of 74% vs 25% (Shimizu et al 1993).

Of the prospective phase III studies, the NCCTG/RTOG/ECOG study randomized 203 adult patients after a biopsy or resection of a low-grade glioma to 50.4 Gy in 28 fractions over 5.5 weeks or 64.8 Gy in 36 fractions over 7 weeks. The majority of patients (70%) had oligodendrogliomas or mixed tumors. Five-year survival was 72% in the low dose arm and 64% in the high dose arm, respectively, which was not significantly different (Shaw et al 2002). An EORTC study in 379 patients compared 45 Gy in 25 fractions and 59.4 Gy in

33 fractions. Only 31% of patients were oligodendrogliomas or mixed tumors but, unlike the previously mentioned study, this was not subject to central review. There was no significant difference in the 5-year progression free (47% and 50%) or overall survival (58 and 59%) between the two arms (Karim et al 1996).

Therefore, for oligodendroglioma, treatment with adjuvant radiation should be delayed except in those patients with clinical, radiological and molecular features of a poor prognosis. These may include normal 1p/19q status, high proliferation index older age, demonstrated growth and progressive symptoms (Ludwig et al 1986; Macdonald 1994; Allison et al 1997; Leighton et al 1997). The recommended dose for low-grade oligodendroglioma and oligoastrocytoma when treatment is indicated is 50 Gy in 2 Gy fractions.

Chemotherapy

For low-grade gliomas, including oligodendroglioma, it is not clear that chemotherapy adds any benefit, although there were positive results reported in early studies (Mason et al 1996). There have been two phase II studies looking at chemotherapy as primary adjuvant therapy after surgery for low-grade oligodendroglioma, rather than radiotherapy, and this is the subject of an ongoing EORTC-led phase III study. In one study, 149 patients with progressive low-grade glioma were treated with temozolomide, correlating response to the presence or absence of 1p/19q deletion. A partial response was achieved in 53% of patients, 37% had stable disease and 10% had progressive disease. The median time to maximal tumor response was 12 months (range 3–30 months) and the median progression free survival was 28 months. The response was significantly higher and lasted longer in those with 1p/19q deletions, who also had longer progression free and overall survival (Kaloshi et al 2007). Another small study of 28 patients looking at combined procarbazine, lomustine and vincristine (PCV) chemotherapy prior to radiotherapy showed a 54% response rate (Buckner et al 2003).

For anaplastic oligodendroglioma and oligoastrocytoma, which in most early studies were grouped with other high-grade gliomas, interest in adjuvant chemotherapy has been intense. This has resulted from several reports of chemosensitivity in anaplastic oligodendrogliomas, with the suggestion that this may be distinct from that of other glial tumors (Cairncross & Macdonald 1988; Macdonald et al 1990; Cairncross & Macdonald 1991; Glass et al 1992). This led to the widespread use and reporting of chemotherapy in high-grade oligodendrogliomas and later in mixed gliomas (Glass et al 1992; Kyritsis et al 1993; Allison et al 1997). The most widely used and studied chemotherapy regimen has been PCV, however a variety of cytotoxic drugs including melphalan, thiotepa, temozolomide, paclitaxel, and platinum-based regimens, the use of chemotherapy prior to radiotherapy and the combination of high dose chemotherapy with autologous bone marrow transplant have also been reported to be beneficial (Cairncross & Macdonald 1988; Levin et al 1990; Saarinen et al 1990; Poisson et al 1991; Cairncross et al 1992; Paleologos et al 1999; Perry et al 1999). A prospective phase II study of 24 patients showed response rates of 75% to PCV in anaplastic

pure oligodendroglioma (Cairncross et al 1994) and a retrospective study of 32 patients using PCV either before or after radiotherapy, showed a response rate of 91% (Kim et al 1996). However, not all studies found benefit from adjuvant chemotherapy in anaplastic oligodendroglioma or oligoastrocytoma (Kyritsis et al 1993).

Subsequently, two randomized studies have been performed looking at the role of adjuvant PCV therapy and relating it to 1p/19q status. EORTC 26951 compared radiotherapy following surgery to radiotherapy followed by standard dose PCV in 368 patients. They were required to have 25% or more oligodendroglial component on histopathology. The median progression free survival was significantly improved in the PCV group (23 vs 13 months), but not overall survival (40 vs 31 months). The 5-year survival for those with 1p/19q deletion with and without chemotherapy was 75% and 74%, respectively and for those with intact 1p/19q was 33% and 28%, respectively (van den Bent et al 2006a). In the RTOG 9402 study, 289 patients were randomized to four cycles of intensive PCV before radiotherapy, or radiotherapy alone. Again, patients with 1p/19q deletion (46%) had much extended survival regardless of randomized therapy. With the intensive PCV regime there was significant chemotherapy-related toxicity. The 5-year survival for those with 1p/19q deletion with and without chemotherapy was 72% and 68%, respectively and for those with intact 1p/19q was 37% and 31%, respectively (Cairncross et al 2006). Both these studies suggest that much of the early enthusiasm for chemotherapy in these tumors was encouraged more by the biology of the tumor than remarkable chemoresponsiveness and addition of PCV chemotherapy to radiotherapy is not supported by the available literature, however practices vary widely (Abrey et al 2007). Alternative chemotherapy protocols are currently being studied, including the use of concomitant and adjuvant radiotherapy and temozolomide, as has become the standard of care for glioblastoma multiforme (Stupp et al 2005; van den Bent et al 2006b). There may still be evidence for the use of chemotherapy in recurrent anaplastic oligodendroglial tumors, particularly those that are chemotherapy naive (van den Bent et al 1998; van den Bent et al 2001; van den Bent et al 2003; Soffietti et al 2004; Triebels et al 2004; Brandes et al 2006; Scopece et al 2006).

Prognosis

Oligodendroglioma (WHO grade II) has a relatively good prognosis compared with other glial neoplasms with median survival often reported to be 10–15 years (Shaw et al 1992; Okamoto et al 2004; Jenkins et al 2006). Five and 10-year survival of 72% and around 50% have been documented (Shaw et al 1992; Leighton et al 1997; Okamoto et al 2004). Significantly shorter survival times are also reported, particularly in older series (Earnest et al 1950; Chin et al 1980; Mork et al 1985; Ludwig et al 1986; Lindegaard et al 1987; Wilkinson et al 1987) and may be related to different criteria for tumor diagnosis and grading. However, despite this extended survival, tumor recurrence with malignant progression (with a median time to progression of 6 to 7 years) is the rule (Winger et al 1989; Shaw et al 1994; Lebrun et al

2004). Factors associated with a good prognosis include those common to all glial tumors, including young age (Helseth & Mork 1989; Kros et al 1994; Lebrun et al 2004; Okamoto et al 2004), higher Karnofsky performance scale score (Leighton et al 1997), and tumor grade. In addition, frontal location (Kros et al 1994), absence of contrast enhancement on imaging (Shaw et al 1992) and complete macroscopic tumor removal (as discussed above) have been implicated. These, of course, may actually be markers for other prognostic factors rather than independent prognostic factors; for instance, contrast enhancement may be dependent on tumor grade and frontal tumors may be more likely to be associated with a good performance score.

A high Ki-67 index (>3–5%) has been associated with a poor prognosis in oligodendroglioma in a number of studies, independent of age, tumor site or grade (Shibata et al 1988; Deckert et al 1989; Heegaard et al 1995; Kros et al 1996; Coons et al 1997; Lebrun et al 2004; Shaffrey et al 2005). A reduction in 5-year survival from 83% to 24% has been documented for patients with a labeling index of greater than 5% (Dehghani et al 1998). In addition, 1p/19q loss is associated with prolonged survival and response to therapy, as discussed above. (Reifenberger et al 1994; Smith et al 2000; Felsberg et al 2004; Walker et al 2004; Kujas et al 2005; Kanner et al 2006; Giannini et al 2008). Both Ki-67 expression and 1p/19q deletion should be assessed at diagnosis of these tumors to guide both prognosis and therapy (Abrey et al 2007).

Anaplastic oligodendroglioma has a relatively good prognosis compared with anaplastic astrocytoma, or glioblastoma multiforme (Winger et al 1989; Cairncross et al 1994). This is related to both the natural history of the tumor and its response to treatment. Median survival of 1–3.5 years has usually been reported (Shaw et al 1992; Dehghani et al 1998; Ohgaki & Kleihues 2005). However, with aggressive combined modality treatment, median survivals of up to 5 years are reported (Cairncross et al 2006; van den Bent et al 2006a). As for low-grade oligodendroglioma, prognosis is strongly linked to 1p/19q deletion (Cairncross et al 1998; van den Bent et al 2006a; Kros et al 2007), with a reported more than 5 years longer median survival for tumors with the deletion than those without (Cairncross et al 2006). Clinical factors associated with prolonged survival include age, performance status and extent of resection (Shaw et al 1992; Cairncross et al 2006; van den Bent et al 2006a).

Prognosis for oligoastrocytoma is probably not as good as for pure oligodendroglial tumors, with median survival times of just over 6 years (Okamoto et al 2004; Ohgaki & Kleihues 2005) and 5- and 10-year survival rates of 58% and 32%, respectively (Shaw et al 1994), although not all studies have agreed (Schiffer et al 1997). A 10-year survival of 49% has also been reported (Okamoto et al 2004). Factors reported to be associated with prolonged survival include age, extent of resection, radiotherapy and Ki-67 proliferation index (Shaw et al 1994; Shaffrey et al 2005). Deletion of 1p/19q is also associated with prolonged survival, including in anaplastic tumors (Eoli et al 2006). Anaplastic oligoastrocytoma has a slightly better prognosis than pure glioblastoma multiforme with a median survival of between 2.8 and 4.2 years with multimodality treatment (Shaw et al 1994; Kim et al 1996).

Key points

- The first description of an oligodendroglioma was published in 1926 by Bailey and Cushing, followed by Bailey and Bucy's classical description of 13 cases in 1929.

- Oligodendrogliomas were previously thought to represent 4–7% of all intracranial gliomas but up to 25% may have oligodendroglial histopathological features. The peak incidence is between the ages of 26 and 46, with anaplastic tumors presenting almost a decade later.

- The tumor occurs within the cerebral hemispheres, most commonly in the frontal lobe.

- Many patients present with seizures.

- Oligodendrogliomas are often calcified on imaging and low-grade tumors usually do not enhance with contrast.

- The characteristic histopathological appearance is of cells with perinuclear halos of clear cytoplasm on a background network composed of distinctive short curvilinear capillaries known as the 'fried egg' or 'chicken wire' appearance.

- A Ki-67 proliferation index of <5% and deletion of 1p/19q are significant prognostic factors and should be assessed in all tumors.

- Most studies demonstrate that patients who undergo gross total resection have an increased survival rate as compared with those who undergo sub-total resection or biopsy alone.

- Postoperative radiotherapy of 50 Gy should be considered in patients who have poor prognostic features, including anaplastic histology, older age, tumor growth on imaging, progression of symptoms, Ki-67 proliferation index >5% or normal 1p/19q status.

- Despite early enthusiasm, the results of phase III trials of chemotherapy in addition to radiotherapy for anaplastic oligodendroglioma have been disappointing. The most widely used regimen has been PCV (procarbazine, lomustine, vincristine), and other trials are ongoing.

REFERENCES

Abrey, L.E., Louis, D.N., Paleologos, N., et al., 2007. Survey of treatment recommendations for anaplastic oligodendroglioma. Neuro. Oncol. 9 (3), 314–318.

Afra, D., Muller, W., Benoist, G., et al., 1978. Supratentorial recurrences of gliomas. Results of reoperations on astrocytomas and oligodendrogliomas. Acta. Neurochir. (Wien) 43 (3–4), 217–227.

Aláminos, M., Davalos, V., Ropero, S., et al., 2005. EMP3, a myelin-related gene located in the critical 19q13. 3 region, is epigenetically silenced and exhibits features of a candidate tumor suppressor in glioma and neuroblastoma. Cancer Res. 65 (7), 2565–2571.

Aldape, K., Burger, P.C., Perry, A., 2007. Clinicopathologic aspects of 1p/19q loss and the diagnosis of oligodendroglioma. Arch. Pathol. Lab. Med. 131 (2), 242–251.

Allison, R.R., Schulsinger, A., Vongtama, V., et al., 1997. Radiation and chemotherapy improve outcome in oligodendroglioma. Int. J. Radiat. Oncol. Biol. Phys. 37 (2), 399–403.

Alvarez, J.A., Cohen, M.L., Hlavin, M.L., 1996. Primary intrinsic brainstem oligodendroglioma in an adult. Case report and review of the literature. J. Neurosurg. 85 (6), 1165–1169.

Andersen, A.P., 1978. Postoperative irradiation of glioblastomas. Results in a randomized series. Acta. Radiol. Oncol. Radiat. Phys. Biol. 17 (6), 475–484.

Aquilina, K., Edwards, P., Strong, A., 2006. Principles and practice of image-guided neurosurgery. In: Moore, A.J., Newell, D.W. (Eds.), Tumor neurosurgery. Principles and practice. Springer Verlag, London, p. 123.

Australian Cancer Network Adult Brain Tumour Guidelines Working Party, 2008. Clinical practice guidelines for the management of adult gliomas: Astrocytomas and oligodendrogliomas. The Cancer Council Australia, Australian Cancer Network and Clinical Oncological Society of Australia, Sydney.

Bailey, P., Bucy, P., 1929. Oligodendrogliomas of the brain. J. Pathol. Bacteriol. 32, 735–751.

Bailey, P., Cushing, H., 1926. Clinical correlation. A classification of the tumors of the glioma group on a histogenetic basis with a correlated study of prognosis. Lippincott, Philadelphia, PA, pp. 105–165.

Balko, M.G., Blisard, K.S., Samaha, F.J., 1992. Oligodendroglial gliomatosis cerebri. Hum. Pathol. 23 (6), 706–707.

Barbashina, V., Salazar, P., Holland, E.C., et al., 2005. Allelic losses at 1p36 and 19q13 in gliomas: correlation with histologic classification, definition of a 150-kb minimal deleted region on 1p36, and evaluation of CAMTA1 as a candidate tumor suppressor gene. Clin. Cancer Res. 11 (3), 1119–1128.

Barker, F.G. 2nd, Chang, S.M., Huhn, S.L., et al., 1997. Age and the risk of anaplasia in magnetic resonance-nonenhancing supratentorial cerebral tumors. Cancer 80 (5), 936–941.

Beckmann, M.J., Prayson, R.A., 1997. A clinicopathologic study of 30 cases of oligoastrocytoma including p53 immunohistochemistry. Pathology 29 (2), 159–164.

Berger, M.S., Ojemann, G.A., 1992. Intraoperative brain mapping techniques in neuro-oncology. Stereotact. Funct. Neurosurg. 58 (1–4), 153–161.

Berman, J.I., Berger, M.S., Mukherjee, P., et al., 2004. Diffusion-tensor imaging-guided tracking of fibers of the pyramidal tract combined with intraoperative cortical stimulation mapping in patients with gliomas. J. Neurosurg. 101 (1), 66–72.

Blumcke, I., Becker, A.J., Normann, S., et al., 2001. Distinct expression pattern of microtubule-associated protein-2 in human oligodendrogliomas and glial precursor cells. J. Neuropathol. Exp. Neurol. 60 (10), 984–993.

Brandes, A.A., Tosoni, A., Cavallo, G., et al., 2006. Correlations between O6-methylguanine DNA methyltransferase promoter methylation status, 1p and 19q deletions, and response to temozolomide in anaplastic and recurrent oligodendroglioma: a prospective GICNO study. J. Clin. Oncol. 24 (29), 4746–4753.

Buckner, J.C., Gesme, D. Jr., O'Fallon, J.R., et al., 2003. Phase II trial of procarbazine, lomustine, and vincristine as initial therapy for patients with low-grade oligodendroglioma or oligoastrocytoma: efficacy and associations with chromosomal abnormalities. J. Clin. Oncol. 21 (2), 251–255.

Burger, P.C., 1990. Classification, grading and patterns of spread of malignant gliomas. In: Apuzzo, M. (Ed.), Malignant cerebral glioma. American Association of Neurological Surgeons, Park Ridge, IL, pp. 3–17.

Burger, P.C., 2002. What is an oligodendroglioma? Brain Pathol. 12 (2), 257–259.

Burger, P.C., Scheithauer, B.W., 1994. Central nervous system. Atlas of tumor pathology. Armed Forces Institute of Pathology, Washington DC, pp. 107–120.

Burger, P.C., Scheithauer, B.W., Vogel, F., 1991. Oligodendroglioma. Surgical pathology of the nervous system and its coverings. John Wiley, New York, pp. 306–327.

Burger, P.C., Vogel, F., 1982. Oligodendroglioma. Surgical pathology of the nervous system and its coverings. John Wiley, New York.

Cairncross, G., Berkey, B., Shaw, E., et al., 2006. Phase III trial of chemotherapy plus radiotherapy compared with radiotherapy alone for pure and mixed anaplastic oligodendroglioma: Intergroup Radiation Therapy Oncology Group Trial 9402. J. Clin. Oncol. 24 (18), 2707–2714.

Cairncross, G., Macdonald, D., Ludwin, S., et al., 1994. Chemotherapy for anaplastic oligodendroglioma. National Cancer Institute of Canada Clinical Trials Group. J. Clin. Oncol. 12 (10), 2013–2021.

Cairncross, J.G., Laperriere, N.J., 1989. Low-grade glioma. To treat or not to treat? Arch. Neurol. 46 (11), 1238–1239.

Cairncross, J.G., Macdonald, D.R., 1988. Successful chemotherapy for recurrent malignant oligodendroglioma. Ann. Neurol. 23 (4), 360–364.

Cairncross, J.G., Macdonald, D.R., 1991. Chemotherapy for oligodendroglioma. Progress report. Arch. Neurol. 48 (2), 225–227.

Cairncross, J.G., Macdonald, D.R., Ramsay, D.A., 1992. Aggressive oligodendroglioma: a chemosensitive tumor. Neurosurgery 31 (1), 78–82.

Cairncross, J.G., Ueki, K., Zlatescu, M.C., et al., 1998. Specific genetic predictors of chemotherapeutic response and survival in patients with anaplastic oligodendrogliomas. J. Natl. Cancer Inst. 90 (19), 1473–1479.

CBTRUS, 2006. Central Brain Tumor Registry of the United States. Available at: www.cbtrus.org.

Celli, P., Nofrone, I., Palma, L., et al., 1994. Cerebral oligodendroglioma: prognostic factors and life history. Neurosurgery 35 (6), 1018–1034; discussion 1034–1015.

Cenacchi, G., Giangaspero, F., Cerasoli, S., et al., 1996. Ultrastructural characterization of oligodendroglial-like cells in central nervous system tumors. Ultrastruct. Pathol. 20 (6), 537–547.

Chan, A.S., Leung, S.Y., Wong, M.P., et al., 1998. Expression of vascular endothelial growth factor and its receptors in the anaplastic progression of astrocytoma, oligodendroglioma, and ependymoma. Am. J. Surg. Pathol. 22 (7), 816–826.

Chang, E.F., Potts, M.B., Keles, G.E., et al., 2008. Seizure characteristics and control following resection in 332 patients with low-grade gliomas. J. Neurosurg. 108 (2), 227–235.

Chin, H.W., Hazel, J.J., Kim, T.H., et al., 1980. Oligodendrogliomas. I. A clinical study of cerebral oligodendrogliomas. Cancer 45 (6), 1458–1466.

Choi, B.H., Kim, R.C., 1984. Expression of glial fibrillary acidic protein in immature oligodendroglia. Science 223 (4634), 407–409.

Christov, C., Adle-Biassette, H., Le Guerinel, C., et al., 1998. Immunohistochemical detection of vascular endothelial growth factor (VEGF) in the vasculature of oligodendrogliomas. Neuropathol. Appl. Neurobiol. 24 (1), 29–35.

Claus, E.B., Horlacher, A., Hsu, L., et al., 2005. Survival rates in patients with low-grade glioma after intraoperative magnetic resonance image guidance. Cancer 103 (6), 1227–1233.

Coons, S.W., Johnson, P.C., Pearl, D.K., 1997. The prognostic significance of Ki-67 labeling indices for oligodendrogliomas. Neurosurgery 41 (4), 878–884; discussion 884–875.

Cooper, E.R., 1935. The relation of oligodendrocytes and astrocytes in cerebral tumours. J. Pathol. Bacteriol. 41, 259–266.

Dam, A.M., Fuglsang-Frederiksen, A., Svarre-Olsen, U., et al., 1985. Late-onset epilepsy: etiologies, types of seizure, and value of clinical investigation, EEG, and computerized tomography scan. Epilepsia 26 (3), 227–231.

Daumas-Duport, C., Tucker, M.L., Kolles, H., et al., 1997. Oligodendrogliomas. Part II: A new grading system based on morphological and imaging criteria. J. Neurooncol 34 (1), 61–78.

Davies, E., Clarke, C., Hopkins, A., 1996. Malignant cerebral glioma II: Perspectives of patients and relatives on the value of radiotherapy. BMJ 313 (7071), 1512–1516.

de la Monte, S.M., 1990. Immunohistochemical diagnosis of nervous system neoplasms. Clin. Lab. Med. 10 (1), 151–178.

Deckert, M., Reifenberger, G., Wechsler, W., 1989. Determination of the proliferative potential of human brain tumors using the monoclonal antibody Ki-67. J. Cancer Res. Clin. Oncol. 115 (2), 179–188.

Dehghani, F., Schachenmayr, W., Laun, A., et al., 1998. Prognostic implication of histopathological, immunohistochemical and clinical features of oligodendrogliomas: a study of 89 cases. Acta. Neuropathol. 95 (5), 493–504.

Derlon, J.M., Cabal, P., Blaizot, X., et al., 2005. [Metabolic imaging for supratentorial oligodendrogliomas]. Neurochirurgie 51 (3–4 Pt 2), 309–322.

Derlon, J.M., Petit-Taboue, M.C., Chapon, F., et al., 1997. The in vivo metabolic pattern of low-grade brain gliomas: a positron emission tomographic study using 18F-fluorodeoxyglucose and 11C-L-methylmethionine. Neurosurgery 40 (2), 276–287; discussion 287–278.

Di Rocco, F., Carroll, R.S., Zhang, J., et al., 1998. Platelet-derived growth factor and its receptor expression in human oligodendrogliomas. Neurosurgery 42 (2), 341–346.

Dohrmann, G.J., Farwell, J.R., Flannery, J.T., 1978. Oligodendrogliomas in children. Surg. Neurol. 10 (1), 21–25.

Dong, S., Pang, J.C., Hu, J., et al., 2002. Transcriptional inactivation of TP73 expression in oligodendroglial tumors. Int. J. Cancer 98 (3), 370–375.

Earnest, F. 3rd, Kernohan, J.W., Craig, W.M., 1950. Oligodendrogliomas; a review of 200 cases. Arch. Neurol. Psychiatry 63 (6), 964–976.

Ekstrand, A.J., James, C.D., Cavenee, W.K., et al., 1991. Genes for epidermal growth factor receptor, transforming growth factor alpha, and epidermal growth factor and their expression in human gliomas in vivo. Cancer Res. 51 (8), 2164–2172.

El-Hateer, H., Souhami, L., Roberge, D., et al., 2009. Low-grade oligodendroglioma: an indolent but incurable disease? Clinical article. J. Neurosurg. 111 (2), 265–271.

Eoli, M., Bissola, L., Bruzzone, M.G., et al., 2006. Reclassification of oligoastrocytomas by loss of heterozygosity studies. Int. J. Cancer 119 (1), 84–90.

Felsberg, J., Erkwoh, A., Sabel, M.C., et al., 2004. Oligodendroglial tumors: refinement of candidate regions on chromosome arm 1p and correlation of 1p/19q status with survival. Brain Pathol. 14 (2), 121–130.

Forsyth, P.A., Posner, J.B., 1993. Headaches in patients with brain tumors: a study of 111 patients. Neurology 43 (9), 1678–1683.

Fortuna, A., Celli, P., Palma, L., 1980. Oligodendrogliomas of the spinal cord. Acta. Neurochir. (Wien) 52 (3–4), 305–329.

Gannett, D.E., Wisbeck, W.M., Silbergeld, D.L., et al., 1994. The role of postoperative irradiation in the treatment of oligodendroglioma. Int. J. Radiat. Oncol. Biol. Phys. 30 (3), 567–573.

Giannini, C., Burger, P.C., Berkey, B.A., et al., 2008. Anaplastic oligodendroglial tumors: refining the correlation among histopathology, 1p 19q deletion and clinical outcome in Intergroup Radiation Therapy Oncology Group Trial 9402. Brain Pathol. 18 (3), 360–369.

Giannini, C., Scheithauer, B.W., Weaver, A.L., et al., 2001. Oligodendrogliomas: reproducibility and prognostic value of histologic diagnosis and grading. J. Neuropathol. Exp. Neurol. 60 (3), 248–262.

Glass, J., Hochberg, F.H., Gruber, M.L., et al., 1992. The treatment of oligodendrogliomas and mixed oligodendroglioma-astrocytomas with PCV chemotherapy. J. Neurosurg. 76 (5), 741–745.

Griffin, C.A., Burger, P., Morsberger, L., et al., 2006. Identification of der(1; 19)(q10; p10) in five oligodendrogliomas suggests mechanism of concurrent 1p and 19q loss. J. Neuropathol. Exp. Neurol. 65 (10), 988–994.

Gugino, L.D., Aglio, L.S., Black, P.M., 2000. Cortical stimulation techniques. In: Kaye, A.H., Black, P.M. Operative neurosurgery. Churchill Livingstone, London, p. 85.

Hart, M.G., Grant, R., Metcalfe, S.E., 2004. Biopsy versus resection for malignant glioma. Cochrane Database of Systematic Reviews CD002034.

Hart, M.N., Petito, C.K., Earle, K.M., 1974. Mixed gliomas. Cancer 33 (1), 134–140.

Heegaard, S., Sommer, H.M., Broholm, H., et al., 1995. Proliferating cell nuclear antigen and Ki-67 immunohistochemistry of oligodendrogliomas with special reference to prognosis. Cancer 76 (10), 1809–1813.

Helseth, A., Mork, S.J., 1989. Neoplasms of the central nervous system in Norway. III. Epidemiological characteristics of intracranial gliomas according to histology. APMIS 97 (6), 547–555.

Henry, R.G., Berman, J.I., Nagarajan, S.S., et al., 2004. Subcortical pathways serving cortical language sites: initial experience with diffusion tensor imaging fiber tracking combined with intraoperative language mapping. Neuroimage 21 (2), 616–622.

Henson, J.W., Gaviani, P., Gonzalez, R.G., 2005. MRI in treatment of adult gliomas. Lancet Oncol. 6 (3), 167–175.

Hildebrand, J., Lecaille, C., Perennes, J., et al., 2005. Epileptic seizures during follow-up of patients treated for primary brain tumors. Neurology 65 (2), 212–215.

Hinton, D.R., Dolan, E., Sima, A.A., 1984. The value of histopathological examination of surgically removed blood clot in determining the etiology of spontaneous intracerebral hemorrhage. Stroke 15 (3), 517–520.

Hirsch, J.F., Sainte Rose, C., Pierre-Kahn, A., et al., 1989. Benign astrocytic and oligodendrocytic tumors of the cerebral hemispheres in children. J. Neurosurg. 70 (4), 568–572.

Hong, C., Bollen, A.W., Costello, J.F., 2003. The contribution of genetic and epigenetic mechanisms to gene silencing in oligodendrogliomas. Cancer Res. 63 (22), 7600–7605.

Horrax, G., Wu, W.Q., 1951. Postoperative survival of patients with intracranial oligodendroglioma with special reference to radical tumor removal; a study of 26 patients. J. Neurosurg. 8 (5), 473–479.

Hsu, Y.Y., Chang, C.N., Wie, K.J., et al., 2004. Proton magnetic resonance spectroscopic imaging of cerebral gliomas: correlation of metabolite ratios with histopathologic grading. Chang Gung Med. J. 27 (6), 399–407.

Jaeckle, K.A., Ballman, K.V., Rao, R.D., et al., 2006. Current strategies in treatment of oligodendroglioma: evolution of molecular signatures of response. J. Clin. Oncol. 24 (8), 1246–1252.

Jaskolsky, D., Zawirski, M., Papierz, W., et al., 1987. Mixed gliomas. Their clinical course and results of surgery. Zentralbl. Neurochir. 48 (2), 120–123.

Jenkins, R.B., Blair, H., Ballman, K.V., et al., 2006. A t(1; 19)(q10; p10) mediates the combined deletions of 1p and 19q and predicts a better prognosis of patients with oligodendroglioma. Cancer Res. 66 (20), 9852–9861.

Jenkinson, M.D., du Plessis, D.G., Smith, T.S., et al., 2006. Histological growth patterns and genotype in oligodendroglial tumours: correlation with MRI features. Brain 129 (Pt 7), 1884–1891.

Jeuken, J.W., von Deimling, A., Wesseling, P., 2004. Molecular pathogenesis of oligodendroglial tumors. J. Neurooncol. 70 (2), 161–181.

Kaloshi, G., Benouaich-Amiel, A., Diakite, F., et al., 2007. Temozolomide for low-grade gliomas: predictive impact of 1p/19q loss on response and outcome. Neurology 68 (21), 1831–1836.

Kanner, A.A., Staugaitis, S.M., Castilla, E.A., et al., 2006. The impact of genotype on outcome in oligodendroglioma: validation of the loss of chromosome arm 1p as an important factor in clinical decision making. J. Neurosurg. 104 (4), 542–550.

Karim, A.B., Maat, B., Hatlevoll, R., et al., 1996. A randomized trial on dose-response in radiation therapy of low-grade cerebral glioma: European Organization for Research and Treatment of Cancer (EORTC) Study 22844. Int. J. Radiat Oncol. Biol. Phys. 36 (3), 549–556.

Keles, G.E., Lamborn, K.R., Berger, M.S., 2001. Low-grade hemispheric gliomas in adults: a critical review of extent of resection as a factor influencing outcome. J. Neurosurg. 95 (5), 735–745.

Kim, L., Hochberg, F.H., Thornton, A.F., et al., 1996. Procarbazine, lomustine, and vincristine (PCV) chemotherapy for grade III and grade IV oligoastrocytomas. J. Neurosurg. 85 (4), 602–607.

Kraus, J.A., Koopmann, J., Kaskel, P., et al., 1995. Shared allelic losses on chromosomes 1p and 19q suggest a common origin of oligodendroglioma and oligoastrocytoma. J. Neuropathol. Exp. Neurol. 54 (1), 91–95.

Kros, J.M., Gorlia, T., Kouwenhoven, M.C., et al., 2007. Panel review of anaplastic oligodendroglioma from European Organization For Research and Treatment of Cancer Trial 26951: assessment of consensus in diagnosis, influence of 1p/19q loss, and correlations with outcome. J. Neuropathol. Exp. Neurol. 66 (6), 545–551.

Kros, J.M., Hop, W.C., Godschalk, J.J., et al., 1996. Prognostic value of the proliferation-related antigen Ki-67 in oligodendrogliomas. Cancer 78 (5), 1107–1113.

Kros, J.M., Pieterman, H., van Eden, C.G., et al., 1994. Oligodendroglioma: the Rotterdam-Dijkzigt experience. Neurosurgery 34 (6), 959–966; discussion 966.

Kros, J.M., Stefanko, S.Z., de Jong, A.A., et al., 1991. Ultrastructural and immunohistochemical segregation of gemistocytic subsets. Hum. Pathol. 22 (1), 33–40.

Kros, J.M., Troost, D., van Eden, C.G., et al., 1988. Oligodendroglioma. A comparison of two grading systems. Cancer 61 (11), 2251–2259.

Kros, J.M., van den Brink, W.A., van Loon-van Luyt, J.J., et al., 1997. Signet-ring cell oligodendroglioma–report of two cases and discussion of the differential diagnosis. Acta. Neuropathol. 93 (6), 638–643.

Kros, J.M., Van Eden, C.G., Stefanko, S.Z., et al., 1990. Prognostic implications of glial fibrillary acidic protein containing cell types in oligodendrogliomas. Cancer 66 (6), 1204–1212.

Kujas, M., Lejeune, J., Benouaich-Amiel, A., et al., 2005. Chromosome 1p loss: a favorable prognostic factor in low-grade gliomas. Ann. Neurol. 58 (2), 322–326.

Kyritsis, A.P., Yung, W.K., Bruner, J., et al., 1993. The treatment of anaplastic oligodendrogliomas and mixed gliomas. Neurosurgery 32 (3), 365–370; discussion 371.

Laack, N.N., Brown, P.D., 2004. Cognitive sequelae of brain radiation in adults. Semin. Oncol. 31 (5), 702–713.

Law, M., Yang, S., Wang, H., et al., 2003. Glioma grading: sensitivity, specificity, and predictive values of perfusion MR imaging and proton MR spectroscopic imaging compared with conventional MR imaging. AJNR. Am. J. Neuroradiol. 24 (10), 1989–1998.

Laws, E.R. Jr., Taylor, W.F., Clifton, M.B., et al., 1984. Neurosurgical management of low-grade astrocytoma of the cerebral hemispheres. J. Neurosurg. 61 (4), 665–673.

Lebrun, C., Fontaine, D., Ramaioli, A., et al., 2004. Long-term outcome of oligodendrogliomas. Neurology 62 (10), 1783–1787.

Lee, C., Duncan, V.W., Young, A.B., 1998. Magnetic resonance features of the enigmatic oligodendroglioma. Invest. Radiol. 33 (4), 222–231.

Lee, T.K., Nakasu, Y., Jeffree, M.A., et al., 1989. Indolent glioma: a cause of epilepsy. Arch. Dis. Child. 64 (12), 1666–1671.

Lee, Y.Y., Van Tassel, P., 1989. Intracranial oligodendrogliomas: imaging findings in 35 untreated cases. AJR Am. J. Roentgenol. 152 (2), 361–369.

Leighton, C., Fisher, B., Bauman, G., et al., 1997. Supratentorial low-grade glioma in adults: an analysis of prognostic factors and timing of radiation. J. Clin. Oncol. 15 (4), 1294–1301.

Lev, M.H., Ozsunar, Y., Henson, J.W., et al., 2004. Glial tumor grading and outcome prediction using dynamic spin-echo MR susceptibility mapping compared with conventional contrast-enhanced MR: confounding effect of elevated rCBV of oligodendrogliomas [corrected]. AJNR Am. J. Neuroradiol. 25 (2), 214–221.

Levin, V.A., Silver, P., Hannigan, J., et al., 1990. Superiority of post-radiotherapy adjuvant chemotherapy with CCNU, procarbazine, and vincristine (PCV) over BCNU for anaplastic gliomas: NCOG 6G61 final report. Int. J. Radiat. Oncol. Biol. Phys. 18 (2), 321–324.

Ligon, K.L., Alberta, J.A., Kho, A.T., et al., 2004. The oligodendroglial lineage marker OLIG2 is universally expressed in diffuse gliomas. J. Neuropathol. Exp. Neurol. 63 (5), 499–509.

Lindegaard, K.F., Mork, S.J., Eide, G.E., et al., 1987. Statistical analysis of clinicopathological features, radiotherapy, and survival in 170 cases of oligodendroglioma. J. Neurosurg. 67 (2), 224–230.

Ludwig, C.L., Smith, M.T., Godfrey, A.D., et al., 1986. A clinicopathological study of 323 patients with oligodendrogliomas. Ann. Neurol. 19 (1), 15–21.

Macdonald, D.R., 1994. Low-grade gliomas, mixed gliomas, and oligodendrogliomas. Semin. Oncol. 21 (2), 236–248.

Macdonald, D.R., Gaspar, L.E., Cairncross, J.G., 1990. Successful chemotherapy for newly diagnosed aggressive oligodendroglioma. Ann. Neurol. 27 (5), 573–574.

Macdonald, D.R., O'Brien, R.A., Gilbert, J.J., et al., 1989. Metastatic anaplastic oligodendroglioma. Neurology 39 (12), 1593–1596.

Magnani, I., Guerneri, S., Pollo, B., et al., 1994. Increasing complexity of the karyotype in 50 human gliomas. Progressive evolution and de novo occurrence of cytogenetic alterations. Cancer Genet Cytogenet 75 (2), 77–89.

Mandonnet, E., Delattre, J.Y., Tanguy, M.L., et al., 2003. Continuous growth of mean tumor diameter in a subset of grade II gliomas. Ann. Neurol. 53 (4), 524–528.

Margain, D., Peretti-Viton, P., Perez-Castillo, A.M., et al., 1991. Oligodendrogliomas. J. Neuroradiol. 18 (2), 153–160.

Mason, W.P., Krol, G.S., DeAngelis, L.M., 1996. Low-grade oligodendroglioma responds to chemotherapy. Neurology 46 (1), 203–207.

McDonald, J.M., Dunlap, S., Cogdell, D., et al., 2006. The SHREW1 gene, frequently deleted in oligodendrogliomas, functions to inhibit cell adhesion and migration. Cancer Biol. Ther. 5 (3), 300–304.

McDonald, J.M., Dunmire, V., Taylor, E., et al., 2005. Attenuated expression of DFFB is a hallmark of oligodendrogliomas with 1p-allelic loss. Mol. Cancer 4, 35.

McGirt, M.J., Chaichana, K.L., Attenello, F.J., et al., 2008. Extent of surgical resection is independently associated with survival in patients with hemispheric infiltrating low-grade gliomas. Neurosurgery 63 (4), 700–707; author reply 707–708.

Megyesi, J.F., Kachur, E., Lee, D.H., et al., 2004. Imaging correlates of molecular signatures in oligodendrogliomas. Clin. Cancer Res. 10 (13), 4303–4306.

Merrell, R., Nabors, L.B., Perry, A., et al., 2006. 1p/19q chromosome deletions in metastatic oligodendroglioma. J. Neurooncol. 80 (2), 203–207.

Miller, C.R., Dunham, C.P., Scheithauer, B.W., et al., 2006. Significance of necrosis in grading of oligodendroglial neoplasms: a clinicopathologic and genetic study of newly diagnosed high-grade gliomas. J. Clin. Oncol. 24 (34), 5419–5426.

Mollemann, M., Wolter, M., Felsberg, J., et al., 2005. Frequent promoter hypermethylation and low expression of the MGMT gene in oligodendroglial tumors. Int. J. Cancer 113 (3), 379–385.

Mork, S.J., Lindegaard, K.F., Halvorsen, T.B., et al., 1985. Oligodendroglioma: incidence and biological behavior in a defined population. J. Neurosurg. 63 (6), 881–889.

Morris, H.H., Estes, M.L., Gilmore, R., et al., 1993. Chronic intractable epilepsy as the only symptom of primary brain tumor. Epilepsia 34 (6), 1038–1043.

Mueller, W., Hartmann, C., Hoffmann, A., et al., 2002. Genetic signature of oligoastrocytomas correlates with tumor location and denotes distinct molecular subsets. Am. J. Pathol. 161 (1), 313–319.

Muller, W., Afra, D., Schroder, R., 1977. Supratentorial recurrences of gliomas. Morphological studies in relation to time intervals with oligodendrogliomas. Acta. Neurochir. (Wien) 39 (1–2), 15–25.

Nakagawa, Y., Perentes, E., Rubinstein, L.J., 1986. Immunohistochemical characterization of oligodendrogliomas: an analysis of multiple markers. Acta. Neuropathol. 72 (1), 15–22.

Nakagawa, Y., Perentes, E., Rubinstein, L.J., 1987. Non-specificity of anti-carbonic anhydrase C antibody as a marker in human neurooncology. J. Neuropathol. Exp. Neurol. 46 (4), 451–460.

Nijjar, T.S., Simpson, W.J., Gadalla, T., et al., 1993. Oligodendroglioma. The Princess Margaret Hospital experience (1958–1984). Cancer 71 (12), 4002–4006.

Nutt, C.L., 2005. Molecular genetics of oligodendrogliomas: a model for improved clinical management in the field of neurooncology. Neurosurg. Focus 19 (5), E2.

Ogasawara, H., Kiya, K., Uozumi, T., et al., 1990. Multiple oligodendroglioma – case report. Neurol. Med. Chir. (Tokyo) 30 (2), 127–131.

Ohgaki, H., Eibl, R.H., Wiestler, O.D., et al., 1991. p53 mutations in nonastrocytic human brain tumors. Cancer Res. 51 (22), 6202–6205.

Ohgaki, H., Kleihues, P., 2005. Population-based studies on incidence, survival rates, and genetic alterations in astrocytic and oligodendroglial gliomas. J. Neuropathol. Exp. Neurol. 64 (6), 479–489.

Okamoto, Y., Di Patre, P.L., Burkhard, C., et al., 2004. Population-based study on incidence, survival rates, and genetic alterations of low-grade diffuse astrocytomas and oligodendrogliomas. Acta. Neuropathol. 108 (1), 49–56.

Olson, J.D., Riedel, E., DeAngelis, L.M., 2000. Long-term outcome of low-grade oligodendroglioma and mixed glioma. Neurology 54 (7), 1442–1448.

Packer, R.J., Sutton, L.N., Rorke, L.B., et al., 1985. Oligodendroglioma of the posterior fossa in childhood. Cancer 56 (1), 195–199.

Pagni, C.A., Canavero, S., Gaidolfi, E., 1991. Intramedullary 'holocord' oligodendroglioma: case report. Acta. Neurochir. (Wien) 113 (1–2), 96–99.

Paleologos, N.A., Macdonald, D.R., Vick, N.A., et al., 1999. Neoadjuvant procarbazine, CCNU, and vincristine for anaplastic and aggressive oligodendroglioma. Neurology 53 (5), 1141–1143.

Perry, A., Scheithauer, B.W., Macaulay, R.J., et al., 2002. Oligodendrogliomas with neurocytic differentiation. A report of 4 cases with diagnostic and histogenetic implications. J. Neuropathol. Exp. Neurol. 61 (11), 947–955.

Perry, J.R., Louis, D.N., Cairncross, J.G., 1999. Current treatment of oligodendrogliomas. Arch. Neurol. 56 (4), 434–436.

Pirotte, B., Goldman, S., Massager, N., et al., 2004. Comparison of 18F-FDG and 11C-methionine for PET-guided stereotactic brain biopsy of gliomas. J. Nucl. Med. 45 (8), 1293–1298.

Poisson, M., Pereon, Y., Chiras, J., et al., 1991. Treatment of recurrent malignant supratentorial gliomas with carboplatin (CBDCA). J. Neurooncol. 10 (2), 139–144.

Postma, T.J., Klein, M., Verstappen, C.C., et al., 2002. Radiotherapy-induced cerebral abnormalities in patients with low-grade glioma. Neurology 59 (1), 121–123.

Ransom, D.T., Ritland, S.R., Kimmel, D.W., et al., 1992. Cytogenetic and loss of heterozygosity studies in ependymomas, pilocytic astrocytomas, and oligodendrogliomas. Genes Chromosomes Cancer 5 (4), 348–356.

Recht, L.D., Lew, R., Smith, T.W., 1992. Suspected low-grade glioma: is deferring treatment safe? Ann. Neurol. 31 (4), 431–436.

Reedy, D.P., Bay, J.W., Hahn, J.F., 1983. Role of radiation therapy in the treatment of cerebral oligodendroglioma: an analysis of 57 cases and a literature review. Neurosurgery 13 (5), 499–503.

Reifenberger, G., Kros, J.M., Louis, D.N., et al., 2007a. Anaplastic oligodendroglioma. In: Louis, D.N., Ohgaki, H., Wiestler, O.D., et al. (Eds.), WHO Classification of Tumours of the Central Nervous System. IARC Press, Lyon, pp. 60–62.

Reifenberger, G., Kros, J.M., Louis, D.N., et al., 2007b. Oligodendroglioma. In: Louis, D.N., Ohgaki, H., Wiestler, O.D., et al. (Eds.), WHO Classification of Tumours of the Central Nervous System. IARC Press, Lyon, pp. 54–59.

Reifenberger, G., Louis, D.N., 2003. Oligodendroglioma: toward molecular definitions in diagnostic neuro-oncology. J. Neuropathol. Exp. Neurol. 62 (2), 111–126.

Reifenberger, G., Szymas, J., Wechsler, W., 1987. Differential expression of glial- and neuronal-associated antigens in human tumors of the central and peripheral nervous system. Acta. Neuropathol. 74 (2), 105–123.

Reifenberger, J., Reifenberger, G., Ichimura, K., et al., 1996. Epidermal growth factor receptor expression in oligodendroglial tumors. Am. J. Pathol. 149 (1), 29–35.

Reifenberger, J., Reifenberger, G., Liu, L., et al., 1994. Molecular genetic analysis of oligodendroglial tumors shows preferential allelic deletions on 19q and 1p. Am. J. Pathol. 145 (5), 1175–1190.

Riemenschneider, M.J., Koy, T.H., Reifenberger, G., 2004. Expression of oligodendrocyte lineage genes in oligodendroglial and astrocytic gliomas. Acta. Neuropathol. 107 (3), 277–282.

Ringertz, N., 1950. Grading of gliomas. Acta. Pathol. Microbiol. Scand. 27 (1), 51–64.

Roberts, M., German, W.J., 1966. A long term study of patients with oligodendrogliomas. Follow-up of 50 cases, including Dr. Harvey Cushing's series. J. Neurosurg. 24 (4), 697–700.

Roerig, P., Nessling, M., Radlwimmer, B., et al., 2005. Molecular classification of human gliomas using matrix-based comparative genomic hybridization. Int. J. Cancer 117 (1), 95–103.

Rubinstein, L.J., 1972. Oligodendrogliomas. Tumors of the Central Nervous System. Armed Forces Institute of Pathology, Washington DC, pp. 85–104.

Russell, D.S., Rubinstein, L.J., 1977. Oligodendroglioma. Pathology of tumors of the central nervous system. Edward Arnold, London.

Saarinen, U.M., Pihko, H., Makipernaa, A., 1990. High-dose thiotepa with autologous bone marrow rescue in recurrent malignant oligodendroglioma: a case report. J. Neurooncol. 9 (1), 57–61.

Sandberg-Wollheim, M., Malmstrom, P., Stromblad, L.G., et al., 1991. A randomized study of chemotherapy with procarbazine, vincristine, and lomustine with and without radiation therapy for astrocytoma grades 3 and/or 4. Cancer 68 (1), 22–29.

Sandeman, D.R., Sandeman, A.P., Buxton, P., et al., 1990. The management of patients with an intrinsic supratentorial brain tumour. Br. J. Neurosurg. 4 (4), 299–312.

Sasaki, H., Zlatescu, M.C., Betensky, R.A., et al., 2001. PTEN is a target of chromosome 10q loss in anaplastic oligodendrogliomas and PTEN alterations are associated with poor prognosis. Am. J. Pathol. 159 (1), 359–367.

Schiffer, D., Dutto, A., Cavalla, P., et al., 1997. Prognostic factors in oligodendroglioma. Can. J. Neurol. Sci. 24 (4), 313–319.

Schwechheimer, K., Gass, P., Berlet, H.H., 1992. Expression of oligodendroglia and Schwann cell markers in human nervous system tumors. An immunomorphological study and western blot analysis. Acta. Neuropathol. 83 (3), 283–291.

Scopece, L., Franceschi, E., Cavallo, G., et al., 2006. Carboplatin and etoposide (CE) chemotherapy in patients with recurrent or progressive oligodendroglial tumors. J. Neurooncol. 79 (3), 299–305.

Shaffrey, M.E., Farace, E., Schiff, D., et al., 2005. The Ki-67 labeling index as a prognostic factor in Grade II oligoastrocytomas. J. Neurosurg. 102 (6), 1033–1039.

Shaw, E., Arusell, R., Scheithauer, B., et al., 2002. Prospective randomized trial of low- versus high-dose radiation therapy in adults with supratentorial low-grade glioma: initial report of a North Central Cancer Treatment Group/Radiation Therapy Oncology Group/Eastern Cooperative Oncology Group study. J. Clin. Oncol. 20 (9), 2267–2276.

Shaw, E.G., Scheithauer, B.W., O'Fallon, J.R., et al., 1994. Mixed oligoastrocytomas: a survival and prognostic factor analysis. Neurosurgery 34 (4), 577–582; discussion 582.

Shaw, E.G., Scheithauer, B.W., O'Fallon, J.R., et al., 1992. Oligodendrogliomas: the Mayo Clinic experience. J. Neurosurg. 76 (3), 428–434.

Shaw, E.G., Tatter, S.B., Lesser, G.J., et al., 2004. Current controversies in the radiotherapeutic management of adult low-grade glioma. Semin. Oncol. 31 (5), 653–658.

Sheline, G.E., Boldrey, E., Karlsberg, P., et al., 1964. Therapeutic considerations in tumors affecting the central nervous system: oligodendrogliomas. Radiology 82, 84–89.

Shibata, T., Burger, P.C., Kleihues, P., 1988. Ki-67 immunoperoxidase stain as marker for the histological grading of nervous system tumours. Acta. Neurochir. Suppl. (Wien) 43, 103–106.

Shih, A.H., Holland, E.C., 2004. Developmental neurobiology and the origin of brain tumors. J. Neurooncol. 70 (2), 125–136.

Shimizu, K.T., Tran, L.M., Mark, R.J., et al., 1993. Management of oligodendrogliomas. Radiology 186 (2), 569–572.

Smith, D.F., Hutton, J.L., Sandemann, D., et al., 1991. The prognosis of primary intracerebral tumours presenting with epilepsy: the outcome of medical and surgical management. J. Neurol. Neurosurg. Psychiatry 54 (10), 915–920.

Smith, J.S., Chang, E.F., Lamborn, K.R., et al., 2008. Role of extent of resection in the long-term outcome of low-grade hemispheric gliomas. J. Clin. Oncol. 26 (8), 1338–1345.

Smith, J.S., Perry, A., Borell, T.J., et al., 2000. Alterations of chromosome arms 1p and 19q as predictors of survival in oligodendrogliomas, astrocytomas, and mixed oligoastrocytomas. J. Clin. Oncol. 18 (3), 636–645.

Smith, M.T., Ludwig, C.L., Godfrey, A.D., et al., 1983. Grading of oligodendrogliomas. Cancer 52 (11), 2107–2114.

Soffietti, R., 1990. Histologic and clinical factors of prognostic significance in astrocytic gliomas. J. Neurosurg. Sci. 34 (3–4), 231–234.

Soffietti, R., Nobile, M., Ruda, R., et al., 2004. Second-line treatment with carboplatin for recurrent or progressive oligodendroglial tumors after PCV (procarbazine, lomustine, and vincristine) chemotherapy: a phase II study. Cancer 100 (4), 807–813.

Spicer, M.A., Apuzzo, M.L., 2005. Image-guided surgery. In: Black, P.M., Loeffler, J.S. Cancer of the nervous system, second ed. Lippincott, Williams and Wilkins, Philadelphia, PA, p. 155.

Stupp, R., Mason, W.P., van den Bent, M.J., et al., 2005. Radiotherapy plus concomitant and adjuvant temozolomide for glioblastoma. N. Engl. J. Med. 352 (10), 987–996.

Sugahara, T., Korogi, Y., Kochi, M., et al., 1998. Correlation of MR imaging-determined cerebral blood volume maps with histologic and angiographic determination of vascularity of gliomas. AJR Am. J. Roentgenol. 171 (6), 1479–1486.

Sun, Z.M., Genka, S., Shitara, N., et al., 1988. Factors possibly influencing the prognosis of oligodendroglioma. Neurosurgery 22 (5), 886–891.

Sung, C.C., Collins, R., Li, J., et al., 1996. Glycolipids and myelin proteins in human oligodendrogliomas. Glycoconj. J. 13 (3), 433–443.

Talos, I.F., Zou, K.H., Ohno-Machado, L., et al., 2006. Supratentorial low-grade glioma resectability: statistical predictive analysis based on anatomic MR features and tumor characteristics. Radiology 239 (2), 506–513.

Taphoorn, M.J., 2003. Neurocognitive sequelae in the treatment of low-grade gliomas. Semin. Oncol. 30 (6 Suppl. 19), 45–48.

Taphoorn, M.J., Klein, M., 2004. Cognitive deficits in adult patients with brain tumours. Lancet Neurol. 3 (3), 159–168.

Taylor, M., Bernstein, M., Perry, J., et al., 2004. Surgical management of malignant glioma. Evidence Summary Report No. 9/8, Program in Evidence Based Care. Cancer Care, Ontario.

Tekkok, I.H., Ayberk, G., Saglam, S., et al., 1992. Primary intraventricular oligodendroglioma. Neurochirurgia. (Stuttg) 35 (2), 63–66.

Thiel, G., Losanowa, T., Kintzel, D., et al., 1992. Karyotypes in 90 human gliomas. Cancer Genet Cytogenet 58 (2), 109–120.

Triebels, V.H., Taphoorn, M.J., Brandes, A.A., et al., 2004. Salvage PCV chemotherapy for temozolomide-resistant oligodendrogliomas. Neurology 63 (5), 904–906.

Trouillard, O., Aguirre-Cruz, L., Hoang-Xuan, K., et al., 2004. Parental 19q loss and PEG3 expression in oligodendrogliomas. Cancer Genet Cytogenet 151 (2), 182–183.

Tucha, O., Smely, C., Preier, M., et al., 2000. Cognitive deficits before treatment among patients with brain tumors. Neurosurgery 47 (2), 324–333; discussion 333–324.

van den Bent, M.J., Afra, D., de Witte, O., et al., 2005. Long-term efficacy of early versus delayed radiotherapy for low-grade astrocytoma and oligodendroglioma in adults: the EORTC 22845 randomised trial. Lancet 366 (9490), 985–990.

van den Bent, M.J., Carpentier, A.F., Brandes, A.A., et al., 2006a. Adjuvant procarbazine, lomustine, and vincristine improves progression-free survival but not overall survival in newly diagnosed anaplastic oligodendrogliomas and oligoastrocytomas: a randomized European Organisation for Research and Treatment of Cancer phase III trial. J. Clin. Oncol. 24 (18), 2715–2722.

van den Bent, M.J., Hegi, M.E., Stupp, R., 2006b Recent developments in the use of chemotherapy in brain tumours. Eur. J. Cancer 42 (5), 582–588.

van den Bent, M.J., Keime-Guibert, F., Brandes, A.A., et al., 2001. Temozolomide chemotherapy in recurrent oligodendroglioma. Neurology 57 (2), 340–342.

van den Bent, M.J., Kros, J.M., Heimans, J.J., et al., 1998. Response rate and prognostic factors of recurrent oligodendroglioma treated with procarbazine, CCNU, and vincristine chemotherapy. Dutch Neuro-oncology Group. Neurology 51 (4), 1140–1145.

van den Bent, M.J., Taphoorn, M.J., Brandes, A.A., et al., 2003. Phase II study of first-line chemotherapy with temozolomide in recurrent oligodendroglial tumors: the European Organization for Research and Treatment of Cancer Brain Tumor Group Study 26971. J. Clin. Oncol. 21 (13), 2525–2528.

Vlieger, E.J., Majoie, C.B., Leenstra, S., et al., 2004. Functional magnetic resonance imaging for neurosurgical planning in neurooncology. Eur. Radiol. 14 (7), 1143–1153.

von Deimling, A., Reifenberger, G., Kros, J.M., et al., 2007a Anaplastic oligoastrocytoma. In: Louis, D.N., Ohgaki, H., Wiestler, O.D., et al. (Eds.), WHO Classification of Tumours of the Central Nervous System. IARC Press, Lyon, pp. 66–67.

von Deimling, A., Reifenberger, G., Kros, J.M., et al., 2007b. Oligoastrocytoma. In: Louis, D.N., Ohgaki, H., Wiestler, O.D., et al. (Eds.), WHO Classification of Tumours of the Central Nervous System. IARC Press, Lyon, pp. 63–65.

Vuorinen, V., Hinkka, S., Farkkila, M., et al., 2003. Debulking or biopsy of malignant glioma in elderly people – a randomised study. Acta. Neurochir. (Wien) 145 (1), 5–10.

Walker, C., du Plessis, D.G., Fildes, D., et al., 2004. Correlation of molecular genetics with molecular and morphological imaging in gliomas with an oligodendroglial component. Clin. Cancer Res. 10 (21), 7182–7191.

Walker, M., Alexander, E. Jr., Hunt, W., et al., 1978. Evaluation of BCNU and/or radiotherapy in the treatment of anaplastic gliomas. A cooperative clinical trial. J. Neurosurg. 49, 333–343.

Walker, M.D., Green, S.B., Byar, D.P., et al., 1980. Randomized comparisons of radiotherapy and nitrosoureas for the treatment of malignant glioma after surgery. N. Engl. J. Med. 303 (23), 1323–1329.

Wallner, K.E., Gonzales, M., Sheline, G.E., 1988. Treatment of oligodendrogliomas with or without postoperative irradiation. J. Neurosurg. 68 (5), 684–688.

Wharton, S.B., Chan, K.K., Hamilton, F.A., et al., 1998a. Expression of neuronal markers in oligodendrogliomas: an immunohistochemical study. Neuropathol. Appl. Neurobiol. 24 (4), 302–308.

Wharton, S.B., Hamilton, F.A., Chan, W.K., et al., 1998b. Proliferation and cell death in oligodendrogliomas. Neuropathol. Appl. Neurobiol. 24 (1), 21–28.

Whitton, A.C., Bloom, H.J., 1990. Low grade glioma of the cerebral hemispheres in adults: a retrospective analysis of 88 cases. Int. J. Radiat. Oncol. Biol. Phys. 18 (4), 783–786.

Wilkinson, I.M., Anderson, J.R., Holmes, A.E., 1987. Oligodendroglioma: an analysis of 42 cases. J. Neurol. Neurosurg. Psychiatry 50 (3), 304–312.

Winger, M.J., Macdonald, D.R., Cairncross, J.G., 1989. Supratentorial anaplastic gliomas in adults. The prognostic importance of extent of resection and prior low-grade glioma. J. Neurosurg. 71 (4), 487–493.

Wolf, R.M., Draghi, N., Liang, X., et al., 2003. p190RhoGAP can act to inhibit PDGF-induced gliomas in mice: a putative tumor suppressor encoded on human chromosome 19q13.3. Genes Dev. 17 (4), 476–487.

Zlatescu, M.C., TehraniYazdi, A., Sasaki, H., et al., 2001. Tumor location and growth pattern correlate with genetic signature in oligodendroglial neoplasms. Cancer Res. 61 (18), 6713–6715.

23 Brainstem tumors

Katherine E. Warren and Russell R. Lonser

Introduction

Tumors involving the brainstem (defined as the anatomic region between the diencephalon and cervicomedullary junction, for the purposes of this chapter), account for 2% of primary brain tumors in adults and 15–20% of primary brain tumors in children (CBTRUS 2008; Smith 1998). Before the routine use of MRI, brainstem tumors were grouped together and were largely associated with a dismal prognosis. Over the past two decades, improved clinical and histologic classification of brainstem tumors have revealed that these neoplasms are heterogeneous and represent very different entities with distinct biological and clinical features. In this chapter, we will discuss the specific clinical, imaging, histologic, and management features of brainstem gliomas.

Epidemiology and etiology

Epidemiology

Although brainstem gliomas can occur at any age, they most frequently occur in children. More than 75% of brainstem gliomas occur in patients under 20 years of age (Hoffman et al 1980; Pollock et al 1991). Overall, males have a slightly higher predominance than females (estimated male:female ratio of 1.3–1.4:1) (Grigsby et al 1989; Fischbein et al 1996).

Etiology

While the etiology for the majority of brainstem gliomas is unknown, a small fraction is associated with familial and hereditary cancer syndromes. Neurofibromatosis type 1 (NF-1), von Hippel-Lindau disease, tuberous sclerosis, Li-Fraumeni and Turcot's neoplasia syndrome patients have an increased incidence of brain tumors, including brainstem neoplasms (Chen 1998; Albers & Gutmann 2009; Farrell & Plotkin 2009). While mutations associated with these syndromes involve tumor suppressor genes (Farrell & Plotkin 2009), the brainstem tumors associated with these syndromes are variable.

In addition to hereditary neoplasia syndromes, other reported possible etiologies for brainstem gliomas include prior radiation therapy, immunologic defects and environmental or chemical exposures. Although there is anecdotal evidence linking these etiologies to the development of brainstem tumors, no definite associations have been confirmed with the exception of prior use of ionizing radiation to the region of the brainstem (Walter et al 1998; Salvatore et al 1996; Kaplan et al 1997; Inskip et al 2001; Varan et al 2004; Klaeboe et al 2005).

Presentation

The clinical presentation of patients with brainstem gliomas can be variable (Table 23.1). Patients with gliomas of the brainstem can present with both general and localizing signs and symptoms, including cranial nerve dysfunction, ataxia, pupillary abnormalities, papilledema, nystagmus, autonomic dysfunction, and/or headache. Approximately 40% of pediatric patients and 15% of adults with brainstem gliomas will have hydrocephalus and related signs/symptoms at presentation (Fisher et al 2000; Guillamo et al 2001b).

While children with diffuse brainstem gliomas typically present with multiple cranial neuropathies, long-tract signs and cerebellar dysfunction, those with focal lesions can present with an array of symptoms ranging from neuropathy of a single cranial nerve to signs and symptoms of increased intracranial pressure secondary to cerebrospinal fluid obstruction. Subtle symptoms, including behavioral changes, nightmares, night terrors, declining school performance, hyperactivity or loss of interest may be present for several months in children prior to diagnosis. Infants may present with failure to thrive, emesis, macrocephaly, irritability, hyperreflexia, and hypotonia (Maria et al 1993; Shah et al 2008). The most common presenting symptoms in adults include gait disturbance, headache, weakness, and diplopia (Guillamo et al 2001b).

Diagnosis

General

Currently, the diagnosis of brainstem glioma is primarily based on MRI findings. The differential diagnosis includes a variety of other posterior fossa tumors and benign lesions (Kratimenos & Thomas 1993) (Table 23.2). Although many of these may be distinguished by MRI (Maria et al 1993), imaging can be non-specific and it may be necessary to confirm the diagnosis with biopsy in select cases.

Role of biopsy

While imaging techniques have high sensitivity, they are not specific. Clinical studies have shown that MRI can delineate pathological tissue but a radiographic diagnosis may be erroneous in up to 20% of brainstem glioma cases (Franzini et al 1988; Giunta et al 1988; Abernathy et al 1989; Kratimenos & Thomas 1993; Schumacher et al 2007). Biopsy for histologic diagnosis is performed in patients with focal brainstem tumors and patients with atypical presentations or findings on MRI. In a study involving 72 patients aged

Table 23.1 Common presenting features of brainstem gliomas

Type	Common signs and symptoms
DIPG	Cranial neuropathies, ataxia, long tract signs
Focal midbrain	Nightmares/night terrors, emesis, failure to thrive, hemiparesis, cranial neuropathies
Cervicomedullary	Lower cranial nerve dysfunction, motor or sensory dysfunction, pyramidal tract symptoms, emesis, headache, decreased use of upper extremities
Dorsal exophytic	Headache, emesis, signs of increased intracranial pressure
Tectal	Late-onset aqueductal stenosis

Table 23.2 Differential diagnosis of brainstem glioma

Posterior fossa tumors	Benign lesions
Embryonal tumors	Vascular malformations
Ependymomas	Histiocytic lesions
Atypical teratoid-rhabdoid tumors (ATRT)	Granulomas
Gangliogliomas	Demyelinating disease
Primitive neuroectodermal tumors (PNET)	Hemangioblastomas
	Infectious etiologies (parasitic cysts, tuberculomas)
	Multiple sclerosis
	Brainstem encephalitis

2–60 years with brainstem lesions, 61% of biopsied lesions were neoplastic (Kratimenos & Thomas 1993).

The value of performing biopsy has been debated because of the perceived surgical risks, the possibility of non-diagnostic sampling and because histologic grading of gliomas has not been prognostic (Barkovich et al 1990; Maria et al 1993). However, recent data demonstrate that image-directed stereotactic biopsies can provide high diagnostic accuracy (Abernathy et al 1989; Cartmill & Punt 1999) with low morbidity (complications of 1–5%) (Rajshekhar & Chandy 1995; Boviatsis et al 2003; Gonçalves-Ferreira et al 2003). Moreover, biopsy of brainstem lesions has shown that non-neoplastic lesions in the brainstem are prevalent (Kratimenos & Thomas 1993). Samadani and Judy (2003) performed a meta-analysis of 293 biopsies of brainstem lesions in children and adults. Some 96% were diagnostic and morbidity (4%)/mortality (3%), was low. In this study, 31% of lesions were high-grade gliomas, 23% low-grade gliomas, and 10% metastatic disease. In addition, 9% were hematomas, 5% lymphomas, and 3% demyelinating disease. Vascular malformations, cysts, radiation necrosis, vasculitis, infarcts and granulomas were also reported. These authors concluded that stereotactic biopsy of patients with brainstem lesions is safe, diagnostic and indicated given the diverse pathology in the brainstem.

Classification and management

While other CNS tumors are typically described by their radiographic appearance, location, tumor cell type and degree of differentiation, brainstem gliomas are classified non-invasively based on MRI radiographic appearance and location (Fig. 23.1). The most useful classification of brainstem tumors is whether they are *diffuse* or *focal* (including dorsal exophytic, cervicomedullary and tectal sub-types) on MRI. Focal and diffuse brainstem tumors have different prognostic and treatment implications. Generally, diffuse infiltrating tumors are associated with a poor prognosis (Sanford et al 1988) and focal tumors are low-grade lesions associated with a good prognosis (Fischbein et al 1996). Below we describe the specific clinical features and management implications of each brainstem glioma classification type.

Diffuse infiltrating brainstem gliomas

Diffuse pontine gliomas

Epidemiology
The majority of diffuse brainstem tumors have their epicenter in the ventral pons and cause diffuse, often symmetrical expansion (Fig. 23.2). Diffuse intrinsic pontine gliomas (DIPGs) represent up to 75–80% of brainstem tumors in children and 45–50% of adult brainstem tumors (Epstein & Farmer 1993; Guillamo et al 2001b; Salmaggi et al 2008). They frequently strike children between 5 and 10 years of age, and adults between 20 and 30 years (Laigle-Donadey et al 2008).

Presentation
Signs and symptoms of DIPG result from its involvement of cranial nerves/nuclei, corticospinal tracts, and cerebellum. The classic triad of symptoms includes cranial neuropathies, long tract signs and ataxia. The cranial nerves most commonly involved at presentation are the abducens (VI) and facial (VII) nerves. Patients frequently have strabismus associated with diplopia, facial weakness and decreased movement of the soft palate. Symptoms are generally present for a short duration (median, 1 month) (Donaldson et al 2006), and are progressive. Adults with DIPG present with similar signs and symptoms, although they commonly have a longer duration of symptoms (Selvapandian et al 1999).

Diagnosis
Since MRI became routinely used in the early 1990s, patients with DIPG have been diagnosed by MRI in the face of a typical clinical presentation. Radiographic findings include a large, poorly demarcated brainstem mass, with its epicenter in the pons, generally involving >50% of the pons, frequently wrapping the basilar artery frequently and exhibiting mass effect on adjacent structures with surrounding edema (Fig. 23.2). DIPGs are hypointense on T1-weighted imaging and hyperintense on T2-weighted imaging. Gadolinium enhancement is variable. In children, DIPGs do not usually enhance significantly on the initial MRI. However, initial enhancement is fairly common in adults, particularly older adults (Guillamo et al 2001b) but the radiographic diagnosis of glioma was incorrect in up to 25% of adult patients with a contrast-enhancing brainstem lesion (Rajshekhar & Chandy 1995; Boviatsis et al 2003). The presence or degree of enhancement at diagnosis does not significantly correlate with prognosis (Fischbein et al 1996).

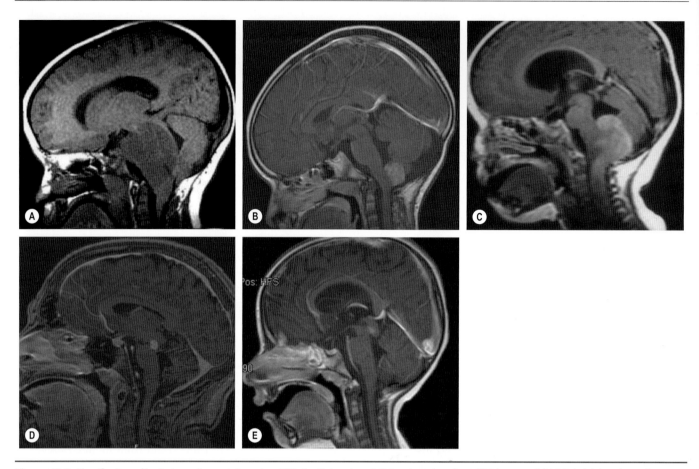

Figure 23.1 Classification of brainstem gliomas is based on MRI. Sagittal post-gadolinium based contrast MRI images of (A) DIPG; (B) dorsal exophytic glioma; (C) cervicomedullary glioma; (D) focal midbrain glioma; (E) tectal glioma.

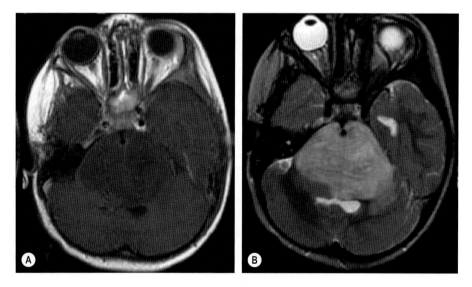

Figure 23.2 Axial MRI demonstrating typical findings of DIPG. (A) T1-weighted post-gadolinium-based contrast image; (B) T2-weighted imaging. Typical findings include a large, often symmetrical expansion of the pons with hypointensity on T1-weighted imaging, hyperintensity on T2-weighted imaging, and lack of significant enhancement. The tumor frequently wraps around the basilar artery. Extension can be seen in the left cerebellar peduncle.

Radiographically and histologically, DIPGs tend to grow preferentially along white matter fiber tracts, spreading contiguously, unhindered by anatomical barriers. They extend rostrally into the midbrain, caudally into the medulla, dorsally into the cerebellar peduncles and can elevate the floor of the fourth ventricle causing obstructive hydrocephalus.

Occasionally, DIPGs spread to distant sites and up to 50% are associated with leptomeningeal dissemination at the time of death (Donahue et al 1998; Gururangan et al 2006; Singh et al 2007). Subsequently, spine MRI is recommended for patients presenting with back pain for institution of palliative radiation therapy if spinal disease is discovered.

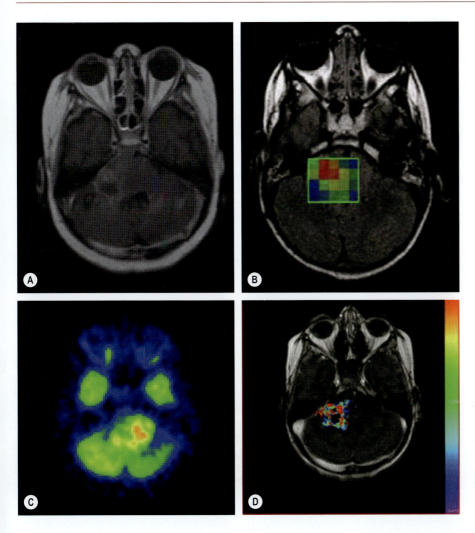

Figure 23.3 DIPG demonstrates biologic and metabolic heterogeneity on imaging. (A) Axial T1-weighted post-contrast MRI. (B) Multivoxel proton spectroscopy with red areas representing high CHO:NAA, blue areas normal CHO:NAA, and yellow-green areas intermediate. (C) FDG PET. (D) Perfusion imaging with red areas indicating increased blood flow.

Histology

Most reports regarding the pathology of brainstem gliomas predate the MRI era and the radiographic sub-classification of brainstem gliomas. In one study of 50 children with diffuse pontine lesions documented by CT, all underwent biopsy and 43 (86%) were found to have astrocytomas (Chico-Ponce de León et al 2003). The remaining children had PNET (two patients); ATRT (two patients); ependymoma (one patient), or were indeterminate (two patients). Many studies report lesions that resemble supratentorial malignant diffuse fibrillary astrocytomas in adults and are histologically classified as WHO grade II, III or grade IV (Louis et al 1993; Fisher et al 2000) (Fig. 23.3), with high-grade gliomas being more commonly diagnosed when biopsied at the time of recurrence (Epstein & McCleary 1986; Cartmill and Punt 1999; Yoshimura et al 2003).

The relevance of histologic grading has been debated, as information at diagnosis is lacking in the majority of cases – the small amount of tissue obtained from biopsy may not be representative of the entire lesion, as these tumors are histologically and metabolically heterogeneous (Fig. 23.4), and they potentially transform to higher-grade lesions after radiation therapy. In one study in which 11 children with diffuse pontine lesions were biopsied at diagnosis, nine were

low-grade lesions (Sanford et al 1988). In comparison, a review of autopsy cases showed that most gliomas with an epicenter in the pons were high-grade gliomas (Mantravadi et al 1982; Fisher et al 2000). More than 80% of adult DIPGs are low-grade tumors (grade II) (Guillamo et al 2001a).

DIPGs are predominantly astrocytic/glial neoplasms with a histologic appearance similar to supratentorial high-grade gliomas, but clinical differences do exist and little information regarding biology or molecular features is available. The median age of presentation is younger for children with DIPG compared with supratentorial high-grade gliomas (7.9 vs 11.4 years), and the tumor grade is more frequently grade III vs grade IV in supratentorial locations (Wolff et al 2008). Only a small number of biologic studies have been performed on biopsy or autopsy material from patients with DIPG, but it is unclear whether these are representative of newly diagnosed pediatric DIPG.

Results of studies do suggest that childhood DIPGs are biologically different from supratentorial high-grade gliomas in children and adult primary and secondary high-grade gliomas, but may share features of each. Adult primary glioblastomas typically arise *de novo* in older patients. *ERBB1* is amplified and overexpressed in up to 50% of specimens (Ekstrand et al 1991; Wong et al 1987) but *TP53* is

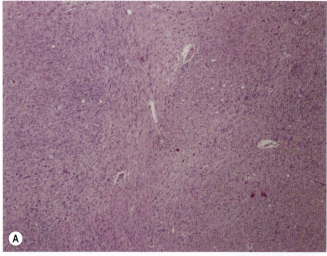

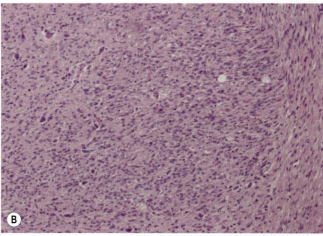

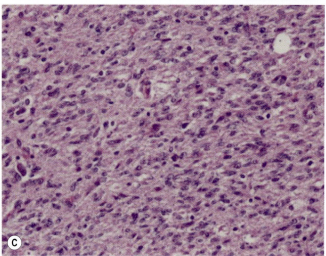

Figure 23.4 Brainstem glioma: An astrocytic neoplasm with increased cellularity and cell atypia partially obscuring normal pons architecture (H&E (A) ×4; (B) ×10; (C) ×20).

generally intact. Secondary glioblastomas typically occur in younger adults, progress from low-grade gliomas, are associated with *TP53* mutations and are rarely associated with *ERBB1* amplification (Wong et al 1987; Ekstrand et al 1991; Lang et al 1994; Watanabe et al 1996; Ichimura et al 2000). Approximately one-third of pediatric supratentorial high-grade gliomas are associated with overexpression of *ERBB1* but gene amplification is not frequently observed (Sure et al 1997; Bredel et al 1999; Sung et al 2000). In comparison, children with DIPG have *ERBB1* expression that appears to correlate with tumor grade. In one study, it was observed in all grade IV tumors, 7 of 9 grade III tumors, 2 of 12 grade II tumors and none of the grade I tumors in a study (Gilbertson et al 2003) suggesting its role in tumor development. Louis and colleagues (1993) demonstrated that DIPG frequently show allelic loss of chromosome 17p and p53 alterations and did not have EGFR amplification, thereby sharing some features of adult secondary glioblastomas. Cheng and colleagues (1999) found that over 70% of pediatric brainstem tumors had *p53* mutations compared with 38% of supratentorial high-grade gliomas.

A recent study using comparative genomic hybridization (CGH) in FFPE autopsy blocks from patients with DIPG (Warren et al 2009) demonstrated that although DNA structural aberrations occurred in areas of known oncogenes and tumor suppressor genes, additional areas were commonly involved. The most frequent DNA structural aberrations included gain of 1q, gain of 7p, gain of 7q and loss of 10q, consistent with prior studies in high-grade gliomas (Burton et al 2002). Although genetic aberrations were identified in all DIPG samples, they were not consistent and extensive variability in the genetic aberrations was noted.

Management

Biopsy is currently not routinely performed for diagnosis of patients with DIPG who present with typical radiographic findings in the face of a typical clinical presentation. This recommendation was primarily based upon review of a study involving 120 children with brainstem glioma who were treated with hyperfractionated radiation therapy (prior to the clinical use of molecular targeted agents) (Albright et al 1993). A total of 24 patients underwent stereotactic biopsy, while 11 underwent craniotomy with biopsy and 10 underwent craniotomy with partial or sub-total resection. All biopsy specimens revealed low-grade or high-grade glioma and treatment was not altered in any patient based in these results (Albright et al 1993). Stereotactic biopsy is currently indicated if the diagnosis is in question (i.e., patients with an atypical history or uncharacteristic findings on MRI).

Because large DIPGs will frequently cause obstructive hydrocephalus, patients may require placement of a ventriculoperitoneal shunt or third ventriculostomy to improve signs and symptoms related to increased intracranial pressure and avoid cerebral herniation. While cerebrospinal fluid diversion may acutely relieve symptoms and temporarily improve quality of life, it has long-term implications as the disease progresses, potentially prolonging survival but not necessarily quality of life (Amano et al 2002; Klimo & Goumnerova 2006). Mild symptoms may alternatively be controlled with steroids and resolve with radiation therapy.

Surgical resection is not possible for DIPG because of their infiltrating nature and functionally eloquent location. Radiation is the only modality that has improved prognosis of patients with DIPG, although tumor control is temporary (Langmoen et al 1991; Halperin et al 2005). Median survival is 20 weeks for children not treated with radiation therapy compared with 40 weeks for those who receive adequate radiation therapy (Langmoen et al 1991). Doses of at least 50 Gy are necessary for maximum benefit (Freeman & Suissa 1986). The standard treatment for both adult and pediatric diffuse brainstem gliomas is 54–60 Gy of focal radiotherapy using conventional external beam radiation with opposed lateral fields, delivered in 180 cGy fractions administered over 6 weeks (Laigle-Donadey et al 2008). Clinical improvement has been reported in up to 70% of patients (Albright et al 1983; Packer et al 1993), although fewer (approximately 50%) have radiographic improvement (Broniscer & Gajjar 2004). Adults with diffuse intrinsic gliomas more frequently respond to radiation therapy compared with children (Laigle-Donadey et al 2008). Clinical progression in children occurs a median of 6–9 months after diagnosis (Korones 2007; Recinos et al 2007).

Intensified doses of radiation have been evaluated in several studies. Initial studies utilizing hyperfractionation with doses of 70–72 Gy suggested improved survival (Edwards et al 1989; Freeman et al 1991; Packer et al 1993) but subsequent trials using doses up to 78 Gy did not confirm this finding (Freeman et al 1993; Packer et al 1994; Prados et al 1995; Mandell et al 1999). Despite a significant number of clinical trials, no chemotherapy or radiosensitizer has ever been shown to significantly improve outcome beyond that achieved with standard radiation therapy alone in a large controlled study of patients with DIPG. A number of obstacles, including insufficient delivery and exposure, tumor heterogeneity, and drug resistance have been proposed. Efforts to overcome these obstacles using high dose chemotherapy and stem cell rescue (Finlay & Zacharoulis 2005), carboplatin following blood–brain barrier disruption (Warren et al 2006), p-glycoprotein inhibition (Greenberg et al 2005), and radiation with concurrent temozolomide (Jalali et al 2009) have not resulted in any significant documented benefit. Consequently, the median survival has not changed in the past three decades.

Prognosis
Median survival of patients with DIPG is less than 1 year. Occasional studies have reported longer survival times, but some were performed in the pre-MRI era, prior to sub-classification of brainstem gliomas. Factors most commonly associated with poor survival are a short duration of symptoms prior to diagnosis, encasement of the basilar artery on MR imaging, and abducens nerve palsy at presentation (Fisher et al 2000). Very young children with DIPG seem to have a better prognosis than older children (Broniscer et al 2008) and there are several reports of spontaneous remissions, particularly in infants (Lenard et al 1998; Schomerus et al 2007). Adults also tend to have a better prognosis with a median survival of 59–83 months and overall survival at 5 and 10 years of 58% and 41%, respectively (Kesari et al 2008; Salmaggi et al 2008).

Challenges
The lack of any significant improvement from chemotherapy is multifactorial. For chemotherapy to be effective, active drug needs to be delivered to the tumor in high enough concentrations for long enough periods of time to exert its effect. Drug delivery to the CNS is hindered by the blood–brain barrier, resulting in inadequate drug concentration and inadequate drug exposure. If molecularly targeted therapy is employed, the target must be present and this is unknown in the majority of DIPG cases. Additional issues for CNS tumors, particularly DIPG, involve drug distribution, drug resistance, lack of tissue diagnosis, and tumor heterogeneity (see Fig. 23.3).

A number of investigational approaches designed to overcome these barriers are underway, including agents designed to block DNA repair mechanisms, molecular targeted therapy and improved delivery techniques such as direct convection-enhanced delivery (CED). IL-13 is a cytokine that inhibits proinflammatory cytokine production and enhances growth and differentiation in a number of cell types. Its effects are mediated via cell surface receptors. IL-13R is overexpressed in >70% of human malignant gliomas and pediatric brain tumor specimens (Joshi et al 2000; Kawakami et al 2004). In a study of formalin fixed tissue sections obtained from diagnosis or at autopsy from children with DIPG, 17 of 28 specimens (61%) expressed varying degrees of IL-13Rα2 by immunohistochemistry (IHC), with a mean percentage of IL-13Rα2 in the immuno-positive specimens of 80% (range, 60–100) (Joshi et al 2008). A clinical trial administering IL13-PE38QQR, a recombinant chimeric cytotoxin that binds to and is internalized by cells expressing the IL-13R (Debinski et al 1995) via CED to children with DIPG is currently underway.

Because of the difficulty and ethical dilemma of obtaining multiple tissue samples, determining the effects of treatment on DIPG is also difficult. For example, changes in the character of the lesion are expected after radiation therapy and radiation necrosis can appear as cystic, enhancing lesions within the pons. Similarly, progressive tumor can appear as a cystic, enhancing mass. It is therefore difficult to distinguish treatment-related effects from tumor progression on standard MRI scans. Other imaging techniques are currently being studied in an effort to define treatment effects.

Focal brainstem gliomas

Focal brainstem gliomas can be distinguished from diffuse brainstem gliomas, by their radiographic appearance and prognosis. They are frequently located in the midbrain or medulla and rarely involve the ventral pons (Fisher et al 2000). Distinct focal tumors including dorsal exophytic, cervicomedullary and tectal gliomas are delineated below, as they have different presentations, radiographic appearances and treatment approaches.

Dorsal exophytic gliomas

Dorsal exophytic gliomas were described by Hoffman and colleagues (1980) as a distinct sub-group of brainstem tumors that may be curable with surgical resection. These tumors are considered intramedullary tumors that grow posteriorly into the fourth ventricle (see Fig. 23.1) (Epstein & Farmer 1993).

Radiographic appearance

Dorsal exophytic gliomas are well-demarcated on MRI and tend to grow along the path of least resistance rather than infiltrate the surrounding tissue. Growth is generally restricted both rostrally and caudally, and the medullary decussation of the corticospinal tracts prevent superior extension into the pons (Epstein & Farmer 1993). They tend to displace rather than invade the pons and upper cervical cord (Epstein & Farmer 1993), although caudal extension into the upper cervical cord has been reported (Abbott et al 1991). It has been hypothesized that dorsal exophytic tumors and diffuse medullary tumors may represent different stages of the same disease (Epstein & Farmer 1993; Fischbein et al 1996) and 5-year survival of both is similar (Fischbein et al 1996).

Presentation

Patients with dorsal exophytic tumors typically present with a long duration of non-specific symptoms that include headache and emesis (Rosemergy & Mossman 2007). While hydrocephalus is frequent and present in approximately 75% of patients, cranial nerve deficits and long tract signs are infrequent (Epstein 1987). On MRI, the lesions are exophytic, expanding into the fourth ventricle or below the cerebellum and frequently enhance after gadolinium-based contrast administration (Laigle-Donadey et al 2008).

Histology

These tumors are usually low-grade astrocytomas, although anaplastic astrocytomas and gangliogliomas have been reported (Epstein & Farmer 1993). The most common histology is pilocytic astrocytoma (Fisher et al 2000). In one study of 76 children with brainstem tumors, in which 21 were dorsal exophytic and biopsied, histologic examination revealed pilocytic astrocytomas ($n = 12$), fibrillary astrocytomas ($n = 4$) or other ($n = 5$) (Fisher et al 2000).

Treatment

The treatment for these lesions is microsurgical resection (Farmer et al 2008) and safe total removal is the goal. A well-defined interface between tumor and white matter tracts frequently permits complete surgical resection (Di Maio et al 2009). When complete resection is not possible, residual tumor is followed with imaging and often remains quiescent or involutes without further therapy. Progression-free survival (PFS) may be prolonged without the need for adjuvant therapy in cases with residual tumor. Two-year overall and PFS is 100% and 67%, respectively (Laigle-Donadey et al 2008).

Cervicomedullary gliomas

Cervicomedullary astrocytomas are a sub-group of brainstem tumors with an epicenter in the medulla or upper cervical cord. They tend to occur in children in the same age group as DIPG (median age, 7 years) (Young Poussaint et al 1999), but overall have a better prognosis. Cervicomedullary gliomas are predominantly low-grade lesions, including pilocytic

astrocytomas, gangliogliomas and WHO grade II astrocytomas (Young Poussaint et al 1999; Di Maio et al 2009). It has been hypothesized (Epstein & Farmer 1993) that growth and expansion of these lesions is guided by secondary structures such as fiber tracts, rather than direct tissue invasion.

Behavior of most cervicomedullary gliomas more closely resembles spinal tumors than brainstem gliomas. However, not all cervicomedullary gliomas demonstrate a benign clinical course, leading to the proposal of two sub-groups. The first group includes those relatively benign tumors that mimic classic spinal tumors, cause symptoms by compression rather than invasion, and possess a clear demarcation between tumor and white matter tracts. The second group includes more malignant tumors that resemble diffuse infiltrating brainstem lesions with an epicenter in the medulla.

Presentation

Patients with lesions involving the cervicomedullary area frequently present with lower cranial nerve dysfunction, motor and/or sensory dysfunction, and pyramidal tract signs (Vandertop et al 1992; Weiner et al 1997). Vomiting, headache, and decreased use of upper extremities have also been noted in a significant number of patients (Young Poussaint et al 1999). Symptoms are generally insidious with a mean duration of symptoms ranging from 24 weeks to 2.3 years prior to diagnosis (Robertson et al 1994; Weiner et al 1997; Young Poussaint et al 1999).

Diagnosis

Cervicomedullary gliomas tend to be hypointense to white matter on T1-weighted MRI (Young Poussaint et al 1999), hyperintense on T2-weighted MRI, and enhance after gadolinium-based contrast administration (Young Poussaint et al 1999).

Treatment

Microsurgical resection is the primary treatment modality for patients with these tumors and may be the only treatment needed. However, surgical morbidity may be significant (Di Maio et al 2009). Successful surgery has been related to a longer duration of symptoms and low-grade pathology (Young Poussaint et al 1999). Distinguishing the infiltrative vs the classic spinal cervicomedullary tumors by MRI before surgical resection is beneficial because a clear tumor-white matter tract interface is not present in the former and may be present in the latter. Di Maio and colleagues (2009) found that patients who had interposed non-enhancing tissue contiguous with normal cervical cord or medulla on MRI and abnormal hypointensity on T1-weighted imaging beyond the obvious tumor had a poorly defined tumor/brainstem interface with increased risk of surgical morbidity. Interestingly, the brainstem/tumor interface definition improved after adjuvant therapy with radiation or chemotherapy. Patients with subtotal or partial resection may be treated adjuvantly with chemotherapy or radiotherapy and a second surgery may be possible (Di Maio et al 2009).

Pattern of spread

Cervicomedullary tumors may appear focal or infiltrative but have a different growth pattern from diffuse intrinsic tumors.

Tumor progression is generally by local extension (Young Poussaint et al 1999). They can grow upwards into the medulla, but tend to be limited by the decussating fibers and pial elements, causing growth in a posterior exophytic pattern (Epstein & Farmer 1993; Squires et al 1997).

Histology
The majority of cervicomedullary gliomas are low-grade gliomas (Epstein & Wisoff 1987) and usually have a slow growth rate, and little/no infiltrative capacity. Epstein and Farmer (1993) reviewed 88 patients with brainstem tumors who underwent radical excision; 50% of the lesions were classified as cervicomedullary gliomas. Of these 44 tumors, 32 (73%) were low-grade astrocytomas, seven were gangliogliomas, four were anaplastic astrocytomas and one was ependymoma. All of these tumors exhibited similar growth patterns with rostral extension limited at the junction of the medulla and upper cervical cord, while expanding posteriorly as a bulge at the caudal medulla.

Prognosis
While cervicomedullary tumors have a better prognosis than DIPG, overall survival is not good for patients with diffuse medullary lesions. In one study which included eight patients with medullary tumors, 50% of the patients died within 2 years (Barkovich et al 1990–1991). However, in a retrospective study of 11 pediatric patients with cervicomedullary astrocytomas, 10 patients survived a mean of 5.2 years (range 0.2–11 years) (Young Poussaint et al 1999). In another study which included 39 patients with cervicomedullary tumors, the overall 5-year PFS and total survivals were 60% and 89%, respectively (Weiner et al 1997). In this study, those patients with a longer preoperative history of symptoms had a more favorable prognosis (Weiner et al 1997).

Tectal gliomas

Tumors of the tectal region are rare, focal, primarily intrinsic gliomas that represent <5% of brainstem gliomas in children (Pollack et al 1994; Bowers et al 2000). Review of several small studies in the literature show that they are essentially comprised of two groups: small, well-circumscribed, indolent tumors or larger, more aggressive lesions. CSF diversion, usually by third ventriculostomy, is frequently the only treatment needed for the indolent group.

Presentation
Because the tectal region is in close proximity to the cerebral aqueduct, the vast majority of patients with tectal gliomas present with late-onset aqueductal stenosis and symptoms related to hydrocephalus, with evidence of increased intracranial pressure, such as headache and emesis. Patients may also present with Parinaud's syndrome (Lazaro & Landeiro 2006), gait disturbance, ataxia, strabismus, vertigo, head bobbing, decline in school performance, tremor and seizures (Grant et al 1999; Ternier et al 2006).

Diagnosis
Symptoms may be present for months to years before diagnosis (Grant et al 1999; Ternier et al 2006). For imaging studies, MRI is the modality of choice. It is not uncommon to have evidence of non-communicating hydrocephalus with distortion or thickening of the tectal plate (Gómez-Gosálvez et al 2001). MRI demonstrates a non-enhancing lesion that is hypointense or isointense on T1-weighted imaging, hyperintense on T2-weighted imaging (Bognar et al 1994; Bowers et al 2000), and rarely enhances after gadolinium-based contrast (see Fig. 23.1) (Bognar et al 1994; Ternier et al 2006). Median age of diagnosis is 10 years in children (Gómez-Gosálvez et al 2001). Surgery (biopsy or resection) may be indicated if a definitive diagnosis is necessary (e.g., in the case of an enlarging tumor).

Histology
Astrocytic tumors are the most common type of tumor found in the tectum, but other tumors, including oligodendroglioma, ependymoma, primitive neuroectodermal tumors, ganglioglioma, metastatic tumors, and periaqueductal gliosis have also been described (Lazaro & Landeiro 2006). Up to 85% of tectal plate lesions are benign gliomas (Lapras et al 1994; Kaku et al 1999; Da lio lu et al 2003) but many lesions are not biopsied. In a study by Ternier and colleagues (2006), smaller lesions (<4 cm^3) were more likely to be hamartomas. Malignant lesions in this area have been reported and up to 31% of tumors in this area can cause symptoms related to the brainstem and will eventually require treatment beyond cerebrospinal fluid diversion (Pollack et al 1994; Oka et al 1999).

Treatment
Cerebrospinal fluid diversion, by shunt or third ventriculostomy, is frequently indicated for the management of hydrocephalus and may be the only treatment needed (Lazaro & Landeiro 2006). Although most agree that surgery should be performed to relieve symptoms, such as hydrocephalus, there is controversy regarding tumor-directed therapy. Some have reported that resection of these lesions can be performed with limited morbidity and good long-term outcomes, although positive outcomes have also been reported with conservative management (Epstein & McCleary 1986; May et al 1991; Gómez-Gosálvez et al 2001). Others believe that treatment of patients with tectal tumors should be decided on a case by case basis (Lazaro & Landeiro 2006). For many, the initial and only treatment is surgery to relieve hydrocephalus. Small lesions may not need tumor-directed therapy. As noted above, smaller lesions are frequently hamartomas (Ternier et al 2006), and several studies have concluded that smaller, non-enhancing lesions confined to the tectal rarely cause radiographic or clinical progression, have a good prognosis, and should be managed conservatively (Grant et al 1999), but most larger lesions at presentation eventually require treatment (Ternier et al 2006).

Vandertop et al reported that debulking could be performed on these patients with minimal morbidity (Vandertop et al 1992). In a report by Lapras et al (1994), 12 patients with tectal gliomas were treated with surgery; one patient died, and four had surgical complications. However, he demonstrated the importance of a tissue diagnosis, particularly for those with malignant gliomas. Focal radiation is frequently reserved for malignant or progressive lesions, but the benefit of radiation in these patients remains unclear (Kihlström et al 1994; Hamilton et al 1996).

Outcomes are similar for surgical resection, biopsy, adjuvant therapy and conservative management (Ternier et al 2006). Although most tectal plate gliomas are low grade and may remain indolent for several years (Lazaro & Landeiro 2006), the natural history is not well-characterized. There is potential for eventual progression and subsequent need for treatment, therefore patients need to be followed long term. The challenge is to identify those patients that will need treatment beyond CSF diversion prior to development of symptoms.

Conclusions

Brainstem gliomas are a heterogeneous group of tumors with different biology and outcome. While MRI has allowed sub-classification of these tumors and identification of focal lesions that are amenable to surgical resection, radiation and chemotherapy, little progress has been made in improving the outcome of those patients with diffuse lesions. Although limited tissue is available for study, results from recent biologic studies have provided hints of diverse biologic features, paving the way for future studies.

Key points

- Brainstem gliomas are a heterogeneous group of tumors, with different presentation, histology, radiographic findings, treatment recommendations and prognosis.

- Tumors are sub-classified as focal (including dorsal exophytic, tectal, and cervicomedullary) or diffuse.

- Patients with focal tumors may have a curative surgical option; radiation and chemotherapy are alternate approaches for unresectable lesions or progressive lesions.

- No progress has been made in the outcome of patients with diffuse intrinsic pontine glioma in over three decades. Little is known about the biology of these tumors due to the limited tissue availability.

- Biology studies performed on DIPG to date have demonstrated significant differences between these tumors and supratentorial gliomas, suggesting a role for the tumor microenvironment.

REFERENCES

Abbott, R., Shiminski-Maher, T., Wisoff, J.H., et al., 1991. Intrinsic tumors of the medulla: surgical complications. Pediatr. Neurosurg. 17, 239–244.

Abernathy, C.D., Camacho, A., Kelly, P.J., 1989. Stereotactic suboccipital transcerebellar biopsy of pontine mass lesions. J. Neurosurg. 70, 195–200.

Albers, A., Gutmann, D., 2009. Gliomas in patients with neurofibromatosis type 1. Expert Rev. Neurother 9 (4), 535–539.

Albright, A.L., Packer, R.J., Zimmerman, R., et al., 1993. Magnetic resonance scans should replace biopsies for the diagnosis of diffuse brain stem gliomas: a report from the Children's Cancer Group. Neurosurgery 33 (6), 1026–1029.

Albright, A.L., Price, R.A., Guthkelch, A.N., 1983. Brain stem gliomas of children. Cancer 52, 2313–2319.

Amano, T., Inamura, T., Nakamizo, A., et al., 2002. Case management of hydrocephalus associated with progression of childhood brain stem gliomas. Childs Nerv. Syst. 18 (11), 599–604.

Barkovich, A.J., Krischer, J., Kun, L.E., et al., 1990. Brain stem gliomas: a classification system based on magnetic resonance imaging. Pediatr. Neurosurg. 16 (2), 73–83.

Bognar, L., Turjman, F., Villanyi, E., et al., 1994. Tectal plate gliomas Part II: CT scans and MRI imaging of tectal gliomas. Acta. Neurochir. 127, 48–54.

Boviatsis, E.J., Kouyialis, A.T., Stranjalis, G., et al., 2003. CT-guided stereotactic biopsies of brain stem lesions: personal experience and literature review. Neurol. Sci. 24, 97–102.

Bowers, D.C., Georgiades, C., Aronson, L.J., et al., 2000. Tectal gliomas: natural history of an indolent lesion in pediatric patients. Pediatr. Neurosurg. 32, 24–29.

Bredel, M., Pollack, I.F., Hamilton, R.L., et al., 1999. Epidermal growth factor receptor expression and gene amplification in high-grade nonbrainstem gliomas of childhood. Clin. Cancer Res. 5, 1786–1792.

Broniscer, A., Gajjar, A., 2004. Supratentorial high-grade astrocytoma and diffuse brainstem glioma: two challenges for the pediatric oncologist. Oncologist 9, 197–206.

Broniscer, A., Laningham, F.H., Sanders, R.P., et al., 2008. Young age may predict a better outcome for children with diffuse pontine glioma. Cancer 113 (3), 566–572.

Burton, E.C., Lamborn, K.R., Feuerstein, B.G., et al., 2002. Genetic aberrations defined by comparative genomic hybridization distinguish long-term from typical survivors of glioblastoma. Cancer Res. 62, 6205–6210.

Cartmill, M., Punt, J., 1999. Diffuse brain stem glioma: a review of stereotactic biopsies. Child's Nerv. Syst. 15, 235–237.

CBTRUS, 2008. Primary brain tumors in the United States, 2000–2004. Central Brain Tumor Registry of the United States, Hinsdale, IL.

Chen, T., 1998. Hereditary neurological tumor syndromes: clues to glioma oncogenesis? Neurosurg. Focus 4 (4), e1.

Cheng, Y., Ng, H.K., Zhang, S.F., et al., 1999. Genetic alterations in pediatric high-grade astrocytomas. Human Pathol. 30, 1284–1290.

Chico-Ponce de León, F., Perezpeña-Diazconti, M., Castro-Sierra, E., et al., 2003. Stereotactically-guided biopsies of brainstem tumors. Childs Nerv. Syst. 19, 305–310.

Da lio lu, E., Cataltepe, O., Akalan, N., et al., 2003. Tectal gliomas in children: The implications for natural history and management strategy. Pediatr. Neurosurg. 38, 223–231.

Debinski, W., Obiri, N.I., Powers, S.K., et al., 1995. Human glioma cells overexpress receptors for interleukin 13 and are extremely sensitive to a novel chimeric protein composed of interleukin 13 and pseudomonas exotoxin. Clin. Cancer Res. 1, 1253–1258.

Di Maio, S., Gul, S.M., Cochrane, D.D., et al., 2009. Clinical, radiologic and pathologic features and outcome following surgery for cervicomedullary gliomas in children. Childs Nerv. Syst. 25 (11), 1401–1410.

Donahue, B., Allen, J., Siffert, J., et al., 1998. Patters of recurrence in brain stem gliomas: evidence for craniospinal dissemination. Int. J. Radiat. Oncol. Biol. Phys. 40 (3), 677–680.

Donaldson, S.S., Laningham, F., Fisher, P.G., 2006. Advances toward an understanding of brainstem gliomas. J. Clin. Oncol. 24 (8), 1266–1272.

Edwards, M.S., Wara, W.M., Urtasun, R.C., et al., 1989. Hyperfractionated radiation therapy for brain stem glioma: a Phase I-II trial. J. Neurosurg. 70, 691–700.

Ekstrand, A.J., James, C.D., Cavenee, W.K., et al., 1991. Genes for epidermal growth factor receptor, transforming growth factor α, and epidermal growth factor and their expression in human gliomas in vivo. Cancer Res. 51, 2164–2172.

Epstein, F., 1987. Intrinsic brainstem tumors of childhood. In: Homberger, F. (Ed.), Progress in experimental tumor research. Karger, Basel, pp. 160–194.

Epstein, F., Farmer, J., 1993. Brainstem glioma growth patterns. J. Neurosurg. 78, 408–412.

Epstein, F., McCleary, E., 1986. Intrinsic brain stem tumors of childhood: surgical indications. J. Neurosurg. 64, 11–15.

Epstein, F., Wisoff, J., 1987. Intra-axial tumors of the cervicomedullary junction. J. Neurosurg. 67, 483–487.

Farmer, J.P., McNeely, P.D., Freeman, C.R., 2008. Brainstem gliomas. In: Albright, A., Pollack, I., Adelson, P. (Eds.), Principles and practice of pediatric neurosurgery. Thieme, New York, pp. 640–654.

Farrell, C., Plotkin, S., 2009. Genetic causes of brain tumors: neurofibromatosis, tuberous sclerosis, von Hippel-Lindau, and other syndromes. Neurol. Clin. 25 (4), 925–946.

Finlay, J., Zacharoulis, S., 2005. The treatment of high grade gliomas and diffuse intrinsic pontine tumors of childhood and adolescence: a historical and futuristic perspective. J. Neurooncol. 75 (3), 253–266.

Fischbein, N.J., Prados, M.D., Wara, W., et al., 1996. Radiologic classification of brain stem tumors: correlation of magnetic resonance imaging appearance with clinical outcome. Pediatr. Neurosurg. 24, 9–23.

Fisher, P.G., Breiter, S.N., Carson, B.S., et al., 2000. A clinicopathologic reappraisal of brain stem tumor classification: identification of pilocytic astrocytoma and fibrillary astrocytoma as distinct entities. Cancer 89, 1569–1576.

Franzini, A., Allegranza, A., Melcarne, A., et al., 1988. Serial stereotactic biopsy of brain stem expanding lesions. Considerations on 45 consecutive cases. Acta. Neurochir. Suppl. 42:S170–S176.

Freeman, C.R., Krischer, J., Sanford, R.A., et al., 1991. Hyperfractionated radiation therapy in brain stem tumors. Results of treatment at the 7020 cGy dose level of POG study 8495. Cancer 68, 474–481.

Freeman, C.R., Krischer, J.P., Sanford, R.A., et al., 1993. Final results of a study of escalating doses of hyperfractionated radiotherapy in brain stem tumors in children: a Pediatric Oncology Group Study. Int. J. Radiat. Oncol. Biol. Phys. 27, 197–206.

Freeman, C., Suissa, S., 1986. Brain stem tumors in children: Results of a survey of 62 patients treated with radiotherapy. Int. J. Radiat. Oncol. Biol. Phys. 12, 1823–1828.

Gilbertson, R.J., Hill, D.A., Hernan, R., et al., 2003. ERBB1 is amplified and overexpressed in high-grade diffusely infiltrating pediatric brain stem glioma. Clin. Cancer Res. 9, 3620–3624.

Giunta, F., Marini, G., Grasso, G., et al., 1988. Stereotactic biopsy for a better therapeutic approach. Acta. Neurochir. 42 (Suppl.), S182–S186.

Gómez-Gosálvez, F.A., Menor, F., Morant, A., et al., 2001. Tectal tumors in paediatrics. A review of eight patients. Rev. Neurol. 33, 605–611.

Gonçalves-Ferreira, A.J., Herculano-Carvalho, M., Pimentel, J., 2003. Stereotactic biopsies of focal brainstem lesions. Surg. Neurol. 60, 311–320.

Grant, G.A., Avellino, A.M., Loeser, J.D., et al., 1999. Management of intrinsic gliomas of the tectal plate in children. Pediatr. Neurosurg. 31, 170–176.

Greenberg, M.L., Fisher, P.G., Freeman, C., et al., 2005. Etoposide, vincristine, and cyclosporin A with standard-dose radiation therapy in newly diagnosed diffuse intrinsic brainstem gliomas: a pediatric oncology group phase I study. Pediatr. Blood Cancer 45 (5), 644–648.

Grigsby, P.W., Thomas, P.R., Schwartz, H.G., et al., 1989. Multivariate analysis of prognostic factors in pediatric and adult thalamic and brainstem tumors. Int. J. Radiat. Oncol. Biol. Phys. 16, 649–655.

Guillamo, J.S., Doz, F., Delattre, J.Y., 2001a. Brain stem gliomas. Curr. Opin. Neurol. 14, 711–715.

Guillamo, J.S., Monjour, A., Taillandier, L., et al.; Association des NeuroOncologues d'Expression Francaise (ANOCEF), 2001b. Brainstem gliomas in adults: prognostic factors and classification. Brain 124, 2528–2539.

Gururangan, S., McLaughlin, C.A., Brashears, J., et al., 2006. Incidence and patterns of neuroaxis metastases in children with diffuse pontine glioma. J. Neurooncol. 77 (2), 207–212.

Halperin, E.C., Constine, L.S., Tarbell, N.J., et al. (Eds.), 2005. Tumors of the posterior fossa and spinal canal. In: Pediatric radiation oncology. Lippincott Williams & Wilkins, London.

Hamilton, M.G., Lauryssen, C., Hagen, N., et al., 1996. Focal midbrain glioma: Long term survival in a cohort of 16 patients and the implications for management. Can. J. Neurol. Sci. 23, 204–207.

Hoffman, H.J., Becker, L., Craven, M.A., 1980. Clinically and pathologically distinct group of benign brainstem gliomas. J. Neurosurg. 7, 243–248.

Ichimura, K., Bolin, M.B., Goike, H.M., et al., 2000. Deregulation of the p14ARF/MDM2/p53 pathway is a prerequisite for human astrocytic gliomas with G1-S transition control gene abnormalities. Cancer Res. 60, 417–424.

Inskip, P.D., Tarone, R.E., Hatch, E.E., et al., 2001. Cellular-telephone use and brain tumours. N. Engl. J. Med. 344, 79–86.

Jalali, R., Raut, N., Arora, B., et al., 2009. Prospective evaluation of radiotherapy with concurrent and adjuvant temozolomide in children with newly diagnosed diffuse intrinsic pontine glioma. Int. J. Radiat. Oncol. Biol. Phys. 77 (1), 113–118.

Joshi, B.H., Plautz, G.E., Puri, R.K., 2000. Interleukin-13 receptor alpha chain: a novel tumor-associated transmembrane protein in primary explants of human malignant gliomas. Cancer Res. 60, 1168–1172.

Joshi, B.H., Puri, R.A., Leland, P., et al., 2008. Identification of interleukin-13 receptor α2 chain overexpression in situ in high-grade diffusely infiltrative pediatric brainstem glioma. Neuro. Oncology 10, 265–274.

Kaku, Y., Yonekawa, Y., Taub, E., 1999. Transcollicular approach to intrinsic tectal lesions. Neurosurgery 44, 338–343.

Kaplan, S., Novikov, I., Modan, B., 1997. Nutritional factors in the etiology of brain tumours: potential role of nitrosamines, fat, and cholesterol. Am. J. Epidemiol. 146, 832–841.

Kawakami, M., Kawakami, K., Takahashi, S., et al., 2004. Analysis of interleukin-13 receptor alpha2 expression in human pediatric brain tumors. Cancer 101, 1036–1042.

Kesari, S., Kim, R.S., Markos, V., et al., 2008. Prognostic factors in adult brainstem gliomas: a multicenter, retrospective analysis of 101 cases. J. Neurooncol. 88, 175–183.

Kihlström, L., Lindquist, C., Lindquist, M., et al., 1994. Stereotactic radiosurgery for tectal low-grade gliomas. Acta. Neurochir. (Wien) 62, 55–57.

Klaeboe, L., Blaasaas, K.G., Haldorsen, T., et al., 2005. Residential and occupational exposure to 50-Hz magnetic fields and brain tumours in Norway: a population-based study. Int. J. Cancer 115 (1), 137–141.

Klimo, P.J., Goumnerova, L., 2006. Endoscopic third ventriculostomy for brainstem tumors. J. Neurosurg. 105 (Suppl. 4), 271–274.

Korones, D., 2007. Treatment of newly diagnosed diffuse brainstem gliomas in children: in search of the Holy Grail. Expert Rev. Anti. Cancer Ther. 7, 663–674.

Kratimenos, G., Thomas, D., 1993. The role of image-directed biopsy in the diagnosis and management of brainstem lesions. Br. J. Neurosurg. 7, 155–164.

Laigle-Donadey, F., Doz, F., Delattre, J.Y., 2008. Brainstem gliomas in children and adults. Curr. Opin. Oncol. 20, 662–667.

Lang, F.F., Miller, D.C., Koslow, M., et al., 1994. Pathways leading to glioblastoma multiforme: a molecular analysis of genetic alterations in 65 astrocytic tumors. J. Neurosurg. 81, 427–436.

Langmoen, I.A., Lundar, T., Storm-Mathisen, I., et al., 1991. Management of pediatric pontine gliomas. Child's Nerv. Syst. 7, 13–15.

Lapras, C., Bognar, L., Turjman, F., et al., 1994. Tectal plate gliomas. Part I: Microsurgery of the tectal plate gliomas. Acta. Neurochir. (Wien) 126, 76–83.

Lazaro, B., Landeiro, J., 2006. Tectal plate tumors. Arq. Neuropsiquiatr. 64 (2-B), 432–436.

Lenard, H.G., Engelbrecht, V., Janssen, G., et al., 1998. Complete remission of a diffuse pontine glioma. Neuropediatrics 29 (6), 328–330.

Louis, D.N., Rubio, M.P., Correa, K.M., et al., 1993. Molecular genetics of pediatric brain stem gliomas. Application of PCR techniques to small and archival brain tumor specimens. J. Neuropathol. Exp. Neurol. 52, 507–515.

Mandell, L.R., Kadota, R., Freeman, C., et al., 1999. There is no role for hyperfractionated radiation in the management of children with newly diagnosed diffuse intrinsic brain stem tumors: results of a Pediatric Oncology Group Phase III trial comparing conventional versus hyperfractionated radiation. Int. J. Radiat. Oncol. Biol. Phys. 43, 959–964.

Mantravadi, R.V., Phatak, R., Bellur, S., et al., 1982. Brain stem gliomas: An autopsy study of 25 cases. Cancer 49, 1294–1296.

Maria, B.L., Rehder, K., Eskin, T.A., et al., 1993. Brainstem glioma: I. Pathology, clinical features, and therapy. J. Child Neurology 8, 112–128.

May, P.L., Blaser, S.I., Hoffman, H.J., et al., 1991. Benign intrinsic tectal tumors in children. J. Neurosurg. 74, 867–871.

Oka, K., Kin, Y., Go, Y., et al., 1999. Neuroendoscopic approach to tectal tumors: a consecutive series. J. Neurosurg. 91, 964–970.

Packer, R., Boyett, J., et al., 1993. Hyperfractionated radiation therapy (72 Gy) for children with brain stem gliomas. A Children's Cancer Group Phase I/II trial. Cancer 72, 1414–1421.

Packer, R., Boyett, J., et al., 1994. Outcome of children with brain stem gliomas after treatment with 7800 cGy of hyperfractionated radiotherapy. A Children's Cancer Group Phase I/II trial. Cancer 74, 1827–1834.

Pollack, I.F., Pang, D., Albright, A.L., et al., 1994. The long-term outcome in children with late onset aqueductal stenosis resulting from benign intrinsic tectal tumors. J. Neurosurg. 80, 681–688.

Pollock, B.H., Krischer, J.P., Vietti, T.J., et al., 1991. Interval between symptom onset and diagnosis of pediatric solid tumors. J. Pediatr. 119, 725–732.

Prados, M.D., Wara, W.M., Edwards, M.S., et al., 1995. The treatment of brain stem and thalamic gliomas with 78 Gy of hyperfractionated radiation. Int. J. Radiat. Oncol. Biol. Phys. 32, 85–91.

Rajshekhar, V., Chandy, M., 1995. Computerized tomography-guided stereotactic surgery for brainstem masses: a risk-benefit analysis in 71 patients. J. Neurosurg. 82, 976–981.

Recinos, P.F., Sciubba, D.M., Jallo, G.I., et al., 2007. Brainstem tumours: Where are we today? Pediatr. Neurosurg. 43, 192–201.

Robertson, P.L., Allen, J.C., Abbott, I.R., et al., 1994. Cervicomedullary tumors in children: a distinct subset of brainstem gliomas. Neurology 44, 1798–1803.

Rosemergy, I., Mossman, S., 2007. Brainstem lesions presenting with nausea and vomiting. N. Z. Med. 120, U253.

Salmaggi, A., Fariselli, L., Milanesi, I., et al., 2008. Natural history and management of brainstem gliomas in adults. A retrospective Italian study. J. Neurol. 255, 171–177.

Salvatore, J.R., Weitberg, A.B., Mehta, S., 1996. Nonionizing electromagnetic fields and cancer: a review. Oncology 10, 563–574.

Samadani, U., Judy, K., 2003. Stereotactic brainstem biopsy is indicated for the diagnosis of a vast array of brainstem pathology. Stereo. Funct. Neurosurg. 81, 5–9.

Sanford, R.A., Freeman, C.R., Burger, P., et al., 1988. Prognostic criteria for experimental protocols in pediatric brain stem gliomas. Surg. Neurol. 30, 276–280.

Schomerus, L., Merkenschlager, A., Kahn, T., et al., 2007. Spontaneous remission of a diffuse brainstem lesion in a neonate. Pediatr. Radiol. 37 (4), 399–402.

Schumacher, M., Schulte-Mönting, J., Stoeter, P., et al., 2007. Magnetic resonance imaging compared with biopsy in the diagnosis of brainstem diseases of childhood: a multicentre review. J. Neurosurg. 106 (Suppl. 2 Pediatr), 111–119.

Selvapandian, S., Rajshekhar, V., Chandy, M.J., 1999. Brainstem glioma: comparative study of clinico-radiological presentation, pathology and outcome in children and adults. Acta. Neurochir. (Wien) 141, 721–727.

Shah, N.C., Ray, A., Bartels, U., et al., 2008. Diffuse intrinsic brainstem tumors in neonates. Report of two cases. J. Neurosurg. Pediatr. 1 (5), 382–385.

Singh, S., Bhutani, R., Jalali, R., 2007. Leptomeninges as a site of relapse in locally controlled, diffuse pontine glioma with review of the literature. Childs Nerv. System 23, 117–121.

Smith, M.A., Freidlin, B., Ries, L., et al., 1998. Trends in reported incidence of primary malignant brain tumors in children in the United States. J. Natl. Cancer Inst. 90 (17), 1269–1277.

Squires, L.A., Constantini, S., Miller, D.C., et al., 1997. Diffuse infiltrating astrocytoma of the cervicomedullary region: clinicopathologic entity. Pediatr. Neurosurg. 27 (3), 153–159.

Sung, T., Miller, D.C., Hayes, R.L., et al., 2000. Preferential inactivation of the p53 tumor suppressor pathway and lack of EGFR amplification distinguish de novo high grade pediatric astrocytomas from de novo adult astrocytomas. Brain Pathol. 10, 249–259.

Sure, U., Rüedi, D., Tachibana, O., et al., 1997. Determination of p53 mutations, EGFR overexpression, and loss of p16 expression in pediatric glioblastomas. J. Neuropathol. Exp. Neurol. 56, 782–789.

Ternier, J., Wray, A., Puget, S., et al., 2006. Tectal plate lesions in children. J. Neurosurg. 104 (Suppl.), 369–376.

Vandertop, W.P., Hoffman, H.J., Drake, J.M., et al., 1992. Focal midbrain tumors in children. Neurosurgery 31 (2), 186–194.

Varan, A., Büyükpamukçu, M., Ersoy, F., et al., 2004. Malignant solid tumors associated with congenital immunodeficiency disorders. Pediatr. Hematol. Oncol. 21 (5), 441–451.

Walter, A.W., Hancock, M.L., Pui, C.H., et al., 1998. Secondary brain tumors in children treated for acute lymphoblastic leukemia at St Jude Children's Research Hospital. J. Clin. Oncol. 16 (12), 3761–3767.

Warren, K., Jakacki, R., Widemann, B., et al., 2006. Phase II trial of intravenous labradimil and carboplatin in childhood brain tumors: a report from the Children's Oncology Group. Cancer Chemother. Pharmacol. 58 (3), 343–347.

Warren, K., Killian, K., Suuriniemi, M., et al., 2009. Genomic DNA analysis of diffuse intrinsic pontine glioma tissue obtained from autopsy. Society of Neuro-Oncology, New Orleans.

Watanabe, K., Tachibana, O., Sata, K., et al., 1996. Overexpression of the EGF receptor and p53 mutations are mutually exclusive in the evolution of primary and secondary glioblastomas. Brain Pathol. 6, 217–223.

Weiner, H.L., Freed, D., Woo, H.H., et al., 1997. Intra-axial tumors of the cervicomedullary junction: surgical results and long-term outcome. Pediatr. Neurosurg. 27 (1), 12–18.

Wolff, J.E., Classen, C.F., Wagner, S., et al., 2008. Subpopulations of malignant gliomas in pediatric patients: analysis of the HIT-GB database. J. Neurooncol. 87, 155–164.

Wong, A.J., Bigner, S.H., Bigner, D.D., et al., 1987. Increased expression of the epidermal growth factor receptor gene in malignant gliomas is invariably associated with gene amplification. Proc. Natl. Acad. Sci. USA 84, 6899–6903.

Yoshimura, J., Onda, K., Tanaka, R., et al., 2003. Autopsy series of 38 pontine gliomas. Neurol. Med. Chir. 43, 375–382.

Young Poussaint, T., Yousuf, N., Barnes, P.D., et al., 1999. Cervicomedullary astrocytomas of childhood: clinical and imaging follow up. Pediatr. Radiol. 29, 662–668.

Intracranial ependymomas

James A. J. King and Abhaya V. Kulkarni

24

Introduction

Ependymomas are tumors of the central nervous system that derive from the ependymal cells that line the ventricles of the brain and the central canal of the spinal cord. This chapter focuses on intracranial ependymomas and therefore, ependymomas that arise in the spinal cord or cauda equina will not be dealt with. While ependymomas are most common in children, they do occasionally arise in adults as well. The first section of this chapter deals with pediatric ependymomas, following which is a section devoted to adult ependymomas.

Ependymomas in children

Epidemiology

Incidence

Ependymomas are relatively uncommon tumors. The annual incidence rate is between 2.2 and 3.4 per million children (Gurney et al 1995; Kuratsu & Ushio 1996; Peris-Bonet et al 2006). Ependymomas are the third most common pediatric brain tumor, behind astrocytomas and primitive neuroectodermal tumors (PNET), which have incidence rates of approximately 16.8 and 5.0 per million children per year, respectively. Ependymomas account for roughly 6–10% of all intracranial tumors of children (Gurney et al 1995; Miller et al 1995; Kuratsu & Ushio 1996; Monteith et al 2006; Mehrazin & Yavari 2007), 30% of those in children younger than 3 years and approximately 1.7% of all childhood cancer (Miller et al 1995).

Age

Ependymomas occur most commonly in younger children, with the median age at diagnosis ranging from 3 to 8 years, depending on the series (Shaw et al 1987; Goldwein et al 1990a,b; Papadopoulos et al 1990; Robertson et al 1998). The incidence rate for ependymomas in children under 5 years of age is approximately 3.9 per million children per year, compared with only 1.1 for older children (Gurney et al 1995). Approximately 70–80% of ependymomas are seen in children under 8 years of age and nearly 40% in children under 4 years of age (Goldwein et al 1990a,b; Nazar et al 1990; Gilles et al 1995; Polednak & Flannery 1995; Peris-Bonet et al 2006; Mehrazin & Yavari 2007).

The very large Childhood Brain Tumor Consortium study reported a large increase in the relative proportion of older children (>11 years) with ependymomas, especially supratentorial ependymomas, over a 50-year period of observation (Gilles et al 1995). This trend was also seen for pilocytic and fibrillary astrocytomas. While there is no clear explanation for this finding, various hypotheses, including a relative decrease in the prenatal exposures that contribute to early childhood cancer or a relative increase in environmental exposures that contribute to later childhood and adolescent cancer, have been proffered.

Gender

Most large pediatric series do not show any consistent gender predilection for ependymomas, arising relatively equally in boys and girls. A number of reports, including a series documenting nearly 2000 cases of pediatric ependymoma from Europe, have shown an increased incidence in boys (Goldwein et al 1990a,b; Papadopoulos et al 1990; Kuratsu & Ushio 1996; Vinchon et al 2005; Peris-Bonet et al 2006), however, this has not held up consistently and it appears that these tumors do not demonstrate a significant gender bias (Shaw et al 1987; Nazar et al 1990; Rousseau et al 1994; Robertson et al 1998).

Location

Ependymomas, being of ependymal origin, almost invariably arise in association with a ventricular surface. In children, the most common site for intracranial ependymomas is in the posterior fossa, associated with the surface of the fourth ventricle. This accounts for the location of roughly two-thirds of childhood ependymomas, with the remainder arising from the supratentorial ventricular system (Pierre-Kahn et al 1983; Goldwein et al 1990a,b; Papadopoulos et al 1990; Sutton et al 1990; Schiffer et al 1991a; Robertson et al 1998). In very rare cases, ependymomas may develop in an ectopic fashion without any direct association to a ventricular surface (Vernet et al 1995; Kojima et al 2003; Miyazawa et al 2007).

Signs and symptoms

Given the predominant location of these tumors in the posterior fossa and their intimate association with the fourth ventricle, the most common presenting signs and symptoms are usually due to raised intracranial pressure from obstructive hydrocephalus. Patients may also display signs and symptoms attributable to direct cerebellar or cranial nerve dysfunction.

Common symptoms, in approximate order of decreasing incidence, include: vomiting, headache (in older children), irritability and lethargy (especially in very young children), and gait disturbance (Goldwein et al 1990a,b; Nazar et al 1990). Clinical signs include: increased head circumference or bulging fontanel (in very young children), papilledema, meningismus, ataxia, cranial nerve palsy, and nystagmus (Goldwein et al 1990a,b; Nazar et al 1990; Maksoud et al 2002). The duration of these symptoms prior to presentation varies greatly and can range from just a few days to several months (Nazar et al 1990). Very rarely, ependymomas may present very acutely following an intratumoral hemorrhage (Ernestus et al 1992; Kojima et al 2003; Miyazawa et al 2007).

A complicating factor in diagnosing young children, is that some may present in a relatively non-specific fashion with, e.g., vomiting and irritability. A high degree of clinical suspicion is needed in such cases. It has been recognized that the diagnosis of brain tumors in children is frequently delayed compared with other childhood tumors (Flores et al 1986).

Pathology

The latest World Health Organization grading of ependymomas defines four major sub-types of the tumor, divided into three grades: subependymoma and myxopapillary ependymoma (grade I), low-grade ependymoma (grade II), and anaplastic ependymoma (grade III) (Louis et al 2007a,b) (Table 24.1). Within the low-grade ependymomas, there are four described histopathological variants: cellular, papillary, tanycytic and clear cell.

Subependymomas are benign, usually asymptomatic, nodules on the walls of the lateral or fourth ventricle. They are most commonly found as an incidental autopsy finding. In very rare cases, they may become clinically evident secondary to obstruction of cerebrospinal fluid (CSF) flow (Rosenblum 1998). Myxopapillary ependymomas are found almost exclusively in the region of the cauda equina, arising from the filum terminale or conus medullaris (Rorke et al 1985). The occurrence of either of these tumors as symptomatic intracranial lesions is exceedingly rare, especially in children (Artico et al 1989; Lombardi et al 1991; Palma et al 1993; Rosenblum 1998). These will not be discussed in this chapter.

Ependymoblastoma was once considered an aggressive form of ependymoma. However, the 2007 WHO classification considers ependymoblastoma among the broader group of embryonal tumors (Louis et al 2007a,b). This group includes

medulloblastomas and other primitive neuroectodermal tumors (PNET), medulloepithelioma, and neuroblastoma. Ependymoblastoma is an aggressive tumor with a propensity for leptomeningeal metastasis (Mørk & Rubinstein 1985; Shyn et al 1986). This tumor will not be discussed in this chapter.

Rosette forming glioneuronal tumor (RGNT) of the fourth ventricle is a newly described WHO grade I glioneuronal tumor, which may have imaging features similar to ependymoma, however, recognition of the characteristic neurocytic rosettes should distinguish it from this entity (Pimentel et al 2008).

Classic low-grade ependymomas, the most common type, have certain histological, ultrastructural, and immunohistochemical features which aid in their diagnosis (Rorke et al 1985; Burger et al 1991). On light microscopy, features include monomorphic nuclear morphology, and round to oval nuclei with 'salt and pepper' speckling of the chromatin (Louis et al 2007a,b). Perivascular pseudo-rosettes, which are clear zones around blood vessels that represent cytoplasmic processes of the tumor cells terminating on vessels, are typical of ependymomas. These are to be distinguished from true ependymal rosettes, in which the lumen of the rosette is circumscribed by the surface of the tumor cells themselves. Ependymomas may also contain structures that resemble central canals or ventricular linings, harking back to their ependymal origin. Although infrequent, they can be diagnostic.

The neoplastic cells may contain eosinophilic cytoplasmic granules. Some of the tumor cells may have the appearance of oligodendrocytes, but these can be distinguished by electron microscopy. Negative OLIG2 immunohistochemistry may also aid in the discrimination of ependymoma from oligodendroglioma and other clear cell CNS neoplasms.

A recent report has documented evidence of ependymoma with neuronal differentiation based on histology, immunohistochemistry and electron microscopy although the significance of this finding is uncertain (Rodriguez et al 2007).

Electron microscopy (EM) typically reveals gland-like lumens with microvilli and cilia, basal bodies, intracytoplasmic intermediate filaments, and long, zipper-like junctional complexes (Burger et al 1991; Sara et al 1994; Rosenblum 1998). EM may also reveal many more true rosettes than might be appreciated on light microscopy (Sara et al 1994). The identification of perivascular elastic fibers on EM in 76% (38 out of 50) of ependymomas in contrast to only 8% (2 out of 25) of choroid plexus papillomas and 0% (0 out of 100) of astrocytomas, has led to the suggestion that this is a useful diagnostic marker in ependymoma, especially in poorly-differentiated examples (Mierau & Goin 2007).

Ependymomas also display varying degrees of immunopositivity to glial fibrillary acid protein (GFAP) and vimentin (Rosenblum 1998). These are rather non-specific and rarely help in the diagnosis. A dot-like perinuclear cytoplasmic reaction to epithelial membrane antigen (EMA) immunostaining is reported and has been shown to be present in approximately 90% of ependymomas but with limited specificity, whereas ring like EMA positive structures may be less sensitive but more specific for ependymoma (Hasselblatt & Paulus 2003; Kawano et al 2004; Takei et al 2007).

Table 24.1 World Health Organization (WHO) Classification of Ependymal Tumors (2007)

Tumor	WHO grade
Subependymoma	I
Myxopapillary ependymoma	I
Ependymoma	II Cellular Papillary Clear cell Tanycytic
Anaplastic ependymoma	III

From Louis, D. N., H. Ohgaki, et al. (2007). 'The 2007 WHO classification of tumours of the central nervous system.' Acta Neuropathol 114(2): 97–109.

CD99 has been suggested to be a reliable marker for ependymoma; in one study, all 38 specimens of ependymoma studied exhibited positive staining (Choi et al 2001; Mahfouz et al 2008).

Histopathological sub-groups of WHO grade II ependymoma
Cellular
The cellular ependymoma is a WHO grade II variant with prominent cellularity without an increase in mitotic rate. It is more common in extraventricular locations (Shuangshoti et al 2005).

Papillary
This variant forms linear, epithelial like surfaces along their sites of exposure to the CSF, with GFAP positive tumor cell processes.

Tanycytic
These tumors are most commonly found in the spinal cord. The tumor is composed of spindly bipolar elements that resemble tanycytes (Flament-Durand & Brion 1985).

Clear cell
Clear cell ependymoma is made up of cells with an oligodendroglial appearance with clear perinuclear halos. It is seen in young patients in the supratentorial compartment and may exhibit more aggressive behavior (Fouladi et al 2003).

The diagnosis of anaplastic ependymoma can be difficult and no clear consensus on the required criteria exists. It is not uncommon for low-grade ependymomas to have occasional mitotic figures, mild cellular pleomorphism, or small scattered areas of necrosis without pseudopalisading. Anaplasia has been variably defined as: increased cellularity, cellular atypia, frequent mitoses (at least 5/10HPF), marked cellular pleomorphism, high nuclear/cytoplasmic ratio, and microvascular proliferation (Rorke et al 1985; Burger et al 1991; Merchant et al 2002a). With the exception of pseudopalisading necrosis, necrosis is generally thought not as ominous as when seen in astrocytomas (Trembath et al 2008). There obviously exists a spectrum of pathological changes and the distinction between low-grade and anaplastic is not always clear. Some authors advocate the use of Ki67 immunohistochemical staining to facilitate identification of mitotic figures (Trembath et al 2008). As well, foci of anaplastic areas may be found scattered in an otherwise bland looking tumor and the significance of this is not known. The difficulty in grading ependymomas becomes especially significant if one is considering different adjuvant treatment options based on tumor grade and also when trying to analyze tumor grade as a prognostic factor for survival.

The difficulty in diagnosing and grading ependymomas can readily be appreciated by noting the inconsistent proportion of allegedly malignant ependymomas in different series, ranging from 12% to as high as 69% (Pierre-Kahn et al 1983; Wallner et al 1986; Shaw et al 1987; Papadopoulos et al 1990; Korshunov et al 2004; Tihan et al 2008). As well, in a prospective randomized trial by the Children's Cancer Group, the pathological diagnosis of the treating institution and the central review was discordant in 69% of cases (Robertson et al 1998). The difficulties in standardizing pathological diagnosis are troublesome in the treatment of the individual child, and also bring into serious question the validity of any of the published series of purported ependymomas.

Progress has been made in characterization of the molecular genetic abnormalities associated with pediatric and adult ependymomas.

The most common cytogenetic abnormalities involve aneuploid karyotypes and abnormalities of chromosomes 6, 9, 17, and 22 (Ransom et al 1992; von Haken et al 1996; Kotylo et al 1997; Kramer et al 1998; Vagner-Capodano et al 1999). The most frequent change in sporadic intracranial ependymoma is loss of chromosome 22q (30–60% of patients) (Hamilton & Pollack 1997), suggesting the presence of an ependymoma tumor suppressor gene on that chromosome (Hulsebos et al 1999; Kraus et al 2001; Suarez-Merino et al 2005; Begnami et al 2007). This also appears to correlate with adult disease and spinal location.

Gains of chromosome 7 have been reported in anaplastic ependymomas but EGFR is not amplified (Santi et al 2005). Pediatric intracranial ependymoma appears to have a differing cytogenetic profile from the adult intracranial disease with loss of 17p seen in approximately 50% and gain of 1q in 26% (Ward et al 2001) and less frequent loss of chromosome 22 (Pezzolo et al 2008).

Clinical observation confirms that spinal intramedullary ependymomas are frequently seen in the inherited cancer syndrome neurofibromatosis type 2 (NF-2), and from this, analysis of NF-2 gene mutations has confirmed mutations in sporadic intramedullary spinal ependymoma, however, not in intracranial or myxopapillary ependymoma (Ebert et al 1999). Ependymoma has also been described in Li Fraumeni syndrome (Metzger et al 1991) although P53 gene pathway disruptions are rare in pediatric ependymomas (Gaspar et al 2006), in Turcot's syndrome, in Klinefelter's (Garre et al 2007) and in the setting of MEN 1. There are several reports of clustering of ependymomas in families (Savard & Gilchrist 1989; Nijssen et al 1994; Dimopoulos et al 2006).

There is emerging evidence for specific genes and cell signaling pathways to be implicated in ependymoma oncogenesis. Microarray experiments of pediatric ependymoma have shown increased expression of the oncogenes, WNT5A and p63, with reduced expression of the NF-2-interacting gene SCHIP-1 and APC. ERB-B2 and ERB-B4 expression is seen in 75% of ependymomas leading to assertion that ERBB receptor signaling results in aggressive disease behavior in ependymoma by promoting tumor cell proliferation (Gilbertson et al 2002).

Perhaps the most significant recent advance is the new hypothesis for the origin of ependymoma: that radial glia in different parts of the CNS are predisposed to acquire distinct genetic abnormalities that transform these cells into cancer stem cells of supratentorial, posterior fossa and spinal ependymoma (Poppleton & Gilbertson 2007).

Taylor et al (2005) have reported that ependymoma gene expression recapitulates that of radial glial cells, and in particular, for supratentorial tumors, CDK4 and Notch signaling pathway genes were over expressed, whereas for infratentorial tumors, IFG-1 and several HOX homeobox genes were over expressed, and for the spinal tumors, the ID genes and the aquaporins were over expressed.

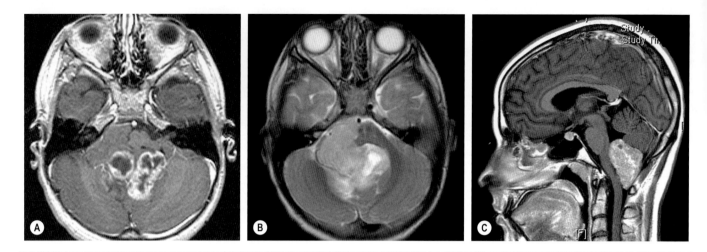

Figure 24.1 Axial T1-weighted MR with gadolinium, (A) demonstrating a large, irregularly enhancing posterior fossa ependymoma with some signal heterogeneity. The tumor is emanating from within the fourth ventricle with a non-enhancing component that extends into the right cerebellopontine angle, better seen on the axial T2-weighted image (B). Sagittal T1-weighted MR with gadolinium (C) from a different patient demonstrating spread of the ependymoma from the fourth ventricle into the foramen magnum and upper cervical cord. These are some of the typical imaging patterns seen with posterior fossa ependymomas.

Neuroimaging

Computerized tomography (CT) imaging usually reveals a mass located within the ventricular system itself, or less commonly, in a periventricular location. The tumor frequently contains cystic areas and calcification and is typically hyperdense. It is well demarcated with contrast enhancement (Centeno et al 1986; Van Tassel et al 1986). Obstructive hydrocephalus is a common accompanying feature that can be quite prominent.

More commonly today, magnetic resonance imaging (MRI) is used to diagnose intracranial mass lesions. On MRI, ependymomas typically display iso- to hypointensity on T1-weighted images and hyper-intensity on T2-weighted images. As well, they enhance with gadolinium injection and may contain areas of signal heterogeneity representing hemorrhage, necrosis, or calcification (Fig. 24.1) (Spoto et al 1990; Comi et al 1998).

The use of proton magnetic resonance spectroscopy, in addition to information gained from diffusion-weighted imaging (DWI), may now allow for the discrimination of the four most frequent posterior fossa tumors in children (Wang et al 1995; Schneider et al 2007; Davies et al 2008).

Differential diagnosis

In the most common situation, the differential diagnosis of interest is that of a posterior fossa mass lesion. Aside from ependymoma, the most common tumors in this location in children include astrocytoma, medulloblastoma, and brainstem glioma. Less common tumors include choroid plexus papilloma, dermoid cyst, and meningioma.

Occasionally, an ependymoma will distinguish itself from these other tumors by way of certain imaging features. For example, their midline location and hyperdensity on CT is typically shared only by medulloblastomas. However, extrusion into the CPA or, especially, into the foramen

magnum or upper cervical spine is much more characteristic of ependymoma than medulloblastoma (Fig. 24.1).

Prognostic factors

Determination of the prognostic factors associated with ependymomas is an area of great interest. However, this process is a very difficult one. One of the major limitations in determining prognostic factors is the difficulty in comparing patient outcomes between, or even within, series. Part of this problem stems from the relatively uncommon nature of this tumor, such that most single institution series report only a limited number of patients who have been accrued over decades. This presents a major limitation, as these patients span many different eras in the treatment of ependymomas. Some of the potentially important milestones include, the exclusion of ependymoblastomas from the ependymoma group; the use and dose of radiotherapy; the use of chemotherapy; the use of CT and MR for diagnosis and postoperative residual tumor assessment; and the improvements in surgical techniques. These all represent potential confounding factors that can occur when comparing results that transgress these milestones. As well, there is much difficulty in standardizing the pathological diagnosis and grading of ependymomas, leading to great inconsistency in the literature. A further limitation is that the vast majority of data comes from retrospective case series. This leads to inevitable biases in the retrieval and analysis of data, particularly with respect to prognostic factors. While the following summarizes the available literature, it should be noted that the quality of the current medical evidence is quite limited.

Age

There are numerous studies that suggest that age is a prognostic factor in children with ependymomas. Most studies show that older children, over the age of 3 or 4 years, have longer survival. In these studies, the 5-year survival rate for the older children ranges from 55% to 83%, compared with 12–48% for the younger age group (Goldwein et al 1990a,b; Nazar et al 1990; Sutton et al 1990; Goldwein et al 1991; Rousseau et al 1994; Pollack et al 1995; Figarella-Branger et al 2000; Shu et al 2007; Tihan et al 2008). Even among children under 3 years old, a prospective study suggested that those >24 months old have a better prognosis (5-year survival of 63% vs 26%) (Duffner et al 1998). Although the verdict on age is not unanimous (some studies have not demonstrated any convincing difference in prognosis (Salazar et al 1983; Robertson et al 1998; Kurt et al 2006), the overall weight of evidence does seem to indicate that older age likely does have some favorable prognostic significance.

Location

Most pediatric ependymomas are located in the posterior fossa and there is some evidence to suggest that this location is associated with a better survival prognosis, although the difference is not as marked as it is for younger vs older children (Marks & Adler 1982; Goldwein et al 1990a,b; Papadopoulos et al 1990; Rousseau et al 1994; Jayawickreme et al 1995; Merchant et al 1997; Mansur et al 2005). The 5-year survivals range from 35% to 59% for infratentorial tumors, compared with 22–46% for supratentorial tumors. However, among posterior fossa tumors, it has been suggested that those with lateral extension into the cerebellopontine angle (CPA) (Ikezaki et al 1993; Figarella-Branger et al 2000) or into the upper cervical region have a worse prognosis (Shu et al 2007). They attribute this to the much greater difficulty in completely removing these tumors due to the involvement of the lower cranial nerves and major vascular structures, e.g., posterior inferior cerebellar artery (PICA).

Tumor sub-type

There were no differences in the clinical outcomes of the four different sub-types of WHO grade II ependymoma (cellular, clear cell, papillary, tanycytic) (Kurt et al 2006).

Tumor grade

There is great controversy regarding the prognostic significance of tumor grade for ependymomas. Numerous retrospective studies have shown that anaplastic ependymomas or, at least, tumors with certain anaplastic features, carry a worse prognosis (Korshunov et al 2004; Salazar et al 1983; Rorke 1987; Shaw et al 1987; Nazar et al 1990; Papadopoulos et al 1990; Figarella-Branger et al 1991; Schiffer et al 1991b; Vanuytsel et al 1992; Rousseau et al 1994; Merchant et al 2002a; Kurt et al 2006). A recent report suggests that histological grade (WHO grade II vs III) is an independent prognostic indicator for event-free survival, but may not be so for overall survival in pediatric posterior fossa ependymomas (Tihan et al 2008).

Other studies have found tumor grade to be a factor for supratentorial tumors only (Ernestus et al 1991; Chiu et al 1992; Palma et al 1993).

While such an association would intuitively make sense (following the pattern that has been well established for different grades of astrocytomas), there are several studies that have found no difference in prognosis based on tumor grade

for ependymomas (Ross & Rubinstein 1989; Goldwein et al 1990a,b; Sutton et al 1990; Bouffet et al 1998; Duffner et al 1998; McLaughlin et al 1998; Robertson et al 1998). Among these series are two prospective studies: a randomized trial from the Children's Cancer Group (Robertson et al 1998) and a prospective cohort study from the Pediatric Oncology Group (Duffner et al 1998). The relatively higher methodological quality of these works needs to be appreciated and taken into account when weighing the overall evidence, especially since there are so few such works in the ependymoma literature. However, it should also be said that these studies were not very large and somewhat limited in scope. Of further note is that in the Children's Cancer Group study, pathological specimens underwent a formal, independent review process (Robertson et al 1998). This process was particularly enlightening, since it demonstrated a discordant pathological diagnosis in 69% of the cases. A more recent report of 258 ependymomas assessed according to the low- and high-grade criteria proposed by Merchant and colleagues (2002a), identified 99% concordance between two independent pathologists. This variation in grading reliability is a rather disturbing finding and significantly limits the conclusions one can infer from most studies that have examined the influence of tumor grade on prognosis.

Molecular markers

A number of studies have now been published attempting to identify molecular markers that correlate with favorable and unfavorable outcome in ependymoma (Lukashova-v Zangen et al 2007; Ridley et al 2008). A recent cytogenetic study of pediatric ependymomas concluded that the combined presence of 6p22-pter and 13q14.3-qter losses predicted significantly reduced survival in this small series (Pezzolo et al 2008). A further report suggested a correlation between 6q loss and longer survival in pediatric intracranial ependymoma (Monoranu et al 2008), whereas loss of regions of chromosome 19 have been shown to correlate with recurrence (Modena et al 2006).

Analysis of human telomere reverse transcriptase expression in 87 pediatric intracranial ependymomas from 65 patients has revealed that the 5-year survival for children with hTERT negative tumors was 84% in contrast to 41% for hTERT positive tumors (Tabori et al 2006). hTERT expression also appears to predict survival in recurrent ependymoma, and analysis of γH2AX expression, a marker of telomere dysfunction allows for further prognostic sub-classification (Tabori et al 2008).

It is likely that further molecular markers will emerge over the coming years and it is anticipated that these will be critical in providing prognostic information regarding individual tumors.

Tumor resection

The extent of tumor resection is a particularly important factor, since it is one that the surgeon has at least some control over. The vast majority of studies do seem to suggest that extent of resection, particularly a gross total resection (GTR), is associated with improved prognosis (Nazar et al 1990; Papadopoulos et al 1990; Sutton et al 1990; Vanuytsel et al 1992; Rousseau et al 1994; Pollack et al 1995; Perilongo et al 1997; Duffner et al 1998; Robertson et al

1998; Figarella-Branger et al 2000; van Veelen-Vincent et al 2002; Jaing et al 2004; Schroeder et al 2008). Reported 5-year survivals range from 60% to 89% after GTR, compared with 21–46% following partial resection. A small number of studies have failed to demonstrate any survival advantage following GTR (Salazar et al 1983; Shaw et al 1987; Goldwein et al 1990a,b).

It is important to determine exactly how one ascertains the degree of surgical resection and, therefore, the amount of postoperative residual tumor. Healey et al (1991) demonstrated in their small series that while postoperative residual tumor, as assessed by radiological imaging, was associated with progression free survival, the assessment by the surgeon of the extent of resection was not prognostically significant. In fact, the surgical assessment of resection was refuted by the postoperative imaging in 32% of cases. It is important to keep in mind that postoperative imaging is mandatory and is the only acceptable means of assessing residual tumor. Even in cases in which a complete resection cannot be obtained, the randomized trial from the Children's Cancer Group suggested that improved survival may be seen in those with <1.5 cm^2 of residual tumor (Robertson et al 1998). With modern operative techniques, GTR rates of between 70% and 84% (van Veelen-Vincent et al 2002; Merchant et al 2004b; Rogers et al 2005) have been reported as assessed by postoperative MRI , in comparison with previous reported rates of between 40% and 60% (Sutton et al 1990; Robertson et al 1998). It is not clear whether this improvement has been accompanied by an increase in perioperative morbidity/mortality.

Miscellaneous factors

While age, tumor location, tumor grade, and extent of surgical resection are by far the most well investigated potential prognostic factors, others have been suggested in the literature. These include factors such as gender, race, and duration of symptoms (Goldwein et al 1990a,b; Vanuytsel et al 1992; Pollack et al 1995). There is very little evidence to suggest that any of these factors is, in fact, significantly prognostic (Shaw et al 1987; Rousseau et al 1994; Robertson et al 1998).

Despite calls for cooperation and evidence to be generated through international randomized prospective trials (Bouffet et al 1998), now a decade on, such data are still lacking in the published literature. Given the small numbers of such cases that are seen at any single institution, a multicenter cooperative effort would be needed in order to prospectively recruit a critical number of patients in a reasonable period of time. Data from such studies would help answer, in a much more definitive way, the many questions that have been asked regarding ependymomas.

Treatment

Surgical therapy

Upon diagnosis of a posterior fossa tumor, any immediate threats to the child's life need to be dealt with urgently. Most commonly, this is severe obstructive hydrocephalus that may warrant rapid ventricular drainage. If the child is severely obtunded as a result of hydrocephalus, urgent external drainage should be performed. However, in most cases, the child will improve, sometimes dramatically, with the urgent administration of steroids, e.g., dexamethasone. This can obviate the need for external ventricular drainage and should be tried first. This usually provides an adequate temporizing measure until the tumor is resected and normal CSF flow patterns are re-established.

Preoperatively, it can be difficult to confirm the exact type of tumor one is dealing with. However, virtually all types of pediatric posterior fossa tumors will benefit, at least in the short term, from surgical decompression. In the previous section, it was stated that complete surgical resection appears to be an important prognostic factor. Therefore, every effort should be made to perform as complete a resection as is safely possible. Some have recommended that if early postoperative imaging reveals residual tumor, second-look surgery is warranted with the goal being GTR (Foreman et al 1997; Korshunov et al 2004). Unfortunately, a complete resection is very frequently extremely difficult, if not impossible. In the randomized trial from the Children's Cancer Group, they followed a standard protocol for postoperative staging and all patients were operated on using relatively recent microsurgical technique (Robertson et al 1998). However, over half their cases (53%) demonstrated residual tumor on postoperative imaging. Rates of between 70% and 83% are now reported for GTR in pediatric intracranial ependymoma (van Veelen-Vincent et al 2002; Merchant et al 2004b; Rogers et al 2005).

An important preoperative investigation is full neuraxis staging with MR. The results of this may have a significant impact on the goals of surgery. Specifically, if distant metastases are clearly observed, this will certainly dampen one's enthusiasm for performing a gross total resection. This can be the deciding factor in determining how aggressively to proceed in resecting a difficult, adherent tumor, for example.

Operative technique

The major challenge in the surgical resection of ependymomas is in resecting the more difficult posterior fossa lesions. A brief description of the operative approach follows, with particular attention to complication avoidance.

The child is placed in a prone position with the neck flexed. Head fixation may be used for older children. A ventricular drain is usually not needed. Mannitol and additional dexamethasone are given. A standard exposure of the posterior fossa is then performed. Ependymomas frequently extend below the foramen magnum and close examination of the preoperative MR will reveal the extent of such extrusion. If there is extension into the upper cervical spine, this will need to be exposed operatively. An excellent exposure is essential in order to maximize the chances of a complete resection and this should not be compromised. Once an adequate bony exposure has been performed, the occipital bone is removed through a bilateral craniotomy. Enough bone must be removed in order to just visualize the transverse sinus bilaterally. The removal of the posterior arch of C1 will be dictated by the extent of tumor seen on the preoperative MR.

Once epidural hemostasis has been obtained, the dura is opened widely in a standard Y-shaped fashion and the dural leaves are carefully reflected back. The brain may be under significant pressure. This pressure can usually be relieved by releasing CSF from the cisterna magna. If this fails, ventricular cannulation may, rarely, be necessary.

Initial inspection of the operative field should be performed to identify evidence of gross arachnoid tumor spread. If present, this should be sent for pathological examination. As well, as CSF is being released, this should be saved and sent for cytological examination.

At this point, it is important to identify the key surgical landmarks. This includes the obex, PICA on both sides and, if possible, the lower cranial nerves. This initial inspection may also demonstrate tumor extrusion into the CPA or upper cervical spine. The tumor is most commonly found in the fourth ventricle itself and to allow for complete exposure, the lower vermis may be split (transvermian approach) in the midline or alternatively a telovelar approach, incorporating incision of the tela choroidea and the inferior medullary velum, may be utilized (Mussi & Rhoton 2000; Tanriover et al 2004). With the tumor exposed, a sample of tumor should be sent for an intraoperative pathology assessment, to confirm the diagnosis.

Tumor location and surgeon familiarity are the most significant factors in determining the type of approach used to access the fourth ventricle. Tanriover et al (2004) performed an anatomic study that suggested that the telovelar approach allowed for greater access to the lateral recesses and the foramen of Luschka, without incision of any part of the cerebellum. As a consequence, this approach may be favored when tumor is identified to be extending out through the foramen of Luschka into the cerebellopontine angle. The transvermian approach provides slightly better visualization of the medial part of the superior half of the roof of the fourth ventricle and thus may be more suitable for primarily midline lesions.

At this critical stage, there are certain key points to be aware of. First, prior to debulking the tumor, it is important to be extremely wary of the floor of the fourth ventricle. The tumor is frequently adherent to this and, unless careful, debulking of the tumor may lead one right into the brainstem. This is to be avoided at all costs. Early visualization of the floor of the fourth ventricle is, therefore, very important. Once identified, a small cottonoid patty should be placed to mark and protect it. One should then see if the tumor separates off the floor of the fourth ventricle. If this reveals an area of adherence to the brainstem, it should be acknowledged that a complete resection of the tumor will not be possible. Attempts to 'shave' tumor off the brainstem are fraught with significant postoperative neurological sequelae and must be avoided.

A second point is to pay close attention to the most lateral extents of the tumor. Having already discussed the ability of ependymomas to extrude into the upper cervical spine, it is also a well-known feature of these tumors to extend through the foramina of Luschka into the CPA. This is another area in which resection of the tumor can present significant challenges. Depending on the extent of the lateral spread, several of the lower cranial nerves, as well as major vascular structures, e.g., vertebral artery and PICA, may be intimately associated with the tumor. Resection at this stage should obviously proceed with great care. Preserving the child's neurological functioning should be the primary goal. Once again, this may necessarily prevent a total resection of the tumor.

Tumor removal is usually performed under microscopic magnification in a piece-meal fashion. An ultrasonic surgical aspirator is frequently quite useful for this. Upon completion of tumor resection, the dura should be closed in a watertight fashion. This usually requires a dural patch graft, which can easily be obtained from the nearby occipital pericranium. The occipital craniotomy bone flap is then replaced.

Postoperatively, the child can usually be extubated, unless there is clear evidence of bulbar dysfunction. Close observation overnight is warranted to rule out the development of postoperative hydrocephalus. A relatively rapid wean off steroids should also be performed.

Surgery for intracranial ependymoma in children is not without morbidity and mortality, with some series reporting up to 7.5% perioperative mortality and a 57% postoperative complication rate of varying severity and duration. The principal complication was transient cranial nerve dysfunction in this and other series (Pollack et al 1995; Doxey et al 1999; van Veelen-Vincent et al 2002). Such accurate reporting of complications is rare in the literature, resulting in difficulties in obtaining of broader appreciation of these rates.

Aside from brainstem or lower cranial nerve dysfunction, a rare, but interesting, postoperative complication is the syndrome of cerebellar mutism (CMS) (Dietze & Mickle 1990; Ferrante et al 1990; Van Calenbergh et al 1995). This consists of varying severity of complete speech arrest, emotional lability, hypotonia and ataxia and is not unique to ependymomas, occurring in children following removal of any midline posterior fossa tumor. There may be a 1- or 2-day delay in the presentation and it may be associated with visual impairment, as well (Liu et al 1998). A total of 24% of 450 children were identified as having some degree of CMS in a prospective questionnaire study linked to CCG and POG studies for children surgically treated for medulloblastoma (Robertson et al 2006). CMS can certainly occur after surgery for posterior fossa ependymoma (García Conde et al 2007), although it is children with large (>5 cm) medulloblastoma who seem at the highest risk (Catsman-Berrevoets et al 1999).

While the mechanism is unclear, it is important to recognize that, while there is clinical improvement, delayed effects are becoming increasingly recognized (Liu et al 1998; Steinbok et al 2003; Grill et al 2004; Robertson et al 2006).

Hydrocephalus is an important concomitant factor in pediatric intracranial ependymoma. Hydrocephalus may be identified at presentation in children with intracranial ependymoma, and may require definitive treatment if primary tumor surgery fails to resolve the issue. In one series of children, 14% went on to require long-term treatment for hydrocephalus (van Veelen-Vincent et al 2002). Children undergoing second surgery for ependymoma are more likely to require the placement of a shunt (Merchant et al 2004a). Adequate treatment of hydrocephalus is imperative in minimizing long-term cognitive deficits and endocrinopathies in these children, especially those undergoing radiation (Merchant et al 2004a; Conklin et al 2008).

Radiation therapy

Radiation therapy has long been used as the primary adjuvant therapy for ependymomas. The evidence for this therapy is derived from several retrospective series (Mork & Loken

1977; Rousseau et al 1994; Perilongo et al 1997; Rogers et al 2005; Massimino et al 2006). Early work has shown that doses below about 4500 cGy to the primary tumor appear not to be as beneficial (Phillips et al 1964; Kim & Fayos 1977; Garrett & Simpson 1983). Because of potentially devastating neurological sequelae, radiation therapy has generally been avoided entirely in children under 3 years of age.

Historically, craniospinal radiotherapy was used for high-grade and infratentorial tumor. However, in the late 1980s, investigators noted that the major cause of treatment failure was local recurrence and that isolated CSF relapse was uncommon. For that reason, many institutions began treating patients with intracranial ependymomas without evidence of CSF spread with conformal radiotherapy to the local site only omitting the craniospinal component. The use of craniospinal radiation is reversed for patients with either microscopic or gross evidence of CSF spread. A report in 1997 (Merchant et al 1997) demonstrated in a retrospective review that there was no benefit from the use of craniospinal radiotherapy for localized ependymomas and that the overwhelming cause of treatment failure was local recurrence in 19 patients, while only one patient suffered recurrence throughout the CSF. Subsequent publications have confirmed this finding and it now represents the standard of care for children with localized intracranial ependymomas (Paulino 2001; Merchant et al 2004b). Originally, the standard dose was 54 Gy in 30 fractions, but preliminary experience from a pilot experience (Merchant et al 2002b) demonstrated increased local control and survival with the use of 59.4 Gy in 33 fractions, which subsequently formed the basis of a phase II study within the Children's Oncology Group (COG protocol ACNS0121) to study the use of this dose in a large cohort of patients, the results of which are awaited.

As a result of newer radiotherapy technologies which allow the precise delivery of high dose radiotherapy to a highly conformal volume, the use of conformal focal radiotherapy is increasingly being utilized in children under the age of 3. This was included in the phase II study of the COG ACNS0121 protocol, and long-term outcomes and risks of adverse effects are awaited from this study. The advances in radiation technology have allowed the use of radiotherapy as retreatment in cases of recurrent ependymoma (Merchant et al 2008), with long-term control in some cases and an acceptable toxicity profile for patients for whom no other useful approaches were available.

There are a number of small studies that have evaluated radiosurgery (SRS) for ependymoma (Stafford et al 2000; Mansur et al 2004; Lo et al 2006), although a recent report has suggested that this modality has a high complication rate (Merchant et al 2008). SRS has been given as a boost following external beam radiotherapy and in attempted salvage, following failed external beam radiation. The use of proton radiotherapy has been reported for ependymoma with favorable results and a suggested benefit of reducing the dose to normal tissues (MacDonald et al 2008).

Chemotherapy

Chemotherapy has been a more recent addition to the adjuvant therapy of intracranial ependymomas (Bouffet &

Foreman 1999). Its use in ependymomas is generally considered in younger patients (under 3 years of age) following initial surgery, and when the disease has recurred (Bouffet & Foreman 1999). Initial results have not been encouraging, with many studies unable to demonstrate any significant beneficial effect (Bouffet et al 1998; Goldwein et al 1990a,b; Sutton et al 1990; Evans et al 1996; Robertson et al 1998; Timmermann et al 2000; Nicholson et al 2007).

Single and multi-agent chemotherapeutic protocols have been used in ependymoma therapy. These include MOPP (van Eys et al 1985; Ater et al 1997), the eight agents in 1-day regimen (8-in-1) (White et al 1993; Geyer et al 1994; Ayan et al 1995; Robertson et al 1998), oral etoposide (Sandri et al 2005), temozolomide (Rehman et al 2006; Nicholson et al 2007), intrathecal cytarabine (Lassaletta et al 2007) and other miscellaneous regimens (Evans et al 1996; Needle et al 1997; Duffner et al 1998; Yoffe et al 2007). While some of these studies have results that may be interpreted as promising, the studies are very small and their results far from conclusive (White et al 1993; Geyer et al 1994; Needle et al 1997; Duffner et al 1998). With single agents, the response rate is 11%, with <5% of complete responses; cisplatin seems to be the most active agent in phase II studies, with modest responses seen to carboplatin, ifosfamide and oral etoposide (Khan et al 1982; Sexauer et al 1985; Gaynon et al 1990; Friedman et al 1992; Needle et al 1997; Bouffet & Foreman 1999).

Merchant et al (2002a) reported that PFS and overall survival were worse in those children receiving pre-RT chemotherapy than in those that did not. The use of high-dose chemotherapy with stem cell rescue has not led to improvement in survival (Grill et al 1996; Mason et al 1998). A study of children under the age of 10 treated with intensive induction chemotherapy followed by myeloablative chemotherapy and autologous stem cell rescue, concluded no benefit over previously reported chemotherapeutic strategies (Zacharoulis et al 2007). These studies also highlight the potentially significant toxicity, sometimes fatal, associated with many of the aggressive chemotherapy regimens.

The greatest potential role for chemotherapy is likely for the group of infants, under 3 years of age, for whom radiation therapy may be withheld following surgical resection. A number of studies have suggested that radiotherapy may be avoided or delayed without compromising overall survival in a substantial proportion of children under the age of 3 (Duffner et al 1998; Grundy et al 2007) or under the age of 5 (Grill et al 2001). These results require further study and in particular, the neurocognitive effects of prolonged chemotherapy in this age group need to be addressed. The use of newer radiation technologies in children less than 3 years of age without evidence of neurocognitive decline and higher progression free survival rates (Merchant et al 2004b), raises questions over the use of such chemotherapeutic regimens (Bouffet et al 2007).

Recurrence and patterns of failure

Ependymomas have a propensity to spread via the cerebrospinal fluid system, and between 5–22% of children present with documented leptomeningeal metastases at diagnosis (Goldwein et al 1990a,b; Vanuytselet al 1992; Polednak & Flannery 1995; Pollack et al 1995; Robertson et al 1998; Horn et al 1999; Merchant et al 2004b; Merchant & Fouladi 2005; Lassaletta et al 2007). Given this fact, full and proper staging of the entire central nervous system is mandatory early in the child's evaluation. This includes full neuraxis MRI and examination of CSF cytology. It has been suggested that the proportion of ependymomas diagnosed with evidence of distant metastases has increased since the early 1970s (Polednak & Flannery 1995). Improvements in preoperative staging technology have likely played a large part in this change.

Although ependymomas do have the capacity for leptomeningeal spread, the vast majority of tumor recurrences occur as a result of lack of local tumor control (Shaw et al 1987; Goldwein et al 1990a,b; Lyons & Kelly 1991; Vanuytsel et al 1992; Kovalic et al 1993). Tumor recurrence presenting as metastatic spread without any evidence of local recurrence is very rare, occurring in only 7–8% of cases (Shaw et al 1987; Robertson et al 1998).

Unfortunately, most childhood ependymomas do recur at some point. The 5- and 10-year progression free survivals range from approximately 36–64% and 46–47%, respectively (Sutton et al 1990; Chiu et al 1992; Kovalic et al 1993; Robertson et al 1998; van Veelen-Vincent et al 2002; Jaing et al 2004). An unresolved issue is exactly what surveillance protocol is optimal in children with ependymomas, in order to maximize detection of recurrence without unduly wasting resources. The Children's Cancer Group has recommended MRI of the brain (and spine if documented metastases) every 3 months for the 1st year (Kramer et al 1994). Others have suggested protocols, based on the pattern and timing of ependymoma recurrences, in which no imaging is performed in the first 18 months following resection. After this period, relatively frequent imaging (every 4–6 months) is performed for 3.5 years and no further surveillance imaging thereafter (Steinbok et al 1996). There is evidence to suggest that those children identified to have asymptomatic recurrence on surveillance MRI have improved survival compared with those children diagnosed with symptomatic recurrence, in excess of what would be expected through earlier diagnosis (Good et al 2001).

Treatment of recurrence

Once tumor recurrence has been identified, treatment options become relatively limited, both in scope and efficacy. Initial consideration should be given to re-operation in cases of local and even metastatic recurrence (Merchant et al 2008), although morbidity related to second surgery has variably been documented to be higher in some series (Massimino et al 2006), yet not as significant in others (Vinchon et al 2005). Since the local area, at least, has already been irradiated, further radiation therapy was thought no longer feasible, other than for isolated areas of remote metastases, however, reports of re-treatment are emerging (Merchant et al 2008). Various chemotherapeutic regimens have been studied, with relatively poor results (Khan et al 1982; Sexauer et al 1985; Ragab et al 1986; Bertolone et al 1989; Goldwein et al 1990a,b; Friedman et al 1992). The agents which show mildly promising results are

cisplatin (also associated with potentially significant renal and otological toxicity), (Khan et al 1982; Sexauer et al 1985; Bertolone et al 1989), and oral etoposide (Chamberlain 2001; Sandri et al 2005; Valera et al 2005), however these are small studies and the results are modest. Temozolomide was recently found to be ineffective in children with recurrent intracranial ependymoma (Nicholson et al 2007). A very aggressive approach of high-dose, intensive chemotherapy with autologous bone marrow transplant rescue has been investigated for recurrent ependymomas (Grill et al 1996; Mason et al 1998). Unfortunately, the children in these small series experienced very little clinical response and there was a high incidence of fatal toxicity. The authors of both series concluded that this was not an effective means of treating recurrent ependymomas.

Outcome

Compared with other childhood brain tumors, the outcome for ependymomas is relatively poor. The 5-year survival rate ranges from 39% to 73% (this series of 83 patients excluded four intraoperative deaths) (Pierre-Kahn et al 1983; Shaw et al 1987; Goldwein et al 1990a,b; Nazar et al 1990; Healey et al 1991; Vanuytsel et al 1992; Ikezaki et al 1993; Robertson et al 1998; Horn et al 1999; Figarella-Branger et al 2000; van Veelen-Vincent et al 2002; Jaing et al 2004; Shu et al 2007). The 10-year survival rate drops to approximately 45–51% (Healey et al 1991; Ikezaki et al 1993; Pollack et al 1995; van Veelen-Vincent et al 2002). Beyond the issue of just absolute survival, there is also the potential impairments that may occur in the quality of life of long-term survivors of childhood brain tumors (Feeny et al 1992; Seaver et al 1994; Hoppe-Hirsch et al 1995; Mulhern et al 2004). These children frequently have relatively low intelligence quotients with poor general academic and psychosocial functioning, even with posterior fossa irradiation alone (Grill et al 1999; Mulhern et al 2004). While current therapeutic modifications must be aimed at improving survival, the issue of quality of life must also be given strong consideration. Future therapeutic directions should be aimed at decreasing the long-term neurological morbidity that otherwise results from surgical-, chemotherapeutic-, and radiation-induced insults to the developing nervous system.

Ependymomas in adults

While ependymomas do occur more commonly in children, they certainly are found in adult patients and make up about 2% of intracranial tumors in adults (Barone & Elvidge 1970; Polednak & Flannery 1995; Guyotat et al 2002). Given the relatively lower incidence, the literature regarding ependymomas in adults is more sparse.

There does not appear to be a clear gender bias in adults, with tumors reported in roughly equal percentages of men and women (Wallner et al 1986; Donahue 1998; Schwartz et al 1999). Adult patients tend to be relatively young, with most series reporting median ages under 45 years (Wallner et al 1986; Shaw et al 1987; Donahue 1998; Schwartz et al 1999). In adults, infratentorial and spinal ependymomas arise with almost equal frequency (Marks & Adler 1982; Read 1984; Kudo 1990; Donahue 1998).

Prognostic factors have not been very well studied within the adult population, although much of what has been said about pediatric ependymomas also likely holds true for adults. There is some evidence to suggest that, overall, adults have a better survival prognosis than children (Garrett & Simpson 1983; Read 1984; Papadopoulos et al 1990; Lyons & Kelly 1991), although this is not a unanimous finding (Shaw et al 1987; Vanuytsel et al 1992). Survival rates have variably been shown to be associated with tumor location, histologic grade, extent of surgery, patient age, and patient Karnofski performance status *but not all studies concur* (Ernestus et al 1997; Guyotat et al 2002; Korshunov et al 2004; Metellus et al 2007). The significance of histologic grade is controversial due to small sample sizes, variability in the definition of anaplasia and discrepancies in histological diagnoses and the variable inclusion of ependymoblastoma in some series. In a retrospective series of 70 patients with adult intracranial ependymoma, only younger patient age was shown to be associated with longer survival. The 5- and 10-year survival rates were 74% ± 8% and 60% ± 10% for patients <40 years of age and 56% ± 11% and 36% ± 12% for those >40 years (Reni et al 2004).

The pathology of the tumor is identical to that described for children and the same difficulties exist in distinguishing anaplastic ependymomas. Anaplastic ependymoma is thought to account for approximately 20% of adult intracranial ependymoma (Reni et al 2004). The imaging features of the tumor also remain the same. However, the differential diagnosis of a posterior fossa mass in an adult is very different from that for children. The most common tumors to consider are metastases from an extracranial primary tumor, hemangioblastoma, vestibular schwannoma, and meningioma. In the absence of other distinguishing features, ependymoma generally falls quite low on the differential diagnosis of a posterior fossa mass in an adult.

Treatment of ependymomas in adults usually follows the management plan outlined for children. The primary therapy consists of surgical resection, with the goal being a gross total resection, with a second surgery offered if resectable residual is identified on postoperative MRI, followed by radiation therapy, usually limited to a localized field (Marks & Adler 1982; Read 1984; Lyons & Kelly 1991; Donahue 1998). Radiotherapy has been found to be beneficial in incompletely resected low-grade ependymomas and to a lesser extent, in completely resected high-grade tumors. The role of radiotherapy in completely resected low-grade tumors remains controversial (Metellus et al 2007). Surgical resection, particularly of the posterior fossa tumors, harbors the same potential complications as described for children and must be well thought out ahead of time. There are exceedingly few reports of chemotherapy use in adult patients and definitive conclusions about its efficacy cannot be made (Read 1984; Lyons & Kelly 1991).

The overall outcome for adult patients with intracranial ependymoma varies, but the 5-year survival rate is approximately 56–84.8% (Garrett & Simpson 1983; Read 1984; Papadopoulos et al 1990; Lyons & Kelly 1991; Vanuytsel et al 1992; Guyotat et al 2001; Metellus et al 2007).

Key points

- Ependymomas occur primarily as posterior fossa masses in children under 8 years of age.
- The distinction between low-grade and anaplastic ependymomas can be difficult and is of questionable prognostic significance.
- Increased age and gross total resection appear to be associated with increased survival, although the quality of the available literature is limited.
- The prognostic significance of other factors, such as tumor location or grade, is not well established.
- Gross total resection should be the operative goal, but is frequently hindered by adherence of the tumor to the floor of the fourth ventricle, lower cranial nerves, or major vascular structures.
- Adjuvant therapy consists of local radiation traditionally in children over 3 years of age and now being considered for those under 3 years of age.
- CSRT may be reserved for patients with dissemination at presentation and at recurrence after second look surgery or metastasectomy.
- The results of chemotherapy have not been encouraging, except in children under the age of 3 years, in whom consideration may be given to withholding or delaying radiation therapy.
- Ependymomas have a 10-year progression-free survival of approximately 45–50%, and usually recur locally, sometimes with evidence of distant spread.
- Treatment of tumor recurrence is limited, but consists of re-operation (if feasible), surgery and radiation for metastatic lesions, and experimental chemotherapeutic regimens.
- The overall 5-year survival for childhood ependymomas is approximately 39–73%.
- The overall 5-year survival for adult ependymomas is approximately 56–84.8%.

REFERENCES

Artico, M., Bardella, L., Ciappetta, P., et al., 1989. Surgical treatment of subependymomas of the central nervous system. Report of 8 cases and review of the literature. Acta. Neurochirurgica 98 (1–2), 25–31.

Ater, J.L., van Eys, J., Woo, S.Y., et al., 1997. MOPP chemotherapy without irradiation as primary postsurgical therapy for brain tumors in infants and young children. J. Neurooncol. 32 (3), 243–252.

Ayan, I., Darendeliler, E., Kebudi, R., et al., 1995. Evaluation of response to postradiation eight in one chemotherapy in childhood brain tumors. J. Neurooncol. 26, 65–72.

Barone, B.M., Elvidge, A.R., 1970. Ependymomas. A clinical survey. J. Neurosurg. 33 (4), 428–438.

Begnami, M.D., Palau, M., Rushing, E.J., et al., 2007. Evaluation of NF2 gene deletion in sporadic schwannomas, meningiomas, and ependymomas by chromogenic in situ hybridization. Hum. Pathol. 38 (9), 1345–1350

Bertolone, S.J., Baum, E.S., Krivit, W., et al., 1989. A phase II study of cisplatin therapy in recurrent childhood brain tumors. A report from the Children's Cancer Study Group. J. Neurooncol. 7 (1), 5–11.

Bouffet, E., Foreman, N., 1999. Chemotherapy for intracranial ependymomas. Childs Nerv. Syst. 15 (10), 563–570.

Bouffet, E., Perilongo, G., Canete, A., et al., 1998. Intracranial ependymomas in children: a critical review of prognostic factors and a plea for cooperation. Med. Pediatr. Oncol. 30 (6), 319–331.

Bouffet, E., Tabori, U., Bartels, U., 2007. Paediatric ependymomas: should we avoid radiotherapy? Lancet Oncol. 8 (8), 665–666.

Burger, P., Scheithauer, B.W., Vogel, F.S., 1991. Surgical pathology of the nervous system and its coverings, third ed. Churchill Livingstone, New York.

Catsman-Berrevoets, C.E., Van Dongen, H.R., Mulder, P., et al., 1999. Tumor type and size are high risk factors for the syndrome of cerebellar mutism and subsequent dysarthria. J. Neurol. Neurosurg. Psychiatry 67 (6), 755–757.

Centeno, R.S., Lee, A.A., Winter, J., et al., 1986. Supratentorial ependymomas. Neuroimaging and clinicopathological correlation. J. Neurosurg. 64 (2), 209–215.

Chamberlain, M.C., 2001. Recurrent intracranial ependymoma in children: salvage therapy with oral etoposide. Pediatr. Neurol. 24 (2), 117–121.

Chiu, J.K., Woo, S.Y., Ater, J., et al., 1992. Intracranial ependymoma in children: analysis of prognostic factors. J. Neurooncol. 13 (3), 283–290.

Choi, Y.L., Chi, J.G., Suh, Y.L., 2001. CD99 immunoreactivity in ependymoma. Appl. Immunohistochem Mol. Morphol. 9 (2), 125–129.

Comi, A.M., Backstrom, J.W., Burger, P.C., et al., 1998. Clinical and neuroradiologic findings in infants with intracranial ependymomas. Pediatric Oncology Group. Pediatr. Neurol. 18 (1), 23–29.

Conklin, H.M., Li, C., Xiong, X., et al., 2008. Predicting change in academic abilities after conformal radiation therapy for localized ependymoma. J. Clin. Oncol. 26 (24), 3965–3970

Davies, N.P., Wilson, M., Harris, L.M., et al., 2008. Identification and characterization of childhood cerebellar tumors by in vivo proton MRS. NMR Biomed. 21 (8), 908–918.

Dietze, D.D. Jr., Mickle, J.P., 1990. Cerebellar mutism after posterior fossa surgery. Pediatr. Neurosurg. 16 (1), 25–31.

Dimopoulos, V.G., Fountas, K.N., Robinson, J.S., 2006. Familial intracranial ependymomas. Report of three cases in a family and review of the literature. Neurosurg. Focus. 20 (1), E8.

Donahue, B.S.A., 1998. Intracranial ependymoma in the adult patient: successful treatment with surgery and radiotherapy. J. Neurooncol. 37 (2), 131–133.

Doxey, D., Bruce, D., Sklar, F., et al., 1999. Posterior fossa syndrome: identifiable risk factors and irreversible complications. Pediatr. Neurosurg. 31 (3), 131–136.

Duffner, P.K., Krischer, J.P., Sanford, R.A., et al., 1998. Prognostic factors in infants and very young children with intracranial ependymoma. Pediatr. Neurosurg. 28 (4), 215–222.

Ebert, C., von Haken, M., Meyer-Puttlitz, B., et al., 1999. Molecular genetic analysis of ependymal tumors. NF2 mutations and chromosome 22q loss occur preferentially in intramedullary spinal ependymomas. Am. J. Pathol. 155 (2), 627–632.

Ernestus, R.I., Wilcke, O., Schröder, R., 1991. Supratentorial ependymomas in childhood: clinicopathological findings and prognosis. Acta. Neurochir. (Wien) 111, 96–102.

Ernestus, R.I., Schröder, R., Klug, J., 1992. Spontaneous intracerebral hemorrhage from an unsuspected ependymoma in early infancy. Childs Nerv. Syst. 8 (6), 357–360.

Ernestus, R.I., Schröder, R., Stützer, H., et al., 1997. The clinical and prognostic relevance of grading in intracranial ependymomas. Br. J. Neurosurg. 11 (5), 421–428.

Evans, A.E., Anderson, J.R., Lefkowitz-Boudreaux, I.B., et al., 1996. Adjuvant chemotherapy of childhood posterior fossa ependymoma: cranio-spinal irradiation with or without adjuvant CCNU, vincristine, and prednisone: a Children's Cancer Group study. Med. Pediatr. Oncol. 27 (1), 8–14.

Feeny, D., Furlong, W., Barr, R.D., et al., 1992. A comprehensive multiattribute system for classifying the health status of survivors of childhood cancer. J. Clin. Oncol. 10 (6), 923–928.

Ferrante, L., Mastronardi, L., Acqui, M., et al., 1990. Mutism after posterior fossa surgery in children. Report of three cases. J. Neurosurg. 72 (6), 959–963.

Figarella-Branger, D., Civatte, M., Bouvier-Labit, C., et al., 2000. Prognostic factors in intracranial ependymomas in children. J. Neurosurg. 93 (4), 605–613.

Figarella-Branger, D., Gambarelli, D., Dollo, C., et al., 1991. Infratentorial ependymomas of childhood. Correlation between histological features, immunohistological phenotype, silver nucleolar organizer region staining values and post-operative survival in 16 cases. Acta. Neuropathol. 82, 208–216.

Flament-Durand, J., Brion, J.P., 1985. Tanycytes: morphology and functions: a review. Int. Rev. Cytol. 96, 121–155.

Flores, L.E., Williams, D.L., Bell, B.A., et al., 1986. Delay in the diagnosis of pediatric brain tumors. Am. J. Dis. Child 140 (7), 684–686.

Foreman, N.K., Love, S., Gill, S.S., et al., 1997. Second-look surgery for incompletely resected fourth ventricle ependymomas: technical case report. Neurosurgery 40, 856–860.

Fouladi, M., Helton, K., Dalton, J., et al., 2003. Clear cell ependymoma: a clinicopathologic and radiographic analysis of 10 patients. Cancer 98 (10), 2232–2244

Friedman, H.S., Krischer, J.P., Burger, P., et al., 1992. Treatment of children with progressive or recurrent brain tumors with carboplatin or iproplatin: a Pediatric Oncology Group randomized phase II study. J. Clin. Oncol. 10, 249–256.

García Conde, M., Martín Viota, L., Febles García, P., et al., 2007. [Severe cerebellar mutism after posterior fossa tumor resection]. Ann. Pediatr. (Barc.) 66 (1), 75–79.

Garre, M.L., Capra, V., Di Battista, E., et al., 2007. Genetic abnormalities and CNS tumors: report of two cases of ependymoma associated with Klinefelter's Syndrome (KS). Childs Nerv. Syst. 23 (2), 219–223.

Garrett, P.G., Simpson, W.J., 1983. Ependymomas: results of radiation therapy. Int. J. Radiation Oncology Biol. Phys. 9, 1121–1124.

Gaspar, N., Grill, J., Geoerger, B., et al., 2006. p53 Pathway dysfunction in primary childhood ependymomas. Pediatr. Blood Cancer 46 (5), 604–613.

Gaynon, P.S., Ettinger, L.J., Baum, E.S., et al., 1990. Carboplatin in childhood brain tumors. A Children's Cancer Study Group Phase II trial. Cancer 66 (12), 2465–2469

Geyer, J.R., Zeltzer, P.M., Boyett, J.M., et al., 1994. Survival of infants with primitive neuroectodermal tumors or malignant ependymomas of the CNS treated with eight drugs in 1 day: a report from the Children's Cancer Group. J. Clin. Oncol. 12 (8), 1607–1615

Gilbertson, R.J., Bentley, L., Hernan, R., et al., 2002. ERBB receptor signaling promotes ependymoma cell proliferation and represents a potential novel therapeutic target for this disease. Clin. Cancer Res. 8 (10), 3054–3064

Gilles, F.H., Sobel, E.L., Tavaré, C.J., et al., 1995. Age-related changes in diagnoses, histological features, and survival in children with brain tumors: 1930–1979 The Childhood Brain Tumor Consortium. Neurosurgery 37 (6), 1056–1068

Goldwein, J.W., Corn, B.W., Finlay, J.L., et al., 1991. Is craniospinal irradiation required to cure children with malignant (anaplastic) intracranial ependymomas? Cancer 67 (11), 2766–2771

● Goldwein, J.W., Glauser, T.A., Packer, R.J., et al., 1990a. Recurrent intracranial ependymomas in children. Survival, patterns of failure, and prognostic factors. Cancer 66 (3), 557–563.

● Goldwein, J.W., Leahy, J.M., Packer, R.J., et al., 1990b. Intracranial ependymomas in children. Int. J. Radiat. Oncol. Biol. Phys. 19 (6), 1497–1502

Good, C.D., Wade, A.M., Hayward, R.D., et al., 2001. Surveillance neuroimaging in childhood intracranial ependymoma: how effective, how often, and for how long? J. Neurosurg. 94 (1), 27–32.

Grill, J., Le Deley, M.C., Gambarelli, D., et al., 2001. Postoperative chemotherapy without irradiation for ependymoma in children under 5 years of age: a multicenter trial of the French Society of Pediatric Oncology. J. Clin. Oncol. 19 (5), 1288–1296

Grill, J., Renaux, V.K., Bulteau, C., et al., 1999. Long-term intellectual outcome in children with posterior fossa tumors according to radiation doses and volumes. Int. J. Radiat. Oncol. Biol. Phys. 45 (1), 137–145.

Grill, J., Viguier, D., Kieffer, V., et al., 2004. Critical risk factors for intellectual impairment in children with posterior fossa tumors: the role of cerebellar damage. J. Neurosurg. 101 (2 Suppl), 152–158.

Grill, J., Kalifa, C., Doz, F., et al., 1996. A high-dose busulfan-thiotepa combination followed by autologous bone marrow transplantation in childhood recurrent ependymoma. A phase-II study. Pediatr. Neurosurg. 25 (1), 7–12.

Grundy, R.G., Wilne, S.A., Weston, C.L., et al., 2007. Primary postoperative chemotherapy without radiotherapy for intracranial ependymoma in children: the UKCCSG/SIOP prospective study. Lancet Oncol. 8 (8), 696–705.

Gurney, J.G., Severson, R.K., Davis, S., et al., 1995. Incidence of cancer in children in the United States. Sex-, race-, and 1-year age-specific rates by histologic type. Cancer 75 (8), 2186–2195

Guyotat, J., Champier, J., Jouvet, A., et al., 2001. Differential expression of somatostatin receptors in ependymoma: implications for diagnosis. Int. J. Cancer 95 (3), 144–151.

Guyotat, J., Signorelli, F., Desme, S., et al., 2002. Intracranial ependymomas in adult patients: analyses of prognostic factors. J. Neurooncol. 60 (3), 255–268.

Hamilton, R.L., Pollack, I.F., 1997. The molecular biology of ependymomas. Brain Pathol. 7 (2), 807–822.

Hasselblatt, M., Paulus, W., 2003. Sensitivity and specificity of epithelial membrane antigen staining patterns in ependymomas. Acta. Neuropathol. 106 (4), 385–388.

• Healey, E.A., Barnes, P.D., Kupsky, W.J., et al., 1991. The prognostic significance of postoperative residual tumor in ependymoma. Neurosurgery 28 (5), 666–671.

Hoppe-Hirsch, E., Brunet, L., Laroussinie, F., et al., 1995. Intellectual outcome in children with malignant tumors of the posterior fossa: influence of the field of irradiation and quality of surgery. Childs Nerv. Syst. 11 (6), 340–346.

• Horn, B., Heideman, R., Geyer, R., et al., 1999. A multi-institutional retrospective study of intracranial ependymoma in children: identification of risk factors. J. Pediatr. Hematol. Oncol. 21 (3), 203–211.

Hulsebos, T.J., Oskam, N.T., Bijleveld, E.H., et al., 1999. Evidence for an ependymoma tumor suppressor gene in chromosome region 22pter-22q11.2. Br. J. Cancer 81 (7), 1150–1154

• Ikezaki, K., Matsushima, T., Inoue, T., et al., 1993. Correlation of microanatomical localization with postoperative survival in posterior fossa ependymomas. Neurosurgery 32, 38–44.

Jaing, T.H., Wang, H.S., Tsay, P.K., et al., 2004. Multivariate analysis of clinical prognostic factors in children with intracranial ependymomas. J. Neurooncol. 68 (3), 255–261.

Jayawickreme, D.P., Hayward, R.D., Harkness, W.F., et al., 1995. Intracranial ependymomas in childhood: a report of 24 cases followed for 5 years. Child's Nerv. Syst. 11, 409–413.

Kawano, N., Yasui, Y., Utsuki, S., et al., 2004. Light microscopic demonstration of the microlumen of ependymoma: a study of the usefulness of antigen retrieval for epithelial membrane antigen (EMA) immunostaining. Brain Tumor. Pathol. 21 (1), 17–21.

Khan, A.B., D'Souza, B.J., Wharam, M.D., et al., 1982. Cisplatin therapy in recurrent childhood brain tumors. Cancer Treat. Rep. 66, 2013–2020.

Kim, Y.H., Fayos, J.V., 1977. Intracranial ependymomas. Radiology 124 (3), 805–808.

Kojima, A., Yamaguchi, N., Okui, S., et al., 2003. Parenchymal anaplastic ependymoma with intratumoral hemorrhage: a case report. Brain Tumor Pathol. 20 (2), 85–88.

Korshunov, A., Golanov, A., Sycheva, R., et al., 2004. The histologic grade is a main prognostic factor for patients with intracranial ependymomas treated in the microneurosurgical era: an analysis of 258 patients. Cancer 100 (6), 1230–1237

Kotylo, P.K., Robertson, P.B., Fineberg, N.S., et al., 1997. Flow cytometric DNA analysis of pediatric intracranial ependymomas. Arch. Pathol. Lab. Med. 121 (12), 1255–1258

Kovalic, J.J., Flaris, N., Grigsby, P.W., et al., 1993. Intracranial ependymoma long term outcome, patterns of failure. J. Neurooncol. 15 (2), 125–131.

Kramer, D.L., Parmiter, A.H., Rorke, L.B., et al., 1998. Molecular cytogenetic studies of pediatric ependymomas. J. Neurooncol. 37 (1), 25–33.

Kramer, E.D., Vezina, L.G., Packer, R.J., et al., 1994. Staging and surveillance of children with central nervous system neoplasms: recommendations of the Neurology and Tumor Imaging Committees of the Children's Cancer Group. Pediatr. Neurosurg. 20, 254–263.

Kraus, J.A., de Millas, W., Sörensen, N., et al., 2001. Indications for a tumor suppressor gene at 22q11 involved in the pathogenesis of ependymal tumors and distinct from hSNF5/INI1. Acta. Neuropathol. 102 (1), 69–74.

Kudo, H., Oi, S., Tamaki, N., et al., 1990. Ependymoma diagnosed in the first year of life in Japan in collaboration with the International Society for Pediatric Neurosurgery. Childs Nerv. Syst. 6 (7), 375–378.

Kuratsu, J., Ushio, Y., 1996. Epidemiological study of primary intracranial tumors in childhood. A population-based survey in Kumamoto Prefecture, Japan. Pediatr. Neurosurg. 25 (5), 240–246; discussion 247.

Kurt, E., Zheng, P.P., Hop, W.C., et al., 2006. Identification of relevant prognostic histopathologic features in 69 intracranial ependymomas, excluding myxopapillary ependymomas and subependymomas. Cancer 106 (2), 388–395.

Lassaletta, A., Perez-Olleros, P., Scaglione, C., et al., 2007. Successful treatment of intracranial ependymoma with leptomeningeal spread with systemic chemotherapy and intrathecal liposomal cytarabine in a two-year-old child. J. Neurooncol. 83 (3), 303–306.

Liu, G.T., Phillips, P.C., Molloy, P.T., et al., 1998. Visual impairment associated with mutism after posterior fossa surgery in children. Neurosurgery 42 (2), 253–256.

Lo, S.S., Abdulrahman, R., Desrosiers, P.M., et al., 2006. The role of Gamma Knife Radiosurgery in the management of unresectable gross disease or gross residual disease after surgery in ependymoma. J. Neurooncol. 79 (1), 51–56.

Lombardi, D., Scheithauer, B.W., Meyer, F.B., et al., 1991. Symptomatic subependymoma: a clinicopathological and flow cytometric study. J. Neurosurg. 75 (4), 583–588.

Louis, D.N., Cavanee, W.K., Ohgaki, H., et al., 2007a. WHO classification of tumors of the central nervous system. IARC, Lyon.

Louis, D.N., Ohgaki, H., Wiestler, O.D., et al., 2007b. The 2007 WHO classification of tumors of the central nervous system. Acta. Neuropathol. 114 (2), 97–109.

Lukashova-v Zangen, I., Kneitz, S., Monoranu, C.M., et al., 2007. Ependymoma gene expression profiles associated with histological subtype, proliferation, and patient survival. Acta. Neuropathol. 113 (3), 325–337.

Lyons, M.K., Kelly, P.J., 1991. Posterior fossa ependymomas: report of 30 cases and review of the literature. Neurosurgery 28 (5), 659–664.

MacDonald, S.M., Safai, S., Trofimov, A., et al., 2008. Proton radiotherapy for childhood ependymoma: initial clinical outcomes and dose comparisons. Int. J. Radiat. Oncol. Biol. Phys. 71 (4), 979–986.

Mahfouz, S., Aziz, A.A., Gabal, S.M., et al., 2008. Immunohistochemical study of CD99 and EMA expression in ependymomas. Medscape J. Med. 10 (2), 41.

Maksoud, Y.A., Hahn, Y.S., Engelhard, H.H., et al., 2002. Intracranial ependymoma. Neurosurg. Focus 13 (3), e4.

Mansur, D.B., Drzymala, R.E., Rich, K.M., et al., 2004. The efficacy of stereotactic radiosurgery in the management of intracranial ependymoma. J. Neurooncol. 66 (1–2), 187–190.

Mansur, D.B., Perry, A., Rajaram, V., et al., 2005. Postoperative radiation therapy for grade II and III intracranial ependymoma. Int. J. Radiat. Oncol. Biol. Phys. 61 (2), 387–391.

Marks, J., Adler, S., 1982. A comparative study of ependymomas by site of origin. Int. J. Radiation Oncology Biol. Phys. 8, 37–43.

Mason, W.P., Goldman, S., Yates, A.J., et al., 1998. Survival following intensive chemotherapy with bone marrow reconstitution for children with recurrent intracranial ependymoma – a report of the Children's Cancer Group. J. Neurooncol. 37 (2), 135–143.

Massimino, M., Giangaspero, F., Garrè, M.L., et al., 2006. Salvage treatment for childhood ependymoma after surgery only: Pitfalls of omitting at once adjuvant treatment. Int. J. Radiat. Oncol. Biol. Phys. 65 (5), 1440–1445

McLaughlin, M.P., Marcus, R.B. Jr, Buatti, J.M., et al., 1998. Ependymoma: results, prognostic factors and treatment recommendations. Int. J. Radiat. Oncol. Biol. Phys. 40 (4), 845–850.

Mehrazin, M., Yavari, P., 2007. Morphological pattern and frequency of intracranial tumors in children. Childs Nerv. Syst. 23 (2), 157–162.

Merchant, T.E., Boop, F.A., Kun, L.E., et al., 2008. A retrospective study of surgery and reirradiation for recurrent ependymoma. Int. J. Radiat. Oncol. Biol. Phys. 71 (1), 87–97.

Merchant, T.E., Fouladi, M., 2005. Ependymoma: new therapeutic approaches including radiation and chemotherapy. J. Neurooncol. 75 (3), 287–299.

Merchant, T.E., Jenkins, J.J., Burger, P.C., et al., 2002a. Influence of tumor grade on time to progression after irradiation for localized ependymoma in children. Int. J. Radiat. Oncol. Biol. Phys. 53 (1), 52–57.

Merchant, T.E., Lee, H., Zhu, J., et al., 2004a. The effects of hydrocephalus on intelligence quotient in children with localized infratentorial ependymoma before and after focal radiation therapy. J. Neurosurg. 101 (2 Suppl), 159–168.

Merchant, T.E., Mulhern, R.K., Krasin, M.J., et al., 2004b. Preliminary results from a phase II trial of conformal radiation therapy and evaluation of radiation-related CNS effects for pediatric patients with localized ependymoma. J. Clin. Oncol. 22 (15), 3156–3162

Merchant, T.E., Zhu, Y., Thompson, S.J., et al., 2002b. Preliminary results from a Phase II trail of conformal radiation therapy for pediatric patients with localised low-grade astrocytoma and ependymoma. Int. J. Radiat. Oncol. Biol. Phys. 52 (2), 325–332.

Merchant, T.E., Haida, T., Wang, M.H., et al., 1997. Anaplastic ependymoma: treatment of pediatric patients with or without craniospinal radiation therapy. J. Neurosurg. 86 (6), 943–949.

Metellus, P., Barrie, M., Figarella-Branger, D., et al., 2007. Multicentric French study on adult intracranial ependymomas: prognostic factors analysis and therapeutic considerations from a cohort of 152 patients. Brain 130 (Pt 5), 1338–1349

Metzger, A.K., Sheffield, V.C., Duyk, G., et al., 1991. Identification of a germ-line mutation in the p53 gene in a patient with an intracranial ependymoma. Proc. Natl. Acad. Sci. U. S. A. 88 (17), 7825–7829

Mierau, G.W., Goin, L., 2007. Perivascular elastic fibers: a diagnostic feature of ependymoma. Ultrastruct Pathol. 31 (4), 251–255.

Miller, R.W., Young, J.L., Novakovic, P.H., 1995. Childhood cancer. Cancer 75 (Suppl), 395–405.

Miyazawa, T., Hirose, T., Nakanishi, K., et al., 2007. Supratentorial ectopic cortical ependymoma occurring with intratumoral hemorrhage. Brain Tumor Pathol. 24 (1), 35–40.

Modena, P., Lualdi, E., Facchinetti, F., et al., 2006. Identification of tumor-specific molecular signatures in intracranial ependymoma and association with clinical characteristics. J. Clin. Oncol. 24 (33), 5223–5233

Monoranu, C.M., Huang, B., Zangen, I.L., et al., 2008. Correlation between 6q25.3 deletion status and survival in pediatric intracranial ependymomas. Cancer Genet. Cytogenet. 182 (1), 18–26.

Monteith, S.J., Heppner, P.A., Woodfield, M.J., et al., 2006. Paediatric central nervous system tumors in a New Zealand population: a 10-year experience of epidemiology, management strategies and outcomes. J. Clin. Neurosci. 13 (7), 722–729.

Mork, S., Loken, A., 1977. Ependymoma. A follow-up study of 101 cases. Cancer 40, 907–915.

Mørk, S.J., Rubinstein, L.J., 1985. Ependymoblastoma. A reappraisal of a rare embryonal tumor. Cancer 55 (7), 1536–1542

Mulhern, R.K., Merchant, T.E., Gajjar, A., et al., 2004. Late neurocognitive sequelae in survivors of brain tumors in childhood. Lancet Oncol. 5 (7), 399–408.

Mussi, A.C., Rhoton, A.L. Jr., 2000. Telovelar approach to the fourth ventricle: microsurgical anatomy. J. Neurosurg. 92 (5), 812–823.

• Nazar, G.B., Hoffman, H.J., Becker, L.E., et al., 1990. Infratentorial ependymomas in childhood: prognostic factors and treatment. J. Neurosurg. 72, 408–417.

Needle, M.N., Goldwein, J.W., Grass, J., et al., 1997. Adjuvant chemotherapy for the treatment of intracranial ependymoma of childhood. Cancer 80 (2), 341–347.

Nicholson, H.S., Kretschmar, C.S., Krailo, M., et al., 2007. Phase 2 study of temozolomide in children and adolescents with recurrent central nervous system tumors: a report from the Children's Oncology Group. Cancer 110 (7), 1542–1550

Nijssen, P.C., Deprez, R.H., Tijssen, C.C., et al., 1994. Familial anaplastic ependymoma: evidence of loss of chromosome 22 in tumor cells. J. Neurol. Neurosurg. Psychiatry 57 (10), 1245–1248

Palma, L., Celli, P., Cantore, G., 1993. Supratentorial ependymomas of the first two decades of life. Long-term follow-up of 20 cases (including two subependymomas). Neurosurgery 32, 169–175.

Papadopoulos, D.P., Giri, S., Evans, R.G., 1990. Prognostic factors and management of intracranial ependymomas. AntiCancer Res. 10 (3), 689–692.

Paulino, A.C., 2001. The local field in infratentorial ependymoma: does the entire posterior fossa need to be treated? Int. J. Radiat. Oncol. Biol. Phys. 49 (3), 757–761.

Perilongo, G., Massimino, M., Sotti, G., et al., 1997. Analyses of prognostic factors in a retrospective review of 92 children with ependymoma: Italian Pediatric Neuro-oncology Group. Med. Pediatr. Oncol. 29 (2), 79–85.

Peris-Bonet, R., Martinez-Garcia, C., Lacour, B., et al., 2006. Childhood central nervous system tumors – incidence and survival in Europe (1978–1997): report from Automated Childhood Cancer Information System project. Eur. J. Cancer 42 (13), 2064–2080

Pezzolo, A., Capra, V., Raso, A., et al., 2008. Identification of novel chromosomal abnormalities and prognostic cytogenetics markers in intracranial pediatric ependymoma. Cancer Lett. 261 (2), 235–243.

Phillips, T.L., Sheline, G.E., Boldrey, E., 1964. Therapeutic considerations in tumors affecting the central nervous system: ependymomas. Radiology. 83, 98–105.

• Pierre-Kahn, A., Hirsch, J.F., Roux, F.X., et al., 1983. Intracranial ependymomas in childhood. Survival and functional results of 47 cases. Child's Brain 10, 145–156.

Pimentel, J., Resende, M., Vaz, A., et al., 2008. Rosette-forming glioneuronal tumor: pathology case report. Neurosurgery 62 (5), E1162–1163; discussion E1163.

Polednak, A.P., Flannery, J.T., 1995. Brain, other central nervous system, and eye cancer. Cancer 75 (1 Suppl), 330–337.

• Pollack, I.F., Gerszten, P.C., Martinez, A.J., et al., 1995. Intracranial ependymomas of childhood: long-term outcome and prognostic factors. Neurosurgery 37 (4), 655–666.

Poppleton, H., Gilbertson, R.J., 2007. Stem cells of ependymoma. Br. J. Cancer 96 (1), 6–10.

Ragab, A.H., Burger, P., Badnitsky, S., et al., 1986. PCNU in the treatment of recurrent medulloblastoma and ependymoma – a POG Study. J. Neurooncol. 3 (4), 341–342.

Ransom, D.T., Ritland, S.R., Kimmel, D.W., et al., 1992. Cytogenetic and loss of heterozygosity studies in ependymomas, pilocytic astrocytomas, and oligodendrogliomas. Genes Chromosomes Cancer 5 (4), 348–356.

Read, G., 1984. The treatment of ependymoma of the brain or spinal canal by radiotherapy: a report of 79 cases. Clin. Radiol. 35 (2), 163–166.

Rehman, S., Brock, C., Newlands, E.S., 2006. A case report of a recurrent intracranial ependymoma treated with temozolomide in remission 10 years after completing chemotherapy. Am. J. Clin. Oncol. 29 (1), 106–107.

Reni, M., Brandes, A.A., Vavassori, V., et al., 2004. A multicenter study of the prognosis and treatment of adult brain ependymal tumors. Cancer 100 (6), 1221–1229

Ridley, L., Rahman, R., Brundler, M.A., et al., 2008. Multifactorial analysis of predictors of outcome in pediatric intracranial ependymoma. Neuro. Oncol. 10 (5), 675–689.

Robertson, P.L., Muraszko, K.M., Holmes, E.J., et al., 2006. Incidence and severity of postoperative cerebellar mutism syndrome in children with medulloblastoma: a prospective study by the Children's Oncology Group. J. Neurosurg. 105 (Suppl), 444–451.

• Robertson, P.L., Zeltzer, P.M., Boyett, J.M., et al., 1998. Survival and prognostic factors following radiation therapy and chemotherapy for ependymomas in children: a report of the Children's Cancer Group. J. Neurosurg. 88 (4), 695–703.

Rodriguez, F.J., Scheithauer, B.W., Robbins, P.D., et al., 2007. Ependymomas with neuronal differentiation: a morphologic and immunohistochemical spectrum. Acta. Neuropathol. 113 (3), 313–324.

Rogers, L., Pueschel, J., Spetzler, R., et al., 2005. Is gross-total resection sufficient treatment for posterior fossa ependymomas? J. Neurosurg. 102 (4), 629–636.

Rorke, L.B., 1987. Relationship of morphology of ependymoma in children to prognosis. Prog. Exp. Tumor. Res. 30, 170–174.

Rorke, L.B., Gilles, F.H., Davis, R.L., et al., 1985. Revision of the World Health Organization classification of brain tumors for childhood brain tumors. Cancer 56 (Suppl), 1869–1886.

1980; Guidetti & Spallone 1981; Pascual-Castroviejo et al 1983; Zhang 1983). The observation that an overproduction of CSF can result from villous hypertrophy of the choroid plexus has since been reported by several investigators (Davis 1924; Ray & Peck 1956; Laurence 1974; Gudeman et al 1979; Welch et al 1983; Hirano et al 1994). Placement of a ventriculostomy and measurement of CSF formation may help in the documentation of overproduction of CSF. Laurence (1974) described six cases of his own but was cautious about the removal of these lesions. However, several surgeons have shown that resection of these rare bilateral choroid plexus lesions results in resolution of the CSF overproduction and alleviation of the concomitant hydrocephalus (Gudeman et al 1979; Welch et al 1983; Hirano et al 1994). Coagulation of this lesion, performed through a minimally invasive endoscopic approach, with the subsequent resolution of CSF overproduction has also been reported (Philips et al 1998).

Imaging

In the current era of imaging, patients are initially diagnosed by computed tomography (CT) and magnetic resonance imaging (MRI). Historically, pneumoencephalography, ventriculography, and angiography were utilized to show these tumors to be intraventricular masses with associated hydrocephalus (Matson 1969). Unfortunately, deaths were associated with the application of pneumoencephalography and ventriculography in the diagnosis of choroid plexus tumors (Laurence 1974; Raimondi & Gutierrez 1975). These deaths probably resulted from the large shifts created by placing a brain needle into large ventricles with a large mass. Plain films, which are rarely used in the modern era, might show marked calcification and non-specific signs of increased pressure such as splayed sutures (Crofton & Matson 1950; Matson 1969; Hawkins 1980).

The introduction of CT improved the safety and accuracy of diagnosis, and ultimately the outcome in children harboring these tumors (Pascual-Castroviejo et al 1983). Both papillomas and carcinomas appear isodense to hyperdense on CT scan, with frequent calcification and usually marked contrast enhancement. Tumors are spherical or multilobular and sometimes cystic. They infrequently extend into another ventricle of CSF cistern, a finding which is not entirely specific for choroid plexus tumors.

MRI is clearly the most accurate and common imaging technique used currently. MRI most often shows a mass which is isointense or slightly hypointense to gray matter on T_1-weighted images, and hyperintense on T_2-weighted images. This tumor is often a lobulated, homogeneous, intraventricular mass on both short T_R/T_E and long T_R/T_E sequences (Vazquez et al 1991). Enhancement with paramagnetic substances such as gadolinium-DTPA is markedly intense and usually homogeneous, although various patterns can be seen including nodular and peripheral enhancement and cyst wall enhancement (Figs 25.1, 25.2) (Naeini et al 2009). A frequent finding is the presence of serpentine signal voids, indicating the presence of an enlarged blood vessel supplying the tumor (Schellhas et al 1988; Coates et al 1989). MRI is the diagnostic imaging study of choice because

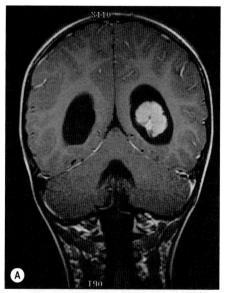

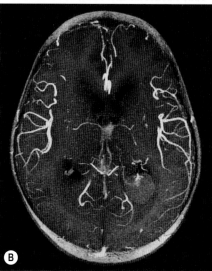

Figure 25.1 (A) This coronal MR scan with gadolinium is of a 4-year-old child who presented for evaluation of headache and lethargy. Note the choroid plexus papilloma in the left lateral ventricle. (B) The same patient underwent a magnetic resonance angiogram (MRA), which showed a hypertrophied posterior choroidal feeding vessel. A high parietal approach was performed with color flow ultrasound guidance. This high approach permitted access to the major arterial feeders anterior to the tumor; these were sacrificed early, shortly after entering the ventricle. The tumor was successfully excised with minimal morbidity (a transient visual field cut).

of its detailed anatomic delineation and triplanar imaging ability. MR angiography (MRA) may provide additional information regarding the vascular supply of the tumor. The advent of MRA is rapidly replacing the need for transfemoral cerebral angiography in the management of these tumors in some patients. Angiography still has a great deal of utility in selected children and adults, especially if preoperative embolization of the feeding vessels is desired. Furthermore, angiography provides the most definitive anatomic configuration of the feeding vessels. The angiogram can provide the

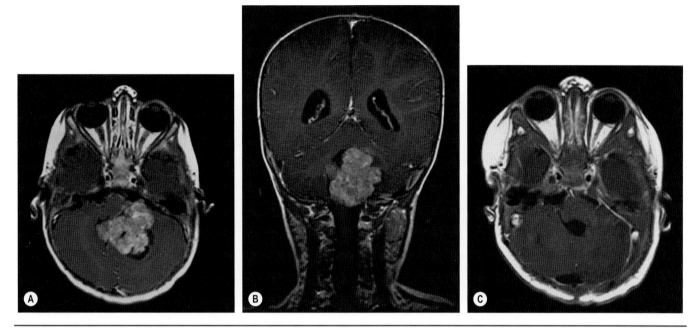

Figure 25.2 Preoperative T1 MR axial (A), coronal (B), and postoperative axial (C) images with gadolinium administration in a 3-year-old child with a choroid plexus carcinoma of the fourth ventricle and left foramen of Luschka. Note how the tumor demonstrates nodular enhancement as it fills the ventricle and creeps out of the foramen. The patient underwent a transcortical approach through the left lateral hemishere with a gross total excision of this carcinoma which was adherent to the seventh to tenth cranial nerves. Despite intraoperative cranial nerve monitoring the patient suffered a temporary, but significant, paresis of the ninth and tenth cranial nerves and required a tracheostomy. The patient underwent postoperative adjuvant chemotherapy and remains tumor free.

surgeon with the most efficacious route to occlude the tumor vessels for a safe resection. We have used preoperative embolization in several children, and it has successfully decreased the transfused quantity of packed red blood cells, as well as rendered challenging operations, less difficult.

Quantitative proton magnetic resonance spectroscopy (MRS) has been used in differentiating papilloma from carcinoma. According to one study, proton MRS shows that carcinoma has higher levels of choline and lactate compared to papilloma, but these studies may have to be repeated at multiple institutions to determine the reproducibility of these findings (Horska et al 2001).

Both papilloma and carcinoma can compress the surrounding brain, although brain invasion is a characteristic of carcinoma (Morrison et al 1984). Some authors have commented on the peritumoral vasogenic edema in the surrounding white matter in carcinoma (Morrison et al 1984; Coates et al 1989). Carcinoma does have a greater tendency to invade the brain, but it can also be found in an entirely intraventricular location.

The radiologic differential diagnosis of choroid plexus tumors includes ependymoma, meningioma, primitive neuroectodermal tumor (PNET), astrocytoma, germinoma, teratoma, and metastases to the choroid plexus. Despite the significant differences in histology most of these tumors on MRI can appear homogeneous and quite similar to choroid plexus tumors. Other unusual tumor-like masses that may have a similar appearance include inflammatory pseudotumor, choroid plexus cysts, and xanthogranulomas.

Pathology and differential diagnosis

On visual inspection, choroid plexus papillomas have cauliflower-like surfaces and are generally well-circumscribed masses arising within a ventricle. The papillomas can extend into the brain parenchyma, compressing it along a broad margin. Heavily calcified tumors may be difficult to section unless they are first decalcified (Burger & Scheithauer 1994). Microscopically, choroid plexus tumors typically appear as a single layer of cuboidal epithelial cells surrounding a delicate fibrovascular stalk, arranged in a papillary configuration with finger-like projections of tissue. A well-formed continuous basement membrane is a prominent feature noted in all cases. Choroid plexus tumors span the histologic spectrum from extremely well-differentiated to anaplastic with minimal epithelial differentiation. Well-differentiated and poorly-differentiated components may be seen in a single tumor (Burger & Scheithauer 1994), however, the majority of choroid plexus neoplasms lie in the well-differentiated part of the spectrum. It is occasionally difficult to differentiate normal choroid plexus from a papilloma, but the latter contains cells that are more crowded, columnar in shape, pleomorphic, and possessing more variation in nuclear size (Fig. 25.3). The nuclear:cytoplasmic ratio is often increased (Burger & Scheithauer 1994).

Ultrastructural observations include apical microvilli, scattered cilia, and interdigitating lateral cell borders sitting atop a basement membrane seated on a delicate fibrovascular stalk. Stromal calcification or xanthomatous changes can be evident.

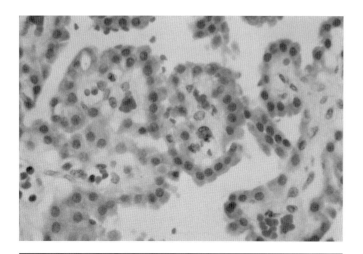

Figure 25.3 This histopathologic section represents the typical papillary appearance of a choroid plexus papilloma completely excised from the lateral ventricle. Note the single layer of columnar cells with organized papillary architecture based on a delicate fibrovascular stroma. The cells are more columnar and pleomorphic than normal choroid plexus cells. (H&E; ×80.)

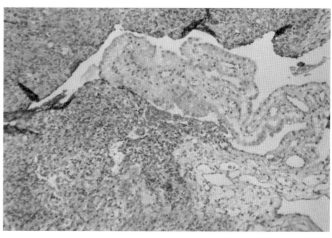

Figure 25.4 This sample is taken from a large choroid plexus carcinoma that invaded the wall of the lateral ventricle. Note the sheet of cells with loss of differentiated papillary architecture (compare Fig. 25.3), and nuclear pleomorphism. This tumor sits adjacent to more normal choroid plexus. (H&E; ×10.)

Atypical microscopic features may be observed in papilloma, and include increased cellularity (two or three cell layers thick as opposed to one), mitoses, nuclear pleomorphism and poorly-formed papillary structures. These intermediate tumors may possess one or two such features and are called atypical papillomas; however, they do not necessarily have a more aggressive natural history and are not classified as carcinoma. Anaplastic transformation of well-differentiated tumors has, however, been reported to occur over time. Although it is uncommon, a lesion that is initially well-differentiated or atypical can become anaplastic, as documented during a subsequent resection (Gullotta & de Melo 1979; Paulus & Janisch 1990).

The histologic features of papilloma vs carcinoma have been subject to close scrutiny and considerable controversy. The focus in diagnosis often centers on this important question: Which particular characteristics differentiate papilloma from carcinoma? Review of the literature reveals that from a historical perspective the criteria for differentiation of papilloma from carcinoma have not been uniform. The definition of choroid plexus carcinoma has varied in several studies based on histologic criteria (Russell & Rubinstein 1971; Dohrmann & Collias 1975; Ellenbogen et al 1989; Matsuda et al 1991; St. Clair et al 1991). Dohrman & Collias (1975), utilizing Russell & Rubinstein's (1971) and Lewis's (1967) criteria of carcinoma reviewed 22 cases of primary choroid plexus carcinoma in the literature from 1844 to 1975 and found that only 11 satisfied their criteria of carcinoma. Similarly, Lewis's review of the literature resulted in the dismissal of many other cases of carcinoma (Lewis 1967).

The consistent histologic features of choroid plexus tumors that unequivocally differentiate carcinoma from papilloma include cellular anaplasia, loss of differentiated papillary choroid architecture, nuclear pleomorphism, mitosis, necrosis, and giant cell formation (Fig. 25.4). At the extreme end of the spectrum are tumors with sheets of anaplastic cells without appreciable papillae. These lesions are very cellular, with complex cribriform structures and a high mitotic index. One issue of contention is whether brain invasion is either required for, or of itself can secure, the diagnosis of carcinoma. Some authors insist that invasion be demonstrated histologically, others do not (St. Clair et al 1991). It is noteworthy that not all surgical specimens will have brain tissue insinuated within tumor projections, especially in cases where the surgeon used ultrasonic aspiration or microsurgical suction to remove the specimen at the brain–tumor interface, and therefore brain has not been included in the surgical specimen. Thus, the absence of finger-like projections invaginating into the brain parenchyma does not necessarily eliminate the diagnosis of carcinoma. Some tumors may invade the stroma but, on careful histopathologic analysis, do not invade the brain. In addition, some choroid tumors with relatively benign histologic features are invasive, while some anaplastic tumors seem to have circumscribed borders (Ausman et al 1984; Ellenbogen et al 1989). Often, the diagnosis of invasion may be inferred by MRI appearance and not by histologic evidence. Thus, while invasion of brain makes the diagnosis of carcinoma highly likely, it is not invariably secured unless there are associated malignant cellular features.

Some authors maintain that, even in choroid plexus papilloma, macro- and microscopic implants can be found in the leptomeninges, the subarachnoid space of the spinal cord, and the ventricular system (Ringertz & Reymond 1949; Russell & Rubinstein 1963). A rare case of pulmonary metastases from a choroid plexus papilloma in an 11-year-old girl was reported in 1950 by Vraa-Jensen. The child developed pulmonary metastasis and lesions in the skull that demonstrated malignant transformation (carcinoma) at autopsy (Vraa-Jensen 1950). Except for case reports, there has been a paucity of clinically symptomatic metastases from papilloma.

The electron microscopic findings are useful for distinguishing choroid plexus carcinoma from ependymoma, which can occasionally demonstrate a similar histologic appearance. The presence of a basal lamina, as seen in choroid plexus tumors, often rules out ependymal origin of a tumor (Hirano 1978).

Some studies have demonstrated the diagnostic utility of immunohistochemistry. Immunohistochemistry of choroid plexus tumors reveals both epithelial and glial characteristics. Choroid neoplasms are positive for cytokeratin (epithelial), S-100 (diffuse staining), and vimentin (Cruz-Sanchez et al 1989; Ang et al 1990). Choroid plexus carcinoma retains cytokeratin positivity but shows decreased S-100 staining (Paulus & Janisch 1990). Positivity for carcinoembryonic antigen is more common in carcinoma, whereas S-100 positivity is more commonly seen in papilloma (Coffin et al 1986).

The differential diagnosis of choroid plexus tumors in children also often focuses on how to differentiate choroid plexus tumors from ependymoma and embryonal tumors. Ependymoma is characterized by non-epithelial glial elements as well as epithelial components. Ependymomas lack the prominent basement membrane possessed by choroid plexus tumors seen on PAS preparations, electron microscopy, or immunohistochemical stains for laminin (Furness et al 1990). Choroid plexus neoplasms are positive for cytokeratin while ependymomas are not; ependymomas are usually GFAP positive, while choroid plexus tumors may be diffusely but not uniformly GFAP positive. In an adult with an intraventricular mass, S-100 protein positivity favors a choroid plexus primary vs a metastatic tumor (Burger & Scheithauer 1994).

In an immunohistochemical study of choroid plexus neoplasms, it was noted that a child who survived with a choroid plexus carcinoma had a tumor that stained positive for S-100 and negative for epithelial membrane antigen, as often seen in papilloma. This immunohistochemical profile was not present in another child, who died with carcinoma (Shirakawa et al 1994). This outcome and staining profile suggested a biologic or genetic variability in carcinoma which may, in part, help us understand why some children do better than others. In addition, DNA sequences similar to those found in SV40 virus have been found in choroid plexus tumors. This provocative finding is supported by the observation that some transgenic mice infected with SV40 have been known to develop choroid plexus neoplasms, indicating the oncogenic properties of polyoma viruses (Bergsagel et al 1992). There is more recent microarray-based evidence that antibodies directed against Kir7.1 and stanniocalcin-1 are both specific and sensitive markers for choroid plexus tumors (Hasselblatt et al 2006). Other microarray-based studies demonstrate that Twist-1 is highly overexpressed in choroid plexus tumors and may be responsible for promoting proliferation and invasion in these tumors (Hasselblatt et al 2009).

However, no clear-cut immunochemical or molecular criteria have emerged with any consistency to separate papilloma from carcinoma or provide for reproducible prognostic significance in choroid plexus tumors.

Preoperative planning and surgical considerations

Many different surgical approaches have been described for the removal of choroid plexus tumors specifically, and intraventricular tumors in general. The location of these lesions in the ventricle makes passage through neural structures mandatory in all surgical approaches, with the possible exception of tumors in the cerebellopontine angle (CPA) (Timurkaynak et al 1986). Choroid plexus tumors are technically challenging not only because of their location but also because their exuberant blood supply is often deep to the tumor bulk and not accessible until much of the tumor is removed. For that reason, we attempt preoperative tumor embolization whenever possible. In small children, this may not always be technically feasible, but the assistance of a skilled interventional neuroradiologist/neurosurgeon can make the tumor resection immeasurably more easy. We have embolized large, highly vascular tumors in children as young as 3 years old and in many adults with large hemispheric lesions. Such embolization, when successful, can markedly lessen the blood loss in these treacherous cases. A similar experience has been reported by other surgeons (Pencalet et al 1998).

Other investigators have commented on the successful use of preoperative chemotherapy to shrink these tumors rather than suffer a large intraoperative blood loss (St. Clair et al 1991; Kumabe et al 1996; Araki et al 1997; Souweidane et al 1999). Souweidane and his colleagues (1991) have demonstrated clearcut volumetric shrinkage of tumor burden with pre-surgical chemotherapy in a patient with a carcinoma. Multiple courses of chemotherapy which was comprised of etoposide (VP16), cyclophosphamide, vincristine, and cisplatin were given prior to staged resections. An overall reduction of nearly 30% of tumor volume was achieved using 3D analysis of tumor volume pre- and post-chemotherapy. Staged surgical approach resulted in a gross total successful resection of her lesion (Souweidane et al 1999).

The importance of the assistance of a skilled perioperative team cannot be overemphasized. The successful excision of a choroid plexus neoplasm takes the concerted efforts of a team that includes members from neuroradiology, neuroanesthesiology, neuro-intensive care, and nursing. Blood loss and hemodynamic instability account for much of the operative morbidity, and judicious and early use of the appropriate blood products is essential. Dependence upon dextran and crystalloid without blood products can lead to coagulation problems. Ventricular drainage will lessen intracranial pressure, and careful monitoring of intravascular volume and mean arterial blood pressure will ensure an adequate cerebral perfusion pressure even during periods of continuous blood loss.

The basic principles of tumor removal are an appropriately placed cortical incision, early isolation of the vascular supply (both arterial and venous), mobilization of the tumor, and microdissection/resection to reduce blood loss. It is sometimes very difficult to mobilize a choroid plexus neoplasm, especially when it has grown to a large size. Vigorous manipulation of an extremely large tumor is unwise, as the arterial supply may be disrupted prior to its visualization. Piecemeal resection must often be performed. Debulking of the tumor's papillary regions with bipolar electrocautery or ultrasonic suction can make a large tumor more manageable. Once the vascular supply is identified, it can be occluded so that the tumor mass can be excised *en bloc* or piecemeal. Endoscopic assistance to find residual, adherent pieces of tumor in the ventricle, or to perform an initial biopsy when the pathology is not apparent, is often quite useful (Cappabianca et al 2008).

An appreciation of the relevant anatomy is extremely helpful in surgical approaches to the ventricles. The primary arteries to the choroid plexus are the anterior and posterior choroidal arteries. The arterial supply of these tumors usually arises from hypertrophied branches of these choroidal arteries. The anterior choroidal artery rises from the internal carotid artery, distal to the posterior communicating artery, and courses posteriorly through the choroidal fissure to lie near the posterior choroid plexus. The anterior choroidal artery is often an important source of supply to tumors in the atrium and temporal horn. The choroidal arteries pass through the choroidal fissure, and opening this fissure will permit proximal control of the feeding vessels.

The posterior choroidal arteries are divided into lateral and medial divisions. The lateral posterior choroidal artery arises from the posterior cerebral artery and pierces the ventricle by traversing the choroidal fissure at the level of the crus of the fornix. This vessel supplies the temporal horn, atrium, and body of the lateral ventricle and tumors contained within those cavities (Timurkaynak et al 1986). The medial posterior choroidal artery, which also originates from the posterior cerebral artery, travels through the velum interpositum sending inconstant branches to the lateral ventricles through the choroidal fissure and foramen of Monro. The medial posterior choroidal artery can supply tumors in the third ventricle and the lateral ventricle, as well as the choroid plexus in the roof of the third ventricle. Tumors may be supplied by one enlarged artery or by multiple feeders from the anterior and posterior choroidal arteries simultaneously (Timurkaynak et al 1986). It is the fact that enlarged tumor arteries may be feeding these hypervascular tumors, which lend the more vascular tumors to preoperative embolization in skilled interventional radiology/neurosurgery hands.

Fourth ventricle tumors are vascularized by choroidal branches of the posterior inferior cerebellar, anterior inferior cerebellar, or superior cerebellar arteries. Venous drainage is often deep, through the subependymal veins, internal cerebral veins, vein of Rosenthal, vein of Galen, and quadrigeminal or precentral cerebellar veins.

There are many important deep veins (lateral and medial), but perhaps the best known for surgical and angiographic orientation in tumor removal in the lateral ventricle is the thalamostriate vein, which runs along the floor of the lateral ventricle from lateral to medial toward the foramen of Monro.

The appropriate choice of approach is determined by the tumor location, vascular supply, and the experience and preference of the surgeon. Extremely large tumors may require a combination of more than one approach so that the cortical excision and retraction are minimal. The different approaches can be grouped according to location in the lateral, third, and fourth ventricles.

The transcortical approaches are powerful ones because they permit access to all five regions of the lateral ventricle through one or a combination of approaches. On the other hand, the low risk of neuropsychologic sequelae and seizure after a well performed callosal section makes this route an attractive and appropriate one in selected patients. Tumors in the frontal horn, although uncommon, can become large and cause obstruction of the foramen of Monro with subsequent ventricular dilatation. The transcortical middle frontal gyrus approach is an excellent approach for tumors in the ipsilateral anterior horn. Tumors extending inferiorly from the lateral ventricle into the third ventricle and requiring a subchoroidal exposure for removal may be resected through either a transcortical approach or a transcallosal approach. Patients who have small ventricles, tumor in both lateral ventricles, or tumor in the body of the lateral ventricle may often be more easily operated on through a transcallosal route.

The superior parietal approach is a natural approach for neurosurgeons because it uses a path to the lateral ventricle that is taken when placing a parietal occipital catheter for CSF diversion. It is a reasonable approach for reaching choroid plexus neoplasms in the collateral trigone, posterior part of the body, atrium, and glomus regions of the ventricle. The lateral posterior choroidal artery, which may be obscured by the tumor mass, should be uncovered in the choroidal fissure between the pulvinar and the crus of the fornix and be isolated and secured to devascularize the tumor. This approach is more risky in the dominant than the non-dominant hemisphere.

No single middle fossa approach will permit early control of both anterior and posterior choroidal arteries initially (Jun & Nutic 1985). The middle temporal gyrus approach provides a direct route to the middle fossa choroid plexus neoplasms with minimal morbidity and early control of the anterior choroidal artery feeding vessels. The lateral temporoparietal junction approach is used in rare cases when a large tumor is harbored in the non-dominant atrium. The risk of a field deficit and damage to the angular gyrus is high but it may be the shortest and most direct route to the tumor below.

Posterior fossa tumors can be removed by a standard posterior fossa craniectomy, retrosigmoid, or extreme lateral approaches. Tumors confined to the IVth ventricle can be reached through a telovelar approach, instead of a vermis splitting approach, even in large IVth ventricular tumors. It has been argued that the telovelar approach through the uvulotonsillar cleft or cerebellomedullary fissure provides excellent superior and lateral exposure as well as complete exposure of the foramen of Luschka. The results of this approach seem to yield a significantly decreased incidence of ataxia and postoperative mutism compared with the vermis splitting approach (Rajesh et al 2007). Tumors that exit through the foramen of Luschka or those that creep anterior to the CPA may require a more laterally placed skull base approach but the telovelar approach often provides adequate exposure through a midline craniotomy. The CPA tumors are challenging to excise because of their location, a complex vascular supply which can include branches of the posterior and anterior inferior cerebellar artery, and the tumor's intimate relationship with the cranial nerves. It sometimes requires hours of meticulous microsurgery to peel the well vascularized tumor off each of the lower cranial nerves (VII–XII) before the tumor exits the foramen of Luschka. Care must be taken not to sacrifice the anterior inferior cerebellar branch adjacent to the seventh/eighth nerve complex or cause vasospasm in any of the small arterial vessels near the brain stem. Papaverine on pledgets placed over these essential vessels may ameliorate the effects of manipulation in this region. Intraoperative cranial nerve monitoring can be used but may have limited utility as stimulation of each cranial nerve occurs often as the tumor is carefully dissected off each nerve.

A 10-year experience with massive blood transfusions was described from one center in Italy encompassing 18 children. Children operated upon in the neonatal period had the highest blood loss (mL/kg) and most related coagulation factor impairment compared to older children (Piastra et al 2006). The operations in neonates and younger children, who have a small blood volume must be approached with careful preoperative planning for transfusion, in our experience, as even appropriate red cell transfusion can lead to a dilutional coagulopathy, unless blood products are given concomitantly.

Prognosis and adjuvant therapy

Prior to 1958, 67 children with choroid plexus neoplasms in all locations were described in the literature. Of these, 24 had been operated upon and only 13 had survived (Matson 1969). Fortuna and co-workers, in 1979, reported a 48% surgical mortality in the literature from their review of 25 cases of choroid plexus neoplasms removed from the third ventricle. The intraventricular location, associated hydrocephalus, and abundant vascular supply are the principal features of all these tumors, and are responsible for their associated morbidity and mortality. These lesions present a formidable challenge even to the experienced neurologic surgeon. In the last three decades, mortality in surgical series has been reported as high as 24% (Hawkins 1980; Guidetti & Spallone 1981), and as low as 0 (Raimondi & Gutierrez 1975).

Improved outcomes were achieved by progressive developments in CSF shunting techniques, imaging technology, and microsurgical technique, and refinements in anesthesiology and perioperative care. Several series report 100% perioperative survival in patients with papilloma undergoing surgery after 1961 (Raimondi & Gutierrez 1975; Tomita et al 1988; Ellenbogen et al 1989).

The complications of transcortical and transcallosal surgery are specific to the approach: preoperative condition of the patient, location of tumor, and difficulty encountered in removing the tumor. The risks and potential complications are well described and include hematoma, hemiparesis, seizure disorders, developmental delay, neuropsychologic deficits, visual field deficits, and cranial nerve deficits (Boyd & Steinbock 1987; Schijman et al 1990).

The series on choroid plexus neoplasms are all too small to make general statements concerning neurologic outcome. Histopathologic features do not always correlate with outcome but, not surprisingly, patients with papilloma tend to have significantly more favorable outcomes compared with patients with less resectable carcinoma. Eight out of 10 infants with choroid plexus papilloma in the third ventricle survived without recurrence after tumor resection in the series reported by Schijman et al in 1990. However, three of the eight survivors had a seizure disorder and mental retardation (Schijman et al 1990). A total of 13 of 17 of Tomita and co-workers patients reported in 1988 exhibited normal neurologic and psychomotor development after removal of choroid plexus papilloma. The majority were under 2 years of age at the time of diagnosis. In a series of 40 choroid plexus neoplasms studied over a 45-year period, only 50% of patients with carcinoma survived compared with 84% with papilloma. The major morbidity in the survivors was hemiparesis (23%) and seizures (25%). However, 18% of the patients presented with a seizure, thus obscuring the precise incidence of postoperative seizures caused by the surgical intervention. Of the patients with papilloma, 23% enjoyed an excellent outcome without neurologic deficit; surprisingly, this was also the outcome for 14% of the carcinoma patients.

There is controversy with regard to the prognosis of choroid plexus carcinoma. There is considerable disagreement on whether the degree of surgical excision extends survival in the malignant lesions. Some groups maintain a pessimistic outlook despite having survivors in their own series, arguing that these tumors possess a uniformly grave outcome (Humphreys et al 1987; St. Clair et al 1991). Other groups who record survivors are no less cautious. Carpenter, in 1982, reviewed 25 patients in the literature with choroid plexus carcinoma and concluded that only 4 of them enjoyed 'relatively good results'. The groups with survivors have simply been impressed that aggressive surgical intervention (multiple if necessary), followed or preceded by adjuvant therapy, has been rewarded by a few long-term survivors, a situation previously thought to be impossible (Ellenbogen et al 1989; Lena et al 1990; Packer et al 1992; Berger et al 1998; McEvoy et al 2000).

The issue of developing second neoplasms after treatment for choroid plexus tumors has been studied by St Jude's Research Hospital. There were 18 patients in their study with choroid plexus tumors and at 10 years follow-up, the estimated cumulative risk of developing a second neoplasm was 20.2% (Broniscer et al 2004). This result must be interpreted with extreme caution because the number of choroid plexus tumors was small and two of the patients at St Jude's had TP53 germline mutations, which had not been noted in choroid plexus carcinomas previously.

The complete removal of a neoplasm of the choroid plexus does not obviate the need for placement of a shunt in all patients (McDonald 1969; Jellinger et al 1970; Raimondi & Gutierrez 1975). One of the more problematic complications of intraventricular surgery for choroid neoplasms is the development of symptomatic subdural fluid collections; this has been discussed in detail by several authors (Matson & Crofton 1960; Shillito & Matson 1982; Boyd & Steinbock 1987). Although this complication is not confined to the removal of choroid plexus tumors, it has occurred with both the transcortical and the transcallosal approaches. Jooma and Grant (1983) reported two cases of a subdural-transcallosal shunt after removal of third ventricular choroid plexus papilloma. In Boyd and Steinbock's (1987) surgical series of 11 choroid plexus neoplasms, two patients developed postoperative subdural collections requiring subdural–peritoneal shunts after transcortical surgery. The authors argued that this complication may possibly be lessened by making a smaller cortical incision, filling the ventricles with physiologic saline prior to dural closure, and placing a fine pial suture or using tissue glue to close the fistula (Boyd & Steinbock 1987).

Extent of surgical resection of choroid plexus tumors remains the most important determinant in providing long-term disease-free survival (McGirr et al 1988; Ellenbogen et al 1989; Johnson 1989; Packer et al 1992; Pierga et al 1993; Sharma et al 1994, McEvoy et al 2000). Adjuvant therapy may be required for tumors that are incompletely resected or malignant, or those that have shown neuraxis/leptomeningeal spread. External beam irradiation remains a potent form of adjuvant therapy in older children, especially craniospinal irradiation for those patients with drop metastases, leptomeningeal spread, and tumors invading the parenchyma (Geerts et al 1996). The role of radiation therapy, both conventional and focused beam, remains undefined in the treatment of this disease. The documentation of neuropsychologic sequelae of radiation therapy on the developing brain (Duffner et al 1985) has led to alternative approaches. Patients under the age of 3 years have received chemotherapy in lieu of radiation, to spare them the cognitive dysfunction and short stature associated with this form of treatment. Gianella-Borradori and associates (1992) successfully treated two children with sub-totally resected malignant carcinomas with 8-drug-in-1-day chemotherapy, without radiation therapy. They concluded that chemotherapy may provide long-term survival but that more trials are needed.

There are more recent reports of aggressive multimodality therapy consisting of combined pre- or post-resection chemotherapy and radiotherapy. This approach is also used on subsequent attempts at radical resection of choroid plexus carcinomas that could not initially be removed. The conclusion is that pretreatment with chemotherapy shrinks the tumor, thus making the subsequent surgery easier and the disease-free survival period longer (St. Clair et al 1991; Kumabe et al 1996; Araki et al 1997).

Gamma Knife® radiosurgery appears to be another management option for patients who progress with choroid plexus neoplasms, despite aggressive surgery. The University of Pittsburgh Gamma Knife Center described Gamma Knife radiosurgery for six papilloma patients whose surgical treatment did not yield a cure. The long-term survival for four of the six patients who did survive, varied from 15 to 120 months. The authors argue that this radiotherapy is well suited for patients with recurrent or residual lesions which are deep seated, and who can receive a high marginal dose to their tumor beds (Kim et al 2008).

A report from the Pediatric Oncology Group in 1995 described eight infants with choroid plexus carcinoma who underwent surgery, successful prolonged postoperative chemotherapy, and delayed radiation. The conclusion was that this aggressive multimodality approach prolonged survival even in children who underwent sub-total resection of a choroid plexus neoplasm. The danger of delayed disease recurrence from meningeal carcinomatosis in carcinoma still exists, despite this aggressive multimodality therapy (Peschgens et al 1995). Wrede and her colleagues (2007) constructed a database of all choroid plexus tumors reported in the literature up to 2004 to understand the prognostic factors in patient survival. Histology was as previously described in the literature and important prognostic factors, with papilloma faring better than carcinoma ($p < 0.0001$; long rank). For carcinoma, both surgery and chemotherapy were linked to a better long-term prognosis. By multivariate analysis, chemotherapy appeared to be significantly linked to better prognosis ($p = 0.0001$), especially in patients with incompletely resected carcinoma (Wrede et al 2007).

However, there appear to be three themes emerging from the use of chemotherapy, although this literature is still evolving: (1) decrease in the volumetric tumor burden with pre-surgical treatment; (2) improvement in the safety profile by decreasing the vascularity of these highly vascular tumors, especially in very young children, and (3) successful delay in the need for radiation therapy in incompletely resected carcinoma.

Key points

- Choroid plexus neoplasms are a diverse group of tumors. They often reach a large size and are associated with hydrocephalus prior to diagnosis. They are most commonly found in the lateral ventricles and, when histologically benign, are surgically curable.

- Regardless of their histology, they are challenging lesions from a surgical point of view, possessing an impressive vascular supply often buried deep to the tumor mass. The anatomy of the ventricles and their relationship to the tumor permits a variety of surgical approaches. The location and size of the lesion, preoperative deficits, associated hydrocephalus, vascularity of the lesion, and experience of the surgeon contribute to the ultimate selection of the surgical approach. A combination of approaches or a staged approach is occasionally required to achieve adequate excision of the lesion with minimal morbidity.

- The treatment of choroid plexus papilloma has yielded excellent results with high survival rates in the microsurgical era. It is curable with surgical extirpation alone in the majority of cases. The treatment of postoperative subdural effusions and hydrocephalus is often the most confounding perioperative challenge in the treatment of these lesions. Significant neurologic deficits can and do occur but have been less common in the microsurgical era.

- Survival after surgical excision of choroid plexus carcinoma was originally thought to be uniformly dismal. In the last two decades, however, there have been small series and scattered case reports of survival after removal of this malignant form of choroid plexus neoplasm (Ellenbogen et al 1989; Lena et al 1990; Packer et al 1992). Some groups report encouraging results based on an aggressive surgical posture, appropriate adjuvant therapy, and vigilant follow-up, and maintain that there is some hope for survival, albeit limited and guarded. The series of choroid plexus carcinoma are too small to derive any conclusive prognostic data on long-term survival. The advent of advances in microsurgical techniques and, use of multiple surgical resections, chemotherapy, radiosurgery and radiation therapy has been in part responsible for a measured improvement over the previously dismal survival statistics. As long as the lesion remains localized and the patient's condition permits, an attempt at an aggressive therapeutic multimodality approach is justified.

REFERENCES

Abbott, K.H., Rollas, Z.H., Meagher, J.N., 1957. Choroid plexus papilloma causing spontaneous subarachnoid hemorrhage. J. Neurosurg. 14, 566–570.

Aicardi, J., Lepintre, J., Cherrie, J.J., et al., 1968. Les papillomes des plexus choroides chez l'enfant. Arch. Fr. Pediatr. 25, 673–686.

Ang, L.C., Taylor, A.R., Bergin, D., et al., 1990. An immunohistochemical study of papillary tumors of the central nervous system. Cancer 65, 2712–2719.

Araki, K., Aori, T., Takahashi, J.A., et al., 1997. A case report of choroid plexus carcinoma. No. Shinkei Geka. 25 (9), 853–857.

Ausman, J.I., Shrontz, C., Chason, J., et al., 1984. Aggressive choroid plexus papilloma. Surg. Neurol. 22, 472–476.

Aziz, A.A., Coleman, L., Morokoff, A., et al., 2005. Diffuse choroid plexus hyperplasia: an under-diagnosed cause of hydrocephalus in children? Pediatr. Radiol. 35 (8), 815–818.

Berger, C., Thiesse, P., Lellouch-Tubiana, A., et al., 1998. Choroid plexus carcinomas in children: clinical features and prognostic factors. Neurosurgery 42 (3), 470–475.

Bergsagel, D.J., Finegold, M.J., Butel, J.S., et al., 1992. DNA sequences similar to those of simian virus 40 in ependymomas and choroid plexus tumors of childhood. N. Engl. J. Med. 326, 988–993.

Bielschowsky, M., Unger, E., 1906. Zur Kenntnis der primaren Epithelgeschwulste der Adergeflechte des Gehirns. Arch. Klin. Chir. 81, 61–82.

Body, G., Darnis, E., Pourcelot, D., et al., 1990. Choroid plexus tumors: antenatal diagnosis and follow-up. J. Clin. Ultrasound 18, 575–578.

Bohm, J., Strange, R., 1961. Choroid plexus papillomas. J. Neurosurg. 18, 493–500.

Boudet, G., Clunet, J., 1910. Contribution a l'etude des tumeurs epitheliales primitives de l'encephale. Arch. Med. Exper. Anat. Pathol. 22, 379–411.

Boyd, M.C., Steinbock, M.B., 1987. Choroid plexus tumors: Problems in diagnosis and management. J. Neurosurg. 66, 800–805.

Broniscer, A., Ke, W., Fuller, C.E., et al., 2004. Second neoplasms in pediatric patients with primary central nervous system tumors: the St. Jude Children's Research Hospital experience. Cancer 100 (10), 2246–2252.

Burger, P.C., Scheithauer, B.W., 1994. Tumors of neuroglia and choroid plexus epithelium. In: Burger, P.C., Scheithauer, B.W. (Eds.), Tumors of the central nervous system, 3rd series. Armed Forces Institute of Pathology, Washington DC, pp. 136–161.

Cappabianca, P., Cinalli, G., Gangemi, M., et al., 2008. Application of neuroendoscopy to intraventricular lesions. Neurosurgery 62 (Suppl 2), 575–597; discussion 597–598.

Carpenter, D.N., Michelsen, W.J., Hays, A.P., 1982. Carcinoma of the choroid plexus. J. Neurosurg. 56, 722–777.

Cassinari, V., 1963. Tumori della parte anteriore del terzo ventricolo. Acta Neurochir. 11, 236–271.

Coates, T.L., Hinshaw, D.B. Jr., Peckman, N., et al., 1989. Pediatric choroid plexus neoplasms: MR, CT, and pathologic correlation. Radiology 173, 81–88.

Coffin, C.M., Wick, M.R., Braun, J.T., et al., 1986. Choroid plexus neoplasms. Clinicopathological and immunohistochemical studies. Am. Surg. Pathol. 10, 394–404.

Crofton, F.D., Matson, D.D., 1950. Roentgenologic study of choroid plexus papillomas in children. Am. J. Roentgenol. Radium Ther. Nucl. Med. 84, 273–311.

Cruz-Sanchez, F.F., Rossi, M.L., Hughes, J.T., et al., 1989. Choroid plexus papillomas: an immunohistological study of 16 cases. Histopathology 15, 61–69.

Cushing, H., 1932. Intracranial tumors. Charles C. Thomas, Springfield, IL.

Dandy, W.E., 1934. Benign encapsulated tumors of the lateral ventricle. Williams & Wilkins, Baltimore.

Davis, L., 1924. A physiopathological study of the choroid plexus with the report of a case of villous hypertrophy. Med. Res. 44, 521–534.

Davis, L.E., Cushing, H., 1925. Papillomas of the choroid plexus. A report of six cases. Arch. Neurol. Psychiatry 13, 681–710.

Dohrmann, G.J., Collias, J.C., 1975. Choroid plexus carcinoma. J. Neurosurg. 43, 225–232.

Duffner, P.K., Cohen, M.E., Thomas, P.R.M., et al., 1985. The long term effects of cranial irradiation in the central nervous system. Cancer 56, 1841–1847.

Eisenberg, H.M., McComb, G., Lorenzo, A.V., 1974. Cerebrospinal fluid overproduction and hydrocephalus associated with choroid plexus papilloma. J. Neurosurg. 40, 380–385.

Ellenbogen, R.G., Winston, K.R., Kupsky, W.J., 1989. Tumors of the choroid plexus in children. Neurosurgery 25 (3), 327–335.

Ernsting, J., 1955. Choroid plexus papilloma causing spontaneous subarachnoid hemorrhage. J. Neurol. Neurosurg. Psychiatry 18, 134–136.

Fairburn, B., 1958. Choroid plexus papilloma and its relationship to hydrocephalus. J. Neurosurg. 17, 166–171.

Fortuna, A., Celli, P., Ferrante, L., et al., 1979. A review of papillomas of the third ventricle. J. Neurosurg. 23, 61–72.

Furness, P.N., Lowe, J., Tarrant, G.S.K., 1990. Subepithelial basement deposition and intermediate filament expression in choroid plexus neoplasms and ependymomas. Histopathology 16, 251–255.

Garrod, 1873. Papillomatous tumor in the fourth ventricle of the brain. Lancet 1, 303.

Geerts, Y., Gabreels, F., Lippens, R., et al., 1996. Choroid plexus carcinoma: a report of two cases and review of the literature. Neuropediatrics 27 (3), 143–148.

Gianella-Borradori, Zeltzer, P.M., Bodey, B., et al., 1992. Choroid plexus tumors in childhood. Cancer 69, 809–816.

Gudeman, S.K., Sullivan, H.G., Rosner, M.J., et al., 1979. Surgical removal of bilateral papillomas of the choroid plexus of the lateral ventricles with resolution of hydrocephalus. J. Neurosurg. 50, 677–681.

Guerard, M., 1832. Tumeur fongeuse dans le ventricle droit du cerveau chez une petite fille de trois ans. Anat. Paris 8, 211–214.

Guidetti, B., Spallone, A., 1981. The surgical treatment of choroid plexus papillomas: The results of 27 years experience. Neurosurgery 6, 380–384.

Gullotta, F., de Melo, A.S., 1979. Plexus chorioideus. Klinishe, light-mikroskopische und elektronenoptische untersuchungen. Neurochirurgia Stuttg. 22, 1–9.

Hammock, M.K., Milhorat, T.H., Breckbill, D.L., 1976. Primary choroid plexus papilloma of the cerebellopontine angle, presenting as brain stem tumor in a child. Childs Brain 2, 132–142.

Hasselblatt, M., Bohm, C., Tatenhorst, L., et al., 2006. Identification of novel diagnostic markers for choroid plexus tumors: a microarray-based approach. Am. J. Surg. Pathol. 30 (1), 66–74.

Hasselblatt, M., Mertsch, S., Koos, B., et al., 2009. TWIST-1 is overexpressed in neoplastic choroid plexus epithelial cells and promotes proliferation and invasion. Cancer Res. 69 (6), 2219–2223.

Hawkins, J.C. III, 1980. Treatment of choroid plexus papillomas in children: a brief analysis of twenty years' experience. Neurosurgery 6, 380–384.

Hirano, A., 1978. Some contributions of electron microscopy to the diagnosis of brain tumors. Acta. Neuropathol. (Berl.) 43, 119–128.

Hirano, H., Hirahara, K., Tetsuhiko, A., et al., 1994. Hydrocephalus due to villous hypertrophy of the choroid plexus in the lateral ventricles. J. Neurosurg. 80, 321–323.

Horska, A., Ulug, A.M., Melhem, E.R., et al., 2001. Proton magnetic resonance spectroscopy of choroid plexus tumors in children. J. Magn. Reson. Imaging 14 (1), 78–82.

Humphreys, R., Nemoto, S., Hendrick, E.B., et al., 1987. Childhood choroid plexus tumors. Concepts Pediatr. Neurosurg. 7, 1–18.

Horska, A., Naidu, S., Herskovits, E.H., 2000. Quantitative 1H MR spectroscopic imaging in early Rett syndrome. Neurology 54 (3), 715–722.

Husag, L., Costabile, G., Probst, C., 1984. Persistent hydrocephalus following removal of choroid plexus papilloma of the lateral ventricle. Neurochirurgia (Stuttg.) 27, 82–85.

Jellinger, K., Grunert, V., Sunder-Plassmann, M., 1970. Choroid plexus papilloma associated with hydrocephalus in infancy. Neuropaediatrics 1, 344–348.

Johnson, D.L., 1989. Management of choroid plexus tumors in children. Pediatr. Neurosci. 15 (4), 195–206.

Johnson, R.T., 1957. Clinicopathological aspects of the cerebrospinal fluid circulation. In: **Wilstenholme, G., O'Conner, M.** (Eds.), Ciba Foundation Symposium on Cerebrospinal Fluid Production, Circulation and Absorption. Little, Brown, Boston, MA, pp. 265–281.

Jooma, R., Grant, D.N., 1983. Third ventricle choroid plexus papillomas. Childs Brain 10, 242–250.

Jun, C., Nutic, S., 1985. Surgical approaches to intraventricular meningiomas of the trigone. Neurosurgery 16, 416–420.

Kahn, E.A., Luros, J.T., 1952. Hydrocephalus from overproduction of cerebrospinal fluid (and experiences with other papilloma of the choroid plexus). J. Neurosurg. 9, 59–67.

Kim, I.Y., Niranjan, A., Kondziolka, D., et al., 2008. Gamma knife radiosurgery for treatment resistant choroid plexus papillomas. J. Neurooncol. 90 (1), 105–110.

Knierim, D.S., 1990. Choroid plexus tumors in infants. Pediatr. Neurosurg. 16, 276–280.

Koos, W.T., Miller, M.H., 1971. Intracranial tumors of infants and children. Mosby, St Louis.

Kumabe, T., Tominaga, T., Kondo, T., et al., 1996. Intraoperative radiation therapy and chemotherapy for huge choroid plexus carcinoma in an infant – case report. Neurol. Med. Chir. 36 (3), 179–184.

Laurence, K., 1974. The biology of choroid plexus papilloma and carcinoma of the lateral ventricle. In: **Vinken, P., Bruyn, G.** (Eds.), Tumors of the brain and skull. Part 2. Handbook of clinical neurology. Elsevier, New York, pp. 555–595.

Lena, G., Genitori, L., Molina, J., et al., 1990. Choroid plexus tumors in children. Review of 24 cases. Acta. Neurochir. 106, 68–72.

Lewis, P., 1967. Carcinoma of the choroid plexus. Brain 90, 177–186.

McDonald, J.V., 1969. Persistent hydrocephalus following the removal of papillomas of the choroid plexus of the lateral ventricles. J. Neurosurg. 30, 736–740.

McEvoy, A.W., Harding, B.N., Phipps, K.P., et al., 2000. Management of choroid plexus tumours in children: 20 years experience at a single neurosurgical centre. Pediatr. Neurosurg. 32 (4), 192–199.

McGirr, S.J., Ebersold, M.J., Scheithauer, B.W., et al., 1988. Choroid plexus papillomas: Long-term follow-up results in a surgically treated series. J. Neurosurg. 69, 843–849.

Masson, C., 1934. Complete removal of two tumors of the third ventricle with recovery. Arch. Surg. 28, 527–537.

Matson, D., 1969. Tumors of the choroid plexus. In: **Matson, D.D.** (Ed.), Neurosurgery of infancy and childhood. Charles C. Thomas, Springfield, IL, pp. 581–595.

Matson, D., Crofton, F., 1960. Papilloma of the choroid plexus in childhood. J. Neurosurg. 17, 1002–1027.

Matsuda, M., Uzura, S., Nakasu, S., et al., 1991. Primary carcinoma of the choroid plexus in the lateral ventricle. Surg. Neurol. 36, 294–299.

Milhorat, T.K., Hammock, M.K., Davis, D.A., et al., 1976. Choroid plexus papilloma. Proof of cerebrospinal overproduction. Childs Brain 2, 273–289.

Morrison, G., Sobel, D.F., Kelly, W.M., et al., 1984. Intraventricular mass lesions. Radiology 153, 435–442.

Naeini, R.M., Yoo, J.H., Hunter, J.V., 2009. Spectrum of choroid plexus lesions in children. AJR. Am. J. Roentgenol. 192 (1), 32–40.

Packer, R.J., Perilongo, G., Johnson, D., et al., 1992. Choroid plexus carcinoma of childhood. Cancer 69, 580–585.

Pascual-Castroviejo, I., Villarejo, F., Perez-Higueras, A., et al., 1983. Childhood choroid plexus neoplasms. A study of 14 cases less than 2 years old. Eur. Pediatr. 140, 51–56.

Paulus, W., Janisch, W., 1990. Clinicopathologic correlations in epithelial choroid plexus neoplasms: a study of 52 cases. Acta. Neuropathol (Berl.) 80, 635–641.

Pecker, J.P., Ferrand, B., Javalet, A., 1966. Tumeurs du troisieme ventricule. Neurochirurgie 12, 1–136.

Pencalet, P., Sainte-Rose, C., Lellouch-Tubiana, A., et al., 1998. Papillomas and carcinomas of the choroid plexus in children. J. Neurosurg. 88 (3), 521–528.

Perthes, G.C., 1919. Entfernung eines Tumors des Plexus Chorioideus an dem Seitenventrikel des Cerebrums. Munch Med. Wochenschr. 66, 677–678.

Peschgens, T., Stollbrink-Peschgens, C., Mertens, R., et al., 1995. Zur Therapie des Plexus-chorioideus-Karzinomas im Kindesalter. Fallbeispiel und Literaturubersicht. Klin. Padiatr. 207 (2), 52–58.

Philips, M., Shanno, G., Duhaime, A., 1998. Treatment of villous hypertrophy of the choroid plexus by endoscopic contact coagulation. Pediatr. Neurosurg. 28 (5), 252–256.

Piastra, M., Di Rocco, C., Tempera, A., et al., 2007. Massive blood transfusion in choroid plexus tumor surgery: 10-years' experience. J. Clin. Anesth. 19 (3), 192–197.

Pierga, J.Y., Kalifa, C., Terrier-Lacombe, M.J., et al., 1993. Carcinoma of the choroid plexus: a pediatric experience. Med. Pediatr. Oncol. 21 (7), 480–487.

Pollack, I.F., Schor, N.F., Martinez, J.A., et al., 1995. Bobble-head doll syndrome and drop attacks in a child with a cystic choroid plexus papilloma of the third ventricle. J. Neurosurg. 83, 729–732.

Portnoy, H.D., Croissant, P.D., 1976. A practical method of measuring hydrodynamics of cerebrospinal fluid. Surg. Neurol. 5, 273–277.

Raimondi, A.J., Gutierrez, F.A., 1975. Diagnosis and surgical treatment of choroid plexus papillomas. Childs Brain 1, 81–115.

Rand, C.W., Reeves, D.L., 1940. Choroid plexus tumors in infancy and childhood. Report of four cases. Bull Los. Angeles Neurol. Soc. 5, 405–410.

Ray, B.S., Peck, F.C. Jr., 1956. Papilloma of the choroid plexus of the lateral ventricles causing hydrocephalus in an infant. J. Neurosurg. 13, 405–410.

Rekate, H.L., Erwood, S., Brodkey, J.A., et al., 1985–1986 Etiology of ventriculomegaly in choroid plexus papilloma. Pediatr. Neurosci. 12, 196–201.

Ringertz, N., Reymond, A., 1949. Ependymomas and choroid plexus papillomas. J. Neuropathol. Exp. Neurol. 8, 355.

Rovit, R.L., Schechter, M.M., Chodroff, P., 1970. Choroid plexus papillomas – observation on radiologic diagnosis. AJR. Am. J. Roentgenol. 110, 608–617.

Rubinstein, L.J., 1972. Tumors of the choroid plexus and related structures. In: **Firminger, H.I.** (Ed.), Tumors of the central nervous system, 2nd series. Armed Forces Institute of Pathology, Washington DC, pp. 257–262.

Russell, D.S., Rubinstein, L.J., 1963. Pathology of tumors of the nervous system. Williams & Wilkins, Baltimore, MD.

Russell, D.S., Rubinstein, L.J., 1971. Pathology of tumors of the nervous system. Edward Arnold, London.

Sachs, E., 1922. Papillomas of the fourth ventricle. Arch. Neurol. Psychiatry 8, 379–382.

Sahar, A., Feinsod, M., Beller, A.J., 1980. Choroid plexus papilloma: hydrocephalus and cerebrospinal fluid dynamics. Surg. Neurol. 13, 476–478.

Schellhas, K.P., Siebert, R.C., Heithoff, K.B., et al., 1988. Congenital choroid plexus papilloma of the third ventricle: diagnosis with real-time sonography and MR imaging. AJNR. Am. J. Neuroradiol. 9, 797–798.

Schijman, E., Monges, J., Raimondi, A.J., et al., 1990. Choroid plexus papillomas of the III ventricle in childhood. Childs Nerv. Syst. 6, 331–334.

Sharma, R., Rout, D., Gupta, A.K., et al., 1994. Choroid plexus papillomas. B. Neurosurg. 8 (2), 169–177.

Shaw, J., 1983. Papilloma of the choroid plexus. In: **Amador, L.** (Ed.), Brain tumors in the young. Thomas, Springfield, pp. 655–670.

Shillito, J., Matson, D.D., 1982. An atlas of pediatric neurosurgical operations. WB Saunders, Philadelphia, PA.

Shirakawa, N., Kannuki, S., Matsumoto, K., 1994. Clinicopathological study on choroid plexus tumors: immunohistochemical features and argyrophilic nucleolar organizer regions values. Noshuyo. Byori. 11 (1), 99–105.

Slaymaker, S.R., Elias, F., 1909. Papilloma of the choroid plexus with hydrocephalus. Report of a case. Arch. Intern. Med. 3, 289–294.

Smith, J.F., 1933. Hydrocephalus associated with choroid plexus papillomas. Neuropathol. Exp. Neurol. 14, 442–449.

Souweidane, M.M., Johnson Jr., J.H., Lis, E., 1999. Volumetric reduction of a choroid plexus carcinoma using preoperative chemotherapy. J. Neuro-Oncol. 43, 167–171.

St. Clair, S.K., Humphreys, R.P., Pillay, P.K., et al., 1991. Current management of choroid plexus carcinoma in children. Pediatr. Neurosurg. 92 (17), 225–233.

Timurkaynak, E., Rhoton, A.L., Barry, M., 1986. Microsurgical anatomy and approaches to the lateral ventricles. Neurosurgery 19, 685–723.

Tomita, T., Naidich, T.P., 1987. Successful resection of choroid plexus papillomas diagnosed at birth: report of two cases. Neurosurgery 20, 774–779.

Tomita, T., McLone, D.G., Flannery, A.M., 1988. Choroid plexus papillomas of neonates, infants and children. Pediatr. Neurosci. 14, 23–30.

Turner, O.A., Simon, M.A., 1937. Malignant papillomas of the choroid plexus. Report of two cases with review of the literature. Am. J. Cancer 30, 289–297.

Van Wagenen, W.P., 1930. Papillomas of the choroid plexus. Report of two cases, one with removal of tumor and one with 'seeding' of the tumor in the ventricular system. Arch. Surg. 20, 199–231.

Vazquez, E., Ball, W.S., Prenger, E.C., et al., 1991. Magnetic resonance imaging of fourth ventricular choroid plexus neoplasms in childhood. Pediatr. Neurosurg. 17, 48–52.

Vigouroux, A., 1970. Ecoulement de liquide cephalorachidien. Hydrocephalie papillome des plexus chorides du IV ventricule. Rev. Neurol. 16, 281–285.

Vraa-Jensen, G., 1950. Papilloma of the choroid plexus with pulmonary metastases. Acta. Psychtr. (Koln.) 25, 299–306.

Welch, K., Strand, R., Bresnan, M., et al., 1983. Congenital hydrocephalus due to villous hypertrophy of the telencephalic choroid plexuses. Case report. J. Neurosurg. 59, 172–175.

Wilkins, R.H., Rutledge, B.J., 1961. Papillomas of the choroid plexus. J. Neurosurg. 18, 14–18.

Wrede, B., Liu, P., Wolff, J.E., 2007. Chemotherapy improves the survival of patients with choroid plexus carcinoma: a meta-analysis of individual cases with choroid plexus tumors. J. Neurooncol. 85 (3), 345–351.

Zhang, W.C., 1983. Clinical significance of anterior inferior cerebellar artery in angiographic diagnosis of choroid plexus papilloma at the cerebellopontine angle. Chin. Med. J. (Engl.) 96, 275–280.

Zülch, K.J., 1956. Biologie und pathologie der hirngeschwulste. In: Olivecrona, H., Tonnis, W. (Eds.), Handbuch. der. Neurochirurgie, Vol. 3. Springer-Verlag, Berlin, pp. 1–702.

Uncommon glial tumors

Thomas C. Chen, James B. Elder, Ignacio Gonzalez-Gomez, and
J. Gordon McComb

Introduction

This chapter's focus is a constellation of neoplastic lesions entitled 'Uncommon glial tumors'. Unlike the tumors covered elsewhere, most of these tumors are rarely encountered. Some tumors (papillary glioneuronal tumor, rosette-forming glioneuronal tumor of the fourth ventricle) have only recently been recognized as independent entities under the World Health Organization classification (Brat et al 2008). Some of the tumors are associated with medical problems such as precocious puberty in patients with hypothalamic hamartomas (Albright & Lee 1993; Stewart et al 1998), and tumors of the kidneys, heart, and lungs in patients with subependymal giant cell astrocytomas (Kaye & Laws 1995). In these, the histopathologic characteristics do not reflect biologic behavior. For example, the appearance of sub-ependymal giant cell astrocytomas is consistent with a malignant astrocytoma, although its growth potential is limited and surgical resection can be curative (Nagib et al 1984). Also, pleomorphic xanthoastrocytoma generally has a good prognosis, despite the appearance of cellular atypia and pleomorphic cells (Kepes et al 1979). Because of these and other unique clinical and histopathologic characteristics, maintaining a current understanding of these rare lesions is important. The tumors discussed in this chapter are classified depending upon whether the predominant cell type is of astrocytic, neuronal, or ganglionic origin (Box 26.1).

Tumors of predominantly astrocytic origin

Astroblastoma

Demographics
Astroblastoma is a rare glial tumor first described by Bailey and Bucy in 1930 (Kaye & Laws 1995). Since then, it has received little formal attention in the literature, largely in the form of isolated case reports (Baka et al 1993; Caroli et al 2004; Alaraj et al 2007; Bannykh et al 2007; Denaro et al 2008; Fathi et al 2008) and case series (Brat et al 2000; Bell et al 2007). It is estimated that astroblastomas make up 0.45–2.8% of all gliomas (Husain & Leestma 1986). The peak age incidence is in the first three decades (Russell & Rubinstein 1989); however, the age distribution in the literature ranges from newborn to 67 years old (Hoag et al 1986; Husain & Leestma 1986). There is no gender, familial or racial predilection (Bonnin & Rubinstein 1989; Kaye & Laws 1995), although congenital forms have been described (Pizer et al 1995). Astroblastomas are most commonly spherical supratentorial tumors, located cortically or sub-cortically (Kaye & Laws 1995). Other reported locations include the cerebellum (Steinberg et al 1985), corpus callosum (De Reuck et al 1975), and brainstem (Notarianni et al 2008).

Diagnosis
The most common presenting symptoms are headaches or seizures (Bell et al 2007). Patients may also present with additional signs and symptoms of cortical dysfunction such as hemiparesis, mental status changes or insomnia (Bonnin & Rubinstein 1989; Kaye & Laws 1995). The tumors are usually supratentorial, most commonly in the frontal or parietal lobes. They may also be extra-axial or intraventricular (Bell et al 2007; Denaro et al 2008).

Computed tomography (CT) appearances of astroblastoma range from hypodense to hyperdense compared with white matter, and some lesions have mixed densities. Calcification within the tumor is common, and may appear as small foci, globular or diffuse calcifications (Bell et al 2007). The tumors can range from a poorly-defined and hypodense tumor with irregular enhancement, to a well-defined tumor with intense enhancement on CT (Hoag et al 1986; Husain & Leestma 1986).

MRI demonstrates a well-demarcated, peripheral mass often with both solid and cystic components that typically display rim enhancement (Bell et al 2007). T1-weighted images show a lesion that is usually either isointense or containing a mixture of hypointense and isointense regions compared with white matter (Bell et al 2007). Administration of gadolinium typically reveals a heterogeneous, mixed solid- and rim-enhancing pattern of contrast uptake. T2-weighted and FLAIR images usually reveal a hyperintense lesion. Imaging may be suggestive of an extra-axial lesion (Baka et al 1993). Tumors may be multi-cystic, often described in the literature as a 'bubbly' appearance on MRI, and may be associated with edema in the surrounding brain. Other features such as a dural tail and intracystic fluid level have also been described but are less common (Bell et al 2007). Skull X-rays are limited value in the diagnostic evaluation of this tumor and others in this chapter, and thus will not be mentioned further. Angiography usually shows a vascular tumor (De Reuck et al 1975).

Pathology
The cell of origin of astroblastoma is unknown. The current classification of astroblastoma is as a glial neoplasm of uncertain origin (Kleihues et al 2000). Bailey and Bucy (1930) believed that they were derived from astroblasts (embryonal unipolar cells with 'sucker' feet attached to vessels), which are the precursors of adult astroglia (Kaye & Laws 1995). Others have proposed the theory that astroblastomas arise by 'dedifferentiation' from mature astroglial cells by an unknown process (Russell & Rubinstein 1989). Rubinstein has further proposed that astroblastomas arise from the tanycyte, a glial precursor cell, which is normally found scattered along the ependymal lining of the embryonal and neonatal mammalian brain (Rubinstein & Herman

1989). Astroblastomas grown in cell culture demonstrate outgrowths of flattened, angulated cells with epithelial features of early developing normal astrocytes (Russell & Rubinstein 1989).

Astroblastomas are typically superficially located, well-circumscribed lesions that may be solid or cystic (Caroli et al 2004). Grossly, astroblastomas appear grayish-pink in color, and range from soft to extremely firm in consistency. Central areas of necrosis, or hemorrhage into cystic cavities may be seen. The size ranges from a few millimeters to >8 cm (Kaye & Laws 1995). Microscopically, astroblastomas have a characteristic appearance. Prominent elongated tumor cells with footplates form pseudo-rosettes around blood vessels. Slight or moderate nuclear pleomorphism with limited mitotic activity is present (Fig. 26.1) (Kaye & Laws 1995). Tumors may display prominent perivascular hyalinization and regional hyaline changes (Brat et al 2000; Kim et al 2004).

Box 26.1

TUMORS OF PREDOMINANTLY ASTROCYTIC ORIGIN

- Astroblastoma
- Gliomatosis cerebri
- Pleomorphic xanthoastrocytoma
- Sub-ependymal giant cell astrocytoma

TUMORS OF MIXED GLIAL AND NEURONAL ORIGIN

- Papillary glioneuronal tumor
- Rosette-forming glioneuronal tumor of the fourth ventricle
- Desmoplastic infantile ganglioglioma
- Dysembryoplastic neuroepithelial tumor
- Ganglioglioma
- Polar spongioblastoma
- Central neurocytoma

TUMORS OF PREDOMINANTLY GANGLIONIC ORIGIN

- Gangliocytoma
- Lhermitte Duclos
- Hypothalamic hamartomas

In one case series of 23 patients, two distinct tumor types were described: high grade, which appeared histologically anaplastic, and low grade, which appeared more differentiated and benign microscopically (Bonnin & Rubinstein 1989). High-grade versions are also described as 'malignant', based on hypercellular regions with high mitotic indices, vascular proliferation and necrotic changes (Bannykh et al 2007). Malignant versions represented 50% of astroblastomas in a recent case series (Brat et al 2000).

Immunohistochemistry demonstrates occasional positivity for glial fibrillary acidic protein (GFAP), and extensive positivity for vimentin, neuron-specific enolase, S-100, and epithelial membrane antigen (Cabello et al 1991; Brat et al 2000; Alaraj et al 2007). Astroblastomas are anti-Leu 7 positive, a natural killer cell antibody positive for cells of neuroepithelial origin, but not for cells of oligodendroglial or embryonal origin (Perentes & Rubinstein 1986). Ultrastructural studies with electron microscopy demonstrate blood vessels with fenestrated endothelial cells, surrounded by a lamellated basal lamina compactly invested by neoplastic cells. Coated vesicles and abundant intermediate filaments are present in tumoral cell cytoplasm (Kubota et al 1985; Cabello et al 1991). Bonnin and Rubinstein (1989) have characterized two types of pathologies, low-grade and high-grade astroblastomas. Low-grade tumors are characterized by a uniform perivascular arrangement of pseudo-rosettes, a low to moderate number of mitotic figures, little cellular atypia, minimal or no vascular endothelial proliferation, and prominent sclerosis of the vascular walls. High-grade tumors have evidence of cytological atypia, compact cellularity, perivascular cells in multiple layers with high mitotic rates, and hypertrophy of the vascular endothelium. Necrosis is seen in up to 70% of the tumors, irrespective of tumor grade, but does not appear to have prognostic significance (Bonnin & Rubinstein 1989).

One series investigated seven tumors for chromosomal alterations using comparative genomic hybridization. The

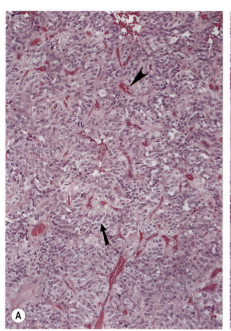
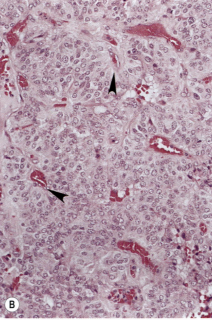

Figure 26.1 (A) Astroblastoma showing the characteristic astroblastic pseudo-rosettes (arrowhead). The cellular population is fairly uniform with occasional mitosis and no endothelial proliferation. The cellularity between the pseudo-rosettes is scanty (arrow) (H&E ×80). (B) Astroblastoma with perivascular pseudo-rosettes; a centrally located blood vessel is surrounded by large cells with the nucleus distant from the vascular core and the cytoplasm extending radially toward the vascular wall (arrowheads). The nucleus is slightly convoluted with coarse granular chromatin and one or more inconspicuous nucleoli (H&E ×160).

gliomatosis cerebri to glioblastoma multiforme has been reported. A one-step silver colloid method for nucleolar organizer region-associated protein (AgNOR) has been used in gliomatosis cerebri to estimate its proliferative potential. AgNOR stain is similar to that of low-grade gliomas, suggesting invasive characteristics, but with a proliferative potential lower than high-grade gliomas.

There has also been interesting work on a molecular level looking at genetic alterations in gliomatosis cerebri tissue, and an attempt to answer the cell of origin. Herrlinger et al (2002) found TP53 mutations in three of seven tumors, and both PTEN mutation and EGFR overexpression in another tumor, leading them to conclude that genetic alterations in gliomatosis cerebri were similar to diffuse astrocytomas. Braeuninger et al (2007) have examined different regions of a gliomatosis cerebri specimen from an 18-year-old patient who had demonstrated progression of gliomatosis cerebri over 7 years. They detected allelic changes in the retinoblastoma and p53 tumor suppressor genes in regions of the tumor that were pathologically similar to glioblastoma multiforme. Increased EGFR expression could also be detected in tumor regions. The authors concluded that the genetic changes could be attributed to malignant progression from a low-grade glioma to a secondary glioblastoma.

Differential diagnosis

The differential diagnosis for gliomatosis cerebri is that of a low-grade glioma, oligodendroglioma, or multifocal glioma. Although it would have been difficult in the past to distinguish gliomatosis cerebri from these forms of glioma without an autopsy, current MR imaging should be able to show an accurate representation. It should be noted that some patients may not have imaging documentation until later in their course. In that case, presentation with increased intracranial pressure without focal radiologic abnormalities may be interpreted initially as pseudotumor cerebri.

Treatment

Because of the diffuse infiltrative nature of this tumor, it is impossible to attempt a surgical resection. Instead, biopsy for a diagnosis followed by radiation is currently the treatment of choice. If hydrocephalus develops, a ventriculoperitoneal shunt for control of intracranial pressure (ICP) may be temporarily helpful. Radiation therapy has been shown to be beneficial in some cases, however the data are still often anecdotal. More recently, Horst et al (2000) reviewed data on 17 patients treated with radiation therapy, in which they documented temporary improvement or stabilization in half of the patients, with duration of improvement of ≥6 months in 50% of the treated patients. Their mean reported survival from onset of symptoms was 24 months. Elshaikh et al (2002) reported treatment using radiation therapy in eight patients with gliomatosis cerebri, with a median survival of 11 months; 1- and 2-year survival rates were 45% and 30%, respectively. The four patients who did not receive radiation therapy all had survival times of ≤2 months. Kim et al (1998) treated 14 patients with whole brain radiation (mean 5780 cGy) and achieved a mean survival time of 38 months after diagnosis.

No dramatic benefit from any chemotherapy regimen has been reported; however, variable responses to PCV (procarbazine, carmustine, vincristine) have been documented (Herrlinger et al 2002). The largest chemotherapy regimen series was reported by Sanson et al (2004) in 63 consecutive patients treated upfront with chemotherapy [PCV or temozolomide (TMZ)]. Clinical objective responses were observed in 21 of 63 (33%) patients, and radiologic responses were seen in 16 of 62 (26%). For all patients combined, the median progression free survival and overall survival were 16 months and 29 months, respectively. Regardless of the regimen, the patients with oligodendroglial GC had a better prognosis than patients with astrocytic or oligoastrocytic GC. TMZ was better tolerated than PVC, although the clinical response was similar in both regimens. Encouraging results with TMZ were also reported by Levin et al (2004) who treated 11 radiotherapy naive patients with a median number of 10 treatment cycles of TMZ, receiving an objective response in 45% of the patients, with a median time to tumor progression of 13 months, and a progression free survival of 55% at 12 months.

Clinical outcome

The outcome is dismal. Although survival periods up to 4 years have been reported from onset of symptoms, most patients die within months. The most comprehensive series of gliomatosis cerebri patients was reported by Taillibert et al (2006) who reported on 296 patients; they reported a median survival of 14.5 years. Positive factors for survival included age younger than 42 years, Karnofsky score >80, low-grade gliomatosis, and oligodendroglial sub-types. Males had an increased survival compared to females, but that may have been secondary to the younger age at presentation, and a greater percentage of oligodendroglial subtypes in males compared to females. Kim et al (1998) reported a mean survival time after diagnosis of 38 months. No effective treatment has been reported.

Pleomorphic xanthoastrocytoma

Demographics

Pleomorphic xanthoastrocytoma (PXA) is a rare glial neoplasm initially reported in 1979 by Kepes et al (1979) in 12 patients. Since then, numerous case reports (Kuhajda et al 1981; Maleki et al 1983; Weldon-Linne et al 1983; Gomez et al 1985; Palma et al 1985; Glasser et al 1995; Yeh et al 2003; Lubansu et al 2004) and clinical series (Jones et al 1983; Davies et al 1994; Petropoulou et al 1995; Tonn et al 1997; Marton et al 2007), with literature reviews, have been published. Currently, nearly 250 cases are represented in the literature (Tekkok & Sav 2004; Marton et al 2007). PXA accounts for <1% of all astrocytic neoplasms (Yin et al 2002). The patients are generally young, usually in their late teens to early 30s. The youngest reported patient was 2 years of age, and the oldest 62 (Heyerdahl Strom & Skullerud 1983; MacKenzie 1987; Davies et al 1994). There does not appear to be a gender, racial or familial predisposition. PXA has been reported throughout the brain, but more commonly on the surface of the temporal or parietal lobes (Russell & Rubinstein 1989).

There have been reported cases of composite PXA-ganglioglioma tumors. In one case, the two tumor cell types were clearly separated. In another report, however, abnormal ganglion cells were clearly demonstrated within the PXA component (Furuta et al 1992; Lindboe et al 1992). A more recent report describes a composite PXA-ganglioglioma in the suprasellar region, which was diagnosed preoperatively as a craniopharyngioma based on radiographic appearance (Yeh et al 2003). Co-existence and possible association of PXA with other neurologic or congenital entities have been reported. For example, a recent report described PXA in the contralateral hemisphere in a patient with Sturge–Weber syndrome (Kilickesmez et al 2005). Another described a multicentric PXA in a patient with neurofibromatosis type I (Saikali et al 2005). Although very rare, leptomeningeal dissemination (Passone et al 2006), spinal cord dissemination (Nakajima et al 2006) and synchronous multicentric disease at presentation (McNatt et al 2005) have been described.

Diagnosis

A history of chronic seizures and headaches is a common presentation (Kepes et al 1979; Goldring et al 1986) (Russell & Rubinstein 1989). Occasionally, increased intracranial pressure with papilledema may be present. Focal neurologic deficit as an initial symptom is uncommon (Maleki et al 1983; Iwaki et al 1987).

CT scans often demonstrate a cystic tumor with nodular enhancement, usually on the surface of the temporal or parietal lobes (Weldon-Linne et al 1983; Blom 1988; Kros et al 1991), although PXA has also been reported in the thalamus and cerebellum (Kros et al 1991; Lindboe et al 1992). Focal calcifications and erosion or remodeling of overlying calvarium may be seen on CT (Maleki et al 1983; Rippe et al 1992).

MRI typically reveals a cystic lesion with enhancing nodular component (Fig. 26.4) (Mascalchi et al 1994). The solid portion of the tumor is isointense to gray matter on T1-weighted images and hyperintense on T2-weighted images (Tonn et al 1997). After administration of gadolinium, the nodular portion of the tumors typically showed marked enhancement. Increased signal intensity on proton-density and T2-weighted images in both the cystic and solid components of the tumors has also been described (Yoshino & Lucio 1992). Most commonly, minimal edema is observed on MRI (Rippe et al 1992). One report described a PXA with radiographic characteristics similar to a meningioma, including location and the presence of a dural tail (Pierallini et al 1999). Cerebral angiography demonstrates an avascular to moderately vascular tumor, with derivation of blood supply from meningeal feeders (Maleki et al 1983; Yoshino & Lucio 1992).

PXA is typically found in superficial locations in the cerebral hemispheres, most commonly the temporal lobe (Giannini et al 1999). Among less common locations, cerebellar PXA is most frequently reported (Chang et al 2006; Hamlat et al 2007). Cerebellar PXA is associated with a slightly older patient group (average age 33 years vs 26 years) compared with supratentorial PXA (Hamlat et al 2007). This tumor may also occur outside of the brain as one case report described a patient with a PXA who presented with a lytic skull lesion (Jea et al 2002).

Pathology

The cell of origin of PXA has been the subject of debate. Kepes initially established the glial nature of xanthoastrocytomas on the basis of their positive GFAP staining, and proposed the subpial astrocyte, which is known to be

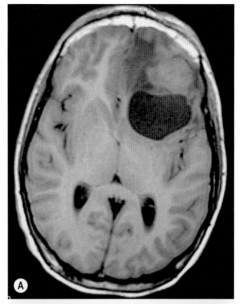

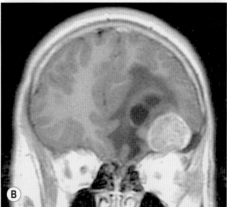

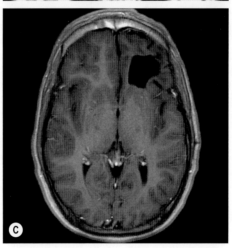

Figure 26.4 Pleomorphic xanthoastrocytoma. This 14-year-old boy presented with developmental delay, seizures and recently developed headaches. MR scan (T1-weighted) without (A) and with (B) contrast shows a uniformly enhancing tumor in the left frontal region with a large cystic component. Diffuse edema is present around the tumor. The patient underwent a total resection of his tumor. He is currently 3 years from his original surgery with T1-weighted image with contrast (C) showing no evidence of remnant tumor. He has not been given any adjuvant therapy and is seizure free on medication.

partially covered by basal lamina, as this neoplasm's cell of origin (Kepes et al 1979). Paulus disputed the astrocytic origin of this tumor, pointing out that not all tumors classified as xanthoastrocytomas were GFAP positive. Moreover, a spectrum of immunostains for mesenchymal tumors, such as α1-antichymotrypsin, tartrate-resistant acid phosphatase, common leukocyte antigen, and OKM-1, were positive in xanthoastrocytomas (Paulus & Peiffer 1988).

The tumor is typically located superficially in the temporal or parietal cortex, involving the leptomeninges, but not the dura mater. A mural nodule of yellowish or reddish tissue, encapsulated by a proteinaceous cyst, is often found (Russell & Rubinstein 1989).

Histologically, PXA shows cellular atypia and nuclear pleomorphism, abundant reticulin and variable lipidization. The tumors are characterized by spindle-shaped cells with elongated nuclei, as well as multinucleated giant cells with intracytoplasmic lipid-containing vacuoles, along with a variable number of lymphocytes and plasma cells (Zorzi et al 1992; Marton et al 2007). Few if any mitoses are present, and there is no evidence of intratumoral necrosis or endothelial proliferation (Fig. 26.5) (Kepes et al 1979; Loiseau et al 1991). Electron microscopy (EM) demonstrates epithelial properties such as intercellular junctions, interdigitations between apposing tumor cells, and a well-defined basal lamina surrounding the tumor nests (Iwaki et al 1987). On the basis of the EM characteristics, Sugita et al (1990) proposed two PXA sub-types: an 'epithelial' form and an 'angiomatous variant'. The angiomatous variant is very vascular, with surrounding desmoplastic reaction secondary to protein leakage from vessels.

Immunohistochemistry is helpful in characterizing these tumors. Most PXA are GFAP-positive; however, some tumors with PXA characteristics have been reported to be GFAP-negative. Reticulin stains show a rich reticulin network (Kepes et al 1979). Ki-67, a marker for actively proliferating cells, is often reported as <1% positive (Sugita et al 1990). Although classified as low-grade astrocytic tumors, both neuronal and glial markers can be detected in tumor cells. Recent work evaluated 40 different PXA specimens for glial and neuronal markers. The authors found 100% immunoreactivity for glial markers GFAP and S-100, and variable positivity for neuronal markers such as class 3 beta-tubulin (73%) and synaptophysin (38%), suggesting that PXA may originate from a bi- or multipotential precursor cell or stem cell (Powell et al 1996; Giannini et al 2002; Saikali et al 2005). Malignant PXAs demonstrate greater mitosis and necrosis (Marton et al 2007).

Cytogenetics performed on one PXA revealed a karyotype of 48 X,Y, with trisomies for chromosomes 3, 5, 7, 15 and monosomy for chromosome 22 (Sawyer et al 1992). Telomeric association, evolving to ring chromosomes, has been reported in a recurrent pleomorphic xanthoastrocytoma (Sawyer et al 1992). Despite the degree of pleomorphism present in the tumor, cytofluorometric analysis of one PXA revealed that the main mode of the tumor was diploid with polyploid classes (no aneuploidy) (Hosokawa et al 1991).

Differential diagnosis

Imaging differential diagnoses for a peripheral enhancing lesion in a child or young adult include glioblastoma,

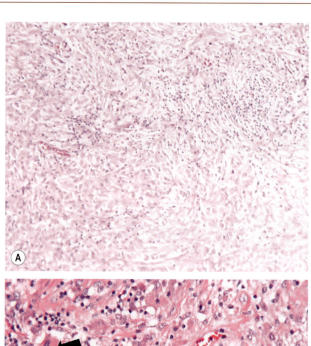

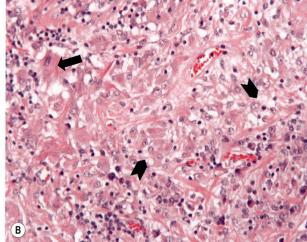

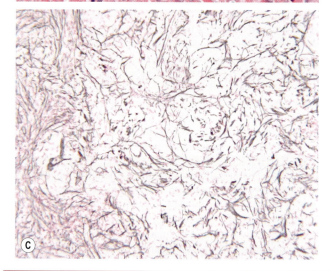

Figure 26.5 (A) Pleomorphic xanthoastrocytoma composed of pleomorphic cells of variable size and shape forming clusters and bundles. An infiltrate of lymphocytes is present (H&E ×10). (B) Pleomorphic xanthoastrocytoma showing the proliferating tumor cells containing a large vesicular nucleus and conspicuous nucleolus some of which are binucleated (arrow). The cytoplasm is abundant and in some cells vacuolated by numerous lipid droplets (arrowheads). (C) Mitotic figures, necrosis, or vascular proliferation are remarkable absent. (H&E ×20.)

ganglioglioma, gangliosarcoma, astrocytoma, meningioma, hemangiosarcoma, oligodendroglioma, juvenile pilocytic astrocytoma, and solitary metastasis (Yoshino & Lucio 1992). Young age, temporal lobe location, a cystic lesion with an enhancing mural nodule and a history of seizures may point towards a diagnosis of PXA (Tonn et al 1997). From a histopathological standpoint, tumors may be distinguished from PXA, based on histological appearance or immunohistochemistry staining properties. Juvenile pilocytic astrocytoma is a common tumor of astrocytic origin which can be readily distinguished from PXA by the numerous hairlike fibrils that abound in the cytoplasm and the processes of the neoplastic cells present in the pilocytic astrocytoma (Gomez et al 1985; Russell & Rubinstein 1989). Fibrous xanthomas have the gross features of a meningioma, but the histological characteristics of a fibrous histiocytoma and all cells are GFAP negative (Kepes et al 1979). PXA must be differentiated from a malignant astrocytoma with xanthomatous changes, as the pleomorphic appearance and bizarre multinucleated giant cells resemble glioblastoma (Grant & Gallagher 1986; Sarkar et al 1990). However, superficial location with leptomeningeal involvement, as well as histopathologic findings such as the relative paucity of mitoses, positive reticulin and neuronal staining, and the absence of intratumoral necrosis point towards the diagnosis of PXA.

Treatment

Surgical excision is the treatment of choice (Tonn et al 1997). Most tumors are superficially located, and gross total resection is usually possible. Seizures and increased intracranial pressure are often successfully treated with tumor removal. Whole brain radiation, using doses ranging from 30–60 Gy, has been used in cases where gross total resection was not achieved. There have not been enough patients with long-term follow-up to determine whether postoperative radiation actually improves the prognosis. Thus far, radiotherapy does not appear to significantly impact clinical outcome (Whittle et al 1989). There also does not appear to be a role for chemotherapy (Marton et al 2007). One study reported the use of ACNU (l-(4-amino-2-methylpyrimidine-5-yl)-methyl-3-(2-chloroethyl)-3-nitrosurea) in one asymptomatic patient with a 2-year follow-up (Sugita et al 1990).

Clinical outcome

The overall outcome is generally good. Seizures, if initially present, are well-controlled with surgery (Kepes et al 1979; Goldring et al 1986). Despite the cellular pleomorphism, long-term survival is the general rule, even in patients who have not received any form of adjunctive therapy. Asymptomatic survival rates of more than 10–20 years are common (Kepes et al 1979; Palma et al 1985; Paulus & Peiffer 1988). The number one prognostic factor in patient survival or future tumor recurrence is the completeness of tumor removal. Local recurrence may occur. After complete resection, the survival rate is 85% at 5 years and 70% at 10 years (Giannini et al 1999). Recurrence rate after total removal is up to 20% with an average time to recurrence of approximately 6 years (Marton et al 2007). For patients with recurrence, surgery is also the treatment of choice as there is little data regarding radiation therapy and chemotherapy. PXA may recur or present with features consistent with composite tumor types. For example, one patient with supratentorial PXA was diagnosed 16 years later with recurrence in her cerebellum (Glasser et al 1995).

Some patients, despite a prolonged period of asymptomatic survival, may undergo rapid deterioration (Weldon-Linne et al 1983). Although most tumors are classified as WHO grade II, anaplastic variants with malignant progression have been described (Tekkok & Sav 2004; Marton et al 2007). A recent report counted 17 anaplastic PXAs and 23 PXAs with malignant transformation among the nearly 250 published cases. Thus, high-grade tumors ultimately comprise approximately 16% of all PXAs, although some authors have questioned whether tumors that undergo rapid malignant deterioration are actually PXAs or histologically misdiagnosed high-grade astrocytomas. The reported time to malignant transformation varies from 7 months to 15 years (Weldon-Linne et al 1983; Marton et al 2007). Kepes (1989) reported three cases of pleomorphic xanthoastrocytoma with malignant degeneration to small cell glioblastoma multiforme (GBM) over a period of 6 years, 15 years, and 6 months. Another series of eight patients with PXA reported malignant transformation in three patients with a mean recurrence time of 5.7 years (Marton et al 2007). In this series, analysis of glioneuronal markers Ki67 and p53 did not help to discriminate those tumors prone to malignancy. The degeneration of these tumors into GBM has been cited as further proof in their astrocytic origin (Kepes 1989).

Subependymal giant cell astrocytoma

Demographics

Tuberous sclerosis complex (TSC) is an autosomal dominant phakomatosis characterized by the classic triad of mental retardation, seizures, and adenoma sebaceum first described by Vogt in 1908. The formation of hamartomatous lesions in many organs, including brain, heart, or kidneys has been attributed to mutations in one of two tumor suppressor genes: TSC1 or TSC2, encoding hamartin and tuberin, respectively (Jozwiak et al 2004). The incidence of tuberous sclerosis has been estimated to range from 1/100 000 to 1/50 000 (Nagib et al 1984). In one large series of 345 tuberous sclerosis patients, 6% of the patients had subependymal giant cell astrocytoma (SGCA). Recently, in a series of 214 patients with TSC who had received a contrast-enhanced CT-scan of the brain, 20% of the patients with TSC had evidence of SGCA. The age range for initial presentation and discovery of SGCA ranges from neonatal (Raju et al 2007) to 50 years old. Most patients have clinical manifestations before the age of 20. In Adriaensen et al's (2009) series, the age of patients with TSC and SGCA was 31 years old; the age of patients with TSC alone (without SGCA) was 37 years old. There is no sex or racial predilection. SGCAs typically arise from subependymal nodules located in the walls of the lateral ventricle adjacent to the foramen of Monro, but may be found at other locations in the ventricles (Nagib et al 1984).

Diagnosis

The initial diagnosis of tuberous sclerosis is based on a multitude of signs and symptoms including dermatological manifestations (adenoma sebaceum, shagreen patches, areas of altered pigmentation, depigmented nevi, subungual fibromas), retinal tumors, seizures, and mental retardation (Fig. 26.6). Other systemic manifestations include tumors of the kidneys, heart, and lung. Lesions of the spleen, pancreas, and genitalia are less common (Nagib et al 1984). Patients' usual presentation with SGCA in an earlier series was with the presence of increased intracranial pressure when the tumor resulted in obstruction at the foramen of Monro (Kapp et al 1967). In one recent series, Sharma et al (2005) reported that the most common location was the lateral ventricle (91%), followed by the third ventricle (9%) in 23 cases of SCGA. Current imaging allows for diagnosis of SGCA before the development of increased intracranial pressure. In neonates, cranial ultrasound can be used initially to establish the presence of the tumor, followed by a CT scan for better anatomical detail. CT scans are useful in following the course of tubers. Fujiwara (1989) followed a 7-month-old child with CT scans until he was 10 years of age, demonstrating sequential growth of subependymal nodules to a SGCA which was subsequently resected. Calcifications can be seen on CT scans both within the SGCA and in tubers adjacent to the ventricular systems. Unlike gliomas, which often have a variable degree of contrast enhancement, SGCAs have fairly uniform enhancement (Nagib et al 1984). The various intracranial manifestations of tuberous sclerosis – including multiple subependymal nodules, tuber (seen as areas of high signal intensity on T2-weighted images), disruption of cortical architecture, and dilated ventricles – are well seen on MR imaging. The current imaging diagnosis of choice for SGCA is MR scanning with and without gadolinium, with coronal sections through the region of the foramen of Monro. SGCAs are isointense to gray matter on T1-weighted images. They are hyperintense to gray matter on T2-weighted images with signal voids secondary to calcification and enhance markedly with contrast (Fig. 26.7). Pulsed perfusion studies have documented that cortical hamartomas are hypoperfused.

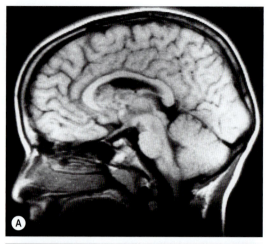

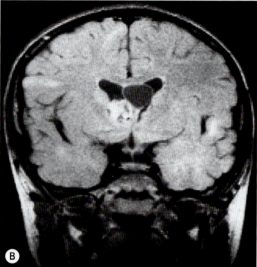

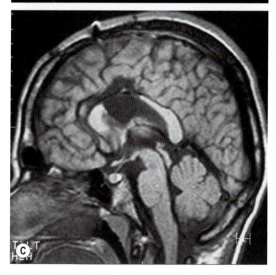

Figure 26.7 Subependymal giant cell astrocytoma. This 9-year-old boy presented with recurrent headaches. (A) MR scan (T1-weighted) without contrast shows a tumor isointense to gray matter in the lateral ventricle. (B) On MR scan (T1-weighted) with contrast the tumor enhances evenly and a cystic component is seen in the coronal section. The patient underwent a gross total resection without further recurrence via an interhemispheric transcallosal approach. (C) MR scan (T1-weighted) with contrast shows no recurrence 2 years later.

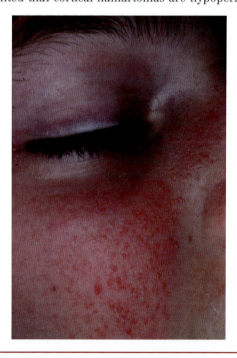

Figure 26.6 Adenoma sebaceum in a child with tuberous sclerosis.

Pathology

Grossly, SGCAs are fairly well circumscribed, gray to pinkish-red in color, and occasionally hemorrhagic because of increased vascularity (Rubinstein 1972). Giant cells, which are also found in cortical tubers, are characteristically seen, with regular nuclei on light microscopy. The cytoplasm is abundant and eosinophilic. Evidence of necrosis and focal areas of mitosis may be present; however, no correlation exists with a poor prognosis in these patients (Fig. 26.8). On electron microscopy, giant cells appear as large cells with abundant cytoplasm and numerous astrocytic filaments. Cytomorphology of SGCA shows spindle and epithelioid

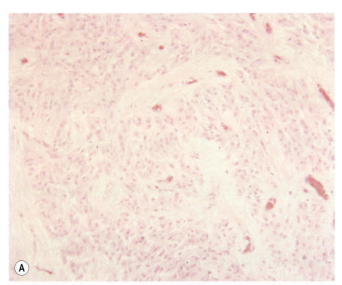

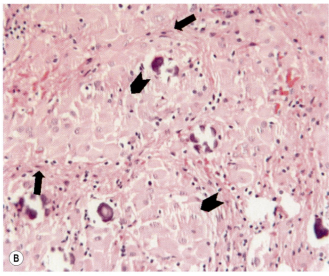

Figure 26.8 (A) Subependymal giant cell astrocytoma exhibiting the typical clusters of gemistocytic cells and fibrillary astrocytic areas. There is a suggestive formation of perivascular pseudo-rosettes reminiscent of ependymoma (H&E ×100). (B) Subependymal giant cell astrocytoma containing a mixed cell population with typical clusters of large gemistocytic cells (arrowheads), surrounded by bundles of fibrillary astrocytes (arrows). Scattered calcifications are also present. (H&E ×200.)

shaped tumor cells with dense eosinophilic cytoplasm, eccentric nuclei, prominent nucleoli, and nuclear cytoplasmic inclusions. In order to determine whether SGCAs are astrocytic or neuronal in origin, Nakamura & Becker (1983) performed glial fibrillary and S-100 stains. They found that half of the tumors were GFAP positive, and six out of seven of the tumors were S-100 positive, suggesting that SGCAs may originate from germinal matrix cells that have not differentiated into astrocytic or neuronal tumors. Bonnin et al (1984) showed that in patients with tuberous sclerosis, most of the tumors were GFAP negative. If the tumors were GFAP positive, they were not associated with tuberous sclerosis. This paper points out that the potential for astrocytic or neuronal differentiation may be incompletely expressed if tuberous sclerosis is present. Other investigators have concluded that both the tumor cells and the giant cells of SGCA demonstrate evidence of both glial and neuronal differentiation (Hirose et al 1995; Lopes et al 1996). More recently, this issue of astrocytic differentiation was revisited by Buccoliero et al (2009). The authors performed immunostaining in nine TSC complex SGCA and reported that all nine tumors were GFAP negative, neurofilament negative (8/9), neuron specific enolase negative (9/9), and synaptophysin positive (8/9). The authors concluded that SGCA was more glioneuronal in nature than astrocytic. Rarely is there an association between malignant glial tumors and patients with tuberous sclerosis. Staining for aB crystallin is positive in subependymal giant cells and in astrocytic tumors among neuroectodermal neoplasms. aB crystallin is negative in ependymal/choroid plexus tumors, suggesting that aB crystallin is selectively secreted by astrocytic tumors. Flow cytometry showed that almost all of the tumors were diploid. No correlation was found between histological features such as atypia, mitoses, endothelial proliferations, or necrosis with flow cytometric characteristics (Shepherd et al 1991).

The biology and genetics of TSC is now better understood. Although the majority of patients with TSC are sporadic (65%), genetic linkage studies of familial cases have led to the discovery of two separate genes linked to the tuberous sclerosis complex: TSC1, located at chromosome 9q34, encoding the tumor suppressor protein called hamartin. The function of hamartin is not clear; it binds to ezrin, a protein involved in the linkage of the cell membrane to the cytoskeleton. TSC2 is located on chromosome 16p13.3 and encodes for a tumor suppressor protein called tuberin. The function of tuberin is most likely in the cellular signaling pathway as it does have a region of homology to rap1GAP, a guanosine triphosphatase activating protein. Tuberin and hamartin interact directly with each other, and the complex function together to regulate specific cellular processes (Narayanan 2003). Moreover, over 50 proteins have been demonstrated to interact with hamartin and/or tuberin. These proteins are varied and include proteins involved in cell cycle regulation such as cyclins; heat shock proteins (HSP 70–1), and oncogenes (Erk, FoxO1). Recently, Jozwiak et al (2004) have immunostained SGCA from nine patients with TSC for expression of the tumor suppressor proteins hamartin and tuberin. They found loss of hamartin expression in all of the SGCA, and loss of tuberin expression in 6/9 SGCA, leading them to propose a two hit disease pathogenesis model for formation of SGCA in TSC patients.

Differential diagnosis

The differential diagnosis for tumors of the lateral ventricle in addition to SGCA includes ependymoma, subependymoma, primary cerebral neuroblastoma, astrocytoma, oligodendroglioma, meningioma, CN, and choroid plexus papilloma. Other tumors commonly described in the tuberous sclerosis complex include cerebral hemangiomas, spongioblastomas, neurinomas, and ependymomas. In one series of 47 pathologically proven lateral ventricular neoplasms, Jelinek et al (1990) found that the clinical characteristics most consistent with SGCA include presentation in the first three decades of life, location at the foramen of Monro, and tumor enhancement with contrast on CT scan. Histologically, the differential diagnosis of a giant cell astrocytoma includes gemistocytic astrocytoma and giant cell glioblastoma. Giant cells may look like the giant cells of GBM or like gemistocytic cells. Gemistocytic astrocytomas are usually non-discrete infiltrating lesions in the white matter of older individuals. Histologically, they are intensely GFAP-positive, with exceptionally large component cells characterized by an eosinophilic cytoplasm (Russell & Rubinstein 1989). Giant cell glioblastomas are not found in the subependymal location, and occur in the older population. Histologically, giant cell glioblastomas are anaplastic tumors with vascular proliferation, necrosis, or pseudopalisading similar to non-giant cell GBM.

Treatment

The treatment of choice is surgical resection, with gross total removal if possible. Sub-total resection is often adequate as these tumors are slow growing and may have limited growth potential in any remaining tumor, similar to that of a pilocytic astrocytoma (Nagib et al 1984). Follow-up imaging should be obtained at regular intervals, however, to rule out tumor re-growth or hydrocephalus. Patients with unresolved hydrocephalus despite tumor removal need to be addressed by a third ventriculostomy or CSF diversion. Neonates suspected of having tuberous sclerosis should have a cardiac evaluation as part of the diagnostic work-up prior to surgical removal of an intraventricular tumor. Painter et al (1984) reported their experience with two neonates who underwent attempted surgical resection but died secondary to refractory intraoperative cardiac arrhythmias. Both were found at autopsy to have multiple cardiac rhabdomyomas. Radiotherapy has been employed in the past, however, there is no evidence documenting any difference in survival. No chemotherapy trials have been conducted.

In summary, the treatment of SGCA is surgical, both for the original tumor and recurrences that might occur, with radiation and chemotherapy playing no role.

Clinical outcome

The clinical outcome for the SGCA alone is generally favorable and patients have been stable at 15-year follow-ups despite sub-total resections (Nagib et al 1984). The prognosis has no bearing on the tumor having focal areas of active mitoses or necrosis. The severity of seizure disorders and degree of mental retardation have no relationship to the status of an SGCA. Adequate treatment of the hydrocephalus present in some of these patients also reflects on outcome.

Tumors of mixed glial and neuronal origin

Multiple distinct glioneuronal tumors have recently been recognized as separate pathologic entities. For some of these neoplasms only scant literature exists, which precludes an in-depth discussion regarding their treatment and prognosis. Others are more established entities and are therefore more amenable to a review of the available literature. The tumors in this section are representative of both scenarios.

Papillary glioneuronal tumor

Demographics

Papillary glioneuronal tumor (PGNT) is a rare neoplasm, with only 37 cases reported in the literature as of 2008 (Williams et al 2008). Initially classified as a variant of ganglioglioma (Kleihues et al 1993), the tumor was recently recognized as a distinct entity (Louis et al 2007; Brat et al 2008). The largest series described nine cases in 1998 and represents the original and most complete description of this neoplasm (Komori et al 1998). In this series, the ages ranged from 11 years to 52 years, with the average age at presentation of 28 years. There is a slight female predilection (Javahery et al 2009), but no obvious racial predilection, although the literature is too scant at this time to determine a trend. Patients most commonly present with headache, but may also present with mild neurologic symptoms such as visual changes, mood disturbances or seizure that are present from 1 day to 2 years prior to diagnosis (Atri et al 2007). Alternatively, the lesion may be asymptomatic and found incidentally (Komori et al 1998).

Since this initial series, multiple case reports have contributed additional information regarding these tumors. PGNT primarily occurs in teens and young adults, but ages reported in the literature range from 4 to 75 years old (Barnes et al 2002; Tsukayama & Arakawa 2002). Although typically low-grade, more aggressive forms have been reported (Newton et al 2008).

Diagnosis

PGNT are commonly located in the parietal, temporal or frontal lobes, often adjacent to the ventricular system (Atri et al 2007; Javahery et al 2009). The tumors are only rarely associated with perilesional edema (Prayson 2000; Atri et al 2007).

MRI demonstrates a well-demarcated, cystic mass with rim enhancement and an associated homogeneously enhancing mural nodule (Figs 26.9, 26.10) (Lamszus et al 2003; Vajtai et al 2006; Edgar & Rosenblum 2007). Cyst fluid is typically similar to cerebrospinal fluid on MRI; hypointense on T1-weighted images, hyperintense on T2-weighted images and no restriction on diffusion-weighted images. Faint septation may be found within the cystic portions of the tumor (Javahery et al 2009). Rarely, the tumor may lack a cystic component (Komori et al 1998). Tumors may appear heterogeneously enhancing when the solid and cystic components are mixed (Komori et al 1998).

Pathology

PGNT is classified as a WHO grade I neoplasm (Brat et al 2008). Histopathologic examination shows a characteristic pseudopapillary arrangement of hyalinized blood vessels

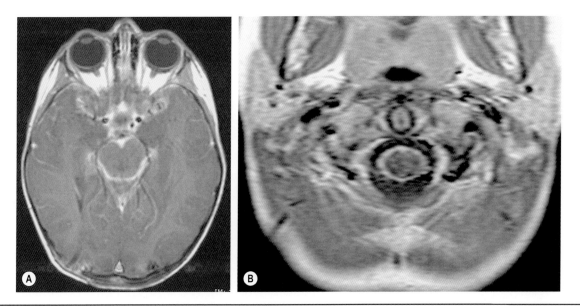

Figure 26.9 (A,B) Enhanced axial T1-weighted MRI showing the basal cisterns and cervical subarachnoid space filled with tumor.

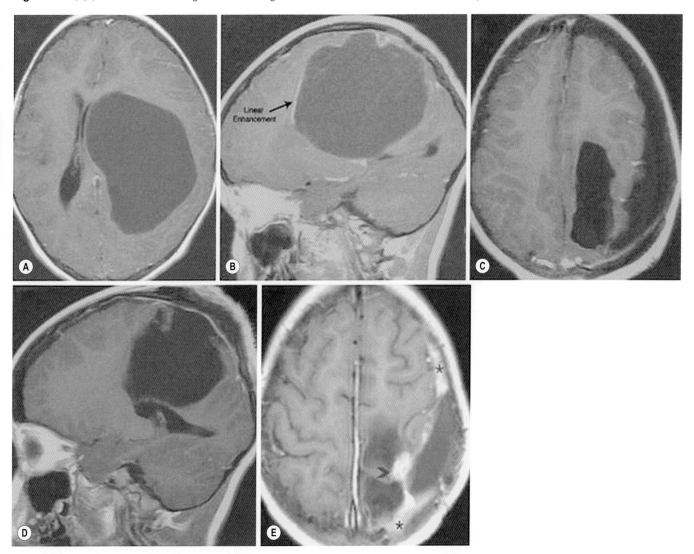

Figure 26.10 Papillary glioneural tumor. Axial (A, C, and E) and sagittal (B and D) T1-weighted contrast-enhanced MR images of the patient. (A, B) Preoperative images show a septated cystic lesion with faint rim enhancement and hypointense fluid. (C, D) Immediate postoperative images show the GTR. (E) Image showing tumor recurrence within the resection cavity (arrowhead) and external to the resection cavity (asterisks). (With permission from Javahery et al. 2009.)

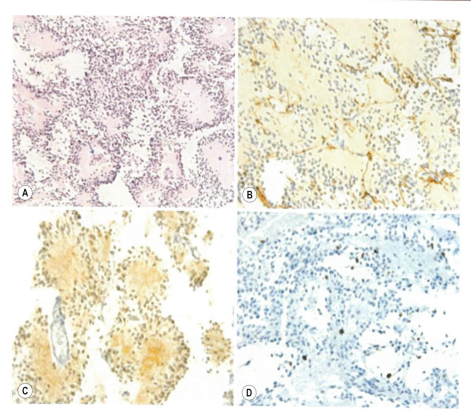

Figure 26.11 Papillary glioneural tumor. Photomicrographs of specimens from the first tumor resection (A–C) and the tumor recurrence (D). (A) Section stained with H&E showing a papillary pattern with either a central vessel (arrow) or neuropil network. (B) Glial fibrillary acidic protein staining shows astrocytic processes. (C) Synaptophysin staining for labeling neuropil and neuronal components. (D) Staining for Ki 67 reveals a Ki 67 proliferative index of 5%. Original magnification ×40. (With permission from Javahery et al. 2009.)

lined by astrocytes, accompanied by focal collections or sheets of neurocytes admixed with ganglion and ganglioid cells in the interpapillary space (Fig. 26.11) (Buccoliero et al 2006). Rare neurons may be found within the tumor (Javahery et al 2009). The tumor cells typically have uniform nuclei, scant cytoplasm and rare mitoses. Pleomorphism, vascular proliferation and necrosis are not typically found. Immunohistochemistry may reveal positivity for GFAP, S-100 and vimentin in the perivascular region, and positivity for synaptophysin in the interpapillary region, although variability exists between case reports (Edgar & Rosenblum 2007; Vaquero & Coca 2007; Javahery et al 2009). The perivascularly arranged cuboidal cells are GFAP and synaptophysin-positive, which is a feature unique to papillary glioneuronal tumors. The histologic examination differs from the well-circumscribed radiographic appearance as the lesions appear to microscopically invade the surrounding brain (Atri et al 2007).

MIB-1 labelling when reported is typically <2% (Komori et al 1998; Bouvier-Labit et al 2000; Prayson 2000; Vajtai et al 2006), although some authors have reported tumors with higher mitotic and proliferative indices, possibly supporting the notion of an atypical variant of PGNT (Atri et al 2007; Vaquero & Coca 2007; Newton et al 2008). Electron microscopy shows a high nuclear to cytoplasmic ratio, and may show membrane-bound granules or cytoplasmic processes such as microfilaments in astrocytic cells lining the vascular pseudopapillae or microtubules in interpapillary cells with neuronal features (Javahery et al 2009). Genetic studies have not revealed chromosomal aberrations such as 1p or 19q deletions (Tanaka et al 2005; Edgar & Rosenblum 2007).

Differential diagnosis

The radiographic appearance of a well-circumscribed cystic lesion with contrast enhancing solid component may mimic pilocytic xanthoastrocytoma, ganglioglioma and juvenile pilocytic astrocytoma (Atri et al 2007). Histologically, hyalinized vessels may be found in other mixed glioneuronal tumors such as ganglioglioma and CN, and low-grade astrocytic tumors such as juvenile pilocytic astrocytoma and pilocytic xanthoastrocytoma. As mentioned above, however, the presence of GFAP and synaptophysin-positive cells in a papillary arrangement around hyalinized blood vessels is a distinguishing feature of papillary glioneuronal tumors. Other tumors with papillary histologic appearance include choroids plexus papilloma, papillary ependymoma, germ cell tumor and metastasis. These may be distinguished based on anatomic location at diagnosis and immunohistochemistry.

Treatment

The treatment of choice is complete surgical resection. The role of chemotherapy or radiation therapy in a patient with recurrence or sub-total resection is unclear, and only a small number of reports document such adjuvant therapy. One recent study described the use of chemotherapy after subtotal resection of a tumor with a MIB-1 labelling index of 12%, although the agent and regimen were not specified (Atri et al 2007). Another patient with a high proliferative index received radiation after surgery and was without evidence of recurrence 5 years after surgery (Vaquero & Coca 2007). A third article reported the use of both conformal radiation and adjuvant chemotherapy (temozolomide) after sub-total resection of an aggressive variant of PGNT (Newton et al 2008). This treatment paradigm is similar to that for a high-grade glioma, and was initiated based on histopathologic findings consistent with a high-grade neoplasm such as regions of mitosis and necrosis, and a Ki-67 of 26%. The authors report stable radiographic appearance of the disease. A fourth report described adjuvant radiation and chemotherapy after resection of recurrent disease described as an aggressive variant of PGNT (Javahery et al 2009). Overall, the literature reports the use of some form of adjuvant therapy for tumor recurrence or for tumors with elevated proliferative indices. Given the small number of cases, however, determining the efficacy of these treatment strategies is difficult.

Clinical outcome
PGNT is most commonly a low-grade lesion with an indolent clinical course (Broholm et al 2002; Williams et al 2008). Most case reports describe gross total resection in patients who are alive with no evidence of recurrence at follow-up times up to 7 years after surgery (Bouvier-Labit et al 2000; Kordek et al 2003; Lamszus et al 2003). Recent reports suggest the presence of an atypical variant of PGNT that has higher mitotic activity and a higher proliferative index, although the reported clinical courses do not reflect these histologic findings (Vaquero & Coca 2007). Other reports describe similar atypical histologic findings in association with more aggressive tumor behavior (Javahery et al 2009). In one case, a patient presented 4 years after gross total resection with recurrent disease at the surgical site (left frontal lobe) as well as in two remote locations (left pulvinar nucleus, medial left thalamus). Histopathologic examination demonstrated positive Ki-67 in 1% of tumor cells from the initial resection, but 5% of cells of the recurrence and the patient received adjuvant radiation therapy and chemotherapy. A second patient in this study demonstrated significant re-growth of residual tumor 3 months after sub-total resection. Ki-67 was positive in 4% of the initial tumor cells and 7% of recurrent tumor cells (Javahery et al 2009). These two cases suggest a possible role for Ki-67 in predicting tumor behavior. Further clinical studies with longer follow-up times will be required to better characterize the clinical course of patients after both total and sub-total resections.

Rosette-forming glioneuronal tumor of the fourth ventricle

Demographics
The rosette-forming glioneuronal tumor (RGNT) of the fourth ventricle is one example of a neoplasm only recently described in the literature (Allende & Prayson 2009). This tumor was not given official WHO status until 2007. Although most of the literature regarding these tumors is in the form of case reports (Preusser et al 2003; Johnson et al 2006; Joseph et al 2008), one study in 2002 reviewed 11 cases (Komori et al 2002). Patient age at diagnosis in this report ranged from 12 to 59 years, and most reports describe cases in young adults.

The scant literature regarding this tumor precludes reliable epidemiologic analysis such as gender or racial predilection. To date, less than 30 cases appear in the literature. In the series from Komori et al (2002), the female to male ratio was 1.75:1 and the mean age at diagnosis was 32 years.

Subsequent case reports and smaller series seem to confirm this gender ratio and mean age at diagnosis (Vajtai et al 2007). One report described the tumor in association with dysgenetic tricho-rhinopharyngeal type I syndrome (Joseph et al 2008). Another report described one of only two examples of a rosette-forming glioneuronal tumor of the fourth ventricle not found in the posterior fossa. This patient had neurofibromatosis type 1 and the tumor was located in the optic chiasm (Scheithauer et al 2009). The other patient was found to have a rosette-forming glioneuronal tumor of the cervico-thoracic spinal cord (Anan et al 2009).

Diagnosis
As the name implies, these tumors are nearly uniformly found in the posterior fossa and typically involve the fourth ventricle or cerebral aqueduct, with frequent focal involvement of the cerebellum. Symptoms at diagnosis are typical of lesions involving cerebrospinal fluid pathways in the posterior fossa, although lesions may be discovered incidentally (Preusser et al 2003; Edgar & Rosenblum 2007). These include headache, nausea, vomiting, and ataxia. Lesions may be large with significant mass effect and hydrocephalus at diagnosis.

Cranial imaging reveals a midline lesion within the fourth ventricle or cerebral aqueduct that commonly involves surrounding structures such as the cerebellar vermis, brainstem, thalamus and pineal region. MRI demonstrates the tumors to be fairly circumscribed with cystic areas. The solid areas are typically isointense on T1-weighted images, hyperintense on T2-weighted images and most tumors show heterogeneous contrast enhancement. The tumors may occasionally be multi-focal or have satellite lesions (Komori et al 2002; Preusser et al 2003; Marhold et al 2008).

Pathology
This tumor is classified as a WHO grade I neoplasm (Rosenblum 2007). Histologically, two components of the tumor can be identified. The first is a population of neuronal cells forming neurocytic and/or perivascular pseudo-rosettes. Immunohistochemistry shows the rosettes staining positive for synaptophysin and MAP-2. The second is an astrocyte population that histologically resembles pilocytic astrocytoma, consisting of fibrillated spindle cells with occasional Rosenthal fibers (Johnson et al 2006). These cells are immunoreactive to S-100 and GFAP (Komori et al 2002). Cellular atypia is minimal, and mitotic activity and MIB-1 labeling indices are low (Komori et al 2002; Edgar & Rosenblum 2007; Vajtai et al 2007). Immunoreactivity for GFAP or synaptophysin is felt to be mutually exclusive (Vajtai et al 2007).

Ultrastructural investigations in one case series confirmed the presence of two cell populations. The neuronal cells contained microtubules, dense core granules and, in a few of the cases, mature synapses. The glial cells contained bundles of intermediate filaments (Komori et al 2002).

Differential diagnosis
The histopathologic features of rosette-forming glioneuronal tumors of the fourth ventricle resemble those of dysembryoplastic neuroepithelial tumors (DNET). However, properties such as rosette formation by neuronal cells and

infratentorial location distinguish this tumor from DNET (Komori et al 2002).

The astrocyte component has a histologic appearance similar to pilocytic astrocytoma. The two can be distinguished based on the presence of neurocytic pseudo-rosettes with positive synaptophysin staining in the rosette-forming glioneuronal tumor of the fourth ventricle. Such unique immunohistochemistry staining properties should help distinguish this tumor from other lesions that may be found in the posterior fossa.

Ependymoma involving the fourth ventricle may be distinguished based on the pattern of synaptophysin and GFAP staining. Specifically, GFAP staining of perivascular pseudo-rosettes distinguishes ependymoma from PGNT of the fourth ventricle (Vajtai et al 2007). Histologically, oligodendroglioma with neurocytic differentiation and CN may appear similar to PGNT, but their appearance in the fourth ventricle or cerebellum is rare.

Treatment

The treatment for these tumors most commonly described in the literature is gross total or sub-total surgical resection (Komori et al 2002; Vajtai et al 2007). Involvement of eloquent areas such as the brain stem may preclude gross total resection. Biopsy without resection has also been described, both via craniotomy and endoscopically (Komori et al 2002; Tan et al 2008). In addition to surgical resection of the lesion, patients may require temporary or permanent CSF diversion.

The role for adjuvant chemotherapy or radiation therapy is unclear. One of the 11 patients in the Komori series received postoperative radiation (Komori et al 2002). Further work is required to determine the natural clinical course of these tumors and to elucidate the roles for surgical resection and adjuvant therapies.

Clinical outcome

The benign histologic appearance of this tumor is reflected by its indolent clinical course (Vajtai et al 2007; Marhold et al 2008). Tumor recurrence is infrequently described after resection, although local invasion into eloquent structures or multi-focality of the tumor may increase the chance of recurrence (Pimentel et al 2008).

Postoperative neurologic deficits, both transient and permanent, are described in up to half of patients who undergo surgical resection. These may include cerebellar signs such as ataxia (Pimentel et al 2008) and/or cranial neuropathies such as CN VII palsy (Albanese et al 2005). The relatively high surgical morbidity and the presumed indolent clinical course have led some authors to question the role of surgical resection and propose consideration of a conservative management approach with continuous clinical and radiographic surveillance (Tan et al 2008).

Desmoplastic infantile ganglioglioma

Demographics

Desmoplastic infantile ganglioglioma (DIG), also known as desmoplastic supratentorial neuroepithelial tumor, is a rare glial tumor of infancy first described by VandenBerg et al (1987b). The tumors were initially characterized by

Taratuto et al (1984) as superficial cerebral astrocytomas with dural attachment, or desmoplastic infantile astrocytoma. The latter is considered a separate entity that is differentiated from DIG due to lack of a neuronal component (Alexiou et al 2008). Both are classified as WHO grade I. Currently, nearly 100 cases have been reported in the literature, mostly in the form of case reports and small case series (Paulus et al 1992; Sperner et al 1994; Tamburrini et al 2003; Lonnrot et al 2007; Alexiou et al 2008; Hoving et al 2008). The tumors represent 1.25% of all intracranial tumors in children and 15.8% of all intracranial tumors in infants (Rout et al 2002). Patient ages range from 2 months to 25 years old, although the tumors usually occur in early childhood (Kuchelmeister et al 1993). There is no familial or racial predilection, but there is a slight male preponderance (Lonnrot et al 2007).

Diagnosis

Most patients present with new onset seizures (Sperner et al 1994; Lonnrot et al 2007). As these tumors often occur in infants, very large tumors may present with progressive increase in head circumference and bulging fontanel. The neurologic exam is usually non-focal, and signs and symptoms of increased intracranial pressure, such as lethargy, may be the only findings. Alternatively, focal neurologic signs such as hemiparesis may be present (Alexiou et al 2008).

The tumors are exclusively supratentorial (Tamburrini et al 2003). CT scans show a large cystic tumor with an enhancing solid component (Taratuto et al 1984; Ng et al 1990). T1-weighted images on MR show the cystic component of the tumor as hypointense to gray matter, with an isointense solid component (Fig. 26.12). The solid component and the cyst rim enhance after gadolinium administration (Sperner et al 1994; Alexiou et al 2008). The tumors are most commonly very large at presentation with a large cystic component (Duffner et al 1994). T2-weighted images demonstrate T2 prolongation in the cyst with variable signal intensity of the solid portion. The tumor usually abuts the meningeal surface, with an intense contrast enhancement pattern (Martin et al 1991). The most common locations are the frontal and parietal lobes, followed by temporal and occipital lobes, and involvement of multiple lobes at presentation is common (Alexiou et al 2008). Less commonly, DIG may involve the locations such as the brainstem, thalamus or pineal region (Fan et al 2001), or present as multifocal disease (Khaddage et al 2004; Lonnrot et al 2007).

Pathology

Grossly, desmoplastic infantile gangliogliomas are large, superficially located lesions that typically involve the cerebral cortex and leptomeninges (Alexiou et al 2008). They are firmly attached to the dura, with a solid component as well as a prominent uni- or multiloculated cysts. The tumors are firm and avascular, with a dense desmoplastic component, superficially resembling a moderately cellular fibroma. No connections with the ventricular system are present.

Microscopically, desmoplastic infantile gangliogliomas show evidence of glial and ganglionic differentiation accompanied by an extreme desmoplastic reaction. The fibroblastic elements are often admixed with variable numbers of

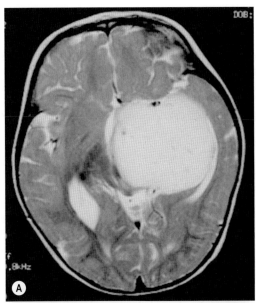

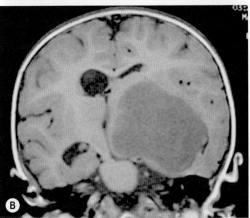

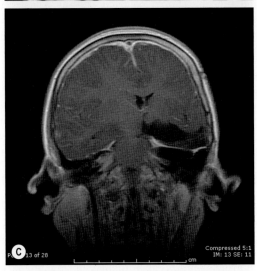

Figure 26.12 Desmoplastic infantile ganglioglioma. This 15-month-old girl infant presented with a progressive right hemiparesis. Preoperative MR scan shows a huge left hemispheric tumor hyperintense to gray matter on T2-weighted image (A) and hypointense in T1-weighted image (B) that extends, to the midline and into the brainstem. (C) 6 years after complete tumor resection, T1-weighted image with contrast demonstrates no evidence of residual tumor. She did receive chemotherapy.

pleomorphic neuroepithelial cells. The tumors are composed of fibroblast-like spindle-shaped cells with elongated nuclei. No necrosis or endothelial proliferation is seen (Fig. 26.13) (VandenBerg et al 1987b; Paulus et al 1992). Electron microscopy studies demonstrate elongated cells with abundant cytoplasm, lobulated nuclei, and prominent nucleoli, partly invested by a pericytoplasmic basal lamina. Tumor cells of both neuronal and glial origin are readily demonstrable by immunohistochemistry in that the cells are typically either GFAP or neurofilament positive, but not both. There is typically a population of undifferentiated, primitive cells in which mitoses and foci of necrosis may be found. A sharp demarcation exists between the tumor and surrounding brain (Tamburrini et al 2003). The cell of origin for these tumors is presumed to be superficial undifferentiated bipotential neuroepithelial cells which can give rise to both neuronal and glial tumor cells (VandenBerg et al 1987a). In one report, Schwann cell differentiation in addition to neuronal and glial differentiation was present (Ng et al 1990).

Mitotic activity is typically low and evidence of necrosis rare (Tamburrini et al 2003; Alexiou et al 2008). If present, necrosis, vascular proliferation or a high Ki-67 index do not necessarily predict a poorer clinical outcome. However, certain imaging and histologic characteristics may suggest a more malignant variant (Trehan et al 2004; Hoving et al 2008). Recent articles have reported tumors with anaplastic radiographic and histologic features that are associated with a more aggressive clinical course. These tumors have aggressive characteristics such as rapid tumor progression after resection, intracerebral and pial metastases, responsiveness to chemotherapy and early death despite aggressive treatment (De Munnynck et al 2002; Hoving et al 2008). The presence of a primitive cell component and elevated MIB-1/Ki-67 may be associated with a more aggressive clinical behavior of the tumor and may warrant consideration of adjuvant chemotherapy, even after gross total resection (Hoving et al 2008).

Differential diagnosis
The differential diagnosis of a large superficially located tumor in infants includes primitive neuroectodermal tumor (PNET), pilocytic xanthoastrocytoma (PXA), supratentorial ependymoma, and astrocytoma (Tamburrini et al 2003; Alexiou et al 2008). Pathologically, desmoplastic infantile gangliogliomas must be distinguished from PXAs, gangliogliomas, and astrocytomas. PXA shares characteristics, including an astrocytic cell population, prominent leptomeningeal involvement with desmoplasia, presence of basal lamina covering part of the cytoplasmic membrane of the tumor cells, and a favorable prognosis. However, PXAs occur in an older age group, are predominantly located in the temporal lobe, and do not have neuronal differentiation (Kepes et al 1979). The name 'desmoplastic infantile ganglioglioma' suggests a kinship to the gangliogliomas. Differences include presentation in infancy, more frequent inclusion of immature neuroepithelial cells, characteristic dense desmoplasia, and lack of a predominant localization in the temporal lobe. Unlike astrocytomas, the presence of a large component of primitive cells, abundant mitoses, and necrosis does not necessarily imply a worse prognosis (VandenBerg et al 1987b).

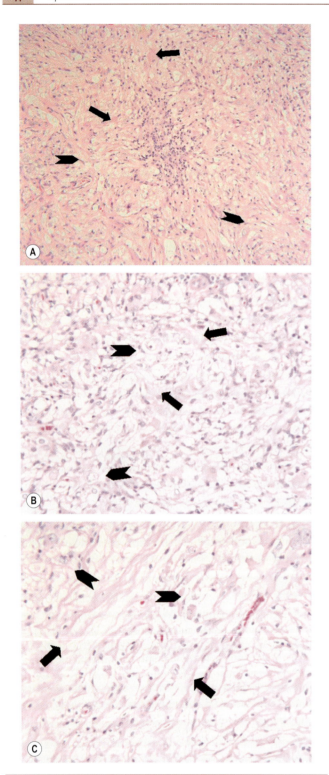

Figure 26.13 (A) Infantile desmoplastic ganglioglioma with a mixture of cellular elements. Most of the elongated cells are fibroblast (arrowheads) intermingled with fibrillary and gemistocytic astrocytes (arrows). There are scattered neurons of varying size. A small lymphocytic infiltrate is also present. (B) Infantile desmoplastic ganglioglioma with irregular bands of fibroconnective tissue (arrows) surrounding neuroglial islands (arrowheads). (C) Infantile desmoplastic ganglioglioma showing a mixture of glial and neuronal elements; these are found scattered and forming clusters (arrowheads) surrounded by prominent fibrous septae (arrows).

Treatment

The treatment of choice is surgery, and the literature suggests that no adjuvant therapy is required if gross total resection is achieved (Tamburrini et al 2003). The tumors are not well vascularized, often have a large cystic component, and are superficially located. If total resection is achieved, adjuvant therapy is not indicated. Long-term survival is possible even if sub-total resection is performed. One report described spontaneous regression of the tumor several months after sub-total resection (Takeshima et al 2003). However, one author found that gross total resection occurred in only 35% of reported cases due to factors such as attachment to eloquent structures and intraoperative hemodynamic instability (Duffner et al 1994).

The role of adjuvant chemotherapy or radiation therapy after sub-total resection is unclear, and some authors doubt there is benefit from either (Bachli et al 2003). Although a number of case reports and series describe adjuvant radiation therapy, the data available have not shown any difference in survival. Case series have also reported the use of adjuvant chemotherapy such as cyclophosphamide, etoposide, vincristine and carboplatinum (Duffner et al 1994). In these cases, chemotherapy appears to be effective, but interpretation of results is difficult given the small number of patients (Duffner et al 1994; Mallucci et al 2000; De Munnynck et al 2002; Nikas et al 2004). One series reported four patients who received chemotherapy after sub-total (three patients) or gross total (one patient) resection. All patients were alive without evidence of tumor progression at 36–60 months follow-up (Duffner et al 1994). Another study showed no difference in survival following chemotherapy (VandenBerg et al 1987b). Recurrent tumor is typically treated with repeat surgical excision. Patients with infiltrative disease or progression after resection may be good candidates for chemotherapy (Tamburrini et al 2003). Radiation therapy should be used only as a last resort in older children. Further data may show a clearer role for adjuvant therapy in the future.

Clinical outcome

Despite the large size of DIG at presentation and malignant histologic features, the clinical outcome after surgery is typically good. Gross total resection is curative in most cases (Nikas et al 2004; Hoving et al 2008). In VandenBerg et al's (1987b) series, eight of nine patients with complete or near-total surgical resection of their tumors have survived 1.5–14 years following surgery. Tumors with a more malignant histologic appearance may not behave aggressively. Also, residual tumor after surgery often does not grow and may regress spontaneously (Tamburrini et al 2003). Deep-seated lesions, such as suprasellar tumors, may be more aggressive and therefore lead to poorer clinical outcome (Bachli et al 2003). Rarely, tumors may display a malignant clinical course (De Munnynck et al 2002). One recent report described a patient who underwent three surgical resections and adjuvant chemotherapy, but died within 9 months of the first operation. A gross total resection had been achieved after the second surgery, and the patient had a partial response to chemotherapy after the third surgery, but died soon thereafter (Hoving et al 2008).

Dysembryoplastic neuroepithelial tumor

Demographics

Dysembryoplastic neuroepithelial tumors (DNETs) were initially described by Daumas-Duport et al (1993). They were incorporated into the World Health Organization (WHO) classification of brain tumors as part of the glioneuronal tumors in 1993. Since then, a total of 72 cases have been reported in the literature (Koeller & Dillon 1992; Daumas-Duport 1993; Kirkpatrick et al 1993). The age range is from 1 year old to 19 years old, with a mean of 9 years. The sex distribution is M:F = 1.5 : 1. There does not seem to be a racial or genetic predisposition.

Diagnosis

The most common presentation is seizures, followed by headaches. Most of the patients have a non-focal neurologic exam. CT scan shows a supratentorial hypodense 'pseudocystic' lesion, especially in the temporal lobe (Daumas-Duport 1993). On MR scanning, the lesion is hypointense to gray matter on T1-weighted images, and hyperintense to gray matter on T2-weighted images, with variable contrast enhancement. Proton-density images demonstrate slightly higher signal intensity in the lesion than in cerebrospinal fluid (Fig. 26.13) (Koeller & Dillon 1992). A variable degree of calcification may be demonstrated by either MR or CT scans (Koeller & Dillon 1992; Daumas-Duport 1993). More recently, Parmar et al (2007) reported on the presence of a hyperintense ring on fluid attenuated inversion recovery (FLAIR) images which they saw in 9/11 patients with pathologically confirmed DNETs. Pathological evaluation of the DNETs suggested that the hyperintense ring might correspond to the presence of peripheral loose neuroglial elements (Parmar et al 2007). Imaging characteristics of DNET may change over time. Jensen et al (2006) reported on a patient with a presumed low grade glioma that had been followed conservatively until the tumor became contrast enhancing. Resection of the tumor demonstrated a DNET with no atypical changes (Jensen et al 2006). Labate et al (2004) analyzed the EEG features of epilepsy patients with a temporal lobe DNET. They found that patients with temporal lobe DNET often had EEG discharges discordant to the tumor; no correlation was found between patients with concordant and/discordant EEG discharges and clinical course (Labate et al 2004). Interestingly, Maehara et al (2004) analyzed [11C] methionine (MET) positron emission tomography (PET) uptake in temporal lobe tumors, and found that DNETs had little or no uptake, compared to other low grade tumors (i.e., ganglioglioma or low-grade gliomas) with similar Ki-67 labeling index. The authors concluded that negative MET uptake in benign temporal lobe tumors with epilepsy is consistent with a preoperative diagnosis of DNET (Maehara et al 2004).

Pathology

Most of the tumors are located in the temporal lobe (both mesial and lateral locations), followed by the frontal, occipital, and parietal lobes. DNETs have also been reported in the insular cortex, brain stem, cerebellum, occipital lobe, and striatum (O'Brien et al 2007). The tumor is macroscopically visible on the surface, well-demarcated in some, and poorly-demarcated in others. There is no uniform tumor consistency. Approximately 40% of DNETs are cystic, but solitary or multinodular forms have been recognized (Whittle et al 1999). Microscopically, DNETs are characterized by a 'specific glioneuronal element', a nodular component, and associated cortical dysplasia (Fig. 26.14). The 'specific glioneuronal element' is composed of both neurons and glial cells, which may range from compact to alveolar in structure, depending upon the degree of extracellular mucoid substance accumulation. While the 'specific glioneuronal element' is similar from one case to another, the nodular component varies. DNET nodules usually look like oligodendroglioma; in between the nodules vertical columns of neurons surrounded by oligodendrocyte-like cells may be seen. These oligodendrocyte-like cells in DNETs are histologically different from oligodendroglioma as they have larger nuclei with frequent nuclear indentations and multiple small nucleoli, while oligodendroglioma cells have round nuclei with only one or two occasional nucleoli (O'Brien et al 2007). It is made up of neurons, astrocytes, and oligodendrocytes, often with evidence of cellular atypia. Foci of cortical dysplasia are also present. Daumas-Duport et al (1988) suggested that DNET results from disorganized embryogenesis, i.e. dysembryoplastic, and the site of origin is most likely from the subpial granular layer. The presence of foci of cortical dysplasia strongly suggests that DNETs arise during the formation of the cortex (Daumas-Duport et al 1988). Recently, Burel-Vandenbos et al (2007) have reported on a DNET with evidence of ependymal differentiation from a right temporal lobe cortical lesion from a girl with refractory seizures (Burel-Vandenbos et al 2007). Whether the 'glioneuronal element' reported in DNETs consist of neuronal elements or mixed neuronal/glial differentiation was evaluated by Raghavan et al (2000) utilizing an antibody to alpha-synuclein, a cytoplasmic protein found predominantly in the brain, and localized in the pre-synaptic nerve terminals, near vesicles. The authors found no evidence of alpha synuclein staining in DNET, compared to other ganglioneuronal tumors such as gangliogliomas, gangliocytomas or ganglioneuroblastomas (Raghavan et al 2000).

Differential diagnosis

The differential diagnoses of DNET include ganglioglioma, mixed oligoastrocytoma, and hamartoma. Histologically, gangliogliomas do not exhibit a multinodular architecture. Unlike DNET, they are not intracortical, but are randomly situated. Bizarre neurons or giant ganglion-like cells are present in gangliogliomas, but not in DNET. The abundant connective tissue stroma and perivascular lymphocytic infiltrates that characterize the ganglion cell-rich part of ganglioglioma are not present in DNET. Lastly, the oligodendroglial component found in DNET is usually not prominent in gangliogliomas (Haddad et al 1992). Oligoastrocytomas may include nodular foci which should not be misinterpreted as DNET. Conversely, cortical infiltration by oligoastrocytoma should not be confused with the characteristic neuroglial component of DNET (Russell & Rubinstein 1989). Hamartomas are characterized only by the presence of neuronal elements, without evidence of astrocytic and oligodendroglial components or cortical dysplasia (Albright & Lee 1993).

Treatment

The treatment is surgical excision. DNETs have a good prognosis whether total or sub-total resection is performed.

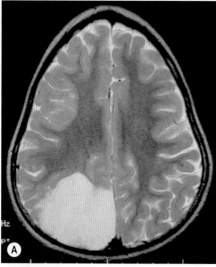

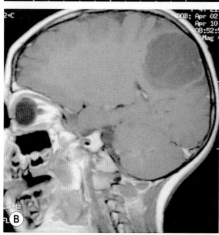

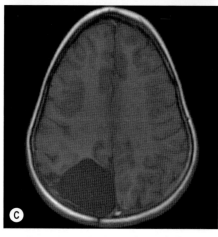

Figure 26.14 Dysembryoblastic neuroepitherial tumor. This 4-year-old girl presented with 1 year history of seizures. A T2-weighted image (A) shows well-circumscribed lobulated parenchymal mass in the right parietal lobe. There is no significant enhancement on T1-weighted image with contrast (B). A contrast enhanced postoperative image (C) reveals no evidence of tumor. She has been seizure free on medication.

Patients with pharmacoresistant seizures may benefit from an extended lesionectomy to remove the seizure focus. In one series of 39 cases, 17 patients underwent sub-total resections with no clinical or radiological evidence of recurrence on long-term follow-up (Daumas-Duport et al 1988). Kirkpatrick et al (1993) found that the pathology in a group of seizure patients was predominantly DNET (27/31 patients). Recently, Chan et al (2006) reported outcomes from seizure surgery in 18 patients with DNETs who either underwent temporal lobectomies or lesionectomies. The authors concluded that temporal lobectomy patients had much better short- and long-term control of seizures than patients who underwent lesionectomies (Chan et al 2006). Patients with gross total resections did not have evidence of recurrence, and there was good seizure control despite sub-total resection in a majority of the patients (Kirkpatrick et al 1993). Tumor resections may be aided by the use of MRI based image guidance (neuronavigation systems) and intraoperative MRI. If possible, an open resection is preferred, as small sample sizes from stereotactic biopsies may generate an unrepresentative tissue sample consisting of an oligodendroglial component, leading to an incorrect diagnosis. Radiotherapy itself does not appear to confer any obvious benefit. There was no difference in survival or recurrence in 13 subjects who had undergone postoperative radiotherapy compared with 26 subjects who had not had postoperative radiotherapy (Daumas-Duport et al 1988). No data on chemotherapy are available. Therefore, the treatment for the original tumor, as well as any recurrence, is surgical.

Clinical outcome

Although newly recognized as a distinct pathological entity, diagnosis of DNET is important as it often has a benign prognosis. However, this indolent course may not be true for all DNETs. Recently, Ray et al (2009) reported on five cases of DNETs with recurrences 2–7 years after a resection. The pathology on the second resection was usually consistent with a benign tumor; however, one patient did develop an anaplastic astrocytoma (Ray et al 2009). Similarly, Josan et al (2007) have recently reported a case of a pilocytic astrocytoma that arose from a DNET. Recognition of DNET will spare young patients the deleterious effects of radio- or chemotherapy. Moreover, DNET is an important etiology of temporal lobe epilepsy, and subsequent removal will result in long-term control of seizures.

Ganglioglioma

Demographics

Gangliogliomas were first named by Courville in 1930 to describe a set of neoplasms with both astrocytic and neuronal components (Kaye & Laws 1995). Gangliogliomas make up 0.4–0.9% of all brain tumors, 1–4 % of all pediatric intracranial tumors and 1% of all intramedullary spinal cord tumors (Kalyan-Raman & Olivero 1987; Miller et al 1990b; Zhang et al 2008). Most patients are <30 years old, and the peak age of incidence is the second decade of life (Safavi-Abbasi et al 2007). However, the age at diagnosis ranges from newborn to 70 years (Benitez et al 1990; Castillo et al 1990; Price et al 1997). There does not appear to be a gender, familial, or racial preference. There are no other associations

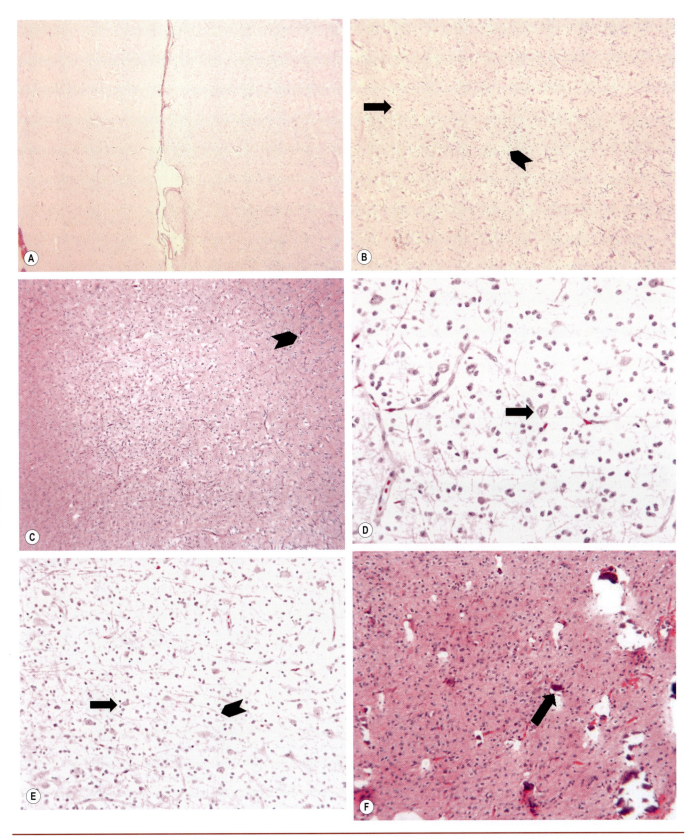

Figure 26.15 (A) Dysembryoplastic neuroepithelial tumor. Sections of two adjacent cortical folia, on the right there is irregular thickening of the cortex and abnormal cortical neuronal lamination due to solid DNET infiltration (H&E ×20). (B) Dysembryoplastic neuroepithelial tumor showing abnormal cortical lamination with scattered large neurons (arrow). There is diffuse infiltration of tumor cells and incipient accumulation of mucopolisaccharide (arrowhead) (H&E ×10). (C) Dysembryoplastic neuroepithelial tumor showing a nodular area of infiltration involving the lower cortical layers. There is early microcystic change with pallor and rarification of the neuropil. The tumor cells are spreading into upper cortical layers surrounding neurons and axons (arrowhead) (H&E ×40). (D) Dysembryoplastic neuroepithelial tumor. Area of diffuse infiltration with scattered large neurons (arrow). There is vacuolation and pale staining of the neuropil due to accumulation of mucopolysaccharide (H&E ×20). (E) Dysembryoplastic neuroepithelial tumor showing the characteristic mixed population of neurons and glial elements. The neurons are large and there is distortion of the neuronal lamination. The glial component consists of astrocytes and oligodendrocytes with mild nuclear pleomorphism proliferating along axons (arrowhead) and surround the neuronal soma (arrow) (H&E ×100). (F) Dysembryoplastic neuroepithelial tumor showing scattered calcifications and solid growth (H&E ×100).

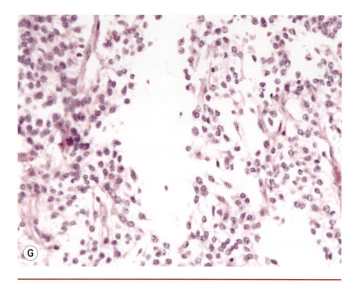

Figure 26.15 cont'd (G) Dysembryoplastic neuroepithelial tumor. Leptomeningeal infiltration is sometimes seen with prominent microcystic change (H&E ×200).

with this tumor, although one patient was reported to have both neurofibromatosis type 1 (NF-1) and a ganglioglioma (Parizel et al 1991). Although gangliogliomas were initially thought by Courville to be located predominantly in the floor of the third ventricle, subsequent series have shown that the majority of gangliogliomas are located in the cerebral hemispheres, most commonly in the temporal lobes, although any part of the brain may be affected (Zentner et al 1994; Kaye and Laws 1995; Lagares et al 2001). In the younger age population, an increased incidence of midline tumors is reported (Haddad et al 1992). Less common locations in the optic nerve, chiasm and tract (Bergin et al 1988; Chilton et al 1990; Sugiyama et al 1992), hypothalamus (Liu et al 1996), trigeminal nerve (Athale et al 1999), brainstem (Garcia et al 1984; Davidson et al 1992), cerebellum (Mizuno et al 1987; Safavi-Abbasi et al 2007), thalamus (Johnson et al 2001), pineal gland (Hunt & Johnson 1989; Johnson et al 1995) and spinal cord (Johannsson et al 1981) have been reported. Although metastatic disease is rare, leptomeningeal and subarachnoid spread have been reported (Tien et al 1992; Wacker et al 1992). Also rarely reported is the composite pleomorphic xanthoastrocytoma-ganglioglioma, which was mentioned in a previous section (Perry et al 1997). In one case report, a patient presented with multicentric disease (Zhang et al 2008).

Diagnosis

The overwhelmingly most common presenting history of a patient with a ganglioglioma is progressive seizure disorder. Seizures may be present from months to several years before the diagnosis is established (Demierre et al 1986; Chamberlain & Press 1990; Diepholder et al 1991). Other presenting signs and symptoms vary depending on patient age, tumor location, and the aggressiveness of the tumor (Fletcher et al 1988). In very young patients, increasing head circumference may be found and would usually indicate increased intracranial pressure (Demierre et al 1986; Hunt & Johnson 1989; Diepholder et al 1991). Patients with intraorbital

gangliogliomas may present with proptosis and visual loss (Bergin et al 1988; Chilton et al 1990), while those with brainstem gangliogliomas may exhibit hemiparesis and cranial nerve deficits (Garcia et al 1984; Nelson et al 1987; Davidson et al 1992). For example, one patient's initial symptoms were hearing loss and ataxia from a left cerebellar mass (Dhillon 1987). The findings are usually longstanding due to the non-aggressive nature of gangliogliomas in most cases. One report described a patient with a ganglioglioma in the superior part of the medulla who had a 46-year history of neurological dysfunction before she finally died from pneumonia (Davidson et al 1992). Gangliogliomas are typically intra-axial lesions, although one report described a ganglioglioma presenting as an extra-axial lesion receiving blood supply primarily from the middle meningeal artery (Siddique et al 2002).

Cerebral angiography does not yield additional information, apart from confirming that these tumors are not vascular (Silver et al 1991). CT scans usually demonstrate a hypodense or isodense lesion with poor contrast enhancement (Rommel & Hamer 1983). Castillo divided gangliogliomas into two groups based on their appearance on CT. Tumors with cystic components were located, with decreasing frequency, in the cerebellum, temporal, frontal, and parietal lobes. Solid tumors, however, were found preferentially in the temporal lobe. Better contrast enhancement was found with the solid tumors (Castillo et al 1990). Calcifications within the tumor are often demonstrated on CT (Dorne et al 1986; Im et al 2002a). Anaplastic tumors may show a heterogeneous appearance on CT, with excellent contrast enhancement (Hall et al 1986). Rarely, local bone erosion due to underlying tumor may be noted on imaging (Zhang et al 2008).

Gangliogliomas have a varied appearance on MRI (Tampieri et al 1991; Berenguer et al 1994). They may have well-defined margins or be poorly-demarcated (Im et al 2002a; Zhang et al 2008). The tumors most often have no peritumoral edema, although mild to moderate edema is present in some lesions (Zhang et al 2008). MR imaging is useful in distinguishing the cystic tumor component (Fig. 26.16) (Furuta et al 1992; Haddad et al 1992). One report divided tumors into three sub-types based on MR appearance: cystic tumors (no solid component), solid-cystic tumors (cysts within a solid tumor) and solid tumors (no cystic component) (Zhang et al 2008). The morphology of the cysts is variable, and the cyst wall may enhance. The cysts are hypointense on T1-weighted MRI and FLAIR, and hyperintense on T2-weighted MRI. The solid portions of most tumors are hypointense relative to gray matter on T1-weighted images, and hyperintense relative to gray matter on T2-weighted images (Benitez et al 1990; Tampieri et al 1991). The solid component displays variable enhancement patterns after gadolinium administration, but can be homogeneous or patchy (Zhang et al 2008). Alternatively, some gangliogliomas do not demonstrate gadolinium enhancement on MRI (Im et al 2002a). As with most tumors, MRI is most sensitive for revealing unique anatomic findings related to the tumor. In one report, for example, MRI was able to demonstrate leptomeningeal and subarachnoid spread along the middle cerebral artery and right Sylvian fissure in a patient with leptomeningeal metastasis (Tien et al 1992). Alternatively, gangliogliomas have been histologically

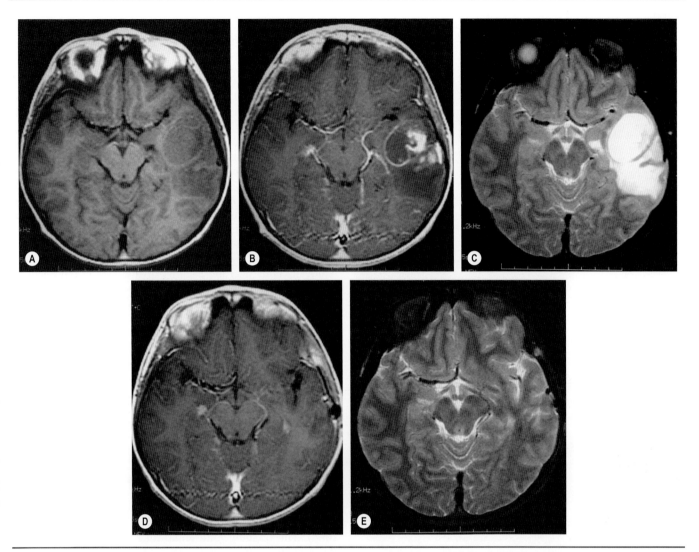

Figure 26.16 Ganglioglioma. This 11-year-old boy had a history of several months of progressive headaches and behavioral changes without any seizure activity or neurologic deficit. The MR scan (T1-weighted) is nearly isointense to gray matter without contrast (A), but irregularly enhances with gadolinium (B). The T2-weighted MR study shows extensive surrounding edema (C). MR scan (T1-weighted) with contrast done 3 months postoperatively shows no evidence of residual tumor (D) and resolution of the surrounding edema on T2-weighted image (E). This patient has not received any adjuvant therapy. He is neurologically normal. The preoperative imaging study was more suggestive of a high-grade glioma than of a ganglioglioma.

diagnosed without an obvious tumor on cranial imaging (Tampieri et al 1991).

Recent work has reported findings from other imaging methodologies for gangliogliomas. For example, positron emission tomography (PET) showed the tumors to be hypometabolic. Single photon emission computed tomography (SPECT) of gangliogliomas has demonstrated tumor hypoperfusion to isoperfusion. Magnetic resonance spectroscopy (MRS) is reported to show a reduced choline/creatine (Cho/Cr) and N-aspartyl-acetate/creatine (NAA/Cr) ratio, and an increased Cho/NAA ratio compared with contralateral normal brain (Im et al 2002a).

Pathology

Grossly, gangliogliomas are firm, grayish tumors which may have cystic components (Kaye & Laws 1995). On light microscopy, both neuronal and glial neoplastic components are readily apparent. Mild to moderate cellularity, minimal pleomorphism, and rare mitotic figures are present (Fig. 26.17). Microcalcifications and desmoplastic changes may be observed (Zhang et al 2008). Anaplastic degeneration, should it occur, is usually detected in the glial component of the tumor (Allegranza et al 1990). Occasionally, other tumors including pleomorphic xanthoastrocytoma (Furuta et al 1992), osteomas (Hori et al 1988), and melanotic cells (Hunt & Johnson 1989) may be interspersed within the ganglioglioma.

On electron microscopy, three main cell types may be seen: ganglion cells with dense core vesicles, glial cells with processes filled with filament, and probable mesenchymal cells adjacent to abundant collagen fibrils (Rubinstein & Herman 1972). Features of neuronal degeneration have been found in gangliogliomas including neurofilament aggregates, and Hirano, Lafora, and zebra bodies (Takahashi et al 1987). Neoplastic ganglion cells show intense immunoreactivity for synaptophysin, a 38 kilodalton (kDa) glycoprotein

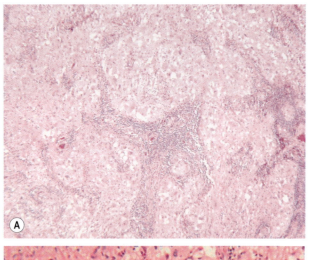

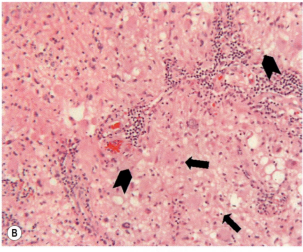

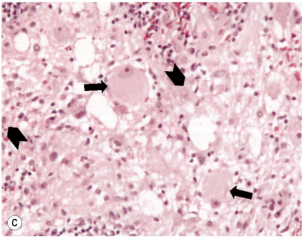

Figure 26.17 (A) Ganglioglioma showing the characteristic mixed composition of neuronal and glial elements divided by fibrovascular septa with lymphocytic aggregates (H&E ×40). (B) Ganglioglioma showing clusters of hapzardly arranged neurons which exhibit marked variation in size and shape (arrowheads). The glial component contains astrocytic and oligodendroglial elements with no atypia (arrows) (H&E ×100). (C) Ganglioglioma showing a neuroglial island. The ganglion cells range from small neuronal elements (arrowheads) to large ganglion cells with Nissl substance and peripheral cytoplasmic vacuolation (arrows). The glial component includes astrocytes and oligodendrocytes (H&E ×200).

located in synaptic vesicle membranes that outlines the borders of cell bodies, and neuron-specific enolase (NSE) (Miller et al 1990a; Diepholder et al 1991; Zhang et al 2008). The glial component stains positive for GFAP (Zhang et al 2008). Approximately 80% of tumors stain positive for the stem cell marker CD34 (Blumcke & Wiestler 2002). Kawai has demonstrated the presence of tyrosine hydroxylase (a rate-limiting enzyme in the catecholamine synthesizing pathway), and numerous dense core vesicles in the neuronal component of gangliogliomas, suggesting that the origin of these cells may have been from ectopic neural crest tissues (Kawai et al 1987; Diepholder et al 1991; Issidorides & Arvanitis 1993). Other neuroendocrine markers including serotonin, somatostatin, met-enkephalin, leu-enkephalin, and substance P have been variably demonstrated in the dense core granules (Takahashi et al 1989).

Flow cytometry of a ganglioglioma demonstrated aneuploidy in both necrotic regions of the tumor and sections with atypical findings (Bowles et al 1988). One study evaluated mRNA expression of various oncogenes including v-sis, v-myc and v-fos, and found increased v-sis and v-fos expression for gangliogliomas and other benign tumors (Fujimoto et al 1988). Another found increased mRNA expression for PFGF-(3 and the ras gene for malignant tumors, but not in benign tumors, including a single case of ganglioglioma (Mapstone et al 1991). Loss of chromosome 17p was recently shown in a child with a malignant ganglioglioma (Wacker et al 1992).

Gangliogliomas may be designated as WHO grade I or III. The grade II designation was recently eliminated (Brat et al 2008).

Differential diagnosis

Most gangliogliomas are preoperatively diagnosed incorrectly as glioma based on CT and MRI findings (Zhang et al 2008). The imaging differential diagnosis of ganglioglioma also includes gangliocytoma, dysembryoplastic neuroepithelial tumor, and oligodendroglioma. Gangliocytomas usually occur in the cerebellum (Lhermitte–Duclos disease), and are characterized by alteration of the normal cerebellar architecture, resulting in hypertrophied neuronal cells in the granule cell layer. Also, a glial component is not present in gangliocytomas (Reznik & Schoenen 1983). Gliomas may be histologically differentiated from gangliogliomas as they do not have neuronal components (Russell & Rubinstein 1989). Radiographically, gliomas are more likely to have peritumoral edema, necrosis, hemorrhage and poor demarcation. Using MRS, gliomas will demonstrate a higher Cho/Cr ratio and lower NAA/Cr ratio than gangliogliomas (Im et al 2002a; Zhang et al 2008). The higher NAA/Cr ratio in gangliogliomas compared to gliomas is reflective of the neoplastic neuronal component of gangliogliomas. Dysembryoplastic neuroepithelial tumors, which also commonly occur in the temporal lobe, have a characteristic glioneuronal element, nodular component, and association with cortical dysplasia (Daumas-Duport et al 1988). Lastly, oligodendrogliomas may be differentiated from gangliogliomas as they do not have neuronal elements, and are derived from oligodendrocytes (Russell & Rubinstein 1989).

Cerebellar ganglioglioma may appear similar to juvenile pilocytic astrocytoma or hemangioblastoma. Cystic components are common to all three tumor types, although the mural nodule of hemangioblastoma is a less common appearance of ganglioglioma.

Treatment

In accessible tumors, the treatment for gangliogliomas is surgical. Gross total removal is the best chance for long-term survival (Haddad et al 1992; Kaye & Laws 1995). An attempt at gross total resection is still the goal even if the ganglioglioma is anaplastic. One report described long-term survival in a 6-month old girl with an anaplastic ganglioglioma after gross total resection (Hall et al 1986). Sub-total resection of exophytic components of gangliogliomas located in the brainstem and optic tracts may be the only option (Garcia et al 1984; Chilton et al 1990). Only partial excisions are usually possible with midline tumors, and these lesions therefore have a greater chance of recurrence (Haddad et al 1992). The results of radiation therapy for gangliogliomas are inconclusive. Radiotherapy (40–60 Gy) is most commonly given to patients with tumors for whom only a sub-total resection could be achieved and who have recurrence, or to patients with anaplastic components to their tumors (Cox et al 1982; Silver et al 1991). One study reported that radiation given after sub-total resection of high-grade lesions reduced the relapse rate (Selch et al 1998). Patients with complete resections and benign histologies should not be given radiotherapy. Consideration of the patient's age should be taken into account as intracranial radiation in younger children may result in substantial deterioration of intellectual and endocrine development (Ellenberg et al 1987). Postoperative radiation has also been suggested by some authors to have a role in the malignant degeneration of gangliogliomas (Kalyan-Raman & Olivero 1987; Jay et al 1994; Sasaki et al 1996). One study found a higher incidence of malignant degeneration among gangliogliomas treated with radiation therapy compared to non-radiated tumors (Rumana & Valadka 1998).

There is scant literature regarding chemotherapy for gangliogliomas, and no clear benefit has been demonstrated (Silver et al 1991). Case reports regarding high-grade lesions or recurrent tumors infrequently describe the use of adjuvant chemotherapy (Kang et al 2007; Liauw et al 2007). Chemotherapy should likely be reserved as a treatment of last resort in patients with unresectable lesions who have already received radiation.

Clinical outcome

Gangliogliomas most commonly appear histologically low-grade and have a benign clinical course (Zhang et al 2008). Long-term survival is excellent if a gross total resection is achieved. Seizure control is much improved in patients with gross total tumor resection (Sutton et al 1983; Sutton et al 1987; Otsubo et al 1990; Silver et al 1991; Haddad et al 1992). A recent case series reported that 76% of patients with epilepsy due to a ganglioglioma were rendered seizure-free after surgical resection of the tumor (Im et al 2002b).

Some gangliogliomas may behave aggressively despite a benign histologic appearance. Also, high-grade gangliogliomas have been described whose clinical behavior is worse than low-grade lesions (Selch et al 1998). Alternatively, histologically high-grade lesions may not behave aggressively (Fig. 26.18) (Kalyan-Raman & Olivero 1987).

Leptomeningeal spread of a tumor with a malignant component has been reported, but is rare (Tien et al 1992; Wacker et al 1992). Dissemination of gangliogliomas may not correlate with histologic grade, and is therefore difficult to predict (Liu et al 1996). If a ganglioglioma undergoes malignant degeneration, it is typically the glial component of the tumor that becomes malignant, possibly due to astrocyte dedifferentiation (Rumana & Valadka 1998). However, malignant transformation with anaplastic neuronal and astrocytic components has also been reported (Jay et al 1994).

Polar spongioblastoma

Demographics

Polar spongioblastomas, first described by Russell & Cairns in 1947, are rare neoplasms involving midline structures. Since then, 12 cases have been reported. The hypothalamus, lateral walls of the third ventricle, fourth ventricle, and optic chiasm are the most commonly involved. It has been reported

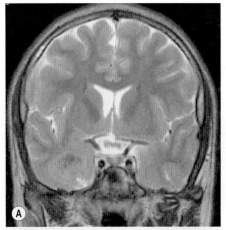

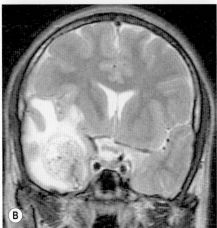

Figure 26.18 Anaplastic ganglioglioma. This 14-year-old boy presented with 4 year history of seizures. (A) MR scan (T2-weighted) shows some heterogeneous low signal intensity in right anterior medial temporal lobe. (B) A year later, he presented increasing seizure frequency. A repeat MR scan demonstrates marked increase in size of the mass associated with significant surrounding edema. The tumor was resected but recurred and required a second excision approximately 6 months later. Whereas the histology from the first excision was consistent with a ganglioglioma, the second had new anaplastic features not seen on the first specimen.

in the frontal lobe, spinal cord, and two cases of cerebro-spinal fluid seeding have been reported. The age range is from 6 months to 46 years, with a median age of 8.5 years. No sexual, familial, or racial predilection can be estimated because of the rarity of the tumor.

Diagnosis

The presenting signs and symptoms, depending on the location of the tumor, range from the diencephalic syndrome to seizures. Information as to the radiological diagnosis is limited. A CT scan in one patient showed a hypodense lesion in the frontal lobe with evidence of calcification. No MR data are available.

Pathology

Grossly, the tumor is grayish-white in color, firm, and usually well-demarcated. If subarachnoid metastasis has occurred, thick sheets of soft gray tissue may be present (Rubinstein 1972). Light microscopy shows tumor cells arranged in characteristic parallel fashion, like a step-ladder, forming compact bands secondary to palisading of the nuclei. The cells are thin, unipolar or bipolar in shape, with dark oval nuclei. Neuroglial fibrils, if present, are more prominent in regions of astrocytic differentiation (Fig. 26.19) (Rubinstein 1972).

Although the polar spongioblastoma has been thought to be cytogenetically related to the embryonal radial glial cell and was considered, therefore, as a primitive glial tumor in the WHO classification of 1979, it has been set aside as a neuroepithelial tumor of uncertain origin in the new WHO classification (Kleihues et al 1993). Ultrastructural studies and immunohistochemistry suggest a neuroendocrine nature. Electron microscopy demonstrates three zones of differentiation: (1) a densely cellular zone corresponding to the palisades seen by light microscopy, (2) a fibrillary zone composed of elongated cytoplasmic processes, intervening between the palisades and the vascular walls, and (3) a perivascular zone with corresponding vessels. This three-sided architecture has led de Chadarevian et al (1984) to propose that the organization is similar to that of the hypothalamic neuroendocrine system, with a perivascular cellular arrangement, intracytoplasmic microtubules, and membrane-bound dense core granules. Jansen et al (1990) have also noted prominent endoplasmic reticulum and microtubules in the tumor cytoplasm, suggesting a neuronal origin. Immunohistochemistry demonstrates that some of the tumor cells are neuron-specific enolase positive. Most of the tumor cells are GFAP negative except in portions of the tumor with more prominent astrocytic differentiation. Bignami et al (1989) have shown that glial hyaluronate binding protein (GHA) is negative in neuroepithelial tumors such as astrocytomas, oligodendrogliomas, medulloblastomas, and ependymomas. Spongioblastomas are GHA positive, however, suggesting that they are derived from a more primitive glial precursor, as immature glial cells forming the periventricular germinal layer are GHA positive in 22-week-old human embryos.

Differential diagnosis

Differential diagnosis of spongioblastomas includes any neuroepithelial tumor which may contain palisades of tumor: ependymomas, oligodendrogliomas, pilocytic astrocytomas, cerebellar astrocytomas, medulloblastomas, and cerebral

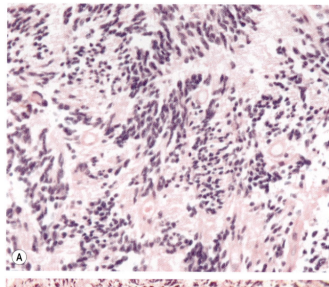

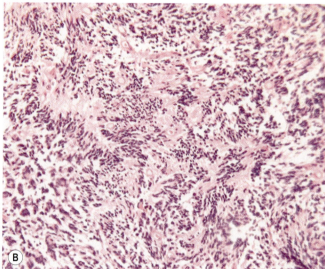

Figure 26.19 (A) Polar spongioblastoma showing the typical pattern of growth characterized by parallel bands of tumor cells and nuclear palisading (H&E ×100). (B) Polar spongioblastoma with compact parallel arrays of primitive neoplastic cells in a loose fibrillary background (H&E ×200).

neuroblastomas. Schiffer et al (1993) believe that polar spongioblastomas should not be considered a tumor entity. They feel that even in cases where nuclear palisading represents the predominant histological characteristic, evidence can be found that it is only an architectural feature of another neuroepithelial tumor. Similar views were echoed by Langford & Camel (1987) and Itoh et al (1987) who felt that tumors such as cerebral astrocytoma or neuroblastoma may have palisades simulating a polar spongioblastoma (Yagashita et al 1996).

Treatment

The treatment of choice is surgical resection. The first cases reported by Russell & Cairns (1947) presented with subarachnoid spread and survived only about a year. Recently long-term survival in patients with frontal or parietal lobe tumors who had undergone a gross total resection has been documented. Steinberg (1985) reported a patient with a sub-totally resected fourth ventricular spongioblastoma who had undergone radiotherapy without recurrence on a 15-year follow-up. The effect of radiotherapy is mixed. Although anecdotal reports suggest that it may be helpful, the survival of some patients has not improved (Jansen et al 1990). No data on chemotherapy are available.

Clinical outcome
Clinical outcome in this small group of patients appears to be varied. Long-term survival even after sub-total resection followed by radiation, may be achieved. Extremely poor outcomes have also been documented. Fuller et al (2006) presented a case of spinal cord spongioblastoma with a fulminant course, with development of necrosis within the tumor and intracranial metastases despite chemotherapy and Decadron, and death less than one month after presentation. Ng et al (1994) presented another case with cerebrospinal metastases and spread in the basal cisterns, contralateral ventricle, and spinal dura metastases.

Central neurocytoma

Demographics
Central neurocytoma (CN) is a rare neuronal tumor of the central nervous system, first described by Hassoun et al in 1982. It constitutes approximately half of all intraventricular tumors in adults, but accounts only for 0.25–0.5% of all CNS tumors. It predominantly affects young adults (usually in the third decade of life, but approximately 20% of cases affect children under 18 years of age) (Schmidt et al 2004). Tumors are usually located in the lateral ventricles, in the region of the foramen of Monro (Hassoun et al 1993; Kerkovsky et al 2008); however, extraventricular CNs have been reported (Cemil et al 2009; Sharma et al 2006; Takao et al 2003; Yang et al 2009). Although the M:F ratio remains unclear, several small series have reported a male dominance.

Diagnosis
CNs are typically intraventricular in localization; almost all tumors are located in either the lateral or third ventricle or both. The typical presentation is a young patient who presents with signs and symptoms of increased intracranial pressure, including headaches, visual changes secondary to papilledema and/or optic nerve/chiasm compression, and occasionally decreased mental status. Endocrine changes secondary to pressure on the sella or suprasellar region can also occur (Chen et al 2008; Dodero et al 2001).

Radiographic diagnoses include CT-scan, which typically demonstrates an isodense mass with uniform contrast enhancement. Calcifications, if present, may be easily demonstrated on CT-scan, and may be visualized as clumped, coarse, or globular nodules in appearance. Acute intra-tumoral hemorrhages may be seen infrequently on CT-scan (Goergen et al 1992; Hanel et al 2001; Kim et al 1992). MRI scan of the brain with and without gadolinium is the diagnostic modality of choice. CNs are usually isointense relative to cortical gray matter on both T1- and T2-weighted images (Fig. 26.20) (McConanchie et al 1994). They usually demonstrate uniform enhancement with gadolinium; patchy areas of intensity may be seen secondary to tumor calcification, cystic spaces, and vascular flow voids within the tumor. Localization of the tumor to the intraventricular space is much easier to visualize with MRI scan than CT-scan (Goergen et al 1992). Recently, MR spectroscopy (MRS) has been applied for spectral analysis of CNs. Kocaoglu et al (2009) retrospectively analyzed seven cases of pathologically documented CNs using MRS and diffusion weighted images (DWI). MRS demonstrated significantly increased choline/creatine and decreased N-acetyl aspartate/choline ratios consistent with the MRS pattern of high grade gliomas. Moreover, the tumors had a heterogenous hyperintense appearance when compared with the contralateral parietal lobe white matter. Recently, Chuang et al (2005) reported a unique glycine peak in one out of three cases of CN that they analyzed by MRS.

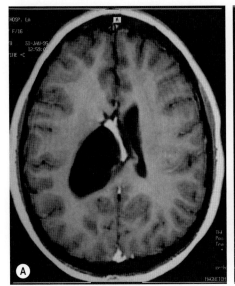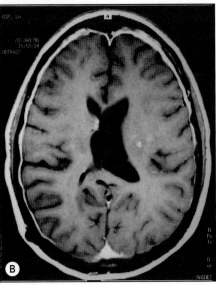

Figure 26.20 Central neurocytoma. This 15-year-old girl presented with symptoms of raised intracranial pressure. MR study showed the presence of a huge contrast enhancing mass engulfing the corpus callosum with extension into both lateral and third ventricles. By an interhemispheric approach, the tumor was resected in two stages leaving no evidence of residual tumor on MR scanning. (A) MR study (T1-weighted) with contrast 6 months later showed evidence of recurrence. The area of gross tumor was resected, however there was extensive diffuse microscopic spread to the parenchyma adjacent to the third ventricle. The patient received a full course of radiation but no chemotherapy. Since treatment, there is no evidence of recurrence, and follow-up MR (T1-weighted) studies with contrast show no evidence of progressive disease (B). However, she is intellectually impaired and has a labile affect.

Pathology

Histologically, CNs are characterized by isomorphous small round or ovoid cells alternating with irregularly shaped patches of fibrillary matrix (Fig. 26.21). The nuclei are amitotic and round, with frequent perinuclear halos, similar to oligodendrogliomas (Patil et al 1990). On immunohistochemistry, CNs have markers of neuronal differentiation, particularly synaptophysin, a 38-kd protein found in the synaptic vesicles (Barbosa et al 1990). Additional markers of neuronal differentiation include neuron specific enolase, Leu-7, and S-100. In addition, loss of neuronal markers, and gain of glial markers (i.e., GFAP), has been demonstrated in recurrent atypical CNs, consistent with a more aggressive tumor (Chen et al 2008). Recently, Soylemezoglu et al (2003) demonstrated that neuronal nuclear antigen (NeuN) may be used in formalin fixed paraffin embedded tissue to distinguish CNs, which are uniformly positive for NeuN in the nuclei of neurocyte, but negative in oligodendrogliomas. Ultrastructural analysis via electron microscopy demonstrate that CNs have neuronal features, including synapses, dense core vesicles, presynaptic clear vesicles, and specialized synaptic junctions. The synapses, whether typical or abortive, have clear and dense core vesicles (Hassoun et al 1982; Kubota et al 1991).

For the most part, CNs are not rapidly growing tumors. Favereaux et al (2000) in a report of 10 cases, reported eight 'classical' central CNs with a MIB-1(proliferation marker) labeling index (LI) of <2.3%, whereas the two 'atypical' CNs had MIB-1 LI of >5.2%. Chen et al (2008) in a series of nine patients had two patients with recurrent CN with increased MIB-1 LI of 2–6.8%, which they classified as atypical CNs. In addition to the high MIB-1 LI, atypical CNs also have histologic evidence of tumor necrosis and loss of neuronal differentiation (Favereaux et al 2000). Sharma et al (1998) compared proliferation markers with silver nucleolar organizer region (AgNOR), proliferating cell nuclear antigen, and MIB-1 LI. The authors did not find any significant advantage of using one proliferation marker versus the other.

Mixed CNs are rare; however, there has been a case of CN intermixed with small ganglionic cells consistent with ganglio CN reported (Buhl et al 2004).

Differential diagnosis

The differential diagnosis of intraventricular tumors includes intraventricular oligodendroglioma, astrocytoma, meningioma, ependymoma, subependymoma, choroid plexus papilloma, colloid cyst, craniopharyngioma, and germ cell tumor (Sharma et al 2006; Tacconi et al 1997). Recently, Iida et al (2008) performed ultrastructural studies of intraventricular tumors, including central CN, oligodendroglioma, cerebral neuroblastoma, and cerebellar neuroblastoma. Central CN and cerebellar neuroblastoma showed synaptic formation, and cerebral neuroblastoma demonstrated immature neurites. On the other hand, oligodendrogliomas showed similar features to oligodendrocytes.

Treatment

The optimal treatment is gross total surgical resection. Approximately 50% of CNs may be gross total resected. CNs that do not have a gross total resection may need a repeat resection, chemotherapy, or radiation therapy. Follow-up

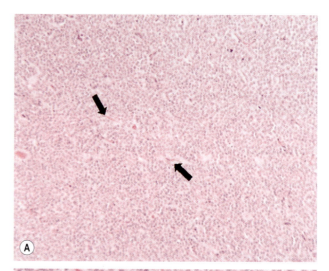

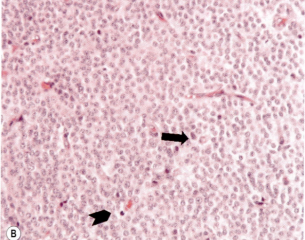

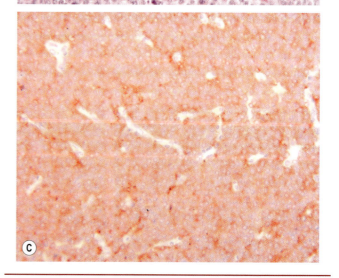

Figure 26.21 (A) Central neurocytoma showing a moderate and monomorphous cellularity. There are scattered thin and arborizing vascular structures (arrows) among tumor cells (H&E ×10). (B) Central neurocytoma showing a uniform cellular population. The tumor cells exhibit a round to oval nucleus, the chromatin is fine granular with delicate nuclear membrane. A small nucleolus is present in scattered cells. The cytoplasm is little and pale eosinophilic. Isolated larger ganglion-like cells are present (arrow). Few mitosis are identified (arrowhead) (H&E ×200). (C) Central neurocytoma. Synaptophysin immunostain showing diffuse cytoplasmic staining supporting its neurocytic lineage (Synaptophysin ×200).

imaging is recommended to determine if there is a change in tumor size. If a gross total resection is possible, that is the patient's best chance for long-term recurrence free survival. Most adjunctive therapies have been used in patients with recurrent CNs. Although there are no large collective experience with chemotherapy for CNs, there have been isolated reports of successful response to chemotherapeutic treatment. Dodds et al (1997) first published a good response of a CN, status-post partial resection, to combination chemotherapy of etoposide, ifosfamide, and carboplatin. Using a similar regimen, Amini et al (2008) have treated a 5-year-old with recurrent central CN with spinal cord drop metastases with combination chemotherapy of topotecan, ifosfamide, and carboplatin with complete response. Nishio et al (1988) reported radiation therapy in five patients with partial or gross total resection of a CN. The radiation was well tolerated, and all patients were free of recurrent tumor at long-term follow-up of 15–227 months after treatment. Rodriguez et al (2004) have used radiosurgery in one patient with good results. Tyler-Kabara et al (2001) have treated four cases of residual CN using radiosurgery with no tumor recurrence.

The largest review of treatment for CNs was recently published by Rades & Schild (2006) using retrospective analysis of a total of 438 patients with CNs (73 children, 365 adults). Children were defined as age ≤18 years old. The authors concluded that patients with complete resections did not need radiation therapy. Patients with sub-total resections benefited from radiation therapy, with treatment doses of 50 Gy for typical lesions and for children; atypical CNs in adults benefited from increased dosage of 55–60 Gy.

Clinical outcome

Patients generally have a good prognosis with treatment. Gross total resections may be potentially curative. Recurrences do occur in spite of gross total resections; however, they are usually local, and respond well to repeat resection or radiation therapy. Recurrent tumors usually have higher tumor proliferation rates, evidence of vascular proliferation, and synaptophysin expression. Soylemezoglu et al (1997) divided 36 cases of biopsied CNs on the basis of MIB-1 labeling index (LI) alone. The authors divided the patients into two groups; those with a MIB-1 LI of <2%, and those with a MIB-1 LI of >2%. Over an observation period of 150 months, there was a 22% relapse rate in patients with MIB LI <2%, and a 63% relapse rate in patients with MIB-1 LI >2%. Recently, Lenzi et al (2006) published an algorithm for treatment of CNs, based on an experience of 20 patients with CNs. They divided the patients into gross total resection or partial resection. Patients with gross total resection and a MIB-1 index <4% were observed only; if the MIB-1 index was >4%, they recommended a course of conformational radiotherapy. If a sub-total resection was performed, conformational radiotherapy with or without chemotherapy was recommended. The investigators felt that atypical histology and a MIB index >4% was significantly associated with a poor prognosis. Whether histological atypia or MIB-1 index was more important from a prognostic standpoint was examined by Mackenzie (1999), who examined 15 cases of CN. The investigator concluded that MIB-1 index >2% was more prognostic of recurrence or poor prognosis than histologic atypia (i.e., cellular pleomorphism, endothelial proliferation, and necrosis). However, recommendation for close follow-up of patients with either elevated proliferation potential or histologic atypia was made.

Rades et al (2004) recently examined the treatment course of 85 patients with atypical CN (MIB-1 LI >2%, atypical histologic features). Patients who underwent a complete resection, but no postoperative adjuvant therapy, had local control rates at 3 years and 5 years of 73% and 57%. Patients who had a complete resection and postoperative radiotherapy had local control rates at 3 and 5 years of 81% and 53%. Patients with incomplete resections had postoperative control rates of 21% and 7%; addition of radiation therapy to these patients increased their control rates to 85% and 70%. Survival rates at 5 years were 93% for complete resection alone, 90% for complete resection and radiation, 43% for incomplete resection alone, and 78% for incomplete resection and radiation.

Primary extraventricular CNs may occur. They are rare, however, occurrence in an extraventricular location does not necessarily imply a poor prognosis. Cemil et al (2009) recently reported a case of a CN in the left frontoparietal lobe. The patient underwent a gross total resection with adjuvant radiotherapy and chemotherapy, with excellent response to therapy. Yang et al (2009) reviewed three cases of extraventricular CN (frontal, parietal, sellar location) with good response to surgery and treatment. Takao et al (2003) reported a case of central CN with craniospinal dissemination, who underwent radiation therapy to his lesion at T4.

Tumors of predominantly ganglionic origin

Gangliocytoma

Demographics

Gangliocytoma is an uncommon central nervous system neoplasm that is predominantly composed of neoplastic mature neuronal cells (Serri et al 2008). The lack of neoplastic glial cells differentiates these tumors from gangliogliomas, which contain neoplastic ganglion and neoplastic glial cells (Kim et al 2001; Jacob et al 2005). The reported incidence of gangliocytoma ranges from 0.1–0.5% of CNS neoplasms (Izukawa et al 1988; Kim et al 2001; Jacob et al 2005). Patients are usually children and adults younger than 30 years old (Tureyen et al 2008). Intracranial gangliocytoma most commonly occurs in the temporal lobe, but may also be found in the frontal lobe, parietal lobe, floor of the third ventricle, sella and cerebellum (Russo et al 1995; Mikami et al 2008; Minkin et al 2008; Serri et al 2008). Supratentorial lesions are typically found in cortical locations, but sub-cortical tumors are also described (Itoh et al 1987). Peripherally located tumors may mimic meningioma (Kim et al 2001). Spinal gangliocytomas account for <10% of gangliocytomas, and are typically found in association with paraspinal sympathetic chain ganglia (Choi et al 2001; Jacob et al 2005).

When isolated to the cerebellum, the diagnosis of Lhermitte–Duclos disease (LDD) is made (Murata et al 1999). LDD is a rarer ganglion cell tumor, and is the primary focus of this subsection. A brief discussion of gangliocytoma that focuses primarily on supratentorial lesions is presented here.

Diagnosis

Patients with supratentorial gangliocytoma most commonly present with seizures (Altman 1988; Minkin et al 2008; Tureyen et al 2008). Other symptoms may include endocrine dysfunction for sellar tumors, headache, focal neurologic deficits and increased intracranial pressure (Sherazi 1998; Mikami et al 2008; Tureyen et al 2008).

Radiology

Radiographic descriptions differ among various case reports. CT may show a hypodense calcified lesion that enhances with contrast administration and is associated with edema and mass effect. On MRI, gangliocytoma may be of low signal intensity on T1-weighted images, hyperintense on T2-weighted images and often demonstrates homogeneous enhancement after gadolinium administration (Peretti-Viton et al 1991; Sherazi 1998; Kim et al 2001). Other reports describe lesions that are hyperdense and non-enhancing on CT, with minimal mass effect. In these cases, MRI shows a lesion without significant mass effect that appears of mixed signal intensities on T1-weighted images and hypointense on T2-weighted images (Altman 1988). Lesions may also be cystic (Tureyen et al 2008).

Pathology

The stem cell marker CD34 is positive in gangliocytomas as well as focal cortical dysplasia (FCD), suggesting a possible relationship between the pathogenesis of the two disease entities, as well as other neoplastic and malformative epileptogenic lesions (Blumcke et al 1999a,b). Gangliocytoma is classified as a WHO grade I neoplasm (Tureyen et al 2008).

Differential diagnosis

The differential diagnosis of gangliocytoma includes glioma, ganglioglioma and meningioma (Kim et al 2001). Ganglioglioma appears similar radiographically, and must be differentiated histologically by the presence or absence of a neoplastic glial component. Hyperintense signal on T2-weighted images may differentiate gangliocytoma from meningioma preoperatively. Gliomas may be distinguished from gangliogliomas based on histopathologic findings of neoplastic glial elements. MAP2 (microtubule associated protein 2) staining and proliferation assays may also assist with histopathologic differentiation by identifying neoplastic neuronal cells (Tureyen et al 2008).

Patients with gangliocytoma commonly present with seizures. However, medically intractable epilepsy may have other causes including cortical dysplasia that may be differentiated based on radiographic findings.

Treatment and clinical outcome

The treatment of choice is surgical resection, which allows long-term progression-free survival (Tureyen et al 2008). In patients with epilepsy, surgical treatment commonly significantly reduces or eliminates seizures. Little data exist regarding radiation therapy or chemotherapy. Gangliocytomas associated with endocrine dysfunction may require medical management of the endocrinopathy (McCowen et al 1999; Isidro et al 2005).

Lhermitte–Duclos disease

Demographics

Lhermitte–Duclos disease (LDD), or dysplastic gangliocytoma of the cerebellum, is a rare tumor first reported in 1920 by Lhermitte & Duclos, with more than 220 cases reported in the literature since then (Sabin et al 1988; Robinson & Cohen 2006; Inoue et al 2007). Although this lesion has been reported in the hypothalamus and spinal cord, the majority arise from the cerebellum (Bevan et al 1989; Azzarelli et al 1991). The age of presentation ranges from birth to the 6th decade, but most commonly the tumor is diagnosed in the 3rd and 4th decades of life with an average age of 34 years (Koch et al 1999). There is no gender or racial predilection (Roessmann & Wongmongkolrit 1984; Faillot et al 1990), unless LDD is found in association with Cowden disease in which case there is a 1:4 male:female preponderance (Murata et al 1999). The disease is most commonly unilateral, and the left cerebellar hemisphere is more often affected than the right (Wolansky et al 1996). There is no hereditary basis for Lhermitte–Duclos disease, but a case of mother and son with the tumor has been reported (Ambler et al 1969). There remains controversy regarding the etiology of the lesion and whether it represents a hamartoma, neoplasm or dysplasia (Koch et al 1999; Nakagawa et al 2007).

Diagnosis

Most patients present with signs and symptoms of cerebellar dysfunction (ataxia, dysdiadochokinesia, nystagmus) or increased intracranial pressure secondary to hydrocephalus (headache, papilledema, nausea, vomiting). Less common clinical presentations, such as loss of consciousness, subarachnoid hemorrhage and hemifacial spasm, have also been reported (Stapleton et al 1992; Inoue et al 2007; Minkin et al 2008). Lhermitte–Duclos disease may be associated with other CNS malformations including hydromyelia, brain heterotopia, and megalencephaly (Reznik & Schoenen 1983). It has been found in association with Cowden disease, an autosomal dominant multiple hamartomatous condition of the skin and mucous membranes, with frequent involvement of the thyroid, breast, colon, and adnexa (Padberg et al 1991; Tan & Ho 2007). Currently, adult onset LDD is considered to be the central nervous system manifestation of Cowden disease (Robinson & Cohen 2006). Approximately 60% of cases of LDD occur sporadically, whereas nearly 40% of cases occur in association with Cowden disease (Murata et al 1999). Case reports have also described patients with LDD found to have other central nervous system pathologies such as neurofibromatosis type I (Yesildag et al 2005), spinal arteriovenous fistula (Akiyama et al 2006), spinal intramedullary ependymoma (Farhadi et al 2007) and anaplastic ganglioglioma (Takei et al 2007).

Radiology

CT scanning shows a hypodense, space-occupying lesion in the cerebellum with minimal contrast enhancement (Fig. 26.22) (Di Lorenzo et al 1984; Smith et al 1989). Areas of calcification may be present. MR scanning demonstrates the characteristic striated pattern of hyperintensity on

T2-weighted imaging, also referred to as 'tiger-striped' (Wolansky et al 1996; Klisch et al 2001). The corresponding areas are hypointense to gray matter on T1-weighted images and display no enhancement after administration of gadolinium (Buhl et al 2003). Diffusion-weighted (DWI) MRI may demonstrate restricted diffusion (Cianfoni et al 2008), or no disturbance of water diffusion (Wu et al 2006). MR spectroscopy (MRS) shows a lactate peak, decreases in the *N*-acetyl-aspartate/creatine (NAA/Cr) and NAA/Choline (NAA/Cho) ratios, and a near normal Cho/Cr ratio (Wu et al 2006; Thomas et al 2007). As with CT, there is minimal enhancement of the tumor on MR. The lamellar appearance of the tumor may be appreciated on T2-weighted images,

corresponding to the pathologic finding of thickened cerebellar folia. As would be expected from CT and MR, the tumor on angiography is an avascular mass (Roski et al 1981; Sabin et al 1988; Faillot et al 1990; Murata et al 1999). MR may also be useful in determining the presence of residual tumor (Marano et al 1988; Reeder et al 1988; Smith et al 1989; Ashley et al 1990; Faillot et al 1990). Fluorodeoxyglucose positron emission tomography (FDG-PET) may reveal a hypermetabolic lesion (Nakagawa et al 2007; Hayasaka et al 2008). 11C-methionine-PET also shows a high uptake area associated with the lesion (Van Calenbergh et al 2006).

Pathology

Grossly, cerebellar gangliocytomas present as widened cerebellar folia (Sabin et al 1988). It is often difficult to establish a surgical plane between the gangliocytoma and normal cerebellum. Microscopically, the normal cerebellar architecture is altered, with the three layers of the cerebellar cortex (molecular, Purkinje, and granular) disrupted. Instead, there is thickening of the molecular layer, widening of the granule cell layer, disappearance of the Purkinje cell layer, and a decrease in the arbor vitae of the cerebellum (Inoue et al 2007). Pleomorphic ganglion cells without invasive characteristics replace the granule cell layer. Neovascular proliferation may be present in areas with the highest neuronal concentration. Excessive numbers of large myelinated axons exist within the molecular layer (Fig. 26.23) (Roski et al 1981; Reznik & Schoenen 1983; Di Lorenzo et al 1984; Reeder et al 1988; Sabin et al 1988; Smith et al 1989; Padberg et al 1991).

Immunohistochemistry shows positive staining for neuron-specific enolase (NSE) and synaptophysin, and negative GFAP staining (Inoue et al 2007). S-100 staining may be positive or negative (Murata et al 1999). MIB-1 is typically low, but reported as high as 5% (Inoue et al 2007). One report described a patient with an intramedullary spinal cord gangliocytoma who experienced a hypertensive episode during surgery. Immunohistochemistry of this patient's tumor demonstrated positive anti-tyrosine hydroxylase antibody staining of dense core vesicles within the mature ganglion cells, suggesting that the transient hypertension was secondary to catecholamine release (Azzarelli et al 1991). Like other gangliocytomas, LDD is considered WHO grade I (Inoue et al 2007).

LDD is associated with germline mutations in the PTEN gene. Recent work has implicated activation of mammalian target of rapamycin (mTOR), a downstream effector in the PTEN/AKT pathway, in the pathogenesis of the granule cell hypertrophy seen in LDD (Abel et al 2005).

Differential diagnosis

The differential diagnosis of LDD includes that for gangliocytomas (discussed above), and includes low-grade gliomas and hamartomas. Histopathologically, the lack of neoplastic glial elements rules out glioma. If obvious, the characteristic radiographic findings of striated and laminar patterns on MRI narrows the differential considerably. Definitive diagnosis is made by the demonstration of disruption of cerebellar architecture with proliferation of ganglion cells in the granule cell layer.

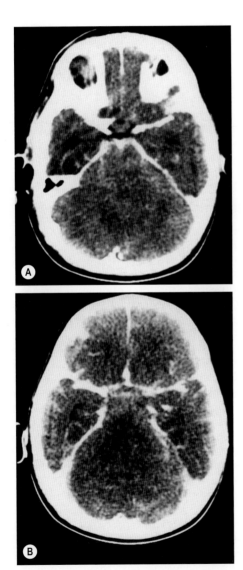

Figure 26.22 Gangliocytoma (Lhermitte–Duclos). This 7-year-old boy with a history of developmental delay expired from acute hydrocephalus. CT scan revealed a non-enhancing hypodense lesion occupying most of the cerebellum with obstruction of the basilar cisterns (A, non-contrast; B, contrast). The diagnosis of gangliocytoma was obtained post mortem.

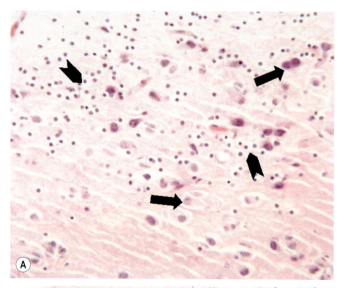

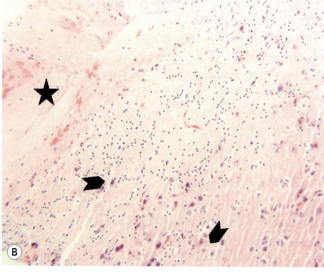

Figure 26.23 (A) Gangliocytoma showing proliferation of pleomorphic large neuronal cells (arrows) that are replacing the small neurons in the internal granular layer (arrowheads) (H&E ×200). (B) Gangliocytoma showing diffuse hypertrophy of the cerebellar folia with proliferating neurons some of which are as large as Purkinje cells (arrowheads). Their arborizations form a thick plexus in the molecular layer (star). (H&E ×100.)

Treatment

The treatment of choice is surgical resection, which should be as radical as possible (Buhl et al 2003). However, total resection is almost never obtained because of the difficulty in obtaining a plane between normal cerebellum and the gangliocytoma, and that this tumor often extends into the cerebellar peduncle and adjacent brainstem (Murata et al 1999). Intraoperative biopsy of the border and intraoperative MRI may help in achieving total tumor removal (Buhl et al 2003). Sub-total resection, however, may be sufficient for diminishing the mass effect, and repeat debulking may be necessary (Marano et al 1988). A treatment strategy involving craniectomy, C1 laminectomy and decompressive duraplasty to treat local compressive symptoms and hydrocephalus

has been described (Tuli et al 1997). Adjunctive radiotherapy and chemotherapy may be considered for recurrent unresectable lesions, however little data exist on the use of such adjuvant therapies and therefore their efficacy is unknown (Buhl et al 2003). Some authors report that radiation therapy may result in an increased risk of malignant transformation (Hayashi et al 2001).

Clinical outcome

The overall outcome in gangliocytomas of the cerebellum is favorable (Buhl et al 2003). Although many reports emphasize sub-total resections only, follow-up of the patients usually shows long-term progression-free survival (Roski et al 1981; Reznik and Schoenen 1983; Marano et al 1988). The tumor is histologically benign, but progression and recurrence are reported up to 20 years after initial diagnosis (Marano et al 1988; Stapleton et al 1992; Inoue et al 2007). Reports of recurrence argue against the origin of LDD as a hamartomatous disorder (Inoue et al 2007). The treatment for recurrence or progression is typically repeat sub-total surgical resection. In patients with histologically proven LDD in association with Cowden disease, serial systemic examinations of other hamartomatous lesions are required to evaluate for malignant degeneration of these systemic lesions (Vantomme et al 2001). The usefulness of radiation and chemotherapy in treating LDD are not known and therefore not recommended for newly diagnosed or recurrent lesions amenable to surgery (Marano et al 1988; Buhl et al 2003).

Hypothalamic hamartoma

Demographics

The first case of hypothalamic hamartoma was reported in 1934 (Le Marquand & Russell 1934). Although the number of cases that have been reported in the world literature is small (<200 cases), the total number of tumors diagnosed and treated greatly exceeds this number (Albright & Lee 1993). The vast majority of the tumors are found in the ventral aspect of the hypothalamus, ranging in position from the tuber cinereum to the mamillary body, and are either sessile or pedunculated in appearance. Although most children present with precocious puberty before the age of 3, patients as old as 8 years of age, have been reported. In one survey of hypothalamic hamartomas, 84% of the children presented with sexual precocity before age 3. There does not appear to be a sexual, familial, or racial predilection. Hypothalamic hamartomas may be associated with midline deformities including callosal agenesis, optic malformations, and hemispheric dysgenesis.

Diagnosis

Most of the patients present with isosexual precocious puberty. Males have voice deepening, muscular development, acne, pubic hair, and enlarged testes and penis. In females, breast development, menses, pubic hair, and excessive muscularity are noted (Albright & Lee 1993). The children are large for their age, and bone age is advanced by at least 3 years. Commonly, the parents will note behavioral changes, complaining of an 'adolescent personality' in their children (Albright & Lee 1993). Neurological findings are often present. Mental retardation is not uncommon.

Boyko et al (1991) believes that pedunculated lesions present with precocious puberty, and sessile lesions present with seizures. Other findings include headaches, visual disturbances, or evidence of autonomic dysfunction (hyperphagia, hyperactivity, or somnolence).

Gelastic seizures or laughing fits occur in up to 21% of the patients. The etiology of gelastic seizures and its subsequent generalization to tonic clonic and partial seizures has been recently studied in detail. Other epilepsy syndromes may occur in patients with hypothalamic hamartomas. Various investigators have documented complex partial seizures (CPS), tonic seizures (TS), and secondarily generalized seizures in these patients. They have all concluded that seizures originate in the hypothalamic hamartomas, with spread from gelastic seizures to tonic clonic seizures or complex partial seizures, but not both (Striano et al 2005; Castro et al 2007; Harvey & Freeman 2007).

Precocious puberty may be confirmed by elevated luteinizing hormone (LH), follicle stimulating hormone (FSH), estradiol, or testosterone levels. Suppression of LH and FSH occurs by gonadotropin releasing hormone (GnRH) continuous stimulation. Prolactin levels may also be elevated, but growth hormone (GH) and thyroid stimulating hormones (TSH) levels are usually normal. The hypothalamic-pituitary axis is usually immature. In one male patient with precocious puberty, the hypothalamic-pituitary axis was found to be unresponsive to clomiphene. A stimulatory response to this drug is found only in the middle to late stages of sexual maturation. The absent stimulatory response suggests a lack of maturation of the usual central nervous system events associated with normal puberty. Negative feedback was intact, but was partially resistant to steroid suppression.

MR is the imaging diagnosis of choice. T1-weighted images show good resolution of the hamartoma from the surrounding brain. No enhancement of the tumor is found with gadolinium (Fig. 26.24). T2-weighted images show the hamartoma to be isointense or hyperintense relative to gray matter. T2-weighted images may be harder to interpret, however, because of the difficulty in distinguishing tumor from the surrounding CSF in the suprasellar cisterns (Albright & Lee 1993). Although there are no large series of hamartomas examined with MR scans, there does not appear to be any difference in MR signal characteristics and histopathology (Boyko et al 1991). MRI imaging studies by Freeman et al (2004) in 72 cases of epileptogenic hypothalamic hamartomas demonstrate that these tumors have intimate relationships with the mammillary body, fornix, and mamillothalamic tract, implicating these structures with seizures in these patients. Recently, Amstutz et al (2006) reported using MR spectroscopy (MRS) to correlate MR spectral patterns with the histology of hypothalamic hamartomas. The authors found a decrease in the N-acetylaspartate (NAA)/ Creatinine (Cr) ratio, increase in myoinositol (mI)/Cr ratio, and increased choline (Cho)/Cr ratio in tumor compared with normal brain. CT scanning has been used in the past, but is no longer needed as these images do not add anything to what can be demonstrated on MRI scan. The tumors appear isodense to gray matter on CT, and do not enhance with contrast. Cerebral angiography does not yield a tumor blush.

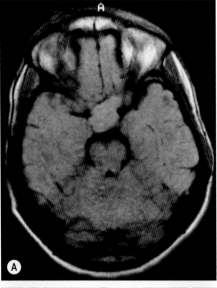

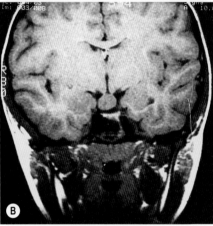

Figure 26.24 MR scan (T1-weighted image) showing the sessile (A) and pedunculated forms (B) of hypothalamic hamartoma, isointense to gray matter.

Pathology

The majority of hamartomas are pedunculated into the interpeduncular cistern, on a stalk containing myelinated fibers. Other hamartomas are sessile, with a wide attachment to the ventral surface of the hypothalamus or embodied in the hypothalamus itself. Hamartomas are usually firm, and vary in size from 0.5–4.0 cm in diameter. In asymptomatic patients, they are usually <1.5 cm in diameter (Albright & Lee 1993). Microscopically, hypothalamic hamartomas are primarily composed of mature neurons interspersed with glial cells. There is moderate glial cellularity over a fibrillar background, without neoplastic differentiation (Fig. 26.25). Independent neuroendocrine units with neurons containing neurosecretory granules, blood vessels with fenestrated endothelium, and double basement membranes may be present. Dense core granules may be seen on electron microscopy. These pathological findings suggest two possible mechanisms for precocious puberty: (1) mechanical compression of inhibitory pathways from the hypothalamus and

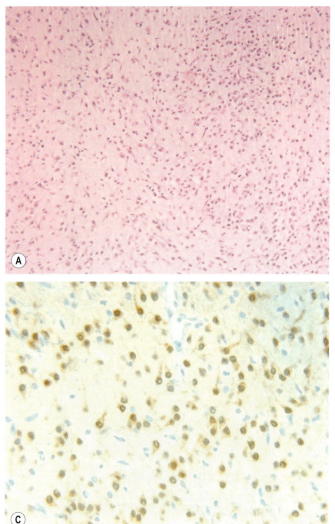

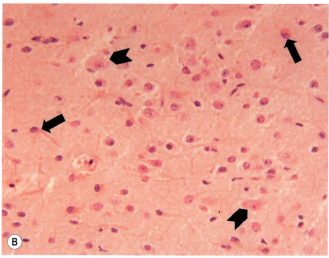

Figure 26.25 (A) Hypothalamic hamartoma with a high and irregularly distributed neuronal density. Clustering of neurons forming a definitive nuclear conglomerate is not present (H&E ×100). (B) Hypothalamic hamartoma composed predominantly of normal appearing neurons varying in size and shape (arrowheads). The glial component exhibit reactive changes represented by increased cytoplasm and prominent astrocytic processes (arrows) (H&E ×200). (C) NeuN immunostaining highlights the range in neuronal size and irregular distribution. The negative glial component is also highlighted (NeuN ×200).

posterior pituitary, and (2) direct neurosecretory function in the hamartomas. In both instances, there is an over-secretion of GnRH, leading to inappropriate production of LH and FSH in the anterior pituitary (Boyko et al 1991). Recently, Beggs et al (2008) examined hypothalamic hamartoma tissue of patients with gelastic seizures with electron microscopy. They found that all samples demonstrated unusual dendritic varicosities, with large and small neurons connected with large numbers of inhibitory and excitatory synapses, consistent with tissue having the substrate to generate seizures. Similar results were demonstrated by Coons et al (2007) who examined 57 cases of hypothalamic hamartomas, demonstrating an increase in small mature neurons, with extensive production of synapse associated proteins, resulting in nodules of these small neurons in the tumor. In contrast to cortical dysplasia, atypical large ganglion-like balloon cells were not seen.

Differential diagnosis

The differential diagnosis of a child presenting with precocious puberty includes hypothalamic astrocytoma, optic nerve/chiasm glioma, germinoma, craniopharyngioma, and a suprasellar cyst. These lesions can usually be distinguished on MR scanning. Pathologically, hamartomas need to be readily differentiated from low-grade gliomas, gangliogliomas, and gangliocytomas. Low-grade gliomas show evidence of astrocytic neoplastic differentiation, without the presence of neuronal elements. Gangliogliomas will show glial neoplastic differentiation, but also have ganglionic components. Gangliocytomas are usually located in the cerebellum (Lhermitte–Duclos disease), however, they have been reported in the hypothalamus (Reznik & Schoenen 1983; Bevan et al 1989). They are distinguished by the presence of pleomorphic ganglionic cells.

Treatment

Treatment of hypothalamic hamartomas may be based on medical therapy or surgical excision. Non-surgical treatment of hamartomas is now possible with long-acting GnRH analogs. Since pulsatile GnRH release is necessary to initiate puberty, continuous GnRH stimulation will inhibit gonadotropin secretion. The disadvantages with GnRH therapy are several-fold: (1) GnRH therapy is expensive (2) it may not reverse the muscularity, increased appetite, and 'adolescent' personality often found in these patients, and (3) it may need to be used for many years depending on the age of the child (Albright & Lee 1993). It should be noted, however, that GnRH has been administered up to 13 years without significant sequelae. In an older patient who may be close to starting puberty, no treatment may be appropriate. Starceski et al (1990) reported an 8 year 7 month-old-boy who was not given any treatment, and was able to obtain an acceptable adult height. Moreover, it should be pointed out that, even without any form of medical treatment in the younger patients, the undesirable side-effects are limited to accelerated growth with tall stature for age, premature sexual childhood development and adult stature shorter than would have been ordinarily obtained.

The ideal surgical candidate is a young patient, who otherwise would need to be on long-term GnRH analog therapy, with precocious puberty but normal pubertal endocrine make-up, in whom a cessation of premature pubertal development is desired. A pedunculated tumor would be ideal for surgical removal (Starceski et al 1990). The original approaches to hypothalamic hamartomas have focused on a variety of basal surgical approaches, including subtemporal, subfrontal, pterional, and frontotemporal. Albright & Lee (1993) have reported good results in the removal of both pedunculated and sessile tumors using a subtemporal approach, which was felt to give the best visualization of the normal anatomy. As the posterior surface of the hamartoma is often adherent to the anterior brainstem with adhesions to the basilar artery, an approach that allows visualization of the basilar artery is needed (Albright & Lee 1993). The anterior transcallosal interforniceal approach has been popularized by Rosenfeld et al (2001). The anterior approach lends itself to direct visualization of the tumor, the ability to debulk and or disconnect the hypothalamic hamartoma from the mamillary bodies, and avoids the cranial nerves and vessels encountered in the basal approaches (Addas et al 2008). Most common complications using this approach come from injury to the hypothalamus on attempting complete removal of the hamartoma; short- or long-term memory loss can occur from injury to the fornices. The anterior approach also lends itself to endoscopic resection which has been successfully implemented for small hypothalamic hamartomas. Although 'minimally invasive', this approach may lead to transient or permanent complications, including forniceal injury and hypothalamic injury. Theoretically, a pedunculated lesion transected at the stalk without removal of the hamartoma should cure the endocrine disturbances, however, removal of the hamartoma allows surgical confirmation of the diagnosis. Sessile lesions are harder to remove, and often a total removal is not possible when they extend into the hypothalamus. In that case, a sub-total removal so that the tumor is flush with the ventral surface of the hypothalamus is the treatment of choice (Albright & Lee 1993). The most likely surgical morbidity from an attempt at removal via the sub-temporal approach is transient oculomotor paresis secondary to oculomotor nerve manipulation. Surgical therapy, on the other hand, has not always been successful (Albright & Lee 1993).

Radiosurgery has also been used to treat hypothalamic hamartomas. The first successful lesioning was described by Arita et al in 1998, and has subsequently been reported in several other small case studies. Régis et al (2006) reported 27 patients treated with gamma knife for seizures secondary to hypothalamic hamartoma. They reported cessation or improvement in seizures in 59% of the patients without significant side effects. Similar to radiosurgery, Schulze-Bonhage & Ostertag (2007) have reported treatment of hypothalamic hamartomas with ^{125}I radioactive seeds in 24 patients. They reported a significant reduction in gelastic seizures in about half of the patients treated. Side-effects included significant weight gain in four of the patients; cognitive side-effects (including lethargy, short-term memory deficits, fatigue) occurred secondary to edema in the hypothalamus from the seed implants in five patients. Most of these side-effects diminished following a decrease in adjacent edema (Schulze-Bonhage & Ostertag 2007). In one series, 7 of 13 male patients underwent radiation after surgery, with no difference in survival. The use of antineoplastic agents is not warranted.

Clinical outcome

The clinical outcome is generally good. Few patients die from hypothalamic hamartomas, even if the lesion is incompletely removed. A cure of the endocrinopathy by surgical intervention is most likely if the lesion is pedunculated, however, partial removal may be sufficient to restore a normal endocrine axis (Albright & Lee 1993). Once a chemical cure is achieved, return to basal endocrine status may be obtained. Previous adolescent bodily changes (i.e., pubic hair, enlarged testes, breast development) will return to normal (Albright & Lee 1993). Operative intervention is only indicated in selected cases where GnRH suppression or no treatment are not viable options.

REFERENCES

Abel, T.W., Baker, S.J., Fraser, M.M., et al., 2005. Lhermitte-Duclos disease: a report of 31 cases with immunohistochemical analysis of the PTEN/AKT/mTOR pathway. J. Neuropathol. Exp. Neurol. 64, 341–349.

Addas, B., Sherman, E.M.S., Hader W.J., 2008. Surgical management of hypothalamic hamartomas in patients with gelastic epilepsy. Neurosurg. Focus 25, E8.

Adriaensen, M.E., Schaefer-Prokop, C.M., Stijnen, T., et al., 2009. Prevalence of subependymal giant cell tumors in patients with tuberous sclerosis and a review of the literature. Eur. J. Neurol. 16, 691–696.

Akiyama, Y., Ikeda, J., Ibayashi, Y., et al., 2006. Lhermitte-Duclos disease with cervical paraspinal arteriovenous fistula. Neurol. Med. Chir. (Tokyo) 46, 446–449.

Alaraj, A., Chan, M., Oh, S., et al., 2007. Astroblastoma presenting with intracerebral hemorrhage misdiagnosed as dural arteriovenous fistula: review of a rare entity. Surg. Neurol. 67, 308–313.

Albanese, A., Mangiola, A., Pompucci, A., et al., 2005. Rosette-forming glioneuronal tumour of the fourth ventricle: report of a case with clinical and surgical implications. J. Neurooncol. 71, 195–197.

Albright, A.L., Lee, P.A., 1993. Neurosurgical treatment of hypothalamic hamartomas causing precocious puberty. J. Neurosurg. 78, 77–82.

Alexiou, G.A., Stefanaki, K., Sfakianos, G., et al., 2008. Desmoplastic infantile ganglioglioma: a report of 2 cases and a review of the literature. Pediatr. Neurosurg. 44, 422–425.

Allegranza, A., Pileri, S., Frank, G., et al., 1990. Cerebral ganglioglioma with anaplastic oligodendroglial component. Histopathology 17, 439–441.

Allende, D.S., Prayson, R.A., 2009. The expanding family of glioneuronal tumors. Adv. Anat. Pathol. 16, 33–39.

Altman, N.R., 1988. MR and CT characteristics of gangliocytoma: a rare cause of epilepsy in children. AJNR Am. J. Neuroradiol. 9, 917–921.

Ambler, M., Pogacar, S., Sidman, R., 1969. Lhermitte-Duclos disease (granule cell hypertrophy of the cerebellum) pathological analysis of the first familial cases. J. Neuropathol. Exp. Neurol. 28, 622–647.

Amini, E., Roffidal, T., Lee, A., et al., 2008. Central neurocytoma responsive to topotecan, ifosfamide, carboplatin. Pediatr. Blood Cancer 51, 137–140.

Amstutz, D.R., Coons, S.W., Kerrigan, J.F., et al., 2006. Hypothalamic hamartomas: Correlation of MR imaging and spectroscopic findings with tumor glial content. AJNR Am. J. Neuroradiol. 27, 794–798.

Anan, M., Inoue, R., Ishii, K., et al., 2009. A rosette-forming glioneuronal tumor of the spinal cord: the first case of a rosette-forming glioneuronal tumor originating from the spinal cord. Hum. Pathol. 40, 898–901.

Arita, K., Kurisu, K., Koji, I., et al., 1998. Subsidence of seizure induced by stereotactic radiation in a patient with hypothalamic hamartoma. J. Neurosurg. 89, 645–648.

Ashley, D.G., Zee, C.S., Chandrasoma, P.T., et al., 1990. Lhermitte-Duclos disease: CT and MR findings. J. Comput. Assist. Tomogr. 14, 984–987.

Athale, S., Hallet, K.K., Jinkins, J.R., 1999. Ganglioglioma of the trigeminal nerve: MRI. Neuroradiology 41, 576–578.

Atri, S., Sharma, M.C., Sarkar, C., et al., 2007. Papillary glioneuronal tumour: a report of a rare case and review of literature. Childs Nerv. Syst. 23, 349–353.

Azzarelli, B., Luerssen, T.G., Wolfe, T.M., 1991. Intramedullary secretory gangliocytoma. Acta Neuropathol. 82, 402–407.

Bachli, H., Avoledo, P., Gratzl, O., et al., 2003. Therapeutic strategies and management of desmoplastic infantile ganglioglioma: two case reports and literature overview. Childs Nerv. Syst. 19, 359–366.

Bignami, A., Adelman, L.S., Perides, G., et al., 1989. Glial hyaluronate-binding protein in polar spongioblastoma. J. Neuropathol. Exp. Neurol. 48, 187–196.

Bailey, P., Bucy, P.C., 1930. Astroblastomas of the brain. Acta Psychiatr. Neurol. 5, 439–461.

Baka, J.J., Patel, S.C., Roebuck, J.R., et al., 1993. Predominantly extraaxial astroblastoma: imaging and proton MR spectroscopy features. AJNR Am. J. Neuroradiol. 14, 946–950.

Bannykh, S.I., Fan, X., Black, K.L., 2007. Malignant astroblastoma with rhabdoid morphology. J. Neurooncol. 83, 277–278.

Barbosa, M.D., Balsitis, M., Jaspan, T.J., et al., 1990. Intraventricular neurocytoma: a clinical and pathological study of three cases and review of the literature. Neurosurgery 26, 1045–1054.

Barnes, N.P., Pollock, J.R., Harding, B., et al., 2002. Papillary glioneuronal tumour in a 4-year-old. Pediatr. Neurosurg. 36, 266–270.

Beggs, J., Nakada, S., Fenoglio, K., et al., 2008. Hypothalamic hamartomas associated with epilepsy: ultrastructural features. J. Neuropathol. Exp. Neurol. 67, 65t7–68.

Bell, J.W., Osborn, A.G., Salzman, K.L., et al., 2007. Neuroradiologic characteristics of astroblastoma. Neuroradiology 49, 203–209.

Benitez, W.I., Glasier, C.M., Husain, M., et al., 1990. MR findings in childhood gangliogliomas. J. Comput. Assist. Tomogr. 14, 712–716.

Berenguer, J., Bargallo, N., Bravo, E., et al., 1994. An unusual frontal ganglioglioma: CT and MRI. Neuroradiology 36, 311–312.

Bergin, D.J., Johnson, T.E., Spencer, W.H., et al., 1988. Ganglioglioma of the optic nerve. Am. J. Ophthalmol. 105, 146–149.

Bevan, J.S., Asa, S.L., Rossi, M.L., et al., 1989. Intrasellar gangliocytoma containing gastrin and growth hormone-releasing hormone associated with a growth hormone-secreting pituitary adenoma. Clin. Endocrinol. (Oxf.) 30, 213–224.

Blom, R.J., 1988. Pleomorphic xanthoastrocytoma: CT appearance. J. Comput. Assist. Tomogr. 12, 351–352.

Blumcke, I., Giencke, K., Wardelmann, E., et al., 1999a. The CD34 epitope is expressed in neoplastic and malformative lesions associated with chronic, focal epilepsies. Acta Neuropathol. 97, 481–490.

Blumcke, I., Lobach, M., Wolf, H.K., et al., 1999b. Evidence for developmental precursor lesions in epilepsy-associated glioneuronal tumors. Microsc. Res. Tech. 46, 53–58.

Blumcke, I., Wiestler, O.D., 2002. Gangliogliomas: an intriguing tumor entity associated with focal epilepsies. J. Neuropathol. Exp. Neurol. 61, 575–584.

Bonnin, J.M., Rubinstein, L.J., 1989. Astroblastomas: a pathological study of 23 tumors, with a postoperative follow-up in 13 patients. Neurosurgery 25, 6–13.

Bonnin, J.M., Rubinstein, L.J., Papasozomenos, S.C., et al., 1984. Subependymal giant cell astrocytoma. Significance and possible cytogenetic implications of an immunohistochemical study. Acta Neuropathol. 62, 185–193.

Bouvier-Labit, C., Daniel, L., Dufour, H., et al., 2000. Papillary glioneuronal tumour: clinicopathological and biochemical study of one case with 7-year follow up. Acta Neuropathol. 99, 321–326.

Bowles, A.P., Jr., Pantazis, C.G., Allen, M.B., Jr., et al., 1988. Ganglioglioma, a malignant tumor? Correlation with flow deoxyribonucleic acid cytometric analysis. Neurosurgery 23, 376–381.

Boyko, O.B., Curnes, J.T., Oakes, W.J., et al., 1991. Hamartomas of the tuber cinerium: CT, MR, and pathologic findings. Am. J. Neuroradiol. 12, 309–314.

Braeuninger, S., Schneider-Stock, R., Kirches, E., et al., 2007. Evaluation of molecular genetic alterations associated with tumor progression in a case of gliomatosis cerebri. J. Neurooncol. 82, 23–27.

Brat, D.J., Hirose, Y., Cohen, K.J., et al., 2000. Astroblastoma: clinicopathologic features and chromosomal abnormalities defined by comparative genomic hybridization. Brain Pathol. 10, 342–352.

Brat, D.J., Parisi, J.E., Kleinschmidt-DeMasters, B.K., et al., 2008. Surgical neuropathology update: a review of changes introduced by the WHO classification of tumours of the central nervous system. Arch. Pathol. Lab. Med. 132, 993–1007.

Broholm, H., Madsen, F.F., Wagner, A.A., et al., 2002. Papillary glioneuronal tumor – a new tumor entity. Clin. Neuropathol. 21, 1–4.

Buccoliero, A.M., Franchi, A., Castiglione, F., et al., 2009. Subependymal giant cell astrocytoma (SEGA): Is it an astrocytoma? Morphological, immunohistochemical and ultrastructural study. Neuropathology 29, 25–30.

Buccoliero, A.M., Giordano, F., Mussa, F., et al., 2006. Papillary glioneuronal tumor radiologically mimicking a cavernous hemangioma with hemorrhagic onset. Neuropathology 26, 206–211.

Buhl, R., Barth, H., Hugo, H.H., et al., 2003. Dysplastic gangliocytoma of the cerebellum: rare differential diagnosis in space occupying lesions of the posterior fossa. Acta Neurochir (Wien) 145, 509–512.

Buhl, R., Huang, H., Hugo, H.H., et al., 2004. Ganglioneurocytoma of the third ventricle. J. Neuro-oncology 66, 341–344.

● Burel-Vandenbos, F., Varlet, P., Lonjon, M., et al., 2007. [Ependymal variant of dysembryoplastic neuro-epithelial tumor]. Ann. Pathol. 27, 320–323.

Cabello, A., Madero, S., Castresana, A., et al., 1991. Astroblastoma: electron microscopy and immunohistochemical findings: case report. Surg. Neurol. 35, 116–121.

Caroli, E., Salvati, M., Esposito, V., et al., 2004. Cerebral astroblastoma. Acta Neurochir (Wien) 146, 629–633.

Castillo, M., Davis, P.C., Takei, Y., et al., 1990. Intracranial ganglioglioma: MR, CT, and clinical findings in 18 patients. AJNR Am. J. Neuroradiol. 11, 109–114.

Castro, L.H., Ferreira, L.K., Teles, L.R., et al., 2007. Epilepsy syndromes associated with hypothalamic hamartomas. Seizure 16, 50–58.

Cemil, B., Tun, K., Guvenc, Y., et al., 2009. Extraventricular neurocytoma: report of a case. Neurol. Neurochir. Pol. 43, 191–194.

Chamberlain, M.C., Press, G.A., 1990. Temporal lobe ganglioglioma in refractory epilepsy: CT and MR in three cases. J. Neurooncol. 9, 81–87.

● Chan, C.H., Bittar, R.G., Davis, G.A., et al., 2006. Long-term seizure outcome following surgery for dysembryoplastic neuroepithelial tumor. J. Neurosurg. 104, 62–69.

Chang, H.T., Latorre, J.G., Hahn, S., et al., 2006. Pediatric cerebellar pleomorphic xanthoastrocytoma with anaplastic features: a case of long-term survival after multimodality therapy. Childs Nerv. Syst. 22, 609–613.

Chen, C.L., Shen, C.C., Wang, J., et al., 2008. Central neurocytoma: a clinical, radiological and pathological study of nine cases. Clin. Neurol. Neurosurg. 110, 129–136.

Chilton, J., Caughron, M.R., Kepes, J.J., 1990. Ganglioglioma of the optic chiasm: case report and review of the literature. Neurosurgery 26, 1042–1045.

Choi, Y.H., Kim, I.O., Cheon, J.E., et al., 2001. Gangliocytoma of the spinal cord: a case report. Pediatr. Radiol. 31, 377–380.

Chuang, M.T., Lin, W.C., Tsai, H.Y., et al., 2005. 3-T proton magnetic resonance spectroscopy of central neurocytoma: 3 case reports and review of the literature. J. Comput. Assist. Tomogr. 29, 683–688.

Cianfoni, A., Wintermark, M., Piludu, F., et al., 2008. Morphological and functional MR imaging of Lhermitte-Duclos disease with pathology correlate. J. Neuroradiol. 35, 297–300.

Coons, S.W., Rekate, H.L., Prenger E.C., et al., 2007. The histopathology of hypothalamic hamartomas: study of 57 cases. J Neuropathol. Exp. Neurol. 66, 131–141.

Cox, J.D., Zimmerman, H.M., Haughton, V.M., 1982. Microcystic ganglioglioma treated by partial removal and radiation therapy. Cancer 50, 473–477.

Daumas-Duport, C., 1993. Dysembryoplastic neuroepithelial tumours. Brain Pathol. 3, 283–295.

Daumas-Duport, C., Scheithauer, B.W., Chodkiewicz, J.P., et al., 1988. Dysembryoplastic neuroepithelial tumor: a surgically curable tumor of young patients with intractable partial seizures. Report of thirty-nine cases. Neurosurgery 23, 545–556.

Davidson, L.A., Graham, D.I., Carey, F.A., 1992. Chronic neurological dysfunction attributable to a ganglioglioma. Histopathology 21, 275–278.

Davies, K.G., Maxwell, R.E., Seljeskog, E., et al., 1994. Pleomorphic xanthoastrocytoma – report of four cases, with MRI scan appearances and literature review. Br. J. Neurosurg. 8, 681–689.

De Chadarevian, J.P., Guyda, H.J., Hollenberg, R.D., 1984. Hypothalamic polar spongioblastoma associated with the diencephalic syndrome. Virchows Arch. 402, 465–474.

De Munnynck, K., Van Gool, S., Van Calenbergh, F., et al., 2002. Desmoplastic infantile ganglioglioma: a potentially malignant tumor? Am. J. Surg. Pathol. 26, 1515–1522.

De Reuck, J., Van de Velde, E., vander Eecken, H., 1975. The angioarchitecture of the astroblastoma. Clin. Neurol. Neurosurg. 78, 89–98.

Demierre, B., Stichnoth, F.A., Hori, A., et al., 1986. Intracerebral ganglioglioma. J. Neurosurg. 65, 177–182.

Denaro, L., Gardiman, M., Calderone, M., et al., 2008. Intraventricular astroblastoma. Case report. J. Neurosurg. Pediatrics 1, 152–155.

Dhillon, R.S., 1987. Posterior fossa ganglioglioma–an unusual cause of hearing loss. J. Laryngol. Otol. 101, 714–717.

Di Lorenzo, N., Lunardi, P., Fortuna, A., 1984. Granulomolecular hypertrophy of the cerebellum (Lhermitte-Duclos disease). Case report. J. Neurosurg. 60, 644–646.

Diepholder, H.M., Schwechheimer, K., Mohadjer, M., et al., 1991. A clinicopathologic and immunomorphologic study of 13 cases of ganglioglioma. Cancer 68, 2192–2201.

Dodds, D., Nonis, J., Mehta, M., et al., 1997. Central neurocytoma: a clinical study of response to chemotherapy. J. Neurooncol. 34, 279–283.

Dodero, F., Alliez, J.R., Metellus, P., et al., 2001. Central neurocytoma: 2 case reports and review of the literature. Acta Neurochir. 142, 1417–1422.

Dorne, H.L., O'Gorman, A.M., Melanson, D., 1986. Computed tomography of intracranial gangliogliomas. AJNR Am. J. Neuroradiol. 7, 281–285.

Duffner, P.K., Burger, P.C., Cohen, M.E., et al., 1994. Desmoplastic infantile gangliogliomas: an approach to therapy. Neurosurgery 34, 583–589.

Edgar, M.A., Rosenblum, M.K., 2007. Mixed glioneuronal tumors: recently described entities. Arch. Pathol. Lab. Med. 131, 228–233.

Ellenberg, L., McComb, J.G., Siegel, S.E., et al., 1987. Factors affecting intellectual outcome in pediatric brain tumor patients. Neurosurgery 21, 638–644.

Elshaikh, M.A., Stevens, G.H., Peereboom, D.M., et al., 2002. Gliomatosis cerebri: treatment results with radiotherapy alone. Cancer 95, 2027–2031.

Faillot, T., Sichez, J.P., Brault, J.L., et al., 1990. Lhermitte-Duclos disease (dysplastic gangliocytoma of the cerebellum). Report of a case and review of the literature. Acta Neurochir (Wien) 105, 44–49.

Fan, X., Larson, T.C., Jennings, M.T., et al., 2001. December 2000:6 month old boy with 2 week history of progressive lethargy. Brain Pathol. 11, 265–266.

Farhadi, M.R., Rittierodt, M., Stan, A., et al., 2007. Intramedullary ependymoma associated with Lhermitte-Duclos disease and Cowden syndrome. Clin. Neurol. Neurosurg. 109, 692–697.

Fathi, A.R., Novoa, E., El-Koussy, M., et al., 2008. Astroblastoma with rhabdoid features and favorable long-term outcome: report of a case with a 12-year follow-up. Pathol. Res. Pract. 204, 345–351.

Favereaux, A., Vital, A., Loiseau, H., et al., 2000. Histopathological variants of central neurocytoma: report of 10 cases. Ann. Pathol. 20, 558–563.

Fletcher, W.A., Hoyt, W.F., Narahara, M.H., 1988. Congenital quadrantanopia with occipital lobe ganglioglioma. Neurology 38, 1892–1894.

Freeman, J.L., Coleman, L.T., Wellard, R.M., et al., 2004. MR imaging and spectroscopic study of epileptogenic hypothalamic hamartomas: analysis of 72 cases. Am. J. Neuroradiol. 25, 450–462.

Freund, M., Hahnel, S., Sommer, C., et al., 2001. CT and MRI findings in gliomatosis cerebri: a neuroradiologic and neuropathologic review of diffuse infiltrating brain neoplasms. Eur. Radiol. 11, 309–316.

Fujimoto, M., Weaker, F.J., Herbert, D.C., et al., 1988. Expression of three viral oncogenes (v-sis, v-myc, v-fos) in primary human brain tumors of neuroectodermal origin. Neurology 38, 289–293.

Fujiwara, S., Takaki, T., Hikita, T., et al., 1989. Subependymal giant-cell astrocytoma associated with tuberous sclerosis. Do subependymal nodules grow? Childs Nerv. Syst. 5, 43–44.

Fuller, C., Helton, K., Dalton, J., et al., 2006. Polar spongioblastoma of the spinal cord: a case report. Pediatr. Dev. Pathol. 9, 75–80.

Furuta, A., Takahashi, H., Ikuta, F., et al., 1992. Temporal lobe tumor demonstrating ganglioglioma and pleomorphic xanthoastrocytoma components. Case report. J. Neurosurg. 77, 143–147.

Garcia, C.A., McGarry, P.A., Collada, M., 1984. Ganglioglioma of the brain stem. Case report. J. Neurosurg. 60, 431–434.

Giannini, C., Scheithauer, B.W., Burger, P.C., et al., 1999. Pleomorphic xanthoastrocytoma: what do we really know about it? Cancer 85, 2033–2045.

Giannini, C., Scheithauer, B.W., Lopes, M.B., et al., 2002. Immunophenotype of pleomorphic xanthoastrocytoma. Am. J. Surg. Pathol. 26, 479–485.

Glasser, R.S., Rojiani, A.M., Mickle, J.P., et al., 1995. Delayed occurrence of cerebellar pleomorphic xanthoastrocytoma after supratentorial pleomorphic xanthoastrocytoma removal. Case report. J. Neurosurg. 82, 116–118.

Goergen, S.K., Gonzales, M.F., McLean, C.A., 1992. Intraventricular CN: radiologic features and review of the literature. Radiology 182, 787–792.

Goldring, S., Rich, K.M., Picker, S., 1986. Experience with gliomas in patients presenting with a chronic seizure disorder. Clin. Neurosurg. 33, 15–42.

Gomez, J.G., Garcia, J.H., Colon, L.E., 1985. A variant of cerebral glioma called pleomorphic xanthoastrocytoma: case report. Neurosurgery 16, 703–706.

Grant, J.W., Gallagher, P.J., 1986. Pleomorphic xanthoastrocytoma. Immunohistochemical methods for differentiation from fibrous histiocytomas with similar morphology. Am. J. Surg. Pathol. 10, 336–341.

Haddad, S.F., Moore, S.A., Menezes, A.H., et al., 1992. Ganglioglioma: 13 years of experience. Neurosurgery 31, 171–178.

Hader, W.J., Ozen, L., Hamiwka L., et al., 2008. Neuropsychological and quality of life outcome after endoscopic resection of hypothalamic hamartomas. Can J. Neurol. Sci. 335, S73.

Hall, W.A., Yunis, E.J., Albright, A.L., 1986. Anaplastic ganglioglioma in an infant: case report and review of the literature. Neurosurgery 19, 1016–1020.

Hamlat, A., Le Strat, A., Guegan, Y., et al., 2007. Cerebellar pleomorphic xanthoastrocytoma: case report and literature review. Surg. Neurol. 68, 89–95.

Hanel, R.A., Montano, J.C., Gasparetto, E., et al., 2001. Uncommon presentation of central neurocytoma causing intraventricular hemorrhage: case report. Arq. Neuropsiquiatr. 59, 628–632.

Harvey, A.S., Freeman J.L., 2007. Epilepsy in hypothalamic hamartoma: clinical and EEG features. Semin. Pediatr. Neurol. 14, 60–64.

Hassoun, J., Gambarelli, D., Grisoli, F., et al., 1982. Central neurocytoma: an electron microscopic study of two cases. Acta Neuropathol. (Berl.) 56, 151–156.

Hassoun, J., Soylemezoglu, F., Gambarelli, D., et al., 1993. Central neurocytoma: a synopsis of clinical and histological features. Brain Pathol. 3, 297–306.

Hayasaka, K., Nihashi, T., Takebayashi, S., et al., 2008. FDG PET in Lhermitte-Duclos disease. Clin. Nucl. Med. 33, 52–54.

Hayashi, Y., Iwato, M., Hasegawa, M., et al., 2001. Malignant transformation of a gangliocytoma/ganglioglioma into a glioblastoma multiforme: a molecular genetic analysis. Case report. J. Neurosurg. 95, 138–142.

Herrlinger, U., Felsberg J., Kuker, W., et al., 2002. Gliomatosis cerebri: molecular pathology and clinical course. Ann. Neurol. 52, 390–399.

Heyerdahl Strom, E., Skullerud, K., 1983. Pleomorphic xanthoastrocytoma: report of 5 cases. Clin. Neuropathol. 2, 188–191.

Hirose, T., Scheithauer, B.W., Lopes, M.B., et al., 1995. Tuber and subependymal giant cell astrocytoma associated with tuberous sclerosis: an immunohistochemical, ultrastructural, and immuno-electron and microscopic study. Acta Neuropathol. 90, 387–399.

Hoag, G., Sima, A.A., Rozdilsky, B., 1986. Astroblastoma revisited: a report of three cases. Acta Neuropathol. 70, 10–16.

Horst, E., Micke, O., Romppainen, M.L., et al., 2000. Radiation therapy approach in gliomatosis cerebri – case reports and literature review. Acta Oncol. 39, 747–751.

Hori, A., Weiss, R., Schaake, T., 1988. Ganglioglioma containing osseous tissue and neurofibrillary tangles. Arch. Pathol. Lab. Med. 112, 653–655.

Hosokawa, Y., Tsuchihashi, Y., Okabe, H., et al., 1991. Pleomorphic xanthoastrocytoma. Ultrastructural, immunohistochemical, and DNA cytofluorometric study of a case. Cancer 68, 853–859.

Hoving, E.W., Kros, J.M., Groninger, E., et al., 2008. Desmoplastic infantile ganglioglioma with a malignant course. J. Neurosurg. Pediatrics 1, 95–98.

Hunt, S.J., Johnson, P.C., 1989. Melanotic ganglioglioma of the pineal region. Acta Neuropathol. 79, 222–225.

Husain, A.N., Leestma, J.E., 1986. Cerebral astroblastoma: immunohistochemical and ultrastructural features. Case report. J. Neurosurg. 64, 657–661.

Iida, M., Tsujimoto, S., Nakayama, H., et al., 2008. Ultrastructural study of neuronal and related tumors in the ventricles. Brain Tumor Pathol. 25, 19–23.

Im, S.H., Chung, C.K., Cho, B.K., et al., 2002a. Intracranial ganglioglioma: preoperative characteristics and oncologic outcome after surgery. J. Neurooncol. 59, 173–183.

Im, S.H., Chung, C.K., Cho, B.K., et al., 2002b. Supratentorial ganglioglioma and epilepsy: postoperative seizure outcome. J. Neurooncol. 57, 59–66.

Inoue, T., Nishimura, S., Hayashi, N., et al., 2007. Ectopic recurrence of dysplastic gangliocytoma of the cerebellum (Lhermitte-Duclos disease): a case report. Brain Tumor. Pathol. 24, 25–29.

Isidro, M.L., Iglesias Diaz, P., Matias-Guiu, X., et al., 2005. Acromegaly due to a growth hormone-releasing hormone-secreting intracranial gangliocytoma. J. Endocrinol. Invest. 28, 162–165.

Issidorides, M.R., Arvanitis, D., 1993. Histochemical marker of human catecholamine neurons in ganglion cells and processes of a temporal lobe ganglioglioma. Surg. Neurol. 39, 66–71.

Itoh, Y., Yagishita, S., Chiba, Y., 1987. Cerebral gangliocytoma. An ultrastructural study. Acta Neuropathol. 74, 169–178.

Iwaki, T., Fukui, M., Kondo, A., et al., 1987. Epithelial properties of pleomorphic xanthoastrocytomas determined in ultrastructural and immunohistochemical studies. Acta Neuropathol. 74, 142–150.

Izukawa, D., Lach, B., Benoit, B., 1988. Gangliocytoma of the cerebellum: ultrastructure and immunohistochemistry. Neurosurgery 22, 576–581.

Jacob, J.T., Cohen-Gadol, A.A., Scheithauer, B.W., et al., 2005. Intramedullary spinal cord gangliocytoma: case report and a review of the literature. Neurosurg. Rev. 28, 326–329.

Jansen, G.H., Troost, D., Dingemans, K.P., 1990. Polar spongioblastoma: an immunohistochemical and electron microscopical study. Acta Neuropathol. 81, 228–232.

Javahery, R.J., Davidson, L., Fangusaro, J., et al., 2009. Aggressive variant of a papillary glioneuronal tumor. Report of 2 cases. J. Neurosurg. Pediatrics 3, 46–52.

Jay, V., Squire, J., Becker, L.E., et al., 1994. Malignant transformation in a ganglioglioma with anaplastic neuronal and astrocytic components. Report of a case with flow cytometric and cytogenetic analysis. Cancer 73, 2862–2868.

Jea, A., Ragheb, J., Morrison, G., 2002. Unique presentation of pleomorphic xanthoastrocytoma as a lytic skull lesion in an eight-year-old girl. Pediatr. Neurosurg. 37, 254–257.

Jelinek, J., Smirniotopoulos, J.G., Paarisi, J.E., et al., 1990. Lateral ventricular neoplasms of the brain: differential diagnosis based on clinical, CT, and MR findings. Am. J. Neuroradiol. 11, 567–574.

• Jensen, R.L., Caamano, E., Jensen, E.M., et al., 2006. Development of contrast enhancement after long-term observation of a dysembryoplastic neuroepithelial tumor. J. Neurooncol. 78, 59–62.

Johannsson, J.H., Rekate, H.L., Roessmann, U., 1981. Gangliogliomas: pathological and clinical correlation. J. Neurosurg. 54, 58–63.

Johnson, M.D., Jennings, M.T., Lavin, P., et al., 1995. Ganglioglioma of the pineal gland: clinical and radiographic response to stereotactic radiosurgical ablation. J. Child. Neurol. 10, 247–249.

Johnson, M.D., Jennings, M.T., Toms, S.T., 2001. Oligodendroglial ganglioglioma with anaplastic features arising from the thalamus. Pediatr. Neurosurg. 34, 301–305.

Johnson, M., Pace, J., Burroughs, J.F., 2006. Fourth ventricle rosette-forming glioneuronal tumor. Case report. J. Neurosurg. 105, 129–131.

Jones, M.C., Drut, R., Raglia, G., 1983. Pleomorphic xanthoastrocytoma: a report of two cases. Pediatr. Pathol. 1, 459–467.

• Josan, V., Smith, P., Kornberg, A., et al., 2007. Development of a pilocytic astrocytoma in a dysembryoplastic neuroepithelial tumor. Case report. J. Neurosurg. 106, 509–512.

Joseph, V., Wells, A., Kuo, Y.H., et al., 2008. The 'rosette-forming glioneuronal tumor' of the fourth ventricle. Neuropathology 29, 309–314.

Jozwiak, S., Kwiatkowski, D., Kotulska, K., et al., 2004. Tuberin and hamartin expression is reduced in the majority of subependymal giant cell astrocytomas in tuberous sclerosis complex consistent with a two-hit model of pathogenesis. J. Child Neurol. 19, 102–106.

Kalyan-Raman, U.P., Olivero, W.C., 1987. Ganglioglioma: a correlative clinicopathological and radiological study of ten surgically treated cases with follow-up. Neurosurgery 20, 428–433.

Kang, D.H., Lee, C.H., Hwang, S.H., et al., 2007. Anaplastic ganglioglioma in a middle-aged woman: a case report with a review of the literature. J. Korean Med. Sci. 22 (Suppl.), S139–S144.

Kawai, K., Takahashi, H., Ikuta, F., et al., 1987. The occurrence of catecholamine neurons in a parietal lobe ganglioglioma. Cancer 60, 1532–1536.

Kaye, A.H., Laws, E.R., 1995. Brain tumors: an encyclopedic approach. Churchill Livingstone, Edinburgh.

Kepes, J.J., Rubinstein, L.J., Eng, L.F., 1979. Pleomorphic xanthoastrocytoma: a distinctive meningocerebral glioma of young subjects with relatively favorable prognosis. A study of 12 cases. Cancer 44, 1839–1852.

Kepes, J.J., 1989. Glioblastoma multiforme masquerading as a pleomorphic xanthoastrocytoma. Childs Nerv. Syst. 5, 127.

Kerkovsky, M., Zitterbart, K., Svoboda, K., et al., 2008. Central neurocytoma: the neuroradiological perspective. Childs Nerv. Syst. 24, 1361–1369.

Khaddage, A., Chambonniere, M.L., Morrison, A.L., et al., 2004. Desmoplastic infantile ganglioglioma: a rare tumor with an unusual presentation. Ann. Diagn. Pathol. 8, 280–283.

Kilickesmez, O., Sanal, H.T., Haholu, A., et al., 2005. Coexistence of pleomorphic xanthoastrocytoma with Sturge-Weber syndrome: MRI features. Pediatr. Radiol. 35, 910–913.

Kim, D.S., Park, S.Y., Lee, S.P., 2004. Astroblastoma: a case report. J. Korean Med. Sci. 19, 772–776.

Kim, D.G., Chi, J.G., Park, S.H., et al., 1992. Intraventricular neurocytoma: clinicopathological analysis of seven cases. J. Neurosurg. 76, 759–765.

Kim, D.G., Yang, H.J., Park, I.A., et al., 1998. Gliomatosis cerebri: clinical features, treatment, and prognosis. Acta Neurochir (Wien) 140, 755–762.

Kim, H.S., Lee, H.K., Jeong, A.K., et al., 2001. Supratentorial ganglio-cytoma mimicking extra-axial tumor: a report of two cases. Korean J. Radiol. 2, 108–112.

Kirkpatrick, P.J., Honavar, M., Janota, I., et al., 1993. Control of temporal lobe epilepsy following en bloc resection of low-grade tumors. J. Neurosurg. 78, 19–25.

Kleihues, P., Burger, P.C., Scheithauer, B.W., et al., 1993. Histological typing of tumours of the central nervous system. Springer-Verlag, Berlin.

Kleihues, P., Cavenee, W.K., and International Agency for Research on Cancer, 2000. Pathology and genetics of tumours of the nervous system. IARC Press, Lyon.

Klisch, J., Juengling, F., Spreer, J., et al., 2001. Lhermitte-Duclos disease: assessment with MR imaging, positron emission tomography, single-photon emission CT, and MR spectroscopy. AJNR Am. J. Neuroradiol. 22, 824–830.

Kocaoglu, M., Ors, F., Bulakbasi, N., et al., 2009. Central neurocytoma: proton MR spectroscopy and diffusion weighted MR imaging findings. Magn. Reson. Imaging 27, 434–440.

Koch, R., Scholz, M., Nelen, M.R., et al., 1999. Lhermitte-Duclos disease as a component of Cowden's syndrome. Case report and review of the literature. J. Neurosurg. 90, 776–779.

Koeller, K.K., Dillon, W.P., 1992. Dysembryoplastic neuroepithelial tumors: MR appearance. AJNR Am. J. Neuroradiol. 13, 1319–1325.

Komori, T., Scheithauer, B.W., Anthony, D.C., et al., 1998. Papillary glioneuronal tumor: a new variant of mixed neuronal-glial neoplasm. Am. J. Surg. Pathol. 22, 1171–1183.

Komori, T., Scheithauer, B.W., Hirose, T., 2002. A rosette-forming glioneuronal tumor of the fourth ventricle: infratentorial form of dysembryoplastic neuroepithelial tumor? Am. J. Surg. Pathol. 26, 582–591.

Kordek, R., Hennig, R., Jacobsen, E., et al., 2003. Papillary glioneuronal tumor–a new variant of benign mixed brain neoplasm. Pol. J. Pathol. 54, 75–78.

Kros, J.M., Vecht, C.J., Stefanko, S.Z., 1991. The pleomorphic xanthoastrocytoma and its differential diagnosis: a study of five cases. Hum. Pathol. 22, 1128–1135.

Kubota, T., Hayashi, M., Kawano, H., et al., 1991. Central neurocytoma: immunohistochemical and ultrastructural study. Acta Neuropathol. 81, 418–427.

Kubota, T., Hirano, A., Sato, K., et al., 1985. The fine structure of astroblastoma. Cancer 55, 745–750.

Kuchelmeister, K., Bergmann, M., von Wild, K., et al., 1993. Desmoplastic ganglioglioma: report of two non-infantile cases. Acta Neuropathol 85, 199–204.

Kuhajda, F.P., Mendelsohn, G., Taxy, J.B., et al., 1981. Pleomorphic xanthoastrocytoma: report of a case with light and electron microscopy. Ultrastruct. Pathol. 2, 25–32.

● Labate, A., Briellmann, R.S., Harvey, A.S., et al., 2004. Temporal lobe dysembryoplastic neuroepithelial tumour: significance of discordant interictal spikes. Epileptic. Disord. 6, 107–114.

Lagares, A., Gomez, P.A., Lobato, R.D., et al., 2001. Ganglioglioma of the brainstem: report of three cases and review of the literature. Surg. Neurol. 56, 315–324.

Lamszus, K., Makrigeorgi-Butera, M., Laas, R., et al., 2003. A 24-year-old female with a 6-month history of seizures. Brain Pathol. 13, 115–117.

Langford, L.A., Camel, M.H., 1987. Palisading patterns in cerebral neuroblastoma mimicking the primitive polar spongioblastoma. An ultrastructural study. Acta Neuropathol. 73, 13–19.

Le Marquand, H.S., Russell, D.S., 1934. A case of pubertas praecox (macrogenitosomia praecox) in a boy associated with a tumor in the floor of the third ventricle. Berkely Hosp. Rep. 3, 31–61.

Lenzi, J., Salvati, M., Raco, A., et al., 2006. Central neurocytoma: a novel appraisal of a polymorphic pathology. Our experience and a review of the literature. Neurosurg. Rev. 29, 286–292.

Levin, N., Gomori, J.M., Siegal, T., 2004. Chemotherapy as initial treatment in gliomatosis cerebri: results with temozolomide. Neurology 63, 354–356.

Liauw, S.L., Byer, J.E., Yachnis, A.T., et al., 2007. Radiotherapy after sub-totally resected or recurrent ganglioglioma. Int. J. Radiat. Oncol. Biol. Phys. 67, 244–247.

Lindboe, C.F., Cappelen, J., Kepes, J.J., 1992. Pleomorphic xanthoastrocytoma as a component of a cerebellar ganglioglioma: case report. Neurosurgery 31, 353–355.

Liu, G.T., Galetta, S.L., Rorke, L.B., et al., 1996. Gangliogliomas involving the optic chiasm. Neurology 46, 1669–1673.

Loiseau, H., Rivel, J., Vital, C., et al., 1991. [Pleomorphic xanthoastrocytoma. Apropos of 3 new cases. Review of the literature]. Neurochirurgie 37, 338–347.

Lonnrot, K., Terho, M., Kahara, V., et al., 2007. Desmoplastic infantile ganglioglioma: novel aspects in clinical presentation and genetics. Surg. Neurol. 68, 304–308.

Lopes, M.B., Altermatt, H.J., Scheithauer, B.W., et al., 1996. Immunohistochemical characterization of subependymal giant cell astrocytomas. Acta Neuropathol. 91, 368–375.

Louis, D.N., Ohgaki, H., Wiestler, O.D., et al., 2007. The 2007 WHO classification of tumours of the central nervous system. Acta Neuropathol. 114, 97–109.

Lubansu, A., Rorive, S., David, P., et al., 2004. Cerebral anaplastic pleomorphic xanthoastrocytoma with meningeal dissemination at first presentation. Childs Nerv. Syst. 20, 119–122.

Mackenzie, I.R., 1999. Central neurocytoma: histologic atypia, proliferation potential, and clinical outcome. Cancer 85, 1606–1610.

MacKenzie, J.M., 1987., Pleomorphic xanthoastrocytoma in a 62-year-old male. Neuropathol. Appl. Neurobiol. 13, 481–487.

● Maehara, T., Nariai, T., Arai, N., et al., 2004. Usefulness of [11C] methionine PET in the diagnosis of dysembryoplastic neuroepithelial tumor with temporal lobe epilepsy. Epilepsia 45, 41–45.

Maleki, M., Robitaille, Y., Bertrand, G., 1983. Atypical xanthoastrocytoma presenting as a meningioma. Surg. Neurol. 20, 235–238.

Mallucci, C., Lellouch-Tubiana, A., Salazar, C., et al., 2000. The management of desmoplastic neuroepithelial tumours in childhood. Childs Nerv. Syst. 16, 8–14.

Mapstone, T., McMichael, M., Goldthwait, D., 1991. Expression of platelet-derived growth factors, transforming growth factors, and the ros gene in a variety of primary human brain tumors. Neurosurgery 28, 216–222.

Marano, S.R., Johnson, P.C., Spetzler, R.F., 1988. Recurrent Lhermitte-Duclos disease in a child. Case report. J. Neurosurg. 69, 599–603.

Marhold, F., Preusser, M., Dietrich, W., et al., 2008. Clinicoradiological features of rosette-forming glioneuronal tumor (RGNT) of the fourth ventricle: report of four cases and literature review. J. Neurooncol. 90, 301–308.

Martin, D.S., Levy, B., Awwad, E.E., et al., 1991. Desmoplastic infantile ganglioglioma: CT and MR features. AJNR Am. J. Neuroradiol. 12, 1195–1197.

Marton, E., Feletti, A., Orvieto, E., et al., 2007. Malignant progression in pleomorphic xanthoastrocytoma: personal experience and review of the literature. J. Neurol. Sci. 252, 144–153.

Mascalchi, M., Muscas, G.C., Galli, C., et al., 1994. MRI of pleomorphic xanthoastrocytoma. Case report. Neuroradiology 36, 446–447.

McConanchie, N.S., Worthington, B.S., Cornford, E.J., et al., 1994. Review article: computed tomography and magnetic resonance in the diagnosis of intraventricular cerebral masses. Br. J. Radiol. 67, 223–243.

McCowen, K.C., Glickman, J.N., Black, P.M., et al., 1999. Gangliocytoma masquerading as a prolactinoma. Case report. J. Neurosurg. 91, 490–495.

McNatt, S.A., Gonzalez-Gomez, I., Nelson, M.D., et al., 2005. Synchronous multicentric pleomorphic xanthoastrocytoma: case report. Neurosurgery 57, E191.

Mikami, S., Kameyama, K., Takahashi, S., et al., 2008. Combined gangliocytoma and prolactinoma of the pituitary gland. Endocr. Pathol. 19, 117–121.

Miller, D.C., Koslow, M., Budzilovich, G.N., et al., 1990a. Synaptophysin: a sensitive and specific marker for ganglion cells in central nervous system neoplasms. Hum. Pathol. 21, 271–276.

Miller, G., Towfighi, J., Page, R.B., 1990b. Spinal cord ganglioglioma presenting as hydrocephalus. J. Neurooncol. 9, 147–152.

Minkin, K., Tzekov, C., Naydenov, E., et al., 2008. Cerebellar gangliocytoma presenting with hemifacial spasms: clinical report, literature review and possible mechanisms. Acta Neurochir (Wien) 150, 719–724.

Mizuno, J., Nishio, S., Barrow, D.L., et al., 1987. Ganglioglioma of the cerebellum: case report. Neurosurgery 21, 584–588.

Murata, J., Tada, M., Sawamura, Y., et al., 1999. Dysplastic gangliocytoma (Lhermitte-Duclos disease) associated with Cowden disease: report of a case and review of the literature for the genetic relationship between the two diseases. J. Neurooncol. 41, 129–136.

Nagib, M.G., Haines, S.J., Erickson, D.L., et al., 1984. Tuberous sclerosis: a review for the neurosurgeon. Neurosurgery 14, 93–98.

Nakagawa, T., Maeda, M., Kato, M., et al., 2007. A case of Lhermitte-Duclos disease presenting high FDG uptake on FDG-PET/CT. J. Neurooncol. 84, 185–188.

Nakajima, T., Kumabe, T., Shamoto, H., et al., 2006. Malignant transformation of pleomorphic xanthoastrocytoma. Acta Neurochir (Wien) 148, 67–71.

Nakamura, Y., Becker, L.E., 1983. Subependymal giant-cell tumor: astrocytic or neuronal? Acta Neuropathol. 60, 271–277.

Narayanan, V., 2003. Tuberous sclerosis complex: genetics to pathogenesis. Pediatr. Neurol. 29, 404–409.

Nelson, J., Frost, J.L., Schochet, S.S., Jr., 1987. Sudden, unexpected death in a 5-year-old boy with an unusual primary intracranial neoplasm. Ganglioglioma of the medulla. Am. J. Forensic Med. Pathol. 8, 148–152.

Newton, H.B., Dalton, J., Ray-Chaudhury, A., et al., 2008. Aggressive papillary glioneuronal tumor: case report and literature review. Clin. Neuropathol. 27, 317–324.

Nishio, S., Takatoshi, T., Takeshita, I., et al., 1988. Intraventricular neurocytoma: clinicopathological features of six cases. J. Neurosurg. 68, 665–670.

Ng, H.K., Tang, N.L., Poon, W.S., 1994. Polar spongioblastoma with cerebrospinal fluid metastases. Surg. Neurol. 41, 137–142.

Ng, T.H., Fung, C.F., Ma, L.T., 1990. The pathological spectrum of desmoplastic infantile ganglioglioma. Histopathology 16, 235–241.

Nikas, I., Anagnostara, A., Theophanopoulou, M., et al., 2004. Desmoplastic infantile ganglioglioma: MRI and histological findings case report. Neuroradiology 46, 1039–1043.

Notarianni, C., Akin, M., Fowler, M., et al., 2008. Brainstem astroblastoma: a case report and review of the literature. Surg. Neurol. 69, 201–205.

• O'Brien, D.F., Farrell, M., Delanty, N., et al., 2007. The Children's Cancer and Leukaemia Group guidelines for the diagnosis and management of dysembryoplastic neuroepithelial tumours. Br. J. Neurosurg. 21, 539–549.

Otsubo, H., Hoffman, H.J., Humphreys, R.P., et al., 1990. Evaluation, surgical approach and outcome of seizure patients with gangliogliomas. Pediatr. Neurosurg. 16, 208–212.

Padberg, G.W., Schot, J.D., Vielvoye, G.J., et al., 1991. Lhermitte-Duclos disease and Cowden disease: a single phakomatosis. Ann. Neurol. 29, 517–523.

Painter, M.J., Pang, D., Ahdab-Barmada, M., et al., 1984. Connatal brain tumors in patients with tuberous sclerosis. Neurosurgery 14, 570–573.

Palma, L., Maleci, A., Di Lorenzo, N., et al., 1985. Pleomorphic xanthoastrocytoma with 18-year survival. Case report. J. Neurosurg. 63, 808–810.

Parizel, P.M., Martin, J.J., Van Vyve, M., et al., 1991. Cerebral ganglioglioma and neurofibromatosis type I. Case report and review of the literature. Neuroradiology 33, 357–359.

Park, S., Suh, Y.L., et al., 2009. Gliomatosis cerebri: clinicopathologic study of 33 cases and comparison of mass forming and diffuse types. Clin. Neuropathol. 28, 73–82.

• Parmar, H.A., Hawkins, C., Ozelame, R., et al., 2007. Fluid-attenuated inversion recovery ring sign as a marker of dysembryoplastic neuroepithelial tumors. J. Comput. Assist. Tomogr. 31, 348–353.

Passone, E., Pizzolitto, S., D'Agostini, S., et al., 2006. Non-anaplastic pleomorphic xanthoastrocytoma with neuroradiological evidences of leptomeningeal dissemination. Childs Nerv. Syst. 22, 614–618.

Patil, A.A., McComb, R.D., Gelber, B., et al., 1990. Intraventricular neurocytoma: a report of two cases. Neurosurgery 26, 140–144.

Paulus, W., Peiffer, J., 1988. Does the pleomorphic xanthoastrocytoma exist? Problems in the application of immunological techniques to the classification of brain tumors. Acta Neuropathol. 76, 245–252.

Paulus, W., Schlote, W., Perentes, E., et al., 1992. Desmoplastic supratentorial neuroepithelial tumours of infancy. Histopathology 21, 43–49.

Perentes, E., Rubinstein, L.J., 1986. Immunohistochemical recognition of human neuroepithelial tumors by anti-Leu 7 (HNK-1) monoclonal antibody. Acta Neuropathol. 69, 227–233.

Peretti-Viton, P., Perez-Castillo A.M., Raybaud, C., et al., 1991. Magnetic resonance imaging in gangliogliomas and gangliocytomas of the nervous system. J. Neuroradiol. 18, 189–199.

Perry, A., Giannini, C., Scheithauer, B.W., et al., 1997. Composite pleomorphic xanthoastrocytoma and ganglioglioma: report of four cases and review of the literature. Am. J. Surg. Pathol. 21, 763–771.

Petropoulou, K., Whiteman, M.L., Altman, N.R., et al., 1995. CT and MRI of pleomorphic xanthoastrocytoma: unusual biologic behavior. J. Comput. Assist. Tomogr. 19, 860–865.

Pierallini, A., Bonamini, M., Di Stefano, et al., 1999. Pleomorphic xanthoastrocytoma with CT and MRI appearance of meningioma. Neuroradiology 41, 30–34.

Pimentel, J., Resende, M., Vaz, A., et al., 2008. Rosette-forming glioneuronal tumor: pathology case report. Neurosurgery 62, E1162–E1163.

Pizer, B.L., Moss, T., Oakhill, A., et al., 1995. Congenital astroblastoma: an immunohistochemical study. Case report. J. Neurosurg. 83, 550–555.

Pollock, J.M., Whitlow, C.T., Tan, H., et al., 2009. Pulsed arterial spin-labeled MR imaging evaluation of tuberous sclerosis. Am. J. Neuroradiol. 30, 815–820.

Powell, S.Z., Yachnis, A.T., Rorke, L.B., et al., 1996. Divergent differentiation in pleomorphic xanthoastrocytoma. Evidence for a neuronal element and possible relationship to ganglion cell tumors. Am. J. Surg. Pathol. 20, 80–85.

Prayson, R.A., 2000. Papillary glioneuronal tumor. Arch. Pathol. Lab. Med. 124, 1820–1823.

Preusser, M., Dietrich, W., Czech, T., et al., 2003. Rosette-forming glioneuronal tumor of the fourth ventricle. Acta Neuropathol. 106, 506–508.

Price, D.B., Miller, L.J., Drexler, S., et al., 1997. Congenital ganglioglioma: report of a case with an unusual imaging appearance. Pediatr. Radiol. 27, 748–749.

Rades, D., Fehlauer, F., Schild, S.E., 2004. Treatment of atypical neurocytomas. Cancer 100, 814–817.

Rades, D., Schild, S.E., 2006. Treatment recommendations for the various subgroups of CNs. J. Neurooncol. 77, 305–309.

Raju, G.P., Urion, D.K., Sahin, M., 2007. Neonatal subependymal giant cell astrocytoma: new case and review of the literature. Pediatr. Neurol. 36, 128–131.

• Raghavan, R., White, C.L., 3rd., Rogers, B., et al., 2000. Alpha-synuclein expression in central nervous system tumors showing neuronal or mixed neuronal/glial differentiation. J. Neuropathol. Exp. Neurol. 59, 490–494.

• Ray, W.Z., Blackburn, S.L., Casavilca-Zambrano S., et al., 2009. Clinicopathologic features of recurrent dysembryoplastic neuroepithelial tumor and rare malignant transformation: a report of 5 cases and review of the literature. J. Neurooncol. 94, 283–292.

Reeder, R.F., Saunders, R.L., Roberts, D.W., et al., 1988. Magnetic resonance imaging in the diagnosis and treatment of Lhermitte-Duclos disease (dysplastic gangliocytoma of the cerebellum). Neurosurgery 23, 240–241.

Regis, J., Bartolomei, F., de Toffol, B., et al., 2000. Gamma knife surgery for epilepsy related to hypothalamic hamartomas. Neurosurgery 47, 1343–1352.

Régis, J., Scavarda, D., Tamura, M., et al., 2006. Epilepsy related to hypothalamic hamartomas: surgical management with special reference to gamma knife surgery. Childs Nerv. Syst. 22, 881–895.

Reznik, M., Schoenen, J., 1983. Lhermitte-Duclos disease. Acta Neuropathol. 59, 88–94.

Rippe, D.J., Boyko, O.B., Radi, M., et al., 1992. MRI of temporal lobe pleomorphic xanthoastrocytoma. J. Comput. Assist. Tomogr. 16, 856–859.

Robinson, S., Cohen, A.R., 2006. Cowden disease and Lhermitte-Duclos disease: an update. Case report and review of the literature. Neurosurg. Focus 20, E6.

Rodriguez, D.L., De La Lama, A., Lopez-Ariztegui, N., et al., 2004. Treatment of central CN. Experience at single institution. Neurocirugia 15, 128–136.

Roessmann, U., Wongmongkolrit, T., 1984. Dysplastic gangliocytoma of cerebellum in a newborn. Case report. J. Neurosurg. 60, 845–847.

Romeike, B.F., Mawrin, C., 2008. Gliomatosis cerebri: growing evidence for diffuse gliomas with wide invasion. Expert Rev. Neurother. 8, 587–597.

Rommel, T., Hamer, J., 1983. Development of ganglioglioma in computed tomography. Neuroradiology 24, 237–239.

Rosenblum, M.K., 2007. The 2007 WHO Classification of Nervous System Tumors: newly recognized members of the mixed glioneuronal group. Brain Pathol. 17, 308–313.

Rosenfeld, J.V., Harvey, A.S., et al., 2001. Transcallosal resection of hypothalamic hamartomas, with control of seizures, in children with gelastic epilepsy. Neurosurgery 48, 108–118.

Roski, R.A., Roessmann, U., Spetzler, R.F., et al., 1981. Clinical and pathological study of dysplastic gangliocytoma. Case report. J. Neurosurg. 55, 318–321.

Rosner, M., Hanneder, M., Siegel, N., et al., 2008. The tuberous sclerosis gene products hamartin and tuberin are multifunctional proteins with a wide spectrum of interacting partners. Mutat. Res. 658, 234–246.

Rout, P., Santosh, V., Mahadevan, A., et al., 2002. Desmoplastic infantile ganglioglioma –clinicopathological and immunohistochemical study of four cases. Childs Nerv. Syst. 18, 463–467.

Rubinstein, L.J., Armed Forces Institute of Pathology (U.S.) and Universities Associated for Research and Education in Pathology, 1972. Tumors of the central nervous system. Armed Forces Institute of Pathology, Washington.

Rubinstein, L.J., Herman, M.M., 1972. A light- and electron-microscopic study of a temporal-lobe ganglioglioma. J. Neurol. Sci. 16, 27–48.

Rubinstein, L.J., Herman, M.M., 1989. The astroblastoma and its possible cytogenic relationship to the tanycyte. An electron microscopic, immunohistochemical, tissue- and organ-culture study. Acta Neuropathol. 78, 472–483.

Rumana, C.S., Valadka, A.B., 1998. Radiation therapy and malignant degeneration of benign supratentorial gangliogliomas. Neurosurgery 42, 1038–1043.

Russell, D.S., Rubinstein, L.J., 1989. Pathology of tumours of the nervous system. Williams & Wilkins, Baltimore, MD.

Russo, C.P., Katz, D.S., Corona, R.J., Jr., et al., 1995. Gangliocytoma of the cervicothoracic spinal cord. AJNR Am. J. Neuroradiol. 16, 889–891.

Sabin, H.I., Lidov, H.G., Kendall, B.E., et al., 1988. Lhermitte-Duclos disease (dysplastic gangliocytoma): a case report with CT, Acta MRI Neurochir (Wien) 93, 149–153.

Safavi-Abbasi, S., Di Rocco, F., Chantra, K., et al., 2007. Posterior cranial fossa gangliogliomas. Skull Base 17, 253–264.

Saikali, S., Le Strat, A., Heckly, A., et al., 2005. Multicentric pleomorphic xanthoastrocytoma in a patient with neurofibromatosis type 1. Case report and review of the literature. J. Neurosurg. 102, 376–381.

Sanson, M., Cartalat-Carel, S., Taillibert, S., et al., 2004. Initial chemotherapy in gliomatosis cerebri. Neurology 63, 2270–2275.

Sarkar, C., Roy, S., Bhatia, S., 1990. Xanthomatous change in tumours of glial origin. Indian J. Med. Res. 92, 324–331.

Sasaki, A., Hirato, J., Nakazato, Y., et al., 1996. Recurrent anaplastic ganglioglioma: pathological characterization of tumor cells. Case report. J. Neurosurg. 84, 1055–1059.

Sawyer, J.R., Thomas, E.L., Roloson, G.J. et al., 1992. Telomeric associations evolving to ring chromosomes in a recurrent pleomorphic xanthoastrocytoma. Cancer Genet. Cytogenet. 60, 152–157.

Scheithauer, B.W., Silva, A.I., Ketterling, R.P., et al., 2009. Rosette-forming glioneuronal tumor: report of a chiasmal-optic nerve example in neurofibromatosis type 1: Special pathology report. Neurosurgery 64, E771–E772.

Schiffer, D., Cravioto, H., Giordana, M.T., et al., 1993. Is polar spongioblastoma a tumor entity? J. Neurosurg. 78, 587–591.

Schmidt, M.H., Gottfried, O.N., von Koch, C.S., et al., 2004. Central neurocytoma: a review. J. Neurooncol. 66, 377–384.

Schulze-Bonhage, A., Ostertag, C., 2007. Treatment options for gelastic epilepsy due to hypothalamic hamartoma: interstitial radiosurgery. Semin. Pediatr. Neurol. 14, 80–87.

Selch, M.T., Goy, B.W., Lee, S.P., et al., 1998. Gangliogliomas: experience with 34 patients and review of the literature. Am. J. Clin. Oncol. 21, 557–564.

Serri, O., Berthelet, F., Belair, M., et al., 2008. An unusual association of a sellar gangliocytoma with a prolactinoma. Pituitary 11, 85–87.

Sharma, M.C., Rathore, A., Karak, A.K., et al., 1998. A study of proliferative markers in central neurocytoma. Pathology 30, 355–359.

Sharma, M.C., Deb, P., Sharma, S., et al., 2006. Neurocytoma: a comprehensive review. Neurosurg. Rev. 29, 270–285.

Sharma, S., Sarkar, C., Gaikwad, S., et al., 2005. Primary neurocytoma of the spinal cord: a case report and review of the literature. J. Neurooncol. 74, 47–52.

Sharma, M.C., Ralte, A.M., Gaekwad, S., et al., 2004. Subependymal giant cell astrocytoma – a clinicopathological study of 23 cases with special emphasis on histogenesis. Pathol. Oncol. Res. 10, 219–224.

Shepherd, C.W.,, Scheithauer, B.W., Gomez, A.K., et al., 1991. Subependymal giant cell astrocytoma: a clinical pathological, and flow cytometric study. Neurosurgery 28, 864–868.

Sherazi, Z.A., 1998. Gangliocytoma–magnetic resonance imaging characteristics. Singapore Med. J. 39, 373–375.

Siddique, K., Zagardo, M., Gujrati, M., et al., 2002. Ganglioglioma presenting as a meningioma: case report and review of the literature. Neurosurgery 50, 1133–1136.

Silver, J.M., Rawlings, C.E., 3rd, Rossitch, E., Jr., et al., 1991. Ganglioglioma: a clinical study with long-term follow-up. Surg. Neurol. 35, 261–266.

Smith, R.R., Grossman, R.I., Goldberg, H.I., et al., 1989. MR imaging of Lhermitte-Duclos disease: a case report. AJNR Am. J. Neuroradiol. 10, 187–189.

Soylemezoglu, F., Scheithauer, B.W., Esteve, J., et al., 1997. Atypical central neurocytoma. J. Neuropathol. Exp. Neurol. 56, 551–556.

Soylemezoglu, F., Onder, S., Tezel, G.G., et al., 2003. Neuronal nuclear antigen (NeuN): a new tool in the diagnosis of central neurocytoma. Pathol. Res. Pract. 199, 463–468.

Sperner, J., Gottschalk, J., Neumann, K., et al., 1994. Clinical, radiological and histological findings in desmoplastic infantile ganglioglioma. Childs Nerv. Syst. 10, 458–463.

Stapleton, S.R., Wilkins, P.R., Bell, B.A., 1992. Recurrent dysplastic cerebellar gangliocytoma (Lhermitte-Duclos disease) presenting with subarachnoid haemorrhage. Br. J. Neurosurg. 6, 153–156.

Starceski, P.J., Lee, P.A., Albright, A.L., et al., 1990. Hypothalamic hamartomas and sexual precosity. Evaluation of treatment options. Am. J. Dis. Childhood 144, 225–228.

Steinberg, G.K., Shuer, L.M., Conley, F.K., et al., 1985. Evolution and outcome in malignant astroglial neoplasms of the cerebellum. J. Neurosurg. 62, 9–17.

Stewart, L., Steinbok, P., Daaboul, J., 1998. Role of surgical resection in the treatment of hypothalamic hamartomas causing precocious puberty. Report of six cases. J. Neurosurg. 88, 340–345.

Striano, S., Striano, P., Sarappa, C., et al., 2005. The clinical spectrum and natural history of gelastic epilepsy-hypothalamic hamartoma syndrome. Seizure 14, 232–239.

Sugita, Y., Kepes, J.J., Shigemori, M., et al., 1990. Pleomorphic xanthoastrocytoma with desmoplastic reaction: angiomatous variant. Report of two cases. Clin. Neuropathol. 9, 271–278.

Sugiyama, K., Goishi, J., Sogabe, T., et al., 1992. Ganglioglioma of the optic pathway. A case report. Surg. Neurol. 37, 22–25.

Sutton, L.N., Packer, R.J., Rorke, L.B., et al., 1983. Cerebral gangliogliomas during childhood. Neurosurgery 13, 124–128.

Sutton, L.N., Packer, R.J., Zimmerman, R.A., et al., 1987. Cerebral gangliogliomas of childhood. Prog. Exp. Tumor. Res. 30, 239–246.

Suzuki, T., Izumoto, S., Fujimoto, Y., et al., 2005. Clinicopathological study of cellular proliferation and invasion in gliomatosis cerebri:

important role of neural cell adhesion molecule L1 in tumor invasion. J. Clin. Pathol. 58, 166–171.

Tacconi, L., Thom, M., Symon, L., 1997. Central neurocytoma: a clinico-pathological study of five cases. Br. J. Neurosurg. 11, 286–291.

Taillibert, S., Chodkiewicz, C., Laigle-Donadey, F., et al., 2006. Gliomatosis cerebri: a review of 296 cases from the ANOCEF database and the literature. J. Neurooncol. 76, 201–205.

Takahashi, H., Ikuta, F., Tsuchida, T., et al., 1987. Ultrastructural alterations of neuronal cells in a brain stem ganglioglioma. Acta Neuropathol. 74, 307–312.

Takahashi, H., Wakabayashi, K., Kawai, K., et al., 1989. Neuroendocrine markers in central nervous system neuronal tumors (gangliocytoma and ganglioglioma). Acta Neuropathol. 77, 237–243.

Takao, H., Nakagawa, K., Ohtomo, K., 2003. Central neurocytoma with craniospinal dissemination. J. Neurooncol. 61, 255–259.

Takei, H., Dauser, R., Su, J., et al., 2007. Anaplastic ganglioglioma arising from a Lhermitte-Duclos-like lesion. J. Neurosurg. 107, 137–142.

Takeshima, H., Kawahara, Y., Hirano, H., et al., 2003. Postoperative regression of desmoplastic infantile gangliogliomas: report of two cases. Neurosurgery 53, 979–984.

Tamburrini, G., Colosimo, C., Jr., Giangaspero, F., et al., 2003. Desmoplastic infantile ganglioglioma. Childs Nerv. Syst. 19, 292–297.

Tampieri, D., Moumdjian, R., Melanson, D., et al., 1991. Intracerebral gangliogliomas in patients with partial complex seizures: CT and MR imaging findings. AJNR Am. J. Neuroradiol. 12, 749–755.

Tan, C.C., Gonzales, M., Veitch, A., 2008. Clinical implications of the infratentorial rosette-forming glioneuronal tumor: case report. Neurosurgery 63, E175–E176.

Tan, T.C., Ho, L.C., 2007. Lhermitte-Duclos disease associated with Cowden syndrome. J. Clin. Neurosci. 14, 801–805.

Tanaka, Y., Yokoo, H., Komori, T., et al., 2005. A distinct pattern of Olig2-positive cellular distribution in papillary glioneuronal tumors: a manifestation of the oligodendroglial phenotype? Acta Neuropathol. 110, 39–47.

Taratuto, A.L., Monges, J., Lylyk, P., et al., 1984. Superficial cerebral astrocytoma attached to dura. Report of six cases in infants. Cancer 54, 2505–2512.

Tekkok, I.H., Sav, A., 2004. Anaplastic pleomorphic xanthoastrocytomas. Review of the literature with reference to malignancy potential. Pediatr. Neurosurg. 40, 171–181.

Thomas, B., Krishnamoorthy, T., Radhakrishnan, V.V., et al., 2007. Advanced MR imaging in Lhermitte-Duclos disease: moving closer to pathology and pathophysiology. Neuroradiology 49, 733–738.

Tien, R.D., Tuori, S.L., Pulkingham, N., et al., 1992. Ganglioglioma with leptomeningeal and subarachnoid spread: results of CT, MR, and PET imaging. AJR Am. J. Roentgenol. 159, 391–393.

Tonn, J.C., Paulus, W., Warmuth-Metz, M., et al., 1997. Pleomorphic xanthoastrocytoma: report of six cases with special consideration of diagnostic and therapeutic pitfalls. Surg. Neurol. 47, 162–169.

Trehan, G., Bruge, H., Vinchon, M., et al., 2004. MR imaging in the diagnosis of desmoplastic infantile tumor: retrospective study of six cases. AJNR Am. J. Neuroradiol. 25, 1028–1033.

Tsukayama, C., Arakawa, Y., 2002. A papillary glioneuronal tumor arising in an elderly woman: a case report. Brain Tumor. Pathol. 19, 35–39.

Tuli, S., Provias, J.P., Bernstein, M., 1997. Lhermitte-Duclos disease: literature review and novel treatment strategy. Can J. Neurol. Sci. 24, 155–160.

Tureyen, K., Senol, N., Sav, A., 2008. Gangliocytoma associated with focal cortical dysplasia in a young-adult: a case report. Turk. Neurosurg. 18, 259–263.

Tyler-Kabara, E., Kondziolka, D., Flickinger, J.C., et al., 2001. Stereotactic radiosurgery for residual neurocytoma. Report of four cases. J. Neurosurg. 95, 879–882.

Vajtai, I., Arnold, M., Kappeler, A., et al., 2007. Rosette-forming glioneuronal tumor of the fourth ventricle: report of two cases with a differential diagnostic overview. Pathol. Res. Pract. 203, 613–619.

Vajtai, I., Kappeler, A., Lukes, A., et al., 2006. Papillary glioneuronal tumor. Pathol. Res. Pract. 202, 107–112.

Van Calenbergh, F., Vantomme, N., Flamen, P., et al., 2006. Lhermitte-Duclos disease: 11C-methionine positron emission tomography data in 4 patients. Surg. Neurol. 65, 293–297.

VandenBerg, S.R., Herman, M.M., Rubinstein, L.J., 1987a. Embryonal central neuroepithelial tumors: current concepts and future challenges. Cancer Metastasis Rev. 5, 343–365.

VandenBerg, S.R., May, E.E., Rubinstein, L.J., et al., 1987b. Desmoplastic supratentorial neuroepithelial tumors of infancy with divergent differentiation potential ('desmoplastic infantile gangliogliomas'). Report on 11 cases of a distinctive embryonal tumor with favorable prognosis. J. Neurosurg. 66, 58–71.

Vantomme, N., Van Calenbergh, F., Goffin, J., et al., 2001. Lhermitte-Duclos disease is a clinical manifestation of Cowden's syndrome. Surg. Neurol. 56, 201–205.

Vaquero, J., Coca, S., 2007. Atypical papillary glioneuronal tumor. J. Neurooncol. 83, 319–323.

Vogt, H., 1908. Zur pathologie und pathologishen Anatomie der verschiedenen idiotie-formen: Tuberose sklerose. Monatsschr. Psychiatry Neurol. 24, 106–150.

Wacker, M.R., Cogen, P.H., Etzell, J.E., et al., 1992. Diffuse leptomeningeal involvement by a ganglioglioma in a child. Case report. J. Neurosurg. 77, 302–306.

Weldon-Linne, C.M., Victor, T.A., Groothuis, D.R., et al., 1983. Pleomorphic xanthoastrocytoma. Ultrastructural and immunohistochemical study of a case with a rapidly fatal outcome following surgery. Cancer 52, 2055–2063.

• Whittle, I.R., Dow, G.R., Lammie, G.A., et al., 1999. Dsyembryoplastic neuroepithelial tumour with discrete bilateral multifocality: further evidence for a germinal origin. Br. J. Neurosurg. 13, 508–511.

Whittle, I.R., Gordon, A., Misra, B.K., et al., 1989. Pleomorphic xanthoastrocytoma. Report of four cases. J. Neurosurg. 70, 463–468.

Williams, S.R., Joos, B.W., Parker, J.C., et al., 2008. Papillary glioneuronal tumor: a case report and review of the literature. Ann. Clin. Lab. Sci. 38, 287–292.

Wolansky, L.J., Malantic, G.P., Heary, R., et al., 1996. Preoperative MRI diagnosis of Lhermitte-Duclos disease: case report with associated enlarged vessel and syrinx. Surg. Neurol. 45, 470–476.

Wu, C.H., Chai, J.W., Lee, C.H., et al., 2006. Assessment with magnetic resonance imaging and spectroscopy in Lhermitte-Duclos disease. J. Chin. Med. Assoc. 69, 338–342.

Yagishita, S., Kawano, N., Oka, H., et al., 1996. Palisades in cerebral astrocytoma simulating the so-called polar spongioblastoma: a histological, immunohistochemical, and electron microscopic study of an adult case. Noshuyo Byori 13, 21–25.

Yang, G.F., Wu, S.Y., Zhang, L.J., et al., 2009. Imaging findings of extraventricular neurocytoma: report of 3 cases and review of the literature. Am. J. Neuroradiol. 30, 581–585.

Yeh, D.J., Hessler, R.B., Stevens, E.A., et al., 2003. Composite pleomorphic xanthoastrocytoma-ganglioglioma presenting as a suprasellar mass: case report. Neurosurgery 52, 1465–1469.

Yesildag, A., Baykal, B., Ayata, A., et al., 2005. Lhermitte-Duclos disease associated with neurofibromatosis type-1 and non-ossifying fibroma. Acta Radiol. 46, 97–100.

Yin, X.L., Hui, A.B., Liong, E.C., et al., 2002. Genetic imbalances in pleomorphic xanthoastrocytoma detected by comparative genomic hybridization and literature review. Cancer Genet. Cytogenet. 132, 14–19.

Yoshino, M.T., Lucio, R., 1992. Pleomorphic xanthoastrocytoma. AJNR Am. J. Neuroradiol. 13, 1330–1332.

Zentner, J., Wolf, H.K., Ostertun, B., et al., 1994. Gangliogliomas: clinical, radiological, and histopathological findings in 51 patients. J. Neurol. Neurosurg. Psychiatry 57, 1497–1502.

Zhang, D., Henning, T.D., Zou, L.G., et al., 2008. Intracranial ganglioglioma: clinicopathological and MRI findings in 16 patients. Clin. Radiol. 63, 80–91.

Zorzi, F., Facchetti, F., Baronchelli, C., et al., 1992. Pleomorphic xanthoastrocytoma: an immunohistochemical study of three cases. Histopathology 20, 267–269.

Medulloblastoma and primitive neuroectodermal tumors

27

Ryan DeMarchi, Michael Ellis, Cynthia Hawkins, and James T. Rutka

Introduction

Medulloblastoma (MB) is a malignant neuroectodermal tumor which arises from the cerebellum. MB, along with other infratentorial primitive neuroectodermal tumors (iPNETs) are among the most common childhood malignancies and are the leading cause of cancer-related deaths in children. Significant advances in diagnostic imaging, surgical management, radiation therapy and chemotherapy regimens in recent decades have shaped the current multi-modal management strategies. More recently, research pertaining to clinical and molecular markers has been used in attempts to predict patient survival as well as delineate novel therapeutic targets. Despite such advances, survival outcomes have improved only slightly in recent years and survivors continue to experience long-term morbidity as a result of our treatments.

Epidemiology

Brain tumors are the second most common malignancy affecting the pediatric population and account for more childhood deaths than any other solid tumor (Gurney 1999; Gurney et al 1999). MB accounts for up to 25% of all brain tumors in children and is the most common malignant pediatric tumor of the posterior fossa (Rutka 1997; Agerlin et al 1999; Davis et al 2001). A recent, large retrospective review found MB to be one of the most common central nervous system tumors diagnosed in the 1st year of life, occurring in 12.2% of children (Larouche et al 2007). Population-based studies from countries in North America, Europe, and Asia have reported highly variable overall incidence rates and while the incidence of MB appears to have been on the decline, this observation has been debated (Helseth & Mørk 1989; Lannering et al 1990; Thorne et al 1994; Kuratsu & Ushio 1996; Farinotti et al 1998; Gjerris et al 1998; Agerlin et al 1999; Hjalmars et al 1999).

The mean age at diagnosis is approximately 6–9 years of age. MB has displayed a male preponderance (M:F ratio 1.5 to 2:1) in most series (Farwell et al 1984; Agerlin et al 1999; Packer et al 1999a; Gurney & Kadan-Lottick 2001). While it is less common to encounter MB in adulthood, up to 30% of all cases occur in this age group (Cervoni et al 1994). The annual incidence of MB in adults is estimated at 0.05/100 000 per year (Farwell & Flannery 1987; Carrie et al 1994; Giordana et al 1999).

Clinical presentation

The clinical presentation of children with MB is variable and depends largely on the child's age, tumor size and rate of growth. Most patients present with a short clinical history of progressive symptoms, which are present for <3 months in approximately 75% of cases and <1.5 months in 50% of cases (Park et al 1983). MB growth leads to obstruction of CSF pathways, and the resultant hydrocephalus is responsible for a significant proportion of clinical presentations. In infants and young children, the diagnosis is suspected in the clinical setting of irritability, loss of appetite, weight loss and failure to thrive. The most common constellation of signs and symptoms of MB is the triad of headache, lethargy and vomiting. These can give rise to other signs of increased intracranial pressure such as drowsiness, sun-setting, full fontanelle, and increasing head circumference. Older children may complain of symptoms such as neck stiffness, dizziness or diplopia and may display ataxia, nystagmus, dysmetria or cranial nerve palsies on examination. A lateral cerebellar syndrome is occasionally seen with desmoplastic MB as they tend to originate more laterally within the cerebellum. A head tilt or abnormal posture signifies descent of the cerebellar tonsils into the foramen magnum with meningeal irritation or compression of the C1 or C2 nerve roots.

Spinal metastasis at initial presentation may present with back or neck pain, focal weakness, numbness or bowel and bladder complaints depending on the level of involvement. Although disseminated disease is common at initial presentation, less than 5% of MB patients present with symptomatic metastasis (Kombogiorgas et al 2007).

Diagnostic evaluation

Multiple diagnostic imaging methods can be used to evaluate MB. The typical appearance of this tumor on non-contrast CT scan of the brain is a homogeneous, well-defined, hyperdense midline lesion with varying subsequent degrees of hydrocephalus and peri-tumoral edema. Radiographic findings such as calcification, necrosis, hemorrhage and intra-tumoral cysts are seen in a minority of MB cases. This tumor typically displays uniform enhancement following contrast administration (Blaser & Harwood-Nash 1996).

MRI is the imaging modality of choice for the diagnosis, preoperative work-up and staging of MB patients (Fig. 27.1). If the diagnosis of MB is suspected, the current standard of care involves obtaining a preoperative non-contrast and contrast-enhanced MRI of the entire cranial-spinal axis (Bartels et al 2006). Furthermore, it is important to obtain an early postoperative MRI (within 48 h) to assess tumor residual and determine subsequent staging as this will guide further management.

The usual MRI appearance of MB is a hypo- to iso-intense mass on T1-weighted images and iso- to hyper-intense on T2-weighted images (Meyers et al 1992; Vézina and Packer 1994). Gadolinium enhancement is typically uniform, but slight heterogeneity is not uncommon (Meyers et al 1992; Mueller et al 1992; Vézina and Packer 1994). MRI detects intra-tumoral cysts in approximately 75% of cases as it is a more sensitive imaging modality compared with CT scan (Mueller et al 1992). Diffusion-weighted imaging (DWI) typically demonstrates restricted diffusion, and in combination with proton MR spectroscopy (MRS) can help to discriminate MB from other posterior fossa tumors (Davies et al 2008; Koral et al 2008). Spinal dissemination and metastasis are identified on contrast enhanced T1-weighted images as foci of enhancement (Fig. 27.2).

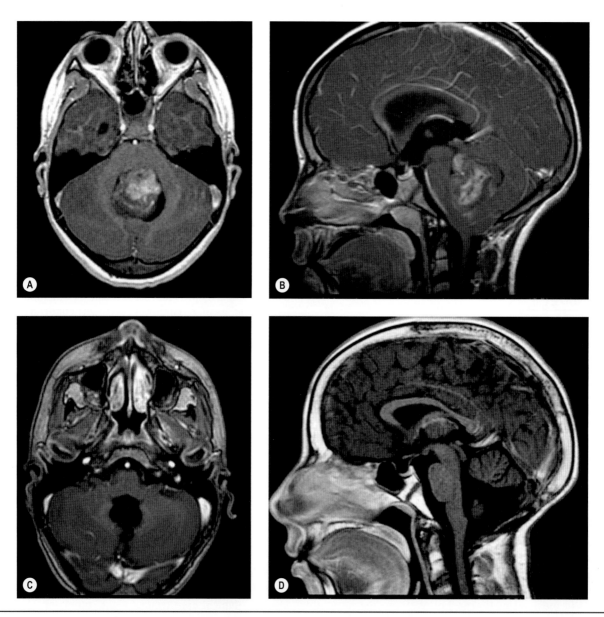

Figure 27.1 A 7-year-old male with a 1 month history of nausea, vomiting, and headache. (A) Axial gadolinium-enhanced MR showing midline posterior fossa tumor filling the fourth ventricle. (B) Sagittal MRI with contrast showing extent of lesion. Note tonsils descending through the foramen magnum. (C) Postoperative axial, contrast-enhanced MRI 5 years after surgery showing complete tumor resection. (D) Postoperative sagittal MRI showing no evidence of residual tumor, and a stable posterior fossa.

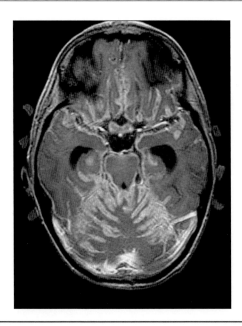

Figure 27.2 Metastatic medulloblastoma with diffuse, leptomeningeal seeding. Contrast-enhanced axial MRI scan.

Pathology

MB was initially included in Rorke's broad classification of PNETs, which included retinoblastoma, neuroblastoma and pineoblastoma (Rorke 1983). This classification system focused largely on the pattern of cellular differentiation, placing less emphasis on tumor location. Subsequent gene expression studies have demonstrated that MB is in fact a separate entity, distinct from supratentorial PNETs (Pomeroy et al 2002). Recent updates to the World Health Organization (WHO) classification of CNS tumors have modified the classification of MB (Louis et al 2007b). The revised classification considers all MB to be WHO grade IV tumors. The five major histologic variants recognized include the classic, desmoplastic/nodular, MB extensive nodularity (MBEN), anaplastic and large-cell sub-types (Fig. 27.3).

On gross pathologic inspection, these tumors appear as pinkish-grey masses arising from the medullary velum and filling the fourth ventricle. Small vessels within the tumor capsule can often be seen, occasionally with associated hemorrhage. If CSF dissemination has occurred by the time of operation, the surface of the cerebellum may appear white and 'sugar coated'. Some MBs are firm, discrete masses, while others are soft and friable.

Immunohistochemical analysis displays neuronal differentiation in a majority of cases, characterized by immunopositivity for synaptophysin, neuron-specific enolase, and class III tubulin (Coffin et al 1990; Maraziotis et al 1992; Washiyama et al 1996; Louis et al 2007b). Glial differentiation and GFAP expression also occur, but this is a less consistent finding (Palmer et al 1981; Keles et al 1992; Maraziotis et al 1992).

The classic sub-type is most common and accounts for up to 80% of all MB. Histopathological examination reveals a highly cellular tumor with round cells, little cytoplasm, and basophilic, hyperchromatic nuclei (Louis et al 2007b). A high mitotic index may be encountered, as can areas of focal necrosis. Homer–Wright rosettes are a characteristic feature, which is often abundant (Louis et al 2007b). Cellular differentiation along glial or neuronal lineage is seen in up to 50% of cases (Packer et al 1984; Janss et al 1996).

Desmoplastic/nodular MB accounts for approximately 15–20% of cases, though this range has shown considerable variation in the literature (McManamy et al 2007). These tumors are often located more laterally within the cerebellum and originate close to the pia-arachnoid surface (Burger & Fuller 1991). Microscopically, they are characterized by interrupted pale, reticulin-free nodules surrounded by reticulin-stained collagen fibers (Louis et al 2007b).

MBEN occurs primarily in children under 3 years of age and is associated with a more favorable prognosis (Giangaspero et al 1999; Suresh et al 2004). It is characterized by a 'grape-like' appearance of expanded reticulin-free nodules. The histopathological appearance of this sub-type is similar to that of the desmoplastic/nodular variant, but has significantly reduced reticulin-stained fibers between nodules (Louis et al 2007b).

Anaplastic MB is associated with a very poor prognosis (Eberhart et al 2002). While a degree of anaplasia may exist in all types of MB, this sub-type is characterized by significant nuclear pleomorphism, nuclear molding, and high mitotic activity (Louis et al 2007a,b).

The large cell variant comprises approximately 4% of all MBs. This variant shares many features with the anaplastic MB, including a poor prognosis. Microscopically, the large cell sub-type is characterized by large round nuclei, prominent nucleoli, nuclear molding and abundant cytoplasm. Clinical studies often combine anaplastic and large cell MB as a single sub-group (LC/A) (Louis et al 2007a,b). In addition to the five histological sub-types described in the most recent WHO classification, on very rare occasions MB can demonstrate focal differentiation along myogenic and melanotic cell lineages. These variants are referred to as medulomyoblastoma and melanotic medulloblastoma, respectively (Er et al 2008; Zanini et al 2008).

Genetics and molecular biology

Deregulation of normal developmental mechanisms has shown to be a major factor in MB formation (Marino 2005; Grimmer & Weiss 2006). The granule cell precursor (GCP) cells of the developing cerebellum represent the most probable cells of origin, but research into exact origins and lineage is ongoing. Some studies have suggested that MB has more than one cell of origin (Behesti & Marino 2009; Gilbertson & Ellison 2008). This finding is supported by MB's heterogeneity at the histologic and molecular levels. Emerging evidence indicates that MB tumorigenesis can be traced back to either neuronal stem cells or GCP lineage-restricted neuronal precursors (Schüller et al 2008; Yang et al 2008).

While most cases of MB occur sporadically, they can also occur in the setting of familial cancer syndromes such as Gorlin syndrome, Turcot syndrome, Li-Fraumeni syndrome, and Rubinstein-Taybi syndrome (Taylor et al 2000). Research into the pathogenesis and molecular basis of these syndromes has provided valuable information on MB.

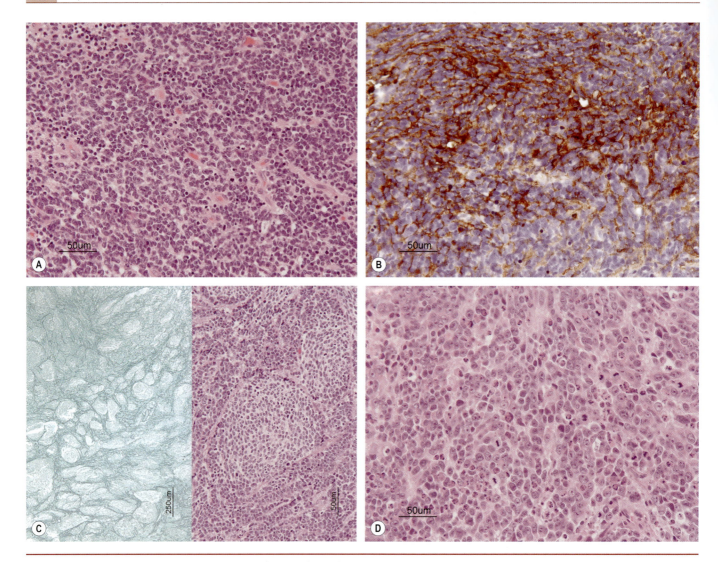

Figure 27.3 (A) Classic medulloblastoma composed of sheets of small blue cells (H&E ×200). (B) Classic medulloblastoma with area GFAP immunopositivity (GFAP ×200). (C) Desmoplastic medulloblastoma. Left panel: reticulin is increased in internodular areas, highlighting the nodular pattern (reticulin ×40). Right panel: Higher power image showing nodules which usually have reduced cellularity compared to the internodular areas (H&E ×200). (D) Large cell medulloblastoma demonstrating increased nuclear size with prominent nucleoli and abundant mitoses and apoptotic bodies (H&E ×200).

Gorlin syndrome, or nevoid basal cell carcinoma syndrome (NBCCS) is an autosomal dominant disorder which predisposes patients to develop multiple cutaneous basal cell carcinomas, along with skeletal abnormalities, mandibular cysts and dural calcifications (Evans et al 1991; Gorlin 1995). Among patients with Gorlin syndrome, 3–5% are expected to develop MB, with the desmoplastic sub-type being over-represented compared with the other variants (Evans et al 1991; Amlashi et al 2003; Kool et al 2008). This syndrome results from germline mutations of the PTCH1 gene, which has been mapped to the chromosome 9q31 locus (Farndon et al 1992; Gailani et al 1992; Johnson et al 1996). This gene encodes the transmembrane receptor involved in the Sonic hedgehog (Shh) signaling pathway, which plays an integral role in cerebellar development (Wallace 1999). PTCH1 acts to inhibit this pathway under normal conditions. Mutations to the PTCH gene lead to subsequent Shh hyperactivity during GCP development and is thought to be a primary event in MB tumorigenesis (Pietsch et al 2004; Dellovade

et al 2006). Other mutations involving this gene, or downstream Shh components (SUFU, PTCH2, SMO) are also seen in up to 25% of sporadic MB (Zurawel et al 2000; Taylor et al 2002; Gilbertson 2004; Taylor et al 2004a; Carlotti et al 2008).

Turcot syndrome is a rare, heritable disorder characterized by the combination of colorectal adenomas and brain tumors (Hamilton et al 1995). This syndrome is heterogeneous, but can be divided into two main sub-types. One sub-type includes patients with mutations in DNA mismatch repair genes, such as hMLH1, hMSH2, and hPMS2 (Lee et al 1998; Carlotti et al 2008). This patient population presents with hereditary non-polyposis colon cancer (HNPCC) and glioblastoma multiforme (GBM) (Hamilton et al 1995; Paraf et al 1997; Carlotti et al 2008). The other sub-type, more relevant to the content of this chapter, includes patients with MB in the setting of familial adenomatosis polypi (FAP) (Hamilton et al 1995; Paraf et al 1997; Hamada et al 1998; Carlotti et al 2008). FAP patients develop hundreds of colonic polyps which are predisposed to malignant progression (Hamilton et al 1995; Carlotti et al 2008). The genetic alteration in this sub-type is a germline mutation in the adenomatous polyposis coli (APC) tumor suppressor gene (Lasser et al 1994; Carlotti et al 2008). The APC protein is part of a polymeric protein complex that regulates the Wnt signaling pathway (Hamilton et al 1995; Paraf et al 1997; Taylor et al 2004a; Polkinghorn & Tarbell 2007; Carlotti et al 2008). Up to 18% of cases of sporadic MB have also identified mutations involving components of this Wnt pathway, with activation of β-catenin being the most common (Zurawel et al 1998; Eberhart et al 2000; Yokota et al 2002; Baeza et al 2003). APC mutations, however, are only identified in a small subset of sporadic MB (Huang et al 2000).

MB is one type of brain tumor which has been associated with Li-Fraumeni syndrome (Adesina et al 1994). Li-Fraumeni syndrome is a rare condition associated with mutations of the p53 tumor suppressor gene (Varley et al 1997; Barel et al 1998). Patients affected by this syndrome are at increased risk of developing several tumors including sarcomas, leukemia, premenopausal breast cancer, brain tumors and adrenocortical carcinoma (Varley et al 1997; Barel et al 1998). Mutations of p53 are rarely seen in sporadic MB (Adesina et al 1994).

An increased risk of MB has also been observed in Rubinstein–Taybi syndrome. This syndrome results from germline mutations of the CREB-binding protein gene on chromosome 16 (Petrij et al 1995). The syndrome is characterized by multiple congenital abnormalities including growth retardation, skeletal anomalies and microcephaly (Allanson & Hennekam 1997). These patients are at increased risk of developing several CNS tumors including MB, oligodendroglioma and meningioma (Taylor et al 2000). MB has also been observed in Aicardi syndrome (Taylor et al 2000).

Recent studies also suggest that pathways not associated with familial syndromes may be implicated in MB pathogenesis (Marino 2005; Sjölund et al 2005; Kelleher et al 2006). The Notch pathway is involved in cell fate determination and differentiation in several cells and tissues (Sjölund et al 2005). The relation between this pathway and cancer was first described in T-cell acute lymphoblastic leukemia (Sjölund et al 2005). Notch receptor deregulation and amplification was found in 15% of MB in one recent review (Sjölund et al 2005).

Non-random chromosomal abnormalities are also seen in MB. The most frequent cytogenetic rearrangement is isochromosome 17, or i(17q), which represents a loss of heterozygosity for the short arm of chromosome 17, occurring in up to 50% of MB (Bigner & Schröck 1997; Bayani et al 2000; Mendrzyk et al 2006). An associated tumor-suppressor gene on chromosome 17 has yet to be identified.

Tumor staging and prognostic factors

Accurate pre- and postoperative staging has shown to be crucial in guiding management and providing estimates of prognosis. The Chang staging system was among the first attempts to stratify children with MB. This system classified patients based on tumor stage (T) and metastasis stage (M) (Chang et al 1969). The tumor stage was based on tumor size, location, and local invasion. This parameter has proven to be of limited utility in estimating prognosis and directing adjuvant treatments. The M stage on the other hand, has shown clinical utility in both regards (Zeltzer et al 1999). The initial Chang system divided the M stage into five subcategories. M0 were cases without evidence of gross, CSF, or hematogenous metastases. M1 referred to patients with positive cytology on CSF analysis. M2 patients had evidence of gross nodular seeding of the subarachnoid or ventricular space, whereas M3 patients showed gross nodular seeding of the spinal subarachnoid space. The M4 stage referred to cases with distant, extra-neural metastases (Zeltzer et al 1999).

Current stratification systems divide MB patients into average or high-risk groups. The average-risk patients are 3 years of age or older, have no evidence of gross or microscopic metastatic disease, and are left with <1.5 cm^2 residual tumor burden after surgical resection. High-risk patients include those <3 years of age, children with evidence of metastatic disease and/or those with significant residual tumor (>1.5 cm^2) post-resection.

Patient age has consistently been found to be associated with prognosis (Raimondi & Tomita 1979; Evans et al 1990; Duffner et al 1993; Albright et al 1996). Age under 3 years at the time of diagnosis has been associated with significantly decreased overall survival (OS) compared with patients ≥3 years of age (36.3% vs 73.4%, respectively) (Kombogiorgas et al 2007). Furthermore, the findings of a recent Canadian Pediatric Brain Tumor Consortium study of adolescent MB patients revealed that time to relapse was linearly proportional to age at diagnosis (Tabori et al 2006). There is no uniform agreement that age per se is the causative factor, however. The poor outcomes seen in younger MB patients may be related to altered therapeutic management patterns, such as withholding or delaying adjuvant radiotherapy (David et al 1997; Grotzer et al 2000). The MBEN variant for example, carries a more favorable prognosis than other sub-types, despite being diagnosed in younger patients.

Absence of metastatic disease at the time of diagnosis is also associated with improved OS and event-free survival (EFS) (Schofield et al 1992; Bouffet et al 1994; Zeltzer et al 1999; Lamont et al 2004; Ray et al 2004; Sanders et al 2008). In average-risk MB patients, M stage has demonstrated prognostic significance with 5-year progression-free survivals (PFS) for patients with M0, M1 and M2 or greater being 70%, 57% and 40%, respectively (Zeltzer et al 1999). The control rates in studies of high-risk patients have been similar (Verlooy et al 2006).

It has traditionally been believed that maximal, safe neurosurgical resection is the optimum initial treatment for MB patients. Patients with minimal residual tumor post-resection, especially those without metastatic disease, have shown prolonged PFS (Raimondi & Tomita 1979; Berry et al 1981; Tomita & McLone 1986; Jenkin et al 1990; Schofield et al 1992; Sure et al 1995; Albright et al 1996; Agerlin et al 1999; Massimino et al 2000). The Children's Cancer Group (CCG) 921 trial showed that patients without metastatic disease at the time of diagnosis with <1.5 cm^2 of residual tumor after resection had a 5-year PFS of 78%, compared with 54% for those with residual tumor burden of ≥1.5 cm^2 (Zeltzer et al 1999). Furthermore, the degree of resection (total vs near total) does not seem to have a significant effect on PFS as long as the residual tumor burden is <1.5 cm^2 (Gajjar et al 1996; Sutton et al 1996).

One of the criticisms of the current staging system is that it is unable to differentiate which average-risk patients might benefit from more aggressive management aimed at prolonging survival compared with less aggressive intervention to minimize the side-effects of therapy. Much research has been directed at attempts to identify additional histologic and molecular prognostic markers which may help to direct risk-adapted therapy for MB patients (Table 27.1). Numerous studies have observed that a high rate of TRKC expression is associated with improved survival (Segal et al 1994; Grotzer et al 2000; Ray et al 2004; Grotzer et al 2007). The 5-year survival rate in those with high expression of TRKC was 89% in one study, compared with 46% for those with low expression (Segal et al 1994). This association has not been duplicated in all studies (Gajjar et al 2004).

MYC oncogene (MYCC and MYCN) amplification has been shown to play a role in MB tumorigenesis (Guessous et al 2008). Low levels of MYCC expression have been identified as a good prognostic marker (de Haas et al 2008). High MYC expression is implicated in both the large cell and anaplastic MB variants, and may be related to the poor survival rates of patients with either of these sub-types (Eberhart et al 2004; Lamont et al 2004). Analysis of combined TRKC and MYC status has also been performed (Grotzer et al 2007). One trial identified patients with elevated TRKC and low MYCC as a 'good risk' group, while the outcome for those patients with low TRKC and high MYCC was less favorable (Grotzer et al 2007). As with TKRC, however, MYC amplification is not consistently identified as a significant prognostic marker (Gajjar et al 2004).

ERBB2 is another oncogene which has been implicated in the pathogenesis of MB (Guessous et al 2008). Overexpression has been shown to be a marker of poor prognosis, and has also been associated with the large cell and anaplastic sub-types (Gilbertson et al 1995; Gajjar et al 2004;

Ray et al 2004). A recent study showed that all average-risk patients with negative ERBB2 status were alive at the 5-year follow-up, whereas only 54% of average-risk patients with positive ERBB2 status had survived (Gajjar et al 2004).

Finally, Wnt/wingless signaling pathway activation has also been suggested as a favorable prognostic factor (Ellison et al 2005; Clifford et al 2006). β-catenin is a marker of Wnt pathway activation and its expression has been associated with improved OS and EFS in all MB sub-types (Ellison et al 2005).

A better understanding of the molecular pathways involved in MB may allow for new therapeutic strategies. Valproic acid, erlotinib, cyclopamine and certain small molecules inhibitors have all shown promise in downregulation of MB molecular pathogenesis under in vitro settings (Taipale et al 2000; Shu et al 2006; Lauth et al 2007; Carlotti et al 2008).

Treatment

The management of MB patients is a collaborative effort between neurosurgeons, oncologists, neuroradiologists and neuropathologists. Most patients undergo multi-modality treatment consisting of a combination of maximal safe surgical resection, cranial-spinal irradiation (CSI), and chemotherapy.

Neurosurgical resection

Neurosurgical resection continues to play a crucial role in the current therapeutic regimens for MB. The goals of surgery include obtaining a tissue diagnosis, achieving maximal safe tumor resection, restoring normal CSF pathways, and decreasing the degree of mass effect on critical neural structures.

The majority of children with posterior fossa MBs will have some degree of hydrocephalus at the time of diagnosis (Rappaport & Shalit 1989; Fritsch et al 2005; Due-Tønnessen and Helseth 2007). Depending on the severity of the patients, symptoms and hydrocephalus, a decision must often be made to treat the hydrocephalus in the early stages. If early management is pursued, then the child with MB may require an external ventricular drain (EVD), a ventriculoperitoneal shunt (VPS) or endoscopic third ventriculostomy (ETV). One must weigh the proposed benefit of VPS or ETV against the fact that permanent CSF diversion is only required in 10–40% of patients after tumor resection (Rappaport & Shalit 1989; Lee et al 1994; Fritsch et al 2005; Morelli et al 2005; Kombogiorgas et al 2008). When compared with other tumors of the posterior fossa, MB patients appear to be more likely to require a VPS for symptomatic hydrocephalus in the postoperative period (Morelli et al 2005; Due-Tønnessen and Helseth 2007). Factors which appear to increase the likelihood of permanent postoperative VPS necessity include younger patient age, larger tumor size, and more severe hydrocephalus at diagnosis (Lee et al 1994; Due-Tønnessen and Helseth 2007; Kombogiorgas et al 2007; Kombogiorgas et al 2008). In our experience, most children with MB do not require early CSF diversion and can be symptomatically controlled with corticosteroids until the time of surgery. For

Table 27.1 Prognostic markers in medulloblastoma

Prognostic marker	Description	Role in MB
TRKC	A receptor tyrosine kinase; mediates neuronal differentiation, survival and other effects of neurotrophic factor	High levels of expression have been associated with improved survival
MYC	A family of genes which encode for transcription factors	High levels of expression have been associated with a poor survival, as seen in large cell and anaplastic MB
ERBB2	A cell membrane, surface-bound receptor tyrosine kinase; involved in signal transduction pathways leading to cell growth and differentiation	High levels of expression have been associated with a poor prognosis, as seen in large cell and anaplastic MB
β-catenin	A cytoplasmic phosphoprotein and a marker of the Wnt signaling pathway; an important regulator of cell–cell adhesion and embryogenesis	High levels of expression have been associated with improved survival

those patients who present with severely impaired neurological status due to hydrocephalus, emergent EVD insertion is the typical initial management.

Patients are usually placed in the prone position at the time of surgical resection. This allows for the use of a pin-based rigid head frame or a padded horseshoe-type holder in very young children in whom pins are generally avoided. Intraoperative adjuncts may be used at the time of surgery, including frameless stereotaxy, ultrasonography, evoked potentials and cranial nerve monitoring. The operating microscope is useful especially for tumors filling the fourth ventricle. A satellite burr hole is placed in children whose ventricles are already quite large, and used to pass a ventricular catheter to reduce intracranial hypertension prior to opening the dura.

Exposure via a standard midline posterior fossa approach is then performed. The skin incision is extended from the inion to the mid-cervical region. Midline dissection in the avascular plane is then performed, followed by lateral mobilization of the cervical musculature from the occiput and cervical laminae. A posterior fossa craniotomy is then performed with care taken to avoid injury to the transverse sinus. Laminectomy of the upper cervical vertebrae is performed if preoperative imaging reveals that the tumor extends caudally into the spinal canal. The dural opening is then fashioned in a Y-shaped manner (Fig. 27.4). Hemostasis of the occipital and circular sinuses must be achieved at this time if any bleeding is present. Suture ligation is the

preferred method of hemostasis if possible, as metal clips can result in artifact on postoperative MRI investigations.

At this point in the operation, the cerebellar tonsils are separated and a transvermian midline approach to the IVth ventricle is undertaken. Cotton patties are used to help develop the plane between the tumor and normal cerebellum. This is done for as great a distance as possible prior to tumor debulking. Adequate exposure often requires that the distal vermis be divided. A cotton patty should be placed on the floor of the IVth ventricle, once identified, to avoid injury to the brainstem and to provide a reference to help guide the depth of resection. The resection is initiated at the dorsal aspect of the tumor with care taken to preserve the posterior inferior cerebellar arteries which are often encountered. Internally debulking the tumor allows for histopathological specimens to be obtained and also helps to develop the lateral plane between tumor and cerebellum.

Upon reaching the IVth ventricle detailed inspection is undertaken to identify areas of possible tumor invasion into the ventricular floor or cerebellar peduncles. Aggressive tumor resection in these areas is not recommended, as the potential postoperative neurological deficits can be profound. As the resection is completed, the neurosurgeon inspects the cerebral aqueduct, foramina of Luschka and obex to confirm that no safely accessible tumor remains.

Other surgical approaches for MB have also been described. The inferior telovelar approach will provide the surgeon with access to the tumor-filled IVth ventricle and does not necessitate a vermian incision (Matsushima et al 1992). In the setting of a more laterally positioned tumor, a corticotomy of the cerebellum over the region of shortest distance to the tumor can be performed (Gök et al 2004).

Prior to initiating the closure meticulous hemostasis is achieved with a combination of judicious bipolar coagulation and gentle tamponade, and can be confirmed through the use of an induced Valsalva maneuver. Dural closure is performed in a watertight fashion, followed by bone flap replacement and multilayer soft tissue and skin closure.

The early postoperative period is characterized by a weaning from and discontinuation of the EVD, if one had been left at the time of operation. Difficulty weaning the ventricular drain or the presence of a pseudomeningocele infers ongoing hydrocephalus and raises the question of whether or not permanent CSF diversion will be required. Within 48 h of resection, all patients should undergo MRI evaluation to assess the degree of residual tumor burden. Significant residual tumor (>1.5 cm^2), as previously mentioned, should prompt discussion regarding the possibility of early repeat surgical resection.

Potential postoperative complications after MB surgery include headache, vomiting, cranial nerve palsies, bulbar symptoms, dysmetria, diplopia, and ataxia (Albright et al 1989; Cochrane et al 1994). Rates of permanent morbidity and mortality after MB resection have significantly declined and are currently 5–10% and 1–3%, respectively (Belza et al 1991; Sutton et al 1996; Helseth et al 1999). The potential postoperative complications are similar to those of other posterior fossa surgeries and include infection, CSF leak, pseudomeningocele, and persistent hydrocephalus.

A unique postoperative complication seen after posterior fossa surgery is cerebellar mutism. This syndrome

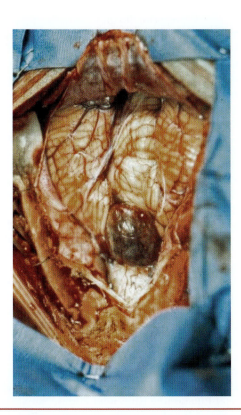

Figure 27.4 Intraoperative photomicrograph of a 7-year-old male at time of surgery. A posterior fossa craniotomy has been performed. The dura has been opened. The medulloblastoma is seen emerging from between the cerebellar tonsils. A midline, trans-vermian approach was used to remove this medulloblastoma.

typically arises within 1–2 days following resection and occurs in 10–25% of cases (Wisoff & Epstein 1984; Pollack et al 1995; Gajjar et al 1996; Robertson et al 2006). The most significant symptoms include mild speech difficulty which progresses to mutism, as well as ataxia. Other associated features which may be seen include emotional lability, neurobehavioral abnormalities, hypotonia, and cranial nerve abnormalities (Pollack et al 1995; Robertson et al 2006). The severity of symptoms is variable and is deemed severe in approximately 43%, moderate in 49% and mild in 8% (Robertson et al 2006). This syndrome usually resolves over weeks to months in the majority of cases (Huber et al 2006). The etiology of cerebellar mutism is unknown, but may relate to edema formation along the superior and middle cerebellar peduncles as a result of splitting the vermis and exerting pressure on the cerebellum intraoperatively (Wisoff & Epstein 1984). Post-surgical cerebellar edema may disrupt the cerebellar motor pathway connections to the dentate nucleus via the middle and superior peduncles (Pollack et al 1995). A recent prospective review identified that the risk of cerebellar mutism was correlated with brainstem invasion, whereas lesion size, length of vermian incision and surgical approach do not appear to display a correlation (Pollack et al 1995; Robertson et al 2006).

Radiation therapy

The introduction of adjuvant CSI in children with MB has led to significant improvements in outcomes and survival (Rutka & Hoffman 1996; Polkinghorn & Tarbell 2007). The 5-year PFS rates in patients receiving local radiotherapy alone compared with those receiving CSI with local boost radiotherapy are <10% and 50%, respectively (Paterson & Farr 1953; Bloom et al 1969; Packer et al 1999b). The postoperative CSI regimen traditionally utilized in the past was 36 Gy to the entire brain and spinal cord with a posterior fossa boost of 54 Gy. High risk patients >3 years of age typically received the standard-dose CSI (36 Gy), a posterior fossa boost of 55.8 Gy, plus adjuvant chemotherapy (Paulino 1997). The adjuvant therapy regimens for average-risk patients have adapted, in-keeping with the advent of risk-adjusted management paradigms.

Due to the potential consequences of radiotherapy, many groups have investigated the safety and efficacy of reducing the dose of CSI for patients with MB (Paulino 1997; Thomas et al 2000). The early studies in this area, which compared CSI doses of 23.4 Gy compared with 36 Gy, in addition to a 54 Gy boost to the posterior fossa, revealed significantly increased relapse rates and lower 5-year PFS rates in the reduced-dose CSI group (Deutsch et al 1996; Thomas et al 2000).

Several recent trials have examined the outcome of average-risk MB patients receiving reduced-dose CSI along with pre-radiation chemotherapy (Oyharcabal-Bourden et al 2005). The 5-year OS and PFS rates were 73.8% and 64.8%, respectively, which are comparable with the outcomes reported for patients who received standard-dose CSI regimens (Bailey et al 1995; Thomas et al 2000). Studies of reduced-dose CSI have similarly been performed examining the role of post-radiation chemotherapy. Outcomes have been at least equivalent to those seen in average-risk patients

receiving standard-dose CSI, with 5-year OS and EFS rates reaching 85% and 83%, respectively in select trials (Packer et al 1994; Packer et al 1999b; Gajjar et al 2006). Reduced-dose CSI in this setting does not lead to an increased rate of disease recurrence (Halberg et al 1991). It therefore appears that average-risk MB patients who receive reduced-dose CSI in addition to either pre- or post-radiation chemotherapy, will achieve similar control rates as those who receive standard-dose CSI. There are on-going studies which attempt to assess the safety and efficacy of even further reductions in the CSI dose (18 Gy). Further attempts to minimize the amount of radiation have led investigators to determine the safety and efficacy of limiting the standard 54 Gy posterior fossa boost to the tumor bed alone (Fukunaga-Johnson et al 1998; Wolden et al 2003).

Studies examining the control rates of MB patients treated with standard-dose CSI and a conformal radiotherapy boost to the tumor bed have reported 5-year PFS and OS rates of 84% and 85%, respectively (Wolden et al 2003). Local control rates at 5 and 10 years appear to be similar to those achieved with boost radiotherapy to the entire posterior fossa (Wolden et al 2003). Furthermore, reducing the CSI dose to 23.4 Gy and providing post-radiation chemotherapy along with a conformal boost to the tumor bed alone, does not appear to alter outcomes or control rates (Douglas et al 2004; Merchant et al 2008). Overall, such studies have demonstrated that patients who receive a limited radiotherapy boost to the tumor bed will achieve control rates comparable to those whose radiotherapy targets the entire posterior fossa.

Investigators have evaluated the most appropriate timing of radiotherapy administration within current treatment paradigms. The preliminary data came from studies which involved neoadjuvant chemotherapy and suggested that it was important to begin radiation within 6–8 weeks of surgical resection (Kühl et al 1998). More recent studies seem to stress that the duration of radiation is the crucial variable, rather than the timing of its initiation (del Charco et al 1998; Taylor et al 2003; Taylor et al 2004b). Both OS and EFS have been shown to improve for patients completing their radiation treatment within the first 50 days of surgical resection (Taylor et al 2004b).

Despite its efficacy, the use of radiation therapy is complicated by both short- and long-term side-effects. The short-term side-effects of CSI are often self-limiting and include headache, fatigue, nausea, irritability, somnolence, and hair loss. The long-term sequelae of CSI often impact neurologic, cognitive, and endocrine function, as well as overall quality of life (Ribi et al 2005). The rate of hypothalamic-pituitary dysfunction was 61% in one study of 51 MB patients, and may result in obesity, hypothyroidism, precocious puberty, and growth retardation (Ribi et al 2005). Spinal irradiation can also contribute to short stature or scoliosis. Neurocognitive deficits are seen in virtually all patients and are manifest as impaired attention, learning, memory, language, executive or social functioning (Ribi et al 2005). Not surprisingly, approximately 72% of patients experience difficulties with academic achievement (Ribi et al 2005). A majority of these long-term side-effects are believed to be dose-dependent but not all studies support the notion of intellectual preservation with reduced CSI dose (Ris et al 2001; Mulhern et al 2005).

Young age appears to be a predictor of neurocognitive sequelae secondary to irradiation (Ris et al 2001; Mabbott et al 2005; Mulhern et al 2005). Finally, radiation-induced neoplasms or vasculopathies must be mentioned here, and will affect up to 10% of patients (Jenkin 1996; Ullrich et al 2007). Secondary tumor development is of particular concern for those MB patients with familial cancer syndromes, as they are at an increased risk (Jenkin 1996).

Chemotherapy

Adjuvant chemotherapy continues to gain importance in the treatment of MB. Previously reserved for patients deemed to be high-risk or those with progressive disease, numerous trials have been performed which have helped to expand its role. A variety of unique chemotherapeutic regimens exist, depending on the providing institution, and while disease response rates have been achieved with single agent therapy, the majority of neurooncologists advocate the use of multi-agent regimens (Packer et al 1994; Kortmann et al 2000; Strother et al 2001; Taylor et al 2003; Matsutani 2004).

The earliest randomized prospective trials, which assessed the efficacy of adjuvant chemotherapy in MB, were performed in the 1970s and 1980s. Patients received standard-dose CSI and were randomized to receive either post-radiotherapy multiagent chemotherapy or radiation alone. The overall results of these trials did not show significant benefits of chemotherapy for average-risk patients. They did, however, suggest that chemotherapy may benefit certain patient sub-groups with poor-risk features such as sub-total resection, brain stem involvement or disseminated disease at diagnosis (Evans et al 1990; Tait et al 1990). Subsequently, studies of high-risk patients were undertaken. The comparison between those high-risk patients receiving surgery and radiation alone vs those additionally receiving adjuvant chemotherapy revealed a survival benefit in the latter group (Krischer et al 1991; Packer et al 1991). Since that time, additional studies have provided evidence to support the use of adjuvant chemotherapy in both average- and high-risk MB patients (Packer et al 1994; Packer et al 1999b; Gajjar et al 2006). Some studies have even questioned the necessity of postoperative radiation therapy in certain MB patients, given the efficacy of newer chemotherapeutic regimens. Rutkowski et al (2005) treated 43 children with postoperative chemotherapy alone and showed 5-year PFS and OS rates of 82% and 93%, respectively, in those patients without metastatic disease who had undergone complete surgical resection.

The timing of chemotherapy administration has also been studied. Neoadjuvant chemotherapy took advantage of the increased permeability of the blood brain barrier during the postoperative period, the enhanced potential for marrow recovery in the absence of prior irradiation, and reduced risks of drug induced toxicity in non-irradiated patients (Kühl et al 1998). The initial experience with pre-radiotherapy chemotherapy showed that it was feasible but that it did not provide a significant benefit over the conventional adjuvant chemotherapeutic strategies (Bailey et al 1995). The 5-year survival rates were approximately 74% in average-risk patients and 57% in those considered high risk (Gentet et al 1995).

Existing data do not seem to support the use of neoadjuvant chemotherapy in high-risk MB patients. Clinical trials have shown that patients who receive chemotherapy prior to radiotherapy achieve similar or worse control rates than those who undergo adjuvant chemotherapy (Zeltzer et al 1999; Taylor et al 2005).

The role of neoadjuvant chemotherapy in average-risk patients has not yet been clearly defined. Prospective, randomized trials have reported 3-year EFS rates of approximately 78% in those patients who received chemotherapy prior to radiotherapy, compared with 65% in patients who did not (Kortmann et al 2000; Taylor et al 2004b). Similar 5-year control rates were observed in the SIOP III study (Taylor et al 2003). In at least one of these trials, however, neoadjuvant chemotherapy was associated with elevated rates of radiation-induced myelotoxicity, and associated treatment interruptions (Kortmann et al 2000). Furthermore, long-term follow-up has revealed significant detriments to quality of life resulting from these treatment regimens (Bull et al 2007).

Another option for MB patients is high-dose, myeloablative chemotherapy followed by hematopoietic stem cell rescue. This strategy initially involved the harvesting of autologous bone marrow-derived stem cells, to be subsequently used for reconstitution of the patient's marrow. Treatment-related mortality rates appear to be in the 10–20% range (Guruangan et al 1998; Finlay 1999; Dhall et al 2008). Early interest in myeloablative chemotherapy and stem cell rescue in MB patients came from the objective responses seen in sub-group analyses from studies investigating its response rate and toxicity profile in children with a variety of recurrent malignant brain tumors (Mahoney et al 1996; Graham et al 1997; Guruangan et al 1998; Mason et al 1998; Finlay 1999). The clinical utility of this strategy in MB has been shown in cases of disease recurrence as well as in the management of young patients without postoperative residual disease (Graham et al 1997). Studies have reported 2-year PFS rates of 93.6% in MB patients receiving CSI and myeloablative chemotherapy followed by stem cell rescue (Strother et al 2001). High-risk patients or those with disseminated disease at the time of diagnosis who underwent a similar treatment protocol achieved 3-year OS and EFS rates of 60% and 49%, respectively. This strategy is an appealing treatment option for patients <3 years of age in whom radiotherapy is preferably avoided. Dhall et al (2008) assessed patients under 36 months of age presenting with MB without dissemination whose treatment consisted of surgical resection and induction chemotherapy, followed by myeloablative chemotherapy and stem cell rescue. In this trial, radiotherapy was not administered as an initial treatment, but was reserved for cases of disease relapse. Patients with gross total resection achieved 5-year OS and EFS rates of 79% and 64%, respectively, while the same control rate measures in patients with residual postoperative tumor were 57% and 29% (Dhall et al 2008).

Chemotherapy has been associated with a broad side-effect profile. Common adverse events, typically arising in the acute post-treatment period, include fatigue, nausea, vomiting, loss of appetite, gastritis, and infections (Kadota et al 2008). Myelosuppression is another complication which tends to occur soon after treatment. The likelihood of this

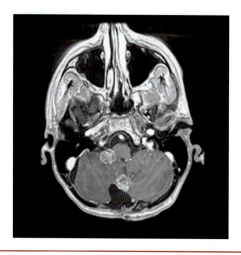

Figure 27.5 Axial gadolinium-enhanced MRI in a 14-year-old male with anaplastic large cell medulloblastoma showing recurrence in the posterior fossa and a separate nodule in the right CP angle 1 year after intensive, high risk protocol treatment.

developing may be increased in those patients who receive chemotherapy in combination with radiotherapy (Krischer et al 1991; Kortmann et al 2000). Less common, but more severe side-effects also occur. Depending on the agent(s) used, care must be taken to determine the presence of nephrotoxicity, hepatotoxicity, cardiomyopathy, sensorineural hearing loss, acute myelogenous leukemia, bladder or pulmonary fibrosis (Blatt et al 1991).

Disease recurrence and surveillance imaging

Despite considerable diagnostic and therapeutic advances in MB management, disease recurrence remains a major concern (Fig. 27.5). Relapse rates of 30–40% have been reported, with many patients experiencing recurrence in the first 2 years (Bouffet et al 1998; Yalçin et al 2002). Disease recurrence at the primary site is most common, but may also be seen within the spinal canal or leptomeninges (Belza et al 1991).

Given the high rate of relapse, most neurosurgeons will advocate close clinical and radiological follow-up after initial treatment. In addition to an early postoperative, baseline MRI (within 48 h of resection), a majority of patients will receive serial MRI investigations every 3–6 months during the first two postoperative years (Friedman & Kun 1995). This may help to detect recurrent disease in the early stage, possibly prior to symptoms, during which an association with improved survival has been observed (Shaw et al 1997; Saunders et al 2003). This surveillance imaging strategy is not universally supported, however, as some studies have shown that it fails to detect asymptomatic disease in a high proportion of cases (Torres et al 1994; Bartels et al 2006). Furthermore, including spinal MR imaging in the absence of documented intracranial progression does not seem to be of significant value (Bartels et al 2006).

Collins' law is often applied to MB patients to predict the time frame during which disease recurrence is most likely. This law suggests that recurrence should occur within a time period equal to the patient's age plus 9 months, and that an

absence of recurrence at that time indicates that the patient is cured of his/her disease (Latchaw et al 1985; Friedberg et al 1997). While some studies have shown that timing of recurrence obeys Collins' law, numerous late recurrences have also been reported (Friedberg et al 1997; Modha et al 2000; Allan et al 2004).

Key points

- Medulloblastoma usually occurs sporadically but may be associated with numerous familial tumor syndromes (e.g., Gorlin syndrome, Rubinstein-Taybi syndrome).

- MRI of the entire neural axis is the diagnostic and staging imaging modality of choice.

- The WHO Classification of CNS tumors identifies five sub-types of medulloblastoma, all of which are considered grade IV.

- The aims of surgical management are maximal safe tumor resection and restoration of CSF pathways. Permanent CSF diversion will be required in 10–40% of children.

- Adjuvant radiotherapy of the entire cranial-spinal axis has been associated with improved outcomes.

- Chemotherapy is most beneficial in younger patients, those with larger tumors and/or those with metastasis at the time of diagnosis.

- Therapies aimed at modulation of molecular signaling pathways involved in medulloblastoma pathogenesis are currently being investigated.

- Treatment failure remains a major concern in medulloblastoma treatment and occurs most commonly in the posterior fossa.

- Late effects of surgical and adjuvant treatments continue to be a significant issue for patients with medulloblastoma.

REFERENCES

Adesina, A.M., Nalbantoglu, J., Cavenee, W.K., 1994. p53 gene mutation and mdm2 gene amplification are uncommon in medulloblastoma. Cancer Res. 54 (21), 5649–5651.

Agerlin, N., Gjerris, F., Brincker, H., et al., 1999. Childhood medulloblastoma in Denmark 1960–1984. A population-based retrospective study. Childs Nerv. Syst. 15 (1), 29–37.

Albright, A.L., Wisoff, J.H., Zeltzer, P.M., et al., 1996. Effects of medulloblastoma resections on outcome in children: a report from the Children's Cancer Group. Neurosurgery 38 (2), 265–271.

Albright, A.L., Wisoff, J.H., Zeltzer, P.M., et al., 1989. Current neurosurgical treatment of medulloblastomas in children. A report from the Children's Cancer Study Group. Pediatr. Neurosci. 15 (6), 276–282.

Allan, R., Gill, A., Spittaler, P., 2004. Recurrent medulloblastoma – violation of Collin's law by 14 years. J. Clin. Neurosci. 11 (7), 756–757.

Allanson, J.E., Hennekam, R.C., 1997. Rubinstein-Taybi syndrome: objective evaluation of craniofacial structure. Am. J. Med. Genet. 71 (4), 414–419.

Amlashi, S.F., Riffaud, L., Brassier, G., et al., 2003. Nevoid basal cell carcinoma syndrome: relation with desmoplastic medulloblastoma in infancy. A population-based study and review of the literature. Cancer 98 (3), 618–624.

Baeza, N., Masuoka, J., Kleihues, P., et al., 2003. AXIN1 mutations but not deletions in cerebellar medulloblastomas. Oncogene 22 (4), 632–636.

Bailey, C.C., Gnekow, A., Wellek, S., et al., 1995. Prospective randomised trial of chemotherapy given before radiotherapy in childhood medulloblastoma. International Society of Paediatric Oncology (SIOP) and the (German) Society of Paediatric Oncology (GPO): SIOP II. Med. Pediatr. Oncol. 25 (3), 166–178.

Barel, D., Avigad, S., Mor, C., et al., 1998. A novel germ-line mutation in the noncoding region of the p53 gene in a Li-Fraumeni family. Cancer Genet. Cytogenet. 103 (1), 1–6.

Bartels, U., Shroff, M., Sung, L., et al., 2006. Role of spinal MRI in the follow-up of children treated for medulloblastoma. Cancer 107 (6), 1340–1347.

Bayani, J., Zielenska, M., Marrano, P., et al., 2000. Molecular cytogenetic analysis of medulloblastomas and supratentorial primitive neuroectodermal tumors by using conventional banding, comparative genomic hybridization, and spectral karyotyping. J. Neurosurg. 93 (3), 437–448.

Behesti, H., Marino, S., 2009. Cerebellar granule cells: Insights into proliferation, differentiation, and role in medulloblastoma pathogenesis. Int. J. Biochem. Cell Biol. 41 (3), 435–445.

Belza, M.G., Donaldson, S.S., Steinberg, G.K., et al., 1991. Medulloblastoma: freedom from relapse longer than 8 years – a therapeutic cure? J. Neurosurg. 75 (4), 575–582.

Berry, M.P., Jenkin, R.D., Keen, C.W., et al., 1981. Radiation treatment for medulloblastoma. A 21-year review. J. Neurosurg. 55 (1), 43–51.

Bigner, S.H., Schröck, E., 1997. Molecular cytogenetics of brain tumors. J. Neuropathol. Exp. Neurol. 56 (11), 1173–1181.

Blaser, S.I., Harwood-Nash, D.C., 1996. Neuroradiology of pediatric posterior fossa medulloblastoma. J. Neurooncol. 29 (1), 23–34.

Blatt, J., Penchansky, L., Phebus, C., et al., 1991. Leukemia in a child with a history of medulloblastoma. Pediatr. Hematol. Oncol. 8 (1), 77–82.

Bloom, H.J., Wallace, E.N., Henk, J.M., 1969. The treatment and prognosis of medulloblastoma in children. A study of 82 verified cases. Am. J. Roentgenol. Radium. Ther. Nucl. Med. 105 (1), 43–62.

Bouffet, E., Doz, F., Demaille, M.C., et al., 1998. Improving survival in recurrent medulloblastoma: earlier detection, better treatment or still an impasse? Br. J. Cancer 77 (8), 1321–1326.

Bouffet, E., Gentet, J.C., Doz, F., et al., 1994. Metastatic medulloblastoma: the experience of the French Cooperative M7 Group. Eur. J. Cancer 30A (10), 1478–1483.

Bull, K.S., Spoudeas, H.A., Yadegarfar, G., et al., 2007. Reduction of health status 7 years after addition of chemotherapy to craniospinal irradiation for medulloblastoma: a follow-up study in PNET 3 trial survivors on behalf of the CCLG (formerly UKCCSG). J. Clin. Oncol. 25 (27), 4239–4245.

Burger, P.C., Fuller, G.N., 1991. Pathology – trends and pitfalls in histologic diagnosis, immunopathology, and applications of oncogene research. Neurol. Clin. 9 (2), 249–271.

Carlotti, C.G., Jr., Smith, C., Rutka, J.T., 2008. The molecular genetics of medulloblastoma: an assessment of new therapeutic targets. Neurosurg. Rev. 31 (4), 359–369.

Carrie, C., Lasset, C., Alapetite, C., et al., 1994. Multivariate analysis of prognostic factors in adult patients with medulloblastoma. Retrospective study of 156 patients. Cancer 74 (8), 2352–2360.

Cervoni, L., Maleci, A., Salvati, M., et al., 1994. Medulloblastoma in late adults: report of two cases and critical review of the literature. J. Neurooncol. 19 (2), 169–173.

Chang, C.H., Housepian, E.M., Herbert, C., Jr., 1969. An operative staging system and a megavoltage radiotherapeutic technic for cerebellar medulloblastomas. Radiology 93 (6), 1351–1359.

Clifford, S.C., Lusher, M.E., Lindsey, J.C., et al., 2006. Wnt/Wingless pathway activation and chromosome 6 loss characterize a distinct molecular sub-group of medulloblastomas associated with a favorable prognosis. Cell Cycle 5 (22), 2666–2670.

Cochrane, D.D., Gustavsson, B., Poskitt, K.P., et al., 1994. The surgical and natural morbidity of aggressive resection for posterior fossa tumors in childhood. Pediatr. Neurosurg. 20 (1), 19–29.

Coffin, C.M., Braun, J.T., Wick, M.R., et al., 1990. A clinicopathologic and immunohistochemical analysis of 53 cases of medulloblastoma with emphasis on synaptophysin expression. Mod. Pathol. 3 (2), 164–170.

David, K.M., Casey, A.T., Hayward, R.D., et al., 1997. Medulloblastoma: is the 5-year survival rate improving? A review of 80 cases from a single institution. J. Neurosurg. 86 (1), 13–21.

Davies, N.P., Wilson, M., Harris, L.M., et al., 2008. Identification and characterisation of childhood cerebellar tumours by in vivo proton MRS. NMR in biomedicine 21 (8), 908–918.

Davis, F.G., Kupelian, V., Freels, S., et al., 2001. Prevalence estimates for primary brain tumors in the United States by behavior and major histology groups. Neuro. Oncology. 3 (3), 152–158.

de Haas, T., Hasselt, N., Troost, D., et al., 2008. Molecular risk stratification of medulloblastoma patients based on immunohistochemical analysis of MYC, LDHB, and CCNB1 expression. Clin. Cancer. Res. 14 (13), 4154–4160.

del Charco, J.O., Bolek, T.W., McCollough, W.M., et al., 1998. Medulloblastoma: time-dose relationship based on a 30-year review. Int. J. Radiat. Oncol. Biol. Phys. 42 (1), 147–154.

Dellovade, T., Romer, J.T., Curran, T., et al., 2006. The hedgehog pathway and neurological disorders. Annu. Rev. Neurosci. 29, 539–563.

Deutsch, M., Thomas, P.R., Krischer, J., et al., 1996. Results of a prospective randomized trial comparing standard dose neuraxis irradiation (3,600 cGy/20) with reduced neuraxis irradiation (2,340 cGy/13) in patients with low-stage medulloblastoma. A Combined Children's Cancer Group-Pediatric Oncology Group Study. Pediatr. Neurosurg. 24 (4), 167–177.

Dhall, G., Grodman, H., Ji, L., et al., 2008. Outcome of children less than three years old at diagnosis with non-metastatic medulloblastoma treated with chemotherapy on the 'Head Start' I and II protocols. Pediatr. Blood Cancer 50 (6), 1169–1175.

Douglas, J.G., Barker, J.L., Ellenbogen, R.G., et al., 2004. Concurrent chemotherapy and reduced-dose cranial spinal irradiation followed by conformal posterior fossa tumor boost for average-risk medulloblastoma: efficacy and patterns of failure. Int. J. Radiat. Oncol. Biol. Phys. 58 (4), 1161–1164.

Due-Tønnessen, B.J., Helseth, E., 2007. Management of hydrocephalus in children with posterior fossa tumors: role of tumor surgery. Pediatr. Neurosurg. 43 (2), 92–96.

Duffner, P.K., Horowitz, M.E., Krischer, J.P., et al., 1993. Postoperative chemotherapy and delayed radiation in children less than three years of age with malignant brain tumors. N. Engl. J. Med. 328 (24), 1725–1731.

Eberhart, C.G., Kratz, J., Wang, Y., et al., 2004. Histopathological and molecular prognostic markers in medulloblastoma: c-myc, N-myc, TrkC, and anaplasia. J. Neuropathol. Exp. Neurol. 63 (5), 441–449.

Eberhart, C.G., Kratz, J.E., Schuster, A., et al., 2002. Comparative genomic hybridization detects an increased number of chromosomal alterations in large cell/anaplastic medulloblastomas. Brain Pathol. 12 (1), 36–44.

Eberhart, C.G., Tihan, T., Burger, P.C., 2000. Nuclear localization and mutation of beta-catenin in medulloblastomas. J. Neuropathol. Exp. Neurol. 59 (4), 333–337.

Ellison, D.W., Onilude, O.E., Lindsey, J.C., et al., 2005. beta-Catenin status predicts a favorable outcome in childhood medulloblastoma: the United Kingdom Children's Cancer Study Group Brain Tumour Committee. J. Clin. Oncol. 23 (31), 7951–7957.

Er, U., Yigitkanli, K., Kazanci, B., et al., 2008. Medullomyoblastoma: teratoid nature of a quite rare neoplasm. Surgical neurology 69 (4), 403–406.

Evans, A.E., Jenkin, R.D., Sposto, R., et al., 1990. The treatment of medulloblastoma. Results of a prospective randomized trial of radiation therapy with and without CCNU, vincristine, and prednisone. J. Neurosurg. 72 (4), 572–582.

Evans, D.G., Farndon, P.A., Burnell, L.D., et al., 1991. The incidence of Gorlin syndrome in 173 consecutive cases of medulloblastoma. Br. J. Cancer 64 (5), 959–961.

Farinotti, M., Ferrarini, M., Solari, A., et al., 1998. Incidence and survival of childhood CNS tumours in the Region of Lombardy, Italy. Brain 121 (Pt 8), 1429–1436.

Farndon, P.A., Del Mastro, R.G., Evans, D.G., et al., 1992. Location of gene for Gorlin syndrome. Lancet 339 (8793), 581–582.

Farwell, J.R., Dohrmann, G.J., Flannery, J.T., 1984. Medulloblastoma in childhood: an epidemiological study. J. Neurosurg. 61 (4), 657–664.

Farwell, J.R., Flannery, J.T., 1987. Adult occurrence of medulloblastoma. Acta. Neurochir. 86 (1–2), 1–5.

Finlay, J.L., 1999. The role of high-dose chemotherapy and stem cell rescue in the treatment of malignant brain tumors: a reappraisal. Pediatr. Transplant. 3 (Suppl), 87–95.

Friedberg, M.H., David, O., Adelman, L.S., et al., 1997. Recurrence of medulloblastoma: violation of Collins' law after two decades. Surg. Neurol. 47 (6), 571–574.

Friedman, H.S., Kun, L.E., 1995. More on surveillance of children with medulloblastoma. N. Engl. J. Med. 332 (3), 191.

Fritsch, M.J., Doerner, L., Kienke, S., et al., 2005. Hydrocephalus in children with posterior fossa tumors: role of endoscopic third ventriculostomy. J. Neurosurg. 103 (Suppl), 40–42.

Fukunaga-Johnson, N., Lee, J.H., Sandler, H.M., et al., 1998. Patterns of failure following treatment for medulloblastoma: is it necessary to treat the entire posterior fossa? Int. J. Radiat. Oncol. Biol. Phys. 42 (1), 143–146.

Gailani, M.R., Bale, S.J., Leffell, D.J., et al., 1992. Developmental defects in Gorlin syndrome related to a putative tumor suppressor gene on chromosome 9. Cell 69 (1), 111–117.

Gajjar, A., Chintagumpala, M., Ashley, D., et al., 2006. Risk-adapted craniospinal radiotherapy followed by high-dose chemotherapy and stem-cell rescue in children with newly diagnosed medulloblastoma (St Jude Medulloblastoma-96): long-term results from a prospective, multicentre trial. Lancet Oncol. 7 (10), 813–820.

Gajjar, A., Hernan, R., Kocak, M., et al., 2004. Clinical, histopathologic, and molecular markers of prognosis: toward a new disease risk stratification system for medulloblastoma. J. Clin. Oncol. 22 (6), 984–993.

Gajjar, A., Sanford, R.A., Bhargava, R., et al., 1996. Medulloblastoma with brain stem involvement: the impact of gross total resection on outcome. Pediatr. Neurosurg. 25 (4), 182–187.

Gentet, J.C., Bouffet, E., Doz, F., et al., 1995. Preirradiation chemotherapy including eight drugs in 1 day regimen and high-dose methotrexate in childhood medulloblastoma: results of the M7 French Cooperative Study. J. Neurosurg. 82 (4), 608–614.

Giangaspero, F., Perilongo, G., Fondelli, M.P., et al., 1999. Medulloblastoma with extensive nodularity: a variant with favorable prognosis. J. Neurosurg. 91 (6), 971–977.

Gilbertson, R.J., 2004. Medulloblastoma: signalling a change in treatment. Lancet Oncol. 5 (4), 209–218.

Gilbertson, R.J., Ellison, D.W., 2008. The origins of medulloblastoma sub-types. Ann. Rev. Pathol. 3, 341–365.

Gilbertson, R.J., Pearson, A.D., Perry, R.H., et al., 1995. Prognostic significance of the c-erbB-2 oncogene product in childhood medulloblastoma. Br. J. Cancer 71 (3), 473–477.

Giordana, M.T., Schiffer, P., Lanotte, M., et al., 1999. Epidemiology of adult medulloblastoma. Int. J. Cancer 80 (5), 689–692.

Gjerris, F., Agerlin, N., Børgesen, S.E., et al., 1998. Epidemiology and prognosis in children treated for intracranial tumours in Denmark 1960–1984. Childs Nerv. Syst. 14 (7), 302–311.

Gök, A., Alptekin, M., Erkutlu, I., 2004. Surgical approach to the fourth ventricle cavity through the cerebellomedullary fissure. Neurosurg. Rev. 27 (1), 50–54.

Gorlin, R.J., 1995. Nevoid basal cell carcinoma syndrome. Dermatologic clinics 13 (1), 113–125.

Graham, M.L., Herndon, J.E., 2nd., Casey, J.R., et al., 1997. High-dose chemotherapy with autologous stem-cell rescue in patients with recurrent and high-risk pediatric brain tumors. J. Clin. Oncol. 15 (5), 1814–1823.

Grimmer, M.R., Weiss, W.A., 2006. Childhood tumors of the nervous system as disorders of normal development. Curr. Opin. Pediatr. 18 (6), 634–638.

Grotzer, M.A., Janss, A.J., Fung, K., et al., 2000. TrkC expression predicts good clinical outcome in primitive neuroectodermal brain tumors. J. Clin. Oncol. 18 (5), 1027–1035.

Grotzer, M.A., von Hoff, K., von Bueren, A.O., et al., 2007. Which clinical and biological tumor markers proved predictive in the prospective multicenter trial HIT'91 – implications for investigating childhood medulloblastoma. Klin. Pädiatr. 219 (6), 312–317.

Guessous, F., Li, Y., Abounader, R., 2008. Signaling pathways in medulloblastoma. J. Cell Physiol. 217 (3), 577–583.

Gurney, J.G., 1999. Topical topics: Brain cancer incidence in children: time to look beyond the trends. Med. Pediatr. Oncol. 33 (2), 110–112.

Gurney, J.G., Kadan-Lottick, N., 2001. Brain and other central nervous system tumors: rates, trends, and epidemiology. Current opinion in oncology 13 (3), 160–166.

Gurney, J.G., Wall, D.A., Jukich, P.J., et al., 1999. The contribution of nonmalignant tumors to CNS tumor incidence rates among children in the United States. Cancer Causes Control 10 (2), 101–105.

Guruangan, S., Dunkel, I.J., Goldman, S., et al., 1998. Myeloablative chemotherapy with autologous bone marrow rescue in young children with recurrent malignant brain tumors. J. Clin. Oncol. 16 (7), 2486–2493.

Halberg, F.E., Wara, W.M., Fippin, L.F., et al., 1991. Low-dose craniospinal radiation therapy for medulloblastoma. Int. J. Radiat. Oncol. Biol. Phys. 20 (4), 651–654.

Hamada, H., Kurimoto, M., Endo, S., et al., 1998. Turcot's syndrome presenting with medulloblastoma and familiar adenomatous polyposis: a case report and review of the literature. Acta. Neurochir. 140 (6), 631–632.

Hamilton, S.R., Liu, B., Parsons, R.E., et al., 1995. The molecular basis of Turcot's syndrome. N. Engl. J. Med. 332 (13), 839–847.

Helseth, A., Mørk, S.J., 1989. Neoplasms of the central nervous system in Norway. III. Epidemiological characteristics of intracranial gliomas according to histology. APMIS 97 (6), 547–555.

Helseth, E., Due-Tonnessen, B., Wesenberg, F., et al., 1999. Posterior fossa medulloblastoma in children and young adults (0–19 years): survival and performance. Childs Nerv. Syst. 15 (9), 451–456.

Hjalmars, U., Kulldorff, M., Wahlqvist, Y., et al., 1999. Increased incidence rates but no space-time clustering of childhood astrocytoma in Sweden, 1973–1992: a population-based study of pediatric brain tumors. Cancer 85 (9), 2077–2090.

Huang, H., Mahler-Araujo, B.M., Sankila, A., et al., 2000. APC mutations in sporadic medulloblastomas. Am. J. Pathol. 156 (2), 433–437.

Huber, J.F., Bradley, K., Spiegler, B.J., et al., 2006. Long-term effects of transient cerebellar mutism after cerebellar astrocytoma or medulloblastoma tumor resection in childhood. Childs Nerv. Syst. 22 (2), 132–138.

Janss, A.J., Yachnis, A.T., Silber, J.H., et al., 1996. Glial differentiation predicts poor clinical outcome in primitive neuroectodermal brain tumors. Ann. Neurol. 39 (4), 481–489.

Jenkin, D., 1996. The radiation treatment of medulloblastoma. J. Neurooncol. 29 (1), 45–54.

Jenkin, D., Goddard, K., Armstrong, D., et al., 1990. Posterior fossa medulloblastoma in childhood: treatment results and a proposal for a new staging system. Int. J. Radiat. Oncol. Biol. Phys. 19 (2), 265–274.

Johnson, R.L., Rothman, A.L., Xie, J., et al., 1996. Human homolog of patched, a candidate gene for the basal cell nevus syndrome. Science 272 (5268), 1668–1671.

Kadota, R.P., Mahoney, D.H., Doyle, J., et al., 2008. Dose intensive melphalan and cyclophosphamide with autologous hematopoietic stem cells for recurrent medulloblastoma or germinoma. Pediatr. Blood Cancer 51 (5), 675–678.

Keles, G.E., Berger, M.S., Lim, R., et al., 1992. Expression of glial fibrillary acidic protein in human medulloblastoma cells treated with recombinant glia maturation factor-beta. Oncol. Res. 4 (10), 431–437.

Kelleher, F.C., Fennelly, D., Rafferty, M., 2006. Common critical pathways in embryogenesis and cancer. Acta. Oncol. (Stockholm, Sweden) 45 (4), 375–388.

Kombogiorgas, D., Natarajan, K., Sgouros, S., 2008. Predictive value of preoperative ventricular volume on the need for permanent hydrocephalus treatment immediately after resection of posterior fossa medulloblastomas in children. J. Neurosurg. Pediatr. 1 (6), 451–455.

Kombogiorgas, D., Sgouros, S., Walsh, A.R., et al., 2007. Outcome of children with posterior fossa medulloblastoma: a single institution experience over the decade 1994–2003. Childs Nerv. Syst. 23 (4), 399–405.

Kool, M., Koster, J., Bunt, J., et al., 2008. Integrated genomics identifies five medulloblastoma sub-types with distinct genetic profiles, pathway signatures and clinicopathological features. PLoS ONE 3 (8), e3088.

Koral, K., Gargan, L., Bowers, D.C., et al., 2008. Imaging characteristics of atypical teratoid-rhabdoid tumor in children compared with medulloblastoma. AJR. Am. J. Roentgenol. 190 (3), 809–814.

Kortmann, R.D., Kühl, J., Timmermann, B., et al., 2000. Postoperative neoadjuvant chemotherapy before radiotherapy as compared to immediate radiotherapy followed by maintenance chemotherapy in the treatment of medulloblastoma in childhood: results of the German prospective randomized trial HIT '91. Int. J. Radiat. Oncol. Biol. Phys. 46 (2), 269–279.

Krischer, J.P., Ragab, A.H., Kun, L., et al., 1991. Nitrogen mustard, vincristine, procarbazine, and prednisone as adjuvant chemotherapy in the treatment of medulloblastoma. A Pediatric Oncology Group study. J. Neurosurg. 74 (6), 905–909.

Kühl, J., Müller, H.L., Berthold, F., et al., 1998. Preradiation chemotherapy of children and young adults with malignant brain tumors: results of the German pilot trial HIT'88/'89. Klin. Pädiatr. 210 (4), 227–233.

Kuratsu, J., Ushio, Y., 1996. Epidemiological study of primary intracranial tumors in childhood. A population-based survey in Kumamoto Prefecture, Japan. Pediatr. Neurosurg. 25 (5), 240–247.

Lamont, J.M., McManamy, C.S., Pearson, A.D., et al., 2004. Combined histopathological and molecular cytogenetic stratification of medulloblastoma patients. Clin. Cancer. Res. 10 (16), 5482–5493.

Lannering, B., Marky, I., Nordborg, C., 1990. Brain tumors in childhood and adolescence in west Sweden 1970–1984. Epidemiology and survival. Cancer 66 (3), 604–609.

Larouche, V., Huang, A., Bartels, U., et al, 2007. Tumors of the central nervous system in the first year of life. Pediatr. Blood Cancer 49 (Suppl), 1074–1082.

Lasser, D.M., DeVivo, D.C., Garvin, J., et al., 1994. Turcot's syndrome: evidence for linkage to the adenomatous polyposis coli (APC) locus. Neurology 44 (6), 1083–1086.

Latchaw, J.P., Hahn, J.F., Moylan, D.J., et al., 1985. Medulloblastoma. Period of risk reviewed. Cancer 55 (1), 186–189.

Lauth, M., Bergström, A., Shimokawa, T., et al., 2007. Inhibition of GLI-mediated transcription and tumor cell growth by small-molecule antagonists. Proc. Natl. Acad. Sci. USA 104 (20), 8455–8460.

Lee, M., Wisoff, J.H., Abbott, R., et al., 1994. Management of hydrocephalus in children with medulloblastoma: prognostic factors for shunting. Pediatr. Neurosurg. 20 (4), 240–247.

Lee, S.E., Johnson, S.P., Hale, L.P., et al., 1998. Analysis of DNA mismatch repair proteins in human medulloblastoma. Clin. Cancer Res. 4 (6), 1415–1419.

Louis, D.N., Ohgaki, H., Wiestler, O.D., et al., 2007a. The 2007 WHO classification of tumours of the central nervous system. Acta. Neuropathol. 114 (2), 97–109.

Louis, D.N., Ohgaki, H., Wiestler, O.D., et al., 2007b. WHO Classification of Tumors of the Central Nervous System, 4th edn. IARC, Lyon.

Mabbott, D.J., Spiegler, B.J., Greenberg, M.L., et al., 2005. Serial evaluation of academic and behavioral outcome after treatment with cranial radiation in childhood. J. Clin. Oncol. 23 (10), 2256–2263.

Mahoney, D.H., Jr., Strother, D., Camitta, B., et al., 1996. High-dose melphalan and cyclophosphamide with autologous bone marrow rescue for recurrent/progressive malignant brain tumors in children: a pilot pediatric oncology group study. J. Clin. Oncol. 14 (2), 382–388.

Maraziotis, T., Perentes, E., Karamitopoulou, E., et al., 1992. Neuron-associated class III beta-tubulin isotype, retinal S-antigen, synaptophysin, and glial fibrillary acidic protein in human medulloblastomas: a clinicopathological analysis of 36 cases. Acta. Neuropathol. 84 (4), 355–363.

Marino, S., 2005. Medulloblastoma: developmental mechanisms out of control. Trends Mol. Med. 11 (1), 17–22.

Mason, W.P., Grovas, A., Halpern, S., et al., 1998. Intensive chemotherapy and bone marrow rescue for young children with newly diagnosed malignant brain tumors. J. Clin. Oncol. 16 (1), 210–221.

Massimino, M., Gandola, L., Cefalo, G., et al., 2000. Management of medulloblastoma and ependymoma in infants: a single-institution long-term retrospective report. Childs. Nerv. Syst. 16 (1), 15–20.

Matsushima, T., Fukui, M., Inoue, T., et al., 1992. Microsurgical and magnetic resonance imaging anatomy of the cerebello-medullary fissure and its application during fourth ventricle surgery. Neurosurgery 30 (3), 325–330.

Matsutani, M., 2004. Chemoradiotherapy for brain tumors: current status and perspectives. Int. J. Clin. Oncol. 9 (6), 471–474.

McManamy, C.S., Pears, J., Weston, C.L., et al., 2007. Nodule formation and desmoplasia in medulloblastomas-defining the nodular/desmoplastic variant and its biological behavior. Brain Pathol. 17 (2), 151–164.

Mendrzyk, F., Korshunov, A., Toedt, G., et al., 2006. Isochromosome breakpoints on 17p in medulloblastoma are flanked by different classes of DNA sequence repeats. Genes Chromosomes Cancer 45 (4), 401–410.

Merchant, T.E., Kun, L.E., Krasin, M.J. et al., 2008. Multi-institution prospective trial of reduced-dose craniospinal irradiation (23.4 Gy) followed by conformal posterior fossa (36 Gy) and primary site irradiation (55.8 Gy) and dose-intensive chemotherapy for average-risk medulloblastoma. Int. J. Radiat. Oncol. Biol. Phys. 70 (3), 782–787.

Meyers, S.P., Kemp, S.S., Tarr, R.W., 1992. MR imaging features of medulloblastomas. AJR. Am. J. Roentgen. 158 (4), 859–865.

Modha, A., Vassilyadi, M., George, A., et al., 2000. Medulloblastoma in children – the Ottawa experience. Childs Nerv. Sys. 16 (6), 341–350.

Morelli, D., Pirotte, B., Lubansu, A., et al., 2005. Persistent hydrocephalus after early surgical management of posterior fossa tumors in children: is routine preoperative endoscopic third ventriculostomy justified? J. Neurosurg. 103 (Suppl), 247–252.

Mueller, D.P., Moore, S.A., Sato, Y., et al., 1992. MRI spectrum of medulloblastoma. Clin. Imaging 16 (4), 250–255.

Mulhern, R.K., Palmer, S.L., Merchant, T.E. et al., 2005. Neurocognitive consequences of risk-adapted therapy for childhood medulloblastoma. J. Clin. Oncol. 23 (24), 5511–5519.

Oyharcabal-Bourden, V., Kalifa, C., Gentet, J.C., et al., 2005. Standard-risk medulloblastoma treated by adjuvant chemotherapy followed by reduced-dose craniospinal radiation therapy: a French Society of Pediatric Oncology Study. J. Clin. Oncol. 23 (21), 4726–4734.

Packer, R.J., Cogen, P., Vezina, G., et al., 1999a. Medulloblastoma: clinical and biologic aspects. Neuro. Oncology 1 (3), 232–250.

Packer, R.J., Goldwein, J., Nicholson, H.S., et al., 1999b. Treatment of children with medulloblastomas with reduced-dose craniospinal radiation therapy and adjuvant chemotherapy: A Children's Cancer Group Study. J. Clin. Oncol. 17 (7), 2127–2136.

Packer, R.J., Sutton, L.N., Elterman, R., et al., 1994. Outcome for children with medulloblastoma treated with radiation and cisplatin, CCNU, and vincristine chemotherapy. J. Neurosurg. 81 (5), 690–698.

Packer, R.J., Sutton, L.N., Goldwein, J.W., et al., 1991. Improved survival with the use of adjuvant chemotherapy in the treatment of medulloblastoma. J. Neurosurg. 74 (3), 433–440.

Packer, R.J., Sutton, L.N., Rorke, L.B., et al., 1984. Prognostic importance of cellular differentiation in medulloblastoma of childhood. J. Neurosurg. 61 (2), 296–301.

Palmer, J.O., Kasselberg, A.G., Netsky, M.G., 1981. Differentiation of Medulloblastoma. Studies including immunohistochemical localization of glial fibrillary acidic protein. J. Neurosurg. 55 (2), 161–169.

Paraf, F., Jothy, S., Van Meir, E.G., 1997. Brain tumor-polyposis syndrome: two genetic diseases? J. Clin. Oncol. 15 (7), 2744–2758.

Park, T.S., Hoffman, H.J., Hendrick, E.B., et al., 1983. Medulloblastoma: clinical presentation and management. Experience at the hospital for sick children, Toronto, 1950–1980. J. Neurosurg. 58 (4), 543–552.

Paterson, E., Farr, R.F., 1953. Cerebellar medulloblastoma: treatment by irradiation of the whole central nervous system. Acta. Radiol. 39 (4), 323–336.

Paulino, A.C., 1997. Radiotherapeutic management of medulloblastoma. Oncology 11 (6), 813–831.

Petrij, F., Giles, R.H., Dauwerse, H.G., et al., 1995. Rubinstein-Taybi syndrome caused by mutations in the transcriptional co-activator CBP. Nature 376 (6538), 348–351.

Pietsch, T., Taylor, M.D., Rutka, J.T., 2004. Molecular pathogenesis of childhood brain tumors. J. Neurooncol. 70 (2), 203–215.

Polkinghorn, W.R., Tarbell, N.J., 2007. Medulloblastoma: tumorigenesis, current clinical paradigm, and efforts to improve risk stratification. Nature clinical practice Oncology 4 (5), 295–304.

Pollack, I.F., Polinko, P., Albright, A.L., et al., 1995. Mutism and pseudobulbar symptoms after resection of posterior fossa tumors in children: incidence and pathophysiology. Neurosurgery 37 (5), 885–893.

Pomeroy, S.L., Tamayo, P., Gaasenbeek, M., et al., 2002. Prediction of central nervous system embryonal tumour outcome based on gene expression. Nature 415 (6870), 436–442.

Raimondi, A.J., Tomita, T., 1979. Medulloblastoma in childhood: comparative results of partial and total resection. Child's brain 5 (3), 310–328.

Rappaport, Z.H., Shalit, M.N., 1989. Perioperative external ventricular drainage in obstructive hydrocephalus secondary to infratentorial brain tumours. Acta. Neurochir. 96 (3–4), 118–121.

Ray, A., Ho, M., Ma, J., et al., 2004. A clinicobiological model predicting survival in medulloblastoma. Clin. Cancer Res. 10 (22), 7613–7620.

Ribi, K., Relly, C., Landolt, M.A., et al., 2005. Outcome of medulloblastoma in children: long-term complications and quality of life. Neuropediatrics 36 (6), 357–365.

Ris, M.D., Packer, R., Goldwein, J., et al., 2001. Intellectual outcome after reduced-dose radiation therapy plus adjuvant chemotherapy for medulloblastoma: a Children's Cancer Group study. J. Clin. Oncol. 19 (15), 3470–3476.

Robertson, P.L., Muraszko, K.M., Holmes, E.J., et al., 2006. Incidence and severity of postoperative cerebellar mutism syndrome in children with medulloblastoma: a prospective study by the Children's Oncology Group. J. Neurosurg. 105 (6 Suppl), 444–451.

Rorke, L.B., 1983. The cerebellar medulloblastoma and its relationship to primitive neuroectodermal tumors. J. Neuropathol. Exp. Neurol. 42 (1), 1–15.

Rutka, J.T., 1997. Medulloblastoma. Clin. Neurosurg. 44, 571–585.

Rutka, J.T., Hoffman, H.J., 1996. Medulloblastoma: a historical perspective and overview. J. Neurooncol. 29 (1), 1–7.

Rutkowski, S., Bode, U., Deinlein, F., et al., 2005. Treatment of early childhood medulloblastoma by postoperative chemotherapy alone. N. Engl. J. Med. 352 (10), 978–986.

Sanders, R.P., Onar, A., Boyett, J.M., et al., 2008. M1 Medulloblastoma: high risk at any age. J. Neurooncol. 90 (3), 351–355.

Saunders, D.E., Hayward, R.D., Phipps, K.P., et al., 2003. Surveillance neuroimaging of intracranial medulloblastoma in children: how effective, how often, and for how long? J. Neurosurg. 99 (2), 280–286.

Schofield, D.E., Yunis, E.J., Geyer, J.R., et al., 1992. DNA content and other prognostic features in childhood medulloblastoma. Proposal of a scoring system. Cancer 69 (5), 1307–1314.

Schüller, U., Heine, V.M., Mao, J., et al., 2008. Acquisition of granule neuron precursor identity is a critical determinant of progenitor cell competence to form Shh-induced medulloblastoma. Cancer Cell 14 (2), 123–134.

Segal, R.A., Goumnerova, L.C., Kwon, Y.K., et al., 1994. Expression of the neurotrophin receptor TrkC is linked to a favorable outcome in medulloblastoma. Proc. Natl. Acad. Sci. USA 91 (26), 12867–12871.

Shaw, D.W., Geyer, J.R., Berger, M.S., et al., 1997. Asymptomatic recurrence detection with surveillance scanning in children with medulloblastoma. J. Clin. Oncol. 15 (5), 1811–1813.

Shu, Q., Antalffy, B., Su, J.M., et al., 2006. Valproic Acid prolongs survival time of severe combined immunodeficient mice bearing intracerebral orthotopic medulloblastoma xenografts. Clin. Cancer Res. 12 (15), 4687–4694.

Sjölund, J., Manetopoulos, C., Stockhausen, M.T., et al., 2005. The Notch pathway in cancer: differentiation gone awry. Eur. J. Cancer 41 (17), 2620–2629.

Strother, D., Ashley, D., Kellie, S.J., et al., 2001. Feasibility of four consecutive high-dose chemotherapy cycles with stem-cell rescue for patients with newly diagnosed medulloblastoma or supratentorial primitive neuroectodermal tumor after craniospinal radiotherapy: results of a collaborative study. J. Clin. Oncol. 19 (10), 2696–2704.

Sure, U., Berghorn, W.J., Bertalanffy, H., et al., 1995. Staging, scoring and grading of medulloblastoma. A postoperative prognosis predicting system based on the cases of a single institute. Acta. Neurochir. 132 (1–3), 59–65.

Suresh, T.N., Santosh, V., Yasha, T.C., et al., 2004. Medulloblastoma with extensive nodularity: a variant occurring in the very young-clinicopathological and immunohistochemical study of four cases. Childs Nerv. Syst. 20 (1), 55–60.

Sutton, L.N., Phillips, P.C., Molloy, P.T., 1996. Surgical management of medulloblastoma. J. Neurooncol. 29 (1), 9–21.

Tabori, U., Sung, L., Hukin, J., et al., 2006. Distinctive clinical course and pattern of relapse in adolescents with medulloblastoma. Int. J. Radiat. Oncol. Biol. Phys. 64 (2), 402–407.

Taipale, J., Chen, J.K., Cooper, M.K., et al., 2000. Effects of oncogenic mutations in Smoothened and Patched can be reversed by cyclopamine. Nature 406 (6799), 1005–1009.

Tait, D.M., Thornton-Jones, H., Bloom, H.J., et al., 1990. Adjuvant chemotherapy for medulloblastoma: the first multi-centre control trial of the International Society of Paediatric Oncology (SIOP I). Eur. J. Cancer 26 (4), 464–469.

Taylor, M.D., Liu, L., Raffel, C., et al., 2002. Mutations in SUFU predispose to medulloblastoma. Nat. Genet. 31 (3), 306–310.

Taylor, M.D., Mainprize, T.G., Rutka, J.T., 2000. Molecular insight into medulloblastoma and central nervous system primitive neuroectodermal tumor biology from hereditary syndromes: a review. Neurosurgery 47 (4), 888–901.

Taylor, M.D., Zhang, X., Liu, L., et al., 2004a. Failure of a medulloblastoma-derived mutant of SUFU to suppress WNT signaling. Oncogene 23 (26), 4577–4583.

Taylor, R.E., Bailey, C.C., Robinson, K. et al., 2003. Results of a randomized study of preradiation chemotherapy versus radiotherapy alone for nonmetastatic medulloblastoma: The International Society of Paediatric Oncology/United Kingdom Children's Cancer Study Group PNET-3 Study. J. Clin. Oncol. 21 (8), 1581–1591.

Taylor, R.E., Bailey, C.C., Robinson, K.J., et al., 2004b. Impact of radiotherapy parameters on outcome in the International Society of Paediatric Oncology/United Kingdom Children's Cancer Study Group PNET-3 study of preradiotherapy chemotherapy for M0-M1 medulloblastoma. Int. J. Radiat. Oncol. Biol. Phys. 58 (4), 1184–1193.

Taylor, R.E., Bailey, C.C., Robinson, K.J., et al., 2005. Outcome for patients with metastatic (M2–M3) medulloblastoma treated with SIOP/UKCCSG PNET-3 chemotherapy. Eur. J. Cancer 41 (5), 727–734.

Thomas, P.R., Deutsch, M., Kepner, J.L., et al., 2000. Low-stage medulloblastoma: final analysis of trial comparing standard-dose with reduced-dose neuraxis irradiation. J. Clin. Oncol. 18 (16), 3004–3011.

Thorne, R.N., Pearson, A.D., Nicoll, J.A., et al., 1994. Decline in incidence of medulloblastoma in children. Cancer 74 (12), 3240–3244.

Tomita, T., McLone, D.G., 1986. Medulloblastoma in childhood: results of radical resection and low-dose neuraxis radiation therapy. J. Neurosurg. 64 (2), 238–242.

Torres, C.F., Rebsamen, S., Silber, J.H., et al., 1994. Surveillance scanning of children with medulloblastoma. N. Engl. J. Med. 330 (13), 892–895.

Ullrich, N.J., Robertson, R., Kinnamon, D.D., et al., 2007. Moyamoya following cranial irradiation for primary brain tumors in children. Neurology 68 (12), 932–938.

Varley, J.M., Evans, D.G., Birch, J.M., 1997. Li-Fraumeni syndrome – a molecular and clinical review. Br. J. Cancer 76 (1), 1–14.

Verlooy, J., Mosseri, V., Bracard, S., et al., 2006. Treatment of high risk medulloblastomas in children above the age of 3 years: a SFOP study. Eur. J. Cancer 42 (17), 3004–3014.

Vézina, L.G., Packer, R.J., 1994. Infratentorial brain tumors of childhood. Neuroimaging Clin. North Am. 4 (2), 423–436.

Wallace, V.A., 1999. Purkinje-cell-derived Sonic hedgehog regulates granule neuron precursor cell proliferation in the developing mouse cerebellum. Curr. Biol. 9 (8), 445–448.

Washiyama, K., Muragaki, Y., Rorke, L.B., et al., 1996. Neurotrophin and neurotrophin receptor proteins in medulloblastomas and other primitive neuroectodermal tumors of the pediatric central nervous system. Am. J. Pathol. 148 (3), 929–940.

Wisoff, J.H., Epstein, F.J., 1984. Pseudobulbar palsy after posterior fossa operation in children. Neurosurgery 15 (5), 707–709.

Wolden, S.L., Dunkel, I.J., Souweidane, M.M., et al., 2003. Patterns of failure using a conformal radiation therapy tumor bed boost for medulloblastoma. J. Clin. Oncol. 21 (16), 3079–3083.

Yalçin, B., Büyükpamukçu, M., Akalan, N., et al., 2002. Value of surveillance imaging in the management of medulloblastoma. Med. Pediatr. Oncol. 38 (2), 91–97.

Yang, Z.J., Ellis, T., Markant, S.L., et al., 2008. Medulloblastoma can be initiated by deletion of Patched in lineage-restricted progenitors or stem cells. Cancer Cell 14 (2), 135–145.

Yokota, N., Nishizawa, S., Ohta, S., et al., 2002. Role of Wnt pathway in medulloblastoma oncogenesis. Int. J. Cancer 101 (2), 198–201.

Zanini, C., Mandili, G., Pulerà, F., et al., 2008. Immunohistochemical and proteomic profile of melanotic medulloblastoma. Pediatr. Blood Cancer 52 (7), 875–877.

Zeltzer, P.M., Boyett, J.M., Finlay, J.L., et al., 1999. Metastasis stage, adjuvant treatment, and residual tumor are prognostic factors for medulloblastoma in children: conclusions from the Children's Cancer Group 921 randomized phase III study. J. Clin. Oncol. 17 (3), 832–845.

Zurawel, R.H., Allen, C., Chiappa, S., et al., 2000. Analysis of PTCH/SMO/SHH pathway genes in medulloblastoma. Genes Chromosomes Cancer 27 (1), 44–51.

Zurawel, R.H., Chiappa, S.A., Allen, C., et al., 1998. Sporadic medulloblastomas contain oncogenic beta-catenin mutations. Cancer Res. 58 (5), 896–899.

NERVE SHEATH TUMORS

28 Acoustic neurinoma (vestibular schwannoma)

Andrew H. Kaye, Robert J. S. Briggs, and Andrew P. Morokoff

Epidemiology

Incidence and prevalence of tumor

Acoustic neurinomas (vestibular schwannomas) account for approximately 6–8% of all primary intracranial tumors, and are responsible for about 78% of lesions developing within the cerebellopontine angle (Cushing 1932; Revilla 1947). However, the percentage differs considerably in more recent series, due probably to variations in the referral base. Tumors are bilateral in around 4–5% of cases.

With one exception, there have been no large studies to determine the incidence of acoustic neurinoma in a well-defined geographic population. Tos et al (1992a) have estimated an annual detection rate of 9.4 tumors per year per million inhabitants of Denmark. This is much lower than estimates based upon anatomic studies of autopsy material. Hardy & Crowe (1936) found six minute and asymptomatic schwannomas in a study of 250 temporal bones, an incidence of 2.4%. In a similar study, Leonard and Talbot (1970) suggested an incidence of around 1.7%. However, post-mortem studies may have overestimated the true incidence of this condition. The fact that audiometry was available in the cadavers studied, and that the specimens were not consecutive, suggests that the material may have been biased to temporal bones with associated pre-existing hearing disorders. In a more recent and unselected post-mortem study of 298 temporal bones, Karjalainen et al (1984) found no occult neurinomas. In a clinical series of 9176 patients investigated for otoneurologic disorders, only 0.76% were found to harbor a cerebellopontine angle tumor, some of which were acoustic neurinomas (Guyot et al 1992). Whatever the true incidence of the condition, the disparity between clinical and pathologic studies does suggest that a substantial number of lesions remain asymptomatic or undiagnosed and that occult neurinomas may follow a benign course (Brackmann & Kwartler 1990a). An increase in the number of tumors treated in the last decade is more likely to represent better awareness of the condition and earlier diagnosis associated with improved imaging modalities, than to suggest a true increase in the prevalence of the disease (Glasscock et al 1987; Tos et al 1992a).

Growth rate

The natural history of acoustic neurinomas is variable, and is reflected in marked differences in the duration of symptoms at the time of presentation. Usually such tumors are slow-growing. In some series, around 40% of tumors treated conservatively did not enlarge at all, or even regressed over the period of observation (Luetje et al 1988; Valvassori & Guzman 1989; Thomsen & Tos 1990; Selesnick & Johnson 1998). On average, lesion diameter will increase at a rate of <2 mm per year in around 78% of patients (Nedzelski et al 1992). In other instances, the rate of growth is more rapid, at between 2.5 and 4 mm per year (Wazen et al 1985; Laasonen & Troupp 1986). The rate of expansion may however, be considerably slower in the elderly, where a mean enlargement of 1.4 mm per year has been reported (Sterkers et al 1992). This is in contrast to a study by Valvassori and Guzman (1989), who concluded that there is no correlation between the rate of tumor growth and patient age. Yet there does exist an inverse relationship between age and tumor size at presentation. Large tumors are significantly more common in the younger age groups (Thomsen et al 1992).

It has been reported that the future behavior of a tumor can be predicted radiologically within a relatively short period of observation. A pattern of slow or absent growth over a period of 18 months to 3 years makes it unlikely that subsequent enlargement will be significant (Nedzelski et al 1992). Valvassori and Guzman (1989) reached a similar conclusion in a study of 35 patients managed expectantly. Any further growth was evident usually within the first year. On the other hand, Noren and Greitz (1992) studied 98 tumors in 93 patients over a period of 12–183 months and observed that 66% of tumors increased in size over 1–2 years, that 86% enlarged when observed for 3–4 years, but that 100% had expanded if follow-up was continued for >4 years. It appears that some tumors may demonstrate significant growth after an initial period of quiescence. Charabi and co-workers (1998) reported a group of 23 patients with acoustic neurinoma: initially no growth was demonstrated for a mean duration of 1.6 years, followed by a period of tumor growth with a mean growth rate of 0.48 cm per year (Charabi et al 1995). In a more recent report on the follow-up of a series of 123 patients observed in Denmark, by the end of a prolonged observation period (mean 3.8 years) tumor growth was observed in 82%, no growth in 12%, and negative growth in 6% of tumors.

Flow cytometric studies have confirmed a variable mitotic rate in acoustic neurinomas, and have shown that this correlates clinically with the speed of tumor growth (Wennerberg & Mercke 1989). DNA cytofluorometric analysis has been used also to establish the proportion of cells in the S-phase of the cell cycle, but this is not linked to tumor size, or to the duration of symptoms at the time of presentation (Rasmussen et al 1984). These data are supported by the results of clinical studies, which have shown no statistical correlation between tumor size at diagnosis and the rate of subsequent growth (Nedzelski et al 1992). Large tumors do not necessarily grow faster than smaller ones. Factors other than mitotic activity which govern the rate of expansion of these lesions include hemorrhage, cystic degeneration, and peritumoral edema. Any of these may, on occasion, result in precipitate enlargement of the tumor (Nager 1969; Lee & Wang 1989).

A hormone closely related closely to bovine pituitary growth factor may play a role in Schwann cell proliferation in acoustic neurinoma (Brockes et al 1986). Other hormone receptors have also been identified in a varying proportion of tumors. Estrogen and progesterone receptors are among them, although neither of these is thought to govern growth behavior, despite a female preponderance of tumors (Markwalder et al 1986; Whittle et al 1987). Estrogen binding receptors are present in 45% of male and 48% of female neurinomas (Martuza et al 1981). There are, however, reports of an increase in size and vascularity of tumors in women, particularly during pregnancy (Allen et al 1974). Recent evidence suggests that a variety of tumors may secrete their own ('autocrine') growth factors, which bind to specific receptors on the cell membrane and stimulate it to traverse the cell cycle more quickly (for review, see Rutka et al 1990).

The growth rate of bilateral tumors is also very variable, but is on average considerably faster than for unilateral lesions (Kasantikul et al 1980a). However, it is uncertain whether this reflects a different biology for these neoplasms, or the fact that they occur in a younger patient population – a sub-group already known to exhibit a more rapid rate of growth (Graham & Sataloff 1984).

Age distribution

Acoustic neurinomas occur most frequently in middle age. In a series of 1113 cases reported by the House group, approximately 50% of patients were in either their 5th or 6th decades, and only 15% of tumors developed in people under the age of 30 (Fig. 28.1). Acoustic neurinomas that develop in patients suffering from neurofibromatosis type 2 tend to present earlier, with a peak incidence around the 3rd decade (Revilla 1947; Eldridge 1981; Evans et al 1992a). It is very rare for acoustic neurinomas to develop in children, except in those who have neurofibromatosis type 2 (Allcutt et al 1991). The youngest recorded patient was 12 months of age (Fabiani et al 1975). Presentation often occurs late in children because unilateral deafness may be overlooked (Allcutt et al 1991). An association between acoustic neurinoma, salivary gland tumors, and childhood cranial irradiation has been reported (Shore-Freedman et al 1983).

Sex distribution

Cumulative results from large series in the literature show a consistent preponderance of tumors in women; women are affected in around 57%, and men in 43% of cases (Fig. 28.2).

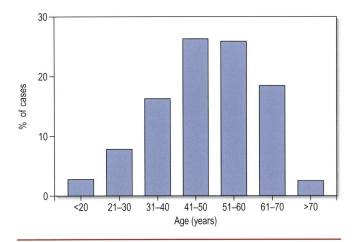

Figure 28.1 Age distribution of a cumulative series of 1113 cases of acoustic neurinoma.

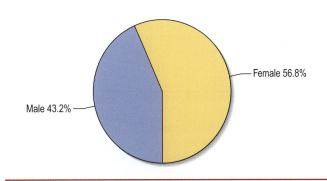

Figure 28.2 Distribution of tumors by sex.

This is not true of tumors in childhood, however, where an equal sex distribution is seen (Hermanz-Schulman et al 1986). A difference in the age distribution of tumors between the sexes was noted by Borcck and Zülch (1951). Men had an earlier peak prevalence (36–42 years) than women (42–56 years), although this finding has not been confirmed by later work.

Racial, national, and geographic considerations

There have, to date, been no large multinational studies to determine demographic factors relating to acoustic neurinoma. However, the proportion which these tumors contribute to the total number of primary intracranial neoplasms varies considerably in different populations. Unfortunately, this does not provide a complete profile of the condition because it depends also on the prevalence of other primary tumors. The incidence of acoustic neurinoma appears to be greatest in the Far East, where they account for 10.6% of primary intracranial neoplasms in India (Dastur et al 1968) and 10.2% of those occurring in China (Huang et al 1982). In the Middle East, a 9% incidence is found in Egypt (Sorour et al 1973). Rates of 4.9% and 4% are reported in England (Barker et al 1976) and the USA, respectively (Kurland et al 1982). The lowest incidence is found in African negroes, figures of 2.6% being recorded in Kenya (Ruberti & Poppi 1971), 0.9% in Nigeria (Adeloye 1979), and 0.5% in what was formerly Rhodesia. The latter can be contrasted with a 3.7% incidence in the white population of the same country (Levy & Auchterlonie 1975). Misdiagnosis may, however, play some part in the low incidence rates reported in Africans. With the use of immunohistochemical markers, Simpson et al (1990) established that some acoustic neurinomas had been misdiagnosed as meningiomas and they concluded that the true incidence in black South Africans was 3.7%. In our experience acoustic neurinomas are very uncommon in negroes, and few if any such families have ever been documented to develop bilateral forms of the disease. Although we are not aware of any studies on social factors, the condition appears to be more common in middle than lower social classes. This may be because the latter are less likely to seek medical attention for relatively minor symptoms.

Genetic factors

Acoustic neurinomas occur in both sporadic and hereditary forms. The vast majority (96%) of tumors are sporadic and unilateral. Hereditary acoustic neurinomas are associated with the condition known as NF-2 (bilateral acoustic neurinomas; central neurofibromatosis). NF-2 was first described in 1822 by the Scottish surgeon Wishart, but bilateral acoustic neurinoma was for a long time regarded as a central form of von Recklinghausen's disease (NF-1). Cushing considered them part of the same disease, however, the two conditions are now known to be distinct in all aspects, clinically and genetically (Kanter et al 1980). NF-1 is much more common than NF-2, and has an incidence of 1/4000 population (Korf 1990). It is characterized by widespread neurofibromas occurring both intra- and extracranially as well as gliomas and other lesions and the NF-1 gene has been localized to chromosome 17 (Barker et al 1987). It is now recognized that there is no increased incidence of schwannomas in NF-1 (Holt 1978; Huson et al 1988) and bilateral tumors are exceptionally rare (Rubenstein 1986).

NF-2 is much more uncommon than NF-1 and has an incidence of about 1 in 33 000–50 000 individuals (Evans et al 2000). The disease is transmitted in an autosomal dominant fashion with high penetrance. The spontaneous mutation rate of the NF-2 gene is high, at around 50% and the hereditary picture is complicated by the high incidence of mosaicism. Bilateral acoustic neurinomas are pathognomonic of this condition, but are not fully penetrant. Other cranial and spinal tumors may also develop. The mean age at onset of symptoms is 22 years, and at diagnosis 28 years. The age at onset of symptoms is significantly younger in maternally than paternally affected cases (18.2 vs 24.5 years). The natural history of NF-2 is variable, and males may sometimes have a milder form of the disease than that which is seen in females. Café-au-lait patches are found in 41% of patients, and presenile lens opacity or subcapsular cataract in 38%. As well as bilateral acoustic neurinomas, the definition of NF-2 also encompasses individuals who have a 1st degree relative suffering from the condition and who have either a unilateral acoustic neurinoma or two of the following: a neurofibroma or schwannoma, meningioma, glioma, or juvenile posterior subcapsular lenticular opacity.

The acoustic neurinomas do not always develop simultaneously, although this is usual. A span of a few months or several years may at times separate them.

The NF-2 gene and Merlin protein

By examining tissue from sporadic tumors, loss of parts of chromosome 22 was recognized early on as a common cytogenetic marker for schwannoma (Seizinger et al 1986) and this was subsequently confirmed by genetic linkage analysis in bilateral acoustic schwannoma patients (Rouleau et al 1987). The chromosome 22 region had previously been found to be abnormal in meningiomas as well (Zang, 1982) and appeared to be commonly mutated in schwannomas, neurofibromas and meningiomas (Seizinger et al 1987b; Jacoby et al 1990; Fontaine et al 1991; Twist et al 1994). Thus, NF-2 associated tumors occur throughout the classic Knudsen 'two-hit' mechanism, whereby a mutation in the second NF-2 allele, on a background of inherited NF-2 gene mutation, leads to abnormalities of both copies of NF-2. The human NF-2 gene located at chromosome 22q12.2 was cloned in 1993 (Rouleau et al 1993; Trofatter et al 1993) and found to have 17 exons encoding a 595 amino acid protein with homology to the Ezrin, Radixin, and Moesin (ERM) superfamily of proteins. The NF-2 gene product was therefore named Merlin (Moesin Ezrin Radixin-like protein) or alternatively, Schwannomin. Alternate splicing of exon 16 which codes for the C-terminus gives rise to two isoforms of Merlin. Isoform 1 is 595 amino acids long, whereas isoform 2 is 590 amino acids long (Bianchi et al 1995). Isoform 1 appears to be the active tumor-suppressing variant and is able to adopt a closed conformation (Sherman et al 1997).

Proteins within the ERM family have a highly conserved amino-terminal region known as the FERM domain (F for 4.1 protein, E for Ezrin, R for Radixin, and M for Moesin) (Chishti et al 1998). The FERM domain forms a 3-part cloverleaf structure that is able to coordinate multiple protein binding partners (McClatchey et al 2009). The second part of the protein consists of a long alpha helical region, followed by a C-terminus, which is less highly conserved (Fig. 28.3). A common feature of proteins having a FERM domain appears to be their involvement in linking the cytoskeleton to the plasma membrane and this appears to be true for Merlin as well. Even although it can be well expected that many regulatory mechanisms applicable to ERM proteins will overlap with those acting on Merlin, in fact none of the ERM proteins, unlike Merlin, have been implicated in a tumor suppressor syndrome and that ERM protein levels are often normal in NF-2 related tumors (Stemmer-Rachamimov et al 1997).

Merlin and cell proliferation

Because it was frequently lost in tumors, the NF-2 gene was suspected early of being a tumor suppressor gene and its protein product, Merlin, was confirmed initially to have a negative effect on cell proliferation, possibly by an anti-Ras action (Tikoo et al 1994; Lutchman et al 1995; Pelton et al 1998). Loss of Merlin has also been linked to cell transformation (Kissil et al 2002). It has been difficult to develop robust cell models for Merlin for a number of reasons, especially because its anti-proliferative action means that establishing

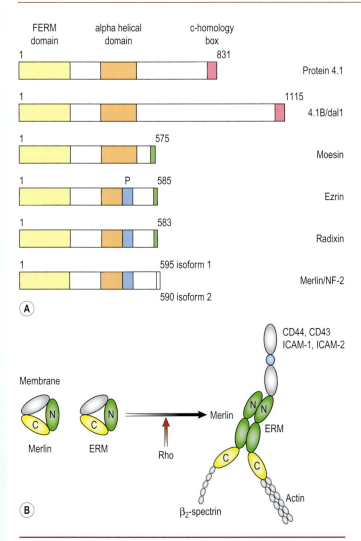

FERM domain   alpha helical domain   c-homology box

Protein 4.1

4.1B/dal1

Moesin

Ezrin

Radixin

Merlin/NF-2

(A)

CD44, CD43
ICAM-1, ICAM-2

Membrane

Merlin

ERM

Rho

Merlin

ERM

Actin

β₂-spectrin

(B)

Figure 28.3 (A) Schematic of the protein band 4.1 superfamily. The structural domains of six members of the family are depicted. Each has a common, conserved N-terminal FERM domain (yellow) and a more centrally located alpha helical domain of unknown function (orange). Merlin, ezrin, and radixin have a proline-rich segment (blue) which may possibly interact with SH3 domain proteins. The C-termini of protein 4.1 and 4.1B/dal 1 are conserved (pink), as are the C-termini of moesin, ezrin, and radixin (green). The two isoforms of Merlin are depicted. (B) A putative interaction model of Merlin associations. The isoform 1 of Merlin is thought to be able to switch between an open and closed state, which is in turn thought to enable its association with other cellular proteins. Stimulated, perhaps, by input from the Rho kinase and secondary messenger pathways, Merlin 'flips' to the open conformation similar to the ERM proteins and thence interacts with the ERM proteins and components of the cytoskeleton and integral membrane receptors.

cell lines with stable Merlin expression is problematic. However, in recent years a number of lines of evidence have slowly built up a coherent picture of the normal function of Merlin, and why loss of function leads to deregulated cell growth and tumorigenesis. For example, Merlin has been shown to downregulate Ras and Rac (Jin et al 2006), inhibit the PI3 kinase pathway by binding to PI3 kinase enhancer long (PIKE-L) (Rong et al 2004b) and decrease STAT function via binding to hepatocyte-growth factor receptor tyrosine kinase substrate (HRS), a molecule which also traffics

growth factor receptors to the degradation pathway (Scoles et al 2002). Merlin also appears to downregulate NF-kappaB activity and to have an anti-apoptotic effect (Utermark et al 2005; Kim et al 2002).

The epithelial growth factor receptor family are an important group of membrane growth factors that includes EGFR (ErbB1), ErbB2 and ErbB3. ErbB2 and ErbB3 and their growth factor ligand neuregulin (NRG), are critical in the proliferation of Schwann cells during development and myelinogenesis where the receptors are activated in response to NRG production by axons (Simons et al 2007). Recently, Merlin has been shown to downregulate ErbB2/3 function and thereby decrease activation of the MAPK pathway, probably by limiting the availability of these receptors at the cell membrane (Lallemand et al 2009). Neuregulin, ErbB2 and ErbB3 expression levels and phosphorylation status have been reported to be increased in schwannomas (Hansen et al 2004) and may confer radio-resistance (Hansen et al 2008). Furthermore, ErbB inhibitors are capable of reducing schwannoma cell proliferation *in vitro* (Hansen et al 2006; Clark et al 2008) prompting some groups to point to this pathway as a potential target for molecular therapy in schwannomas (Stonecypher et al 2006; Doherty et al 2008). Merlin also downregulates EGFR (Curto et al 2007) as well as other growth factors such insulin-like growth factor-1 receptor (IGF1R) and platelet-derived growth factor receptor (PDGFR) (Lallemand et al 2009). In addition, the degradation of PDGFR is increased by Merlin (Fraenzer et al 2003).

Merlin: role in cytoskeletal organization

An important realization in the last few years has been that, although it is a moderate suppressor of cell proliferation, the more important tumor-suppressor function of Merlin is its role in membrane organization and cell contact inhibition. In fact, this property makes it unique among tumor suppressor genes. Contact inhibition of growth is a feature of cells that grow to confluence and is mediated by cell-cell protein complexes known as adherens junctions that contain cadherins, and function to limit proliferation once a solid cell sheet has been formed. Cells grown on ECM under subconfluent conditions on the other hand, as well as tumor cells, form multiple focal contacts that help the cell to migrate. The migration is achieved by the cell making actin-rich protrusions at its leading edge called lamellipodia. Focal contacts involve the proteins β-integrins, focal adhesion kinase (FAK) and paxillin. Multiple lines of evidence implicate Merlin in the adhesive cytoskeleton organization of the Schwann cell. Merlin is found is the actin-rich cell protrusions such as lamellipodia and membrane ruffles (Gonzalez-Agosti et al 1996; Schmucker et al 1997) as well as in cell-cell and cell-matrix contacts which are formed by focal adhesion and focal contact proteins respectively (Fernandez-Valle et al 2002; Lallemand et al 2003). Loss of Merlin can result in loss of contact inhibition, a more spread out shape and more adhesion and motility along the extracellular matrix – all features which can be reversed upon re-expression of the protein (Gutmann et al 1999; Bashour et al 2002). Schwannoma cells are known to have increased adhesion via activation of integrins α6, β1 and β4 and Schwann cells that lack Merlin have increased numbers of focal contacts, allowing them to adhere more strongly to extracellular matrix and presumably migrate abnormally (Utermark et al 2003).

The FERM domain of Merlin can also bind the membrane glycoproteins CD43 and CD44. During growth arrest and when cells become confluent, Merlin exists in a complex with CD44 and the other ERM proteins (Morrison et al 2001) and is able to negatively regulate CD44 binding to hyaluronan, thus reducing ECM adhesion (Bai et al 2007).

Merlin is also able to bind other proteins involved in cell adhesion such as Na+/H+ exchanger regulatory factor-1 and 2 (NHERF1/2), FAK, paxillin and β1-integrin (Stemmer-Rachamimov et al 2001; Poulikakos et al 2006; Obremski et al 1998; Fernandez-Valle et al 2002). Additionally, Merlin coordinates the downregulation of EGFR with contact inhibition by sequestering EGFR into a non-signaling membrane compartment (Curto et al 2007). The adaptor PDZ domain containing protein Erbin, has been found to be a possible link between Merlin, the adherens junction and MAPK activation as well (Rangwala et al 2005).

Unlike the other ERM proteins which contain an actin-binding site in their C-terminus, the N-terminus of Merlin is able to directly bind F-actin, the key component of the cytoskeleton, albeit somewhat more weakly than the other members of the ERM family (James et al 2001). Merlin also binds and thereby inhibits N-WASP (Wiskott–Aldrich Syndrome Protein), which polymerizes actin via Arp2/3 (Manchanda et al 2005).Thus, Merlin is probably involved in stabilization of the cytoskeleton, but it is not entirely clear what role it plays.

The C-terminus of Merlin can fold back on itself (self-associate) and block both the N-terminal (FERM) and C-terminal binding sites. In ERM proteins, this self-association appears to switch off the function of the protein, whereas current evidence suggests that the tumor-suppressor function of Merlin is active in the closed conformation, although this is somewhat controversial (McClatchey et al 2005). It is notable that most NF-2 missense mutations affect exon 2, causing protein substitution in the FERM domain, which is likely to disrupt this self-association (Okada et al 2007).

Merlin has a tyrosine phosphorylation site (T230) as well as a serine phosphorylation site (S518) in its C-terminus, the latter of which plays a critical role in its function. Phosphorylation of Merlin appears to keep the protein in an open (growth permissive) state, whereas when dephosphorylated it can self-associate and become closed (Rong et al 2004a). In this respect, Merlin is the opposite of the other ERM proteins. The Rho family of GTPases (Rho, Rac and cdc42) which are critical membrane-cytoskeletal regulatory molecules that promote focal contact formation upon integrin binding, appear to be prominently involved in the function and activation of Merlin. Merlin is phosphorylated at S518 by p21-activated kinase (PAK1) which is a downstream effector of Rac and cdc42 (Sherman et al 1997; Xiao et al 2002; Kissil et al 2003; Alfthan et al 2004). Furthermore, Merlin participates in a negative feedback loop with Rac, PAK1 and PI3K (Shaw et al 2001; Kaempchen et al 2003; Kissil et al 2003; Hirokawa et al 2004; Okada et al 2007) and thus when Merlin is lost or phosphorylated, Rac is activated at the cell membrane, promoting increased membrane ruffling and immature adherens junctions (Flaiz et al 2007; Lallemand

et al 2003). In addition, Merlin can be phosphorylated by protein kinase A (PKA) in response to NRG binding to ErbB2/ErbB3 (Alfthan et al 2004; Thaxton et al 2008) and by PI3-Kinase (Ye, 2007; Okada et al 2009). On the other hand, increase in dephosphorylated Merlin is necessary for cells undergoing growth arrest and contact inhibition (Shaw et al 1998b). Merlin is dephosphorylated by myosin phosphatase (MYPT-1-PP1δ). For example, hyaluronan binding by CD44 and adherens junction formation can both activate MYPT1 which dephosphorylates Merlin leading to an accumulation of the growth-suppressing closed form (Okada et al 2007). The MYPT inhibitor protein CPI-17, has also been shown to participate in tumorigenesis by promoting phosphorylation of Merlin (Jin et al 2006).

Overall, Merlin appears to be a key regulator of contact-mediated inhibition of cell proliferation, as well as ECM adhesion. This may explain why schwannoma cells that lack functional Merlin continue to grow despite confluent cell density and form a 'pseudomesaxon' in which the cells wrap around the perineural extracellular matrix rather than properly myelinate the axon (Dickersin 1987). Overall Merlin is known to bind over 30 different proteins (Scoles 2008), not all of which are fully understood in terms of its cellular function, but these are slowly being elucidated. A better understanding of these pathways might highlight areas for targeted molecular drug therapy for schwannomas in the future.

Mouse models of NF-2

Insights into the cell-specific function, and possible role in tumorigenesis of the NF-2 gene have been obtained from knockout mouse models developed in recent years. These models have shown that NF-2/Merlin is essential for normal embryonic development. Mice that are NF-2 –/– die prior to gastrulation due to lack of development of extra-embryonic structures that are required for mesoderm formation (McClatchey et al 2005) During development, NF-2 expression appears to be upregulated during the final stages of tissue fusion after cell-cell adhesion has been established, at the time of neural tube closure and in migratory neural crest cells (Akhmametyeva et al 2006). Merlin seems to play an essential role in tissue adherence and fusion, especially in the nervous system, which is consistent with its role in stabilizing cell-cell adherens junctions (Lallemand et al 2003).

In contrast to the narrow spectrum of benign tumors in NF-2 patients, NF-2 heterozygous mice (NF2 +/–) develop a variety of malignant tumors, mainly osteosarcomas, fibrosarcomas and liver carcinomas, that display additional loss of the wild type allele (McClatchey et al 1998). There is a lower incidence of other tumors in these heterozygous mice, as well as increased sensitivity to asbestos, but they do not develop the classical features of NF-2. However, when both alleles of NF-2 are conditionally knocked-out in Schwann cells and neural crest cells using the flox-cre system in mice, schwannomas, Schwann cell hyperplasia, cataracts and cerebral calcifications do occur (Giovannini et al 2000) suggesting that there is an insufficient rate of second NF-2 allele mutation in the heterozygous mouse models compared to that in human NF-2 patients. Similarly, when NF-2 is knocked out in arachnoid cells in mice, different subtypes of meningiomas develop (Kalamarides et al 2002).

An important distinction, however, is that the schwannomas in these mouse models of NF-2 do not have a predilection for the vestibular nerve. The schwannomas also tend to behave more aggressively in mice (Stemmer-Rachamimov et al 2004). Two possible explanations as to why mouse models differ from human schwannomas include differences in the background expression of Merlin binding partners between mouse and human tissues, and differences in the timing of Merlin mutations. The fact that mice in the animal models develop tumors later in life suggest another mutant 'hit' is occurring in addition to the wild type NF-2 allele, however no additional genetic or epigenetic events have been found in tumors in NF-2 patients. A recent report demonstrated that *NF-2 –/–* glial cells result in upregulated Src, FAK and paxillin activity and that ErbB2 inhibition can reduce the effects of Merlin loss on proliferation (Houshmandi et al 2009). Although these models are instructive, further work needs to be done to understand and develop models more accurately representing acoustic schwannomas and NF-2.

Molecular alterations in schwannomas

Most sporadically occurring schwannomas have bi-allelic loss of NF-2 (Stemmer-Rachamimov et al 1997) as well as many meningiomas and also sporadic mesotheliomas of the lung associated with asbestos exposure (Bianchi et al 1995), thyroid carcinoma, hepatocellular carcinoma cell lines and perineural tumors, suggesting a common role in tumorigenesis. Missense mutations in the *NF-2* gene occur at an extremely low frequency, with nearly all the mutations being nonsense, frameshift, or splice site mutations that would all lead to the production of N-terminally truncated Merlin. Strikingly, truncated Merlin species are rarely detected in primary tumor samples, suggesting that mutant Merlin proteins are unstable and actively degraded. In one study mutation of both NF-2 alleles occurred in 65% of sporadic schwannomas with a relatively high frequency of mosaicism within the tumors themselves (Mohyuddin et al 2002). It has now become apparent that attempts to correlate *NF-2*-gene mutation frequency with NF-2-associated tumor types only provides an incomplete picture of Merlin involvement in these tumors. Even although genetic loss of NF-2 material is not found in all schwannomas, loss of expression of Merlin has been reported in 100% of tumors (Stemmer-Rachamimov et al 1997). Similarly, Merlin protein is also reduced or absent in most sporadically occurring meningiomas, schwannomas, and ependymomas (Kimura et al 1998; Gutmann 1997; Lee 1997). This suggests that there are frequent post-translational mechanisms downregulating Merlin expression in these tumors. As discussed above, phosphorylation of Merlin at its S518 site is an important physiological mechanism to switch off the growth suppression activity of the protein and lending support to this, increased levels of phosphorylated Merlin have been found in schwannomas (Cai et al 2008; Wang et al 2009). Cleavage by calpain has been proposed as another possibly important mechanism of Merlin downregulation (Kimura et al 1998; Kaneko 2001).

It is likely that other gene or protein alterations are involved in schwannoma formation besides NF-2/Merlin alone. Micro-array cDNA analysis has been used to screen the differential expression of genes in schwannomas and cultured Schwann cells and found altered regulation of 41 genes, 13 of which were confirmed after real-time PCR analysis (Hanemann et al 2006). Some of these genes play a role in other types of tumors and warrant further investigation in schwannoma molecular pathogenesis.

Vestibular schwannomas are also a component of the Carney complex – a unique multiple endocrine neoplasia syndrome comprising myxomas, spotty pigmentation, and endocrine overactivity (Carney et al 1985, 1986; Mansell et al 1991). This syndrome is usually sporadic, although autosomal dominant inheritance has been reported (Carney et al 1986). Interestingly, mutations in the protein kinase A1α regulatory sub-unit (PRKAR1A) gene have been found in these tumors (Boikos et al 2006) and Protein Kinase A is one of the major proteins interacting with Merlin (phosphorylating it at the C-terminus), suggesting that mutations in other parts of the molecular signalling pathway that involves Merlin could lead to the development of schwannomas. Much work still needs to be done to elucidate fully the function of Merlin and how it promotes schwannoma formation, but a clearer picture of this fascinating tumor-suppressor molecule has been slowly emerging in recent years. Better understanding may lead to the development of novel targeted therapies for schwannoma and NF-2, directed at one or more of the molecules described.

Sites of predilection

Acoustic neurinomas are thought to arise at the point where glial (central) nerve sheaths are replaced by those of Schwann (peripheral) cells and fibroblasts. This transition (the Obersteiner–Redlich zone) is located usually within the internal auditory canal. The variability of this demarcation, however, means that some tumors arise laterally within the internal auditory meatus, while others lie entirely within the cerebellopontine angle (Neely & Hough 1986). It was at one time believed that tumors arose primarily from the superior vestibular nerve, but evidence now suggests an almost equal incidence of superior and inferior vestibular nerve lesions (Clemis et al 1986). Only rarely is the cochlear division involved (Bebin 1979). Clemis et al (1986) concluded that 50–60% of tumors arose from the superior vestibular nerve, 40–50% from the inferior vestibular nerve, and <10% from the cochlear nerve. Neurinomas can arise from other nerves within the temporal bone, and at times it may be impossible to determine their nerve of origin (Best 1968).

The reason why this neoplasm should arise so frequently from the vestibular nerve is unknown, but it does contain an excess of the embryonic precursors of Schwann cells (SC) (Bebin 1979). It has been suggested that schwannomas express key markers of immature Schwann cells (Hung et al 2002) whereas other studies have observed dedifferentiation (Harrisingh et al 2004). SC precursors originate from the neural crest and migrate along peripheral and cranial nerves. During embryogenesis a genetically distinct, transient population of neral-crest derived cells known as boundary cap cells is formed that are thought to give rise to SC precursors and immature SC which go on to migrate along and myelinate nerve roots (Coulpier et al 2009; Maro et al

2004). These boundary cap cells are situated at the margin between the CNS and PNS, where neurinomas are thought to arise (Feltri et al 2008). The question of whether schwannomas, like gliomas, may actually arise from a type of stem cell such as the boundary cap cells is, however, yet to be answered.

Presenting features

Unilateral sensorineural hearing loss, tinnitus, and disequilibrium are the most common presenting symptoms, although only about 10% of patients with such features will be found on investigation to harbor an acoustic neurinoma (Valvassori & Potter 1982). The mode of presentation is dependent on tumor size, and whether or not early symptoms are overlooked. In the past four decades, there has been a steady increase in the proportion of small tumors detected and, therefore, a shift in the pattern of symptoms away from those due to mass effect (Symon et al 1989). The most common symptoms of acoustic neurinoma are unilateral sensorineural hearing loss (96%), unsteadiness (77%), tinnitus (71%), mastoid pain or otalgia (28%), headache (29%), facial numbness (7%), and diplopia (7%) (Hardy et al 1989a). Only around one-third of patients first seek medical attention for non-audiologic complaints (Hart et al 1983) and, at the time of presentation, only around 50% of patients will have objective neurologic findings other than from the 8th nerve.

Unilateral or asymmetric sensorineural hearing loss is almost always the initial symptom, and has been present usually for a median of 1–3 years at the time of diagnosis (Johnson 1977). If hearing loss is neglected, however, there follows a 'silent' interval, usually of 1–4 years, although it may be much longer, while the tumor expands into the cerebellopontine angle cistern. Symptoms then ensue from compression of the cerebellum, adjacent cranial nerves, or brain stem. With lesions >4 cm, 58% of patients will exhibit cerebellar dysfunction, and 53% will have corneal or facial hypoesthesia (Thomsen et al 1983).

Hearing loss

Patients with unilateral or bilateral asymmetric sensorineural deafness or with unexplained unilateral tinnitus should be investigated to exclude an acoustic neurinoma. Speech discrimination is typically affected more than the pure tone loss, and can cause difficulty when using the telephone. Loudness recruitment is uncommon. Although hearing loss is most often progressive, it can on occasion be sudden, due perhaps to compromise of the inner ear vasculature. The incidence of sudden hearing loss varies between series, but is around 10–20% (Sataloff et al 1985). Yet, of patients who present with sudden hearing loss, in only around 1% will the cause be found to be an acoustic neurinoma (Shaia & Sheehy 1976). More recent reports suggest that magnetic resonance imaging will detect acoustic neuromas in a greater number of patients who present with sudden hearing loss (Chaimoff et al 1999). Rarely, hearing loss fluctuates (Pensak et al 1985; Berg et al 1986). Only about 5% of patients with acoustic neurinoma will have normal hearing. This is more likely to occur if the tumor is very small, or if it is confined

to the cerebellopontine angle cistern and there is no significant intracanalicular component (Beck et al 1986). These tumors have been shown to present with balance disturbance or trigeminal or facial nerve dysfunction, headache, or unilateral subjective hearing difficulty (Lustig et al 1998).

Delayed or missed diagnosis is more likely if the presentation is atypical, or if hearing loss is attributed by the patient to a specific event. It is particularly likely if the patient suffers already from a longstanding ear disorder such as Ménière's disease. The other group likely to be missed is those with normal results in investigations which are almost always abnormal in cases of acoustic neurinoma (pure tone audiometry and auditory evoked brain stem responses, see below). Rarely, a cochlear rather than a retrocochlear pattern of hearing loss develops (Flood & Brightwell 1984).

Disequilibrium

Disequilibrium and vertigo are common because the tumor origin is nearly always from the vestibular nerve. True paroxysmal vertigo is rare (6.3%) (Morrison 1975), and is only occasionally accompanied by nausea. The onset is not usually abrupt, as it is in Ménière's disease, although 5% of acoustic neurinoma patients will give a history that would be accepted as typical of that condition. While mild chronic disequilibrium has often been present for some years before diagnosis, it is unusual for either ataxia or vertigo to be the presenting complaint. The reason why destruction of the vestibular nerve is not often disabling lies with the brain stem and contralateral vestibular apparatus, which compensate for the loss. The elderly, however, appear less well able to adapt to this change.

Clinically, mild abnormalities of balance may be detected by Unterberger's stepping test (Moffat et al 1989a). The patient is asked to stand upright with eyes closed, with the arms outstretched at 90° to the trunk, and then to mark time on the spot (i.e. to raise the legs alternately, bringing the thigh to a horizontal position). The result is positive if the patient deviates >50 cm from the spot, or rotates by >30° within 50 steps. The presence of severe ataxia more likely suggests that the patient has developed compression of the cerebellum, or has obstructive hydrocephalus secondary to distortion of the brain stem. Involvement of the cerebellum causes incoordination, primarily of the lower limbs, and a tendency for the patient to deviate to the side of the tumor. Brain stem compression may also involve the sensory and motor tracts, usually of the contralateral side.

Tinnitus

Tinnitus is the presenting symptom in around 3% of patients (Wiegand & Fickel 1989), and is occasionally the sole manifestation of acoustic neurinoma. Preoperative tinnitus affects 57–83% of patients, but is troublesome in only 13–38% (Brow 1979; Wiegand & Fickel 1989). Symptoms are usually low-grade, constant, and confined to the affected ear. There is great variation in the type of sounds experienced.

Raised intracranial pressure

Papilledema is almost exclusive to lesions >3 cm in diameter, and is present in around 7–15% of patients (Hardy et al

1989a; Boesen et al 1992). Large tumors displace the cerebellum and deform the brain stem, compressing the fourth ventricle or aqueduct. Associated features of spontaneous nystagmus, opticokinetic nystagmus, and trigeminal nerve dysfunction are significantly more common in patients with papilledema than in cases in which the tumor is of a comparable size but where swelling of the optic discs is absent (Boesen et al 1992). Very large tumors may result in herniation of the cerebellar tonsils.

Nystagmus

Nystagmus may be spontaneous, positional (when the neck is hyperextended and the head turned to right or left), or opticokinetic (driven in response to an image slip on the retina from a rotating target). The latter may be evident if there is significant compression of the gaze center in the pons (Thomsen et al 1983). The most common type is unilateral labyrinthine nystagmus, which is evident as fine horizontal beats directed away from the side of the lesion. It is of peripheral vestibular origin, and is enhanced by abolition of ocular fixation using Frenzel's glasses. In about 16% of patients, nystagmus will be of Bruns type, which is indicative of a large tumor producing significant brain stem distortion. It comprises bidirectional nystagmus with a coarse gaze-evoked nystagmus on looking to the ipsilateral side and a high frequency small amplitude vestibular nystagmus on looking to the contralateral side (Croxson et al 1988). Electronystagmography will demonstrate impaired vestibular function in over 80% of cases, but this is a non-specific finding and, therefore, of limited diagnostic value.

Cranial nerve palsy

Trigeminal nerve involvement manifests usually as corneal or lower facial hypoesthesia. Only rarely is the whole face affected, and the motor division is spared. Facial weakness is uncommon, and is almost exclusive to large tumors (Portmann & Sterkers 1975). Minor degrees of facial weakness can be detected by delay or absence of the blink reflex (Pulec & House 1964) and may be preceded by subtle facial twitching, particularly involving the orbicularis oculi muscle (Jackler & Pitts 1990). Hemifacial spasm is another rare presentation, affecting only 1% of patients. Epidermoid tumor, aneurysm, and facial neurinoma should, in particular, be considered in the differential diagnosis when hemifacial spasm is evident. Altered sensation over the posterior aspect of the external auditory canal, which is innervated by the nervus intermedius, is said to occur in 95% of patients (Hitselberger 1966). Alteration in taste is reported rarely. Facial nerve dysfunction in the presence of a small tumor is much more likely to suggest that the lesion is a facial neurinoma or a meningioma rather than an acoustic neurinoma.

Several classifications have been devised to grade pre- and postoperative facial nerve function. The system of House and Brackmann (1985) has gained wide support, and is shown in Table 28.1.

On occasions, very large tumors will compress the nerves in the jugular foramen causing dysphagia, dysphonia and, in late cases, complete bulbar palsy. However, loss of the pharyngeal reflex or the presence of vocal cord palsy

Table 28.1 Facial nerve grading system (House & Brackmann 1985)

Grade	Description	Characteristics
I	Normal	Normal facial function in all areas
II	Mild dysfunction	Gross: slight weakness noticeable on close inspection; may have very slight synkinesis. At rest: normal symmetry and tone. Motion: Forehead: moderate to good function; Eye: complete closure with minimum effort; Mouth: slight asymmetry
III	Moderate dysfunction	Gross: obvious but not disfiguring difference between two sides; noticeable but not severe synkinesis, contracture, and/or hemifacial spasm. At rest: normal symmetry and tone. Motion: Forehead: slight to moderate movement; Eye: complete closure with effort; Mouth: slightly weak with maximum effort
IV	Moderately severe dysfunction	Gross: obvious weakness and/or disfiguring asymmetry. At rest: normal symmetry and tone. Motion: Forehead: none; Eye: incomplete closure; Mouth: asymmetric with maximum effort
V	Severe dysfunction	Gross: only barely perceptible motion. At rest: asymmetry. Motion: Forehead: none; Eye: incomplete closure; Mouth: slight movement
VI	Total paralysis	No movement

From House J W & Brackmann D E (1985) Facial nerve grading system. Otolaryngol Head Neck Surg 93: 146–147.

may indicate a second neurinoma in the jugular foramen if the patient suffers from neurofibromatosis.

Rarely is the abducent nerve involved directly, except by the largest of lesions. Occasionally an increase in intracranial pressure may displace the brain stem caudally, and thereby cause distortion of the 6th nerve by the anterior cerebellar artery, which overlies it (Bebin 1979).

Other presenting features

Several case reports have documented exceptional presentations, including subarachnoid hemorrhage (Gleeson et al 1978; Yonemitsu et al 1983), and tumor within the external auditory canal (Tran Ba Huy et al 1987) or middle ear (Amoils et al 1992). Intralabyrinthine schwannomas have also been reported. These may arise from either the cochlear or vestibular nerves. Here, tumor is present in the inner ear but is absent from either the internal auditory canal or the cerebellopontine angle (for review, see Amoils et al 1992). Very occasionally, brain stem compression may produce symptoms contralateral to the side of the tumor. This may manifest as contralateral trigeminal nerve dysfunction (Koenig et al 1984), facial pain, or hemifacial spasm (Nishi et al 1987; Snow & Fraser 1987), although such features are much more common with meningiomas than acoustic neurinoma.

Although they are usually slow-growing, acoustic neurinomas can present with acute neurologic deterioration due

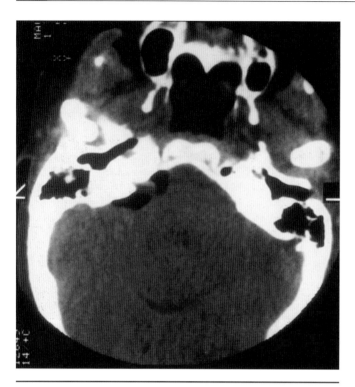

Figure 28.8 CT air contrast cisternogram demonstrating a small acoustic neurinoma.

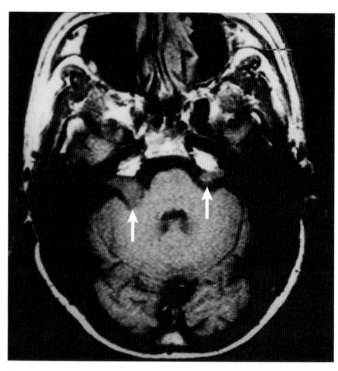

Figure 28.9 T1-weighted axial MR scan showing bilateral acoustic neurinomas (arrows).

House et al 1986; Stack et al 1988). Most acoustic neurinomas are visible on non-contrasted T1-weighted images (Fig. 28.9), but not on T2-weighted images, where the tumor may be isointense with CSF. Intravenous contrast enhancement with gadolinium-DTPA improves the detection rate of small neurinomas, which may otherwise have a signal intensity similar to that of brain parenchyma (Glasscock et al 1988; Brackmann & Kwartler 1990a). Tumors enhance markedly after gadolinium (Fig. 28.10), with which it becomes possible to detect lesions as small as 2–3 mm (Welling et al 1990). The major advantages of MRI over CT are superior contrast resolution, lack of beam-hardening artifact, the facility to image the tumor in multiple planes, and the ability to identify vascular structures and therefore assess vessel displacement or encasement. However, because cortical bone emits no signal, MRI is inferior to CT for delineation of the anatomy of the petrous temporal bone. Newer MRI techniques such as T2 fast spin echo (FSE) and three dimensional Fourier transformation-constructive interference in steady state sequence (3DFT-CISS) allow high resolution imaging of labyrinthine and cerebrospinal fluid interface with bone and soft tissue (Casselman et al 1993; Phelps 1994). These techniques outline acoustic tumors, nerves, and vessels in the cerebellopontine angle and internal auditory canal without paramagnetic contrast (Fig. 28.11). The relationship of the tumor to the lateral end of the internal auditory canal (IAC) can be assessed, as can the relationship of the posterior semicircular canal to the fundus of the IAC. The remaining advantage of CT over MR imaging is the accurate preoperative assessment of petrous apex and perilabyrinthine pneumatization and jugular bulb position. False positive MRI has

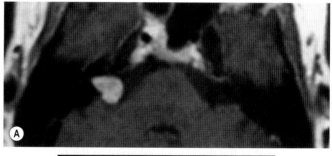
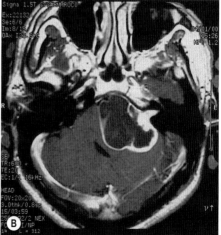

Figure 28.10 (A) Gadolinium enhanced MR scan of a small acoustic neurinoma. (B) Cystic acoustic neurinoma, note peripheral enhancement.

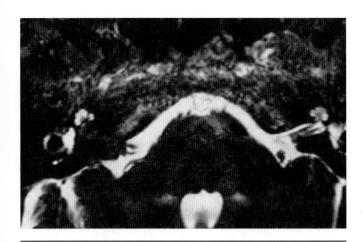

Figure 28.11 Magnetic resonance T2-weighted 'CISS' sequences demonstrating the acoustic neurinoma as a filling defect in the right internal auditory canal.

been reported occasionally as a consequence of arachnoiditis or adhesions (Haberman & Kramer 1989; Von Glass et al 1991).

Arteriography

The indications for arteriography have diminished considerably with the advent of CT and MRI, but it is necessary if an aneurysm or AVM is suspected in the differential diagnosis (Dalley et al 1986). Some surgeons still advocate angiography to define the vascular anatomy in relation to very large lesions. On occasions, it may aid in differentiating a large acoustic neurinoma from a meningioma, particularly if a dilated tentorial artery of Bernasconi is demonstrated in the case of the latter. Angiography has been advocated also for childhood tumors, which may be extremely vascular, and where preoperative embolization is said to be beneficial (Allcutt et al 1991).

Assessment of tumor size

CT and MRI are used routinely to measure tumor size. Unfortunately there are many different classifications in current usage, none of which is universally accepted. Tumors have been classified by Pulec et al (1971) into three groups: small (intracanalicular), medium-sized (extending beyond the internal meatus but by <2.5 cm), and large (>2.5 cm). This, and the Koos (1988) classification, are probably used more widely than most. At the First International Conference on Acoustic Neuroma, however, Tos & Thomsen (1992) made a plea that the following classification be adopted universally, so that reporting of results could be standardized. They have proposed that the intrameatal component (usually about 1–1.5 cm) not be included in the measurement. Size instead is measured as the largest extrameatal diameter. Tumors are classified as intrameatal, small (1–10 mm), medium (11–25 mm), large (26–40 mm), and extra large (>40 mm). It remains to be seen whether this becomes the accepted scheme or just one more to add to the bewildering myriad already in existence. It appears likely that, with the advent of computerized three-dimensional reconstruction

imaging, tumor volume rather than maximum diameter will become ultimately the measurement upon which these lesions are graded.

Laboratory diagnosis

Audiometry

Air, bone, and speech hearing tests are the mainstay screening procedures for acoustic neurinoma. High frequency hearing loss is the most common abnormality seen on pure tone audiometry (PTA) (Johnson 1977). Only 5% of patients will have normal hearing with good speech discrimination (Beck et al 1986), making PTA an important and reliable test in routine neuro-otologic investigation. The pattern of hearing loss is variable. In several large series hearing loss was reported variously as being primarily of a high frequency in 35–66% of patients and low frequency in 4–9%, while the audiogram was flat in 13–18% (pure tone pattern differing by not >10 dB throughout the speech range) and trough-shaped in 4–12%, and in 16–27% of patients the ear was dead (Johnson 1977; Bebin 1979; Hardy et al 1989a). The likelihood of abnormal audiometry correlates with tumor size (Johnson 1977). However, even when the pure tone audiogram is normal, speech discrimination is often impaired, and almost all such patients will exhibit abnormalities also on auditory evoked brain stem response testing (Musiek et al 1986). Tone, decay, and the absence of recruitment are also characteristic audiologic findings (Johnson 1977). Other audiometric parameters include Bekesey audiometry, the SISI test, alternate bilateral loudness balance (ABLB) tests, and the acoustic reflex test. A full account can be found in Johnson (1979), although these 'site of lesion' tests are applied only rarely in modern practice.

Speech discrimination

Speech discrimination is not related simply to the degree of pure tone hearing loss. Some patients may have exceptionally poor speech discrimination despite near normal pure tone audiometry. Speech discrimination scores in a series of 425 cases of acoustic neurinoma were 0% in 35% of patients, very poor (2–30% discrimination score) in 21%, moderate to poor (32–60% discrimination) in 16%, and moderate to good (62–100%) in the remaining 28% of cases (Johnson 1977). In total, only 20% of patients with acoustic neurinoma had good speech discrimination.

The speech discrimination score is an important consideration when contemplating hearing preservation procedures. When hearing is normal in the contralateral ear, residual hearing on the operated side is useful socially only if speech discrimination is good and the pure tone audiogram is within 30 dB of the normal side.

Caloric testing

Over the years, much time and effort has been invested in examination of the vestibular system of patients suspected of harboring an acoustic neurinoma. The object was to find a simple and inexpensive screening test for the condition. Caloric testing was pioneered by Barany, for which he was awarded the Nobel Prize in 1914. In the era before modern neurosurgical imaging, the differentiation of labyrinthine from cerebellar ataxia was of considerable importance. Vestibular assessment by caloric testing often reveals an ipsilateral canal paresis in acoustic neurinoma, but this is a non-specific finding which is often absent in small tumors (Dix 1974). The detection rate for lesions larger than 4.5 cm is considerably better. In this group, Hallpike's caloric test will be normal in <4%, diminished in 33%, and absent in the remaining 70% (Boesen et al 1992). Electronystagmography has now superseded bithermal caloric testing in many centers (Linthicum & Churchill 1968).

In a prospective study of 409 patients with asymmetric hearing loss or tinnitus, caloric testing had a sensitivity of 80% for the detection of acoustic neurinoma, but achieved a specificity of only 50% (Swan & Gatehouse 1992). This makes it inappropriate as a screening test, both on the grounds of an unacceptable number of missed tumors and because of the high false positive rate. Other conditions that may produce abnormal caloric results include vestibular neuronitis and Ménière's disease. One of the reasons for the poor sensitivity of this investigation is that it stimulates the lateral semicircular canal and, therefore, only the superior vestibular nerve.

Auditory brain stem evoked responses

Auditory brain stem evoked responses (ABRs) are the most sensitive indicator of a retrocochlear lesion, and have both a higher detection rate and a lower false positive rate than other non-radiologic screening tests (Selters & Brackmann 1977). Unlike lesions of the cochlea, compression or stretching of the cochlear nerve produces a delay in the response latency which may be detected even when hearing is normal. The stimulus applied is a click from an earphone, and this elicits an electrical response which is recorded from scalp electrodes sited over the mastoids and vertex. The non-test ear is masked with white noise, and an averaging computer extracts the auditory response from the random signal. Generally, ABR testing is applicable only if hearing is better than 70 dB.

Patients with retrocochlear hearing loss show a consistent interaural difference in the latency of wave V during ABRs (Selters & Brackmann 1977). The upper limit of normal is 0.2 ms. Other algorithms used to detect a retrocochlear lesion include the absolute latency of wave V, and the intervals between waves I and V (upper limit of normal = 4.5 ms). ABRs are reported to be abnormal in 95% of patients with acoustic neurinoma (Josey et al 1980), and the false positive rate is said to be about 10% (Brackmann & Kwartler 1990a). Other series, however, have found that ABRs are considerably less specific than this. Weiss et al (1990) reported that the probability of finding a cerebellopontine angle tumor in the presence of an abnormal result was only around 15%. This is perhaps not surprising because ABRs test the function of the auditory system as a whole. Despite this shortcoming, the ABR is still used widely as a screening procedure, even though a negative result does not exclude the diagnosis. A recent study reports the sensitivity of ABR for detection of extracanalicular tumors to be 94% but only 77% for intracanalicular tumors (Godey et al 1998). Tumor size cannot be predicted from the degree of latency delay. However,

large lesions may cause sufficient brain stem compression to affect contralateral latencies as well (Selters & Brackmann 1977). It is of interest that ABRs are abnormal in more than 30% of patients with NF-1, even though acoustic neurinomas are rare in this group of patients (Schorry et al 1989).

Stapedial reflex testing

Stapedial reflex testing is a further test of retrocochlear pathology, but is less sensitive than ABR. Abnormalities are found in around 80% of patients.

Electrocochleography

Transtympanic electrocochleography (EcoG) is usually non-specific, although the presence of an action potential complex in the absence of subjective hearing is said to be pathognomonic (Morrison et al 1976). EcoG and ABR may be combined, particularly as the former is more sensitive for the detection of wave I. This increases the number of instances when the wave I–V interval can be measured (Prasher & Gibson 1983).

Electroneuronography

Electroneuronography (EnoG) has been used preoperatively to assess facial nerve involvement in temporal bone tumors. A compound action potential is measured in response to supramaximal bipolar stimulation of the main trunk of the facial nerve, and its amplitude compared with that of the contralateral side. Amplitude reduction is said to relate to tumor size, but cannot predict postoperative facial nerve function (Kartush et al 1987).

Screening tests

Moffat & Hardy (1989) have justified the early diagnosis and treatment of acoustic neurinomas on both economic and humanitarian grounds. Unfortunately MRI, and even CT, are too expensive in most countries to use as a routine screening test for patients with asymmetric hearing loss or other features which may represent a cerebellopontine angle tumor. Over the years many different test results have been proposed as being almost pathognomonic of retrocochlear hearing loss, only to be found wanting on closer examination. Examples include the phenomenon of loudness recruitment, abnormally rapid tone decay, disproportionately poor speech discrimination, and the stapedial reflex threshold.

In order to reduce the financial burden from radiologic imaging of large numbers of patients and yet avoid missing a significant number of tumors, several non-diagnostic investigations have been combined to provide a screening battery. The necessary trade-off in every case is between sensitivity and specificity. Of patients with an acoustic neurinoma, over 98% will manifest an abnormality in at least two out of three of the following: caloric testing, ABR, and plain radiology of the internal auditory meatus (Moffat et al 1989b). Other workers have proposed combining pure tone audiometry, ABR, caloric testing, and the stapedial reflex test (Thomsen et al 1992). If the results are abnormal or equivocal, radiologic assessment is then undertaken. In a study of 82 cerebellopontine angle tumor suspects, Barrs & Olsson (1987) found that the interaural wave V (IT5) latency difference on ABR testing had a sensitivity of 100% and a specificity of 80%. One tumor was diagnosed for every three abnormal IT5 results. Although the sensitivity from non-radiologic screening is high, it is inevitable that a few tumors will be missed using such algorithms. This may have medicolegal implications.

It is clear that the sensitivity of auditory brain stem response testing has fallen as the ability to image smaller acoustic neurinomas has improved. The cost of screening with MRI can be reduced substantially if the fast spin echo magnetic resonance imaging techniques without gadolinium enhancement are used. A limited non-enhanced fast spin echo MRI can be used to image the internal auditory canal and cerebellopontine angle. This technique currently provides maximal sensitivity for acoustic neurinoma detection with minimal cost (Daniels et al 1998).

Gross morphologic features

Acoustic neurinomas typically are firm, well circumscribed, and encapsulated. They distort and compress rather than invade brain. The tumor, which is invested in a sheet of arachnoid, is of a yellowish white appearance and has a rubbery consistency. These lesions are relatively avascular except in childhood, or when very large (Kasantikul et al 1980a). The presence of areas of red or brown discoloration indicates old or recent hemorrhage. The surface of large tumors in particular is often irregular and lobulated. Usually the neoplasm is solid, although small thin-walled cysts may be evident. On occasion the greater part of the lesion will be found to be cystic (Fig. 28.10B). Large tumors compress and deform the cerebellum and the lateral aspect of the pons, the upper medulla, and the brachium pontis. Very large lesions may displace the cerebellum inferiorly, causing tonsillar herniation.

Histopathology

In 1842, Cruveilhier (1842) produced a detailed report of the clinical and pathologic features of a 26-year-old patient who died from an acoustic neurinoma. Intracranial schwannomas have a marked preponderance for sensory nerves, particularly the eighth cranial nerve. Although the tumor is usually confined to the vestibular division, invasion of the cochlear (Neely 1981; Marquet et al 1990) and facial nerves has been described (Luetje et al 1983). Tumors arise at the neurilemmal–glial junction, or anywhere between this and the origin of the nerves within the labyrinth (Stewart et al 1975). There have been no reports of primary tumors occurring in the neuroglial portion of the nerve.

It was Virchow who called these tumors 'neuromas', based upon their macroscopic appearance. Microscopy revealed many parallel fibers, which were mistaken for axons, hence the later term 'neurinoma'. However, Murray & Stout (1940) identified the cell of origin correctly as the Schwann cell, using *in vitro* tissue culture techniques. Despite this, some controversy still remains as to whether the Schwann cell or the related perineural fibroblast is indeed the true source of this neoplasm.

Microscopically, the tumor consists of two distinct patterns of architecture which, in any individual lesion, are intermingled but well demarcated. These are known as Antoni types A and B, and are fundamental to the diagnosis (Antoni 1920). Antoni type A tissue predominates, and consists of groups of spindle-shaped cells with elongated hyperchromatic nuclei. The cytoplasm is pale and has a stringy appearance due to numerous hairlike argyrophilic fibers which lie parallel to the long axis of the cell (Fig. 28.12) (Russell & Rubinstein 1989). Characteristic of schwannomas in general, although frequently absent in acoustic neurinomas, is the presence of palisading. The cells are grouped together in bundles (Verocay bodies). Within each bundle the cells lie roughly parallel with their nuclei aligned in rows, separated by clear hyaline bands. The fibers interlace with those of other bundles, which are orientated at different angles.

Antoni type B tissue has a less compact structure. The cells are pleomorphic, vacuolated, and separated by a loose eosinophilic matrix (Fig. 28.13). Microcystic change is

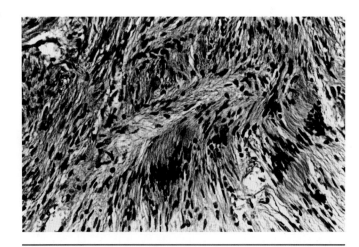

Figure 28.12 Acoustic neurinoma containing bundles of spindle-shaped cells forming Antoni type A tissue. A Verocay body is present. (H&E ×380.)

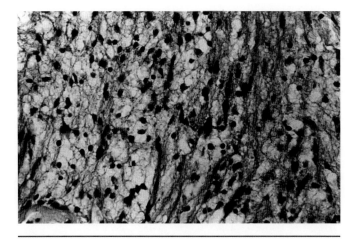

Figure 28.13 Microscopic appearance of Antoni type B tissue in an acoustic neurinoma. The cells are more pleomorphic than Antoni A, and are separated by a loose eosinophilic matrix. (H&E ×380.)

frequent, although Antoni type B tissue does not represent degeneration of type A (Murray & Stout 1940). Confluence of these areas is responsible for the cysts which are sometimes a feature of these tumors. Type B tissue may also become xanthomatous, due to lipid accumulation; this gives rise to a yellowish naked eye appearance.

The degree of tumor cellularity may be quite variable. Secondary changes occur in some schwannomas. Areas of infarction or hemorrhage may be seen, particularly in tumors with excessive vascularization. On occasion, angiomas may be combined with neurinomas, particularly in women (Kasantikul et al 1980b). Hemosiderin-filled macrophages may be evident within foci of degeneration, and areas of necrosis may be present. Other tumors may contain foci of calcification. The term 'ancient schwannoma' has been given to lesions where the nuclei are atypical, hyperchromatic, and enlarged, and the tumor is associated with a dense fibrous stroma. Mitotic activity is not increased in ancient schwannomas, however, and neither this appearance, nor the presence of pleomorphism, by itself signifies malignant change. Other neoplasms have been reported occasionally to metastasize to an acoustic neurinoma (le Blanc 1974) and melanotic acoustic neurinomas have been described on very rare occasions (Russell & Rubinstein 1989).

Benign schwannomas rarely present a diagnostic challenge histologically, although meningiomas may on occasion have similar features, including the presence of Verocay bodies (Sobel & Michaud 1985). Immunohistochemical markers are therefore generally of rather limited value. Acoustic neurinomas stain strongly positive for the S-100 protein (Fig. 28.14). This is a cytoplasmic protein but it is not specific to this condition. Its uses primarily are for the identification of nerve sheath tumors, amelanotic melanoma, and myoepithelial cells. Meningiomas by contrast, stain positively only weakly with S-100, but can be differentiated further by their reaction to HMFG (epithelial membrane antigen) (Schnitt & Vogel, 1986; Simpson et al 1990). A proportion of acoustic neurinomas stain positively for glial fibrillary acidic protein (GFAP) (Stanton et al 1987).

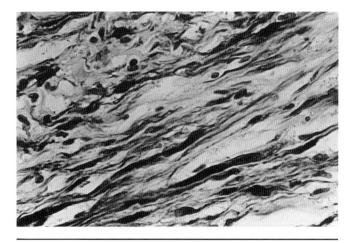

Figure 28.14 Positivity of an acoustic neurinoma for the S-100 protein. (H&E ×620.)

The bilateral acoustic neurinomas of NF-2 do not differ microscopically from those that occur sporadically. They do, however, show a tendency to be more adherent to adjacent structures (Linthicum & Brackmann 1980). Rarely, meningioma has been observed to be intermixed microscopically with schwannoma (Gruskin & Carberry 1979).

Under the electron microscope, Antoni type A tissue has a lamellar pattern composed of thin elongated cell processes covered by a basal lamina, which are separated by intercellular basement membrane material. Antoni B tissue contains large numbers of organelles and vacuoles, consistent with high metabolic activity (Russell & Rubinstein 1989). Other typical electron microscopic features include long-spaced collagen fibrils and the development of whorls and lamellae composed of stacks of double membranes grouped tightly together.

Malignancy

Malignancy is far more common in peripheral than in cranial neurinomas. The vast majority present *de novo* rather than as malignant change in a pre-existing benign lesion (Yousem et al 1985). Around 50–70% are associated with von Recklinghausen's disease, and the age at presentation in these cases is considerably younger than for those that occur sporadically (for review, see Russell & Rubinstein 1989).

Malignant acoustic neurinomas are exceptionally rare, and only a handful have been reported in the world literature. Russell & Rubinstein (1989) collected a series of only six, in patients ranging from 26 to 72 years of age. In one there was considerable bony erosion by tumor, while three manifested themselves as recurrence after previous surgical excision. Histologically, the features were similar to neurofibrosarcoma, with increased cellularity and numerous mitoses. Initially the tumors were encapsulated, but later they became locally invasive. Recurrence is common after surgery and these tumors may become progressively more anaplastic with the passage of time. The risk of recurrence entails a poor long-term prognosis, although the rarity of malignant change means that precise details of tumor behavior are lacking. Studies of large numbers of malignant peripheral schwannomas indicate that metastases are uncommon and occur late. The degree of mitotic activity and anaplasia is said not to predict survival (Ducatman et al 1986). Nager (1969) was unable to find any report of malignant degeneration within a pre-existing acoustic neurinoma. Such a case was documented by McLean et al (1990) although, in retrospect, the original specimen did exhibit some atypical features.

A malignant schwannoma with rhabdomyoblastic differentiation is otherwise known as a malignant triton tumor. This very rare soft tissue sarcoma arises almost exclusively from peripheral nerves, usually in patients with von Recklinghausen's disease. Few cases of acoustic nerve triton tumors have been reported (Best 1987; Han et al 1992; Comey et al 1998). Total excision with adjuvant chemotherapy and radiotherapy has been advocated, however the prognosis in all cases was poor. Concerns have been raised that radiation therapy for acoustic neuromas may induce malignant transformation. The 5-year survival for this tumor in peripheral nerves is 12% (Brooks et al 1985).

General management plan

Differential diagnosis

Acoustic neurinomas are by far the most common tumors occurring within the cerebellopontine angle. In a review of 205 tumors, Revilla (1948) found that 78% were neurinomas (mostly acoustic), 6% meningioma, 6% cholesteatoma, 6% gliomas, and the remaining 4% miscellaneous. The presenting features of meningioma can be similar to acoustic neurinoma but, because the tumor arises frequently from the anterior or superior lip of the internal auditory meatus, there may be early involvement of the facial and trigeminal nerves with relative sparing of hearing (Sekhar & Jannetta 1984). Similarly, inferior extension may involve the cranial nerves in the jugular foramen. The relationship between the cranial nerves and the tumor is much less predictable than with acoustic neurinoma, but the success of hearing preservation is greater, particularly for larger lesions (Maurer & Okawara 1988). Schwannomas of adjacent cranial nerves, in particular of the trigeminal, facial, glossopharyngeal, or vagus nerves, can also involve the cerebellopontine angle. Facial neurinomas, which account for about 1% of cerebellopontine angle tumors, may be difficult to differentiate from an acoustic neurinoma preoperatively. However, facial neurinomas sometimes arise from the region of the geniculate ganglion and may extend into the middle cranial fossa via erosion of the petrous temporal bone (King & Morrison 1990). Very large acoustic neurinomas, by contrast, are more likely to extend into the middle cranial fossa via the tentorial hiatus, although this is uncommon. The presence of contrast enhancement in the region of the genicular ganglion, despite features otherwise typical of an acoustic neurinoma, can also aid in the differential diagnosis. Facial neurinomas may also evolve from the tympanic or mastoid segments of the nerve. Other schwannomas of the temporal bone include those arising from the chorda tympani nerve, the auricular branch of the glossopharyngeal (Jacobson's) nerve, and the auricular branch of the vagus (Arnold's) nerve (Amoils et al 1992). At times it may not be possible to ascertain from which nerve a neurinoma of the petrous temporal bone has arisen (Best 1968).

As well as meningioma and neurinoma of adjacent cranial nerves, the differential diagnosis of acoustic neurinoma includes epidermoid, aneurysm, arteriovenous malformation, glomus jugulare tumor, choroid plexus papilloma, hemangioma, lipoma, lymphoma, medulloblastoma, enterogenous cyst, and metastatic tumor within the temporal bone (Schisano & Olivecrona 1960; Brackmann & Bartels 1980; Robinson & Rudge 1983; Wakabayashi et al 1983; Yoshi et al 1989; Umezu et al 1991; Yamada et al 1993). Differentiation of these lesions is not usually difficult on radiologic grounds.

Conservative treatment and the timing of surgery

The question of the timing of acoustic neurinoma surgery remains unresolved and, in many respects, has become less clear with the passage of time. Age by itself is not a contraindication to successful surgery (Samii et al 1992), although an expectant policy with careful follow-up may be a reasonable alternative to surgery when the tumor is small and the patient is infirm or perhaps reluctant to contemplate excision for other reasons.

The difficulty in assessing tumor growth rates in the pre-CT era, and the dramatic reduction in mortality and morbidity from surgery in the 1960s to 1980s suggested that all tumors, with a few notable exceptions, should be removed at diagnosis. This view was strengthened by the knowledge that larger tumor size is associated undoubtedly with an increase in morbidity and, in particular, poorer prospects for facial nerve recovery, preservation of residual hearing, and good quality of life. Yet despite this, the decision to offer immediate treatment is not always clear cut. Better awareness among clinicians, coupled with improvements in diagnostic screening, has resulted in greater numbers of tumors being diagnosed at an early or even asymptomatic stage. Although the surgical results for facial nerve function and overall morbidity are likely to be excellent under these circumstances, unfortunately this is not yet true for preservation of hearing. With the advent of MRI, and subsequent reports which suggest that up to 50% of untreated patients with small lesions will display no further tumor growth, expectant treatment has become a viable alternative to surgery in some cases. It can be argued that small tumors should be managed conservatively in the first instance, excision not being contemplated until it has been established that the lesion is actually expanding. In a study of 35 patients, Valvassori & Guzman (1989) determined that any further tumor growth was evident usually within the first 12 months of follow-up. A relatively short observation period may therefore allow patients with indolent forms of the disease to be selected out. Lifelong follow-up will be necessary, as demonstrated by Charabi et al (1995, 1998).

This is not to suggest that delayed treatment is applicable for any but a minority of patients. Conservative management is probably unwise in the younger age groups because the rate of tumor growth is possibly more rapid. Similarly, an expectant policy is unsuitable for lesions larger than 2.0 cm because any further expansion is liable to have a significant influence upon surgical morbidity. In our experience, the great majority of patients are far more concerned about their facial nerve function and prospects for a good outcome in general than they are about preservation of hearing in the affected ear. We believe that early surgery remains the treatment of choice for most patients because outcome relates so strongly to tumor size. If patients are to be managed conservatively in the first instance, repeat MRI at 8 months, 18 months, and subsequently at 2-yearly intervals has been recommended (Valvassori & Guzman 1989).

Neurofibromatosis type 2

NF-2 is particularly challenging to manage satisfactorily. As well as bilateral acoustic neurinomas other tumors may occur, notably cranial and spinal neurinomas, meningiomas, and ependymomas. Any patient under the age of 30 years who presents with an acoustic neurinoma or meningioma should be suspected of suffering from NF-2. MRI with gadolinium enhancement should be performed to screen both for a small contralateral lesion and for the presence of other intracranial tumors.

The major objective of treatment is to preserve functional hearing for as long as possible. Unfortunately, auditory symptoms often occur late in the disease (Linthicum & Brackmann 1980; Bess et al 1984). Furthermore, deterioration of hearing in a series of nine patients with bilateral tumors treated conservatively was rapid in every case, and ranged from 11 to 16 dB per year (Kitamura et al 1992). However, as with sporadic tumors, the speed of progression does appear to be highly variable (Baldwin et al 1991). The combination of rapid tumor growth and poorer prognosis as the tumor enlarges argues for these lesions being treated promptly. However, examination of the temporal bone in NF-2 patients shows that minor infiltration of the cochlear nerve and inner ear is more common than with sporadic tumors (Linthicum & Brackmann 1980). The prognosis for hearing preservation is likely therefore to be correspondingly less favorable (Brackmann 1979). The dilemma is whether to offer early treatment, which provides the only hope of preserving long-term hearing, albeit a small one, or to delay surgery until useful hearing has been lost or tumor size mandates surgery, and to train the patient to cope with impending deafness in the interim. Hearing loss is not the only difficulty when treating this patient subgroup. Involvement of the facial nerve is more common (Martuza & Ojemann 1982; Baldwin et al 1991), and facial nerve preservation rates are correspondingly less good.

A large symptomatic tumor will require treatment, regardless of the risk of total deafness. In every case surgery should aim to conserve residual hearing, unless the tumor is very large. If the tumors are small and hearing is good, the National Institutes of Health consensus document (1988) proposes that an attempt should be made to excise one tumor. The authors' preference is to remove first the tumor on the side of poorer hearing (usually, but not invariably, the larger of the two). In the fortunate circumstance where useful hearing remains intact, the contralateral lesion may be explored later. However, if hearing is lost at the first operation, there are four options. Treatment of the contralateral neurinoma can be delayed until useful hearing is lost, since hearing at even very low levels may assist the patient with lip reading. Alternatively, the remaining tumor can be excised macroscopically or the patient offered stereotactic radiosurgery. The fourth option is to undertake sub-total tumor removal with decompression of the internal auditory canal, which may delay the progression of hearing loss (Miyamoto et al 1991). However, even elective sub-total tumor removal can result in total deafness (Wigand et al 1988; Baldwin et al 1991), and total excision with hearing preservation is very unlikely if the lesion is >2 cm in diameter (Hughes et al 1982). Sub-total excision that fails to preserve hearing should be followed shortly by total removal. In a report of 19 patients with bilateral tumors, 65% retained facial function after surgery, but the outlook for hearing in both the operated and unoperated groups was dismal (Baldwin et al 1991). In a recent report of hearing preservation in patients with NF-2, using the middle fossa approach, 23 procedures were performed on 18 patients

and measurable hearing was preserved in 65% (Slattery et al 1998). The mean tumor size in this group was 1.1 cm; this reinforces the importance of early diagnosis and family screening in NF-2 patients. Since the results for hearing preservation by both surgery and stereotactic radiosurgery are poor, and the course of untreated disease is variable, we do not believe that operation is justified at present on a solitary hearing ear with a small tumor.

If bilateral excision is contemplated, the second operation should, where possible, be delayed until there has been recovery of facial nerve function. Although the likelihood is very small, it should be remembered that surgery carries with it the risk of bilateral rather than just unilateral deafness (Linthicum & Brackmann 1980; Miyamoto et al 1990). Sometimes removal of tumor on one side will result in some improvement in residual hearing in the contralateral ear.

Stereotactic radiosurgery is an alternative to surgery in NF-2 patients. However, this technique also may result in both delayed hearing loss and facial palsy. Progressive hearing deterioration or deafness will ensue in 64% of such patients (Hirsch & Noren 1988). More recent reports claim better hearing preservation rates when the mean tumor margin radiation dosage is reduced and studies in non-NF-2 related tumors have shown adequate long-term control rates. Similarly, high rates of hearing preservation have been claimed with the use of fractionated stereotactic radiation therapy rather than single fraction stereotactic radiation (Lederman et al 1997). If long-term tumor growth control rates are demonstrated then fractionated stereotactic radiation therapy may have a significant role in the management of NF-2 patients.

On rare occasions a cerebellopontine angle tumor in neurofibromatosis will be a facial rather than an acoustic tumor, and theoretically may permit total tumor removal with preservation of hearing (Piffko & Pasztor 1981). King & Morrison (1990) found that 21% of their cases of facial neurinoma developed in patients with NF-2. Unfortunately the translabyrinthine operation, involving destruction of hearing, is often more favorable than a retrosigmoid approach to these tumors because of improved access to the petrous segment of the lesion, and to normal facial nerve beyond it.

Tumor in a solitary hearing ear

Such a patient presents a challenge similar to that faced when dealing with NF-2. Whether or not to operate at the time of diagnosis remains controversial, and is a matter of personal judgment. Some authors advocate early surgery, arguing that the success of hearing preservation will only diminish as the tumor enlarges (Pensak et al 1991). Yet hearing preservation is successful currently in around only one-third of patients. We think that the risk of deafness is too high, particularly when the natural history of the condition is uncertain. Initially we favor conservative treatment, unless the tumor is large and exerting mass effect. Large tumors we treat by radical subcapsular excision. The results of hearing preservation with stereotactic radiosurgery have improved with lower tumor margin doses and this form of treatment is now a first-line option in many centers.

Surgical management

Historical perspective

The first successful operation to remove a cerebellopontine angle tumor is credited to Sir Charles Ballance in 1894. Unfortunately the patient required enucleation of the eye subsequently as a consequence of complications secondary to trigeminal and facial nerve palsy. Krause described the retrosigmoid suboccipital approach in 1903, but mortality at the time was very high, ranging from 67% to 84% (Dandy 1925). Tumor removal was achieved usually by extraction with a finger inserted into the posterior fossa, a practice which carried with it a high risk of injury to branches of the basilar artery as well as to the cranial nerves and brain stem. As a consequence of the poor results, Cushing proposed sub-total tumor removal. This he achieved by scooping out the center of the lesion, and by the application of Zinker's solution to the cavity for hemostasis. This technique, which was combined with a generous decompressive suboccipital craniectomy and uncapping of the cerebellum, reduced mortality to about 25% by 1917, and 4% by 1931 (Cushing 1917, 1931). However, 40% of patients died within 5 years from tumor recurrence (Cushing 1931). An excellent account summarizing Cushing's techniques and surgical results can be found in German (1961). The first successful attempt at total tumor excision with preservation of the facial nerve was reported by Sir Hugh Cairns in 1932. Recognition that the anterior inferior cerebellar artery was often adherent to the tumor capsule, that changes in vital signs were often related to brain stem ischemia, and that preservation of the arteries within the cerebellopontine angle was essential to a good outcome were further milestones in the surgery of this disease (Adams 1943; Atkinson 1949). Elliott & McKissock (1954) were perhaps the first to report successful preservation of hearing. In 1961, McKissock (1961) reported a remarkable series of patients with small tumors undergoing surgery, without the aid of magnification. In each case the facial and cochlear nerves remained intact, and residual hearing was present in some cases.

The translabyrinthine operation was proposed by Panse (1904). A radical mastoidectomy was performed, which included removal of the labyrinth, the cochlea, and the facial nerve. The procedure quickly fell into disrepute because of limited access, sub-total tumor excision, destruction of the facial nerve, hemorrhage from the venous sinuses, cerebrospinal fluid leakage, and the resultant high mortality (Dandy 1925). Later the translabyrinthine and suboccipital approaches were combined, but mortality remained high, mainly because of meningitis secondary to cerebrospinal fluid fistula. The operation was reintroduced by House (1964a), using modern microsurgical techniques. In his monograph, which was to become a landmark in the surgery of acoustic neurinoma, a series of 41 cases was reported in which there were no deaths, and almost all patients achieved some return of facial function. The results from House's group stimulated a great striving for better and better technical excellence. Mortality is now very low, and attention has turned to the preservation of hearing and of normal facial function.

Surgical anatomy

A detailed account of the surgical anatomy can be found in Rhoton (1986) and Rhoton & Tedeschi (1992). In brief, the cerebellopontine angle cistern is bounded laterally by the petrous face, medially by the pons, and superiorly by the tentorium cerebelli. It contains the trigeminal, facial, and vestibulocochlear nerves, together with the anterior inferior cerebellar artery (AICA), and superior petrosal vein. Although the facial and vestibulocochlear nerves may at first sight appear to pass as a single bundle from the pontomedullary junction to the internal auditory meatus, they are separate. The superior and inferior vestibular nerves lie posteriorly and superiorly, and the cochlear nerve posteriorly and inferiorly. A shallow groove marks the boundary between them. The facial nerve lies anteriorly and slightly superiorly, with the nervus intermedius lying between the facial and vestibular nerves. The labyrinthine artery (and occasionally the main trunk of the anterior inferior cerebellar artery) lies usually between the facial and vestibular nerves. However, in all except the smallest lesions, the neural relationships will be distorted as the tumor enlarges; because of its position, the facial nerve is usually displaced anteriorly and superiorly, although in around 5% of cases the nerve will lie over the posterior tumor capsule.

The constant landmarks for identification of the neural structures during tumor excision are their medial and lateral extents. Within the internal auditory meatus each of the nerves is separated from the others by two bony septa, the transverse crest and the vertical crest (Bill's bar, named after William House). Within the porus acousticus the superior and inferior vestibular nerves lie posteriorly, the facial nerve anterosuperiorly, and the cochlear nerve anteroinferiorly. Identification of Bill's bar will therefore allow the nerves anterior to it (the facial and cochlear) to be delineated with confidence from those posterior to it (the superior and inferior vestibular).

At the brain stem, the facial, cochlear, and vestibular nerves are more widely separated. The most important structures to identify here are the flocculus and the tuft of choroid plexus which emerges from the foramen of Luschka at the lateral margin of the pontomedullary sulcus. The foramen of Luschka is situated just dorsal to the glossopharyngeal root entry zone (Rhoton 1986). Immediately anterosuperior to the choroid plexus lies the entry of the vestibulocochlear nerve. The facial nerve arises in the pontomedullary sulcus a further 1–2 mm anterior to the vestibulocochlear nerve.

The anterior inferior cerebellar artery may pass around the brain stem either anterior to, ventral to (the most common finding), or between the facial and vestibulocochlear nerves; in only 23% of 132 subjects was the AICA not related significantly to the nerves (Sunderland 1945). The degree to which it loops laterally toward the internal auditory meatus is variable. On occasion the artery may actually enter the meatus (around 14%) and it is particularly vulnerable to injury in this instance. In the majority of cases the artery loops laterally almost to the internal meatus (50%), while in 16% of patients there is no loop, and the AICA lies close to the brain stem. After passing the nerves, the artery loops back consistently to the surface of the middle cerebellar peduncle above the flocculus (Rhoton 1986).

Occasionally, the AICA may be substituted by a branch of the posterior inferior cerebellar artery. Penetrating branches of the AICA enter the pons and upper medulla to supply the facial and vestibular nuclei, the spinal tract of the trigeminal nucleus, part of the medial lemniscus, and much of the middle and inferior cerebellar peduncles.

The superior petrosal vein (vein of Dandy) drains the upper aspect of the cerebellum into the superior petrosal sinus. The vein (or group of veins) may be divided to improve exposure if necessary, or if there is a risk of avulsion during retraction of the cerebellum. It has been suggested, however, that this may, on occasion, exacerbate postoperative cerebellar swelling, particularly if the suboccipital route has been employed for tumor excision.

Knowledge of the arachnoid is important because it provides the key to dissection of the tumor from the surrounding structures. Within the internal meatus the nerves and internal auditory artery are covered in a sleeve of arachnoid. A tumor arising from the vestibular nerve, therefore, will also be invested in arachnoid. As the lesion grows from the porus acousticus into the cerebellopontine angle, the arachnoid which covers it comes into contact with the arachnoid which overlies the cerebellum and the adjacent nerves and vessels of the angle cistern (Tos et al 1988). The only structures not separated from the tumor by arachnoid are the facial and cochlear nerves, and the brain stem end of the vestibulocochlear complex. As a result, when the tumor encroaches on the medially placed structures there is a double layer of arachnoid separating it from the brain stem and cerebellum. This arachnoidal cap provides an important cleavage plane during tumor dissection.

The tumor obtains its blood supply from two sources. The principal supply is via the dura of the petrous pyramid at the margins of the internal auditory meatus. Bleeding in this region may be tedious and troublesome during tumor removal. Medially the tumor is supplied by the labyrinthine artery and by the other branches of the anterior inferior cerebellar artery.

As well as encroaching upon the cerebellum and brain stem, large tumors may be related to the abducent nerve and basilar artery. The superior pole of large tumors will involve the trigeminal nerve, and may abut on the undersurface of the tentorium cerebelli. It is exceptional for the trochlear nerve to be involved at the incisural notch. Inferiorly, large tumors may become adherent to structures in the region of the jugular foramen.

The height of the jugular bulb is variable, and may on occasion lie above the level of the lower border of the internal auditory canal (Shao et al 1993). This has important consequences during surgery because it limits exposure in the translabyrinthine operation, and there is a risk of injury when the posterior wall of the internal auditory meatus is removed via a suboccipital approach. The relationship between the jugular bulb and the internal meatus should be determined preoperatively by high resolution CT scan of the temporal bones.

Intraoperative monitoring

The use of constant electromyographic (EMG) facial nerve monitoring is now accepted as essential during acoustic neurinoma surgery. Electrodes are placed in the ipsilateral orbicularis oculi and orbicularis oris for the detection of muscle action potentials in response to surgical manipulation or monopolar or bipolar electrical stimulation of the facial nerve. Although objections that the current may harm the nerve have been raised, this is not borne out in clinical practice. For optimal benefit from the facial nerve EMG monitoring it is preferable that a non-muscle relaxant anesthetic technique is used.

In a study of 108 patients, Dickins & Graham (1991) concluded that facial nerve monitoring does improve functional results. The stimulator is used to identify the anatomic configuration of the facial nerve, to warn the surgeon if the nerve is being traumatized by manipulation or by traction, and to confirm physiologic as well as anatomic integrity at the completion of the procedure. The early postoperative facial nerve function after tumor removal can be predicted by measurement of the stimulation threshold and the response amplitude to proximal facial nerve stimulation (Mandpe et al 1998). During tumor dissection, the stimulus intensity should be reduced as much as possible, particularly when a unipolar device is in use (~0.25 m/A), or current may leak to the facial nerve when adjacent non-neural tissue is stimulated and produce a false positive response. Care must be taken also not to confuse a masseter contraction from stimulation of the trigeminal nerve with movement of the facial musculature. Dissection of the nerve in a medial to lateral direction is likely to maximize the usefulness of monitoring. Clearly, if physiologic function is lost at any stage, the stimulator is of no further use to aid dissection proximal to that point. Dealing with the region just medial to the porus is usually the most difficult part of the procedure. However, the manner in which the tumor is dissected from the nerve must be tempered by the clinical situation, because a lateral to medial dissection is often easier technically, particularly when the translabyrinthine operation is used.

Intraoperative audiometric monitoring has been employed during hearing preservation procedures (Ojemann et al 1984). The methods available currently are monitoring of the electrocochleogram (EcoG) via a transtympanic electrode placed through the inferior part of the tympanic membrane to rest on the promontory of the medial wall of the middle ear, or extratympanic electrode, recording of brain stem auditory evoked potentials (BAEPs) using scalp electrodes, direct monitoring of the cochlear nerve, or measurement of oto-acoustic emissions. EcoG has a larger signal to noise ratio than BAEP, making it more sensitive. A significant reduction in wave V amplitude on BAEP, or a shift in latency, warns the surgeon to moderate dissection, retraction, or the use of bipolar cautery. When wave V is unchanged at the end of surgery useful hearing will be preserved, even if it was lost transiently at some stage (Nadol et al 1992). However, the value of such monitoring remains uncertain. In many instances changes are abrupt, dramatic, and irreversible, and reflect compromise to inner ear vascularity or damage to the labyrinth (Ojemann et al 1984). Unlike monitoring of the facial nerve, there is a delay in response because the measurements require averaging. This is reduced with the use of direct 8th nerve monitoring where changes are closer to real time. In only a few cases does a change in operative technique, such as modification of cerebellar retraction (Sekiya & Moller 1987) lead to a recovery of monitored potentials. However, identification of the event that caused hearing loss may still be of benefit if it allows the surgeon to modify operative technique in future cases. In a series of 28 patients, Kveton & Book (1992) found no advantage for intraoperative BAEP monitoring in terms of final outcome, although this has not been the experience of other groups (Ebersold et al 1992; Fischer et al 1992).

Instrumentation

In addition to the usual array of microsurgical instruments, a fenestrated sucker of the Brackmann type is a useful aid to dissection and minimizes risk of injury to the nerves and vessels. It has been suggested that sucker-induced trauma contributes significantly to postoperative facial neurapraxia (Tos et al 1992c). The Cavitron ultrasonic surgical aspirator (CUSA) or House–Urban rotary dissector may be used to debulk large tumors. We have no experience with either the CO2 or NdYAG lasers, which are reported by some authors to be more advantageous still (Takeuchi et al 1982; Cerullo & Mardichian 1987). The major benefit is said to be rapid tumor debulking with minimal manipulation of the tumor or neurovascular structures (Gardner et al 1983). Use of lasers has not become popular because of the lack of precision associated with uncontrolled heating of adjacent tissue and potential for neural injury.

Surgical approach

There are three basic approaches to the cerebellopontine angle: by excision of the labyrinth (translabyrinthine); through a posterior fossa craniectomy (suboccipital/retrosigmoid); or via the middle cranial fossa. On occasion, more than one approach may be combined at the same or separate operations.

No clear consensus has emerged from the literature as to which is the procedure of choice. There are definite advantages and disadvantages associated with each surgical approach. The route chosen is governed by tumor size, the degree of hearing loss, the hearing level in the contralateral ear, and the surgical preference and expertise of the operator. There have, in particular, been many publications recently that compare and contrast the suboccipital and translabyrinthine operations (Di Tullio et al 1978; Tos & Thomsen 1982; Glasscock et al 1986; Mangham 1988; Hardy et al 1989a). Good results are reported with each method and a surgeon can expect progressive improvement in results with experience. It has been proposed that a surgeon should perform the operation at least 10 times a year to remain proficient.

The major advantage of the translabyrinthine operation is that the facial nerve can be identified lateral to the tumor at an early stage in the dissection, and access to the fundus of the internal auditory meatus is excellent. Furthermore, retraction of the cerebellum is minimal and the risk of postoperative edema is consequently less. The major disadvantage of this route is that residual hearing is irrevocably destroyed. The approach is unfamiliar to neurosurgeons, and requires the close cooperation of a neurootologist experienced in dissection of the temporal bone. Access is confined,

but even the largest of tumors can be removed safely via this approach (Briggs et al 1994; Lanman et al 1999).

As a consequence of progressive improvements in operative results, particularly in mortality and facial nerve outcome, attention has turned more recently to the ability to preserve useful hearing. The suboccipital operation provides good access to the cerebellopontine angle but, if hearing is to be conserved, tumor at the fundus of the internal auditory meatus may be difficult to expose under direct vision. This is true particularly when the posterior semicircular canal is medially placed. Theoretically, this may increase the risk of sub-total tumor excision when compared with the translabyrinthine operation. This limitation can be reduced by use of the middle fossa exposure which unroofs the internal auditory canal from above, although the falciform crest still obscures the inferior half of the IAC fundus (Haberkamp et al 1998). Recently there has been renewed interest in the middle fossa approach for removal of intracanalicular tumors or those with a small cerebellopontine angle component, particularly where the IAC portion extends to the fundus. Higher rates of hearing preservation have been reported without any compromise of facial nerve function (Brackmann et al 1994; Weber & Gantz 1996). However, this route provides more limited access to the cerebellopontine angle, and is therefore restricted to the treatment of small lesions.

The question of hearing conservation deserves careful consideration when selecting the surgical approach. Anatomic preservation of the inner ear and cochlear nerve does not guarantee function, and it is exceptional for hearing to improve on its preoperative level (Telian et al 1988). Whether such hearing is useful depends upon the level of hearing in the contralateral ear. Hearing loss need not be profound before it is socially useless when the other ear is normal. For hearing to be useful socially there must be both good speech discrimination, and a pure tone audiogram within 20–40 dB of the contralateral ear (House & Nelson 1979). Anything less is the equivalent of deafness because there is no balance between the good and impaired ears, directional hearing becomes difficult, and there are problems in coping with noisy environments. In one unselected series, only 16% of patients with an intact cochlear nerve were able to use a telephone with the operated side – 4.4% of the entire group who had undergone suboccipital tumor excision (Bentivoglio et al 1988a). As well as the poor success rate for hearing preservation, there is also the issue of whether such attempts compromise the likelihood of complete tumor removal. Neely (1981, 1984) has shown that the cochlear nerve may be involved with tumor, and that attempts to preserve hearing may not be consistent with one of the major goals of surgery, namely macroscopic tumor excision.

We favor the translabyrinthine operation for large tumors, regardless of hearing level, and for medium-sized lesions with poor hearing. It provides a more direct approach to the cerebellopontine angle, and retraction of the cerebellum is negligible. In our hands the morbidity is lower and hospital stay generally a little shorter than after a suboccipital approach. For hearing preservation removal, two of the authors (AK and RB) prefer the retrosigmoid approach for tumors with up to 2 cm CPA extension, particularly where cerebrospinal fluid can be seen lateral to the tumors within the IAC. The middle fossa approach is preferred for intracanalicular tumors and those with up to 1 cm CPA extension where tumor completely fills the IAC. The merits of the different approaches will be considered further in the section dealing with results.

Staged resection

Excision of large lesions is difficult and time-consuming. Although planned two-stage resection was described by Ojemann et al (1972), Ojemann and Crowell (1978), and Sheptak and Jannetta (1979), for dealing with very large tumors (>4 cm), one-stage removal is now the norm. Hitselberger and House (1979) observed that when surgery was abandoned because of persistent vital sign changes, a second operation was often tolerated better than the first. They have proposed that the tumor may disengage itself from the brain stem and major vessels in the interim, and thereby reduce vascular compression. In contrast, Mangham (1988) found that the morbidity of planned two-stage operations was significantly higher than for one-stage resection, particularly in relation to facial nerve function. However, if technical difficulties do force abandonment of the procedure short of total removal, a second operation should be undertaken unless there are strong reasons for not doing so. A second operation is best performed within 2–4 days of the initial exploration, before adhesions start to form and the operative site becomes hyperemic.

Sub-total excision

Elective sub-total removal may be indicated in the elderly, or the infirm, where the aim is to achieve safe brain stem decompression with preservation of facial nerve function, or in patients with bilateral tumors in whom the aim is to preserve residual hearing for as long as possible. More contentious is the issue of achieving the twin aims of total tumor excision and hearing preservation, particularly in the light of the histologic study by Neely (1984), in which he showed that microscopic invasion of the cochlear nerve by tumor was common. However, his work has not been confirmed by Perre et al (1990), who found no infiltration of the cochlear nerve by acoustic neurinoma, except in NF-2 patients. Yet recurrence is not an inevitable sequel, even if tumor is left behind at operation. Capsule remnant may be of no clinical significance, and indeed can atrophy. We will return to this issue later.

Suboccipital/retrosigmoid operation

Although many neurosurgeons utilize solely the suboccipital approach for excision of vestibular schwannoma our preference is that this is used only for those in which hearing preservation is attempted. The suboccipital approach does provide a wide visualization and the ability to save hearing. Good results have been reported by many groups. (Ojemann et al 1972; Ojemann 1978, 1979, 1980, 1990, 1992, 1993, 1996; Ojemann & Crowell 1978; Ojemann et al 1984; Nadol et al 1987; Ojemann & Black 1988; Ojemann & Martuza 1990; Nadol et al 1992; Rhoton 1986; Symon et al 1989; Klemink et al 1990; Ebersold et al 1992; Samii et al 1992; Gormley et al 1997; Samii & Matthies 1997a,b; Koos et al 1998) The operative approach and techniques have been reported and illustrated in detail in other publications (Ojemann et al 1984; Ojemann & Martuza 1990; Ojemann 1992, 1993, 1996, 2001). The operation is done in collaboration with an otologic surgeon, who exposes the internal auditory canal and dissects the tumor within that region.

Preoperative medical therapy

Steroids are usually commenced prior to the operation if the tumor is large and there is edema of the cerebellum. The steroid dose is continued postoperatively and tapered over 3–7 days, depending on the size of the tumor and facial nerve function. We do not use steroid therapy for smaller tumors. Antibiotics are given intravenously and continue for 24 h postoperatively.

Management of preoperative hydrocephalus

Symptomatic hydrocephalus is now uncommon in patients presenting with vestibular schwannoma, but if present will usually improve with steroid therapy. A ventricular drain may occasionally be needed at surgery, and for a few days postoperatively. Only rarely does a patient need a ventricular peritoneal shunt as a preliminary procedure.

Patients with acoustic neuroma may have enlarged ventricles with no symptoms, and no special treatment is needed. Occasionally an elderly patient with a tumor and large ventricles has symptoms suggestive of normal pressure hydrocephalus. If the only symptom is hearing loss, a ventricular peritoneal shunt may be the only treatment needed. If there are also symptoms of brain stem or cerebellar compression, treatment of the tumor will also be necessary.

Positioning

Numerous positions have been utilized for this operation, including semi-sitting, prone, supine/oblique, lateral or park bench and a lateral oblique position. In general, we have utilized the lateral or park bench position, preserving the semi-sitting position for very large patients with short necks. The patient is placed on the table with the operative side superiorly with a pad and axillary roll under the torso. Both legs are flexed and two pillows placed between them. The hips are taped for stability and an armrest and back support are placed. The head is held in a three-pin head holder, and flexed and rotated 10–15° towards the floor. The ipsilateral shoulder is taped to hold it away from the surgeon's access to the craniotomy. The Frameless Stereotactic System may be used to help guide the approach, particularly to mark out the position of the transverse and sigmoid sinus.

Continuous electrophysiological monitoring for facial nerve function during the operation is essential and some surgeons use auditory evoked responses in an attempt to help preserve hearing.

Incision and exposure

A linear or slightly sigmoid shaped incision is made one figure breadth posterior to the transverse-sigmoid sinus junction. The inferior end of the incision is curved medially. The muscles are divided longitudinally and dissected off the bone using monopolar cautery until the root of the digastric groove is visible. Care must be taken to avoid diathermy injury to the extracranial facial nerve which exits the stylomastoid foramen anteriorly in the groove. Pericranium may be harvested at this stage for use in closure of the dura at the end of the procedure. Special care is taken to include the arterial vessels as they are encountered in the muscle. The occipital nerve may be divided during the opening. An emissary vein is usually exposed in the region of the medial mastoid area, and is usually controlled with bone wax. The bone over the lateral half of the cerebellar hemisphere is exposed.

The initial burr hole is made near the asterion to expose the 'corner' of the transverse-sigmoid sinus junction and the bone flap is elevated using the high speed drill. A large emissary vein frequently arises from the sigmoid sinus and should be skeletonized with the drill, dissected free of the bone flap and coagulated before division. Small tears in the venous sinus should be covered with a patch of Gelfoam and cottonoid patties. Further bone can be removed anteriorly over the edge of the sigmoid sinus to improve exposure, but this often necessitates opening the mastoid air cells, which must be waxed thoroughly.

We have generally utilized a craniotomy, with three burr holes being inserted, the first being in the region of the asterion anteriorly and superiorly, the second being approximately 2 cm posteriorly along the border of the transverse sinus and the third being through the very thin bone inferiorly. However, in elderly patients with very adherent dura it may be more prudent to perform a craniectomy, as it is essential to preserve the dura to enable a watertight closure at the end of the procedure. It is essential to remove the bone laterally and superiorly to expose the edges of the transverse and sigmoid sinuses, as this will allow them to be retracted with sutures to hold the dural flaps and allow a direct line of site down the posterior surface of the petrous temporal bone.

The dura is opened in an asymmetrical Y-shaped fashion, with the larger flap hinged anteriorly on the sigmoid sinus, and the smaller flap hinged superiorly on the transverse sinus edge. A critical next step is to open the arachnoid membrane over the infero-lateral cerebellar cisterns and drain CSF to allow the cerebellum to relax. This process is made easier by the preoperative institution of a lumbar drain, and it is essential in larger tumors. A Greenberg retractor system is attached and the retractor blade is used to gently retract the cerebellum. At this stage the operating microscope is brought in, the cerebellopontine angle exposed and the tumor is identified.

It is essential to identify the arachnoid plane around the tumor; this greatly facilitates dissection of the surrounding neurovascular structures, which must be preserved. The petrosal vein, which s usually coming off the cerebellum or middle cerebellar peduncle to the petrosal sinus just above the tumor, is preserved if possible, but it may be necessary to take the vein to improve access. It is far better to coagulate and divide this vein rather than inadvertently avulse it from the superior petrosal sinus.

The posterior capsule of the tumor is stimulated to locate the facial nerve. In the majority of patients the facial nerve will be on the anterior surface of the tumor and there will be no response on this first stimulation. However, in some patients the nerve is displaced more superiorly, particularly in its lateral course just before it enters the internal auditory canal. In this situation a response may be seen on the initial stimulation. The facial nerve can also be displaced antero-medially along the brain stem and over the anterior superior aspect of the tumor and in this circumstance the facial nerve may be displaced against the 5th nerve. On rare occasions, the facial nerve is on the inferior or posterior surface of the tumor capsule (Ojemann 2001).

The 9th, 10th and 11th cranial nerves must be identified and the arachnoid adjacent to the cerebellum is carefully dissected to aid exposure of the inferior medial capsule. The arachnoid in this area may need to be opened over these nerves to aid the exposure and prevent traction on the nerves. There is frequently an arterial loop in this region, arising from the anterior inferior cerebellar artery. With large tumors the 9th and 10th nerves are carefully reflected off the tumor and arterial branches going to the capsule are diathermied and divided. It is essential to protect the lower cranial nerves during the remainder of the operation.

Except in the largest tumors, it is usually possible to continue the dissection between the tumor capsule and cerebellum down to the brain stem before opening the tumor capsule. This aids in the careful identification and preservation of the plane between the tumor capsule and the adjacent neural structures.

Following dissection of the tumor capsule away from the cerebellum, and identification of the lower cranial nerves the posterior capsule is then opened through a linear incision and internal decompression of the tumor is performed utilizing a combination of sharp dissection, bipolar coagulation and the ultrasonic aspirator. It is essential to realize that heat transmission from the bipolar can damage the cranial nerves, therefore the lowest effective voltage must be used. Irrigating or non-stick 'cool' bipolars are helpful. Further debulking of the tumor will allow identification and dissection of the tumor- arachnoid plane. It is then possible to retract the tumor capsule laterally, away from the cerebellum and in medium size tumors the 8th nerve complex can usually be defined with minimal dissection. In larger tumors these nerves will usually not be seen initially, and only become apparent after removal of more tumor.

Internal decompression of the tumor superiorly will allow the tumor to be reflected laterally away from the cerebellum and inferiorly from the tentorium above, displaying the 5th nerve which may be splayed superiorly and anteriorly across the brainstem. Generally, it is best to continue the dissection on a 'broad' front along the whole line of the tumor, rather than just restricted the resection to one section.

If hearing preservation is *not* an aim of the surgery, the vestibular and cochlear fibres entering the tumor can be divided using bipolar coagulation and sharp dissection. The surgeon must carefully look for a branch of the anterior inferior cerebellar artery which may loop behind or between these nerves. The facial nerve is located just under the 8th nerve complex, or may be a few millimeters away. It is usually recognized by its 'whitish' color, which is different to the adjacent brain stem. Intermittent stimulation with the facial nerve monitor may help localize the nerve. A further aid to identification of the facial nerve is to follow the 9th nerve to the root entry zone, with the facial nerve arising just adjacent to this region.

Following further debulking, the tumor capsule is then gently dissected away from the brain stem and cranial nerves, including the 7th nerve. There is usually a good plane between the brain stem and the tumor capsule, but at times the tumor may be adherent within the brain stem and the dissection must proceed with meticulous care. The edge of the 7th nerve is carefully identified, with the arachnoid between the tumor and the capsule being dissected with a sharp arachnoid knife or microscissors. It is usually best to dissect the tumor capsule from the 7th nerve 'side to side', rather than along the length of the nerve in order to prevent stretching and damage to the nerve.

For those tumors in which hearing preservation is an aim of the surgery it is essential to identify the vestibular and cochlear nerves and the relationship to the capsule prior to significant debulking of the tumor. This will help to preserve the plane between the nerves and the tumor capsule. The arachnoid between the nerves and the tumor is opened with sharp dissection, a plane identified and then the tumor can be internally decompressed to allow further dissection of the capsule away from the nerves.

Following resection of the tumor from within the cerebellopontine angle the next step is to expose the tumor in the internal auditory canal. Gelatine sponge (Gelfoam) is placed in the subarachnoid space so as to prevent dissemination of bone dust in the cerebrospinal fluid A dural flap, with the base lying along the posterior lip of the internal auditory canal, is lifted from the posterior aspect of the petrous temporal bone over the region of the internal auditory canal and the bone is then carefully removed using the high speed air drill with constant suction irrigation for cooling. Occasionally, a high jugular bulb will be exposed during the bone removal. The surgeon must avoid entering the labyrinth, as this would cause loss of hearing. After the internal auditory canal is exposed the dura is opened and an internal decompression may be performed using sharp dissection so that the capsule can be mobilized with minimal pressure.

Dissection then depends on assessment of the relationship of the tumor to the vestibular and cochlear nerves and the facial nerve. In some patients the vestibular nerves entering the medial edge of the tumor are divided and the cochlear and facial nerves are identified and the dissection proceeds from medial to lateral. In other patients it may be difficult to define the cochlear nerve medially. In those cases the tumor is carefully rotated near the lateral end of the canal, looking for the 7th nerve anterosuperiorly and the cochlear nerve anteroinferiorly. Again, it is important to avoid stretching or putting tension on the cochlear or facial nerves so that the fibres are not avulsed. The position of the 7th nerve can be confirmed with stimulation. An internal decompression of the tumor may be performed with sharp dissection to facilitate the exposure. Dissection along the facial and cochlear nerves is undertaken with micro dissectors and a sharp arachnoid knife. The dissection is alternated from different directions, depending on what seems to give the best exposure, the easiest plane of dissection and the least traction on the nerves.

In some patients, the lateral end of the tumor may not be exposed because of the limitations in the bone canal. In these patients, and routinely at the end of all procedures we are now using the 70° endoscope to either confirm the complete excision of tumor within the canal, or to aid in resection of the last fragments of the tumor lying laterally within the canal.

Closure

Following resection of the tumor the dural flap over the posterior petrous temporal bone is then laid back over the exposed bone, which has previously been carefully waxed to prevent CSF leakage. The dural flap is held in place with oxycellulose. Meticulous hemostasis is essential at the end of the procedure. The aim to achieve a watertight dural closure in all cases; in most cases this requires sewing in a dural patch either pericranium or artificial material. The bone flap is replaced, being held in place by small titanium plates and any bone defects repaired using bone substitute. A complete bone repair may reduce the incidence of postoperative headache. The wound is closed in layers.

Postoperative care

The patient is nursed in the high dependency neurosurgery care unit for the first 24–48 h postoperatively. Intravenous antibiotics are given for 24 h. Particular attention is given to control of postoperative hypertension. We aim to minimize the use of postoperative steroids unless there is brain stem or cerebellar edema. The patient is mobilized early and anti-thromboembolism management is instituted. A non contrast CT scan is performed routinely on day 1 postoperatively to exclude hematoma and hydrocephalus. Delayed facial palsy can occur after 14 days postoperatively. This is usually managed with a short course of oral steroids and frequently resolves.

Translabyrinthine operation

The translabyrinthine operation was reintroduced to neurosurgery by William House (1964a). The posterior fossa dura is opened in Trautmann's triangle, bounded by the sigmoid sinus, jugular bulb, and superior petrosal sinus. This exposure provides a more direct route to the cerebellopontine angle than does suboccipital craniectomy, and access is at the expense of bone rather than cerebellar retraction. The surgical field is confined, particularly in the region of the inferior pole of large tumors, but the apex of the cerebellopontine angle is more readily exposed than via the suboccipital route. The presence of an anteriorly placed sigmoid sinus or a high jugular bulb may render access slightly more difficult, but rarely does this cause undue problems. A high jugular bulb occurs in around 9–18% of temporal bones and can be anticipated in petrous bones that are poorly pneumatized (Turgut & Tos 1992; Shao et al 1993). Translabyrinthine exposure can, however, be increased in three ways: (1) superiorly, by opening the middle fossa dura and dividing the tentorium; (2) posteriorly, with or without division of the sigmoid sinus (venous phase angiography should be undertaken to establish the dominance of the sinus and to assess the size of the torcular herophili if ligation is contemplated); or (3) anteriorly, via a transotic approach.

The transotic approach was proposed by Jenkins and Fisch (1980) as a modification of House and Hitselberger's transcochlear operation (1976). This is essentially a sub-total petrosectomy, but with skeletonization rather than translocation of the facial nerve. Access is thus provided circumferentially around the internal auditory meatus. We have never found this extension to the translabyrinthine approach necessary when dealing with primary tumors.

Sacrifice of residual hearing is the major disadvantage of the translabyrinthine operation. However, only 1% of affected ears will have normal hearing after suboccipital surgery (Harner et al 1984), and it is rare for hearing to improve on preoperative levels (Telian et al 1988). The question of hearing preservation will be discussed later. Translabyrinthine surgery is contraindicated in the presence of chronic perforation of the tympanic membrane or acute infection of the middle ear or mastoid, because of the risk of meningitis. The operation requires close cooperation between neurosurgeon and neurootologist. House (1979) suggests that both should be thoroughly proficient in all phases of the procedure and be able to act interchangeably. We think that this is unnecessary, and that each specialist should utilize the skill in which (s)he has the greater expertise.

Occasionally, the preoperative diagnosis of acoustic neurinoma is found at surgery to be incorrect. Although access is more confined via the labyrinth, King and Morrison (1980) removed three jugular neurinomas successfully via this route. Meningiomas with an origin anterior to the porus may however prove more problematic because the angle of approach to the petrous face is less acute than with suboccipital surgery, although access to the petrous apex is unquestionably better. In these cases exposure can be extended by opening the dura over the temporal lobe and dividing the superior petrosal sinus and tentorium. This exposure is best planned in advance, a small temporal craniectomy being used in addition to the usual translabyrinthine exposure. However, it can be done as an *ad hoc* procedure by extending the mastoid incision upwards onto the temporal squamosa.

Technique

The patient is anesthetized, prepared, and placed in the supine position. The operation is conducted under general anesthesia with endotracheal intubation and continuous facial nerve EMG monitoring. Although spontaneous ventilation was at one time popular to identify potential brain stem compromise, mechanical ventilation is now the norm because of the ability to lower intracranial tension. Continuous monitoring of arterial blood pressure, electrocardiogram, and central venous pressure is established, together with adequate venous access. Changes in blood pressure (hypertension) or heart rate (bradycardia or arrhythmia) during tumor dissection warn the surgeon of pressure or traction effects to the brain stem, or impairment of its blood supply. The bladder is drained via a urethral catheter. The head is rotated around 45°, avoiding obstruction to the great veins of the neck. Dissection of the petrous bone adds a further 1.5–2 h to the duration of the procedure, so that attempts to avoid pressure sores and to keep the patient warm are essential. Fat and fascia lata are taken from the lateral aspect of the right thigh and are soaked in antibiotic solution until required. Mannitol may be useful if the tumor is large.

An inverted hockey stick incision commences just below the mastoid tip, runs about 2 cm behind and parallel to the root of the pinna, and curves anteriorly to end about 1 cm above the external auditory meatus. The exposure from this incision is larger than necessary, but keeps the hemostats away from the operative field. In addition, it allows access to the middle cranial fossa with division of the superior petrosal sinus and tentorium should it be required. This is not necessary for acoustic neurinoma surgery, but may be appropriate when dealing with other lesions of the cerebellopontine angle.

The scalp flap is reflected anteriorly. Using cutting diathermy, a pericranial flap is raised in a similar fashion, and turned anteriorly to expose the posterior bony rim of the external meatus. Two of the authors (AK and RB), prefer to secure the patient's head using a three-pin fixation. This allows use of the Greenberg retractor for subsequent sigmoid sinus compression and dural retraction during the temporal bone dissection. Abdominal fat is harvested immediately prior to use at completion of the procedure rather than tissue from the thigh. We also prefer a more generous C-shaped incision which is placed well behind the mastoid and sigmoid sinus. After the scalp flap is elevated, fibroperiosteal flaps are created with a T-shaped incision which can be securely closed over the fat packing (Fig. 28.15).

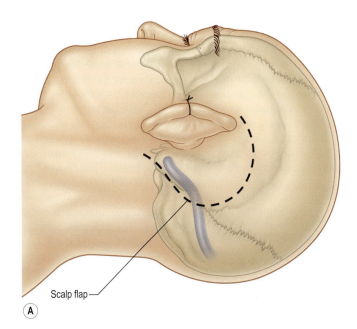

Scalp flap

(A)

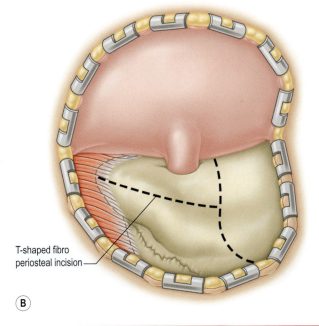

T-shaped fibro periosteal incision

(B)

Figure 28.15 (A) Skin incision for the translabyrinthine operation. (B) Fibroperiosteal incisions to expose mastoid cortex.

Next the neurootologist performs an extensive cortical mastoidectomy using an air drill with a cutting burr. The bone dust is collected for use later. The initial dissection is conducted under direct vision, resorting to the operating microscope as the exposure deepens. The opening is roughly the shape of a large keyhole. The external opening should be as large as possible, to permit extradural retraction of the cerebellum and temporal lobe if necessary, particularly if the sigmoid sinus is anteriorly placed or the middle fossa dura low. Anteriorly, the posterior wall of the external meatus is thinned. Superiorly, the dissection should expose the edge of the middle fossa dura and superior petrosal sinus. The dissection is carried anteriorly above the external meatus as far as possible. The sigmoid sinus is exposed posteriorly, and approximately 1 cm of dura exposed behind the sinus, but a small island of bone may be left over the sinus, allowing it to be depressed without risk of injury (Bill's island) (Fig. 28.16). Inferiorly, the mastoid process is hollowed out. It is particularly important to remove sufficient bone posteriorly and superiorly to improve access by retraction of the dura. The margins of the bony defect should be smoothed and beveled to avoid overhanging edges, and perhaps to lessen the risk of postoperative chronic wound pain.

The dissection is deepened in the space between the middle fossa dura and superior margin of the meatus, to open the mastoid antrum and aditus. The incus and head of the malleus are exposed, and the incus is removed. The lateral semicircular canal is identified on the medial wall of the epitympanic recess. This is the key landmark for the horizontal portion of the facial nerve, which lies below and parallel to the anterior part. Once the position of the facial nerve has been established, its descending portion can be skeletonized and this marks the anterior limit of the exposure inferiorly (Fig. 28.17A). Even when covered with a thin plate of bone, the stimulator may still be used to identify the location of the intrapetrous portion of the facial nerve,

although the stimulus current will have to be increased temporarily.

Dense bone marks the otic capsule surrounding the semicircular canals. The lateral canal is removed first, and its anterior limb leads into the vestibule. The posterior and superior canals are followed to the crus commune, but the ampullated end of the posterior canal is not removed because it lies deep to the second genu of the facial nerve. The labyrinthine vein traverses the arc of the superior semicircular canal, and is a useful landmark (Fig. 28.17B). The posterior fossa dura is skeletonized and the vestibular aqueduct and endolymphatic sac removed. The jugular bulb is identified. Exposure here must be adequate to allow mobilization of the lower pole of the tumor later. Removal of bone in the angle between the jugular bulb and dura is particularly useful in this regard. The position of the jugular bulb is variable. It

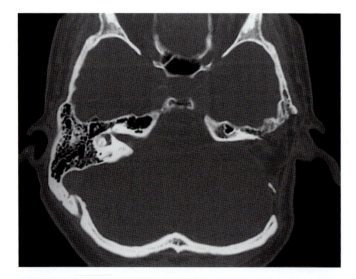

Figure 28.16 Postoperative CT demonstrating the left temporal bone defect following translabyrinthine removal of a large acoustic neurinoma. Exposure of the cerebellopontine angle and internal auditory meatus is more direct than via a suboccipital approach.

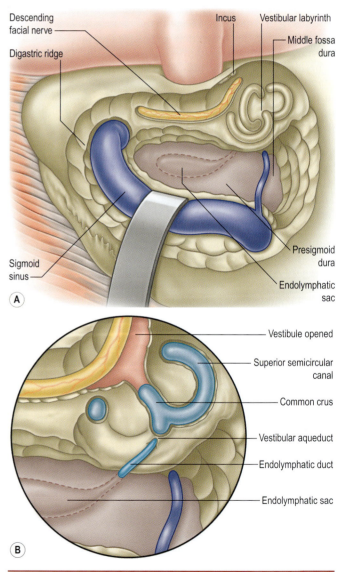

Figure 28.17 (A) Extended mastoidectomy completed with skeletonization of the semicircular canals and descending facial nerve. (B) Labyrinthectomy completed.

may be quite high, on occasion almost reaching the ampulla of the posterior semicircular canal (House 1979). Bleeding from injury to the jugular bulb can be controlled by hemostatic gauze or with a muscle pack. After completion of the labyrinthectomy the descending and horizontal segments of the facial nerve should be skeletonized on the medial aspect to allow maximal access to the vestibule and internal auditory canal.

The internal auditory meatus lies immediately deep to the vestibule. The most satisfactory way of entering the internal meatus is to remove the utricle and saccule, to identify the stump of the superior vestibular nerve, and to follow it through the thin bone into the internal auditory meatus. Once exposed, the entire posterior wall, and as much of the superior and inferior walls as possible, are removed. A diamond burr is used at this stage. Initially bone removal is performed inferiorly between the jugular bulb and internal auditory canal. The cochlear aqueduct is opened and followed medially to the posterior fossa dura. This forms the most inferior aspect of the bony dissection to prevent injury to the lower cranial nerves. Further bone is removed anteriorly above the cochlear aqueduct at least until the anterior wall of the internal auditory canal can be palpated. Great care is needed when drilling away the anterior aspect of the superior margin of the meatus, as the facial nerve lies directly beneath the dura. A burr should be selected to fit between the middle fossa dura and the dura of the IAC, where if possible the direction of rotation of the drill should be changed such that, should the drill tip run off, it will be directed away from the nerve. The bone dissection is completed by removing the lateral lip of the porus acousticus. If necessary, the intrapetrous portion of the facial nerve lying between the internal meatus and geniculate ganglion can

also be exposed with a diamond burr. In the lateral end of the meatus the facial and superior vestibular nerves are separated by a vertical crest (Bill's bar), which provides a constant landmark for the identification of the facial nerve lateral to the tumor (Fig. 28.18).

The resultant cavity in the temporal bone is roughly pyramidal, bounded posteriorly by the sigmoid sinus and posterior fossa dura, superiorly by the middle fossa dura and superior petrosal sinus, and anteriorly by the petrous bone, middle ear cavity and facial nerve, and with the internal auditory meatus as its apex. The otologic dissection is completed using an elevator to remove the remaining bone flakes left behind on the dura.

The neurosurgeon starts the next phase of the procedure by opening the dura, first of the posterior fossa, and then of the meatus. The extent of the dural incision in the posterior fossa is dependent upon the tumor size. For large lesions the incision runs posteriorly from the meatus and divides into upper and lower limbs. The superior limb extends to the junction of the sigmoid and superior petrosal sinuses, and the inferior limb down toward the jugular bulb. Retraction sutures are placed on each of the dural flaps (Fig. 28.19). The incision is then extended into the porus. Here the dura forms a rough fibrous ring, which is often quite vascular. Once divided, the dura is freed from the vestibular nerves using a blunt hook or dissector, and the thin dura of the internal meatus is divided up to the fundus of the canal. The tumor and superior vestibular nerve are gently displaced inferiorly until the facial nerve is identified anterior to it and Bill's bar, and confirmed with the nerve stimulator. The superior and inferior vestibular nerves are then divided lateral to the tumor. A blunt hook can be passed behind them to assist with division, if required. The apex of the

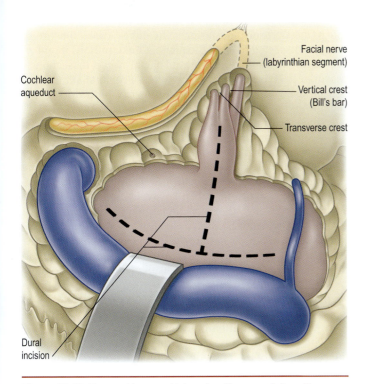

Figure 28.18 Temporal bone and internal auditory canal dissection complete: lines for dural incision shown.

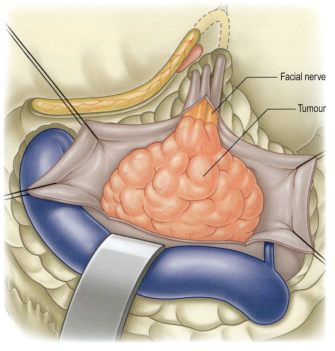

Figure 28.19 Initial tumor exposure following dural incision and retraction.

intracanalicular component of the tumor is then displaced posteriorly, and the plane between tumor and facial nerve is developed by sharp dissection. It is necessary to divide the arachnoid lying either side of the facial nerve. Care should be taken not to apply traction to the nerve. The tumor is freed progressively from its attachment to the arachnoid and dura. If the tumor is very small this plane can be continued and the tumor freed from the attachment at the porus, at which point it is always densely adherent to the dura. However, this is not the best strategy for large tumors, for two reasons. First, the facial nerve usually deviates acutely just medial to the porus (almost always either anteriorly or upward), and it is very easy to lose the correct plane and become subcapsular. Second, if the attachment of the tumor to the porus is divided completely, the weight of the tumor is suspended from the facial nerve and may cause a traction neurapraxia. For these reasons, large tumors occupying the cerebellopontine angle should be mobilized and debulked before the dissection is completed at the porus. Particular care should be taken when dissecting along the inferior margin of the porus, as it is here that the anterior inferior cerebellar artery is most likely to be encountered.

The dissection begins in the cerebellopontine angle by incision of the arachnoidal cap between the cerebellum and the posterior tumor capsule. The medullary CSF cistern is opened in the region of the jugular foramen and the 9th to 11th nerves are freed from the mass. The anterior inferior cerebellar and vertebral arteries may at times be visible at this point. The plane between tumor and cerebellum is then developed progressively. Only vessels actually entering the lesion can be coagulated. Gentle retraction using a sucker tip held against a pattie will prevent the capsule of more friable tumors from breaking up. Once the limit of mobilization is reached, or when any of the major landmarks are identified, a pattie or small silastic sheet is placed to mark their position, and the point of attack is then shifted to another direction. However, it is a mistake to line the dissection with too much material, and a conscious effort should be made to keep it to a minimum. Larger neurinomas must be debulked to continue the dissection; the Cavitron ultrasonic aspirator (CUSA) is ideal for this purpose. Care must be taken not to breach the tumor capsule or apply excessive movement to it, which might injure the nerves or induce spasm in adjacent arteries. Progressively more of the arachnoidal plane can be developed as the tumor is debulked until, ultimately, the brain stem is exposed. Rarely, induced hypotension may be useful if the tumor is excessively vascular, or a small piece of wool soaked in saline, thrombin, or hydrogen peroxide can be left temporarily within the tumor cavity. A systolic blood pressure of 80–100 mmHg can be sustained for long periods without adverse consequences.

The white surface of the brain stem is readily distinguishable from the more yellowish appearance of the cerebellum. The flocculus and the choroid plexus emerging from the foramen of Luschka should be identified, and are important landmarks for the adjacent cranial nerves. With larger tumors, exposure of the facial nerve entry zone is difficult until nearly all of the tumor has been debulked. Adhesions between tumor and brain stem are rarely dense, but a number of veins are usually encountered here, and bleeding may be troublesome. It is absolutely essential that all arteries

are preserved because they may supply not only the tumor but the brain stem.

Any arterial bleeding should be treated by patient, gentle pressure on a piece of appropriately placed hemostatic gauze. If the anesthetist reports changes in vital signs during this or at any other point in the dissection, traction on the tumor should be discontinued. It may be necessary also to remove some of the packing in order to reduce compression of the adjacent vessels. The vestibular and cochlear nerves are divided once they have been differentiated from the facial nerve, remembering that the anterior inferior cerebellar and/or labyrinthine arteries may on occasion lie directly anterior to the vestibular nerve.

The upper and lower poles of the tumor can be mobilized only when the position of the facial nerve has been established. Usually it is displaced anterior to the tumor mass or, less commonly, over the superior surface. During dissection of the upper pole, the trigeminal nerve is encountered deep down as a white band passing across the subarachnoid space to enter Meckel's cave. The nerve is often adherent to the tumor capsule near the pons, and the basilar artery and abducent nerve may be visible deep to them.

The dissection is completed by working from lateral to, medial to, or above the facial nerve. Sharp dissection is less traumatic to the nerve than blunt, and traction must be avoided. Throughout the dissection the nerve should be irrigated with saline, both to wash away any bleeding which will otherwise obscure the field, and to keep it moist. It is often easier to dissect the facial nerve from the tumor in a lateral to medial direction. However, if the plane has been lost medial to the porus, the facial nerve can usually be identified by displacing the tumor inferiorly with the sucker. The nerve is exposed deep to and slightly above the porus, and is separated from it by sharp dissection. The facial nerve is most vulnerable to injury if it lies on the superior pole or, much more rarely, posteriorly. In either case, the tumor must be dissected deep to the nerve. Constant EMG monitoring during tumor debulking and facial nerve dissection is essential to reduce injury to the nerve. Proximal stimulation can be used to assess functional integrity both during dissection and at the completion of the tumor removal.

Once the tumor has been removed (Fig. 28.20), the facial nerve and porus acousticus should be inspected carefully for capsular remnants or residual neurinoma. If it is necessary to leave tumor fragments behind, bipolar coagulation of the remnants may make regrowth less likely (Lye et al 1992), although care must be taken to avoid heat injury to the structure to which they are adherent. In general, neural integrity should not be jeopardized in an attempt to excise every last vestige of tumor capsule. This occasions some agonizing at operation, and the alternative is resection and nerve grafting. However, the likelihood of symptomatic recurrence from small capsular remnants appears to be slight (Lye et al 1992), The least satisfactory outcome is to leave tumor attached to the nerve, having already damaged it irrevocably in an attempt at total tumor excision.

The physiologic integrity of the facial nerve is tested at the conclusion of the procedure. Although non-function does not preclude a good final outcome, success almost guarantees it (Mandpe et al 1998). The technique for dealing with a divided facial nerve is given below. All cottonoids and

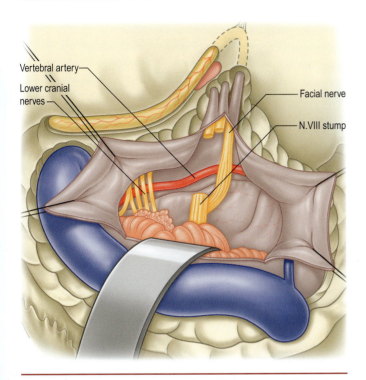

Vertebral artery

Lower cranial nerves

Facial nerve

N.VIII stump

Figure 28.20 The tumor bed at completion of the resection. The facial nerve is shown in its most usual position displaced medially and upwards.

silastic sheeting are then removed from the wound, and any small clots are evacuated. Meticulous hemostasis must be obtained, and the blood pressure should be restored to pre-operative levels before the wound is closed. Some surgeons may choose to line the cerebellum and brain stem with hemostatic gauze. This, however, should not be used to excess because it swells over a period of hours by absorption of fluid into the cellulose, and can itself induce pressure effects. Careful attention is required during wound closure if cerebrospinal fluid leakage, the most common complication of acoustic neurinoma surgery, is to be avoided. The bone dust collected during labyrinthectomy is made into a thick paste (bone pate) by mixing it with a small amount of autologous blood.

During excision of the labyrinth the incus is removed, and a posterior tympanotomy slot is cut to expose the middle ear cavity and the mesotympanic end of the eustachian tube. Small pieces of fat, each about the size of a grain of wheat, are packed into the eustachian tube and middle ear cavity. Particular attention is paid to the region of the aditus, the head of the malleus, and the stapes footplate. The drilled surface of the petrous bone, posterior canal wall, aditus, and any exposed mastoid air cells are then covered with bone pate. A patch of fascia late (~2.5 cm × 2 cm), or abdominal fascial flap, is then applied to the area and sealed with fibrin glue. No attempt is made to close the dural defect. The temporal bone is filled with two or three finger-sized fat strips, which are positioned through the dural defect, just into the cerebellopontine angle. These are sealed laterally with the remaining fibrin glue. The remainder of the wound closure technique is the same as that used for a retrosigmoid approach. If the skin has been elevated from the posterior wall of the external auditory canal, a BIPP pack should be

placed in the ear for 7 days. The authors (AK and RB) repair the dural defect with interrupted proline sutures and if necessary place a patch graft of fascia or dermis sutured into position if the dura is very fragmented. This does not provide a watertight seal as no attempt is made to close the defect at the porus, but rather a secure bed for the abdominal fat graft is created. For extensively pneumatized temporal bones the incus is removed and the eustachian tube occluded in the protympanum as described above. For less pneumatized temporal bones the incus is not removed. Muscle is packed around the incus in the aditus and then the translabyrinthine defect is obliterated with longitudinal strips of fat. The fibroperiosteal flaps are then securely closed to hold the fat packing in position.

Middle cranial fossa approach

The middle cranial fossa approach was described by House in 1961. It is unique in allowing access to the labyrinthine segment of the facial nerve without sacrifice of hearing. On its own it has been used for hearing preservation operations on tumors confined to the internal auditory canal or extending less than 5 mm into the cerebellopontine angle (Glasscock et al 1986). In addition, it may be combined with either the translabyrinthine or suboccipital approaches for the removal of larger lesions (Glasscock et al 1986). It has been criticized on the grounds of its restricted exposure, and because of potential complications which include temporal lobe epilepsy, dysphasia, intracerebral hematoma, and a greater risk to the facial nerve (Gantz et al 1986). Access to the posterior fossa is very limited, and this may give rise to problems in securing adequate hemostasis. With this approach the facial nerve lies superior to the tumor, requiring the surgeon to work around it. Manipulation of the nerve is therefore likely to be greater than with either the suboccipital or translabyrinthine approaches and is reflected in slightly poorer early facial nerve results. Despite these potential limitations the middle fossa approach is now favored in a number of centers for tumor removal where hearing preservation is attempted, particularly where preoperative imaging demonstrates that tumor extends to the fundus of the IAC (Brackmann et al 1994; Weber & Gantz 1996).

Technique

The technique described here is that currently used by the authors RB and AK. The patient is positioned supine with the head rotated into a full lateral position and secured with three-pin fixation. A lumbar spinal drain is initially inserted to facilitate subsequent dural and temporal lobe elevation. An area of abdomen is prepared for harvesting of a fat graft. The surgeon sits at the head of the table.

A variety of incisions have been described, such as a vertical preauricular muscle splitting or an inverted U-shaped flap. We prefer a curved incision with an inferior vertical limb placed just anterior to the helix to allow elevation of an anteriorly based scalp flap. Temporalis muscle is then elevated separately as an anteroinferiorly based flap. A generous rectangular craniotomy measuring approximately 5 × 4 cm is then made in the squamous portion of the temporal bone (Fig. 28.21). The base of the craniotomy should be level with the middle fossa floor as identified by the temporal root of the zygomatic arch, and the opening is placed two-thirds

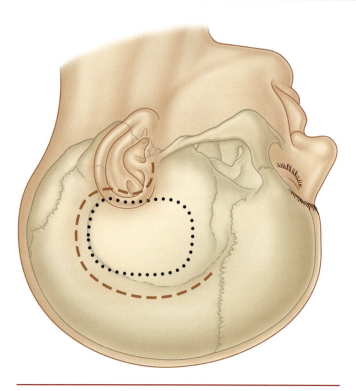

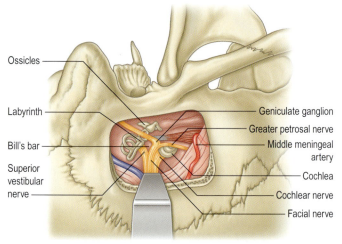

Figure 28.22 Middle fossa craniotomy with dural elevation and outline of intratemporal structures.

anterior and one-third posterior to the external auditory meatus. The lumbar spinal drain is opened while the craniotomy is being performed. The dura is initially separated from both the lateral and inferior borders of the craniotomy. Inferiorly, further bone may be removed using a rongeur or burr to the level of the surface of the temporal bone. Any mastoid cells which are opened posteriorly should be occluded with bone wax. Dural elevation should commence posteriorly with progressive exposure of the tegmen mastoideum, tegmen tympani, and arcuate eminence. Elevation in an anterior direction will avoid elevation of the greater superficial petrosal nerve and therefore inadvertent traction to the facial nerve. In approximately 5% of cases the bony covering of the greater superficial petrosal nerve and geniculate ganglion is dehiscent at the facial hiatus (Rhoton et al 1968; Buchheit & Rosenwasser, 1988). Dura is elevated forward until the foramen spinosum and middle meningeal artery are exposed (Fig. 28.22). Medially the superior petrosal sinus is identified and carefully elevated from its groove to identify the true posterior surface of the temporal bone. Dural retraction can be achieved using the specifically designed House–Urban middle fossa retractor, which is secured to the craniotomy margins. We prefer to use the Greenberg retractor with a 1 cm wide metal blade. The blade is bent to avoid the projection that occurs with the self-retaining device. The blade of the retractor is inserted to the apex of dural elevation and is progressively advanced as elevation proceeds. If at any stage the dura is torn the defect should be repaired immediately to prevent herniation of the temporal lobe. Anteromedial to the arcuate eminence the surface of the temporal bone is somewhat flattened and this has been termed the 'meatal plane' as it lies above the

region of the internal auditory canal. The line of the IAC bisects the angle between the superior semicircular canal (SSC) arcuate eminence and the greater superficial petrosal nerve (GSPN). Bleeding may be troublesome during dural elevation. Bleeding of small dural vessels is easily controlled by bipolar cautery and venous bleeding from the bone surface by bone wax. Venous sinus bleeding, e.g., around the foramen spinosum, is controlled by Surgicel packing.

A variety of techniques have been described for identification of the internal auditory canal (IAC). The early techniques used the GSPN and SSC as landmarks to define the internal canal. The GSPN was identified as it exited the facial hiatus and then bone was removed posteriorly along the course of the nerve until the geniculate ganglion was uncovered. The labyrinthine portion of the facial nerve was then identified medial to the ganglion and hence the IAC exposed further medially. The superior semicircular canal was bluelined by removal of bone over the arcuate eminence to provide a further posterior landmark. These methods required meticulous technique with little margin for error as the ampullated end of the SSC and the cochlea lie within millimeters of the labyrinthine segment of the facial nerve. We prefer the method of identifying and dissecting the IAC that is described by Garcia-Ibanez and Garcia-Ibanez (1980) and more recently by Brackmann et al (1994). Bone removal is commenced at the medial aspect of the meatal plane where both the SSC and cochlea are at greatest distance. Drilling begins directly over the bisection of the angle between GSPN and SSC until the dura of the IAC is exposed beneath the petrous bridge. To facilitate safe tumor removal, wide bone removal is required and so dissection extends anteriorly into the petrous apex medial to the otic capsule of the cochlea and posteriorly to the level of the SSC. Bone is progressively removed around the medial IAC until the posterior fossa dura and IAC dura is exposed over 270°. After medial exposure of the internal canal, bone is gradually removed in a lateral direction. The semicircular canal is skeletonized and the labyrinthine segment of the facial nerve identified. Bill's bar is identified laterally, however care is

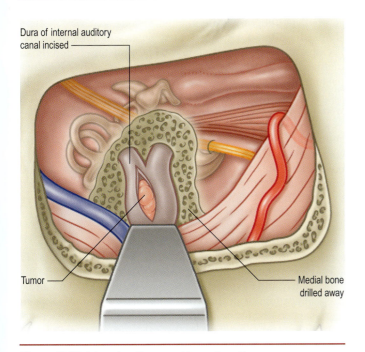

Dura of internal auditory canal incised

Tumor

Medial bone drilled away

Figure 28.23 Internal auditory canal bony dissection.

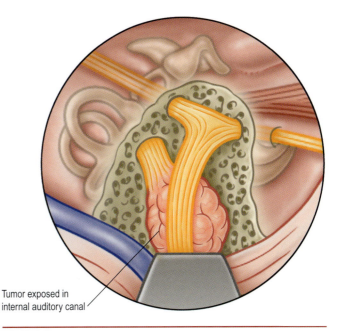

Tumor exposed in internal auditory canal

Figure 28.24 Tumor exposure within the internal auditory canal following dural incisions.

taken not to remove bone >120° at the lateral IAC to avoid entering the cochlea or SSC ampulla. As the dura of the IAC is exposed, the exact extent of the canal can be assessed by extradural palpation with a small hook or elevator. Continuous facial nerve EMG monitoring is essential to ensure atraumatic bony dissection as the dura and fallopian canal is exposed. Separation of the IAC dura from the bony canal also helps to prevent accidental injury to the dura and underlying facial nerve. Bill's bar, the vertical crest of bone at the fundus, marks the lateral extent of the IAC and also the clear anatomic division between the superior vestibular nerve and the facial nerve (Fig. 28.23).

At the completion of bone removal, the cerebellopontine angle is initially opened by incising the posterior fossa dura between the posterior aspect of the porus acousticus and the superior petrosal sinus. Cerebrospinal fluid is released by dividing the arachnoid, and the dural incision is continued laterally along the posterior aspect of the IAC. The dura is elevated and reflected anteriorly to expose the facial nerve overlying the anterior aspect of the tumor (Fig. 28.24). Great care must be taken where the dura is adherent to the tumor and the nerves at the porus acousticus. At the fundus of the IAC the dura is carefully divided posterior to Bill's bar and then over the facial nerve until the separation of superior vestibular nerve and facial nerve is clearly displayed. The electrode for continuous 8th nerve monitoring can now be placed beneath the reflected dural flap anteriorly or on the cochlear nerve medially within the cerebellopontine angle.

Tumor removal with successful facial nerve preservation is accomplished by initial separation of the facial nerve from the superior vestibular nerve (SVN) and from the tumor. If the tumor has arisen from the superior vestibular nerve the lateral fibers of the nerve blend into the tumor and the posterior border of the facial nerve must be sharply dissected

from tumor capsule. The line of anatomic dissection is easily identified laterally. With inferior vestibular nerve tumors the facial nerve must be separated from the SVN along its length and then separated from the tumor capsule beneath. A normal preoperative caloric response may provide indirect evidence that the tumor arises from the inferior vestibular nerve, and this may be considered as a relative contraindication to this approach (House & Luetje 1979). The principles of tumor dissection are the same as those outlined above. The superior vestibular nerve is divided laterally and, unless the tumor is small and only involving the superior vestibular nerve, the inferior vestibular nerve is likewise divided. After initial separation of the facial nerve from the tumor, debulking is performed unless the tumor is very small. Debulking allows subsequent manipulation within the IAC without stretching of the facial or cochlear nerves. The previous anterior bone removal medial to the cochlea allows displacement of the facial nerve towards the petrous apex, thereby facilitating dissection of the tumor from the cochlear nerve. The facial nerve will be most densely adherent to the tumor at the level of the porus, and the exact direction of the course of the nerve must be established as sharp dissection proceeds. For successful hearing preservation, the arterial supply to the cochlea must be preserved and so bipolar cautery is only used when absolutely necessary. The arterial supply to the cochlea consists of vessels which run between the facial and cochlear nerves in the anterior half of the canal so the utmost care must be taken to preserve vessels anteriorly within the IAC. Similarly, during medial dissection of the tumor, care must be taken to identify and preserve the anterior inferior cerebellar artery, which may loop between the facial and vestibulocochlear nerves at the porus. After initial debulking of the tumor progressive dissection from the cochlear nerve should be performed in a medial to lateral dissection direction. This avoids traction on the fragile

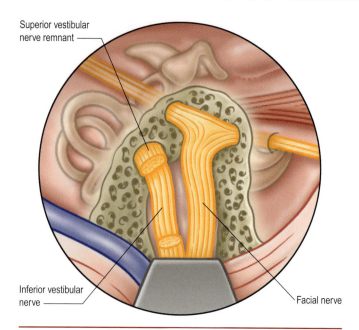

Superior vestibular
nerve remnant

Inferior vestibular
nerve

Facial nerve

Figure 28.25 Tumor removal complete. Superior vestibular nerve divided. Cochlear nerve beneath facial nerve.

nerve fibers entering the cochlea laterally at the spiral foramina and is important in preserving hearing (Fig. 28.25).

After total tumor removal is achieved and hemostasis is noted to be secure, the anterior dural flap is replaced to protect the facial nerve. A watertight dural repair is not possible, however a single suture may be used to re-approximate the posterior fossa dura. This provides support for a piece of abdominal fat which is used to occlude the bony IAC defect. Any air cells opened on the temporal bone surface are occluded with bone wax and if necessary reinforced with a sheet of temporalis fascia. The dura is secured to the margins of the craniotomy, the bone flap is replaced and secured with rigid fixation, and the wound is then closed in layers in the usual fashion. The spinal drain is removed at the completion of the procedure.

Combined approaches

Should exposure prove to be inadequate, the translabyrinthine approach may be combined with the transtentorial or suboccipital routes, as may be suboccipital and middle fossa operations. Although we have undertaken combined approaches in the past, and still do so on occasion for other tumors of the cerebellopontine angle, particularly meningiomas, we no longer find them necessary for excision of acoustic neurinomas.

Postoperative care

Patients are extubated at completion of the procedure and after perioperative recovery are nursed in a neurosurgical intensive care unit for 24 h. A brief period of postoperative ventilation may be appropriate after long procedures, particularly if the patient has become hypothermic during surgery. Although this has the advantage that intracranial pressure is kept low, one major disadvantage is that early signs of neurologic deterioration from an impending

cerebellopontine angle hematoma are masked. The patient should be nursed 15° head-up to reduce venous pressure. Perioperative antibiotics should be administered, and dexamethasone may be of limited benefit, not only to reduce postoperative edema in the cerebellum, but to reduce swelling of the facial nerve and resultant delayed facial weakness.

When large tumors have been excised, the patient should be assessed for bulbar palsy before oral fluids are commenced. The consequences of facial palsy are dealt with below. Vestibular sedatives may be required if dizziness and vomiting are troublesome, but their use should be restricted to a minimum. Scalp sutures and the BIPP ear pack are removed on the 7th day.

Results

Most of the complications that may befall a patient after surgery are common to all three approaches. The exceptions are epilepsy and dysphasia, which are confined to the middle fossa operation, or in the exceptional case when it has been necessary to divide the tentorium. In unselected series mortality figures for the different surgical approaches are almost identical and range from 0 to 2% in the hands of experienced surgeons in specialist centers. Almost all fatalities occur in patients with very large tumors. The major causes of death are brain stem infarction and hematoma in the cerebellopontine angle. Most other deaths follow cardiovascular or respiratory complications.

Tumor size is by far the most important single determinant of outcome, in terms of mortality, facial nerve outcome, and the prospect for a good general recovery (Olivecrona 1967; House & Luetje 1979). Several large series have documented surgical results as they relate to tumor size. Outcome is regarded as excellent if patients are able to resume their previous employment, fair if they remain independent but unable to work, and poor if their independence has been lost. This classification excludes facial nerve function. The results of five series are summarized in Table 28.2.

There has been much discussion in the literature comparing and contrasting the merits and disadvantages of the suboccipital, translabyrinthine, and middle fossa approaches to the cerebellopontine angle. Good results are reported with each method, which indicates that experience, operative microsurgical technique, and postoperative management are more important determinants of outcome than the surgical approach *per se*. Direct comparisons between large series employing different surgical techniques are often misleading for two reasons. First, tumor size is the most important predictor of outcome, yet there is no single accepted classification to enable standardization of reporting of results. Second, the suboccipital and middle fossa approaches are often selected for hearing preservation procedures. Inevitably such patients have a higher proportion of small tumors and therefore a better prognosis than with the translabyrinthine operation, which is more appropriate for larger lesions with poor residual hearing. Patients with small or medium-sized tumors also have a significantly shorter mean hospital stay than those with larger lesions (Mangham 1988).

When considering the approach of choice for any one lesion, we agree with Chen & Fisch (1992) that 'most patients are far more concerned about the complete removal of their

Table 28.2 Surgical results by tumor size

Author	Cases (n)	Operation	Tumor size	(%)[a]	Mortality (%)	Facial nerve result (%)[b]	Outcome in survivors Excellent (%)	Fair (%)	Poor (%)
Yasargil & Fox 1974	100	SO	Small	4	0		95	5	0
			Medium	19	0	85	82	13	5
			Large	77	4		56	37	7
Ojemann et al 1984	123	SO	Small	15	0		100	0	0
			Medium	30	0		100	0	0
			Large	55	1		91	7	2
King & Morrison 1980	150	TL[c]	Small	11	0	100	94	6	0
			Medium	42	2	80	100	0	0
			Large	47	3	20	93	5	2
Bentivoglio et al 1988a	94	SO	Small	14	0	100	100	0	0
			Medium	28	0	85	92	4	4
			Large	58	4	45	66	28	8
Hardy et al 1989a	100	TL	Small	4	0		100	0	0
			Medium	30	0	82	83	17	0
			Large	66	4		66	29	5

SO, suboccipital; TL, translabyrinthine.
[a]The results of the different series are not strictly comparable as the definitions of tumor size varied. Small, medium, and large approximate to the Pulec classification.
[b]Facial nerve figures in some series are anatomic preservation rates, while others relate to functional outcome.
[c]Denotes primary surgical approach, although series mixed.

tumor and their facial function postoperatively than about hearing'. It is primarily for this reason that we favor the translabyrinthine operation for the majority of patients. Postoperative morbidity and hospital stay are generally shorter after translabyrinthine surgery (Tos & Thomsen 1982; Gardner et al 1983; Tator & Nedzelski 1985), although the incidence of postoperative meningitis may be slightly higher because of a more direct route for contamination of the CSF by nasopharyngeal organisms (Mangham 1988). Sterkers et al (1984) initially favored the translabyrinthine operation but used the suboccipital approach subsequently for hearing preservation. They have since reverted to the translabyrinthine operation as a result of higher morbidity and an increased incidence of facial nerve palsy. Although the results reported in the literature are excellent with each of the approaches, it should be remembered that they represent the best in the field. For the less experienced surgeon the translabyrinthine approach is probably more likely to produce a good result because of improved access to the fundus of the tumor and the ability to identify the facial nerve lateral to it at an early stage of the dissection, but it is unfamiliar to most neurosurgeons, who may be uncomfortable with it, at least to start with.

Facial nerve function

In unselected series, anatomic preservation rates for the facial nerve are generally around 71–90% using the suboccipital route (Yasargil et al 1977; Sugita & Kobayashi 1982; Harner & Ebersold 1985; Bentivoglio et al 1988a) and 80–96% for the translabyrinthine group (House & Luetje 1979; Whittaker & Luetje 1985; Hardy et al 1989a). In neither group was anatomic preservation of the nerve achieved at the expense of sub-total tumor excision, as previously suggested by Di Tullio et al (1978). Success at preservation is highly dependent on tumor size (Table 28.2). In a series of 444 patients, House & Luetje (1979) reported complete facial

paralysis in 0% of patients with small tumors, in 10.4% of those with medium-sized lesions, and in 21.4% of those with large tumors.

In a report of 43 patients with small tumors operated on through the middle fossa, Gantz et al (1986) were able to preserve the facial nerve in all but one case. However, 60% had some facial nerve dysfunction immediately after surgery and 38% experienced complete paralysis. Ultimately, 86% achieved near normal function. Improved results, both in terms of hearing preservation and facial nerve function, have been reported in a subsequent series of patients from the same institution (Weber & Gantz 1996). Shelton et al (1989a) reported their experience of 106 cases operated via the middle fossa, with near normal facial nerve function in 89% of patients, and with some residual hearing in 59%. The increased trauma to the facial nerve via the middle fossa approach is probably the reason for the higher incidence of early facial weakness.

Anatomic integrity of the facial nerve does not guarantee facial function, either in the short or long term. If the nerve is intact anatomically but facial paralysis is complete postoperatively, then some return of function can be anticipated in 90% of cases (Hitselberger 1979), although it is unlikely to be complete. The rate at which the nerve recovers also predicts the final outcome. While recovery may continue for up to 3 years, Hitselberger (1979) found that it was always less than perfect if >4 months had elapsed from the time of surgery. Return of facial function may be heralded by transient facial pain. Facial nerve dysfunction does not usually affect all regions of the face to the same degree. Adequate movement of the oral commissure is more than twice as likely to occur than complete eye closure, and asymmetry of the forehead is particularly common (Wiegand & Fickel 1989). The presence of preoperative facial weakness increases the probability of facial nerve injury at surgery, but does not predict the final outcome if the nerve is spared anatomically (Lye et al 1982). These authors were able to preserve the nerve in 91% of cases with normal preoperative facial nerve function, but in only 67% of patients with preoperative weakness. However, it is not clear whether some of the disparity between the two groups is the result of differences in tumor size.

The degree of facial nerve weakness in the early postoperative period may be predicted at surgery from a comparison of the amplitude of the compound muscle action potential obtained by facial nerve stimulation proximal and distal to the site of tumor excision. If the percentage amplitude is >90% then very good early facial function may be anticipated. If the amplitude lies between 50% and 90% then temporary weakness may occur, but the final outcome is likely to be good. An amplitude of <50% suggests that a temporary lateral tarsorrhaphy may be advisable under the same anesthetic, and that some degree of permanent facial weakness is probable (Ebersold et al 1992). We prefer to assess facial nerve function postoperatively in order to determine the most effective and cosmetic measures appropriate for eye protection.

Hearing preservation
In only around 30–50% of hearing preservation operations will functional hearing remain, despite anatomic preservation of the auditory apparatus (Tatagiba et al 1992). This figure may be significantly higher for selected small tumors, particularly when a middle fossa approach is used. In an analysis of the English language literature from 1954 to 1986, the overall success with hearing preservation was 33% in series with a preponderance of small tumors (Gardner & Robertson 1988). The causes of such high failure rates are thought to be multifactorial. Possible factors include nerve manipulation with disruption of the myelin sheath (Sekiya & Moller 1987), impairment to the vasculature of the inner ear or cochlear nerve (Ebersold et al 1992), heat or vibration injury to the nerve and cochlea during removal of the posterior wall of the internal auditory canal, and damage to the labyrinth (Tatagiba et al 1992). From their experience with intraoperative monitoring, Ojemann et al (1984) observed that one of the critical stages in terms of hearing preservation was removal of tumor from the lateral aspect of the internal auditory canal. They proposed that dissection avulses some of the cochlear nerve fibers at the cribriform area, where they enter the modiolus. The most frequently injured labyrinthine structures are the crus commune of the posterior and superior semicircular canals, and the posterior semicircular canal (Tatagiba et al 1992). Hearing loss after labyrinthine injury is ascribed to loss of perilymph from the inner ear, although total deafness is not an inevitable sequel to it, particularly if the opening into the labyrinth is occluded quickly (Tatagiba et al 1992).

It is generally accepted that hearing preservation is deemed successful only if that which remains is of serviceable quality. The 50/50 rule is often applied: that there is less than a 50 dB hearing loss in the pure tone range, and that speech discrimination is >50%. Yet this is not sufficient to be useful socially if contralateral hearing is normal. A pure tone average (PTA) of 30 dB and a speech discrimination score (SDS) of >70% is required.

As with tumor size and facial nerve function, there is no single accepted classification for the reporting of hearing

Table 28.3 Classification for hearing for the evaluation of hearing preservation in acoustic neuroma

Classification	Pure tone threshold	Speech discrimination (%)
A	<30 dB	>70 dB
B	>30 dB and <50 dB	>50 dB
C	>50 dB	>50 dB
D	Any level	<50 dB

American Academy of Otolaryngology Head and Neck Surgery, (Committee on Hearing and Equilibrium (1995).

results. The Shelton–Brackmann classification (Shelton et al 1989b) is, however, gaining support. Hearing is classified as good (PTA <30 dB, SDS >70%), serviceable (PTA <50 dB, SDS >50%), measurable (any residual hearing), or anacusis. More recently, the American Academy of Otolaryngology Head and Neck Surgery Committee on Hearing and Equilibrium have proposed a classification for hearing for the evaluation of hearing preservation in acoustic neuroma (Committee on Hearing and Equilibrium 1995). Hearing threshold should be reported as the average of the pure tone hearing thresholds by air conduction at 0.5, 1.0, 2.0, and 3.0 kHz. The best word recognition (speech discrimination) scores at presentation levels of up to 40 dB sensation level should be recorded before and after treatment. Hearing is classified according to the classes in Table 28.3. Formal testing is necessary. Great caution must be exercised in believing the patient's evaluation of his/her residual hearing. Some patients have claimed that hearing in the operated ear was unchanged after translabyrinthine surgery. Clearly this is not the case, and the contralateral ear is responding to the auditory stimulus. For this reason, evaluation must insure adequate masking of the unoperated ear. Success at preservation varies considerably between series, but Wigand et al (1991) reported a success rate of 51% in a series which included tumors as large as 3 cm. Using the middle fossa approach, Brackmann et al (1994) retained hearing at or near the preoperative level in 71% of a series of 24 consecutive patients with small tumors. Nadol et al (1992) were able to retain useful hearing in 50% of cases in which the tumor extended <5 mm into the cerebellopontine angle, but in only 12% of tumors >25 mm.

It is exceptional for hearing to improve upon the preoperative level. Nadol et al (1992) reported this in only 5% of patients, and Gardner & Robertson (1988) in 6%. This is probably because atrophy of the organ of Corti occurs secondary to denervation, because the elevated protein concentration in the perilymph damages the outer hair cells, and because of inner ear ischemia caused by compression of the labyrinthine artery within the porus acousticus. Perlman & Kimura (1955) demonstrated that temporary vascular occlusion of only 30 min was sufficient to produce permanent impairment of hearing as a consequence of severe hair cell and spiral ganglion cell loss. Finally, the cochlear nerve itself may be invaded by tumor (Neely 1981). Kveton (1990) hypothesized that improvement in hearing was the result of reversal of conduction block. Small tumor size, good preoperative speech discrimination, and male sex correlate significantly with a good hearing outcome (Nadol et al 1992). Similarly, the topical application of papaverine to the cochlear nerve after tumor removal has been recommended (Brackmann et al 1994).

Hearing may worsen or fluctuate months or even years after surgery. The formation of scar tissue around the cochlear nerve as a consequence of packing the drilled surface of the porus may be a contributory factor (Shelton et al 1990). However, because the tumor may on occasion invade the cochlear nerve, delayed hearing loss can represent tumor recurrence (Neely 1984). Delayed edema is a further etiologic factor in early hearing loss, and may respond to corticosteroids (Goel et al 1992). Prophylactic nimodipine administration has been suggested in order to prevent vasospasm of the internal auditory artery and also because of its neural protective effects (Nadol et al 1987).

In >50% of patients in whom hearing preservation has been successful there will be a significant decline in function as follow-up lengthens, even in the absence of recurrent disease (Shelton et al 1990). In an 8-year follow-up study of 25 patients the unoperated side remained the better hearing ear in all patients over the entire period (Shelton et al 1992). This argues that the philosophy of preserving any measurable hearing in order to safeguard against the possibility of deafness developing in the contralateral ear is unjustified. Taking into account late deterioration, it has been estimated that only 7–9% of the total group who undergo hearing preservation procedures will have useful hearing in the long term (Whittaker & Luetje 1992).

It may be anticipated that medially placed tumors, that is those which do not occupy the fundus of the internal auditory meatus, might have a better prognosis for both facial nerve function and for hearing preservation than tumors which fill the porus. Although it is much easier to identify the nerves lateral to the tumor, the surgical results are no better in this subgroup of patients, either in terms of facial nerve recovery or hearing preservation. This is because these lesions often present late, and when the tumor is correspondingly of a greater size (Tos et al 1992b).

Complications of surgery
Hematoma in the operative cavity
Hematoma is a rare but potentially fatal consequence of surgery. If hemostasis has been meticulous, this complication should occur in <2% of cases. Profound unconsciousness, respiratory failure, and pulmonary edema can develop very rapidly and temperature elevation may be evident. Prompt action is required if the diagnosis is suspected. The patient should be ventilated to protect the airway and, if a frontal burr hole has been placed, intracranial pressure should be lowered by tapping the lateral ventricles. The patient should be transferred with the greatest speed to the operating room. If the patient's state is perilous, the wound can be opened in the ward; however, this should be avoided if at all possible as the hematoma may lie deep in the cavity, adherent to the pons. Optimal conditions are required if the clot is to be evacuated without risk to the cranial nerves and brain stem vasculature, and this is unlikely to be achieved without proper illumination, magnification, and instrumentation. Copious irrigation and a fine sucker will help to evacuate the hematoma and lessen the risk of nerve injury. A period of postoperative ventilation is recommended if re-exploration has been necessary.

Brain stem infarction
Devastating neurologic sequelae may follow injury to the anterior inferior cerebellar artery. It is a fundamental principle of this type of surgery that arteries of any size within the cerebellopontine angle are preserved, even if they are firmly adherent to the tumor capsule. Only small branches actually entering the substance of the tumor may be cauterized and divided. Larger vessels must be mobilized from the capsule or, if this proves impossible, capsular remnants should be left attached to the vessel. For the same reason, some surgeons have found it necessary on very rare occasions to leave capsular remnants adherent to the brain stem, since subpial dissection in this region may be equally catastrophic. Bleeding from a brain stem vessel should be controlled by gentle pressure on a piece of crushed muscle or hemostatic gauze.

Cerebrospinal fluid leakage
With the exception of facial nerve palsy, cerebrospinal fluid leakage from the wound or middle ear cavity (rhinorrhea) is the most common postoperative complication of acoustic neurinoma surgery (House et al 1982; Tos & Thomsen 1985; Gordon & Kerr 1986; Brackmann & Kwartler 1990a). An incidence of around 10–15% is reported in most major series (Di Tullio et al 1978; King & Morrison 1980; Glasscock et al 1986; Hardy et al 1989a; Ebersold et al 1992). The major contributing factors are poor wound healing, hydrocephalus, and failure to obliterate air cells opened in the porus acousticus or mastoid. After translabyrinthine or suboccipital surgery CSF may leak into the permeatal or retrofacial air cells, or via the dural defect into the mastoid air cells, and thence gain access to the middle ear cavity and eustachian tube. In addition to CSF leakage, symptomatic aerocele may develop.

Meticulous attention to the technique of wound closure can dramatically diminish the incidence of this complication. Using the method described in the operative section above, Hardy et al (1993) reduced their CSF leakage rate to 1.6% in a recent series of 230 patients. Some authors have argued that fat should not be used in wound closure because it may make subsequent MRI studies difficult to interpret (Ebersold et al 1992), but their CSF leakage rate using bone wax alone is unacceptably high. Current MRI techniques using fat suppression sequences in combination with gadolinium enhancement allow very sensitive identification of residual or recurrent tumor. We have no experience with synthetic bone replacement materials pioneered recently; ionomeric cement has the ability to adhere even to moist surfaces, and is reported to be a significant advance over other synthetic cements such as polymethyl methacrylate (Ramsden et al 1992). Apparently there is concern, however, about toxicity when ionomeric cement is in contact with CSF. Hydroxyapatite cement has been used successfully to repair the bone defect after suboccipital craniotomy, however it can only be applied in a relatively dry site.

If CSF leakage does occur, conservative measures such as lumbar drain insertion or the placement of additional sutures in the wound are successful in around 25% of patients (Hardy et al 1989a), but the remainder will require re-exploration. In general, CSF leakage from the wound is much more likely to settle with conservative treatment than is rhinorrhea. The value of prophylactic antibiotics is questionable. The technique used to seal the defect should be the same as described above. Bone pate is used to fill the exposed air cells, and is reinforced with a fascia lata patch sealed in place with fibrin glue. Fat is used to fill the bony defect, and this too is sealed with fibrin glue. A persistent CSF fistula after the translabyrinthine approach may be managed by permanent closure of the external auditory meatus, removal of the bony external auditory canal and middle ear cleft, and direct closure of the eustachian tube in the protympanum. This achieves very secure closure; however, the removal of squamous epithelium from the external canal and tympanic membrane must be meticulous. A lumbar drain may be placed for a few days to maintain a low CSF pressure until the wound has had the opportunity to heal.

Meningitis
The risk of postoperative meningitis relates not only to the development of CSF leakage. The protracted nature of the operation and the communication of the operative site with the eustachian tube are other important factors. Infection rates in the literature are generally around 3–6% (Di Tullio et al 1978; King & Morrison 1980; Bentivoglio et al 1988b; Hardy et al 1989a).

Diplopia
Postoperative unilateral abducent nerve paresis must be differentiated from a gaze palsy secondary to involvement of the lateral gaze center in the pons. The latter usually resolves within a few days of surgery, whereas injury to the abducent nerve may take considerably longer. Diplopia can be treated by an eye patch although, if the patient has a concomitant facial palsy, a more than adequate tarsorrhaphy will achieve the same result. Meningitis should be considered in the differential diagnosis of a delayed 6th nerve palsy.

Hearing loss
It is quite common for hearing to be decreased transiently after any surgery to the posterior fossa. The current hypothesis is that the low CSF pressure is transmitted via the cochlear aqueduct to the perilymph, producing perilymphatic hypotonia (Walstead et al 1991). Hearing loss in the contralateral ear after acoustic neurinoma removal has also been attributed to an autoimmune response (Harris et al 1985). Clemis et al (1982) reported three such patients, all of whom recovered spontaneously.

Special considerations
TUMORS IN THE ELDERLY AND INFIRM
In view of the slow growth rate in the majority of tumors, a conservative approach to management may be appropriate for very elderly or infirm patients, particularly if the tumor is small. However, the value of an expectant policy in aged but otherwise fit patients is less clear. Nedzelski et al (1986) studied the growth behavior of 50 untreated acoustic neurinomas in elderly patients followed up for between 12 and 144 months. They reported that around 20% of such patients required surgery within a third of their life expectancy. Yet even quite old patients will tolerate surgical excision of tumors. Two recent series, one suboccipital, the other translabyrinthine, have emphasized that age is not a contraindication to successful surgery. House et al (1987) reported a series of 116 patients over the age of 65 years

with only one death, and functional preservation of the facial nerve in 91% of cases. Samii et al (1992) recorded 61 patients operated on without mortality, with anatomic preservation of the facial nerve in 95%, and with residual hearing in 41%. In both series the majority of excisions were macroscopic (91% and 97%, respectively). As well as tumor size and evidence of mass effect, the presence of disabling symptoms such as vertigo is an indication for early intervention. Predictive factors for a poor outcome are ASA (American Society of Anesthesiologists) grading of physical status >3, a Karnofsky score <80, and tumor size >3 cm (Samii et al 1992). In the case of surgery for a symptomatic tumor in a frail patient, it may be appropriate to reduce the duration of the operation, either by elective sub-total excision or, rarely, by macroscopic removal with no attempt at preservation of the facial nerve.

Sub-total excision
Sub-total excision may be a planned procedure in, for example, a patient with a large tumor in a solitary hearing ear, or if facial weakness would be completely unacceptable. On other occasions it may be necessary to leave a rim of capsule adherent to the brain stem or adjacent vessels. Olivecrona (1967) observed that half of his 83 patients remained asymptomatic after partial tumor removal. This was also the experience of Wazen et al (1985): 11 of 13 elderly patients who had residual tumor after surgery showed no significant expansion over an average period of 6 years. In a series of 12 patients who underwent radical intracapsular removal of large tumors, and who were followed for up to 22 years, Lownie and Drake (1991) reported recurrence in only two cases, both within 3 years of surgery. However, Hitselberger and House (1979) found that the late recurrence rate necessitating re-exploration in their series was high, and that surgery on the second occasion was more hazardous. Ransohoff et al (1961) noted ultimately that 60% of patients treated in the 1930s by sub-total excision either died from recurrent disease or required a second operation. In Cushing's series of 182 patients, those who underwent sub-total excision but died eventually from tumor recurrence lived for an average of 5 years after the initial operation (German 1961).

With the exception of NF-2 patients, elective sub-total excision is unsatisfactory and illogical for small or medium-sized tumors. If a cure is not to be effected when the tumor is of a favorable size, then treatment should be delayed until symptoms become more serious. A more vexing issue is whether it is preferable to excise every last remnant of tumor at the risk of compromise to neural integrity, or to minimize the possibility of nerve or brain stem injury by leaving capsular or tumor remnants behind. Recent studies suggest that it is very reasonable to leave a small volume of tumor capsule along the course of the facial nerve in order to preserve anatomic and functional continuity of the nerve. Ohta and co-workers (1998) demonstrated tumor regrowth in only one of 8 patients with residual tumor along the facial nerve and suggested that removal of tumor in the internal auditory meatus may make regrowth unlikely. This issue is particularly relevant to attempts at hearing preservation. The success rate is generally poor, and any residual hearing may not be socially useful. In order to answer this question fully it is clear that longitudinal MRI studies are required, given that the growth potential of residual tumor appears at present to be unpredictable. Lye et al (1992) reported recently the results of a follow-up MRI study of 14 patients with capsular remnants left attached to vital structures at the time of otherwise total tumor removal. Over a mean period of 70 months, half the patients had radiologic evidence of persistent neurinomas. Four of these showed signs of progressive enlargement, although none was symptomatic and CT was normal in each. Persistence of tumor was more common if the residual fragment had not been cauterized at the time of operation (Lye et al 1992).

Facial nerve neurinoma
Facial nerve neurinomas account for <2% of lesions thought preoperatively to be acoustic neurinomas (House & Luetje 1979). The radiologic differential diagnosis has been discussed. At operation the facial nerve fibers are found to enter the tumor, and cannot be separated from it. The lateral extent of the tumor is often considerably greater than that of tumors of vestibular origin, and may involve the entire intratemporal course of the facial nerve. The basic principles of excision are the same as for removal of an acoustic neurinoma, although the facial nerve will be divided. Direct end-to-end anastomosis may be possible, or a primary graft may be fashioned from the greater auricular or sural nerves.

Indications for and results of radiotherapy

Conventional external beam radiotherapy has been used as an adjuvant therapy for patients with sub-total tumor resection, or in cases of advanced disease (Cushing 1921). In a series of 31 patients receiving postoperative irradiation, Wallner et al (1987) reported that a dose of 50–55 Gy was well tolerated, and reduced the probability of recurrence from 46% to 6%. Treatment was administered in 1.8 Gy fractions, 5 days per week. However, irradiation did not influence recurrence rates if >90% of the tumor had been excised, and radiation therapy for tumor recurrence after a previous surgical resection was associated with a poor prognosis. Irradiation is reported also to reduce tumor vascularity (Wallner et al 1987) and has been used in the preoperative management of highly vascular tumors (Ikeda et al 1988). Sequelae of radiation therapy include multiple cranial nerve palsies, brain stem edema, and brain stem ischemia (Brackmann & Kwartler 1990a).

Stereotactic radiosurgery

Since the first treatment of a vestibular schwannoma in 1967 by Lars Leksell using a 201 source Co[60] Gamma Knife for stereotactic delivery of radiation, a large experience has been obtained in treating acoustic neurinomas in a number of centers (Leksell 1971). Generally, only lesions <3 cm are suitable for this form of treatment. The principle of the technique is that multiple converging gamma beams are collimated to a focus, targeted on the lesion via a stereotactic frame applied to the skull. A dose of 10–15 Gy is delivered to the tumor periphery and a maximum of 15–25 Gy to the center (Noren et al 1992). The entire dose is delivered as a single fraction over 10–20 min. The dose gradient of the radiation is extremely steep at the edge of the target tissue.

The mechanism by which tumor growth is inhibited remains uncertain. *In vitro* studies suggest that Schwann cells suffer irreversible damage after single fraction doses of 30 Gy (Anniko et al 1981). Histopathology reveals interstitial fibrosis, tumor necrosis, vascular hyperplasia, and hyalinization (Lunsford et al 1992a). Apoptosis has been reported in the tumor cells (Fukuoka et al 1998).

Tumor control

Following initial experience with poor hearing preservation and high rates of trigeminal and facial nerve dysfunction, it was recognized that the incidence of cranial neuropathy is directly related to the radiation dose at the tumor margin. Between 1987 and 1992, the marginal tumor dose was therefore reduced from around 16 Gy to 12–13 Gy (Flickinger et al 1996; Miller et al 1999). A number of centers have now published series with follow-up of ≥5 years (Table 28.4). In most large series, the tumor control rate, usually defined as absence from further treatment) was between 90% and 100% at the end of the follow-up period. The Pittsburgh group has reported on 252 patients who received 12–13 Gy margin dose Gamma Knife radiosurgery between 1991 and 2001 and who had at least 10 years of follow-up (Lunsford et al 2005; Chopra et al 2007). The tumor control rate (absence of any further intervention) was 98%. A 99% tumor control rate at 5 years was reported by the Gainesville, Florida center (Friedman 2008; Friedman et al 2006). The first report to include very long-term follow-up (317 patients receiving a median margin dose of 13.2 Gy with a mean follow up of 7.8 years at the Komaki City Gamma Knife Center in Japan showed a 10-year actuarial control rate of only 92% (Hasegawa et al 2005). Despite this, the results displayed little or no difference between the 5- and 10-year PFS; the authors point of that most failures occurred within the first 3 years. It may be that further very long-term follow-up data may not reveal an increasing late recurrence rate compared to what we know already.

There is still debate about the exact dose that achieves control. In the Komaki City series, there was a difference between those treated with >13 Gy and those with ≤13 Gy margin dose, with 97% and 89% PFS, respectively (Hasegawa et al 2005). In another series, however, there

Table 28.4 Recent published series of radiosurgical treatment of small to moderate sized VS with lower margin doses

Author	Year	Patients	Margin dose (Gy)	Median f/up (years)	Tumor control rate (%) (at time)
Flickinger et al	2004	313	12–13	2	98 (6 years)
Chung et al	2005	195	12–13	3	95 (7 years)
Wowra et al	2005	111	13	7	95
Hasegawa et al	2005a	317	13.2	7.8	92 (10 years)
Hasegawa et al	2005b	73	14.6	11	87
Chopra et al	2007	216	12–13	5.7	98
Friedman et al	2008	450	12.5	5	99
Pollock et al	2009	293	13	5	94 (7 years)

of the round window or promontory is predictive for likely success with a cochlear implant (Waltzman et al 1990; Friedman et al 1998). This is an electronic device placed in the inner ear to stimulate the cochlear nerve. If the cochlear nerve is lost, however, or if the hair cells and spiral ganglion cells have been destroyed, the only other option is direct electrical stimulation of the cochlear nucleus with an auditory brain stem implant (Hitselberger et al 1984). A fully implantable multi-electrode prosthesis has been developed based on the nucleus 22 channel cochlear implant. Experience in Europe has been with a 21 electrode array and in the USA and Australia with an 8 electrode array. The electrode array is placed over the surface of the cochlear nucleus within the lateral recess of the fourth ventricle, usually at the time of translabyrinthine acoustic neurinoma removal. The translabyrinthine approach provides the most direct lateral access with visualization of the foramen of Luschka, although a retrosigmoid approach has been successfully used in some centers for electrode placement. Stimulation is via a transcutaneous coil system with a variety of processing strategies available, depending on the results of electrode mapping. In most cases, multiple channels have been available for stimulation (Brackmann et al 1993; Laszig et al 1999). The multichannel auditory brain stem implant is still in experimental use; it appears that the majority of subjects achieve a significant aid to lipreading and useful perception of environmental sounds. Only a very occasional patient (1%) has achieved open set speech understanding. Patients may get non-auditory sensation with stimulation of some electrodes, but in the majority this can be avoided when using the device by selective programming of electrodes (Shannon et al 1993). Auditory brain stem implantation should now be considered in all patients with neurofibromatosis type 2 when non-hearing preservation surgical removal of an acoustic neurinoma is performed. Suitable candidates are those patients with non-aidable hearing and any size tumor, or patients with serviceable hearing where hearing preservation is unlikely due to tumor size. Implantation at the time of first side tumor removal is a reasonable option if there is a bilateral profound hearing loss, but can also be considered in a patient with serviceable hearing in the contralateral ear, particularly if the contralateral tumor is large and further hearing loss is likely in the near future.

Bulbar palsy

Transient bulbar palsy may develop after removal of large tumors. Provided that the nerves are intact, the prognosis for recovery appears good (Hardy et al 1989a). To reduce the risk of aspiration, patients should undergo formal assessment of swallowing to ensure bulbar competence before oral fluids are commenced postoperatively.

Patterns of failure

House (1968) noted that, when tumor regrowth does occur, it does so within 4 years of the initial resection. Incomplete tumor resection may be a conscious decision at the time of surgery; the most common indications are adherence of the

capsule to the brain stem or other vital structures (e.g., AICA), and preservation of good facial nerve function. The behavior of the tumor remnant is unpredictable. Recurrence is not an inevitable sequel, and spontaneous involution of the remnant is well documented (Shea et al 1985). However, in a study of 33 patients with residual tumor followed up for a mean of 5.5 years, 36.5% required surgery for symptomatic recurrent tumor, and 9% died (Shea et al 1985). After 'total' tumor excision, recurrence rates in most large series are less than 1–2%. Inadvertent sub-total excision has been discussed in the preceding sections, but is most likely if visualization of the fundus of the internal auditory canal has been inadequate. Recurrence rates as high as 15% have been reported for retrosigmoid tumor removal where hearing preservation is attempted (Cerullo et al 1998). Continued tumor expansion can be expected in 5–15% of patients treated with stereotactic radiosurgery.

Management of recurrent disease

The growth rate of recurrent tumors is said to be more rapid than that of *de novo* lesions (Sterkers et al 1992). The rarity of recurrence means that there are no large series to quantify accurately the risks of reoperation. Many large series include a few recurrent tumors, and the risks of reexploration and tumor removal may not differ substantially from those of the treatment of primary tumors (Ebersold et al 1992). Shea et al (1985), however, did note that morbidity for second operations is substantially higher than for primary tumors; they reported a 25% mortality. Arachnoidal adhesions resulting from previous exploration hinder identification of the nerves, and may make the lesion more difficult to free from the brain stem and adjacent vessels. Yet this is not the experience of Hitselberger & House (1979), who have commented that surgical planes are not obscured after a previous translabyrinthine operation. Tos et al (1988) reoperated on four patients through the labyrinth between 1 and 6 months after previous translabyrinthine surgery, without apparent difficulty. The interval between operations is likely to have a significant bearing on the density of adhesions.

The treatment options for recurrent disease are similar to those for a primary tumor. If the facial nerve is non-functional as a consequence of the first operation, further surgery may be considerably less difficult. The translabyrinthine approach is ideal if the previous exploration was via a retrosigmoid or middle fossa route. The facial nerve can then be identified lateral to the tumor before any scar tissue is encountered. After translabyrinthine surgery a second operation may be via a retrosigmoid or transcochlear approach, so that at least some of the important landmarks may be identified before approaching the area of the tumor, where normal anatomic planes will be obscured by the previous surgery. Hearing preservation is very unlikely in this group, and the results of facial nerve preservation are also likely to be correspondingly less good than for primary tumors.

Management outcome

The results of surgery as they relate to death, facial nerve function, and hearing are discussed in the section dealing with the results of surgery.

Headache

It is our experience, and that of others (Schessel et al 1992), that postoperative headache is much more common with the suboccipital than translabyrinthine operation. Symptoms may last for years after surgery. The etiology remains unclear, but may be related to dissection of the nuchal musculature, scarring around the greater and lesser occipital nerves, or traction on the dura by adherence of the musculature. Replacement of the posterior fossa bone flap and reduction of muscle dissection to a minimum may help to reduce the incidence of this complication. A further factor which merits consideration is that, during the translabyrinthine operation, drilling of the temporal bone is completed before the dura is opened. In contrast during suboccipital surgery bone dust enters the basal cisterns when the posterior wall of the internal auditory canal is removed and thereby may precipitate chemical meningitis.

Tinnitus

Tinnitus is thought to be generated by the cochlea (Moller 1984), the cochlear nerve (Shea et al 1981), or the brain stem (Pulec et al 1978). Tinnitus may not be able to be abolished even by section of the cochlear nerve. After tumor removal there is only a 40–60% chance that tinnitus will improve, and a 6–40% likelihood that it will worsen (Silverstein et al 1986; Goel et al 1992). The probability of this is determined in part by the severity of preoperative symptoms. Baguley et al (1992) reported recently the effect of translabyrinthine surgery on tinnitus in a series of 129 patients. If tinnitus was not present preoperatively there was a 27% chance that it would develop after surgery, but it was very unlikely to be troublesome. If mild or moderate tinnitus was present before surgery there was a 25% chance that it would be abolished and a 37% chance that it would worsen. However, the risk that it would be severe under such circumstances was only around 2.5%. Severe tinnitus was very likely to improve after surgery, and was abolished entirely in one-fifth of patients.

Vestibular rehabilitation

Initially, after labyrinthectomy or vestibular nerve section there is ataxia, with the patient veering to the operated side. Horizontal nystagmus, with the slow phase toward the ablated side, may also be evident. Although it may be anticipated that symptoms and signs are likely to be greatest in patients with small tumors and normal preoperative vestibular function, this is not in fact the case. Jenkins (1985) found that age, sex, tumor size, or the presence of brain stem compression did not alter significantly the rate of postoperative vestibular compensation. In most patients symptoms will be short-lived and, within a few weeks, nystagmus will be abolished and ataxia minimal (Fisch 1973). A recent study found that 31% of patients had disequilibrium lasting longer than 3 months after surgical removal of an acoustic neurinoma. Age >55.5 years, female gender, constant preoperative disequilibrium present for >3.5 months and central findings on electronystagmography were associated with a worse outcome (Driscoll et al 1998).

Animal studies have shown that early visual and somatosensory stimulation determines both the speed and ultimate recovery after vestibular injury (Igarashi et al 1979). For this reason, vestibular exercises are important in the early postoperative period, and patients with bilateral vestibular nerve loss, impaired vision, or altered proprioception are less likely to make a good recovery. Healthy patients with unilateral vestibular loss should have a structured program of exercise, with emphasis on head movement. Initially the patient will experience feelings of instability, but labyrinthine sedatives should be avoided if possible, as these are likely to delay the compensatory process. An exercise strategy for rehabilitation following vestibular injury can be found in Goebel (1992). However, despite good compensation, all patients will have some chronic disturbance of postural equilibrium after labyrinthectomy, albeit insignificant clinically (House & Nelson 1979).

Quality of life

Figures for quality of life as they relate to tumor size are given in Table 28.2. Although it is customary to exclude facial nerve outcome from this analysis, a poor functional result in this regard may have profound social implications for the patient, because of the disfiguring appearance. In particular, the combination of hearing loss and cosmetic deformity may lead to a reluctance to resume social contacts (Wiegand & Fickel 1989). For others, the psychological impact of surgery is less but the physical aspects are more debilitating, particularly loss of balance. A detailed account of the patient's perspective of his or her illness and recovery can be found in Wiegand and Fickel (1989). Recently, more objective studies of quality of life following acoustic neurinoma surgery have been performed and have demonstrated that the surgery can have a significant impact on patients' overall quality of life (Nickolopoulos et al 1998).

Key points

- The results of treatment have improved dramatically since the pioneering days of surgery in the early 1900s, and House's landmark monograph of 1964. During that time mortality has fallen from 80% to <5%, primarily as a result of the introduction of modern anesthesia and the operating microscope.

- Reduction of morbidity is now the major goal, particularly the preservation of good facial function and the salvage of residual hearing.

- Incremental modifications of operative technique, the introduction of new technology such as stereotactic radiosurgery, and understanding of molecular genetics provide the prospect for further improvements in outcome during the coming decade.

REFERENCES

Adams, R.D., 1943. Occlusion of the anterior inferior cerebellar artery. Arch. Neurol. Psychiatry 49, 765–770.

Adeloye, A., 1979. Neoplasms of the brain in the African. Surg. Neurol. 11, 247–255.

Akhmametyeva, E.M., Mihaylova, M.M., Luo, H., et al., 2006. Regulation of the neurofibromatosis 2 gene promoter expression during embryonic development. Dev. Dyn. 235, 2771–2785.

Alfthan, K., Heiska, L., Gronholm, M., et al., 2004. Cyclic AMP-dependent protein kinase phosphorylates merlin at serine 518

Fisch, U., Dobie, R.A., Gmur, A., et al., 1987. Intracranial facial nerve anastomosis. Am. J. Otol. 8, 23–29.

Fischer, G., Fischer, C., Remond, J., 1992. Hearing preservation in acoustic neuroma surgery. J. Neurosurg. 76, 910–917.

Flaiz, C., Kaempchen, K., Matthies, C., et al., 2007. Actin-rich protrusions and nonlocalized GTPase activation in Merlin-deficient schwannomas. J. Neuropathol. Exp. Neurol. 66, 608–616.

Flickinger, J.C., Kondziolka, D., Pollock, B.E., et al., 1996. Evolution in technique for vestibular schwannoma radiosurgery and effect on outcome. Int. J. Radiat. Oncol. Biol. Phys. 36, 275–280.

Flood, L.M., Brightwell, A.P., 1984. Cochlear deafness in the presentation of a large acoustic neuroma. J. Laryngol. Otol. 98, 87–92.

Fontaine, B., Rouleau, G.A., Seizinger, B.R., et al., 1991. Molecular genetics of neurofibromatosis 2 and related tumors (acoustic neuroma and meningioma). Ann. NY Acad. Sci. 615, 338–343.

Fraenzer, J.T., Pan, H., Minimo, L. Jr., et al., 2003. Overexpression of the NF2 gene inhibits schwannoma cell proliferation through promoting PDGFR degradation. Int. J. Oncol. 23, 1493–1500.

Friedman, R.A., Brackmann, D.E., Mills, D., 1998. Auditory nerve integrity after middle fossa acoustic tumor removal. Otolaryngol. Head Neck Surg. 119 (6), 588–592.

Friedman, R.A., Brackmann, D.E., Hitselberger, W.E., et al., 2005. Surgical salvage after failed irradiation for vestibular schwannoma. Laryngoscope 115, 1827–1832.

Friedman, W.A., 2008. Linear accelerator radiosurgery for vestibular schwannomas. Prog. Neurol. Surg. 21, 228–237.

Friedman, W.A., Bradshaw, P., Myers, A., et al., 2006. Linear accelerator radiosurgery for vestibular schwannomas. J. Neurosurg. 105, 657–661.

Fukuoka, S., Oka, K., Seo, Y., et al., 1998. Apoptosis following gamma knife radiosurgery in a case of acoustic schwannoma. Stereotact. Funct. Neurosurg. 70 (Suppl. 1), 88–94.

Gantz, B.J., Gmuer, A.A., Holliday, M., 1984. Electroneurographic evaluation of the facial nerve. Method and technical problems. Ann. Otol. Rhinol. Laryngol. 93, 394–398.

Gantz, B.J., Parnes, L.S., Harker, L.A., et al., 1986. Middle cranial fossa acoustic neuroma excision: results and complications. Ann. Otol. Rhinol. Laryngol. 95, 454–459.

Garcia-Ibanez, E., Garcia-Ibanez, J.L., 1980. Middle fossa neurectomy: A report of 373 cases. Otolaryngol. Head Neck Surg. 88, 486–490.

Gardner, G., Robertson, J.H., 1988. Hearing preservation in unilateral acoustic neuroma surgery. Ann. Otol. Rhinol. Laryngol. 97, 55–66.

Gardner, G., Robertson, J.H., Clark, W.C., 1983. 105 patients operated upon for cerebellopontine angle tumors – experience using combined approach and CO2 laser. Laryngoscope 93, 1049–1055.

German, W.J., 1961. Acoustic neurinomas: A follow-up. Clin. Neurosurg. 7, 21–39.

Giovannini, M., Robanus-Maandag, E., Van Der Valk, M., et al., 2000. Conditional biallelic Nf2 mutation in the mouse promotes manifestations of human neurofibromatosis type 2. Genes Dev. 14, 1617–1630.

Glasscock, M.E. III, Devine, S.C., McKennan, K.X., 1987. The changing characteristics of acoustic neuroma patients over the last ten years. Laryngoscope 97, 1164–1167.

Glasscock, M.E. III, McKennan, K.X., Levine, S.C., 1988. False negative M R I scan in an acoustic neuroma. Otolaryngol. Head Neck Surg. 98, 612–614.

Glasscock, M.E., Kveton, J.F., Jackson, C.G., et al., 1986. A systemic approach to the surgical management of acoustic neuroma. Laryngoscope 96, 1088–1094.

Gleeson, R.K., Butzer, J.F., Grin, O.D. Jr., 1978. Acoustic neuroma presenting as subarachnoid hemorrhage: Case report. J. Neurosurg. 49, 602–604.

Godey, B., Morandi, X., Beust, L., et al., 1998. Sensitivity of auditory brainstem response in acoustic neuroma screening. Acta Otolaryngol. (Stockh) 118, 501–504.

Goebel, J.A., 1992. Experimental and practical considerations for rehabilitation following vestibular injury. In: Tos, M., Thomsen, J. (Eds.), Acoustic neuroma. Kugler, Amsterdam, pp. 905–911.

Goel, A., Sekhar, L.N., Langheinrich, W., et al., 1992. Late course of preserved hearing and tinnitus after acoustic neurilemmoma surgery. J. Neurosurg. 77, 685–689.

Goetting, M.G., Swanson, S.E., 1987. Massive hemorrhage into intracranial neurinomas. Surg. Neurol. 27, 168–172.

Gonzalez-Agosti, C., Xu, L., Pinney, D., et al., 1996. The merlin tumor suppressor localizes preferentially in membrane ruffles. Oncogene 13, 1239–1247.

Gordon, D.S., Kerr, A.G., 1986. Cerebrospinal fluid rhinorrhea following surgery for acoustic neuroma. J. Neurosurg. 64, 676–678.

Gormley, W.B., Sekhar, L.N., Wright, D.C., et al., 1997. Acoustic neuromas: Results of current surgical management. Neurosurgery 41, 50–58.

Graham, M.D., 1975. The jugular bulb in anatomic and clinical considerations in contemporary otology. Arch. Otolaryngol. 101, 560–564.

Graham, M.D., Sataloff, R.T., 1984. Acoustic tumors in the young adult. Arch. Otolaryngol. 110, 405–407.

Gruskin, P., Carberry, J.N., 1979. Pathology of acoustic tumors. In: House, W.F., Luetje, C.M. (Eds.), Acoustic Tumors, vol. I. Diagnosis. University Park Press, Baltimore, pp. 85–148.

Gutmann, D.H., Giordano, M.J., Fishback, A.S., Guha, A., 1997. Loss of merlin expression in sporadic meningiomas, ependymomas and schwannomas. Neurology 49, 267–270.

Gutmann, D.H., Haipek, C.A., Hoang Lu, K., 1999. Neurofibromatosis 2 tumor suppressor protein, merlin, forms two functionally important intramolecular associations. J. Neurosci. Res. 58, 706–716.

Guyot, J.P., Hausler, R., Reverdin, A., et al., 1992. The value of otoneurologic diagnosis procedures compared with radiology and operative findings. In: Tos, M., Thomsen, J. (Eds.), Acoustic neuroma. Kugler, Amsterdam, pp. 31–37.

Haberkamp, T.J., Meyer, G.A., Fox, M., 1998. Surgical exposure of the fundus of the internal auditory canal: Anatomic limits of the middle fossa versus the retrosigmoid transcanal approach. Laryngoscope 108, 1190–1194.

Haberman, R.S. II, Kramer, M.B., 1989. False positive MRI and CT findings of an acoustic neuroma. Am. J. Otol. 10, 301–303.

Hammerschlag, P.E., Cohen, N.L., Brundy, J., 1992. Rehabilitation of facial paralysis following acoustic neuroma excision with jump interpositional graft hypoglossal facial anastomosis and gold weight lid implantation. In: Tos, M., Thomsen, J., (Eds.) Acoustic neuroma. Kugler, Amsterdam, pp. 789–792.

Han, D.H., Kim, D.G., Chi, J.B., et al., 1992. Malignant triton tumor of the acoustic nerve: Case report. J. Neurosurg. 76, 874–877.

Hanemann, C.O., Bartelt-Kirbach, B., Diebold, R., et al., 2006. Differential gene expression between human schwannoma and control Schwann cells. Neuropathol. Appl. Neurobiol. 32, 605–614.

Hansen, M.R., Linthicum, F.H. Jr., 2004. Expression of neuregulin and activation of erbB receptors in vestibular schwannomas: possible autocrine loop stimulation. Otol. Neurotol. 25, 155–159.

Hansen, M.R., Clark, J.J., Gantz, B.J., et al., 2008. Effects of ErbB2 signaling on the response of vestibular schwannoma cells to gamma-irradiation. Laryngoscope 118, 1023–1030.

Hansen, M.R., Roehm, P.C., Chatterjee, P., et al., 2006. Constitutive neuregulin-1/ErbB signaling contributes to human vestibular schwannoma. Proliferation Glia 53, 593–600.

Hardy, D.G., Macfarlane, R., Moffat, D.A., 1993. Wound closure after acoustic neuroma surgery. Br. J. Neurosurg. 7, 171–174.

Hardy, D.G., Macfarlane, R., Baguley, D., et al., 1989a. Surgery for acoustic neurinoma. An analysis of 100 translabyrinthine operations. J. Neurosurg. 71, 799–804.

Hardy, D.G., Macfarlane, R., Baguley, D., et al., 1989b. Facial nerve recovery following acoustic neuroma surgery. Br. J. Neurosurg. 3, 675–680.

Hardy, M., Crowe, S.J., 1936. Early asymptomatic acoustic tumors. Arch. Surg. 32, 292–301.

Harner, S.G., Ebersold, M.J., 1985. Management of acoustic neuromas, 1978–1983. J. Neurosurg. 63, 175–179.

Harner, S.G., Reese, D.F., 1984. Roentgenographic diagnosis of acoustic neurinoma. Laryngoscope 94, 306–309.

Harner, S.G., Laws, E.R. Jr., Onofrio, B.M., 1984. Hearing preservation after removal of acoustic neuroma. Laryngoscope 94, 1431–1434.

Harris, J.P., Low, N.C., House, W.F., 1985. Contralateral hearing loss following inner ear injury, sympathetic cochleolabyrinthitis? Am. J. Otol. 6, 371–377.

Harrisingh, M.C., Perez-Nadales, E., Parkinson, D.B., et al., 2004. The Ras/Raf/ERK signalling pathway drives Schwann cell dedifferentiation. The EMBO J. 23, 3061–3071.

Hart, R.G., Gardner, D.P., Howieson, J., 1983. Acoustic tumors – atypical features and recent diagnostic tests. Neurology 33, 211–221.

Hasegawa, T., Fujitani, S., Katsumata, S., et al., 2005a. Stereotactic radiosurgery for vestibular schwannomas: analysis of 317 patients followed more than 5 years. Neurosurgery 57, 257–265.

Hermanz-Schulman, M., Welch, K., Strand, R., et al., 1986. Acoustic neuromas in children. AJNR Am. J. Neuroradiol. 7, 519–521.

Hirokawa, Y., Tikoo, A., Huynh, J., et al., 2004. A clue to the therapy of neurofibromatosis type 2: NF2/merlin is a PAK1 inhibitor. Cancer J 10, 20–26.

Hirsch, A., Noren, G., 1988. Audiological findings after stereotactic radiosurgery in acoustic neurinoma. Acta. Otolaryngol. (Stockh) 106, 244–251.

Hitselberger, W.E., 1966. External auditory canal hypesthesia. An early sign of acoustic neuroma. Am. Surg. 32, 741–743.

Hitselberger, W.E., 1979. Hypoglossal facial anastomosis. In: House, W.F., Luetje, C.M. (Eds.) Acoustic tumors, vol. II. Management. University Park Press, Baltimore, MD, pp. 97–103.

Hitselberger, W.E., House, W.F., 1979. Partial versus total removal of acoustic tumors. In: House, W.F., Luetje, C.M. (Eds.), Acoustic tumors, vol. II. Management. University Park Press, Baltimore, MD, pp. 265–268.

Hitselberger, W., House, W., Edgerton, B., et al., 1984. Cochlear nucleus implant. Otolaryngol. Head Neck Surg. 92, 52–54.

Holt, G., 1978. ENT manifestations of von Recklinghausen's disease. Laryngoscope 88, 1617–1632.

House, J.W., Brackmann, D.E., 1985. Facial nerve grading system. Otolaryngol. Head Neck Surg. 93, 146–147.

House, J.W., Hitselberger, W.E., House, W.F., 1982. Wound closure and cerebrospinal fluid leak after translabyrinthine surgery. Am. J. Otol. 4, 126–128.

House, J.W., Nissen, R.L., Hitselberger, W.E., 1987. Acoustic tumor management in senior citizens. Laryngoscope 97, 129–130.

House, J.W., Waluch, V., Jachler, R.K., 1986. Magnetic resonance imaging in acoustic neuroma diagnosis. Ann. Otol. Rhinol. Laryngol 95, 16–20.

House, W.F., 1961. Surgical exposure of the internal auditory canal and its contents through the middle cranial fossa. Laryngoscope 71, 1363–1385.

House, W.F., 1964a. Evolution of transtemporal bone removal of acoustic tumors. Laryngoscope 94, 731–742.

House, W.F., 1968. Partial tumor removal and recurrence in acoustic tumor surgery. Arch. Otolaryngol. 88, 644–654.

House, W.F., 1979. The translabyrinthine approach. In: House, W.F., Luetje, C.M. (Eds.), Acoustic tumors, vol. II. Management. University Park Press, Baltimore, MD, pp. 43–89.

House, W.F., Hitselberger, W.E., 1976. The transcochlear approach to the skull base. Arch. Otolaryngol. 102, 334–342.

House, W.F., Luetje, C.M., 1979. Evaluation and preservation of facial function. In: House, W.F., Luetje, C.M. (Eds.), Acoustic tumors. University Park Press, Baltimore, pp. 89–94.

House, W.F., Nelson, J.R., 1979. Long-term cochleo-vestibular effects of acoustic tumor surgery. In: House, W.F., Luetje, C.M. (Eds.), Acoustic tumors, vol. II. Management. University Park Press, Baltimore, MD, pp. 207–234.

Houshmandi, S.S., Emnett, R.J., Giovannini, M., et al., 2009. The neurofibromatosis 2 protein, merlin, regulates glial cell growth in an ErbB2- and Src-dependent manner. Mol. Cell Biol. 29, 1472–1486.

Huang, W.-Q., Zheng, S.-J., Tian, Q.-S., et al., 1982. Statistical analysis of central nervous system tumors in China. J. Neurosurg. 56, 555–564.

Hughes, G.B., Sismanis, A., Glasscock, M.E. III, et al., 1982. Management of bilateral acoustic tumors. Laryngoscope 92, 1351–1359.

Hung, G., Colton, J., Fisher, L., et al., 2002. Immunohistochemistry study of human vestibular nerve schwannoma differentiation. Glia 38, 363–370.

Huson, S.M., Harper, P.S., Compston, D.A.S., 1988. Von Recklinghausen neurofibromatosis: a clinical and population study in south east Wales. Brain 111, 355–381.

Igarashi, M., Levy, J.K., Takahashi, M., et al., 1979. Effect of exercise upon locomotor balance modification after peripheral vestibular lesions (unilateral utricular neurotomy) in squirrel monkeys. Adv. Otorhinolaryngol. 25, 82–87.

Ikeda, K., Ito, H., Kashihara, K., et al., 1988. Effective preoperative irradiation of highly vascular cerebellopontine angle neurinoma. Neurosurgery 22, 566–573.

Ishihara, H., Saito, K., Nishizaki, T., et al., 2004. CyberKnife radiosurgery for vestibular schwannoma. Minim. Invasive Neurosurg. 47, 290–293.

Jääskeläinen, J., Pyykkö, I., Blomstedt, G., et al., 1990. Functional results of facial nerve suture after removal of acoustic neurinoma: an analysis of 25 cases. Neurosurgery 27, 408–411.

Jackler, R.K., Pitts, L.H., 1990. Acoustic neuroma. Neurosurg. Clin. N. Am. 1, 199–223.

Jacoby, L.B., Pulaski, K., Rouleau, G.A., et al., 1990. Clonal analysis of human meningiomas and schwannomas. Cancer Res. 50, 6783–6786.

Jahrsdoerfer, R.A., Benjamin, R.S., 1988. Chemotherapy of bilateral acoustic neuromas. Otolaryngol. Head Neck Surg. 98, 273–282.

James, M.F., Manchanda, N., Gonzalez-Agosti, C., et al., 2001. The neurofibromatosis 2 protein product merlin selectively binds F-actin but not G-actin, and stabilizes the filaments through a lateral association. Biochem. J. 356, 377–386.

Jenkins, H.A., 1985. Long-term adaptive changes of the vestibulo-ocular reflex in patients following acoustic neuroma surgery. Laryngoscope 95, 1224–1234.

Jenkins, H.A., Fisch, U., 1980. The transotic approach to resection of difficult acoustic tumors of the cerebellopontine angle. Am. J. Otol. 2, 70–76.

Jin, H., Sperka, T., Herrlich, P., Morrison, H., 2006. Tumorigenic transformation by CPI-17 through inhibition of a merlin phosphatase. Nature 442, 576–579.

Johnson, E.W., 1977. Auditory test results in 500 cases of acoustic neuroma. Arch. Otolaryngol. 103, 152–158.

Johnson, E.W., 1979. Results of audiometric tests in acoustic tumor patients. In: House, W.F., Luetje, C.M. (Eds.), Acoustic tumors, vol. I. Diagnosis. University Park Press, Baltimore, MD, pp. 209–224.

Josey, A.F., Jackson, C.G., Glasscock, M.E., 1980. Brainstem evoked audiometry in confirmed 8th nerve tumors. Am. J. Otolaryngol. 1, 285–290.

Kaempchen, K., Mielke, K., Utermark, T., et al., 2003. Upregulation of the Rac1/JNK signaling pathway in primary human schwannoma cells. Hum. Mol. Genet. 12, 1211–1221.

Kalamarides, M., Niwa-Kawakita, M., Leblois, H., et al., 2002. Nf2 gene inactivation in arachnoidal cells is rate-limiting for meningioma development in the mouse. Genes Dev. 16, 1060–1065.

Kaneko, T., Yamashima, T., Tohma, Y., et al., 2001. Calpain-dependent proteolysis of merlin occurs by oxidative stress in meningiomas: a novel hypothesis of tumorigenesis. Cancer 92, 2662–2672.

Kano, H., Kondziolka, D., Khan, A., et al., 2009. Predictors of hearing preservation after stereotactic radiosurgery for acoustic neuroma. J. Neurosurg. 111, 863–873.

Kanter, W.R., Eldridge, R., Fabricans, R., et al., 1980. Central neurofibromatosis with bilateral acoustic neuroma. Genetic, clinical and biochemical distinctions from peripheral neurofibromatosis. Neurology 30, 851–859.

Karjalainen, S., Nuutinen, J., Neitaammaki, H., et al., 1984. The incidence of acoustic neuroma in autopsy material. Arch. Otorhinolaryngol. 240, 91–93.

Kartush, J.M., Niparko, J.K., Graham, M.D., et al., 1987. Electroneuronography: preoperative facial nerve assessment for tumors of the temporal bone. Otolaryngol. Head Neck Surg. 97, 257–261.

Kasantikul, V., Netsky, M.G., Glasscock, M.E. III, et al., 1980a. Acoustic neurilemmoma, clinicoanatomical study of 103 patients. J. Neurosurg. 52, 28–35.

Kasantikul, V., Netsky, M.G., Glasscock, M.E. III, et al., 1980b. Intracanalicular neurilemmomas: clinicopathologic study. Ann. Otol. Rhinol. Laryngol 89, 29–32.

Khangure, M.S., Moijtahedi, S., 1983. Air C T cisternography of anterior inferior cerebellar artery loop simulating an intracanalicular acoustic neuroma. Am. J. Neuroradiol. 4, 994–995.

Kim, J.Y., Kim, H., Jeun, S.S., et al., 2002. Inhibition of NF-kappaB activation by merlin. Biochem. Biophys. Res. Commun. 296, 1295–1302.

Kimura, Y., Koga, H., Araki, N., et al., 1998. The involvement of calpain-dependent proteolysis of the tumor suppressor NF-2 (merlin) in schwannomas and meningiomas. Nat. Med. 4, 915–922.

King, T.T., Morrison, A., 1980. Translabyrinthine and transtentorial removal of acoustic nerve tumors. Results of 150 cases. J. Neurosurg. 52, 210–216.

King, T.T., Morrison, A.W., 1990. Primary facial nerve tumors within the skull. J. Neurosurg. 72, 1–8.

King, T.T., Sparrow, O.C., Arias, J.M., et al., 1993. Repair of facial nerve after removal of cerebellopontine angle tumors: a comparative study. J. Neurosurg. 78, 720–725.

Kissil, J.L., Johnson, K.C., Eckman, M.S., et al., 2002. Merlin phosphorylation by p21-activated kinase 2 and effects of phosphorylation on merlin localization. J. Biol. Chem. 277, 10394–10399.

Kissil, J.L., Wilker, E.W., Johnson, K.C., et al., 2003. Merlin, the product of the Nf2 tumor suppressor gene, is an inhibitor of the p21-activated kinase, Pak1. Mol. Cell. 12, 841–849.

Kitamura, K., Kakoi, H., Ishida, T., 1992. Audiological assessment of bilateral acoustic tumors during conservative management. In: Tos, M., Thomsen, J. (Eds.), Acoustic neuroma. Kugler, Amsterdam, pp. 835–838.

Klemink, J.L., laRouare, M.J., Kileny, P.R., et al., 1990. Hearing preservation following suboccipital removal of acoustic neuromas. Laryngoscope 100, 597–601.

Koenig, M., Kalyan-Raman, K., Sureka, O.N., 1984. Contralateral trigeminal nerve dysfunction as a false localizing sign in acoustic neurinoma: a clinical and electrophysiological study. Neurosurgery 14, 335–337.

Koh, E.S., Millar, B.A., Menard, C., et al., 2007. Fractionated stereotactic radiotherapy for acoustic neuroma: single-institution experience at The Princess Margaret Hospital. Cancer 109, 1203–1210.

Kondziolka, D., Mathieu, D., Lunsford, L.D., et al., 2008. Radiosurgery as definitive management of intracranial meningiomas. Neurosurgery 62, 53–58; discussion 58–60.

Koos, W.T., 1988. Criteria for preservation of vestibulo-cochlear nerve function during microsurgical removal of acoustic neurinomas. Acta Neurochir. 92, 55–66.

Koos, W.T., Day, J.D., Matula, C., et al., 1998. Neurotopographic considerations in microsurgical treatment of small acoustic neuromas. J. Neurosurg. 88, 506–512.

Korf, B.R., 1990. The genetic basis of neurofibromatosis. Neurol. Forum 2, 2–7.

Krause, F., 1903. Zur Freilegung der hinteren Felsenheinflache und des Kleinhims. Beitr. Klin. Chir. 37, 728–764.

Kurland, L.T., Schoenberg, B.S., Annegers, J.F., et al., 1982. The incidence of primary intracranial neoplasms in Rochester, Minnesota 1935–1977. Ann. NY Acad. Sci. 381, 6–16.

Kveton, J.F., 1990. Delayed spontaneous return of hearing after acoustic tumor surgery: evidence for cochlear nerve conduction block. Laryngoscope 100, 473–476.

Kveton, J.F., Book, J., 1992. A comparison of auditory nerve monitoring techniques in acoustic tumor surgery. In: Tos, M., Thomsen, J., (Eds.) Acoustic neuroma. Kugler, Amsterdam, pp. 537–542.

Laasonen, E.M., Troupp, H., 1986. Volume growth rate of acoustic neurinomas. Neuroradiology 28, 203–207.

Lallemand, D., Curto, M., Saotome, I., et al., 2003. NF2 deficiency promotes tumorigenesis and metastasis by destabilizing adherens junctions. Genes Dev. 17, 1090–1100.

Lallemand, D., Manent, J., Couvelard, A., et al., 2009. Merlin regulates transmembrane receptor accumulation and signaling at the plasma membrane in primary mouse Schwann cells and in human schwannomas. Oncogene 28, 854–865.

Lanman, T.H., Brackmann, D.E., Hitselberger, W.E., et al., 1999. Report of 190 consecutive cases of large acoustic tumors (vestibular schwannoma) removed via the translabyrinthine approach. J. Neurosurg. 90 (4), 617–623.

Lanser, M.J., 1992. The genetics of acoustic neuromas: a linkage and physical map of chromosome 22. In: Tos, M., Thomsen, J. (Eds.), Acoustic neuroma. Kugler, Amsterdam, pp. 165–171.

Lanser, M.J., Jackler, R.K., Pitts, L.H., 1992. Intratumoral hemorrhage and cyst expansion as causes of acute neurological deterioration in acoustic neuroma patients. In: Tos, M., Thomsen, J. (Eds.), Acoustic neuroma. Kugler, Amsterdam, pp. 229–234.

Larsson, E.M., Holtas, S., 1986. False diagnosis of acoustic neuroma due to subdural injection during gas CT cisternogram. J. Comput. Assist. Tomogr. 10, 1025–1026.

Laszig, R., Marangos, N., Sollmann, W.P., et al., 1999. Central electrical stimulation of the auditory pathway in neurofibromatosis type 2. Ear Nose Throat. J. 78, 110–111, 115–117.

Le Blanc, R.A., 1974. Metastasis of bronchogenic carcinoma to acoustic neurinoma. Case report. J. Neurosurg. 41, 614–617.

Lederman, G., Lowry, J., Wertheim, S., et al., 1997. Acoustic neuroma: Potential benefits of fractionated stereotactic radiosurgery. Stereotact. Funct. Neurosurgery 69, 175–182.

Lee, D.J., Westra, W.H., Staecker, H., Long, D., Niparko, J.K., Slattery, W.H., 3rd., 2003. Clinical and histopathologic features of recurrent vestibular schwannoma (acoustic neuroma) after stereotactic radiosurgery. Otol. Neurotol. 24, 650–660; discussion 660.

Lee, J.H., Sundaram, V., Stein, D.J., Kinney, S.E., Stacey, D.W., Golubic, M., 1997. Reduced expression of schwannomin/merlin in human sporadic meningiomas. Neurosurgery 40, 578–587.

Lee, J.P., Wang, A.D., 1989. Acoustic neurinoma presenting as intratumoral bleeding. Neurosurgery 24, 764–768.

Leksell, L., 1971. A note on the treatment of acoustic tumors. Acta Chir. Scand. 137, 763–765.

Leonard, J.R., Talbot, M.L., 1970. Asymptomatic acoustic neurilemmoma. Arch. Otolaryngol. 91, 171–224.

Levine, R.E., 1994. Eye lid reanimation. In: Brackmann, D.E., Shelton, C.E., Aviaga, A. (Eds.), Otologic surgery. WB Saunders, Philadelphia, PA, pp. 717–740.

Levy, L.F., Auchterlonie, W.C., 1975. Primary cerebral neoplasia in Rhodesia. Int. Surg. 60, 286–293.

Linskey, M.E., 2008. Hearing preservation in vestibular schwannoma stereotactic radiosurgery: what really matters? J. Neurosurg. 109 (Suppl.), 129–136.

Linthicum, F.H., Brackmann, D.E., 1980. Bilateral acoustic tumors. A diagnostic and surgical challenge. Arch. Otolaryngol. 106, 729–733.

Linthicum, F.H., Churchill, D., 1968. Vestibular test results in acoustic tumor cases. Arch. Otolaryngol. 88, 604–607.

Lownie, S.P., Drake, C.G., 1991. Radical intracapsular removal of acoustic neurinomas. Long-term follow-up of 11 patients. J. Neurosurg. 74, 422–425.

Luetje, C.M., Whittaker, C.K., Callaway, L.A., et al., 1983. Histological acoustic tumor involvement of the VIIth nerve and multicentric origin in the VIIIth nerve. Laryngoscope 93, 1133–1139.

Luetje, C.M., Whittaker, C.K., Davidson, K.C., et al., 1988. Spontaneous acoustic tumor involution: a case report. Otolaryngol. Head Neck Surg. 98, 95–97.

Lunsford, L.D., Linskey, M.E., Flickinger, J.C., 1992a.. Stereotactic radiosurgery for acoustic nerve sheath tumors. In: Tos, M., Thomsen, J. (Eds.), Acoustic neuroma. Kugler, Amsterdam, pp. 279–287.

Lunsford, L.D., Niranjan, A., Flickinger, J.C., et al., 2005. Radiosurgery of vestibular schwannomas: summary of experience in 829 cases. J. Neurosurg. 102 (Suppl.), 195–199.

Lustig, L.R., Rifkin, S., Jackler, R.K., et al., 1998. Acoustic neuromas presenting with normal or symmetrical hearing: Factors associated with diagnosis and outcome. Am. J. Otol. 19 (2), 212–218.

Lutchman, M., Rouleau, G.A., 1995. The neurofibromatosis type 2 gene product, schwannomin, suppresses growth of NIH 3T3 cells. Cancer Res. 55, 2270–2274.

Lye, R.H., Dutton, J., Ramsden, R.T., et al., 1982. Facial nerve preservation during surgery for removal of acoustic nerve tumors. J. Neurosurg. 57, 739–746.

Lye, R.H., Pace-Balzan, A., Rasden, R.T., et al., 1992. The fate of tumor rests following removal of acoustic neuromas: an MRI Gd-DTPA study. Br. J .Neurosurg. 6, 195–201.

Manchanda, N., Lyubimova, A., Ho, H.Y., et al., 2005. The NF2 tumor suppressor Merlin and the E R M proteins interact with N-WASP and regulate its actin polymerization function J. Biol. Chem. 280, 12517–12522.

Mandpe, A.H., Mikulse, A., Jackler, R.K., et al., 1998. Am. J. Otol. 19 (1), 112–117.

Mangham, C.A., 1988. Complications of translabyrinthine vs. suboccipital approach for acoustic tumor surgery. Otolaryngol. Head Neck Surg. 99, 396–400.

Mansell, P.I., Higgs, E., Reckless, J.P., 1991. A young woman with spotty pigmentation, acromegaly, acoustic neuroma and cardiac myxoma: Carney's complex. J. R. Soc. Med. 84, 496–497.

Markwalder, T.M., Waelti, E., Markwalder, R.V., 1986. Estrogen and progestin receptors in acoustic and spinal neurilemmomas. Clinicopathologic correlation. Surg. Neurol. 26, 142–148.

Maro, G.S., Vermeren, M., Voiculescu, O., et al., 2004. Neural crest boundary cap cells constitute a source of neuronal and glial cells of the PNS. Nat. Neurosci. 7, 930–938.

Marquet, J.F.E., Fotton, G.E.J., Offeciers, F.E., et al., 1990. The solitary Schwannoma of the eighth cranial nerve. An immunohistochemical study of the cochlear nerve–tumor interface. Arch. Otolaryngol. Head Neck Surg. 116, 1023–1025.

Martuza, R.L., Ojemann, R.G., 1982. Bilateral acoustic neuroma: clinical aspects, pathogenesis and treatment. Neurosurgery 10, 1–22.

Martuza, R.L., MacLaughlin, D.T., Ojemann, R.G., 1981. Specific estradiol binding in Schwannomas, meningiomas and neurofibromatosis. Neurosurgery 9, 665–671.

Mattox, D.E., 1992. Infratemporal fossa approaches (Fisch) to the clivus. In: Long, D.M. (Ed.), Surgery for skull base tumors. Blackwell, Oxford, pp. 204–210.

Maurer, P.K., Okawara, S.H., 1988. Restoration of hearing after removal of cerebellopontine angle meningioma: diagnostic and therapeutic implications. Neurosurgery 22, 573–575.

McClatchey, A.I., Fehon, R.G., 2009. Merlin and the ERM proteins – regulators of receptor distribution and signaling at the cell cortex. Trends Cell Biol. 19, 198–206.

McClatchey, A.I., Giovannini, M., 2005. Membrane organization and tumorigenesis – the NF2 tumor suppressor, Merlin. Genes Dev. 19, 2265–2277.

McClatchey, A.I., Saotome, I., Mercer, K., et al., 1998. Mice heterozygous for a mutation at the NF2 tumor suppressor locus develop a range of highly metastatic tumors. Genes Dev. 12, 1121–1133.

McKenzie, K.G., Alexander, E. Jr., 1950. Restoration of facial function by nerve anastomosis. Ann. Surg. 132, 411–415.

McKissock, W., 1961, cited by Walsh L., 1965. Acoustic tumors. Proc. R. Soc. Med. 58, 1033–1037.

McLean, C.A., Laidlaw, J.D., Brownbill, D.S.B., et al., 1990. Recurrence of acoustic neurilemmoma as a malignant spindle-cell neoplasm. Case report. J. Neurosurg. 73, 946–950.

Mendenhall, W.M., Friedman, W.A., Bova, F.J., 1994. Linear accelerated based radiosurgery for acoustic schwannoma. Int. J. Radiat. Oncol. Bio. Phys. 28, 803–810.

Migliavacca, F., 1967. Facial nerve anastomosis for facial paralysis following acoustic neuroma surgery. Acta Neurochir. 17, 274–279.

Miller, R.C., Foote, R.L., Coffey, R.J., et al., 1999. Decreasing cranial nerve complications after radiosurgery for acoustic neuromas: A prospective study of dose and volume. Int. J. Radiat. Oncol. Biol. Phys. 43, 305–311.

Mingrino, S., Zuccarello, M., 1981. Anastomosis of the facial nerve with accessory or hypoglossal nerves. In: Samii, M., Jannetta, P.J. (Eds.), The cranial nerves. Springer-Verlag, Berlin, pp. 512–514.

Miyamoto, R.T., Campbell, R.L., Fritsch, M., et al., 1990. Preservation of hearing in neurofibromatosis 2. Otolaryngol. Head Neck Surg. 103, 619–624.

Miyamoto, R.T., Roos, K.L., Campbell, R.L., et al., 1991. Contemporary management of neurofibromatosis. Ann. Otol. Rhinol. Laryngol. 100, 38–43.

Moffat, D.A., Hardy, D.G., 1989. Early diagnosis and surgical management of acoustic neuroma: is it cost effective? J. R. Soc. Med. 82, 329–332.

Moffat, D.A., Croxson, G.R., Baguley, D.M., et al., 1989c. Facial nerve recovery after acoustic neuroma removal. J. Laryngol. Otol. 103, 169–172.

Moffat, D.A., Hardy, D.G., Baguley, D.M., 1989b. The strategy and benefits of acoustic neuroma searching. J. Laryngol. Otol. 103, 51–59.

Moffat, D.A., Harries, M.L., Baguley, D.M., et al., 1989a. Unterberger's stepping test in acoustic neuroma. J. Laryngol. Otol. 103, 839–841.

Mohyuddin, A., Neary, W.J., Wallace, A., et al., 2002. Molecular genetic analysis of the NF2 gene in young patients with unilateral vestibular schwannomas J. Med. Genet. 39, 315–322.

Moller, A.R., 1984. Pathophysiology of tinnitus. Ann. Otol. Rhinol. Laryngol. 93, 39–44.

Moller, A.R., Hattam, H., Olivecrona, H., 1978. The differential diagnosis of pontine angle meningioma and acoustic neuroma with computed tomography. Neuroradiology 17, 21–23.

Morgon, A., Disant, F., Fischer G., et al., 1985. In: Portmann, M. (Ed.), Facial nerve. Masso, New York, pp. 445–450.

Morrison, A.W., 1975. Management of sensorineural deafness. Butterworths, London.

Morrison, H., Sherman, L.S., Legg, J., et al., 2001. The NF2 tumor suppressor gene product, merlin, mediates contact inhibition of growth through interactions with CD44. Genes Dev. 15, 968–980.

Morrison, Q.W., Gibson, W.P.R., Beagley, H., 1976. Transtympanic electrocochleography in the diagnosis of retrocochlear tumors. Clin. Otolaryngol. 1, 153–167.

Murray, M.R., Stout, A.P., 1940. Schwann cell versus fibroblast as origin of specific nerve sheath tumor, observations upon normal nerve sheaths and neurilemomas in vitro. Am. J. Pathol. 16, 41–60.

Musiek, F.E., Kibbe-Michal, K., Guerkink, N.A., et al., 1986. ABR results in patients with posterior fossa tumors and normal pure tone hearing. Otolaryngol. Head Neck Surg. 94, 568–573.

Myrseth, E., Moller, P., Pedersen, P.H., et al., 2009. Vestibular schwannoma: surgery or gamma knife radiosurgery? A prospective, nonrandomized study. Neurosurgery 64, 654–661; discussion 661–663.

Nadol, J.B. Jr., Chiong, C.M., Ojemann, R.G., et al., 1992. Preservation of hearing and facial nerve function in resection of acoustic neuroma. Laryngoscope 102, 1153–1158.

Nadol, J.B. Jr., Levine, R.A., Ojemann, R.G., et al., 1987. Preservation of hearing in surgical removal of acoustic neuromas of the internal auditory canal and cerebellar pontine angle. Laryngoscope 97, 1287–1294.

Nager, G.T., 1969. Acoustic neuromas: pathology and differential diagnosis. Arch. Otolaryngol. 89, 252–279.

National Institutes of Health, 1988. Consensus Development Conference. Neurofibromatosis. Conference Statement. Arch. Neurol. 45, 575–578.

Nedzelski, J.M., Canter, R.J., Kassel, E.E., et al., 1986. Is no treatment good treatment in the management of acoustic neuromas in the elderly. Laryngoscope 96, 825–829.

Nedzelski, J.M., Schessel, D.A., Pfleiderer, A., et al., 1992. The natural history of growth of acoustic neuroma and the role in non-operative management. In: Tos, M., Thomsen, J. (Eds) Acoustic neuroma. Kugler, Amsterdam, pp. 149–158.

Neely, J.G., 1981. Gross and microscopic anatomy of the eighth cranial nerve in relationship to the solitary schwannoma. Laryngoscope 91, 1512–1531.

Neely, J.G., 1984. Is it possible to totally resect an acoustic tumor and preserve hearing? Otolaryngol. Head Neck Surg. 92, 162–167.

Neely, J.G., Hough, J., 1986. Histologic findings in two very small intracanalicular solitary schwannomas of the eighth nerve. Ann. Otol. Rhinol. Otolaryngol. 95, 460–465.

Nickolopoulos, T.P., Johnson, I., O'Donoghue, G.M., 1998. Quality of life after acoustic neuroma surgery. Laryngoscope 108, 1382–1385.

Nishi, T., Matsukado, Y., Nagaturo, S., et al., 1987. Hemifacial spasm due to contralateral acoustic neuroma: case report. Neurology 37, 339–342.

Noren, G., Greitz, D., 1992. The natural history of acoustic neurinomas. In: Tos, M., Thomsen, J. (Eds.), Acoustic neuroma. Kugler, Amsterdam, pp. 191–192.

Noren, G., Greitz, D., Hirsch, A., et al., 1992. Gamma Knife radiosurgery in acoustic neurinomas. In: Tos, M., Thomsen, J. (Eds.) Acoustic neuroma. Kugler, Amsterdam, pp. 289–292.

Obremski, V.J., Hall, A.M., Fernandez-Valle, C., 1998. Merlin, the neurofibromatosis type 2 gene product, and beta1 integrin associate in isolated and differentiating Schwann cells. J. Neurobiol. 37, 487–501.

Ohta, S., Yokayama, T., Nishizawa, S., et al., 1998. Regrowth of the residual tumor after acoustic neurinoma surgery. Br. J. Neurosurg. 12 (5), 419–422.

Ojemann, R., Crowell, R.C., 1978. Acoustic neuromas treated by microsurgical suboccital operations. Prog. Neurol. Surg. 9, 337–373.

Ojemann, R.G., Martuza, R., 1990. Acoustic neuroma, In: Youmans, J.R. (Ed.), Neurological surgery, 3rd edn. WB Saunders, Philadelphia, PA, pp. 3316–3350.

Ojemann, R.G., 1978. Microsurgical suboccipital approach to cerebellopontine angle tumors. Clin. Neurosurg. 25, 461–479.

Ojemann, R.G., 1979. Acoustic neuroma. Contemp. Neurosurg. 20, 1–6.

Ojemann, R.G., 1980. Comments on Fischer G, Costantini JL, Mercier P: Improvement of hearing after microsurgical removal of acoustic neuroma. Neurosurgery 7, 158.

Ojemann, R.G., 1990. Strategies to preserve hearing during resection of acoustic neuroma. In: Wilkins, R.H., Rengachary, S.S. (Eds.), Neurosurgery update I. McGraw Hill, New York, pp. 424–427.

Ojemann, R.G., 1992. Suboccipital approach to acoustic neurinomas. In: Wilson, C.B. (Ed.), Neurosurgical procedures: personal approaches to classic techniques. Williams and Wilkins, Baltimore, MD, pp. 78–87.

Ojemann, R.G., 1993. Management of acoustic neuroma (vestibular schwannoma). Clin. Neurosurg. 40, 498–535.

Ojemann, R.G., 1996. Acoustic neurinoma (vestibular schwannomas). In: Youmans, J.R. (Ed.), Neurological surgery, 4th edn. WB Saunders, Philadelphia, PA, p. 2841.

Ojemann, R.G., 2001. Acoustic neurinoma (vestibular schwannomas) – the suboccipital approach. In: Kaye, A.H., Laws, E.R. (Eds.), Brain tumors, 2nd edn. Churchill Livingstone, Edinburgh, pp. 671–686.

Ojemann, R.G., Black, P.McL., 1988. Difficult decisions in managing patients with benign brain tumors. Clin. Neurosurg. 35, 254–284.

Ojemann, R.G., Levine, R.A., Montgomery, W.M., et al., 1984. Use of intraoperative auditory evoked potentials to preserve hearing in unilateral acoustic neuroma removal. J. Neurosurg. 61, 938–948.

Ojemann, R.G., Montgomery, W.W., Weiss, A.D., 1972. Evaluation and surgical treatment of acoustic neuroma. N. Engl. J. Med. 287, 895–899.

Okada, M., Wang, Y., Jang, S.W., et al., 2009. Akt phosphorylation of merlin enhances its binding to phosphatidylinositols and inhibits the tumor-suppressive activities of merlin. Cancer Res. 69, 4043–4051.

Okada, T., You, L., Giancotti, F.G., 2007. Shedding light on Merlin's wizardry. Trends Cell. Biol. 17, 222–229.

Olivecrona, H., 1967. Acoustic tumors. J. Neurosurg. 26, 6–13.

Panse, R., 1904. Ein Gliom des Akustikus. Arch. Ohrenheilk. 61, 251–255.

Pelton, P.D., Sherman L.S., Rizvi T.A., et al., 1998. Ruffling membrane, stress fiber, cell spreading and proliferation abnormalities in human Schwannoma cells. Oncogene 17, 2195–2209.

Pensak, J.L., Glasscock, M.E. III, Josey, A.F., et al., 1985. Sudden hearing loss and cerebellopontine angle tumors. Laryngoscope 95, 1188–1193.

Pensak, M., Tew, J., Keith, R., et al., 1991. Management of acoustic neuroma in an only hearing ear. Skull Base Surg. 1, 93–96.

Perlman, H., Kimura, R., 1955. Observation of the living blood vessels of the cochlea. Ann. Oto. Rhinol. Laryngol. 64, 1176–1192.

Perre, J., Viala, P., Foncin, J.F., 1990. Involvement of the cochlear nerve in acoustic tumors. Acta Otolaryngol. (Stockh) 110, 245–252.

Phelps, P.E., 1994. Fast spin echo in otology. J. Laryngol. Otol. 108, 385–394.

Piffko, P., Pasztor, E., 1981. Operated bilateral acoustic neuromas with preservation of hearing and facial nerve function. Otol. Rhinol. Laryngol. 43, 255–261.

Pitty, L.F., Tator, C.H., 1992. Hypoglossal–facial nerve anastomosis for facial nerve palsy following surgery for cerebellopontine angle tumors. J. Neurosurg. 77, 724–731.

Pollock, B.E., 2008. Vestibular schwannoma management: an evidence-based comparison of stereotactic radiosurgery and microsurgical resection. Prog. Neurol. Surg. 21, 222–227.

Pollock, B.E., Driscoll, C.L., Foote, R.L., et al., 2006. Patient outcomes after vestibular schwannoma management: a prospective comparison of microsurgical resection and stereotactic radiosurgery. Neurosurgery 59, 77–85; discussion 77–85.

Pollock, B.E., Lunsford, L.D., Flickinger, J.C., et al., 1998a. Vestibular schwannoma management. Part I. Failed microsurgery and the role of delayed stereotactic radiosurgery. J. Neurosurg. 89, 944–948.

Pollock, B.E., Lunsford, L.D., Kondziolka, D., et al., 1998b. Vestibular schwannoma management. Part II. Failed radiosurgery and the role of delayed microsurgery. J. Neurosurg. 89, 949–955.

Portmann, M., Sterkers, J.M., 1975. The internal auditory meatus. In: Portmann, M., Sterkers, J.M., Charaction, R., et al. (Eds.), Tumors of the internal auditory meatus and surrounding structures. Churchill Livingstone, Edinburgh, pp. 193–232.

Poulikakos, P.I., Xiao, G.H., Gallagher, R., et al., 2006. Re-expression of the tumor suppressor NF2/merlin inhibits invasiveness in mesothelioma cells and negatively regulates FAK. Oncogene 25, 5960–5968.

Prasher, D.K., Gibson, W.P., 1983. Brainstem auditory-evoked potentials and electrocochleography: comparison of different criteria for detection of acoustic neuroma and other cerebellopontine angle tumors. Br. J. Audiol. 17, 163–174.

Pulec, J.L., House, W.F., 1964. Facial nerve involvement and testing in acoustic neuroma. Arch. Otolaryngol. 80, 685–692.

Pulec, J.L., Hodel, S.F., Anthony, P.F., 1978. Tinnitus: diagnosis and treatment. Ann. Otol. Rhinol. Laryngol. 87, 821–839.

Pulec, J.L., House, W.F., Britton, B.H. Jr., et al., 1971. A system of management of acoustic neuroma based on 364 cases. Trans. Am. Acad. Ophthalmol. Otolaryngol. 75, 48–55.

Ramsden, R.T., Panizza, F., Lye, R.H., 1992. The use of ionomeric bone cement in the prevention of CSF leakage following acoustic neuroma surgery. In: Tos, M., Thomsen, J. (Eds.), Acoustic neuroma. Kugler, Amsterdam, pp. 725–727.

Rangwala, R., Banine, F., Borg, J.P., et al., 2005. Erbin regulates mitogen-activated protein (MAP) kinase activation and MAP kinase-dependent interactions between Merlin and adherens junction protein complexes in Schwann cells. J. Biol. Chem. 280, 11790–11797.

Ransohoff, J., Potanos, J., Boschenstein, F., et al., 1961. Total removal of recurrent acoustic tumor. J. Neurosurg. 18, 804–810.

Rasmussen, N., Tribukait, B., Thomsen, J., et al., 1984. Implications of D N A characterization of human acoustic neuromas. Acta Otolaryngol. Suppl. (Stockh) 406, 278–281.

Regis, J., Tamura, M., Delsanti, C., et al., 2008. Hearing preservation in patients with unilateral vestibular schwannoma after gamma knife surgery. Prog. Neurol. Surg. 21, 142–151.

Revilla, A.G., 1947. Neurinoma of the cerebellopontine angle recess. Clinical study of 160 cases including operative mortality and end results. Bull. Johns Hopkins Hosp. 80, 254–296.

Revilla, A.G., 1948. Differential diagnosis of tumors at the cerebellopontine recess. Bull. Johns Hopkins Hosp. 83, 187.

Rhoton, A. Jr., 1986. Microsurgical anatomy of the brainstem surface facing an acoustic neuroma. Surg. Neurol. 25, 326–339.

Rhoton, A.L., Tedeschi, H., 1992. Microsurgical anatomy of acoustic neuroma. Otolaryngol. Clin. N. Am. 25 (2), 257–294.

Rhoton, A.L., Pulec, J.L., Hall, G.M., et al., 1968. Absence of bone over the geniculate ganglion. J. Neurosurg. 28, 48–53.

Robinson, K., Rudge, P., 1983. The differential diagnosis of cerebellopontine angle lesions. J. Neurol. Sci. 60, 1–21.

Roche, P.H., Khalil, M., Soumare, O., et al 2008a. Hydrocephalus and vestibular schwannomas: considerations about the impact of gamma knife radiosurgery. Prog. Neurol. Surg. 21, 200–206.

Roche, P.H., Khalil, M., Thomassin, J.M., et al., 2008b. Surgical removal of vestibular schwannoma after failed gamma knife radiosurgery. Prog. Neurol. Surg. 21, 152–157.

Rogg, J.M., Ahn, S.H., Tung, G.A., et al., 2005. Prevalence of hydrocephalus in 157 patients with vestibular schwannoma. Neuroradiology 47, 344–351.

Rong, R., Surace, E.I., Haipek, C.A., et al., 2004a. Serine 518 phosphorylation modulates merlin intramolecular association and binding to critical effectors important for NF2 growth suppression. Oncogene 23, 8447–8454.

Rong, R., Tang, X., Gutmann, D.H., et al., 2004b. Neurofibromatosis 2 (NF2) tumor suppressor merlin inhibits phosphatidylinositol 3-kinase through binding to PIKE-L. Proc. Natl. Acad. Sci. U. S. A. 101, 18200–18205.

Rouleau, G.A., Merel, P., Lutchman, M., et al., 1993. Alteration in a new gene encoding a putative membrane-organizing protein causes neurofibromatosis type 2. Nature 363, 515–521.

Rouleau, G.A., Wertelecki, W., Haines, J.L., et al., 1987. Genetic linkage of bilateral acoustic neurofibromatosis to a DNA marker on chromosome 22. Nature 329, 246–248.

Rubenstein, A.E., 1986. Neurofibromatosis: A review of the clinical problem. Ann. NY Acad. Sci. 486, 1–13.

Ruberti, R.F., Poppi, M., 1971. Tumors of the central nervous system in the African. East Afr. Med. J. 48, 576–584.

Russell, D.S., Rubinstein, L.J., 1989. Pathology of tumors of the nervous system, 5th edn. Edward Arnold, London, pp. 541–545.

Rutka, J.T., Trent, J.M., Rosenblum M.L., 1990. Molecular probes in neuro-oncology: a review. Cancer Invest 8, 419–432.

Sakamoto, G.T., Blevins, N., Gibbs, I.C., 2009. Cyberknife radiotherapy for vestibular schwannoma. Otolaryngol. Clin. North Am. 42, 665–675.

Samii, M., Matthies, C., 1997a. Management of 1000 vestibular schwannomas (acoustic neuromas): Surgical management and results with an emphasis on complications and how to avoid them. Neurosurgery 40, 11–21.

Samii, M., Matthies, C., 1997b. Management of 1000 vestibular schwannomas (acoustic neuromas): Hearing function in 1000 tumor resections. Neurosurgery 40, 248–260.

Samii, M., Tatagiba, M., Matthies, C., 1992. Acoustic neurinoma in the elderly: factors predictive of postoperative outcome. Neurosurgery 31, 615–620.

Sataloff, R.T., Davies, B., Myers, D.L., 1985. Acoustic neuromas presenting as sudden deafness. Am. J. Otol. 6, 349–352.

Schessel, D.A., Nedzelski, J.M., Rowed, D.W., et al., 1992. Pain after surgery for acoustic neuroma. Otolaryngol. Head Neck Surg. 107, 424–429.

Schisano, G., Olivecrona, H., 1960. Neurinomas of the gasserian ganglion and trigeminal root. J. Neurosurg. 17, 306–322.

Schmucker, B., Ballhausen, W.G., Kressel, M., 1997. Subcellular localization and expression pattern of the neurofibromatosis type 2 protein merlin/schwannomin. Eur. J. Cell Biol. 72, 46–53.

Schnitt, S.J., Vogel, H., 1986. Meningiomas: Diagnostic value of immunoperoxidase staining for epithelial membrane antigen. Am. J. Surg. Pathol. 10, 640–649.

Schorry, E.K., Stowens, D.W., Crawford, A.H., et al., 1989. Summary of patient data from a multidisciplinary neurofibromatosis clinic. Neurofibromatosis 2, 129–134.

Scoles, D.R., 2008. The merlin interacting proteins reveal multiple targets for NF2 therapy. Biochim. Biophys. Acta 1785, 32–54.

Scoles, D.R., Nguyen, V.D., Qin, Y., et al., 2002. Neurofibromatosis 2 (NF2) tumor suppressor schwannomin and its interacting protein HRS regulate STAT signaling. Hum. Mol. Genet. 11, 3179–3189.

Seizinger, B.R., Martuza, R.L., Gusella, J.F., 1986. Loss of genes on chromosome 22 in tumorigenesis of human acoustic neuroma. Nature 322, 644–647.

Seizinger, B.R., Rouleau, G., Ozelius, L.J., et al., 1987b. Common pathogenetic mechanism for three tumor types in bilateral acoustic neurofibromatosis. Science 236, 317–319.

Sekhar, L.N., Jannetta, P.J., 1984. Cerebellopontine angle meningiomas. Microsurgical excision and follow-up results. J. Neurosurg. 60, 500–505.

Sekiya, T., Moller, A.R., 1987. Cochlear nerve injuries caused by cerebellopontine angle manipulation. An electrophysiology and morphological study in dogs. J. Neurosurg. 67, 244–249.

Selesnick, S.H., Johnson, G., 1998. Radiologic surveillance of acoustic neuromas. Am. J. Otol. 19, 846–849.

Selters, W.A., Brackmann, D.E., 1977. Acoustic tumor detection with brainstem evoked electric response audiometry. Arch. Otolaryngol. 103, 181–187.

Shaia, F.T., Sheehy, J.L., 1976. Sudden sensorineural hearing impairment; a report of 1220 cases. Laryngoscope 86, 389–398.

Shannon, R.V., Fayad, J., Moore, J., et al., 1993. Auditory brain stem implant. II. Post surgical issues and performance. Otolaryngol. Head Neck Surg. 108, 634–642.

Shao, K.-N., Tatagiba, M., Samii, M., 1993. Surgical management of high jugular bulb in acoustic neurinoma via retrosigmoid approach. Neurosurgery 32, 32–37.

Shaw, R.J., McClatchey, A.I., Jacks, T., 1998b. Localization and functional domains of the neurofibromatosis type II tumor suppressor, merlin. Cell Growth Differ. 9, 287–296.

Shaw, R.J., Paez, J.G., Curto, M., et al., 2001. The Nf2 tumor suppressor, merlin, functions in Rac-dependent signaling. Dev. Cell 1, 63–72.

Shea, J.J., Emmett, J.R., Orchik, D.J., et al., 1981. Medical treatment of tinnitus. Ann. Otol. Rhinol. Otolaryngol. 90, 601–606.

Shea, J.J. 3rd, Hitselberger, W.E., Benecke, J.E., et al., 1985. Recurrence rate of partially resected acoustic tumors. Am. J. Otol. Nov. (Suppl.), 107–109.

Shelton, C., Brackmann, D.E., House, W.F., et al., 1989a. Middle fossa acoustic tumor surgery: results in 106 cases. Laryngoscope 99, 405–408.

Shelton, C., Brackmann, D.E., House, W.F., et al., 1989b. Acoustic tumor surgery: prognostic factors in hearing preservation. Arch. Otolaryngol. Head Neck Surg. 115, 1213–1216.

Shelton, C., Hitselberger, W.E., House, W.F., et al., 1990. Hearing preservation after acoustic tumor removal: longterm results. Laryngoscope 100, 115–119.

Shelton, C., Hitselberger, W.E., House, W.F., et al., 1992. Long-term results of hearing preservation after acoustic tumor removal. In: Tos, M., Thomsen, J. (Eds.) Acoustic neuroma. Kugler, Amsterdam, pp. 661–664.

Sheptak, P.E., Jannetta, P.J., 1979. The two-stage excision of huge acoustic neurinomas. J. Neurosurg. 51, 37–41.

Sherman, L., Xu, H.M., Geist, R.T., et al., 1997. Interdomain binding mediates tumor growth suppression by the NF2 gene product. Oncogene 15, 2505–2509.

Shirato, H., Sakamoto, T., Sawamura, Y., et al., 1999. Comparison between observation policy and fractionated stereotactic radiotherapy (SRT) as an initial management for vestibular schwannoma. Int. J. Radiat. Oncol. Biol. Phys. 44, 545–550.

Shore-Freedman, E., Abraham, C., Recant, W., et al., 1983. Neurilemmoma and salivary gland tumors of the head and neck following childhood irradiation. Cancer 51, 2159–2163.

Silverstein, H., Haberkamp, T., Smouha, E., 1986. The state of tinnitus after inner ear surgery. Otolaryngol. Head Neck Surg. 99, 438–441.

Simons, M., Trotter, J., 2007. Wrapping it up: the cell biology of myelination. Curr. Opin. Neurobiol. 17, 533–540.

Simpson, R.H.W., Sparrow, O.C., Duffield, M.S., 1990. Cerebellopontine angle tumors in black South Africans – how rare are acoustic schwannomas? S. Afr. Med. J. 78, 11–14.

Slattery, W.H. III, Brackmann, D.E., Hitselberger, W., 1998. Hearing preservation in neurofibromatosis type 2. Am. J. Otol. 19 (5), 638–643.

Smith, J.W., 1979. Treatment of facial palsy by cross-face nerve grafting. In: Buchheit, W.A., Truex, R.C., Jr. (Eds.), Surgery of the posterior fossa. Raven Press, New York, pp. 173–179.

Snow, R.B., Fraser, R.A., 1987. Cerebellopontine angle tumor causing contralateral trigeminal neuralgia: a case report. Neurosurgery 21, 84–86.

Sobel, R.A., Michaud, J., 1985. Microcystic meningioma of the falx cerebri with numerous palisaded structures: an unusual

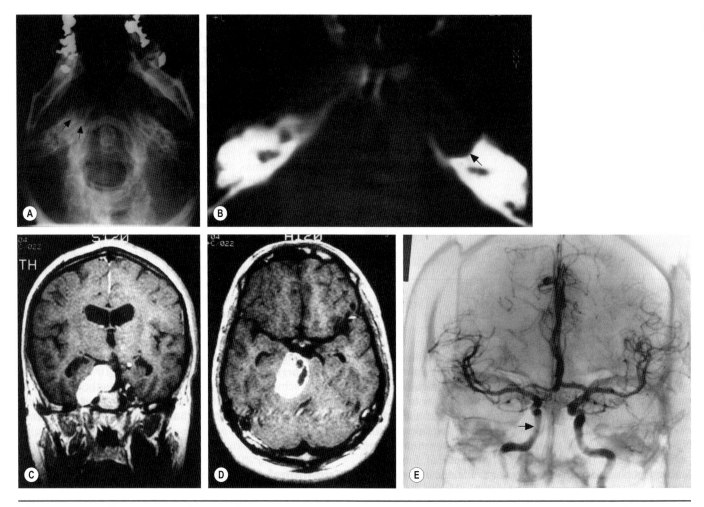

Figure 29.2 (A) Skull roentgenogram; base view demonstrates amputation of the right petrous apex (arrows). (B) Axial CT correlate on a different patient demonstrates similar erosion of the left petrous apex (arrow). (C) T1-weighted coronal MR image demonstrates an extra-axial mass eroding through the floor of the middle fossa into the pterygoid fossa. The tumor is inhomogeneous in signal intensity and somewhat hyperintense with respect to the surrounding brain. (D) T1-weighted axial MR image demonstrates the relationship of the tumor to the cavernous sinus. Note the integrity of the dura which clearly demarcates the tumor from the cavernous sinus. Note the atrophy of the masticatory muscles innervated by V. (E) Subtraction film from bilateral carotid artery arteriogram (superimposed) demonstrating medial displacement of the precavernous segment of the right internal carotid artery (arrow).

The ganglion and third division are extradural in the middle fossa. The first and second divisions pass within the lateral wall of the cavernous sinus. The trochlear nerve lies above the trigeminal root, the 7th and 8th nerves below it, and the oculomotor and 6th nerves lie anteromedial to the ganglion in the cavernous sinus. The posterior cerebral and superior cerebellar arteries pass over the root, while the anterior inferior cerebellar artery passes under. The horizontal portion of the precavernous internal carotid artery, the eustachian tube, and the greater superficial petrosal nerve course below the distal part of the ganglion. There is often a bony defect in the floor of the middle cranial fossa such that a dural membrane alone separates the precavernous carotid from the ganglion. The petrosal vein lies lateral and posterior to the root, which enters the porus trigeminus just below the superior petrosal sinus. The motor fibers are situated medially along the root, but come to lie inferiorly at the level of the ganglion as the sensory fibers rotate anteromedially. The motor fibers pass through the foramen ovale with the mandibular division (Fig. 29.3).

Trigeminal schwannomas most commonly arise from the gasserian ganglion, but may also arise in a more proximal location from the trigeminal root or more distally from one of the three post-ganglionic divisions. The ophthalmic branch is more frequently involved than either the maxillary of mandibular branches. Jefferson (1955) proposed the original classification system according to location includes three different types. Type A refers to tumors contained predominantly in the middle fossa. Type B refers to tumors in the posterior fossa and the Type C tumor is a dumbbell tumor with elements in both the posterior and middle fossa and is contiguous through the porus trigeminus. Approximately

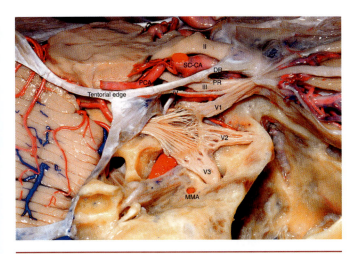

Figure 29.3 Dissection demonstrating the anatomy about Meckel's cave. Gasserian ganglion is well defined with the three major sensory branches clearly dissected. Cranial Nerves II, III, IV, V1, V2, V3 are marked. (MMA) Middle Meningeal Artery, (SC-CA) Supraclinoid Carotid Artery, (PCA) Posterior Cerebral Artery, (DR) Dural Ring, (PR) Proximal Ring.

Table 29.1 Initial symptoms in 120 patients with trigeminal neuroma[a]

Symptom	Cases	
	n	%
Trigeminal nerve dysfunction	72	55
Numbness	35	27
Pain	30	23
Paresthesias	7	5
Headache	19	15
Diplopia	13	10
Hearing loss/tinnitus	10	8
Visual loss	7	5
Ear pain	4	3
Other	10	8

[a]Other symptoms: Subarachnoid hemorrhage, vertigo, seizure, exophthalmos, gait difficulty, hemifacial spasm. Two patients had more than one initial symptom.

50% arise predominantly within the middle cranial fossa, 30% within the posterior fossa, and 20% are dumb-bell shaped with significant extension into both cranial fossae. The predominant symptoms and signs, and the surgical approach, will vary somewhat according to the location of the tumor. The predominant symptom is trigeminal hypesthesia, but can also include hearing disturbance, focal seizures, hemiparesis, gait disturbance, increased intracranial pressure (Yasui 1989; McCormick 1988), otalgia, exophthalmos, paralysis of the 3rd, 4th and 6th cranial nerves and signs of posterior fossa involvement (Nager 1984). The most common complaint at the time of presentation is that of a sensory disturbance in the ipsilateral face (McCormick 1988) (Table 29.1). The duration of symptoms may vary from a few months to >15 years (McCormick 1988; Pollack 1989). The disturbance is most often described as numbness, but may include pain or paresthesias. It may be confined to the distribution of one division, but more commonly involves all three to a variable degree. Complete anesthesia in all three divisions is distinctly uncommon, and suggests malignant invasion of the gasserian ganglion (Jefferson 1955). The pain associated with a schwannoma differs from that seen in trigeminal neuralgia in the duration of the paroxysms (often hours) and the lack of trigger zones. Sensory disturbance is especially common in middle fossa tumors. Tumors in this location can compress adjacent nerves within the cavernous sinus, resulting in diplopia. They may extend into the orbital apex producing exophthalmos and visual loss. Tumors located primarily within the posterior fossa more often present with hearing loss, tinnitus or a gait disturbance (Pollack 1989). Dumb-bell shaped tumors can present with a combination of middle and posterior fossa-type symptoms. Other complaints, in descending order of relative frequency, include headache, seizure, and hemifacial spasm (McCormick 1988).

Objective findings are common and usually referable to the involved trigeminal nerve. Decreased sensation in one or more dermatomes along with a diminished or absent corneal is seen in 80–90% of patients (Lesois 1986). Mild weakness in the muscles of mastication is found in 30–40% (Bordi 1989; McCormick 1988). Findings referable to adjacent cranial nerves are found in 75% of cases (McCormick 1988). Middle fossa tumors can produce a conductive hearing loss from eustachian tube destruction, and a facial paresis secondary to compression of the nerve in the fallopian canal or traction on the greater superficial petrosal nerve (Jefferson 1955; Nager 1984). Large tumors arising in the root usually produce signs of a cerebellopontine angle syndrome. This consists of hearing loss and facial weakness secondary to distortion of cranial nerves VIII and VII, as well as ataxia and spasticity secondary to cerebellar and brainstem compression. They also may extend downwards and cause dysfunction of the lower cranial nerves resulting in abnormal phonation, deglutition, and an absent palatal reflex. The large dumbbell-shaped tumors often produce a combination of middle and posterior fossa signs. Although objective findings are common, 10–20% of patients will have a normal neurologic exam (Jefferson 1955; Mello 1972) (Table 29.2).

Plain films will often demonstrate amputation of the petrous apex (Holman 1961; Palacios 1972). The margins are smooth and without sclerosis, unlike the more common malignant and primary bone lesions in this region (Fig. 29.2A). The middle fossa floor may be eroded, and one or more foramina at the skull base enlarged (Fig. 29.2B). A ganglion tumor that extends anteriorly may erode the lateral aspect and dorsum of the sella or the clinoid processes. It may enlarge the superior orbital fissure or optic foramen. Alternatively, it may extend extracranially and erode the pterygoid plates. Isolated posterior fossa tumors may produce very little bony changes and be impossible to detect on plain films. Conversely, they may erode the anterior lip of the internal acoustic meatus and be mistaken for acoustic tumors. They may also produce non-specific changes within the sella and calvarium associated with increased intracranial pressure.

Cerebral angiography will most often show inferomedial displacement of the precavernous portion of the petrous carotid (Chase 1963; McCormick 1988) (Fig. 29.2E). This

Table 29.2 Abnormal findings on admission examination in 136 patients with trigeminal neurinoma[a]

Neurologic abnormality	Cases	
	n	%
Trigeminal nerve		
Decreased sensation	100	74
Diminished or absent corneal reflex	93	68
Pain	52	38
Motor weakness	53	39
Other cranial nerve deficits		
II	14	10
III	19	14
IV	9	7
VI	47	35
VII	31	23
VIII	44	32
IX, X	11	8
XI	2	1
XII	4	3
Cerebellar signs	31	23
Long tract signs	22	16
Papilledema	14	10

[a]Only 27 patients (21%) had abnormal findings limited to the trigeminal nerve.

finding is characteristic of middle fossa tumors. Tumors in the posterior fossa will often elevate and medially displace the posterior cerebral and superior cerebellar arteries. The basilar artery may be displaced posteriorly and contralaterally. The petrosal vein may be elevated, or may fail to fill with contrast. The tumors are usually relatively avascular, although a blush from feeders off the precavernous carotid or the external circulation is noted in 20–25% (McCormick 1988; Mello 1972; Palacios 1972; Westberg 1963). At the time of angiography a balloon occlusion test of the ipsilateral internal carotid may be performed in order to evaluate the extent of cross circulation should the carotid have to be sacrificed intraoperatively (Pollack 1989).

The bony changes seen on plain film are exquisitely demonstrated on CT bone windows (Fig. 29.2B). The soft tissue mass itself usually appears iso- to hyperdense relative to surrounding brain (Goldberg 1980). Cystic changes within the tumor may be present (Fig. 29.4A–C). Following the administration of iodinated contrast, the tumors usually enhance homogeneously and intensely (Goldberg 1980; Nager 1984). However, ring-like or irregular enhancement is not uncommon. With MR the soft tissue mass usually appears hypointense on T1 weighted images and hyperintense on T2 (Rigamonti 1987). The enhancement pattern following the administration of gadolinium is similar to that seen with enhanced CT: usually homogeneous and intense (Fig. 29.2C,D). CT and MR are critical in defining the extent of the tumor and planning the surgical approach (Fig. 29.4). Techniques involving dynamic spin-echo (TR/TE 200/15 ms) MRI offer an advantage in differentiating meningiomas from schwannomas (Ikushima 1997). In dynamic MRI, meningiomas had more varied dynamic patterns than schwannomas. The utilization of newer radiological studies such as these can assist in surgical management.

The clinical and neuroradiologic evaluation should allow accurate preoperative diagnosis in most cases. Bilateral neurinomas are a manifestation of the central form of neurofibromatosis (Nager 1984). The differential includes skull base metastases, primary bone tumors, meningiomas, epidermoids, and acoustic schwannomas. Metastases and primary bone tumors, such as chondrosarcomas and chordomas, usually produce a pattern of irregular bony destruction rather than a smooth scalloping of bone. Meningiomas more often produce hyperostosis than erosion, and there is often intratumoral calcification, which is uncommon in schwannomas. Epidermoids often show a sclerotic margin in areas of bony erosion not usually seen in schwannomas and exhibit a characteristic diffusion restriction on diffusion-weighted imaging. Acoustic schwannomas almost always produce asymmetric enlargement of the internal auditory canal. In addition, hearing loss is an earlier and more prominent complaint in the acoustic schwannoma. Other recent reported cases of lesions mimicking trigeminal schwannomas include: idiopathic trigeminal neuropathy (Dominguez 1999) and primary lymphoma of Meckel's cave (Abdel 1999).

The surgical approach is principally dependent on the location and extension of the tumor, and thus the need for detailed preoperative neuroradiologic evaluation. The tumors are removed through an intracapsular debulking procedure using either the bipolar cautery or the ultrasonic aspirator. After debulking, the capsule must be carefully dissected away from surrounding structures. In large tumors, the trochlear nerve will usually be found on the superior pole of the capsule, the auditory and facial nerves along the inferior pole. The oculomotor and abducens nerves will usually be found medially along with the carotid artery. Part or all of the trigeminal complex may have to be excised because of tumor involvement. In the past many of these tumors were subtotally resected, as they were adherent to the cavernous sinus, the internal carotid artery, or the brainstem. Long-term results following subtotal resection are controversial. Some authors report an inevitable symptomatic recurrence, usually within 3 years (Pollack 1989). Others report a satisfactory clinical outcome with very few symptomatic recurrences (Bordi 1989; Pollack 1989). The rate of recurrence as in most tumors, appears to be dependent on the tumor location and the degree of surgical resection. Recent studies have shown a high percentage of lesions amenable to complete surgical resection with reported total resection achieved in 76–81% of cases (Sharma 2008; Zhang 2008). The ability to achieve a total resection is strongly influenced by invasion of the cavernous sinus with one series demonstrating total resection in 81% of trigeminal schwannomas not involving the cavernous sinus but only 40% when the cavernous sinus was involved (Zhang 2008).

The original literature divided trigeminal schwannoma locations into three categories (Lesois 1986; McCormick 1988). More recent reviews have added a fourth category, consisting of tumors extending into multiple fossae (Dolenc 1994; Konovalov 1996; Samii 1995a; Yoshida 1999). Anywhere from 36–59% of trigeminal schwannomas involve multiple fossae. The four groups of trigeminal schwannomas are: (1) posterior fossa tumors; (2) tumors of the Gasserian ganglion; (3) dumbbell-shaped and supra-subtentorial tumors, and (4) neurinomas of the peripheral branches

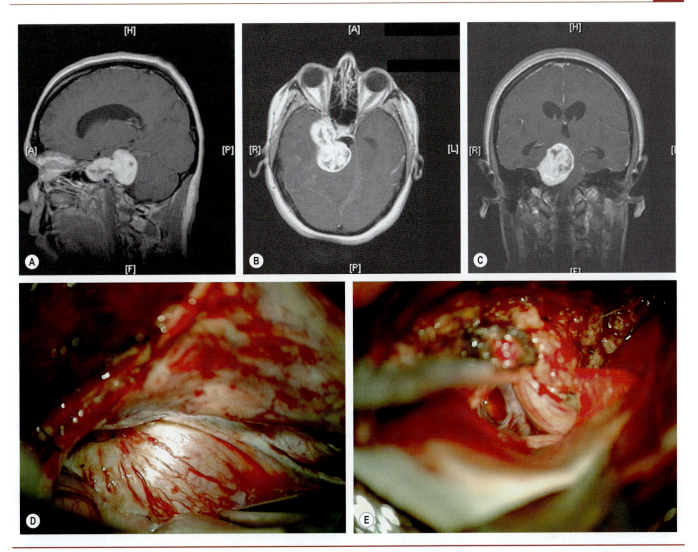

Figure 29.4 (A) Gadolinium enhanced sagittal MRI of a dumbbell-shaped tumor shows areas of decreased attenuation representing either necrosis or cystic degeneration. (B) Gadolinium enhanced axial MRI of a dumbbell-shaped tumor with extension through Meckel's cave and some erosion of the posterior clinoid. (C) Gadolinium enhanced coronal MRI of the relatively homogenously enhancing mass with cystic components. (D) Intraoperative photograph demonstrating a right trigeminal schwannoma in the middle cranial fossa. (E) Intraoperative photograph demonstrating a preserved mandibular division of the trigeminal nerve after resection of the schwannoma seen in (D).

(Konovalov 1996). The extension of the categories to include multiple fossae has combined the middle and posterior fossae, middle and extracranial space and middle and posterior fossae and extracranial space (Yoshida 1999). The most common approach in the literature is the subtemporal intradural approach through the middle cranial fossa, since the majority of these tumors arise from the ganglion and lie predominantly in the middle cranial fossa (Fig. 29.4D,E). In addition, tumors which straddle the middle and posterior cranial fossae, and do not extend below the internal auditory canal, can be removed through a middle fossa approach. This is accomplished by incising the free margin of the tentorium and ligating the superior petrosal sinus. In contrast, very little access can be gained to the middle cranial fossa through a standard suboccipital approach. This is therefore confined to those tumors which lie exclusively within the posterior fossa. The combined or petrosal

approach is employed in the large dumbbell-shaped tumors that extend ventral to the lower brainstem and below the internal acoustic meatus. Tumors often can grow along the course of the trigeminal nerve from the brainstem into Meckel's cave (Fig. 29.5).

Skull base procedures used for large middle fossa tumors incorporate the use of an orbitozygomatic osteotomy to facilitate exposure of the cavernous sinus and minimize temporal lobe retraction (Sekhar 1987). The advent of skull base techniques has dramatically improved surgical resection results and decreased postoperative morbidity. A review of the surgical management of trigeminal schwannomas separated the surgical approach used based on the location of the tumor: patients with peripheral and ganglion type lesions were treated via an entirely extradural temporopolar approach (Day 1998). In addition to the more traditional subtemporal intradural approach, other extra-dural approaches including

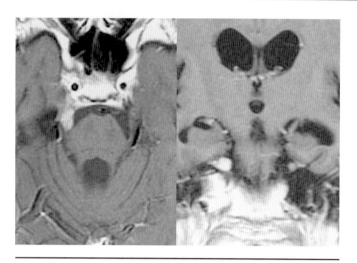

Figure 29.5 Gadolinium enhanced MRI demonstrating a small trigeminal schwannoma predominantly in the posterior fossa following the course of the trigeminal from the brainstem into Meckel's cave. The normal left 5th nerve is well seen.

orbitozygomatic infratemporal, zygomatic infratemporal, zygomatic transpetrosal, and presigmoid transpetrosal-transtentorial approaches can be utilized (Zhang 2009). Lesions confined to the posterior fossa are generally approached via a lateral suboccipital approach. Dumbbell-shaped lesions required a combined petrosal approach. Advocates of the skull-base approaches cite the advantage of decreased temporal lobe retraction and improved access to the anterior cranial fossa.

With modern microsurgical techniques mortalities have been drastically reduced. A recent series comprising a total of 41 patients contained only one operative death; a mortality rate of 2.2% (Bordi 1989; McCormick 1988; Pollack 1989). Morbidity includes cranial nerve injury, CSF leak, meningitis, and hydrocephalus. Many patients will be left with some degree of permanent trigeminal dysfunction. The most common symptom after surgery is the persistence of trigeminal hypesthesia (Day 1998), which patients should be informed may never resolve. There is often the need for tarsorrhaphy to prevent neurotropic keratitis. New onset postoperative cranial nerve dysfunction, such as abducens and oculomotor palsies, will usually resolve within 4 months. Some preoperative neurologic deficits, such as cerebellar and brainstem compression syndromes, diplopia, facial pain and weakness, and hearing loss may improve postoperatively. CSF leak and/or hydrocephalus may require shunt placement.

There is increasing evidence of a role for stereotactic radiosurgery in the treatment of trigeminal schwannomas (Wang et al 2005; Pan et al 2005). One study examined 16 patients over 44 months, six of which had undergone previous surgical resection before radiosurgery (Huang et al 1999). The tumor control rate was 100% with regression in nine patients and no tumor growth in seven patients. Eleven patients had no improvement in their presenting clinical symptoms, although no patient suffered any new cranial nerve deficits. The exact role and indications for the use of stereotactic radiosurgery have yet to be completely defined

especially when larger tumors are encountered. Wang et al (2005) evaluated 30 patients who had undergone stereotactic radiosurgery for trigeminal schwannomas ranging in size from 3.1–5.3 cm with a reported tumor growth rate control of 90% but two patients required urgent surgery secondary to tumor swelling or cyst formation.

Of significant concern in the recent literature is the increasing incidence of malignancy in trigeminal schwannomas. A previous review (Dolenc 1994) reported no malignancies, while a more recent review has a malignancy incidence of 7.9% (Day 1998).

Facial schwannomas

Schwannomas arising from the facial nerve account for approximately 1.9% of all intracranial schwannomas (Symon et al 1993). The facial nerve is the third most common nerve to be affected by schwannomas (after acoustic and trigeminal neuromas). The first such case was described by Schmidt in 1931. Since then, a number of isolated reports and a few large series have been published, totaling more than 180 cases (Murata et al 1985; Neely et al 1974; Rosenblum et al 1987; Saito et al 1972). The incidence of facial schwannoma may actually be much higher, as autopsy reports have found incidental tumors in up to 0.8% of petrous bones (Saito et al 1972). These tumors most commonly present in the fourth and fifth decades of life, although pediatric cases as young as one year have been reported (O'Donoghue et al 1989). There is a distinct female predilection in most of the larger series. From 15–21% of patients have been known to have neurofibromatosis (Isamat et al 1975; Symon et al 1993).

The facial nerve has a rather long and complex course from the brainstem to the stylomastoid foramen. Schwannomas can occur anywhere along the course of the facial nerve although they most commonly arise from the sensory fibers of the nerve. The course of the facial nerve may be divided on an anatomical and clinical basis into five segments (Schuknecht et al 1986). As it emerges from the lateral aspect of the brainstem just above the pontomedullary junction, it courses superiorly and laterally toward the internal acoustic meatus. Here it is cradled in a groove on the superior surface of the cochlear division of the eighth cranial nerve. This first segment lies within the cerebellopontine angle cistern. The second segment of the nerve travels approximately 7–8 mm within the internal auditory canal, where it occupies the anterosuperior quadrant. At the lateral end of the canal it passes above the transverse crest to enter the fallopian canal within the petrous bone. The third or labyrinthine segment travels anteriorly and laterally, superior to the cochlea and vestibule. This is the shortest segment, only 3–4 mm in length, and is perpendicular to the long axis of the petrous pyramid. This segment terminates at the geniculate ganglion, which contains the cell bodies of the parasympathetic fibers of the nervus intermedius. The geniculate ganglion lies just below the middle cranial fossa, from which it is sometimes separated by only dura. Schwannomas often occur in this region of the geniculate ganglion secondary to the structural reorganization that occurs in this part of the facial nerve. The greater superficial petrosal nerve carries some of the autonomic fibers forward into the middle fossa through the facial hiatus on the anterior surface of the petrous pyramid. The remaining facial fibers turn sharply backward and run posterolaterally along the medial wall of the tympanic cavity. This horizontal or tympanic segment of the nerve runs parallel to the long axis of the petrous bone. After crossing the medial wall of the tympanic cavity a second genu is present as the nerve turns sharply downward. In this vertical or mastoid segment the nerve runs along the posterior aspect of the middle ear cavity. Here the parasympathetic fibers of the chorda tympani and the branch to the stapedius muscle are given off. Finally, the nerve exits the skull base at the stylomastoid foramen (Fig. 29.6).

The facial nerve acquires a Schwann cell sheath approximately 2 mm after exiting the brainstem (Nadich et al 2009). Therefore, tumors of Schwann cell origin may arise anywhere along the aforementioned course. The older literature indicated a predilection for the vertical or mastoid segment of the nerve (Lipkin 1987). However, more recent work implicates the region of the geniculate ganglion as the most common epicenter (Fisch et al 1977; Horn et al 1981; O'Donoghue et al 1989; Symon et al 1993). The clinical symptoms and signs will vary according to the site of origin, and the direction and degree of spread to adjacent segments. Schwannomas can also be multicentric, with involvement of many different branches and segments of the facial nerve.

The most common presenting symptoms are hearing loss, facial paralysis, facial pain, hemifacial spasm, tinnitus, vertigo, otorrhea, and otalgia. The majority of tumors will involve two or more segments of the nerve. The earliest symptom is hearing loss, occurring in 41–91% of cases (King et al 1990; Symon et al 1993; Yamaki et al 1998). The hearing loss is sensorineural if the mass is predominantly in the cisternal or intracanalicular segment of the nerve, and conductive if the tympanic or mastoid segment is involved. Tinnitus occurs in up to 60% of cases and vertigo in as many as 34% (Symon et al 1993). Facial weakness is common at the time of presentation, though not usually the first symptom. From 46–90% of patients will have weakness, twitching, or both (King et al 1990; O'Donoghue et al 1989;

Symon et al 1993). The facial palsy usually develops slowly and gradually, indicating neoplastic rather than inflammatory involvement. A slowly progressive facial palsy should be considered the result of a nerve tumor until proven otherwise. However, up to 20% of patients will develop sudden onset of facial weakness which may be mistaken for a Bell's palsy (Fisch 1977; Pulec 1969) Recurrent attacks of facial weakness with incomplete recovery between episodes may also occur. Although facial weakness is a very frequent finding in this group of patients, only about 5% of cases of peripheral facial palsy are found to be attributable to a schwannoma of the facial nerve (Neely et al 1974). Other symptoms and signs include mass in the middle ear cavity, otalgia, otorrhea, facial pain or sensory loss, headache, seizures, ataxia, and dry eye (Symon et al 1993) (Table 29.3).

CT and MR are the most useful preoperative tests. The diagnosis is based on the recognition of one or more enlarged segments of the fallopian canal filled with homogeneously enhancing soft tissue (Fig. 29.7). CT is superior for demonstrating bony changes, while MR is more sensitive in detecting small tumors and defining extension. Improvements in the diagnostic imaging of the temporal bone have increased the possibility of a correct pre-operative diagnosis (Yamaki et al 1998). Tumors which arise primarily in the cisternal or canalicular segment of the nerve may be extremely hard to distinguish from the much more common acoustic schwannoma, and as many as 36% will be misdiagnosed as such (O'Donoghue 1989). Large tumors that extend into the middle cranial fossa may be distinguished from acoustic and trigeminal schwannomas based on their pattern of extension. Facial schwannomas extend through the mid-petrosal area, whereas trigeminal tumors erode the petrous apex and acoustic tumors extend through the tentorial incisura (Inouye et al 1987). Preoperative neurootological testing has been largely supplanted by detailed neuroradiologic imaging.

The approach to these tumors is determined by the location and extent of the mass and the patient's preoperative level of neurologic function. The surgical strategy itself is unique for each case and is tailored to: (1) the site of main tumor mass; (2) its extension along the facial nerve, and (3) involvement of the auditory organs (Yamaki et al 1998).

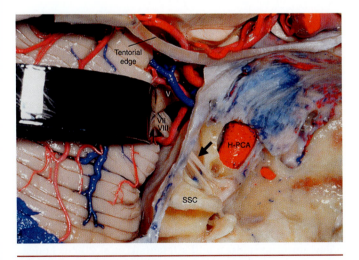

Figure 29.6 Anatomical dissection demonstrating the course of the facial nerve. Cranial Nerves VII and VII. (SSC) Superior Semicircular Canal, (H-PCA) Horizontal-Petrous Carotid Artery.

Table 29.3 Signs and symptoms of VII nerve schwannomas

Hearing loss	41–91%
Sensorineural – intracanalicular	
Conductive – tympanic or mastoid	
Tinnitus	60%
Vertigo	34%
Facial weakness	46–90%
Sudden onset	20%
Other	
Mass in middle ear	
Otalgia	
Otorrhea	
Facial pain	
Sensory loss	
Dry eye	

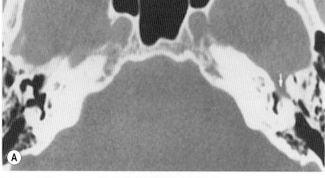

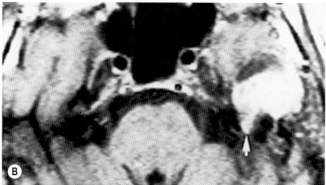

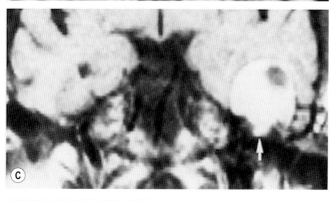

Figure 29.7 (A) Axial CT demonstrating petrosal erosion with a widened fallopian canal secondary to a large facial schwannoma. (B) Axial gadolinium enhanced MRI demonstrating a left facial schwannoma. (C) Coronal gadolinium enhanced MRI demonstrating a large homogenously enhancing mass involving the left petrous portion of the temporal bone. (Courtesy of Dr Peter Som.)

Tumors lying proximal to the geniculate ganglion may be approached through the middle fossa, the posterior fossa, or through the labyrinth. If functional hearing is not present, the translabyrinthine approach allows for excellent visualization and mobilization of the proximal and distal segments of the nerve, as well as access to both the middle and posterior fossae (Fisch et al 1977; Lipkin et al 1987; O'Donoghue et al 1989; Pulec 1972). If hearing preservation is to be attempted a sub-temporal/middle fossa approach is preferable unless the tumor lies predominantly within the cerebellopontine angle. In these cases a lateral suboccipital approach is employed (Symon et al 1993). Nerve repair is more

difficult with either the subtemporal or suboccipital exposure, and the latter has the additional disadvantage of offering minimal access to the middle fossa. Tumors involving the tympanic or mastoid segment of the nerve may be removed via a simple mastoidectomy. Some have advocated a conservative approach in those cases in which facial function remains intact and no intracranial extension exists (King et al 1990). Others have argued that in order to maximize the chances of successful nerve grafting, surgery should be performed before the onset of facial weakness whenever possible (Fisch 1977; Symon et al 1993).

The technique involved in removing these tumors is the same as in the acoustic and trigeminal schwannomas. First, an intracapsular debulking is performed followed by stripping of the capsule from adjacent neurovascular structures. The extent of resection varies from debulking to an aggressive resection with nerve reconstruction (McMonagle et al 2008). Even in those cases in which >50% of the nerve was preserved, post-operative facial function was extremely poor. Consideration must therefore be given to the possibility of an immediate nerve grafting procedure. If the proximal and distal ends of the nerve can be brought in apposition, either *in situ* or after distal re-routing, a primary anastomosis can be accomplished with suture or fibrin glue. Alternatively, an interpositional graft using the sural or greater auricular nerve can be performed. Both techniques result in similar postoperative facial function. The primary determinant is the duration of preoperative facial paralysis (O'Donoghue et al 1989; Symon et al 1993). When paralysis has been present for >2 years, nerve grafting is probably not indicated. Successful grafts can be expected to take from 6 months to 1 year to function. In those patients without long-standing preoperative facial paralysis in whom immediate nerve grafting was either not possible or unsuccessful, a facial-hypoglossal anastomosis can be considered. Regardless of the reanimation procedure performed, House-Brackmann (House & Brackmann 1985) grade III is the best level of facial function to be expected (Table 29.4). During the period of recovery, care must be taken to protect the involved eye. This may include tarsorrhaphy, gold weight insertion, or the use of an eye bubble.

Facial nerve schwannomas are curable if completely excised. The mortality rate using modern microsurgical technique has been extremely low. Morbidity, other than the expected facial paralysis, includes hearing loss. This occurs in up to 33% of patients, and is permanent in approximately half of these cases (Symon et al 1993). Other complications include CSF leak, meningitis, and/or hydrocephalus. Care must be taken to completely seal the mastoid air cells, the external auditory canal, and the eustachian tube when these structures are opened.

Significant advances have been made in the treatment of facial schwannomas with radiosurgery. In a recent series of six patients with facial schwannomas undergoing radiosurgery with a marginal dose of 12–12.5 Gy, promising results were achieved. All patients maintained the pre-radiosurgery level of facial function and hearing with a mean follow-up of over 46 months (Madhok et al 2009). Longer follow-up is needed to determine the role of radiosurgery in the treatment of facial schwannomas but initial results are promising.

Table 29.4 Facial nerve grading system (House & Brackmann 1985)

Grade	Description	Characteristics
I	Normal	Normal facial function in all areas

II	Mild dysfunction	Gross: slight weakness noticeable on close inspection; may have very slight synkinesis
		At rest: normal symmetry and tone
		Motion:
		    Forehead: moderate to good function
		    Eye: complete closure with minimum effort
		    Mouth: slight asymmetry

III	Moderate dysfunction	Gross: obvious but not disfiguring difference between two sides; noticeable but not severe synkinesis, contracture, and/or hemifacial spasm
		At rest: normal symmetry and tone
		Motion:
		    Forehead: slight to moderate movement
		    Eye: complete closure with effort
		    Mouth: slightly weak with maximum effort

IV	Moderately severe	Gross: obvious weakness and/or dysfunction disfiguring asymmetry
		At rest: normal symmetry and tone
		Motion:
		    Forehead: none
		    Eye: incomplete closure
		    Mouth: asymmetric with maximum effort

V	Severe dysfunction	Gross: only barely perceptible motion
		At rest: asymmetry
		Motion:
		    Forehead: none
		    Eye: incomplete closure
		    Mouth: slight movement

VI	Total paralysis	No movement

Jugular foramen schwannomas

Schwannomas have been known to arise from the nerve roots exiting the jugular foramen since the report by Gerhardt in 1878 (Gerhardt 1878). These tumors are characterized by palsy of the 9th, 10th, and 11th cranial nerves. The first successful surgical removal was described by Cairns in 1935 (see Cohen 1937). Since that initial description just over 200 cases of schwannomas arising from the jugular foramen have been described (Bakar et al 2008). As with most schwannomas, these tumors usually present in the 3rd to 5th decades of life, with a slight female predilection. Most reports do not identify the specific root of origin. However, the glossopharyngeal nerve appears to be most commonly affected, with approximately 28 cases cited (Samii et al 1995b).

The glossopharyngeal, vagus, and cranial accessory nerves emerge as a series of rootlets from the retro-olivary sulcus of the medulla and pass inferolaterally towards the jugular foramen. A Schwann cell sheath is acquired within 1.1 mm of the root entry zone, with the more caudal rootlets exhibiting the shortest glial segments (Suzuki et al 1989; Nadich et al 2009). The jugular foramen itself is divided into a pars nervosa and a pars vascularis by a fibrous or bony septum (DiChiro et al 1964). The former contains the glossopharyngeal nerve and the inferior petrosal sinus, the latter the vagus and accessory nerves, the jugular vein, and the posterior meningeal artery (Fig. 29.8).

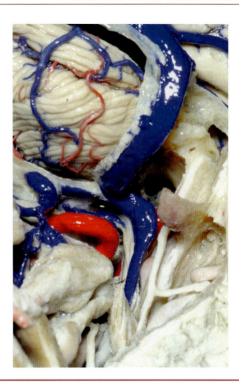

Figure 29.8 Anatomical dissection of the jugular fossa region.

Kaye et al (1984) classified jugular foramen schwannomas into three types according to their primary location: within the posterior fossa in the cerebellopontine angle cistern, within the skull base, or extending inferiorly from the jugular foramen into the neck. Recently the largest series to date was published including 53 patients and proposed a modification to Kaye's classification system (Bulsara et al 2008). Bulsara and colleagues (2008) divided the patients into three types of jugular foramen schwannomas, based primarily on the preoperative imaging. Type A tumors are as in Kaye's classification intracranial and amenable to either a retromastoid approach if there is no bony involvement or an extreme lateral infrajugular transtubercular approach (ELITE) with osseous involvement. Type B tumors are composed of dumbbell shaped tumors with limited cervical extension and are accessible through an ELITE approach. Type C tumors are dumbbell shaped tumors with high cervical extension and are approached with the ELITE or transjugular approach couple with a high cervical approach.

The clinical presentation will vary somewhat according to this classification scheme. In general, symptoms and signs associated with jugular foramen schwannomas may be present for many years before diagnosis, with an average duration of about 2.7 years (Hakuba et al 1979). Blurred vision was a frequent complaint amongst jugular foramen schwannomas as a whole (Hakuba et al 1979). Tumors confined to the posterior fossa most commonly present with ipsilateral sensorineural hearing loss, sometimes accompanied by tinnitus. This is especially common in glossopharyngeal tumors, in which over 90% of the cases presented in such a fashion (Fink et al 1978; Kadri et al 2004; Samii et al 1995b; Shiroyama et al 1988). Facial numbness, weakness, or hemifacial spasm may also be present. Large tumors in this location may present with symptoms and signs of brainstem and/or cerebellar compression such as nystagmus and ataxia, along with evidence of raised intracranial pressure such as headache, nausea, vomiting, and papilledema. Palsies of the nerves of the jugular foramen are distinctly uncommon amongst these tumors (Shiroyama et al 1988). Schwannomas confined to the jugular foramen and those with extension into the neck are more likely to present with evidence of lower cranial nerve palsies such as hoarseness, swallowing difficulties and/or weakness and atrophy of the sternomastoid and trapezius muscles. Diminished gag reflex with a unilateral vocal cord paralysis is common. Loss of taste is a notably uncommon complaint and rarely found on exam.

Detailed neuroimaging, including contrast enhanced MR and CT, is the most important preoperative evaluation. The jugular foramen is usually enlarged, and CT bone windows will show scalloping of the margins. MR is the most sensitive imaging modality for discovering small tumors and demonstrating tumor extension (Fig. 29.9). Angiography will demonstrate an avascular mass that displaces the anterior inferior cerebellar artery superomedially and the posterior inferior cerebellar artery inferomedially (Hakuba et al 1979). The venous phase is especially important for evaluating the jugular bulb and vein, which are often occluded. The differential diagnosis includes acoustic schwannoma, meningioma, metastasis, and glomus jugulare tumor. Acoustic schwannomas will usually enlarge the internal auditory canal rather than the jugular foramen. Meningiomas more often produce hyperostosis than bone erosion or scalloping, and demonstrate a much more prominent blush on angiography. Metastases and glomus jugulare tumors tend to irregularly destroy bone rather than smoothly erode or scallop. In addition, the latter have a very prominent blush on angiography and invade rather than compress the jugular bulb and vein.

The surgical approach to these lesions is determined by their location and extension. Those tumors confined to the posterior fossa can be removed through a standard lateral suboccipital craniectomy as performed for the more common acoustic schwannoma (Shiroyama et al 1988) (Fig. 29.10). For tumors located primarily within the jugular foramen, a pre-sigmoid inferolabyrinthine mastoidectomy combined with a retro-sigmoid craniectomy allows for ligation of the sigmoid sinus and direct exposure of the lateral margin of the jugular foramen (Hakuba et al 1979; Kadri et al 2004). This exposure minimizes the distance between the surgeon and the tumor. Alternatively, the jugular foramen may be opened intracranially through a standard lateral suboccipital craniectomy by removing a triangular-shaped wedge of bone between the foramen and the internal auditory canal (Hakuba et al 1979). Significant extension into the neck usually requires a combined approach with the aid of an otolaryngologist, either simultaneously or in a staged procedure (Kadri et al 2004). The neck dissection allows for control of the carotid artery, jugular vein, and adjacent lower cranial nerves below the skull base. Bulsara et al (2008) recently described the aforementioned approaches including ELITE and retromastoid with or without a high cervical exposure based on the tumor's classification providing a reasonable paradigm based on the extent of the tumor.

As with all intracranial schwannomas, complete surgical excision is curative. In general, tumors which are sub-totally resected tend to regrow and produce symptoms (Samii et al 1995b; Shiroyama et al 1988). However, there are patients who have been observed for long periods after subtotal resection without neurologic deterioration (Samii et al 1995b). No reliable information is available on the effectiveness of radiation in reducing the incidence or time to recurrence. Since schwannomas tend to be slow growing tumors follow-up needs to be of a significant duration to demonstrate treatment effect.

Complications following surgical removal of these tumors might be expected to involve the swallowing mechanism. While this has been noted in some series (Hakuba et al 1979; Kadri et al 2004; Samii et al 1995b) and early tracheostomy has been recommended by some authors (Naunton et al 1969), the most recent reports have demonstrated a remarkably low incidence of serious dysphagia and aspiration (Bulsara et al 2008). Many patients can be managed with temporary nasogastric feedings and meticulous pulmonary toilet. Most will eventually adapt and tolerate a regular diet. Other complications include CSF leak, meningitis, and hydrocephalus.

Accessory nerve schwannomas

Schwannomas of the 11th nerve are very rare with only 12 cases reported in the literature (Ohkawa et al 1996). Spinal

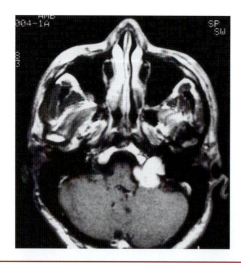

Figure 29.9 Axial and coronal gadolinium enhanced MRI demonstrating a IX nerve schwannoma.

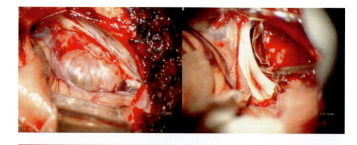

Figure 29.10 Intraoperative photograph demonstrating a schwannoma of the 9th and 10th nerve complex before and after complete resection through a suboccipital approach.

accessory neuromas often present in conjunction with jugular foramen schwannomas, but can occur independently as chronic neck or shoulder pain, associated with muscular spasms. The tumor itself can often originate from the spinal root of the accessory nerve (Caputi et al 1997). On CT and MRI imaging there is a heterogenously enhancing cisternal mass. Accessory nerve neuromas have also presented as jugular foramen syndromes, involving the 9th, 10th, and 11th cranial nerves, with the mass originating in the jugular foramen itself (Sawada et al 1992). Accessory neuromas have also presented as subarachnoid bleeding (Caputi et al 1997). The standard approach to these tumors involves a suboccipital craniectomy and C1 laminectomy.

Hypoglossal schwannomas

In 1933, de Martel described the first case of a schwannoma arising from the intracranial portion of the hypoglossal nerve. Since then, approximately 70 cases have been reported in the literature (Ho et al 2005). As a purely motor nerve, the hypoglossal would be expected to be an unusual site for the development of a schwannoma. There is usually an association with von Recklinghausen's disease if a motor nerve is affected. Approximately 14% or five cases out of 35 of hypoglossal neuromas in a review series arose in patients afflicted with central neurofibromatosis (Fujiwara et al 1980; Morelli 1966). The age range of the patients was from 17 to 62 years, with a mean age at diagnosis of 41 years. The female predilection noted in most series of schwannomas is even stronger for the hypoglossal; 23 of the 30 patients without neurofibromatosis were female.

The hypoglossal nerve arises as a series of rootlets from the rostral medulla in the pre-olivary sulcus between the inferior olive and the pyramid. The rootlets coalesce and usually form two motor roots which acquire a Schwann cell sheath within 0.1 mm of the brainstem (Tarlov et al 1937; Nadich et al 2009). The roots pass anteriorly, inferiorly, and laterally through the cerebellomedullary cistern towards the hypoglossal canal. Within the cisternal segment the nerve passes over the vertebral artery at the level of the origin of the posterior inferior cerebellar artery. The hypoglossal canal lies inferomedial to the jugular foramen within the occipital bone. In addition to the hypoglossal nerve, the canal usually contains a meningeal artery and a venous plexus. The postero-lateral aspect of the canal is bordered by the anteromedial aspect of the occipital condyle. This becomes important in the surgical removal of dumbbell-shaped tumors with extracranial extension. After passing through the canal the nerve lies between the jugular vein and the carotid artery. It is the only cranial nerve which crosses both the internal and external branches of the carotid artery.

Dysfunction of the hypoglossal nerve alone rarely produces symptoms of concern to the patient. Most patients present with symptoms related to raised intracranial pressure, or mass effects on the brainstem, cerebellum or adjacent lower cranial nerves. Thus headache, often suboccipital or nuchal, is the most common presenting complaint occurring in 73% of cases (Morelli et al 1966). This may be associated with nausea, vomiting, or papilledema. This clinical description is especially common in the older literature when the tumors often grew to large size before diagnosis. Dysfunction of the nerves of the adjacent jugular foramen is common (67%) (Odake 1989) resulting in swallowing difficulty, hoarseness, or hypesthesia of the pharynx. There may be ipsilateral palatal deviation and diminished gag reflex. Limb weakness with spasticity resulting from pyramidal tract compression is present in up to 66% of patients (Odake 1989). Vestibulocerebellar symptoms such as ataxia, dizziness, vertigo and nystagmus are common. Other symptoms can include facial numbness or weakness, sensorineural hearing loss, or weakness and atrophy of the ipsilateral sternomastoid and trapezius muscles (Table 29.5). The classic finding on exam is that of hemiatrophy of the tongue with fasciculations and ipsilateral deviation on protrusion. This finding may be present for many years, but as it produces little difficulty for the patient it is often ignored.

Plain skull radiographs are not helpful. Special tomographic projections of the skull base have been largely replaced with the use of computed tomography, which will sometimes demonstrate enlargement of the hypoglossal canal. However, the hypoglossal or condylar canal lies in an especially thick region of the occipital bone. Therefore, widening of this skull base foramen is not as common as elsewhere. In some instances, the adjacent jugular foramen is eroded, making the differential diagnosis almost impossible (Fig. 29.11A) (Morelli 1966). CT will usually demonstrate an iso- to hyperdense mass ventral to the lower brainstem which enhances homogeneously and intensely following contrast administration. Together with gadolinium-enhanced magnetic resonance, which is the most sensitive means of demonstrating the shape and extent of the soft-tissue mass, the surgical approach can be effectively planned (Fig. 29.11A–C). Angiography will demonstrate local vascular displacement, usually elevation of the ipsilateral vertebral artery, by an avascular mass. The jugular bulb and vein are usually not obstructed or infiltrated. This helps to distinguish the hypoglossal from the jugular foramen schwannoma, and from other lesions such as the glomus jugulare.

The surgical approach is dictated largely by the extent of the tumor. Those tumors which appear purely intracranial may be approached through a standard lateral suboccipital craniectomy, as for the acoustic schwannoma (Bartal et al 1973; Morelli et al 1966; Scott et al 1949). A more direct exposure of the region of the hypoglossal canal can be gained by performing a mastoidectomy and retrolabyrinthine petrosectomy as described by Hakuba et al (1979) for tumors of the jugular foramen (Dolan et al 1982; Odake et al 1989). Dumbbell-shaped tumors with significant extracranial extension can be removed via an extreme lateral approach, as described by Sen & Sekhar (1990). This includes removal of

Table 29.5 Signs and symptoms of XII nerve schwannomas

Symptom	(%)
Tongue hemiatrophy	
Headache	73
IX, X, XI nerve dysfunction	67
Limb weakness (spastic)	66
Ataxia, vertigo, nystagmus	
Facial weakness, hearing loss	

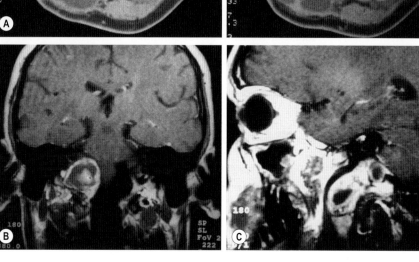

Figure 29.11 (A) Axial CT scan demonstrating erosion of the hypoglossal foramen and adjacent skull base secondary to a XII nerve schwannoma. (B) Coronal gadolinium enhanced MRI demonstrating the same XII nerve schwannoma. Note extension through the skull base. (C) Sagittal gadolinium enhanced MRI demonstrating the XII nerve schwannoma. The extracranial extension is well visualized.

the posterior half of the occipital condyle and lateral mass of C1. Alternatively, dumb-bell shaped tumors can be removed in two-stages by combining a standard retrosigmoid craniectomy with a neck dissection. A report of a large dumbbell neuroma used a single stage surgery employing a lateral suboccipital craniectomy with partial mastoidectomy and removal of the posterior arch of atlas on the side of the tumor. The posterior arch of the atlas was removed up to the foramen transversarium where the vertebral artery emerged. Total excision of the condyle was not done so as not to destabilize the atlas articulation (Kachhara et al 1999). As with schwannomas occurring elsewhere, the tumors are internally debulked prior to any attempt at dissection of the capsule from adjacent neurovascular structures. Most of the cases cited have required the sacrifice of the involved hypoglossal nerve.

Hypoglossal neuromas can present as skull base lesions, requiring extensive surgical resection. A case of a hypoglossal neurilemmoma occurring in the right skull base was resected via a posterolateral approach (Myatt et al 1998). In this technique, a suboccipital craniectomy, mastoidectomy and removal of the lateral process of the atlas was performed. This exposure thereby also provides an

inferior approach to the jugular foramen and hypoglossal canal that allows the lower cranial nerves to be identified as they exit from their skull base foramina. A supracondylar approach provides lower morbidity, but only allows for a minimal surgical exposure (Gilsbach et al 1998). This approach is useful to gain access to benign lesions of the hypoglossal canal and of the jugular tubercle to decompress tumors or cysts. The surgical field in this approach is restricted laterally by the jugular bulb, medially and basally by the residual occipital condyle and dorsally by the dura. This approach may therefore prove useful for removing small lesions or to perform extended biopsies.

Complete surgical extirpation is curative; subtotal resection can be expected to result in recurrence, although long-term follow-up in many of the cases is lacking. A mortality rate of approximately 7% exists among the older reported cases (Odake 1989). Respiratory difficulties with aspiration and pneumonia appeared to be the cause. However, most of these cases preceded the microsurgical era. Morbidity includes CSF leak, meningitis and hydrocephalus. Pre-existing associated lower cranial nerve palsies often do not improve, but brainstem and cerebellar findings can be expected to do so (Odake 1989).

Extraocular nerve schwannomas

Schwann cell tumors arising on the intracranial component of the oculomotor, trochlear, or abducens nerve are extremely rare. Being purely motor nerves, neurinomas arising from the ocular nerves are very uncommon, unless associated with von Recklinghausen's disease. Kovacs (1927) was probably the first to report an isolated oculomotor nerve sheath tumor at autopsy, in 1927. As with schwannomas arising elsewhere, the tumors tend to occur during middle age, with a peak incidence in the 4th and 5th decades. There is a slight female predilection (58% vs 42%) (Celli et al 1992).

The oculomotor nerve arises from the oculomotor sulcus along the medial surface of the cerebral peduncle at the level of the mesencephalon. It passes through the interpeduncular cistern, acquiring a Schwann cell sheath within approximately 0.6 mm of it's emergence from the brainstem (Tarlov 1937; Nadich et al 2009). It passes inferolaterally, between the posterior cerebral and superior cerebellar arteries towards the cavernous sinus. It enters the roof of the sinus in a triangular-shaped fold of dura formed by the anterior, posterior, and inter-clinoid ligaments. Passing forwards in the superior aspect of the lateral wall of the cavernous sinus it exits the intracranial cavity through the superior orbital fissure (Fig. 29.3). The transition of the oculomotor nerve from central to the peripheral nervous system is approximately 0.6 mm distal to the brain stem (Tarlov 1937; Nadich et al 2009). Anywhere distal to this point schwannomas can occur, i.e. in the interpeduncular, prepontine, parasellar, cavernous region, or the orbital apex.

The trochlear nerve arises from the dorsal aspect of the brainstem at the level of the pontomesencephalic junction. It emerges from the superior medullary velum just below the inferior colliculus, and acquires a Schwann cell sheath within approximately 0.6 mm (Tarlov 1937; Nadich et al 2009). It swings around the brainstem in the ambient cistern, adjacent to the superior cerebellar and cerebral peduncles. Running anteriorly below the free margin of the tentorium, it pierces the dura of the cavernous sinus just behind the posterior clinoid process. It travels forwards in the lateral wall of the cavernous sinus below the oculomotor nerve towards the superior orbital fissure.

The abducens nerve emerges from the ventral aspect of the pontomedullary sulcus and heads anteriorly through the prepontine cistern to pierce the dura overlying the dorsum sellae. The glial segment of the nerve is approximately 0.5 mm long (Tarlov 1937). It ascends the rostral clivus between the meningeal and periosteal layers of the dura. It passes through a notch at the base of the posterior clinoid process, below the Gruber's ligament, to enter the back of the cavernous sinus. Within the cavernous sinus, the nerve lies lateral to the internal carotid artery. It enters the orbit through the superior orbital fissure.

Celli et al (1992) divided this group of tumors into three categories according to their anatomic extent. This classification scheme is analogous to that devised by Jefferson (1955) for the trigeminal schwannomas. Tumors may be considered cisternal, cavernous, or cisternocavernous (dumbbell-shaped). Unlike schwannomas developing along the other cranial nerves, extraocular schwannomas usually arise far from the glial-Schwann cell junction. Those tumors which lie predominantly in the subarachnoid space around the brainstem are considered cisternal. Those which lie predominantly in the cavernous sinus are considered cavernous. Those tumors which have a significant component in both regions are considered cisternocavernous. Symptoms, signs, and surgical approaches will vary according to the class of tumor.

The majority of oculomotor schwannomas (70%) (Celli et al 1992) will present with a third nerve palsy as the initial symptom. Some authors have even gone so far as to say that oculomotor palsy as the initial symptom may be pathognomonic in neurinomas originating from the oculomotor nerve (Okamoto et al 1985). When left untreated the oculomotor palsy progresses to complete ophthalmoplegia. Preceding the oculomotor nerve paresis or simultaneously is a functional loss of the homolateral optic nerve sometimes progressing to amaurosis (Leunda et al 1982). Unilateral exophthalmos as well as frontal or orbital neuralgic pain with or without sensory disorders in the area of V1 of trigeminal nerve are characteristic for the clinical picture in later stages. The differential diagnosis of these associated neurological symptoms includes sphenoid ridge meningiomas, trigeminal neurinomas, any of the tumors within the cavernous sinus, aneurysms, chondromas, giant pituitary adenomas, and metastatic carcinomas.

Oculomotor schwannomas tend to be evenly divided between the cisternal and cavernous types. When cisternal they tend to spread upwards into the interpeduncular and suprasellar cisterns resulting in compression of the brainstem, third ventricle and hypothalamus. Patients present with either an isolated parent nerve palsy, or a combination of a parent nerve palsy with signs of brainstem compression. The cavernous variety produce compression of the nerves of the cavernous sinus and occasionally, in addition, the optic nerve, resulting in a cavernous sinus syndrome or orbital apex syndrome, respectively.

Trochlear nerve schwannomas are most often cisternal. They tend to grow upwards into the tentorial incisura, or medially into the prepontine or interpeduncular cisterns. Palsy of the parent nerve is an unusually uncommon presenting symptom, occurring in less than half (44%) of patients (Celli et al 1992). There is no preoperative trochlear nerve involvement in at least 45% of cases reviewed (Santorenos et al 1997). Up to one-third of patients will actually present with an isolated oculomotor palsy. When the tumors grow to a large size within the ambient cistern, a characteristic clinical syndrome may result which has been called 'ataxic hemiparesis' (Bendheim & Berg 1981). As a consequence of compression of the superior cerebellar and cerebral peduncles an ipsilateral limb ataxia combined with a contralateral spastic hemiparesis is present.

Abducens schwannomas are most often cisternocavernous. Most will present with a combination of a parent nerve palsy and symptom/signs of raised intracranial pressure. In addition, there may be a hemiparesis secondary to brainstem compression, or palsies of other nerves within the cavernous sinus. These tumors may be difficult to distinguish from the more common trigeminal schwannoma, which often presents with a sixth nerve palsy.

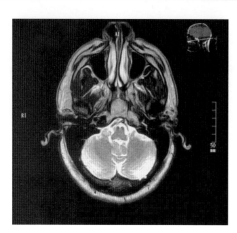

Figure 29.12 Example of an incidental lower cranial nerve schwannoma not producing significant mass effect that we would choose to observe.

Plain film and CT bone windows will demonstrate scalloping of the clinoids, sella, and petrous apex in cisternocavernous tumors. In cavernous lesions there may be widening of the superior orbital fissure or erosion of the middle fossa floor. Cisternal tumors may produce non-specific changes within the sella if intracranial pressure is elevated. As with schwannomas elsewhere, these tumors tend to enhance following contrast administration. MR may be helpful in distinguishing cisternal schwannomas from intrinsic tumors of the brainstem, and is the most sensitive imaging modality for detecting small lesions (Garen et al 1987) (Fig. 29.12). MRI also provides information about the displacement of the cavernous carotid artery. Trochlear nerve tumors are characteristically isointense on T1- and T2-weighted MR images and enhances brightly with gadolinium (Santorenos et al 1997).

Cisternal schwannomas of the oculomotor nerve may be approached through a frontotemporal craniotomy as these tumors tend to grow up into the suprasellar cistern. Those of the trochlear nerve may require a subtemporal/transtentorial approach. Occasionally, a cisternal tumor of the trochlear or abducens nerve will lie entirely within the posterior fossa and may be removed via a lateral suboccipital approach. The majority of cisternal tumors can be entirely removed, and the parent nerve clearly identified. Cisternocavernous tumors may be approached either subtemporally or frontotemporally, while cavernous tumors are usually removed via a frontotemporal approach. Newer skull base approaches incorporating an orbitozygomatic osteotomy may prove useful in the management of tumors with a significant cavernous component. The orbitozygomatic osteotomy can provide an optimal approach to the cavernous sinus and the interpeduncular cisterns. To date, only about 50% of these tumors have been completely resected, and the parent nerve has been identified in only half of the cases (Celli et al 1992). It is not always possible to determine the nerve of origin at operation, especially in large tumors, because these cranial nerves as well as the ophthalmic nerve come close together in the parasellar region. Intraoperative observations of characteristically pale and thickened nerve

segments may not truly indicate schwannoma origination, as such segmental thickening can also be seen as a 'pseudo-neuromatous' reaction to the nerve proximal to a localized and severe chronic compression (Kachara et al 1998).

Only one operative mortality has been reported. However, resection nearly always requires sacrifice of the parent nerve resulting in a permanent extraocular palsy. Despite the large proportion of sub-total resections, there has been only one documented symptomatic recurrence (Vaquero et al 1985). However, at present insufficient follow-up exists to provide reliable information regarding the incidence or time to recurrence after subtotal resection.

Recent experience with stereotactic radiosurgery has demonstrated good results in both tumor control and symptomatic improvement. Kim et al (2008) evaluated eight patients with schwannomas of the oculomotor, trochlear, and abducens nerves. In seven of the patients, GammaKnife surgery was the primary treatment modality and in one patient, radiosurgery was performed after sub-total resection. Tumor regression was demonstrated in all patients on follow-up MRI with a mean progression-free period of 21 months. In addition, 80% of patients with diplopia secondary to a trochlear schwannoma experienced symptomatic improvement (Kim et al 2008). Radiosurgery is likely to play an increasingly important role in the treatment of extraocular nerve schwannomas.

Olfactory schwannomas

Approximately 23–26 cases of schwannomas arising from the olfactory nerve exist in the literature (Christin et al 1920; Molter 1920; Sehrbundt et al 1973; Spiller et al 1903; Sturm et al 1968; Ulrich et al 1978; Kanaan et al 2008). The tumors are believed to have arisen on the fila olfactoria, which acquire a Schwann cell sheath approximately 0.5 mm beyond the olfactory bulbs (Tarlov 1937; Nadich et al 2009). Very little is known about the epidemiology and clinical manifestations of these tumors. To date the solitary cases cited have occurred in young males. The tumors have been very large with anosmia, decreased visual acuity, seizures and evidence of raised intracranial pressure being common findings at the time of presentation. The MRI findings are similar to other schwannomas with homogenous enhancement and variable cystic contents. Computed tomography is helpful in distinguishing whether the tumor has surrounding scalloping of bone more consistent with a schwannoma or the hyperostosis seen in an olfactory groove meningioma. Given the large size of the tumors at the time of surgery or autopsy it is difficult to prove an olfactory origin in all the cases cited. The standard approach is generally a subfrontal approach although recently alternative approaches have been described. Kanaan et al (2008) recently described an expanded endoscopic endonasal technique in a case of an anterior cranial fossa olfactory schwannoma (Kanaan et al 2008).

REFERENCES

Abdel Aziz, K.M., van Loveren, H.R., 1999. Primary lymphoma of Meckel's cave mimicking trigeminal schwannoma: case report. Neurosurgery 44, 859–862.

Bakar, B., Percin, A.K., Tekkok, I.H., 2008. Retro-tympanic pulsatile mass originating from dumb-bell jugular foramen schwannoma. Acta. Neurochir. (Wien). 150, 291–293.

Bartal, A.D., Djaldetti, M.M., Mandel, E.M., et al., 1973. Dumb-bell neurinoma of the hypoglossal nerve. J. Neurol. Neurosurg. Psychiatry 36, 592–595.

Bendheim, P.E., Berg, B.O., 1981. Ataxic hemiparesis from a midbrain mass. Ann. Neurol. 9, 405–406.

• Bordi, L., Compton, J., Symon, L., 1989. Trigeminal neuroma. Surg. Neurol. 31, 272–276.

Bulsara, K.R., Sameshima, T., Friedman, A.H., et al., 2008. Microsurgical management of 53 jugular foramen schwannomas: lessons learned incorporated into a modified grading system. J. Neurosurg. 109, 794–803.

Burger, P.C., Scheithauer, B.W., Vogel, F.S., 1991. Surgical pathology of the nervous system and its coverings, 3rd edn. Churchill Livingstone, New York.

Caputi, F., de Sanctis, S., Gazzeri, G., et al., 1997. Neuroma of the spinal accessory nerve disclosed by a subarachnoid hemorrhage: case report. Neurosurgery 41, 946–950.

• Celli, P., Ferrante, L., Acqui, M., et al., 1992. Surgical Neurinoma of the third, fourth, and sixth cranial nerves: a survey and report of a new fourth nerve case. Neurology 38, 216–224.

Chase, N.E., Taveras, J.M., 1963. Carotid angiography in the diagnosis of extradural parasellar tumors. Acta Radiologica (Diagn) 1, 214–224.

Christin, E., Naville, F., 1920. A propos de neurofibromatoses centrales. Leurs formes familiales et hereditaires. Les neurofibromes des nerfs optiques. Cas a evolution atypique. Diversites des structures histologiques (etude clinique et anatomique). Anna. Med. 8, 30–50.

Cohen, H., 1937. Glosso-pharyngeal neuralgia. J. Laryngol. Otol. 52, 527–536.

Das Gupta, T.K., Brasfield, R.D., Strong, E.W., et al., 1969. Benign solitary schwannomas (neurilemmomas). Cancer 24, 355–366.

Dastur, D.K., Sinh, G., Pandya, S.K., 1967. Melanotic tumor of the acoustic nerve. J. Neurosurg. 27:166–170.

• Day, J.D., Fukushima, T., 1998. The surgical management of trigeminal neuromas. Neurosurgery 42, 233–240.

de Martel, T., Subirana, A., Guillaume, J., 1933. Los tumores de la fossa cerebral posterior: voluminos neurinoma del hipogloso con desarrollojuxta-bulbo-protuberancial. Operacion-curacion. Ars. Medicina 9, 416–419.

DiChiro, G., Fisher, R.L., Nelson, K.B., 1964. The jugular foramen. J. Neurosurg. 21, 447–460.

Dolan, E.J., Tucker, W.S., Rotenberg, D., et al., 1982. Intracranial hypoglossal schwannoma as an unusual cause of facial nerve palsy. J. Neurosurg. 56, 420–423.

Dolenc, V.V., 1994. Frontotemporal epidural approach to trigeminal neurinomas. Acta Neurochirurgica 130, 55–65.

Dominguez, J., Lobato, R.D., Madero, S., et al., 1999. Surgical findings in idiopathic trigeminal neuropathy mimicking a trigeminal neurinoma. Acta Neurochirurgica 141, 269–272.

Erlandson. R.A., Woodruff, J.M., 1982. Peripheral nerve-sheath tumors: an electron micro-scopic Study of 43 cases. Cancer 49, 273–287.

Fernandez-Valle, C., Tang, Y., Richard, J., et al., 2002. Paxillin binds schwannomin and regulates its density- dependent localization and effect on cell morphology. Nat. Genet. 31, 354–362.

Fink, K.H., Early, C.B., Bryan, R.N., 1978. Glossopharyngeal schwannomas. Surg. Neurol. 9, 239–245.

Fisch, V., Ruttner, J., 1977. Pathology of intratemporal tumours involving the facial nerve. In: Fisch, V. (Ed.), Facial nerve surgery. Aesculapius, Birmingham, pp. 448–456.

• Flickinger, J.C., Kondziolka, D., Niranjan, A., et al., 2004. Acoustic neuroma radiosurgery with marginal tumor doses of 12 to 13 Gy. Int. J. Radiat. Oncol. Biol. Phys. 60 (1), 225–230.

Frazier, C.H., 1918. An operable tumor involving the gasserian ganglion. Am. J. Med. Sci. 156, 483–490.

Fujiwara, M., Hachisuga, S., Numaguchi, Y., 1980. Intracranial hypoglossal neurinoma; report of a case. Neuroradiology 20, 87–90.

Garen, P.D., Harper, C.G., Teo, C., et al., 1987. Cystic schwannoma of the trochlear nerve mimicking a brain-stem tumor. Case report. J. Neurosurg. 67, 928–930.

Gerhardt, C., 1878. Zur diagnostik multipler nerombildung. Deutsh Arch. Klin. Med. 21, 268–289.

• Ghatak, N.R., Norwood, C.W., Davis, C.H., 1975. Intracerebral schwannoma. Surg. Neurol. 3, 45–47.

Gibson, A.A., Hendrick, E.B., Cowen, P.E., 1966. Intracerebral schwannoma: a report of a case. J. Neurosurg. 24, 552–557.

Gilsbach, J.M., Sure, U., Mann, W., 1998. The supracondylar approach to the jugular tubercle and hypoglossal canal. Surg. Neurol. 50, 563–570.

Goldberg, R., Byrd, S., Winter, J., 1980. Varied appearance of trigeminal neuromas on CT. Am. J. Radiol. 134, 57–60.

• Hakuba, A., Hashi, K., Fujita, K., et al., 1979. Jugular foramen neurinomas. Surg. Neurol. 11, 83–94.

Hanada, M., Tanaka, T., Kanayama, S., et al., 1982. Malignant transformation of intrathoracic ancient neurilemmoma in a patient without von Recklinghausen's disease. Acta Pathologica Japonica 32, 527–536.

Ho, C.L., Deruytter, M.J., 2005. Navigated dorsolateral suboccipital transcondylar (NADOSTA) approach for treatment of hypoglossal schwannoma. Case report and review of the literature. Clin. Neurol. Neurosurg. 107 (3), 236–242.

Holman, C.B., Olive, I., Svien, H.J., 1961. Roentgenologic features of neurofibromas involving the gasserian ganglion. Am. J. Radiol. 86, 148–153.

Horn, K.L., Crumley, R.L., Schindler, R.A., 1981. Facial neurilemmomas. Laryngoscope 91, 1326–1331.

House, J.W., Brackmann, D.E., 1985. Facial nerve grading systems. Otolaryngol. Head Neck Surg. 93, 146–147.

• Huang, C.F., Kondziolka, D., Flickinger, J.C., et al., 1999. Stereotactic radiosurgery for trigeminal schwannomas. Neurosurgery 45, 11–16.

Ikushima, I., Korogi, Y., Kuratsu, J., et al., 1997. Dynamic M R I of meningiomas and schwannomas: is differential diagnosis possible? Neuroradiology 39, 633–638.

• Inouye, Y., Tabuchi, T., Hakuba, A., et al., 1987. Facial nerve neuromas: CT findings. J. Comp. Assist. Tomogr. 11, 942–947.

Isamat, F., Bartumeus, F., Mirand, A.M., et al., 1975. Neurinomas of the facial nerve: report of three cases. J. Neurosurg. 43, 600–613.

Jefferson, G., 1955. The trigeminal neurinomas with some remarks on malignant invasion of the gasserian ganglion. Clin. Neurosurg. 1, 11–54.

Johnson, M.D., Glick, A.D., Davis, B.N., 1988. Immunohistochemical evaluation of Leu-7, myelin basic- protein, S100-protein, glial fibrillary acidic-protein, and LN3 immunoreactivity in nerve sheath tumors and sarcomas. Arch. Pathol. Lab. Med. 112, 155–160.

Kachara, R., Nair, S., Radhakrishnan, V.V., 1998. Oculomotor nerve neurinoma: Report of two cases. Acta Neurochirurgica 140, 1147–1151.

Kachhara, R., Nair, S., Radhakrishnan, V.V., 1999. Large dumbbell neurinoma of hypoglossal nerve: case report. Br. J. Neurosurg. 13, 338–340.

Kadri, P.A., Al-Mefty, O., 2004. Surgical treatment of dumbbell-shaped jugular foramen schwannomas. Neurosurg. Focus 17 (2), E9.

Kanaan, H.A., Gardner, P.A., Yeaney, G., et al., 2008. Expanded endoscopic endonasal resection of an olfactory schwannoma. J. Neurosurg. Pediatr. 2, 261–265.

Kanter, W.R., Eldridge, R., Fabricant, R., 1980. Central neurofibromatosis with bilateral acoustic neuroma: genetic, clinical and biochemical distinctions from peripheral neurofibromatosis. Neurology 30, 851–859.

Kawahara, E., Oda, Y., Ooi, Y., et al., 1988. Expression of glial fibrillary acidic protein (GFAP) in peripheral nerve sheath tumors. Am. J. Surg. Pathol. 12, 115–120.

• Kaye, A.H., Hahn, J.F., Kinney, S.E., et al., 1984. Jugular foramen schwannomas. J. Neurosurg. 60, 1045–1053.

Kim, I.Y., Kondziolka, D., Niranjan, A., et al., 2008. Gamma Knife surgery for schwannomas originating from cranial nerves III, IV, and VI. J. Neurosurg. 109 (Suppl.), 149–153.

King, T.T., Morrison, A.W., 1990. Primary facial nerve tumors within the skull. J. Neurosurg. 72, 1–8.

Konovalov, A.N., Spallone, A., Mukhamedjanov, D.J., et al., 1996. Trigeminal neurinomas. A series of 111 surgical cases from a single institution. Acta Neurochirurgica 138, 1027–1035.

Kovacs, W., 1927. Ueber ein solitares neuinom des nervus oculomotorius. Zentralbl. Allg. Pathol. 40, 518–522.

Lesois, F., Rousseaux, M., Villette, L., 1986. Neurinomas of the trigeminal nerve. Acta Neurochirurgica 82, 118–122.

Leunda, G., Vaquero, J., Cabezudo, J., et al., 1982. Schwannoma of the oculomotor nerve. Report of four cases. J. Neurosurg. 57, 563–565.

Lipkin, A.F., Coker, N.J., Jenkins, H.A., et al., 1987. Intracranial and intratemporal facial neuroma. Otolaryngol-Head Neck Surg. 96, 71–79.

• Madhok, R., Kondziolka, D., Flickinger, J.C., et al., 2009. Gamma knife radiosurgery for facial schwannomas. Neurosurgery 64 (6), 1102–1105.

• McCormick, P.C., Bello, J.A., Post, K.D., 1988. Trigeminal schwannoma: surgical series of 14 patients and a review of the literature. J. Neurosurg. 70, 737–745.

McLean, C.A., Laidlaw, J.D., Brownbill, D.S., et al., 1990. Recurrence of acoustic neurilemmoma as a malignant spindle-cell neoplasm. J. Neurosurg. 73, 946–950.

• McMonagle, B., Al-Sanosi, A., Croxson, G., et al., 2008. Facial schwannoma: results of a large case series and review. J. Laryngol. Otol. 122 (11), 1139–1150.

Mello, L.R., Tanzer, A., 1972. Some aspects of trigeminal neurinomas. Neuroradiology 4, 215–221.

Molter, K., 1920. Uber gleichzeitige cerebrale, medullare und periphere. Neurofibromatosis naugural dissertation, Universitat zu Jena). Wendt und Klauwell, Jena.

Morelli, R.J., 1966. Intracranial neurilemmoma of the hypoglossal nerve: review and case report. Neurology 158, 709–713.

Murata, T., Hakuba, A., Okumura, T., et al., 1985. Intrapetrous neurinomas of the facial nerve: report of three cases. J. Neurosurg. 23, 507–512.

Myatt, H.M., Holland, N.J., Cheesman, A.D., 1998. A skull base extradural hypoglossal neurilemmoma resected via an extended posterolateral approach. J. Laryngol. Otol. 112, 1052–1057.

Nadich, T.P., Duvernoy, H.M., Delman, B.N., et al., 2009. Duvernoy's atlas of the human brain stem and cerebellum. Springer Wien, New York.

Nager, G.T., 1984. Neurinomas of the trigeminal nerve. Am. J. Otolaryngol. 5, 301–331.

Naunton, R.F., Proctor, L., Elpern, B.S., 1969. The audiologic signs of ninth nerve neurinoma. Arch. Otolaryngol. 87, 20–25.

Neely, J.G., Alford, B.R., 1974. Facial nerve neuromas. Arch. Otolaryngol. 100, 298–301.

New, P.F.J., 1972. Intracerebral schwannoma: case report. J. Neurosurg. 36, 795–797.

O'Donoghue, G.M., Brackmann, D.E., House, J.W., et al., 1989. Neuromas of the facial nerve. Am. J. Otol. 10, 49–54.

Odake, G., 1989. Intracranial hypoglossal neurinoma with extracranial extension: review and case report. Neurosurgery 24, 583–587.

Ohkawa, M., Fujiwara, N., Takashima, H., et al., 1996. Radiologic manifestation of spinal accessory neurinoma: a case report. Radiat. Med. 14, 269–273.

Okamoto, S., Handa, H., Yamashita, J., 1985. Neurinoma of the oculomotor nerve. Surg. Neurol. 24, 275–278.

Palacios, E., MacGee, E.E., 1972. The radiographic diagnosis of trigeminal neurinomas. J. Neurosurg. 36, 153–156.

Pan, L., Wang, E.M., Zhang, N., et al., 2005. Long-term results of Leksell gamma knife surgery for trigeminal schwannomas. J. Neurosurg. 102 (Suppl.), 220–224.

Peet, M.M., 1927. Tumor of the gasserian ganglion. With the report of two cases of extra-cranial carcinoma infiltrating the ganglion by direct extension through the maxillary division. Surg. Gynecol. Obstet. 44, 202–207.

Phi, J.H., Paek, S.H., Chung, H.T., et al., 2007. Gamma Knife surgery and trigeminal schwannoma: is it possible to preserve cranial nerve function? J. Neurosurg. 107, 727–732.

Pollack, I.F., Sekhar, L.N., Janetta, P.J., et al., 1989. Neurilemmomas of the trigeminal nerve. J. Neurosurg. 17, 306–322.

Pool, J.L., Pava, A.A., 1970. Acoustic nerve tumors. Charles C Thomas, Springfield, IL.

Prakash, B., Roy, S., Tandon, P.N., 1980. Schwannoma of the brain stem. Case report. J. Neurosurg. 53, 121–123.

Pulec, J.L., 1969. Facial nerve tumors. Ann. Otol. Rhinol. Laryngol. 78, 962–982.

Pulec, J.L., 1972. Symposium on ear surgery. II. Facial nerve neuroma. Laryngoscope 82, 1160–1176.

Rigamonti, D., Spetzler, R.F., Shetter, A., et al., 1987. Magnetic resonance imaging and trigeminal schwannoma. Surg. Neurol. 28, 67–70.

Robey, S.S., deMent, S.H., Eaton, K.K., et al., 1987. Malignant epithelioid peripheral nerve sheath tumor arising in a benign schwannoma. Surg. Neurol. 28, 441–446.

Rosenblum, B., Davis, R., Camins, M., 1987. Middle fossa facial schwannoma removed via the intracranial extradural approach: case report and review of the literature. Neurosurgery 21, 739–741.

Rubinstein, L.J., 1972. Tumors of the central nervous system. Armed Forces Institute of Pathology, Washington.

Saito, H., Baxter, H., 1972. Undiagnosed intratemporal facial nerve neurilemmomas. Arch. Otolaryngol. 95:415–419.

Salvati, M., Ciapetta, P., Raco, A., et al., 1992. Radiation-induced schwannomas of the neuraxis. Report of three cases. Tumori 78, 143–146.

• Samii, M., Migliori, M.M., Tatagiba, M., et al., 1995a. Surgical treatment of trigeminal schwannomas. J. Neurosurg. 82, 711–718.

Samii, M., Babu, R.P., Tatagiba, M., et al., 1995b. Surgical treatment of jugular foramen schwannomas. J. Neurosurg. 82, 924–932.

Santorenos, S., Hanieh, A., Jorgensen, R.E., 1997. Trochlear nerve schwannomas occurring in patients without neurofibromatosis: case report and review of the literature. Neurosurgery 41, 28–34.

Sawada, H., Udaka, F., Kameyama, M., et al., 1992. Accessory nerve neuroma presenting as recurrent jugular foramen syndrome. Neuroradiology 34, 417–419.

Schmidt, C., 1931. Neurinom des nervus facialis. Zentralblatt Hals Nas-Ohrenheilk 16, 329.

Schuknecht, H.F., Gulya, A.J., 1986. Anatomy of the temporal bone with surgical implications. Lea & Febiger, Philadelphia, PA.

Scott, M., Wycis, H., 1949. Intracranial neurinoma of the hypoglossal nerve, successful removal, case report. J. Neurosurg. 6, 333–336.

• Sehrbundt, V., Pau, A., Turtas, S., 1973. Olfactory groove neurinomas. J. Neurosurg. Sci. 17, 193–196.

Sekhar, L.N., 1987. Operative management of tumors involving the cavernous sinus. In: Sekhar, L.N., Schramm, V.S., Jr. (Eds.), 1987 Tumors of the cranial base: diagnosis and treatment. Futura Publishing, Mt. Kisco, New York, pp. 393–419.

• Sen, C.N., Sekhar, L.N., 1990. An extreme lateral approach to intradural lesions of the cervical spine and foramen magnum. Neurosurgery 27, 197–204.

Sharma, B.S., Ahmad, F.U., Chandra, P.S., et al., 2008. Trigeminal schwannomas: experience with 68 cases. J. Clin. Neurosci. 15 (7), 738–743.

Shiroyama, Y., Inoue, S., Tshua, M., et al., 1988. Intracranial neurinomas of the jugular foramen and hypoglossal canal. No Shinkei Geka 16, 313–319.

Spiller, W.G., Hendrickson, W.F., 1903. A report of two cases of multiple sarcomatosis of the central nervous system and one case of intramedullary primary sarcoma of the spinal cord. Am. J. Med. Sci. 126, 10–33.

Stout, A.P., 1935. Peripheral manifestations of a specific nerve sheath tumor (neurilemmoma). Am. J. Cancer 24, 751–796.

Sturm, K., Bohnis, G., Kosmaoglu, V., 1968. Uber ein Neurinom der Lamina cribrosa. Zentralblatt Fur Neurochirurgiebl 29, 217–222.

Suzuki, F., Hanada, J., Todo, G., 1989. Intracranial glossopharyngeal neurinomas. Report of two cases with special emphasis on computer tomography and magnetic resonance imaging findings. Surg. Neurol. 13, 390–394.

• Symon, L., Cheesman, A.D., Kawauchi, M., et al., 1993. Neuromas of the facial nerve: a report of 12 cases. Br. J. Neurosurg. 7, 13–22.

Tarlov, I.M., 1937. Structure of the nerve root. II. Differentiation of sensory from motor roots; observations on identification of function in roots of mixed cranial nerves. Arch. Neurol. Psychiatry 37, 1338–1355.

Twist, E.C., Ruttledge, M.H., Rousseau, M., et al., 1994. The neurofibromatosis type 2 gene is inactivated in schwannomas. Hum. Molec. Genet. 3, 147–151.

Ulrich, J., Levy, A., Pfister, C., 1978. Schwannoma of the olfactory groove. Case report and review of previous cases. Acta Neurochirurgica 40, 315–321.

VanRensberg, M.J., Proctor, N.S., Danzinger, J., et al., 1975. Temporal lobe epilepsy due to an intracerebral schwannoma: case report. J. Neurol. Neurosurg. Psychiatry 38, 703–709.

Vaquero, J., Martinez, R., Salazar, J., 1985. Suprasellar recurrnce of a third nerve neurinoma (letter). J. Neurosurg. 62, 317.

Verocay, J., 1910. Zur kenntnis der neurofibrome. Beitrage Zur Pathologischen Anatomie und Zur Allgemeinen Pathologie 48, 1–69.

Wallner, K.E., Sheline, G.E., Pitts, L.H., et al., 1987. Efficacy of irradiation for incompletely excised acoustic neurilemmomas. J. Neurosurg. 67, 858–863.

Wang, E.M., Pan, L., Wang, B.J., et al., 2005. Gamma knife radiosurgery for large trigeminal schwannomas. Zhonghua Yi Xue Za Zhi 85 (18), 1266–1269.

Westberg, G., 1963. Angiographic changes in neurinoma of the trigeminal nerve. Acta Radiologica (Diagn) 1, 513–520.

White, W., Shiu, M.H., Rosenblum, M.K., et al., 1990. Cellular schwannoma: a clinicopathologic study of 57 patients and 58 tumors. Cancer 66, 1266–1275.

• Woodruff, J.M., Godwin, T.A., Erlandson, R.A., et al., 1981. Cellular schwannoma. Am. J. Surg. Pathol. 5, 733–744.

Yamaki, T., Morimoto, S., Ohtaki, M., et al., 1998. Intracranial facial nerve neurinoma: surgical strategy of tumor removal and functional reconstruction. Surg. Neurol. 49 (5), 538–546.

Yasui, T., Hakuba, A., Kim, S.H., et al., 1989. Trigeminal neurinomas: operative approach in eight cases. J. Neurosurg. 71, 506–511.

• Yoshida, K., Kawase, T., 1999. Trigeminal neurinomas extending into multiple fossae: surgical methods and review of the literature. J. Neurosurg. 91, 202–211.

• Zhang, L., Yang, Y., Xu, S., et al., 2009. Trigeminal schwannomas: a report of 42 cases and review of the relevant surgical approaches. Clin. Neurol. Neurosurg. 111 (3), 261–269.

Zulch, K.J., 1962. Brain tumors: their biology and pathology. Springer-Verlag, New York.

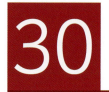

30 Brain tumors associated with neurofibromatosis

Ashok R. Asthagiri, Katherine E. Warren, and Russell R. Lonser

Introduction

The neurofibromatoses include three genetically distinct tumor predisposition syndromes that affect the nervous system. Because of the significant influence of Harvey Cushing and their common proclivity to develop nerve sheath tumors, the neurofibromatoses remained inextricably intertwined as one diagnostic entity until the late twentieth century (Cushing 1917). Despite reports delineating the clinical features distinct to neurofibromatosis type I (NF-1) and neurofibromatosis type II (NF-2), it was not until 1987 that these syndromes were formally separated by nomenclature and unique diagnostic criteria established for each (NIH 1987). More recently, a third clinically and genetically distinct tumor predisposition syndrome has been distinguished from NF-2, termed schwannomatosis. In this chapter, we discuss the genetics and molecular pathobiology underlying these tumor predisposition syndromes, diagnostic schema used to clinically identify the disorders and how management of intracranial tumors in these patient populations differ from analogous tumors found in the general population.

Neurofibromatosis type 1

Mark Akenside, an English poet and physician, published the first case of NF-1 (von Recklinghausen's disease, peripheral neurofibromatosis) in 1768 (Akenside 1768). In this report, he described a 60-year-old man who inherited from his father the propensity to develop multiple pedunculated cutaneous tumors (dermal neurofibromas). The eponym for the disease is named after Friedrich Daniel von Recklinghausen, a German pathologist who labeled the characteristic tumors 'neurofibromas' and systematically described their histopathologic appearance (Von Recklinghausen 1882). NF-1 is the most common of the neurofibromatoses, occurring approximately 1 in 3000 live births (Huson et al 1989; Lammert et al 2005). No gender, race or ethnic specificity has been identified.

Genetics and molecular biology

NF-1 is inherited as an autosomal dominant trait with nearly 100% penetrance by 20 years of age, although significant variability in expressivity may be present between family members carrying the same mutation (Obringer et al 1989; DeBella et al 1999). Approximately 50% of cases are caused by new mutations (Friedman 1999). These sporadic cases may be the result of a germline mutation or, less commonly, a mutation of the *NF-1* gene occurring during the postzygotic stage of embryogenesis. The latter results in somatic mosaicism. In patients with somatic mosaicism, the proportion of affected cells and tissue types affected varies with timing of the mutational event during embryogenesis and the cell type in which change occurs. Thus, the clinical phenotype can range from generalized disease to localized (segmental) disease (Ruggieri & Huson 2001).

NF-1 is a multiple neoplasia syndrome resulting from a mutation in the *NF-1 tumor suppressor gene* located on chromosome 17q. The *NF-1* gene, isolated and sequenced in 1990, encompasses a 350 kb region of genomic DNA that encodes for a 220 to 250 kDa protein product, termed 'neurofibromin' (Wallace et al 1990; DeClue et al 1991; Gutmann et al 1991). Analysis of the protein sequence revealed a 360 amino acid region with significant similarity to guanosine triphosphatase (GTPase)-activating proteins (GAP) catalytic domains (Xu et al 1990). Subsequently, it was shown that neurofibromin mediates tumor suppression through inhibition of Ras, a key regulator of signal transduction, proliferation and malignant transformation (DeClue et al 1992). Consistent with Knudson's two hit model of tumorigenesis, brain tumors that develop in NF-1 patients demonstrate loss of heterozygosity (LOH) at the NF-1 locus (Gutmann et al 2000). Interestingly, NF-1 haploinsufficiency has been shown to result in a cell-autonomous growth advantage for astrocytes, suggesting that some of the non-neoplastic neurologic manifestations in NF-1 patients may be the result of their heterozygous, haploinsufficient condition (Bajenaru et al 2001).

Clinical characteristics and diagnosis

Patients with neurofibromatosis type I develop both benign and malignant tumors affecting the nervous system as well as other neurologic, vascular, dermatologic, skeletal, and ophthalmologic manifestations. The NIH criteria for diagnosis of NF-1 remains based on the identification of at least two characteristic clinical features, or one in a patient with a 1st degree relative with NF-1. The clinical features include the presence of: (1) six or more café-au-lait macules (>5 mm in greatest diameter in pre-pubertal individuals and >15 mm in greatest diameter in post-pubertal individuals); (2) two or more neurofibromas of any type or one plexiform neurofibroma; (3) freckling in the axillary or inguinal regions; (4) an optic pathway glioma; (5) two or more iris hamartomas (Lisch nodules); and (6) a distinctive osseous lesion, such as sphenoid wing dysplasia or thinning of the long bone cortex, with or without pseudarthrosis (Table 30.1) (Stumpf et al 1988).

Clinical features of NF-1 are apparent in most affected individuals by 8 years of age, although these may not be sufficient to satisfy NIH criteria for diagnosis in infants and young children carrying the NF-1 mutation (Korf 1992). Although the clinical manifestations of NF-1 may be

Table 30.1 Diagnostic criteria of neurofibromatoses

NF-1 (NIH 1988) Must have two or more of the following:	NF-2 (Evans et al 2005a) Principal finding		Additional findings needed for diagnosis	Schwannomatosis (Baser et al 2006) • Must not fulfill diagnostic criteria for NF-2; • have no evidence of vestibular schwannoma by MR-imaging; • no 1st-degree relative with NF-2; • and no known constitutional NF-2 mutation		
≥6 café-au-lait macules (0.5 cm in children or >1.5 cm in adults)	Bilateral vestibular schwannomas	+	None	*Definite*		
≥2 cutaneous/subcutaneous neurofibromas or one plexiform neurofibroma	Family history	+	Unilateral vestibular schwannoma or two NF-2-associated lesions (meningioma, glioma, neurofibroma, schwannoma, or cataract)	Age >30 years	+	≥2 non-intradermal schwannomas, at least one with histologic confirmation
Axillary or groin freckling	Unilateral vestibular schwannoma	+	Two NF-2-associated lesions associated with the disorder (meningioma, glioma, neurofibroma, schwannoma, or cataract)	One pathologically confirmed schwannoma	+	A 1st-degree relative who meets the above criteria
Optic pathway glioma	Multiple meningiomas	+	Unilateral vestibular schwannoma or two other NF-2-associated lesions (glioma, neurofibromas, schwannoma, or cataract)	*Possible*		
≥2 Lisch nodules (iris hamartomas seen on slit lamp examination)				Age <30 years	+	Two or more non-intradermal schwannomas, at least one with histologic confirmation
Bony dysplasia (sphenoid wing dysplasia, bowing of long bone, pseudarthrosis)				Age >45 years	+	Two or more non-intradermal schwannomas, at least one with histologic confirmation
1st degree relative with NF-1				Radiographic evidence of a schwannoma	+	1st-degree relative meeting the criteria for definite schwannomatosis
				Segmental Meets criteria for either definite or possible schwannomatosis but limited to one limb or ≤5 contiguous segments of the spine		

protean, the overall course of disease is generally progressive. Although disfigurement caused by dermal neurofibromas and plexiform neurofibromas are the most overt feature of NF-1, histologically benign gliomas of the optic pathway and brainstem may be associated with significant morbidity and mortality. By 70 years of age, the cumulative risk for development of brain and central nervous system tumors among NF-1 patients is 7.9%, compared with 4.6% among the general population (Walker et al 2006). There is also an increased risk (2.7 times higher) of developing cancer among NF-1 patients when compared with the general population (Walker et al 2006). Cumulative morbidity from systemic manifestations and NF-1-associated malignancies results in a significant decrease in life expectancy. A retrospective review of US death certificates from 1983 through 1997 performed by the National Center for Health Statistics, reported mean and median ages at death for persons with NF-1 was 54.4 and 59 years, compared with 70.1 and 74 years among the general population (Rasmussen et al 2001).

Brain tumor types

Optic pathway gliomas

Optic pathway tumors account for 2–5% of all brain tumors in childhood, of which the majority (70%) are NF-1-associated

(Listernick et al 1999a; Czyzyk et al 2003). The prevalence of optic pathway gliomas in NF-1 may be as high as 15–21% (Lewis et al 1984; Lund & Skovby 1991). NF-1-associated optic pathway gliomas are generally pilocytic astrocytomas (World Health Organization grade I). Pilocytic astrocytomas are the most common (17%) primary brain tumor among children, but sporadic cases are most frequently identified in an infratentorial location (CBTRUS 2008).

Optic pathway gliomas in NF-1 typically involve the optic nerve, but may also affect the chiasm and post-chiasmal extension of the afferent optic pathway (Fig. 30.1). Bilateral optic nerve tumors are exclusive to NF-1. The majority of optic pathway gliomas in NF-1 present in early childhood, with a peak incidence between ages 4–6 years (Listernick et al 1994). When symptomatic, patients may present secondary to endocrinopathy (precocious puberty), ophthalmologic symptoms (proptosis, decreased visual acuity, strabismus), raised intracranial pressure, and/or other neurologic signs (motor deficits, psychomotor retardation, seizures). Proptosis and painless unilateral visual loss accompany intraorbital lesions. Due to their anatomic location, chiasmatic and post-chiasmal lesions are more commonly associated with bilateral visual loss, endocrinopathy (involvement of hypothalamus) and raised intracranial pressure (hydrocephalus).

age (Abaza et al 1996; Baser et al 2002c; Mautner et al 2002; Slattery et al 2004; Baser et al 2005b).

Vestibular schwannomas are best visualized by high resolution contrast-enhanced T1-weighted MR imaging (Fig. 30.2). These tumors tend to assume a more lobular growth pattern than sporadic vestibular schwannomas, appearing as 'grape-like' clusters by MR-imaging (Cushing 1917; Sobel & Wang 1993). Fat saturation protocols are critical in the assessment of tumor burden in the setting of previous surgery, as many surgical interventions employ the use of autologous fat grafting. T2-weighted or FLAIR sequences are used to quantify peritumoral edema and cysts, and may help characterize the course of the cranial nerves within the cerebrospinal cisterns with a high level of accuracy.

Since no significant relationship between mutation type, vestibular schwannoma size, vestibular schwannoma growth rate and hearing loss has been established in NF-2, proposed treatment paradigms reflect regional treatment patterns and experience. The Gold Standard for management of vestibular schwannomas in NF-2 remains surgical removal of the lesion, although timing of intervention is controversial. Surgical resection of vestibular schwannomas in NF-2 are associated with increased morbidity because they tend to invade the cochlear and facial nerves, compared with sporadic vestibular schwannomas that commonly displace and compress the neighboring neural elements (Sobel & Wang 1993; Jääskeläinen et al 1994). Early proactive surgical management of smaller vestibular schwannomas (<3 cm) can preserve measurable hearing and normal facial nerve function in 57–70% and 75–92% of patients, respectively (Brackmann et al 2001; Samii et al 1997).

Another option for the treatment of vestibular schwannomas in NF-2 is stereotactic radiosurgery. Utilizing current radiation doses (14 Gy or less to margin, maximum dose <28 Gy), gadolinium-enhanced MRI planning and stereotactic delivery, local control was observed in 74–100% of tumors over an average follow-up period of 54 months. Measurable hearing and normal facial nerve function was maintained in 33–57% and 92–100% of patients, respectively, in this treatment group (Kida et al 2000; Roche et al 2000; Rowe et al 2003; Mathieu et al 2007). Longer-term follow-up revealing sustained low risk for malignant transformation in a neoplasia predisposition disease and durable local control are still needed (Baser et al 2000; Rowe et al 2007). Other concerns include increased difficulty of post-radiotherapy operation due to scar formation and maintaining viability of the cochlear nerve for future hearing rehabilitation procedures.

In patients with hearing loss, where the cochlear nerve is anatomically preserved and physiologic integrity is confirmed with promontory stimulation, cochlear implantation may afford sustained improvement in hearing (Hoffman et al 1992; Neff et al 2007). When the physiologic integrity of the nerve is compromised, the only current option for hearing rehabilitation is the auditory brainstem implant (ABI). NF-2 patients with multi-channel ABIs obtain environmental sound and significant lip reading assistance, but few obtain significant open-set speech understanding (Otto et al 2002; Schwartz et al 2008).

Currently, chemotherapeutic agents, including anti-angiogenic drugs (bevacizumab, PTC2999) and tyrosine kinase inhibitors (lapatinib) are entering early phase clinical trials after preliminary salvage-therapy based investigation revealed improved hearing in 57% of patients and imaging response (vestibular schwannoma volume reduction by 20%) in 60% of NF-2 patients after treatment with bevacizumab (Plotkin et al 2009). Further study into the chronic effects of long-term use and durability of effect will be needed before it can be determined which patients may benefit from these forms of therapy.

Meningiomas

Meningiomas are the second most frequently encountered tumor associated with NF-2. Intracranial meningiomas are present in 45–58% of patients (Evans et al 1992a; Parry et al 1994; Mautner et al 1996). NF-2-associated cranial meningiomas occur earlier in life than sporadic tumors and are frequently multiple (Parry et al 1994; Mautner et al 1996; Evans et al 1999; Nunes & MacCollin 2003). A diagnosis of NF-2 may occur in 10–18% of children who initially present with a 'sporadic' meningioma, and therefore full screening and longitudinal follow-up should be performed in these patients (Evans et al 1999; Evans et al 2005b).

Meningiomas in NF-2 produce clinical symptoms due to compression of adjacent neural structures, the sequelae of which are determined by tumor location. Convexity tumors may enlarge to great proportions before the onset of headaches, changes in visual acuity or seizures develop. On the contrary, smaller tumors of the optic nerve sheath, skull base and spinal canal may cause profound symptoms. Their location in the cerebellopontine angle may be masked by the presence of large vestibular schwannomas. The natural history of meningiomas in NF-2 has not been extensively studied, but their presence marks a more clinically severe form of NF-2.

Cranial meningiomas are best visualized by contrast-enhanced T1-weighted MRI (Fig. 30.2). These lesions typically show homogenous contrast uptake, delineating them from adjacent neural structures. T2-weighted or FLAIR sequences highlight the extent of edema in adjacent neural tissues. Characteristically, a region of enhancement may be appreciated trailing away from the central mass of the tumor along the dura, referred to as the 'dural tail' (Goldsher et al 1990). Difficulties in radiologic evaluation are most evident in identifying early optic nerve sheath meningiomas, where dedicated coronal, high spatial resolution fat-saturated gadolinium enhanced sections of the orbit may need to be performed (Jackson et al 2003; Wichmann 2004). Additionally, meningiomas of the cavernous sinus and cerebellopontine angle may be difficult to discern from large, robustly enhancing schwannomas in the same location.

Meningiomas located on the cerebral convexities are typically well-defined extra-axial lesions that typically respect arachnoidal planes. There is an increased risk for recurrence when adjacent brain-invasion is present (Perry et al 1997). Skull base tumors may encompass and incorporate cranial nerves passing through cranial foramina or the cavernous sinus. All major histologic subtypes of meningiomas occur in NF-2 patients, although the fibroblastic variant appears overrepresented (Goldsher et al 1990; Antinheimo et al 1995). A more aggressive clinical phenotype in NF-2 patients is supported by the presence of an increased proliferative activity and a greater frequency of atypical (WHO grade II) and anaplastic (WHO grade III) tumors (Antinheimo et al 1997; Perry et al 2001).

Because of the limited risk and curative nature of complete excision, surgery remains the mainstay of treatment of symptomatic NF-2 lesions of the cerebral convexity and spinal canal. Tumors of the skull base, including those of the cavernous sinus, cerebello-pontine angle, clinoid process and petrous apex may receive benefit in cranial nerve function and relief of mass effect with debulking procedures, but complete resection may be associated with high morbidity (Larson et al 1995; Couldwell et al 1996). Optic nerve sheath meningiomas may be successfully operated upon if detected at a stage when the tumor tissue has not yet advanced far into the optic canal. The limited operability of these 'high-risk' meningiomas among sporadic cases has led to the utilization of adjuvant stereotactic radiosurgery to promote local control of tumor residual (Kondziolka et al 1999). Studies reporting on the safety and efficacy of this combined approach in the management of high-risk meningiomas in the NF-2 population has not been reported upon (Couldwell et al 2006).

Non-vestibular, cranial nerve schwannomas and gliomas

Schwannomas may occur along the course of other cranial nerves (Fig. 30.3). Up to half of patients with NF-2 may harbor non-vestibular cranial nerve schwannomas which usually arise from cranial nerves III, V, and VII, although lesions of the lower cranial nerves are more frequently associated with symptom development (Mautner et al 1996; Samii et al 1997; Fisher et al 2007). Gliomas (primarily ependymomas) are present in 18–53% of NF-2 patients but cause clinical symptoms in fewer than 20% (Asthagiri et al 2009). Although the majority of these tumors are located within the spinal cord, a small proportion may be positioned rostrally within the brainstem. The natural history of non-vestibular schwannomas and gliomas in NF-2 remains unknown; therefore, management remains based on symptom development and is primarily surgical.

Schwannomatosis

Because a clear understanding of the clinical spectra of NF-2 was not delineated until the mid-1990s and the clinical phenotypes of NF-2 and schwannomatosis partially overlap, early reports that identified patients with multiple schwannomas often included an admixture of patients (Shishiba et al 1984; Purcell & Dixon 1989). As more reports accumulated identifying a sub-group of patients who developed multiple schwannomas of the peripheral nerves without the remaining clinical manifestations associated with NF-2, it became clear that a third nerve sheath tumor predisposition

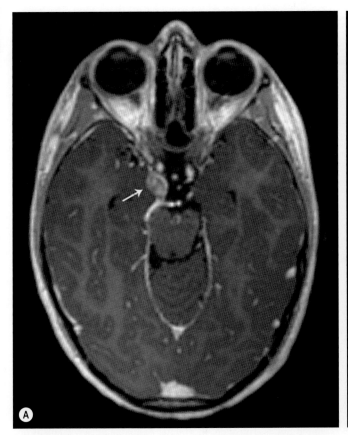
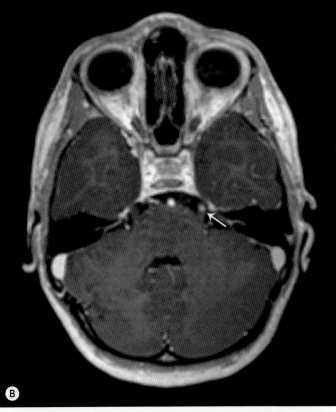

Figure 30.3 Gadolinium enhanced T1-weighted MR-imaging reveals non-vestibular nerve schwannomas of the (A) oculomotor nerve (arrow) and (B) trigeminal nerve (arrow). These may be identified in patients with either neurofibromatosis type 2 or schwannomatosis. Patients with non-vestibular schwannomas and a suspected diagnosis of schwannomatosis should be thoroughly screened for the presence of other NF-2-associated lesions.

syndrome phenotype had been identified ('schwannomatosis', 'multiple neurilemmomas', and 'multiple schwannomas') (Tanabe et al 1997; Shin et al 1998; Pandit et al 2000). Subsequently, the NF-2 locus was excluded as the germline event in cases of familial schwannomatosis, and the tumor suppressor gene *INI1/SMARCB1* was identified as the predisposing gene in familial and sporadic cases of schwannomatosis (MacCollin et al 2003; Buckley et al 2005; Hulsebos et al 2007; Hadfield et al 2008). No published data report the prevalence or birth incidence, but a population-based study in Finland estimated the annual incidence of newly identified cases of schwannomatosis was similar to that of NF-2 (Antinheimo et al 2000).

Several features distinguish schwannomatosis from NF-2. Indeed, the diagnostic criteria for schwannomatosis require exclusion of a diagnosis of NF-2, lack of vestibular nerve involvement by MR-imaging, no family history of NF-2 and the patient must not have a *known* (genetic testing to exclude NF-2 is not required) constitutional mutation of the *NF-2* gene (MacCollin et al 2005; Baser et al 2006). Characteristic ocular findings of NF-2 (presenile cataracts, retinal hematoma) and NF-1 (Lisch nodules) are also notably absent in schwannomatosis. Therefore, early evaluation of the patient with suspected schwannomatosis should include ophthalmologic examination and high resolution MR-imaging of the internal auditory canal.

Although schwannomatosis can be inherited in an autosomal dominant manner, the majority of cases are de novo and risk of transmission to offspring is significantly reduced in patients with de novo disease (15%) (MacCollin et al 2003) The most common presenting symptom of schwannomatosis is intractable pain, often associated with a peripheral nerve tumor mass (MacCollin et al 2005). Patients with schwannomatosis may develop non-vestibular nerve cranial nerve schwannomas that may become symptomatic due to functional motor deficit, numbness, pain, or local mass effect (Westhout et al 2007). Treatment of intracranial tumors associated with schwannomatosis is primarily symptom-driven and remains surgical for lesions causing significant mass effect.

Key points

- The neurofibromatoses are composed of three genetically and phenotypically distinct disorders: NF-1, NF-2, and schwannomatosis.

- Neurofibromatosis type 1 is associated with the development of brain tumors, including optic pathway gliomas and brainstem gliomas. These tumors, when compared to their sporadic counterparts, have a more favorable natural history and do not require treatment unless clinical and/or radiographic progression is clearly identified.

- In addition to bilateral vestibular schwannomas, patients with neurofibromatosis type 2 may develop other brain tumors including: intracranial meningiomas, non-vestibular nerve cranial nerve schwannomas, and brainstem ependymomas. Treatment of intracranial tumors associated with NF-2 typically remains symptom driven.

- Patients with schwannomatosis may develop non-vestibular nerve cranial nerve schwannomas in addition to schwannomas of other peripheral nerves. A diagnosis of schwannomatosis requires exclusion of a diagnosis of NF-2.

REFERENCES

Abaza, M.M., Makariou, E., Armstrong, M., et al., 1996. Growth rate characteristics of acoustic neuromas associated with neurofibromatosis type 2. Laryngoscope 106 (6), 694–699.

Akenside, M., 1768. Observations on cancers. Med. Trans. Coll. Phys. Lond. 1, 64–92.

Alfthan, K., Heiska, L., Grönholm, M., et al., 2004. Cyclic AMP-dependent protein kinase phosphorylates merlin at serine 518 independently of p21-activated kinase and promotes merlin-ezrin heterodimerization. J. Biol. Chem. 279 (18), 18559–18566.

Antinheimo, J., Haapasalo, H., Haltia, M., et al., 1997. Proliferation potential and histological features in neurofibromatosis 2-associated and sporadic meningiomas. J. Neurosurg. 87 (4), 610–614.

Antinheimo, J., Haapasalo, H., Seppälä, M., et al., 1995. Proliferative potential of sporadic and neurofibromatosis-2-associated Schwannomas as studied by MIB-1 (Ki-67) and PCNA labeling. J. Neuropathol. Exp. Neurol. 54 (6), 776–782.

Antinheimo, J., Sankila, R., Carpén, O., et al., 2000. Population-based analysis of sporadic and type 2 neurofibromatosis-associated meningiomas and schwannomas. Neurology 54 (1), 71–76.

Aoki, S., Barkovich, A.J., Nishimura, K., et al., 1989. Neurofibromatosis types 1 and 2: Cranial MR findings. Radiology 172 (2), 527–534.

Asthagiri, A.R., Parry, D.M., Butman, J.A., et al., 2009. Neurofibromatosis type 2. Lancet 373 (9679), 1974–1986.

Bajenaru, M.L., Donahoe, J., Corral, T., et al., 2001. Neurofibromatosis 1 (NF-1) heterozygosity results in a cell-autonomous growth advantage for astrocytes. Glia 33 (4), 314–323.

Barkovich, A.J., Krischer, J., Kun, L.E., et al., 1990. Brain stem gliomas: A classification system based on magnetic resonance imaging. Pediatr. Neurosurg. 16 (2), 73–83.

Baser, M.E., Evans, D.G., Jackler, R.K., et al., 2000. Neurofibromatosis 2, radiosurgery and malignant nervous system tumours. Br. J. Cancer 82 (4), 998.

Baser, M.E., Friedman, J.M., Aeschliman, D., et al., 2002a. Predictors of the risk of mortality in neurofibromatosis 2. Am. J. Hum. Genet. 71 (4), 715–723.

Baser, M.E., Friedman, J.M., Evans, D.G., 2006. Increasing the specificity of diagnostic criteria for schwannomatosis. Neurology 66 (5), 730–732.

Baser, M.E., Friedman, J.M., Wallace, A.J., et al., 2002b. Evaluation of clinical diagnostic criteria for neurofibromatosis 2. Neurology 59 (11), 1759–1765.

Baser, M.E., Kuramoto, L., Woods, R., et al., 2005a. The location of constitutional neurofibromatosis 2 (NF-2) splice site mutations is associated with the severity of NF-2. J. Med. Genet. 42 (7), 540–546.

Baser, M.E., Makariou, E.V., Parry, D.M., 2002c. Predictors of vestibular schwannoma growth in patients with neurofibromatosis Type 2. J. Neurosurg. 96 (2), 217–222.

Baser, M.E., Mautner, V.F., Parry, D.M., et al., 2005b. Methodological issues in longitudinal studies: Vestibular schwannoma growth rates in neurofibromatosis 2. J. Med. Genet. 42 (12), 903–906.

Bianchi, A.B., Hara, T., Ramesh, V., et al., 1994. Mutations in transcript isoforms of the neurofibromatosis 2 gene in multiple human tumour types. Nat. Genet. 6 (2), 185–192.

Bourn, D., Carter, S.A., Evans, D.G., et al., 1994. A mutation in the neurofibromatosis type 2 tumor-suppressor gene, giving rise to widely different clinical phenotypes in two unrelated individuals. Am. J. Hum. Genet. 55 (1), 69–73.

Brackmann, D.E., Fayad, J.N., Slattery, W.H. 3rd, et al., 2001. Early proactive management of vestibular schwannomas in neurofibromatosis Type 2. Neurosurgery 49 (2), 274–283.

Buckley, P.G., Mantripragada, K.K., Díaz de Ståhl, T., et al., 2005. Identification of genetic aberrations on chromosome 22 outside the NF-2 locus in schwannomatosis and neurofibromatosis type 2. Hum. Mutat. 26 (6), 540–549.

CBTRUS, 2008. Statistical Report: Primary brain tumors in the United States, 2000–2004. Central Brain Tumor Registry of the United States, Hinsdale, IL. Online. Available at: www.cbtrus.org

Cohen, M.E., Duffner, P.K., Heffner, R.R., et al., 1986. Prognostic factors in brainstem gliomas. Neurology 36 (5), 602–605.

Cohen, M.E., Duffner, P.K., Heffner, R.R., et al., 2005. Fractionated stereotactic radiotherapy of optic pathway gliomas: tolerance and long-term outcome. Int. J. Radiat. Oncol. Biol. Phys. 62 (3), 814–819.

Couldwell, W.T., Fukushima, T., Giannotta, S.L., et al., 1996. Petroclival meningiomas: Surgical experience in 109 cases. J. Neurosurg. 84 (1), 20–28.

Couldwell, W.T., Kan, P., Liu, J.K., et al., 2006. Decompression of cavernous sinus meningioma for preservation and improvement of cranial nerve function: Technical note. J. Neurosurg. 105 (1), 148–152.

Cushing, H., 1917. Tumors of the nervus acusticus and the syndrome of the cerebellopontine angle. WE Dandy, Philadelphia, PA.

Czyzyk, E., Jóźwiak, S., Roszkowski, M., et al., 2003. Optic pathway gliomas in children with and without neurofibromatosis 1. J. Child Neurol. 18 (7), 471–478.

DeBella, K., Szudek, J., Friedman, J.M., 1999. Use of the N I H criteria for diagnosis of NF-1 in children. Pediatrics 105, 608–614.

DeClue, J.E., Cohen, B.D., Lowy, D.R., 1991. Identification and characterization of the neurofibromatosis type 1 protein product. Proc. Natl. Acad. Sci. USA 88 (22), 9914–9918.

DeClue, J.E., Papageorge, A.G., Fletcher, J.A., et al., 1992. Abnormal regulation of mammalian p21(ras) contributes to malignant tumor growth in von Recklinghausen (type 1) neurofibromatosis. Cell 69 (2), 265–273.

Degen, J.W., Walbridge, S., Vortmeyer, A.O., et al., 2003. Safety and efficacy of convection-enhanced delivery of gemcitabine or carboplatin in a malignant glioma model in rats. J. Neurosurg. 99 (5), 893–898.

Duffner, P.K., Cohen, M.E., Seidel, F.G., et al., 1989. The significance of M R I abnormalities in children with neurofibromatosis. Neurology 39 (3), 373–378.

Dumanski, J.P., Carlbom, E., Collins, V.P., et al., 1987. Deletion mapping of a locus on human chromosome 22 involved in the oncogenesis of meningioma. Proc. Natl. Acad. Sci. USA 84 (24), 9275–9279.

Eldridge, R., Parry, D.M., Kaiser-Kupfer, M.I., 1991. Neurofibromatosis 2 (NF-2): Clinical heterogeneity and natural history based on 39 individuals in 9 families and 16 sporadic cases. Am. J. Hum. Genet. 49 (Suppl.), 133.

Epstein, F., McCleary, E.L., 1986. Intrinsic brain-stem tumors of childhood: surgical indications. J. Neurosurg. 64 (1), 11–15.

Evans, D.G., Birch, J.M., Ramsden, R.T., 1999. Paediatric presentation of type 2 neurofibromatosis. Arch. Dis. Childh. 81 (6), 496–499.

Evans, D.G., Huson, S.M., Donnai, D., et al., 1992a. A clinical study of type 2 neurofibromatosis. Q. J. Med. 84 (304), 603–618.

Evans, D.G., Huson, S.M., Donnai, D., et al., 1992b. A genetic study of type 2 neurofibromatosis in the United Kingdom. I. Prevalence, mutation rate, fitness, and confirmation of maternal transmission effect on severity. J. Med. Genet. 29 (12), 841–846.

Evans, D.G., Ramsden, R.T., Shenton, A., et al., 2007. Mosaicism in neurofibromatosis type 2: An update of risk based on uni/bilaterality of vestibular schwannoma at presentation and sensitive mutation analysis including multiple ligation-dependent probe amplification. J. Med. Genet. 44 (7), 424–428.

Evans, D.G., Trueman, L., Wallace, A., et al., 1998. Genotype/phenotype correlations in type 2 neurofibromatosis (NF-2): Evidence for more severe disease associated with truncating mutations. J. Med. Genet. 35 (6), 450–455.

Evans, D.G., Baser, M.E., O'Reilly, B., et al., 2005a. Management of the patient and family with neurofibromatosis 2: a consensus conference statement. Br. J. Neurosurg. 19 (1), 5–12.

Evans, D.G., Watson, C., King, A., et al., 2005b. Multiple meningiomas: differential involvement of the NF-2 gene in children and adults. J. Med. Genet. 42 (1), 45–48.

Evans, D.G., Moran, A., King, A., et al., 2005c. Incidence of vestibular schwannoma and neurofibromatosis 2 in the North West of England over a 10-year period: Higher incidence than previously thought. Otol. Neurotol. 26 (1), 93–97.

Feiling, A., Ward, E., 1920. A familial form of acoustic tumour. BMJ 10, 496–497.

Fischbein, N.J., Prados, M.D., Wara, W., et al., 1996. Radiologic classification of brain stem tumors: Correlation of magnetic resonance imaging appearance with clinical outcome. Pediatr. Neurosurg. 24 (1), 9–23.

Fisher, L.M., Doherty, J.K., Lev, M.H., et al., 2007. Distribution of nonvestibular cranial nerve schwannomas in neurofibromatosis 2. Otol. Neurotol. 28 (8), 1083–1090.

Frazier, J.L., Lee, J., Thomale, U.W., et al., 2009. Treatment of diffuse intrinsic brainstem gliomas: Failed approaches and future strategies – A review. J. Neurosurg. Pediatr. 3 (4), 259–269.

Friedman, J.M., 1999. Epidemiology of neurofibromatosis type 1. Am. J. Med. Genet. 89 (1), 1–6.

Gardner, W.J., Frazier, C.H., 1930. Bilateral acoustic neurofibromas: A clinical study and field survey of a family of five generations with bilateral deafness in thirty-eight members. Arch. Neurol. Psychiatr. 23, 266–302.

Goldsher, D., Litt, A.W., Pinto, R.S., et al., 1990. Dural 'tail' associated with meningiomas on Gd-DTPA-enhanced M R images: Characteristics, differential diagnostic value, and possible implications for treatment. Radiology 176 (2), 447–450.

Gutmann, D.H., Donahoe, J., Brown, T., et al., 2000. Loss of neurofibromatosis 1 (NF-1) gene expression in NF-1-associated pilocytic astrocytomas. Neuropathol. Appl. Neurobiol. 26 (4), 361–367.

Gutmann, D.H., Wood, D.L., Collins, F.S., 1991. Identification of the neurofibromatosis type 1 gene product. Proc. Natl. Acad. Sci. USA 88 (21), 9658–9662.

Hadfield, K.D., Newman, W.G., Bowers, N.L., et al., 2008. Molecular characterisation of SMARCB1 and NF-2 in familial and sporadic schwannomatosis. J. Med. Genet. 45 (6), 332–339.

Hoffman, R.A., Kohan, D., Cohen, N.L., 1992. Cochlear implants in the management of bilateral acoustic neuromas. Am. J. Otol. 13 (6), 525–528.

Hulsebos, T.J., Plomp, A.S., Wolterman, R.A., et al., 2007. Germline mutation of INI1/SMARCB1 in familial schwannomatosis. Am. J. Hum. Genet. 80 (4), 805–810.

Huson, S.M., Compston, D.A., Clark, P., et al., 1989. A genetic study of von Recklinghausen neurofibromatosis in south east Wales. I prevalence, fitness, mutation rate, and effect of parental transmission on severity. J. Med. Genet. 26 (11), 704–711.

Itoh, T., Magnaldi, S., White, R.M., et al., 1994. Neurofibromatosis type 1: The evolution of deep gray and white matter M R abnormalities. AJNR Am. J. Neuroradiol. 15 (8), 1513–1519.

Jääskeläinen, J., Paetau, A., Pyykkö, I., et al., 1994. Interface between the facial nerve and large acoustic neurinomas. Immunohistochemical study of the cleavage plane in NF-2 and non-NF-2 cases. J. Neurosurg. 80 (3), 541–547.

Jackson, A., Patankar, T., Laitt, R.D., 2003. Intracanalicular optic nerve meningioma: A serious diagnostic pitfall. AJNR. Am. J. Neuroradiol. 24 (6), 1167–1170.

Jahraus, C.D., Tarbell, N.J., 2006. Optic pathway gliomas. Pediatr. Blood Cancer 46 (5), 586–596.

Jallo, G., 2006. Brainstem gliomas. Childs Nerv. Syst. 22 (1), 1–2.

Kanter, W.R., Eldridge, R., Fabricant, R., et al., 1980. Central neurofibromatosis with bilateral acoustic neuroma: genetic, clinical and biochemical distinctions from peripheral neurofibromatosis. Neurology 30 (8), 851–859.

Kaplan, A.M., Albright, A.L., Zimmerman, R.A., et al., 1996. Brainstem gliomas in children. A children's cancer group review of 119 cases. Pediatr. Neurosurg. 24 (4), 185–192.

Kestle, J.R., Hoffman, H.J., Mock, A.R., 1993. Moyamoya phenomenon after radiation for optic glioma. J. Neurosurg. 79 (1), 32–35.

Kida, Y., Kobayashi, T., Tanaka, T., et al., 2000. Radiosurgery for bilateral neurinomas associated with neurofibromatosis type 2. Surg. Neurol. 53 (4), 383–390.

King, A., Listernick, R., Charrow, J., et al., 2003. Optic pathway gliomas in neurofibromatosis type 1: The effect of presenting symptoms on outcome. Am. J. Med. Genet. 122 A(2), 95–99.

Kissil, J.L., Johnson, K.C., Eckman, M.S., et al., 2002. Merlin phosphorylation by p21-activated kinase 2 and effects of phosphorylation on merlin localization. J. Biol. Chem. 277 (12), 10394–10399.

Kluwe, L., Mautner, V.F., 1998. Mosaicism in sporadic neurofibromatosis 2 patients. Hum. Mol. Genet. 7 (13), 2051–2055.

Knudson, A.G. Jr., 1971. Mutation and cancer: statistical study of retinoblastoma. Proc. Natl. Acad. Sci. U. S. A. 68 (4), 820–823.

Kondziolka, D., Levy, E.I., Niranjan, A., et al., 1999. Long-term outcomes after meningioma radiosurgery: Physician and patient perspectives. J. Neurosurg. 91 (1), 44–50.

Korf, B.R., 1992. Diagnostic outcome in children with multiple cafe au lait spots. Pediatrics 90 (6), 924–927.

Kortmann, R.D., Timmermann, B., Paulsen, F., et al., 2002. The role of radiotherapy in the management of low grade glioma of the visual pathway in children. Neuro-Ophthalmol. 27 (1–3), 17–37.

Lafay-Cousin, L., Holm, S., Qaddoumi, I., et al., 2005. Weekly vinblastine in pediatric low-grade glioma patients with carboplatin allergic reaction. Cancer 103 (12), 2636–2642.

Lammert, M., Friedman, J.M., Kluwe, L., et al., 2005. Prevalence of neurofibromatosis 1 in German children at elementary school enrollment. Arch. Dermatol. 141 (1), 71–74.

Larson, J.J., van Loveren, H.R., Balko, M.G., et al., 1995. Evidence of meningioma infiltration into cranial nerves: Clinical implications for cavernous sinus meningiomas. J. Neurosurg. 83 (4), 596–599.

Lewis, R.A., Gerson, L.P., Axelson, K.A., et al., 1984. Von Recklinghausen neurofibromatosis. II. Incidence of optic gliomata. Ophthalmology 91 (8), 929–935.

Listernick, R., Charrow, J., Greenwald, M., et al., 1994. Natural history of optic pathway tumors in children with neurofibromatosis type 1: A longitudinal study. J. Pediatr. 125 (1), 63–66.

Listernick, R., Charrow, J., Gutmann, D.H., 1999a. Intracranial gliomas in neurofibromatosis type 1. Am. J. Med. Genet. 89 (1), 38–44.

Listernick, R., Charrow, J., Tomita, T., et al., 1999b. Carboplatin therapy for optic pathway tumors in children with neurofibromatosis type-1. J. Neurooncol. 45 (2), 185–190.

Listernick, R., Darling, C., Greenwald, M., et al., 1995. Optic pathway tumors in children: The effect of neurofibromatosis type 1 on clinical manifestations and natural history. J. Pediatr. 127 (5), 718–722.

Listernick, R., Ferner, R.E., Liu, G.T., et al., 2007. Optic pathway gliomas in neurofibromatosis-1: Controversies and recommendations. Ann. Neurol. 61 (3), 189–198.

Listernick, R., Ferner, R.E., Piersall, L., et al., 2004. Late-onset optic pathway tumors in children with neurofibromatosis 1. Neurology 63 (10), 1944–1946.

Liu, G.T., 2006. Optic gliomas of the anterior visual pathway. Curr. Opin. Ophthalmol. 17 (5), 427–431.

Lund, A.M., Skovby, F., 1991. Optic gliomas in children with neurofibromatosis type 1. Eur. J. Pediatr. 150 (12), 835–838.

MacCollin, M., Chiocca, E.A., Evans, D.G., et al., 2005. Diagnostic criteria for schwannomatosis. Neurology 64 (11), 1838–1845.

Maccollin, M., Mautner, V.F., 1998. The diagnosis and management of neurofibromatosis 2 in childhood. Semin. Pediatr. Neurol. 5 (4), 243–252.

MacCollin, M., Willett, C., Heinrich, B., et al., 2003. Familial schwannomatosis: Exclusion of the NF-2 locus as the germline event. Neurology 60 (12), 1968–1974.

Mahoney, D.H. Jr., Cohen, M.E., Friedman, H.S., et al., 2000. Carboplatin is effective therapy for young children with progressive optic pathway tumors: A Pediatric Oncology Group phase II study. Neuro-Oncology 2 (4), 213–220.

Masuda, A., Fisher, L.M., Oppenheimer, M.L., et al., 2004. Hearing changes after diagnosis in neurofibromatosis Type 2. Otol. Neurotol. 25 (2), 150–154.

Mathieu, D., Kondziolka, D., Flickinger, J.C., et al., 2007. Stereotactic radiosurgery for vestibular schwannomas in patients with neurofibromatosis Type 2: An analysis of tumor control, complications, and hearing preservation rates. Neurosurgery 60 (3), 460–468.

Mautner, V.F., Baser, M.E., Thakkar, S.D., et al., 2002. Vestibular schwannoma growth in patients with neurofibromatosis Type 2: A longitudinal study. J. Neurosurg. 96 (2), 223–228.

Mautner, V.F., Lindenau, M., Baser, M.E., et al., 1996. The neuroimaging and clinical spectrum of neurofibromatosis 2. Neurosurgery 38 (5), 880–886.

Milstein, J.M., Geyer, J.R., Berger, M.S., et al., 1989. Favorable prognosis for brainstem gliomas in neurofibromatosis. J. Neurooncol. 7 (4), 367–371.

Molloy, P.T., Bilaniuk, L.T., Vaughan, S.N., et al., 1995. Brainstem tumors in patients with neurofibromatosis type 1: A distinct clinical entity. Neurology 45 (10), 1897–1902.

Moyhuddin, A., Baser, M.E., Watson, C., et al., 2003. Somatic mosaicism in neurofibromatosis 2: Prevalence and risk of disease transmission to offspring. J. Med. Genet. 40 (6), 459–463.

Murad, G.J., Walbridge, S., Morrison, P.F., et al., 2007. Image-guided convection-enhanced delivery of gemcitabine to the brainstem. J. Neurosurg. 106 (2), 351–356.

Neff, B.A., Wiet, R.M., Lasak, J.M., et al., 2007. Cochlear implantation in the neurofibromatosis type 2 patient: Long-term follow-up. Laryngoscope 117 (6), 1069–1072.

NIH, 1987. National Institutes of Health Consensus Development Conference Statement on Neurofibromatosis. Neurofibromatosis Res. Newsl. 3, 3–6.

NIH, 1988. Neurofibromatosis. Conference statement. National Institutes of Health Consensus Development Conference. Arch. Neurol. 45, 575–578.

NIH, 1991. NIH Consensus development conference: Acoustic neuroma. NIH. Consensus Statement 9, 1–24.

Nunes, F., MacCollin, M., 2003. Neurofibromatosis 2 in the pediatric population. J. Child Neurol. 18 (10), 718–724.

Obringer, A.C., Meadows, A.T., Zackai, E.H., 1989. The diagnosis of neurofibromatosis-1 in the child under the age of 6 years. Am. J. Dis. Child 143 (6), 717–719.

Otto, S.R., Brackmann, D.E., Hitselberger, W.E., et al., 2002. Multichannel auditory brainstem implant: Update on performance in 61 patients. J. Neurosurg. 96 (6), 1063–1071.

Packer, R.J., Ater, J., Allen, J., et al., 1997. Carboplatin and vincristine chemotherapy for children with newly diagnosed progressive low-grade gliomas. J. Neurosurg. 86 (5), 747–754.

Pandit, S.K., Rattan, K.N., Gupta, U., et al., 2000. Multiple neurilemmomas of the penis. Pediatr. Surg. Int. 16 (5–6), 457.

Parry, D.M., Eldridge, R., Kaiser-Kupfer, M.I., et al., 1994. Neurofibromatosis 2 (NF-2): Clinical characteristics of 63 affected individuals and clinical evidence for heterogeneity. Am. J. Med. Genet. 52 (4), 450–461.

Parry, D.M., MacCollin, M.M., Kaiser-Kupfer, M.I., et al., 1996. Germline mutations in the neurofibromatosis 2 gene: Correlations with disease severity and retinal abnormalities. Am. J. Hum. Genet. 59 (3), 529–539.

Perry, A., Giannini, C., Raghavan, R., et al., 2001. Aggressive phenotypic and genotypic features in pediatric and NF-2-associated meningiomas: A clinicopathologic study of 53 cases. J. Neuropathol. Exp. Neurol. 60 (1), 994–1003.

Perry, A., Stafford, S.L., Scheithauer, B.W., et al., 1997. Meningioma grading: an analysis of histologic parameters. Am. J. Surg. Pathol. 21 (12), 1455–1465.

Plotkin, S.R., Stemmer-Rachamimov, A.O., Barker, F.G. 2nd, et al., 2009. Hearing improvement after bevacizumab in patients with neurofibromatosis type 2. N. Engl. J. Med. 361 (4), 358–367.

Pollack, I.F., Shultz, B., Mulvihill, J.J., 1996. The management of brainstem gliomas in patients with neurofibromatosis 1. Neurology 46 (6), 1652–1660.

Purcell, S.M., Dixon, S.L., 1989. Schwannomatosis: An unusual variant of neurofibromatosis or a distinct clinical entity? Arch. Dermatol. 125 (3), 390–393.

Pykett, M.J., Murphy, M., Harnish, P.R., et al., 1994. The neurofibromatosis 2 (NF-2) tumor suppressor gene encodes multiple alternatively spliced transcripts. Hum. Mol. Genet. 3 (4), 559–564.

Raffel, C., McComb, J.G., Bodner, S., et al., 1989. Benign brain stem lesions in pediatric patients with neurofibromatosis: Case reports. Neurosurgery 25 (6), 959–964.

Rasmussen, S.A., Yang, Q., Friedman, J.M., 2001. Mortality in neurofibromatosis 1: An analysis using U.S. death certificates. Am. J. Hum. Genet. 68 (5), 1110–1118.

Roche, P.H., Régis, J., Pellet, W., et al., 2000. Neurofibromatosis type 2. Preliminary results of gamma knife radiosurgery of vestibular schwannomas. Neurochirurgie 46 (4), 339–354.

Rouleau, G.A., Merel, P., Lutchman, M., et al., 1993. Alteration in a new gene encoding a putative membrane-organizing protein causes neuro-fibromatosis type 2. Nature 363 (6429), 515–521.

Rowe, J., Grainger, A., Walton, L., et al., 2007. Safety of radiosurgery applied to conditions with abnormal tumor suppressor genes. Neurosurgery 60 (5), 860–863.

Rowe, J.G., Radatz, M.W., Walton, L., et al., 2003. Clinical experience with gamma knife stereotactic radiosurgery in the management of vestibular schwannomas secondary to type 2 neurofibromatosis. J. Neurol. Neurosurg. Psychiatry 74 (9), 1288–1293.

Ruggieri, M., Huson, S.M., 2001. The clinical and diagnostic implications of mosaicism in the neurofibromatoses. Neurology 56 (11), 1433–1443.

Ruggieri, M., Iannetti, P., Polizzi, A., et al., 2005. Earliest clinical manifestations and natural history of neurofibromatosis type 2 (NF2) in childhood: A study of 24 patients. Neuropediatrics 36 (1), 21–34.

Ruttledge, M.H., Andermann, A.A., Phelan, C.M., et al., 1996. Type of mutation in the neurofibromatosis type 2 gene (NF-2) frequently determines severity of disease. Am. J. Hum. Genet. 59 (2), 331–342.

Samii, M., Matthies, C., Tatagiba, M., 1997. Management of vestibular schwannomas (acoustic neuromas): Auditory and facial nerve function after resection of 120 vestibular schwannomas in patients with neurofibromatosis 2. Neurosurgery 40 (4), 696–706.

Schwartz, M.S., Otto, S.R., Shannon, R.V., et al., 2008. Auditory brainstem implants. Neurotherapeutics 5 (1), 128–136.

Scoles, D.R., 2008. The merlin interacting proteins reveal multiple targets for NF-2 therapy. Biochimica et Biophysica Acta – Reviews on Cancer 1785 (1), 32–54.

Seizinger, B.R., Martuza, R.L., Gusella, J.F., 1986. Loss of genes on chromosome 22 in tumorigenesis of human acoustic neuroma. Nature 322 (6080), 644–647.

Seizinger, B.R., Rouleau, G., Ozelius, L.J., et al., 1987. Common pathogenetic mechanism for three tumor types in bilateral acoustic neurofibromatosis. Science 236 (4799), 317–319.

Sevick, R.J., Barkovich, A.J., Edwards, M.S., et al., 1992. Evolution of white matter lesions in neurofibromatosis type 1: MR findings. AJR. Am. J. Roentgenol. 159 (1), 171–175.

Sharif, S., Ferner, R., Birch, J.M., et al., 2006. Second primary tumors in neurofibromatosis 1 patients treated for optic glioma: Substantial risks after radiotherapy. J. Clin. Oncol. 24 (16), 2570–2575.

Sherman, L., Xu, H.M., Geist, R.T., et al., 1997. Interdomain binding mediates tumor growth suppression by the NF-2 gene product. Oncogene 15 (20), 2505–2509.

Shin, K.H., Moon, S.H., Suh, J.S., et al., 1998. Multiple neurilemmomas: A case report. Clin. Orthop. Relat. Res. (357), 171–175.

Shishiba, T., Niimura, M., Ohtsuka, F., et al., 1984. Multiple cutaneous neurilemmomas as a skin manifestation of neurilemmomatosis. J. Am. Acad. Dermatol. 10 (5 I), 744–754.

Slattery, W.H. 3rd, Fisher, L.M., Iqbal, Z., et al., 2004. Vestibular schwannoma growth rates in Neurofibromatosis type 2 Natural History Consortium subjects. Otol. Neurotol. 25 (5), 811–817.

Sobel, R.A., Wang, Y., 1993. Vestibular (acoustic) schwannomas: Histologic features in neurofibromatosis 2 and in unilateral cases. J. Neuropathol. Exp. Neurol. 52 (2), 106–113.

Stroink, A.R., Hoffman, H.J., Hendrick, E.B., et al., 1986. Diagnosis and management of pediatric brain-stem gliomas. J. Neurosurg. 65 (6), 745–750.

Stumpf, D.A., Alksne, J.F., Annegers, J.F., 1988. National Institutes of Health consensus development statement on neurofibromatosis. Arch. Neurol. 45 (5), 575–578.

Sun, C.X., Robb, V.A., Gutmann, D.H., et al., 2002. Protein 4.1 tumor suppressors: Getting a FERM grip on growth regulation. J. Cell Sci. 115 (21), 3991–4000.

Tanabe, K., Tada, K., Ninomiya, H., 1997. Multiple schwannomas in the radial nerve. J. Hand Surg. 22B (5), 664–666.

Taveras, J.M., Mount, L.A., Wood, E.H., 1956. The value of radiation therapy in the management of glioma of the optic nerves and chiasm. Radiology 66, 518–528.

Tenny, R.T., Laws, E.R. Jr., Younge, B.R., et al., 1982. The neurosurgical management of optic glioma. Results in 104 patients. J. Neurosurg. 57 (4), 452–458.

Trofatter, J.A., MacCollin, M.M., Rutter, J.L., et al., 1993. A novel moesin-, ezrin-, radixin-like gene is a candidate for the neurofibromatosis 2 tumor suppressor. Cell 75 (4), 826.

Ullrich, N.J., Raja, A.I., Irons, M.B., et al., 2007a. Brainstem lesions in neurofibromatosis type 1. Neurosurgery 61 (4), 762–766.

Ullrich, N.J., Robertson, R., Kinnamon, D.D., et al., 2007b. Moyamoya following cranial irradiation for primary brain tumors in children. Neurology 68 (12), 932–938.

Von Recklinghausen, F., 1882. Ueber die multiplen Fibrome der Haut und ihre Beziehung zu den multiplen Neuromen. Festschrift für Rudolf Virchow, Berlin.

Walker, L., Thompson, D., Easton, D., et al., 2006. A prospective study of neurofibromatosis type 1 cancer incidence in the UK. Br. J. Cancer 95 (2), 233–238.

Wallace, M.R., Marchuk, D.A., Andersen, L.B., et al., 1990. Type 1 neurofibromatosis gene: Identification of a large transcript disrupted in three NF-1 patients. Science 249 (4965), 181–186.

Westhout, F.D., Mathews, M., Paré, L.S., et al., 2007. Recognizing schwannomatosis and distinguishing it from neurofibromatosis type 1 or 2. J. Spinal. Disord. Tech. 20 (4), 329–332.

Wichmann, W., 2004. Reflexions about imaging technique and examination protocol: 2. MR-examination protocol. Eur. J. Radiol. 49 (1), 6–7.

Wishart, J.H., 1822. Case of tumours in the skull, dura mater and brain. Edinburgh Med. Surg. J. 18, 393–397.

Xu, G.F., O'Connell, P., Viskochil, D., et al., 1990. The neurofibromatosis type 1 gene encodes a protein related to GAP. Cell 62 (3), 599–608.

Zhao, Y., Kumar, R.A., Baser, M.E., et al., 2002. Intrafamilial correlation of clinical manifestations in neurofibromatosis 2 (NF-2). Gene. Epidemiol. 23 (3), 245–259.

31 Meningiomas

Samer Ayoubi, Ian F. Dunn, and Ossama Al-Mefty

Introduction

Surgery has the potential to cure meningiomas. Therefore it is not surprising that progress in meningioma treatment and advancements in neurosurgery mirror one another as surgeons seek to treat meningiomas in difficult locations the same way they are treated in more accessible locations: with total removal of the tumor and its origin without inflicting neurologic deficits.

Meningiomas left their mark on prehistoric skulls as hyperostosis, and were diagnosed during a patient's life in the eighteenth and nineteenth centuries only if they caused changes in the overlying skull. Thirteen operations with known outcome were performed between 1743 and 1896, with nine ending in death (Al-Rodhan et al 1991). John Cleland, Professor of Anatomy in Glasgow, was the first to notice, in 1864, that these tumors take their origin from the arachnoid rather than the dura, and that in structure, they resemble the Pacchionian granulations in a number of points (Cushing 1922). In 1915, Cushing and Weed reasserted Cleland's opinion that meningiomas were derived from arachnoid cell clusters. Cushing would go on to coin the term 'meningioma' to refer to a tumor histopathology that was, at the time, the subject of great controversy (Cushing 1922). In 1938, he published with Eisenhardt their classic monograph, *Meningiomas: Their Classification, Regional Behaviour, Life History, and Surgical End Results*, in which they reported in detail the cases of 313 patients encountered between 1903 and 1932 (Cushing & Eisenhardt 1938).

Pathology

Cell of origin

The meningioma cell of origin is believed to be specialized meningothelial cells called arachnoid cap cells (Kepes 1982; Haines & Frederickson 1991; Ragel & Jensen 2005). The arachnoid villi protrude into the venous sinuses. The venous endothelium is in contact with all or a portion of the arachnoid villi. In the latter case, these cells are referred to as arachnoid cap cells. The rest of the granulation is covered by a fibrous capsule. Arachnoid villi are most numerous in the area of the superior sagittal sinus, followed by the cavernous sinus, tuberculum sellae, lamina cribrosa, foramen magnum, and torcular herophili. Arachnoid granulations and pacchionian bodies are larger and more pronounced versions of arachnoid villi (Fig. 31.1).

WHO classification

The 2007 World Health Organization (WHO) classification of tumors of the nervous system lists meningiomas under the heading of 'meningeal tumors' and the sub-heading 'meningiomas' (Louis et al 2000; Perry et al 2007). WHO recognizes three grades based on pathologic criteria which reflect their risk of recurrence and aggressive growth (Table 31.1).

Macroscopic appearance

Meningiomas are typically globular, often multiloculated tumors attached to the dura. The cut surface of a meningioma is pale and translucent or homogeneous and reddish-brown, depending on the degree of vascularity. A gritty consistency is common. A whorled pattern may be apparent on the cut surface after fixation of the specimen. Intratumoral hemorrhage is rare, and necrosis is generally absent. Although invasion of the dura and dural sinuses is common, meningiomas are usually easily separated from the pia mater. The cleavage plane may not encompass the whole surface of the tumor (Sindou & Alaywan 1998). Meningioma 'en plaque' refers to meningiomas that occur as a flattened sheath of tumor, taking the shape of the underlying bone. It is more common in the sphenoid bone area, where it is often associated with hyperostosis. The extent of peritumoral brain edema associated with meningiomas can be highly variable; it is postulated that venous stasis occurs not as a result of the compression of an adjacent cortical vein but from the poor development of the tumor's venous drainage system. If a meningioma has a well-developed efferent draining vein, even with the regional production of vascular endothelial growth factor, which is thought to play a role in edema formation, such a tumor might not induce peritumoral brain edema, because the transit time of the blood passing through the channel in the tumor is short, resulting in a relatively rapid washout of vascular endothelial growth factor (Tanaka et al 2006). It is also suggested that perilesional edematous areas are ischemic. The measured mean cerebral blood flow and cerebral blood volume are lower in the peritumoral edema than normal area of brain, while the time to peak is greater in the perilesional edema when compared with areas of normal brain (Sergides et al 2009).

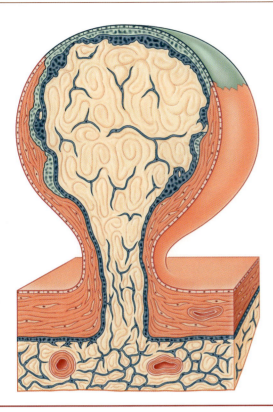

Figure 31.1 Diagrammatic representation of the arachnoid granulation shows the continuity of its layers and spaces with those of the meninges on the surface of the brain. (From Kida S, Yamashima T, Kubota T, Ito H, Yamamoto S. A light and electron microscopic and immunohistochemical study of human arachnoid villi. J Neurosurg. 1988 Sep;69(3): 429–435.)

Table 31.1 Meningiomas grouped by likelihood of recurrence and grade

Grade I
  Meningothelial meningioma
  Fibrous (fibroblastic) meningioma
  Transitional (mixed) meningioma
  Psammomatous meningioma
  Angiomatous meningioma
  Microcystic meningioma
  Secretory meningioma
  Lymphoplasmacyte-rich meningioma
  Metaplastic meningioma

Grade II
  Atypical meningioma
  Clear cell meningioma (intracranial)
  Chordoid meningioma

Grade III
  Rhabdoid meningioma
  Papillary meningioma
  Anaplastic (malignant) meningioma

Adapted from Louis DN, Scheithauer BW, Budka H, et al. Meningiomas. In: Kleihues P, Cavenee WK, editors: Pathology and Genetics of Tumours of the Nervous System. Lyon: IARC Press; 2000. 176–180.

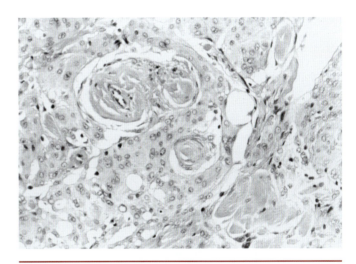

Figure 31.2 Hematoxylin and eosin (H&E) staining shows the histologic pattern of meningothelial meningiomas and polygonal cells with ill-defined cytoplasm.

Distribution

The most common sites are the parasagittal or falcine region (20–25%), convexity (19–35%), sphenoid ridge (17–20%), intraventricular (5%), tuberculum sellae (3–10%), infratentorial (13%), and others (4%). In children, meningiomas occur more commonly within the posterior fossa and ventricular system. In the more unusual locations such as in the ventricles or in the cerebral parenchyma, they probably arise from perivascular arachnoidal cells (Drummond et al 2004). Meningiomas at the convexity, particularly the parasagittal location, tend to be significantly more aggressive with a higher tendency for recurrence while meningiomas of the cranial base are more benign with fewer tendencies for recurrence (Ketter et al 2008).

Electron microscope

Benign meningiomas mimic the appearance of normal arachnoid villi in their ultrastructural features seen on electron microscopy: prominent interdigitation of the plasma membrane, abundant cytoplasmic intermediate filaments (10 nm) immunocytochemically consistent with vimentin, frequent hemidesmosomes to which the intermediate filaments anchor, and focal intercellular deposits of electron-dense granular material. Arachnoid and meningioma cells are connected by epithelial-cadherins (Ca^{2+}-dependent adhesion molecules),

and both express glutathione-independent prostaglandin D_2 synthase (Yamashima et al 1997).

Microscopic appearance

Histologically, meningothelial (syncytial) meningiomas are characterized by densely packed cells arranged in sheets with no clearly discernible cytoplasmic borders (Fig. 31.2). Microscopically, they mimic normal arachnoidal cells. Whorls can be found but are not prominent. Mineralized whorls, containing calcium apatite and collagen, are called *psammoma bodies* (from the Greek word *psammos*, meaning *sand*). Distinctive features of meningiomas include intranuclear cytoplasmic pseudoinclusion, in which an invaginated cytoplasmic remnant occupies the interior of the nucleus and displaces the nuclear chromatin. Another useful feature is the presence of so-called Orphan Annie's eye nuclei. These

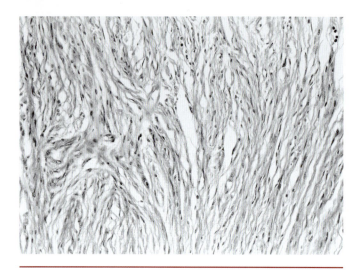

Figure 31.3 Hematoxylin and eosin (H&E) staining shows a fibroblastic meningioma formed of sheets of elongated spindle meningothelial cells.

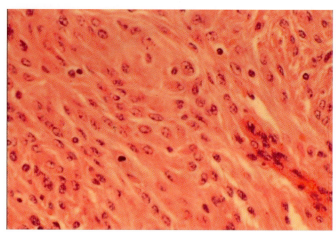

Figure 31.4 Hematoxylin and eosin (H&E) staining shows atypical meningioma. A mitotic figure is seen in the middle.

are target-like nuclei with central clearing and peripheral margination of the chromatin.

Microscopically, fibroblastic (fibrous) meningiomas reveal multilaminated sheets of interlacing elongated spindle cells. The intervening stroma is composed of reticulin fibers and collagen (Fig. 31.3). Transitional meningiomas represent a combination of the meningotheliomatous and fibroblastic types. Characteristically, cellular whorls are seen, separated by elongated spindle cells. Variations in meningioma histology may reflect mutations at separate genetic loci, in that the loss of heterozygosity (LOH) on chromosome 22 is much more common in fibroblastic than in meningothelial variants (Wellenreuther et al 1997).

One important variant to discuss is the so-called hemangiopericytic variety. Sometimes, meningiomas are composed partly or totally of small cells that focally grow in a hemangiopericytic pattern. The biologic behavior of this variant has not been well characterized. It is important to differentiate these so-called hemangiopericytic meningiomas (of meningothelial origin) from true hemangiopericytomas, which are mesenchymal tumors of non-meningothelial origin. True hemangiopericytomas of the meninges are similar to those occurring in other parts of the body. Their behavior is characterized by early recurrence and a tendency to metastasize.

Atypical meningioma

Atypical meningioma is associated with a higher rate of recurrence and aggressive growth. The criteria used to diagnose atypical meningioma are independent of meningioma subtype. Atypical meningioma is associated with increased mitotic activity or three or more of the following features: increased cellularity, small cells with a high nucleus-to-cytoplasm ratio, prominent nucleoli, uninterrupted patternless or sheetlike growth, and foci of spontaneous or geographic necrosis. For this variant, increased mitotic activity has been defined as four or more mitoses per 10 high-power fields (Louis et al 2000) (Fig. 31.4). Osseous involvement is associated with a poor outcome in patients with atypical

meningiomas. This may reflect more aggressive tumor biological characteristics compared to those that do not invade bone, although alternatively, poor outcomes may result from failure to treat diseased bone (Gabeau-Lacet et al 2009).

Anaplastic meningiomas

The exact definition of anaplastic and malignant meningiomas is still open to discussion (Perry et al 1999). One feature undoubtedly labels a meningioma as malignant: distant extraneural metastasis (Figueroa et al 1999). The most common sites for metastasis are the liver, lungs, pleura, and lymph nodes. Frank parenchymal invasion of the underlying brain also carries an ominous prognosis. Anaplastic meningioma is a meningioma exhibiting histologic features of frank malignancy far in excess of the abnormalities present in atypical meningiomas. Such features include obviously malignant cytology (e.g., having an appearance similar to sarcoma, carcinoma, or melanoma) or a high mitotic index (≥20 mitoses per 10 high-power fields) (Fig. 31.5). A correlation has been shown between MIB-1 labeling index and the histological grade of the meningiomas. Poor prognosis may be associated with a high MIB-1 labeling index, although significant overlap exists in the MIB-1 labeling ranges for benign, atypical and anaplastic meningiomas (Yang et al 2008). The rate of p53 overexpression is observed in 10% of benign meningiomas, 25% of atypical meningiomas, and 79% of anaplastic meningiomas, and it becomes significantly higher as histological malignancy increases (Yang et al 2008).

Immunohistochemistry

Epithelial membrane antigen (EMA) is positive in 80% of meningiomas. The results of S-100 staining are quite variable. Meningiomas also express markers for fibroblasts (i.e., vimentin) and epithelial cells (i.e., EMA and cytokeratins). Antileu 7, an antibody positive in schwannomas, is uniformly negative in meningiomas. Although results of glial fibrillary acidic protein (GFAP) stains are negative in meningiomas, a few cases of GFAP-positive meningiomas have been reported in the world literature (Su et al 1997).

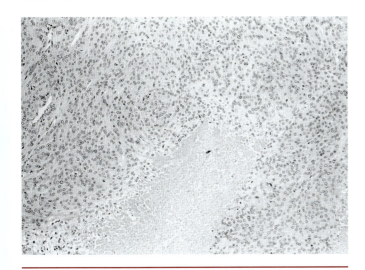

Figure 31.5 Hematoxylin and eosin (H&E) staining shows a meningioma with obvious malignant cytology and a very high mitotic index.

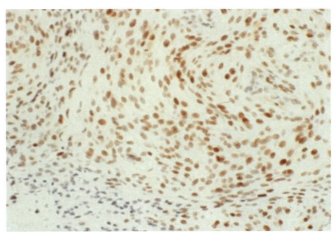

Figure 31.6 Immunohistochemical staining of a meningioma for proliferating cell nuclear antigen. Notice the high labeling index, which portends aggressive behavior. Unstained cells are in the inferior aspect of the slide, in blue.

Syncytial and transitional meningiomas express E (epithelial)-cadherin, a Ca^{2+}-dependent cell adhesion molecule (Yamashima et al 1992). Another use of immunohistochemistry lies in differentiating atypical meningiomas from similar but pathologically distinct tumors, such as secretory meningioma versus metastatic carcinoma (Assi et al 1999).

Hyperostosis

This feature is a characteristic finding in meningiomas, especially in *en plaque* meningiomas. In most cases, histologic studies of hyperostotic bone reveal tumor cells in the diploë and haversian canals (Pieper et al 1999).

Tumor progression

Meningiomas also go through tumor progression (Al-Mefty et al 2004a; Yang et al 2008). Tumor progression is defined by irreversible change in the tumor characteristics reflecting the sequential appearance of a genetically altered subpopulation of cells with the new characteristics (Nowell 1986). In some instances, the properties of advanced malignancy may be established before the neoplasm reaches macroscopic size, in other cases, well differentiated and slow growing tumors may persist for years before shifting to more aggressive behavior. De novo atypical and anaplastic meningiomas differ from atypical and anaplastic meningiomas that have progressed from benign meningiomas in clinical behavior, hormone receptor status, proliferative indices, and cytogenetic profile (Krayenbühl et al 2007). Transformed atypical meningiomas, which have a negative progesterone receptor (PR) and higher proliferative index, seem to have much more aggressive behavior than the de novo sub-group (Krayenbühl et al 2007). Genetic alterations associated with aggressive behavior, loss of part or monosomy of chromosome 10 and an increased monosomy or derivative chromosome 1 in combination with monosomy of chromosome 14, occur mainly in the groups with malignant transformation that have a worse outcome (Krayenbühl et al 2007). The overexpression of p53, likely representing mutant forms of the protein, is associated with the malignant progression of a meningioma (Yang et al 2008).

Clinical behavior

Extensive efforts have been made to determine the clinical behavior and malignant potential of meningiomas. These efforts have focused on different aspects of meningioma pathology: histology, labeling, karyotype and genetics, radiology, and hormone receptors. Some histologic features portend aggressive behavior. These features include hypercellularity, loss of architecture, nuclear pleomorphism, an increased mitotic index, focal necrosis, hypervascularity, hemosiderin deposition, and small cell formation (Perry et al 1999). Labeling techniques have been devised to quantify the mitotic rate of meningiomas and therefore predict their behavior. Bromodeoxy-uridine (BUdR) labeling allows the examiner to determine the percentage of cells in the S phase of mitosis. An alternative to BUdR labeling is immunohistochemical staining for proliferating cell nuclear antigen (PCNA) (Fig. 31.6). Fresh specimens can also be labeled for the monoclonal antibody Ki-67 or MIB-1 which can be done on any paraffin-embedded specimen. A high labeling index indicated by either method denotes a more aggressive tumor (Cobb et al 1996; Hsu et al 1998; Yang et al 2008). However, an elevated Ki-67 labeling index can be paradoxically seen in tumors that were previously irradiated (Jennelle et al 1999). Ki-67 labeling index is an independent predictor of both tumor recurrence and overall survival in patients with atypical and anaplastic meningiomas (Bruna et al 2007). Immunoreactivity for transforming growth factor-α has also been correlated with an increased level of malignant behavior (Schwechheimer et al 1998). Positive E-cadherin immunoreactivity is seen in benign meningiomas regardless of the histomorphologic sub-type or of the tumor's invasion into dura, bone, brain, or muscle, while it is absent from most morphologically-malignant meningiomas (Schwechheimer et al 1998). SPARC, a secreted, extracellular matrix-associated protein implicated in the modulation of cell adhesion and migration is highly expressed in invasive tumors, regardless of grade. SPARC may be used to assess the invasiveness of histologically benign meningiomas in the absence of the tumor-brain interface (Rempel et al 1999). The Ets-1 transcription factor is thought to play an important role in the invasive process of tumor cells through the induction of urokinase-type plasminogen activator (u-PA). A significant difference is observed between Ets-1 and u-PA expression in benign and high-grade meningiomas (Kitange et al 2000). Complex karyotypes increase progressively from benign (34%) to atypical (45%) to anaplastic (70%) meningiomas (Cerda-Nicolas et al 2000).

Multiple meningiomas

These are defined as two or more meningiomas appearing simultaneously or sequentially in the same patient (Rosa & Luessenhop 1991). The reporting of multiple meningiomas has increased with the advent of new imaging techniques such as computed tomography (CT) and magnetic resonance imaging (MRI). The incidence of multiple meningiomas is in the range of 1% to 16% of meningiomas. Between 60% and 90% of patients with multiple meningiomas are women. Multiple meningiomas occur in association with neurofibromatosis type 2. They have also been described in families with no evidence of neurofibromatosis (Maxwell et al 1998). Multiple meningiomas may be secondary to a recurrence at the edge of the surgical resection or to postoperative seeding through the CSF. This possibility is further supported by the fact that recurrent meningiomas were found to be clonal with respect to the primary tumors (Von Deimling et al 1999).

Intraosseous meningiomas and extraneuraxial meningiomas

These are uncommon. All the reported intraosseous meningiomas have been in cranial bones. Extraneuraxial meningiomas can involve the orbit, paranasal sinuses, nasopharynx, skin and subcutis, lungs, mediastinum, and adrenal gland.

Metastasis

Tumors of the CNS may metastasize to a primary intracranial tumor. Three-quarters of these metastases target meningiomas, although meningiomas represent only 32% of intracranial tumors. There probably are many reasons for this propensity, including the fact that patients with meningiomas, which are slow growing tumors, are more at risk for metastasis than patients with other brain tumors. Other factors may be the increased vascularity of meningiomas and the peculiar microenvironment in these tumors.

Epidemiology

Data published by the central brain tumor registry of the USA show that meningiomas account for 32% of all brain tumors, with incidence rate of 5.3 per 100 000 person–years, the incidence was twice as common in women (3.17 for males; 7.19 for females) and was as common in blacks as in whites (CBTRUS 2008). The incidence in Nordic countries is 1.9 per 100 000 person–years for males and 4.5 per 100 000 person–years for females (Klaeboe et al 2005; Larjavaara et al 2008).

The incidence in Japan is 1.82 per 100 000 person–years for males and 3.95 per 100 000 person–years for females (Kuratsu et al 2001; Kaneko et al 2002). The incidence of meningioma in Africa is similar (Ruberti 1995) although old reports indicated higher incidence (Froman & Lipschitz 1970; Giordano & Lamouche 1973; Levy 1973; Manfredonia 1973; Odeku & Adeloye 1973). But the incidence of meningiomas is probably considerably underestimated (Larjavaara et al 2008). The rates for meningiomas increase dramatically after age 65 and continue to be high even among the population aged 85 and older (Kurland et al 1982; Preston-Martin et al 1982; Sutherland et al 1987; CBTRUS 2008). The incidence has been stable or even declined over the last 15 years. Increases in the incidence during the late 1970s and early 1980s coincided with improved diagnostic methods (Kaneko et al 2002, Klaeboe et al 2005). The overall incidence was 2.6/100 000 population in the combined results of three large studies of intracranial neoplasms in the 80s (Kurland et al 1982; Preston-Martin et al 1982; Sutherland et al 1987). Incidental meningiomas were found in 0.9% in the general population in an MRI study. The meningiomas ranged from 5 to 60 mm in diameter, and their prevalence was 1.1% in women and 0.7% in men (Vernooij 2007). Prevalence rate (new patients and former patients who are survivors) in the year 2000 was 50.4% per 100 000 with an expected 138 388 meningioma patients in the USA. This emphasizes the need for quality-of-life (QoL) considerations, particularly for those long-term survivors of this benign tumor (Davis et al 2001). Meningiomas in the pediatric population are rare, accounting for less than 1–2% of brain tumors in this cohort, with a majority (71%) of these tumors occurring in males (Bondy & Ligon 1996).

Etiology

Trauma

Trauma was suggested by Cushing in the 1930s as a significant etiologic factor in the development of meningiomas (Cushing & Eisenhardt 1938), with evidence for this association from isolated reports (Barnett et al 1986; Kotzen et al 1999). Case–control studies have suggested otherwise. Some studies suggested that head trauma may exert a modest influence on the risk of meningioma (Preston-Martin et al 1980; Phillips et al 2002). If head trauma is a cause of meningioma, the population attributable risk percentage would be no higher than 23% (Phillips et al 2002). Evidence supporting a causal relationship in Phillips's study included temporal sequence of head trauma occurring prior to meningioma diagnosis, the greatest risk being 10–19 years prior to reference date, a plausible induction period for this slow-growing tumor and the risk increasing with number of traumas (Phillips et al 2002). Possible causal mechanisms include neoplastic change in meningeal tissue with healing, inflammation, and the release of growth factors (Barnett et al 1986; Phillips et al 2002). Other studies did not find this association (Choi et al 1970; Annegers et al 1979; Inskip et al 1998). Furthermore, it has been argued that invoking an association between head trauma and meningiomas would not explain the increased incidence of these tumors in females as head trauma is much more common among males (Longstreth et al 1993).

Viruses

The presence of viral protein, RNA or DNA, in human meningioma cells suggests a possible role in tumor induction, and maintenance of transformation. The implicated viruses may act alone or in a permissive manner with other mutagens. Some genomic viral sequences have been found in neoplastic brain tissue (Fisher et al 1999; Cuomo et al 2001; Del Valle et al 2001; Wrensch et al 2001). Attention was placed on the family Polyomaviridae because these viruses appear to be involved in tumor pathogenesis (Delbue et al 2005). Several recent reports indicate a possible association between brain tumors and the human polyoma viruses: JC virus, BK virus, and Simian virus 40 (De Mattei et al 1995; Krynska et al 1999; Arrington et al 2000; Caldarelli-Stefano et al 2000), but their role has not yet been well-defined (Delbue et al 2005). JCV and BKV usually infect the human population during early childhood and primary infection is often asymptomatic. These viruses can remain latent in the kidney cells of the host until reactivation, which occurs in the event of immunodepression. SV40 does not naturally infect humans, but was introduced in the human population through contaminated poliovirus vaccine in the late 1950s (Delbue et al 2005). Coinfection with JCV and BKV was found in two patients with meningiomas suggesting a possible interaction of both viruses with cellular factors. In addition, the effects of each polyoma virus on cellular transformation could be enhanced by the presence of the other one (Delbue et al 2005). But it is difficult to demonstrate the oncogenic role of the virus and the role of BKV in human neoplasias remains unclear (Delbue et al 2005). Marked interest in polyoma viruses is also due to the fact that >75% of the worldwide adult population is infected latently with these viruses, without any apparent complications. It thus follows that an understanding of the interaction of the virus with the host, which leads to tumorigenesis, is of interest and of pressing urgency for consideration of JCV and BKV as oncogenic risk factors (Delbue et al 2005). Inoue-Melnick virus (IMV), a deoxyribonucleic acid (DNA) virus linked to subacute myelo-opticoneuropathy was isolated from six of seven human meningioma-derived cell cultures but was not isolated from six other brain tumor cell cultures (Inoue 1991). Although there is strong biochemical evidence associating DNA tumor viruses with human meningiomas, the role of the virus in the development of the tumor remains undefined (Rachlin & Rosenblum 1991). It is known that some viruses, when inoculated into laboratory animals, will produce central nervous system (CNS) tumors. All of the polyoma viruses (polyoma, SV40), a sub-group of papovaviruses, are capable of producing CNS tumors in animals, as are several types of adenoviruses (human, simian, and avian) (Rachlin & Rosenblum 1991). Immunocytochemical techniques have identified papovavirus antigen in human meningiomas (Weiss et al 1975). Likewise, DNA hybridization techniques have found SV40 viral DNA (both papovaviruses) and adenovirus DNA within meningiomas, but the viral DNA material was not integrated into the tumor cell DNA in all cases (Fiori & Di Mayorca 1976; Ibelgaufts & Jones 1982). The presence of viral protein, RNA or DNA, in human meningioma cells suggests a possible role in tumor induction, maintenance of transformation, or both, in which case the implicated viruses may act alone or in a permissive manner with other mutagens. Of course, the presence of viral material is not *prima facie* evidence that it is causally related to meningioma formation, and the actual role, if any, of viruses in human brain tumor formation is as yet undefined.

Radiation

In 1953, Mann and colleagues were the first to report a radiation-induced meningioma. The patient, a 6-year-old girl, received 6500 rad after resection of an optic nerve glioma. A meningioma was diagnosed 4 years later within the radiotherapy field. There is no doubt that radiation injury is a factor in the development of meningiomas. The criteria for radiation-induced meningiomas include: (1) the tumor must arise in the irradiated field; (2) histological features must differ from those of any previous neoplasm; (3) a sufficient latency or induction period following radiation must elapse before meningioma is diagnosed (usually >5 years); (4) no family history of phakomatosis; (5) the tumor must not be recurrent or metastatic; (6) the tumor must not be present prior to radiation therapy (Al-Mefty et al 2004b). Numerous reports show that meningiomas have occurred following low levels of irradiation such as were given in the past for tinea capitis (1000 cGy) (Modan et al 1974; Sadetzki et al 2002), following the high doses of radiation given for the treatment of primary head and neck malignancies (5500–7500 cGy) (Mack et al 1993; Al-Mefty 2004a), and following intermediate levels of radiation (Bogdanowicz & Sachs 1974; Waga & Handa 1976). Al-Mefty et al (2004b) found a latency period of 6–58 years (mean 24.6 years) in high-dose irradiation induced meningiomas (Fig. 31.7) and 34–46 years (mean 40 years) in low-dose irradiation induced meningiomas. A similar latency period of 36 years for low-dose radiation induced meningiomas was found in other studies (Sadetzki et al 2002). In addition, analysis of the Nagasaki and Hiroshima atomic bomb survivors showed that the incidence in exposed persons is higher than in non-exposed and gradually increased with time (Shibata et al 1994; Sadamori et al 1996; Shintani et al 1999). The incidence increased in Nagasaki survivors 6 years later than survivors in Hiroshima (Shintani et al 1999). The incidence was dependent on the dose of radiation received. Malignant aggressive meningiomas were not common in survivors of either bomb, indicating that single exposure vs frequent long-term exposure might have influenced the histology of the tumor (Shibata et al 1994; Sadamori et al 1996; Shintani et al 1999). Radiation induced meningiomas possess chromosome alterations different from non-radiation induced meningiomas (Al-Mefty et al 2004b) (Fig. 31.8). It appears that in radiation-induced meningiomas, there is karyotypic instability or the presence of multiple chromosome rearrangements (Kleinschmidt-DeMasters & Lillehei 1995; Chauveinc et al 1997; Al-Mefty et al 2004b). In radiation-induced meningioma, unlike sporadic meningiomas, *NF-2* gene inactivation and loss of chromosome 22 are less frequent (Shoshan et al 2000; Al-Mefty et al 2004b). Other aberrations include loss of all or part of chromosome 1p or loss of heterozygosity on chromosome 1p (Shoshan et al 2000; Zattara-Cannoni et al 2001; Al-Mefty et al 2004b) and structural abnormalities of chromosome 6 (Al-Mefty et al

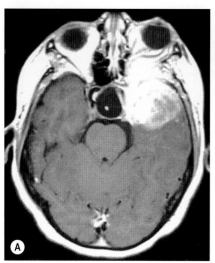 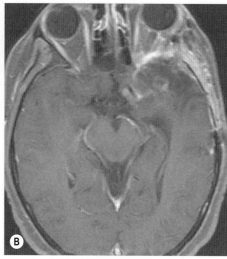 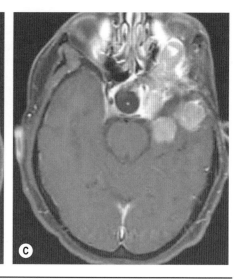

Figure 31.7 Magnetic resonance imaging of a radiation-induced meningioma in the left cavernous sinus, orbit, and frontal lobe after radiation therapy for pituitary adenoma showing initial tumor (A); after one of several resections (B); and eventual re-recurrence (C).

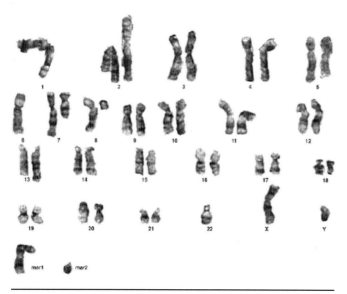

Figure 31.8 Karyotyping demonstrates monosomy of chromosomes 1, 16, and 22 in a radiation-induced meningioma.

2004b). These are associated with aggressive behavior. Several studies are being carried out to determine whether the use of mobile phones increases the risk of developing brain neoplasms. There is no evidence to date to support a relation between the use of mobile phones and development of brain tumors (Inskip et al 2001; Kan et al 2008). The overall incidence of meningiomas has remained stable during the period after the introduction and widespread use of mobile phones (Lonn et al 2004).

Genetics and molecular biology

Meningiomas were among the first solid tumors analyzed for genetic abnormalities. Giemsa staining, FISH, comparative genomic hybridization, and spectral karyotyping have been

used to elucidate the most common chromosomal abnormalities associated with meningiomas (Ragel & Jensen 2005).

Chromosome 22

The link between abnormalities in the long arm of chromosome 22 (22q) and meningiomas was first suspected in patients with neurofibromatosis type 2 (NF-2) (Ragel & Jensen 2005; Keller et al 2009). The *NF-2* tumor suppressor gene is located on chromosome 22q12.1. Its protein product is called schwannomin or Merlin, a moesin-, ezrin-, radixin-like protein, and is a part of the band 4.1 families of cytoskeleton-associated proteins. Overexpression of Merlin significantly inhibits the proliferation of human meningioma cells relative to the proliferation of cells transduced with a control vector (Ikeda et al 1999). Although a reduced expression of schwannomin/Merlin has been demonstrated in sporadic meningiomas, Merlin loss alone, usually caused by an alteration in the *NF-2* gene, is not sufficient for meningioma development (Ragel & Jensen 2005). It is now generally accepted that meningiomas arise when there is a loss of *NF-2* or other tumor suppressor genes in combination with the activation of proto-oncogenes (Zankl & Zang 1980; Collins et al 1990; Khan et al 1998; Maxwell et al 1998; Ragel & Jensen 2005). The majority of meningiomas occur as isolated, sporadic tumors. Nevertheless, deletions of chromosome 22 are found in all NF-2-associated meningiomas, and in 54–78% of sporadic meningiomas (Seizinger et al 1987; Ruttledge et al 1994; Ragel & Jensen 2005). *NF-2* gene mutations are higher in fibroblastic and transitional meningiomas than the meningothelial subtype, and are similar in both atypical and anaplastic meningiomas to the frequency of *NF-2* gene mutations in fibroblastic and transitional meningiomas suggesting that *NF-2* gene mutations are probably involved with tumorigenesis but not tumor progression. The fact that there is a higher incidence of chromosome 22 loss of heterozygosity and a lower frequency of *NF-2* gene mutations in meningiomas has led to the search for a second tumor suppressor gene on 22q, in proximity to but distinct from the *NF-2* gene (Peyrard et al 1994; Lekanne-Deprez et al 1995, Ragel & Jensen 2005). Possible candidates include the *BAM22*, *LARGE*, *MN1*, and *INI1* genes (Ragel & Jensen 2005). The *BAM22* gene on chromosome 22q12 is a member of the human β-adaptin gene family that may have a role in intracellular transport of proteins in the trans-Golgi network. The *LARGE* gene was identified in the 22q12.3-q13.1 region. Its protein is structurally similar to members of the *N*-acetylglucosaminyltransferase family which may have a role in tumorigenesis. *LARGE* gene is implicated in meningioma tumorigenesis because of its location on chromosome 22, but no evidence exists to implicate this gene directly. The *MN1* gene has a possible role in tumor suppression. The function of the MN1 protein is unknown, although based on its amino acid structure, it most likely plays a role in transcription. The *INI1* gene is located on chromosome 22q. The function of the INI1 protein is unknown, but its structure suggests that it functions in transcriptional regulation (Ragel & Jensen 2005). *INI1* (*SMARCB1/hSNF5*) gene is involved in the pathogenesis of rhabdoid tumors, and is important with the addition of the rhabdoid variety of meningiomas to the WHO classification (Schmitz et al 2001).

Chromosome 1
Deletions of the short arm of chromosome 1 are the second most frequent alteration detected showing monosomy 1p in 70% of atypical and almost 100% of anaplastic meningiomas. This indicates a correlation between loss of chromosome 1p and meningioma progression (Muller et al 1999; Bello et al 2000; Ragel & Jensen 2005, Keller et al 2009). Loss of 1p also correlates also with tumor recurrence (Ragel & Jensen 2005). Alkaline phosphatase is a possible tumor suppressor, whose location on chromosome 1p (1p34–1p36.1) and loss of function is correlated with higher-grade meningiomas (Ragel & Jensen 2005, Keller et al 2009).

Other chromosomes
Many cytogenetic alterations are associated with meningioma progression and typical or anaplastic histology, including the presence of dicentric or ring chromosomes; losses of chromosome arms 1p, 6q, 7, 9p, 10, 14q, 18q, 19, or 20; as well as gains/amplifications of 1q, 9q, 12q, 15q, 17q, or 20q (Weber et al 1997; Khan et al 1998; Lamszus et al 1999; Leone et al 1999; Ozaki et al 1999; Ragel & Jensen 2005). Alteration in cell-cycle checkpoint tumor suppressor genes located on chromosome 9p, including *CDKN2A* and *CDKN2B* is seen in anaplastic meningiomas (Ragel & Jensen 2005). The membrane-associated 4.1 protein family *DAL-1*, located on chromosome 18p11.3, has also been suggested as a tumor suppressor (Gutmann et al 2000; Ragel & Jensen 2005).

Oncogene expression
Although no single oncogene has been directly implicated in meningioma development, it is possible that either one or multiple oncogenes may contribute to this process. These include *myc*, *ras*, *ROS1* oncogene for tyrosine receptor kinase, and the *bcl-2* protooncogene, which are correlated with higher-grade meningiomas (Ragel & Jensen 2005).

Meningioma clonality
There is evidence to support the idea that although meningiomas are monoclonal in origin, a small number of meningiomas may be polyclonal in origin (Zhu et al 1999). In regard to multiple meningiomas, X-chromosomal analysis and mutational *NF-2* gene analysis suggest that multiple tumors are monoclonal in origin supporting dural dissemination through the subarachnoid space. Nevertheless, approximately 50% of multiple meningiomas exhibit different *NF-2* gene mutations, indicating independent tumorigenesis origins (Ragel & Jensen 2005).

Gonadal steroid hormones and other receptors
The preponderance of female patients harboring meningiomas, the acceleration of meningiomas during pregnancy and menses and after the insertion of subcutaneous hormonal contraceptive implants, and the association with breast cancer have implicated sex steroids in the growth of meningiomas, and the increased risk for meningiomas among women exposed to either endogenous or exogenous sex hormones especially with increasing age at menarche (Bickerstaff et al 1958; Roelvink et al 1987; Michelsen & New 1969; Longstreth et al 1993; Piper et al 1994; Bondy & Ligon 1996; Jhawar et al 2003; Claus et al 2005).

Progesterone and estrogen receptors
Progesterone receptors are identified in normal arachnoid tissue, while normal adult meninges express low levels of progesterone receptors. They are expressed in meningiomas, in which they are functional (Pravdenkova et al 2006). Normal meningeal tissues do not have estrogen receptors and controversy still surrounds the presence of estrogen receptors in meningiomas (Pravdenkova et al 2006). Most estrogen receptors identified in meningiomas are type II receptors, which have a lower affinity and specificity for estrogen than the type I receptors classically found in breast cancers (McCutcheon 1996). It is believed that estrogen binds in <30% of meningiomas, with the majority of these receptors being the type II sub-type (Smith & Cahill 1994; McCutcheon 1996). The expression of progesterone receptors alone in a meningioma is a favorable sign for the clinical and biological behavior of the tumor (Brandis et al 1993; Nagashima et al 1995; Hsu et al 1997; Fewings et al 2000; Pravdenkova et al 2006). An absence of both progesterone receptors and estrogen receptors or the presence of estrogen receptors with or without progesterone receptors are associated with aggressive histopathological characteristics as well as qualitative and quantitative accumulations of abnormal karyotypes, especially in de novo tumors and in tumors in women. The initial receptor status might change in any progression or recurrence of the tumor (Pravdenkova et al 2006).

Androgen receptors
Androgen receptors are found in meningiomas with approximately the same frequency as progesterone receptors (Smith & Cahill 1994). These receptors are found more frequently in meningiomas in women, and it has been speculated that they may help to modulate progesterone receptor activity (Carroll et al 1995).

Somatostatin receptors
Somatostatin receptors are found in meningioma tissue and in normal human leptomeninges as well (Reubi et al 1986,

1989; Lamberts et al 1992a). The functional significance of these receptors is unknown; however, somatostatin receptor scintigraphy has been found to be a useful diagnostic instrument in identifying meningiomas and differentiating residual tumor from other changes seen in the postoperative setting (Klutmann et al 1998).

Dopamine D₁ receptor

The dopamine D_1 receptor has also been demonstrated in meningiomas. The function of these receptors in meningiomas remains unclear, but they may provide an alternative means by which surgically unresectable meningiomas can be treated with specific D_1 receptor antagonists (Carroll et al 1996). The epidermal growth factor (EGF) receptors, which may play a role in neoplastic transformation of normal cells and tumor growth, are found in meningiomas (Westphal & Herrmann 1986; Horsfall et al 1989; Reubi et al 1989). There is a positive modulatory effect on the receptor by platelet derived growth factor (PDGF) (Weisman et al 1986). The co-expression of PDGF-2 (a potent mitogen) and PDGF-R suggests an autocrine loop that may contribute to the growth and maintenance of these tumors. Other growth factors, including insulin-like growth factors (Glick et al 1992; Tsutsumi et al 1994), and fibroblast growth factors (Takahashi et al 1990; Takahashi et al 1991) are thought to influence meningioma cell growth by acting in an autocrine manner. Growth hormone receptor mRNA has been found to be ubiquitously expressed in meningiomas (Friend et al 1999). Furthermore, blocking the growth hormone receptor decreased, while administration of insulin-like growth factor I increased, the growth rates of many primary meningioma cultures (Friend et al 1999). The therapeutic implications of these findings for adjunctive treatment of meningiomas remain to be investigated.

Presenting features: symptoms and signs

There is no single symptom or sign that alone identifies which patients harbor an intracranial meningioma. Indeed, some tumors are identified fortuitously in patients who have no symptoms or signs of intracranial disease. Other patients have a variety of presenting features, including headache, paresis, seizures, personality change/confusion, and visual impairment. Rohringer and co-workers (1989), in a population based study of 193 patients with intracranial meningioma, found headache and paresis to be the most common symptoms and signs, occurring in 36% and 30% of patients, respectively, and an increased incidence of abnormal physical findings in those patients with malignant meningiomas.

Meningiomas in specific locations may have, more or less, a typical clinical presentation. Examples include tumors of the olfactory groove, which historically have been associated with anosmia and the Foster Kennedy syndrome (optic atrophy and scotoma in the ipsilateral eye with papilledema in the other eye); tuberculum sellae meningiomas, which cause early significant visual loss (usually a 'chiasmal syndrome' with ipsilateral optic atrophy and an incongruous bitemporal hemianopia) (Al-Mefty & Smith 1991); cavernous sinus meningiomas, which may result in proptosis, diplopia, or primary aberrant oculomotor regeneration (Schatz et al

1977); and foramen magnum tumors, which have associated nuchal and suboccipital pain and stepwise appendicular sensory and motor deficits (Meyer et al 1984). In contradistinction to the multitude of signs and symptoms that may occur in adults, children may present with signs of increased intracranial pressure without further localizing features.

Diagnostic imaging

Computed tomography of intracranial meningiomas

Computed tomography (CT) scanning can detect the majority of meningiomas and can, in most instances, determine their extent (Latchaw & Hirsch 1991). On non-enhanced CT scans, the typical meningioma is isodense to slightly hyperdense to brain and of homogeneous density, although calcification may be present and may range from tiny punctate areas to dense calcification of the entire lesion (Latchaw & Hirsch 1991) (Fig. 31.9). Edema, which appears as low density on CT, is often evident to various degrees, the extent of which has few predictable correlates (Ginsberg 1996). CT perfusion can be used to measure mean cerebral blood flow and cerebral blood volume in the peritumoral edema to assess levels of ischemia in brain areas around intracranial meningiomas (Sergides et al 2009). CT optimally identifies either hyperostosis or bone lysis. Osseous changes associated with a meningioma usually represent tumor involvement as opposed to bony reactive changes (Bikmaz et al 2007). Intravenous contrast usually shows intense, homogeneous enhancement, and morphologic features, such as sharp demarcation and a broad base against bone or free dural margins, are easily seen. On CT, approximately 15% of benign meningiomas have an unusual appearance (Russell et al 1980). Areas of hyperdensity, hypodensity, and non-uniform enhancement may be seen and may represent hemorrhage, cystic

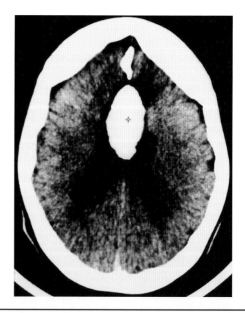

Figure 31.9 Axial CT scan. A large, densely and completely calcified falcine meningioma is present.

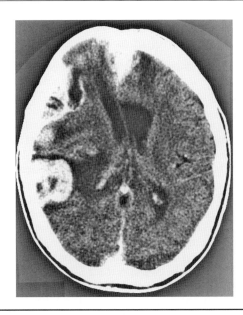

Figure 31.10 Axial CT scan, post-contrast. This axial contrast enhanced CT scan of a multiply recurrent malignant meningioma demonstrates the radiologic sign known as mushrooming. Irregular projections from the main mass of the tumor are seen. A previous craniectomy has been performed.

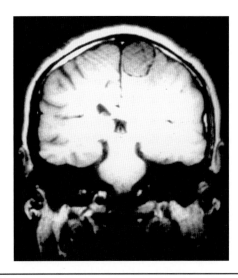

Figure 31.11 Coronal T1-weighted magnetic resonance image. A parasagittal meningioma is seen. It is isointense to slightly hypointense with respect to the gray matter. Note the low intensity signal surrounding the tumor, thus confirming its extraparenchymal origin.

degeneration, or necrosis, respectively. Aggressive meningiomas may at times be distinguished by preoperative imaging findings of indistinct or irregular margins or mushroom-like projections from the main tumor mass (Fig. 31.10). Brain single-photon emission computed tomography (SPECT) by (99m)Tc-Tetrofosmin ((99m)Tc-TF) shows a significant correlation between (99m)Tc-TF uptake and both tumor grade and Ki-67 expression which may imply that (99m)Tc-TF brain SPECT can be useful in differentiating benign from anaplastic meningiomas and is a potential indicator of their proliferative activity (Fotopoulos et al 2008). Positron emission tomography/computed tomography (PET/CT) with C-11 choline may also be used for grading and follow-up of meningiomas as 11 choline uptake is increased in all meningiomas and is higher in patients with grade II than in grade I meningiomas (Giovacchini et al 2009).

Angiography of intracranial meningiomas

Angiography, which once played a pre-eminent role in the diagnosis of intracranial meningioma, has, to a large extent, been supplanted by high resolution CT, magnetic resonance imaging (MRI), and magnetic resonance angiography (MRA). Indeed, the determination of venous sinus patency, historically the purview of the angiogram, can be well visualized on MRA, thus eliminating this as an indication for angiography. Angiography remains a vital means by which the feasibility and safety of preoperative embolization can be determined. Furthermore, pertinent collateral circulation can be identified.

As they grow, meningiomas first access the adjacent meningeal arterial supply. These initial nutrient arteries remain as the supply to the center of the tumor. From this central site, there is usually a radiant spread of branches towards the periphery of the tumor. As the angiogram

extends into the middle to late venous phase, a uniform blush can be seen. Venous drainage tends to occur in the usual temporal sequence typical of the brain. Large meningiomas will also parasitize the pial arterioles, which can be visualized in the arterial phase of the angiogram (Jacobs & Harnsberger 1991). Visualization of pial supply has been shown to predict a decreased likelihood of an extrapial dissection being possible (Sindou & Alaywan 1998). The impact, however, of this foreknowledge on microsurgical technique is unclear (DeMonte & Sawaya 1998).

Magnetic resonance imaging of intracranial meningiomas

The high-field MR imaging characteristics of meningiomas are relatively consistent. On T1-weighted images, 60–90% of meningiomas are isointense, whereas 10–30% are mildly hypointense when compared with gray matter (Spagnoli et al 1986; Elster et al 1989; Demaerel et al 1991a; Zimmerman 1991) (Fig. 31.11). T2-weighted imaging reveals that 30–45% of meningiomas are of increased signal intensity, whereas approximately 50% are isointense to gray matter (Spagnoli et al 1986; Elster et al 1989; Demaerel et al 1991a; Zimmerman 1991).

Vascular distortion or encasement and tumor vascularity are better assessed by MR imaging than by CT scanning. Flow voids produced by flowing blood identify the vasculature local to the tumor. The ability to decide on an extra-axial localization of a neoplasm is also heightened on MR imaging. Spagnoli and co-workers (1986) identified one or more marginating characteristics in all of their reported cases imaged at 1.5T. Typical marginating characteristics include displacement of blood vessels, the presence of CSF clefts between the tumor and the brain, and inward displacement of the gray–white junction (Ginsberg 1996).

The ability of T2-weighted images to subtype meningiomas is controversial, with some studies reporting 75–96% accuracy and others finding no correlation (Spagnoli et al

1986; Elster et al 1989; Demaerel et al 1991a; Kaplan et al 1992). The amount of cerebral edema present in association with the meningioma may also help to sub-type some of these tumors (Elster et al 1989; Demaerel et al 1991a; Chen et al 1992; Kaplan et al 1992). However, making such distinctions is of little clinical value in the treatment of meningiomas. High signal intensity on T2-weighted images has also been correlated with microscopic hypervascularity and soft tumor consistency (Chen et al 1992). It may also help to predict the ease with which the tumor can be resected from the surrounding brain (Ildan et al 1999). Contrast-enhanced MRI provides the highest level of detection of meningiomas (Zimmerman 1991). Diagnostic classification of meningiomas using MR imaging has a high specificity. Sensitivity is maximal in the low-grade meningioma class and minimal in the high-grade meningioma (Julià-sapé et al 2006). Most meningiomas enhance intensely and homogeneously with intravenous paramagnetic contrast material, and in approximately 10% of cases small additional meningiomas are encountered that are missed on unenhanced MR images (Fig. 31.12). Likewise, contrast enhancement of the dura extending away from the margins of the mass is typical of meningioma, although it can be seen with other dural-based lesions. This 'dural tail' can represent tumor extension, and its resection is important to lessen the risk of recurrence. Postoperative enhanced MRI has also been found to be more sensitive and specific in the detection of residual or recurrent meningioma. Thick and nodular enhancement has a high correlation with recurrent or residual neoplasm (Weingarten et al 1992). Several clinicoradiological features relate to the proliferative potential of meningiomas. Low proliferative indices meningiomas exhibit several features, such as diffuse calcification, small size, round shape, and no perifocal edema. On the contrary, meningiomas with high proliferative indices show a lobulated shape, edema, an unclear border against the brain, and no calcification (Nakasu et al 1995).

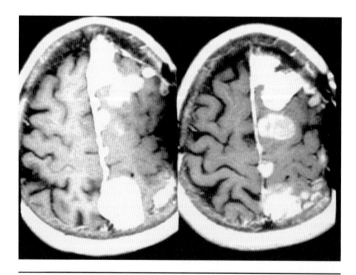

Figure 31.12 Axial post-gadolinium enhanced T1-weighted magnetic resonance image. Multiple meningiomas are clearly seen. Prior to contrast enhancement the extent and number of meningiomas were grossly underestimated.

Magnetic resonance spectroscopy of intracranial meningiomas

Proton MR spectroscopy (1H MR spectroscopy) is a non-invasive technique that is acquiring an important role in the diagnosis of brain tumors before surgery. This technique provides metabolic information regarding the tissue being studied that complements the anatomic information obtained with MR imaging (Majós et al 2004; Roda et al 2000). Different parameters may be varied to optimize 1H MR spectroscopy data acquisition. These parameters determine not only the appearance of the spectrum but also the information that can be extracted from it. One of the most relevant is TE (spin echo at a time) (Majós et al 2004). Short TE 1H MR spectroscopy (TE = 30) produces a slightly more accurate diagnostic outcome in general, whereas long TE (TE = 136) is preferable when meningioma is suspected. (Majós et al 2004). The normal ^{1}H MR spectrum for brain tissue is displayed in Figure 31.13A. Well defined peaks occur at 3.2 ppm for choline, 3.0 ppm for phosphocreatine/creatine (PCr/Cr), and 2.0 ppm for N-acetylaspartate (NAA). A less well defined peak for lactate occurs at 1.3 ppm A typical proton MR spectrum for meningioma is shown in Figure 31.13B. Note the marked increase in choline signal, which may reflect an elevated concentration of mobile membrane precursors. Such an increased pool of membrane components would be necessary during increased cell proliferation, but because the increased choline peak is common to most neoplasms studied, it is not specific for meningioma (Demaerel et al 1991b; Kugel et al 1992), but provides some differentiation between meningiomas and both glioblastomas and metastases (Majós et al 2004).

A marked reduction of both the NAA and PCr/Cr peaks is typically seen in meningioma. As NAA is essentially confined to neurons, this is not a surprising finding. The reason for the marked reduction of the PCr/Cr peak in meningiomas is less clear, although it has been confirmed by *in vivo* phosphorus MRS and *in vitro* ^{1}H MRS, as well as biochemically (Lowry et al 1977). This reduction is greater than that seen in astrocytomas (Kugel et al 1992; Peeling & Sutherland 1992). An additional peak seen in some meningiomas at 1.47 ppm has been assigned to alanine (Kugel et al 1992; Ott et al 1993) (Fig. 31.13B). Alanine (Ala) helps to separate meningiomas from gliomas and metastasis (Majós et al 2004). *In vitro* studies have shown that ^{1}H MRS can differentiate various low-grade tumors, including meningiomas (Tugnoli et al 1998). Furthermore, Preul and his colleagues (1996) were able correctly to diagnose 90–91 tumors examined *in vivo* using ^{1}H MRS including all nine meningiomas. There is also evidence that ^{1}H MRS may be useful in the grading of tumor aggressiveness and in the differentiation of recurrent tumor growth from treatment effects (Ott et al 1993).

Management

Surgery

The mainstay of treatment for meningiomas remains surgical resection. Critical parameters that affect the ease of surgical removal include tumor location, size, consistency, vascular and neural involvement, and, in the case of recurrence, prior

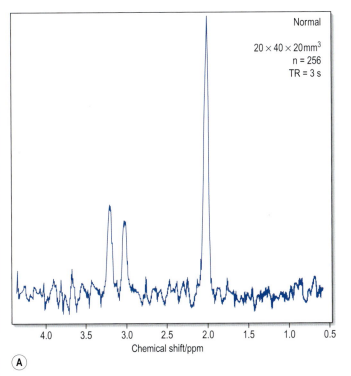
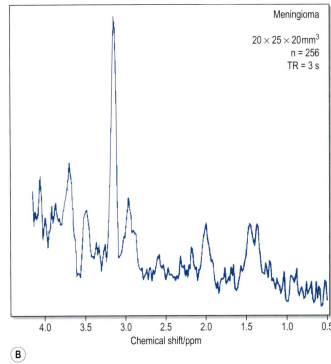

Figure 31.13 (A) Normal proton MR spectrum for brain tissue. Note the well defined peaks at 3.2 ppm for choline, 3.0 ppm for phosphocreatine/creatine, and 2.0 ppm for *N*-acetylaspartate. A less well defined peak for lactate occurs at 1.3 ppm. (B) Typical proton MR spectrum for meningioma. Note the marked increase in the choline signal and decreases in both the phosphocreatine/creatine and *N*-acetylaspartate peaks. A fourth peak is seen at just under 1.5 ppm and has been attributed to alanine. (Reproduced with permission from Demaerel P, Johannik K, Van Hecke P, et al. (1991b) Localized 1H NMR spectroscopy in fifty cases of newly diagnosed intracranial tumors. J Comput Assist Tomogr 1991b; 15(1): 67–76.)

surgery and/or radiotherapy. To reduce the chances of recurrence, it is necessary to resect not only all of the neoplasm but all of the involved dura, soft tissue, and bone.

In 1957, Simpson introduced a 5-grade classification of the surgical removal of meningiomas (Simpson 1957). The higher the Simpson grade, the higher the rate recurrence. Kobayashi and associates (1992) revised the Simpson grading system from a microsurgical perspective by introducing a classification based on the extent of microscopic resection (Table 31.2). The inclusion of an additional 2-cm dural margin has been denoted as a grade 0 removal. This further decreases the rate of recurrence (Kinjo et al 1993). This is possible not only in convexity meningiomas, but also in small medial sphenoid wing meningiomas after dissecting the dura from the floor of the middle fossa and the lateral wall of the cavernous sinus. New and innovative approaches have been devised to reach and widely expose meningiomas in any location.

Preoperative care

All patients have preoperative MRI and a bony window CT scan, which are integrated in the neuronavigation system in use. MRA or CT scan angiography are used to delineate the vascular system. The patient is put on anticonvulsant therapy, dexamethasone, antibiotics and an H_2 antagonist. Pneumatic compression devices are placed on the legs. The spinal needle is inserted to drain cerebrospinal fluid during the operation when needed. Electrodes for electromyography, motor evoked potentials, sensory evoked potentials and auditory evoked potentials are inserted as appropriate to

Table 31.2 Modified Shinshu grade or Okudesa-Kobayashi grade

Grade I	Complete microscopic removal of tumor and dural attachment with any abnormal bone
Grade II	Complete microscopic removal of tumor with diathermy coagulation of its dural attachment
Grade IIIA	Complete microscopic removal of intradural and extradural tumor without resection or coagulation of its dural attachment
Grade IIIB	Complete microscopic removal of intradural tumor without resection or coagulation of its dural attachment or of any extradural extensions
Grade IVA	Intentional subtotal removal to preserve cranial nerves or blood vessels with complete microscopic removal of dural attachment
Grade IVB	Partial removal, leaving tumor of <10% in volume
Grade V	Partial removal, leaving tumor of >10% in volume, or decompression with or without biopsy

Adapted from Kobayashi K, Okudera H, Tanaka Y: Surgical considerations on skull base meningioma. Paper presented at the First International Skull Base Congress, June 18, 1992, Hanover, Germany.

monitor the nerves in the operative fields, as are leads for specific cranial nerves.

General operative procedures

Positioning of the patient should be done in a fashion that maximizes the patient's safety, the accessibility of the tumor, the allowance for unimpeded venous drainage, the beneficial effects of gravity, and the surgeon's comfort.

As well as taking advantage of the effects of gravity, several methods are employed to minimize brain retraction, among which is spinal drainage. However, contraindications, such as large tumors or obstructive hydrocephalus, should be considered. Hyperventilation to a P_{CO_2} of 25–30 and a 20% solution of mannitol at a dosage of 0.25 g/kg contribute to the degree of brain relaxation.

The best means of reducing brain retraction, however, is to eliminate the need to do so by using one of the basal approaches. Since these approaches utilize orbital and zygomatic osteotomies and increase removal of the bony skull base, they allow a low flat route to basally located tumors (Jane et al 1982; Al-Mefty et al 1988; Sen & Sekhar 1990; Al-Mefty et al 1991; DeMonte & Al-Mefty 1993a).

Scalp flaps, which should be wide-based to allow for a rich blood supply and designed to facilitate any subsequent reoperation, should be linear, gently curvilinear, or bicoronal incisions (rather than 'horseshoe' flaps).

In the vast majority of first operations for meningiomas, a layer of arachnoid separates the tumor from the brain parenchyma, cranial nerves, and blood vessels. When it does, the chances of neural and/or vascular injury can be greatly reduced by defining and staying within this surgical plane. One maneuver that facilitates the definition of the arachnoidal borders is the extensive debulking of the tumor, thus allowing the tumor capsule to collapse inward. The method used to debulk the tumor, which may be suction, coagulation, sharp excision, or use of the ultrasonic aspirator or the surgical laser, depends on the tumor consistency, vascularity, and location.

Once the mass of the meningioma is resected, careful attention must be given to removing the involved dura and bone. The extent of bone that must be removed can be determined by inspection of the preoperative CT scan's 'bone windows'. All of the hyperostotic bone should be considered contaminated by neoplastic cells: the fear of entering the mastoid air cells or paranasal sinuses is not cause for failing to remove this diseased bone. A wide margin of dura should be resected, and the defect should be repaired with pericranium, temporalis fascia, or fascia lata.

Cranio-orbital zygomatic approach

This approach is most suitable for large lesions in the suprasellar, parasellar, and retrosellar areas and for those extending into the cavernous sinus or the orbit and along the tentorial notch. Deep lesions can be handled through subfrontal, trans-sylvian, or sub-temporal routes during the same operation.

Patient position
The patient is placed supine. The head is rotated 30–40° to the opposite side and is slightly tilted toward the floor. The head is fixed in position using the Mayfield head holder.

Craniotomy techniques
A curvilinear incision is made behind the hairline and extends from the zygomatic arch on the ipsilateral side to pass the midline toward to the superior temporal line of the opposite side. The superficial and deep fascia of the temporalis muscle are cut parallel to the zygomatic arch, preserving the frontal branches of the facial nerve. A large, vascularized pericranial flap is reflected. The zygomatic arch is incised obliquely anteriorly and posteriorly. The zygoma

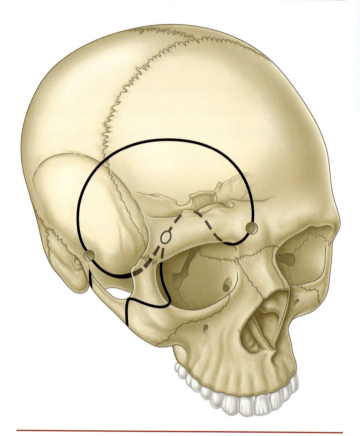

Figure 31.14 Artist's representation of the osteotomies and areas of bone removal required to perform a cranio-orbital-zygomatic craniotomy.

is then reflected inferiorly. The temporalis muscle is detached from its insertions and retracted inferiorly. A burr hole is place in the anatomic key hole. This allows access to the anterior cranial fossa and the periorbita. Burr holes are then placed on the floor of the middle fossa. Using a high-speed drill, the burr holes are connected. The orbital roof is cut using a v-shaped osteotome. The bone flap is reflected as one piece. The lateral wall and roof of the orbit are removed in a separate osteotomy (Fig. 31.14).

Further steps depend on the size and extent of the lesion. Extradural removal of the anterior clinoid process, exposure of the subclinoid internal carotid artery, and exposure of the petrous internal carotid artery are key steps to unlocking the cavernous sinus. The avenue and site of entering into the cavernous sinus depend on the anatomy of the tumor within it.

Zygomatic extended middle fossa approach

This approach can be combined with an anterior petrosectomy for lesions extending posteriorly into the upper petroclival area above the level of the internal auditory meatus.

Patient position
The patient's head is rotated approximately 30–40° to the contralateral side and tilted slightly contralaterally. The head is fixed in this position using the Mayfield head holder. A spinal drain is placed.

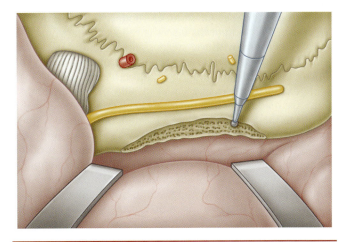

Figure 31.16 Zygomatic anterior petrosal approach with drilling of the petrous apex behind V3 after sectioning the middle meningeal.

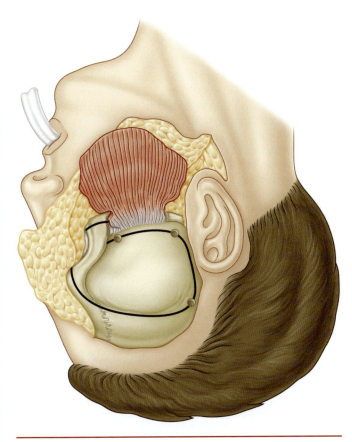

Figure 31.15 Zygomatic middle fossa flap of the anterior petrosal approach.

Surgical technique

A preauricular, curvilinear incision is made starting at the inferior margin of the root of the zygoma, anterior to the tragus, encircling posteriorly just above the external auditory meatus, and then curved anteriorly and medially toward the midline just behind the hairline. The skin flap is separated from the underlying temporalis fascia. The superficial and deep temporalis fascia layers are cut sharply anteriorly, preserving the frontal branches of the facial nerve. The zygoma root and arch are dissected in the subperiosteal plane and cut obliquely anteriorly and posteriorly. The zygoma with its masseter muscle attachment is reflected inferiorly. The temporalis muscle is sharply separated from the underlying bone and is retracted inferiorly. Two burr holes are placed low in the middle fossa. One or two additional burr holes can be placed at the superficial temporal line (Fig. 31.15). The burr holes are connected using a high-speed drill. An additional craniectomy is done to ensure maximal access to the inferior middle fossa.

For sphenopetroclival meningiomas with extension along the tentorium, the anterior petrosal approach may be needed. The dura of the middle fossa is separated under the operative microscope. Spinal drainage is useful during this portion of the procedure. The second and third divisions of cranial nerve V are identified. The middle meningeal artery is identified at its entrance from the foramen spinosum and is coagulated and cut. The greater petrosal nerve is identified posteriorly. Inferior and medial to the greater petrosal nerve is the petrous internal carotid artery. In most cases, the petrous internal carotid artery is separated from the middle fossa only by a thin, fibrous layer of tissue. Exposure of the petrous internal carotid artery is done when lateral entry into the cavernous sinus is anticipated. Detailed understanding of the anatomy of the temporal bone is required for performing an anterior petrosectomy (Fig. 31.16). The dural opening for the standard extended middle fossa approach or in combination with the anterior petrosal approach can be performed more medially to avoid excessive direct manipulation of the temporal lobe and its underlying veins.

Petrosal approach and extended petrosal approach

Tumors involving the petroclival area and extension into perimesencephalic or peripontine structures can be approached using the petrosal approach. For more extensive lesions involving anteriorly the clinoidal area and carotid cistern area, the extended petrosal approach should be considered. To access these regions, the petrosal approach offers a number of advantages. The surgeon's operative distance to these regions is shorter than with the retrosigmoid approaches; there is minimal retraction of the cerebellum and temporal lobe; the neural structures (i.e., cranial nerves VII and VIII) are preserved; the otologic structures (i.e., cochlea, labyrinth, and semicircular canals) are preserved; and the major venous sinuses (i.e., transverse and sigmoid), along with the vein of Labbe and other temporal and basal veins, are preserved.

Patient position

The patient is placed in the supine position on the operating table. The table is flexed approximately 20° to allow head and trunk elevation. The patient's ipsilateral shoulder is slightly elevated using a shoulder roll. The head is rotated away from the side of the tumor (approximately 50°) and is flexed slightly toward the floor. The head is fixed in a three-point Mayfield headrest.

Surgical technique

The incision starts at the zygoma, anterior to the tragus, and is carried to approximately 2–3 cm above and encircling the ear, where it descends behind the mastoid process. The skin flap is sharply dissected from the underlying pericranium and fascia. The temporalis fascia is reflected sharply and is kept in continuity with the sternocleidomastoid muscle; the temporalis muscle itself is subsequently sharply dissected off the bone and reflected anteriorly and inferiorly.

Four burr holes, two on each side of the transverse sinus, are made. The first burr hole is placed just medial and inferior to the asterion, which is located at the inferior junction of the transverse and sigmoid sinuses. The second burr hole is placed at the squamous and mastoid junction of the temporal bone, along the projection of the superior temporal line, which opens into the supratentorial compartment. The final two holes are placed approximately 2–3 cm more medially and closer together on either side of the transverse sinus. A temporoparietal craniotomy and lateral occipital craniotomy are performed without connecting the burr holes across the sinus. The holes across the sinus are then connected using the B-1 attachment (without a footplate) of the Midas Rex drill (Midas-Rex, Fort Worth, TX). After meticulous separation of the wall of the sinus from the flap, the bone plate is elevated.

This stage of the operation requires that the surgeon must be familiar with the anatomy of the temporal bone and its surrounding structures. A complete mastoidectomy is performed using a high-speed air drill. The diamond bit should be used when drilling around near vital neural and otologic structures. The sigmoid sinus is skeletonized down to the jugular bulb. The sinodural angle, Citelli's angle, which identifies the location of the superior petrosal sinus, is exposed. The surgeon next drills the superficial mastoid air cells and the deep (retrofacial) air cells. The facial canal and the lateral and posterior semicircular canals are identified. The petrous bone is thinned by drilling along the pyramid toward the apex (Fig. 31.17).

The posterior fossa dura just anterior to the sigmoid sinus is opened. The dura at the floor of temporal fossa is

also opened to the drainage point of the superior petrosal sinus. Depending on the specific anatomy of the vein of Labbe, it may need to be dissected along its course to avoid injury during temporal lobe exposure. The superior petrosal sinus is coagulated or ligated and then transected. The tentorium incision is extended parallel to the pyramid toward the incisura. Care must be taken to avoid injury to cranial nerve IV by cutting the tentorial edge posterior to the insertion of the nerve. For larger tumors with extensive extension into the posterior fossa and CPA, the dura posterior to the sigmoid sinus can be opened, allowing wider and more inferiorly directed access. Access to the transverse sinus is achieved above and below the sinus. We advocate the avoidance of sinus sacrifice in this and all other approaches.

Transcondylar approach

Patient position

Although called by different names: far lateral, posterolateral, extreme lateral, or transcondylar – it is in essence one approach with variations in the patient's position, skin incision, muscle reflection, and craniotomy. We describe our use of the transcondylar approach.

The head and neck are kept in a neutral position to maintain the anatomic course of the vertebral artery and for easier stabilization, if necessary. The patient is then log-rolled and rotated 45°. The patient's head is fixed in position with a Mayfield headrest. The ipsilateral shoulder is gradually pulled downward and taped to keep it from obstructing the field. The ipsilateral thigh is also prepared and draped for the removal of fat and fascia lata if needed.

Craniotomy technique

The skin is incised behind the ear in a curvilinear fashion two fingerbreadths behind the mastoid. The curved incision begins at the level of the external auditory canal and turns downward to the level of the C4 vertebra, where it gradually curves anteriorly into the horizontal neck crease. The skin flap is then retracted laterally and secured with fishhook retractors. This skin flap is well vascularized and can easily be tailored to accommodate other approaches if necessary.

The muscles are presented in three layers. First, the sternocleidomastoid muscle is detached from its origin at the occipital bone. Its innervation by the accessory nerve should be preserved and freed as it enters the medial aspect of the muscle at the level of the C3 vertebra. The splenius capitis, longissimus capitis, and semispinalis muscles – the muscles of the second muscular layer – are also detached along with the sternocleidomastoid muscle and retracted inferiorly and medially.

The muscles of the third, deep layer create two triangles: the superior and inferior suboccipital triangles. The superior suboccipital triangle is delineated by the rectus capitis posterior major, obliquus capitis superior, and obliquus capitis inferior muscles. In the depth of this triangle is the venous compartment, which cushions the horizontal part of the suboccipital vertebral artery, its branches, and the C1 nerve. The inferior suboccipital triangle is delineated by the obliquus capitis inferior, semispinalis cervicis, and longissimus cervicis muscles. In the depth of this triangle is the vertical part of the suboccipital vertebral artery, its branches, its

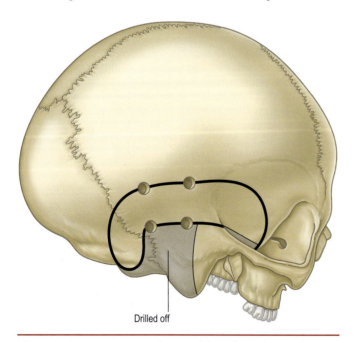

Figure 31.17 Posterior petrosal approach bone flap and mastoidectomy (inset).

Drilled off

surrounding venous plexus, and the C2 nerve with its anterior and posterior rami. The lateral corners of both triangles meet at the transverse process of the atlas, which is located 1 cm below the mastoid tip.

The muscles of this third layer are detached and reflected medially or resected. To improve exposure, the posterior belly of the digastric muscle can also be detached and reflected laterally.

The vertebral artery usually is larger on the left side. During surgery on foramen magnum meningiomas, two segments of the vertebral artery are encountered: the suboccipital (V_3) and the intracranial (V_4). Exposing and mobilizing the V_3 complex allows full proximal control of the artery. Transposing the V_3 complex allows drilling of the condyle, ventral exposure of the tumor, and safe dissection. The V_3 segment is subdivided into two parts: vertical (V_{3v}) and horizontal (V_{3h}).

Opening of the posterior atlanto-occipital membrane is followed by drilling of the posterior wall of the transverse foramen of the atlas and careful, subperiosteal dissection. This dissection spares the lateral (periosteal) ring, which is used to manipulate the V_3 complex.

The posterior ramus of the C2 nerve (i.e., suboccipital nerve) must be sacrificed. The fibrous membrane around the sinus along with the areolar tissue on it must be kept intact to prevent bleeding and the possibility of an air embolus. For bony resection, a lateral, posterior fossa craniotomy is done, and the mastoid tip is drilled to expose the occipital condyle (Fig. 31.18). The sigmoid sinus and jugular bulb are fully exposed, and the atlantal and occipital condyles are drilled. Drilling of the condyle must be tailored to suit the needs of each case. Ventrally located tumors require more extensive drilling of the condyle. Laterally placed tumors need only partial drilling of the condyle. Laminectomy of the atlas and sometimes of the axis must often be done.

The dural incision is centered on the dural ring surrounding the vertebral artery. Opening the dural ring leaves a dural cuff of sufficient size around the artery. An incision along the sigmoid sinus is extended inferiorly to the dural ring. This incision extends further inferiorly and laterally to the level of the atlas or lower if necessary. The dura is tented laterally.

Closure and reconstruction

Skull base approaches require especially meticulous closure. CSF leaks must be avoided by achieving watertight dural closure. The dura may be expanded using autologous fascia lata grafts. A vascularized pericranial graft provides the principal protective layer for skull base reconstruction. A vascularized temporalis muscle graft can also provide an additional strong reconstructive element for the larger, temporally based approaches.

Surgical approaches and techniques by tumor location
Convexity meningiomas

Meningiomas having the greatest potential for total removal and cure are those that overlie the cerebral convexities since they allow for excision with a wide dural margin. Even in instances of transdural bone and soft tissue invasion, an *en bloc* removal is still possible in a procedure that is termed a 'grade zero' removal (Kinjo et al 1993) (Fig. 31.19).

There is usually a long clinical history in the majority of patients. Depending on the location of the tumor, the patient may experience mental deterioration, contralateral limb weakness, sensory aberration, or visual loss, or disturbances of speech when the dominant hemisphere is affected. Seizures are especially frequent when the central or temporal cortices are compressed. Occasionally a bump on the patient's head is the only finding.

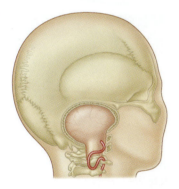

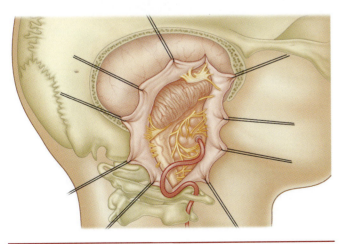

Figure 31.18 Transcondylar flap and mobilization of the vertebral artery.

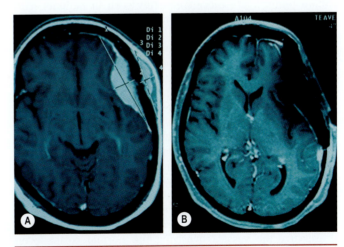

Figure 31.19 Grade 0 removal that includes the tumor, a margin of normal dura, and the involved bone. (A) This axial cut shows the extension of the tumor through the bone under the galea. (B) Postoperative scan shows grade 0 removal.

The initial vital step for the resection of any meningioma is identification of the arachnoidal dissection plane. This should be developed circumferentially for convexity meningiomas by using sharp dissection and inserting non-adhering surgical cottonoids between the arachnoid layer and the tumor capsule. Although the initial isolation of the arachnoidal dissection plane is generally difficult superficially, it usually becomes apparent within the first few millimeters from the surface. Recurrent tumors and some aggressive meningiomas do not have the normal anatomical layers and require careful sharp dissection under the operative microscope to minimize cortical injury.

If the tumor involved the bone, a series of burr holes circumscribe the tumor completely and are made far from the margin of the tumor to obtain healthy dura around the tumor. The dura is opened circumferentially around the tumor 2 cm from the margin of the lesion and the tumor is then removed en bloc (Fig. 31.20).

A consideration for convexity meningiomas that overlie the sylvian fissure is the possibility that branches of the middle cerebral artery have adhered to the tumor capsule. The best procedure for freeing these branches is to begin at points where they are uninvolved and follow them through the tumor. The branches can usually be dissected free in a straightforward fashion, unless the surgical plane is incorrect or the case is a reoperation.

Once the meningioma and a wide dural margin have been resected, the dural defect is repaired with pericranium, temporalis fascia, or fascia lata in a watertight fashion. If excision of bone was required, an acrylic or titanium cranioplasty may be fashioned.

Parasagittal and falcine meningiomas

The signs and symptoms associated with meningiomas arising from the parasagittal and falcine areas are related to where the tumor mass lies along the anteroposterior plane. Anteriorly situated tumors may cause headache, slowly progressive mental decline, visual deterioration secondary to increased intracranial pressure, or generalized seizures. In contradistinction, focal seizures, at times following a Jacksonian pattern, are more frequently seen in patients with meningiomas localized in the middle third. These seizures, as with any motor findings, are generally first evident in the contralateral foot and leg. Symptoms from tumors of the posterior third can, like those in the anterior third, be of insidious onset. Headache, mental symptoms, and intracranial hypertension are common. A distinguishing feature, however, is the finding of visual field loss.

A bicoronal incision allows maximal vascularity to the skin, especially if subsequent craniotomies are performed. The pericranial flap is reflected separately. Multiple burr holes, put in close approximation to each other, are made at the periphery of the tumor. Burr holes straddling the superior sagittal sinus allow safe separation of the dura from the bone. Microsurgical separation of the tumor capsule from surrounding cortex is performed. Most important is preserving the vessels overlying the normal cortex even small ones as the venous drainage of the brain might depend on them. Sacrificing these small draining veins might prove fatal. Decisions regarding the sinus should be individualized for each case according to several factors: the age and

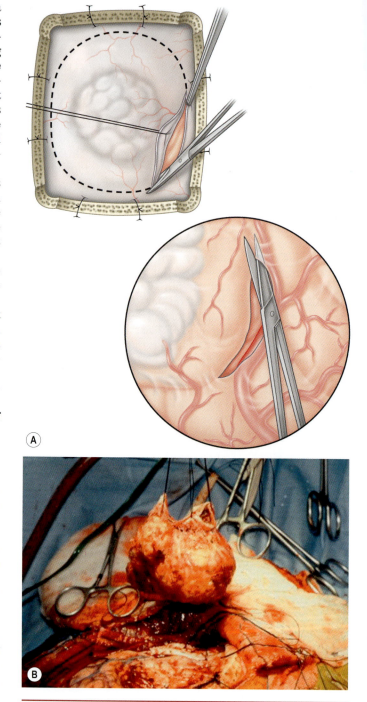

Figure 31.20 After the arachnoidal plane around the tumor is established, dissection should take place in this plane outside the pia (A). The arterial and cortical veins are separated, and surgical patties are gently introduced. This technique, which is used circumferentially around the lesion, delivers the tumor en bloc with little blood loss. The most important technical point is to preserve all cortical veins and arteries and avoid violating the pia. The tumor is then lifted from its bed (B).

symptoms of the patient, the patency of the sinus, the location of the tumor, and the cortical venous collaterals (Fig. 31.21). A truly occluded sinus can be totally excised at any point. Tumor infiltration of one wall can be repaired primarily after the tumor is removed from the sinus. The presence of a cleavage plane between the venous channels per se and

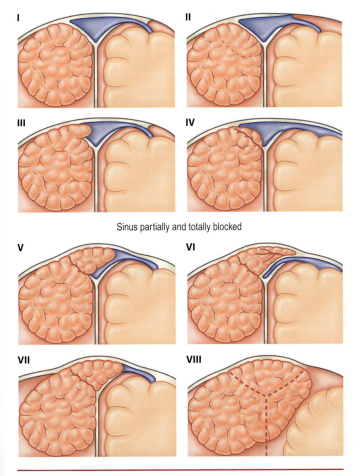

Figure 31.21 Artist's representation of the classification of superior sagittal sinus involvement by parasagittal meningiomas.

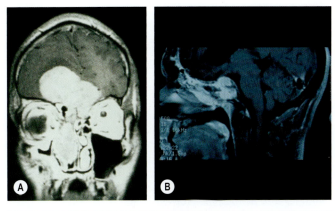

Figure 31.22 Olfactory groove meningioma. (A) Preoperative MRI demonstrates the giant size and displacement of the anterior cerebral artery. (B) MRI after total removal and reconstruction of the floor with pericranial flap.

the invaded outer sinus wall allows tumor removal with preservation of the venous conduit. One or two walls of the sinus can be excised, and reconstruction still provides a good percentage of patency. Technically, total sinus replacement with a venous graft can also be successful; however, the long-term results of this maneuver show patency of only 50%. The potential for delayed occlusion of a totally replaced sinus graft makes us hesitant to excise and replace a patent sinus in the posterior third or the posterior part of the middle third. During reconstruction of the superior sagittal sinus, the blood flow through the sinus may be maintained using an intraluminal shunt (Hakuba et al 1979). This may be essential in posterior third involvement, since even temporary occlusion may result in cerebral engorgement and swelling. The relatively low recurrence rate in the present study (4%) favors attempts at complete tumor removal, including the portion invading the sinus.

Ligating the sinus has the risk of venous infarction and can be performed only in the anterior third. The subgroup of patients without venous reconstruction displays statistically significant clinical deterioration after surgery compared with the group which has a venous reconstruction. Therefore, venous flow restoration seems justified when not too risky (Chernov 2007).

Large parasagittal meningiomas that extend deep into the interhemispheric fissure and, especially, falcine

meningiomas often have anterior cerebral artery branches that have adhered to the bottom edge of the tumor near the free edge of the falx.

Meningiomas of the falx cerebri are less common (20–50% less) than parasagittal tumors, more commonly bilateral, and rarely involve the superior sagittal sinus (Gautier-Smith 1970). As in the case of parasagittal meningiomas, extensive central debulking decreases the need for cerebral retraction. Excision of the falx allows complete removal, as well as access to the opposite side for removal of contralateral tumor extension. The inferior sagittal sinus, which is usually involved by the meningioma, can usually be excised with the tumor unless it provides an essential avenue for venous drainage.

Olfactory groove and tuberculum sellae

Surgical approaches to meningiomas arising from the olfactory groove and to those of the tuberculum sellae (TS) are similar in many respects (Fig. 31.22). Since both tumors are midline lesions that, to a variable degree, derive their blood supply from the ethmoidal branches of the ophthalmic artery, the anterior branch of the middle meningeal artery, and the meningeal branches of the ICA, interruption of this transbasal blood supply is the initial step (Al-Mefty & Smith 1991). Following devascularization, the tumor is debulked with the CUSA or laser, and, finally, the capsule is dissected free and removed (Fig. 31.23)

A unilateral supraorbital craniotomy is usually sufficient for removal of these tumors, but it can easily be extended bilaterally if required. The olfactory nerves are dissected free from the frontal lobes and can be functionally preserved in the case of smaller tumors.

Both tuberculum sellae and large olfactory groove meningiomas displace the optic nerves (ONs) posterolaterally, at times moving them lateral to the carotid arteries. Since the ONs may be quite attenuated and their distinction from the tumor capsule may be quite difficult, extreme caution and piecemeal removal of the tumor using fine tipped bipolars and microdissection are required. At times, it may be necessary to start the dissection at the chiasm to locate and dissect an obscure optic nerve on the contralateral side. Also, the optic nerves are fixed at their entrance into the optic canal,

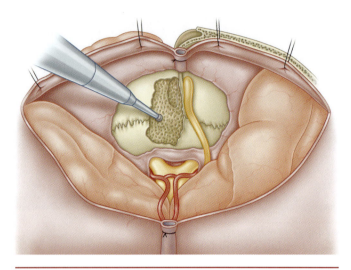

Figure 31.23 Exposure of an olfactory groove meningioma through supraorbital bifrontal approach. After devascularization, the tumor is debulked to a thin capsule that is then dissected carefully from the anterior cerebral artery, optic apparatus, and cortex, and the offending dura and bone removed.

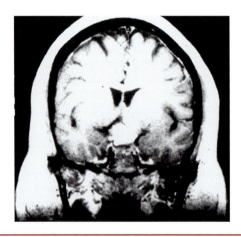

Figure 31.24 T1-weighted MRI post-gadolinium. The signal void representing the left A1 segment of the anterior cerebral artery can be seen encased by this tuberculum sellae meningioma. Careful dissection is required to preserve perforating arteries arising from this vessel and the anterior communicating complex.

and their dissection may begin there. Operative inspection of both optic canals, especially in cases of TS meningiomas, is essential since a tongue of tumor may extend into this area and be missed if efforts are not made to determine its existence.

The anterior cerebral arteries (ACAs) and their branches are the vascular structures most at risk during removal of TS or olfactory groove meningiomas. The A1 segments tend to be particularly stretched or adherent (Fig. 31.24). Further, the arterial twigs arising from the ACAs may be a source of vascular supply for the tumor. These vessels should be carefully followed, prior to occlusion, to ascertain that they are not hypothalamic perforators or optic apparatus supply.

The pituitary stalk, which is generally displaced posteriorly and to one side, can be identified by its characteristic vascular pattern and distinctive color.

Liliequist's membrane is virtually always intact in primary operations and, therefore, dissection of a posteriorly extending tumor from the upper basilar artery is usually straightforward. These tumors may extend into the ethmoid and down into the nasal cavity. Although removal of the extracranial portion can be staged for a second operation, it is frequently preferable to remove intracranial and extracranial parts of the tumor in one operation.

If the sphenoid sinus or nasal cavity is entered during surgery, the mucosa is exenterated, the sinus is packed with fat, the dura is grafted, and a pericranial flap is laid on the floor of the frontal fossa to prevent leakage of CSF. Late recurrence of olfactory groove meningioma is significant and believed to be due to the conservative handling of the underlying invaded bone (Obeid & Al-Mefty 2003).

The diaphragma sellae meningioma is a separate clinico-anatomic entity, although in the literature, they are largely grouped with the tuberculum sellae tumors. They usually grow retro-chiasmatically and manifest with hypothalamic dysfunction. Diaphragma sellae meningiomas are technically more difficult than tuberculum sellae meningiomas because of the deep location and the difficulty of dissecting these tumors from the pituitary stalk. Surgical resection of tuberculum sellae meningiomas is based on a supraorbital approach that allows minimal brain retraction and early control of arterial feeders.

A purely endoscopic endonasal approach to suprasellar supradiaphragmatic lesions with multilayer closure is promoted as a feasible minimally invasive alternative to craniotomy (Laufer et al 2007). With the ability to achieve total removal with minimal morbidity through the skull base approach, the purely endoscopic approach is still inferior to surgery, especially in large and calcified tumors. The ability to decompress the optic nerves inside the optic canals remains a limitation in endoscopic approaches compared to direct surgical decompression. Besides, the risk of CSF leak has not yet been eliminated. However, the use of the endoscope in combination with the microscope to see the concealed corners is proving very useful in certain situations.

Sphenoid wing meningiomas

Sphenoid wing and clinoidal meningiomas are classified based on their origin along the sphenoid wing as clinoidal, middle, and lateral sphenoid wing lesions (Cushing & Eisenhardt 1938; Bonnal et al 1980; Al-Mefty 1990). Meningiomas *en plaque* also occur in the area of the sphenoid wing. Those meningiomas have no significant intracranial component and are characterized by marked hyperostosis of the sphenoid bone, a result of diffuse tumor invasion that causes progressive painless proptosis and, occasionally, diverse cranial neuropathies (due to foraminal encroachment). The dural involvement is widespread, affecting the frontal, temporal, orbital, and sphenoidal regions. The surgical approach to this type of pathology is the complete removal of the greater and lesser sphenoid wings (including the anterior clinoid), the opening of the basal foramina, and the removal of the superior and lateral orbital walls, which then facilitates the removal of the involved dura. Resection of the dura of the superior orbital fissure and the lateral wall of the cavernous sinus can be included. Careful dural repair with fascia lata is reinforced with autologous fat and/or pericranium or temporalis muscle and/or fascia, as needed.

En masse lesions of the pterional third of the sphenoid ridge can be associated with relatively localized head pain and bulging of the frontal and temporal bones. Seizures and contralateral hemiparesis are not uncommon. These tumors can be resected in a fashion similar to convexity meningiomas once the sphenoid ridge is drilled away to allow for the circumferential dural resection needed to remove the tumor's attachment. Drilling away the sphenoid ridge causes interruption of the blood supply to these tumors, which is from the branches of the internal maxillary artery, and leaves a less vascular tumor, thus aiding its removal and minimizing blood loss. Meningiomas in this location spread the sylvian fissure apart and may adhere to or, at times, encase the MCA branches. An arachnoidal plane is invariably present, however, and, with care, the vessels can be freed.

The extradural removal of the sphenoid ridge devascularizes more medially located meningiomas, as well. Furthermore, it allows the optic canal to be opened to decompress the optic nerve. The subclinoid carotid artery can be isolated, which provides distal control of the cavernous carotid artery and facilitates opening and dissecting the tumor from the cavernous sinus. If dissection is planned in the cavernous sinus, proximal ICA control in either the petrous canal or the neck is necessary.

A cranio-orbital-zygomatic approach meets all the requirements for an optimal approach to meningiomas of the sphenoid ridge and can easily be tailored to fit the needs of each patient.

During removal of middle and inner third (alar and clinoidal) meningiomas, the internal carotid, the middle and anterior cerebral arteries and their branches, as well as the optic, oculomotor, and olfactory nerves, are the neurovascular structures at greatest risk. Additionally, anterior clinoidal meningiomas (ACMs), which commonly invade the cavernous sinus, put the third to the sixth cranial nerves at risk (Bonnal et al 1980; Al-Mefty 1990). Group 1 anterior clinoid meningiomas carry an especial risk of carotid injury because of their direct adventitial adherence to the supraclinoid carotid artery (Fig. 31.25).

The surrounding arachnoidal layer allows for these meningiomas to be separated from the neurovascular structures by careful dissection (with the exception of the group 1 anterior clinoid meningiomas), although the tumor may cause marked distortion of the normal anatomy. Initially, the

distal MCA branches are identified in the sylvian fissure and followed back to the tumor. In a similar fashion, the olfactory nerve is dissected from the inferior frontal lobe and followed back to the optic nerve and carotid artery. Identification of the opposite optic nerve allows identification of the optic chiasm. Following the chiasm will allow the identification of the ipsilateral optic nerve (Fig. 31.26).

As in all cases of meningioma surgery, intratumoral debulking facilitates removal, but care must be taken in the opticocarotid triangle and posterior to the carotid bifurcation where injury to perforating arteries may lead to visual loss and hemiparesis, respectively. The location of the ophthalmic artery, which crosses the anterior corner of the opticocarotid triangle, must be anticipated.

Clinoidal meningiomas, which usually present with unilateral loss of vision and optic atrophy, require opening the optic canal and sheath since tumor ingrowth occurs with a high frequency and leaving residual meningioma in this area may contribute to lack of visual improvement postoperatively. As mentioned, clinoidal meningiomas frequently involve the cavernous sinus, which they invade through the superior wall (Bonnal et al 1980; Al-Mefty 1990). Entry through the superior wall may be made via the medial, anteromedial, and paramedial triangles, thereby exposing the anterior loop of the cavernous ICA to allow dissection of the tumor from this space.

Cavernous sinus meningiomas

Meningiomas involving the cavernous sinus may start primarily within it, or the cavernous sinus may be involved by extension from a clinoidal, sphenoid wing, tuberculum sellae, or sphenopetroclival meningioma. Involvement by meningioma of the cavernous sinus (CS) does not preclude aggressive tumor removal. Progressive neurologic deficit and/or progressive enlargement of the tumor, as shown by serial MR

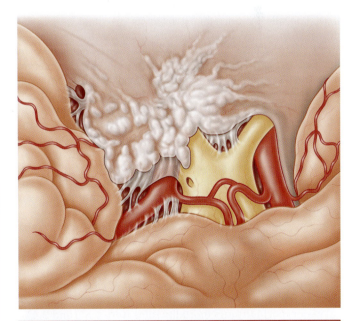

Figure 31.26 Exposure of a clinoidal meningioma through the cranio-orbital zygomatic approach. After splitting the sylvian fissure, the distal branches of the middle cerebral artery are identified and followed toward the encased carotid bifurcation.

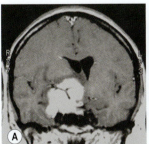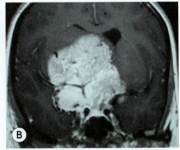

Figure 31.25 An anterior clinoid meningioma encases the carotid artery. (A) Type I with serve adherence to the carotid. (B) Type II with presence of interfacing arachnoid plane.

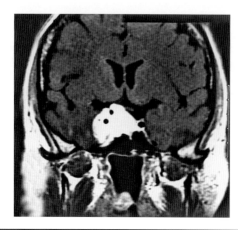

Figure 31.27 Coronal T1-weighted post-contrast MRI. This large cavernous sinus meningioma was completely asymptomatic in this patient even though there is clearly compression of the right optic nerve.

images, are indicators for resection of cavernous sinus meningioma (Fig. 31.27). Extensive evaluation of the available anatomic and physiologic collateral circulation should be made prior to surgery in order to predict the potential risk of cerebral ischemia in the event of carotid artery occlusion. Proximal and distal ICA control, which must be established prior to dissection within the cavernous sinus space, may be achieved by exposing the ICA in the cervical or intrapetrous portions. Entry into the CS may be either through the medial or lateral triangles. Dissection of the tumor progresses in a stepwise fashion, beginning by opening of the dura propria of the optic nerve sheath longitudinally along the length of the optic canal (DeMonte & Al-Mefty 1993a). The distal dural ring is opened next, with the opening extending posteriorly to the oculomotor trigone, and, thereby, also opening the proximal dural ring and allowing a wide entry into the anterior and superior CS space. The carotid artery can be mobilized laterally by releasing it from its proximal and distal dural rings, which then allows dissection in the medial CS space. Lateral entry into the cavernous sinus begins by an incision beneath the projected course of the third nerve, allowing elevation of the outer dural layer of the lateral wall of the cavernous sinus, which is peeled away. The ICA can be located by dissection between the 3rd and 4th nerves and the first division of the trigeminal nerve (Parkinson's triangle). The course of the 6th nerve, which runs lateral to the ICA and is usually directly opposed to it, is usually parallel, but deep to V_1. The tumor is removed from within the cavernous sinus space by suction, bipolar coagulation, and microdissection. A plane of cleavage along the carotid artery can usually be developed. Venous bleeding, typically not a problem when the tumor fills the sinus, may occur as the venous plexus is decompressed by tumor removal. In that event, hemostasis can be obtained by packing the CS space with oxidized cellulose or another similar hemostatic agent.

In the author's series, total removal of cavernous sinus meningioma has been possible in 76% of patients. The surgical major morbidity and mortality rates were 4.8% and 2.4%, respectively. Preoperative CN deficits improved in 14%, remained unchanged in 80%, and permanently worsened in 6%. Seven patients experienced 10 new CN deficits (DeMonte et al 1994).

Posterior fossa meningiomas

A total of 10% of all intracranial meningiomas arise in the posterior fossa. Almost half of these meningiomas are located in the cerebellopontine angle (CPA), 40% are tentorial or cerebellar convexity, and 9% and 6% are clival or at the foramen magnum, respectively (Castellano & Ruggiero 1953; Yasargil et al 1980; Martinez et al 1983). Meningiomas arising medial to the trigeminal nerve (petroclival meningiomas) must be differentiated from those arising lateral to it (CPA or posterior petrous pyramid meningiomas) because petroclival meningiomas carry a significantly higher rate of surgical morbidity (Castellano & Ruggiero 1953; Sekhar & Jannetta 1984; Al-Mefty et al 1988).

CPA (posterior petrous pyramid) meningiomas

Cranial nerve findings are quite common with meningiomas in this location. Hearing loss, facial pain or numbness, and facial weakness or spasm are common, as are headache and cerebellar hemispheric signs (DeMonte & Al-Mefty 1993a).

The cranial nerves of the posterior fossa have a relatively constant relationship to CPA meningiomas: the trochlear nerve is usually superior and lateral to the tumor, whereas the trigeminal nerve is superior and anterior; the abducens nerve is found anteriorly, whereas the 7th and 8th cranial nerves are posterior and the 9th through 11th cranial nerves are inferior (DeMonte & Al-Mefty 1993b).

A standard retrosigmoid approach usually allows sufficient exposure for removal of these tumors (Sekhar & Jannetta 1984; Samii & Ammirati 1991); exposure of the presigmoid dura is, nevertheless, performed to allow retraction of the sigmoid sinus laterally and thus decrease its obstruction of the surgeon's view. The meningioma's dural attachment to the posterior pyramid, which is progressively coagulated and divided to devascularize the tumor, must be done with care to avoid injury to the exiting cranial nerves. If the size of the tumor precludes safe removal, the tumor capsule should be opened and the tumor centrally debulked. After the tumor has been debulked and devascularized, the capsule is carefully dissected from the surrounding cranial nerves, the brain stem, the superior cerebellar artery (SCA; superior and medial), the anterior inferior cerebellar artery (AICA; medial), and posterior inferior cerebellar artery (PICA; inferior and medial). Once the tumor is removed, the dural attachment should be removed or coagulated (either with the bipolar or laser) and any hyperostotic bone drilled away, keeping in mind the location of the nearby inner ear structures.

Petroclival meningiomas

Like CPA meningiomas, these tumors cause diverse cranial neuropathies. Facial hyperesthesia may occur in upward of 80% of patients, while hearing loss and facial weakness occur in 50% and 40%, respectively. The lower cranial nerves and the ocular motor nerves (usually the abducens nerve) are affected in approximately one-third of the patients. Headache and ataxia are common (DeMonte & Al-Mefty 1993b).

For petroclival meningiomas (Fig. 31.28), which require a more lateral approach to maximize visualization and decrease the need for cerebellar retraction, the petrosal approach is an ideal choice (Fig. 31.29). The relationship of the cranial nerves to petroclival meningiomas is similar to

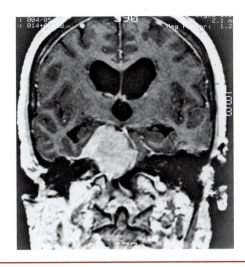

Figure 31.28 Coronal T1-weighted post-contrast MRI. Obstructive hydrocephalus and hyperesthesia in the distribution of the right trigeminal nerve were the only symptoms of this large petroclival meningioma.

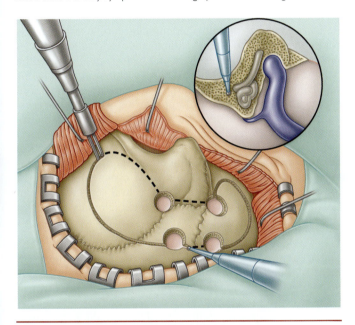

Figure 31.29 Artist's representation of the osteotomies and areas of bone removal required to perform a petrosal craniotomy.

CPA meningiomas except that in the former, the 6th cranial nerve is usually anterior and inferior and may be encased by the tumor (DeMonte & Al-Mefty 1993b). The basilar artery may be displaced posteriorly or to the opposite side, or it may be encased. The posterior cerebral artery (PCA), SCA, AICA, and PICA are usually posterior and medial to the tumor, but they, too, may be encased by it.

Tumor removal begins with progressive devascularization of the tumor by coagulating and dividing its vascular supply from the tentorium and from its insertion on the petrous pyramid and clivus. The arachnoid over the tumor is opened to allow entry through the capsule and central debulking. As noted above, neurovascular structures may be embedded in the meningioma, requiring that great care be taken, especially when using tools such as the ultrasonic aspirator or laser. The tumor capsule is then dissected free

from the surrounding structures, but this must be done gently to avoid hypotension and bradycardia from vagal stimulation. The need to preserve the small perforating arteries to the brain stem and cranial nerves cannot be overemphasized.

As for CPA meningiomas, the point of dural attachment is vaporized and the hyperostotic bone removed with a high speed diamond-tipped drill working under constant irrigation between the cranial nerves. After the dura is closed in a watertight manner, the drilled petrous bone is covered with autologous fat, the temporalis muscle is rotated over the defect and sewn to the sternocleidomastoid muscle, and the soft tissues are closed in multiple layers.

Tentorial and cerebellar convexity meningiomas
Intracranial hypertension, headache, and progressive cerebellar signs (dysmetria, ataxia, hypotonia, and nystagmus) are the usual clinical features associated with either cerebellar convexity meningiomas or those tentorial meningiomas with a large posterior fossa component. If the supratentorial component of a tentorial meningioma is large, visual field defects may also be present.

In many respects, cerebellar convexity and tentorial meningiomas are quite similar to their supratentorial counterparts, the parasagittal and falcine meningiomas. The major area of concern is the status of the transverse sinus: a totally occluded transverse sinus may be excised with the rest of the meningioma, whereas the management of an incompletely occluded transverse sinus is similar to that used for the superior sagittal sinus. When the two transverse sinuses are proven to be interconnected at the torcula, occlusion of the transverse sinus may be accomplished by a temporary vascular clip to measure its filling pressures. If there is no swelling, venous engorgement, or rise in filling pressures of >7–10 mmHg, the transverse sinus may be divided if invaded by meningioma (Spetzler et al 1992). If the sinus is not involved, it should not be sacrificed; rather, the surgeon should alternate the field of vision from the supratentorial to the infratentorial compartments. The technique for removing the tumor is the same as that described for supratentorial parasagittal and falcine meningiomas.

Foramen magnum meningiomas
Foramen magnum tumors, the least common of the posterior fossa meningiomas, are located anterior or anterolateral to the cervicomedullary junction, and are usually intimately involved with the lower cranial nerves (IX–XII), the cervicomedullary junction, and the vertebral artery and its branches (especially PICA). The typical clinical syndrome consists of suboccipital and neck pain (usually in the C2 dermatome), ipsilateral upper extremity dysesthesias, contralateral dissociated sensory loss, progressive limb weakness beginning in the ipsilateral upper extremity and progressing in a counterclockwise fashion, and wasting of the intrinsic muscles of the hand (DeMonte & Al-Mefty 1993b). Since the traditional posterior approach to meningiomas in this location does not address the anterior location of the tumors, the transcondylar or far lateral approach has been devised (Sen & Sekhar 1990; DeMonte & Al-Mefty 1993b) (Fig. 31.18).

The tumor capsule is opened carefully, particular care being given to avoid injury to the cranial nerves or blood vessels, and debulked. It may be detached from its clival base to decrease the vascularity. Careful separation of the tumor from the medulla and upper cervical spinal cord, the lower cranial nerves, and the vertebral artery may be accomplished by dissection in the arachnoidal plane surrounding the tumor. The area of dural attachment is removed, as is any hyperostotic bone, and the dura is closed in a watertight manner to prevent CSF leakage. If the entire occipital condyle has been removed, an occipital–cervical fusion should be performed. Postoperatively, the patient is managed in either a stiff collar or a halo-thoracic brace, depending on the nature of the fusion construct. Injury to the lower cranial nerves, the main cause of operative morbidity, has led to the routine use, in some centers, of electromyographic monitoring of the muscles supplied by the vagus, accessory, and hypoglossal nerves (DeMonte et al 1993).

Dysfunction of the lower cranial nerves is the primary cause of postoperative morbidity. Hence, careful assessment of the patient's ability to protect the airway is mandatory, and, in some cases, early tracheostomy may be warranted to avoid the complication of aspiration pneumonitis.

Intraventricular meningiomas

Meningiomas of the lateral ventricles, which arise from arachnoid cells contained in the choroid plexus and tela choroidea, account for a mere 1% of all intracranial meningiomas. They are almost always (90% of cases) located in the trigone of the lateral ventricle. The vascular supply is from the anterior choroidal artery; in larger lesions, the posterior choroidal artery will also contribute (Konovalov et al 1991).

Numerous approaches to this region have been described and include cortical incisions in the middle temporal gyrus, the posterior paramedian parietal cortex, and the lateral temporal-parietal lobe (Fornari et al 1981; Guidetti et al 1985; Criscuolo & Symon 1986). Access following a temporal or occipital lobectomy has also been proposed (Spencer et al 1991). Since all of these incisions and approaches traverse the cerebral cortex, the possibility of postoperative epilepsy is increased, as is secondary local cortical dysfunction resulting from the vigor of the cerebral retraction required for these routes. Kempe and Blaylock (1976) have described removal of trigonal meningiomas through a midline section of the corpus callosum, which does not require a cortical incision and, with modification, requires little cerebral retraction (McComb & Apuzzo 1987). However, it may be contraindicated for patients with a right homonymous hemianopia since complete splenial section in this circumstance results in alexia without agraphia, a highly morbid condition. This limits the use of this approach as preoperative visual field defects are present in 40–70% of cases (Fornari et al 1981; Konovalov et al 1991). In these patients, and in those with very large tumors, a middle temporal gyrus or posterior paramedian parieto-occipital approach may be better.

The preferred route, however, remains the transcallosal approach. The patient is positioned in the lateral, park bench, or three-quarter prone position, with the side harboring the lateral ventricular meningioma placed inferiorly (McComb & Apuzzo 1987). The head is laterally flexed upward and the table angled such that the falx is placed 30° above the horizontal. A craniotomy straddling the superior sagittal sinus is fashioned, the dura is flapped over the sinus, and any bridging veins are dissected from the cortical surface. The arachnoidal adhesions to the falx are divided, allowing the dependent hemisphere to fall away from the midline, with the rigid falx acting as a retractor and supporting the opposite hemisphere. Once the corpus callosum and the pericallosal arteries are identified, an incision 1.5–2.0 cm in length is made in the corpus callosum between the pericallosal arteries and carried into the tumor-containing lateral ventricle. If the arterial supply to the tumor can be reached, it is divided and then the meningioma is removed in a piecemeal fashion. In cases of large tumors the arterial supply is often inaccessible. The tumor is carefully dissected from the ventricular walls and the choroidal fissure. The internal cerebral veins, which run in the velum interpositum of the transverse cerebral fissure, may adhere to any inferomedial extension of the meningioma into the choroidal fissure.

Pineal region meningiomas

Meningiomas of the pineal region, which arise from either the posterior velum interpositum or more commonly from the dura at the falcotentorial junction, are quite rare (Tung & Apuzzo 1991). Neuro-ophthalmologic symptoms and signs (impaired upgaze, diminished pupillary reflexes) are less common than with other pathologies. Generally, signs of increased intracranial pressure and hydrocephalus bring the patient to medical attention. The two chief approaches for removing these tumors are the supracerebellar-infratentorial route and the supratentorial approaches. The latter is most appropriate for falcotentorial meningiomas as it allows options for tentorial or falcine incisions to increase exposure or to devascularize the neoplasm (Tung & Apuzzo 1991). The infratentorial approach, on the other hand, has the advantages of being the shortest and most direct route, and, in most cases, of having the internal cerebral veins and vein of Galen anterior and superior to the meningioma.

Radiotherapy

The use of traditional external beam irradiation in the treatment of small and medium size meningiomas has largely been replaced by stereotactic radiosurgery in the form of focused-beam radiation delivered in one session and involving the use of spatially defined localization and a rigid head fixation device, or in the form of fractionated, smaller-dose radiation delivered stereotactically and is called stereotactic radiotherapy (Elia et al 2007). Various energy sources are used. The most common of which are photons from ^{60}Co gamma ray sources (GammaKnife) or linear accelerators (LINAC) and heavy particles (protons, helium ions) from cyclotrons. Radiosurgery is an excellent treatment for asymptomatic, small- to moderate-sized meningiomas. It is also ideal for patients with incompletely resected meningiomas, recurrent meningiomas, and risk factors precluding conventional surgery (Kondziolka et al 1999a; Chin et al 2003; Iwai et al 2008). The first use of the GammaKnife to treat a patient with a meningioma was in 1970 (Steiner et al 1991).

Factors that determine dose prescription include: tumor volume, proximity to sensitive structures such as optic nerve, facial nerve, brainstem, and eloquent brain, and previous or future irradiation (Chin et al 2003). The traditional optimal radiosurgery treatment size is less than 3 cm in diameter (Chin et al 2003; Iwai et al 2008). A larger treatment volume requires a lower dose to prevent undue risk of radiation necrosis. (Chin et al 2003) large-volume tumors up to 47.2 mm in diameter can be treated with 2-staged radiosurgery (volume fraction) (Hasegawa et al 2007; Kollová et al 2007; Iwai et al 2008).

An optimum radiosurgical dose for meningioma is still under debate. Doses <12 Gy are a reportedly significant factor in the failure to control meningioma growth (Kollová et al 2007). There is a significantly higher incidence of a tumor volume decrease with a maximum radiosurgical dose >22 Gy and tumor margin dose ≥12 Gy (Davidson et al 2007; Hasegawa et al 2007; Kollová et al 2007). The prescription dose suggested for tumor margins is 12–16 Gy (Chin et al 2003; Davidson et al 2007; Hasegawa et al 2007; Kollová et al 2007). A higher margin doses are associated with higher treatment risks but not an improved tumor control rate (Hasegawa et al 2007; Kollová et al 2007). The size of the tumor can also be a factor in determining the marginal dose. The suggested dose at the tumor margin for meningiomas is 18 Gy (<1 cm), 16 Gy (1–3 cm), and 12–14 Gy (>3 cm) (Chin et al 2003).

The accepted safe dose to the optic nerve is 8 Gy (Chin et al 2003; Kollová et al 2007; Iwai et al 2008; Kondziolka et al 2008), although doses up to 10 Gy have been reported without causing optic nerve injury if only a short (<9–12 mm) segment is placed at risk (Morita et al 1999, Kondziolka et al 1999b). The mean dose to the hypophysis should not exceed 15 Gy, which is considered a safe limit to avoid hypopituitarism caused by radiosurgery (Kollová et al 2007). Depending on the volume, meningiomas along the skull base in the posterior fossa should receive a maximum of 12–16 Gy to avoid injury to the brain stem and facial nerve (Chin et al 2003). The dose to the brain stem should not exceed 14–15 Gy (Chin et al 2003; Kollová et al 2007; Kondziolka et al 2008). Location of the 7th to 8th cranial nerve complex should be identified so that the radiation dose in this area does not exceed 12 Gy (Chin et al 2003; Kondziolka et al 2008).

In contrast to other cranial nerves, the motor cranial nerves in the cavernous sinus appear most resistant to radiation (Tishler et al 1993; Leber et al 1998; Chin et al 2003; Kondziolka et al 2008). 19 Gy appears to be a threshold for injury of the trigeminal nerve (Chin et al 2003).

Overall treatment results for meningiomas are excellent. Tumor growth control is 83–95% of the cases (Steiner et al 1991; Kondziolka et al 1999a; Chin et al 2003), and the actuarial progression-free survival rate is 93–100% at 5 years (Davidson et al 2007; Kollová et al 2007; Iwai et al 2008) and 83–97% at 10 years (Davidson et al 2007; Hasegawa et al 2007; Iwai et al 2008).

The volume of treated tumors decreases in 13.9–69.7% of cases, remains unchanged in 27.8–83.3% and increases in 2.5–12% (Davidson et al 2007; Hasegawa et al 2007; Kollová et al 2007; Iwai et al 2008). Treatment is not without side-effects. The temporary morbidity rate was 10.2% and the permanent morbidity rate was 5.7% (Kollová et al 2007). Local recurrence is reported to occur in 6% and recurrence outside the treatment field is reported to occur in 10% (Iwai et al 2008).

Treatment of parasagittal and convexity meningiomas with radiosurgery results in a higher incidence of perilesional edema and treatment of parasagittal tumors exposes a larger volume of brain to radiation compared with skull base tumors (Chin et al 2003). Radiosurgery can be considered a sole treatment for tumors <3 cm that do not cause neurological deficits. Symptomatic tumors and those >3 cm should be treated by resection and then by radiosurgery targeting areas of residual tumor (Chin et al 2003). Radiosurgery is an effective and safe treatment for cavernous sinus meningiomas especially in tumors <3 cm (Chin et al 2003; Davidson et al 2007; Hasegawa et al 2007), but craniotomy is needed for debulking and decompressing the optic apparatus in larger tumors and those that compromise vision or tumors that abut the optic pathways but do not cause compression or visual loss to allow an appropriate radiosurgical dose, while limiting radiation to the optic apparatus dose to <8–10 Gy (Chin et al 2003). Only small petroclival meningiomas may be appropriately treated with SRS alone. Radiosurgery in larger tumors could be undertaken postoperatively if there are remnants (Chin et al 2003).

The incidence of radiosurgically induced neoplasms is low. However, few of the large GKS series have sufficiently long follow-up review periods to establish the true incidence of radiosurgically induced neoplasia. Both physicians and patients need to be aware of this possibility (Sheehan et al 2006). Malignant transformation after stereotactic irradiation can occur, but it is not evident if the cause is intrinsic transformation or radiation induced (Kunert et al 2009; Iwai et al 2008) this potential complication is much lower than that known for conventional fractionated radiotherapy (Chin et al 2003). Aggressive regrowth can follow failed radiosurgery, even in a substantially delayed fashion several years after radiosurgical treatment (up to 14 years), indicating that consistent and extended follow-up evaluations should be performed in all cases of even benign meningiomas after radiosurgery (Couldwell et al 2007).

Experience with the LINAC is more limited. Tumor control at 5 years was achieved in 89.3–100% (Chang et al 1998; Hakim et al 1998; Shafron et al 1999). No definitive study has been done comparing the efficacy of the LINAC to that of the GammaKnife in treating meningiomas.

Brachytherapy

The stereotactic and direct microsurgical implantation of radioactive seeds into meningiomas has been reported by several groups who have found these procedures to be beneficial, but so far the number of patients treated is low and the length of follow-up is short (Gutin et al 1987; Kumar et al 1991). The concern with tumor size is not as great as it is with stereotactic irradiation since the radiation dose is slowly delivered by the decay of the radioisotope (usually ^{125}I).

Accurate and precise planning of dosimetry is crucial. Marked changes in tumor sizes that can be seen with treatment indicate a concern that seed migration and the delivery of unwanted radiation to nearby neurovascular structures might occur (Al-Mefty 1991). If this concern can be successfully dealt with, then brachytherapy may become a very valuable adjunct for treating meningiomas.

Chemotherapy

The role of adjuvant chemotherapy in patients with meningiomas remains unclear and continues to evolve (Newton

2007). Chemotherapy has been applied mainly to inoperable lesions, especially in the setting of tumor progression or recurrence after some form of radiotherapy (Newton 2007). Numerous approaches have been taken, including the use of traditional cytotoxic drugs, molecular agents, immunomodulators, and hormone-manipulating drugs. Although none of these drugs has been particularly effective, a modest activity in sub-groups of patients has been demonstrated with some agents (Newton 2007). Conventional chemotherapy (5-fluorouracil, folinic acid, levamisole, cyclophosphamide, Adriamycin and vincristine) (Bernstein et al 1994; Chamberlain 1996; Newton 2007), and interferon a-2B showed modest response (Kaba et al 1997; Newton 2007), while other drugs such as the topoisomerase inhibitor irinotecan are under investigation for their effect on malignant and benign meningiomas (Gupta et al 2007). Antiestrogenic agents (tamoxifen) (Goodwin et al 1993) and antiprogesterone agents (agent RU-486) (Grunberg et al 1991; Lamberts et al 1992b) has been generally ineffective (Newton 2007). Drugs that inhibit the growth factor receptors involved in the oncogenesis of meningiomas (imatinib and erlotinib) are under study (Newton 2007).

Hydroxyurea works by inhibition of the enzyme ribonucleotide reductase which is a tightly regulated enzyme working on either de novo DNA synthesis or DNA repair processes (Newton 2007). Hydroxyurea remains one of the most promising agents in treating meningioma, it has demonstrated modest clinical activity against inoperable and recurrent meningiomas and can often induce clinical and radiological stabilization (Schrell et al 1997a,b; Cusimano 1998; Newton 2007).

REFERENCES

Al-Mefty, O., 1990. Clinoidal meningiomas. J. Neurosurg. 73 (6), 840–849.

Al-Mefty, O., 1991. Comment on Kumar, P.P., Patil, A.A., Liebrock, L.G., et al. Brachytherapy: a viable alternative in the management of basal meningiomas. Neurosurgery 29 (5), 680.

Al-Mefty, O., Fox, J.L., Smith, R.R., 1988. Petrosal approach for petroclival meningiomas. Neurosurgery 22 (3), 510–517.

Al-Mefty, O., Kadri, P., Pravdenkova, S., et al., 2004a. Malignant progression in meningioma: Documentation of a series and analysis of cytogenetic findings. J. Neurosurg. 101 (2), 210–218.

Al-Mefty, O., Smith, R.R., 1991. Tuberculum sellae meningiomas. In: Al-Mefty, O. (Ed.), Meningiomas. Raven Press, New York, pp. 397–398.

Al-Mefty, O., Topsakal, C., Pravdenkova, S., et al., 2004b. Radiation-induced meningiomas: Clinical, pathological, cytokinetic, and cytogenetic characteristics. J. Neurosurg. 100 (6), 1002–1013.

Al-Rodhan, N.R.F., Laws, E.R. Jr., 1991. The history of intracranial meningiomas. In: Al-Mefty, O. (Ed.), Meningiomas. Raven Press, New York, pp. 1–7.

Annegers, J.F., Laws, E.R. Jr., Kurland, L.T., et al., 1979. Head trauma and subsequent brain tumors. Neurosurgery 4 (3), 203–206.

Arrington, A.S., Lednicky, J.A., Butel, J.S., 2000. Molecular characterisation of SV40 DNA in multiple samples from a human mesothelioma. Anticancer Res. 20 (2A), 879–884.

Assi, A., Declich, P., Iacobellis, M., et al., 1999. Secretory meningioma, a rare meningioma subtype with characteristic glandular differentiation: an histological and immunohistochemical study of 9 cases. Adv. Clin. Pathol. 3 (3), 47–53.

Barnett, G.H., Chou, S.M., Bay, J.W., 1986. Posttraumatic intracranial meningioma: a case report and review of the literature. Neurosurgery 18 (1), 75–78.

Bello, M.J., de Campos, J.M., Vaquero, J., et al., 2000. High-resolution analysis of chromosome arm 1p alterations in meningioma. Cancer Genet. Cytogenet. 120 (1), 30–36.

Bernstein, M., Villamil, A., Davidson, G., et al., 1994. Necrosis in a meningioma following systemic chemotherapy. J. Neurosurg. 81 (2), 284–287.

Bickerstaff, E.R., Small, J.M., Guest, I.A., 1958. The relapsing course of certain meningiomas in relation to pregnancy and menstruation. J. Neurol. Neurosurg. Psychiatry 21 (2), 89–91.

Bikmaz, K., Mrak, R., Al-Mefty, O., 2007. Management of bone-invasive, hyperostotic sphenoid wing meningiomas. J. Neurosurg. 107 (5), 905–912.

Bogdanowicz, W.M., Sachs, E., 1974. The possible role of radiation in oncogenesis of meningioma. Surg. Neurol. 2 (6), 379–383.

Bondy, M., Ligon, B.L., 1996. Epidemiology and etiology of intracranial meningiomas: A review. J. Neurooncol. 29 (3), 197–205.

Bonnal, J., Thibaut, A., Brotchi, J., et al., 1980. Invading meningiomas of the sphenoid ridge. J. Neurosurg. 53 (3), 587–599.

Brandis, A., Mirzai, S., Tatagiba, M., et al., 1993. Immunohistochemical detection of female sex hormone receptors in meningiomas: correlation with clinical and histological features. Neurosurgery 33 (2), 212–218.

Bruna, J., Brell, M., Ferrer, I., et al., 2007. Ki-67 proliferative index predicts clinical outcome in patients with atypical or anaplastic meningioma. Neuropathology 27 (2), 114–120.

Caldarelli-Stefano, R., Boldorini, R., Monga, G., et al., 2000. JC virus in human glial-derived tumours. Hum. Pathol. 31 (3), 394–395.

Carroll, R.S., Schrell, U.M., Zhang, J., et al., 1996. Dopamine D1, dopamine D2, and prolactin receptor messenger ribonucleic acid expression by the polymerase chain reaction in human meningiomas. Neurosurgery 38 (2), 367–375.

Carroll, R.S., Zhang, J., Dashner, K., et al., 1995. Androgen receptor expression in meningiomas. J. Neurosurg. 82 (3), 453–460.

Castellano, F., Ruggiero, G., 1953. Meningiomas of the posterior fossa. Acta Radiol. 104 (Suppl.), 1–177.

CBTRUS, 2008. Statistical Report: Primary brain tumors in the United States, 2000–2004. Central Brain Tumor Registry of the United States, Hinsdale, IL.

Cerda-Nicolas, M., Lopez-Gines, C., Perez-Bacete, M., et al., 2000. Histopathological and cytogenetic findings in benign, a typical and anaplastic human meningiomas: A study of 60 tumors. Clin. Neuropathol. 19 (6), 259–267.

Chamberlain, M.C., 1996. Adjuvant combined modality therapy for malignant meningiomas. J. Neurosurg. 84 (5), 733–736.

Chang, S.D., Adler, J.R., Martin, D.P., 1998. LINAC radiosurgery for cavernous sinus meningiomas. Stereotact. Funct. Neurosurg. 71 (1), 43–50.

Chauveinc, L., Ricoul, M., Sabatier, L., et al., 1997. Dosimetric and cytogenetic studies of multiple radiation induced meningiomas for a single patient. Radiother. Oncol. 43 (3), 285–288.

Chen, T.C., Zee, C.S., Miller, C.A., et al., 1992. Magnetic resonance imaging and pathological correlates of meningiomas. Neurosurgery 31 (6), 1015–1022.

Chernov, M., 2007. Meningiomas of the superior sagittal sinus. J. Neurosurg. 106 (4), 736–737.

Chin, L.S., Szerlip, N.J., Regine, W.F., 2003. Stereotactic radiosurgery for meningiomas. Neurosurg. Focus 14 (5), E6–1–E6-E6–1–E6.

Choi, N.W., Schuman, L.M., Gullen, W.H., 1970. Epidemiology of primary central nervous system neoplasms II. Case-control study. Am. J. Epidemiol. 91 (5), 467–485.

Claus, E.B., Bondy, M.L., Schildkraut, J.M., et al., 2005. Epidemiology of intracranial meningioma. Neurosurgery 57 (6), 1088–1095.

Cobb, M.A., Husain, M., Andersen, B.J., et al., 1996. Significance of proliferating cell nuclear antigen in predicting recurrence of intracranial meningiomas. J. Neurosurg. 84 (1), 85–90.

Collins, V.P., Nordenskjöld, M., Dumanski, J.P., 1990. The molecular genetics of meningiomas. Brain Pathol. 1 (1), 19–24.

Couldwell, W.T., Cole, C.D., Al-Mefty, O., 2007. Patterns of skull base meningioma progression after failed radiosurgery. J. Neurosurg. 106 (1), 30–35.

Criscuolo, G.R., Symon, L., 1986. Intraventricular meningioma. A review of 10 cases of the National Hospital, Queen Square (1974–1985) with reference to the literature. Acta Neurochir. (Wien) 83 (3–4), 83–91.

Cuomo, L., Trivedi, P., Cardillo, M.R., et al., 2001. Human herpesvirus 6 infection in neoplastic and normal brain tissue. J. Med. Virol. 63 (1), 45–51.

Cushing, H., 1922. The meningiomas (dural endotheliomas): their source, and favoured seats of origin. Brain 45, 282–316.

Cushing, H., Eisenhardt, L., 1938. Meningiomas: Their classification, regional behavior, life history, and surgical end results. Charles, C. Thomas, Springfield, IL.

Cushing, H., Weed, L.H., 1915. Studies on the cerebrospinal fluid and its pathway. No. IX. Calcareous and osseous deposits in the arachnoidea. Bull. Johns Hopkins Hosp. 26, 367.

Cusimano, M.D., 1998. Hydroxyurea for treatment of meningioma (letter). J. Neurosury. 88 (5), 938–939.

Davidson, L., Fishback, D., Russin, J.J., 2007. Postoperative Gamma Knife surgery for benign meningiomas of the cranial base. Neurosurg. Focus 23 (4), E6.

Davis, F.G., Kupelian, V., Freels, S., et al., 2001. Prevalence estimates for primary brain tumors in the United States by behavior and major histology groups. Neuro. Oncol. 3 (3), 152–158.

Del Valle, L., Gordon, J., Assimakopolou, M., et al., 2001. Detection of JC virus DNA sequences and expression of the viral regulatory protein T-antigen in tumors of the central nervous system. Cancer Res. 61 (10), 4287–4293.

Delbue, S., Pagani, E., Gucrini, F.R., et al., 2005. Distribution, characterization and significance of polyomavirus genomic sequences in tumors of the brain and its covering. J. Med. Virol. 77 (3), 447–454.

Demaerel, P., Wilms, G., Lammens, M., et al., 1991a. Intracranial meningiomas: correlation between MR imaging and histology in fifty patients. J. Comput. Assist. Tomogr. 15 (1), 45–51.

Demaerel, P., Johannik, K., Van Hecke, P., et al., 1991b. Localized ^{1}H NMR spectroscopy in fifty cases of newly diagnosed intracranial tumors. J. Comput. Assist. Tomogr. 15 (1), 67–76.

De Mattei, M., Martini, F., Corallini, A., et al., 1995. High incidence of BK virus large T-antigen-coding sequences in normal human tissues and tumors of different histotypes. Int. J. Cancer 61 (6), 756–760.

DeMonte, F., Al-Mefty, O., 1993a. Anterior clinoidal meningiomas. In: Rengachary, S.S., Wilkins, R.H. (Eds.), Neurosurgical operative atlas, vol. 3. Williams & Wilkins, Baltimore, MD, pp. 49–61.

DeMonte, F., Al-Mefty, O., 1993b. Neoplasms and the cranial nerves of the posterior fossa. In: Barrow, D.L. (Ed.), Surgery of the cranial nerves of the posterior fossa. American Association of Neurological Surgeons, Park Ridge, IL, pp. 253–274.

DeMonte, F., Sawaya, R.E., 1998. Comments on Sindou, M.P. & Alaywan, M. Most intracranial meningiomas are not cleavable tumors: Anatomic-surgical evidence and angiographic predictability. Neurosurgery 42 (3), 480.

DeMonte, F., Smith, H.K., Al-Mefty, O., 1994. Outcome of aggressive removal of cavernous sinus meningiomas. J. Neurosurg. 81 (2), 245–251.

DeMonte, F., Warf, P., Al-Mefty, O., 1993. Intraoperative monitoring of the lower cranial nerves during surgery of the jugular foramen and lower clivus. In: Loftus, C., Traynelis, V. (Eds.), Intraoperative monitoring techniques in neurosurgery. McGraw-Hill, New York, pp. 205–212.

Drummond, K.J., Zhu, J.J., Black, P.M., 2004. Meningiomas: updating basic science, management, and outcome. Neurologist 10 (3), 113–130.

Elia, A.E., Shih, H.A., Loeffler, J.S., 2007. Stereotactic radiation treatment for benign meningiomas. Neurosurg. Focus 23 (4), E5.

Elster, A.D., Challa, V.R., Gilbert, T.H., et al., 1989. Meningiomas: MR and histopathologic features. Radiology 170 (3 pt. 1), 857–862.

Fewings, P.E., Battersby, R.D., Timperley, W.R., et al., 2000. Long-term follow up of progesterone receptor status in benign meningioma: a prognostic indicator of recurrence. J. Neurosurg. 92 (3), 401–405.

Figueroa, B.E., Quint, D.J., McKeever, P.E., et al., 1999. Extracranial metastatic meningioma. Br. J. Radiol. 72 (857), 513–516.

Fiori, M., Di Mayorca, G., 1976. Occurrence of BK virus DNA in DNA obtained from certain human tumors. Proc. Natl. Acad. Sci. USA 73 (12), 4662–4666.

Fisher, S.G., Weber, L., Carbone, M., 1999. Cancer risk associated with simian virus 40 contaminated polio vaccine. Anticancer Res. 19 (3B), 2173–2180.

Fornari, M., Savoiardo, M., Morello, G., et al., 1981. Meningiomas of the lateral ventricles: neuroradiological and surgical considerations in 18 cases. J. Neurosurg. 54 (1), 64–74.

Fotopoulos, A.D., Alexiou, G.A., Goussia, A., et al., 2008. (99m) Tc-Tetrofosmin brain SPECT in the assessment of meningiomas-correlation with histological grade and proliferation index. J Neurooncol. 89 (2), 225–230.

Friend, K.E., Radinsky, R., McCutcheon, I.E., 1999. Growth hormone receptor expression and function in meningiomas: effect of a specific receptor antagonist. J. Neurosurg. 91 (1), 93–99.

Froman, C., Lipschitz, R., 1970. Demography of tumors of the central nervous system among the Bantu (African) population of the Transvaal, South Africa. J. Neurosurg. 32 (6), 660–664.

Gabeau-Lacet, D., Aghi, M., Betensky, R.A., et al., 2009. Bone involvement predicts poor outcome in atypical meningioma. J. Neurosurg. 111 (3), 464–471.

Gautier-Smith, P.C., 1970. Parasagittal and falx meningiomas. Butterworths, London.

Ginsberg, L.E., 1996. Radiology of meningiomas. J. Neurooncol. 29 (3), 229–238.

Giordano, C., Lamouche, M., 1973. Méningiomes en Côte D'Ivoire. Afr. J. Med. Sci. 4 (2), 259–263.

Giovacchini, G., Fallanca, F., Landoni, C., et al., 2009. C-11 choline versus F-18 fluorodeoxyglucose for imaging meningiomas: an initial experience. Clin. Nucl. Med. 34 (1), 7–10.

Glick, R.P., Unterman, T.G., Van der Woude, M., et al., 1992. Insulin and insulin-like growth factors in central nervous system tumors. Part V: Production of insulin-like growth factors I and II in vitro. J. Neurosurg. 77 (3), 445–450.

Goodwin, J.W., Crowley, J., Stafford, B., et al., 1993. A phase II evaluation of tamoxifen in unresectable or refractory meningiomas: a southwest oncology group study. J. Neurooncol. 15 (1), 75–77.

Grunberg, S.M., Weiss, M.H., Spitz, I.M., et al., 1991. Treatment of unresectable meningiomas with the antiprogesterone agent mifepristone. J. Neurosurg. 74 (6), 861–866.

Guidetti, B., Delfini, R., Gagliardi, F.M., et al., 1985. Meningiomas of the lateral ventricles. Clinical, neuroradiologic and surgical consideration in 19 cases. Surg. Neurol. 24 (4), 364–370.

Gupta, V., Su, Y.S., Samuelson, C.G., et al., 2007. Irinotecan: a potential new chemotherapeutic agent for atypical or malignant meningiomas. J. Neurosurg. 106, 455–462.

Gutin, P., Leibel, S.A., Hosobuchi, Y., et al., 1987. Brachytherapy of recurrent tumors of the skull base and spine with iodine-125 sources. Neurosurgery 20 (6), 938–945.

Gutmann, D.H., Donahoe, J., Perry, A., et al., 2000. Loss of DAL-1, a protein 4. 1-related tumor suppressor, is an important early event in the pathogenesis of meningiomas. Hum. Mol. Genet. 9 (10), 1495–1500.

Haines, D.E., Frederickson, R.G., 1991. The meninges. In: Al-Mefty, O. (Ed.), Meningiomas. Raven Press, New York, p. 9.

Hakim, R., Alexander, E., Loeffler, J.S., et al., 1998. Results of linear accelerator-based radiosurgery for intracranial meningiomas. Neurosurgery 42 (3), 446–454.

Hakuba, A., Huh, C.W., Tsujikawa, S., et al., 1979. Total removal of a parasagittal meningioma of the posterior third of the sagittal sinus and its repair by autogenous vein graft: case report. J. Neurosurg. 51, 379–382.

Hasegawa, T., Kida, Y., Yoshimoto, M., et al., 2007. Long-term outcomes of Gamma Knife surgery for cavernous sinus meningioma. J. Neurosurg. 107 (4), 745–751.

Horsfall, D.J., Goldsmith, K.G., Ricciardelli, C., et al., 1989. Steroid hormone and epidermal growth factor receptors in meningiomas. Aust. N. Z. J. Surg. 59 (11), 881–888.

Hsu, D.W., Efird, J.T., Hedley-Whyte, E.T., 1997. Progesterone and estrogen receptors in meningiomas: prognostic considerations. J. Neurosurg. 86 (1), 113–120.

Hsu, D.W., Efird, J.T., Hedley-Whyte, E.T., 1998. MIB-1 (Ki-67) index and transforming growth factor-alpha (TGF alpha) immunoreactivity are significant prognostic predictors for meningiomas. Neuropathol. Appl. Neurobiol. 24 (6), 441–452.

Ibelgaufts, H., Jones, K.W., 1982. Papovavirus-related RNA sequences in human neurogenic tumours. Acta Neuropathol. 56 (2), 118–122.

Ikeda, K., Saeki, Y., Gonzalez-Agosti, C., et al., 1999. Inhibition of NF-2-negative and NF-2-positive primary human meningioma cell proliferation by overexpression of merlin due to vector-mediated gene transfer. J. Neurosurg. 91 (1), 85–92.

Ildan, F., Tuna, M., Göçer, A.P., et al., 1999. Correlation of the relationships of brain–tumor interfaces, magnetic resonance imaging, and angiographic findings to predict cleavage of meningiomas. J. Neurosurg. 91 (3), 384–390.

Inoue, Y.K., 1991. Inoue-Melnick virus and associated diseases in man: Recent advances. Prog. Med. Virol. 38, 167–179.

Inskip, P.D., Mellemkjaer, L., Gridley, G., et al., 1998. Incidence of intracranial tumors following hospitalization for head injury (Denmark). Cancer Causes Control 9 (1), 106–116.

Inskip, P.D., Tarone, R.E., Hatch, E.E., et al., 2001. Cellular-telephone use and brain tumors. N. Engl. J. Med. 344 (2), 79–86.

Iwai, Y., Yamanaka, K., Ikeda, H., 2008. Gamma Knife radiosurgery for skull base meningioma: long-term results of low-dose treatment. J. Neurosurg. 109 (5), 804–810.

Jacobs, J.M., Harnsberger, H.R., 1991. Diagnostic angiography and meningiomas. In: Al-Mefty, O. (Ed.), Meningiomas. Raven Press, New York, pp. 225–241.

Jane, J.A., Park, T.S., Pobereskin, L.H., et al., 1982. The supraorbital approach: Technical note. Neurosurgery 11 (4), 537–542.

Jennelle, R., Gladson, C., Palmer, C., et al., 1999. Paradoxical labeling of radiosurgically treated quiescent tumors with Ki67, a marker of cellular proliferation. Stereotact. Funct. Neurosurg. 72 (Suppl. 1), 45–52.

Jhawar, B.S., Fuchs, C.S., Colditz, G.A., et al., 2003. Sex steroid hormone exposures and risk for meningioma. J. Neurosurg. 99 (5), 848–853.

Julià-sapé, M., Acosta, D., Majós, C., et al., 2006. Comparison between neuroimaging classifications and histopathological diagnoses using an international multicenter brain tumor magnetic resonance imaging database. J. Neurosurg. 105 (1), 6–14.

Kaba, S.E., DeMonte, F., Bruner, J.M., et al., 1997. The treatment of recurrent unresectable and malignant meningiomas with interferon alpha-2B. Neurosurgery 40 (2), 271–275.

Kan, P., Simonsen, S.E., Lyon, J.L., et al., 2008. Cellular phone use and brain tumor: A meta-analysis. J. Neurooncol. 86 (1), 71–78.

Kaneko, S., Nomura, K., Yoshimura, T., et al., 2002. Trend of brain tumor incidence by histological subtypes in Japan: estimation from the Brain Tumor Registry of Japan, 1973–1993. J. Neurooncology 60 (1), 61–69.

Kaplan, R.D., Coons, S., Drayer, B.P., et al., 1992. MR characteristics of meningioma subtypes at 1.5 Tesla. J. Comput. Assist. Tomogr. 16 (3), 366–371.

Keller, A., Ludwig, N., Backes, C., et al., 2009. Genome wide expression profiling identifies specific deregulated pathways in meningioma. Int. J. Cancer 124 (2), 346–351.

Kempe, L.G., Blaylock, R., 1976. Lateral-trigonal intraventricular tumors: a new operative approach. Acta Neurochir. (Wien) 35 (4), 233–242.

Kepes, J.J., 1982. Meningiomas: Biology, pathology and differential diagnosis. Masson, New York.

Ketter, R., Rahnenfuhrer, J., Henn, W., et al., 2008. Correspondence of tumor localization with tumor recurrence and cytogenetic progression in meningiomas. Neurosurgery 62 (1), 61–69.

Khan, J., Parsa, N.Z., Harada, T., et al., 1998. Detection of gains and losses in 18 meningiomas by comparative genomic hybridization. Cancer Genet. Cytogenet. 103 (2), 95–100.

Kida, S., Yamashima, T., Kubota, T., Ito, H., Yamamoto, S., 1988. A light and electron microscopic and immunohistochemical study of human arachnoid villi. J. Neurosurg. 69 (3), 429–435.

Kinjo, T., Al-Mefty, O., Kanaan, I., 1993. Grade zero removal of supratentorial convexity meningiomas. Neurosurgery 33 (3), 394–399.

Kitange, G., Tsunoda, K., Anda, T., et al., 2000. Immunohistochemical expression of Ets-1 transcription factor and the urokinase-type plasminogen activator is correlated with the malignant and invasive potential in meningiomas. Cancer 89 (11), 2292–2300.

Klaeboe, L., Lonn, S., Scheie, D., et al., 2005. Incidence of intracranial meningiomas in Denmark, Finland, Norway and Sweden, 1968–1997. Int. J. Cancer 117 (6), 996–1001.

Kleinschmidt-DeMasters, B.K., Lillehei, K.O., 1995. Radiation-induced meningioma with a 63-year latency period. Case report. J. Neurosurg. 82 (3), 487–488.

Klutmann, S., Bohuslavizki, K.H., Brenner, W., et al., 1998. Somatostatin receptor scintigraphy in postsurgical follow-up examinations of meningioma. J. Nucl. Med. 39 (11), 1913–1917.

Kobayashi, K., Okudera, H., Tanaka, Y., 1992. Surgical considerations on skull base meningioma. Presented at the First International Skull Base Congress, June 18, Hanover, Germany.

Kollová, A., Liscák, R., Novotný, J., Jr., et al., 2007. Gamma Knife surgery for benign meningioma. J. Neurosurg. 107 (2), 325–336.

Kondziolka, D., Levy, E.I., Niranjan, A., et al., 1999a. Long-term outcomes after meningioma radiosurgery: physician and patient perspectives. J. Neurosurg. 91 (1), 44–50.

Kondziolka, D., Niranjan, A., Lunsford, L.D., et al., 1999b. Stereotactic radiosurgery for meningiomas. Neurosurg. Clin. N. Am. 10 (2), 317–325.

Kondziolka, D., Flickinger, J.C., Lunsford, L.D., 2008. The principles of skull base radiosurgery. Neurosurg. Focus 24 (5), E11.

Konovalov, A.N., Filatov, Y.M., Belousova, O.B., 1991. Intraventricular meningiomas. In: Schmidek, H.H. (Ed.), Meningiomas and their surgical management. WB Saunders, Philadelphia, PA, p. 364.

Kotzen, R.M., Swanson, R.M., Milhorat, T.H., et al., 1999. Post-traumatic meningioma: case report and historical perspective. J. Neurol. Neurosurg. Psychiatry 66 (6), 796–798.

Krayenbühl, N., Pravdenkova, S., Al-Mefty, O., 2007. De novo versus transformed atypical and anaplastic meningiomas: Comparisons of clinical course, cytogenetics, cytokinetics, and outcome. Neurosurgery 61 (3), 494–504.

Krynska, B., Del Valle, L., Croul, S., et al., 1999. Detection of human neurotropic JC virus DNA sequence and expression of the viral oncogenic protein in pediatric medulloblastomas. Proc. Natl. Acad. Sci. 96 (20), 11519–11524.

Kugel, H., Heindel, W., Ernestus, R.I., et al., 1992. Human brain tumors: spectral patterns detected with localized H_1 MR spectroscopy. Radiology 183 (3), 701–709.

Kumar, P.P., Patil, A.A., Leibrock, L.G., et al., 1991. Brachytherapy: a viable alternative in the management of basal meningiomas. Neurosurgery 29 (5), 676–680.

Kunert, P., Matyja, E., Janowski, M., 2009. Rapid growth of small, asymptomatic meningioma following Radiosurgery. Br. J. Neurosurg. 23 (2), 206–208.

Kuratsu, J., Takeshima, H., Ushio, Y., 2001. Trends in the incidence of primary intracranial tumors in Kumamoto, Japan. Int. J. Clin. Oncol. 6 (4), 183–191.

Kurland, L.T., Schoenberg, B.S., Annegers, J.F., et al., 1982. The incidence of primary intracranial neoplasms in Rochester, Minnesota. Ann. N. Y. Acad. Sci. 381, 6–16.

Lamberts, S.W., Reubi, J.C., Krenning, E.P., 1992a. Somatostatin receptor imaging in the diagnosis and treatment of neuroendocrine tumors. J. Steroid. Biochem. Mol. Biol. 43 (1–3), 185–188.

Lamberts, S.W., Tanghe, H.L., Avezaat, C.J., et al., 1992b. Mifepristone (RU 486) treatment of meningiomas. J. Neurol. Neurosurg. Psychiatry 55 (6), 486–490.

Lamszus, K., Kluwe, L., Matschke, J., et al., 1999. Allelic losses at 1p, 9q, 10q, 14q and 22q in the progression of aggressive meningiomas and undifferentiated meningeal sarcomas. Cancer Genet. Cytogenet. 110 (2), 103–110.

Larjavaara, S., Haapasalo, H., Sankila, R., et al., 2008. Is the incidence of meningiomas underestimated? A regional survey. Br. J. Cancer 99 (1), 182–184.

Latchaw, R.E., Hirsch, W.L., 1991. Computerized tomography of intracranial meningiomas. In: Al-Mefty, O. (Ed.), Meningiomas. Raven Press, New York, pp. 195–207.

Laufer, I., Anand, V.K., Schwartz, T.H., 2007. Endoscopic, endonasal extended transsphenoidal, transplanum transtuberculum approach for resection of suprasellar lesions. J. Neurosurg. 106 (3), 400–406.

Leber, K.A., Bergloff, J., Pendl, G., 1998. Dose response tolerance of the visual pathways and cranial nerves of the cavernous sinus to stereotactic radiosurgery. J. Neurosurg. 88 (1), 43–50.

Lekanne-Deprez, R.H., Riegman, P.H., Groen, N.A., et al., 1995. Cloning and characterization of MN 1, a gene from chromosome 22q11, which is disrupted by a balanced translocation in a meningioma. Oncogene. 10, 1521–1528.

Leone, P.E., Bello, M.J., de Campos, J.M., et al., 1999. NF-2 mutations and allelic status of 1p, 14q and 22q in sporadic meningiomas. Oncogene 18 (13), 2231–2239.

Levy, L.F., 1973. Brain tumors in Malawi, Rhodesia and Zambia. Afr. J. Med. Sci. 4 (4), 393–397

Longstreth, W.T., Dennis, L.K., McGuire, V.M., et al., 1993. Epidemiology of intracranial meningioma. Cancer 72 (3), 639–648.

Lonn, S., Klaeboe, L., Hall, P., et al., 2004. Incidence trends of adult primary intracerebral tumors in four Nordic countries. Int. J. Cancer 108 (3), 450–455.

Louis, D.N., Scheithauer, B.W., Budka, H., et al., 2000. Meningiomas. In: Kleihues, P., Cavenee, W.K. (Eds.), Pathology and genetics of tumours of the nervous system. IARC Press, Lyon, pp. 176–180.

Lowry, O.H., Bergers, S.J., Chi, M.M., et al., 1977. Diversity of metabolic patterns in human brain tumors. I. High energy phosphate compounds and basic composition. J. Neurochem. 29 (6), 959–977.

Mack, E.E., Wilson, C.B., 1993. Meningiomas induced by high-dose cranial irradiation. J. Neurosurg. 79 (1), 28–31.

Majós, C., Julia-Sape, M., Alonso, J., et al., 2004. Brain tumor classification by proton MR spectroscopy: comparison of diagnostic accuracy at short and long TE. AJNR: Am. J. Neuroradiol. 25 (10), 1696–1704.

Manfredonia, M., 1973. Tumors of the nervous system in the African in Eritrea (Ethiopia). Afr. J. Med. Sci. 4 (4), 383–387.

Mann, I., Yates, P.C., Ainslie, J.P., 1953. Unusual case of double primary orbital tumour. Br. J. Ophthalmol. 37 (12), 758–762.

Martinez, R., Vaquero, J., Areitio, E., et al., 1983. Meningiomas of the posterior fossa. Surg. Neurol. 19, 237–243.

Maxwell, M., Shih, S.D., Galanopoulos, T., et al., 1998. Familial meningioma: Analysis of expression of neurofibromatosis 2 protein merlin. Report of two cases. J. Neurosurg. 88 (3), 562–569.

McComb, J.G., Apuzzo, M.L., 1987. Posterior interhemispheric retrocallosal and transcallosal approaches. In: Apuzzo, M.L. (Ed.), Surgery of the third ventricle. Williams & Wilkins, Baltimore, pp. 623–626.

McCutcheon, I.E., 1996. The biology of meningiomas. J. Neurooncol. 29 (3), 207–216.

Meyer, F.B., Ebersold, M.J., Reese, D.F., 1984. Benign tumors of the foramen magnum. J. Neurosurg. 61 (1), 136–142.

Michelsen, J.J., New, P.F., 1969. Brain tumour and pregnancy. J. Neurol. Neurosurg. Psychiatry 32 (4), 305–307.

Modan, B., Baidatz, D., Mart, H., 1974. Radiation-induced head and neck tumors. Lancet 1 (7852), 277–279.

Morita, A., Coffey, R.J., Foote, R.L., et al., 1999. Risk of injury to cranial nerves after gamma knife radiosurgery for skull base meningiomas: experience in 88 patients. J. Neurosurg. 90 (1), 42–49.

Muller, P., Henn, W., Niedermayer, I., et al., 1999. Deletion of chromosome 1p and loss of expression of alkaline phosphatase indicate progression of meningiomas. Clin. Cancer Res. 5 (11), 3569–3577.

Nagashima, G., Aoyagi, M., Wakimoto, H., et al., 1995. Immunohistochemical detection of progesterone receptors and the correlation with Ki-67 labeling indices in paraffin-embedded sections of meningiomas. Neurosurgery 37 (3), 478–483.

Nakasu, S., Nakajima, M., Matsumura, K., et al., 1995. Meningioma: Proliferating potential and Clinicoradiological features. Neurosurgery 37 (6), 1049–1055.

Newton, H.B., 2007. Hydroxyurea chemotherapy in the treatment of meningiomas. Neurosurg. Focus 23 (4), E11, 1–8.

Nowell, P.C., 1986. Mechanisms of tumor progression. Cancer Res. 46 (5), 2203–2207.

Obeid, F., Al-Mefty, O., 2003. Recurrence of olfactory groove meningioma. Neurosurgery 53 (3), 534–542.

Odeku, E.L., Adeloye, A., 1973. Cranial meningiomas in the Nigerian Africans. Afr. J. Med. Sci. 4 (2), 275–287.

Ott, D., Hennig, J., Ernst, T., 1993. Human brain tumors: assessment with in vivo proton M R spectroscopy. Radiology 186 (3), 745–752.

Ozaki, S., Nishizaki, T., Ito, H., et al., 1999. Comparative genomic hybridization analysis of genetic alterations associated with malignant progression of meningioma. J. Neurooncol. 41 (2), 167–174.

Peeling, J., Sutherland, G., 1992. High-resolution ^{1}H NMR spectroscopy studies of extracts of human cerebral neoplasms. Magn. Reson. Med. 24, 123–136.

Perry, A., Louis, D.N., Scheithauer, B.W., et al., 2007. Meningiomas. In: Louis, D.N., Ohgaki, H., Wiestler, O.D., et al. (Eds.), WHO classification of tumors of the central nervous system. IARC Press, Lyon, pp. 164–172.

Perry, A., Scheithauer, B.W., Stafford, S.L., et al., 1999. 'Malignancy' in meningiomas: A clinicopathologic study of 116 patients, with grading implications. Cancer 85 (9), 2046–2056.

Peyrard, M., Fransson, I., Xie, Y.G., et al., 1994. Characterization of a new member of the human beta-adaptin gene family from chromosome 22q12, a candidate meningioma gene. Hum. Mol. Genet. 3 (8), 1393 1399.

Phillips, L.E., Koepsell, T.D., van Belle, G., et al., 2002. History of head trauma and risk of intracranial meningioma: population-based case-control study. Neurology 58 (12), 1849–1852.

Pieper, D.R., Al-Mefty, O., Hanada, Y., et al., 1999. Hyperostosis associated with meningioma of the cranial base: Secondary changes or tumor invasion. Neurosurgery 44 (4), 742–746.

Piper, J.G., Follett, K.A., Fantin, A., 1994. Sphenoid wing meningioma progression after placement of a subcutaneous progesterone agonist contraceptive implant. Neurosurgery 34 (4), 723–725.

Pravdenkova, S., Al-Mefty, O., Sawyer, J., et al., 2006. Progesterone and estrogen receptors: Opposing prognostic indicators in meningioma. J. Neurosurg. 105 (2), 163–173.

Preston-Martin, S., Henderson, B.E., Peters, J.M., 1982. Descriptive epidemiology of central nervous system neoplasms in Los Angeles County. Ann. NY. Acad. Sci. 381, 202–208.

Preston-Martin, S., Paganini-Hill, A., Henderson, B.E., et al., 1980. Case-control study of intracranial meningiomas in women in Los Angeles County, California. J. Natl. Cancer Inst. 65 (1), 67–73.

Preul, M.C., Caramanos, Z., Collins, D.L., et al., 1996. Accurate, noninvasive diagnosis of human brain tumors by using proton magnetic resonance spectroscopy. Nat. Med. 2 (3), 323–325.

Rachlin, J.R., Rosenblum, M.L., 1991. Etiology and biology of meningiomas. In: Al-Mefty, O. (Ed.), Meningiomas. Raven Press, New York, p. 27.

Ragel, B.T., Jensen, R.L., 2005. Molecular genetics of meningiomas. Neurosurg. Focus 19 (5), E9, 1–8.

Rempel, S.A., Ge, S., Gutierrez, J.A., 1999. SPARC: A potential diagnostic marker of invasive meningiomas. Clin. Cancer Res. 5 (2), 237–241.

Reubi, J.C., Horisberger, U., Lang, W., et al., 1989. Coincidence of E G F receptors and somatostatin receptors in meningiomas but inverse, differentiation-dependent relationship in glial tumors. Am. J. Pathol. 134 (2), 337–344.

Reubi, J.C., Maurer, R., Klijn, J.G., et al., 1986. High incidence of somatostatin receptors in human meningiomas: biochemical characterization. J. Clin. Endocrinol. Metab. 63 (2), 433–438.

Rohringer, M., Sutherland, G.R., Louw, D.F., et al., 1989. Incidence and clinicopathological features of meningioma. J. Neurosurg. 71 (5 pt. 1), 665–672.

Roda, J.M., Pascual, J.M., Carceller, F., et al., 2000. Nonhistological diagnosis of human cerebral tumors by ^{1}H magnetic resonance spectroscopy and amino acid analysis. Clin. Cancer Res. 6 (10), 3983–3993.

Roelvink, N.C., Kamphorst, W., van Alphen, H.A., et al., 1987. Pregnancy-related primary brain and spinal tumors. Arch. Neurol. 44 (2), 209–215.

Rosa, L., Luessenhop, A.J., 1991. Multiple meningiomas. In: Schmidek, H.H. (Ed.), Meningiomas and their surgical management. WB Saunders, Philadelphia, p. 83.

Ruberti, R.F., 1995. The surgery of meningiomas: a review of 215 cases. Afr. J. Neurol. Sci. 14 (1), 1.

Russell, E.J., George, A.E., Kricheff, I.I., et al., 1980. Atypical computed tomographic features of intracranial meningioma: radiological-pathological correlation in a series of 131 consecutive cases. Radiology 135, 673–682.

Ruttledge, M.H., Sarrazin, J., Rangaratnam, S., et al., 1994. Evidence for the complete inactivation of the NF-2 gene in the majority of sporadic meningiomas. Nat. Genet. 6 (2), 180–184.

Sadamori, N., Shibata, S., Mine, M., et al., 1996. Incidence of intracranial meningiomas in Nagasaki atomic-bomb survivors. Int. J. Cancer 67 (3), 318–322.

Sadetzki, S., Flint-Richter, P., Ben-Tal, T., et al., 2002. Radiation-induced meningioma: a descriptive study of 253 cases. J. Neurosurg. 97 (5), 1078–1082.

Samii, M., Ammirati, M., 1991. Cerebellopontine angle meningiomas (posterior pyramid meningiomas). In: Al-Mefty, O. (Ed.), Meningiomas. Raven Press, New York, pp. 508–511.

Schatz, N.J., Savino, P.J., Corbett, J.J., 1977. Primary aberrant oculomotor regeneration. A sign of intracavernous meningioma. Arch. Neurol. 34 (1), 29–32.

Schmitz, U., Mueller, W., Weber, M., et al., 2001. INI1 mutations in meningiomas at a potential hotspot in exon 9. Br. J. Cancer 84 (2), 199–201.

Schrell, U.M., Rittig, M.G., Anders, M., et al., 1997a. Hydroxyurea for treatment of unresectable and recurrent meningiomas. II. Decrease in the size of meningiomas in patients treated with hydroxyurea. J. Neurosurg. 86 (5), 840–844.

Schrell, U.M., Rittig, M.G., Anders, M., et al., 1997b. Hydroxyurea for treatment of unresectable and recurrent meningiomas. I. Inhibition of primary human meningioma cells in culture and in meningioma transplants by induction of the apoptotic pathway. J. Neurosurg. 86 (5), 845–852.

Schwechheimer, K., Zhou, L., Birchmeier, W., 1998. E-Cadherin in human brain tumours: Loss of immunoreactivity in malignant meningiomas. Virchows Arch. 432 (2), 163–167.

Seizinger, B.R., De la Monte, S., Atkins, L., et al., 1987. Molecular genetic approach to human meningioma: Loss of genes on chromosome 22. Proc. Natl. Acad. Sci. USA. 84 (15), 5419–5423.

Sekhar, L.N., Jannetta, P.J., 1984. Cerebellopontine angle meningiomas. Microsurgical excision and follow-up results. J. Neurosurg. 60 (3), 500–505.

Sen, C.N., Sekhar, L.N., 1990. An extreme lateral approach to intradural lesions of the cervical spine and foramen magnum. Neurosurgery 27 (2), 197–204.

Sergides, I., Hussain, Z., Naik, S., et al., 2009. Utilization of dynamic C T perfusion in the study of intracranial meningiomas and their surrounding tissue. Neurol. Res. 31 (1), 84–89.

Shafron, D.H., Friedman, W.A., Buatti, J.M., et al., 1999. LINAC radiosurgery for benign meningiomas. Int. J. Radiat. Oncol. Biol. Phys. 43 (2), 321–327.

Sheehan, J., Yen, C.P., Steiner, L., 2006. Gamma Knife surgery-induced meningioma. Report of two cases and review of the literature. J. Neurosurg. 105 (2), 325–329.

Shoshan, Y., Chernova, O., Juen, S.S., et al., 2000. Radiation-induced meningioma: a distinct molecular genetic pattern? J. Neuropathol. Exp. Neurol. 59 (7), 614–620.

Shibata, S., Sadamori, N., Mine, M., et al., 1994. Intracranial meningiomas among Nagasaki atomic bomb survivors. Lancet 344 (8939–8940), 1770.

Simpson, D., 1957. The recurrence of intracranial meningiomas after surgical treatment. J. Neurol. Neurosurg. Psychiatry 20, 22–39.

Shintani, T., Hayakawa, N., Hoshi, M., et al., 1999. High incidence of meningioma among Hiroshima atomic bomb survivors. J. Radiat. Res. 40 (1), 49–57.

Sindou, M.P., Alaywan, M., 1998. Most intracranial meningiomas are not cleavable tumors: Anatomic-surgical evidence and angiographic predictability. Neurosurgery 42 (3), 476–480.

Smith, D.A., Cahill, D.W., 1994. The biology of meningiomas. Neurosurg. Clin. N. Am. 5 (2), 201–215.

Spagnoli, M.V., Goldberg, H.I., Grossman, R.I., et al., 1986. Intracranial meningiomas: high-field MR imaging. Radiology 161 (2), 369–375.

Spencer, D.D., Collins, W., Sass, K.J., 1991. Surgical management of lateral intraventricular tumors. In: Schmidek, H.H. (Ed.),

Meningiomas and their surgical management. WB Saunders, Philadelphia, pp. 345–348.

Spetzler, R.F., Daspit, C.P., Pappas, C.T., 1992. The combined supra- and infratentorial approach for lesions of the petrous and clival regions, experience with 46 cases. J. Neurosurg. 76 (4), 588–599.

Steiner, L., Lindquist, C., Steiner, M., 1991. Meningiomas and gamma knife radiosurgery. In: Al-Mefty, O. (Ed.), Meningiomas. Raven Press, New York, pp. 263–272.

Su, M., Ono, K., Tanaka, R., et al., 1997. An unusual meningioma variant with glial fibrillary acidic protein expression. Acta Neuropathol. 94 (5), 499–503.

Sutherland, G.R., Florell, R., Louw, D., et al., 1987. Epidemiology of primary intracranial neoplasms in Manitoba, Canada. Can. J. Neurol. Sci. 14 (4), 586–592.

Takahashi, J.A., Mori, H., Fukumoto, M., et al., 1990. Gene expression of fibroblast growth factors in human gliomas and meningiomas: demonstration of cellular source of basic fibroblast growth factor mRNA and peptide in tumor tissue. Proc. Natl. Acad. Sci. USA 87 (15), 5710–5714.

Takahashi, J.A., Suzui, H., Yasuda, Y., et al., 1991. Gene expression of fibroblast growth factor receptors in the tissues of human gliomas and meningiomas. Biochem. Biophys. Res. Commun. 177 (1), 1–7.

Tanaka, M., Imhof, H.G., Schucknecht, B., et al., 2006. Correlation between the efferent venous drainage of the tumor and peritumoral edema in intracranial meningiomas: superselective angiographic analysis of 25 cases. J. Neurosurg. 104 (3), 382–388.

Tishler, R.B., Loeffler, J.S., Lunsford, L.D., et al., 1993. Tolerance of cranial nerves of the cavernous sinus to radiosurgery. Int. J. Radiat. Oncol. Biol. Phys. 27 (2), 215–221.

Tsutsumi, K., Kitagawa, N., Niwa, M., et al., 1994. Effect of suramin on ^{125}I-insulin-like growth factor-I binding to human meningiomas and on proliferation of meningioma cells. J. Neurosurg. 80 (3), 502–509.

Tugnoli, V., Tosi, M.R., Barbarella, G., et al., 1998. Magnetic resonance spectroscopy study of low grade extra and intracerebral human neoplasms. Oncol. Rep. 5 (5), 1199–1203.

Tung, H., Apuzzo, M.L., 1991. Meningiomas of the third ventricle and pineal region. In: Al-Mefty, O. (Ed.), Meningiomas. Raven Press, New York, pp. 583–591.

Vernooij, M.W., Ikram, M.A., Tanghe, H.L., et al., 2007. Incidental findings on brain MRI in the general population. N. Engl. J. Med. 357 (18), 1821–1828.

von Deimling, A., Larson, J., Wellenreuther, R., et al., 1999. Clonal origin of recurrent meningiomas. Brain Pathol. 9 (4), 645–650.

Waga, S., Handa, H., 1976. Radiation-induced meningioma: with review of literature. Surg. Neurol. 5 (4), 215–219.

Weber, R.G., Bostrom, J., Wolter, M., et al., 1997. Analysis of genomic alterations in benign, atypical, and anaplastic meningiomas: toward a genetic model of meningioma progression. Proc. Natl. Acad. Sci. USA 94 (26), 14719–14724.

Weingarten, K., Ernst, R.J., Jahre, C., et al., 1992. Detection of residual or recurrent meningioma after surgery: value of enhanced vs unenhanced M R imaging. Am J. Radiol. 158 (3), 645–650.

Weisman, A.S., Villemure, J.G., Kelly, P.A., 1986. Regulation of D N A synthesis and growth of cells derived from primary human meningiomas. Cancer Res. 46 (5), 2545–2550.

Weiss, A.F., Portmann, R., Fischer, H., et al., 1975. Simian virus 40-related antigens in three human meningiomas with defined chromosome loss. Proc. Natl. Acad. Sci. USA 72 (2), 609–613.

Wellenreuther, R., Waha, A., Vogel, Y., et al., 1997. Quantitative analysis of neurofibromatosis type 2 gene transcripts in meningiomas supports the concept of distinct molecular variants. Lab. Invest. 77 (6), 601–606.

Westphal, M., Herrmann, H.D., 1986. Epidermal growth factor-receptors on cultured meningioma cells. Acta Neurochir. (Wien) 83 (1–2), 62–66.

Wrensch, M., Weinberg, A., Wiencke, J., et al., 2001. Prevalence of antibodies to four herpesviruses among adults with glioma and controls. Am. J. Epidemiol. 154 (2), 161–165.

Yamashima, T., Sakuda, K., Tohma, Y., et al., 1997. Prostaglandin D synthase (beta-trace) in human arachnoid and meningioma cells: Roles as a cell marker or in cerebrospinal fluid absorption, tumorigenesis, and calcification process. J. Neurosci. 17 (7), 2376–2382.

Yamashima, T., Tohma, Y., Junkoh, Y., 1992. Expression of cell adhesion molecule: Epithelial-cadherin in meningiomas. Noshuyo. Byori. Brain Tumor Pathol. 9, 33–50.

Yang, S.Y., Park, C.K., Park, S.H., 2008. Atypical and anaplastic meningiomas: prognostic implications of clinicopathological features. J. Neurol. Neurosurg. Psychiatry 79 (5), 574–580.

Yasargil, M.G., Mortara, R.W., Curcic, M., 1980. Meningiomas of basal posterior cranial fossa. Adv. Tech. Stand. Neurosurg. 7, 3–115.

Zankl, H., Zang, K.D., 1980. Correlations between clinical and cytogenetical data in 180 human meningiomas. Cancer Genet. Cytogenet. 1, 351–356.

Zattara-Cannoni, H., Roll, P., Figarella-Branger, D., et al., 2001. Cytogenetic study of six cases of radiation-induced meningiomas. Cancer Genet. Cytogenet. 126 (2), 81–84.

Zhu, J.J., Maruyama, T., Jacoby, L.B., et al., 1999. Clonal analysis of a case of multiple meningiomas using multiple molecular genetic approaches: Pathology case report. Neurosurgery 45 (2), 409–416.

Zimmerman, R.D., 1991. MRI of intracranial meningiomas. In: Al-Mefty, O. (Ed.), Meningiomas. Raven Press, New York, pp. 209–223.

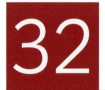

Meningeal hemangiopericytomas

Charles S. Cobbs and Barton L. Guthrie

Introduction

Meningeal hemangiopericytoma is a malignant neoplasm with sarcoma-like behavior. It is postulated to arise from meningeal capillary pericyte or precursor cells with angioblastic tendencies (Stout & Murray 1942a; Horten et al 1977). Information about this tumor comes from approximately 300 cases, reported variably as 'angioblastic meningiomas' within large series of meningiomas (Simpson 1957; Skullerud & Loken 1974; Jellinger & Slowik 1975; Kepes 1982; de la Monte et al 1986; Dziuk et al 1998) and series devoted exclusively to meningeal hemangiopericytomas (Pitkethly et al 1970; Goellner et al 1978; Fabiani et al 1980. Thomas et al 1981; Jääskeläinen et al 1985; Kochanek et al 1986; Guthrie et al 1989; Chiechi et al 1996; Uttley et al 1995; Brunori et al 1997; Galanis et al 1998).

The classification of nomenclature of this lesion is interesting. Cushing & Eisenhardt, in their 1938 classification of meningiomas, identified a vascular form of the tumor that they called angioblastic meningioma. They recognized three variants of the angioblastic meningioma: a vascular, but otherwise ordinary, meningioma (angiomatous meningioma); a tumor occurring primarily in the posterior fossa that is essentially a hemangioblastoma; and a third variety that appeared to have arisen from meningothelial cells with angioblastic features. This latter tumor was noted to behave in a malignant fashion with a tendency for local recurrence, despite aggressive resection. It is this tumor to which the term angioblastic is generally applied (Bailey et al 1928; Cushing & Eisenhardt 1938). In 1942, Stout & Murray (1942a) described a malignant and vascular tumor of the soft tissues (thigh, buttock, retroperitoneum) made of cells resembling capillary pericytes. They called it hemangiopericytoma, and it has since become a well-recognized soft tissue sarcoma (Enzinger & Smith 1976). In a later series, they reported a case that involved the meninges (Stout & Murray 1942b) but was felt to have invaded the meninges rather than to have had a primary meningeal origin. Begg & Garret (1954) first reported a primary cranial meningeal hemangiopericytoma. Significantly, they noted that it was histologically identical to both the soft tissue hemangiopericytoma of Stout & Murray (1942a) and the aggressive variant of angioblastic meningioma originally described by Cushing & Eisenhardt in 1938. They proposed that this variant of Cushing & Eisenhardt's angioblastic meningioma was actually a meningeal hemangiopericytoma, which was compatible with the known aggressive behavior of systematic hemangiopericytoma.

Since these early reports, various investigators have argued whether meningeal hemangiopericytoma is a form of meningioma. Popoff et al (1974) found that meningeal hemangiopericytomas were histologically and ultrastructurally identical to the hemangiopericytomas arising in soft tissues elsewhere, and proposed that the meningeal tumor should not be classified as a meningioma. On the other hand, Horten et al (1977), reviewing 79 cases of vascular (angioblastic) meningiomas, found areas within these tumors that appeared to be transitional between hemangiopericytomas and fibrous meningiomas and/or hemangioblastomas. They concluded that these tumors and ordinary meningiomas arise from multipotential precursor cells, and so classification of meningeal hemangiopericytomas as angioblastic meningiomas was not inconsistent with their postulated origin from capillary pericyte. Meningeal hemangiopericytomas are currently differentiated from meningiomas according to the new WHO II classification (Kleihues et al 1993). Certainly, these tumors must be recognized as a distinct entity since they are biologically more malignant than benign meningiomas, with which they may be confused.

Gross and microscopic pathology

Meningeal hemangiopericytomas are lobulated and vary from pink-gray to red in color. Their texture is usually firm, but they may occasionally be soft in their consistency (Fig. 32.1). They are extremely vascular and have a distressing tendency to bleed at surgery. They often adhere to the dura but usually do not invade the brain, so a plane of dissection is evident (Jääskeläinen et al 1985; Guthrie et al 1989). It is of note that they do not spread *en plaque* and rarely, if ever, do they contain calcification.

Microscopically, the tumors are very cellular, with round to oval cells (Fig. 32.2). The architecture may vary from field to field and occasionally resemble either meningotheliomatous or fibrous meningiomas (Horten et al 1977; Guthrie et al 1989). The tumor cells are arranged around thin-walled vascular spaces lined by a non-neoplastic endothelium. These sinusoidal 'staghorn' shaped capillaries are a distinguishing feature and can be quite numerous (Rubinstein 1972; Horten et al 1977; Kochanek et al 1986).

Mitoses are frequent and are regionally variable, numbering from one to several per high-power field (Kochanek et al 1986; Guthrie et al 1989). Microcysts, necrosis, and papillary architecture may be seen (Guthrie et al 1989) and have been reported in up to 50% of the tumors (Kochanek et al 1986). Whorls and psammoma bodies are not seen (Kochanek et al 1986; Guthrie et al 1989). Reticulin, which is usually abundant, tends to envelop individual cells, as opposed to meningiomas, which exhibit reticulin enveloping cell groups, giving the typical lobulated appearance of meningiomas.

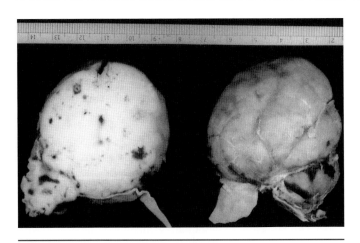

Figure 32.1 This meningeal hemangiopericytoma was removed *in toto*. Notice the dural attachment and lobular appearance.

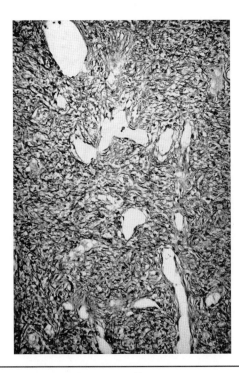

Figure 32.2 Microscopically, meningeal hemangiopericytomas appear as sheets of cells with numerous vascular spaces that can assume a 'staghorn' configuration.

Meningeal hemangiopericytomas almost always contain subpopulations of cells that express factor XIIIa, which may be used to confirm the diagnosis (Probst-Cousin et al 1996). Expression of factor XIIIa reactivity implies that these cells have fibrohistiocytic differentiation, distinguishing them from meningioma and other soft tissue tumors (Nemes 1992; Molnar & Nemes 1995). Other markers that may be expressed in hemangiopericytic tumor cells include vimentin, HLD-DR, CD34, Leu 7, and S-100 protein (Probst-Cousin et al 1996). Tumor cells are negative for the immunohistochemical markers fVIII-RA, epithelial membrane antigen (EMA), and GFAP (Nakamura et al 1987). With transmission electron microscopy, hemangiopericytoma cells exhibit leiomyoblas-

tic differentiation and secretion of basement membrane-like material, while surface membrane specializations (interdigitations, desmosomes, zonulae adherentes, and gap junctions) are absent (Pena 1977; Brunori et al 1997). A thorough description of the histology of this tumor can be found in the review by Kochanek et al (1986).

These tumors typically recur after surgical therapy, and the histology does not change from one recurrence to the next. Likewise, primary and metastatic hemangiopericytomas are histologically identical (Guthrie et al 1989). Meningeal hemangiopericytomas are distinct from atypical or malignant meningiomas. The latter display a meningothelial architecture not usually present in hemangiopericytomas, but show varying degrees of atypical or anaplastic features, such as loss of architecture, increased cellularity, nuclear pleomorphism, mitosis, necrosis, or brain infiltration (Jääskeläinen et al 1986).

Molecular characteristics and biologic behavior

Molecular studies indicate that hemangiopericytomas are genetically distinct from meningiomas. In one study, homozygous deletions of the *CDKN2*/p16 gene were detected in seven of 28 meningeal hemangiopericytomas and in only one of 26 meningiomas ($p = 0.03$) (Ono et al 1996). Rearrangements of chromosome 12q13 are common in hemangiopericytoma, and several oncogenes are located in this region including *MDM2*, *CDK4*, and *CHOP/GADD153*. Other chromosomal regions are less consistently altered cytogenetically in hemangiopericytomas, including 19q13, 6p21, and 7p15 (Henn et al 1993; Mandahl et al 1993). Thus, loss of function of the tumor suppressor *p16* or activation of oncogenes on chromosome 12q13 may be involved in the oncogenesis of meningeal hemangiopericytoma. In contrast, cytogenetic alterations of chromosomes 12q13, 19q13, 6p21, and 7p15 are not common in meningiomas (Joseph et al 1995). Mutation of the *NF-2* tumor suppressor gene, which is frequently associated with meningiomas, is not found in hemangiopericytomas. *NF-2* mutations were not detected in 28 meningeal hemangiopericytomas, whereas nine of 26 sporadic meningiomas had *NF-2* mutations when analyzed by polymerase chain reaction ($p < 0.001$) (Joseph et al 1995).

The histologic appearance of hemangiopericytoma does not allow accurate assessment of the prognosis, and hence tumors with malignant histologic features may have a more benign course and vice-versa (Enzinger & Smith 1976). Unfortunately, attempts to predict prognosis based on mitotic potential have not proven statistically significant. The MIB-1 and Ki-67 indices of 62 meningeal hemangiopericytomas ranged from 1.24% to 39% in one study (Probst-Cousin et al 1996). Statistical analyses of these tumors indicated no significant correlation between the staining index and recurrence-free survival. Long-term observation (>100 months) did, however, reveal a tendency to longer survival in the group with a staining index <5%. Evaluation of DNA ploidy with flow cytometry in hemangiopericytomas showed that only 1 of 7 tumors had a DNA aneuploid stem line (Zellner et al 1998). These results were in contrast to the results seen in meningiomas, where degree of DNA ploidy correlated with histopathologic features such as necrosis, infiltration, and mitotic activity (Zellner et al 1998). Thus, mitotic indices and studies of DNA ploidy do not appear to be useful indicators of biologic behavior in hemangiopericytomas.

Incidence

Meningeal hemangiopericytomas are rare. In large series of meningiomas, their incidence ranges from 2% to 4% of that of meningiomas, thus comprising far less than 1% of intracranial neoplasms (Simpson 1957; Pitkethly et al 1970; Jellinger & Slowik 1975; Wara et al 1975; Fabiani et al 1980; Chan & Thompson 1985; Jääskeläinen et al 1985; Mirimanoff et al 1985; Guthrie et al 1989). About 10% of meningeal hemangiopericytomas occur in children (Herzog et al 1995). Their rarity undoubtedly accounts for the fact that they are frequently misdiagnosed.

Clinical findings

Several studies have shown that meningeal hemangiopericytoma as opposed to meningioma is more common in males (56–75%) than females, even in the spinal location (Jääskeläinen et al 1985; Schroder et al 1986; Guthrie et al 1989). A more recent study showed a slight female preponderance (Chiechi et al 1996). The average age at diagnosis is 38–42 years (Kochanek et al 1986; Schroder et al 1986; Guthrie et al 1989; Chiechi et al 1996). The anatomic location is similar to that of meningiomas, with approximately 15% located in the posterior fossa and 15% located in the spine (Cappabianca et al 1981; Schroder et al 1986; Guthrie et al 1989). Of the spinal tumors, about half have been in the cervical region (Schroder et al 1986). While the vast majority of these tumors are based in the meninges, at least three have been reported in the pineal region (Stone et al 1983; Lesoin et al 1984; Sell et al 1996). Primary multifocal meningeal hemangiopericytomas have not been reported (Schroder et al 1986; Guthrie et al 1989).

The average patient is symptomatic for <1 year, particularly in the CT and MRI era (Guthrie et al 1989). Presenting symptoms are related to tumor location (Jääskeläinen et al 1985; Kochanek et al 1986; Schroder et al 1986; Guthrie et al 1989). The most frequent presenting symptom is headache (Goellner et al 1978; Chiechi et al 1996). Seizures are initially present in only about 16% of patients with supratentorial tumors (Guthrie et al 1989), which is compatible with the fact that they do not infiltrate the brain and grow rather rapidly.

Imaging

Meningeal hemangiopericytomas resemble meningiomas on imaging studies. Plain films are of interest only, in that no hyperostosis has been reported, and, if there is bone change, it is erosion (Osborne et al 1981; Jääskeläinen et al 1985; Guthrie et al 1989).

Computed tomography typically shows a narrow or broad-based meningeal attachment. Most often the tumors appear hyperdense with focal areas of hypodensity on unenhanced CT scans, and have areas of heterogeneous enhancement with the administration of contrast (Chiechi et al 1996). They may show features suggesting malignancy (macroscopic brain invasion of 'mushrooming' inhomogeneous contrast enhancement or irregular borders) (New et al 1982). Bone erosion is seen in >50% of hemangiopericytomas (Chiechi et al 1996).

Hemangiopericytomas are usually isointense with gray matter and display prominent vascular flow voids on T1- and T2-weighted MR images (Chiechi et al 1996; Akiyama et al 2004). Heterogeneous enhancement is the most common appearance on T1-weighted gadolinium enhanced images. About half of the tumors will have a dural tail sign. CT and MRI characteristics that may help to differentiate hemangiopericytomas from meningiomas include a narrow-based dural attachment (seen more frequently in hemangiopericytomas) and hyperostosis of adjacent bone (commonly seen in meningiomas but very rare in hemangiopericytomas) (Chiechi et al 1996; Akiyama et al 2004). Two reports have demonstrated the use of MR spectroscopy to help distinguish hemangiopericytoma from a benign meningioma (Cho et al 2003; Hattingen et al 2003). In these cases, the hemangiopericytoma had increased choline peak compared with meningiomas.

The tumors frequently show characteristic arteriographic features including a 'corkscrew' vascular configuration and a long-lasting venous strain (Fig. 32.3) (Marc et al 1975). As many as half have a significant internal carotid blood supply (Marc et al 1975; Jääskeläinen et al 1985; Guthrie et al 1989), and few show early venous drainage, another factor which distinguishes them from ordinary meningiomas (Jääskeläinen et al 1985; Guthrie et al 1989).

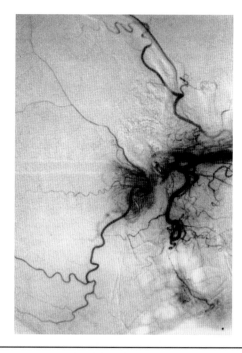

Figure 32.3 Arteriography of this tuberculum meningeal hemangiopericytoma illustrates the early filling vessels in a corkscrew configuration. Notice also the early draining vein.

Despite these features, Guthrie et al (1989) found that, of 20 angiographic studies, only one was diagnosed preoperatively as a meningeal hemangiopericytoma. Jääskeläinen et al (1985) reported that, in hindsight, with knowledge of the above characteristics, at least 8 of their 17 meningeal hemangiopericytomas could have been diagnosed as such by angiography.

Gadolinium-enhanced MRI is helpful in delineating anatomy but is non-specific with regard to differentiation from ordinary meningiomas (Guthrie et al 1989). DiChiro et al (1987) have shown that metabolically active meningiomas, including angioblastic, meningiomas (hemangiopericytomas), may be differentiated by hypermetabolic activity on positron emission tomography (PET) and that such 'hot spots' on PET are of prognostic significance.

Treatment

Management of patients with meningeal hemangiopericytoma is difficult. At initial presentation, these patients are often thought to have meningioma. However, meningeal hemangiopericytoma should be suspected if the history is brief and the lesion appears extremely vascular by CT, MRI, or MRA. Surgery, if possible, is the treatment of choice. If hemangiopericytoma is suspected, arteriography should be considered for the possibility of embolization, which can markedly reduce intraoperative bleeding. It should be remembered that these tumors can invade cerebral vasculature, with the result that embolization of meningeal feeders may not be as effective in stopping bleeding as it is for ordinary meningioma. Likewise, during surgery, amputation of the meningeal attachment of this tumor may not adequately devascularize it, and significant blood loss may occur.

These tumors have a propensity for recurrence, and every attempt should therefore be made to achieve a complete removal at the time of the initial surgery. In large series reporting surgery for these tumors however, this has been possible in only 50–67% of the cases (Jääskeläinen et al 1985; Schroder et al 1986; Guthrie et al 1989). If a complete (Simpson grade I) resection is achieved, then the likelihood of definitive cure is high (Soyuer et al 2004; Bassiouni et al 2007). If complete removal is not possible, adjuvant radiation therapy is recommended (Soyuer et al 2004). Some authors have suggested giving preoperative radiation and waiting several months for a response in order to simplify the surgery (Wara et al 1975; Fuki et al 1980). Given the difficulties of a previously irradiated surgical field however, radiation should not be routinely used in an attempt to reduce the difficulty of resection.

Radiosurgery

The availability and attractiveness of radiosurgery have forced consideration of this as a treatment option. Radiosurgery has been reported as probably effective against inoperable meningiomas (Duma et al 1993). Its efficacy for hemangiopericytoma has not been formally delineated. It would seem that this tumor, with its relatively discrete margins and known radiosensitivity, should be susceptible to radiosurgery. Galanis et al (1998) reported that they treated 10 patients with recurrent lesions with stereotactic radiosurgery. Of these, three previously non-irradiated patients (all with lesions <25 mm) achieved complete responses, which persisted at a median of 3 years. In 14 lesions (70%), a partial response occurred with a median duration of 12 months, whereas three lesions (15%) remained stable. Other studies have shown that surgery followed by focal radiosurgery prevents recurrent local disease but not metastatic disease (Dufour et al 2001). In a more recent study, 11 of 14 patients with recurrent hemangiopericytomas demonstrated local tumor control after radiosurgery (Sheehan et al 2002). A total of 12 of 15 tumors (80%) dramatically decreased in size on follow-up imaging scans. Gamma Knife radiosurgery provided local tumor control for 80% of recurrent hemangiopericytomas. Thus, when residual tumor is identified after resection or radiotherapy, early radiosurgery should be considered as a feasible treatment modality. Nevertheless, despite local tumor control, patients are still at risk for distant metastasis.

These authors have experience with only one such patient, for whom the short-term response has been dramatic. However, as with any new treatment modality, recommendation for radiosurgery as a primary treatment must be made with caution and probably should be used for patients for whom surgery is not an option.

Chemotherapy

Little information exists with respect to the utility of chemotherapy for intracranial hemangiopericytoma. One report discussed the use of chemotherapy in patients who had recurred after surgery and radiation therapy (Chamberlain & Glantz 2008). In these patients, a combination of four cycles of cyclophosphamide, doxorubicin, and vincristine, followed by α-IFN and two cycles of ifosfamide, cisplatin, and etoposide, was administered. In this setting of recurrent disease, the median overall survival after chemotherapy was 14 months. These authors suggested that salvage chemotherapy demonstrated modest efficacy with acceptable toxicity in this cohort of adult patients with recurrent surgery- and radiotherapy-refractory intracranial HPC.

Surgical mortality

Operative mortality for meningeal hemangiopericytomas has ranged from 9% to 27%, with many deaths attributable to exsanguination (Jääskeläinen et al 1985; Schroder et al 1986; Guthrie et al 1989). Using current technology, including embolization, Guthrie et al (1989) report no surgical deaths since 1974, and, that with care, surgical complications should be minimal. As with most tumors, operation for recurrence is more hazardous both in terms of morbidity and mortality (Guthrie et al 1989).

Recurrence

Meningeal hemangiopericytomas have a relentless tendency to recur. The reported recurrence-free interval after the first operation varies due to the variable measures of tumor recurrence. In an exhaustive review of the literature to 1985, Schroder et al (1986) found a median recurrence-free interval of 50 months (range 1 month to 26 years).

Table 32.1 Prognosis of patients with meningeal hemangiopericytoma (%)

	5 years	10 years	15 years
Rate of recurrence	65	76	87
Rate of metastasis	13	33	64
Survival	67	40	23

Compiled from Guthrie B L, Ebersold M J, Scheithauer B W et al. (1989) Meningeal hemangiopericytoma: histopathological features, treatment, and long-term followup of 44 cases. Neurosurgery 25: 514–522.

Table 32.2 Effect of postoperative radiation for meningeal hemangiopericytoma

	Probability of recurrence (%)		
	3 years	5 years	10 years
Radiation	30	50	70
No radiation	50	100	100

Jääskeläinen et al (1985) found a mean time to recurrence of 78 months in 18 patients. Guthrie et al (1989), diagnosing recurrence as a progression of symptoms with radiographic or operative confirmation, found a median recurrence-free interval of 40 months (mean 47 months). In seven patients, Brunori et al (1997) reported five recurrences with a mean time to recurrence of 85 months, while the other two patients had only been followed for 3 years and 1 year, respectively. After reviewing the literature, Schroder et al (1986) found the 5-year recurrence to be around 60%. From an actuarial standpoint, Guthrie et al (1989) calculated 5-, 10-, and 15-year recurrence rates of 65%, 76%, and 87%, respectively (Table 32.1). From these data, it is obvious that meningeal hemangiopericytomas are much more aggressive than meningiomas and that recurrence is likely if a patient survives for 5 years, and becomes more likely with extended survival. The fact is that if the patient lives long enough, the tumor will recur.

After the first recurrence, meningeal hemangiopericytomas tend to recur at shorter intervals. Guthrie et al (1989) reported a series of 44 patients operated 79 times in whom the average interval to subsequent recurrences tended to shorten. The average time to second, third, and fourth operations for recurrence was 38, 35, and 17 months, respectively. In addition, these investigators found that 53% of patients improved and 3% worsened after the first operation, whereas only 33% improved and 13% worsened after subsequent operation, suggesting that the time for optimal surgical removal is at the first operation.

Metastasis

Unlike any other primary intracranial tumor, meningeal hemangiopericytoma frequently metastasizes outside the CNS. The most common sites of metastasis in descending frequency are bone, lung, and liver (Simpson 1957; Kruse 1961; Pitkethly et al 1970; Horten et al 1977; Thomas et al 1981; Kepes 1982; Inoue et al 1984; Jääskeläinen et al 1985; Schroder et al 1986; Guthrie et al 1989). Realization that distant metastasis can occur after years of apparent tumor-free life is crucial for appropriate long-term management of these patients.

Survival

Guthrie et al (1989) found that the median survival after the first operation was 60 months, with actuarial 5-, 10-, and 15-year survival of 67%, 40%, and 23%, respectively (Table 32.1). This is comparable with the cumulative survival of approximately 65%, 45%, and 15% compiled by Schroder et al (1986), from reviewing 118 cases in the literature to 1985.

Factors affecting prognosis

As with any intracranial tumor, there are clinical and pathologic features that are important in predicting a patient's clinical course. In a detailed review of this disease, Guthrie et al (1989) studied the relationship of multiple factors to the long-term prognosis of their 44 patients. Age and sex were not important, nor were the histologic characteristics of the tumor, including mitotic activity. Kochanek et al (1986), on the other hand, reported that tumors with a higher mitotic rate tend to recur faster. It seems reasonable that tumors with a higher mitotic rate should be more aggressive, but actual evidence that this is the case for hemangiopericytoma is lacking (see above). The extent of tumor removal is less clearly correlated with the recurrence of meningeal hemangiopericytoma than it is for meningiomas (Kochanek et al 1986). Guthrie et al (1989) found an average survival of 109 months after apparent complete removal versus 65 months after incomplete removal. Oddly enough, the recurrence-free interval was unrelated to the extent of removal, possibly because patients with significant residual tumor tended to be irradiated (Jääskeläinen et al 1985; Guthrie et al 1989).

Extraneural metastasis is a devastating occurrence and significantly shortens survival. In the Mayo Clinic series, 10 of 44 patients experienced extraneural metastasis at an average time of 99 months. The average survival after metastasis was 24 months. Five patients alive at 99 months who did not develop metastasis survived an additional 76 months (Guthrie et al 1989).

The treatment variable most strongly related to prognosis is postoperative radiation therapy. Chan & Thompson (1985) found that 12 patients with 'malignant meningiomas' (most likely unrecognized hemangiopericytomas) receiving postoperative radiation therapy survived an average of 4.6 useful years, while those not irradiated survived less than 1 year. Guthrie et al (1989) found that patients irradiated after the first operation experienced recurrence at an average of 74 months, with a 5- and 10-year recurrence rate of 38% and 64%, respectively. Those patients not irradiated suffered recurrence at an average of 29 months, with a 5- and 10-year recurrence of 90% (Guthrie et al 1989; Table 32.2). These authors found a dose effect in that patients receiving <4500 cGy tended to experience recurrence sooner than those receiving 5000 cGy or more. In this same series, patients irradiated after the first operation survived an average of 92 months, but those not irradiated lived 62 months. This response by a hemangiopericytoma to radiation has been observed by others for intracranial as well as peripheral locations (Friedman & Egan 1960; Lal et al 1976; Mira et al 1977; Fuki et al 1980; Schroder et al 1986).

Discussion

The malignant nature of meningeal hemangiopericytoma has long been recognized and, regardless of whether it is categorized as a meningioma (Rubinstein 1972; Horten et al 1977; Zülch 1979) or not (Popoff et al 1974; Pena 1977; Goellner et al 1978; Fabiani et al 1980; Kochanek et al 1986), the treating physician must realize that its behavior is drastically different than that of meningiomas. Meningiomas afflict females at a ratio of 1.5 : 1 to 3 : 1 over males (Cushing & Eisenhardt 1938; Simpson 1957; Jellinger & Slowik 1975; MacCarty & Taylor 1979; Adegbite et al 1983; Chan & Thompson 1985), but meningeal hemangiopericytomas show a slight male predominance. The average age of patients with meningeal hemangiopericytomas is 38–42 years, younger than that of 50 years for patients with meningioma (Skullerud & Loken 1974; Jellinger & Slowik 1975; Yamashita et al 1980; Chan & Thompson 1985; Mirimanoff et al 1985). Most hemangiopericytomas are symptomatic for less than 1 year, while patients with meningiomas may be symptomatic for several years. Patients with meningeal hemangiopericytomas tend not to present with seizures. The two lesions arise in similar areas; however, meningeal hemangiopericytomas are never multifocal, whereas up to 16% of meningiomas may be (Kepes 1982).

Meningeal hemangiopericytomas are much more aggressive than ordinary meningiomas, with 5- and 10-year recurrence rates of 65% and 76%, respectively (Guthrie et al 1989), while those for meningiomas are 20% and 30%, respectively (Adegbite et al 1983; Mirimanoff et al 1985). As with many malignant vs benign tumors, meningeal hemangiopericytomas are relatively more responsive to radiation (King et al 1966; Carella et al 1982; Guthrie et al 1989). Perhaps the most striking difference from meningiomas is the tendency for meningeal hemangiopericytomas to metastasize. Kepes (1982), in his thorough monograph on meningiomas, found very few ordinary meningiomas that metastasized. In contrast, the rate of metastasis of meningeal hemangiopericytomas at 5, 10, and 15 years is 13%, 33%, and 64%, respectively (Guthrie et al 1989), making metastasis likely with prolonged survival.

Meningeal hemangiopericytomas should not be equated with atypical or malignant meningiomas. The latter tumors show loss of architecture, increased cellularity, nuclear atypia, and mitoses, but remain recognizable as meningiomas. Jääskeläinen et al (1986) studied a series of atypical and anaplastic meningiomas and found them to be more aggressive than ordinary meningiomas, but less so than meningeal hemangiopericytomas. In particular, malignant meningiomas have little or no tendency to metastasize.

In summary, a meningeal hemangiopericytoma is an aggressive extra-axial central nervous system tumor that behaves like a soft tissue sarcoma. It has a relentless tendency for local recurrence and, even if local control can be achieved, distant metastasis remains a threat. Optimal management is aggressive local excision at the time of the first operation, followed by radiation therapy (and/or radiosurgery) of at least 5000–5500 cGy. Diligent, long-term observation with periodic chest X-rays and work-up of bone pain and abnormal liver function studies to rule out metastasis, is required in all patients.

Key points

- Meningeal hemangiopericytomas are malignant tumors comprising <1% of intracranial neoplasms. They arise in the same areas as meningiomas and behave like soft tissue sarcomas.

- Pathologically, these tumors may resemble meningiomas, but they are derived from fibrohistiocytic precursor cells. On a molecular level, they are distinct from meningiomas, and often have rearrangements of chromosome 12q13.

- The average age at diagnosis is 40 years, and most patients present with symptoms related to tumor location, with the most common presenting symptom being headache.

- MRI with gadolinium is the imaging technique of choice.

- These tumors are very vascular and may have large tumor blood vessels.

- Surgery is the treatment of choice, and preoperative embolization may be helpful.

- Tumor recurrence is the rule, and adjuvant radiation is recommended. Radiosurgery is an excellent treatment for recurrent local disease.

- The 5- and 10-year recurrence rates are around 65% and 75%, respectively.

- The median survival at 5 and 10 years is around 65% and 40%, respectively. The treatment modality most strongly related to prognosis is postoperative radiation therapy of at least 5000–5500 cGy.

- Diligent follow-up with a keen suspicion of distant metastases is required.

REFERENCES

Adegbite, A.B., Khan, M.I., Paine, K.W.E., et al., 1983. The recurrence of intracranial meningiomas after surgical treatment. J. Neurosurg. 58, 51–56.

Akiyama, M., Sakai, H., Onoue, H., et al., 2004. Imaging intracranial haemangiopericytomas: study of seven cases. Neuroradiology 46 (3), 194–197.

Bailey, P., Cushing, H., Eisenhardt, L., 1928. Angioblastic meningiomas. Arch. Pathol. 6, 953–990.

Bassiouni, H., Asgari, S., Hübschen, U., et al., 2007. Intracranial hemangiopericytoma: treatment outcomes in a consecutive series. Zentralbl. Neurochir. 68 (3), 111–118.

Begg, C.F., Garret, R., 1954. Hemangiopericytoma occurring in the meninges. Cancer 7, 602–606.

Brunori, A., Delitala, A., Oddi, G., et al., 1997. Recent experience in the management of meningeal hemangiopericytomas. Tumori. 83, 856–860.

Cappabianca, P., Mauri, F., Pettinato, G., et al., 1981. Hemangiopericytoma of the spinal canal. Surg. Neurol. 15, 298–302.

Carella, R.J., Ransohoff, J., Newal, J., 1982. Role of radiation therapy in the management of meningioma. Neurosurgery 10, 332–339.

Chamberlain, M.C., Glantz, M.J., 2008. Sequential salvage chemotherapy for recurrent intracranial hemangiopericytoma. Neurosurgery 63 (4), 720–727.

Chan, R.C., Thompson, G.B., 1985. Morbidity, mortality, and quality of life following surgery for intracranial meningiomas. A retrospective study in 257 cases. J. Neurosurg. 62, 18–24.

Chiechi, M.V., Smirniotopoulos, J.G., Mena, H., 1996. Intracranial hemangiopericytomas: MR and CT features. AJNR Am. J. Neuroradiol. 17 (7), 1365–1371.

Cho, Y.D., Choi, G.H., Lee, S.P., et al., 2003. (1)H-MRS metabolic patterns for distinguishing between meningiomas and other brain tumors. Magn. Reson. Imaging 21 (6), 663–672.

33 Meningeal sarcomas

Georges F. Haddad, Ian F. Dunn, and Ossama Al-Mefty

Sarcoma, autrement dit fungus, est une excroissance de chair qui vient de l'aliment propre de la partie où elle naist.

Ambroise Paré (1517–1590)
(quoted by Bailey 1929)

Introduction

The word sarcoma was coined by adjoining the Greek terms 'sarx' (denoting flesh) and 'oma', thus describing the fleshy appearance of these tumors which usually have very little connective tissue stroma (*Churchill's Medical Dictionary* 1989). Pathologically, sarcomas are defined as malignant tumors arising from mesenchymal tissue (Cotran et al 1999).

History

Virchow is credited with the first systematic classification of cerebral tumors (Virchow 1869, quoted in Rubinstein 1971). He used the term 'sarcoma' to refer to primary fleshy malignant neoplasms of the central nervous system and the term 'glioma' to refer to their more benign counterparts. Rubinstein (1971) thought that these 'sarcomas' most probably represented glioblastoma multiforme. Virchow's classification explains why older statistics list sarcomas as comprising 30–40% of brain tumors (Zülch 1986), whereas recent studies quote the occurrence of cerebral sarcomas to be <3% of all brain tumors.

In 1929, Bailey reported on eight sarcomas that he classified into five categories. Subsequently, several classification schemes were devised; some were based on site of origin within the cranial vault (dural, leptomeningeal), others on histologic architecture (perivascular, perithelial, alveolar), and others according to histologic sub-type (Rubinstein 1971). Christensen & Lara (1953) adopted this latter classification; they reviewed 24 cases of primary intracranial sarcomas and classified them as fibrous, spindle cell, and polymorphocellular, in increasing degrees of malignancy.

The study of intracranial sarcomas was hampered by the lack of agreement on a single classification scheme and by the fact that not all major investigators could agree on whether some specific tumors were actually of mesenchymal origin and thus sarcomas, or of neuroectodermal origin and thus gliomas. Examples of these are monstrocellular sarcomas, regarded by Kernohan & Uihlein (1962) as true sarcomas, but considered by Rubinstein (1971) to be giant cell glioblastoma multiforme. Another such tumor is the so-called circumscribed arachnoidal cerebellar sarcoma, first mentioned by Foerster & Gagel (1939) but believed, by Rubinstein & Northfield (1964), to be a desmoplastic variant of medulloblastoma. Difficulties also arose in classifying the medullomyoblastoma: sarcoma vs primitive neuroectodermal tumor (PNET), with rhabdomyoblastic differentiation (Burger et al 1991; Coons & Johnson 1994). In view of the rarity of primary meningeal sarcomas, the following discussion will contain some references and findings related to primary cerebral sarcomas in general, including both deep and superficial cerebral sarcomas.

Classification

Whereas meningiomas, the most prevalent meningeal tumors, arise from meningothelial cells, sarcomas issue from mesenchymal cells. According to Bruner et al (1998), the sources of these mesenchymal cells may be as follows: dura, leptomeninges, pial or adventitial fibroblasts covering perforating blood vessels deep in the cerebral matter, tela choroidea, and the stroma of the choroid plexus. Thus, primary intracranial sarcomas may be superficial and involve the meninges (i.e. meningeal sarcomas) or they may be deep and arise within the brain parenchyma or within the ventricles. Bruner et al (1998) make the distinction between primary meningeal sarcomas arising *de novo* from intracranial mesenchymal cells and secondary meningeal sarcomas arising in a pre-existing meningioma. Sarcomas can also involve the meninges via direct extension (the skull base, the cranial vault, the sinuses, or intracerebral sarcoma) or by distant metastasis.

According to the most recent classification scheme of the World Health Organization, the diagnostic term 'meningeal sarcoma' is not specifically used, given its ascription to both sarcoma and malignant meningioma in past literature (Paulus et al 2007). For the sake of this chapter, meningeal sarcomas are thus included under the general heading of 'mesenchymal, non-meningothelial tumors'. This group also includes other entities that will not be discussed in this chapter, namely:

1. Hemangiopericytomas
2. Sarcogliomas: sarcomas eliciting a neoplastic reaction from enclosed glial islands
3. Melanocytic meningeal tumors
4. Lipoma.

We will not deal with other entities that were included, at one time or another, under the heading of intracranial sarcomas, namely:

1. CNS lymphoma, reported as reticulum cell sarcoma (Zülch 1971; Paulus & Scheithauer 1997)

2. Desmoplastic medulloblastoma, reported as cerebellar arachnoidal sarcoma (Zülch 1971; Paulus & Scheithauer 1997)

3. Giant cell glioblastoma, reported as monstrocellular sarcoma (Zülch 1971; Paulus & Scheithauer 1997)

4. Meningeal granulocytic sarcoma, denoting infiltration of the dura by granulocytic cells, usually as a late complication of acute myelogenous leukemia (Guthrie et al 1990); this has also been reported in the context of other myeloproliferative disorders (Roy et al 1989).

Enzinger & Weiss, writing about sarcomas in 1988, stated that, 'earlier classifications have been largely descriptive … More recent classifications have been based principally on the line of differentiation of the tumor, that is, the type of tissue formed by the tumor rather than the type of tissue from which the tumor arose'. In 1990, Scheithauer (1990) echoed this sentiment, writing that, 'instead of our historical tendency to focus upon histogenesis and to apply "cell-of-origin" thinking in our efforts at classification, we might be better served to concentrate our diagnostic efforts upon demonstrating specific cellular differentiation'.

Major advances in studying the genetics of sarcomas affecting the soft tissues may be applicable to sarcomas affecting the brain or the meninges. In general, molecular characteristics of intracranial sarcoma mimic their systemic counterparts. Two consistent chromosomal translocations are found in alveolar rhabdomyosarcoma: t(2,13) and, less often, t(1,13) (Bell 1999). Even although a t(11,22) translocation is often considered diagnostic of Ewing's sarcoma and peripheral primitive neuroectodermal tumors (pPNETs), it has also been reported in alveolar rhabdomyosarcoma (Thorner 1996). Further research in the molecular and genetic substrates of sarcomas will undoubtedly lead to further refinements in their classification.

The headings 'spindle cell' sarcoma and 'polymorphocellular' sarcoma used in previous editions of this chapter seem to have become outmoded at the present time (Haddad & Al-Mefty 1995). We shall therefore discuss meningeal sarcomas under headings related to their cellular differentiation: fibrosarcoma, leiomyosarcoma, rhabdomyosarcoma, chondrosarcoma, and malignant fibrous histiocytomas.

Incidence

Zülch believes that the average frequency of intracranial sarcomas may be between 2.5% and 3%. Tomita & Gonzalez-Crussi (1984) found eight primary sarcomas in a review of 402 children with intracranial tumors, giving a rate of about 2% in a pediatric population. Bruner et al (1998), adjusting the figures of Kernohan & Uihlein (1962), estimated that the true incidence is around 1.2% of intracranial tumors. Coons & Johnson (1994) reported the incidence of primary sarcomas to be <1% of all intracranial tumors. Paulus et al (1991) reported 19 primary intracranial sarcomas out of 25 000 cases of brain tumor biopsies, yielding an incidence of <0.1%. These authors, however, did not include meningeal sarcomatosis in their tally. Bigner & Johnston (1994) stated that primary intracranial sarcomas are more common than sarcomas metastatic to the CNS. The most common tumor types include fibrosarcoma, malignant fibrous histiocytoma, and undifferentiated sarcoma (Paulus et al 1991; Oliveira et al 2002).

Pathology

Meningeal sarcoma usually presents as a massive growth. Tumors arising from the dura are often firmer than those originating from the leptomeninges or from within the brain. The tumors are sharply demarcated from the adjacent brain in places but they lack a capsule and often infiltrate the brain in other areas. They sometimes spread over the cortex in a sheath, following the gyri and sulci (Russell & Rubinstein 1989). The cut surface is usually firm but may reveal areas of necrosis and hemorrhage (Coons & Johnson 1994).

The microscopy of meningeal sarcomas mimics the microscopy of their systemic counterparts. Rather than describe every possible differentiation of mesenchymal cells and quote in detail the few reviews and case reports that deal with each sub-group, we will just point out that meningeal sarcomas can differentiate along several lines. They can produce fibrous tissue (fibrosarcoma); cartilage (chondromas, chondrosarcomas, and mesenchymal chondrosarcomas); smooth muscle (leiomyosarcomas); striated muscle (rhabdomyosarcomas); bone (osteosarcomas); adipose tissue (liposarcoma); or blood vessels (angiosarcomas). Poorly-differentiated cells may give rise to tumors termed 'malignant fibrous histiocytomas'.

Fibrosarcomas are characterized by interlacing bundles of spindle cells giving a 'herringbone' appearance, frequent mitoses, and areas of necrosis (Paulus & Scheithauer 1997). The tumors stain abundantly for reticulin. They may also be positive for vimentin, but this feature does not distinguish them from other intracranial sarcomas (Bruner et al 1998).

Most primary intracranial malignant fibrous histiocytomas arise from the meninges (Burger et al 1991), although the extremely rare parenchymal variant is described (reviewed in Mitsuhashi et al 2004). They are composed of several morphologic cell types: fibroblasts, xanthomatous cells, histiocytic-type cells, and multinucleated giant cells (Tomita & Gonzalez-Crussi 1984; Ho et al 1992). They are characterized by numerous mitoses and frequent necrosis (Paulus & Scheithauer 1997). They accounted for 6 of 19 sarcomas reported by Paulus et al (1991). These authors stated, 'While fibrosarcoma has previously been the most frequently diagnosed intracranial sarcoma, most of these tumors are nowadays differently diagnosed, particularly as malignant fibrous histiocytomas'; on the other hand, McKeever et al (1997) suggested that most malignant fibrous histiocytomas should be classified as fibrosarcomas. As is apparent from the two previous sentences, the classification of intracranial sarcomas remains in a state of flux.

Cartilage-producing sarcomas can be classified either as chondrosarcomas or as mesenchymal chondrosarcomas (Tomita & Gonzalez-Crussi 1984; Cybulski et al 1985; Katayama et al 1987). In chondrosarcomas, only the cartilaginous elements are neoplastic (Fig. 33.1), whereas both cartilaginous and mesenchymal elements are neoplastic in mesenchymal chondrosarcomas (Fig. 33.2) (Harsh & Wilson 1984; Shuangshoti & Kasantikul 1989). The latter reveal, on

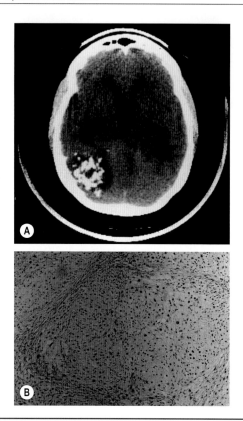

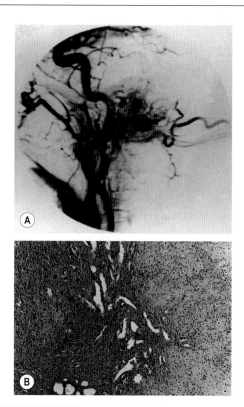

Figure 33.1 (A) Plain CT scan of a 33-year-old woman with a chondrosarcoma. Note the hypodense tumor with areas of calcification. The mass was avascular on cerebral angiography. (B) Photomicrograph of the neoplasm showing a lobulated pattern. The tumor cells are stellate-shaped and surrounded by abundant mucoid intercellular material (H&E ×150). (Reproduced with permission from Hassounah M, Al-Mefty O, Akhtar M et al. (1985) Primary cranial and intracranial chondrosarcomas: a survey. Acta Neurochir 78: 123–132.)

Figure 33.2 (A) Lateral arterial DSA showing marked tumor hypervascularity in a mesenchymal chondrosarcoma. The patient is a 65-year-old man. (B) Photomicrograph of a mesenchymal chondrosarcoma showing a biphasic pattern. Part of the tumor is composed of undifferentiated spindle-shaped cells, while the other part reveals moderately well-differentiated cartilage (H&E ×150). (Reproduced with permission from Hassounah M, Al-Mefty O, Akhtar M et al. (1985) Primary cranial and intracranial chondrosarcomas: a survey. Acta Neurochir 78: 123–132.)

light microscopy, areas of atypical chondroid differentiation intermixed with areas of dense mesenchymal neoplastic tissue (Burger et al 1991; Bruner et al 1998). This appearance has been likened to 'clouds in the sky' (Burger et al 1991). Some authors have reported that malignant chondrocytes may stain positively for glial fibrillary acidic protein (GFAP) (Shuangshoti & Kasantikul 1989). The tumors previously reported under the name 'chondroid chordoma' are presently thought to represent low-grade chondrosarcomas (Coons & Johnson 1994). More recently, immunopositivity for the D2–40 antigen has been described in identifying extraskeletal myxoid chondrosarcoma (Sangoi et al 2009). Forbes & Eljamel (1998) reviewed the subject of meningeal chondrosarcomas in 1998. They culled 29 cases from the world literature and added two cases of their own. There were 20 cranial and 11 spinal tumors. A total of 22 cases were defined as mesenchymal chondrosarcomas. All the non-mesenchymal chondrosarcomas (nine cases) occurred in the cranium. The authors stated that the most common extraskeletal site for mesenchymal chondrosarcomas was the meninges, and that the falx cerebri was the most common intracranial site. They reported only two metastases. The mean survival was 4.5 years.

Intracranial cells can also differentiate along a muscle lineage. Sarcomas originating from smooth muscle are

termed leiomyosarcomas; those originating from striated muscle are termed rhabdomyosarcomas. The demonstration of microfilaments with dense bodies is generally considered conclusive proof of smooth muscle differentiation (Table 33.1). Smooth muscle differentiation is different from smooth muscle origination, however, because of the fact that fibroblasts may also differentiate along smooth muscle lines. The Epstein–Barr virus was demonstrated within the nuclei of a dural leiomyosarcoma in an HIV-positive patient (Morgello et al 1997; Zevallos-Giampietri et al 2004); indeed, an immunocompromised state is associated with just under half of reported cases of cerebral leiomyosarcoma (reviewed in Mathieson et al 2009).

Most meningeal rhabdomyosarcomas consist of small non-specific cells on H&E staining. Immunohistologic techniques and electron microscopy are often used to make the diagnosis (Paulus & Scheithauer 1997). A 10-year survival has been reported in a case of meningeal sarcoma with rhabdomyoblastic differentiation. It was unclear, however, if this was a *de novo* sarcoma or a malignant transformation of a meningioma (Ferracini et al 1992). Survival beyond 2 years is rare (Celli et al 1998). Intracranial liposarcomas are exceedingly rare (Paulus & Scheithauer 1997).

We should also mention that several case reports of primary central nervous system Ewing sarcomas have been reported (Russell & Rubinstein 1989). It is important to distinguish intracranial Ewing's sarcomas from PNET, and this is often done by definitively showing evidence of any one of several *EWS* gene translocations (Navarro et al 2007).

Primary meningeal sarcomatosis refers to involvement of the leptomeninges by sarcomatous spread in the absence of a localized tumor. This process may lead to total encasement of the spinal cord (Russell & Rubinstein 1989). The protein content of cerebrospinal fluid is usually high, while the glucose concentration is low (Guthrie et al 1990). Cerebrospinal fluid cytology is usually positive for malignant cells. A considerable number of cases reported as meningeal sarcomatosis seem to have actually represented seeding of medulloblastomas or metastatic meningeal carcinomatosis (Stanley 1997). Sarcomas, especially the least-differentiated group, may seed the subarachnoid space (Bishop et al 1983; Russell & Rubinstein 1989). Extraneural metastases have also been reported (Bishop et al 1983; Russell & Rubinstein 1989; Gaspar et al 1993; Younis et al 1995). Previous surgery or shunting of cerebrospinal fluid may play a role in systemic seeding of these tumors. These are extremely rare lesions, accounting in some reports for only 10% of intracranial sarcomas (Bruner et al 1998), and the prognosis is typically poor (reviewed in Uluc et al 2004).

The intermixing of glial and mesenchymal components in a tumor may be seen in a variety of cases. At times, the edges of a meningeal sarcoma might encompass islands of reactive hypertrophied fibrillary glia (Rubinstein 1971; Russell & Rubinstein 1989). These islands may remain non-neoplastic or may become malignant, thus giving rise to a sarcoglioma. In contradistinction, the term 'gliosarcoma' refers to a glial tumor that induces secondarily malignant changes in surrounding mesenchymal cells. It is sometimes difficult to differentiate between these two entities.

Every meningeal sarcoma should be subjected to a battery of tests to determine into which sub-group it fits. Some differentiating factors may be apparent on light microscopy (cartilage islands, osseous elements). Special stains may also be helpful, such as the use of PAS stain to denote glycogen in rhabdomyosarcoma or the use of fat stains in liposarcomas. The use of immunohistochemistry and electron microscopy is often needed, however, to clarify the issue. The technical details related to these two techniques are beyond the scope of this chapter, but the reader should be aware that specimens submitted for these techniques should be handled in specific ways, that results must be interpreted within the context of all other findings, and that false positive and false negative results may occur. Having said that, immunohistochemistry and electron microscopy remain very powerful tools in the study of meningeal sarcomas (Tables 33.1 and 33.2).

Age and gender

Meningeal sarcomas can occur at any age but are more common in the first decade of life, the notable exceptions being malignant fibrous histiocytoma and fibrosarcomas that occur preferentially in adults and sarcomas showing muscle differentiation that tend to occur in children (Malat et al 1986; Russell & Rubinstein 1989; Paulus et al 1991; Coons & Johnson 1994). Primary meningeal sarcomatosis is

Table 33.1 Ultrastructural findings in selected intracranial tumors

Tumor	Ultrastructural findings
Meningioma	Complex interdigitation of cell processes Well formed desmosome junctions Cytoplasmic filaments that may attach to desmosomes and have a loose architecture in contradistinction to GFAP filaments that densely fill the cytoplasm No basal lamina
Schwannoma	Complex interdigitation of thin cytoplasmic processes Basal lamina Luse bodies (thick collagen fibers with long periodicity in their banding structure)
Smooth muscle tumors	Actin-containing microfilaments usually arranged longitudinally, with periodic small oval, or spindle shaped electron dense patches (dense bodies) in contact with the filaments. These dense bodies distinguish smooth muscle filaments from the ubiquitous and non-specific intermediate filaments that can be found in almost any cell Attachment plaques: similar to the dense bodies except for their location near the plasma membrane Pericellular basal lamina and prominent pinocytotic activity: less specific but helpful

Fibroblastic tumors	Spindle shaped cells with moderate cytoplasmic accumulations of rough endoplastic reticulum cisterns containing material of moderate electron density
	No diagnostic ultrastructural feature. Diagnosis of exclusion
	No: 1. Basal lamina
	        2. Pinocytotic vesicles
	        3. Complex intertwining cell processes

Melanoma	Cytoplasmic melanin granules (melanosomes) Junctional devices are rare
Rhabdomyosarcoma	Thick and thin filaments, arranged in parallel array on longitudinal section and in hexagonal array on cross-section May have basal lamina

Data from Mrak R (1997) Tumors: Application of ultrastructural methods. In: Garcia J (ed.) Neuropathology: The Diagnostic Approach. St. Louis: Mosby, 2007. With permission of Elsevier.

more frequent in infants and children (Russell & Rubinstein 1989) and may have a male predominance. In most meningeal sarcomas, no difference in incidence according to gender has been reported (Zülch 1986; Russell & Rubinstein 1989; Paulus et al 1991).

Site

Paulus et al (1991) reported on 19 intracranial sarcomas: 12 involved the meninges; the rest were located exclusively within the brain. Meningeal sarcomas have no preferential site of involvement (Zülch 1986; Russell & Rubinstein 1989). Russell & Rubinstein (1989) report that most rhabdomyosarcomas arise in the midline. A review of fibrosarcomas has shown a parietal predilection for these tumors (Cai & Kahn 2004).

Etiology

Several reports have emphasized the finding of meningothelial elements within sarcomas (Russell & Rubinstein 1989; Ferracini et al 1992). In these cases, it is sometimes difficult

Table 33.2 Selected immunohistochemical stains useful in the diagnosis of meningeal sarcomas

GFAP	Excellent marker of glial differentiation in CNS tumors
Neurofilament proteins (NFP)	In neoplastic neurons and their cytoplasm
Microtubule-associated protein 2	Sensitive marker for neuroblastic differentiation
Epidermal growth factor	Positive immunoreactivity in meningiomas
Leu 7 monoclonal antibody	Reacts with oligodendroglioma and peripheral nerve tumors May be positive in neurofibrosarcomas
Cytokeratins	Positive in some metastatic carcinomas and in chordomas May be positive in intracranial germ tumors May also be present in some gliomas (e.g., GBM), in rhabdoid tumors, leiomyosarcomas, and rhabdomyosarcoma
Epithelial membrane antigen	Positive in meningiomas, chordomas, and neurofibromas Negative in hemangiopericytomas
Desmin	Intermediate filament of all muscle cells
Actin	In all muscle cells
Myoglobin	Skeletal muscles. Positive in <50% of rhabdomyosarcomas. More specific but less sensitive than desmin stain
Vimentin	Positive in mesenchymal cells but also in numerous meningiomas, schwannomas, hemangioblastomas, chordomas, and sarcomas
S-100	Positive in astrocytomas, oligodendrogliomas, ependymomas, GBM, schwannoma, chordomas, chondrosarcomas, liposarcomas, and melanomas

Data from Cáccamo D & Rubinstein L, Tumors: Application of immunocytological methods. In: Garcia J (ed.) Neuropathology: The Diagnostic Approach. St. Louis: Mosby, 1997, With permission of Elsevier, and Wikstrand C, Fung K, Trojanowski J et al. (1998) Antibodies and molecular biology. In: Bigner D, McLendon R & Bruner J (eds) Russell & Rubinstein's Pathology of Tumors of the Nervous System, 6th edn. London: Edward Arnold.

to ascertain which tumor is primary and which is secondary. Russell & Rubinstein (1989) concede that the distinction between secondary sarcomatous changes in a pre-existing meningioma and primary sarcomas is not always clear. On the other hand, Zülch (1986) believes that there is no indication that sarcomas arise as an anaplastic variant of a pre-existing meningioma.

Trauma has been cited as a possible factor in the development of sarcomas. Zülch (1986) cites a case recorded by Reinhardt in 1928 in which a metal wire was found embedded within 'a sarcomatous meningeal tumor (meningioma?) [sic]'. Kristoferitsch & Jellinger (1986) reported on a case of angiosarcoma occurring at the site of a cordotomy performed 5 years earlier. Ho et al (1992) reported on an intracerebral malignant fibrous histiocytoma diagnosed at the operative site of a posterior communicating artery aneurysm clipped 3 months earlier. Meningeal sarcomas may be associated with subdural effusions diagnosed at the same time as the tumors, or they may occur within the beds of subdural hematomas drained several years earlier (Kothandaram 1970; Cinalli et al 1997; Nussbaum et al 1995).

Several reports have linked meningeal sarcomas to previous irradiation of the brain, for brain tumors, pituitary adenoma, or leukemia (Russell & Rubinstein 1989). Meningeal sarcomas have also been diagnosed in the setting of AIDS (leiomyosarcoma and Kaposi sarcoma) (Ariza & Kim 1988; Morgello et al 1997; Paulus & Scheithauer 1997).

A higher incidence of fibrosarcomas has been reported in neurofibromatosis (Malat et al 1986). Intracranial chondrosarcomas are associated with Maffucci syndrome, whereas osteosarcomas are associated with Paget's disease (Paulus & Scheithauer 1997). Familial occurrence of cerebral sarcomas has also been reported (Gainer et al 1975).

Differential diagnosis

The differential diagnosis of primary meningeal sarcomas comprises the following (Paulus et al 1991):

1. Meningeal metastasis from an extracranial sarcoma
2. An intracranial extension from the skull or other parameningeal site (rhabdomyosarcoma, chondrosarcoma)
3. Other malignant mesenchymal tumors such as hemangiopericytomas, embryonal tumors with mesenchymal differentiation (e.g., rhabdomyoblastic differentiation) or chordomas
4. A neoplastic mesenchymal component in the context of a neuroectodermal tumor (gliosarcoma; medulloblastoma with rhabdomyoblastic, leiomyoblastic or cartilaginous differentiation; and islands of cartilage produced by astrocytoma)
5. A malignant meningioma
6. Non-malignant tumors that may simulate sarcomas because of pleomorphism (pleomorphic xanthoastrocytoma, benign fibrous histiocytoma) or because of fascicular arrangement of spindle cells with desmoplasia (superficial cerebral astrocytoma).

In a case where the diagnosis of primary sarcomatous meningitis is entertained, it is imperative to rule out the following entities: seeding medulloblastomas, myelogenous infiltration, and metastatic carcinomatosis.

Presentation

Meningeal sarcomas can present as space-occupying lesions (Katayama et al 1987; Reusche et al 1990), or with new-onset seizures (Cybulski et al 1985), hydrocephalus, or symptoms referable to the spinal cord (Bishop et al 1983).

Radiology

There is no pathognomonic radiologic picture of meningeal sarcomas. On computed tomography and magnetic resonance images, they enhance as solitary or multiple lesions. The mass may enhance heterogeneously (Cybulski et al 1985; Katayama et al 1987) or in a ring-like fashion (Lee et al 1988). The tumor may appear cystic at times (Reusche et al 1990). On magnetic resonance, the mass is usually hypointense on T1-weighted images and hyperintense on T2-weighted images (Lee et al 1988). Liposarcomas may appear hyperintense on T1-weighted sequences due to the fat content of the tumor. Meningeal sarcomas may elicit severe edema from the adjacent brain (Wang et al 1986), or no parenchymal edema may be seen (Lee et al 1988). Skull erosion is seen in 25% of patients (Guthrie et al 1990), but there is no evidence of hyperostosis. On angiography, meningeal sarcomas may present either as an avascular area (Lee et al 1988), a vascular blush (Wang et al 1986), or as a mass with neovascularity (Guthrie et al 1990). Their blood supply may be either from the internal or from the external carotid artery (Guthrie et al 1990). The intracranial arteries may be encased by tumor (Tomita & Gonzalez-Crussi 1984)

Prognosis

The 5-year postoperative survival rate is quoted as 16%, with an average survival of 32 months (Guthrie et al 1990); however, long-term survivals after radical removal have been reported (Christensen & Lara 1953; Rubinstein 1971; Harsh & Wilson 1984; Ferracini et al 1992). Some patients have survived for up to 20 years after surgery and radiation therapy (Rubinstein 1971). A favorable outcome is most likely after radical excision of a better-differentiated, well-circumscribed tumor (Rubinstein 1971). Gaspar et al (1993) reported on nine patients with primary cerebral fibrosarcomas. The tumors were superficially located in five patients. No patient had a history of prior radiation therapy. The rates of meningeal seeding and of distant metastasis were 44%. The median survival was 6 months.

Treatment

Most authors agree that radical resection offers the best chance for long-term survival (Tomita & Gonzalez-Crussi 1984). The roles of radiotherapy and chemotherapy are still not clearly defined (Reynier et al 1984; Tomita & Gonzalez-Crussi 1984). Although some authors have questioned the efficacy of radiotherapy (Gasparini et al 1990), the benefits of chemotherapy and radiotherapy in the treatment of parameningeal sarcomas seem to be proven (Raney et al 1987; Alert et al 1988), especially for more undifferentiated forms. One should keep in mind, however, that chemotherapy may precipitate the demise of the patient, as reported in a case of intracranial osteosarcoma, where intravenous methotrexate caused massive edema leading to fatal herniation (Villareal et al 1990).

Recommendations

Even although some authors have used the term 'aggressive meningeal tumors' to refer to meningeal sarcomas, atypical meningiomas, malignant meningiomas, and hemangiopericytomas as a group, we think that all efforts should be made to further characterize these rare tumors. Advances in the prognostication and treatment of meningeal sarcomas will only be achieved after a thorough study of each and every case. All suspected meningeal sarcomas should therefore be investigated by a multidisciplinary team of physicians including a neurosurgeon, a pathologist, an oncologist, a

radiologist, a radiotherapist and, if needed, a pediatrician. The radiologic findings should be carefully reviewed. A possible primary sarcoma that may have metastasized to the meninges should be ruled out. The pathologist should sample the tumor extensively and make use of a battery of tests using light microscopy, immunohistochemistry, and electron microscopy. Whenever feasible, the underlying molecular and genomic alterations should be investigated in these usually aggressive tumors.

> **Key points**
>
> - Meningeal sarcomas represent <3% of all brain tumors.
> - They arise from mesenchymal cells.
> - More recent classifications have been based principally on the line of differentiation of the tumor, i.e. the type of tissue formed by the tumor rather than the type of tissue from which the tumor arose. The microscopy of meningeal sarcomas mimics the microscopy of their systemic counterparts. They can produce fibrous tissue (fibrosarcomas), cartilage (chondromas, chondrosarcomas, and mesenchymal chondrosarcomas), smooth muscle (leiomyosarcomas), striated muscle (rhabdomyosarcomas), bone (osteosarcomas), adipose tissue (liposarcoma), or blood vessels (angiosarcomas). Poorly-differentiated cells may give rise to tumors termed malignant fibrous histiocytoma.
> - Meningeal sarcomas usually present as a massive growth. Tumors arising from the dura are often firmer than those originating from the leptomeninges or from within the brain. The tumors are sharply demarcated from the adjacent brain in places but they lack a capsule and often infiltrate the brain in other areas.
> - Sarcomas, especially the least differentiated group, may seed the subarachnoid space.
> - The intermixing of glial and mesenchymal components in a tumor may be seen in a variety of cases.
> - Meningeal sarcomas can occur at any age but are more common in the first decade of life, the notable exceptions being malignant fibrous histiocytoma and fibrosarcomas that occur preferentially in adults and sarcomas showing muscle differentiation that tend to occur in children.

REFERENCES

Alert, J., Longchong, M., Valdés, M., et al., 1988. Cranial irradiation of children with soft-tissue sarcomas arising in parameningeal sites. Neoplasma. 35, 627–633.

Ariza, A., Kim, J., 1988. Kaposi's sarcoma of the dura mater. Hum. Pathol. 19 (12), 1461–1462.

Bailey, P., 1929. Intracranial sarcomatous tumors of leptomeningeal origin. Arch. Surg. 18, 1359–1402.

Bell, R., Winder, J., Andrulis, I., 1999. Molecular alterations in bone and soft tissue sarcoma. Can. J. Surg. 42, 259–266.

Bigner, S., Johnston, W., 1994. Cytopathology of the central nervous system. American Society of Clinical Pathologists, Chicago.

Bishop, N., Chakrabarti, A., Piercy, D., et al., 1983. A case of sarcoma of the central nervous system presenting as a Guillain–Barré syndrome. J. Neurol. Neurosurg. Psychiatry 46, 352–354.

- Bruner, J., Tien, R., Enterline, D., 1998. Tumors of the meninges and related tissues. In: Bigner, D., McLendon, R., Bruner, J. (Eds.), Russell & Rubinstein's pathology of tumors of the nervous system, sixth ed. Edward Arnold, London.

- Burger, P., Scheithauer, B., Vogel, S., 1991. Surgical pathology of the nervous system and its coverings. Churchill Livingstone, New York.

Cáccamo, D., Rubinstein, L., 1997. Tumors: Application of immunocytological methods. In: Garcia, J. (Ed.), Neuropathology: The diagnostic approach. Mosby, St. Louis.

34 Pineal cell and germ cell tumors

Jeffrey N. Bruce, E. Sander Connolly, and Adam M. Sonabend

Introduction

A complete understanding of pineal cell and germ cell tumors is hindered by the often confusing nomenclature that has evolved around them. Although most pineal cell and germ cell tumors occur in the pineal region, tumors of the pineal region can encompass a wide variety of tumor histologies, including astrocytomas, meningiomas, ependymomas, and metastatic tumors. It is important to recognize that, in references to 'pineal region tumors', not all tumors are of pineal or germ cell origin. Furthermore, although all pineal cell tumors originate within the pineal gland, many intracranial germ cell tumors may originate in areas other than the pineal region, particularly the suprasellar region.

Germ cell tumors refer to a group of pluripotential tumors of germ cell origin spanning a wide range of differentiation and malignant characteristics. At the benign end of the spectrum, these include teratomas, dermoid tumors, and epidermoid tumors. Endodermal sinus tumors, embryonal cell tumors, and choriocarcinomas are at the malignant end of the spectrum, with germinomas and immature teratomas falling somewhere in between. Although most intracranial germ cell tumors occur in the pineal region, a sizeable number can be found in the suprasellar region as well.

Pineal cell tumors, otherwise known as pineal parenchymal tumors, are derived from pineal parenchymal cells within the pineal gland, and therefore primarily occur in the pineal region. They are categorized as either pineocytomas or pineoblastomas, although mixed tumor forms can occur.

The term 'pinealoma' was originally used by Krabbe in 1923 to refer to pineal parenchymal tumors (Krabbe 1923). Gradually this term assumed a more general meaning and was used to refer to any tumor of the pineal region, regardless of its histology. This term is now obsolete and the preferred term is 'pineal region tumor' when referring to tumors of unspecified pathology in the pineal region. Since this term encompasses all tumors of the pineal region, the histology should be specified to avoid confusion (e.g., 'pineal region teratoma').

Similarly, the nomenclature regarding germinomas can be confusing. These particular germ cell tumors are known as seminomas when they occur in the testes or as dysgerminomas when the ovaries are involved. Although histologically identical to their gonadal counterparts, 'germinoma' is the preferred term for an intracranial occurrence. Older literature sometimes uses the outdated term 'atypical teratoma'. Finally, other tumors such as meningioma, hemangioblastoma, choroid plexus papilloma, papillary tumor of the pineal region, metastatic tumor, chemotectoma, adenocarcinoma, and lymphoma can also be found on the pineal region (Bruce 1993b, Jouvet et al 2003; Kashiwagi et al 1989; Pluchino et al 1989, Smith et al 1966). Additionally, a variety of vascular lesions can occur, including cavernous malformations, arteriovenous malformations, and vein of Galen malformations (Fukui et al 1983; Ventureyra 1981).

Incidence and prevalence

Estimating the true incidence and prevalence of pineal cell and germ cell tumors is problematic for several reasons. Historically, many presumed pineal cell tumors and germ cell tumors of the pineal or suprasellar region were treated empirically without definitive histologic confirmation. Furthermore, pathologic terminology has changed over the years, making studies from past eras difficult to analyze. Additionally, estimates of proportional representation of a given tumor type are subject to natural bias due to the referral patterns of the specialized institutions that often treat these rare tumors. Most case series report the relative frequency of tumors based as a percentage of brain tumors, which does not necessarily reflect the actual incidence within a given population. Although incidence and prevalence are useful estimates, accurate figures must await prospective population-based studies using modern pathologic classification.

Pineal region tumors

When analyzing epidemiologic data on pineal region tumors, it is important to realize that these tumors encompass a wide variety of histopathology. Tumors of pineal cell and germ cell origin are not always reported separately, and so statistics for pineal region tumors cannot always be extrapolated to make generalizations about specific histologic subtypes. Nevertheless, certain trends are apparent from the available epidemiologic data, which has historically been drawn from series of pineal region tumors. An epidemiologic study of The Central Brain Tumor Registry of the United States, including data from 20 675 tumors found that 0.5% of the CNS tumors were localized in the pineal region (Surawicz et al 1999). Another comprehensive series analyzing pineal

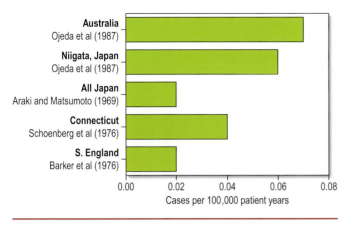

Figure 34.1 Incidence of pineal region tumors by geographic location.

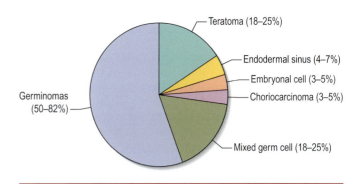

Figure 34.2 Relative percentages of histologic sub-types among intracranial germ cell tumors (total incidence 0.1/100000 per year) (Bruce et al 2000; Horowitz & Hall 1991; Jennings et al 1985; Russell & Rubinstein 1989b; Stein & Bruce 1992).

region tumor incidence is the study by Zimmerman, comparing his brain tumor series (4865 cases) to that of Cushing (2141 cases), Dastar of India (774 cases), Ito of Japan (1365 cases) and Zülch of Germany (5955 cases), and determining the incidence of 'pinealoma' to be 0.6%, 0.7%, 0.9%, 5.9%, and 0.4%, respectively (Zimmerman & Bilaniuk 1982). Zülch's and Ito's series also make mention of a separate category of teratoma (0.2% and 1.6%, respectively). The terms 'pinealoma' and 'teratoma' in these series are never clearly defined, but it is likely that pinealoma refers to pineal cell neoplasms, whereas teratoma refers to germ cell neoplasms. This interpretation of the terminology is responsible for the traditional teaching that pineal region tumors (including both germ cell & pineal cell tumors) are more common in Japan than elsewhere. The Japanese predilection is supported by both Sano's series, in which pineal tumors accounted for 4% of the overall total (Sano 1984), and the annual report of pathologic autopsy cases in Japan for 1965–1974, which shows 6.23% of 3382 brain tumors to be of the pineal region (Koide et al 1980).

The validity of this presumed Japanese predilection has been questioned as possibly biased by selective case reporting (Ojeda et al 1987). No statistically significant difference was demonstrated between the number of pineal region tumors seen in Niigata Prefecture, Japan (0.07/100000 person-years) and Western Australia (0.06) in a prospective study of actual population-based incidence. Furthermore, other population-based figures from southern England (0.02) (Barker et al 1976), Connecticut (0.03) (Schoenberg et al 1976), and all Japan (0.02) (Araki & Matsumoto 1969), failed to demonstrate an excessively increased incidence in Japan (Fig. 34.1). It should be emphasized once again that these figures refer to pineal region tumors of all histologies, and not only to those pineal cell or germ cell origin.

Germ cell tumors

Intracranial germ cell tumors are a heterogeneous group of tumors which include germinomas, teratomas, embryonal cell tumors, endodermal sinus (yolk sac) tumors, choriocarcinomas, dermoid tumors, and epidermoid tumors. Germ cell tumors account for 0.4–3.4% of the intracranial neoplasms seen each year in both the USA and Europe (Jennings et al 1985; Surawicz et al 1999). The incidence of germ cell tumors and cysts in the CNS is 0.09/100000 person-years in the US population (Surawicz et al 1999). Considerable geographic variation exists among germ cell tumors; the highest incidence is in Japan, varying between 2.1% and 4.8% (Arita et al 1980; Sano 1976b, Takakura 1985).

Germinomas are the most common intracranial germ cell tumor. Among large series, pure germinomas comprise between 40% and 65% of all germ cell tumors, giving an average US incidence of 0.1/100000 (Bruce et al 2000; Horowitz & Hall 1991). Teratomas (18–20%), endodermal sinus tumors (4–7%), embryonal cell tumors (3–5%), and choriocarcinomas (3–5%) are correspondingly less frequent (Fig. 34.2) (Jennings et al 1985). Moreover, large series with extensive tissue sampling have shown mixed germ cell tumors to comprise 25% of germ cell tumors (Bruce et al 2000; Russell & Rubinstein 1989b; Stein & Bruce 1992). The percentage of pure germinomas among germ cell tumors varies between populations, with the Taiwanese showing 82% germinomas compared with approximately 50% in an unselected western series and 16% in a western pediatric series (Ho & Liu 1992; Jennings et al 1985).

Most germ cell tumors occur before the third decade of life, with regional differences among pediatric populations. In the US population, the mean age of diagnosis for germ cell tumors is 22 years (Surawicz et al 1999). In Japanese children, germ cell tumors account for between 4.8% and 15% of all brain tumors (Matsutani et al 1987; Sano 1976b; Takakura 1985). In western countries, the incidence in the pediatric population is between 0.3% and 3.4% (Hoffman et al 1984; Jenkin et al 1978; Jennings et al 1985; Wara et al 1979). Ho and Lu (1992) have also shown increased incidence among the children of Taiwan (11%), but Taiwanese adults seem to be affected no more often than European adults (0.6%).

Pineal cell tumors

The true incidence of pineal cell tumors is unknown, but indirect calculations based on data from Schild and co-workers (1993) estimate 0.01/100000 persons per year in the USA. They also found that pineal region neoplasms, 15–30% of which are of pineal cell origin, account for 0.4–1.0% of the 17000 cerebral neoplasms diagnosed each year. More recently, in a US-based epidemiologic study of

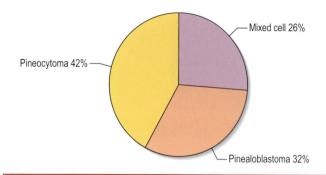

Figure 34.3 Relative percentages of histologic sub-types among pineal cell tumors in the USA (total incidence 0.1/100 000 per year). Based on 90 tumors from the series of Herrick & Rubinstein (1979); Bruce (1993a,b); Schild et al (1993). (Courtesy of Oxford University Press.)

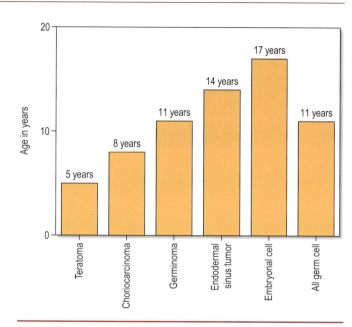

Figure 34.4 Most common age of onset for intracranial germ cell tumors. (From Jennings et al 1985.)

20 765 CNS tumors, pineal parenchymal tumors accounted for 0.2% of all CNS tumors (Surawicz et al 1999).

Schild's study of 30 pineal parenchymal tumors found approximately 50% pineoblastomas, 30% pineocytomas, and 20% mixed tumors. However, in the same publication, 110 cases reviewed in the literature showed a slightly greater percentage of pineocytomas at 53%, compared with 47% pineoblastomas. In Russell and Rubinstein's (1989b) series of 53 pineal cell tumors, pineocytomas accounted for 57%. In the New York Neurological Institute, in an operative series of 135 cases of pineal region tumors, 57% were pineocytomas, 23% were pineoblastomas, and 20% were mixed tumors (Bruce & Stein 1995b) (see Fig. 34.3 for relative percentages from various studies).

Although the incidence of pineal region tumors is four to five times higher in Japan than in the USA, pineal cell tumors make up only about 11% of these tumors compared with 30% in the USA. Thus, the overall incidence of pineal cell tumors is about the same in both countries (Koide et al 1980). As mentioned previously, Ojeda et al (1987) showed that, in comparison to Western Australia, Niigata (Japan) has a similar 10-year prevalence.

Age distribution

Germ cell tumors

Intracranial germ cell tumors occur most frequently between the ages of 10 and 12 (27%), with 70% occurring between 10 and 21 years, and 95% before age 33 (Fig. 34.4) (Jennings et al 1985), with a mean age at diagnosis of 22 years (Surawicz et al 1999). These rates are similar for both sexes. Germinomas occur with relatively the same frequency by age, with 26% between 10 and 12, 65% between 10 and 21, and 95% before age 27. Only 11% occur before the age of 9, although a 16-month-old boy with germinoma has been reported (Ammar et al 1991). Although not statistically significant, women are affected at slightly younger ages than men. Overall, the age distribution of non-germinomatous germ cell tumors resembles that seen for germinomas, except that twice as many occur in children less than 9 years of age (24%). The large number of cases in very young children is mainly due to teratomas and choriocarcinomas. Both

of these tumor types have one-third of their presentations in early childhood.

Teratomas have two incidence peaks: the greatest number occur in children less than 9 years of age, but 20% occur between ages 16 and 18. Overall, 66% of teratomas occur between ages 4 and 18, and 95% before age 36. Choriocarcinomas also show a proclivity for younger groups: 35% before the age of 9 years; 25% between ages 7 and 9; 70% between ages 7 and 15; and 95% between ages 1 and 21. By contrast, endodermal sinus tumors and embryonal cell tumors tend to occur in middle and late adolescence, respectively. Of endodermal sinus tumors: 40% occur between ages 13 and 15; 65% between ages 10 and 15; and 95% between the ages of 4 and 21. Only 12% occur in children less than 9 years of age. A total of 30% of embryonal cell tumors occur between the ages of 16 and 18; 70% between ages 10 and 18; and 95% between ages 7 and 27. Only 10% of cases occur in very young children.

In summary, germ cell tumors occur almost exclusively during the first three decades of life. Germinomas are most common in early adolescence around the time of puberty but may occur at any time during youth. Non-germinomatous tumors show a similar pattern, with choriocarcinomas and teratomas being especially prevalent in early childhood and endodermal sinus tumors and embryonal carcinomas being more common in late adolescence.

Pineal cell tumors

In Schild's series, the mean age of presentation for all pineal cell tumors was 22, ranging from 11 months to 77 years (Fig. 34.5) (Schild et al 1993). Surawicz et al (1999), in the prospective study of 20 765 patients with brain tumors, found a mean age at diagnosis for pineal cell tumors of 28 years. In 50 patients with pineal cell tumors at the New York Neurological Institute, the mean age of presentation was 36 years,

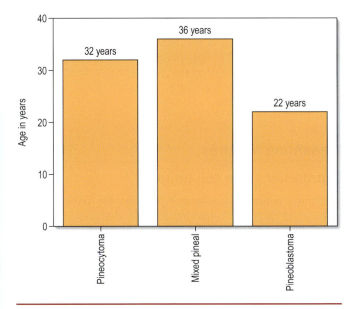

40

36 years

32 years

30

22 years

Age in years

20

10

0

Pineocytoma

Mixed pineal

Pineoblastoma

Figure 34.5 Average age of onset for pineal cell tumors, based on 90 tumors from the series of Herrick & Rubinstein (1979); Bruce (1993b); Schild et al (1993). (Courtesy of Oxford University Press.)

with a range from 7 to 70 years (Bruce et al 2000). The nine cases of pineocytoma in Schild's study occurred between ages 17 and 72, with a mean age of 36. Of Russell and Rubinstein's (1989b) 30 cases of pineocytoma, 25 occurred in adulthood and only five (17%) in children, all in the first decade of life. In 20 adult patients at the New York Neurological Institute, the mean age of presentation was 40, with a range of 21–57 years.

All 15 cases of pineoblastoma reviewed by Schild et al (1993) presented between the ages of 11 months and 66 years, with an average age of 18 years. Russell and Rubinstein (1989b) also found this more malignant variety of pineal cell tumor in a younger population, evidenced by 14 of their 23 cases (61%) occurring in the first decade of life and all the remaining cases occurring before the age of 40. In the eight adult patients at the Neurological Institute, a mean age of presentation at 33 years was found, which dropped to 27 years if the unusual case of a 70-year-old male is disregarded.

In summary, pineal cell neoplasms generally occur in the 3rd and 4th decades of life. Nonetheless, they may occur earlier, especially with the more malignant pineoblastoma (61% present in the first decade) of life. Isolated cases may present in old age.

Sex distribution

Germ cell tumors

Intracranial germ cell tumors are overwhelmingly more likely to occur in males. An epidemiologic study by The Central Brain Tumor Registry of the United States found a higher incidence of germ cell tumor in males (0.14/100 000 person-years) than in females (0.04 per 100 000 person-

years) (Surawicz et al 1999). In addition, within the English language literature, Jennings and co-workers (1985) showed that, for all intracranial germ cell tumors, males are 2.24 times more likely to be affected. A similar male predominance of 1.88:1 exists for pure germinomas but is stronger for non-germinomatous germ cell tumors, which show a slightly stronger male preponderance of 3.25:1. Men were more likely to have pineal involvement (65%), while women were more likely to have suprasellar involvement (75%). Several studies, however, showed equal gender representation for suprasellar germ cell tumors (Hoffman et al 1991; Jennings et al 1985; Takeuchi et al 1978).

Pineal cell tumors

Among large series of pineal cell tumors, there seems to be either no gender preference for these tumors or a very small one in favor of men (Bruce et al 2000; Russell & Rubinstein 1989b; Schild et al 1993). A slight male predominance has been shown in the Japanese literature (7:5 male to female) (Koide et al 1980).

Family history and genetic factors

Germ cell tumors

A familial tendency for germ cell tumors has not been found, although one exceptional mixed germ cell tumor in two brothers has been reported (Wakai et al 1980). Hereditary features have been demonstrated in presacral teratomas, however these are also exceptional (Hunt et al 1977).

Pineal cell tumors

Heritable examples of pineal cell tumors are rare, although the occurrence of pineoblastoma in a 12-year-old girl and her 43-year-old mother has been reported (Lesnick et al 1985). A more striking familial association involves the 30 or so documented cases of the childhood syndrome known as 'trilateral retinoblastoma', consisting of simultaneous pineoblastoma and bilateral retinoblastoma (Bader et al 1982). Interestingly, pediatric patients bearing familial mutation of Rb gene that developed pinealoblastomas appear to bear worse prognosis than a similar population of pediatric patients with sporadic pinealoblastomas that did not have Rb mutation (Plowman et al 2004). Retinoblastomas, especially in the bilateral form, are genetically inherited and have been associated with gene deletions (Murphree & Benedict 1984; Russell & Rubinstein 1989b). In trilateral retinoblastoma, the pineoblastoma is thought to represent an additional neoplastic focus originating in the vestigial photoreceptors of the pineal gland. Photoreceptor morphology in the human pineal gland demonstrates an embryologic origin common to that of the retinal photoreceptor, although the function within the pineal gland has been lost through evolution (Bader et al 1982). Studies have demonstrated common immunostaining for neuron specific enolase, S-antigen, and rhodopsin in patients with trilateral retinoblastoma (Rodrigues et al 1987).

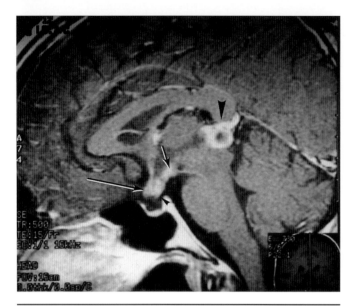

Figure 34.6 Gadolinium enhanced MRI of a 33-year-old woman who presented with visual loss, amenorrhea, and diabetes insipidus. MRI shows germinomatous invasion of the pineal gland (large arrowhead), optic chiasm (long arrow), pituitary stalk (small arrowhead), and floor of the third ventricle (short arrow).

Sites of predilection

Germ cell tumors

Germ cell tumors may arise in a variety of midline sites, the gonads and mediastinum being most common, but also in the sacrococcygeum, retroperitoneum, nasopharynx, and orbit (Gonzalez-Crussi 1982). Within the central nervous system, the pineal gland is the main site of predilection, followed by the suprasellar region; synchronous lesions at both sites are also possible (Fig. 34.6) (Jennings et al 1985; Russell & Rubinstein 1989a, Sugiyama et al 1992). Other less common locations involve the central neuraxis in the midline as included in Russell & Rubinstein's (189a) review of 120 germ cell tumors: pineal (45 cases); suprasellar (33 cases); intrasellar (3 cases); fourth ventricle (18 cases); spinal (5 cases); massive intracranial (3 cases), and other sites (13 cases). Bjornsson's series of 41 germinomas consisted of 25 situated anteriorly and 16 posteriorly in the third ventricle (Bjornsson et al 1985). Jennings and co-workers (1985) reviewed 389 intracranial germ cell tumors and found that 95% arose from the midline, with 37% in the suprasellar cistern, 48% in the pineal gland, and an additional 6% involving both. In this large series, which may reflect referral bias, germinomas were more likely to arise in the suprasellar region and non-germinomatous germ cell tumors were more likely to involve the pineal gland.

Several other rare sites of intracranial germ cell tumor have been reported, including the thalamus, basal ganglia, ventricular system, cerebellum, frontal region, and septum pellucidum (Jennings et al 1985; Ogata et al 1964; Tanaka & Ueki 1979). Germinoma of the infundibulum and of the optic chiasm has also been described (Manor et al 1990).

Pineal cell tumors

Pineal cell tumors are derived from the pinealocytes of the pineal gland (Russell & Rubinstein 1989a; Russell & Rubinstein 1989b). Although they may spread anywhere throughout the cerebrospinal pathways, the primary site is always within the pineal gland.

Presenting features

Suprasellar germ cell tumors

The most common presenting features for patients with suprasellar germ cell tumors include diabetes insipidus, visual field defects and other hypothalamic–pituitary abnormalities (Fig. 34.6) (Hoffman et al 1991; Jennings et al 1985; Sakai et al 1988). Neuroendocrine dysfunction can include hypopituitarism, delayed sexual development, growth failure, and precocious puberty. Less commonly, hypothalamic dysfunction can cause obtundation, behavioral disturbance, anorexia, and obesity. Tumors of sufficiently large size may present with hydrocephalus.

Pineal region tumors

Tumors in the pineal region, regardless of their histology, may become symptomatic by three possible mechanisms: (1) increased intracranial pressure from hydrocephalus; (2) direct compression of brain stem or cerebellum; or (3) endocrine dysfunction (Bruce et al 2000; Bruce 1993b; Sawaya et al 1990). Headache is the most common presenting symptom and occurs following obstruction of the third ventricle outflow at the aqueduct of Sylvius. More advanced hydrocephalus can result in nausea, vomiting, papilledema, obtundation, and other cognitive deficits.

Direct brain stem compression may lead to disturbances of extraocular movements, classically known as Parinaud syndrome (Parinaud 1886; Posner & Horrax 1946). This can include paralysis of upgaze or convergence, retraction nystagmus, and light-near pupillary dissociation. Compression or infiltration of the dorsal midbrain and periaqueductal area can cause paralysis of downgaze, ptosis, and lid retraction. Double vision from fourth nerve palsy is rare but may occur. Eye movement dysfunction may also be caused by hydrocephalus, in which case improvement would be expected following ventricular shunting. Involvement of the superior cerebellar peduncles can lead to ataxia and dysmetria. Hearing disturbances can occasionally occur, probably from compression of the inferior colliculi (DeMonte et al 1993; Missori et al 1995).

Endocrine dysfunction is rare and may be caused by direct tumor involvement in the hypothalamus or result from secondary effects of hydrocephalus (Bruce et al 2000; Fetell & Stein 1986). In general, diabetes insipidus and other neuroendocrine disturbances are indicative of hypothalamic infiltration by tumor, even when not radiographically visualized (Jennings et al 1985). Precocious puberty has been historically associated with pineal region tumors; however, true documented cases are rare (Borit 1981; Fetell & Stein 1986; Krabbe 1923; Zondek et al 1953). This syndrome is limited to boys with ectopic β-hCG (beta-human chorionic

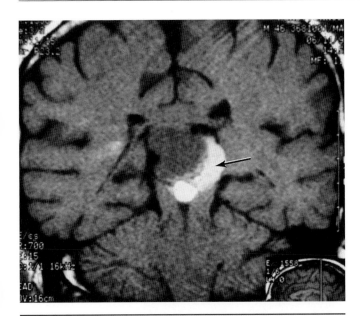

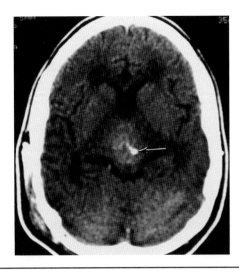

Figure 34.8 Non-contrast CT scan in an 18-year-old man with a germinoma. The tumor can be seen engulfing the calcification (arrow).

Figure 34.7 Non-contrast MRI of a pineocytoma in a 40-year-old man presenting with acute hydrocephalus. At surgery the high signal area (arrow) turned out to be acute hemorrhage.

gonadotropin) secretion from choriocarcinomas or germinomas with syncytiotrophoblastic cells (Fetell & Stein 1986; Jennings et al 1985). The β-hCG secondarily stimulates androgen secretion by the Leydig cells of the testes resulting in the premature sexual maturation characteristics of what is more appropriately termed pseudopuberty.

A rare, but notable, presentation is pineal apoplexy from hemorrhage into a pineal tumor or a pineal cyst (Fig. 34.7) (Burres & Hamilton 1979; Herrick & Rubinstein 1979; Higashi et al 1979; Patel et al 2005; Steinbok et al 1977). Pineal cell tumors in particular, and choriocarcinomas to a lesser extent, are associated with this phenomenon, probably because of their prominent vascularity. These same characteristics may also predispose to postoperative hemorrhage (Bruce & Stein 1993a). The clinical manifestation can include severe headache of sudden onset or acute worsening, with or without the existence of other signs of hydrocephalus (Patel et al 2005).

Imaging diagnosis

MRI has replaced CT as the diagnostic method of choice for all pineal tumors. High resolution MRI with gadolinium can visualize the tumor size, vascularity and homogeneity, and its relationship with surrounding structures. Besides detecting the presence of hydrocephalus, MRI provides useful anatomic information necessary for planning operative approaches including the tumor's position within the third ventricle, its extension laterally and supratentorially, its degree of brain stem involvement, and its position relative to the deep venous system. Indeed, pineal tumors generally displace the vessels of the deep venous system superiorly along the dorsal periphery of the tumor. This is an important point when planning surgical approaches, because most tumors are separable from the surrounding veins and mid-

brain (Stein & Bruce 1992). Notable exceptions are meningiomas arising from the velum interpositum and epidermoid or other tumors originating in the corpus callosum. These tumors displace the deep venous system ventrally and inferiorly, providing a diagnostic clue on the MRI scan. The position of the tumor relative to the deep venous system is important, because it may influence the choice between an infratentorial and a supratentorial approach. Although the location of the deep venous system may be conspicuous with MRI, magnetic resonance venography may be desirable to better delineate it.

The diagnostic utility of MRI has limitations. Despite advances in radiographic imaging, accurate prediction of tumor histology based solely on radiographic characteristics remains unreliable (Bruce 1993b; Ganti et al 1986; Müller-Forell et al 1988; Tien et al 1990; Zimmerman 1985). CT scans may be complementary by providing details of calcification, blood–brain barrier breakdown, and degree of vascularity. On the other hand, the margination pattern and irregularities of the tumor border depicted on MRI can provide some idea of tumor invasiveness; however, the true degree of encapsulation is best defined at surgery (Stein & Bruce 1992). Angiograms are generally not helpful unless a vascular anomaly is suspected.

Germ cell tumors

On CT scans, germinomas tend to be homogeneous and either isointense or of slightly higher attenuation than gray matter while exhibiting moderate to marked contrast enhancement. Calcification is likely to occur in both suprasellar and pineal region germinomas, with the tumor tending to surround and engulf the calcification (Fig. 34.8) (Chang et al 1981; Ganti et al 1986; Smirniotopoulos et al 1992). On MRI, germinomas are relatively isointense to normal white matter on T1-weighted images and slightly hyperintense on T2-weighted images (Fig. 34.9A,B). Cystic areas can occasionally be seen (Tien et al 1990; Zee et al 1991). Gadolinium helps to define the tumor well, as germinomas enhance markedly and homogeneously (Fig. 34.9C).

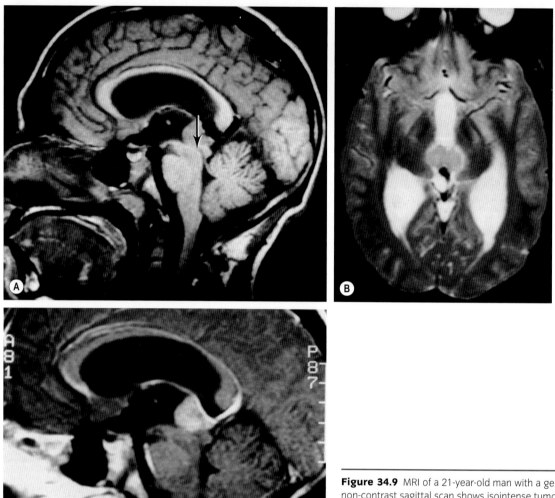

Figure 34.9 MRI of a 21-year-old man with a germinoma. (A) T1-weighted non-contrast sagittal scan shows isointense tumor which has obstructed the aqueduct of Sylvius (arrow) to cause hydrocephalus. (B) T2-weighted non-contrast axial scan: tumor hyperintense to brain matter but hypointense to CSF. (C) Homogeneous gadolinium enhancement of the tumor on T1-weighted sagittal scan.

The heterogenic histologic composition of teratomas is reflected in their radiographic appearance, which is notable for heterogeneity, multilocularity, and irregular enhancement (Fig. 34.10). Various signal characteristics reflect lipid content, soft tissue components, calcification, and cystic elements. Malignant teratomas have similar characteristics but are distinguished by invasion into surrounding structures (Tien et al 1990). On CT scanning, teratomas are generally well circumscribed and, unlike most other pineal tumors, contain areas of low attenuation due to their adipose tissue. Contrast enhancement with both CT and MRI can be irregular, heterogeneous, or ring-enhancing.

Accurate description of the radiographic features of malignant non-germinomatous germ cell tumors is difficult because of their rarity in any clinical series. The heterogeneity that is often described may represent mixed germ cell elements. In general, malignant germ cell tumors tend to have infiltrating borders with varying degrees of enhancement. Areas of prior hemorrhage can be seen, particularly with choriocarcinoma.

Epidermoid tumors have decreased signal intensity on T1 and increased signal on T2 (Tien et al 1990). They are distinguished from dermoid tumors which have increased signal on both T1 and T2, although isointensity on T2 has been described (Hudgins et al 1987; Tien et al 1990).

Pineal cell tumors

Both pineocytomas and pineoblastomas tend to be hypo- or isointense on T1-weighted imaging and hyperintense on T2 (Fig. 34.11). In general, pineal cell tumors tend to be homogeneous and have uniform enhancement (Chiechi et al 1995). Hemorrhage and necrosis are more common in pineoblastomas, which also tend to be larger, while cysts are occasionally seen in pineocytomas (Smirniotopoulos et al 1992). Pineocytomas are not encapsulated, yet tend to be well-defined. Calcifications can be present, although usually in a pattern different from germinomas (Fig. 34.11D). With pineal cell tumors, this is usually in the form of intratumoral calcifications, whereas the germinoma often engulfs a calcified pineal gland (Ganti et al 1986; Smirniotopoulos et al 1992).

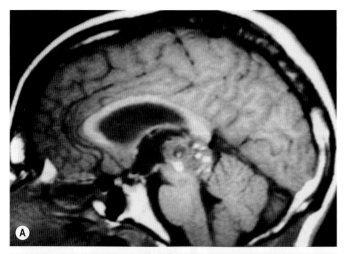

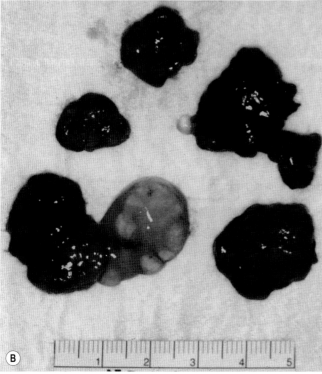

Figure 34.10 (A) Sagittal MRI of a heterogeneous mixed germ cell tumor of the pineal region in a 21-year-old man who presented with hydrocephalus. After pathologic examination following complete surgical resection, the tumor was found to have multiple components including endodermal sinus tumor, embryonal cell carcinoma, immature teratoma, and mature teratoma. (B) Gross tissue specimens, reflecting heterogeneity of various germ cell components.

Laboratory diagnosis

The tumor markers α-fetoprotein (AFP) and β-hCG are specific for malignant germ cell elements and should be measured in all patients with pineal region tumors (Allen et al 1979; Bruce & Stein 1990; Sawaya et al 1990). Because they are reliable indicators of malignant germ cell elements, the presence of malignant germ cell markers makes surgery and biopsy unnecessary, and such patients should be

managed with radiation and chemotherapy. Measurement of germ cell markers can be helpful not only for diagnostic purposes but also for monitoring response to therapy or as an early sign of tumor recurrence. Marker levels should be measured in both blood and CSF, as CSF measurements are generally more sensitive (Allen et al 1979; Arita et al 1980; Chan et al 1984; Ono et al 1982; Sano 1984; Sawaya et al 1990).

AFP is a glycoprotein normally produced by fetal yolk sac elements and has a biologic half-life of approximately 5 days (Sawaya et al 1990). AFP is markedly elevated with endodermal sinus tumors, while smaller elevations may occur with embryonal cell carcinomas and immature teratomas (Allen et al 1985; Allen et al 1979; Arita et al 1980; Jennings et al 1985; Jooma & Kendall 1983; Sawaya et al 1990; Wilson et al 1979). Although elevated AFP has been reported with germinomas (Arita et al 1980), this may reflect sampling error of what are actually mixed germ cell tumors. Teratomas do not secrete AFP or β-hCG; however, immature teratomas may have slightly elevated AFP levels (Bruce 1993b; Ho & Liu 1992; Jooma & Kendall 1983).

β-hCG is a glycoprotein that is normally secreted by placental trophoblastic tissue and has a biologic half-life of 15–20 h (Sawaya et al 1990). Markedly elevated levels are found with choriocarcinomas, while mild elevations can sometimes be seen with embryonal cell carcinomas and germinomas (Allen et al 1979; Arita et al 1980; Bruce 1993b, Haase & Norgaard-Pedersen 1979; Jennings et al 1985; Jooma & Kendall 1983; Neuwelt & Smith 1979; Page et al 1986; Sawaya et al 1990; Takeuchi et al 1978). Most germinomas are nonsecretory, however a small percentage will contain low levels of β-hCG if syncytiotrophoblastic giant cells are present (Arita et al 1980; Bloom 1983; Bruce 1993b, Jennings et al 1985; Neuwelt et al 1979; Takeuchi et al 1978). Elevations of β-hCG in germinomas may correlate with a less favorable prognosis (Uematsu et al 1992; Yoshida et al 1993). The absence of AFP or β-hCG elevation should be interpreted with caution since it does not necessarily rule out the presence of a germinoma or embryonal cell carcinoma. Similarly, elevated AFP associated with a germinoma should be cause for suspecting the additional presence of mixed tumor elements containing either embryonal cell carcinoma or endodermal sinus tumor (Russell & Rubinstein 1989a). Other biologic markers for germ cell tumors include lactate dehydrogenase isoenzymes and placental alkaline phosphatase (Metcalfe & Sikora 1985; Sawaya et al 1990; Shinoda et al 1988). These germ cell markers have diagnostic value when used in the immunohistochemical analysis of histologic specimens but are not useful as serum or CSF markers.

No reliable markers exist for pineal parenchymal tumors, although several have been investigated. Melatonin, as the primary secretory protein of the pineal gland and the one responsible for its association with circadian rhythm in humans (Bruce et al 1991; Erlich & Apuzzo 1985), has been measured in pineal tumors, usually with inconsistent results (Arendt 1978; Barber et al 1978; Miles et al 1985; Vorkapic et al 1987; Wurtman & Kammer 1966). Curiously, abnormal melatonin levels have also been seen in patients with other intracranial or systemic malignancies, but the significance is unknown (Dempsey & Chandler 1984; Erlich & Apuzzo 1985; Tamarkin et al 1982; Vaughan 1984).

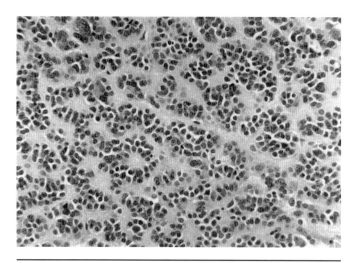

Figure 34.19 Pineocytoma consisting of benign, well-differentiated cells forming rosettes.

1987). Rare cases of melanin pigment have been found (Herrick & Rubinstein 1979). The ultrastructure has not been described in a systematic fashion, however reports suggest some commonality between these tumors and the photosensory cells of pineals in lower vertebrates as evidenced by cytoplasmic protrusions resembling the end bulbs of the human fetal gland and giant club-shaped cilia with the 9+0 pattern (Markesbery et al 1981; Russell & Rubinstein 1989b).

Pineocytomas can be quite cellular, but are generally less so than pineoblastomas. The tumor cells are benign, mature cells that may be indistinguishable from normal pinealocytes and are arranged in sheets or diffuse lobules (Fig. 34.19). Giant cells may be present, but mitotic figures are not common. Perivascular bulbous cellular terminations can often be seen with Bielschowski stain (Schild et al 1993). Pineocytomas may exhibit neuronal or astrocytomatous differentiation (Borit & Blackwood 1979; Borit et al 1980; Herrick & Rubinstein 1979). Whether these differentiation patterns reflect the multipotentiality of pineal parenchymal tumors or the simultaneous transformation of adjacent astrocytic and neuronal cells is not clear. Neuronal differentiation is often accompanied by the formation of rosettes, the centers of which contain the tangles of small knobbed terminations of delicate argyrophilic processes. A separate designation as 'pineocytomatous rosettes' has been given to distinguish them from the more primitive Homer Wright rosettes (Borit et al 1980; Schild et al 1993). Antibody staining to synaptophysin, neurofilaments, or chromogranin A may be positive, reflecting neural differentiation (Jouvet et al 1994; Schild et al 1993). Pineocytomas may stain positive for the S-antigen (Korf et al 1986; Perentes et al 1986; Rodrigues et al 1987). As viewed with electron microscopy, pineocytomas may contain dense core vesicles in the tumor cell processes, cilia with characteristic 9+0 filament complex, synaptic ribbons, bulbous cell process endings with microtubules, and occasional clear-centered vesicles with synapse formation (Herrick & Rubinstein 1979; Markesbery et al 1981; Russell & Rubinstein 1989b).

Alternating electron-dense and electron-lucent cells joined by zonulae adherentes and a complex system of vacuoles and organelles similar to normal mammalian pinealocytes have also been described (Hassoun et al 1983). Tumor cells may show the presence of either vesicle-crowned rodlets or fibrous filaments if differentiation along neurosensory pathways has occurred, while the presence of dense core vesicles is indicative of neuroendocrine differentiation (Jouvet et al 1994).

Despite the characteristic appearances of pineocytomas or pineoblastomas, the intermediately-differentiated tumors are more variable and therefore more difficult to characterize. Tumors may contain features of both pineocytomas and pineoblastomas, although no consensus exists on where the transition from well-differentiated pineocytoma to undifferentiated pineoblastoma occurs. Mixed tumors have been designated when divergent differentiation exists along neuronal, glial, or glioneuronal lines (Borit et al 1980); however currently, the designation is more applicable to tumors showing co-existent pineocytoma and pineoblastoma elements (Schild et al 1993). Such lack of uniformity in defining mixed tumors makes it difficult to correlate clinical behavior among the different reported series of pineal cell tumors.

Papillary tumor of the pineal region

Papillary tumor of the pineal region (PTPR) is a recently recognized tumor that was first described in 2003 (Jouvet et al 2003), and was introduced as a distinct tumor entity in the 2007 WHO classification of brain tumors. These lesions are thought to arise from the specialized ependyma of the subcommissural organ (Hasselblatt et al 2006; Jouvet et al 2003; Shibahara et al 2004). Due to its relatively recent recognition, the clinical behavior of this tumor is not well described. Fevre-Montange et al's (2006b) retrospective study of 31 patients is the largest published series of these tumors to date. This study reported an age range from 5 to 66 years (median age, 29 years) and slight female predominance. A total of 21 out of 31 patients underwent gross total resection and 15 patients received radiation therapy in addition to the tumor resection. In spite of this, the majority of patients had recurrences. With regard to prognosis, the 5-year survival was 73% and progression free survival 27% (Fevre-Montange et al 2006b). The histology of PTPR consists of an epithelial-like growth pattern in which the vessels are covered by layers of columnar or cuboidal tumor cells forming perivascular pseudorosettes (Fevre-Montange et al 2006b; Jouvet et al 2003). The immunohistochemical profile of PTPR is characterized by the expression of transthyretin (TTR) and cytokeratin (CK) 18 and with poor to absent expression of CK7 and CK20, markers that are commonly found in metastatic carcinomas and thus provide a useful means to differentiate these two entities (Fevre-Montange et al 2006a,b). Interestingly, CK18 and TTR are also expressed by the subcommissural organ, supporting the hypothesis that PTPR derives from it (Kasper et al 1990; Montecinos et al 2005). Immunohistochemical differentiation of PTPR from choroid plexus papillomas is possible since most of the former lack expression of Kir7.1 which is abundantly found in choroid plexus tumors (Hasselblatt et al 2006).

Definition and incidence of malignancy

Germ cell tumors

Malignant germ cell tumors are capable of systemic and CSF metastases. Dissemination may occur through a variety of mechanisms including hematogenous spread (Borden et al 1973; Galassi et al 1984; Stowell et al 1945; Tompkins et al 1950), direct paraspinal extension (Dayan et al 1966; Rubery & Wheeler 1980), and via ventriculo-peritoneal shunts (Dayan et al 1966; Jennings et al 1985; Kun et al 1981; Neuwelt et al 1979; Rubery & Wheeler 1980; Salazar et al 1979; Takei & Pearl 1981; Wilson et al 1979). Extraneural metastasis to various sites has been reported in up to 3% of all germ cell tumors with lung and bone the most common sites, but also kidney, bladder, mediastinum, gastrointestinal tract, breast, and mesentery (Borden et al 1973; Dayan et al 1966; Galassi et al 1984; Jennings et al 1985; Rubery & Wheeler 1980; Salazar et al 1979; Stowell et al 1945; Tompkins et al 1950). Various estimates, ranging from 5% to 57%, have been given for the incidence of CSF seeding, with large series giving around 10% (Brada & Rajan 1990; Bruce et al 1990; Chapman & Linggood 1980; Jenkin et al 1978; Jennings et al 1985; Sano & Matsutani 1981). Although positive CSF cytology has been cited as evidence of spinal seeding, this assumption has not been convincingly proven (Jennings et al 1985). Likewise, a negative CSF cytology does not preclude leptomeningeal dissemination (Chapman & Linggood 1980; Jooma & Kendall 1983; Sung et al 1978). Surgical intervention does not appear to increase the risk of spinal dissemination (Brada & Rajan 1990).

Germinomas can spread directly along the floor and walls of the third ventricle or alternatively via CSF pathways (Jennings et al 1985). Seeding and infiltration of a germinoma into the optic nerve sheath has also been reported (Manor et al 1990; Stefanko et al 1979). In general, the non-germinomatous malignant germ cell tumors have a higher incidence of metastatic dissemination compared with germinomas. Jennings and co-workers (1985) found correlations between: (1) hypothalamic involvement and third ventricle involvement simultaneously; (2) involvement of the third ventricle and dissemination through a non-contiguous site; and (3) the presence of spinal cord extension with additional metastasis in other sites. Spinal cord metastases were more likely to occur with germ cell tumors in the pineal region compared with other locations (Jennings et al 1985).

Pineal cell tumors

Pineal parenchymal tumors are capable of spread along the CSF pathways (Fig. 34.20) (Borit et al 1980; Herrick & Rubinstein 1979; Schild et al 1993). Remote spread is unusual, although dissemination through a ventriculo-peritoneal shunt is possible (Lesoin et al 1987; Pfletschinger et al 1986). In general, pineoblastomas have more malignant potential and propensity for CSF dissemination compared with pineocytomas (Borit et al 1980; Schild et al 1993). Herrick & Rubinstein (1979) reported evidence of lepto-meningeal dissemination at autopsy in all 11 patients with pineoblastoma, whereas Hoffman and co-workers (1984) reported metastases in 6 of 13 pineoblastomas.

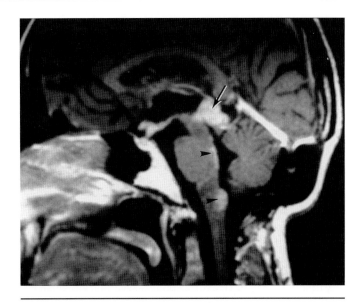

Figure 34.20 MRI scan of a 44-year-old woman, 10 years after resection of a mixed pineal cell tumor. The tumor has recurred in the pineal region (arrow) and has seeded the fourth ventricle (arrowheads).

Pineocytomas, despite decreased growth rate and malignant potential, do have the propensity for CSF dissemination, although to a much lesser degree (Bruce et al 1990; D'Andrea et al 1987; Disclafani et al 1989; Herrick & Rubinstein 1979).

Schild and co-workers (1993) reported leptomeningeal failure following radiation therapy in 0 of 4 pineocytomas; 0 of 4 intermediately-differentiated pineal parenchymal tumors; 1 of 2 mixed pineal parenchymal tumors; and 4 of 9 pineoblastomas. Leptomeningeal failure occurred only in the presence of persistent primary tumor. In this same series of 21 pineal parenchymal tumors, radiographic seeding at the time of diagnosis was present in only one of the 11 patients with pineoblastoma. Malignant cells were present in the CSF in three of the 21 tumors (one intermediately-differentiated pineal parenchymal tumor and two pineoblastomas), however it is debatable whether the presence of a positive cytology is associated with spinal seeding. Considerable controversy exists regarding the correlation of neuronal differentiation with prognosis and malignant features (Herrick & Rubinstein 1979; Schild et al 1993). Differentiating between pineocytoma and pineoblastoma is more useful for predicting CSF dissemination than local tumor recurrence (Schild et al 1993).

General management plan

All patients with suspected germ cell or pineal cell tumors should have the following work-up:

1. High resolution MR scan with gadolinium of the head, with particular attention to possible multicentric disease within the CSF pathways

2. Measurement of AFP and β-hCG in the serum and CSF to detect malignant germ cell elements

3. Cytologic examination of CSF of patients undergoing third ventricular shunt placement or ventriculostomy

4. Evaluation of pituitary function if endocrine abnormalities are suspected

5. Formal visual field examination for suprasellar tumors.

Following the preoperative work-up, a histopathologic diagnosis must be made, preferably by craniotomy, although stereotactic biopsy may be indicated under certain circumstances. Most patients derive benefit from aggressive tumor resection.

Postoperative adjuvant therapy depends upon the tumor histology. Surgical resection is usually curative for benign tumors. Most malignant germ cell or pineal cell tumors will require radiation therapy. Malignant non-germinomatous germ cell tumors will usually require chemotherapy prior to radiation.

Surgical management

Management of hydrocephalus

Most patients will have hydrocephalus secondary to obstruction of the aqueduct, and it may therefore be best to wait until third ventriculostomy or shunt placement to obtain CSF for cytology and measurement of tumor markers. A procedure for CSF diversion is necessary prior to tumor resection in most cases of pineal region tumor. Symptomatic patients are best managed initially with a stereotactic-guided endoscopic third ventriculostomy to allow a gradual reduction in intracranial pressure and resolution of symptoms prior to tumor resection (Goodman 1993). This method is preferable to ventriculoperitoneal shunting, as it eliminates potential complications such as infection, over shunting, and peritoneal seeding of malignant cells. Mildly symptomatic patients in whom a gross total resection is anticipated at surgery can be managed with a ventricular drain placed at the time of surgical resection (Bruce & Ogden 2004; Edwards et al 1988). The drain can be removed or converted to a shunt in the postoperative period as the circumstances dictate.

Tissue diagnosis: biopsy vs open resection

Given the diverse pathology that can occur in the pineal region, a histologic diagnosis is necessary to optimize management decisions (Bruce & Ogden 2004; Calaminus et al 2004; Fevre-Montange et al 2006b; Konovalov & Pitskhelauri 2003; Stein & Bruce 1992; Villano et al 2008). An individual tumor's histology strongly influences the choice of postoperative adjuvant therapy, need for metastatic work-up, estimation of prognosis, and planning of long-term follow-up. Although CSF cytology and radiographic examination provide insight into the histologic diagnosis, they are not sufficiently sensitive to supplant a tissue diagnosis (D'Andrea et al 1987; Fujimaki et al 1994; Kersh et al 1988; Liang et al 2002; Satoh et al 1995; Wood et al 1981; Zee et al 1991). CSF cytology occasionally reveals malignant cells but is rarely diagnostic. The only time a tissue diagnosis is unnecessary, is in the presence of malignant germ cell markers; in these cases, chemotherapy and radiation should proceed without a biopsy (Bruce & Ogden 2004; Choi et al 1998; Kersh et al 1988).

Tissue diagnosis can be obtained by either a stereotactic biopsy or an open procedure. This decision is influenced by clinical features of the patient, radiographic features of the tumor, and the surgeon's degree of experience with the procedures. Inflexible or dogmatic dedication to either procedure is not appropriate. In general, patients with known primary systemic tumors, multiple lesions, or medical conditions that make open resection dangerous are good candidates for stereotactic biopsy (Bruce et al 2001; Bruce & Ogden 2004). Radiographic evidence of brainstem invasion might make stereotactic biopsy an attractive choice; however, the degree of invasion seen radiographically can be misleading and may not reflect a dissectible tumor capsule at surgery. The advantage of open resection is the ability to obtain larger amounts of tissue and more extensive tissue sampling. This is particularly important for pineal region lesions in general and germ cell tumors in particular, where heterogeneity and mixed cell populations are common. This diversity makes it difficult for neuropathologists to appreciate the subtleties of histologic diagnosis, when only small specimens are available (Bruce & Ogden 2004; Chandrasoma et al 1989; Edwards et al 1988; Ho & Liu 1992; Kraichoke et al 1988).

Additionally, a clinical advantage is gained when the tumor burden is reduced via an open procedure. For the one-third of tumors that are benign, resection is usually complete and curative, making it the clear procedure of choice (Bruce & Ogden 2004; Bruce & Stein 1995b; Stein & Bruce 1992). The advantages of tumor debulking are less apparent with malignant tumors; however, anecdotal evidence favors more radical resection, when possible, to improve the response to adjuvant therapy (Bruce & Ogden 2004; Bruce & Stein 1995b; Lapras et al 1987; Sawamura et al 1997; Schild et al 1996). Additionally, for certain patients with mild hydrocephalus whose tumors can be completely resected, shunting can be avoided (Bruce & Ogden 2004; Edwards et al 1988).

Stereotactic biopsy offers the advantages of relative ease of performance and reduced complications compared with an open procedure (Dempsey et al 1992; Kreth et al 1996; Pecker et al 1979; Pluchino et al 1989; Regis et al 1996). Usually only local anesthesia is necessary. However, stereotactic biopsy carries a risk of hemorrhage from several mechanisms, including bleeding in highly vascular tumors, damage to the deep venous system, and bleeding into the ventricle where the tissue turgor is insufficient to tamponade minor bleeding (Bruce & Ogden 2004; Chandrasoma et al 1989; Edwards et al 1988; Pecker et al 1979; Peragut et al 1987). These risks notwithstanding, several large series have validated the relative safety of stereotactic biopsies for these tumors, despite their rather hazardous location (Dempsey et al 1992; Kreth et al 1996). Of minor concern, but worth mentioning, is a report of metastatic seeding along the biopsy tract following biopsy of a pineoblastoma (Rosenfeld et al 1990).

Stereotactic procedures

The relative technical ease of performing stereotactic biopsy procedures should be viewed cautiously with regard to pineal region lesions. Numerous pitfalls must be avoided to complete a successful biopsy. An appreciation of the complex anatomy at the biopsy site and through the potential trajectory is critical.

Most target-centered stereotactic frame systems are adequate for biopsies. Computed tomographic images are sufficient to provide accurate targeting information and to track the trajectory in three dimensions. MRI provides more sensitive soft tissue visualization and current software has minimized any spatial inaccuracy. Volumetric treatment planning should be used to identify the trajectory track in all the axial, sagittal, and coronal planes. Two possible approaches are favored for stereotactic surgical trajectories (Dempsey et al 1992; Maciunas 2000; Pluchino et al 1989; Sawaya et al 1990). The most common is through a prec-oronal entry point, reaching the tumor through an anterolaterosuperior approach that avoids the interior surface of the lateral ventricle and comes inferior and lateral to the internal cerebral veins to reduce the risk of bleeding. The alternative approach is through a posterolaterosuperior approach near the parieto-occipital junction, which can be useful for tumors that extend laterally or superiorly.

Serial biopsies are desirable whenever possible; however, this is often prohibited by the small size of the tumors commonly encountered (Dempsey et al 1992; Kreth et al 1996). The side-cutting cannula type of biopsy needle is preferred over a cup forceps instrument, which can tear a blood vessel. If bleeding is encountered, continuous suction and irrigation for up to 15 min may be necessary. When bleeding is suspected, an immediate scan should be obtained to assess intraventricular blood and the degree of hydrocephalus to determine the need for ventricular drainage.

Endoscopic biopsy

Endoscopic biopsy of pineal tumors through the ventricles has been reported as an alternative method for securing a tissue diagnosis (Chernov et al 2006; Ferrer et al 1997; Gaab & Schroeder 1998; Pople et al 2001; Yamini et al 2004). In addition to sampling error, a major drawback of this procedure is that the tumor is biopsied along its ventricular surface where there is no tissue turgor to tamponade the bleeding. Even minor bleeding within the CSF space can be problematic, a problem that is compounded by the highly vascular properties of many pineal tumors. Typically, this procedure is combined with a ventriculostomy. However, even with flexible endoscopes, it is difficult to perform a biopsy simultaneously with a ventriculostomy, because the trajectory required is different for each procedure. Transventricular endoscopic biopsy has an approximately 75% diagnostic sensitivity and a morbidity of 15% (reversible in the cited series) (Al-Tamimi et al 2008). The rigid endoscope is not easily maneuverable without risk of damage to the fornix and the septal and thalamostriate veins at the foramen of Monro. The suitable entry point through the forehead might allow use of a rigid scope, but this offers no advantage over a simple stereotactic biopsy.

More typically, endoscopes have been used to aspirate pineal cysts; however, the benefits of this approach are equivocal. In fact, recently there have been reports of infratentorial supracerebellar endoscopic approach to the pineal region for aspiration of pineal cysts (Cardia et al 2006; Gore et al 2008). Whereas endoscopic access to the infratentorial supracerebellar corridor poses a novel tool that is 'minimally invasive', the application of such a technique to tumors might be more complex than its use for fenestration of cysts. To date, the infratentorial supracerebellar endoscopic approach remains experimental and lacks evidence suggesting any advantage to the standard craniotomy approach.

Approaches to the pineal region

Surgery has assumed an increasingly more important role coinciding with improvements in surgical technique and neuroanesthesia, along with a better appreciation of the value of aggressive resection and accurate diagnosis in the subsequent management of pineal region tumors. In view of the wide variety of tumor subtypes and mixed tumors that occur in the pineal region, the foremost consideration among surgical goals is the accurate establishment of a histologic diagnosis (Bruce & Stein 1990; Chapman & Linggood 1980; Dempsey et al 1992; Edwards et al 1988; Fuller et al 1993; Graziano et al 1987; Hoffman et al 1983; Neuwelt 1985; Packer et al 1984b; Pluchino et al 1989; Rout et al 1984; Shokry et al 1985; Stein 1971; Stein & Bruce 1992; Suzuki & Iwabuchi 1965; Ventureyra 1981). The establishment of an accurate histologic diagnosis has implications for the choice of postoperative adjuvant therapy, necessity for metastatic work-up, planning of optimal long-term follow-up, and prediction of long-term prognosis. Radiographic features, tumor marker measurement, and CSF cytologic examination can lead to educated predictions of tumor histology; however, accurate histologic diagnosis can only be established with pathologic examination of a surgical specimen (D'Andrea et al 1987; Ganti et al 1986; Kersh et al 1988; Wood et al 1981; Zimmerman 1985).

The role of surgery extends beyond providing a histologic diagnosis, as there is a growing appreciation of the value of aggressive tumor removal for improving the prognosis of patients. With benign tumors, complete resection is usually curative (Stein & Bruce 1992). With malignant tumors, radical debulking is thought to improve the outcome and response to adjuvant therapy (Hoffman et al 1991; Lapras & Patet 1987; Sano 1976a; Schild et al 1996; Shokry et al 1985; Stein & Bruce 1992). In some instances, complete resection of a malignant tumor may be possible, although it is not necessarily considered curative (Neuwelt 1985; Stein & Bruce 1992).

Pineal region tumors may be approached through one of the several variations of either an infratentorial or supratentorial approach. Supratentorial approaches include the parietal-interhemispheric approach popularized by Dandy (1921) and the occipital-transtentorial approach originally described by Horrax (1937) and later modified by Poppen (1966). The supratentorial approaches are useful for tumors with a significant supratentorial extension or lateral extension to the trigone of the lateral ventricle (Bruce 1993b). Supratentorial approaches offer the advantage of wide exposure but have the disadvantage of encountering the tumor beneath the convergence of the deep venous system where they interfere with tumor removal. The transcallosal-interhemispheric approach involves a paramedian trajectory between the falx and the right parietal lobe with partial resection of the corpus callosum (Dandy 1936; Lapras & Patet 1987). Complications may result from parietal lobe retraction or venous infarction from sacrifice of a bridging vein (Bruce & Stein 1993b). The occipital-transtentorial approach involves retraction of the occipital lobe and division of the tentorium for adequate exposure. This provides a good view of the quadrigeminal plate but may result in visual field defects (Nazzaro et al 1992; Reid & Clark 1978).

The infratentorial-supracerebellar approach provides a midline trajectory between the tentorium and cerebellum (Bruce & Stein 1992; Krause 1926; Stein 1971). The tumor is encountered below the deep venous system, where it is less likely to interfere with resection. Gravity works in the surgeon's favor by allowing the cerebellum to fall away to expose the pineal region, by minimizing pooling of venous blood in the operative field, and by assisting with the dissection of the tumor off the deep venous system. Although this can often involve a long reach, tumors extending to the foramen of Monro can be removed.

Various positions have been described for these different approaches. The sitting slouch position is generally used for the infratentorial-supracerebellar and transcallosal-interhemispheric approaches. Potential complications include ventricular and cortical collapse with subdural hematoma, pneumocephalus, and air embolus (Bruce & Stein 1993a; Bruce & Stein 1993b). Use of this position, however, facilitates surgery by allowing gravity to assist in the tumor dissection from the roof of the third ventricle and it avoids venous blood pooling. The three-quarter prone lateral decubitus position is designed to avoid many of the above complications and is often used for the occipital-transtentorial approach, however gravity does not work in the surgeon's favor (Ausman et al 1988; McComb & Apuzzo 1988). The Concorde position has been proposed to combine the benefits of both positions, while minimizing the risks (Kobayashi et al 1983).

The most common complications following pineal region surgery are extraocular movement dysfunction, altered mental status, and ataxia (Bruce & Stein 1993a; Bruce & Stein 1993b). Less common complications include shunt malfunction and aseptic meningitis. Many neurologic deficits are present preoperatively and may be temporarily worse following surgery. Most postoperative deficits tend to be transient and improve spontaneously with time. Several factors correlate with a higher incidence and severity of deficits including prior radiation therapy, advanced preoperative symptoms, higher degree of malignant features, and invasive tumor characteristics (Bruce & Stein 1993a; Bruce & Stein 1993b; Stein 1979). Supratentorial approaches can result in seizures, hemianopsia, or hemiparesis (Bruce & Stein 1993b; Hoffman et al 1984; Nazzaro et al 1992). The most significant complication of pineal region surgery is hemorrhage into a partially resected tumor bed (Bruce & Stein 1993b; Bruce & Stein 1995a). Hemorrhage is a common associated phenomenon with pineal region tumors and pineal parenchymal tumors in particular (Fig. 34.7) (Bruce & Stein 1993a; Bruce & Stein 1993b; Dempsey et al 1992; Herrick & Rubinstein 1979; Peragut et al 1987). Hemorrhage may occur up to several days postoperatively and may be related to tumor vascularity or malignant characteristics. Tumors may also hemorrhage prior to surgery, presenting with pineal apoplexy (Higashi et al 1979; Steinbok et al 1977).

Most large series in the microsurgical era, each reporting on >20 patients and involving all types of pineal region pathology, have an operative mortality from 0 to 8% and permanent morbidity from 0 to 12% (Bruce & Stein 1995b;

Jooma & Kendall 1983; Lapras et al 1987; Neuwelt 1985; Pendl 1985; Rout et al 1984; Sano 1987; Wood et al 1981). In the largest reported series of surgery for pineal region tumors, gross total removal was possible in 87% of benign tumors and 29% of malignant tumors (Bruce & Stein 1995b).

The long-term outcome for malignant tumors following surgery depends on tumor histology and the effects of adjuvant therapy. Gross total resection of a malignant tumor may be associated with a more favorable prognosis (Lapras et al 1987; Sano 1987; Stein & Bruce 1992). For benign tumors (teratomas, dermoid tumors, epidermoid tumors, and lipomas) the long-term prognosis following surgical resection is excellent, and surgery is usually curative (Bruce & Stein 1990; Stein & Bruce 1992). There is a small subset of pineocytomas (up to 16% of all pineal cell tumors) that are discrete, histologically benign, and fully resectable (Stein & Bruce 1992; Vaquero et al 1990). These patients have an excellent prognosis, are likely cured with surgery alone, and are optimally managed by careful monitoring without any adjuvant therapy (Rubinstein 1981).

Approaches for suprasellar germ cell tumors
Suprasellar tumors can usually be approached through a subfrontal or pterional route (Bruce 1993a; Hoffman 1987). Resection is limited by the extent of invasion of the optic structures and hypothalamus. A subfrontal approach allows access to the third ventricle through the lamina terminalis, depending upon whether the chiasm is prefixed. Pterional approaches provide access to the suprasellar and parasellar regions, but exposure of the third ventricle is insufficient unless combined with a sub-frontal approach. All approaches to the suprasellar region carry a risk of visual loss from injury to the optic structures; endocrine disturbance, particularly diabetes insipidus, from hypothalamic or pituitary stalk injury; or cognitive deficits and memory loss from damage to the fornices and anterior commissure (Apuzzo & Litofsky 1993). A transcallosal approach may be preferable for large tumors that extend to the foramen of Monro, although direct visualization of the optic structures is limited (Bruce 1993a; Hoffman 1987). Ideally, such tumors are removed through a dilated foramen of Monro; however, if exposure is insufficient, an interforniceal or subchoroidal transvelum interpositum approach may be used (Apuzzo & Litofsky 1993; Cossu et al 1984; Sawaya et al 1990). The transcallosal approaches carry an increased risk of memory loss, presumably due to forniceal damage.

Complications
Patients frequently have some impairment of extraocular movements in the immediate postoperative period, particularly limited up-gaze and convergence (Bruce & Stein 1993a; Bruce & Stein 1995b; Little et al 2001). Some degree of pupillary impairment with difficulty focusing may also occur. Many of these extraocular problems are transient and resolve within the first few days, although they can persist for several months. Permanent major impairment is rare, although some mild limitation of up-gaze is not unusual and has little clinical significance. As with most neurological deficits, their persistence and magnitude are proportional to the degree to which they were present preoperatively

(Bruce & Stein 1993a; Lapras & Patet 1987). Similarly, ataxia is often present but resolves within a few days after surgery.

More severe morbidity is rare but can be a caused by overzealous brainstem manipulation. This can lead to cognitive impairment or even, in its extreme form, akinetic mutism. Complications are more common in previously irradiated patients, patients with invasive tumors, and patients who were progressively symptomatic preoperatively (Bruce & Stein 1993a; Lapras & Patet 1987).

One of the most devastating complications is hemorrhage into an incompletely resected tumor bed. Patients with highly vascular, invasive tumors such as malignant pineal parenchymal tumors are at greatest risk for this complication (Bruce & Stein 1993a; Dempsey et al 1992; Herrick & Rubinstein 1979; Peragut et al). Small hemorrhages can be managed conservatively, but a large hemorrhage may require immediate evacuation. Such decisions must consider the possibility of obstructive hydrocephalus.

Complications of supratentorial approaches include hemiparesis from brain retraction or from sacrifice of bridging veins (Apuzzo & Litofsky 1993; Bruce & Stein 1993a; Bruce & Stein 1993b). Fortunately, these deficits usually resolve spontaneously, and infarction and permanent deficits are rare. Seizure prophylaxis is desirable in the immediate postoperative period, although long-term use is not necessary. Parietal lobe retraction can cause sensory or stereognostic deficits on the opposite side (Apuzzo & Tung 1993). Occipital lobe retraction during the transtentorial approach can cause visual field defects (Apuzzo & Tung 1993; Lapras et al 1987; Nazzaro et al 1992). Although disconnection syndromes have been reported with corpus callosum incisions, this has been rare in our experience, even when the splenium is divided (Apuzzo & Tung 1993; Bruce 2000).

Complications related to the sitting position include subdural hematoma, hygroma, and ventricular collapse (Bruce & Stein 1993b; Bruce & Stein 1995b; Stein & Bruce 1992). These conditions are generally self-limited. Air embolus is rarely a problem but can be anticipated by a drop in the end-tidal carbon dioxide levels or Doppler monitoring.

Pineal tumor patients are generally young and have relatively few medical problems. Consequently, the incidence of medical complications such as cardiac or respiratory problems is low.

Surgical outcome

Pineal region surgery is among the most arduous of microsurgical challenges, and outcomes vary substantially with the expertise of individual surgeons. With modern microsurgical techniques, surgical series including >20 patients report operative mortality from 0 to 8% and permanent morbidity from 0 to 12% (Bruce & Ogden 2004; Bruce & Stein 1995b; Chandy & Damaraju 1998; Edwards et al 1988; Konovalov & Pitskhelauri 2003). The impact of surgery on long-term outcome depends on the tumor's histology and responsiveness to adjuvant therapy. With benign tumors, such as teratomas, cystic pilocytic astrocytomas, dermoid tumors, epidermoid tumors, and low-grade pineocytomas, expectations include complete surgical removal, excellent long-term follow-up, and probable cure (Bruce & Ogden 2004; Bruce

& Stein 1995a; Deshmukh et al 2004; Rubinstein 1981; Stein & Bruce 1992; Vaquero et al 1990).

With malignant tumors, the paucity of surgical series reported in the literature makes it difficult to draw conclusions regarding the effect of degree of resection on outcome. The anecdotal evidence, however, is that, except for germinomas, greater resection improves the prognosis and the response to adjuvant therapy (Bruce & Ogden 2004; Lapras & Patet 1987; Sano 1984; Sawamura et al 1997; Stein & Bruce 1992). A small subset of pineocytomas, representing approximately 16% of all pineal cell tumors, are discrete, encapsulated, histologically benign and fully resectable (Bruce & Ogden 2004; Dandy 1936; Peragut et al 1987; Rubinstein 1981; Stein & Bruce 1992; van Wagenen 1931; Vaquero et al 1990). Surgery alone may lead to long-term recurrence-free periods without any additional therapy. Such patients, however, should be monitored closely with serial MRI.

Radiation therapy

All patients with malignant germ cell or pineal cell tumors require radiation therapy consisting of 4000 cGy to the ventricular system with an additional 1500 cGy to the tumor bed. The total radiation dose of 5500 cGy should be given in 180 cGy daily fractions. Recent studies suggest that a more limited field of radiation may be equally efficacious while avoiding the adverse side-effects of ventricular exposure (Dattoli & Newall 1990).

Radiation therapy may be withheld for the rare, histologically benign pineocytoma which has been completely resected (Stein & Bruce 1992; Vaquero et al 1990). Identification of these exceptions is based on intraoperative observation of a well circumscribed tumor and histologic analysis. These tumors can have good long-term control with surgery alone, although careful follow-up is necessary.

Germinomas are among the most radiosensitive of any malignant brain tumors and a significant majority are cured with radiation. With germinomas, surgery and radiation of 5000 cGy to 6000 cGy has achieved 5-year survival of above 75% and 10-year survival as high as 69% (Edwards et al 1988; Sano & Matsutani 1981; Sung et al 1978; Wolden et al 1995). Dosages of <5000 cGy have been correlated with a higher incidence of local failure in both pineal cell tumors (Schild et al 1993) and germ cell tumors (Kreth et al 1996; Sung et al 1978).

Long-term complications from radiation therapy are of particular concern in pineal tumor patients since many of them can expect extended long-term survival and even cure. Delayed complications of cranial radiation therapy include cognitive deficits, hypothalamic and endocrine dysfunction, cerebral necrosis, and *de novo* tumor formation (Bruce 1993b; Duffner et al 1985; Edwards et al 1988; Hodges et al 1992; Nighoghossian et al 1988; Noell & Herskovic 1985; Sakai et al 1988). Pediatric patients are particularly vulnerable to adverse radiation effects (Bendersky et al 1988; Donahue 1992; Rowland et al 1984). In a series of 27 pediatric patients with pineal germinomas treated with radiation therapy, 26% had no improvement in preoperative diabetes insipidus, 22% developed hypopituitarism, all had minor growth defects, and nearly all had some degree of mild cognitive dysfunction (Jenkin et al 1990). In another series, seven of 26 patients irradiated for germ cell tumors developed intellectual retardation or cerebral dullness (Sakai et al 1988).

All patients with malignant germ cell or pineal cell tumors should have postoperative staging with spinal MRI to look for evidence of tumor seeding (Bruce & Stein 1993b). MRI has supplanted CT myelography as the procedure of choice for this screening (Rippe et al 1990; Stein & Bruce 1992). Early studies recommended CSF cytologic examination as a diagnostic test for spinal metastases, however the correlation between metastases and CSF cytology is not strong (DeGirolami & Schmidek 1973; Shibamoto et al 1988; Ueki & Tanaka 1980; Waga et al 1979). Definitive documentation of spinal metastases is important since the use of prophylactic spinal radiation is controversial. Previously, craniospinal irradiation was recommended routinely for malignant pineal tumors (Griffin et al 1981; Jenkin et al 1978; Rich et al 1985; Sung et al 1978). Several reports, however, have noted the actual incidence of spinal metastasis to be relatively low and therefore recommend that prophylactic spinal radiation not be given (Bruce et al 1990; Bruce & Stein 1990; Dattoli & Newall 1990; Disclafani et al 1989; Edwards et al 1988; Linstadt et al 1988; Wood et al 1981). In Jennings review of intracranial germ cell tumors, the incidence of spinal seeding was 10% (Jennings et al 1985). This study noted a higher incidence of spinal cord metastasis with germinomas (11%) and endodermal sinus tumors (23%), and a higher incidence among pineal vs suprasellar tumors. Estimates of spinal seeding with pineal cell tumors have been variable and complicated by the difficulty in uniformly distinguishing between pineocytomas and pineoblastomas. Overall estimates are in the range of 10–20% with markedly increased rates for pineoblastoma compared with pineocytoma (Bruce & Stein 1995b; Schild et al 1993). The prevailing recommendation is currently to give spinal radiation only for documented seeding, using a dose of 3500 cGy (Bruce et al 1990; Bruce & Stein 1990; Disclafani et al 1989; Edwards et al 1988; Rao et al 1981; Rippe et al 1990; Wood et al 1981).

Chemotherapy

Chemotherapy has been most beneficial for patients with non-germinomatous malignant germ cell tumors; significant improvement in long-term follow-up has been demonstrated with current regimens. Patients with germinomas containing syncytiotrophoblastic giant cells have a less favorable prognosis and may benefit from more aggressive treatment with chemotherapy in addition to radiotherapy (Bruce et al 1995; Bruce & Ogden 2004; Stein & Bruce 1992).

Most of the germ cell chemotherapy regimens have been extrapolated from experience treating germ cell tumors of extracranial origin, where success has been remarkable (Einhorn 1981; Hainsworth & Greco 1983; Logothetis et al 1985; McLeod et al 1988). Unfortunately, these regimens have not been as successful in treating intracranial tumors (Edwards et al 1988; Haase & Norgaard-Pedersen 1979; Jennings et al 1985; Kobayashi et al 1989; Packer et al 1984b; Parsa et al 2001; Patel et al 1992; Prioleau & Wilson 1976; Takakura 1985; Yoshida et al 1993). Most successful

chemotherapy regimens are derived from the protocols for testicular cancer using the Einhorn regimen of cisplatin, vinblastine, and bleomycin, although other combinations involving cyclophosphamide or etoposide have been investigated (Calaminus et al 2004; Einhorn & Donohue 1977; Parsa et al 2001). Recent studies using VP-16 (etoposide) in place of vinblastine and bleomycin to avoid the pulmonary toxicity have shown improved response rate with less morbidity (Kobayashi et al 1989; Patel et al 1992; Yoshida et al 1993). Currently, a regimen of cisplatin or carboplatin with etoposide is among the most widely used.

The role of radiation therapy combined with chemotherapy in these tumors is unclear (Merchant et al 1998). Although radiation therapy is generally given before chemotherapy, the optimal timing has not been defined. An aggressive approach seems reasonable, given the poor prognosis of these tumors. Whether radiation therapy improves survival over chemotherapy alone is not clear, although several reports show increased survival in aggressively treated patients using a combination of chemotherapy, radiation, and surgery (Bamberg et al 1984; Bruce et al 2001; Calaminus et al 2004; Chan et al 1984; Herrmann et al 1994; Hoffman et al 1991; Jennings et al 1985; Robertson et al 1997; Takakura 1985). Delayed surgery after radiation and chemotherapy is indicated for patients with residual tumors whose germ cell markers have normalized (Friedman et al 2001; Weiner et al 2002). The residual tumor is likely to be benign germ cell elements that are resistant to radiation and chemotherapy. For pure germinomas, the exquisite radiosensitivity of these tumors has made chemotherapy less compelling, except for patients with recurring or metastatic disease. This success has spurred interest in the use of chemotherapy as a means of reducing the overall dosage of radiation (Allen et al 1994; Allen et al 1987; Aoyama et al 2002; Kochi et al 2003; Sawamura et al 1998; Silvani et al 2005). Although this is a sound philosophy, the long-term results have not withstood the same test of time that radiation therapy alone has for these tumors.

Chemotherapy has been used mostly for recurrent or disseminated pineal cell tumors. (Jakacki et al 1995; Packer et al 1984b, Sawaya et al 1990; Schild et al 1993). There have been some positive responses with various combinations of vincristine, lomustine, cisplatin, etoposide, cyclophosphamide, actinomycin D, and methotrexate. Success with these various regimens has been limited, however, so no clear-cut recommendations can be given (Chang et al 1995).

Radiosurgery

One of the more recent developments in pineal region treatment is the application of radiosurgical techniques (Backlund et al 1974; Casentini et al 1990; Dempsey et al 1992; Kobayashi et al 2001). Several studies have clearly documented the relative safety of this method, although long-term follow-up results are currently lacking. The problem with radiosurgery is not the response of the targeted mass, but the recurrence of tumor outside of the treatment volume. Radiosurgery is generally limited to tumors <3 cm in diameter.

Distinct differences in the radiobiologic effects of radiosurgery and conventional fractionated radiation must be considered when choosing optimal therapeutic strategies. Germinomas, for example, have an excellent long-term response to fractionated radiation, and it is unlikely that radiosurgery can improve on these results. Additionally, because radiosurgery provides no therapeutic coverage to the ventricular system, tumors such as pineal cell and germ cell tumors are particularly vulnerable to ventricular recurrence. Radiosurgery may have its greatest benefit in providing a local boost to the tumor bed so that radiation exposure to the ventricles and surrounding brain can be reduced (Casentini et al 1990; Hasegawa et al 2003). It may also be useful for tumors that recur locally.

Patterns of failure

Germ cell tumors

Germ cell tumors most often fail locally (Dearnaley et al 1990; Sano & Matsutani 1981). Spinal failure generally does not occur without simultaneous local failure (Shokry et al 1985). Systemic metastases are rare but can occur to bone with germinomas or lung with malignant teratomas (Dearnaley et al 1990; Farwell & Flannery 1989). Recurrence of germinomas outside radiation ports has been described (Uematsu et al 1992).

Pineal cell tumors

Pineal cell tumors are most likely to fail locally, and spinal failures, when they occur, are nearly always in the setting of residual or recurrent local tumor (Schild et al 1993). At autopsy, nearly all fatal pineoblastomas and to a lesser extent pineocytomas have evidence of leptomeningeal and ependymal spread (Fig. 34.20) (Borit & Blackwood 1979; Herrick & Rubinstein 1979; Packer et al 1984b).

Management of recurrent disease

Management of recurrences is generally handled on an individual basis because of the scarcity of these tumors. Possible therapeutic options include radiosurgery, chemotherapy, or additional external beam radiation, particularly if not given to its maximum (Merchant et al 1998). Reoperation is reserved for patients with relatively slow growing tumors who are in a stable condition with reasonable expectation for longevity and a favorable outcome following prior surgery (Bruce & Stein 1990). Chemotherapy may be useful for germ cell and pineal cell tumors that have recurred following radiation (Allen et al 1985; Edwards et al 1988, Einhorn & Donohue 1977; Neuwelt et al 1980; Sawaya et al 1990; Schild et al 1993; Siegal et al 1983). The relative success of high dose chemotherapy combined with stem cell rescue holds some promise for these otherwise poor risk tumors (Bosl & Motzer 1997; Graham et al 1997).

Long-term outcome

Germ cell tumors

Long-term expectations for germ cell tumors are most dependent on tumor histology. Benign germ cell tumors such as teratoma, dermoid and epidermoid tumors are generally associated with 100% 5- and 10-year survivals following surgical treatment alone (Bjornsson et al 1985; Stein & Bruce 1992).

Among the malignant germ cell tumors, an important distinction is made between germinomas and non-germinomatous tumors. The 5-year survival for germinomas is generally in the 80–90% range following surgery and radiation (Bruce 1993b; Hoffman et al 1991; Matsutani et al 1997; Wolden et al 1995). Whether survival is improved for patients with suprasellar germinomas compared with pineal region germinomas is unclear. Takakura (1985) reported survival rates of 65% at both 5 and 10 years in 49 pineal germinomas, while corresponding rates were 90% and 84%, respectively for 22 suprasellar germinomas. Other reports have shown as high as 100% 5-year survival for patients with suprasellar germinomas following surgery and radiation (Legido et al 1988; Sano & Matsutani 1981). Germinomas with syncytiotrophoblastic giant cells may have higher recurrence rates (Uematsu et al 1992; Yoshida et al 1993). Germinomas in children tend to have a better prognosis than those in adults (Jenkin et al 1978; Sano & Matsutani 1981).

Patients with malignant non-germinomatous germ cell tumors have the worst prognosis and rarely survive beyond 2 years (Chan et al 1984; Edwards et al 1988; Jennings et al 1985; Packer et al 1984a; Page et al 1986; Tavcar et al 1980). Improvements in chemotherapy, however, could improve on these results (Kobayashi et al 1989; Matsutani et al 1997; Neuwelt 1985; Patel et al 1992; Yoshida et al 1993). Among malignant non-germinomatous germ cell tumors, immature teratomas have a slightly better prognosis, with a 5-year survival of approximately 25%. A worse prognosis is associated with the presence of elevated tumor markers in these patients (Takakura 1985). Factors correlating with increased survival include greater extent of resection, higher dose of radiation therapy, and use of chemotherapy (Schild et al 1996).

Pineal cell tumors

It is difficult to establish specific outcome parameters for pineal cell tumors because of small series size, lack of uniform histologic classification, and lack of uniform treatment regimens. The largest series project a 5-year survival between 55% and 62% for tumors treated primarily with surgery and radiation, although a small number included chemotherapy as well (Schild et al 1993; Stein & Bruce 1992). The long-term prognosis is significantly improved when radiation doses >50Gy are given (Schild et al 1996). The prognosis is particularly favorable for pineocytomas, where 5-year survivals can be >80% (Schild et al 1996). There is even a small sub-group of discrete, histologically benign, and completely resectable pineocytomas, which can be treated with surgery alone and have an excellent prognosis (Stein & Bruce 1992; Vaquero et al 1990). For pineoblastomas, the prognosis correlates with the extent of disease at the time of diagnosis (Chang et al 1995).

Conclusion

The tumors of the pineal region constitute an uncommon but complex group of neoplasms that are heterogeneous as far as histology, demographics, and prognosis. For the most part, the clinical manifestations of these tumors are more consistent and include symptoms related to hydrocephalus and those that arise as a product of brainstem compression (including Parinaud Syndrome). The initial approach to a patient with a suspected pineal region tumor is sampling for tumor markers to rule out the possibility of germ cell tumors, which can be treated with radiation with good outcome. In the absence of tumor markers, the need for tissue for diagnosis and the benefits associated with maximizing surgical resection make this the following step in the treatment of these lesions for the vast majority of patients. Once histological diagnosis is made, further adjuvant treatment such as chemotherapy and radiation are tailored to the particular tumor and patient characteristics. The management of tumors of the pineal region represent a challenging field that is evolving, novel surgical and medical modalities are being tested and might alter the standard of care for these lesions.

Key points

- Tumors of the pineal region encompass a broad spectrum of histologic subtypes, ranging from benign to malignant with many tumors of intermediate cell types and mixed cell types.

- Germ cell tumors in the pineal region are more common in men. Pineal cell tumors and suprasellar germ cell tumors are found equally in men and women.

- Tumors in the pineal region are generally associated with obstructive hydrocephalus and therefore present with signs of increased intracranial pressure. Compression of the midbrain and cerebellum can cause disturbances of extraocular movements and ataxia.

- General work-up for pineal region tumors includes MRI and measurement of germ cell markers (α-fetoprotein and β-hCG).

- Malignant germ cell or pineal cell tumors can spread into the ventricles or spinal cord through CSF pathways.

- Due to the wide variety of possible tumor sub-types, a histologic diagnosis is mandatory for optimal clinical management of pineal region tumors. The only exception is in the setting of elevated germ cell markers which, by definition, indicate the presence of a malignant germ cell tumor.

- Surgical resection is difficult, although morbidity and mortality results are acceptable with current microsurgical techniques. Surgery is generally curative for benign pineal and germ cell tumors, and correlates positively with survival for many malignant tumors.

- Radiation therapy is indicated for malignant germ cell and pineal cell tumors. Chemotherapy is particularly useful for malignant germ cell tumors.

REFERENCES

Allen, J., DaRosso, R., Donahue, B., et al., 1994. A phase II trial of preirradiation carboplatin in newly diagnosed germinoma of the central nervous system. Cancer 74, 940–944.

Allen, J.C., Bosl, G., Walker, R., 1985. Chemotherapy trials in recurrent primary intracranial germ cell tumors. J. Neurooncol. 3, 147–152.

Allen, J.C., Kim, J.H., Packer, R.J., 1987. Neoadjuvant chemotherapy for newly diagnosed germ-cell tumors of the central nervous system. J. Neurosurg. 67, 65–70.

Allen, J.C., Nisselbaum, J., Epstein, F., et al., 1979. Alphafetoprotein and human chorionic gonadotropin determination in cerebrospinal fluid. An aid to the diagnosis and management of intracranial germ-cell tumors. J. Neurosurg. 51, 368–374.

Al-Tamimi, Y.Z., Bhargava, D., Surash, S., et al., 2008. Endoscopic biopsy during third ventriculostomy in paediatric pineal region tumours. Childs Nerv. Syst. 24, 1323–1326.

Ammar, A., Al-Majid, H., Kutty, M., 1991. Germinoma in a 16-month old baby: A case report and brief review of the literature. Acta. Neurochir. (Wien) 110, 189–192.

Aoyama, H., Shirato, H., Ikeda, J., et al., 2002. Induction chemotherapy followed by low-dose involved-field radiotherapy for intracranial germ cell tumors. J. Clin. Oncol. 20, 857–865.

Apuzzo, M., Litofsky, N., 1993. Surgery in and around the anterior third ventricle. In: Apuzzo, M. (Ed.), Brain surgery: complication avoidance and management, Vol 1. Churchill Livingstone, New York, pp. 541–579.

Apuzzo, M., Tung, H., 1993. Supratentorial approaches to the pineal region. In: Apuzzo, M. (Ed.), Brain surgery: Complication avoidance and management. Churchill-Livingstone, New York, pp. 486–511.

Araki, C., Matsumoto, S., 1969. Statistical re-evaluation of pinealoma and related tumours in Japan. Prog. Exp. Tumor. Res. 30, 307–312.

Arendt, J., 1978. Melatonin as a tumour marker in a patient with pineal tumour. BMJ 2, 635–636.

Arita, N., Ushio, Y., Hayakawa, T., et al., 1980. Serum levels of alphafetoprotein, human chorionic gonadotropin and carcinoembryonic antigen in patients with primary intracranial germ cell tumors. Oncodev. Biol. Med. (Amsterdam) 1, 235–240.

Ausman, J.I., Malik, G.M., Dujovny, M., et al., 1988. Three-quarter prone approach to the pineal-tentorial region. Surg. Neurol. 29, 298–306.

Backlund, E.-O., Rahn, T., Sarby, B., 1974. Treatment of pinealomas by stereotaxic radiation surgery. Acta. Radiol. Ther. Phys. Biol. 13, 368–376.

Bader, J.L., Meadows, A.T., Zimmerman, L.E., et al., 1982. Bilateral retinoblastoma with ectopic intracranial retinoblastoma: trilateral retinoblastoma. Cancer Genet Cytogenet 5, 201–213.

Bamberg, M., Metz, K., Alberti, W., et al., 1984. Endodermal sinus tumor of the pineal region. Metastasis through a ventriculoperitoneal shunt. Cancer 54, 903–906.

Barber, S., Smith, J., Hughes, R., 1978. Melatonin as a tumour marker in a patient with pineal tumour. Lancet ii, 328.

Barker, D., Weller, R., Garfield, J., 1976. Epidemiology of primary tumors of the brain and spinal cord: a regional survey in southern England. J. Neurol. Neurosurg. Psychiatry 39, 290–296.

Becker, L.E., Hinton, D., 1983. Primitive neuroectodermal tumors of the central nervous system. Hum. Pathol. 14, 538–550.

Bendersky, M., Lewis., M., Mandelbaum, D.E., et al., 1988. Serial neuropsychological follow-up of a child following craniospinal irradiation. Dev. Med. Child Neurol. 30, 808–820.

Bjornsson, J., Scheithauer, B., Okazaki, H., et al., 1985. Intracranial germ cell tumors: Pathobiological and immunohistochemical aspects of 70 cases. J. Neuropathol. Exp. Neurol. 44, 32–46.

Bloom, H., 1983. Primary intracranial germ cell tumours. Clin. Oncol. 2, 233–257.

Borden, S., Weber, A.L., Toch, R., et al., 1973. Pineal germinoma. Long term survival despite hematogenous metastases. J. Pathol. 114, 9–12.

Borit, A., 1981. History of tumors of the pineal region. Am. J. Surg. Pathol. 5, 613–620.

Borit, A., Blackwood, W., 1979. Pineocytoma with astrocytomatous differentiation. J. Neuropathol. Exp. Neurol. 38, 253–258.

Borit, A., Blackwood, W., Mair, W.G., 1980. The separation of pineocytoma from pineoblastoma. Cancer 45, 1408–1418.

Bosl, G., Motzer, R., 1997. Testicular germ-cell cancer. New Engl. J. Med. 337, 242–253.

Brada, M., Rajan, B., 1990. Spinal seeding in cranial germinoma. Br. J. Cancer 61, 339–340.

Bruce, J.N., 1993a. Intracranial germinomas. Neurosurgical Consultations 4, 1–8.

Bruce, J.N., 1993b. Management of pineal region tumors. Neurosurg. Q. 3, 103–119.

Bruce, J.N., 2000. Posterior third ventricular tumors. In: Kaye, A.H., Black, P.M. (Eds.), Operative neurosurgery, Vol 1. Churchill Livingstone, London, pp. 769–775.

Bruce, J.N., Balmaceda, C., Stein, B., et al., 2000. Pineal region tumors. In: Rowland, L. (Ed.), Merritt's textbook of neurology, 10th edn. Williams & Wilkins, Baltimore, pp. 341–347.

Bruce, J.N., Connolly, E.S., Stein, B.M., 1995. Pineal and germ cell tumors. In: Kaye, A.H., Laws, E.R. (Eds.), Brain tumors. Churchill Livingstone, London, pp. 725–755.

Bruce, J.N., Connolly, E.S., Stein, B.M., 2001. Pineal and germ cell tumors. In: Kaye, A.H., Laws, E.R. (Eds.), Brain tumors, 2nd edn. Churchill Livingstone, London, pp. 771–800.

Bruce, J.N., Fetell, M.R., Stein, B.M., 1990. Incidence of spinal metastases in patients with malignant pineal region tumors: Avoidance of prophylactic spinal irradiation. J. Neurosurg. 72, 354A.

Bruce, J.N., Ogden, A.T., 2004. Surgical strategies for treating patients with pineal region tumors. J. Neurooncol. 69, 221–236.

Bruce, J.N., Stein, B.M., 1990. Pineal tumors. In: Rosenblum, M. (Ed.), The role of surgery in brain tumor management. WB Saunders, Philadelphia, PA, pp. 123–138.

Bruce, J.N., Stein, B.M., 1992. Infratentorial approach to pineal tumors. In: Wilson, C.B. (Ed.), Neurosurgical procedures: Personal approaches to classic operations. Williams & Wilkins, Baltimore, MD, pp. 63–76.

Bruce, J.N., Stein, B.M., 1993a. Supracerebellar approaches in the pineal region. In: Apuzzo, M. (Ed.) Brain surgery: Complication avoidance and management. Churchill-Livingstone, New York, pp. 511–536.

Bruce, J.N., Stein, B.M., 1993b. Complications of surgery for pineal region tumors. In: Post, K.D., Friedman, E.D., McCormick, P.C. (Eds.). Postoperative complications in intracranial neurosurgery. Thieme, New York, pp. 74–86.

Bruce, J.N., Stein, B.M., 1995a. Supracerebellar approach for pineal region neoplasms. In: Schmidek, H.H., Sweet, W.H. (Eds.). Operative neurosurgical techniques, 3rd edn. W B Saunders, Philadelphia, PA, pp. 755–763.

Bruce, J.N., Stein, B.M., 1995b. Surgical management of pineal region tumors. Acta. Neurochir. 134, 130–135.

Bruce, J.N., Tamarkin, L., Riedel., C., et al., 1991. Sequential cerebrospinal fluid and plasma sampling in humans: 24-hour melatonin measurements in normal subjects and after peripheral sympathectomy. J. Clin. Endo. Metab. 72, 819–823.

Burres, K.P., Hamilton, R.D., 1979. Pineal apoplexy. Neurosurgery 4, 264–268.

Calaminus, G., Bamberg, M., Jurgens, H., et al., 2004. Impact of surgery, chemotherapy and irradiation on long term outcome of intracranial malignant non-germinomatous germ cell tumors: results of the German Cooperative Trial MAKEI 89. Klin. Padiatr. 216, 141–149.

Cardia, A., Caroli, M., Pluderi, M., et al., 2006. Endoscope-assisted infratentorial-supracerebellar approach to the third ventricle: an anatomical study. J. Neurosurg. 104, 409–414.

Casentini, L., Colombo, F., Pozza, F., et al., 1990. Combined radiosurgery and external radiotherapy of intracranial germinomas. Surg. Neurol. 34, 79–86.

Chan, H., Humphreys, R., Hendrick, E., et al., 1984. Primary intracranial choriocarcinoma. A report of two cases and a review of the literature. Neurosurgery 15, 540–545.

Chandrasoma, P.T., Smith, M.M., Apuzzo, M.L., 1989. Stereotactic biopsy in the diagnosis of brain masses: comparison of results of biopsy and resected surgical specimen. Neurosurgery 24, 160–165.

Chandy, M.J., Damaraju, S.C., 1998. Benign tumours of the pineal region: a prospective study from 1983. to 1997. Br. J. Neurosurg. 12, 228–233.

Chang, C., Kageyama, T., Yoshida, J., et al., 1981. Pineal tumors: Clinical diagnosis, with special emphasis on the significance of pineal calcification. Neurosurgery 8, 656–668.

Chang, S.M., Lillis-Hearne, P.K., Larson, D.A., et al., 1995. Pineoblastoma in adults. Neurosurgery 37, 383–391.

Chapman, P.H., Linggood, R.M., 1980. The management of pineal area tumors: a recent reappraisal. Cancer 46, 1253–1257.

Chernov, M.F., Kamikawa, S., Yamane, F., et al., 2006. Neurofiberscopic biopsy of tumors of the pineal region and posterior third ventricle: indications, technique, complications, and results. Neurosurgery 59, 267–277.

Chiechi, M.V., Smirniotopoulos, J.G., Mena, H., 1995. Pineal parenchymal tumors: CT and MR features. J. Comput. Assist. Tomogr. 19, 509–517.

Choi, J.U., Kim, D.S., Chung, S.S., et al., 1998. Treatment of germ cell tumors in the pineal region. Childs Nerv. Syst. 14, 41–48.

Cossu, M., Labinu, M., Orunesu, M., et al., 1984. Subchoroidal approach to the third ventricle: Microsurgical anatomy. Surg. Neurol. 21, 552–565.

Cravioto, H., Dart, D., 1973. The ultrastructure of 'pinealoma' (Seminoma-like tumor of the pineal region). J. Neuropathol. Exp. Neurol. 32, 552–564.

D'Andrea, A.D., Packer, R.J., Rorke, L.B., et al., 1987. Pineocytomas of childhood. A reappraisal of natural history and response to therapy. Cancer 59, 1353–1357.

Dandy, W.E., 1921. An operation for the removal of pineal tumors. Surg. Gynecol. Obstet. XXXIII, 113–119.

Dandy, W.E., 1936. Operative experience in cases of pineal tumor. Arch. Surg. 33, 19–46.

Dattoli, M.J., Newall, J., 1990. Radiation therapy for intracranial germinoma: the case for limited volume treatment. Int. J. Radiat. Oncol. Biol. Phys. 19, 429–433.

Dayan, A., Marshall, A., Miler, A., et al., 1966. Atypical teratomas of the pineal and hypothalamus. J. Pathol. Bacteriol. 92, 1–25.

Dearnaley, D.P., A'Hern, R.P., Whittaker, S., et al., 1990. Pineal and CNS germ cell tumors: Royal Marsden Hospital experience 1962–1987. Int. J. Radiat. Oncol. Biol. Phys. 18, 773–781.

DeGirolami, U., Schmidek, H., 1973. Clinicopathological study of 53 tumors of the pineal region. J. Neurosurg. 39, 455–462.

DeMonte, F., Zelby, A., Al-Mefty, O., 1993. Hearing impairment resulting from a pineal region meningioma. Neurosurgery 32, 665–668.

Dempsey, P.K., Kondziolka, D., Lunsford, L.D., 1992. Stereotactic diagnosis and treatment of pineal region tumours and vascular malformations. Acta. Neurochir. (Wien) 116, 14–22.

Dempsey, R., Chandler, W., 1984. Abnormal serum melatonin levels in patients with intrasellar tumors. Neurosurgery 15, 815–819.

Deshmukh, V.R., Smith, K.A., Rekate, H.L., et al., 2004. Diagnosis and management of pineocytomas. Neurosurgery 55, 349–357.

Disclafani, A., Hudgins, R.J., Edwards, S.B., et al., 1989. Pineocytomas. Cancer 63, 302–304.

Donahue, B., 1992. Short- and long-term complications of radiation therapy for pediatric brain tumors. Pediatr. Neurosurg. 18, 207–217.

Duffner, P., Cohen, M., Thomas, P., et al., 1985. The long-term effects of cranial irradiation on the central nervous system. Cancer 56, 1841–1846.

Eberts, T.J., Ransburg, R.C., 1979. Primary intracranial endodermal sinus tumor. J. Neurosurg. 50, 246–252.

Edwards, M.S., Hudgins, R.J., Wilson, C.B., et al., 1988. Pineal region tumors in children. J. Neurosurg. 68, 689–697.

Einhorn, L.H., 1981. Testicular cancer as a model for curable neoplasm. Cancer Res. 41, 3275–3280.

Einhorn, L.H., Donohue, J., 1977. Cis-Diaminedichloroplatinum, Vinblastine, and Bleomycin combination therapy in disseminated testicular cancer. Ann. Intern. Med. 87, 293–298.

Erlich, S., Apuzzo, M., 1985. The pineal gland: Anatomy, physiology and clinical significance. J. Neurosurg. 63, 321–341.

Farwell, J.R., Flannery, J.T., 1989. Pinealomas and germinomas in children. J. Neurooncol. 7, 13–19.

Ferrer, E., Santamarta, D., Garcia-Fructuoso, G., et al., 1997. Neuroendoscopic management of pineal region tumours. Acta. Neurochir. (Wien) 139, 12–21.

Fetell, M.R., Stein, B.M., 1986. Neuroendocrine aspects of pineal tumors. In: Zimmeman, E.A., Abrams, G.M. (Eds.), Neurologic clinics: Neuroendocrinology and brain peptides, Vol 4. WB Saunders, Philadelphia, PA, pp. 877–905.

Fevre-Montange, M., Champier, J., Szathmari, A., et al., 2006a. Microarray analysis reveals differential gene expression patterns in tumors of the pineal region. J. Neuropathol. Exp. Neurol. 65, 675–684.

Fevre-Montange, M., Hasselblatt, M., Figarella-Branger, D., et al., 2006b. Prognosis and histopathologic features in papillary tumors of the pineal region: a retrospective multicenter study of 31 cases. J. Neuropathol. Exp. Neurol. 65, 1004–1011.

Friedman, J.A., Lynch, J.J., Buckner, J.C., et al., 2001. Management of malignant pineal germ cell tumors with residual mature teratoma. Neurosurgery 48, 518–523.

Fujimaki, T., Matsutani, M., Funada, N., et al., 1994. CT and MRI features of intracranial germ cell tumors. J. Neurooncol. 19, 217–226.

Fukui, M., Matsuoka, S., Hasuo, K., et al., 1983. Cavernous hemangioma in the pineal region. Surg. Neurol. 20, 209–215.

Fuller, B., Kapp, D., Cox, R., 1993. Radiation therapy of pineal region tumors: 25 new cases and a review of 208 previously reported cases. Int. J. Radiat. Oncol. Biol. Phys. 28, 229–245.

Gaab, M.R., Schroeder, H.W., 1998. Neuroendoscopic approach to intraventricular lesions. J. Neurosurg. 88, 496–505.

Galassi, E., Tognetti, F., Frank, F., et al., 1984. Extraneural metastases from primary pineal tumors. Review of the literature. Surg. Neurol. 21, 497–504.

Ganti, S.R., Hilal, S.K., Silver, A.J., et al., 1986. CT of pineal region tumors. AJNR Am. J. Neuroradiol. 7, 97–104.

Glass, R., Culbertson, C., 1946. Teratoma of the pineal gland with choriocarcinoma and rhabdomyosarcoma. Arch. Pathol. 41, 552–555.

Gonzalez-Crussi, F., 1982. Extragonadal teratomas. Armed Forces Institute of Pathology, Washington, DC.

Goodman, R., 1993. Magnetic resonance imaging-directed stereotactic endoscopic third ventriculostomy. Neurosurgery 32, 1043–1047.

Gore, P.A., Gonzalez, L.F., Rekate, H.L., et al., 2008. Endoscopic supracerebellar infratentorial approach for pineal cyst resection: technical case report. Neurosurgery 62, 108–109.

Graham, M.L., Herndon, J.E., 2nd., Casey, J.R., et al., 1997. High-dose chemotherapy with autologous stem-cell rescue in patients with recurrent and high-risk pediatric brain tumors. J. Clin. Oncol. 15, 1814–1823.

Graziano, S.L., Paolozzi, F.P., Rudolph, A.R., et al., 1987. Mixed germ-cell tumor of the pineal region. J. Neurosurg. 66, 300–304.

Griffin, B., Griffin, T., Tong, D., et al., 1981. Pineal region tumors: results of radiation therapy and indications for elective spinal irradiation. Int. J. Radiat. Oncol. Biol. Phys. 66, 300–304.

Haase, J., Norgaard-Pedersen, B., 1979. Alpha-fetoprotein (AFP) and human chorionic gonadotropin (HCG) as biochemical markers of intracranial germ cell tumors. Acta. Neurochir. 53, 269–274.

Hainsworth, J., Greco, F., 1983. Testicular germ cell neoplasms. Am. J. Med. 75, 817–832.

Hasegawa, T., Kondziolka, D., Hadjipanayis, C.G., et al., 2003. Stereotactic radiosurgery for CNS nongerminomatous germ cell tumors. Report of four cases. Pediatr. Neurosurg. 38, 329–333.

Hasselblatt, M., Blumcke, I., Jeibmann, A., et al., 2006. Immunohistochemical profile and chromosomal imbalances in papillary tumours of the pineal region. Neuropathol. Appl. Neurobiol. 32, 278–283.

Hassoun, J., Gambarelli, D., Peragut, J.C., et al., 1983. Specific ultrastructural markers of human pinealomas. A study of four cases. Acta. Neuropathol. 62, 31–40.

Herrick, M.K., Rubinstein, L.J., 1979. The cytological differentiating potential of pineal parenchymal neoplasms (true pinealomas). A clinicopathological study of 28 tumours. Brain 102, 289–320.

Herrmann, H.D., Westphal, M., Winkler, K., et al., 1994. Treatment of nongerminomatous germ-cell tumors of the pineal region. Neurosurgery 34, 524–529.

Higashi, K., Katayama, S., Orita, T., 1979. Pineal apoplexy. J. Neurol. Neurosurg. Psychiatry 42, 1050–1053.

Ho, D.M., Liu, H.-C., 1992. Primary intracranial germ cell tumor: pathologic study of 51 patients. Cancer 70, 1577–1584.

Hodges, L.C., Smith, L.J., Garrett, A., et al., 1992. Prevalence of glioblastoma multiforme in subjects prior to therapeutic radiation. J. Neurosci. Nurs. 24, 79–83.

Hoffman, H., 1987. Considerations and techniques in the pediatric age group. In: Apuzzo, M., (Ed.) Surgery of the third ventricle. Williams and Wilkins, Baltimore, MD, pp. 727–750.

Hoffman, H.J., Otsubo, H., Bruce, E., et al., 1991. Intracranial germ-cell tumors in children. J. Neurosurg. 74, 545–551.

Hoffman, H., Yoshida, M., Becker, L., et al., 1983. Pineal region tumors in childhood. Experience at the Hospital for Sick Children. In: Humphreys, R. (Ed.) Concepts in pediatric neurosurgery 4. Karger, Basel, pp. 360–386.

Hoffman, H.J., Yoshida, M., Becker, L.E., et al., 1984. Experience with pineal region tumors in childhood. Neurol. Res. 6, 107–112.

Horowitz, M.B., Hall, W.A., 1991. Central nervous system germinomas. Arch. Neurol. 48, 652–657.

Horrax, G., 1937. Extirpation of a huge pinealoma from a patient with pubertas praecox. Arch. Neurol. Psychiatry 37, 385–397.

Hudgins, R.J., Rhyner, P.A., Edwards, M.S., 1987. Magnetic resonance imaging and management of pineal region dermoid. Surg. Neurol. 27, 558–562.

Hunt, P., Davidson, K., Ashcraft, K., 1977. Radiography of hereditary presacral teratoma. Radiology 122, 187–191.

Jakacki, R.I., Zeltzer, P.M., Boyett, J.M., et al., 1995. Survival and prognostic factors following radiation and/or chemotherapy for primitive neuroectodermal tumors of the pineal region in infants and children: a report of the Children's Cancer Group. J. Clin. Oncol. 13, 1377–1383.

Jenkin, D., Berry, M., Chan, H., et al., 1990. Pineal region germinomas in childhood treatment considerations. Int. J. Radiat. Oncol. Biol. Phys. 18, 541–545.

Jenkin, R.D., Simpson, W.J., Keen, C.W., 1978. Pineal and suprasellar germinomas. Results of radiation treatment. J. Neurosurg. 48, 99–107.

Jennings, M.T., Gelman, R., Hochberg, F., 1985. Intracranial germ-cell tumors: natural history and pathogenesis. J. Neurosurg. 63, 155–167.

Jooma, R., Kendall, B.E., 1983. Diagnosis and management of pineal tumors. J. Neurosurg. 58, 654–665.

Jouvet, A., Fauchon, F., Liberski, P., et al., 2003. Papillary tumor of the pineal region. Am. J. Surg. Pathol. 27, 505–512.

Jouvet, A., Fevre-Montange, M., Besancon, R., et al., 1994. Structural and ultrastructural characteristics of human pineal gland, and pineal parenchymal tumors. Acta. Neuropathol. 88, 334–348.

Kashiwagi, S., Hatano, M., Yokoyama, T., 1989. Metastatic small cell carcinoma to the pineal body: case report. Neurosurgery 25, 810–813.

Kasper, M., Terpe, H.J., Perry, G., 1990. Age-dependent pattern of intermediate filament protein expression in the human pineal gland. J. Hirnforsch. 31, 215–221.

Kersh, C.R., Constable, W.C., Eisert, D.R., et al., 1988. Primary central nervous system germ cell tumors: effect of histologic confirmation on radiotherapy. Cancer 61, 2148–2152.

Kobayashi, T., Kida, Y., Mori, Y., 2001. Stereotactic gamma radiosurgery for pineal and related tumors. J. Neurooncol. 54, 301–309.

Kobayashi, S., Sugita, K., Tanaka, Y., et al., 1983. Infratentorial approach to the pineal region in the prone position: Concorde position. J. Neurosurg. 58, 141–143.

Kobayashi, T., Yoshida, J., Ishiyama, J., et al., 1989. Combination chemotherapy with cisplatin and etoposide for malignant intracranial germ-cell tumors. An experimental and clinical study. J. Neurosurg. 70, 676–681.

Kochi, M., Itoyama, Y., Shiraishi, S., et al., 2003. Successful treatment of intracranial nongerminomatous malignant germ cell tumors by administering neoadjuvant chemotherapy and radiotherapy before excision of residual tumors. J. Neurosurg. 99, 106–114.

Koide, O., Watanabe, Y., Sato, K., 1980. A pathological survey of intracranial germinoma and pinealoma in Japan. Cancer 45, 2119–2130.

Konovalov, A.N., Pitskhelauri, D.I., 2003. Principles of treatment of the pineal region tumors. Surg. Neurol. 59, 250–268.

Korf, H.W., Klein, D.C., Zigler, J.S., et al., 1986. S-antigen-like immunoreactivity in a human pineocytoma. Acta. Neuropathol. (Berl) 69, 165–167.

Krabbe, K.H., 1923. The pineal gland, especially in relation to the problem on its supposed significance in sexual development. Endocrinology 7, 379–414.

Kraichoke, S., Cosgrove, M., Chandrasoma, P.T., 1988. Granulomatous inflammation in pineal germinoma. A cause of diagnostic failure at stereotaxic brain biopsy. Am. J. Surg. Pathol. 12, 655–660.

Krause, F., 1926. Operative Frielegung der Vierhugel, nebst Beobachtungen uber Hirndruck und Dekompression. Zentrabl. Chir. 53, 2812–2819.

Kreth, F.W., Schatz, C.R., Pagenstecher, A., et al., 1996. Stereotactic management of lesions of the pineal region. Neurosurgery 39, 280–291.

Kun, L.E., Tang, T.T., Sty, J.R., et al., 1981. Primary cerebral germinoma and ventriculoperitoneal shunt metastasis. Cancer 48, 213–215.

Lapras, C., Patet, J.D., 1987. Controversies, techniques and strategies for pineal tumor surgery. In: **Apuzzo, M.L.** (Ed.), Surgery of the third ventricle. Williams and Wilkins, Baltimore, MD, pp. 649–662.

Lapras, C., Patet, J.D., Mottolese, C., et al., 1987. Direct surgery for pineal tumors: occipital-transtentorial approach. Prog. Exp. Tumor. Res. 30, 268–280.

Legido, A., Packer, R.J., Sutton, L.N., et al., 1988. Suprasellar germinomas in childhood. A reappraisal. Cancer 63, 340–344.

Lesnick, J.E., Chayt, K.J., Bruce, D.A., et al., 1985. Familial pineoblastoma. Report of two cases. J. Neurosurg. 62, 930–932.

Lesoin, F., Cama, A., Dhellemes, P., et al., 1987. Extraneural metastasis of a pineal tumor. Report of 3 cases and review of the literature. Eur. Neurol. 27, 55–61.

Liang, L., Korogi, Y., Sugahara, T., et al., 2002. MRI of intracranial germ-cell tumours. Neuroradiology 44, 382–388.

Linstadt, D., Wara, W.M., Edwards, M.S.B., et al., 1988. Radiotherapy of primary intracranial germinomas: the case against routine craniospinal irradiation. Int. J. Radiat. Oncol. Biol. Phys. 15, 291–297.

Little, K.M., Friedman, A.H., Fukushima, T., 2001. Surgical approaches to pineal region tumors. J. Neurooncol. 54, 287–299.

Logothetis, C.J., Samuels, M.L., Selig, D.E., et al., 1985. Chemotherapy of extragonadal germ cell tumors. J. Clin. Oncol. 3, 316–325.

Maciunas, R., 2000. Stereotactic biopsy of pineal region lesions. In: **Kaye, A., Black, P.** (Eds.) Operative neurosurgery, Vol 1. Churchill Livingstone, London, pp. 841–848.

Manor, R.S., Bar-Ziv, J., Tadmor, R., et al., 1990. Pineal germinoma with unilateral blindness. Seeding of germinoma cells with optic nerve sheath. J. Clin. Neuro. Ophthalmol. 10, 239–243.

Markesbery, W.R., Brooks, W.H., Milsow, L., et al., 1976. Ultrastructural study of the pineal germinoma in vivo and in vitro. Cancer 37, 327–337.

Markesbery, W.R., Haugh, R.M., Young, A.B., 1981. Ultrastructure of pineal parenchymal neoplasms. Acta. Neuropathol. (Berl) 55, 145–149.

Marshall, A., Dayan, A., 1964. An immune reaction against seminomas, dysgerminomas, pinealomas and mediastinal tumours of similar histological appearance. Lancet 2, 1102–1104.

Masuzawa, T., Shimabukuro, H., Nakahara, N., et al., 1986. Germ cell tumors (germinoma and yolk sac tumor) in unusual sites in the brain. Clin. Neuropathol. 5, 190–202.

Matsutani, M., Sano, K., Takakura, K., et al., 1997. Primary intracranial germ cell tumors: a clinical analysis of 153 histologically verified cases. J. Neurosurg. 86, 446–455.

Matsutani, M., Takakura, K., Sano, K., 1987. Primary intracranial germ cell tumors: pathology and treatment. Prog. Exp. Tumor. Res. 30, 307–312.

McComb, J.G., Apuzzo, M.L.J., 1988. The lateral decubitus position for the surgical approach to pineal location tumors. Concepts. pediat. Neurosurg. 8, 186–199.

McLeod, D.G., Taylor, H.G., Skoog, S.J., et al., 1988. Extragonadal germ cell tumors. Clinicopathologic findings and treatment experience in 12 patients. Cancer 61, 1187–1191.

Merchant, T.E., Davis, B.J., Sheldon, J.M., et al., 1998. Radiation therapy for relapsed CNS germinoma after primary chemotherapy. J. Clin. Oncol. 16, 204–209.

Metcalfe, S., Sikora, K., 1985. A new marker for testicular cancer. Brit. J. Cancer 52, 127–129.

Miles, A., Tidmarsh, S., Philbrick, D., et al., 1985. Diagnostic potential of melatonin analysis in pineal tumors. N. Engl. J. Med. 313, 329–330.

Missori, P., Delfini, R., Cantore, G., 1995. Tinnitus and hearing loss in pineal region tumours. Acta. Neurochir. 135, 154–158.

Montecinos, H.A., Richter, H., Caprile, T., et al., 2005. Synthesis of transthyretin by the ependymal cells of the subcommissural organ. Cell Tissue Res. 320, 487–499.

Müller-Forell, W., Schroth, G., Egan, P.J., 1988. MR imaging in tumors of the pineal region. Neuroradiology 30, 224–231.

Murphree, A., Benedict, W., 1984. Retinoblastoma: Clues to human oncogenesis. Science 223, 1028–1033.

Naganuma, H., Inoue, H., Misumi, S., et al., 1984. Intracranial germ-cell tumors. Immunohistochemical study of three autopsy cases. J. Neurosurg .61, 931–937.

Nazzaro, J.M., Shults, W.T., Neuwelt, E.A., 1992. Neuro-ophthalmological function of patients with pineal region tumors approached transtentorially in the semisitting position. J. Neurosurg. 76, 746–751.

Neuwelt, E., 1985. An update on the surgical treatment of malignant pineal region tumors. Clin. Neurosurg. 32, 397–428.

Neuwelt, E., Frenkel, E., Smith, R., 1980. Suprasellar germinomas (ectopic pinealomas): Aspects of immunological characterization and successful chemotherapeutic responses in recurrent disease. Neurosurgery 7, 352–358.

Neuwelt, E., Glasberg, M., Frenkel, E., et al., 1979. Malignant pineal region tumors. J. Neurosurg. 51, 597–607.

Neuwelt, E., Smith, R., 1979. Presence of lymphocyte membrane surface markers on 'small cells' in a pineal germinoma. Ann. Neurol. 6, 133–136.

Nighoghossian, N., Confavreaux, C., Sassolas, G., et al., 1988. Insufisance hypothalamique apres irradiation demence tardive, subaigue et curable. Rev. Neurol. (Paris) 144, 215–218.

Noell, K., Herskovic, A., 1985. Principles of radiotherapy of CNS tumors. In: Wilkins, R., Rengachary, S. (Eds.) Neurosurgery, Vol 1. McGraw-Hill, New York, pp. 1084–1095.

Ogata, M., Yamashita, T., Ishikawa, T., et al., 1964. Report on treatment results on ectopic pinealoma apparently arising from septum pellucidum. No To Shinkei 16, 615–618.

Ojeda, V.J., Ohama, E., English, D.R., 1987. Pineal neoplasms and third-ventricular teratomas in Niigata (Japan) and Western Australia. A comparative study of their incidence and clinicopathological features. Med. J. Aust. (Sydney) 146, 357–359.

Ono, N., Takeda, F., Uki, J., et al., 1982. A suprasellar embryonal carcinoma producing alpha-fetoprotein and human chorionic gonadotropin; treated with combined chemotherapy followed by radiotherapy. Surg. Neurol. 18, 435–443.

Packer, R.J., Sutton, L.N., Rorke, L.B., et al., 1984a. Intracranial embryonal cell carcinoma. Cancer 54, 520–524.

Packer, R.J., Sutton, L.N., Rosenstock, J.G., et al., 1984b. Pineal region tumors of childhood. Pediatrics 74, 97–101.

Page, R., Doshi, B., Sharr, M., 1986. Primary intracranial choriocarcinoma. J. Neurol. Neurosurg. Psych. 49, 93–95.

Parinaud, H, 1886. Paralysis of the movement of convergence of the eyes. Brain 9, 330–341.

Parsa, A.T., Pincus, D.W., Feldstein, N., et al., 2001. Pineal region tumors. In: **Keating, R.F., Goodrich, J.T., Packer, R.** (Eds.), Tumors of the pediatric central nervous system. Thieme, New York, pp. 308–325.

Patel, A.J., Fuller, G.N., Wildrick, D.M., et al., 2005. Pineal cyst apoplexy: case report and review of the literature. Neurosurgery 57, E1066.

Patel, S.R., Buckner, J.C., Smithson, W.A., et al., 1992. Cisplatin-based chemotherapy in primary central nervous system germ cell tumors. J. Neurooncol. 12, 47–52.

Pecker, J., Scarabin, J.-M., Vallee, B., et al., 1979. Treatment in tumours of the pineal region: value of stereotaxic biopsy. Surg. Neurol. 12, 341–348.

Pendl, G., (Ed.), 1985. Case material. Pineal and midbrain lesions. Springer-Verlag, Wien, pp. 128–207.

Peragut, J.C., Dupard, T., Graziani, N., et al., 1987. De la prévention des risques de la biopsie stéréotaxique de certaines tumeurs de la région pinéale: a propos de 3 observations. Neurochirurgie 33, 23–27.

Perentes, E., Rubinstein, L.J., Herman, M.D., et al., 1986. S-antigen immunoreactivity in human pineal glands and pineal parenchymal tumors. A monoclonal antibody study. Acta. Neuropathol. (Berl) 71, 224–227.

Pfletschinger, J., Olive, D., Czorny, A., et al., 1986. Metastases peritoneales d'un pinealoblastome chez une patiente porteuse d'une derivation ventriculo-peritoneale. Pediatritrie XXXXI, 231–236.

Plowman, P.N., Pizer, B., Kingston, J.E., 2004. Pineal parenchymal tumours: II. On the aggressive behaviour of pineoblastoma in patients with an inherited mutation of the RB1 gene. Clin. Oncol. (R Coll Radiol) 16, 244–247.

Pluchino, F., Broggi, G., Fornari, M., et al., 1989. Surgical approach to pineal tumours. Acta. Neurochir. (Wien) 96, 26–31.

Pople, I.K., Athanasiou, T.C., Sandeman, D.R., et al., 2001. The role of endoscopic biopsy and third ventriculostomy in the management of pineal region tumours. Br. J. Neurosurg. 15, 305–311.

Poppen, J.L., 1966. The right occipital approach to a pinealoma. J. Neurosurg. 25, 706–710.

Posner, M., Horrax, G., 1946. Eye signs in pineal tumors. J. Neurosurg. 3, 15–24.

Preissig, S., Smith, M., Huntington, H., 1979. Rhabdomyosarcoma arising in a pineal teratoma. Cancer 44, 281–284.

Prioleau, G., Wilson, C., 1976. Endodermal sinus tumor of the pineal region. Cancer 38, 2489–2493.

Rao, Y., Medini, E., Haselow, R., et al., 1981. Pineal and ectopic pineal tumors: the role of radiation therapy. Cancer 48, 708–713.

Regis, J., Bouillot, P., Rouby-Volot, F., et al., 1996. Pineal region tumors and the role of stereotactic biopsy: review of the mortality, morbidity, and diagnostic rates in 370 cases. Neurosurgery 39, 907–914.

Reid, W.S., Clark, W.K., 1978. Comparison of the infratentorial and transtentorial approaches to the pineal region. Neurosurgery 3, 1–8.

Rich, T., Cassady, J., Strand, R., et al., 1985. Radiation therapy for tumors of the pineal region. Cancer 55, 932–940.

Rippe, J.D., Boyko, O.B., Friedman, H.S., et al., 1990. Gd-DTPA-enhanced MR imaging of leptomeningeal spread of primary intracranial CNS tumor in children. AJNR Am. J. Neuroradiol. 11, 329–332.

Robertson, P.L., DaRosso, R.C., Allen, J.C., 1997. Improved prognosis of intracranial non-germinoma germ cell tumors with multimodality therapy. J. Neurooncol. 32, 71–80.

Rodrigues, M.M., Bardenstein, D.S., Donoso, L.A., et al., 1987. An immunohistopathologic study of trilateral retinoblastoma. Am. J. Ophthalmol. 103, 776–781.

Rosenfeld, J.V., Murphy, M.A., Chow, C.W., 1990. Implantation metastasis of pineoblastoma after stereotactic biopsy. J. Neurosurg. 73, 287–290.

Rout, D., Sharma, A., Radhakrishnan, V.V., et al., 1984. Exploration of the pineal region: observations and results. Surg. Neurol. 21, 135–140.

Rowland, J.H., Glidewell,O.J., Sibley, R.F., et al., 1984. Effects of different forms of central nervous system prophylaxis on neuropsychologic function in childhood leukemia. J. Clin. Oncol. 2, 1327–1335.

Rubery, E., Wheeler, T., 1980. Metastases outside of the central nervous system from a presumed pineal germinoma. Case report. J. Neurosurg. 53, 562–565.

Rubinstein, L.J., 1981. Cytogenesis and differentiation of pineal neoplasms. Hum. Pathol. 12, 441–448.

Rubinstein, L.J., 1985. Embryonal central neuroepithelial tumors and their differentiating potential. A cytogenetic view of a complex neuro-oncological problem. J. Neurosurg. 62, 795–805.

Russell, D.S., Rubinstein, L.J., (Eds.), 1989a. Tumours and tumour-like lesions of maldevelopmental origin. In: Pathology of tumours of the nervous system. Williams and Wilkins, Baltimore, MD, pp. 664–765.

Russell, D.S., Rubinstein, L.J. (Eds.), 1989b. Tumours of specialized tissues of central neuroepithelial origin. In: Pathology of tumours of the nervous system. Williams and Wilkins, Baltimore, MS, pp. 351–420.

Sakai, N., Yamada, H., Andoh, T., et al., 1988. Primary intrcranial germ-cell tumors. A retrospective analysis with special reference to long-term results of treatments and the behavior of rare types of tumors. Acta. Oncol. 27, 43–50.

Salazar, O.M., Castro-Vita, H., Bakos, R.S., et al., 1979. Radiation therapy for tumors of the pineal region. Int. J. Radiat. Oncol. Biol. Phys. 5, 491–499.

Sano, K., 1976a. Diagnosis and treatment of tumours in the pineal region. Acta. Neurochir. 34, 153–157.

Sano, K., 1976b. Pinealoma in children. Childs Brain 2, 67–72.

Sano, K., 1984. Pineal region tumors: problems in pathology and treatment. Clin. Neurosurg. 30, 59–89.

Sano, K., 1987. Pineal region and posterior third ventricular tumors: a surgical overview. In: Apuzzo, M. (Ed.), Surgery of the third ventricle. Williams and Wilkins, Baltimore, MD, pp. 663–683.

Sano, K., 1999. Pathogenesis of intracranial germ cell tumors reconsidered. J. Neurosurg. 90, 258–264.

Sano, K., Matsutani, M., 1981. Pinealoma (germinoma) treated by direct surgery and postoperative irradiation. Childs Brain 8, 81–97.

Satoh, H., Uozumi, T., Kiya, K., et al., 1995. MRI of pineal region tumours: relationship between tumours and adjacent structures. Neuroradiology 37, 624–630.

Sawamura, Y., de Tribolet, N., Ishii, N., et al., 1997. Management of primary intracranial germinomas: diagnostic surgery or radical resection? J. Neurosurg. 87, 262–266.

Sawamura, Y., Shirato, H., Ikeda, J., et al., 1998. Induction chemotherapy followed by reduced-volume radiation therapy for newly diagnosed central nervous system germinoma. J. Neurosurg. 88, 66–72.

Sawaya, R., Hawley, D.K., Tobler, W.D., et al., 1990. Pineal and third ventricular tumors. In: Youmans, J. (ed.) Neurological surgery. WB Saunders, Philadelphia, PA, pp. 3171–3203.

Schild, S.E., Scheithauer, B.W., Haddock, M.G., et al., 1996. Histologically confirmed pineal tumors and other germ cell tumors of the brain. Cancer 78, 2564–2571.

Schild, S.E., Scheithauer, B.W., Schomberg, P.J., et al., 1993. Pineal parenchymal tumors. Clinical, pathologic, and therapeutic aspects. Cancer 72, 870–880.

Schoenberg, B., Christine, B., Whisnant, J., 1976. The descriptive epidemiology of primary intracranial neoplasms: the Connecticut experience. Am. J. Epidemiology 104, 499–510.

Shibahara, J., Todo, T., Morita, A., et al., 2004. Papillary neuroepithelial tumor of the pineal region. A case report. Acta. Neuropathol. 108, 337–340.

Shibamoto, Y., Abe, M., Yamashita, J., et al., 1988. Treatment results of intracranial germinoma as a function of irradiated volume. Int. J. Radiat. Oncol. Biol. Phys. 15, 285–290.

Shinoda, J., Yamada, H., Sakai, N., et al., 1988. Placental alkaline phosphatase as a tumor marker for primary intracranial germinoma. J. Neurosurg. 68, 710–720.

Shokry, A., Janzer, R.C., Von Hochstetter, A.R., et al., 1985. Primary intracranial germ-cell tumors. A clinicopathological study of 14 cases. J. Neurosurg. 62, 826–830.

Siegal, T., Pfeffer, M.R., Catane, R., et al., 1983. Successful chemotherapy of recurrent intracranial germinoma with spinal metastases. Neurology. 33, 631–633.

Silvani, A., Eoli, M., Salmaggi, A., et al., 2005. Combined chemotherapy and radiotherapy for intracranial germinomas in adult patients: a single-institution study. J. Neurooncol. 71, 271–276.

Smirniotopoulos, J.G., Rushing, E.J., Mena, H., 1992. Pineal region masses: differential diagnosis. Radiographics 12, 577–596.

Smith, W.T., Hughes, B., Ermocilla, R., 1966. Chemodectoma of the pineal region, with observations of the pineal body and chemoreceptor tissue. J. Path. Bact. 92, 69–76.

Stachura, I., Mendelow, H., 1980. Endodermal sinus tumor originating in the region of the pineal gland. Cancer 45, 2131–2137.

Stefanko, S.Z., Talerman, A., Mackay, W.M., et al., 1979. Infundibular germinoma. Acta. Neurochir. (Wien) 50, 71–78.

Stein, B.M., 1971. The infratentorial supracerebellar approach to pineal lesions. J. Neurosurg. 35, 197–202.

Stein, B.M., 1979. Surgical treatment of pineal region tumors. Clin. Neurosurg. 26, 490–510.

Stein, B.M., Bruce, J.N., 1992. Surgical management of pineal region tumors (honored guest lecture). Clin. Neurosurg. 39, 509–532.

Steinbok, P., Dolmen, C., Kaan, K., 1977. Pineocytomas presenting as subarachnoid hemorrhage. Report of 2 cases. J. Neurosurg. 47, 776–780.

Stowell, R., Sachs, E., Russell, W., 1945. Primary intracranial chorioepithelioma with metastases to lung. Am. J. Pathol. 21, 787–801.

Sugiyama, K., Uozumi, T., Kiya, K., et al., 1992. Intracranial germ-cell tumor with synchronous lesions in the pineal and suprasellar regions: report of six cases and review of the literature. Surg. Neurol. 38, 114–120.

Sung, D.I., Harisiadis, L., Chang, C.H., 1978. Midline pineal tumors and suprasellar germinomas: highly curable by irradiation. Radiology 128, 745–751.

Surawicz, T.S., McCarthy, B.J., Kupelian, V., et al., 1999. Descriptive epidemiology of primary brain and CNS tumors: results from the Central Brain Tumor Registry of the United States, 1990–1994. Neuro. Oncol. 1, 14–25.

Suzuki, J., Iwabuchi, T., 1965. Surgical removal of pineal tumors (pinealomas & teratomas). Experience in a series of 19 cases. J. Neurosurg. 23, 565–571.

Takakura, K., 1985. Intracranial germ cell tumors. Clin. Neurosurg. 32, 429–444.

Takei, Y., Pearl, G.S., 1981. Ultrastructural study of intracranial yolk sac tumor: with special reference to oncologic phylogeny of germ cell tumors. Cancer 48, 2038–2046.

Takeuchi, J., Handa, H., Nagata, I., 1978. Suprasellar germinoma. J. Neurosurg. 49, 41–48.

Tamarkin, L., Danforth, D., Lichter, A., 1982. Decreased nocturnal plasma meltonin peak in patients with estrogen positive breast cancer. Science 216, 1003–1005.

Tanaka, R., Ueki, K., 1979. Germinomas in the cerebral hemisphere. Surg. Neurol. 12, 239–241.

Tavcar, D., Robboy, S.J., Chapman, P., 1980. Endodermal sinus tumor of the pineal region. Cancer 45, 2646–2651.

Tien, R.D., Barkovich, A.J., Edwards, M.S.B., 1990. M. R. Imaging of pineal tumors. AJNR Am. J. Neuroradiol. 11, 557–565.

Tompkins, V., Haymaker, W., Campbell, E., 1950. Metastatic pineal tumors. A clinicopathological report of two cases. J. Neurosurg. 7, 159–169.

Ueki, K., Tanaka, R., 1980. Treatment and prognoses of pineal tumors – experience of 110 cases. Neurol. Med. Chir. 20, 1–26.

Uematsu, Y., Tsuura, Y., Miyamoto, K., et al., 1992. The recurrence of primary intracranial germinomas. Special reference to germinoma with STGC (syncytiotrophoblastic giant cell). J. Neurooncol. 13, 247–256.

Van Wagenen, W.P., 1931. A surgical approach for the removal of certain pineal tumors. Surg. Gynecol. Obstet. 53, 216–220.

Vaquero, J., Ramiro, J., Martinez, R., et al., 1990. Clinicopathological experience with pineocytomas: report of five surgically treated cases. Neurosurgery 27, 612–619.

Vaughan, G., 1984. Melatonin in humans. Pineal. Res. Rev. 2, 141–201.

Ventureyra, E.C., 1981. Pineal region: surgical management of tumours and vascular malformations. Surg. Neurol. 16, 77–84.

Villano, J.L., Propp, J.M., Porter, K.R., et al., 2008. Malignant pineal germ-cell tumors: an analysis of cases from three tumor registries. Neuro. Oncol. 10, 121–130.

Vorkapic, P., Waldhauser, F., Bruckner, R., et al., 1987. Serum melatonin levels: a new neurodiagnostic tool in pineal region tumors? Neurosurgery 21, 817–824.

Waga, S, Handa, H., Yamashita, J., 1979. Intracranial germinomas: treatment and results. Surg. Neurol. II, 167–172.

Wakai, W., Segawa, H., Kithara, S., et al., 1980. Teratoma in the pineal region in two brothers. Case reports. J. Neurosurg. 53, 239–243.

Wara, W.M., Jenkin, R.T.D., Evans, A., et al., 1979. Tumors of the pineal and suprasellar region: Children's cancer study group treatment results 1960–1975. Cancer 43, 698–701.

Weiner, H.L., Lichtenbaum, R.A., Wisoff, J.H., et al., 2002. Delayed surgical resection of central nervous system germ cell tumors. Neurosurgery 50, 727–734.

Wilson, E.R., Takei, Y., Bikoff, W.T., et al., 1979. Abdominal metastases of primary intracranial yolk sac tumors through ventriculoperitoneal shunts: report of three cases. Neurosurgery 5, 356–364.

Wolden, S.L., Wara, W.M., Larson, D.A., et al., 1995. Radiation therapy for primary intracranial germ-cell tumors. Int. J. Radiat. Oncol. Biol. Phys. 32, 943–949.

Wood, J.H., Zimmerman, R.A., Bruce, D.A., et al., 1981. Assessment and management of pineal-region and related tumors. Surg. Neurol. 16, 192–210.

Wurtman, R.J., Kammer, H., 1966. Melatonin synthesis by an ectopic pinealoma. N. Engl. J. Med. 274, 1233–1237.

Yamini, B., Refai, D., Rubin, C.M., et al., 2004. Initial endoscopic management of pineal region tumors and associated hydrocephalus: clinical series and literature review. J. Neurosurg. 100, 437–441.

Yoshida, J., Sugita, K., Kobayashi, T., et al., 1993. Prognosis of intracranial germ cell tumours: effectiveness of chemotherapy with cisplatin and etoposide (CDDP & VP-16). Acta. Neurochir. (Wien) 120, 111–117.

Zee, C.-S., Segall, H., Apuzzo, M., et al., 1991. MR imaging of pineal region neoplasms. J. Comput. Assist. Tomogr. 15, 56–63.

Zimmerman, R., 1985. Pineal region masses: Radiology. In: Wilkins, R., Rengachary, S., (Eds.) Neurosurgery, Vol 1. McGraw-Hill, New York, pp. 680–686.

Zimmerman, R.A., Bilaniuk, L.T., 1982. Age-related incidence of pineal calcification detected by computed tomography. Neuroradiology 142, 659–662.

Zondek, H., Kaatz, A., Unger, H., 1953. Precocious puberty and choriepithelioma of the pineal gland with report of a case. J. Endocrinol. 10, 12–16.

PITUITARY TUMORS

PART 6

35 Non-functional pituitary tumors

Rudolf Fahlbusch and Venelin M. Gerganov

Introduction

Approximately one-third of pituitary adenomas are not associated with either clinical endocrinopathy or elevated levels of circulating hormone. These are designated non-functioning adenomas (NFA) and are sub-divided into two categories – silent adenomas and null cell adenomas. NFA account, however, for approximately 60–80% of all operated pituitary macroadenomas (Table 35.1). Cells of NFA either synthesize biologically inactive peptides or glycoproteins or there is defective secretion of hormone. The pathological diagnosis of silent adenoma is usually made on the basis of immunostaining for a specific transcription factor, e.g., steroidogenic factor (SF-1) in a silent gonadotroph cell adenoma, in combination with staining for a hormone – FSH or LH in a silent gonadotroph cell adenoma or ACTH in a silent corticotroph cell adenoma. The majority of clinically silent adenomas are composed of gonadotroph cells (Table 35.2) (Asa et al 1996; Asa & Ezzat 2009; de Oliveira Machado et al 2005).

Two sub-types of silent corticotroph cell adenoma are recognized – subtypes I and II. These are distinguished on the basis of ultrastructural features. Subtype I is usually densely granulated, whereas subtype II is sparsely granulated. Recently, a subtype III silent adenoma was defined – an uncommon tumor that displays aggressive behaviour (Erickson et al 2009). This subtype is usually clinically silent but may present with features of growth hormone or prolactin excess. Immunohistochemistry may be completely negative or there may be variable staining for growth hormone, prolactin and TSH, either singly or in combination (Erickson et al 2009). The pathological diagnosis relies on electron microscopy (Horvath et al 1980).

True hormone-negative or null cell adenomas account for approximately 5% of all pituitary adenomas. Like silent adenomas, these usually present with features of local mass effect. The oncocytic sub-type is distinguished on the basis of large numbers of mitochondria in the cytoplasm of tumor cells. The histogenesis of null cells is unclear. However, some investigations have demonstrated common transcription factors in null cell adenomas and gonadotroph cells (Ishii et al 2006) and expression of glycoprotein hormone genes in null cells (Jameson et al 1987). These data suggest that null cells may represent poorly-differentiated gonadotroph cells.

Diagnosis

The diagnosis of NFA is based mainly on assessment of the endocrinological deficits, of the ophthalmological symptoms that they cause, and, mainly, on the MR imaging findings (Fahlbusch et al 1999). In our series of 721 surgically treated patients with NFA, 48% presented with endocrinological disturbances, 31% presented with visual disturbances, 10% with headache, while in 10% a pituitary apoplexy occurred (Nomikos et al 2004). In 4% of the patients the adenoma was an incidental finding.

NFA originate from the pituitary gland and extend within the sella, to the suprasellar space, and/or to the cavernous sinus, leading to compression of the normal pituitary gland or of the pituitary stalk. Major intrasellar extension leads to early pituitary insufficiency, generally beginning with GH and gonadotrophin deficits (loss of libido and potency, respectively oligomenorrhea and amenorrhea), followed by secondary hypothyroidism (cold intolerance) and secondary adrenalism (adynamia). In the case of primary suprasellar development, pituitary deficiency may occur later, if at all. Diabetes insipidus is extremely rarely present in such patients, regardless of tumor size. It typically may occur in patients with a craniopharyngioma, or an infiltrative pituitary disease, such as lymphocytic hypophysitis, sarcoidosis or lymphoma (Vance 2004).

In our series, the most frequent endocrinological deficit was secondary hypogonadism. Partial or complete secondary adrenocortical failure occurred in 35% and 18% had features of hypothyroidism. A total of 28% of the patients (199/721) presented with hyperprolactinemia; 36 of them had been treated with dopamine agonists. In the literature a higher incidence of hyperprolactinemia has been reported: 48% in the series of Marazuela et al (1994) and 65% in that of Comtois et al (1991). Mildly elevated prolactin levels up to six-fold and not higher than 3150 µU/mL, were regarded in our series as non-tumorous or 'functional' hyperprolactinemia, caused by displacement and/or damage of the pituitary stalk. This has to be differentiated from true excessive hyperprolactinemia, caused by prolactin production in adenoma cells. No patients presented with diabetes insipidus.

The importance of hypopituitarism is emphasized by the fact that in patients with pituitary deficit, there is a clear tendency towards reduced quality of life and reduced life

672

©2011 Elsevier Ltd

Table 35.1 Senior authors experience with 3299 pituitary adenomas, operated in the period 1982–2005 and classified according to their endocrinological type

Endocrinological type	Transsphenoidal	Approach Transcranial	Transsphenoidal/ transcranial
NFA	1413	170	72
Prolactinomas	589	19	6
GH-secreting	781	25	16
ACTH			
Cushing's disease	452	5	1
Nelson's syndrome	37	4	0
TSH-secreting	27	3	1
Total	3299	226	96

Table 35.2 Non-functioning pituitary adenomas

Adenoma type	*n*	(%)
Hormone negative/null cell adenomas		
Null cell adenoma	668	33.2
Oncocytic adenoma	216	10.7
Silent adenomas		
FSH-/LH cell adenoma	865	43
Prolactin cell adenoma, sparsely granulated	31	1.5
Prolactin cell adenoma, densely granulated	3	0.15
GH cell adenoma, sparsely granulated	19	0.94
Mixed GH/Prolactin cell adenoma	1	0.05
Acidophilic stem cell adenoma	1	0.05
TSH cell adenoma	18	0.9
Alpha-subunit-only adenoma	10	0.5
Plurihormonal adenoma	36	1.8
Unclassified adenoma	33	1.6
ACTH cell adenoma, sparsely granulated[a]	89	4.4
ACTH cell adenoma, densely granulated[a]	22	1.1
Sum	2011	100

Data from the German Pituitary Tumor Registry. Modified from Saeger W, Lüdecke DK, Buchfelder M, Fahlbusch R, Quabbe HJ, Petersenn S Pathohistological classification of pituitary tumors: 10 years of experience with the German Pituitary Tumor Registry. Eur J Endocrinol. 2007 Feb;156(2): 203–16.
[a]Silent and non-silent ACTH cell adenomas are separate groups according to the new WHO classification.

expectancy (Bevan & Burke 1986; Bülow et al 1997; Rosen & Bengtsson 1990). Even in patients on adequate replacement therapy, related cardiovascular and cerebrovascular diseases contribute significantly to the increased mortality (Bülow et al 1997; Rosen & Bengtsson 1990).

Depending on the localization of the optic chiasm (prefixed, normal position or post-fixed position), the tumor extension eventually causes a chiasmal syndrome. This includes initial visual field defects, followed by loss of visual acuity, and finally optic nerve atrophy (see Ch. 11). The typical bitemporal hemianopia is seen only in half of the patients, while homonymously located scotomas occur in cases of superior and posterior tumor extension, below the optic tract. Lateral tumor extension with displacement and/ or invasion of the cavernous sinus can cause ocular motor disturbances, due to injury of CNs III, IV and VI, or periorbital pain, mediated by the V nerve (see Ch. 11 for details).

Giant adenomas (>4 cm in diameter), which composed 5% of our cases, may cause various vegetative symptoms due to compression of the diencephalon. They may reach and compress the Foramina Monroi and thus cause obstructive hydrocephalus with increased intracranial pressure symptoms, which is another life-threatening scenario in pituitary adenomas (Mortini et al 2007; Thapar & Laws 2001). Epileptic seizures may occur when the tumor extends laterally towards the temporal lobe.

Pituitary apoplexy

Ocular motor disturbances are typically observed in pituitary apoplexy, an acute potentially life-threatening event caused by the rapid enlargement of a pituitary adenoma, attributed, in more than half of the cases, to intratumoral haemorrhage and in the rest, to intratumoral infarction. Pituitary apoplexy occurs in 0.6–9% of all pituitary adenomas (Bills et al 1993; Liu & Weiss 2003; Sherman et al 2008). It has a slight male predominance and occurs at a mean age of 46.7 years. This syndrome may be the initial presentation of undiagnosed pituitary tumor; in the study of Semple et al (2005), 81% of patients presenting with pituitary apoplexy did not have a known pituitary tumor. The apoplexy occurs without any identifiable predisposing factors (Liu & Weiss 2003; Rovit & Fein 1972). Furthermore, no adenoma subtype has been recognized to confer a higher risk of apoplexy. Such patients present clinically with acute headache, nausea, vomiting, altered consciousness, and/or visual disturbances, mainly ocular motor deficits, combined with complete or, rarely, partial pituitary insufficiency. The ocular motor deficits are most frequently due to oculomotor nerve involvement (Cardoso & Peterson 1984). Acute adrenal insufficiency, accompanied by hyponatremia is requires urgent treatment with high-dose corticosteroid replacement therapy and treatment of the hyponatremia. If the hemorrhage extends through the arachnoid membrane into the cerebrospinal fluid, the presentation is similar to and should be distinguished from an aneurysmal subarachnoid hemorrhage (Liu & Weiss 2003). The diagnosis of pituitary apoplexy is confirmed with MRI, which is reported to have almost 100% sensitivity in detecting both the tumor and the associated hemorrhage or infarct (Bills et al 1993; Piotin et al 1999). Pituitary apoplexy has to be distinguished from intratumoral hemorrhage, which also may be associated with acute headache and visual deterioration; however, it is much less dramatic clinically.

Failure to recognize and treat this life-threatening syndrome may lead to blindness and poor outcome. The dominating opinion is that such patients should be treated surgically via the transsphenoidal approach, which is mandatory in case of existing visual loss or neurological deficits (Bills et al 1993; Cardoso & Peterson 1984; da Motta et al 1999; Onesti & Wisniewski 1990; Randeva et al 1999; Rovit & Fein 1972). Emergency surgery is required when there is deteriorating vision, sudden onset of blindness, or diminished level of consciousness (Sherman et al 2008). However, the stabilization of the patient's general condition before surgery is of primary importance. The initial management step should always be to achieve homeostasis for electrolytes and anterior pituitary functions. We agree with Sibal et al (2004) that patients presenting without neuroophthalmological signs or having mild and non-progressive signs should be managed conservatively in the acute phase. The hemorrhage can destroy an active endocrine disease such as acromegaly; however, tiny solid remnants can be overlooked and can be the reason for a later recurrence (Kamiya et al 2000). Therefore, subsequent careful follow-up of the patients is necessary.

Preoperative evaluation

The management of a patient with NFA begins with the establishing of an accurate diagnosis, which is based on endocrine, ophthalmological, and neuroradiological examinations. The goal is to correlate ultimately the clinical, anatomical, and endocrine findings (Fahlbusch & Thapar 1999; Vance 2004) and select a personalized management plan.

Endocrine functional tests

The endocrinological screening is aimed at revealing any hormonal deficits or hypersecretion. The following basal serum hormone values should be examined: prolactin- to exclude true prolactinomas; LH, FSH, oestrogen, and – respectively – testosterone, for evaluation of the gonadal axis; TSH, T3 and T4 for evaluation of the thyroid axis; and cortisol for evaluation of the adrenal function. In case of suspected adrenal insufficiency, an ACTH (Synacthen) test with blood samples taken at 0 min, 30 min, and 60 min is indicated. The insulin hypoglycemia test (IHT-Test) discovers initial pituitary deficiency (hyposomatotropism) by evaluating GH level; blood samples are taken at −15 min, 0 min (injection of 0.15 U/kg insulin), 30 min, 60 min, and 90 min and stress insufficiency by evaluating cortisol and ACTH.

Ophthalmological examination

A formal neuroophthalmological examination is essential in all patients (see Ch. 11). The examination includes visual field testing (perimetry), both to confrontation and with Goldmann perimetry and/or semiautomatic perimetry. Evaluation of visual acuity without and with correction is essential. Fundoscopy must be undertaken to evaluate the presence of optic nerve atrophy. Primary diseases of the optic system, such as glaucoma-induced scotomas, diabetic retinopathy or changes due to arterial hypertonia, should be excluded.

Neuroradiology

Currently, MRI is the modality of choice for the diagnosis and characterization of a pituitary lesion. The standard protocol for MRI of the pituitary and parasellar region consists of sagittal T1- and T1-weighted images performed with and without intravenous contrast (Kucharczyk et al 1994; Zee et al 2003). The native T1- and T2-weighted images are usually diagnostic of pituitary macroadenomas. These tumors are usually hypointense to isointense to gray matter on T1-weighted images and have variable signal intensity on T2-weighted images (Zee et al 2003). About 20–30% of them show evidence of previous hemorrhage (Fig. 35.1). Sellar enlargement is seen in 94–100% of pituitary macroadenomas. Macroadenomas exhibit heterogeneous enhancement after gadolinium administration. Contrast enhancement may differentiate the adenoma from the displaced pituitary gland, may detect cavernous sinus invasion, and is helpful in the differential diagnosis of sellar and parasellar lesions (Cottier et al 2000; Elster 1994; Kucharczyk et al 1994).

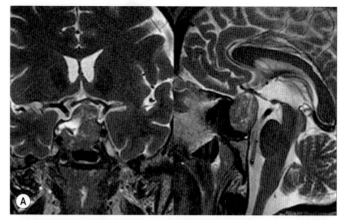
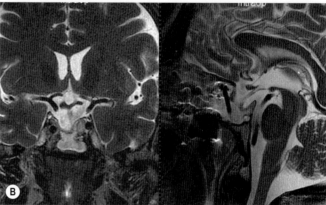

Figure 35.1 (A) T2-weighted MRI image, acquired with a high-field 1.5T iopMRI, of a 45-year-old female patient with a large NFA, showing evidence of previous intratumoral hemorrhage; (B) following the complete tumor removal, the preserved pituitary stalk and gland are well seen on the final iopMRI image acquisition.

It may be difficult to determine if the cavernous sinus is involved by the adenoma, a situation that occurs in 6–10% of pituitary adenomas (Daita et al 1995). Frequently, the macroadenoma displaces the medial wall of the cavernous sinus laterally without actually invading it. In other patients, who usually have oculomotor deficits, the tumor may penetrate into the sinus (Visot et al 2006). The radiological signs of cavernous sinus invasion are: encasement of the intracavernous ICA (Scotti et al 1988), replacement of the medial cavernous sinus compartment by tumor tissue (Cottier et al 2000), or tumor growth beyond tangents joining the intracavernous and supraclinoid segments of the ICA (Knosp et al 1993). The detection of cavernous sinus invasion may be more readily determined using higher MR field strength. In a study on the value of high-field MR imaging for diagnosis of sellar lesions, Wolfsberger et al (2004a,b) showed that this technique could predict tumor invasion through the medial cavernous sinus border by direct delineation of the medial border as a distinct line between the sellar lesion and the venous spaces. A positive correlation to surgical findings was found on 84% of 3-tesla MR images with a sensitivity of 83% and a specificity of 84%.

The MRI angiography demonstrates tumor relationship to the carotid arteries, to the basilar artery and their branches, as well as vessel changes, such as displacement or narrowing, so convincingly that traditional angiographies are rarely indicated in differential diagnosis, e.g., for excluding a thrombosed aneurysm. In case of bone invasiveness, when the sellar floor is disrupted and the tumor infiltrates the sphenoid sinus, CT with bony window can be very helpful. The CT remains an alternative to MRI if a ferromagnetic intracranial aneurysm clip or cardiac pacing device exists.

Indications for surgery

The goal of surgery is to achieve selective morphological and endocrinological tumor excision without complications, thus curing the patient. There is a generally accepted trend towards early surgery in case of NFA (Karavitaki et al 2007; Thapar & Laws 2001). Surgery is indicated if there is radiological or clinical evidence of chiasmal compression, extension into the sphenoid sinus or temporal lobe and/or hypopituitarism.

Contraindications for early primary surgery are: irreversible peritumoral edema, a very uncommon situation observed mainly in giant and invasive adenomas; and irreversible hypothalamic dysfunctions, presenting with disturbed sleep/wake rhythm, severe electrolyte disturbances (hypo- or hypernatremia), caloric and temperature disturbances. These categories of patients should be operated following correction of their disturbance or should receive alternative symptomatic treatment. The same is true for patients in poor general condition (ASA III and IV).

Role of incidentalomas

Incidentalomas are defined as pathological findings in the sellar area, observed during head imaging performed in patients for reasons, unrelated to ophthalmological and/or endocrinological symptoms. The great majority of these incidentalomas are NFA. It is still controversial if they should be operated early after their discovery, should be operated at a later stage, or should simply be followed-up.

Some autopsy studies showed that incidentally discovered pituitary adenomas, mainly inactive adenomas, were found in up to 10% of the cases (Buurman & Saeger 2006). Arita et al (2006) observed 45 incidentalomas over a period of 5 years: 40% of them increased in size and 20% became symptomatic. According to several published studies on the natural evolution of untreated nonfunctioning macroadenomas, 7–51% of them showed further growth tendency (Dekkers et al 2006; Dekkers et al 2007; Fainstein et al 2004; Molitch 1993, 2008; Sanno et al 2003). However, during the follow-up period of about 5 years, the rate exceeded 50%. These findings, as well as the very low operative morbidity related to surgery for incidentalomas, are further argument for their active management. Another indication for surgery is the evidence of hyposomatotropism and/or hypogonadism. Karavitaki et al (2007) described the natural history of 24 diagnosed and only observed NFA. Half of them grew further; in 57% visual field defects occurred and additional 21% developed a contact to the optic chiasm, respectively to the optic nerves. This observation would strongly support the tendency to a more aggressive early indication for surgery. From the 16 observed

microadenomas, only 12% increased in size, which substantiated the conservative management strategy in such adenomas.

At present, it remains impossible to predict the natural evolution of incidentalomas. Therefore, it is difficult to formulate clear guidelines for neurosurgeons and each individual patient requires a personalized decision. In the case of endocrine hyper- or hypofunction, symptoms due to the mass effect of the adenoma, or documented growth tendency, surgery is indicated. In completely asymptomatic patients, follow-up with regular MRI, ophthalmological, and endocrine control, may be recommended (Visot et al 2006).

Choice of approach

Approximately 90–97% of all NFA can be removed via the transsphenoidal approach (Fahlbusch & Marguth 1981; Honegger et al 2007; Laws & Thapar 1999; Nomikos et al 2004; Visot et al 2006) (Fig. 35.2). It is suitable for: all intrasellar tumors with and without invasion of the sphenoid sinus; for parasellar adenomas extending towards the cavernous sinus, regardless if it is displaced or focally invaded; and in most adenomas with suprasellar extension. The approach is not suitable in the case of asymmetrical suprasellar development, when major tumor parts are localized between the carotid artery and the optic chiasm/optic nerve tract, as well as in case of sphenoid sinusitis (Maartens & Kaye 2006). Ectatic midline ('kissing') carotid arteries have been also considered as a contraindication for transsphenoidal surgery (Liu & Weiss 2003). However, in experienced hands with the use of navigational control, this procedure is also possible.

Transcranial surgery should be selected in adenomas that are unresectable by the transsphenoidal route: in the case of subfrontal, retrosellar, or subtemporal tumor extension; in tumors whose suprasellar part is larger than their intrasellar part; and/or present with a narrow sellar entrance, preventing total descent of the suprasellar tumor part. Even in such adenomas, the transcranial surgery is usually performed as a second stage of a two-step procedure after transsphenoidal surgery. Large suprasellar adenomas, reaching the level of the optic chiasm or extending even higher that do not present with chiasmal syndrome, are suspicious for developing without capsule. They may surround the optic nerves and chiasm and – if approached transsphenoidally – have a greater operative risk of hemorrhage or damage to the visual apparatus. Therefore, in some of these cases, complete tumor removal should not be attempted.

If complete tumor removal cannot be achieved by either of the approaches alone, a two-stage procedure may be required (Fig. 35.3). In such tumors, we prefer as a first stage, the transsphenoidal approach: it allows safe sellar closure and less risk of CSF leak, provided the transcranial surgery is performed after at least 8–10 days. Depending on the severity of chiasmal compression and the degree of improvement after the transsphenoidal surgery, the second stage can be postponed for 2–3 months. In the meantime, the pituitary and optic nerve functions recover. Although some authors recommend performing combined transsphenoidal-transcranial surgeries in the case of giant

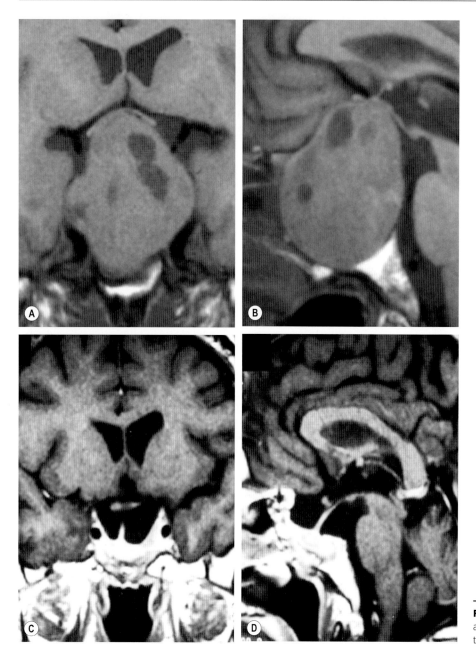

Figure 35.2 Giant non-functioning adenoma in a 57-year-old male patient (A,B); complete transsphenoidal removal (C,D).

adenomas (D'Ambrosio et al 2009), it is not well tolerated, especially in the elderly, and should be an exception.

Transsphenoidal approach

The sphenoid sinus has been approached in earlier years via a sublabial incision, which is still preferred in patients with small nostrils, especially in children; via a pernasal, or via a paraseptal approach. The advantage of the transsphenoidal approaches is that they are more physiological and use the nasal cavity as an anatomical passage to the sphenoid sinus (Fahlbusch & Marguth 1981; Fahlbusch & Thapar 1999; Laws & Thapar 1999; Thapar & Laws 2001). The disadvantage, when performed with an operative microscope, is the limited visualization, especially of the

more caudal clivus area, as well as the need of nasal tamponade.

The direct pernasal approach was propagated by Griffith and Veerapen (1987) who performed it via one nostril with operative microscope and used a C-arm fluoroscopy for defining the sagittal plane. The midline is defined by detecting the nasal spine (spina nasalis) and the vomer position in one line towards the sella or with the help of neuronavigation.

Endoscopy allows a direct pernasal surgery via one or two nostrils, performed as pure endoscopic or as endoscope-assisted transsphenoidal surgery.

The first author (RF) has performed all transsphenoidal approaches for nearly 20 years, as endoscopic-assisted procedures. Initially, the middle turbinate and the choanae are

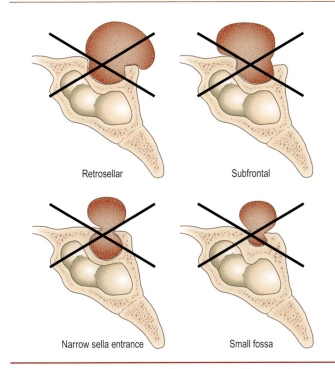

Retrosellar

Subfrontal

Narrow sella entrance

Small fossa

Figure 35.3 Contraindications for the transsphenoidal approach.

identified with a 0-degree endoscope. The mucosal incision is then preformed under microscopic control approximately 1.5 cm anterior to the choanae (Fig. 35.4). The posterior bony septum at the level of the vomer is drilled off with a diamond drill, avoiding injury to the contralateral mucosa, and the sphenoid sinus is entered. A speculum is introduced to enlarge the working avenue and to protect the nasal mucosa from injury, during the hundreds of in- and out-movements of the instruments.

Early within this procedure, the endoscope is used to inspect the sella and visualize the protuberances of the carotid artery on both sides, which are not so easily visible with the microscope. Thus, the midline is identified with certainty. The mucosa of the sphenoid sinus should be removed as much as possible to avoid postoperative mucocele formation.

Tumor removal

NFA constitute the great majority of macroadenomas. In the case of supra- and parasellar extension, we remove initially the tumor portion dorsally and lateral from the midline, followed by the retro- and the suprasellar parts. Thus, a too early descent of the diaphragm in folds is prevented, which could hinder the complete tumor removal. In case of soft tumor invasion of the cavernous sinus, the tumor can be followed to the carotid artery via the perforation in the medial cavernous wall. Additional exposure in such cases is gained by removal of the turbinate and drilling the bony wall of the cavernous sinus. The tumor is then approached, either with (Frank & Pasquini 2006) or without endoscopic control.

In the case of firm tumor consistency, successive tumor removal is not possible and the only option for complete removal is to perform an en-block resection.

Preservation of the pituitary gland

The pituitary body is normally compressed and displaced to a postero-lateral location under the elevated diaphragm. It is very rarely located anterior – in this case it should be displaced to reach the adenoma. A median or paramedian location, as a septum within the tumor, is seen exceedingly rare, usually after previous intratumoral hemorrhages.

Sellar closure

In case of a CSF leak, caused by a rupture and/or damage of the occasionally invaded suprasellar capsule, a watertight closure is mandatory. Autologous material is still preferred, although a tendency to use artificial material is observed. The experience with the use of artificial materials is enlarging; the early results are, from the authors' point of view, impressive (Dusick et al 2006; Semple et al 2005). However, the series was not homogenous enough, including patients without observed CSF leak, and long-term follow-up is still missing.

We prefer subcutaneous fat tissue and fascia lata, harvested from the thigh or from the abdomen. The material should cover the place of the defect or – if it is not directly visible – the whole diaphragma sellae with overlapping of the adjacent structures. In the case of intrasellar tumors it is placed at the level of the sella entrance or at the sella floor. Tiny pieces of fat tissue should be used in addition: either as a first cover in the case of multiple or wider defects, or as an additional layer in the sphenoid sinus as a support to the fascia. Tiny pieces of fat tissue can be placed intra-as extra-durally in a sandglass form. Human fibrin glue can provide additional safety against continuous CSF leak. If major intraoperative CSF leak is observed, a lumbar drainage is inserted. Depending on the severity of the leak, 10–20 mL CSF are drained 3–4 times daily for 3–5 days.

If no CSF leak is observed, a piece of Tachocomb (collagen fleece coated with fibrin glue) may be placed for safety reasons (prevention of 'delayed leak') on the sella floor. Gelfoam pieces do not have the same occluding effectiveness; however, they serve as place-holder, separating the intrasellar space from the sphenoid sinus. The sphenoid sinus should not be completely occluded by tamponades, otherwise the fluid outflow from the sinus may be precluded, thus causing headache or even infection.

We have never found it necessary to reconstruct the bony sellar floor – with bone or cartilage taken from the nasal septum – as recommend by some authors, performing endoscopic surgery (Cappabianca & Cavallo 2004). From our earlier experience with early reoperations, we have learned that the sellar floor regenerates completely or nearly completely within 8–10 months, provided it has not been too extensively enlarged by the tumor. Covering the sellar area with mucosa or with a pedicled mucosal flap from the nasal septum is not necessary in pituitary adenomas and is mainly indicated in case of large dura defects, e.g., following the endonasal removal of skull base tumors (Fernandez-Miranda et al 2009; Hadad et al 2006). Principally, any technique of closure and reconstruction of the sella is welcomed, provided the rate of CSF fistulas, requiring reoperations, as well as that of meningitis, remain under 1% (Nomikos et al 2004).

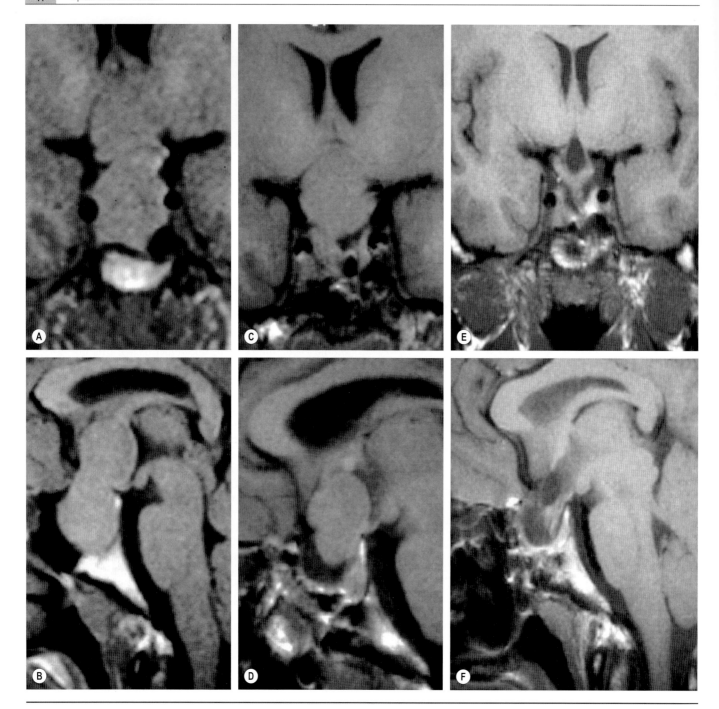

Figure 35.4 Two-stage removal of a very large NFA. (A,B) Preoperative images; (C,D) MRI images after the transsphenoidal surgery; (E,F) MRI images after the transcranial surgery, revealing the complete tumor removal.

At the end of surgery, any bleeding points from the nasal mucosa should be detected and controlled, which is best done under endoscopic control. The nasal septum and the middle turbinate are repositioned. In the great majority of cases, nasal tamponade is not required. If the surgeon has some difficulties, especially in patients with hypertension or in case of previous nasal bleeding, a smaller tamponade is placed in one or in both nostrils, parallel to the septum, and removed after 1 day.

Despite this careful management, re-bleeding can occur even days after surgery. In milder forms a (re-)tamponade for 3–5 days is sufficient. In more severe cases, a re-operation with tailored coagulation of the ethmoidal artery at the level of the medial wall of the orbit can be indicated. Sometimes the cause for recurrent bleeding is a tiny bone piece that has penetrated the mucosa. In exceptionally rare cases, vascular malformations of the mucosa, even outside the area of the operative approach, can be discovered angiographically and, respectively, closed by embolization.

Endoscopy

In the modern era of transsphenoidal surgery, the pure endoscopy for pituitary adenomas has been increasingly proposed (Cappabianca & Cavallo 2004; Fernandez-Miranda et al 2009; Jho & Alfieri 2001). In general, rigid endoscopes with 4 mm outer diameter and 0° and 30° lens angle are used. Different companies offer a variety of equipment, including instruments for tumor removal, irrigation, and suckers for single and bimanual procedures through one or two nostrils. The rigid long endoscopes can be fixed with a special holding device on the operating table. Efforts have been undertaken to move such endoscopes by robotic systems, with the opportunity for simultaneous navigation (Bumm et al 2005).

The major advantage of the endoscope is that, in contrast to the microscope, it allows for a much wider overview of the sphenoid sinus, which is possible due to the fish-eye effect of the endoscopic optic. In case of a wide sphenoid sinus and lack of complex bony septi, a panoramic view of the entire sinus, approximately 120°, is acquired, including visualization of the optic nerve canal and of the canals of the carotid arteries. Thereby, the midline can be precisely determined and fluoroscopic or navigational control is not required. The possibility to look around the corner and visualize the lateral parts of sphenoid sinus and of the cavernous sinus are other major advantages of this technique. With the endoscope tip positioned closer to the medial cavernous sinus wall, following sella opening and removal of the intrasellar tumor part, a much better visualization of the eventual tumor remnants within the sinus is possible. Further, it allows for detection of even tiny lesions of the descending diaphragm, which may be a source of CSF leak. The usefulness of the endoscope is limited in case of an extensive sellar floor expansion towards the roof of the sphenoid sinus or if a major tumor part propagates into the sinus. The control of extensive hemorrhages into the sinus can be time-consuming. The insertion of nasal septi mainly on the carotid prominence may present additional problems if a pure endoscopic technique is applied.

The use of a microscope or of an endoscope is a matter of personal preference, although they are both only tools for observation. The ultimate success of the surgery is still related to the experience of the pituitary surgeon. Future developments are expected to be far beyond these classical techniques.

Navigation

The neuronavigational guidance in transsphenoidal surgeries is promoted by many neurosurgeons as a means to increase their accuracy and safety. It was supported before the time of CT and MRI control, even by one of the pioneers of transsphenoidal surgery, Jules Hardy (1999). It can be performed with CT-guidance, MRI-guidance, fluoroscopy guidance, or as a combination thereof (Elias et al 1999; Fox

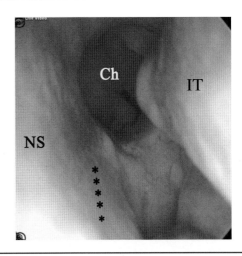

Figure 35.5 Initial endoscopic view of the nasal cavity. Ch, choanae; IT, inferior turbinate; NS, nasal septum; dotted line, mucosal incision, 1.5 cm anterior to the choanae.

& Wawrzyniak 2008; Jagannathan et al 2006; Jane et al 2001), depending on the particular case and the preferences of the surgeon. The navigation is either pointer-related or microscope-based (Figs 35.5, 35.6). The latter allows for direct visualization of the segmented structures, such as the carotid or basilar artery, as well as the tumor. It is not so technically demanding for the surgeon and easier to handle than the pointer-guided navigation.

Most pituitary surgeons agree that the main indication for navigation is repeated operations for recurrence or of a growing remnant (Jagannathan et al 2006; Lasio et al 2002). In such cases, the normal nasal and sellar anatomy can be disrupted and the landmarks of the nasal sinuses, the sphenoid, and anterior skull base may be damaged, obliterated, or obscured by postoperative scars (Jagannathan et al 2006). The navigation allows for a reliable identification of the midline. In such cases, a good alternative may be the fluoroscopic control. The navigation is definitely of great value in the case of 'kissing' carotid arteries, which can narrow the transverse diameter of the sella to 6–8 mm; or tumor invasion of the cavernous sinuses with encasement of the carotid arteries. Another indication, although more disputed, is in microadenomas when the sella is of normal size (Fox & Wawrzyniak 2008).

In summary, in NFA, microscope-based navigation is indicated in the case of: a narrow space between the carotid arteries; encased carotid arteries by an invasive tumor, and in repeated surgeries when the normal landmarks are absent.

Intraoperative MRI

The classical intraoperative imaging modality is the X-ray fluoroscopy with the C-shaped mobile set-up, which provides reliable and very accurate images, usually in the sagittal plane, of the bony structures or metal surgical instruments placed in the operating field. The introduction of intraoperative MR imaging (iopMRI) was a recent major introduction. It allows for immediate intraoperative quality control and,

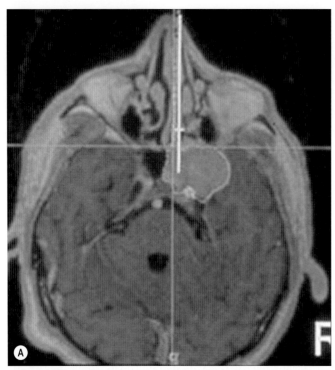

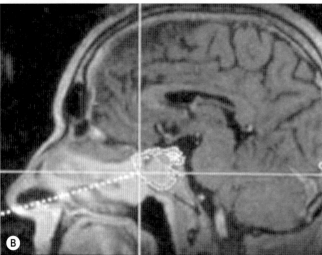

Figure 35.6 (A,B) Navigational guidance during a sublabial transsphenoidal removal of a NFA involving the left cavernous sinus.

descending sella diaphragm, can be detected in up to one-third of pituitary macroadenomas even with the low-field strength iopMRI setup (Fahlbusch & Thapar 1999). With the high-field MRI, in contrast with the low-field one, the intrasellar and parasellar spaces may also be visualized precisely and the invasion of the cavernous sinus can be directly estimated. Furthermore, the better image quality provided by the high-field iopMRI, allows circumventing the interpretation difficulties encountered with the low-field MR systems, which are caused usually by artifacts from metal debris of the diamond drills or by blood.

In a study of 106 patients with hormonally inactive pituitary macroadenomas operated transsphenoidally, the role of the high-field iopMRI was evaluated (Nimsky et al 2006). The technique proved to be safe and highly reliable. The decision to perform a scan is taken by the surgeon; either to control the completeness of tumor removal or in the case of incomplete removal, for determining the consequent surgical strategy. The surgical workflow is interrupted for the image acquisition for about 15 min; the whole transsphenoidal procedure is identical to that performed in regular operating rooms. We use the regular microinstruments at the 5 G line. It is advisable to use porcelain-coated drills in order to avoid metal-related artifacts. We proceed with tumor removal whenever some remnant is seen that is deemed accessible for further resection. A last MRI scanning is performed prior to closure.

In this group, tumor remnants were detected in 57 patients and the resection was continued in 37 (Fig. 35.8). In the 85 patients, in whom complete tumor removal was intended, intraoperative imaging revealed definite tumor remnants or at least suspicious findings in 36 patients (42%). Thus, the rate of complete tumor removal could be increased from 58% to 82%.

A further advantage of the iopMRI is the acquisition of immediate post-resectional imaging control. Thus, even if a remnant exists that cannot be removed safely, the images allow for planning of the consequent stages of its management without delay, e.g., transcranial surgery, follow-up, or radiotherapy (Dina et al 1993).

Other methods for identification of the sellar content

Ultrasound

Ultrasound was introduced to visualize and localize smaller microadenomas in the sella, usually in Cushing syndrome, in which it may be difficult for the surgeon to identify the adenoma (Ram & Bruck 1999). Later on, its application has been expanded to macroadenomas as a means for determining the extent of tumor resection. Doppler ultrasound was used to identify the carotid artery in the cavernous sinus, in order to prevent its injury during tumor removal within the cavernous sinus (Arita et al 1998). Suzuki et al (2004) used an echo probe inserted in a right frontal trephination hole in order to obtain brightness-mode echo images and Doppler color flow images. These images allowed for real-time visualization of the tumor and surrounding brain structures, including major arteries and the cisterns during the removal of macroadenomas, thus enhancing the safety of this surgery and maximizing the removal of the tumor. It must be

where remnants are depicted, for achieving more complete tumor resection (Fig. 35.7) (Bohinski et al 2001; Fahlbusch & Thapar 1999; Fahlbusch et al 2001; Martin et al 1999; Nimsky et al 2006; Pergolizzi et al 2001). The significance of intraoperative imaging is highlighted by the results of a comparison of the iopMRI findings with the estimation of the surgeon with regard to the extent of resection (Fahlbusch & Thapar 1999). It revealed a discrepancy in 42% of the cases: the iopMRI showed some remaining tumor, whereas the surgeon either did not suspect any remnant or thought the tumor location prohibited further resection (Nimsky et al 2006). Suprasellar tumor remnants, which had been too small or hidden from the surgeon's eye in folds of the

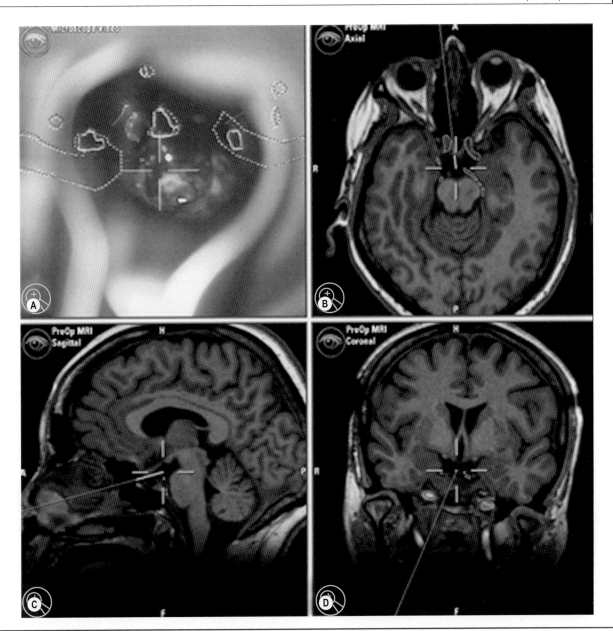

Figure 35.7 (A–D) In contrast to the sublabial approach, the direct pernasal approach allows only for a limited opening of the speculum. This leads to technical difficulties and inaccuracy of the navigation, as presented on (C).

discussed how far this invasive procedure is valuable regarding the poor tumor visualization obtained with the low resolution US, when compared with iopMRI.

From a historical point of view, it is of interest to mention that other indirect methods for identification of the sellar pathology were less useful. Laser-Doppler flowmetry has been introduced as a method for identification of the anterior and posterior pituitary lobe and their differentiation from the adenoma, which normally has displaced these structures within and outside the sella (Steinmeier et al 1991). Another technique, assessed in a cooperative study between Liverpool and Erlangen, was the monitoring of the intrasellar pressure (Lees et al 1994). The goal was to predict invasion of adenomas into the cavernous sinus, which at that time could not be diagnosed from CT and early MRI examinations.

The pressure values were found to be highest in cases with major cavernous sinus invasion.

Transcranial approaches
Frontolateral approach

The favorite approach of the authors in the last years is the frontolateral one. It is a safe and flexible technique that provides sufficient access to the sellar, suprasellar, and parasellar areas with direct visualization of the tumor between the optic nerves (Samii & Gerganov 2008). A curved skin incision is made frontotemporal behind the hairline. The craniotomy is made just above the supraorbital margin and usually measures 30–35 mm in width and 20–25 mm in height. The medial extension of the craniotomy is modified according to the size of the frontal sinus but should reach

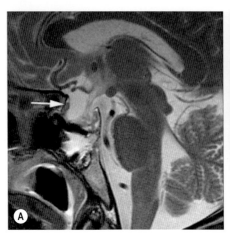 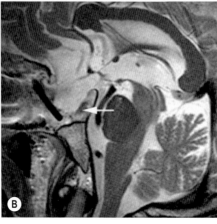 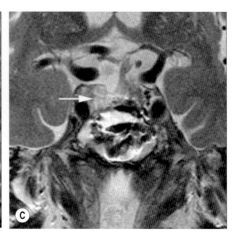

Figure 35.8 Tumor remnants, detected with iopMR imaging. (A) Anterior located remnant (arrow); reason: fear of CSF leak; (B) posteriorly located remnant (arrow); reason: insufficient drilling and exposure; (C) lateral located remnant (arrow); reason: bleeding from the cavernous sinus. The wax plate used to separate the sphenoid sinus from the sellar space is well seen on all images.

the supraorbital notch. With a large frontal sinus, the craniotomy is made slightly more laterally. Following a semicircular frontal based dural incision, the basal cisterns are opened and a sufficient amount of CSF is allowed to egress. Thus, the need of frontal lobe retraction is obviated. The olfaction even on the side of the approach can be preserved if a careful and sharply dissection of the olfactory nerve within the arachnoid plane is performed. In case of a prefixed optic chiasm, however, the access to the adenoma is limited and the frontotemporal approach may be preferred.

The exposure provided by the frontolateral approach is similar to that achieved with a unilateral frontal or bifrontal craniotomy. The disadvantages of the latter techniques, however, are avoided: violation of the frontal sinus, venous, or sinus-related complications, bilateral frontal lobe injuries, and damage to olfactory nerves (Liu & Weiss 2003).

Frontotemporal approach
The technique of the frontotemporal approach is well known. It provides the shortest trajectory to the suprasellar cistern and allows removal of laterally extending adenomas via several working corridors: lateral to the carotid artery, between the carotid artery and the optic nerve, and between the two optic nerves (Buchfelder & Kreutzer 2008; Maartens & Kaye 2006). Of paramount importance is the preservation of the tiny perforators (Liu & Weiss 2003). The major disadvantage of the frontotemporal approach is that the surgeon's view of the left optic nerve and intrasellar contents is compromised (Visot et al 2006). The approach is usually selected in case of adenomas with major lateral extension.

Sub-temporal approach
This is a rarely utilized approach, usually in adenomas with a significant parasellar, sub-temporal and retrochiasmatic extension (Buchfelder & Kreutzer 2008). A major problem is the complete removal of the intrasellar portion of the tumor.

Superior approach
The superior approach is indicated in the more rare giant adenomas, which reach the Foramina of Monroe or even

extend into the lateral ventricle(s) (Maartens & Kaye 2006). In such tumors, however, usually a decompressive removal is possible in order not to induce delayed life threatening hemorrhages into the tumor and its periphery.

Cranial base techniques
Some authors promoted different skull base approaches, such as the cranio-orbito-zygomatic approach, the transbasal approach, the pretemporal extradural skull base approach, the extended transsphenoidal approach, the sublabial transseptal approach with nasomaxillary osteotomy, the transethmoidal approaches, and the sublabial transantral approach (Dolenc 1997; Youssef & Agazzi 2005). However, these are rarely, if ever, necessary. Similarly, the approaches to the cavernous sinus (Dolenc 1997) are indicated in exceptional cases.

The complications, related to all transcranial approaches are usually due to elevation of the frontal or temporal lobes; to the dissection of major vessels, and to manipulations of the optic nerve (Visot et al 2006). Especially dangerous, is the manipulation of the optic nerve, chiasm, or tract because it may lead to injury of the small feeding arteries and to postoperative worsening of vision.

Operative results

In the series of the first author, mentioned above, the adenoma was removed completely transsphenoidally in 275/500 cases. A suspicious finding on postoperative MRI was seen in 120 cases; a small remnant in 25 cases; and a larger remnant that necessitated additional surgery or radiotherapy, in 80 cases. The analysis of the prognostic factors for outcome of transsphenoidal surgery, showed that the outcome correlated with the age of the patient, the size of the adenoma, its invasiveness, and immunohistochemical characteristics. Best results were achieved in the middle-aged patients with tumors <3 cm (87% complete resection vs 46.5% in those >3 cm). In the case of radiologically determined invasiveness, the rate of complete resection was 42%, compared with 95% in those without invasive features.

Interestingly, the histologically determined invasiveness was not found to correlate significantly.

Endocrinological results

The pituitary function can be preserved in almost all cases (Sibal et al 2004): in the authors' series only 4% of the patients operated transsphenoidally had new postoperative endocrine deficit (Nomikos et al 2004). The endocrinological outcome is related to the approach used and is considerably worse if a transcranial surgery is performed: 62.5% of those operated transcranially had some new endocrine deficit. The function of the adenohypophysis at 1 year normalized in 19.6%, improved in 30.1%, remained unchanged in 48.9% and worsened in 1.4% of the patients with some degree of preoperative hypopituitarism, operated transsphenoidally. Similar rates have been published by different authors: improvement is observed in 35.7–65.3% and unchanged function is observed in 32.1–54% (Arafah 1986; Marazuela et al 1994; Nelson & Tucker 1984; Webb et al 1999). The outcome was considerably worse in the group operated transcranially: normalization of the function was not observed in any patient, some improvement had 11.3%, unchanged remained in 73.7% and worsened in 15%.

Generally, the results 3 months after surgery are predictive in regard to the long-term outcome. The hyperprolactinemia resolved completely 1 year after the surgery in 95.5% of the patients. In the majority (80%), it normalized within 1 week, while in 16% it normalized within 3 months. Secondary adrenocortical failure, either partial or complete, had 34.8% of the patients operated transsphenoidally. After the surgery, it normalized in 40.8%, improved in 31.1%, remained unchanged in 23.6%, and worsened in 4.5%. Newly acquired deficit was observed in 0.8%. The adrenocortical failure did not resolve in any of the patients operated transcranially, although it improved in 11.7%; new deficits were found in 29.6%. The secondary hypogonadism resolved in 16% and remained unchanged in 84% at 1 year in the transsphenoidal group, while in the transcranial group, normalization was observed in only 4%. New deficits were found in 2.1% in the first and in 50% of the later groups. The secondary hypothyroidism resolved in 34% and remained unchanged in 66%; new deficit had 1.5%. The rate in the transcranial group was: resolution 28.5%; unchanged 71.5%; new deficit 7.3%. Although 34% of the patients had diabetes insipidus early after surgery, only in four of them (0.5%) did it persist at 1 year. Similar rates have been reported by other experienced groups: permanent diabetes insipidus have 3–5% of the patients (Comtois 1991; Ebersold et al 1986).

Ophthalmological results

The first formal neuroophthalmological control examination should be performed within 7 days of surgery and repeated at 3 months and at 12 months (see Ch. 11 for details). Immediately after surgery, the monitoring of the visual function is especially important. Any alteration of the vision should be detected as early as possible and treatable causes, such as bleeding or compression of the optic nerve, chiasm, or tract should be excluded. With the transsphenoidal approach, the

Table 35.3 Visual outcome in the senior author series of 3299 pituitary adenomas, operated in the period 1982–2005.

	1 week post-op	3 months post-op	12 months post-op
Normal	9.4	25.3	26.1
Improved	77.4	69.5	69.5
Unchanged	2.4	2.4	1.6
Deteriorated	10.8	2.8	2.8

risk of damage of the optic system structures and visual deterioration is very low and improvement occurs in >85% of the patients (Bevan & Burke 1986; Ebersold et al 1986; Losa et al 2008; Thapar & Laws 2001; Zhang et al 1999). In our series, lasting visual deterioration developed in one patient, who already had a preoperative chiasmal syndrome. The deterioration was found to be due to bleeding in a suprasellar tumor remnant. The visual function normalized in 26%, improved in 70%, and remained unchanged in 2% at 1 year (Table 35.3). Similar data were presented by Thapar and Laws (2001): postoperative improvement occurred in 87%; stabilization was achieved in 9%; and in 4% the vision deteriorated. In the series by Losa et al (2008) visual function normalized in 39% and improved in 51% of 279 patients who had a preoperative deficit. The preoperative existing oculomotor nerve palsy resolved in 18 of 22 patients. In the case of blindness, caused by a solid NFA, full recovery of vision is an exception. If the vision is lost after an apoplexy, however, early surgery may lead to significant improvement. The visual function starts to recover within 2 weeks in one-third of the cases, within 3 months in approximately two-thirds, and within 1 year in <5% (Erickson et al 2009). The extent of recovery is further related to the age of the patient: in those over 65 years, it very rarely normalizes completely.

We have very rarely observed new postoperative ocular motor nerve deterioration. Careful handling within the sinus should avoid permanent dysfunction, which we have never observed in our series. In the case of preoperative existing dysfunction, as in apoplexy cases and more rarely in the case of cavernous sinus displacement by solid tumors, a complete recovery may be generally expected.

Invasiveness

Pituitary tumors are often invasive, in particular to the cavernous sinus and/or to the sphenoid sinus (Knosp et al 1993). Microadenomas and giant invasive pituitary adenomas have different biological structure, as shown by recent studies. The expression of the P-53 gene is more commonly encountered in invasive adenomas and pituitary carcinomas (Lasio et al 2002). More studies exist that have found a positive correlation between the increased KI-67 – a marker of cellular proliferation – labeling index and aggressive biological behavior (Salehi et al 2009). The specificity of this parameter, however, is not so high: a considerable overlap in the Ki-labeling has been found between non-invasive and invasive adenomas. Moreover, such overlapping also exists between adenomas and pituitary carcinomas. The index is significantly higher in hormonally active than in non-functioning tumors (Thapar et al 1996; Webb et al 1999); however, the clinical significance of this finding is unclear.

Salehi and the leading pituitary neuropathologic research group of Kovacs and Scheithauer (Salehi et al 2009) point that although many studies found a significant association of Ki-67 index with invasiveness, the findings are inconsistent (Mastronardi et al 1999; Thapar et al 1996).

The invasion may involve the sellar floor, the diaphragm, or the cavernous sinus. One should distinguish between 'invasion' from a radiological, surgical intraoperative and histological points of view. The histological invasion of the sellar floor has no practical significance, while the invasion of the cavernous sinus can be confirmed only intraoperatively. In our series, invasion occurred in nearly all giant adenomas (>4 cm), 40% of the macroadenomas, and just 5% of microadenomas.

Recurrences/remnants

The rate of complete removal of NFA in experienced hands is 61.4–70.2% (Losa et al 2008; Nomikos et al 2004; Zhang et al 1999). In a recently published study on the intraoperative application of high-field MRI, we showed that this modality allowed us to increase the rate of complete removal to 82% (Nomikos et al 2004). The factors, found by Lasio et al (2002) to correlate with less than complete removal were invasion of the cavernous sinus, increased largest tumor diameter, and absence of tumor apoplexy at presentation (Losa et al 2008).

Following a complete removal of an NFA, the recurrence rate is usually low. In our experience, the recurrence rate at 10 years follow-up was 5.1% after initial complete tumor removal; 28.3% in the case of a suspicious residual existing on postoperative MR imaging; and 52% in the case of initial incomplete removal (Fig. 35.9). Interestingly, most of the recurrences occurred in the first 5 years: 4% in the first, 22.5% in the second, and 40% in the third group (Figs 35.10–35.12). The study of different proliferation and molecular biology, such as Ki-67 labeling index, flow cytometry for DNA ploidy indexes, could not confirm their prognostic value relative to a potential recurrence (Tanaka et al 2003).

The generally accepted indications for re-operations for both recurrences and growing remnants are: increase of tumor size, new endocrinological deficits, and new ophthalmological symptoms. The management of a patient with a recurrence should be individualized with consideration of a number of factors: time of recurrence, size and location of the recurrence, age of the patient, general condition, ophthalmological and neurological functions, and endocrine findings (Ciric et al 2000). In a young patient with a symptomatic recurrence, a transsphenoidal reoperation would be justified. Similar management would be recommended in young and healthy patients with a non-symptomatic recurrence. The time after the initial surgery is also an important issue: if the recurrence occurred within a relatively short period after complete resection, radiotherapy may be recommended following the reoperation (Figs 35.13 & Fig. 35.14). Small asymptomatic recurrences, occurring late after surgery, may best be followed-up with regular MRI and ophthalmological examinations. A conservative follow-up would be the best option in the case of adults or those with severe systemic diseases (Fig. 35.15).

The immunohistochemical type of the adenoma was found to correlate to the risk of recurrence (Table 35.4): those tumors staining positive for ACTH have the highest rate of recurrences (23%), followed by null-cell adenomas (12%). In such cases, a more careful follow-up is, therefore, mandatory.

Radiotherapy

Although the role of postoperative radiotherapy is controversial, most authors do not recommend its prophylactic application in cases of complete or near-complete tumor removal. Postoperative radiotherapy might be considered in selected patients with large tumor remnants that cannot be removed surgically and those with panhypopituitarism, as well as in patients with early recurrence following initial complete tumor removal (Minniti et al 2007; Nelson et al 1989). Generally, radiotherapy is reserved as an adjuvant treatment in case the reoperation of the recurrence does not accomplish

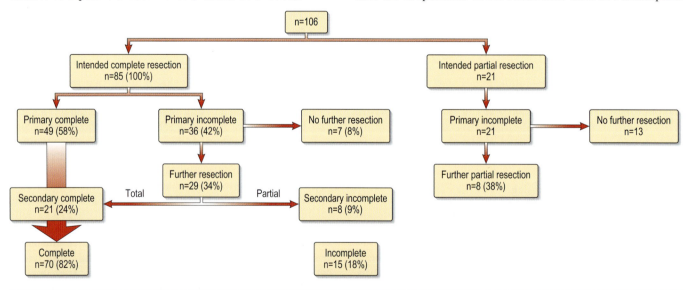

Figure 35.9 Tumor removal rates in NFA, operated with a 1.5 T iopMRI control. (From Nimsky C, von Keller B, Ganslandt O, Fahlbusch R. Intraoperative high-field magnetic resonance imaging in transsphenoidal surgery of hormonally inactive pituitary macroadenomas. Neurosurgery. 2006;59: 105–114).

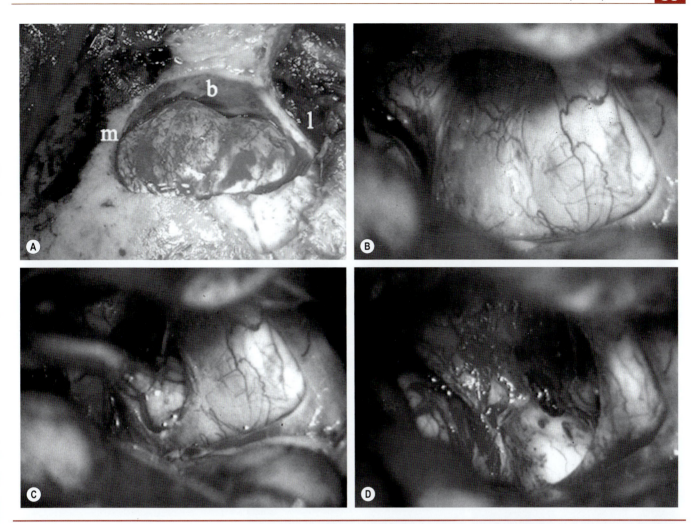

Figure 35.10 Frontolateral craniotomy (A) and microscopic view of the suprasellar area (b, skull base; m, midline; l, lateral); (B) initial view of the tumor; (C) tumor removal; (D) the image shows the completely removed tumor and the preservation of all feeding vessels to the optic structures.

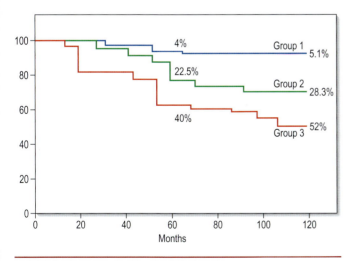

Figure 35.11 Recurrence-free survival after 10 years (120 months) follow-up. Group 1: initial complete tumor removal; Group 2: suspicious tumor remnant; Group 3: initial complete removal.

a desired reduction in its size. The long-term side-effects associated with radiotherapy in the area, such as an up to 50% incidence of pituitary deficiencies (Nomikos et al 2004) or the much rarer optic nerve atrophy and visual deterioration (Brada et al 1993; Brada & Jankowska 2008), should always be considered when recommending this treatment (Minniti et al 2005). These side-effects are frequently emphasized by the endocrinologists, who favor the medical treatment and disregard all alternatives. Moreover, with the new technological developments, such as conformal radiotherapy, the complication rate was further reduced (Prasad 2006).

Stereotactic techniques that allow a more precise delivery of a higher dose of radiation to the target has been introduced recently (Ghostine & Ghostine 2008; Sheehan et al 2005). The radiation dose is delivered either as a single dose or in several fractionated doses: Gamma Knife-based, LINAC-based or proton beams-based. These techniques are increasingly utilized for the management of residual or recurrent tumors that are not too large or close to the optic

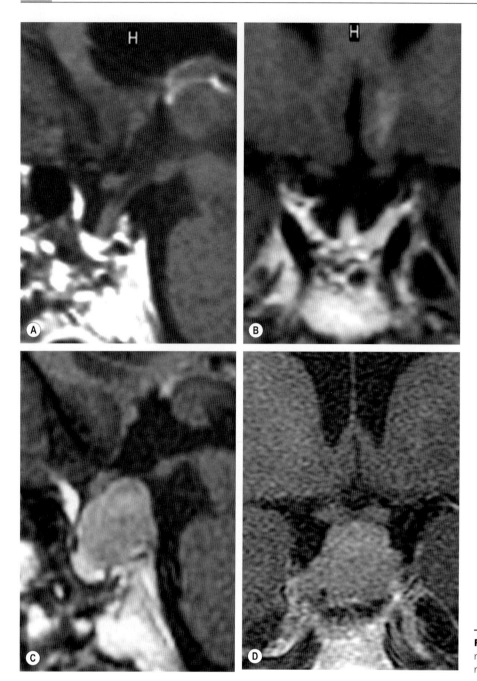

Figure 35.12 Although the adenoma was removed completely (A,B) in this case, a recurrence was detected 6 years later (C,D).

structures (at least 5 mm). The achieved tumor control rate is 87–100% with a follow-up of 6–60 months and the 5-year progression-free survival rate reaches 90% (Brada & Ajithkumar 2004; Pollock et al 2008; Sherman et al 2008). Furthermore, it is related to a lesser risk of anterior pituitary insufficiency. The long-term effects of stereotactic radiosurgery on pituitary function and visual function remain to be determined, since most patient series have only a relatively short duration of follow-up. Some authors have reported a higher pituitary deficiency rate 5 years after radiosurgery (Pollock et al 2008). Another recently developed option is the intensity-modulated radiation therapy, which leads to a local control rate of 89% with a median follow-up of 42.5 months (Mackley et al 2007). The results have to be, however, validated over a longer follow-up.

The long-term outcome, in terms of tumor control and morbidity, of radiosurgery, conventional, and conformal radiotherapy, have yet to be determined, as no comparative studies on these methods exist (Minniti et al 2006). In macroadenomas causing visual field defects, surgery is the first-line of treatment because, with any type of radiotherapy, several months may be needed to achieve volume reduction and alleviation of the compressive effect (Pamir et al 2007).

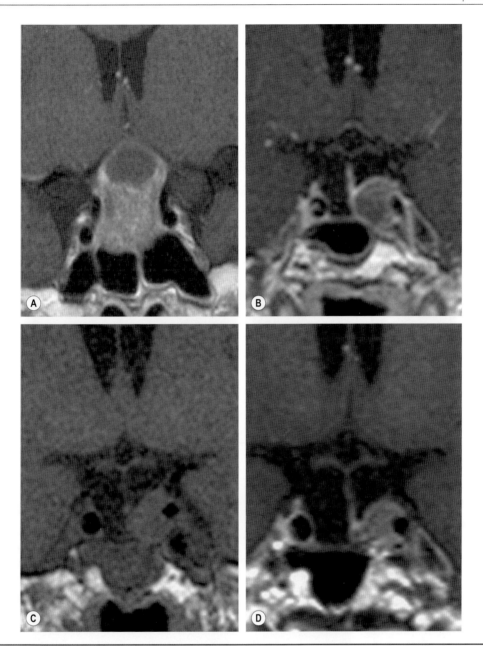

Figure 35.13 Small remnant of an NFA was seen after transsphenoidal surgery (A) that over a follow-up period of more than 10 years did not show any change in size (B–D).

Dekkers, O.M., Perreira, A.M., Roelfsma, F., et al., 2006. Observation alone after transsphenoidal surgery for non-functioning pituitary adenomas. J. Clin. Endocr. Metab. 91, 1796–1801.

Dekkers, O.M., Hammer, S., de Keizer, R.J., et al., 2007. The natural course of non-functioning pituitary macroadenomas. Eur. J. Endocrinol. 156, 217–224.

de Oliveira Machado, A.L., Adams, E.F., Schott, W., et al., 2005. Analysis of secretory, immunostaining and clinical characteristics of Human 'functionless' pituitary adenomas: Transdifferentiation or gonadotropinomas? Exp. Clin. Endocrinol. Diabetes 113, 344–349.

Dina, T.S., Feaster, S.H., Laws, E.R. Jr., et al., 1993. MR of the pituitary gland postsurgery: serial M R studies following transsphenoidal resection. AJNR. Am. J. Neuroradiol. 14, 763–769.

Dolenc, V.V., 1997. Transcranial epidural approach to pituitary tumors extending beyond the sella. Neurosurgery 41, 542–550.

Dusick, J.R., Mattozo, C.A., Esposito, F., et al., 2006. BioGlue for prevention of postoperative cerebrospinal fluid leaks in transsphenoidal surgery: A case series. Surg. Neurol. 66, 371–376.

Ebersold, M.J., Quast, L.M., Laws, E.R. Jr., et al., 1986. Long-term results in transsphenoidal removal of nonfunctioning pituitary adenomas. J. Neurosurg. 64, 713–719.

Elster, A.D., 1994. High-resolution, dynamic pituitary M R imaging: standard of care or academic pastime? AJR. Am. J. Roentgenol. 163, 680–682.

Elias, W.J., Chadduck, J.B., Alden, T.D., et al., 1999. Frameless stereotaxy for transsphenoidal surgery. Neurosurgery 45, 271–277.

Erickson, D., Scheithauer, B., Atkinson, J., et al., 2009. Silent subtype 3 pituitary adenoma: a clinicopathological analysis of the Mayo Clinic experience. Clin. Endocrinol. (Oxf.) 71, 92–99.

Fahlbusch, R., Marguth, F., 1981. Optic nerve compression by pituitary adenomas. In: Samii, M., Janetta, P.J. (Eds.), Cranial nerves. Springer Verlag, Berlin, pp. 140–147.

Fahlbusch, R., Thapar, K., 1999. New developments in pituitary surgical techniques. Baillière's Best Pract. Res. Clin. Endocrinol. Metab. 13, 471–484.

Fahlbusch, R., Ganslandt, O., Buchfelder, M., et al., 2001. Intraoperative magnetic resonance imaging during transsphenoidal surgery. J. Neurosurg. 95, 381–390.

Fahlbusch, R., Buchfelder, M., Honegger, J., et al., 1999. Nonfunctional pituitary adenomas In: Krisht, A.F., Tindall, G. (Eds.), Pituitary disorders. Lippincott, Williams and Wilkins.

Fainstein Day, P., Guitelman, M., Artese, R., et al., 2004. Retrospective multicentric study of pituitary incidentalomas. Pituitary 7, 145–148.

• Fernandez-Miranda, J.C., Prevedello, D.M., Gardner, P., et al., 2009. Endonasal endoscopic pituitary surgery: is it a matter of fashion? Acta. Neurochir. (Wien) 152 (8), 1281–1282.

Fox, W.C., Wawrzyniak, S., Chandler, W.F., 2008. Intraoperative acquisition of three-dimensional imaging for frameless stereotactic guidance during transsphenoidal pituitary surgery using the Arcadis Orbic System. J. Neurosurg. 108, 746–750.

Frank, G., Pasquini, E., 2006. Endoscopic endonasal cavernous sinus surgery, with special reference to pituitary adenomas. Front Horm. Res. 34, 64–82.

Ghostine, S., Ghostine, M.S., Johnson, W.D., 2008. Radiation therapy in the treatment of pituitary tumors. Neurosurg. Focus 24, E8.

• Griffith, H.B., Veerapen, R., 1987. A direct transnasal approach to the sphenoid sinus. Technical note. J. Neurosurg. 66, 140–142.

Hadad, G., Bassagasteguy, L., Carrau, R.L., et al., 2006. A novel reconstructive technique after endoscopic expanded endonasal approaches: vascular pedicle nasoseptal flap. Laryngoscope 116, 1882–1886.

Hardy, J., 1999. Neuronavigation in pituitary surgery. Surg. Neurol. 52, 648–649.

Honegger, J., Ernemann, U., Psaras, T., et al., 2007. Objective criteria for successful transsphenoidal removal of suprasellar Nonfunctioning pituitary adenomas. A prospective study. Acta Neurochir. 149, 21–29.

Horvath, E., Kovacs, K., Killinger, D.W., et al., 1980. Silent corticotropic adenomas of the human pituitary gland: a histologic, immunocytologic and ultrastructural study. Am. J. Pathol. 98, 617–638.

Jagannathan, J., Prevedello, D.M., Ayer, V.S., et al., 2006. Computer-assisted frameless stereotaxy in transsphenoidal surgery at a single institution: review of 176 cases. Neurosurg. Focus 20, E9.

Ishii, Y., Suzuki, M., Takekoshi, S., et al., 2006. Immunonegative 'null cell' adenomas and gonadotropin (Gn) subunit (SUs) immunopositive adenomas share frequent expression of multiple transcription factors. Endocr. Pathol. 17 (1), 35–43.

Jameson, J.L., Klibanski, A., Black, P.M., et al., 1987. Glycoprotein hormone genes are expressed in clinically non-functioning pituitary adenomas. J. Clin. Invest. 80, 1472–1478.

Jane, J.A. Jr., Thapar, K., Alden, T.D., et al., 2001. Fluoroscopic frameless stereotaxy for transsphenoidal surgery. Neurosurgery 48, 1302–1308.

Jho, H.D., Alfieri, A., 2001. Endoscopic endonasal pituitary surgery: evolution of surgical technique and equipment in 150 operations. Minim. Invasive Neurosurg. 44, 1–12.

Kamiya, Y., Jin-No, Y., Tomita, K., et al., 2000. Recurrence of Cushing's disease after long-term remission due to pituitary apoplexy. Endocr. J. 47, 793–797.

Karavitaki, H., Collison, K., Halliday, J., et al., 2007. What is the natural history of non operated nonfunctioning pituitary adenomas? Clin. Endocrinol. (Oxford) 67 (6), 938–943.

• Knosp, E., Steiner, E., Kitz, K., et al., 1993. Pituitary adenomas with invasion of the cavernous sinus space: a magnetic resonance imaging classification compared with surgical findings. Neurosurgery 33, 610–618.

Kucharczyk, W., Bishop, J.E., Plewes, D.B., et al., 1994. Detection of pituitary microadenomas: Comparison of dynamic keyhole fast spin echo, unenhanced, and conventional contrast enhanced MR imaging. AJR. Am. J. Roentgenol. 163, 671–679.

Lasio, G., Ferroli, P., Felisati, G., et al., 2002. Image-guided endoscopic transnasal removal of recurrent pituitary adenomas. Neurosurgery 51, 132–137.

• Laws, E.R. Jr., Thapar, K., 1999. Pituitary surgery. Endocrinol. Metab. Clin. North. Am. 28, 119–131.

Lees, P.D., Fahlbusch, R., Zrinzo, A., et al., 1994. Intrasellar pituitary tissue pressure, tumor size and endocrine status–an international comparison in 107 patients. Br. J. Neurosurg. 8 (3), 313–318.

Liu, J.K., Weiss, M.H., Couldwell, W.T., 2003. Surgical approaches to pituitary tumors. Neurosurg. Clin. N. Am. 14, 93–107.

Losa, M., Mortini, P., Barzaghi, R., et al., 2008. Early results of surgery in patients with nonfunctioning pituitary adenoma and analysis of the risk of tumor recurrence. J. Neurosurg. 108 (3), 525–532.

Mackley, H.B., Reddy, C.A., Lee, S.Y., et al., 2007. Intensity-modulated radiotherapy for pituitary adenomas: the preliminary report of the Cleveland Clinic experience. Int. J. Radiat. Oncol. Biol. Phys. 67, 232–239.

Marazuela, M., Astigarraga, B., Vicente, A., et al., 1994. Recovery of visual and endocrine function following transsphenoidal surgery of large non-functioning pituitary adenomas. J. Endocrinol. Invest. 17, 703–707.

Maartens, N.F., Kaye, A.H., 2006. Role of transcranial approaches in the treatment of sellar and suprasellar lesions. Front Horm. Res. 34, 1–28.

Martin, C.H., Schwartz, R., Jolesz, F., et al., 1999. Transsphenoidal resection of pituitary adenomas in an intraoperative M R I unit. Pituitary 2, 155–162.

Mastronardi, L., Guiducci, A., Spera, C., et al., 1999. Ki-67 labelling index and invasiveness among anterior pituitary adenomas: analysis of 103 cases using the MIB-1 monoclonal antibody. J. Clin. Pathol. 52, 107–111.

Minniti, G., Traish, D., Ashley, S., et al., 2005. Risk of second brain tumor after conservative surgery and radiotherapy for pituitary adenoma: update after an additional 10 years. J. Clin. Endocrinol. Metab. 90, 800–804.

Minniti, G., Traish, D., Ashley, S., et al., 2006. Fractionated stereotactic conformal radiotherapy for secreting and nonsecreting pituitary adenomas. Clin. Endocrinol. (Oxf.) 64, 542–548.

Minniti, G., Jaffrain-Rea, M.L., Osti, M., et al., 2007. Radiotherapy for nonfunctioning pituitary adenomas: from conventional to modern stereotactic radiation techniques. Neurosurg. Rev. 30, 167–175.

Molitch, M.E., 1993. Incidental pituitary adenomas. Am. J. Med. Sci. 306, 262–264.

Molitch, M.E., 2008. Nonfunctioning pituitary tumors and pituitary incidentalomas. Endocrinol. Metab. Clin. North Am. 37, 151–171.

Mortini, P., Barzaghi, R., Losa, M., et al., 2007. Surgical treatment of giant pituitary adenomas: strategies and results in a series of 95 consecutive patients. Neurosurgery 60, 993–1002.

Nelson, A.T. Jr., Tucker, H.S. Jr., Becker, D.P., 1984. Residual anterior pituitary function following transsphenoidal resection of pituitary macroadenomas. J. Neurosurg. 61, 577–580.

Nelson, P.B., Goodman, M.L., Flickenger, J.C., et al., 1989. Endocrine function in patients with large pituitary tumors treated with operative decompression and radiation therapy. Neurosurgery 24, 398–400.

Nimsky, C., von Keller, B., Ganslandt, O., et al., 2006. Intraoperative high-field magnetic resonance imaging in transsphenoidal surgery of hormonally inactive pituitary macroadenomas. Neurosurgery 59, 105–114.

Nomikos, P., Ladar, C., Fahlbusch, R., et al., 2004. Impact of primary surgery on pituitary function in patients with nonfunctioning pituitary adenomas-a study on 721 patients. Acta Neurochir. 146, 27–35.

Onesti, S.T., Wisniewski, T., Post, K.D., 1990. Clinical versus subclinical pituitary apoplexy: presentation, surgical management, and outcome in 21 patients. Neurosurgery 26, 980–986.

Pamir, M.N., Kilic, T., Belirgen, M., et al., 2007. Pituitary adenomas treated with gamma knife radiosurgery: volumetric analysis of 100 cases with minimum 3 year follow-up. Neurosurgery 61, 270–280.

Pergolizzi, R.S. Jr., Nabavi, A., Schwartz, R.B., et al., 2001. Intraoperative M R guidance during trans-sphenoidal pituitary resection: preliminary results. J. Magn. Reson. Imaging 13, 136–141.

Piotin, M., Tampieri, D., Rufenacht, D.A., et al., 1999. The various MRI patterns of pituitary apoplexy. Eur. Radiol. 9, 918–923.

Pollock, B.E., Cochran, J., Natt, N., et al., 2008. Knife radiosurgery for patients with nonfunctioning pituitary adenomas: results from a 15-year experience. Int. J. Radiat. Oncol. Biol. Phys. 70, 1325–1329.

Prasad, D., 2006. Clinical results of conformal radiotherapy and radiosurgery for pituitary adenoma. Neurosurg. Clin. N. Am. 17, 129–141.

Ram, Z., Bruck, B., Hadani, M., 1999. Pituitary. Ultrasound in Pituitary Tumor Surgery 2, 133–138.

Randeva, H.S., Schoebel, J., Byrne, J., et al., 1999. Classical pituitary apoplexy: clinical features, management and outcome. Clin. Endocrinol. 51, 181–188.

Rovit, R.L., Fein, J.M., 1972. Pituitary apoplexy: a review and reappraisal. J. Neurosurg. 37, 280–288.

Rosen, T., Bengtsson, B.A., 1990. Premature mortality due to cardiovascular disease in hypopituitarism. Lancet 336, 285–288.

Saeger, W., Lüdecke, D.K., Buchfelder, M., et al., 2007. Pathohistological classification of pituitary tumors: 10 years of experience with the German Pituitary Tumor Registry. Eur. J. Endocrinol. 156 (2), 203–216.

Salehi, F., Agur, A., Scheithauer, B.W., et al., 2009. Ki-67 in pituitary neoplasms: a review – part I. Neurosurgery 65, 429–437.

Samii, M., Gerganov, V.M., 2008. Surgery of extra-axial tumors of the cerebral base. Neurosurgery 62 (6 Suppl. 3), 1153–1166.

Sanno, N., Oyama, K., Tahara, S., et al., 2003. A survey of pituitary incidentaloma in Japan. Eur. J. Endocrinol. 149, 123–127.

Scotti, G., Yu, C.Y., Dillon, W.P., et al., 1988. MR imaging of cavernous sinus involvement by pituitary adenomas. AJR. Am. J. Roentgenol. 151, 799–806.

Sheehan, J.P., Niranjan, A., Sheehan, J.M., et al., 2005. Stereotactic radiosurgery for pituitary adenomas: an intermediate review of its safety, efficacy, and role in the neurosurgical treatment armamentarium. J. Neurosurg. 102, 678–691.

Sherman, J.H., Pouratian, N., Okonkwo, D.O., et al., 2008. Reconstruction of the sellar dura in transsphenoidal surgery using an expanded polytetrafluoroethylene dural substitute. Surg. Neurol. 69, 73–76.

Semple, P.L., Webb, M.K., de Villiers, J.C., et al., 2005. Pituitary apoplexy. Neurosurgery 56, 65–73.

Sibal, L., Ball, S.G., Connolly, V., et al., 2004. Pituitary apoplexy: a review of clinical presentation, management and outcome in 45 cases. Pituitary 7, 157–163.

Steinmeier, R., Fahlbusch, R., Powers, A.D., et al., 1991. Pituitary microcirculation: physiological aspects and clinical implications. A laser-Doppler flow study during transsphenoidal adenomectomy. Neurosurgery 29, 47–54.

Suzuki, R., Asai, J., Nagashima, G., et al., 2004. Transcranial echoguided transsphenoidal surgical approach for the removal of large macroadenomas. J. Neurosurg. 100, 68–72.

Thapar, K., Scheithaner, W., Kovacs, K., et al., 1996. P53 expression in pituitary adenomas and carcinomas: correlation with invasiveness and tumor growth fractions. Neurosurg. 38, 763–770.

Thapar, K., Laws, E.R. Jr., 2001. Pituitary tumors. In: Kaye, A.H., Laws, E.R. Jr. (Eds.), Brain tumors. An encyclopedic approach, 2nd edn. Churchill Livingstone, Edinburgh, pp. 803–856.

Tanaka, Y., Hongo, K., Tada, T., et al., 2003. Growth pattern and rate in residual nonfunctioning pituitary adenomas: correlations among tumor volume doubling time, patient age and MIB-1 index. J. Neurosurg. 98, 359–365.

Vance, M.L., 2004. Treatment of patients with a pituitary adenoma: one clinician's experience. Neurosurg. Focus 16, Article 1.

Visot, A., Pencalet, P., Boulin, A., et al., 2006. Surgical management of endocrinologically silent pituitary tumors. In: Schmidek, Roberts (Ed.), Schmidek and Sweet's operative neurosurgical techniques. Elsevier, p 355–371.

Webb, S.M., Rigla, M., Wägner, A., et al., 1999. Recovery of hypopituitarism after neurosurgical treatment of pituitary adenomas. Clin. Endocrinol. Metab. 84, 3696–3700.

Wolfsberger, S., Ba-Ssalamah, A., Pinker, K., et al., 2004a. Application of three-tesla magnetic resonance imaging for diagnosis and surgery of sellar lesions. J. Neurosurg. 100, 278–286.

Wolfsberger, S., Kitz, K., Wunderer, J., et al., 2004b. Multiregional sampling reveals a homogenous distribution of Ki-67 proliferation rate in pituitary adenomas. Acta Neurochir. (Wien) 146, 1323–1327.

Youssef, A.S., Agazzi, S., van Loveren, H.R., 2005. Transcranial surgery for pituitary adenomas. Neurosurgery 57, 168–175.

Zee, C.S., Go, J.L., Kim, P.E., et al., 2003. Imaging of the pituitary and parasellar region. Neurosurg. Clin. N. Am. 14, 55–80.

Zhang, X., Fei, Z., Zhang, J., et al., 1999. Management of nonfunctioning pituitary adenomas with suprasellar extensions by transsphenoidal microsurgery. Surg. Neurol. 52, 380–385.

36

Diagnostic considerations and surgical results for hyperfunctioning pituitary adenomas

Edward R. Laws Jr, John A. Jane Jr, and Kamal Thapar

Introduction

Just as pituitary tumors are pathologically, endocrinologically, and biologically a heterogeneous group of lesions, so too are the results of surgery, which vary among the different pituitary tumor sub-types. The results of our series of over 3000 pituitary adenomas are summarized in Table 36.1 (Jane & Laws 2001). The results of surgery and special considerations for each major type of functioning pituitary tumor are discussed below (Figs 36.1–36.3).

Prolactin-producing pituitary adenomas

The prolactinoma is the most common primary tumor of the adenohypophysis and accounts for approximately 30% of all pituitary adenomas encountered in clinical practice. Much has been learned of the natural history of prolactinomas, particularly with regard to their growth potential. From a practical standpoint, prolactinomas can be viewed as having one of two biologic profiles, although this divergence is not reflected in their histopathology (Fig. 36.4). On the one hand, some prolactinomas appear to exist only as microadenomas; they maintain a well defined margin, show little growth potential over time, and appear quite amenable to gross total excision (Fig. 36.5). In contrast, a second and more aggressive phenotype of prolactinoma also exists, one with a definite capacity for progressive growth. Almost always macroadenomas when detected, these latter variants appear far more subject to aggressive, invasive, and recurrent local growth, so much so that attempts at their complete operative removal are frequently ineffective (Figs 36.6, 36.7). Admittedly, these are two extreme forms of the disease, and although the behavior of some prolactinomas can be expected to fall somewhere in between, the clinical profiles of most prolactinomas encountered in clinical practice frequently do assume one of these two phenotypes.

Based on the foregoing clinical observations, together with the almost exclusive presence of microadenomas among autopsy-encountered prolactinomas, it can be inferred that, although all PRL-secreting macroadenomas were once microadenomas, not all microprolactinomas are destined to become macroadenomas. This is an important clinical and conceptual point which has been repeatedly validated by a number of natural history studies. In an early report, wherein 43 patients with microprolactinomas were followed by polytomography and/or early generation CT scanning for a mean duration of 4 years, tumor progression was demonstrated in only two (March et al 1981). Similar results were shown by Weiss and co-workers (1983a) in a 6-year follow-up of 27 untreated patients with microprolactinomas. In this report,

radiologically evident tumor growth was present in only three cases. Sisam and co-workers (1987), using only high resolution CT scanning in all subjects, performed serial scans in 38 patients with microprolactinomas and could not demonstrate progression in a single instance during a mean interval of 50 months. Moreover, in 21 of these 38 patients, the prolactin level fell over the course of the study. In another study, only 2 of 13 patients with a microprolactinoma demonstrated tumor progression over a period of >5 years (Schlechte et al 1989). The conclusions from these and other similar studies is that risk of progression of a micro- to a macroprolactinoma is small, somewhere in the order of 3–7%. Once established, however, the natural history of a macroprolactinoma is unknown, as virtually all such tumors will require therapy of one form or another. There remains a concern about the possibility of a macroprolactinoma enlarging during pregnancy, a phenomenon observed in 5–15% of such patients.

Clinical presentation

Whereas elements of the amenorrhea-galactorrhea syndrome had been known since antiquity, it was not until the twentieth century that clinicians (Forbes and associates in 1954) linked the syndrome with the presence of a pituitary tumor. The eventual isolation and physiologic characterization of prolactin as a distinct pituitary hormone almost two decades later served to validate these prescient observations, providing the pathophysiologic role of prolactin in the genesis of this disease.

The clinical features of PRL-secreting pituitary adenomas relate to the endocrinologic consequences of sustained hyperprolactinemia and/or the neurologic sequelae of an expansile sellar mass. Elevations of PRL appear to affect the pulsatile secretory activity of gonadotrophin-releasing hormone (GnRH) neurons, and so the primary endocrinologic consequence of hyperprolactinemia is hypogonadism. Among women of reproductive age, some form of menstrual dysfunction is almost always the most prominent presenting feature. Typically manifesting as secondary amenorrhea, menstrual dysfunction may also take the form of oligomenorrhea, delayed menarche, and primary amenorrhea, or even regular menses with infertility. Galactorrhea is variably present in 30–80% of these patients. Signs of estrogen deficiency, such as decreased libido and dyspareunia may also be observed, depending on the chronicity of the condition, and osteoporosis may occur. Almost half of affected women also complain of headache, but because most tumors in women are microadenomas, the occurrence of headache does not correlate with tumor size. Similarly unexplained are various psychologic and vegetative symptoms that

Table 36.1 Summary of postoperative remission and recurrence after transsphenoidal surgery for pituitary adenomas. (Authors' series, 1972–2000, n = 3093)

Clinical entity	n[a]	Remission rate[b]	Recurrence[c]
Acromegaly	537	Microadenoma 88%; Macroadenoma 65%	1.3%
Prolactinoma	889	Microadenoma 87%; Macroadenoma 56%	13%
Cushing's disease	490	Microadenoma 91%; Macroadenoma 65%	12% (adults); 42% (children)
Nelson–Salassa syndrome	65	Microadenoma 70%; Macroadenoma 40%	40%
Clinically non-functioning[d] and miscellaneous pituitary adenomas	1073		16% (radiographic); 6% (symptomatic)

[a]Includes total number of cases in each category (micro- and macroadenomas).
[b]Remission criteria as follows: (i) *acromegaly*: basal GH <2.5 ng/mL; GH <1.0 ng/mL on oral glucose tolerance test; and normalization of serum IGF-1 level; (ii) *prolactinoma*: serum PRL level <20 ng/mL; (iii) *Cushing's disease*: normalization of 24 h urinary free cortisol; (iv) *Nelson–Salassa syndrome*: normalization of serum ACTH level.
[c]Recurrence rates based on a cohort of 100 patients in each category, each of whom was followed for a period of 10 or more years.
[d]Among clinically non-functioning tumors, recovery of vision was used as one end point of therapeutic success. Objective changes in visual status were as follows: improved 87%; unchanged 9%; deterioration 4%.

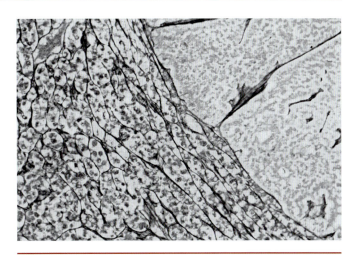

Figure 36.2 Pituitary adenomas: histology. Note the monomorphous population of cells comprising the adenoma and its discrete interface with the normal gland. (Original magnification ×200; reticulin stain.)

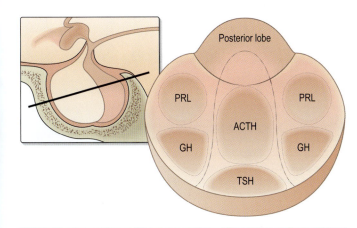

Figure 36.1 Topologic organization of the anterior pituitary gland. The distribution of the various secretory cells in the pituitary is not random – different hormone-secreting cells preferentially accumulate at different intraglandular sites. These locations also roughly correspond to the intraglandular sites of origin for the respective types of pituitary adenomas. Gonadotrophs are diffusely distributed throughout the gland, their tumors arising anywhere within the gland.

occasionally affect women with prolactinomas; these include hostility, depression, anxiety, and weight gain.

Lacking the conspicuous feature of menstrual disturbance to herald their presence, prolactinomas in men and postmenopausal women produce few early symptoms. Most will remain undetected until they become sufficiently large to produce mass effects. Accordingly, men and postmenopausal women typically present with headache and visual dysfunction. Depending on the extent of the tumor, ophthalmoplegia and other neurologic findings may also be present. The frequent large size of these tumors and their

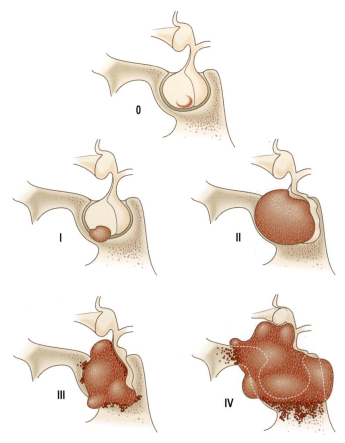

Figure 36.3 Radiologic classification of pituitary adenomas. Pituitary tumors are commonly classified on the basis of their size, invasion status, and growth patterns as proposed by Hardy (1973). Tumors less than 1 cm in diameter are designated as microadenomas whereas larger tumors are designated as macroadenomas. Grade 0: Intrapituitary microadenoma; normal sellar appearance. Grade I: Intrapituitary microadenoma; focal bulging of sellar wall. Grade II: Intrasellar macroadenoma; diffusely enlarged sella; no invasion. Grade III: Macroadenoma; localized sellar invasion and/or destruction. Grade IV: Macroadenoma; extensive sellar invasion and/or destruction. Tumors are further subclassified on the basis of their extrasellar extensions, whether suprasellar or parasellar.

compression of the normal pituitary gland means that hypo-pituitarism of varying degrees is a common accompaniment. As it does in women, PRL excess also produces hypogonad-ism in men; however, seldom does this symptom alone prompt men to seek medical attention. Although reduced libido, impotence, and relative infertility are common and early features of prolactinomas in men, these symptoms are often dismissed as being 'functional' or related to aging by both patient and physician, thus delaying diagnosis until mass effects or hypopituitarism supervene. Galactorrhea may be present in a small proportion of men with hyperpro-

lactinemia, although its demonstration may require vigorous breast manipulation.

A complication common to both men and women with hyperprolactinemia is bone demineralization (Klibanski & Greenspan 1986; Klibanski & Zervas 1991; Schlechte 1995). Once considered a direct consequence of sustained hyperpro-lactinemia, osteoporosis occurring in this setting has been more convincingly correlated with hypogonadism than hyper-prolactinemia per se, and to estrogen deficiency in women.

Laboratory evaluation

The endocrine evaluation of a suspected prolactinoma begins with confirmation of an elevated serum PRL level. In the absence of pregnancy or postpartum lactation, serum PRL levels are normally <20 ng/mL. When markedly elevated (i.e., >200 ng/mL), a single serum PRL determination may

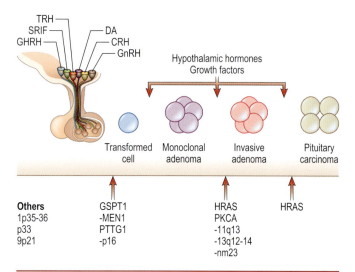

Figure 36.4 Multistep model of pituitary tumorigenesis. The events currently considered important to pituitary tumorigenesis and their presumed temporal occurrence are depicted. This theoretical model assumes a linear progression from indolence to aggressive behavior, but this may not be the case. Biologically aggressive tumors may be aggressive from the outset and may not require staged escalation from indolence. Still, the model is useful in providing some context to data from the literature. If hypothalamic hormones contribute to the process, they most likely do so in the growth/progression of the transformed clone.

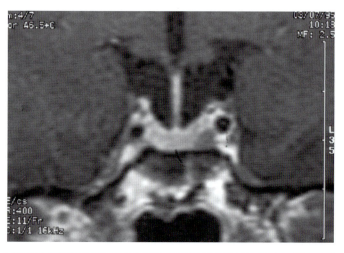

Figure 36.5 Microprolactinoma. Contrast-enhanced coronal MR image showing a discrete low signal area on the left-hand side of the gland corresponding to a microprolactinoma.

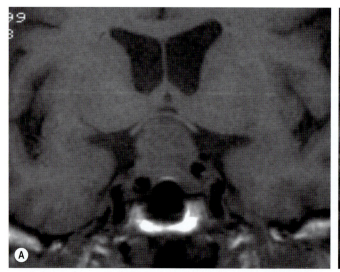

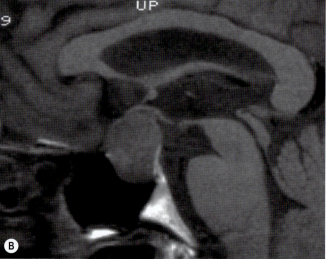

Figure 36.6 Chiasmal compression. Coronal (A) and saggital (B) MR images showing suprasellar extension of a pituitary adenoma with chiasmal compression.

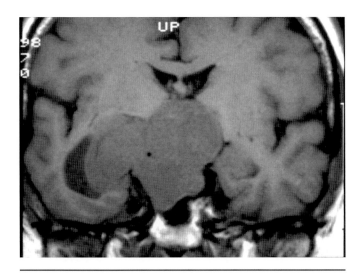

Figure 36.7 Pituitary adenoma. MR image of a giant pituitary adenoma with suprasellar, middle fossa, and infrasellar extension. In a healthy patient in whom gross total resection is the goal, this lesion would require both a transcranial and a transsphenoidal approach.

be diagnostic of prolactinoma; however, lesser elevations often require careful interpretation, as a variety of intrasellar lesions, various systemic disorders, and numerous drugs (i.e., chlorpromazine, haloperidol, metoclopramide, verapamil, cimetidine, and many others) may be associated with moderate hyperprolactinemia. When interpreting serum PRL levels, particular attention should be given to exclude hypothyroidism, chronic renal failure, and cirrhosis, all of which may be accompanied by moderate hyperprolactinemia (Molitch 1992b). In particular, hypothyroidism may be associated with significant pituitary enlargement as the result of thyrotroph hyperplasia, mimicking a tumor. Similarly, a careful history of drug ingestion may also obviate the need for further investigation.

When medical and pharmacologic causes of hyperprolactinemia have been excluded, a lesion involving the sella and/or hypothalamus can generally be inferred and the degree of hyperprolactinemia assumes critical diagnostic importance in discerning the nature of the pathologic process. As a practical rule, serum PRL levels exceeding 200 ng/mL are almost always due to a pure prolactinoma or a mixed pituitary adenoma with a lactotrophic component; PRL levels exceeding 1000 ng/mL indicate an invasive prolactinoma. One caveat must be mentioned regarding the prolactin assay. Prolactin assays are subject to falsely low values when performed on samples with very high prolactin levels. This so-called 'hook effect' generally occurs with large prolactinomas and is resolved by performing the assay with serial dilutions (St-Jean et al 1996).

When PRL levels are <200 ng/mL, the responsible lesion may be a small prolactinoma, but a non-PRL secreting pituitary adenoma, or any of a variety of other neoplastic, inflammatory, or structural lesions in the vicinity of the sella must also be considered in the differential diagnosis (Smith & Laws 1994). Commonly referred to as 'pseudoprolactinomas' these lesions generate moderate hyperprolactinemia on the basis of the 'stalk section effect'. It is important to recognize that the magnitude of PRL elevations produced by prolactinomas is roughly proportional to their size. Accordingly, in the setting of a macroadenoma accompanied by only moderately elevated PRL values, the lesion is most apt to be a pseudoprolactinoma; a true macroprolactinoma would be expected to have much higher PRL levels, well above the 200 ng/mL threshold.

Treatment

Therapeutic options for prolactinomas include pharmacologic control, surgical resection, and radiation therapy. As a result of substantial clinical experience, particularly during the past decade, each of these treatment modalities has been subjected to comprehensive study. What has emerged is a fairly accurate appraisal of their individual merits and limitations, and some consensus on the clinical indications for each. Still, factors such as tumor size, degree of hyperprolactinemia, clinical presentation, and patient preference all afford the treating physician some latitude in selecting therapeutic strategies, particularly from the standpoint of medical versus surgical therapy.

Medical therapy

Prolactinomas were the first pituitary tumors for which medical therapy had a proven and primary role. In fact, the consistency with which dopamine agonists normalize PRL levels, restore fertility, and reduce tumor mass, has legitimized their use as the initial therapy for most patients with prolactinomas.

The mechanism of action of dopaminergic agents – bromocriptine being the prototypical example – involves selective activation of type 2 (D2) dopamine receptors located on the lactotroph cell surface. The resultant intracellular response includes suppression of adenylate cyclase activity, reduction in cAMP levels, and quenching of intracellular calcium levels, events which all appear directly coupled to inhibition of prolactin synthesis and release. Additional mechanistic insights into the action of these agents are provided by histopathologic and ultrastructural studies of prolactinomas preoperatively treated with bromocriptine or other dopaminergic drugs. Among responsive tumors, a marked reduction in cellular cytoplasmic volume is readily seen, indicating that cytoplasmic loss is the prime factor accounting for tumor shrinkage induced by such therapy. An additional cellular target is the secretory apparatus, as evidenced by involution of the rough endoplasmic reticulum and Golgi complexes (Kovacs & Horvath 1986; Tindall et al 1982). At a sub-cellular level, dopaminergic agents reduce PRL gene transcription and translation, as demonstrated by diminished expression of PRL mRNA transcripts and the loss of PRL immunoreactivity, respectively (Kovacs et al 1991). Finally, as revealed by PET scanning *in vivo*, the overall metabolic activity of responsive tumors is dramatically reduced (Muhr et al 1991). With protracted use, dopaminergic agents may induce varying degrees of calcification, amyloid deposition, and both perivascular and interstitial fibrosis. The latter, if extensive, may adversely affect future attempts at operative removal (Bevan et al 1987; Landolt et al 1982).

With regard to the aforementioned pharmacologic effects, two additional points merit specific attention. First, although a favorable response to dopaminergic agents can be expected in most patients, there is a spectrum of therapeutic responsiveness. Among the most dramatically responsive tumors, a significant reduction in serum PRL levels, objective visual improvement, and radiologically evident tumor shrinkage may be demonstrated within hours (Spark & Dickstein 1979), days (Chiodini et al 1981), and weeks (Fahlbusch et al 1987) of initiating therapy. Alternatively, a small proportion of tumors are fully resistant to dopaminergic agents, showing a reduction neither in PRL levels nor in tumor size. In some such examples, dopamine receptor or post-receptor defects have been demonstrated (Pellegrini et al 1989). The second important issue is that all the pharmacologic effects of these agents, perhaps with the exception of fibrotic change, are fully reversible upon cessation of dopaminergic therapy. Accordingly, such pharmacotherapy cannot be regarded as tumoricidal. Instead, such therapy provides a means for pharmacologic control; the long-term effectiveness of dopaminergic therapy requires its ongoing use. Almost without exception, withdrawal of therapy virtually guarantees a prompt return to the pretreatment state, both in terms of tumor re-expansion and recurrence of hyperprolactinemia. There are reports, however, of regression and apparent cure of microprolactinomas after some years of successful dopamine agonist therapy (Colao et al 2003).

Numerous reports have established the effectiveness of bromocriptine and related dopaminergic agents (pergolide mesylate, lisuride, cabergoline, and the non-ergot agent, quinagolide) in the treatment of prolactinomas. Pergolide is no longer recommended for this indication and lisuride is not being used. Some concern is present regarding cardiac valvular disease produced by cabergoline (Horvath et al 2004), but it is still considered the most effective agent, and normal recommended doses have been considered safe.

In a cumulative review of 13 reported series involving 286 hyperprolactinemic women treated with primary bromocriptine therapy, 64–100% experienced normalization of PRL levels, and 57–100% had resumption of menses and documented ovulation (Vance et al 1984; Vance & Thorner 1987). In another comprehensive review in which data were compiled from 19 published series involving 236 patients, Molitch (1992b) observed that bromocriptine reduced tumor size to some extent in 77% of patients. Cabergoline is equally if not more effective in producing prolactinoma shrinkage (Webster et al 1994).

Given the proven effectiveness of dopaminergic therapy in a wide range of clinical settings, the indications for its use in prolactinoma management are both broad and comprehensive. In fact, in all but a few selected instances of prolactinoma, dopaminergic therapy is often the most appropriate first choice (Klibanski & Zervas 1991). Among macroadenomas, its immediate effectiveness is, at the least, comparable to surgical therapy, and its long-term effectiveness may even be better. Various reports have shown that 70–100% of microprolactinomas will respond favorably to bromocriptine, with normalization of PRL levels, diminished galactorrhea, restored fertility, and reduction in tumor size (Corenblum & Taylor 1983; Johnston et al 1983; Jordan & Kohler 1987; Klibanski & Zervas 1991; Molitch 1992b; Vance et al 1984; Vance & Thorner 1987; Winfield et al

1984). Among macroadenomas, dopamine agonists have clearly eclipsed operative treatment as the most effective form of therapy. In a prospective trial of 27 patients with macroprolactinomas receiving only bromocriptine, PRL levels were normalized in 67%, and a ≥50% reduction in tumor volume was achieved in half of all patients (Molitch et al 1985).

Surgical treatment

Once the primary mode of therapy for prolactinomas, operative treatment has been justifiably usurped by dopaminergic therapy. Despite its secondary and more selective role in prolactinoma management, surgery remains an essential component of the therapeutic armamentarium against these tumors, as there are a number of situations in which surgery will be the most appropriate first-line option and, in some instances, the only effective option (Figs 36.8–36.14) (Hamilton et al 2005; Thapar & Laws 1998).

The indications for surgical management of prolactinomas are several (Box 36.1). One of the clearest indications

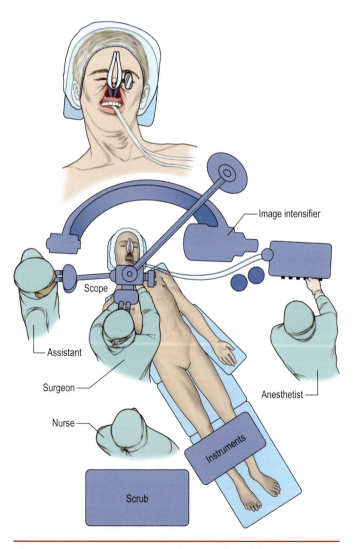

Figure 36.8 Operating room set up for transsphenoidal surgery.

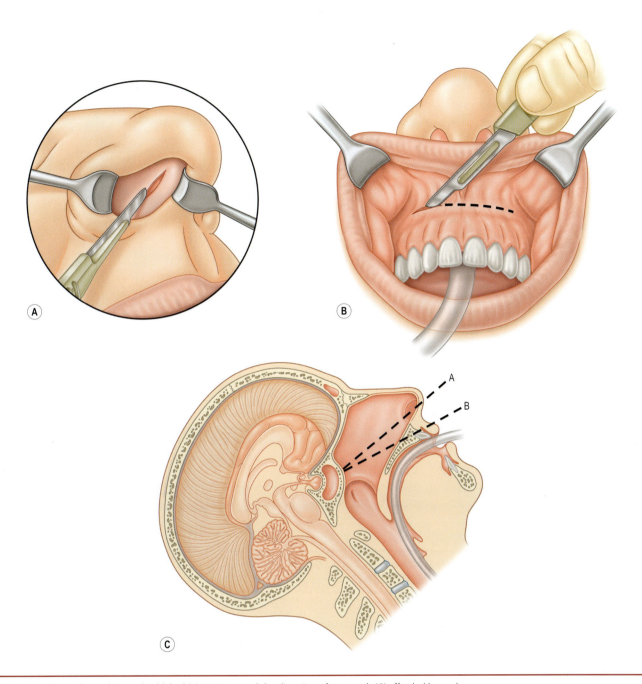

Figure 36.9 The endonasal (A) and sublabial (B) incisions and the direction of approach (C) afforded by each.

for operative intervention is pituitary apoplexy. When MRI indicates that the bulk of the tumor is composed of hemorrhagic and/or necrotic material, dopamine agonists are unlikely to provide a satisfactory reduction in tumor volume. Cystic prolactinomas, sharing a similarly poor volumetric response to dopaminergic agents, are often best treated surgically (Fig 36.15). A small percentage of patients will be intolerant of the side-effects of dopamine agonist agents. In these situations, surgery is indicated and can be highly successful.

Another indication is resistance to dopaminergic therapy. Resistance usually manifests in one of two ways. The first is when the prolactin levels fail to normalize. In such a situation, there is still a risk that the patient may suffer the adverse effects of hyperprolactinemia and there is the threat that the tumor may continue to enlarge despite continued pharmacologic management (Fig. 36.16). The second type of hyporesponder is the patient who has a good response to medical management in terms of normalization of hyperprolactinemia; however, there is little or no volumetric response and mass effects remain. Included in such situations are the pseudoprolactinomas, sellar masses other than genuine prolactinomas that produce hyperprolactinemia on the basis of stalk compression. Both types of hyporesponders represent legitimate indications for surgical management. Analysis of the results of surgical management of hyporesponders in our

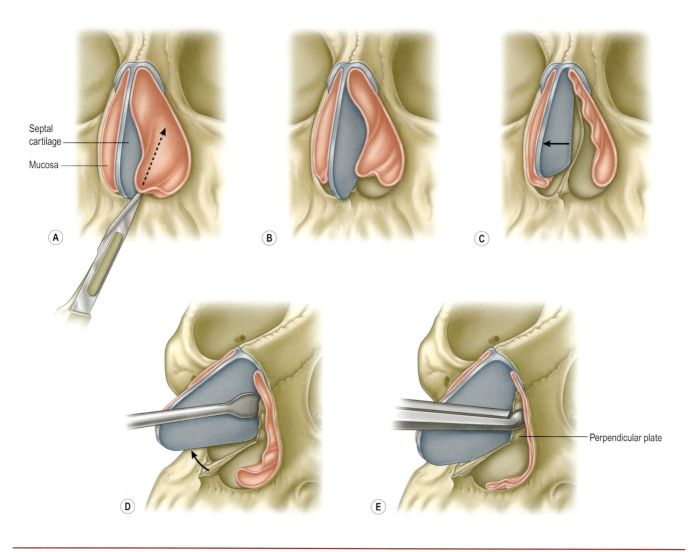

Septal
cartilage

Mucosa

Perpendicular plate

Figure 36.10 The nasal tunnels are connected (A) and elevated (B). Displacement of the nasal septum to the right (C) and disarticulation from the maxillary ridge (D). Removal of the perpendicular plate of the ethmoid (E).

Box 36.1 Surgical indications for prolactinomas

MICROPROLACTINOMAS

- Resistance or suboptimal response to dopamine agonist therapy
- Intolerance to dopamine agonist therapy
- Patient preference against long-term dopamine agonist therapy

MACROPROLACTINOMAS

- Pituitary apoplexy
- Cystic prolactinoma
- Resistance or suboptimal response to dopamine agonist therapy
- Reduction of tumor burden as an adjuvant to enhancing the effectiveness of dopamine agonist therapy, radiotherapy, or radiosurgery
- A prolactinoma with extensive erosion into the sphenoid sinus, wherein the risk of a CSF leak is high with dopamine agonist-induced tumor shrinkage
- In the female patient desiring pregnancy, surgery is undertaken with the objective of reducing the eventual risk of pregnancy-induced tumor enlargement
- Mass effects presenting during pregnancy
- When the diagnosis of prolactinoma is uncertain and a tissue diagnosis is required.

series has shown encouraging effectiveness in up to 36% of such patients (Hamilton et al 2005).

Surgery may also be indicated in the patient with a large invasive prolactinoma in whom a successful response to dopaminergic therapy can be anticipated, but in whom extensive erosion of the skull base may be the source of a CSF leak with pharmacologic tumor shrinkage. As discussed below, surgical issues and indications also arise in the context of infertility and planned or established pregnancy; these are discussed in a subsequent section.

The strongest argument in favor of surgical resection for prolactinomas has been, and continues to be, that surgery is potentially a definitive mode of therapy which, in contradistinction to medical therapy, provides the only opportunity for potential 'cure'. In actual fact, however, long-term curative resections are achieved in only a minority of patients with macroprolactinomas, and among all prolactinomas of all sizes, 'curative' resections are associated with a progressive recurrence rate over time.

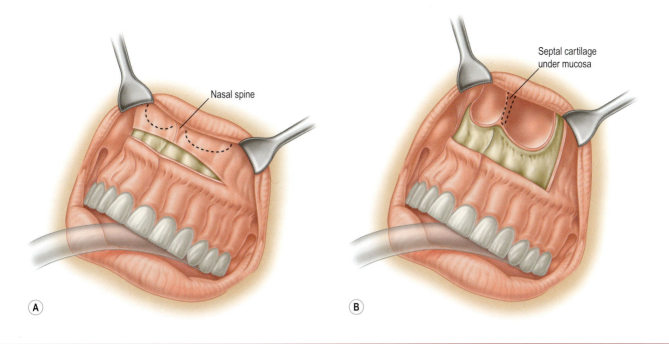

Figure 36.11 The sublabial approach. Relationships of the initial incision (A) and exposure of the pyriform aperture and the cartilaginous septum (B).

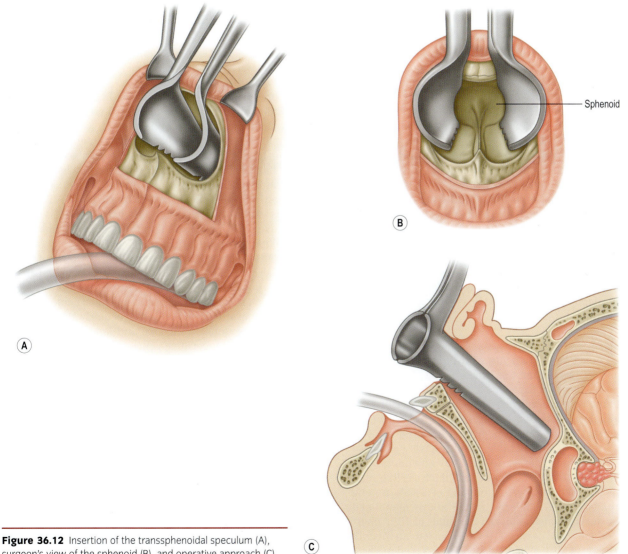

Figure 36.12 Insertion of the transsphenoidal speculum (A), surgeon's view of the sphenoid (B), and operative approach (C).

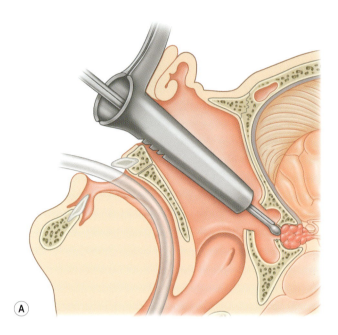
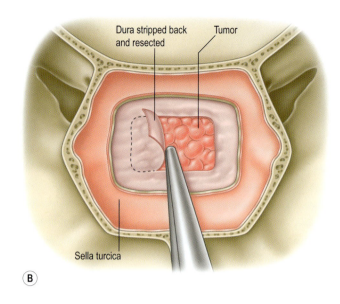

Figure 36.13 Removal of the floor of the sella (A), and opening of the dural window (B).

Microadenomas

The rate of curative resections, as defined by postoperative normalization of PRL levels, is highest among microadenomas, particularly those accompanied by PRL levels <100 ng/mL. In the Mayo Clinic series involving 100 patients with prolactinomas, 32 of which met these criteria, normalization of PRL levels was achieved in 88% (Randall et al 1983). Larger tumors and/or those accompanied by higher PRL elevations suffered a dramatic reduction in surgical cure rate. Among microadenomas having preoperative PRL levels in excess of 100 ng/mL, a curative result was observed in only 50%. Similar results have been reported by others (Landolt 1981). In his summary of 31 published series involving 1224 patients with microprolactinomas, Molitch (1992b) calculated an overall endocrinologic cure rate of 71.2%, independent of preoperative PRL levels. Similarly, in a multicenter international survey involving 1518 patients with microprolactinomas, Zervas (1984) reported an overall surgical cure rate of 74%.

Macroadenomas

The surgical outcome for patients with PRL-secreting macroadenomas has proved far less encouraging. In a second report of the Mayo Clinic experience, only 53% of surgically treated patients with macroadenomas experienced normalization of PRL levels. Among locally invasive macroadenomas, the surgical cure rate was further reduced to 28% (Randall et al 1985). Comparable results have been also shown in other surgical series. In the above-mentioned literature review of 31 published series, Molitch (1992b) calculated an overall curative resection rate of 31.8% among 1256 macroadenomas. Similarly, in the above mentioned international survey which analyzed outcomes of 1022 operated macroadenomas, Zervas (1984) reported an overall surgical cure rate of 30%. Of patients who have failed medical therapy, relief of mass effects can be expected in the overwhelming majority, even though biochemical remission is not easily achieved.

The preoperative serum PRL level has proven an especially reliable predictor of surgical outcome as the degree of hyperprolactinemia reflects both the size and invasiveness of the tumor. As a general rule, curative resection rates drop precipitously when preoperative PRL levels exceed 200 ng/mL. This has been validated by several series wherein surgical cure rates varied between 74% and 88% when PRL levels were below this threshold, but dropped to 18–47% when PRL levels exceeded 200 ng/mL (Molitch 1992b). When the preoperative PRL level exceeds 1000 ng/mL, seldom does surgery alone result in cure.

Whereas preoperative PRL levels are predictive of potential surgical curability, PRL determinations obtained in the immediate postoperative period are useful indicators of whether or not surgical cure actually has been achieved. Subnormal postoperative PRL levels, particularly those <10 ng/mL, virtually guarantee a durable and long-lasting curative result. Although postoperative values between 11 and 20 ng/mL also qualify as 'curative', these patients appear to be at some risk for future tumor recurrence (Serri et al 1983).

As a strategy to improve surgical outcomes in prolactinomas, some have suggested that preoperative treatment with dopamine agonists may improve operative results. In one retrospective report examining the surgical outcomes of 20 patients with bromocriptine pretreatment and 20 patients treated with surgery alone, bromocriptine treatment was associated with more favorable outcomes among both microprolactinomas (87% vs 50%) and macroadenomas (33% vs 17%) (Perrin et al 1991). The report of Weiss and co-workers (1983b) suggests a similar trend. In 10 of 19 macroadenomas pretreated with bromocriptine, tumor shrinkage of >30% was noted, and subsequent surgery resulted in

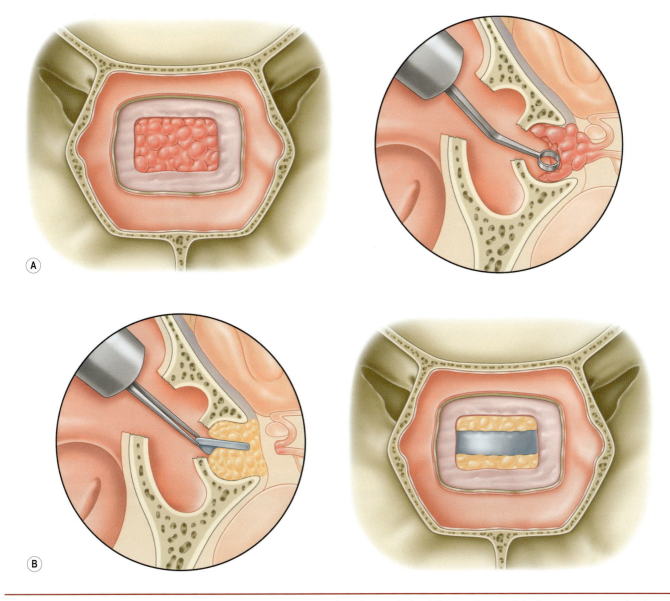

Figure 36.14 Removal of the adenoma with a ring curette (A). At closure, the sella is packed with fat or Gelfoam and the floor is reconstructed with a stent of nasal cartilage (B).

normalization of PRL levels in 70%. Of the remaining nine patients in whom bromocriptine failed to induce shrinkage of this degree, only 22% had normalization of PRL levels with surgery. In other reports, no beneficial effect of bromocriptine pretreatment has been observed (Hubbard et al 1987; Wilson 1984). Although this concept of medical pretreatment has theoretical appeal, our experience suggests that improvements in surgical results with this strategy, if they occur at all, are modest at best.

Postoperative recurrence

In evaluating the overall effectiveness of surgical therapy, some consideration must be given to the issue of tumor recurrence (Laws & Thapar 1996; Thomson et al 1994; Thomson et al 2002). Ordinarily, tumor recurrence manifests endocrinologically with return of hyperprolactinemia;

radiologically evident tumor regrowth is neither necessarily, nor, for that matter, commonly present. The reported frequency of biochemical recurrence has varied greatly. Serri and co-workers (1983) reported recurrence rates of 50% for microadenomas and 80% for macroadenomas, following mean remission periods of 4 years and 2.5 years, respectively. Although this is one of the most carefully performed and most frequently quoted studies to date, these recurrence rates are among the highest in the literature. In his review, Molitch (1992b) observed more favorable results; recurrent hyperprolactinemia was observed in 17.4% (82/471) of microadenomas and in 18.6% (48/235) of macroadenomas. Similarly, Post and Habas (1990) reported 17% and 20% recurrence rates for microadenomas and macroadenomas, respectively, for patients followed longer than 5 years. These data more accurately approximate our own experience.

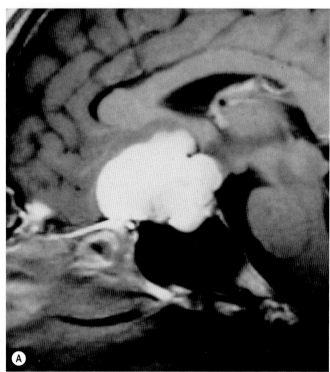
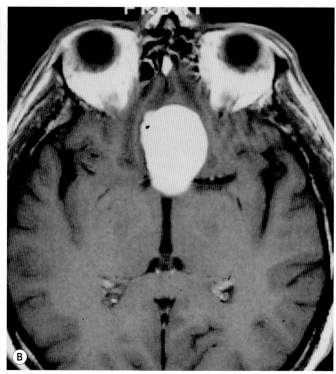

Figure 36.15 Pituitary adenoma. MR images of a cystic non-functioning pituitary adenoma for which a transcranial approach is preferable to a transsphenoidal approach. The large suprasellar component with an anterior extension, the relatively small sella, and preoperative uncertainty of the pathologic diagnosis are all indications for a transcranial approach to this lesion.

Worthy of reiteration is the fact that, in the majority of 'recurrences', particularly in the setting of microprolactinomas, the relapse tends to be biochemical rather than radiologic. For example, in a 10-year follow-up study of 58 women with macroprolactinomas, all of whom were successfully treated with transsphenoidal surgery, 43% experienced a relapse of moderate hyperprolactinemia; only two patients showed imaging evidence of tumor recurrence (Massoud et al 1996). This peculiar phenomenon of delayed hyperprolactinemia is poorly understood and is believed to be a variant of the 'stalk section effect'. In most instances, the hyperprolactinemia is only of a modest degree, is not always symptomatic, may spontaneously resolve, is only rarely associated with radiologically evident recurrence, and does not necessarily warrant therapy.

Surgical issues relating to fertility and pregnancy

Prolactinomas pose three basic problems with regard to planned or established pregnancy: (Alexander et al 1980) infertility; (Arafah et al 1980) risk of tumor growth during pregnancy; and (Assie et al 2007) effects of therapy on fetal development. Hyperplasia of normal pituitary lactotrophs is a normal physiologic response during pregnancy and one that is associated with a doubling in size of the normal pituitary. It follows that a corresponding response may also occur in neoplastic lactotrophs, producing an increase in tumor size. For microadenomas, the risk of tumor enlargement is small, symptomatic enlargement occurring in 1.6% of cases and radiologically evident enlargement occurring in 4.5% (Molitch 1985). In contrast, macroadenomas have

a significantly greater propensity for pregnancy induced growth, as symptomatic and asymptomatic enlargement occurs in 15.5% and 8.5% of cases, respectively (Molitch 1985). Among macroadenomas that have previously undergone surgical or radiotherapeutic ablation prior to pregnancy, the risk of regrowth during pregnancy is significantly less (4.3%).

In the patient with a microprolactinoma who desires pregnancy, both bromocriptine and surgery have comparable rates (80–85%) of restoring fertility. In patients treated with bromocriptine, therapy should be stopped at the first sign of pregnancy. Cabergoline is not approved for women desiring pregnancy. Such patients should have careful clinical examinations throughout pregnancy to identify the very exceptional microadenoma that might enlarge. Because PRL levels normally rise during the first trimester, these are not informative with regard to the status of the tumor.

In the patient with a macroprolactinoma who desires pregnancy, several management options exist, each of which is directed at avoiding the 15–35% risk of tumor enlargement that occurs during pregnancy. The more conservative approach, one preferable in our opinion, begins with primary resection of the macroprolactinoma with the objective of a curative resection. Should hyperprolactinemia and ovulatory failure persist postoperatively, bromocriptine is used to restore fertility. Pregnancy in this setting will be associated with a greatly reduced risk (4.5%) of tumor expansion. A second approach involves treating the patient initially with dopamine agonists to restore fertility, withdrawing therapy at the first sign of pregnancy, and carefully monitoring the

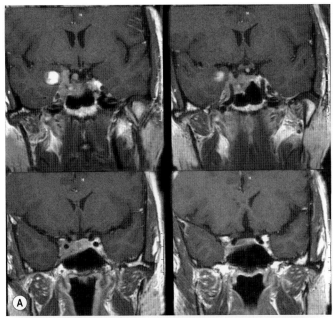

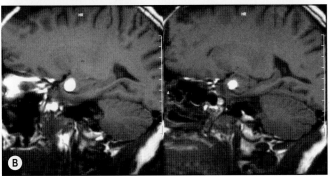

Figure 36.16 Prolactinoma. MR images of a prolactin-secreting macroadenoma which failed to respond to maximal therapy with dopamine agonists, necessitating transcranial decompression.

patient throughout the pregnancy with serial clinical and neuro-ophthalmologic evaluations. Should symptomatic tumor enlargement occur, the options include urgent surgical resection or reinstitution of bromocriptine for the duration of the pregnancy.

Growth hormone-secreting pituitary adenomas

Clinical features

Somatotroph adenomas affect men and women with roughly similar frequency, most cases being diagnosed within the 4th and 5th decades. Their clinical features are referable to either tumor mass effect or the endocrinologic sequelae of GH excess. Local effects are of particular concern in acromegaly because the relative proportion of macroadenomas (>60%) is substantially higher than that observed with other hormonally active pituitary tumors (Scheithauer et al 1986; Thapar et al 1995). Endocrine manifestations are, however,

the most conspicuous feature of the disease and provide the usual basis for presentation. The endocrinopathy of pathologic GH excess assumes one of two clinically related phenotypes. The first and more common of the two is acromegaly, the result of sustained GH excess, which begins or persists beyond puberty. Should GH excess manifest prior to epiphyseal closure, a more proportioned increase in linear growth termed 'gigantism' is the result.

Growth hormone has a wide spectrum of physiologic action, and the endocrine manifestations of acromegaly are correspondingly diverse. Major areas of pathologic involvement include changes in skin and connective tissues, abnormalities of musculoskeletal, cardiovascular, and respiratory systems, and impaired glucose tolerance. Despite the multisystem nature of the process and the often dramatic physical transformation that eventually typifies active acromegaly, the disease is seldom diagnosed at an early stage. Instead, acromegaly is an insidiously progressive condition wherein the mean interval between disease onset and diagnosis is approximately 8.7 years (Molitch 1992a).

Virtually all patients at presentation have some overgrowth of bone and soft tissues, usually occurring at characteristic body locations. Facial features become classically coarse, with thickening of the lips, exaggeration of the nasolabial folds, fleshy enlargement of the nose, and the development of a corrugated and highly furrowed scalp. Frontal bossing, prognathism, maxillary widening, and dental malocclusion and increased spacing between the teeth render the appearance unmistakable. The voice assumes a low and deeply resonant pitch, a finding related to laryngeal hypertrophy and enlargement of paranasal sinuses, which may also contribute to snoring and sleep apnea. Macroglossia, a common accompaniment, is also the result of soft tissue overgrowth and reflects the generalized visceromegaly seen with acromegaly. Exuberant soft tissue hypertrophy also accounts for the fleshy spade-like enlargement of the hands and feet, as evidenced by increased hand volume and heel pad thickness, respectively. Hypertrophy of sweat and sebaceous glands results in excessively oily and malodorous perspiration. Musculoskeletal abnormalities, particularly arthropathies, are prominent and among the more disabling components of acromegaly. Periosteal new bone formation leads to elongation and widening of vertebral bodies which, together with osteophyte formation and degeneration of intervertebral discs, leads to kyphotic deformity and crippling spinal stenosis. The epiphyses of costochondral junctions fail to close, resulting in elongation of a characteristic barrel chest deformity. Arthropathy occurs in approximately 70% of acromegalic patients. In up to half of these, symptoms are sufficiently severe that normal daily activities are limited. Weight-bearing joints such as the knees and hips are most often involved. Proliferation of articular cartilage, ulceration and fissuring at weight bearing points, new bone formation, and synovial thickening eventually give way to a crippling and often irreversible osteoarthritis. Cardiovascular complications, present in about one-third of acromegalic patients, can be sources of significant morbidity and mortality. Hypertension, cardiomyopathy, and arrhythmia are the processes responsible. A possible association between acromegaly and the development of malignant tumors, particularly colonic carcinomas, has been a smoldering concern for some time. Although two large retrospective reviews of acromegalic patients failed to show any increase risk of malignancy (Mustacchi & Shimkin 1957; Nabarro 1987), several reports have established a potential link (Ezzat & Melmed 1991; Ezzat et al 1991). There is now some consensus that acromegaly is in fact associated with an increased risk of colon cancer or premalignant polyps, perhaps in the order of a 3–8-fold excess risk. Skin tags are believed to be a peripheral marker of colonic polyps; they are present in virtually all patients in whom colonic polyps have been demonstrated. It has been suggested that important risk factors for colon cancer in acromegaly include: male gender, age >50 years, a positive family history for colon cancer, more than three skin tags, and a prior history of colonic polyps (Ezzat & Melmed 1991; Ezzat et al 1991).

That acromegaly is a condition which reduces life expectancy has been validated by three detailed epidemiologic studies (Alexander et al 1980; Bengtsson et al 1988; Wright et al 1970). Over the period of one study, Wright and co-workers (1970) observed that the death rate among acromegalic patients was more than twice that of a control population. Cardiovascular disease, cerebrovascular disease, malignant tumors, and respiratory disease accounted for 24%, 15%, 15.5%, and 15.5% of deaths, respectively. Comparable results were obtained from a second study from the Newcastle region of the UK, wherein the respective mortality rates among male and female acromegalics were 4.8 and 2.4 times those of a control population (Alexander et al 1980). In the Göteborg region of Sweden, acromegalic patients suffered a three-fold increase in mortality. Again, vascular disease and malignancy figured prominently as causes of premature death (Bengtsson et al 1988). It appears that prevention or reversal of the cardiovascular complications associated with acromegaly requires therapy that reduces circulating GH levels to <2.5 ng/mL (Bates et al 1993; Swearingen et al 1998).

Endocrine diagnosis

Although the clinical phenotype is often characteristic, GH excess must be documented on careful endocrine testing. Consensus diagnostic endocrine criteria include: (Alexander et al 1980) elevated basal GH level (>2.5 ng/mL); (Arafah et al 1980) insufficient GH suppressibility on oral glucose tolerance testing (>0.8 ng/mL) ; and (Assie et al 2007) elevation of serum insulin-like growth factor 1 (IGF-1) levels (Bonadonna et al 2005; Force 2004; Freda et al 1998a,b; Giustina et al 2000; Growth Hormone Research Society & Pituitary Society 2004; Melmed et al 2002). Whereas fulfillment of these criteria does establish a state of GH excess which, in the overwhelming majority of instances will imply the presence of a somatotroph adenoma, one is wise to not automatically make this assumption, even in the presence of a radiologically evident sellar mass. As a rule, one should always consider the remote possibility of ectopic acromegaly wherein GH excess is the result of a rare extrapituitary growth hormone-releasing hormone (GHRH) producing tumor. Although numerically quite insignificant in the broader context of acromegaly, this rare cohort of GHRH-producing lesions is diagnostically important. These include

GHRH-producing carcinoid tumors in the gastrointestinal tract or lung, pancreatic islet cell tumors, small cell carcinoma of the lung, and, rarely, pheochromocytomas (Faglia et al 1992). As a result of their GHRH production, these lesions induce somatotroph hyperplasia with resultant sellar enlargement, GH excess, and clinical acromegaly that is phenotypically indistinguishable from that due to a somatotroph adenoma. Hypothalamic hamartomas and gangliocytomas may also induce elevated GH levels and acromegaly (Scheithauer et al 1986). Failure to consider and exclude these ectopically secreting variants as potential causes of acromegaly can lead to inappropriate therapy, delaying recognition of an underlying and potentially aggressive neoplasm for which acromegaly may be the only early manifestation (Faglia et al 1992). If suspected, the diagnosis of an ectopic GHRH-producing lesion can be confirmed by radioimmunoassay; such lesions will produce measurable elevations in plasma GHRH levels (Thorner 1999).

In approximately one-third of patients, modest elevations of serum prolactin levels will also be seen. In some instances the elevation represents a 'stalk section effect' whereas, in others, it will reflect prolactin hypersecretion from a plurihormonal somatotroph adenoma. Finally, since somatotroph adenomas are a well known component of several genetic syndromes (the autosomal dominant multiple endocrine neoplasia type 1 syndrome [pituitary, parathyroid, and pancreatic islet cell tumors], Carney complex, McCune-Albright syndrome, and familial acromegaly), the endocrine evaluation should be directed at identifying or excluding these conditions (Horvath & Stratakis 2008; O'Brien et al 1996; Scheithauer et al 1987).

Treatment

The menu of potential treatment options for somatotroph adenomas is more extensive than that for any other type of pituitary tumor. Each effective to varying degrees in various situations, surgical resection, medical therapy with somatostatin analogs, dopamine agonists, growth hormone receptor antagonists, radiation therapy, and radiosurgery, all afford the treating physician some latitude in providing a comprehensive, and frequently sequential, management plan for the acromegalic patient. No one form of therapy is uniformly effective, and so combination therapy figures prominently in the management of this disease.

Surgery

For the majority of patients presenting with acromegaly, surgical resection will represent the initial treatment of choice. The effectiveness of surgery will depend on a number of factors, including tumor size and invasion status, and preoperative GH levels. In the most favorable circumstances, such as those involving non-invasive intrasellar microadenomas with basal GH levels <45 ng/mL, surgery alone can prove curative (Fig. 36.17). In other instances, such as those involving some invasive macroadenomas and those with preoperative GH levels in excess of 50 ng/mL, curative resection may still represent a reasonable operative goal, although the possibility of inaccessible tumor remnants, persistent GH hypersecretion, and the potential need for eventual adjuvant therapy is recognized from the outset (Laws et al 1979;

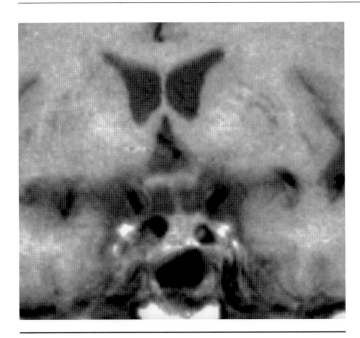

Figure 36.17 Somatotroph microadenoma. In the coronal MR image in an acromegalic patient, a small microadenoma adjacent to the carotid artery is seen, as well as the narrow interval between the two carotid arteries which represents a potential operative hazard for the transsphenoidal approach.

Shimon et al 2001). Finally, there is the least favorable situation wherein one is confronted with a tumor whose size and invasiveness have clearly exceeded the limits of surgical resectability. For such tumors, surgical resection is undertaken primarily for the relief of mass effects. In doing so, tumor burden is also reduced, thus possibly enhancing the effectiveness of adjuvant pharmacologic and/or radiation therapies.

In the overwhelming majority of surgically treated acromegalic patients, including all those in whom biochemical remission has been achieved, as well as those in whom GH levels have been significantly reduced but not normalized, prompt regression of several symptoms can be expected postoperatively. Headache frequently improves immediately and, over the next few days, is followed by improvements in hyperhydrosis, paresthesias, and regression of soft tissue swelling. Such responses tend to be the rule, being observed to some degree in 97% of surgically treated patients (Laws 1990). Diabetes mellitus also responds to surgery in a predictably favorable fashion; for patients in whom GH levels are normalized, resolution of diabetes and/or glucose intolerance has been reported in up to 80–100% of cases (Balagura et al 1981; Tucker et al 1980). Significant improvements in glucose tolerance can also be expected in patients in whom surgery reduces, but fails to normalize, GH levels. Hypertension tends to be considerably less responsive to surgery than other acromegalic features (Balagura et al 1981; Tucker et al 1980). Although some improvement in blood pressure has been noted postoperatively, hypertension often persists, sometimes even after successful surgery.

Hyperprolactinemia, accompanying some 40–50% of somatotroph adenomas, is frequently the result of a bihormonal tumor capable of both GH and PRL hypersecretion.

In acromegalic women of child bearing age, approximately half will have amenorrhea (Nabarro 1987). We previously reported on series of six such amenorrheic females, of whom four experienced postoperative resumption of menses; two of these eventually conceived (Laws et al 1979). A comparable response has been reported by others (Arafah et al 1980).

Symptomatic mass effects can be expected to respond to surgery in the majority of instances. Improvements in visual fields have been reported in 90–100% of patients (Grisoli et al 1985; Laws et al 1977).

Defining endocrinologic remission

Although it has been recognized for some time that the completeness of surgical resection must ultimately be judged on the basis of measurable endocrinologic parameters, there has been a distinct lack of uniformity in the specific endocrinologic criteria that investigators have used to define remission or 'cure'. This concept of 'cure' in acromegaly has evolved considerably, and some consensus now exists as to the minimum biochemical criteria that must underlie its definition (Bonadonna et al 2005; Force 2004; Freda et al 1998a,b; Giustina et al 2000; Growth Hormone Research Society & Pituitary Society 2004; Melmed et al 2002). First, it is preferable to speak in terms of remission rather than 'cure', as the long-term outcome of surgically treated somatotroph adenomas is still not definitively known and no endocrinologic criteria, however stringent, can absolutely guarantee that the patient will remain permanently free of disease. Currently, and in addition to a favorable clinical response, the operational definition of endocrinologic remission in acromegaly requires normalization of age-adjusted plasma IGF-1 levels. Those who also achieve a normal nadir GH level during an OGTT (<0.14 µg/mL) appear to have a significantly lower rate of recurrent elevation in IGF-1 levels compared with those whose nadir remains above 0.14 µg/mL (Freda et al 2004; Freda et al 1998a). In virtually all instances, patients fulfilling these criteria will also have basal GH levels of <2.5 ng/mL, but since the converse is often, but not necessarily true, there has been a move away from using the latter, or for that matter, any specific basal or random GH level as the sole remission criterion (Kreutzer et al 2001). If remission is to be based on any critical GH level, the only prognostically justifiable criterion is a mean GH level <2.5 ng/mL. As discussed previously, reductions of mean GH levels below this threshold have been identified as the most important factor associated with reducing mortality in acromegaly (Bates et al 1993). Accordingly, if lowering of GH levels is to be used as a measure of surgical success, reduction below this value would, in this context, represent a reasonable therapeutic end point.

Reported rates of endocrine remission

These are summarized in Table 36.2, which includes only studies that use current consensus biochemical criteria (Beauregard et al 2003; Biermasz et al 2000b; De et al 2003; Freda et al 1998b; Gittoes et al 1999; Kreutzer et al 2001; Labat-Moleur et al 1991; Losa et al 1989; Nomikos et al 2005; Shimon et al 2001; Swearingen et al 1998; Tindall et al 1993; Trepp et al 2005). Tumor size and invasion status

Table 36.2 Results of primary transsphenoidal surgery for GH-secreting pituitary adenomas (remission rates)

Series	n	Total series	Microadenoma	Macroadenoma	Remission criteria
Losa et al 1989	29	16/29 (55%)	N/A	N/A	Nadir GH <1 ng/mL with OGTT *and* normal IGF-1 level
Tindall et al 1993[a]	91	75/91 (82%)	N/A	N/A	GH ≤5 ng/mL *and/or* normal IGF-1 level
Freda et al 1998[b]	115	61%	88%	53%	Nadir GH ≤2 ng/mL with OGTT and/or normal IGF-1
Swearingen et al 1998	162	57%	91%	48%	IGF-1 or nadir GH <2 ng/mL with OGTT
Gittoes et al 1999	66	64%	86%	52%	Random GH <2.5 ng/mL or nadir GH <1 ng/mL with OGTT
Biermasz et al 2000b	59	67%	6/8 (75%)	33/50 (66%)	Nadir GH <1 ng/mL with OGTT
Kreutzer et al 2001	57	61.1% OGTT; 70.2% IGF-1			Nadir GH <1 ng/mL with OGTT or normal IGF-1
Shimon et al 2001	98	74%	84%	64%	Repeated fasting or nadir GH <2 ng/mL with OGTT or normal IGF-1
Beauregard et al 2003	99	56/99 (57%)	82%	Macro: 60% Invasive: 24%	Random GH <2.5 µg/L or nadir GH <1 ng/mL with OGTT or normal IGF-1
De et al 2003	90	57/90 (63%)	79%	56%	Serial GH <2.5 µg/L or nadir GH <1 ng/mL with OGTT or normal IGF-1
Trepp et al 2005	94		80%	1–2 cm: 65% ≥2 cm: 27%	Random GH <2.5 µg/L, nadir GH <1 ng/mL with OGTT or normal IGF-1
Nomikos et al 2005	506	290/506 (57.3%)	75.3%	Intrasellar: 74.2% Other: 41.8% Giant: 10%	Random GH <2.5 µg/L, nadir GH <1 ng/mL with OGTT, normal IGF-1
Authors' series 1988–1997	117	64/117 (55%)	16/22 (73%)	48/95 (50.5%)	GH ≤2.5 ng/mL; GH <1 ng/mL with OGTT; normal IGF-1 level

[a]Results from 91 patients who did not have prior therapy from a total series of 103 patients are included here.
[b]10 of the patients in remission postoperatively received radiotherapy.

have a clear influence on surgical outcome. Understandably, remission rates will be highest for microadenomas, tending to drop somewhat for diffuse macroadenomas, and dropping very significantly for invasive macroadenomas and those with extrasellar extension. For microadenomas, postoperative endocrine remission has been variably reported in 73–91% of somatotroph microadenomas (Table 36.2). When all macroadenomas are considered, including all grades of invasion and extrasellar extension, postoperative remission has been reported in 48–66% of patients. When remission rates of diffuse (i.e., grade II) and invasive (i.e., grade III–IV) macroadenomas are separated, however, the outcomes among the latter are considerably less favorable. Among grades II, III, and IV tumors, Tindall and co-workers (1993) reported remission rates of 60%, 23.1%, and 0%, respectively. Interestingly, a relationship between tumor size/grade and outcome was less obvious in the series of Ross and Wilson (1988). Aside from grade IV tumors, which had a remission rate of 23%, the remission rates for grade II and III tumors in that series were similar (57%). In our series of 445 acromegalic patients using GH <2 ng/mL as the remission criterion, remission rates for microadenomas, diffuse macroadenomas, and invasive macroadenomas were 65%, 55%, and 52%, respectively.

Pharmacologic therapy

Three classes of agents are available for reducing GH levels in acromegaly: dopamine agonists, somatostatin analogs, and the growth hormone receptor antagonist, pegvisomant (Bush & Vance 2008).

Dopamine agonists

Although dopamine agonists have been used as both a primary and adjuvant treatment for acromegaly, the response is at best modest; GH levels will normalize in only a minority of patients and even fewer will experience a significant reduction in tumor size. In their review of the literature, Jaffe and Barkan (1992) noted that suppression of GH levels to <5 ng/mL is observed in only 20% of bromocriptine treated patients; normalization of IGF-1 levels occurred in 10% of cases. In the same analysis, reduction in tumor size was observed in approximately 30% of treated cases, although the change was often negligible. The best responses to dopamine agonists tend to occur in patients with tumors that express both GH and PRL. Concomitant use of both dopamine agonists and octreotide is sometimes effective in some patients who have had a suboptimal response to either drug alone.

Somatostatin analogs

The therapeutic rationale for somatostatin analogs in acromegaly stems from the fact that somatostatin is the physiologic inhibitor of GH secretion by pituitary somatotrophs. Of these agents, octreotide is the most well studied example, having been the subject of nearly two decades of comprehensive clinical testing. This 8-amino acid compound inhibits GH secretion with 45 times the potency of native somatostatin. Unlike dopamine agonists which induce cellular shrinkage and conspicuous alterations in the tumor histology, no consistent morphologic changes are seen in tumors treated with somatostatin analogs. However, these agents exert a potent antiproliferative effect, inducing highly significant reductions in tumor growth fractions (Thapar et al 1997).

Results from the International Multicenter Acromegaly Study Group demonstrated reductions in GH levels among 94% of 189 patients; normalization of GH and IGF-1 levels occurred in 47% and 46% of cases, respectively (Vance & Harris 1991). In a double-blind, placebo-controlled trial involving 116 acromegalic patients, octreotide administered for 6 months decreased GH and IGF-1 levels in 71% and 93% of patients, respectively (Ezzat et al 1992). In a sub-set of 39 patients in whom integrated GH secretion was evaluated, GH levels were suppressed to <5 ng/mL in 49% of patients, and to <2 ng/mL in 26%. In addition to biochemical improvement, the majority of patients experience prompt and sometimes dramatic relief from acromegalic symptomatology. Headache and arthralgias disappear rapidly, and regression of soft tissue swelling, paresthesias, and hyperhydrosis is a fairly uniform occurrence. The reduction in tumor size is often far less impressive, being observed in only about one-third of all patients (Ezzat et al 1992). The degree of shrinkage is also variable, being minimal in most cases, but dramatic in a few instances (Lamberts et al 1992; Lamberts et al 1996). As a rule of thumb, 30% of patients will experience a reduction in tumor size and of those that do, the size reduction will be <30%.

One initial limitation of octreotide had been the need for administration by multiple daily subcutaneous injections (100–500 μg every 8 h), but this inconvenience has been overcome with long-acting octreotide preparations, octreotide LAR. Requiring depot intramuscular injections at 28-day intervals, this agent has also been shown to be effective in reducing GH levels and stabilizing tumor size (Davies et al 1998; Flogstad et al 1997; Stewart et al 1995). Other long-acting somatostatin analogs, such as lanreotide, have also been found effective (Cannavo et al 2000; Caron et al 1997; Morange et al 1994; Turner et al 1999).

Although somatostatin analogs are generally well tolerated, gastrointestinal side-effects such as loose stools, abdominal pain, nausea, mild malabsorption, and gallstone formation can be a nuisance. In particular, gallstones may develop up to 10–20% of patients and are related to an inhibitory effect on gallbladder motility. There has been some interest in the preoperative treatment of somatotroph adenomas as a means of improving surgical remission rates, however, a significant benefit has yet to be proven, and remains debatable (Cappabianca et al 2003; Colao et al 1997; Kristof et al 1999; Wasko et al 2000). Patients who are resistant to somatostatin analogs may respond to pegvisomant, a growth hormone receptor antagonist. This newer class of agent effectively normalizes IGF-1 levels and improves insulin sensitivity and glucose tolerance (Jawiarczyk et al 2008). It is not associated with the negative effects on gallbladder motility, but can cause temporary elevations in liver enzymes. Although growth hormone levels remain elevated, the medication does not appear to promote tumor growth (Jimenez et al 2008). More recent data suggest that pegvisomant benefits patients not only as a second tier therapy after failed somatostatin analog treatment but also when given as an adjunct in the setting of successful somatostatin analog therapy. The addition of pegvisomant to patients with already normal IGF-1 levels on somatostatin analog therapy, significantly improved quality-of-life measures and acromegalic symptoms (Neggers et al 2008).

Radiation therapy

Radiation therapy is ordinarily considered in acromegalic patients suffering from persistent or recurrent disease following surgery. The radiotherapeutic response of somatotroph adenomas has been well studied and is quite predictable (Eastman et al 1992; Eastman et al 1979). GH levels drop to 50% of baseline in the first 2 years and to 75%

of baseline after 5 years. Still, the latent interval required to suppress GH levels to <5 ng/mL in the majority of patients is at least 10 years. In view of what is now recognized concerning the need for prompt normalization of GH levels in the prevention of premature mortality in acromegaly, interim control of GH hypersecretion with somatostatin analogs and dopaminergic agents is indicated while awaiting a radiotherapeutic response. Fortunately, radiotherapy offers a more immediate response with respect to tumor growth. In almost all instances, including the case of rapidly growing and locally aggressive tumors, radiation therapy will effectively halt tumor progression (Eastman et al 1992). Radiation induced hypopituitarism occurs as a time-related consequence of radiotherapy, as does the development of cerebrovascular changes (Biermasz et al 2000a; Eastman et al 1992; Eastman et al 1979; Feek et al 1984; Gutt et al 2001; Guy et al 1991; Hasegawa et al 2000; Peck & McGovern 1966; Rauhut et al 2002; Tsang et al 1996).

Data confirming the long-term efficacy of radiosurgery as compared to standard fractionated radiotherapy are promising (Castinetti et al 2007; Jagannathan et al 2008b; Jezkova et al 2006; Landolt et al 1998; Laws et al 2004; Pollock et al 2007; Roberts et al 2007; Sheehan et al 2005). Landolt and co-workers (1998) compared the outcomes of 16 refractory acromegalics treated with GammaKnife radiosurgery with those of 50 acromegalics treated with standard radiotherapy. Although there was no difference in the frequency with which hormone hypersecretion was eventually normalized between the two groups (~70–80%), the mean time to normalization in the radiosurgery group was 1.4 years, as compared with 7.1 years in the conventional radiotherapy group. Complications, including hypopituitarism, were more frequent in the conventional radiotherapy group as well. Jagannathan and co-workers (2008b) reported normalization in IGF-1 levels in 53% of 95 patients at a mean of 29.8 months after GammaKnife radiosurgery. Similar results have been reported using Cyberknife radiosurgery (Roberts et al 2007).

Tumor recurrence

The rate of recurrence in acromegaly will depend upon the stringency of the criteria with which remission was originally defined, as well as the period of follow-up. When strict criteria are used to define remission, such as suppression of GH levels to <1 ng/mL on an OGTT and normalization of IGF-1 levels, a durable remission is usually achieved and recurrence tends to be infrequent. The rate of recurrence in several large series has ranged from 0 to 18.5% during mean follow-up periods of 2.9–16 years (Table 36.3); the mean rate of recurrence is approximately 6% (Biermasz et al 2000b; Buchfelder et al 1991; Davis et al 1993; Freda et al 1998b; Losa et al 1989; Shimon et al 2001; Swearingen et al 1998). Of surgically treated acromegalic patients in whom endocrine remission had been achieved, we have encountered an 8% recurrence rate during a 10-year follow-up period, with a remission criterion of GH <5 ng/mL (Laws et al 1996). The series by Davis et al (1993) emphasizes the importance of long-term follow-up and the tendency of recurrences to increase with time. Risk of recurrence can be predicted using a postoperative OGTT in

Table 36.3 Rates of somatotroph adenoma recurrence after prior successful surgery

Series	Patients in remission (n)	Recurrence rate	Mean follow-up (years)	Original remission criteria
Losa et al 1989	16	0.0%	2.9	GH <1 ng/mL with OGTT *and* normal IGF-1 level
Buchfelder et al 1991	61	6.6%	6.0	GH <5 ng/mL
Buchfelder et al 1991	63	0.0%	6.5	GH <2 ng/mL with OGTT
Davis et al 1993	90[a]	17.8%	5.8	GH <2 ng/mL (fasting or on OGTT)
Freda et al 1998b[a]	61	5.4%	5.4	GH <2 ng/mL with OGTT and/or normal IGF-1
Swearingen et al 1998[b]	124	6% at 10 years; 10% at 15 years	7.8	IGF-1 or GH <2 ng/mL with OGTT
Biermasz et al 2000b	27	18.5%	16	GH <1 ng/mL or IGF-1
Shimon et al 2001	73	1.4%	3.9	Repeated fasting or nadir GH <2 ng/mL or normal IGF-1

[a]32% received postoperative radiation therapy (10/32 were in remission with surgery alone at the time of radiotherapy).
[b]40% received postoperative radiation therapy.

patients with normal postoperative IGF-1 levels. Patients who suppress to GH levels <0.14 µg/mL appear have a significantly lower risk of recurrence than those who do not (Freda et al 2004).

Many recurrent acromegalics will be candidates for repeat surgery, however, the need for reoperation and its role among the alternatives of surgical management should be carefully individualized. The tendency to consider both recurrent and persistent acromegaly under the general category of 'recurrence', means that few data are available concerning the surgical outcomes of genuinely recurrent somatotroph adenomas. Of 29 acromegalic patients with recurrent tumors, we recently reported a 48% rate of secondary remission with reoperation (Laws et al 1996). Similar results were reported by Nicola et al (1991) (any recurrent acromegalics will be candidates for repeat surgery) in their operative series of 10 recurrent tumors. For tumors in which remission cannot be achieved surgically, adjuvant radiotherapy has been and continues to be the usual next step, particularly in the presence of macroscopic or radiologically evident residual disease.

Corticotroph adenomas: Cushing's disease and Nelson's syndrome

From the standpoints of both diagnosis and therapy, no pituitary tumor presents a greater management challenge than does the corticotroph adenoma. Secreting ACTH in excess, these tumors are responsible for the well known hypercortisolemic state, Cushing's disease. Of immediate practical importance is the distinction between Cushing's disease and Cushing's syndrome. The latter designation is somewhat non-specific etiologically, and refers to any pathologic or iatrogenic state of glucocorticoid excess. Cushing's disease, on the other hand, is a more precise clinicopathologic designation, referring specifically to those hypercortisolemic states generated in response to an ACTH-secreting pituitary tumor. Since both Cushing's disease and Cushing's syndrome share an identical clinical phenotype, the diagnostic challenge lies in distinguishing those patients harboring a pituitary tumor from those whose glucocorticoid excess is due to other causes. Although this is seldom easy, the distinction can and must be made, for it is a necessary prerequisite to appropriate therapeutic intervention.

Box 36.2 Differential diagnosis of Cushing's syndrome

CUSHING'S SYNDROME

- ACTH-dependent (80%)
- Pituitary lesions (85%):
  - Corticotroph adenoma
  - Corticotroph carcinoma (rare)
  - Primary corticotroph hyperplasia (rare)
- Ectopic ACTH lesions (15%):
  - Small cell carcinoma of lung
  - Carcinoid tumors
  - Islet cell tumors
  - Medullary thyroid carcinoma
  - Pheochromocytoma
  - Other rare tumors
- Ectopic CRH-producing lesions (rare)
- ACTH-independent (20%)
- Adrenal adenoma
- Adrenal carcinoma
- Nodular adrenal hyperplasia (rare)
- Exogenous steroids

PSEUDO-CUSHINGOID STATES

- Depression
- Alcoholism
- Obesity
- Diabetes

Cushing's syndrome: etiologic considerations

It is convenient to classify hypercortisolemic states on the basis of ACTH-dependent and ACTH-independent etiologies (Box 36.2). Foremost among the ACTH-dependent causes are corticotroph adenomas, which also account for 70% of all non-iatrogenic cases of Cushing's syndrome in the adult. Less common ACTH-dependent causes include the ectopic ACTH syndrome which includes various ACTH-secreting lesions such as small cell carcinoma of the lung, bronchial and foregut carcinoids, medullary carcinoma of the thyroid, pancreatic islet cell tumors, pheochromocytoma, and rare ovarian and testicular tumors. Also included in this group are a rare collection of corticotropin-releasing hormone (CRH) secreting tumors including hypothalamic gangliocytomas, small cell lung cancers, prostatic tumors, colonic carcinomas, nephroblastomas, thyroid medullary carcinomas, and bronchial carcinoids. ACTH-independent causes of Cushing's syndrome include various primary adrenal lesions, such as benign adrenal adenomas, adrenal carcinomas, and rarely, adrenal nodular hyperplasia.

Also considered in the differential diagnosis of Cushing's syndrome are polycystic ovary syndrome and other non-neoplastic conditions which either mimic the Cushingoid phenotype or are associated with low level glucocorticoid excess. Often referred to as 'pseudocushingoid states', the more common of these conditions include obesity, depression, alcoholism, exogenous glucocorticoid ingestion, and various states of physiologic stress.

Cushing's disease

Corticotroph adenomas represent approximately 10–16% of all surgically resected pituitary tumors (Jane & Laws 2001; Kovacs & Horvath 1986). Women are affected far more frequently than men; female-to-male ratios varying from 3:1 to 10:1 have been reported. Although corticotroph adenomas can occur at any age, their peak incidence occurs between the 3rd and 5th decades. Whereas these tumors are responsible for fully 70% of all cases of non-iatrogenic Cushing's syndrome in the adult, they account for only 30% of hypercortisolemic states in the pediatric population; primary adrenal tumors are the dominant etiology in this age group.

Clinical features

Most patients with corticotroph adenomas come to medical attention on an endocrine basis. Since these tumors are typically small and confined to the sella, symptoms referable to mass effect are seldom presenting complaints. The clinical features of Cushing's disease are well known and are directly attributable to chronic glucocorticoid excess. The most conspicuous feature of the condition is weight gain with centripetal fat deposition, a common and characteristic presenting complaint. Fat accumulates in the face and in the supraclavicular and dorsocervical fat pads, giving rise to the typical 'moon facies' and 'buffalo hump'. Accumulations of fat on the thorax and abdomen (truncal obesity) round out the remaining changes in body habitus. Skin changes are commonly present in Cushing's disease. Skin thinning, due to atrophy of the epidermis and underlying connective tissue, renders the skin highly susceptible to injury with even the most minor trauma. This, together with capillary fragility, often leads to easy bruising and an overall plethoric appearance to the skin and face. Wide purple striae are present in many patients, typically over the abdomen and flanks. Additional dermatologic findings can include hirsutism and, rarely, hyperpigmentation.

Metabolic aberrations figure prominently in Cushing's disease and account for the high mortality rates that once accompanied this condition. Hypertension and varying degrees of glucose intolerance are common features, ones which contribute to accelerated atherosclerosis and other cardiovascular complications, particularly in patients with longstanding disease. Osteoporosis of some degree is present in virtually all patients. Bone demineralization is especially prominent in the vertebral bodies; compression fractures can be identified in a significant proportion of asymptomatic patients and in almost half of patients with back pain. Pathologic fractures also occur elsewhere, notably the ribs, feet, and the pelvis. Demineralization of the dorsum sellae is

frequently apparent on skull X-rays, being the consequence of cortisol action rather than the result of an expanding sellar tumor. An additional common musculoskeletal problem is steroid myopathy. Although only about half of all patients complain of muscle weakness, the majority will have demonstrable proximal myopathy on formal testing.

Reproductive function is commonly impaired in both sexes. In females, menstrual dysfunction and infertility result from a direct antigonadal effect of cortisol and androgen excess. Men can suffer from decreased libido and relative infertility. As is true of all hypercortisolemic states, patients with Cushing's disease also suffer from impaired host defenses. Patients are especially prone to superficial fungal infections, notably tinea versicolor and mucocutaneous candidiasis. Other infections, such as ordinary respiratory infections which would be otherwise uncomplicated in normal individuals, can often assume an aggressive and life-threatening course in these patients. Finally, psychiatric disturbances are extremely common in patients with Cushing's disease. Ranging from depressed mood and emotional lability to mania and psychosis, these manifestations contribute heavily to the morbidity of the condition.

In its most florid form, the clinical phenotype is unmistakable; however, subtle, cyclic, and generally less obvious versions of the condition do occur. That many patients experience years of symptoms prior to diagnosis underscores the ease with which the condition can be overlooked or misdiagnosed. Worthy of emphasis is the fact that Cushing's disease is a life-threatening condition.

Historical data indicate that the natural history of Cushing's syndrome was once quite ominous, with the case-fatality rate approaching 50% at 5 years following the onset of symptoms (Plotz et al 1952). Cardiovascular complications were the predominant causes of death, followed by infection and suicide. For this reason, Cushing's disease is accompanied by therapeutic imperatives that are somewhat more compelling than those posed by other hypersecretory states.

Laboratory evaluation

In contrast to other pituitary tumors, wherein imaging studies assume foremost diagnostic importance, the diagnosis of corticotroph adenomas rests primarily on carefully interpreted endocrine studies performed in basal and dynamic states. The need for a coordinated, comprehensive, and somewhat compulsive endocrine approach to these lesions cannot be overemphasized (Newell-Price et al 1998; Thorner et al 1992). Even today, failed therapy for these lesions can often be traced back to interventions prematurely initiated and undertaken without the benefit of a thorough and complete endocrine assessment. On the other hand, a confirmatory endocrine diagnosis of a corticotroph adenoma provides a high degree of assurance that an adenoma is present and can be selectively removed.

There are three essential steps in the diagnosis of corticotroph adenomas: (Alexander et al 1980) establishing hypercortisolism; (Arafah et al 1980) distinguishing ACTH-dependent from ACTH-independent causes of hypercortisolemia; and (Assie et al 2007) distinguishing Cushing's disease from ectopic states of ACTH excess. As discussed below, the endocrine profile of ACTH adenomas/Cushing's disease includes elevation of urinary free cortisol levels; no cortisol suppression on low dose dexamethasone testing; cortisol suppression on high dose dexamethasone testing; and moderately elevated ACTH levels.

Step 1: Establishing hypercortisolemia

Measurement of free cortisol in a 24-h urine specimen is a simple, sensitive, and first choice means of establishing hypercortisolemia. Urinary free cortisol is a biologically relevant marker, reflecting the plasma free cortisol activity during the previous 24-h period. The urinary free cortisol increases exponentially for quantum increments in plasma cortisol levels, rendering the test extremely sensitive: elevations are virtually always detected in non-iatrogenic Cushing's syndrome. Demonstrable elevation in basal plasma cortisol levels also occurs in endogenous hypercortisolemic states but the range of observed values from isolated samples overlaps sufficiently with normal individuals, thus limiting the discriminating value of the test. The development of reliable salivary cortisol measurements provides another effective means of determining cortisol excess and the alteration of the normal diurnal variation in cortisol production, accomplished by obtaining salivary samples at 11 p.m. (Findling & Raff 1999).

A second screening test, the low dose dexamethasone suppression test, should also be routinely used to verify hypercortisolemia. In normal individuals, by way of negative feedback inhibition on the hypothalamus and pituitary, low doses of dexamethasone (1–4 mg) will suppress ACTH secretion, reducing a.m. cortisol levels to less <5 µg/dL. In hypercortisolemic states of all etiologies, sensitivity to low dose dexamethasone suppression is lost and reduction in cortisol levels does not occur. As originally designed, the test requires dexamethasone administration over a 48-h period (0.5 mg, every 6 h). Variations of the test are now performed over shorter periods of time, such as the overnight dexamethasone suppression test (1 mg dexamethasone at 11 p.m. with measurement of plasma cortisol at 8 a.m.). Although this latter variation is an excellent outpatient screening tool, it is subject to a higher false-positive rate in a number of circumstances (depression, transient stress, obesity, alcoholism, hyperthyroidism, and with the use of certain medications).

Step 2: Distinguishing ACTH-dependent from ACTH-independent causes of hypercortisolemia

Once hypercortisolism has been established, subsequent studies are aimed at identifying the source of hormonal excess. A logical first step involves determining whether the process is ACTH dependent or ACTH independent. Measurement of plasma ACTH levels provides an initial clue, as levels are suppressed in primary adrenal pathologies, but are elevated in the case of corticotroph adenomas, ectopic ACTH syndrome, and in some CRH-producing tumors. Ordinarily, corticotroph adenomas produce only moderate elevations of ACTH (80–200 pg/mL), whereas marked elevations are typical of ectopic ACTH-producing lesions (>200 pg/mL). There is, however, considerable overlap in ACTH levels between corticotroph adenomas and ectopic lesions, and the two are seldom definitively separable on the basis of ACTH levels alone.

Step 3: Distinguishing Cushing's disease from ectopic ACTH states

It is important to recognize that the secretory activity of corticotroph adenomas, unlike that of ectopic ACTH-producing lesions, is not autonomous. In most instances, corticotroph adenomas retain responsiveness to the negative feedback effects of glucocorticoids, although their sensitivity to the effect is reset to a higher than normal threshold. Accordingly, in response to a sufficiently large glucocorticoid challenge, the secretory activity of corticotroph adenomas can be suppressed. This forms the basis of the high dose dexamethasone test. As classically described, the standard high dose test involves administration of dexamethasone over a 48-h period (2 mg every 6 h) and measurement of urinary cortisol or 17-hydroxycorticosteroids. A 50% reduction in urinary steroid excretion is taken as an appropriate suppressive response and is strongly suggestive of a corticotroph adenoma; ectopic ACTH-producing lesions are resistant to suppression. An abbreviated and more time-efficient version of this test can be performed overnight; a single 8 mg dose of dexamethasone is given at 11 p.m. and plasma cortisol levels are measured in the morning. Again, a 50% reduction in the plasma cortisol level indicates a normal suppressive response. Although most corticotroph adenomas will suppress with an 8 mg dose, some will require doses of up to 32 mg for suppression; whether or not suppression occurs appears to be diagnostically more important than the actual dose used. It has been suggested that the sensitivity, specificity, and diagnostic accuracy of the overnight test for Cushing's disease is 89%, 100%, and 91%, respectively (Luciano & Oldfield 1990). It is important to acknowledge that, although suppression on high dose testing is compatible with the endocrine profile of corticotroph adenomas, the test is not infallible; occasionally ectopic ACTH-producing lesions will exhibit a similar suppressive response. Additional corroborative proof of a corticotroph adenoma is often desired.

The corticotropin-releasing hormone (CRH) stimulation test provides an additional means of distinguishing corticotroph adenomas from ectopic ACTH-producing lesions. The theoretical premise of this test is that corticotroph adenomas express CRH receptors, rendering them responsive to intravenously administered ovine CRH. It has been observed that patients with corticotroph adenomas have an exaggerated response to CRH stimulation, resulting in a prompt, dramatic, and measurable increase in ACTH and cortisol levels. The criteria for a positive response include a 50% increase in plasma ACTH levels or a 20% increase in plasma cortisol levels above baseline. As a rule, this response should be absent with ectopic ACTH-producing lesions because the hypercortisolemic state induced by the latter renders normal pituitary corticotrophs chronically and functionally suppressed, resistant to the stimulatory effects of CRH. There are, however, occasional exceptions; unresponsive corticotroph adenomas and responsive ACTH-producing peripheral tumors are both known to occur. Still, when the results of the CRH testing are integrated with high dose suppression testing, the diagnostic accuracy in favor of a corticotroph adenoma approaches 98% (Kaye & Crapo 1990).

In many cases, the aforementioned studies will be sufficient to secure an endocrine diagnosis of Cushing's disease.

In a small proportion of patients, however, the results of these studies will be atypical, conflicting, or otherwise inconclusive, necessitating additional investigations. In these less straightforward instances, bilateral inferior petrosal sinus (IPS) sampling can be a helpful means of confirming or excluding a pituitary source of ACTH excess (Oldfield et al 1991). The procedure is based on the premise that the venous drainage of corticotroph adenomas lateralizes into the ipsilateral inferior petrosal sinus. Accordingly, if a pituitary adenoma is the source of ACTH excess, ACTH concentrations within the IPS should be higher than those present in the peripheral blood. The procedure involves bilateral transfemoral retrograde catheterization of both inferior petrosal sinuses. In patients with a corticotroph adenoma, the basal central to peripheral ACTH concentration gradient is almost always >2.0. In patients with ectopic ACTH-producing lesions, this gradient is <1.7. The diagnostic accuracy of this procedure has been further increased by measuring ACTH levels during CRH stimulation; central to peripheral gradients of >3.0 are diagnostic of Cushing's disease. In addition to confirming a pituitary source for ACTH, IPS sampling has the secondary merit of being able to determine on which side of the pituitary gland the adenoma is located. When the ACTH concentration in one IPS exceeds that in the other by a factor of more than 1.5, the adenoma is likely situated on the side having the higher IPS ACTH concentration. This information can facilitate the intraoperative identification of small adenomas, ones too small to be seen radiologically. In our experience with IPS sampling, we have found the procedure to be helpful but by no means uniformly conclusive in definitively establishing a pituitary etiology for hypercortisolism or in correctly identifying on which side of the gland an adenoma is likely to be situated. In their recent literature review, Newell-Price and co-workers (1998) concluded that IPS sampling has a sensitivity and specificity of 96% and 100%, respectively for Cushing's disease, and a diagnostic accuracy of 78% with respect to lateralization of the adenoma.

Imaging

Ordinarily, the diagnosis of a corticotroph adenoma will be established by endocrine investigations; imaging studies, although essential, should be considered of secondary diagnostic importance. Gadolinium enhanced MR imaging is the most sensitive means of identifying these lesions. They appear as hypointense defects which become more obvious and most easily discerned following gadolinium enhancement. In the evaluation of Cushing's disease, MR imaging has a sensitivity of approximately 70% and a specificity of 87% in detecting corticotroph adenomas (Klibanski & Zervas 1991). These figures can be improved with the use of dynamic pituitary imaging (Friedman et al 2007; Tabarin et al 1998). In addition to dynamic imaging, spoiled gradient recalled acquisition in the steady stage (SPGR) sequences, not ordinarily used in standard pituitary protocols, can improve the diagnostic accuracy (Patronas et al 2003). It has become our norm to re-image patients with apparent negative scans using this protocol.

It should be kept in mind that incidental microadenomas, many of which are non-functioning, are not uncommon in the pituitary. Thus, an adenoma detected on pituitary imaging should only be considered causal if the results of endocrine studies are fully compatible with a diagnosis of Cushing's disease (Fig. 36.18). Alternatively, even if the responsible tumor is not visualized by MRI, a confirmatory endocrine diagnosis of Cushing's disease ensures a high level of confidence that a corticotroph adenoma is indeed present.

The extent to which extracranial imaging (i.e., CT or MRI of the chest and abdomen) should be undertaken will depend primarily on how secure the endocrine diagnosis of a corticotroph adenoma is. Atypical results on endocrine testing that fail to exclude adrenal pathology or an ectopic ACTH or CRH producing lesion may necessitate extracranial imaging.

Treatment

Once it has been established that the etiology for hypercortisolism is a corticotroph adenoma, surgery remains the undisputed therapy of first choice (Blevins et al 1998; Bochicchio et al 1995; Chandler et al 1987; Guilhaume et al 1988; Mampalam et al 1988; Nakane et al 1987; Petruson et al 1997; Semple et al 2000; Tindall et al 1990). In fact, the merits of transsphenoidal surgery are well exemplified in treatment of corticotroph adenomas, wherein selective removal of the adenoma, cure of hypercortisolemia, and preservation of normal glandular function are all reasonable therapeutic expectations of the procedure. With most adenomas being only a few millimeters in size, together with their frequent deep location within the gland, simply finding the adenoma is perhaps the greatest operative challenge. This is especially true when the tumor is not visualized on preoperative imaging studies. What is generally required is a careful and systematic dissection of the sellar contents. If a tumor is not evident upon opening the dura, or after examining all glandular surfaces, the gland must be incised and systematically explored. Subtle changes in tissue color or texture, or in the contour of the gland will aid in the identification of an adenoma, and in distinguishing it from the normal gland. If no adenoma is found, excisional biopsies from within the substance of the gland are obtained, beginning with the central mucoid wedge. If an adenoma is not evident in the resected material, the lateral wings of the gland are carefully inspected and resected as necessary. In the adult patient in whom an adenoma cannot be identified by this stage, and for whom fertility is not an issue, a subtotal hypophysectomy is generously performed, leaving only a stump of residual anterior lobe tissue attached to the stalk. If careful examination of the resected tissues still fails to reveal an adenoma, both cavernous sinuses must be evaluated as well as the posterior lobe; the latter has, on rare occasion, been known to harbor a minute adenomatous nodule. Failing to see an adenoma by now, the surgeon must at least consider the possibility of a supradiaphragmatic tumor nodule. Given the additional operative risks of a diaphragmatic breach, one would not ordinarily contemplate transdiaphragmatic exploration without clear imaging evidence pointing to such a possibility.

In our experience of some 380 patients with Cushing's disease, remission can be achieved in >90% of microadenomas and in 60% of macroadenomas (Jane & Laws 2001).

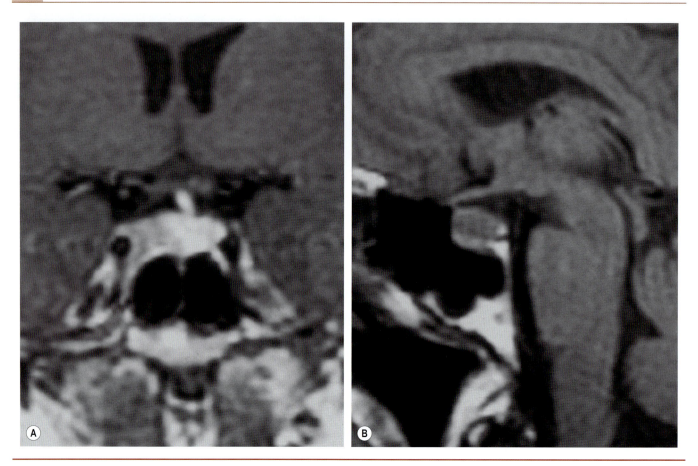

Figure 36.18 Cushing's disease. MR images of the sella in a patient with Cushing's disease. Note the adenoma on the patient's right, appearing as a hypointense area, shifting the gland and the stalk to the patient's left. A corticotroph microadenoma was identified on the right-hand side of the gland at the time of transsphenoidal exploration.

Surgical remission can be achieved in 89% of patients presenting with microadenomas (Prevedello et al 2008). Patients presenting with normal (or negative) preoperative MRI scans can achieve similar results (Semple et al 2000). For macroadenomas and patients undergoing reoperation, a combined remission rate of 46% was achieved (Thapar & Laws 2000). In pediatric Cushing's disease surgical remission can be expected in 76% (Kanter et al 2005). Comparable results have been reported by others (Table 36.4) (Blevins et al 1998; Bochicchio et al 1995; Chee et al 2001; Chen et al 2003; Esposito et al 2006; Flitsch et al 2003; Guilhaume et al 1988; Hammer et al 2004; Mampalam et al 1988; Nakane et al 1987; Patil et al 2008; Prevedello et al 2008; Semple & Laws 1999; Tindall et al 1990; Yap et al 2002).

Whether or not surgical cure has been achieved is generally evident by the 2nd or 3rd postoperative day. Morning cortisol levels should be <3 µg/dL and serum ACTH levels should be undetectable if the procedure is to be considered curative. In the occasional patient in whom a curative result has also been obtained, the decline in cortisol levels may be less precipitous, with subnormal cortisol levels being evident only after several days. As a rule, a postoperative a.m. cortisol level that persists within the 'normal' range, even if it represents a dramatic decrease from the pretreatment level,

Table 36.4 Results of primary transsphenoidal surgery for Cushing's disease (remission rates)

Series	Patients (n)	Remission rate (%)	Recurrence rate (%)	Follow-up period (years)
Nakane et al 1987	100	86	9	3.2
Guilhaume et al 1988	64	66	14	2
Mampalam et al 1988	216	79	5	3.9
Tindall et al 1990	53	85	2	4.8
Bochicchio et al 1995[a]	668	76	8	3.8
Blevins et al 1998[b]	21	67	36	5.2
Semple & Laws 1999	105	75.2	Not stated	Not stated
Chee et al 2001	61	78.7	14.6	7.3
Yap et al 2002	97	68.5	11.5	7.7
Chen et al 2003	174	74	7	>5 years minimum
Flitsch et al 2003	147	98	6.1	Not stated
Hammer et al 2004	289	82	9	11.1
Esposito et al 2006	100	79.5	3	2.7
Patil et al 2008	215	85.6	17.4	3.75
Prevedello et al 2008[c]	167	88.6	12.8	3.25

[a]Data based on a multicenter retrospective survey of the European Cushing's Disease Survey Group.
[b]Series consisted of macroadenomas only.
[c]Series consisted of MRI-positive microadenomas.

almost always indicates incomplete removal and persistent disease. For those patients successfully treated, regression of Cushingoid features and restitution of the pituitary-adrenal axis occur within months. Patients routinely relate feelings of full rejuvenation, both physically and emotionally. Depending on the extent of glandular resection, hormonal replacement may be required, although this will be a long-term requirement for only a minority of patients.

Once remission has been achieved, biochemical or radiologic recurrence is unfortunately relatively common; approximately 12% of patients can be expected to experience recurrence within 10 years, and others do so many years after successful surgery, with incidence rising steadily over time (Blevins et al 1998; Bochicchio et al 1995; Chandler et al 1987; Guilhaume et al 1988; Jane & Laws 2001; Laws & Thapar 1996; Mampalam et al 1988; Nakane et al 1987; Patil et al 2008; Petruson et al 1997; Tindall et al 1990).

Management of persistent/recurrent disease

In patients not initially cured by surgery, four options remain: (Alexander et al 1980) repeat transsphenoidal exploration; (Arafah et al 1980) medical therapy; (Assie et al 2007) radiation therapy; and (Balagura et al 1981) bilateral adrenalectomy. When confronted with such a situation, the surgeon must first ascertain the cause of failed surgery. In some situations, such as with laterally extending invasive adenomas, complete excision is not a reasonable expectation of the procedure, thus the issue of repeat exploration does not arise. A more common scenario, however, relates to an inability to definitively find and remove the tumor, either as the result of technical issues or because of a diagnostic error (e.g., the cause of hypercortisolemia is not a pituitary tumor). At this point, all preoperative diagnostic studies should be carefully re-evaluated and the diagnosis of pituitary-dependent disease must be reaffirmed. If bilateral IPS sampling was not performed preoperatively, then it would clearly be indicated at this time. Finally, the surgical specimen must be evaluated by an experienced pathologist to determine whether it contains normal gland, an ACTH immunoreactive adenoma, or corticotroph hyperplasia. Assuming that all studies continue to point to a pituitary tumor, some consideration of sellar re-exploration should be given, although the viability and effectiveness of this option will depend on the surgeon's impression of the thoroughness of the initial exploration. In one series, repeat sellar exploration led to remission in approximately 70% of cases (Ram et al 1994). We tend to recommend repeat surgery in several clinical situations: (1) if the histopathology confirms removal of an ACTH adenoma and imaging does not suggest cavernous sinus invasion and (2) if pathology is negative but we had performed a limited exploration of the gland. However, adjuvant therapy is recommended for invasive tumors and those patients with Cushing's disease in whom another surgery is not felt to be indicated.

Radiation therapy

For patients unresponsive to sellar exploration, the most effective next step is some form of radiation therapy. Tsang and co-workers (1996) achieved remission in 53% of 29 patients with postoperative persistent/recurrent Cushing's disease at 10 years following a 50 Gy dose. In another recent series of 30 patients with persistent or recurrent Cushing's disease, Estrada and co-workers (1997) reported remission in 83% during a median follow-up period of 42 months after conventional radiotherapy (mean dose 50 Gy). Of those patients experiencing remission, most did so within 2 years; in some, remission occurred as late as 60 months.

Radiosurgery also appears to be an effective option for refractory corticotroph adenomas. One of the earliest long-term experiences with radiosurgery was reported by Degerblad and co-workers (1986), where radiosurgery normalized cortisol levels in 76% of patients. In approximately half of 'cured' patients, normalization was achieved within 1 year and, in the remainder, within 3 years. The response also appeared to be a durable one, as no instance of biochemical recurrence was observed during a 3–9-year follow-up period. Others have achieved comparable results, normalizing hypercortisolemia in 50–66% of patients and doing so within 12–20 months (Jagannathan et al 2008a; Jagannathan et al 2007b; Mauermann et al 2007; Pollock 2007; Sheehan et al 2000). In our experience, surveillance for recurrence remains necessary after apparently successful radiosurgery. In a recent study, recurrence occurred in 20% of patients at a mean of 27 months (Jagannathan et al 2007). In this same study, a second GammaKnife procedure achieved remission in three of seven patients who underwent repeat radiosurgery. However, repeated GammaKnife radiosurgery was associated with new cranial neuropathy in four of seven patients. New endocrinopathy was seen in one-fifth of the patients within a mean follow-up period of 45 months. While awaiting remission, patients with active Cushing's are managed medically to decrease circulating cortisol levels. The most common regimen includes steroid synthesis inhibitors such as Ketokonazole (Chou & Lin 2000; Sonino & Boscaro 1999; Sonino et al 1991).

Medical therapy

Pharmacologic therapy is perhaps the least attractive therapeutic option for corticotroph adenomas. Although a somewhat exhaustive collection of agents has been used against these tumors, problems of variable efficacy, potential toxicity, and the need for life-long, closely monitored therapy all serve to establish this modality as a clear third choice. Still, there are a few circumstances in which there is little alternative but to exercise this medical option. One example concerns the occasional extremely ill patient in whom the sequelae of hypercortisolemia are so debilitating that preoperative reductions in cortisol are necessary in assuring a safe anesthetic and operative procedure. A second and more common practice concerns the use of pharmacologic agents in controlling hypercortisolemia while awaiting a radiotherapeutic response. In both situations, these agents retain a temporary role. Finally, in the rare refractory patient in whom all therapies short of bilateral adrenalectomy have failed, medical therapy may be required on a long-term basis.

Two basic classes of agents are available for treating Cushing's disease. The first class includes centrally acting agents which, through diverse mechanisms, are directed at suppressing ACTH secretion. Cyproheptadine, bromocriptine, somatostatin analogs, and sodium valproate fall into this category. Although each of these agents has shown varying effectiveness in individual patients, response consistency and durability have proven sufficiently poor that they cannot be regarded as viable options for most patients.

The second and more effective class of agents are peripherally acting adrenal blockers which inhibit adrenal steroidogenesis, producing a pharmacologically adrenalectomized state. Included in this group is the adrenolytic agent mitotane, and the inhibitors of cortisol synthesis ketoconazole, etomidate, metyrapone, aminoglutethimide, and trilostane. Whereas each of these agents has been shown to be effective in reducing cortisol levels, each is accompanied by a spectrum of variably tolerated side-effects. When they are used, diligent supervision is required because accompanying adrenal blockade, whether partial or complete, is the ever present risk of adrenal insufficiency.

Bilateral adrenalectomy

Total bilateral adrenalectomy followed by lifelong glucocorticoid and mineralocorticoid replacement is generally regarded as an option of last resort, reserved for the occasional patient in whom all other therapies have failed. Ordinarily, such patients will have already undergone multiple attempts at transsphenoidal resection for a tumor which was either never found, or whose invasive growth had defied complete resection. Some of these patients will be awaiting a radiotherapeutic response, and many will have proven too intolerant of long-term pharmacologic therapy. For such patients, particularly those too fragile to tolerate ongoing hypercortisolemia, total bilateral adrenalectomy is a definitive option that provides immediate relief. The high morbidity and mortality rates that once accompanied this procedure have lessened substantially, particularly with the development of laparoscopic adrenalectomy approaches. Pituitary irradiation is routinely recommended in all patients undergoing bilateral adrenalectomy as a measure for reducing the occurrence of Nelson's syndrome (Liu et al 2007; Mauermann et al 2007; McCutcheon & McCutcheon 2002; Pollock et al 2002).

Nelson's syndrome

Nelson's syndrome refers to the clinical situation wherein a corticotroph adenoma will manifest or, more commonly, will progress following bilateral adrenalectomy. An iatrogenic condition, the syndrome will eventually develop in at least 10–15% of Cushing's disease patients who undergo bilateral adrenalectomy (Assie et al 2007; Fleseriu et al 2007; Gil-Cardenas et al 2007; Kasperlik-Zaluska et al 2006; Thompson et al 2007). Although corticotroph adenomas occurring in the setting of Nelson's syndrome are morphologically indistinguishable from those responsible for Cushing's disease, the former are notoriously more aggressive. Most are macroadenomas, typically fast growing and grossly invasive of surrounding structures. The syndrome is easily recognizable, beginning with a history of hypercortisolemia in which the corticotroph adenoma was either unsuspected, undetected, or incompletely resected. Thereafter, hypercortisolemia would have been treated with bilateral adrenalectomy, producing a temporary remission, only to be followed by aggressive tumor growth and the neurologic sequelae of

an expanding sellar mass. Typically, these tumors exhibit tremendous secretory activity, producing dramatic elevations in ACTH levels, together with elevations of other proopiomelanocortin related peptides, such as melanocyte-stimulating hormone. Elevations of the latter are presumably responsible for the hyperpigmentation that typifies the syndrome.

Although only a proportion of adrenalectomized patients with Cushing's disease will progress to Nelson's syndrome, it is impossible to predict if and when the progression will take place in any given patient. In some patients, Nelson's syndrome will manifest within months to years of the adrenalectomy; in others, decades will pass until it occurs. When it does manifest, however, the management of the condition is virtually always difficult. Curative resections are seldom a realistic goal because most patients will have invasive macroadenomas. Transsphenoidal surgery for Nelson's syndrome remains primarily a palliative procedure. Surgical resection and re-resections are, however, sometimes necessary to control mass effect among the larger tumors. Our surgical experience with Nelson's syndrome includes some 60 patients (Jane & Laws 2001). In approximately half of these, surgical resection was followed by lessening of hyperpigmentation and significant reductions in serum ACTH levels. In a more recent review of our series, only 17% of patients experienced postoperative remission (De Tommasi et al 2005). For patients not controlled by surgery and in those not previously irradiated, radiotherapy is recommended. The aggressive nature of the tumor means that as many as 20% of patients will eventually succumb to uncontrolled local tumor growth in spite of all therapeutic interventions possible.

Thyrotroph pituitary adenomas

Accounting for <1% of all pituitary adenomas, the thyrotroph adenoma is the least common type of hormonally active pituitary adenoma. Beck-Peccoz and co-workers (1996), in a comprehensive literature review, identified some 280 examples. It was once believed that most thyrotroph adenomas arose in the setting of longstanding hypothyroidism, presumably by way of feedback inhibitory loss, induction of thyrotroph hyperplasia, and eventual adenomatous transformation. Whereas such a perspective was compatible with early experimental studies wherein thyroidectomy regularly induced thyrotroph pituitary adenomas in rodents, careful clinicopathologic analysis of human thyrotroph adenomas has suggested an alternative sequence of events (Furth et al 1973). In fact, in the majority of reported cases, the initial manifestations were those of hyperthyroidism and goiter, events wholly compatible with tumoral hypersecretion of TSH. With a presentation indistinguishable from the far more common occurrence of primary hyperthyroidism, many such patients were incorrectly diagnosed as suffering from a primary thyroid condition and were subjected to some form of thyroid ablation. This intervention served to ameliorate symptoms for a time but was eventually followed by progressive symptoms of an expanding sellar mass. Only then was the pituitary correctly recognized as the primary site of pathology. As a result of this diagnostic delay, most reported tumors had attained considerable size when definitively detected, with many exhibiting invasive and destructive extrasellar growth.

Thyrotroph adenomas can occur in all age groups (range 11–84 years) and exhibit no gender preference. Most thyrotroph adenomas will present with the classic signs and symptoms of hyperthyroidism. Ordinarily, a diffusely enlarged thyroid gland will be demonstrable. These tumors can also co-secrete GH, and a small proportion of patients will present with true acromegaly. Depending on the tumor size and degree of glandular and/or stalk compression, hypopituitarism and moderate hyperprolactinemia may be additional features of an endocrine presentation. Neurologic symptomatology is also common, particularly in those having undergone prior thyroidectomy, in whom it may be the dominant mode of presentation. In one literature review, more than half of all patients had demonstrable visual field defects at presentation (Greenman & Melmed 1995). Of cases cited in the literature, approximately one-third of tumors were confined to the sella, one-third extended beyond the sella, and one-third exhibited gross invasion of parasellar structures (Beck-Peccoz et al 1996).

The key endocrinologic feature of these tumors is the presence of detectable TSH levels in the presence of high levels of circulating thyroid hormones. Although there are a number of uncommon medical states associated with inappropriate TSH secretion, including familial dysalbuminemia, certain drugs (amiodarone, amphetamines, oral contrast agents), peripheral resistance to thyroid hormones, and states exhibiting an increase in transport proteins (thyroid binding globin, albumin, transthyretin), most can be excluded on the basis of clinical history and examination (Beck-Peccoz et al 1996). In as many as 80% of thyrotroph adenomas, the glycoprotein hormone alpha subunit is produced in measurable excess. An alpha sub-unit to TSH ratio that exceeds 1 provides additional evidence in favor of a thyrotroph adenoma. Measurable elevations in GH and/or PRL may occur in as many as a third of patients; FSH and LH elevations are much less frequent.

Surgical resection, radiotherapy, and medical therapy with somatostatin analogs are all therapeutic options for thyrotroph adenomas (Laws et al 2006). Surgery is the clear first choice and should be initially considered in all patients in whom a thyrotroph adenoma is suspected. In that the majority of cases reported to date have been large and/or invasive lesions that had often been subject to considerable diagnostic delay and possible disinhibiting effects of thyroidectomy, biochemical remission can be achieved in only a minority of patients. Of 177 cases reviewed by Beck-Peccoz et al (1996) surgery alone was curative in only 33%; the majority also required adjuvant radiotherapy to control thyrotropin hypersecretion (Beck-Peccoz et al 1996). Similarly, in the single institution study reported by the National Institutes of Health, involving the treatment and follow-up of 22 surgically treated patients, a 35% surgical remission rate was achieved (Brucker-Davis et al 1999). Of patients in whom surgery does not induce remission, somatostatin analogs and radiation alone or in combination represent important adjuvants. The effectiveness of octreotide against thyrotroph adenomas has also been shown (Chanson et al 1993). Among 33 treated patients, normalization of thyroid hormones and TSH levels was achieved in 78% and 72% of patients, respectively. Variable reductions in tumor size were observed in 10 of 25 patients receiving long-term therapy (Chanson et al 1993).

Atypical pituitary adenomas and pituitary carcinomas

Despite the regularity with which many pituitary adenomas exhibit aggressive local behavior, it is intriguing why so few of these epithelial tumors are capable of metastatic dissemination. In fact, metastasizing pituitary tumors, i.e., pituitary carcinomas, are very rare; Pernicone and co-workers (1997), in their recent review of the English literature, identified 52 published examples, to which they added 12 new cases (Pernicone et al 1997). Pituitary carcinoma is a precisely defined entity, one that includes only those tumors of adenohypophyseal origin accompanied by demonstrated craniospinal and/or systemic metastases. In contrast to most human carcinomas, the usual histologic criteria of malignancy (nuclear atypia and pleomorphism, mitotic activity, necrosis, hemorrhage, invasiveness) are insufficient to permit an unqualified diagnosis of pituitary carcinoma, in that these features may be seen in benign pituitary adenomas. Instead, the diagnosis is predicated upon tumor behavior and is relatively independent of histology. Metastatic dissemination more commonly involves the CSF axis, including virtually any site within the supratentorial, infratentorial, and/or spinal compartments. Extraneural dissemination occurs less frequently and also exhibits less geographic restraint; bone, liver, lymph nodes, lung, kidney, and heart have all been reported as recipient sites. Brain invasion by a pituitary tumor is generally regarded as evidence of malignancy. From a diagnostic standpoint, however, this criterion can seldom be invoked in that no radiologic indicators reliably distinguish brain displacement from actual invasion and because the brain is almost never sampled at the time of pituitary surgery. As a result, brain invasion is, with rare exception, an autopsy finding rather than a consideration in the diagnosis of biopsies.

Pituitary carcinomas primarily affect adults, although given their occurrence in individuals as young as 1.5 years or as old as 75 years, it appears that no age group is exempt. Like benign adenomas, pituitary carcinomas appear to be more frequent among females. Their clinical presentation is variable, both from endocrinologic and oncologic points of view. With regard to the former, the majority (75%) of reported pituitary carcinomas have been hormonally actively tumors, most producing either prolactin or ACTH and accompanied by their corresponding endocrinopathy. Of the ACTH-producing carcinomas, it is both interesting and understandable that a disproportionate number have occurred in the setting of Nelson's syndrome. Acromegaly associated GH-producing carcinomas are considerably less common, and thyrotroph carcinomas are distinct rarities, only a single example having been reported (Mixon et al 1993; Stewart et al 1992). Approximately one-quarter of all pituitary carcinomas are clinically non-functioning. From an oncologic standpoint, the initial clinical course of many patients will be indistinguishable from that in patients with a benign pituitary adenoma. Local invasion may, or may not be present, and tumor histology may be entirely benign. A protracted clinical course, often punctuated by multiple local recurrences, is then followed by metastatic dissemination. In some, but not all such cases, a clear escalation in histologic aggressiveness is observed when comparing primary tumors to metastatic deposits. In this setting, the process appears to be one of malignant transformation in a previously benign tumor. Less frequently, the behavior of other pituitary carcinomas suggests de novo malignancy. Such tumors are biologically malignant from the outset, beginning as locally invasive, relentlessly destructive, cytologically atypical sellar masses which promptly give way to metastatic dissemination. To date, the primary tumor in all instances has been a macroadenoma; no accounts of metastases emanating from a pituitary microadenoma have been reported. The interval between initial presentation and documentation of metastatic dissemination ranged from months to many years (mean ~ 7 years) (Pernicone et al 1995).

Although the factors that confer on pituitary carcinomas their capacity for metastatic dissemination are unknown, the mechanisms underlying metastatic spread appear more fully understood. Depending on the site of the metastatic deposit, propulsion of tumor cells via CSF pathways, hematogenous dissemination, and lymphatic spread will, in isolation or in combination, be the responsible mechanism(s). As mentioned, the majority of metastases occur within the craniospinal axis. Such involvement appears to begin with invasion of the subarachnoid space, providing a reservoir from which tumor cells are continually percolated and disseminated by CSF flow. Most craniospinal deposits tend to be superficially situated, either subpial or periventricular in distribution. Deeper deposits, particularly those involving brain parenchyma, are considered to be the result of tumor cells permeating the perivascular (Virchow–Robin) spaces, or perhaps the result of venous sinus invasion.

Extracranial spread of pituitary carcinomas involves both hematogenous and lymphatic routes. Invasion of the cavernous sinus provides the necessary venous access for transport to the internal jugular vein via the petrosal system. Although the pituitary itself lacks lymphatic drainage, invasion of the tumor into the skull base provides access to the rich lymphatic network present in the latter, one which in turn mediates systemic dissemination. The conclusive diagnosis of a pituitary carcinoma rests upon the morphologic examination of a metastatic deposit in a patient with a known history of a pituitary tumor. As a rule, the metastatic deposit will retain the immunotype of the primary tumor. The pituitary is not infrequently the recipient to metastasizing carcinomas originating systemically, and one must, therefore, by careful clinical and pathological examination, exclude the far more common occurrence of metastatic deposits to the pituitary gland before arriving at a diagnosis of primary pituitary carcinoma.

As a result of their rarity, specific management guidelines do not exist for these unusual cancers. Since the primary lesion is ordinarily the most symptomatic component of the disease, these tumors will be treated in a fashion similar to that of an aggressive pituitary adenoma. One or more surgical resections, radiation therapy, and, if responsive, pharmacologic therapy may all be required in an attempt to control the primary tumor, although as evidenced by published experience, this seldom appears to have been achieved. Recent case reports suggest a role for the alkylating chemotherapeutic agent Temozolomide in the management of these patients (Fadul et al 2006; Kovacs et al 2007; Lim et al 2006; Neff et al 2007; Syro et al 2006). However, patient numbers are too small to draw definitive conclusions. Metastatic deposits, particularly those involving the craniospinal axis, may require resection as is symptomatically necessary. In most cases, death from pituitary carcinoma results from the mass effects of uncontrollable local disease. In that neither the presence nor treatment of systemic metastases appears to significantly affect the prognosis of pituitary carcinomas, the frequency of metastases, particularly nonfunctioning ones, is likely underreported. Thus the true incidence of metastasizing pituitary tumors may be more common than is currently held. The prognosis for pituitary carcinomas is usually poor. In the series of Pernicone and co-workers (1997), 66% of 15 patients died within one year of diagnosis, and no patient survived longer than 8 years (Pernicone et al 1997).

Pituitary apoplexy

As classically defined, pituitary apoplexy refers to the abrupt and occasionally catastrophic occurrence of acute hemorrhagic infarction of a pituitary adenoma (Fig. 36.19). The clinical syndrome is easily recognized, consisting of acute headache, meningismus, visual impairment, ophthalmoplegia, and alterations in consciousness. Without timely intervention, patients are subject to die of subarachnoid hemorrhage and increased intracranial pressure, or succumb to acute, life-threatening hypopituitarism. Of particular importance is the realization that most patients will not, at the time of their ictus, be aware that they harbor a pituitary adenoma; apoplexy itself is often the presenting manifestation. As defined herein, pituitary apoplexy is a complication in 1–2% of all pituitary adenomas. Sub-clinical hemorrhage into a pituitary adenoma with accompanying hemorrhage, necrosis, or cystic change is evident in up to 20% of all surgical specimens without an antecedent history of an apoplectic event. Pituitary apoplexy has been the subject of a number of comprehensive reviews (Bills et al 1993; Bonicki et al 1993; Cardoso & Peterson 1984; Ebersold et al 1983; Laws 1997; Mohr & Hardy 1982; Semple et al 2006, 2007, 2008). There is little consensus in the literature as to which tumor types, if any, are most vulnerable to apoplectic hemorrhage. Some have suggested that hormonally active tumors associated with acromegaly and Cushing's disease are especially prone to apoplexy, whereas others have found large non-functioning tumors to bear substantial risk.

The pathophysiologic basis of pituitary apoplexy remains speculative. Ischemic necrosis of a rapidly growing tumor, intrinsic vascular abnormalities peculiar to pituitary tumors, and compression of the superior hypophyseal artery against the sellar diaphragm have all been suggested as mechanisms contributing to apoplectic hemorrhage (Cardoso & Peterson 1984). Predisposing factors also loosely associated with apoplexy include bromocriptine therapy, anticoagulation,

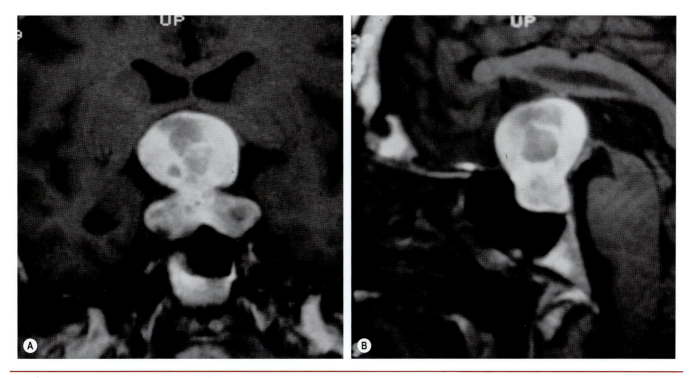

Figure 36.19 Pituitary apoplexy. Sagittal and coronal MR images of a hemorrhagic pituitary adenoma in a patient with acute headache and visual loss.

diabetic ketoacidosis, head trauma, estrogen therapy, and pituitary irradiation. Most cases occur in the absence of any known predisposing condition.

Chronologically, the pathologic profile of apoplexy begins with infarction of the tumor and the surrounding gland, followed by hemorrhage and edema. This sudden increase in intratumoral pressure and volume causes precipitous expansion of the tumor, followed by mechanical compression of the optic apparatus and of structures within the cavernous sinus. The bulk of the hemorrhage is generally contained within a tense tumor wall, although extravasation of blood into the subarachnoid space is a frequent occurrence. Obstructive hydrocephalus may further complicate apoplexy in large macroadenomas having a significant suprasellar component. Glandular destruction of varying degree is a regular pathologic feature of apoplexy, one accounting for partial, total, transient, or permanent hypopituitarism. The posterior pituitary, having its own blood supply, generally escapes injury. Accordingly, diabetes insipidus is rarely a complication of pituitary apoplexy.

Acute hemorrhagic infarction of a pituitary tumor constitutes a true neurosurgical emergency for which prompt recognition and glucocorticoid replacement are the most important first management steps. Acute adrenal insufficiency from operative or non-operative stress may frequently be present and can readily result in collapse or even fatality if not appropriately treated in a timely manner. Despite occasional reports to the contrary, it has been our position that urgent and effective surgical decompression of the sella with removal of the lesion constitutes the most appropriate management for this condition. Whereas historical accounts of pituitary apoplexy were often associated with a fatal outcome, current management protocols with steroid replacement and urgent decompression have led to a good prognosis in most instances. Recovery of vision and oculomotor palsies, although somewhat unpredictable and by no means guaranteed, frequently occurs with time. Our more recent review would suggest that recovery occurs more often after an infarctive event instead of a hemorrhagic (Semple et al 2006).

Key points

- Pituitary tumors are common lesions, accounting for 10–15% of all primary intracranial tumors.

- The normal pituitary gland consists of lactotrophs, somatotrophs, corticotrophs, thyrotrophs, and gonadotrophs, any of which may be subject to neoplastic transformation, giving rise to a neoplasm which retains the secretory capacity, morphologic characteristics, and nomenclature of the cell of origin.

- Pituitary tumors are believed to be monoclonal neoplasms that arise as the result of specific somatic mutations, of which several genomic alterations have been cataloged to date.

- Pituitary tumors can present on the basis of pituitary hypersecretion (amenorrhea-galactorrhea syndrome, acromegaly, Cushing's disease, or secondary hyperthyroidism) or highly characteristic mass effects which also include hypopituitarism.

- Their diagnosis requires both an endocrine diagnosis and an anatomic diagnosis, the former being provided by specific basal and provocative hormone assays, and the latter being provided by MR imaging.

- The goals of therapy include: (1) reversal of endocrinopathy and restoration of normal pituitary function; (2) elimination of mass effect and restoration of normal neurologic function; (3) eliminating or minimizing the possibility of tumor recurrence; and (4) obtain a definitive histologic diagnosis.

- Therapeutic options include surgery, medical therapy, conventional radiotherapy, and stereotactic radiosurgery. Each patient requires an individualized program of management, which frequently begins with transsphenoidal surgery, and may also include other options depending on the responsiveness to surgery.

- Prolactin-producing pituitary adenomas are best managed by dopamine agonist therapy, with surgery being reserved for those patients poorly responsive or intolerant to medical therapy.

- For growth hormone-producing pituitary tumors, transsphenoidal surgery is the treatment of choice. Depending on the size and invasion status of the tumor, surgery can induce remission in 50–75% of patients. For patients in whom remission is not achieved surgically and GH levels remain in excess of 2.5 ng/mL, adjuvant therapy with somatostatin analogs, GH receptor antagonists, radiosurgery, or conventional radiation is advisable.

- The diagnosis of corticotroph adenomas responsible for Cushing's disease requires a comprehensive endocrine evaluation to establish the pituitary as the source of cortisol excess. Most are microadenomas whose removal requires careful transsphenoidal exploration of the normal pituitary gland. In the majority of instances, a corticotroph adenoma can be identified intraoperatively and a durable remission can be achieved in approximately 90% of cases.

- Clinically non-functioning pituitary adenomas typically present when sufficiently large to produce mass effects. Transsphenoidal removal will reverse compressive symptoms in the majority of patients, without the need of adjuvant therapy. Progressive lesions exhibiting rapid regrowth are candidates for radiotherapy. So treated, approximately 75% of patients experience symptom free and/or progression free survival during long-term follow-up.

- All patients with pituitary tumors, particularly those having undergone surgery, require periodic surveillance for hormone deficiencies, as careful replacement therapy can very significantly lessen the morbidity associated with these lesions.

REFERENCES

Alexander, L., Appleton, D., Hall, R., et al., 1980. Epidemiology of acromegaly in the Newcastle region. Clin. Endocr. 12, 71–79.

Arafah, B.M., Brodkey, J.S., Kaufman, B., et al., 1980. Transsphenoidal microsurgery in the treatment of acromegaly and gigantism. J. Clin. Endocrinol. Metab. 50, 578–585.

Assie, G., Bahurel, H., Coste, J., et al., 2007. Corticotroph tumor progression after adrenalectomy in Cushing's Disease: A reappraisal of Nelson's Syndrome. J. Clin. Endocrinol. Metab. 92, 172–179.

Balagura, S., Derome, P., Guiot, G., 1981. Acromegaly: analysis of 132 cases treated surgically. Neurosurgery 8, 413–416.

Bates, A.S., Van't Hoff, W., Jones, J.M., et al., 1993. An audit of outcome of treatment in acromegaly. Q. J. Med. 86, 293–299.

Beauregard, C., Truong, U., Hardy, J., et al., 2003. Long-term outcome and mortality after transsphenoidal adenomectomy for acromegaly. Clin. Endocrinol. 58, 86–91.

Beck-Peccoz, P., Brucker-Davis, F., Persani, L., et al., 1996. Thyrotropin-secreting pituitary tumors. Endocr. Rev. 17, 610–638.

Bengtsson, B.A., Eden, S., Ernest, I., et al., 1988. Epidemiology and long-term survival in acromegaly. A study of 166 cases diagnosed between 1955 and 1984. Acta Medica Scandinavica 223, 327–335.

Bevan, J.S., Adams, C.B., Burke, C.W., 1987. Factors in the outcome of transsphenoidal surgery for prolactinoma and non-functioning pituitary tumor, including pre-operative bromocriptine therapy. Clin. Endocrinol. 26, 541–546.

Biermasz, N.R., van Dulken, H., Roelfsema, F., 2000a. Postoperative radiotherapy in acromegaly is effective in reducing GH concentration to safe levels. Clin. Endocrinol. 53, 321–327.

Biermasz, N.R., van Dulken, H., Roelfsema, F., 2000b. Ten-year follow-up results of transsphenoidal microsurgery in acromegaly. J. Clin. Endocrinol. Metab. 85, 4596–4602.

Bills, D., Meyer, F., Laws, E.R. Jr., et al., 1993. A retrospective analysis of pituitary apoplexy. Neurosurgery 33, 602–609.

Blevins, L.S., Christy, J.H., Khajavi, M., et al., 1998. Outcomes of therapy for Cushing's disease due to adrenocorticotropin-secreting pituitary macroadenomas. J. Clin. Endocrinol. Metab. 83, 63–67.

Bochicchio, D., Losa, M., Buchfelder, M., 1995. Factors influencing the immediate and late outcome of Cushing's disease treated by transsphenoidal surgery: A retrospective study by the European Cushing's disease survey group. J. Clin. Endocrinol. Metab. 80, 3114–3120.

Bonadonna, S., Doga, M., Gola, M., et al., 2005. Diagnosis and treatment of acromegaly and its complications: consensus guidelines. J. Endocrinol. Invest. 28, 43–47.

Bonicki, W., Kasperlik-Zaluska, A., Koszewski, W., 1993. Pituitary apoplexy: endocrine, surgical and oncological emergency. Incidence, clinical course and treatment with reference to 799 cases of pituitary adenomas. Acta Neurochirurgica 120, 118–122.

Brucker-Davis, F., Oldfield, E.H., Skarulis, M.C., et al., 1999. Thyrotropin-secreting pituitary tumors: diagnostic criteria, thyroid hormone sensitivity, and treatment outcome in 25 patients followed at the National Institutes of Health. J. Clin. Endocrinol. Metab. 84, 476–486.

Buchfelder, M., Brockmeier, S., Fahlbusch, R., 1991. Recurrence following transsphenoidal surgery for acromegaly. Horm. Res. 35, 113–118.

Bush, Z.M., Vance, M.L., 2008. Management of acromegaly: Is there a role for primary medical therapy? Rev. Endocrinol. Metab. Disord. 9, 83–94.

Cannavo, S., Squadrito, S., Curto, L., et al., 2000. Results of a two-year treatment with slow release lanreotide in acromegaly. Horm. Metab. Res. 32, 224–229.

Cappabianca, P., Cavallo, L.M., Esposito, F., et al., 2003. Rationale of pre-surgical medical treatment with somatostatin analogs in acromegaly. J. Endocrinol. Invest. 26, 55–58.

Cardoso, E., Peterson, E., 1984. Pituitary apoplexy: a review. Neurosurgery 14, 363–373.

Caron, P., Morange-Ramos, I., Cogne, M., et al., 1997. Three year follow-up of acromegalic patients treated with intramuscular slow-release lanreotide. J. Clin. Endocrinol. Metab. 82, 18–22.

Castinetti, F., Morange, I., Dufour, H., et al., 2007. Radiotherapy and radiosurgery in acromegaly. Pituitary 1–8.

Chandler, W.F., Schteingart, D., Lloyd, R., et al., 1987. Surgical treatment of Cushing's disease. J. Neurosurg. 66, 204–212.

Chanson, P., Weintraub, B.D., Harris, A.G., 1993. Octreotide therapy for thyroid-stimulating hormone-secreting pituitary adenomas. A follow-up of 52 patients. Ann. Intern. Med. 119, 236–240.

Chee, G.H., Mathias, D.B., James, R.A., et al., 2001. Transsphenoidal pituitary surgery in Cushing's disease: can we predict outcome? Clin. Endocrinol. 54, 617–626.

Chen, J.C., Amar, A.P., Choi, S., et al., 2003. Transsphenoidal microsurgical treatment of Cushing disease: postoperative assessment of surgical efficacy by application of an overnight low-dose dexamethasone suppression test. J. Neurosurg. 98, 967–973.

Chiodini, P., Liuzzi, A., Cozzi, R., 1981. Size reduction of macroprolactinomas by bromocriptine or lisuride treatment. J. Clin. Endocrinol. Metab. 53, 737–743.

Chou, S.C., Lin, J.D., 2000. Long-term effects of ketoconazole in the treatment of residual or recurrent Cushing's disease. Endocrinol. J. 47, 401–406.

Colao, A., Di Sarno, A., Cappabianca, P., et al., 2003. Withdrawal of long-term cabergoline therapy for tumoral and nontumoral hyperprolactinemia. N. Engl. J. Med. 349, 2023–2033.

Colao, A., Ferone, D., Cappabianca, P., et al., 1997. Effect of octreotide pretreatment on surgical outcome in acromegaly. J. Clin. Endocrinol. Metab. 82, 3308–3314.

Corenblum, B., Taylor, P.J., 1983. Long-term follow-up of hyperprolactinemic women treated with bromocriptine. Fertil. Steril. 40, 596–599.

Davies, P.H., Stewart, S.E., Lancranjan, L., et al., 1998. Long-term therapy with long-acting octreotide (Sandostatin-LAR) for the management of acromegaly [published erratum appears in Clin. Endocrinol. (Oxf.) 1998 May;48(5):673]. Clin. Endocrinol. 48, 311–316.

Davis, D.H., Laws, E.R. Jr., Ilstrup, D.M., et al., 1993. Results of surgical treatment for growth hormone-secreting pituitary adenomas. J. Neurosurg. 79, 70–75.

De, P., Rees, D.A., Davies, N., et al., 2003. Transsphenoidal surgery for acromegaly in Wales: Results based on stringent criteria of remission. J. Clin. Endocrinol. Metab. 88, 3567–3572.

De Tommasi, C., Vance, M.L., Okonkwo, D.O., et al., 2005. Surgical management of adrenocorticotropic hormone-secreting macroadenomas: outcome and challenges in patients with Cushing's disease or Nelson's syndrome. J. Neurosurg. 103, 825–830.

Degerblad, M., Rahn, T., Bergstrand, G., et al., 1986. Long-term results of stereotactic radiosurgery to the pituitary gland in Cushing's disease. Acta Endocrinologica 112, 310–314.

Eastman, R.C., Gorden, P., Glatstein, E., et al., 1992. Radiation therapy of acromegaly. Endocrinol. Metab. Clin. North Am. 21, 693–712.

Eastman, R.C., Gorden, P., Roth, J., 1979. Conventional supervoltage irradiation is an effective treatment for acromegaly. J. Clin. Endocrinol. Metab. 48, 931–940.

Ebersold, M.J., Laws, E.R. Jr., Scheitauer, B.W., et al., 1983. Pituitary apoplexy treated by transsphenoidal surgery: A clinicopathological and immunocytochemical study. J. Neurosurg. 58, 315–320.

Esposito, F., Dusick, J.R., Cohan, P., et al., 2006. Clinical review: Early morning cortisol levels as a predictor of remission after transsphenoidal surgery for Cushing's disease. J. Clin. Endocrinol. Metab. 91, 7–13.

Estrada, J., Boronat, M., Mielgo, M., et al., 1997. The long-term outcome of pituitary irradiation after unsuccessful transsphenoidal surgery in Cushing's disease. N. Engl. J. Med. 336, 172–177.

Ezzat, S., Melmed, S., 1991. Are patients with acromegaly at increased risk for neoplasia? J. Clin. Endocrinol. Metab. 72, 245–249.

Ezzat, S., Snyder, P., Young, W.F. Jr., et al., 1992. Octreotide treatment of acromegaly. A randomized, multicenter study. Ann. Intern. Med. 117, 711–718.

Ezzat, S., Strom, C., Melmed, S., 1991. Colon polyps in acromegaly. Ann. Intern. Med. 114, 754–755.

Fadul, C.E., Kominsky, A.L., Meyer, L.P., et al., 2006. Long-term response of pituitary carcinoma to temozolomide. Report of two cases. J. Neurosurg. 105, 621–626.

Faglia, G., Arosio, M., Bazzoni, N., 1992. Ectopic acromegaly. Endocrinol. Metab. Clin. North Am. 21, 575–595.

Fahlbusch, R., Buchfelder, M., Schrell, U., 1987. Short-term preoperative treatment of macroprolactinomas by dopamine agonists. J. Neurosurg. 67, 807–815.

Feek, C.M., McLelland, J., Seth, J., et al., 1984. How effective is external pituitary irradiation for growth hormone-secreting pituitary tumors? Clin. Endocrinol. 20, 401–408.

Findling, J.W., Raff, H., 1999. Newer diagnostic techniques and problems in Cushing's disease. Endocrinol. Metab. Clin. North. Am. 28, 191–210.

Fleseriu, M., Loriaux, D.L., Ludlam, W.H., et al., 2007. Second-line treatment for Cushing's disease when initial pituitary surgery is unsuccessful. Curr. Opin. Endocrinol. Diabetes Obes. 14, 323–328.

Flitsch, J., Knappe, U.J., Ludecke, D.K., 2003. The use of postoperative A C T H levels as a marker for successful transsphenoidal microsurgery in Cushing's disease. Zentralblatt Neurochirurgie 64, 6–11.

Flogstad, A.K., Halse, J., Bakke, S., et al., 1997. Sandostatin L A R in acromegalic patients: long-term treatment. J. Clin. Endocrinol. Metab. 82, 23–28.

Forbes, A.P., Henneman, P.H., Griswold, G.C., et al., 1954. Syndrome characterized by galactorrhea, amenorrhea and low urinary FSH: comparison with acromegaly and normal lactation. J. Clin. Endocrinol. Metab. 14, 265–271.

Force, A.A.G.T., 2004. AACE Medical Guidelines for Clinical Practice for the diagnosis and treatment of acromegaly. [erratum appears in Endocrinol. Pract. 2005 11(2):144]. Endocr. Pract. 10, 213–225.

Freda, P.U., Nuruzzaman, A.T., Reyes, C.M., et al., 2004. Significance of 'abnormal' nadir growth hormone levels after oral glucose in postoperative patients with acromegaly in remission with normal insulin-like growth factor-I levels. J. Clin. Endocrinol. Metab. 89, 495–500.

Freda, P.U., Post, K.D., Powell, J.S., et al., 1998a. Evaluation of disease status with sensitive measures of growth hormone secretion in 60 postoperative patients with acromegaly. J. Clin. Endocrinol. Metab. 83, 3808–3816.

Freda, P.U., Wardlaw, S.L., Post, K.D., 1998b. Long-term endocrinological follow-up evaluation in 115 patients who underwent transsphenoidal surgery for acromegaly. J. Neurosurg. 89, 353–358.

Friedman, T.C., Zuckerbraun, E., Lee, M.L., et al., 2007. Dynamic pituitary M R I has high sensitivity and specificity for the diagnosis of mild Cushing's syndrome and should be part of the initial workup. Horm. Metab. Res. 39, 451–456.

Furth, J., Ueda, G., Clifton, K., 1973. The pathophysiology of pituitaries and their tumors. Methodological advances. Methods Cancer Res. 10, 201–277.

Gil-Cardenas, A., Herrera, M.F., Diaz-Polanco, A., et al., 2007. Nelson's syndrome after bilateral adrenalectomy for Cushing's disease. Surgery 141, 147–151; discussion 151–142.

Gittoes, N.J., Sheppard, M.C., Johnson, A.P., et al., 1999. Outcome of surgery for acromegaly–the experience of a dedicated pituitary surgeon. Q. J. Med. 92, 741–745.

Giustina, A., Barkan, A., Casanueva, F.F., et al., 2000. Criteria for cure of acromegaly: a consensus statement. J. Clin. Endocrinol. Metab. 85, 526–529.

Greenman, Y., Melmed, S., 1995. Thyrotropin-secreting pituitary tumors. In: Melmed, S. (Ed.), The pituitary. Blackwell Science, Cambridge, M A, pp. 546–558.

Grisoli, F., Leclercq, T., Jaquet, P., 1985. Transsphenoidal surgery for acromegaly. Long-term results in 100 patients. Surg. Neurol. 23, 513–519.

Growth Hormone Research Society, Pituitary Society, 2004. Biochemical assessment and long-term monitoring in patients with acromegaly: statement from a joint consensus conference of the Growth Hormone Research Society and the Pituitary Society. J. Clin. Endocrinol. Metab. 89, 3099–3102.

Guilhaume, B., Bertagna, X., Thomsen, M., 1988. Transsphenoidal pituitary surgery for the treatment of Cushing's disease: Results in 64 patients and long term follow-up studies. J. Clin. Endocrinol. Metab. 66, 1056–1064.

Gutt, B., Hatzack, C., Morrison, K., et al., 2001. Conventional pituitary irradiation is effective in normalising plasma IGF-I in patients with acromegaly. Eur. J. Endocrinol. 144, 109–116.

Guy, J., Mancuso, A., Beck, R., et al., 1991. Radiation-induced optic neuropathy: a magnetic resonance imaging study. J. Neurosurg. 74, 426–432.

Hamilton, D.K., Vance, M.L., Boulos, P.T., et al., 2005. Surgical outcomes in hyporesponsive prolactinomas: analysis of patients with resistance or intolerance to dopamine agonists. Pituitary 8, 53–60.

Hammer, G.D., Tyrrell, J.B., Lamborn, K.R., et al., 2004. Transsphenoidal microsurgery for Cushing's disease: initial outcome and long-term results. J. Clin. Endocrinol. Metab. 89, 6348–6357.

Hardy, J., 1973. Transsphenoidal surgery of hypersecreting pituitary adenomas. In: Kohler, P.O., Ross, G.T. (Eds.), Diagnosis and treatment of pituitary tumors. Elsevier, New York, pp. 179–194.

Hasegawa, S., Hamada, J., Morioka, M., et al., 2000. Radiation-induced cerebrovasculopathy of the distal middle cerebral artery and distal posterior cerebral artery. Case report. Neurol. Medico-Chirurgica. 40, 220–223.

Horvath, A., Stratakis, C.A., 2008. Clinical and molecular genetics of acromegaly: MEN1, Carney complex, McCune-Albright syndrome, familial acromegaly and genetic defects in sporadic tumors. Rev. Endocr. Metab. Disord. 9, 1–11.

Horvath, J., Fross, R.D., Kleiner-Fisman, G., et al., 2004. Severe multivalvular heart disease: a new complication of the ergot derivative dopamine agonists. Mov. Disord. 19, 656–662.

Hubbard, J.L., Scheithauer, B.W., Abboud, C.F., et al., 1987. Prolactin-secreting adenomas: the preoperative response to bromocriptine treatment and surgical outcome. J. Neurosurg. 67, 816–821.

Jaffe, C.A., Barkan, A.L., 1992. Treatment of acromegaly with dopamine agonists. Endocrinol. Metab. Clin. North. Am. 21, 713–735.

Jagannathan, J., Kanter, A.S., Olson, C., et al., 2008. Applications of radiotherapy and radiosurgery in the management of pediatric Cushing's disease: a review of the literature and our experience. J. Neurooncol. 90, 117–124.

Jagannathan, J., Sheehan, J.P., Pouratian, N., et al., 2008a. Gamma knife radiosurgery for acromegaly: outcomes after failed transsphenoidal surgery. Neurosurgery 62, 1262–1269; discussion 1269–1270.

Jagannathan, J., Sheehan, J.P., Pouratian, N., et al., 2007b. Gamma Knife surgery for Cushing's disease. J. Neurosurg. 106, 980–987.

Jane, J.A. Jr., Laws, E.R. Jr., 2001. The surgical management of pituitary adenomas in a series of 3,093 patients. J. Am. Coll. Surg. 193, 651–659.

Jawiarczyk, A., Kaluzny, M., Bolanowski, M., et al., 2008. Additional metabolic effects of adding G H receptor antagonist to long-acting somatostatin analog in patients with active acromegaly. Neuroendocrinol. Lett. 29, 571–576.

Jezkova, J., Marek, J., Hana, V., et al., 2006. Gamma knife radiosurgery for acromegaly – long-term experience. Clin. Endocrinol. 64, 588–595.

Jimenez, C., Burman, P., Abs, R., et al., 2008. Follow-up of pituitary tumor volume in patients with acromegaly treated with pegvisomant in clinical trials. Eur. J. Endocrinol. 159, 517–523.

Johnston, D.G., Prescot, R., Kendall-Taylor, P., et al., 1983. Hyperprolactinemia: Long-term effects of bromocriptine. Am. J. Med. 75, 868–874.

Jordan, R.M., Kohler, P.O., 1987. Recent advances in diagnosis and treatment of pituitary tumors. Adv. Intern. Med. 32, 299–323.

Kanter, A.S., Diallo, A.O., Jane, J.A., et al., 2005. Single-center experience with pediatric Cushing's disease. J. Neurosurg. 103, 413–420.

Kasperlik-Zaluska, A.A., Bonicki, W., Jeske, W., et al., 2006. Nelson's syndrome – 46 years later: clinical experience with 37 patients. Zentralbl. Neurochirurg. 67, 14–20.

Kaye, T.B., Crapo, L., 1990. The Cushing syndrome: an update on diagnostic tests. Ann. Intern. Med. 112, 434–444.

Klibanski, A., Greenspan, S.L., 1986. Increase in bone mass after treatment of hyperprolactinemic amenorrhea. N. Engl. J. Med. 315, 542–546.

Klibanski, A., Zervas, N.T., 1991. Diagnosis and management of hormone-secreting pituitary adenomas. N. Engl. J. Med. 324, 822–831.

Kovacs, K., Horvath, E., 1986. Tumors of the pituitary gland. Armed Forces Institute of Pathology, Washington, D C.

Kovacs, K., Horvath, E., Syro, L.V., et al., 2007. Temozolomide therapy in a man with an aggressive prolactin-secreting pituitary neoplasm: Morphological findings. [erratum appears in Hum. Pathol. 38(3):526]. Hum. Pathol. 38, 185–189.

Kovacs, K., Stefaneanu, L., Horvath, E., et al., 1991. Effect of dopamine agonist medication on prolactin-producing pituitary adenomas. A morphological study including immunocytochemistry, electron microscopy, and in situ hybridization. Virchows Arch. Pathol. Anat. 418, 439–446.

Kreutzer, J., Vance, M.L., Lopes, M.B., et al., 2001. Surgical management of GH-secreting pituitary adenomas: an outcome study using modern remission criteria. J. Clin. Endocrinol. Metab. 86, 4072–4077.

Kristof, R.A., Stoffel-Wagner, B., Klingmuller, D., et al., 1999. Does octreotide treatment improve the surgical results of macroadenomas in acromegaly? A randomized study. Acta Neurochirurgica 141, 399–405.

Labat-Moleur, F., Trouillas, J., Seret-Begue, D., et al., 1991. Evaluation of 29 monoclonal and polyclonal antibodies used in the diagnosis of pituitary adenomas. A collaborative study from pathologists of the Club Francais de l'Hypophyse. Pathol. Res. Pract. 187, 534–538.

Lamberts, S.W., Reubi, J.C., Krenning, E.P., 1992. Somatostatin analogs in the treatment of acromegaly. Endocrinol. Metab. Clin. North. Am. 21, 737–752.

Lamberts, S.W., Van der Lely, A.J., De Herder, W.W., et al., 1996. Octreotide. N. Engl. J. Med. 334, 246–254.

Landolt, A.M., 1981. Surgical treatment of pituitary prolactinomas: postoperative prolactin and fertility in seventy patients. Fertil. Steril. 36, 620–625.

Landolt, A.M., Haller, D., Lomax, N., et al., 1998. Stereotactic radiosurgery for recurrent surgically treated acromegaly: comparison with fractionated radiotherapy. J. Neurosurg. 88, 1002–1008.

Landolt, A.M., Keller, P., Froesch, E., et al., 1982. Bromocriptine: does it jeopardise the result of later surgery for prolactinomas? Lancet 2, 657–658.

Laws, E.R. Jr., Piepgras, D.G., Randall, R.V., et al., 1979. Neurosurgical management of acromegaly. Results in 82 patients treated between 1972 and 1977. J. Neurosurg. 50, 454–461.

Laws, E.R. Jr., Trautmann, J.C., Hollenhorst, R.W. Jr., 1977. Transsphenoidal decompression of the optic nerve and chiasm. Visual results in 62 patients. J. Neurosurg. 46, 717–722.

Laws, E.R. Jr., Sheehan, J.P., Sheehan, J.M., et al., 2004. Stereotactic radiosurgery for pituitary adenomas: a review of the literature. J. Neurooncol. 69, 257–272.

Laws, E.R. Jr., Vance, M.L., Jane, J.A. Jr., 2006. TSH adenomas. Pituitary 9, 313–315.

Laws, E.R. Jr., 1990. Neurosurgical management of acromegaly. In: Cooper, P.R. (Ed.), Contemporary diagnosis and management of pituitary adenomas. American Association of Neurological Surgeons, Park Ridge, pp. 53–59.

Laws, E.R. Jr., 1997. Surgical management of pituitary apoplexy. In: Welch, K., Caplan, L., Reis, D. (Eds.), Primer on cerebrovascular diseases. Academic Press, New York, pp. 508–510.

Laws, E.R. Jr., Chennelle, A., Thapar, K., et al., 1996. Recurrence after transsphenoidal surgery for pituitary adenomas: clinical and basic science aspects. In: von Werder, K., Fahlbusch, R. (Eds.), Pituitary adenomas. Elsevier, Amsterdam, pp. 3–9.

Laws, E.R. Jr., Thapar, K., 1996. Recurrent pituitary adenomas. In: Landolt, A.M., Vance, M.L., Reilly, P.L. (Eds.), Pituitary adenomas. Churchill Livingstone, Edinburgh, pp. 385–394.

Lim, S., Shahinian, H., Maya, M.M., et al., 2006. Temozolomide: a novel treatment for pituitary carcinoma. Lancet. Oncol. 7, 518–520.

Liu, J.K., Fleseriu, M., Delashaw, J.B., et al., 2007. Treatment options for Cushing disease after unsuccessful transsphenoidal surgery. Neurosurg. Focus 23, E8.

Losa, M., Oeckler, R., Schopohl, J., et al., 1989. Evaluation of selective transsphenoidal adenomectomy by endocrinological testing and somatostatin-C measurement in acromegaly. J. Neurosurg. 70, 561–567.

Luciano, M., Oldfield, E.H., 1990. The diagnosis of Cushing's disease. In: Cooper, P.R. (Ed.), Contemporary diagnosis and management of pituitary adenomas. Association of Neurological Surgeons, Park Ridge, pp. 101–123.

Mampalam, T.J., Tyrrell, J.B., Wilson, C., 1988. Transsphenoidal microsurgery for Cushing's disease. A report of 216 cases. Ann. Intern. Med. 109, 487–493.

March, C., Kletzky, O., Danavan, V., 1981. Longitudinal evaluation of patients with untreated prolactin-secreting pituitary adenomas. Am. J. Obstet. Gynecol. 139, 835–844.

Massoud, F., Serri, O., Hardy, J., et al., 1996. Transsphenoidal adenomectomy for microprolactinomas: 10 to 20 years of follow-up. Surg. Neurol. 45, 341–346.

Mauermann, W.J., Sheehan, J.P., Chernavvsky, D.R., et al., 2007. Gamma Knife surgery for adrenocorticotropic hormone-producing pituitary adenomas after bilateral adrenalectomy. J. Neurosurg. 106, 988–993.

McCutcheon, I.E., McCutcheon, I.E., 2002. Stereotactic radiosurgery for patients with ACTH-producing pituitary adenomas after prior adrenalectomy. Int. J. Radiat. Oncol. Biol. Physics 54, 640–641.

Melmed, S., Casanueva, F.F., Cavagnini, F., et al., 2002. Guidelines for acromegaly management. J. Clin. Endocrinol. Metab. 87, 4054–4058.

Mixon, A., Frieman, T., Katz, D., et al., 1993. Thyrotropin secreting pituitary carcinoma. J. Clin. Endocrinol. Metab. 76, 529–533.

Mohr, G., Hardy, J., 1982. Hemorrhage, necrosis, and apoplexy in pituitary adenomas. Surg. Neurol. 18, 181–189.

Molitch, M.E., 1992a. Clinical manifestations of acromegaly. Endocrinol. Metab. Clin. North. Am. 21, 597–614.

Molitch, M.E., 1992b. Pathologic hyperprolactinemia. Endocrinol. Metab. Clin. North. Am. 21, 877–901.

Molitch, M.E., 1985. Pregnancy in the hyperprolactinemic woman. N. Engl. J. Med. 312, 1365–1370.

Molitch, M.E., Elton, R.L., Blackwell, R.E., et al., 1985. Bromocriptine as primary therapy for prolactin-secreting macroadenomas: results of a prospective multicenter study. J. Clin. Endocrinology Metab. 60, 698–705.

Morange, I., De Boisvilliers, F., Chanson, P., et al., 1994. Slow release lanreotide treatment in acromegalic patients previously normalized by octreotide. J. Clin. Endocrinol. Metab. 79, 145–151.

Muhr, C., Bergstrom, M., Lundberg, P., et al., 1991. PET imaging of pituitary adenomas. Exerpta. Med. Int. Congr. Ser. 961, 237–244.

Mustacchi, P., Shimkin, M.B., 1957. Occurrence of cancer in acromegaly and hypopituitarism. Cancer 10, 100–104.

Nabarro, J.D., 1987. Acromegaly. Clin. Endocrinol. 26, 481–512.

Nakane, T., Kuwayama, A., Watanabe, M., et al., 1987. Long term results of transsphenoidal adenomectomy in patients with Cushing's disease. Neurosurgery 21, 218–222.

Neff, L.M., Weil, M., Cole, A., et al., 2007. Temozolomide in the treatment of an invasive prolactinoma resistant to dopamine agonists. Pituitary 10, 81–86.

Neggers, S.J., van Aken, M.O., de Herder, W.W., et al., 2008. Quality of life in acromegalic patients during long-term somatostatin analog treatment with and without pegvisomant. J. Clin. Endocrinol. Metab. 93, 3853–3859.

Newell-Price, J., Trainer, P., Besser, M., et al., 1998. The diagnosis and differential diagnosis of Cushing's syndrome and pseudo-Cushing's states. Endocr. Rev. 19, 647–672.

Nicola, G.C., Tonnarelli, G., Griner, A.C., 1991. Surgery for recurrence of pituitary adenomas. In: Faglia, G., Beck-Peccoz, P., Ambrosi, B. (Eds.), Pituitary adenomas: New trends in basic and clinical research. Excerpta Medica, Amsterdam, pp. 329–338.

Nomikos, P., Buchfelder, M., Fahlbusch, R., et al., 2005. The outcome of surgery in 668 patients with acromegaly using current criteria of biochemical 'cure'. Eur. J. Endocrinol. 152, 379–387.

O'Brien, T., O'Riordan, S.D., Gharib, H., et al., 1996. Results of treatment of pituitary disease in multiple endocrine neoplasia, type 1. Neurosurgery 39, 273–279.

Oldfield, E.H., Doppman, J.L., Nieman, L.K., et al., 1991. Petrosal sinus sampling with and without corticotropin-releasing hormone for the differential diagnosis of Cushing's syndrome. N. Engl. J. Med. 325, 897–905.

Patil, C.G., Prevedello, D.M., Lad, S.P., et al., 2008. Late recurrences of Cushing's disease after initial successful transsphenoidal surgery. J. Clin. Endocrinol. Metab. 93, 358–362.

Patronas, N., Bulakbasi, N., Stratakis, C.A., et al., 2003. Spoiled gradient recalled acquisition in the steady state technique is superior to conventional postcontrast spin echo technique for magnetic resonance imaging detection of adrenocorticotropin-secreting pituitary tumors. J. Clin. Endocrinol. Metab. 88, 1565–1569.

Peck, F.C. Jr., McGovern, E.R., 1966. Radiation necrosis of the brain in acromegaly. J. Neurosurg. 25, 536–542.

Pellegrini, I., Gunz, G., Bertran, P., et al., 1989. Resistance to bromocriptine in prolactinomas. J. Clin. Endocrinol. Metab. 69, 500–509.

Pernicone, P., Scheithauer, B., Sebo, T.J., 1995. Pituitary carcinoma: a clinicopathologic study of fifteen cases. J. Neuropathol. Exp. Neurol. 54, 456.

Pernicone, P.J., Scheithauer, B.W., Sebo, T.J., et al., 1997. Pituitary carcinoma: A clinicopathologic study of 15 cases. Cancer 79, 804–812.

Perrin, G., Treluyer, C., Trouillas, J., 1991. Surgical outcome and pathological effects of bromocriptine pretreatment in prolactinomas. Pathol. Res. Pract. 187, 587–592.

Petruson, K., Jakobsson, K., Oetryseib, B., et al., 1997. Transsphenoidal adenomectomy in Cushing's disease via a lateral rhinotomy approach. Surg. Neurol. 48, 37–45.

Plotz, C.M., Knowlton, A.I., Ragan, C., 1952. The natural history of Cushing's syndrome. Am. J. Med. 13, 597–614.

Pollock, B.E., 2007. Radiosurgery for pituitary adenomas. Prog. Neurol. Surg. 20, 164–171.

Pollock, B.E., Jacob, J.T., Brown, P.D., et al., 2007. Radiosurgery of growth hormone-producing pituitary adenomas: Factors associated with biochemical remission. J. Neurosurg. 106, 833–838.

Pollock, B.E., Young, W.F. Jr., Pollock, B.E., et al., 2002. Stereotactic radiosurgery for patients with ACTH-producing pituitary adenomas after prior adrenalectomy. Int. J. Radiat. Oncol. Biol. Physics 54, 839–841.

Post, K., Habas, J.E., 1990. Comparison of long term results between prolactin secreting adenomas and A C T H secreting adenomas. Can. J. Neurol. Sci. 17, 74–77.

Prevedello, D.M., Pouratian, N., Sherman, J., et al., 2008. Management of Cushing's disease: outcome in patients with microadenoma detected on pituitary magnetic resonance imaging. J. Neurosurg. 109, 751–759.

Ram, Z., Nieman, L.K., Cutler, G.B. Jr., et al., 1994. Early repeat surgery for persistent Cushing's disease. J. Neurosurg. 80, 37–45.

Randall, R.V., Laws, E.R. Jr., Abboud, C.F., et al., 1983. Transsphenoidal microsurgical treatment of prolactin-producing pituitary adenomas. Results in 100 patients. Mayo Clin. Proc. 58, 108–121.

Randall, R.V., Scheithauer, B.W., Laws, E.R. Jr., 1985. Pituitary adenomas associated with hyperprolactinemia: A clinical and immunohistochemical study of 97 patients operated on transsphenoidally. Mayo Clin. Proc. 53, 24–28.

Rauhut, F., Stuschke, M., Sack, H., et al., 2002. Dependence of the risk of encephalopathy on the radiotherapy volume after combined surgery and radiotherapy of invasive pituitary tumours. Acta Neurochirurgica 144, 37–45; discussion 45–36.

Roberts, B.K., Ouyang, D.L., Lad, S.P., et al., 2007. Efficacy and safety of CyberKnife radiosurgery for acromegaly. Pituitary 10, 19–25.

Ross, D.A., Wilson, C.B., 1988. Results of transsphenoidal microsurgery for growth hormone-secreting pituitary adenoma in a series of 214 patients. J. Neurosurg. 68, 854–867.

Scheithauer, B.W., Kovacs, K., Randall, R.V., et al., 1986. Pathology of excessive production of growth hormone. Clin. Endocrinol. Metab. 15, 655–681.

Scheithauer, B.W., Laws, E.R. Jr., Kovacs, K., et al., 1987. Pituitary adenomas of the multiple endocrine neoplasia type I syndrome. Semin. Diagn. Pathol. 4, 205–211.

Schlechte, J., 1995. Clinical impact of hyperprolactinemia. Baillière's. Clinical Endocrinol. Metab. 9, 359–366.

Schlechte, J., Dolan, K., Sherman, B., et al., 1989. The natural history of untreated hyperprolactinemia: a prospective analysis. J. Clin. Endocrinol. Metab. 68, 412–418.

Semple, P.L., De Villiers, J.C., Bowen, R.M., et al., 2006. Pituitary apoplexy: do histological features influence the clinical presentation and outcome? J. Neurosurg. 104, 931–937.

Semple, P.L., Jane, J.A. Jr., Laws, E.R. Jr., 2007. Clinical relevance of precipitating factors in pituitary apoplexy. Neurosurgery 61, 956–961; discussion 961–952.

Semple, P.L., Jane, J.A., Lopes, M.B., et al., 2008. Pituitary apoplexy: correlation between magnetic resonance imaging and histopathological results. J. Neurosurg. 108, 909–915.

Semple, P.L., Laws, E.R. Jr., 1999. Complications in a contemporary series of patients who underwent transsphenoidal surgery for Cushing's disease. J. Neurosurg. 91, 175–179.

Semple, P.L., Vance, M.L., Findling, J., et al., 2000. Transsphenoidal surgery for Cushing's disease: outcome in patients with a normal magnetic resonance imaging scan. Neurosurgery 46, 553–558; discussion 558–559.

Serri, O., Rasio, E., Beauregard, H., et al., 1983. Recurrence of hyperprolactinemia after selective transsphenoidal adenomectomy in women with prolactinoma. N. Engl. J. Med. 309, 280–283.

Sheehan, J.M., Vance, M.L., Sheehan, J.P., et al., 2000. Radiosurgery for Cushing's disease after failed transsphenoidal surgery. J. Neurosurg. 93, 738–742.

Sheehan, J.P., Niranjan, A., Sheehan, J.M., et al., 2005. Stereotactic radiosurgery for pituitary adenomas: an intermediate review of its safety, efficacy, and role in the neurosurgical treatment armamentarium. J. Neurosurg. 102, 678–691.

Shimon, I., Cohen, Z.R., Ram, Z., et al., 2001. Transsphenoidal surgery for acromegaly: endocrinological follow-up of 98 patients. Neurosurgery 48, 1239–1243; discussion 1244–1235.

Sisam, D., Sheehan, J., Sheeler, L., 1987. The natural history of untreated microprolactinoma. Fertil. Steril. 48, 67–71.

Smith, M., Laws, E.R. Jr., 1994. Magnetic resonance imaging measurements of pituitary stalk compression and deviation in patients with nonprolactin-secreting intrasellar and parasellar tumors: lack of correlation with serum prolactin levels. Neurosurgery 34, 834–839.

Sonino, N., Boscaro, M., 1999. Medical therapy for Cushing's disease. Endocrinol. Metab. Clin. North. Am. 28, 211–222.

Sonino, N., Boscaro, M., Paoletta, A., et al., 1991. Ketoconazole treatment in Cushing's syndrome: experience in 34 patients. Clin. Endocrinol. 35, 347–352.

Spark, R.F., Dickstein, G., 1979. Bromocriptine and endocrine disorders. Ann. Intern. Med. 90, 949–956.

St-Jean, E., Blain, F., Comtois, R., 1996. High prolactin levels may be missed by immunoradiometric assay in patients with macroprolactinomas. Clin. Endocrinol. 44, 305–309.

Stewart, P., Carey, M., Graham, C., et al., 1992. Growth hormone secreting pituitary carcinoma: a case report and literature review. Clin. Endocrinol. 37, 189–195.

Stewart, P.M., Kane, K.F., Stewart, S.E., et al., 1995. Depot long-acting somatostatin analog (Sandostatin-LAR) is an effective treatment for acromegaly. J. Clin. Endocrinol. Metab. 80, 3267–3272.

Swearingen, B., Barker, F.G. 2nd., Katznelson, L., et al., 1998. Long-term mortality after transsphenoidal surgery and adjunctive therapy for acromegaly. J. Clin. Endocrinol. Metab. 83, 3419–3426.

Syro, L.V., Uribe, H., Penagos, L.C., et al., 2006. Antitumour effects of temozolomide in a man with a large, invasive prolactin-producing pituitary neoplasm. Clin. Endocrinol. 65, 552–553.

Tabarin, A., Laurent, F., Catargi, B., et al., 1998. Comparative evaluation of conventional and dynamic magnetic resonance imaging of the pituitary gland for the diagnosis of Cushing's disease. Clin. Endocrinol. 49, 293–300.

Thapar, K., Kovacs, K., Muller, P.J., 1995. Clinical-pathological correlations of pituitary tumours. Baillière's Clin. Endocrinol. Metab. 9, 243–270.

Thapar, K., Kovacs, K.T., Stefaneanu, L., et al., 1997. Antiproliferative effect of the somatostatin analogue octreotide on growth hormone-producing pituitary tumors: results of a multicenter randomized trial. Mayo Clin. Proc. 72, 893–900.

Thapar, K., Laws, E.R. Jr., 1998. Current management of prolactin-secreting tumors. In: Salcman, M. (Ed.), Current techniques in neurosurgery. Current Medicine, Philadelphia, P A, pp. 175–190.

Thapar, K., Laws, E.R. Jr., 2000. Transsphenoidal surgery for recurrent pituitary tumors. In: Kaye, A.H., Black, P.M. (Eds.), Operative neurosurgery. Churchill Livingstone, New York, pp. 685–707.

Thompson, S.K., Hayman, A.V., Ludlam, W.H., et al., 2007. Improved quality of life after bilateral laparoscopic adrenalectomy for Cushing's disease: a 10-year experience. Ann. Surg. 245, 790–794.

Thomson, J.A., Davies, D.L., McLaren, E.H., et al., 1994. Ten year follow up of microprolactinoma treated by transsphenoidal surgery. Br. Med. J. 309, 1409–1410.

Thomson, J.A., Gray, C.E., Teasdale, G.M., et al., 2002. Relapse of hyperprolactinemia after transsphenoidal surgery for microprol-

actinoma: lessons from long-term follow-up. Neurosurgery 50, 36–39; discussion 39–40.

Thorner, M.O., 1999. The discovery of growth hormone-releasing hormone. J. Clin. Endocrinol. Metab. 84, 4671–4676.

Thorner, M.O., Vance, M.L., Horvath, E., 1992. The anterior pituitary. In: Wilson, J.D., Foster, D.W. (Eds.), Williams textbook of endocrinology, eighth ed. WB Saunders, Philadelphia, P A, pp. 221–310.

Tindall, G.T., Herring, C.J., Clark, R.V., et al., 1990. Cushing's disease: results of transsphenoidal microsurgery with emphasis on surgical failures. J. Neurosurg. 72, 363–369.

Tindall, G.T., Kovacs, K., Horvath, E., et al., 1982. Human prolactin-producing adenomas and bromocriptine: a histological, immuno-cytochemical, ultrastructural, and morphometric study. J. Clin. Endocrinol. Metab. 55, 1178–1183.

Tindall, G.T., Oyesiku, N., Watts, N., et al., 1993. Transsphenoidal adenomectomy for growth hormone secreting pituitary adenomas in acromegaly: outcome analysis and determinants of failure. J. Neurosurg. 78, 205–215.

Trepp, R., Stettler, C., Zwahlen, M., et al., 2005. Treatment outcomes and mortality of 94 patients with acromegaly. Acta Neurochirurgica 147, 243–251; discussion 250–241.

Tsang, R.W., Brierley, J.D., Panzarella, T., et al., 1996. Role of radiation therapy in clinical hormonally-active pituitary adenomas. Radiother. Oncol. 41, 45–53.

Tucker, H., Grubb, S., Wigand, J., et al., 1980. The treatment of acromegaly by transsphenoidal surgery. Arch. Intern. Med. 140, 795–802.

Turner, H.E., Vadivale, A., Keenan, J., et al., 1999. A comparison of lanreotide and octreotide L A R for treatment of acromegaly. Clin. Endocrinol. 51, 275–280.

Vance, M.L., Evans, W., Thorner, M., 1984. Drugs five years later: Bromocriptine. Ann. Intern. Med. 100, 78–91.

Vance, M.L., Harris, A.G., 1991. Long-term treatment of 189 acromegalic patients with the somatostatin analog octreotide. Results of the International Multicenter Acromegaly Study Group. Arch. Intern. Med. 151, 1573–1578.

Vance, M.L., Thorner, M.O., 1987. Prolactinomas. Endocrinol. Metab. Clin. North. Am. 16, 731–753.

Wasko, R., Ruchala, M., Sawicka, J., et al., 2000. Short-term pre-surgical treatment with somatostatin analogues, octreotide and lanreotide, in acromegaly. J. Endocrinol. Invest. 23, 12–18.

Webster, J., Piscitelli, G., Polli, A., et al., 1994. A comparison of cabergoline and bromocriptine in the treatment of hyperprol-actinemic amenorrhea. Cabergoline Comparative Study Group. N. Engl. J. Med. 331, 904–909.

Weiss, M.H., Teal, J., Gott, P., 1983a. Natural history of microprol-actinomas: six-year followup. Neurosurgery 12, 640–642.

Weiss, M.H., Wycoff, R.R., Yadley, R., et al., 1983b. Bromocriptine treatment of prolactin-secreting tumors: surgical implications. Neurosurgery 12, 640–642.

Wilson, C.B., 1984. A decade of pituitary microsurgery. The Herbert Olivecrona lecture. J. Neurosurg. 61, 814–833.

Winfield, A., Finkel, D.M., Schatz, N.J., et al., 1984. Bromocriptine treatment of prolactin-secreting pituitary adenomas may restore pituitary function. Ann. Intern. Med. 101, 783–785.

Wright, A.D., Hill, D.M., Lowy, C., et al., 1970. Mortality in acromegaly. Quarterly Journal of Medicine 39, 1–16.

Yap, L.B., Turner, H.E., Adams, C.B., et al., 2002. Undetectable post-operative cortisol does not always predict long-term remission in Cushing's disease: a single centre audit. Clin. Endocrinol. 56, 25–31.

Zervas, N.T., 1984. Surgical results for pituitary adenomas: Results of an international survey. In: Black, P.M., Zervas, N.T., Ridgeway, E.C., et al., (Eds.), Secretory tumors of the pituitary gland, Vol 1. Raven Press, New York, pp. 377–385.

Chordomas and chondrosarcomas of the skull base

37

Griffith R. Harsh IV

Introduction

Chordomas and chondrosarcomas are osseous tumors of the skull base and spine. Although they are often grouped together by virtue of origin within bone and their location, they have distinct embryology, pathology, biologic behavior, clinical features, and responses to treatment. Chordomas arise from remnants of the embryonal notochord to form osseous tumors found more commonly at the skull base and sacrum than in the mobile spine. Although many initially behave as low-grade malignancies, growing slowly but invasively, in most cases, this growth accelerates and often proves fatal. Chondrosarcomas originate within chondral elements of bone throughout the body; within the skull they have a predilection for the sphenoid bone and the clival basiocciput. Most chondrosarcomas have a slowly progressive course marked by locally invasive growth which may not threaten function or survival for decades.

Chordomas and chondrosarcomas of the skull base can present formidable challenges to effective treatment. These challenges include the relative inaccessibility of the skull base, tumor involvement of critical neural and vascular structures, invasive growth predisposing to local recurrence, and possible metastatic dissemination. Despite such challenges, the combination of surgical resection and high dose radiation can cure almost all low grade chondrosarcomas and provide meaningful intervals of disease control of both chordomas and high-grade chondrosarcomas. Informative trials of treatment, however, have been difficult because of the rarity and relatively long clinical courses of chordomas and chondrosarcomas. This chapter will review the clinical and pathologic aspects of chordomas and chondrosarcomas, the currently preferred treatments and their outcomes, and potential future advances.

Incidence and epidemiology

Chordomas and chondrosarcomas together account for approximately 0.2% of all intracranial tumors and 6% of all primary skull base tumors (Heffelfinger et al 1973; Volpe & Mazabraud 1983; O'Neill et al 1985).

Chordomas

Chordomas are the most common extradural clival tumors. The overall incidence of chordomas is <0.1/100 000 persons per year (McMaster et al 2001), and they account for about 0.15% of all intracranial tumors (Berkmen & Blatt 1968; McMaster et al 2001). Chordomas occur in all age groups. The peak incidence is in the 4th or 5th decade of life (Unni 1996); the median age at diagnosis in a large series was 46 years (Unni 1996). Although <5% of these tumors arise in children, pediatric cases are prominent in the literature (Bartal & Heilbronn 1970; Bourdial et al 1970; Scuotto et al 1980; Wold & Laws 1983; Fink et al 1987; Handa et al 1987; Matsumoto et al 1989; Kaneko et al 1991; Inagaki et al 1992; Yadav et al 1992; Niida et al 1994; Borba et al 1996). Chordomas also occur in the elderly. Some authors have reported a male preponderance (Dahlin & MacCarty 1952; Heffelfinger et al 1973; Ariel & Verdu 1975; Kendall 1977), while others have found an even gender distribution (Krayenbühl & Yasargil 1975; O'Neill et al 1985; Muzenrider 1992, O'Connell et al 1994; Forsyth et al 1993; Watkins et al 1993). There is no known association between the development of chordomas and potential risk factors such as radiation or other environmental carcinogens. Chordomas occur in isolation and are not part of any known systemic syndrome. Although chordoma occurrence in one family has been linked to chromosome 7q33 (Yang et al 2005), no gene mutation specific to chordoma has been identified.

Chondrosarcomas

Chondrosarcomas are very rare. They account for 0.02% of all intracranial neoplasms (Borba & Al-Mefty 1998; Hassounah 1985; Cianfriglia et al 1978). Although skull base chondrosarcomas can occur in any age group, most patients are between 20 and 50 years old (Kamrin et al 1964; Evans et al 1977; Hassounah et al 1985; Oguro et al 1989) and the mean age at diagnosis is 40.7 years (Gay et al 1995). Chondrosarcomas are slightly more common in men (Koch et al 2000).

Although chondrosarcomas are usually isolated tumors, they may occur as part of a systemic syndrome, such as Paget's disease, Ollier's disease, and Maffucci's syndrome (Rosenberg et al 1999; Korten et al 1998). Ollier's disease involves multiple enchondral bone cysts and Maffucci's syndrome involves multiple enchondromas and cutaneous and visceral hemangiomas. Ploidy ranges from hyperhaploidy to pentaploidy (Mandahl et al 2002). Although loss (and gain) of genetic material from many different chromosomes occurs, cytogenetic studies have identified no single characteristic aberration (Mandahl et al 2002).

Location

Chordomas

Chordomas were first recognized at autopsy by Luschka in 1856 and Virchow in 1857. Believing that these tumors were cartilaginous in origin, Virchow named them 'ecchondrosis physaliphora' (Virchow 1857). In 1858, Muller proposed that these tumors were related to the notochord. In 1864, Klebs described the first symptomatic case. In 1894, Ribbert coined the term 'chordoma' after he found these tumors in the nucleus pulposus and correctly surmised their notochordal origin.

Chordomas are found where remnants of notochord are left: the clivus, sella, parasellar regions, foramen magnum, first cervical vertebra, spine, sacrum, and mediastinum. Some 35% arise in the skull base, 15% in the mobile spine, and 50% in the sacrococcyx (Heffelfinger et al 1973; Borba & Al-Mefty 1998). The most common site of skull base chordomas is the clival midline. Various classification schemes based on location have been proposed: clival, parasellar, and sellar (Krayenbühl & Yasargil 1975); basiocciput (caudal) and, less commonly, basisphenoid (rostral) (Schisano & Tovi 1962; Raffel et al 1985); and, of greatest help in the choice of surgical approach, superior, middle, and inferior clival (Sekhar et al 1992).

In all locations, chordomas expand and destroy bone. They extend invasively to involve extra- and intra-axial structures. Chordomas from the rostral notochord often extend into the dorsum sellae and present as sellar, supra-sellar, or cavernous sinus tumors which compress the pituitary gland, optic nerves and chiasm, and the midbrain (Thodou et al 2000). Chordomas extending ventrally through the clivus can present as nasopharyngeal masses causing nasal obstruction or dysphagia (Campbell et al 1980). Chordomas extending from the dorsal clivus can compress the pons and medulla; dorsolaterally extending tumors can involve the spheno-occiput or petrosal temporal bone. Although chordomas usually arise outside the dura, they may infiltrate and penetrate the cranial or spinal dura. Dural invasion usually occurs late in the course of aggressive tumors. Chordomas can also extend intradurally through surgical durotomies. There are rare reports of primary intra-dural intracranial chordomas (Steenberghs et al 2002; Nishi-gaya et al 1998).

Metastases, which become clinically evident in 10–20% of patients, usually occur late in the course of the disease (Laws & Thapar 1996). Metastasis is more common with sacral and vertebral tumors than with chordomas of the skull base (Chambers & Schwinn 1979; Markwalder et al 1979; Volpe & Mazabraud 1983). Neither histologic nor clinical features are closely correlated with metastatic potential. When metastases do occur, the most common sites are skin, bone, lung, and lymph nodes. Intradural metastases of skull base chordomas are rare; most occur following surgery (Krol et al 1989). New deposits of tumor are not infrequently found along routes of surgical access. Although, metastases can be found in up to 40% of patients at autopsy (Laws & Thapar 1996), local recurrence and invasiveness pose the greatest threat to patient function and survival.

Chondrosarcomas

Chondrosarcomas are mesenchymal, but their origin is controversial; possibilities include embryonal cartilaginous rests, mesenchymal pluripotent cells, and metaplasia of fibroblasts (Neff et al 2002: Gay et al 1995). They may arise within bone anywhere in the body, but they have a predilection for the central skeleton. Most cranial chondrosarcomas occur at skull base synchondroses, sites of fusion of separate cartilages forming the chondrocranium (Hassounah et al 1985). Embryologically, the skull base forms from a cartilaginous matrix (Ariel & Verdu 1975). During ossification, some cartilage may fail to form bone and remain as a rest. These cartilaginous rests may transform into chondrosarcomas. Although chondrosarcomas can arise from cartilage forming the anterior, middle or posterior fossa, most skull base chondrosarcomas arise near the clivus. Sixty-six percent arise from the petro-occipital junction (the petro-clival synchondrosis), 28% from the clivus itself, and 6% from the sphenoethmoid complex (Rosenberg et al 1999). Isolated chondrosarcomas are usually paramedian. However, when part of Ollier's or Maffucci's syndrome, chondrosarcomas may be midline (Tachibana et al 2000).

Chondrosarcomas, too, originate as extradural tumors. Most grow slowly, destroy bone, and extend into surrounding soft tissue. Most chondrosarcomas are low-grade malignancies (Rosenberg et al 1999), and thus have a better prognosis than chordomas (Crockard et al 2001a,b). The main threat after treatment is local recurrence (Stapleton et al 1993). Metastases occur in 7–12% of patients (Hassounah et al 1985; Koch et al 2000) and are a late occurrence.

Pathology

Small chordomas and chondrosarcomas lie within the middle table of the bone from which they arise. As they expand within this space, they erode normal bone structures, from which they are not clearly demarcated. Further growth thins and expands cortex and displaces overlying periosteum and dura. They then develop a nodular surface. Although these tumors are, strictly speaking, unencapsulated, attenuated periosteum and dura often form a pseudocapsule that grossly delimits tumor. By eroding cranial foramina and by expanding, displacing, and traversing bone, these tumors compress cranial nerves, brain, and basal arteries.

Chordomas

Chordomas are grayish-tan to bluish white tumors. Their consistency varies from gelatinous to leathery and their texture from smooth to gritty. There may be soft foci of hemorrhagic necrosis or firm areas of dense calcification. The tumor's size varies greatly. In bone, the tumor infiltrates the marrow space and expands the cortex to form a well-demarcated mass. Larger tumors penetrate the cortex and grow into neighboring soft tissue.

Histologically, chordomas are composed of lobules and nests of large epithelial-appearing cells separated by fibrous bands. The neoplastic cells are arranged in sheets or cords, or float individually, amidst the myxoid stroma. The nuclei are of moderate size and show mild to moderate atypia.

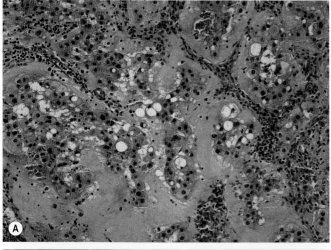

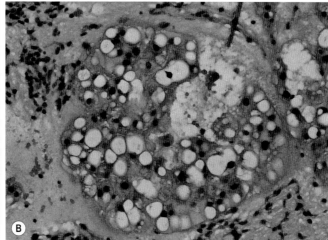

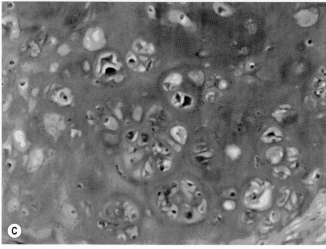

Figure 37.1 Chordoma and chondrosarcoma – pathology. (A) A low-power view of a chordoma demonstrates lobulation and mucinous background material. (B) A high-power view of the same tumor shows a lobule to be composed of typical vacuolated (physaliphorous) cells. (C) A high-power view of a chondrosarcoma demonstrates atypical chondrocytes arranged in a background hyaline cartilage matrix.

They have abundant pink cytoplasm. Variable numbers of cells have clear vacuoles, which impart a 'bubbly' appearance to the cytoplasm (Fig. 37.1A,B). These physaliferous cells are large, vacuolated, mucus-containing cells that are similar to cells of the primitive notochord. Mitoses are limited and foci of necrosis are common. The neoplastic cells contain periodic acid-Schiff diastase-sensitive glycogen.

Chordomas are immunoreactive with epithelial markers, such as cytokeratin and epithelial membrane antigen, and with oncofetal markers, such as carcinoembryonic antigen and α-fetoprotein. Some chordomas stain for S-100 protein, a feature that differentiates them from other sarcomatoid round cell or myxoid neoplasms (Heffelfinger et al 1973). Staining for brachyury, SOX-9, and podoplanin, markers for primitive notochord, helps distinguish chordoma from chondrosarcoma (Oakley et al 2008).

Chondrosarcomas

Chondrosarcomas are cartilaginous tumors of different grades of malignancy (Ewing 1939). Macroscopically, they consist of gray to tan-white nodules. The tumor consistency ranges from mucinous to firm and gritty. Additionally, there may be large, yellow-white chalky chunks of calcification.

Chondrosarcomas infiltrate the normal marrow and encase cancellous bone. They may transgress the cortex and form a soft tissue mass.

Microscopically, four primary types of chondrosarcoma have been described: conventional, clear cell, dedifferentiated, and mesenchymal (Rosenberg et al 1999; Richardson 2001). Almost all skull base chondrosarcomas are of the conventional type. The dedifferentiated and mesenchymal variants are more aggressive tumors (Unni 1996) and rarely affect the skull base.

Conventional chondrosarcoma is composed of hyaline, myxoid, or a combination of hyaline and myxoid cartilage. Mixed hyaline and myxoid chondrosarcomas contain variable amounts of both matrices. Hyaline chondrosarcomas are characterized by hypercellular hyaline cartilage. The neoplastic chondrocytes lie in clear lacunae within the hyaline matrix (Fig. 37.1C). The chondrocytes vary in size and shape. The chondrocyte nuclei have fine chromatin and small nucleoli and vary in size and shape from small and round to medium size and ovoid. The cytoplasm may be clear or eosinophilic. The cytoplasm may also have a bubbly appearance which mimics that of the physaliphorous cells of a chordoma (Rosenberg et al 1999). Mitotic activity is usually very low and foci of necrosis may be present.

cavernous sinus and petroclival areas. Bone lesions meriting consideration include chondroma, osteoma, osteoblastoma, fibrous dysplasia, eosinophilic granuloma, giant cell tumor, and plasmacytoma/multiple myeloma. Nasopharyngeal carcinoma, mucinous adenocarcinoma, and salivary gland tumors extending intracranially also enter into the differential diagnosis (Box 37.1) (Menezes et al 1994; Meyer et al 1984).

Pituitary adenomas arise within the sella, which is usually expanded. The calcification of craniopharyngiomas can resemble that of chordoma or chondrosarcoma, but these tumors rarely destroy bone and often have cysts. Metastases to the bone, particularly those from breast, lung, and prostate cancer, may both destroy bone and calcify.

Meningiomas in this region arise from the dura of the clivus (0.6–0.8%) (Castellano & Ruggiero 1953), sella, cavernous sinus, petrous apex, or the foramen magnum (2–3%) (Meyer et al 1984; Castellano & Ruggiero 1953). They occur more frequently in women. Clival meningiomas and cranial nerve schwannomas may present with cranial nerve palsies or myelopathy. Foramen magnum meningiomas may also cause local pain. Lymphomas are more likely to involve adjacent soft tissue.

Chondromas are benign tumors composed of mature hyaline cartilage. They grow and usually become symptomatic during adolescence. Osteomas and osteoblastomas are blastic lesions that rarely involve the skull base. Osteoid osteomas are smaller than osteoblastomas and present with pain that is relieved by aspirin. Osteoblastomas present with pain that is often nocturnal. In fibrous dysplasia, normal bone matrix is replaced with abnormal calcified tissue containing collagen and fibroblasts (Levy et al 1991). Fibrous dysplasia normally presents in late childhood or adolescence. The monostotic form is more common; the polyostotic form is associated with Albright's syndrome.

Eosinophilic granulomas usually occur during childhood and present as an enlarging tender mass that appears lytic without a rim of sclerosis on skull X-rays or CT scan (Brisman et al 1997). Eosinophilic granulomas rarely affect the skull base, but those that do can cause otorrhea and cranial nerve palsies (Brisman et al 1997). Giant cell tumors can arise within the bone of the skull base. Plasmacytomas and multiple myeloma are malignant plasma cell tumors that grow within bone.

Natural history

The prognosis for patients with chordomas left untreated is poor. Mean duration of patient survival from various series ranges from 6 to 28 months (Kamrin et al 1964; Heffelfinger et al 1973). Patient age and gender, the histologic appearance of the tumor, the therapy received, and tumor recurrence carry prognostic significance. Older patients do worse than younger ones (Forsyth et al 1993). One series showed a strong relation between age at diagnosis and survival. All patients younger than 40 years with a chordoma were alive 5 years later. In contrast, the survival rate at 5 years for patients older than 40 years when diagnosed was 22% (Mitchell et al 1993). Women have a poorer outcome than men. Some studies show shorter survival (Halperin 1997); others show briefer progression-free intervals but similar overall survival (Thieblemont et al 1995). A high mitotic rate suggests rapid growth and poor outcome. Radiation therapy improves local tumor control. Both surgery and radiation therapy increase the duration of survival. The interval of tumor control after treatment of recurrence is much shorter than that after the initial therapy.

The natural history for patients with chondrosarcomas, particularly those of lower grade, is better, but most patients without treatment still die as a result of their tumor (Gay et al 1995). Evans and co-workers (1977) reviewed 71 cases of chondrosarcoma from all body regions. They found that histologic grade, based on mitotic rate, cellularity, and nuclear atypia, was strongly correlated with survival and recurrence rates. Patients with grades, I, II, and III tumors had 5-year survival rates of 90%, 81%, and 43%, respectively.

In most cases of either tumor type, the combination of surgery and radiation offers the possibility of improved survival and longer maintenance of neurologic function. Almost all patients, regardless of their individual set of prognostic factors, warrant comprehensive evaluation, and most require aggressive treatment.

Treatment

Options for the management of skull base chordomas and chondrosarcomas include: clinical and radiological observation, biopsy followed by observation, biopsy followed by radiation, surgical removal, and surgery followed by radiation; chemotherapy has also been used. The appropriate choice of treatment of a patient with a chordoma or chondrosarcoma of the skull base requires confidence in the diagnosis, familiarity with the various combinations of treatments and their outcomes, and consideration of potential outcomes in the context of the demographics and neurologic function of the individual patient.

Numerous reports suggest the value to both tumor control and patient survival of extensive resection and high-dose radiotherapy for both chordomas and chondrosarcomas (Al-Mefty & Borba 1997; Crockard et al 2001a,b; Forsyth et al 1993; Gay et al 1995). The multidisciplinary treatment team of neurosurgeon, otolaryngologist, and radiation oncologist should develop a comprehensive treatment plan that maximizes tumor control and patient survival while limiting the risk of iatrogenic complications. The surgeons and radiation therapists together should determine the target of treatment, the benefit to survival, and the risk to the patient. Surgery is also often indicated for the restoration or preservation of neurologic function.

The surgical approach should be tailored to the goal chosen for each individual patient. The goals of surgical resection may vary: en-bloc excision of tumor, piecemeal gross total resection of the tumor, or a radical subtotal removal to decompress critical neurovascular structures or to improve tumor geometry for postoperative radiotherapy. Choice of surgical approach should also consider tumor size, site of origin, direction of expansion, relationships with cranial nerves and arteries, extent of tumor invasion, the patient's preoperative health, the surgeon's familiarity with the approach, and prior treatments. For instance, a chordoma of the lower clivus, extending posteriorly to invaginate the brain stem and laterally to envelop the nerves of the jugular foramen, might best be treated by a combined approach. The surgeons might remove the central tumor, so as to reduce the exposure of the brain stem to radiation, but leave the tumor in the jugular foramen for radiotherapy, so as to minimize the risk of surgically iatrogenic bulbar neuropathy.

Occasionally, preliminary biopsy is indicated: (1) if the patient's age, medical condition, or neurologic deficits or the tumor's size and location argue against extensive surgery and only radiation therapy is planned; or (2) if other diagnostic possibilities, such as metastasis, pituitary adenoma, and lymphoma, which might not warrant resection, cannot be excluded. In the latter case, biopsy can often be performed at the start of an intended resection. Since these lesions are predominantly extradural, standard stereotactic needle biopsy techniques may not be useful and biopsy is more likely to be performed through the nose, mouth or mastoid. Usually, however, the radiographic appearance of a skull base lesion is sufficiently characteristic of chordoma or chondrosarcoma that preliminary biopsy can be eschewed.

Surgery

Surgery then is usually the initial treatment, to confirm the diagnosis, relieve neurologic symptoms, and remove as much of the tumor as possible without causing either new neurologic deficit or unacceptable cosmetic deformity. Advances in skull base surgery have improved the surgical outcome for these challenging lesions. The surgical strategy depends on the goals of the surgery and the location and extent of tumor. In some cases, intentionally staged operations via multiple approaches may be required to obtain satisfactory tumor exposure, especially for larger tumors. Microscopic and endoscopic visualization may both be helpful (Frank et al 2006). In the case of reoperation, the results of the earlier operation must be considered. Previous surgical traverse may have left scarred, distorted tissue planes that are difficult to define. A fresh route is often preferred.

Chordomas and chondrosarcomas of the skull base usually pose significant challenges to attempts at complete resection. Obstacles include the critical neural and vascular structures of the region; craniospinal bone, possibly essential to structural integrity; and dura, important to CSF retention and prevention of infection. The basic strategy of skull base surgery is to maximize the exposure of the interface of tumor with critical structures while minimizing brain retraction, usually by removing bone. Within the last 20 years, new approaches to the central skull base have followed the improved definition of its complex anatomy by multiplanar cross-sectional CT and MR imaging. In the last decade, intraoperative frameless navigation systems have made this imaging even more useful; the immobility of tumors attached to the skull base reduces the inaccuracies from brain shift that can arise with parenchymal tumors. Increased cooperation between neurosurgeons and their otolaryngologic colleagues has facilitated both improved exposure of these lesions by more aggressive removal of bone and better prevention of CSF leakage and infection by vascularized soft tissue repair.

Surgical approaches

In general, chordomas and chondrosarcomas of the central skull base can be grouped for choice of surgical access by the portion of the clivus involved, whether they breach the dura, and whether they are exclusively midline or also have lateral extension (Harsh et al 1996) (Table 37.1). Since most chordomas and chondrosarcomas are predominantly extradural, an extradural approach is usually preferred (Sen & Sekhar 1990). This allows direct access to affected bone. Often involved bone is removed in the approach to infiltrated dura; examples include a transclival approach to a chordoma compressing the pons and a retrolabyrinthine approach to a petroclival chondrosarcoma. Even if it is not restricting access to dural and intradural tumor, tumor-infiltrated bone should be drilled away.

Tumors limited to the sella can be resected by a simple transsphenoidal approach (Laws 1984; Fraioli et al 1995). A combination of transnasal and transoral approaches, performed with either microscope or endoscope, can access midline tumors from the tuberculum and dorsum sellae superiorly to C1 inferiorly, even when tumor traverses the dura to displace the brain stem (Figs 37.3, 37.4). Extension of tumor superior or inferior from the sella, if in the midline (between the supraclinoidal, cavernous, and petrous internal carotid arteries) can be accessed by extending the transsphenoidal approach by removing the tuberculum sella and adjacent planum above and the midclivus below. Often substantial intracranial extension posteriorly of soft tumor can be removed by such extended transsphenoidal approaches, which were initially employed using the microscope but are now commonly facilitated by the endoscope (Fig. 37.5). (Cavallo et al 2007; Couldwell et al 2004; Dehdashti et al 2008; Fatemi et al 2008; Hong Jiang et al 2008; Jho & Ha 2004; Laws et al 2005; Stippler et al 2009). The endoscope's wide-angled view, excellent illumination, high magnification, and use of bilateral nasal surgical corridors permits surgical maneuvers, such as mobilization of the internal carotid artery and superior transposition of the pituitary gland (Fig. 37.6).

Suprasellar extension of firm tumor usually requires a craniotomy; this is particularly true of densely calcified tumors which extend lateral to the internal carotid arteries or incorporate cranial nerves or intracranial vessels. Usually

Table 37.1 Operative approaches to chordomas and chondrosarcomas

Tumor location	Approach	Structures at risk	Complications
Sellar (midline)	T-S (E/M)	Optic apparatus; ICA; pituitary; CSF	Blindness; stroke; hypopit; CSF fistula
Clival midline	T-S ext, extended subfrontal	Optic; ICA; CN VI, XII; pituitary; CSF; frontal lobe	Blindness; stroke; diplopia; hypopit; CSF fistula; frontal hematoma
Sellar + suprasellar midline	T-S ext	Optic; ICA; pituitary; CSF	Blindness; stroke; hypopit; CSF fistula
Sellar + infrasellar midline	T-S ext, T-E (lat rhin), T-O	Optic; ICA; CN VI, XII; pituitary; CSF	Blindness; stroke; diplopia; hypopit; CSF fistula
Sellar + inf clival midline	T-S ± T-O	Optic; ICA; CV VI, XII; Pituitary; CSF	Blindness, stroke, diplopia; hypopit; CSF fistula
Parasellar	F-T, transcav; T-N-Mx	Optic; ICA; CN III, IV,VI, XII; pituitary; CSF	Blindness; stroke; diplopia; hypopit; CSF fistula
Lateral sinus-pterygopalatine	Transfacial; T-N-Mx	Optic apparatus; ICA; CN VI, XII; pituitary; CSF	Blindness; stroke; diplopia; hypopituitarism; CSF fistula
Petro (anterior)-clival (mid)			
Petro (posterior)-clival (mid)	Anterior transpetrosal (subtemporal)	Temporal lobe; ICA; CN III–VI	Temporal hematoma; stroke; CN palsies
Petrous (posterior)	Posterior transpetrosal (presigmoid)	CN VI–XI; AICA; temporal lobe; brain stem	CN palsies; stroke; temporal hematoma; brain stem injury
Petroclival ant-inf-paramed			
Petroclival ant-inf-lateral	Suboccipital craniotomy	CN VII–XII; VA, AICA, PICA; cerebellum; brain stem	CN palsies; stroke; cerebellar hematoma; brain stem injury
	T-O (extradural)	CN VI, XII; bran stem; CSF; O-C1	Diplopia, bran stem injury; CSF fistula; instability
	Far /extreme lateral (intradural)	Vertebral artery, PICA; CN IX–XII; brain stem	Stroke; lower cranial nerve palsies; brain stem injury

AICA, anterior inferior cerebellar artery; C2, second cervical vertebra; Cl, first cervical vertebra; CN, cranial nerve; CSF, cerebrospinal fluid; F-T, frontotemporal; ICA, internal carotid artery; M, maxillary; O, occiput; PICA, posterior inferior cerebellar artery; T-E, transethmoid; T-O, transoral; T-S ext, extended transsphenoidal; T-S, transsphenoidal.

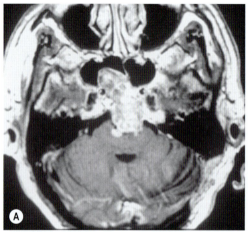
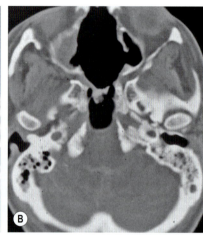

Figure 37.3 Clival chordoma – extended transsphenoidal approach. (A) An axial contrast enhanced T1-weighted MR image demonstrates a tumor of the upper and midclivus accessed transsphenoidally. The chordoma has eroded the clivus and displaces the pons posteriorly. (B) An axial non-contrast CT scan demonstrates the surgical corridor between the petrous and intracavernous internal carotid arteries.

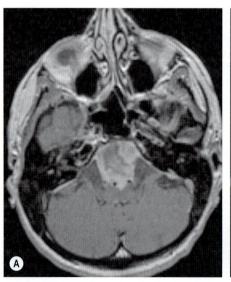
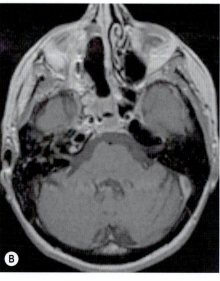

Figure 37.4 Clival chordoma – transnasal transclival approach. (A) Preoperative and (B) postoperative contrast. T1-weighted enhanced axial MRI scans demonstrate removal of a midclival chordoma invaginating the pontomedullary junction and enveloping the vertebro-basilar junction.

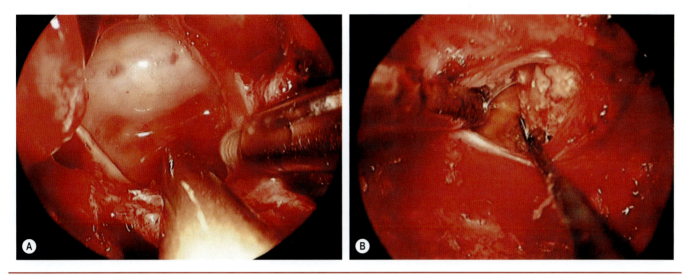

Figure 37.5 Endoscopic endonasal transsphenoidal resection of the intradural extension of an infrasellar calcified clival tumor. (A) A high speed drill is used to create a window through the clivus just beneath the sella. (B) Dura is opened and intradural calcified tumor is dissected from the brainstem and removed.

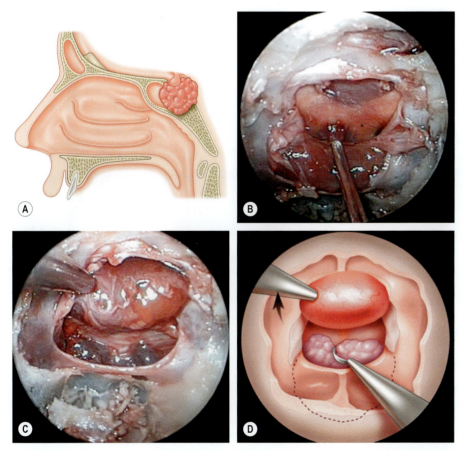

Figure 37.6 Superior transposition of the pituitary gland. Tumor posterior to the pituitary gland (A) may be exposed, by removing the bone of the sellar face, tuberculum sella, and posterior planum sphenoidale (cadaveric dissection, B), such that the pituitary gland can be transposed superiorly (cadaveric dissection, C), and then the tumor is removed (D).

such tumors warrant a craniofacial procedure, combining the suprasellar exposure of a frontal craniotomy with the clival access of a transnasal, trans-spheno-ethmoid approach, which can often be endoscopic. The transbasal and extended subfrontal approaches are attempts to achieve this exposure from a single perspective (Fig. 37.7) (Derome 1985; Sekhar et al 1992).

Exposure of lateral extension of parasellar and midclival tumors anterior to the internal carotid arteries may be achieved by adding various degrees of maxillotomy to a more midline transnasal (endoscopic) or transfacial (microscopic or endoscopic) approach (Kassam et al 2008). More posterior tumors with parasellar extension, especially when superior or lateral to the cavernous internal carotid artery,

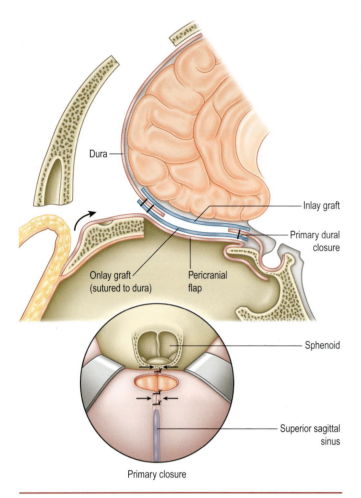

Figure 37.7 Transbasal approach and repair of the anterior cranial fossa floor. A low bifrontal craniotomy (with or without orbito-nasal osteotomies) permits transgression of the cribriform plate, planum sphenoidale, and ethmoid and sphenoid sinuses *en-route* to clival tumor. The defect in the anterior cranial fossa floor should be repaired in multilayered fashion with primary suture of dura where possible, an inlay graft of fascia or dural substitute, and a vascularized pericranial flap.

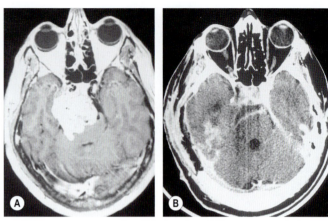

Figure 37.8 Transpetrosal approaches. Contrast enhanced axial preoperative MRI (A) and postoperative CT (B) scans of a chondrosarcoma of the right petrous apex and postero-inferior cavernous sinus invaginating the pons and enveloping the basilar artery in a patient with intact hearing removed by a transpetrosal retrolabyrinthine approach.

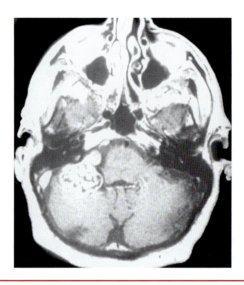

Figure 37.9 Suboccipital retrosigmoid approach. Chondrosarcomas of the mid-petrous face can be removed by a suboccipital craniotomy.

usually require a frontotemporal craniotomy, which may include dissection of involved cavernous sinus (Van Loveren et al 1996; Dolenc 1997).

Tumors arising from the midclivus and petrous apex and involving the tentorium and subjacent posterior fossa can be exposed by a subtemporal, anterior transpetrosal route (Harsh & Sekhar 1992; Kawase et al 1994). Larger tumors arising in this region with greater extension medially, inferiorly, and posteriorly usually require one of the posterior transpetrosal approaches. Presigmoid exposure is common to this group, but the extent of labyrinthectomy differs as required by the location, size, and consistency of the tumor and the status of the patient's hearing (Lawton et al 1996) (Fig. 37.8). Chondrosarcomas of the petrous bone that are primarily intradural may arise sufficiently posterior to the internal auditory canal that a suboccipital craniotomy suffices (Fig. 37.9). These lateral approaches have the advantage of avoiding contaminated nasal sinuses and oropharynx. In some cases, the risks of CSF leakage and infection can be reduced by using a two-stage procedure: transdural

removal of intradural tumor and dural repair by a lateral approach followed by an anterior approach for extradural tumor.

Chordomas and chondrosarcomas involving the midline and paramedian lower clivus and the craniovertebral junction are accessible through a transoral approach. This is ideal for midline, extradural tumors involving the tip of the clivus and the dens (Crockard 1985). For intradural tumors and extradural tumors with significant lateral extension requiring a more oblique approach, the posterolateral and far lateral approaches are preferred (Babu et al 1994). These have in common unilateral removal of the foramen magnum, suboccipital bone, and the C1 lamina. The posterolateral approach uses a retromastoid to midline cervical incision and exposes the vertebral artery at its dural entry and along the C1 lamina. It suffices for removal of predominantly intradural tumor anterior to the cervicomedullary junction. The far lateral approach uses a retromastoid incision extended beneath the mastoid process into the lateral neck to dissect muscles of the suboccipital and C1 transverse process and to mobilize the vertebral artery from the foramen transversarium of C1 (Sen & Sekhar 1991). Additional removal of the posterior third of the atlantal and occipital condyles (up to the hypoglossal canal) and their atlanto-occipital joint provides a slightly more anteriorly directed view of an inferior clival, superior cervical tumor than does the basic far lateral approach. This is sometimes helpful in removing tumor within the clivus. At the craniocervical junction, the combination of tumor erosion and surgical removal of involved bone may cause instability which warrants fusion. Instrumentation is then often needed because most patients will receive radiotherapy which will retard bone fusion.

Surgical technique

Chordomas, grossly, often have two intermixed components: a soft, gelatinous portion within expanded bone or dura and a more sinewy infiltration and expansion of dura or extracranial soft tissue. The gelatinous part can be easily removed by suction or gentle dissection and curettage; often thickened arachnoid protects cranial nerves, brainstem, and vessels. The exception occurs in reoperations in which this protection has been violated by prior dissection. Then, tumor may surround cranial nerves and extend between brainstem arteries and the pia. Inappropriately aggressive resection then risks cranial neuropathies and brainstem stroke from injury to perforating arteries. The sinewy portion requires more sharp dissection. The plane between tumor and surrounding soft tissue is often obscure. Where possible, thickened, potentially infiltrated dura and extradural soft tissue should be excised.

Chondrosarcomas tend to be more discrete and thus more completely resectable than chordomas. Some chondrosarcomas, however, may be so heavily calcified and incorporated into the skull base that they can be removed only by fragmenting them into dense parcels or drilling. In manipulating these calcified fragments, it is essential to first identify and then dissect tumor from nearby cranial nerves and critical vessels. Incorporation of fine cranial nerves or vessels within a calcified mass may preclude safe tumor removal and warrant subtotal resection (Fig. 37.10). This portion of the tumor is often relatively indolent and long term tumor control rates with adjuvant radiotherapy are quite high.

Adherence to several basic principles helps to reduce the incidence of complications following operations to remove chordomas and chondrosarcomas of the skull base. First, although removal of bone is almost always preferable to retraction of brain as a means of gaining exposure, the exposure should be no larger than that required to remove the tumor. Usually, the larger the dissection, the greater the risk to cranial nerves, blood vessels, and dural integrity.

Second, for tumors that extend intradurally, either traverse of the naso-oro-pharynx must be avoided or the dural defect must be closed securely. Often, removal of involved bone and dura creates a large fistula for leakage of CSF. With transnasal, expanded transsphenoidal approaches, CSF rhinorrhea and meningitis can be a significant problem

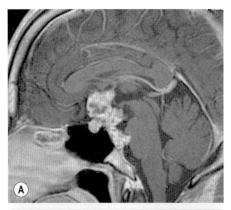

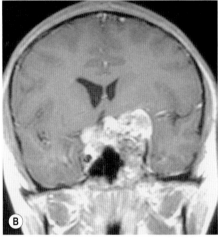

Figure 37.10 Chondrosarcoma of the clivus, sella, bilateral cavernous sinuses, and suprasellar, premesensephalic, and prepontine cisterns. Investment of the vertebral, basilar, and internal carotid arteries and their perforating branches as well as multiple cranial nerves argue against attempted resection. (A) Sagittal, (B) coronal.

(Stippler et al 2009). Historically, they have occurred in 10–50% of cases of transoral and transnasal resection of tumors with a significant intradural component. This incidence can be diminished by multilayered closure in which at least one layer is vascularized.

Dural openings should be sutured closed, primarily if possible, or by using autologous fascia or dural substitute, if needed. If a graft cannot be sewn in, the defect should be spanned by an inlay graft of dural substitute whose edges are placed deep to the margins of the dura. Repaired dura should then be covered by an onlay graft of fascia or dural substitute held snugly in gasket seal fashion by a firm strut (thin bone or cartilage, polyethylene glycol plate, or titanium wire mesh) wedged beneath the margins of the bone opening (Leng et al 2008) (Fig. 37.11). This can then be covered by more tissue adhesive, fat, and a vascularized soft tissue pedicle flap such as septal nasal mucosa fed by the posterior nasal artery for an extended transsphenoidal approach (Hadad et al 2006), pericranium for sub-frontal craniotomies, or temporalis fascia and muscle for lateral approaches (see Figs 37.7, 37.11). With large, insecurely repaired openings, temporary drainage of CSF through a ventriculostomy or lumbar drain is indicated.

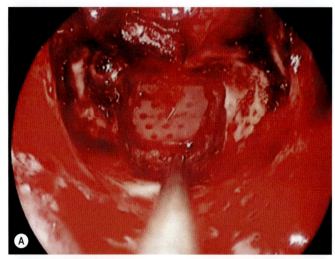

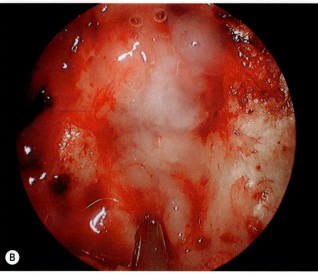

Figure 37.11 Repair of a transclival dural opening. Closure is multilayered: an inlay graft (of fascia or dural substitute, 1) held anteriorly by a central suture (held taut by a Weck clip, (A)) through a bone replacement plate and/or by gasket seal trapping by the edges of a bone replacement plate (cartilage, titanium wire mesh, or absorbable polyethylene glycol, 2) wedged beneath the bone edges and covered by tissue sealant, 3, (B) and a vascularized nasal mucosal flap (4, pedicled on a branch of the posterior nasal artery) and held superior and posterior by gelfoam or a small Foley balloon (5) within the sphenoid sinus.

Third, dissection should be meticulous. Approaches to these tumors frequently require maneuvering around internal carotid and vertebral arteries and cranial nerves. Although a lateral approach can provide a view angle parallel to the plane between tumor and brain stem advantageous for dissection, adherence to microsurgical techniques, often best facilitated by endoscopic illumination, magnification and angulation, permits safe tumor removal through a direct anterior approach as well.

Inadvertent injury to either the internal carotid artery or its branches perfusing the optic apparatus, diencephalon, brain stem, or upper cervical cord can prove catastrophic. Similarly, the greatest care must be taken to avoid injury to the cranial nerves. Close attention to anatomic keys is essen-

tial (Kassam et al 2008); neuronavigation techniques may prove helpful (Hwang & Ho 2007); and fortunately, the pseudoencapsulated structure of both chordomas and chondrosarcomas and the frequently encountered soft consistency of the intradural extensions of chordomas facilitate separation of tumor from nerves and blood vessels. These structures are more likely to be displaced than invaded. The exception occurs at the neural foramina where nerves, surrounded by tumor-infiltrated bone, are most vulnerable to injury. Here, and in the cavernous sinus, it is sometimes preferable to leave small deposits of tumor, treatable by radiation therapy, than to incur high risk of injury to a cranial nerve. Intentional sacrifice of a cranial nerve is almost never justified by a desire to obtain a complete resection of tumor.

Fourth, the intent of surgery, formulated preoperatively, must be kept in mind. Not infrequently, the goal of surgery is to remove sufficient tumor to optimize the geometry of the tumor bed for subsequent radiation therapy. Since radiation exposure of the brain stem or optic pathways is the most common factor limiting the dose that can be given to these tumors, the primary requirement of surgery is often removal of tumor invaginating the brain stem and in proximity to the nerves or chiasm (Fig. 37.12). Reduction of tumor mass is generally helpful to the extent that it reduces radiation target volume, but the advantage conferred by reducing tumor burden decreases at low tumor volumes (Hug et al 1999). This diminishing return, the relatively indolent growth of low-grade chondrosarcomas, and the microscopically invasive nature of chordomas and of higher grade chondrosarcomas often render aggressive efforts at microscopic total resection of these tumors ill advised.

Surgical outcome

Most surgical series of chordomas and chondrosarcomas have suggested that resection extends survival (Krayenbühl & Yasargil 1975; Volpe & Mazabraud 1983; Derome 1985; Hassounah et al 1985; O'Neill et al 1985; Arnold & Herrmann 1986; Brooks et al 1987; Sen et al 1989; Rabadan & Conesa 1992; Forsyth et al 1993; Crockard 1996). One study of 51 patients with intracranial chordomas showed that the 40 whose tumors were resected (partially or completely) were more likely to survive 5 years (55% vs 36%) than the 11 whose tumors were only biopsied (Forsyth et al 1993).

A more complete resection may yield a better outcome than a less aggressive one (Sen et al 1989; Gay et al 1995) (Table 37.2). There are reports of long-term disease-free survival following radical resection alone (Kveton et al 1986; Gay et al 1995). These results have led some surgeons to advocate radical surgical resection in most cases. Some surgical series in which radical resection was followed by radiation therapy report impressive rates of tumor control among those patients surviving the operation. In one series of 60 patients (46 chordomas and 14 low-grade chondrosarcomas) no tumor recurrence was found in 80% at 3 years and 76% at 5 years after surgery (Gay et al 1995). Patients with chondrosarcomas did better than those with chordomas (5-year recurrence-free survival rates of 90% and 65%, respectively). However, 11 patients died during the postoperative follow-up period: three from systemic complications within 3 months of surgery; five from tumor recurrence; one from unrelated causes, and two from late complications of radiotherapy.

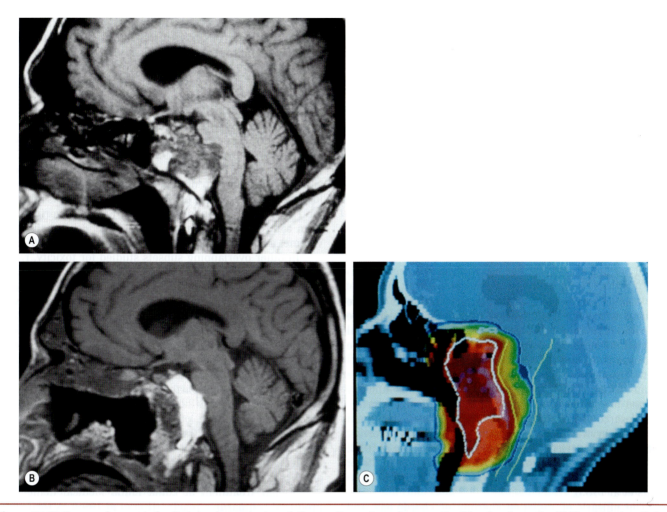

Figure 37.12 Transnasal removal of a clival chordoma prior to radiotherapy. Comparison of preoperative (A) and postoperative (B) T1-weighted sagittal MRI scans shows removal of tumor invaginating the brainstem and repair of the surgical corridor with hyperintense fat. This interposition of fat increases the distance between the tumor's clival origin and the brainstem and can significantly improve the safety of subsequent high dose irradiation (C).

Table 37.2 Surgical series

Patients (n)	Tumor type(s)	Surgical resection	Radiation therapy	Complications	Outcome	Reference
38	Chordomas					Watkins et al 1993
17	8 chordomas; 9 CS	GTR 53%	XRT 59%			Sen et al 1989
60	46 chordomas; 14 CS	67% GTR or NTR	XRT 8%; P–P 10%; SRS 2%	30% CSF leak; 10% meningitis; 40% decreased Karnofsky score	84% recurrence-free for 5 years in TR; 64% in STR	Gay et al 1995
51	51 chordomas (19 chondroid)	11 BX; 40 STR	XRT 76%		51% 5-year survival	Forsyth et al 1993
25	Chordomas	GTR 43%; NTR 48%; STR 9%	P–P 74%; XRT 9%	Stroke; CN III palsy; hemianopia	4 died; 5 with recurrence; 16 recurrence-free	Al-Mefty & Borba 1997
11	10 chordomas, 1 CS	Pedicled rhinotomy, sub-total	P–P	Palatal tear; CSF leak ± meningitis; lacrimal sac injury		Ojemann et al 1995
36	Chordomas	GTR or NTR in 62%	22%	no CSF leak, meningitis, or new CN deficit	14% 5-year mortality; 19% recurrence	Menezes et al 1997

BX, biopsy; CN, cranial nerve; GTR, gross total resection; NTR, near total resection; P–P, proton–photon radiotherapy; SRS, stereotactic radiosurgery; STR, sub-total resection; XRT, conventional radiotherapy.

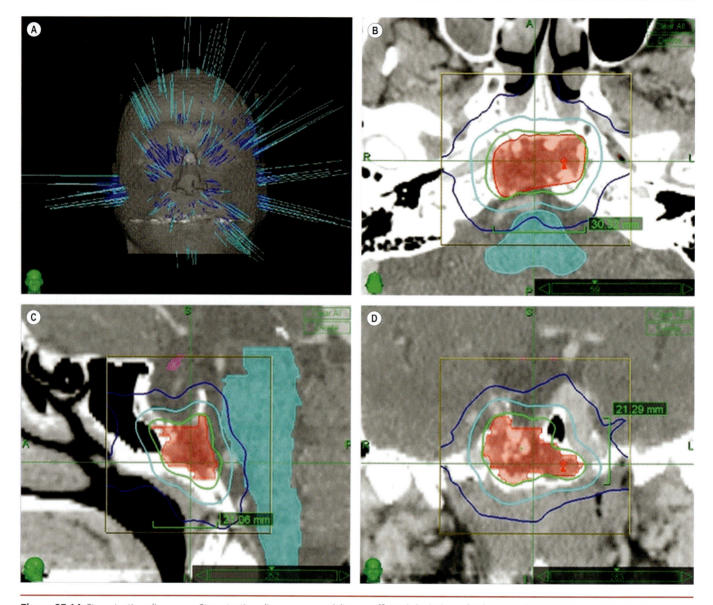

Figure 37.14 Stereotactic radiosurgery. Stereotactic radiosurgery may deliver a sufficiently high dose of radiation without excessive exposure of the brainstem that it may supplement or even substitute for fractionated radiation. This treatment plan shows convergence of 120 beams (A) to deliver high doses to the tumor (shown in axial (B), sagittal (C), and coronal (D) planes), and tolerated doses to the optic nerves and chiasm, brainstem, and temporal lobes.

effect on survival than primary surgery, may be of value to the majority of patients with surgically accessible tumor recurrence.

Chemotherapy

Chemotherapy is an option for surgically inaccessible, previously irradiated recurrent local, or metastatic tumor. As surgery and radiotherapy have improved the local control of chordomas and chondrosarcomas, effective treatment of metastatic disease has become increasingly important. Approximately 30–40% of patients with chordomas develop metastases (Chambers & Schwinn 1979; Sundaresan et al 1979) most commonly to the lungs, liver and bone (O'Neill et al 1985).

Historically, chemotherapy has had poor efficacy (Castellano & Ruggiero 1953). Newer agents with tumor specific rationales, such as imatinib mesylate, a tyrosine kinase inhibitor which targets several enzymes and a growth factor expressed in chordomas, may be an improvement (Casali et al 2004).

Conclusion

Chordomas and chondrosarcomas of the skull base are rare and challenging tumors. The relative inaccessibility of the skull base, the tumors' proximity to critical neurovascular structures, their relative radioresistance to standard doses, their lack of chemosensitivity, and their tendency to recur locally require thoughtful choice and meticulous administration of therapy. Despite these challenges, the combination of surgical resection and high-dose radiation can cure almost all low-grade chondrosarcomas and provide meaningful intervals of control of both chordomas and high-grade chondrosarcomas.

Key points

- Chordomas and chondrosarcomas are tumors of the skull base which, although often grouped together by virtue of origin within bone and their location, have distinct embryology, pathology, biologic behavior, clinical features, and responses to treatment.

- Initially, most behave as low-grade malignancies, growing slowly but invasively. Local recurrence is common, and, for most chordomas and high-grade chondrosarcomas, eventually proves lethal.

- Surgery followed by radiation therapy is the preferred treatment for both pathologies. Advances in skull base surgery, when used with discretion, have improved the surgical outcome. Newer, more conformal radiation treatments have greater effectiveness and lower morbidity than previous strategies. No effective chemotherapy is known.

REFERENCES

Al-Mefty, O., Borba, L.A., 1997. Skull base chordomas: a management challenge. J. Neurosurg. 86 (2), 182–189.

Ariel, I.M., Verdu, C., 1975. Chordoma: an analysis of twenty cases treated over a twenty-year span. J. Surg. Oncol. 7 (1), 27–44.

Arnold, H., Herrmann, H.D., 1986. Skull base chordoma with cavernous sinus involvement. Partial or radical tumour-removal? Acta Neurochir. (Wien) 83 (1–2), 31–37.

Babu, R.P., Sekhar, L.N., Wright, D.C., 1994. Extreme lateral transcondylar approach: technical improvements and lessons learned. J. Neurosurg. 81 (1), 49–59.

Bartal, A.D., Heilbronn, Y.D., 1970. Transcervical removal of a clivus chordoma in a 2-year-old child. Reversal of quadriplegia and bulbar paralysis. Acta Neurochir. (Wien) 23 (2), 127–133.

Berkmen, Y.M., Blatt, E.S., 1968. Cranial and intracranial cartilaginous tumours. Clin. Radiol. 19 (3), 327–333.

Berson, A.M., Castro, J.R., Petti, P., et al., 1988. Charged particle irradiation of chordoma and chondrosarcoma of the base of skull and cervical spine: the Lawrence Berkeley Laboratory experience. Int. J. Radiat. Oncol. Biol. Phys. 15 (3), 559–565.

Borba, L., Al-Mefty, O., 1998. Skull-base chordomas. Contemp. Neurosurg. 20, 1–6.

Borba, L.A., Al-Mefty, O., Mrak, R.E., et al., 1996. Cranial chordomas in children and adolescents. J. Neurosurg. 84 (4), 584–591.

Bourdial, J., Vergnon, L., Laffolee, P., et al., 1970. [A case of chordoma of the clivus with cervical extension in a child]. Ann. Otolaryngol. Chir. Cervicofac. 87 (12), 820–822.

Bourgouin, P.M., Tampieri, D., Robitaille, Y., et al., 1992. Low-grade myxoid chondrosarcoma of the base of the skull: C T, M R, and histopathology. J. Comput. Assist. Tomogr. 16 (2), 268–273.

Bouropoulou, V., Bosse, A., Roessner, A., et al., 1989. Immunohistochemical investigation of chordomas: histogenetic and differential diagnostic aspects. Curr. Top Pathol. 80, 183–203.

Brisman, J.L., Feldstein, N.A., Tarbell, N.J., et al., 1997. Eosinophilic granuloma of the clivus: case report, follow-up of two previously reported cases, and review of the literature on cranial base eosinophilic granuloma. Neurosurgery 41 (1), 273–279.

Brooks, J.J., LiVolsi, V.A., Trojanowski, J.Q., 1987. Does chondroid chordoma exist? Acta Neuropathol. (Berl.) 72 (3), 229–235.

Brooks, J.J., Trojanowski, J.Q., LiVolsi, V.A., 1989. Chondroid chordoma: a low-grade chondrosarcoma and its differential diagnosis. Curr. Top Pathol. 80, 165–181.

Campbell, W.M., McDonald, T.J., Unni, K.K., et al., 1980. Nasal and paranasal presentations of chordomas. Laryngoscope 90 (4), 612–618.

Casali, P.G., Messina, A., Stacchiotti, S., et al., 2004. Imatinib mesylate in chordoma. Cancer 101 (9), 2086–2097.

Castellano, F., Ruggiero, G., 1953. Meningiomas of the posterior fossa. Acta Radiol. 104 (Suppl.), 1–177.

Castro, J.R., Linstadt, D.E., Bahary, J.P., et al., 1994. Experience in charged particle irradiation of tumors of the skull base: 1977–1992. Int. J. Radiat. Oncol. Biol. Phys. 29 (4), 647–655.

Catton, C., O'Sullivan, B., Bell, R., et al., 1996. Chordoma: long-term follow-up after radical photon irradiation. Radiother. Oncol. 41 (1), 67–72.

Cavallo, L.M., Cappabianca, P., Messina, A., et al., 2007. The extended endoscopic endonasal approach to the clivus and craniovertebral junction: anatomical study. Childs Nerv. Syst. 23, 665–671.

Chambers, P.W., Schwinn, C.P., 1979. Chordoma. A clinicopathologic study of metastasis. Am. J. Clin. Pathol. 72 (5), 765–776.

Cianfriglia, F., Pompili, A., Occhipinti, E., 1978. Intracranial malignant cartilaginous tumours. Report of two cases and review of literature. Acta Neurochir. (Wien) 45 (1–2), 163–175.

Coltrera, M.D., Googe, P.B., Harrist, T.J., et al., 1986. Chondrosarcoma of the temporal bone. Diagnosis and treatment of 13 cases and review of the literature. Cancer 58 (12), 2689–2696.

Couldwell, W.T., Weiss, M.H., Rabb, C., et al., 2004. Variations on the standard transsphenoidal approach to the sellar region, with emphasis on the extended approaches and parasellar approaches: Surgical experience in 105 cases. Neurosurgery 55, 539–550.

Crockard, A., 1996. Chordomas and chondrosarcomas of the cranial base: results and follow-up of 60 patients. Neurosurgery 38 (2), 420.

Crockard, H.A., 1985. The transoral approach to the base of the brain and upper cervical cord. Ann. R. Coll. Surg. Engl. 67 (5), 321–325.

Crockard, H.A., Cheeseman, A., Steel, T., et al., 2001a. A multidisciplinary team approach to skull base chondrosarcomas. J. Neurosurg. 95 (2), 184–189.

Crockard, H.A., Steel, T., Plowman, N., et al., 2001b. A multidisciplinary team approach to skull base chordomas. J. Neurosurg. 95 (2), 175–183.

Cummings, B.J., Hodson, D.I., Bush, R.S., 1983. Chordoma: the results of megavoltage radiation therapy. Int. J. Radiat. Oncol. Biol. Phys. 9 (5), 633–642.

Dahlin, D., MacCarty, C., 1952. Chordoma, a study of fifty-nine cases. Cancer 5, 1170–1178.

Debus, J., Hug, E.B., Liebsch, N.J., et al., 1997. Brainstem tolerance to conformal radiotherapy of skull base tumors. Int. J. Radiat. Oncol. Biol. Phys. 39 (5), 967–975.

Debus, J., Schulz-Ertner, D., Schad, L., et al., 2000. Stereotactic fractionated radiotherapy for chordomas and chondrosarcomas of the skull base. Int. J. Radiat. Oncol. Biol. Phys. 47 (3), 591–596.

Dehdashti, A.R., Karabatsou, K., Ganna, A., et al., 2008. Expanded endoscopic endonasal approach for treatment of clival chordomas: early results in 12 patients. Neurosurgery 63, 299–309.

Derome, P.J., 1985. Surgical management of tumours invading the skull base. Can. J. Neurol. Sci. 12 (4), 345–347.

Dolenc, V.V., 1997. Transcranial epidural approach to pituitary tumors extending beyond the sella. Neurosurgery 41 (3), 542–552.

Doucet, V., Peretti-Viton, P., Figarella-Branger, D., et al., 1997. MRI of intracranial chordomas. Extent of tumour and contrast enhancement: criteria for differential diagnosis. Neuroradiology 39 (8), 571–576.

Evans, H., Ayala, A., Romsdahl, M., 1977. Prognostic factors in chondrosarcomas of bone. A clinico-pathologic analysis with emphasis on histologic grading. Cancer 40, 818–831.

Ewing, J.A., 1939. review of the classification of bone tumors. Surg. Gynecol. Obstet. 68, 971–976.

Fatemi, N., Dusick, J.R., Gorgulho, A.A., et al., 2008. Endonasal microscopic removal of clival chordomas. Surg. Neurol. 69, 331–338.

Fagundes, M.A., Hug, E.B., Liebsch, N.J., et al., 1995. Radiation therapy for chordomas of the base of skull and cervical spine: patterns of failure and outcome after relapse. Int. J. Radiat. Oncol. Biol. Phys. 33 (3), 579–584.

Fink, F.M., Ausserer, B., Schrocksnadel, W., et al., 1987. Clivus chordoma in a 9-year-old child: case report and review of the literature. Pediatr. Hematol. Oncol. 4 (2), 91–100.

Finn, D.G., Goepfert, H., Batsakis, J.G., 1984. Chondrosarcoma of the head and neck. Laryngoscope 94 (12 Pt 1), 1539–1544.

Forsyth, P.A., Cascino, T.L., Shaw, E.G., et al., 1993. Intracranial chordomas: a clinicopathological and prognostic study of 51 cases. J. Neurosurg. 78 (5), 741–747.

Fraioli, B., Esposito, V., Santoro, A., et al., 1995. Transmaxillosphenoidal approach to tumors invading the medial compartment of the cavernous sinus. J. Neurosurg. 82 (1), 63–69.

Frank, G., Sciarretta, V., Calbucci, F., et al., 2006. The endoscopic transnasal transsphenoidal approach for the treatment of cranial base chordomas and chondrosarcomas. Neurosurgery 59 (Suppl. 1), ONS50–ONS57.

Gay, E., Sekharn, L.N., Rubinstein, E., et al., 1995. Chordomas and chondrosarcomas of the cranial base: results and follow-up of 60 patients. Neurosurgery 36 (5), 887–897.

Goel, A., 1995. Chordoma and chondrosarcoma: relationship to the internal carotid artery. Acta Neurochir. (Wien) 133 (1–2), 30–35.

Habrand, I.L., Austin-Seymour, M., Birnbaum, S., et al., 1989. Neurovisual outcome following proton radiation therapy. Int. J. Radiat. Oncol. Biol. Phys. 16 (6), 1601–1606.

Hadad, G., Bassagasteguy, L., Carrau, R.L., et al., 2006. A novel reconstructive technique after endoscopic expanded endonasal approaches: vascular pedicle nasoseptal flap. Laryngoscope 116, 1882–1886.

Halperin, E.C., 1997. Why is female sex an independent predictor of shortened overall survival after proton/photon radiation therapy for skull base chordomas? Int. J. Radiat. Oncol. Biol. Phys. 38 (2), 225–230.

Handa, J., Suzuki, F., Nioka, H., et al., 1987. Clivus chordoma in childhood. Surg. Neurol. 28 (1), 58–62.

Harsh, G.R. IV, Sekhar, L.N., 1992. The subtemporal, transcavernous, anterior transpetrosal approach to the upper brain stem and clivus. J. Neurosurg. 77 (5), 709–717.

Harsh, G.R. IV, Joseph, M.P., Swearingen, B., et al., 1996. Anterior midline approaches to the central skull base. Clin. Neurosurg. 43, 15–43.

Hassounah, M., Al-Mefty, O., Akhtar, M., et al., 1985. Primary cranial and intracranial chondrosarcoma: a survey. Acta Neurochir. (Wien) 78, 123–132.

Heffelfinger, M.J., Dahlin, D.C., MacCarty, C.S., et al., 1973. Chordomas and cartilaginous tumors at the skull base. Cancer 32 (2), 410–420.

Higinbotham, N.L., Phillips, R.F., Farr, H.W., et al., 1967. Chordoma. Thirty-five-year study at Memorial Hospital. Cancer 20 (11), 1841–1850.

Hong Jiang, W., Ping Zhao, S., Hai Xie, Z., et al., 2008. Endoscopic resection of chordomas in different clival regions. Acta Otolaryngol. 129, 71–83.

Hug, E.B., Loredo, L.N., Slater, J.D., et al., 1999. Proton radiation therapy for chordomas and chondrosarcomas of the skull base. J. Neurosurg. 91 (3), 432–439.

Hug, E.B., 2001. Review of skull base chordomas: prognostic factors and long-term results of proton-beam radiotherapy. Neurosurg. Focus 10 (3), E11.

Hwang, P.Y., Ho, C.L., 2007. Neuronavigation using an image-guided endoscopic transnasalsphenoethmoidal approach to clival chordomas. Neurosurgery 61, 212–218.

Inagaki, H., Anno, Y., Hori, T., et al., 1992. [Clival chordoma in an infant; case report and review of the literature]. No Shinkei Geka 20 (7), 809–813.

Jho, H.D., Ha, H.G., 2004. Endoscopic endonasal skull base surgery: Part 3 –The clivus and posterior fossa. Minim. Invasive Neurosurg. 47, 16–23.

Kamrin, R., Potanos, J., Pool, J., 1964. An evaluation of the diagnosis and treatment of chordoma. J. Neurol. Neurosurg. Psychiatry 27, 157–165.

Kaneko, Y., Sato, Y., Iwaki, T., et al., 1991. Chordoma in early childhood: a clinicopathological study. Neurosurgery 29 (3), 442–446.

Kassam, A.B., Vescan, A.D., Carrau, R.L., et al., 2008. Expanded endonasal approach: vidian canal as a landmark to the petrous internal carotid artery. Technical Note. J. Neurosurg. 108, 177–183.

Kawase, T., Shiobara, R., Toya, S., 1994. Middle fossa transpetrosal-transtentorial approaches for petroclival meningiomas. Selective

pyramid resection and radicality. Acta Neurochir. (Wien) 129 (3–4), 113–120.

Kendall, B.E., 1977. Cranial chordomas. Br. J. Radiol. 50 (598), 687–698.

Klebs, E., 1864. Ein Fall von Ecchondrosis spheno-occipitalise amylacea. Virchows Arch. Path. Anat. 31, 396–399.

Koch, B.B., Karnell, L.H., Hoffman, H.T., et al., 2000. National cancer database report on chondrosarcoma of the head and neck. Head Neck 22 (4), 408–425.

Korten, A.G., ter Berg, H.J., Spincemaille, G.H., et al., 1998. Intracranial chondrosarcoma: review of the literature and report of 15 cases. J. Neurol. Neurosurg. Psychiatry 65 (1), 88–92.

Krayenbühl, H., Yasargil, M., 1975. Cranial chordomas. Prog. Neurol. Surg. 6, 380–434.

Krol, G., Sze, G., Arbit, E., et al., 1989. Intradural metastases of chordoma. AJNR Am. J. Neuroradiol. 10 (1), 193–195.

Kveton, J., Brackmann, D., Glasscock, M., 1986. Chondrosarcoma of the skull base. Otolaryngol. Head Neck Surg. 94, 23–32.

Larson, T.C. III, Houser, O.W., Laws, E.R. Jr., 1987. Imaging of cranial chordomas. Mayo Clin. Proc. 62 (10), 886–893.

Laws, E.R. Jr., 1984. Transsphenoidal surgery for tumors of the clivus. Otolaryngol. Head Neck Surg. 92 (1), 100–101.

Laws, E., Thapar, K., 1996. Parasellar lesions other than pituitary adenomas. In: Powell, M., Lightman, S.L. (Eds.), Management of pituitary tumors: A handbook. Churchill Livingstone, New York, pp., 175–222.

Laws, E.R., Kanter, A.S., Jane, J.A. Jr., 2005. Extended transsphenoidal approach. J. Neurosurg. 102, 825–828.

Lawton, M.T., Daspit, C.P., Spetzler, R.F., 1996. Transpetrosal and combination approaches to skull base lesions. Clin. Neurosurg. 43, 91–112.

Liebsch, N.J., Munzenrider, J.E., 2003. Proton radiotherapy for cranial base chordomas. In: Harsh, G. (Ed.), Chordomas and chondrosarcomas of the skull base and spine. Thieme, New York, pp., 307–314.

Leng, L.Z., Brown, S., Anand, V.K., et al., 2008. 'Gasket-Seal' watertight closure in minimal-access endoscopic cranial base surgery. Neurosurgery 62, 342–343.

Levy, M.L., Chen, T.C., Weiss, M.H., 1991. Monostotic fibrous dysplasia of the clivus. Case report. J. Neurosurg. 75 (5), 800–803.

Luschka, H., 1856. Die Altersveranderungen der Zwischenwirbelknorpel. Virchows Arch. Path Anat. 9, 312–327.

Mandahl, N., Gustafson, P., Mertens, F., et al., 2002. Cytogenetic aberrations and their prognostic impact in chondrosarcoma. Genes Chromosomes Cancer 33 (2), 188–200.

Markwalder, T.M., Markwalder, R.V., Robert, J.L., et al., 1979. Metastatic chordoma. Surg. Neurol. 12 (6), 473–478.

Matsumoto, J., Towbin, R.B., Ball, W.S. Jr., 1989. Cranial chordomas in infancy and childhood. A report of two cases and review of the literature. Pediatr. Radiol. 20 (1–2), 28–32.

McMaster, M.L., Goldstein, A.M., Bromley, C.M., et al., 2001. Chordoma: incidence and survival patterns in the United States, 1973–1995. Cancer Causes Control 12, 1–11.

Menezes, A.H., Gantz, B.J., Traynelis, V.C., et al., 1997. Cranial base chordomas. Clin. Neurosurg. 44, 491–509.

Menezes, A.H., Traynelis, V.C., Gantz, B.J., 1994. Surgical approaches to the craniovertebral junction. Clin. Neurosurg. 41, 187–203.

Meyer, J.E., Oot, R.F., Lindfors, K.K., 1986. CT appearance of clival chordomas. J. Comput. Assist. Tomogr. 10 (1), 34–38.

Meyer, F.B., Ebersold, M.J., Reese, D.F., 1984. Benign tumors of the foramen magnum. J. Neurosurg. 61 (1), 136–142.

Meyers, S.P., Hirsch, W.L. Jr., Curtin, H.D., et al., 1992. Chordomas of the skull base: MR features. AJNR Am. J. Neuroradiol. 13 (6), 1627–1636.

Mitchell, A., Scheithauer, B.W., Unni, K.K., et al., 1993. Chordoma and chondroid neoplasms of the spheno-occiput. An immunohistochemical study of 41 cases with prognostic and nosologic implications. Cancer 72 (10), 2943–2949.

Muller, H., 1858. Ueber das vorkommen von resten der chorda dorsalis bei mecschen nach der geburt und uber ihr verhaltnis zu den gallertgeschwulsten am clivus. Ztschr. Rat. Med. 2, 202–229.

Muthukumar, N., Kondziolka, D., Lunsford, L.D., et al., 1998. Stereotactic radiosurgery for chordoma and chondrosarcoma: further experiences. Int. J. Radiat. Oncol. Biol. Phys. 41 (2), 387–392.

Muzenrider, J., 1992. Proton beam radiation and chordomas and chondrosarcomas. Third International Conference on Head and Neck Tumors, San Francisco, CA.

Munzenrider, J.E., Liebsch, N.J., 1999. Proton therapy for tumors of the skull base. Strahlenther Onkol 175 (Suppl.), 57–63.

Neff, B., Sataloff, R.T., Storey, L., et al., 2002. Chondrosarcoma of the skull base. Laryngoscope 112 (1), 134–139.

Nguyen, Q.N., Chang, E.L., 2008. Emerging role of proton beam radiation therapy for chordoma and chondrosarcoma of the skull base. Curr. Oncol. Rep. 10, 338–343.

Niida, H., Tanaka, R., Tamura, T., et al., 1994. Clival chordoma in early childhood without bone involvement. Childs Nerv. Syst. 10 (8), 533–535.

Nishigaya, K., et al., 1998. Intradural retroclival chordoma without bone involvement: no tumor regrowth 5 years after operation. Case report. J. Neurosurg. 88 (4), 764–768.

Oakley, G.J., Fuhrer, K., Seethala, R.R., 2008. Brachyury, SOX-9, and podoplanin, new markers in the skull base chordoma vs chondrosarcoma differential: a tissue microarray-based comparative analysis. Mod. Pathol. 21 (12), 1461–1469.

Oguro, K., Nakahara, N., Yamaguchi, Y., et al., 1989. Chondrosarcoma of the posterior fossa–case report. Neurol. Med. Chir. (Tokyo) 29 (11), 1030–1038.

Ojemann, R.G., Thornton, A.F., Harsh, G.R., 1995. Management of anterior cranial base and cavernous sinus neoplasms with conservative surgery alone or in combination with fractionated photon or stereotactic proton radiotherapy. Clin. Neurosurg. 42, 71–98.

O'Connell, J.X., Renard, L.G., Liebsch, N.J., et al., 1994. Base of skull chordoma. A correlative study of histologic and clinical features of 62 cases. Cancer 74 (8), 2261–2267.

O'Neill, P., Bell, B.A., Miller, J.D., et al., 1985. Fifty years of experience with chordomas in southeast Scotland. Neurosurgery 16 (2), 166–170.

Oot, R.F., Melville, G.E., New, P.F., et al., 1988. The role of MR and CT in evaluating clival chordomas and chondrosarcomas. AJR Am. J. Roentgenol. 151 (3), 567–575.

Pai, H.H., Thornton, A., Katznelson, L., et al., 2001. Hypothalamic/pituitary function following high-dose conformal radiotherapy to the base of skull: demonstration of a dose-effect relationship using dose-volume histogram analysis. Int. J. Radiat. Oncol. Biol. Phys. 49 (4), 1079–1092.

Pearlman, A.W., Friedman, M., 1970. Radical radiation therapy of chordoma. Am. J. Roentgenol. Radium. Ther. Nucl. Med. 108 (2), 332–341.

Rabadan, A., Conesa, H., 1992. Transmaxillary-transnasal approach to the anterior clivus: a microsurgical anatomical model. Neurosurgery 30 (4), 473–482.

Raffel, C., Wright, D.C., Gutin, P.H., et al., 1985. Cranial chordomas: clinical presentation and results of operative and radiation therapy in twenty-six patients. Neurosurgery 17 (5), 703–710.

Rhomberg, W., Eiter, H., Böhler, F., et al., 2006. Combined radiotherapy and razoxane in the treatment of chondrosarcomas and chordomas. Anticancer Res. 26 (3B), 2407–2411.

Ribbert, H., 1894. Ueber die Ecchondrosis physalifora sphenooccipitalis. Centralbl. Allg. Path Path Anat. 5, 457–461.

Richardson, M.S., 2001. Pathology of skull base tumors. Otolaryngol. Clin. North Am. 34 (6), 1025–1042, vii.

Rosenberg, A.E., Nielsen, G.P., Keel, S.B., et al., 1999. Chondrosarcoma of the base of the skull: a clinicopathologic study of 200 cases with emphasis on its distinction from chordoma. Am. J. Surg. Pathol. 23 (11), 1370–1378.

Santoni, R., Liebsch, N., Finkelstein, D.M., et al., 1998. Temporal lobe (TL) damage following surgery and high-dose photon and proton irradiation in 96 patients affected by chordomas and chondrosarcomas of the base of the skull. Int. J. Radiat. Oncol. Biol. Phys. 41 (1), 59–68.

Saunders, W.M., Chen, G.T., Austin-Seymour, M., et al., 1985. Precision, high dose radiotherapy. II. Helium ion treatment of tumors adjacent to critical central nervous system structures. Int. J. Radiat. Oncol. Biol. Phys. 11 (7), 1339–1347.

Schisano, G., Tovi, D., 1962. Clivus chordomas. Neurochirurgia (Stuttg.) 5, 99–120.

Schulz-Ertner, D., Nikoghosyan, A., Didinger, B., et al., 2004a. Carbon ion radiation therapy for chordomas and low grade chondrosarcomas – current status of the clinical trials at GSI. Radiother. Oncol. 73 (Suppl.), S53–S56.

Schulz-Ertner, D., Nikoghosyan, A., Thilmann, C., et al., 2004b. Results of carbon ion radiotherapy in 152 patients. Int. J. Radiat. Oncol. Biol. Phys. 58 (2), 631–640.

Scuotto, A., Albanese, V., Tomasello, F., 1980. Clival chordomas in children. Acta Neurol. (Napoli) 2 (2), 121–127.

Sekhar, L.N., Nanda, A., Sen, C.N., et al., 1992. The extended frontal approach to tumors of the anterior, middle, and posterior skull base. J. Neurosurg. 76 (2), 198–206.

Sen, C.N., Sekhar, L.N., 1991. Surgical management of anteriorly placed lesions at the craniocervical junction – an alternative approach. Acta Neurochir. (Wien) 108 (1–2), 70–77.

Sen, C.N., Sekhar, L.N., 1990. An extreme lateral approach to intradural lesions of the cervical spine and foramen magnum. Neurosurgery 27 (2), 197–204.

Sen, C.N., Sekhar, L.N., Schramm, V.L., et al., 1989. Chordoma and chondrosarcoma of the cranial base: an 8-year experience. Neurosurgery 25 (6), 931–941.

Slater, J.D., Austin-Seymour, M., Munzenrider, J., et al., 1988. Endocrine function following high dose proton therapy for tumors of the upper clivus. Int. J. Radiat. Oncol. Biol. Phys. 15 (3), 607–611.

Stapleton, S.R., Wilkins, P.R., Archer, D.J., et al., 1993. Chondrosarcoma of the skull base: a series of eight cases. Neurosurgery 32 (3), 348–356.

Steenberghs, J., Kiekens, C., Menten, J., et al., 2002. Intradural chordoma without bone involvement. Case report and review of the literature. J. Neurosurg. 97 (Suppl.), 94–97.

Stippler, M., Gardner, P.A., Snyderman, C.H., et al., 2009. Endoscopic endonasal approach for clival chordomas. Neurosurgery 64, 268–278. •

Sundaresan, N., Galicich, J.H., Chu, F.C., et al., 1979. Spinal chordomas. J. Neurosurg. 50 (3), 312–319.

Tachibana, E., Saito, K., Takahashi, M., et al., 2000. Surgical treatment of a massive chondrosarcoma in the skull base associated with Maffucci's syndrome: a case report. Surg. Neurol. 54 (2), 165–170.

Tai, P.T., Craighead, P., Bagdon, F., 1995. Optimization of radiotherapy for patients with cranial chordoma. A review of dose-response ratios for photon techniques. Cancer 75 (3), 749–756.

Terahara, A., Niemierko, A., Goitein, M., et al., 1999. Analysis of the relationship between tumor dose inhomogeneity and local control in patients with skull base chordoma. Int. J. Radiat. Oncol. Biol. Phys. 45 (2), 351–358.

Thieblemont, C., Biron, P., Rocher, F., et al., 1995. Prognostic factors in chordoma: role of postoperative radiotherapy. Eur. J. Cancer 31A (13–14), 2255–2259.

Thodou, E., Kontogeorgos, G., Scheithauer, B.W., et al., 2000. Intrasellar chordomas mimicking pituitary adenoma. J. Neurosurg. 92 (6), 976–982.

Tzortzidis, F., Elahi, F., Wright, D.C., et al., 2006. Patient outcome at long-term follow-up after aggressive microsurgical resection of cranial base chondrosarcomas. Neurosurgery 58 (6), 1090–1098.

Unni, K., 1996. Dahlin's bone tumors: General aspects and data on 11,087 cases, 5th edn. Lippincott-Raven, Philadelphia, pp., 291–303.

Van Loveren, H.R., Mahmood, A., Liu, S.S., et al., 1996. Innovations in cranial approaches and exposures: anterolateral approaches. Clin. Neurosurg. 43, 44–52.

Virchow, R., 1857. Untersuchungen uber die entwickelung des schadelgrundes im gesunden und krankhaften zustande, und uber den einfluss derselben auf schadelform, gesichtsbildung und gehirnbau. Virchows, Berlin.

Volpe, R., Mazabraud, A., 1983. A clinicopathologic review of 25 cases of chordoma (a pleomorphic and metastasizing neoplasm). Am. J. Surg. Pathol. 7 (2), 161–170.

Wanebo, J.E., Bristol, R.E., Porter, R.R., et al., 2006. Management of cranial base chondrosarcomas. Neurosurgery 58 (2), 249–255.

Watkins, L., Khudados, E.S., Kaleoglu, M., et al., 1993. Skull base chordomas: a review of 38 patients, 1958–1988. Br. J. Neurosurg. 7 (3), 241–248.

Wold, L.E., Laws, E.R. Jr., 1983. Cranial chordomas in children and young adults. J. Neurosurg. 59 (6), 1043–1047.

Yadav, Y.R., Kak, V.K., Khosla, V.K., et al., 1992. Cranial chordoma in the first decade. Clin. Neurol. Neurosurg. 94 (3), 241–246.

Yang, X.R., Beerman, M., Bergen, A.W., et al., 2005. Corroboration of a familial chordoma locus on chromosome 7q and evidence of genetic heterogeneity using single nucleotide polymorphisms (SNPs). Int. J. Cancer 116 (3), 487–491.

Glomus jugulare tumors

Rashid M. Janjua and Harry R. Van Loveren

Introduction

Glomus tumors are tumors derived from the paraganglionic cells that comprise the sympathetic and parasympathetic system. Other names for this group of tumors include paragangliomas, non-chromaffin paragangliomas and chemodectomas. Paraganglionic tissue is most prominent in the embryonic phase (embryonic neuroepithelium) and after birth, associated with the sympathetic and the parasympathetic system. Nevertheless, it can undergo tumorous transformation, with sympathetic tumors arising from the superior cervical ganglion, para-aortic bodies and adrenal gland and parasympathetic tissue surrounding the glossopharyngeal and vagus nerves (Semaan & Megerian 2008).

This chapter serves to provide an overview in the diagnosis and management of these tumors and provides an 8-step approach to their surgical removal.

Physiology

Paraganglia contain two cell types, the chief cells and the supporting sustentacular cells, which are arranged in 'cell balls' surrounded by a prominent capillary network. The chief cells belong to the diffuse neuroendocrine system (DNES) and contain secretory granules as found in the carotid body and adrenal medulla. Physiologically, they are chemoreceptors sensitive to changes in serum pH, pCO_2 and pO_2 (Semaan & Megerian 2008), thereby affecting regulation of the respiratory center in the medulla oblongata.

Tumors arising from the paraganglionic tissue in the tympanic branch of the glossopharyngeal nerve (Jacobson's nerve) are called 'Glomus tympanicum' for their location in the middle ear. Paraganglionic cells in the adventitia of the jugular bulb give rise to the same tumors and at that location, are referred to as 'Glomus jugulare' tumors. Tumors associated with the vagus nerve are referred to as 'Glomus vagale' and when arising from the carotid body referred to as 'carotid body' tumors (Semaan & Megerian 2008). When their exact origin cannot be ascertained, they are called 'jugulotympanic paragangliomas' (JTP).

Genetics

Some 80% of paragangliomas are sporadic, with the remainder inherited as an autosomal dominant trait. Inherited forms tend to be multicentric, bilateral and display earlier onset of symptoms (Grufferman et al 1980; Sobol & Dailey 1990). Multicentric tumors are found in 3–10% of sporadic cases and in 25–50% of familial cases. Malignant forms are

rare, with an incidence ranging from 6.4% for carotid body tumors, to 17% for glomus vagale (Shamblin et al 1971; Sniezek et al 2001). Currently, there are no histologic or cytochemical predictors of malignant behavior and the diagnosis of malignancy is dependent upon the presence of nodal or distant metastasis (Semaan & Megerian 2008).

Contrary to sympathetic paragangliomas (adrenal and extra-adrenal), head and neck parasympathetic paragangliomas may be inherited in a familial pattern without other tumors. These familial tumors are caused by germline mutations in the genes encoding for the subunits B, C, and D of the mitochondrial complex II enzyme (succinate-ubiquinone-oxidoreductase or succinyl dehydrogenase (SDH) (sub-units SDHB, SDHC and SDHD, respectively). This enzyme plays a key role in the mitochondrial electron transport chain of the Krebs cycle. Recent studies suggest screening for SDHD in all patients with head and neck paragangliomas, as 11% of the patients with the non-familial form may carry this deletion (Baysal 2008) and require lifelong screening for pheochromocytomas and extra-adrenal paragangliomas (Fakhry et al 2008; Havekes et al 2009).

Malignancy of the tumor is probably related to p53 and p16INK4A mutations. Additional studies have shown malignant tumors to be characterized by the presence of a high MIB-1 index, p53, Bcl-2 and CD34 (Rodriguez-Justo et al 2001). No single test or combination of tests has thus far yielded sufficiently high sensitivity and specificity to result in widespread acceptance in every day clinical practice.

Clinical presentation

Early stage paragangliomas present with symptoms related to close approximation of the tumor vessels to the tympanic membrane producing pulsatile tinnitus or to involvement of the middle ear, resulting in conductive hearing loss. Additionally, they result in lower cranial neuropathy secondary to compression and invasion at the jugular foramen. Paragangliomas of the jugular foramen are locally expansile and spread superiorly into the posterior fossa and inferiorly along the jugular vein. This expansile growth results gradually in obliteration of the jugular bulb. Erosion through the floor of the hypotympanum presents as a middle ear mass. The color of a middle ear mass is critical in the differential diagnosis with white masses representing cholesteatomas, gray masses adenomas, or neuromas and dark masses representing vascular tumors, a high-riding jugular bulb or an aberrant carotid artery. Blanching of the mass from application of positive pressure with a pneumatic otoscope (Brown's sign) should caution the examiner to refrain from a biopsy (Roland et al 1997). Encasement of the facial nerve may result from invasion of the facial recess and retro-facial air cells.

These tumors usually contain catecholamines but clinically significant secretion occurs in only 2% of the cases (Farr 1967). When this occurs, patients complain of facial flushing and palpitations with labile hypertension and tachycardia. At our institution, all patients are screened by determination of plasma catecholamines, (nor)metanephrines, and urine vanillylmandelic acid (VMA) and if elevated, a pheochromocytoma is excluded with abdominal computed tomography (CT). The sensitivity of blood tests is higher than that in urine (Semaan & Megerian 2008), with an overall diagnostic sensitivity of 98% and specificity of 92% for metanephrines (Eisenhofer et al 2008).

On cranial CT, these tumors are seen as soft tissue masses with erosion of the hypotympanum, with a characteristic 'salt and pepper' appearance. The tumor follows the path of least resistance into the air cell network of the mastoid bone eventually eroding through their septae. This fluffy edge appearance is distinctly different from benign masses, like schwannomas, which expand smoothly with intact cortical bone defining their border in the mastoid and the expanded jugular foramen. Magnetic resonance imaging (MRI) is superior in evaluating tumor vascularity, extension along neural foramina and multicentricity. On T1-weighted images, glomus tumors appear hypointense with a speckled appearance with early and pronounced enhancement on gadolinium enhanced images due to the hypervascular nature of the tumor. Four-vessel conventional angiography confirms the vascular nature of these tumors.

Preoperatively, all patients are evaluated for specific lower cranial nerve function: direct laryngoscopy for evaluation of vocal cord function, swallowing evaluation and an audiogram are routinely obtained. In some patients, the nerve deficit may not be clinically evident to the patient but detectable on detailed examination and diagnostic studies. This information is of importance in the preoperative discussion with the patients. In treating skull base tumors, the role of cognitive scripting to implant into the patient's mind reasonable expectation of surgical outcome is of immense importance. In this approach, the patient and family are focused on the possibility of postoperative deficits and their resulting consequences. These can be as severe as tracheostomy, placement of a percutaneous gastric tube and hoarseness, all temporary or permanent. This allows the patient preparation time before surgery, which results in better cooperation in rehabilitation, as well as a milder psychological impact. Having patients anticipate an alteration in their neurological status allows them to cope better with the result and improves their recovery effort.

Treatment

Embolization

All patients undergo four-vessel cerebral angiography to evaluate their vascular anatomy as well as the blood supply to the tumor. In tumors that encase the carotid artery with a possibility of surgical sacrifice, cross compression and the Alcock's test (compression of the carotid artery during vertebral injection) may be performed during the angiography.

This provides information on the ability of the contralateral carotid artery and one or both vertebral arteries to supply the ipsilateral hemisphere in case of a carotid sacrifice.

The initial description of a method of embolization was by Brooks who injected pieces of autologous muscle into the surgically exposed cervical carotid, with the hope that they would be carried by orthograde flow into carotid-cavernous fistulae and occlude them (Brooks 1930). Luessenhop and Spence (1960) used steel particles covered with methylmethacrylate introduced into the surgically exposed internal carotid artery in order to block feeding arteries supplying a brain arteriovenous malformation (AVM), which they called 'artificial embolization'. Since then, techniques and indications have been improved and until recently, glues and polyvinyl particles of different sizes were being used (Tasar & Yetiser 2004) with Onyx® being the latest embolization glue used successfully for glomus tumors (Rimbot et al 2007). As the glomus jugulare tumors are fed by branches of the external carotid artery, safe preoperative embolization can usually be attained, however, embolization of the ascending pharyngeal artery carries with it a small risk of facial nerve paralysis. Embolization can be safely performed to decrease the risk of intraoperative bleeding or in addition to radiation to diminish the size of the tumor. It also provides considerable symptomatic relief and improves the quality of life of those for whom surgery is not available or not indicated (Kingsley & O'Connor 1982).

Often, an 80–90% reduction in tumor vascularity can be obtained with embolization. There is no standard of measuring the technical success angiographically but the benefit of preoperative embolization is often touted by quoting diminished intraoperative blood loss volumes Some studies have concluded that there is no surgical advantage to performing preoperative embolization (Fisch 1982; Kumar et al 1982), while others have found that, even if the blood loss is diminished, the requirement for transfusion is not affected (Leonetti et al 1997; Litle et al 1996). Nevertheless, Murphy and Brackmann (1989) analyzed their results of preoperative embolization in 35 patients with glomus jugulare tumors and found that the embolized patients ($n = 18$) had less intraoperative blood loss (mean = 1 122 mL) and shorter operation time as compared with the non-embolized patients ($n = 17$) who had a longer operative time and greater blood loss (mean = 2769 mL).

At our institution, embolization is routinely attempted for the reasons mentioned and the presumption that a less bloody operative field leads to more precise dissection and protection of cranial nerves. We have not used it as a standalone treatment modality, since the tumor is only partially devitalized and smaller feeding arteries still persist.

Surgical treatment

The multidisciplinary team approach, as pioneered by Gardner (1977), is the preferred approach to glomus jugulare tumors at our center. This 'divide and conquer' strategy brings the full expertise and skill of each of the three specialties (neurosurgery, neurootology, head and neck surgery) to bear in each step of the operative approach. This enhanced execution along with diminished surgeon fatigue facilitates a better outcome.

A well-conceived team-oriented plan is only effective if it is well communicated. A well-informed anesthesia team should be prepared for possible hypertensive crisis during tumor dissection. This is a diminishing issue with advances in neuro-anesthesia and the introduction of rapid onset hypotensive agents that can rapidly respond to and control intraoperative hypertension secondary to catecholamine release directly into the blood stream.

The neuro-otology literature has proposed multiple classifications for glomus tumors. Alford and Guilford's classification from 1962 classified extracranial tumors, whereas the revised Jenkins and Fisch (1981) classification accounted for intracranial extension. Jackson et al (1982) further revised the classification and divided the glomus tumors into 'glomus tympanicum' and 'glomus jugulare'. None of these have found universal acceptance or application.

Glomus jugulare tumors that come to the attention of a neurosurgeon generally do so because they straddle the jugular foramen with a posterior fossa component. The presence or absence of cranial nerve deficit will influence the decision to operate, the surgical strategy and intraoperative decision-making.

Like many processes in industry, business or medicine, a multi-step process that is simultaneously complex and seldom undertaken, is best served by reverting as often as possible to acceptable 'default settings'. Within the context of these defaults, the approach is also tailored to the individual patient and tumor. Our default approach to achieve success in glomus jugulare surgery consists of an '8-step-approach' that helps surgeons diminish the mystery and the fear normally associated with surgery in or around the jugular foramen.

The patient is positioned supine to allow the head and neck surgeon with unrestricted access to and normal orientation of the vessels and nerves in the neck. The head is turned to the contralateral side until the sagittal sinus in nearly parallel to the floor to facilitate the trajectory of view through the mastoid and into the posterior fossa. An ipsilateral shoulder roll should be considered to decrease torsion of the neck with special attention to the possibility of kinking the contralateral and generally the only remaining jugular vein. The head can be free on a padded horseshoe headrest as is the preference of most head and neck surgeons and neurootologists, or fixed in a Mayfield® headholder (Integra, Plainsboro, NJ), which facilitates the neurosurgeon's desire for a retractor system in the posterior fossa and the occasional use of frameless-guidance technology. Hair is removed using surgical clippers. Nerve monitoring electrodes are placed for registration of cranial nerves VII through XII, including a special endotracheal tube with incorporated EMG leads for vocal cord monitoring (Medtronic Xomed®, Jacksonville, FL).

After prep and drape, a C-shaped incision is made that exposes the entire mastoid, suboccipital area, and continues into the neck crossing over the sternocleidomastoid muscle to its anterior border.

Step 1: Neck dissection

This step is performed by the head/neck surgeon. In sequential fashion, the hypoglossal, vagus, glossopharyngeal and accessory nerves are identified and tagged with vessel loops.

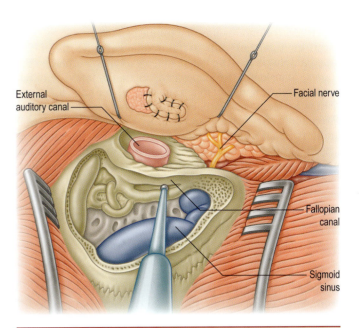

Figure 38.1 The mastoidectomy is performed and facial recess air cells drilled out. If the middle ear is involved, it can now be opened and the ossicles removed.

The facial nerve is also identified along its course into the parotid gland from behind the styloid process, up to its entry on the deep surface of the parotid gland. The internal jugular vein (IJV) and the internal carotid artery (ICA) are isolated in the neck.

Step 2: Mastoidectomy (Fig. 38.1)

A mastoidectomy is performed with preservation of the semicircular canals. Although partial resection of the semicircular canals (Horgan et al 2001; Taplin et al 2006) can be achieved with hearing preservation, major resection will produce deafness.

FOR TUMORS INVADING THE MIDDLE EAR, ADDITIONAL EXPOSURE IS REQUIRED:

After achieving proximal vascular control, the surgeon retracts the skin flap and transects the external ear canal with a scalpel deep into the bony canal. The muscles over the mastoid are split, starting at the supramastoid crest and continuing toward the mastoid tip where the sternocleidomastoid muscle is detached. A posterior extension is required if a posterior fossa exposure is necessary. All soft tissue in the ear canal, including the tympanic membrane and its annulus, malleus, and the incus are removed. The transected ear canal is closed in three layers: the canal edges are closed with continuous suture, soft tissues are brought over and closed and a periosteal flap excavated from the skin flap is oversewn.

The facial nerve is identified emerging from the stylomastoid foramen. A partial superficial parotidectomy is used to expose the pes (branching point) of the facial nerve.

The facial canal and recess are defined and after exposure and sacrifice of the chorda tympani nerve, the middle ear cavity can be appreciated. This area is defined inferiorly by the jugular bulb, laterally by the annulus of the tympanic membrane and medially by the descending facial nerve. The hypotympanum and retro-facial air cells are hereby exposed which are common routes for tumor extension.

If the tumor extends to the middle ear, then the incostapedial joint is disarticulated sharply avoiding injury to the stapes. Avulsion of the stapes can violate the integrity of the round window and lead to a route of perilymphatic fluid leak with subsequent semicircular canal dysfunction and vertigo. The middle ear cavity is accessed by removing the external auditory canal wall. The anterior mastoid wall is thinned to eggshell thickness. Next, the skin of the external auditory ear meatus and the tympanum are freed from the posterior wall of the canal. The canal wall dividing the mastoid and the middle ear is drilled away and any tumor identified in the middle ear and surrounding areas is removed in a piecemeal fashion.

Step 3: Suboccipital/retrosigmoid craniotomy

The cortical bone of the sigmoid plate overlying the sigmoid sinus is removed and a retrosigmoid suboccipital craniectomy or craniotomy is performed. The size of craniectomy/craniotomy is tailored to the size and location of the posterior fossa component of the tumor. In the standard case, only one finger-breadth of retrosigmoid bone is removed to facilitate ligation of the sigmoid sinus superior to the tumor. Bone removal continues down to the foramen magnum which is opened ipsilateral to the tumor.

Step 4: Venous ligation

The jugular vein, which was previously tagged in the neck, is ligated just distal to the tumor using three 0-silk sutures. The vein is then cut leaving two sutures on the residual cervical stump. Thereafter, the retrosigmoid dura distal to the entry of the vein of Labbe into the sigmoid sinus is opened enough to accommodate a curved needle. The 0-silk suture on a needle is passed through the dural opening and exited from the presigmoid dura encircling the vessel and tied. Two additional sutures are applied and the sinus cut leaving two sutures proximally. At this point, and depending on the patient's anatomy, the only inflow to the jugular bulb complex comes from the one or more drainage sites of the inferior petrosal sinus into the back wall of the jugular bulb which will be visualized only at the time of tumor removal from the jugular bulb itself.

Step 5: Unroofing of the jugular bulb (Figs 38.2, 38.3)

Once the tumor is removed from the retrofacial air cells, attention is turned to the jugular bulb. The residual mastoid tip is removed with a high speed drill. Mastoid tip resection continues right through the digastric groove/ridge to expose the lateral wall of the jugular bulb and the jugular bulb–jugular vein transition. Bone resection across the jugular bulb–jugular vein transition has been a relative mystery to neurosurgeons and consists of remnant inferior mastoid bone and occipital bone posterolateral to the occipital condyle. This can be resected with relative impunity as the facial nerve is located anterior to this trajectory and the glossopharyngeal, vagus and accessory nerves are protected medial to the tumor.

Step 6: Extracranial tumor removal (Fig. 38.4)

Tumor extending into the neck is dissected from the cranial nerves. The tumor is mobilized toward the skull base along with the transected jugular vein, until reaching the jugular

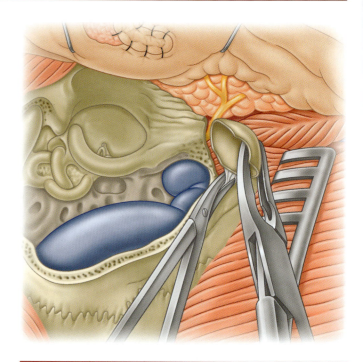

Figure 38.2 After the venous ligation on both ends of the tumor has been accomplished the mastoid tip is removed with rongeurs. This eposes the jugular process which is covered by the rectus capitis lateralis muscle.

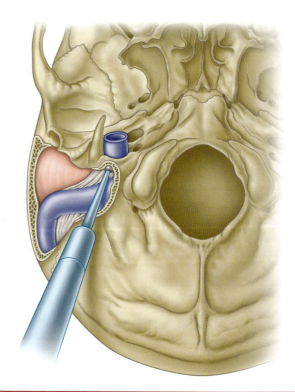

Figure 38.3 After detaching the muscle, the jugular process is drilled which is located postero-lateral to the jugular foramen.

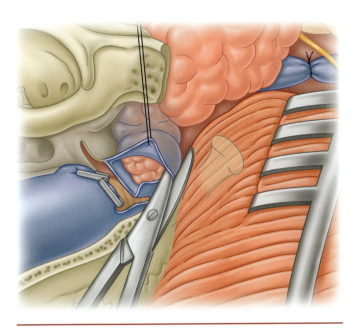

Figure 38.4 The lateral sigmoid sinus wall is opened distal to the proximal ligation exposing the tumor which is debulked in a piecemeal fashion.

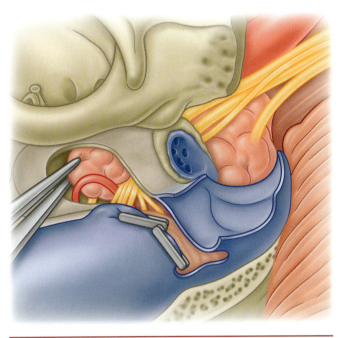

Figure 38.5 The intracranial part of the tumor can usually be dissected from the tumor with ease. In this illustration, the back wall of the jugular bulb has been removed.

bulb. Turning attention above, the sigmoid sinus is incised longitudinally along its lateral surface from the site of its ligation down toward the jugular bulb. The tumor is then excavated from the jugular vein and bulb while preserving the deep venous wall. The deep venous wall of the jugular bulb covers and therefore protects the cranial nerves (IX, X, XI) that traverse the jugular foramen. When the last bit of tumor within the jugular bulb is removed, a gush of venous bleeding is encountered from the multiple orifices of the inferior petrosal sinus. These are gently packed with Oxycel® and bone wax, with awareness that the cranial nerves of the jugular foramen lie interspersed beneath the deep venous wall of the jugular bulb in this area. The tumor from the neck can be amputated at the bulb along with the jugular vein.

Step 7: Intracranial tumor removal (Fig. 38.5)
With the pre-sigmoid as well as the retro-sigmoid dura exposed, the intradural space can be exposed. Often, the exposure from the pre-sigmoid opening is sufficient and the surgical technique for removal of the intracranial portion of the tumor is similar to that used for vestibular schwannomas. The tumor surface is stimulated with a Prass probe to identify any overlying cranial nerves. Hereafter, the superficial capsule is coagulated with bipolar diathermy and intracapsular debulking performed using an ultrasonic aspirator. Finally, the capsule is resected leaving the tumor attached to the nerves if salvage of their function is attempted.

Step 8: Exploration of the jugular foramen (Fig. 38.6)
Aside from patient selection for surgery, exploration of the jugular foramen represents the most important decision made by the glomus surgeon and team. Resection of the back wall of the jugular bulb and removal of the remnants of

tumor deep to it in the pars nervosa of the jugular foramen offers the opportunity of radical tumor resection and cure, but also introduces the risk of cranial nerve paralysis in those patients who retained function prior to surgery. Although patients who have gradually lost swallowing function over a number of years and developed compensatory swallowing mechanisms related to subconsciously shifting food at the posterior pharynx, sudden loss of function at surgery is difficult and sometimes impossible to adequately compensate for. In patients with preserved IX, X, XI function, we do not remove tumor from the jugular foramen but rather leave it for surveillance or radiosurgery depending upon the patient's age both chronologically and physiologically. At the conclusion of tumor removal, the dura is closed in a watertight fashion, possibly requiring a regionally harvested or synthetic graft and the mastoidectomy cavity filled with a fat graft. After copious irrigation, the skin flap is re-approximated and closed.

Adjuvant therapy

Conformal radiation
Traditional external beam radiation was the first employed adjuvant treatment given to patients after sub-total resection of glomus tumors (Li et al 2007). A meta-analysis by Springate and Weichselbaum (1990) reviewed 19 studies in which traditional radiation was used. This indicated glomus tumors to be radiosensitive, as local control was found in 349 of 384 patients with a low morbidity of 2–3% serious sequelae. Tumor control rates after surgery alone, after surgery and conventional radiation, and after conventional radiation alone, were cited as 86%, 90% and 93%, respectively. External beam radiation requires large field sizes that extend into

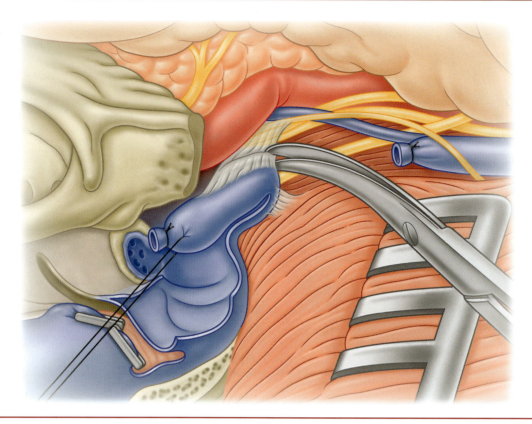

Figure 38.6 The back wall of the jugular bulb can be dissected away from the cranial nerves IX, X and XI. In patients with (partially) intact function, this back wall may need to be retained in order to preserve nerve function.

the neck and can lead to radionecrosis of the bone, xerostomia and induction of secondary tumors. The authors, citing high tumor control rates and a comparatively higher post-treatment cranial nerve morbidity and cerebrospinal fluid leak rate with surgery, advocated radiation as the primary treatment for glomus tumors. However, as meta-analysis based upon several small studies, it lacked the validity to alter the treatment algorithm.

Radiosurgery

The field of stereotactic radiosurgery has emerged as an effective means with which to address many of the pitfalls of traditional external beam radiation applied to glomus tumors and its use has increased steadily in recent years with high response rates. A compelling argument has been made for the use of radiosurgery as the only treatment modality for glomus jugulare tumors. Elshaikh et al (2002) reported a 100% 5-year tumor control rate with conventional radiation and radiosurgery in their retrospective review of patients with recurrent glomus tumors, compared with 62% for surgery alone. Foote et al's (2002) review of patients treated with radiosurgery alone after a median 37-month follow-up showed stabilized tumor in 17, decreased size in eight and symptom resolution in 15 patients. The largest series reviewed consists of 104 patients with 121 paragangliomas (Hinerman et al 2008), followed for a median of 8.5 years after various modalities, 6% of which were radiosurgery. Of the 104

patients, only six patients had a recurrence, resulting in a 96% control rate. The data are incomplete and inconclusive but it appears reasonable to include radiosurgery in the treatment paradigm for glomus tumors as a primary or adjunct strategy depending upon patient age, condition, tumor size, location, growth history, cranial nerve status, and the skills and experience of available surgical teams.

REFERENCES

Alford, B.R., Guilford, F.R., 1962. A comprehensive study of tumors of the glomus jugulare. Laryngoscope 72, 765–805.

Baysal, B.E., 2008. Clinical and molecular progress in hereditary paraganglioma. J. Med. Genet. 45, 689–694.

Brooks, B., 1930. The treatment of traumatic arteriovenous fistula. South Med. J. 23, 100–106.

Eisenhofer, G., Siegert, G., Kotzerke J., et al., 2008. Current progress and future challenges in the biochemical diagnosis and treatment of pheochromocytomas and paragangliomas. Horm. Metab. Res. 40, 329–337.

Elshaikh, M.A., Mahmoud-Ahmed, A.S., Kinney, S.E., et al., 2002. Recurrent head-and-neck chemodectomas: a comparison of surgical and radiotherapeutic results. Int. J. Radiat. Oncol. Biol. Phys. 52, 953–956.

Fakhry, N., Niccoli-Sire, P., Barlier-Seti A., et al., 2008. Cervical paragangliomas: is SDH genetic analysis systematically required? Eur. Arch. Otorhinolaryngol. 265, 557–563.

Farr, H.W., 1967. Carotid body tumors. A thirty year experience at Memorial Hospital. Am. J. Surg. 114, 614–619.

Fisch, U., 1982. Infratemporal fossa approach for glomus tumors of the temporal bone. Ann. Otol. Rhinol. Laryngol. 91, 474–479.

Foote, R.L., Pollock, B.E., Gorman, D.A., et al., 2002. Glomus jugulare tumor: tumor control and complications after stereotactic radiosurgery. Head Neck 24, 332–339.

Gardner, G., Cocke, E.W. Jr., Robertson, J.T., et al., 1977. Combined approach surgery for removal of glomus jugulare tumors. Laryngoscope 87, 665–688.

Grufferman, S., Gillman, M.W., Pasternak, L.R., et al., 1980. Familial carotid body tumors: case report and epidemiologic review. Cancer 46, 2116–2122.

Havekes, B., van der Klaauw, A.A., Weiss, M.M., et al., 2009. Pheochromocytomas and extra-adrenal paragangliomas detected by screening in patients with SDHD-associated head-and-neck paragangliomas. Endocr. Relat. Cancer 16 (2), 527–536.

Hinerman, R.W., Amdur, R.J., Morris, C.G., et al., 2008. Definitive radiotherapy in the management of paragangliomas arising in the head and neck: a 35-year experience. Head Neck 30, 1431–1438.

Horgan, M.A., Delashaw, J.B., Schwartz, M.S., et al., 2001. Transcrusal approach to the petroclival region with hearing preservation. Technical note and illustrative cases. J. Neurosurg. 94, 660–666.

Jackson, C.G., Glasscock, M.E. 3rd, Harris, P.F., 1982. Glomus tumors. Diagnosis, classification, and management of large lesions. Arch. Otolaryngol. 108, 401–410.

Jenkins, H.A., Fisch, U., 1981. Glomus tumors of the temporal region. Technique of surgical resection. Arch. Otolaryngol. 107, 209–214.

Kingsley, D., O'Connor, A.F., 1982. Embolization in otolaryngology. J. Laryngol. Otol. 96, 439–450.

Kumar, A.J., Kaufman, S.L., Patt J., et al., 1982. Preoperative embolization of hypervascular head and neck neoplasms using microfibrillar collagen. AJNR Am. J. Neuroradiol. 3, 163–168.

Leonetti, J.P., Donzelli, J.J., Littooy, F.N., et al., 1997. Perioperative strategies in the management of carotid body tumors. Otolaryngol. Head Neck Surg. 117, 111–115.

Li, G., Chang, S., Adler, J.R., et al., 2007. Irradiation of glomus jugulare tumors: a historical perspective. Neurosurgical Focus 23, E13.

Litle, V.R., Reilly, L.M., Ramos, T.K., 1996. Preoperative embolization of carotid body tumors: when is it appropriate? Ann. Vasc. Surg. 10, 464–468.

Luessenhop, A.J., Spence, W.T., 1960. Artificial embolization of cerebral arteries. Report of use in a case of arteriovenous malformation. J. Am. Med. Assoc. 172, 1153–1155.

Murphy, T.P., Brackmann, D.E., 1989. Effects of preoperative embolization on glomus jugulare tumors. Laryngoscope 99, 1244–1247.

Rimbot, A., Mounayer, C., Loureiro C., et al., 2007. [Preoperative mixed embolization of a paraganglioma using Onyx]. J. Neuroradiol. 34, 334–339.

Rodriguez-Justo, M., Aramburu-Gonzalez, J.A., Santonja, C., 2001. Glomangiosarcoma of abdominal wall. Virchows Arch. 438, 418–420.

Roland, P., Meyerhoff, W., Marple, B., 1997. Hearing loss. Thieme, New York.

Semaan, M.T., Megerian, C.A., 2008. Current assessment and management of glomus tumors. Curr. Opin. Otolaryngol. Head Neck Surg. 16 (5), 420–426.

Shamblin, W.R., ReMine, W.H., Sheps, S.G., 1971. Carotid body tumor (chemodectoma). Clinicopathologic analysis of ninety cases. Am. J. Surg. 122, 732–739.

Sniezek, J.C., Netterville, J.L., Sabri, A.N., 2001. Vagal paragangliomas. Otolaryngol. Clin. North. Am. 34, 925–939.

Sobol, S.M., Dailey, J.C., 1990. Familial multiple cervical paragangliomas: report of a kindred and review of the literature. Otolaryngol. Head Neck Surg. 102, 382–390.

Springate, S.C., Weichselbaum, R.R., 1990. Radiation or surgery for chemodectoma of the temporal bone: a review of local control and complications. Head Neck 12, 303–307.

Taplin, M.A., Anthony, R., Tymianski M., et al., 2006. Transmastoid partial labyrinthectomy for brainstem vascular lesions: clinical outcomes and assessment of postoperative cochleovestibular function. Skull Base 16, 133–143.

Tasar, M., Yetiser, S., 2004. Glomus tumors: therapeutic role of selective embolization. J. Craniofac. Surg. 15, 497–505.

It would appear that a crucial factor in the risk of PNC is the type of wood dust to which the workers are exposed. At least 48 woods are known to have been used in workshops in which workers have developed these tumors; these woods are derived from both deciduous and evergreen trees and from trees native to both the northern and southern hemispheres. Hardwood species tend to be the wood types most associated with PNC. Hardwoods, by definition, come from deciduous trees, in contrast to softwoods, which derive from conifer trees; generally the prefix 'hard' or 'soft' connotes the density of the wood but there are notable exceptions, e.g., the well known light balsa wood is actually from a deciduous tree and is therefore a hardwood. Since dusts from several different species are generally present in most workplaces, it is difficult to pinpoint the particular woods that are the cause (Wills 1982). Nonetheless, there is evidence to implicate beech, oak, walnut, and eucalyptus woods in particular (Ironside & Matthews 1975; Franklin 1982; Mohtashamipur et al 1989).

Wood dust contains many biologically active chemicals of botanic origin as well as fungal proteins from fungi affecting the wood. The biologic chemicals include alkaloids, saponins, aldehydes, quinones, flavonoids, tropolones, oils, cardiotoxic steroids, stilbenes, resins, and proteins (Roush 1979). Although extrinsic materials such as pesticides and preservatives may be applied to the wood, the British and Australian data tend to point away from these as the cause for the disease. Such chemicals were not used in the British furniture industry at the time of greatest risk, which was between the two world wars (Acheson et al 1968, 1982), nor have they been applied to machining in the Australian lumber industry. Survey of workers in the furniture industry revealed that precancerous squamous metaplasia was found in the nasal mucosa of 64% of woodworkers, but in only 18% of other workers in the industry (Hadfield & MacBeth 1971). Impaired mucociliary clearance secondary to the wood dust exposure was found to be associated with these changes. These effects would lead to impaired clearance of dust from the noses of these workers, thus prolonging contact between the carcinogen and the nasal mucosa.

There is some epidemiologic evidence indicating an increased incidence of other types of tumors such as gastrointestinal lung cancers and lymphomas in workers exposed to inhalation of wood dusts, but these data are somewhat conflicting (Mohtashamipur et al 1989). Organic dusts arising in other situations have also been found to be associated with ethmoid adenocarcinoma. Dust arising during the machining of the soles of shoes was found to be associated with a 35-fold increase in the risk of PNC (Acheson et al 1970). Less well-defined associations have been made, linking adenocarcinoma with exposure to flour dust, polyaromatic hydrocarbons and asbestos exposure (Roush 1979).

Clinical features

Patients are most commonly in the 6th to 8th decade at the time of presentation. The common presenting symptoms of PNC are nasal obstruction, often unilateral, epistaxis, and nasal discharge. There is often a preceding history of chronic rhinitis causing similar symptoms which contributes to the

> **Box 39.2** Clinical features of PNC
>
> - Nasal obstruction (often unilateral)
> - Nasal discharge and epistaxis
> - Facial pain or sensory disturbance
> - Proptosis
> - Facial swelling or invasion
> - Visual disturbance or diplopia
> - Anosmia (often unilateral)

common delay in diagnosis. Less frequently patients present with facial pain, facial sensory disturbance, swelling of the cheek, proptosis, diplopia, or visual disturbance (Lund 1983). Presentation with symptoms referable to intracranial involvement is rare. Esthesioneuroblastoma has been reported to present with ectopic ACTH syndrome (Kanno et al 2005) or Cushing's syndrome (Yu et al 2004) due to functional ACTH-producing cells within the tumor. Lymph node involvement or metastatic disease at presentation are unusual, occurring in 10–15% of patients at presentation (Waldron et al 2003). Anosmia, usually unilateral, is a common presenting sign in patients with ethmoid sinus or nasal involvement (Box 39.2).

The diagnosis was delayed by between 3 and 14 months in an American series (Sisson et al 1989). The authors recommended vigorous examination in all adults presenting with sinonasal complaints of >6 weeks duration, including telescopic endonasal examination and biopsy of all suspicious areas. If the symptoms do not resolve within 2 weeks of vigorous medical therapy, a limited computed tomographic (CT) examination of the sinuses was recommended. Using this regimen, the authors were able to reduce the mean diagnostic delay in their practice from 8 to 4 months, with 33% of the tumors in their series being diagnosed at a relatively early stage (T1 or T2); this is much earlier than in other series and the authors suggested that this reflected their more vigorous investigation of suspicious presenting complaints. Cancers of the nasal cavity tend to present earlier due to more pronounced early symptoms and easier diagnosis, and this is reflected in the better prognosis of these lesions (Hyams et al 1988).

Imaging diagnosis

CT scanning and magnetic resonance imaging (MRI) are the investigations of choice for assessment of PNC. Typical CT findings include a soft tissue density tumor mass with erosion of the bony walls around the sinus of origin with invasion into adjacent anatomic structures. The tumor enhances nonuniformly with contrast. Multiple fine cuts using window settings for bone and soft tissue are required for detailed presurgical assessment, allowing assessment of tumor extent and bony erosion (Figs 39.2, 39.3). Direct coronal scans are useful and are particularly valuable in assessment of orbital roof, cribriform plate, olfactory groove, and intracranial involvement (Fig. 39.4). CT assessment of sinus involvement may be misleading as inspissated mucus in an obstructed sinus may mimic the appearances of tumor; this is particularly crucial when assessing the sphenoid sinus, as tumor involvement there may dictate whether the tumor is

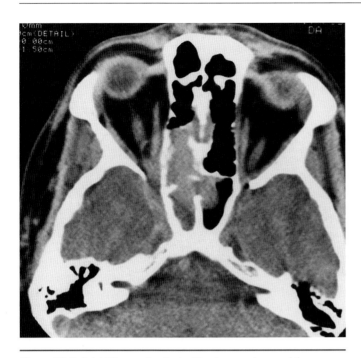

Figure 39.2 Axial CT scan of patient with adenocarcinoma of the ethmoid, displayed on soft tissue window settings. There is a soft tissue mass in the sphenoid sinus, but one cannot be sure if this is tumor or only mucus trapped there.

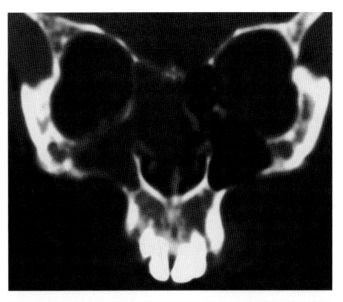

Figure 39.4 Coronal CT scan of another case, again using bone windows. This displays tumor involvement of the maxilla and ethmoid sinuses, erosion of the orbital wall, and tumor extending right up to the olfactory groove but with no erosion evident there. Nevertheless, microscopic dural involvement was present.

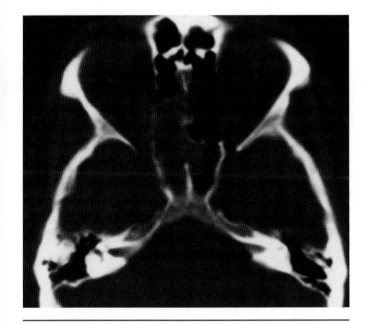

Figure 39.3 Axial CT scan of the same patient with bone windows to display bony erosion.

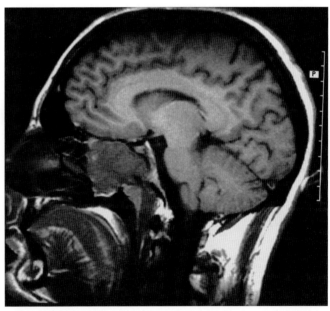

Figure 39.5 Parasagittal MRI scan of the same patient in Figures 39.2 and 39.3 slightly to the right of the midline, showing the tumor involvement of the sphenoid sinus. The bony floor of the anterior cranial fossa appears intact as a black line in this section.

resectable in its entirety. MRI can usually differentiate between tumor and inspissated mucus (Maroldi et al 1997) (Figs 39.5, 39.6) and may demonstrate invasion of tumor along the perineural space (Pandolfo et al 1989). MRI may show orbital apex or small intracranial deposits better than CT. Inspissated mucus is variable in its MRI signal intensity but is often different from tumor on T1- or T2-weighted images. Most commonly, entrapped mucus is seen as high signal on T2-weighted images (Fig. 39.6). Tumors usually appear as hypointense on T1, variably hyperintense on T2 and with heterogeneous contrast enhancement (Yu et al 2009; Derdeyn et al 1994) but signal characteristics are not specific for any particular type of histopathology (Kairemo et al 1998). MRI appears to be the most useful imaging modality for postoperative surveillance (Lund et al 1996). Appearance of recurrences does not differ significantly from the

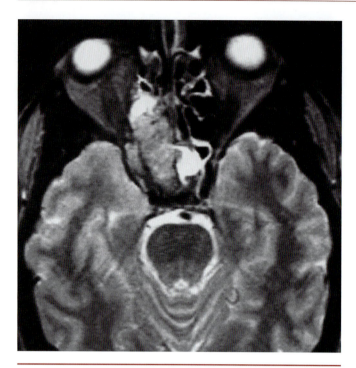

Figure 39.6 Axial MRI scan of a patient showing tumor involvement of the right side of the sphenoid sinus, but mucus accumulation on the left, as shown by the high signal there.

Tumor type	Occurrence (%)
Squamous cell carcinoma	51
Anaplastic carcinoma	10
Transitional cell carcinoma	8
Adenocarcinoma	6
Salivary carcinoma	4
Lymphoma	5
Melanoma	3
Sarcoma	6
Other	2

Table 39.1 Histologic distribution of PNC in a registry series

initial tumor (Pickuth et al 1999). It is recommended that patients be followed for several years after treatment, as early detection of recurrence is associated with a better prognosis.

Positron-emission tomography (PET) utilizing [18F]-FDG has been investigated and may provide useful information, especially in the setting of recurrence (Fatterpekar et al 2008). However, increased uptake on PET is also seen in inflammatory and granulation tissue, so differentiation of tumor can often be difficult. PET images can be co-registered to CT, making interpretation easier.

Laboratory diagnosis

Endoscopic or open examination of the nasal cavity and nasal sinuses, with biopsy of suspicious areas, is the key method of confirming the diagnosis, which is essential before major surgery is undertaken. Cytologic diagnosis of maxillary sinus disease has been suggested by examination of washings of the sinus; although malignancy may be diagnosed by this method, there were two false negative cytology reports among the seven cases of malignant tumor in one Japanese series (Nishioka et al 1989). Systemic investigations will be required to assess the general condition of the patient. No other specific investigations are required except that we find it useful to perform preoperative nasal swabs to guide antibiotic prophylaxis during craniofacial resection.

Gross morphologic features

PNC commences in one cavity but then invades the bony walls to involve adjacent structures. Often tumors grow extraperiosteally before invading further into the invaded cavity,

particularly with respect to the orbit where some surgeons have selectively resected periosteum in an attempt to avoid orbital exenteration (Perry et al 1988). When the tumor arises in or involves the ethmoid sinus, early spread to the dura of the olfactory groove is the rule rather than the exception (Danks et al 1994); gross intradural disease is less common, reflecting the barrier provided by the dura. The majority of the tumors are gray to pink or red, friable fungating growths that are susceptible to contact bleeding (Hyams et al 1988). Some tumors may have a papillomatous appearance or be found in a papilloma after removal. Papillomas are benign but may be bulky and even cause bony erosion by pressure on occasion, and tend to be firm or rubbery in texture. Maxillary cancers typically invade into the hard palate, facial skin, and nose as well as into the ethmoid and sphenoid sinuses, the intracranial cavity, the orbit, and posteriorly into the pterygopalatine fossa. Adenoid cystic carcinomas are notorious for their diffuse infiltration, which is difficult to demarcate, as well as their tendency to spread along neural pathways. These features contribute to the very high recurrence rate of this tumor type (Hyams et al 1988).

Histopathologic features

A number of different tumor types are grouped under the generic heading of cancer of the paranasal sinuses (Table 39.1) (Robin et al 1979); 50–75% of cases are SCC. Anaplastic carcinoma, transitional cell carcinoma, and adenocarcinoma each has an incidence of about 5–10%. Salivary carcinoma (principally adenoid cystic), lymphoma, melanoma, sarcoma, and esthesioneuroblastoma are less common (Robin et al 1979); these are more common in the AFIP series, but this may reflect a secondary referral bias (Hyams et al 1988).

The relative incidence of the different histologies varies in different regions; for instance, adenocarcinoma makes up 35% of the cases in the state of Victoria, Australia, due to a large hardwood-based industry (Giles et al 1992). The distribution of histologies in the authors' surgical experience is shown in Table 39.2. Adenocarcinoma is very strongly represented, reflecting both its high incidence in that region and also a referral bias in patients referred for craniofacial resection. Meningioma, hemangiopericytoma, and basal cell carcinoma are rare as primary paranasal sinus tumors but may invade the sinuses by direct spread from adjacent sites and present similar management problems. A large number of rare tumor types may involve the paranasal sinus region (Hyams et al 1988).

Table 39.2 Histologic distribution of PNC in the RMH series of 82 patients treated by craniofacial resection

Tumor type	Occurrence	
	n	(%)
Squamous cell carcinoma	38	46
Adenocarcinoma	30	37
Adenoid cystic carcinoma	9	11
Esthesioneuroblastoma	5	6

On microscopic examination, SCC has the typical appearance of these tumors elsewhere in the body, with areas of keratin formation either as sheets or as epithelial pearls. Stromal invasion and destruction confirm the malignant nature of the lesion. In the nasal cavity, a well-differentiated tumor may mimic a papilloma because of its regular cellular pattern, exophytic growth, and lack of stromal invasion. The diagnosis is made on the basis of cellular abnormalities, such as loss of polarity and atypical nuclear changes.

Adenocarcinomas generally arise in the upper nasal cavity or in the ethmoid sinuses, from either the surface epithelium or the minor salivary gland tissue (Wax et al 1995). There are papillary and sessile forms. Microscopically, the sessile tumors often bear a strong resemblance to carcinomas of the colon which is accentuated by the presence of goblet cells. The tumors can be graded as low or high grade on histologic grounds, and this correlates well with prognosis (Hyams et al 1988). Adenocarcinomas have been reported to have a better prognosis than squamous or undifferentiated tumors.

Anaplastic carcinomas have all the features of invasive cancer but no features typical of a particular type. They have a poor prognosis with a high rate of early metastasis. Very rare types of aggressive tumor, such as sinonasal undifferentiated carcinoma (SNUC) also occur and probably arise from the Schneiderian epithelium (mucoperiosteum) (Frierson et al 1986). The etiology of this type of tumor likely involves EBV infection (Gallo et al 1995).

Transitional cell carcinomas have the appearance of an irregular and excessively thick columnar epithelium with multiple mitotic figures in the closely packed nuclei. The base is irregular with invasion into surrounding stroma. The transitional cell papilloma is a benign form of tumor which may be locally recurrent and progress to carcinoma. Prediction of clinical behavior can be difficult and even the carcinoma has a somewhat better prognosis than that of other forms of PNC (Robin et al 1979). These tumors are relatively evenly distributed among the different sinuses and the nasal cavity.

Adenoid cystic carcinomas arise from the minor salivary glands in the mucosa and are most common in the maxillary antrum. They have the characteristic appearance of a mixture of microcystic pseudoluminal spaces and tubular epithelial lined structures but may include solid areas. Their biologic behavior is good in the short term, but in later years, the pattern is one of relentless progression, local recurrence and late metastasis, such that their long-term survival is similar to SCC (Hyams et al 1988; Waldron et al 2003).

Esthesioneuroblastoma, or olfactory neuroblastoma, is a variant of neuroblastoma arising from the olfactory apparatus, specifically the basal progenitor cells, tending to arise in the upper nasal cavity and ethmoid sinuses. Derivation from nerve cells in the olfactory mucosa (pattern I of Mendelhoff) or supporting epithelial cells (pattern II of Mendelhoff) has been described but does not appear to correlate with patient outcome (Mills & Freison 1985). Several patterns have been described, the most common being that of a cellular tumor comprising uniform small cells with round nuclei, scanty cytoplasm, and a prominent reticular or fibrillary background. Homer Wright rosettes may be present. Fibrovascular stroma may be abundant. The differential diagnosis includes lymphoma and embryonal rhabdomyosarcoma. Immunohistochemistry is positive for neuron-specific enolase and S-100 (O'Connor et al 1989) and negative for epithelial and lymphoid antigens. Electron microscopy demonstrates neurofilaments, neurotubules, and neurosecretory granules (Rosai 1981). RT-PCR for HASH-1 expression might be a specific marker (Dulguerov et al 2001). This tumor occurs throughout life with bimodal peaks in the 2nd and 6th decades. Grading and staging systems have been proposed and correlate with prognosis where grade I tumors have good prognosis and grade IV tumors are uniformly fatal (Hyams et al 1988).

Lymphomas in the paranasal sinuses tend to be high grade, both histologically and in their clinical behavior. They can be typed histochemically for B and T cell markers (Ratech et al 1989).

Staging

PNC are typically locally malignant on the basis of continuing destructive local invasion and involvement of vital local structures. Esthetic considerations weigh heavily in the consequences of untreated disease as well as in the planning of treatment options. Distal spread to regional lymph nodes or other organs is uncommon but may occur in the more malignant tumors. Patients with PNC often present to the neurosurgeon at an advanced stage when radical resection is difficult or impossible. Adverse outcome has been associated with extension of tumor into the orbit, infratemporal or pterygopalatine fossas and intracranially. It has been difficult to determine whether each of these sites represents an independent prognostic sign or whether extension of tumor is merely a surrogate marker for generally advanced bulky disease.

The results of treatment are highly dependent on the stage of the disease at presentation. In most series, the 5-year survival for T1 or T2 disease is 3–5 times better than that for T4 disease. Unfortunately, the vast majority of patients present with stage T3 or T4 disease. There are at least six classification systems currently in use to stage maxillary sinus tumors. The use of different systems in the various series obscures the interpretation of results and makes it difficult to compare different treatment strategies. All systems are based on the TNM system. The T stage is of paramount importance because nodal and distant spread are relatively uncommon and occur late in the disease. A review of 205 patients revealed Harrison's classification to be the most valid of the six classification systems (Willatt et al 1987). This system allowed a balanced distribution of cases with good correlation with treatment and survival in the different stages. Another, similar review (Har-El et al 1988) of 70 patients, found that Harrison's classification and

Table 39.3 Staging of carcinoma of the maxillary sinus

	American Joint Committee	Japanese Joint Committee	Harrison's
T1	Tumor confined to antral mucosa of infrastructure with no bony erosion or destruction	Tumor confined to the maxillary sinus with no evidence of bony involvement	Tumor confined to maxillary sinus with no evidence of bony involvement
T2	Tumor confined to suprastructure without bony destruction or to infrastructure with destruction of medial or inferior walls only	Tumor causing destruction of bony wall with external periosteum remaining intact as the capsule and surrounding tissue not invaded but only compressed. Minimal invasion into the ethmoid cells and the exophytic tumor in the middle nasal meatus included	Bony erosion without evidence of involvement of facial skin, orbit, pterygopalatine fossa, or ethmoid labyrinth
T3	More extensive tumor invading skin of cheek, orbit, anterior ethmoid sinuses, or pterygoid muscles	Tumor infiltrated deeply into the surrounding tissue by penetration of external periosteum	Involvement of orbit, ethmoid labyrinth, or facial skin
T4	Massive tumor with invasion of cribriform plate, posterior ethmoids, sphenoid, nasopharynx, pterygoid plates, or base of skull	Tumor extending to the base of skull, nasopharynx, maxilla of opposite side, and/or facial skin with ulceration. This includes deep infiltration into the orbit with limited eye movement or visual impairment or extension into the temporal fossa or invasion of the pterygoid muscles	Tumor extension to nasal pharynx, sphenoidal sinus, cribriform plate, or pterygopalatine fossa

also that of the Japanese Joint Committee were the most practical and appropriate for staging PNC. Harrison's classification and those of the American and Japanese Joint Committees are shown in Table 39.3. There are no widely accepted staging systems of ethmoid carcinoma, although a three-stage system has been proposed (Parsons et al 1988). Stage 1 tumor is limited to the sinus of origin. Stage 2 includes extension to adjacent areas such as the upper nasal cavity, the orbit, or the sphenoid sinus. Stage 3 includes destruction of the skull base, pterygoid plates, or intracranial extension. On the basis of our experience with patients treated by craniofacial resection and radiotherapy, we consider sphenoid sinus and orbital apex involvement to be the worst prognostic indicators, while dural involvement correlated less strongly with a poor outcome (Danks et al 1994). Thus, we do not entirely concur with Parsons et al's classification; however, others have found dural involvement to be a significant prognostic factor for survival (Bilsky et al 1997).

For esthesioneuroblastoma, the Kadish classification system has been quite widely used (Kadish et al 1976). Kadish stage A tumors are confined to the nasal cavity, stage B lesions involve the sinuses, and stage C masses involve the middle cranial fossa. Both the Kadish and the Hyams system of classification have been demonstrated to correlate with prognosis (Miyamoto et al 2000).

Management outline

The ideal management of PNC incorporates early diagnosis by vigorous investigation of presenting complaints. However, most cases of PNC are generally far advanced at the time of presentation. The emphasis in this chapter will be on the treatment of advanced PNC, as it is these tumors that usually involve the neurosurgeon.

The results of conventional local removal by transnasal or lateral rhinotomy have proven to be disappointing; conventional radiotherapy alone has also led to poor results. The 5-year survival rate with either modality alone did not exceed 25% and was often less (Terz et al 1980). Similar results have been reported for esthesioneuroblastoma (Gruber et al 2002). Subsequently, management has utilized

different combinations of radiotherapy and surgery, generally using radiotherapy doses above 50 Gy. Ten large mixed series from 1968 to 1983 were reviewed (Knegt et al 1985); the mean 5-year survival with these treatments was a disappointing 35%, only a modest improvement on either radiotherapy or surgery alone.

Other authors (Ketcham et al 1973; Millar et al 1973; Terz et al 1980) developed craniofacial resection for the adequate excision of tumors, with some apparent improvement in long-term results. Japanese groups developed different approaches using multimodal therapy; they combined chemotherapy and radiotherapy with surgery but the surgery was often less radical than in other series; chemotherapy was often intra-arterial and also applied topically inside the tumor cavity. More interesting advances include the concurrent use of intravenous infusions of *cis*-platinum and 5-fluorouracil (5FU) during radiotherapy and the use of three-dimensional computer planning and semi-stereotactic methods of delivering high-dose radiotherapy. These modalities will be discussed in detail later in this chapter.

Unfortunately, meaningful comparison between the different published series is extremely difficult for several reasons. Most series are small or extend over many years because PNC are uncommon. Several series span the period before and after the introduction of CT. Many series are retrospective and draw conclusions between treatment groups who were selected using various criteria and thus cannot be easily compared. The series all include different mixtures of tumors, histologies, site and stage, and also differ considerably in the ratio of recurrent to previously untreated cases. In many series, the follow-up period is quite short. Recurrences may occur after 5 years; of the patients in one large series who died, 8% did so >5 years after treatment (Lund 1983). This delayed recurrence is especially marked with adenoid cystic carcinoma where the 10-year cure rate may be as low as 7% (Hyams et al 1988); to a lesser degree this also applies to adenocarcinoma. A patient who survives 5 years cannot be regarded as cured. Finally, many series do not adequately discuss the treatment morbidity and mortality.

Despite a detailed and exhaustive review of the literature, conclusions as to the relative merits of different modalities of treatment can only be inferential. Many authors appropriately conclude their papers by recommending a properly constructed prospective multicenter trial of the different treatment modalities available but, unfortunately, no such studies have been performed to this time.

Surgical management

The goal of surgery is to achieve a radical tumor resection with a margin of normal tissue; this margin is necessarily limited by the close confines and important relationships of PNC. Orbital resection is required where tumor invasion has occurred, although this is controversial and will be discussed below. When a tumor involves the ethmoid sinuses, the resection will usually be inadequate unless craniofacial resection is employed to fully resect the roof of the ethmoid sinuses. Posterior extension into the pterygopalatine fossa or nasopharynx may make radical resection difficult or impossible. In our experience, extensive sphenoid or cavernous sinus involvement has precluded radical curative resection; this may often be suspected on preoperative imaging, but it is often only at surgery that direct inspection and frozen section biopsies can definitively establish resectability. Some authors report radical resection involving the cavernous sinus, but detailed results of this group have not been reported (Perry et al 1988). On the other hand, a large mass of intracranial tumor extending superiorly from the olfactory groove has not precluded successful radical resection; these tumors can be resected by conventional neurosurgical techniques, along with the cranial base which is then grafted (Sundaresan & Shah 1988; Danks et al 1994). However, in some cases, multiple intradural nodules of tumor spreading over the anterior cranial fossa floor may prevent curative resection. In the RMH series of 82 cases of PNC treated by craniofacial resection, sphenoid sinus involvement was the major predictor of later tumor recurrence. Dural or orbital involvement, however, correlated more weakly with the risk of later recurrence, indicating adequate treatment of these sites by this operative strategy (see also Danks et al 1994).

The decision to undertake orbital resection is controversial and certainly this should not be undertaken unless all other tumor can be adequately resected. The conventional wisdom is that orbital exenteration is required if there is invasion of the bony walls of the orbit. However, in a detailed retrospective analysis of a series of 41 patients where there was a strong commitment to preserving the eye (Perry et al 1988), local recurrence did not occur in the orbit; however, 10 of these 14 tumors were esthesioneuroblastomas, an otherwise uncommon tumor. Ketcham's experience in a series dominated by advanced SCC was that there was a 30% survival rate in those who had preservation of the orbit, compared with a 50% survival rate in those who had orbital resection (Ketcham & van Buren 1985). In a large series of 209 patients followed for over 10 years, Lund and co-workers (1998) adopted a policy of orbital sacrifice only if the periosteum was breached by tumor; their figures showed no survival difference for orbital involvement with or without periosteal invasion. Our policy is to preserve the orbit where there is extensive bilateral orbital invasion or other involvement that precludes radical resection. We prefer to exenterate the orbit if there is breach of the bony orbital walls by

tumor in cases where a radical and complete tumor clearance can be achieved. Perhaps the more conservative option would be appropriate in cases of esthesioneuroblastoma because of its known sensitivity to radiotherapy and chemotherapy.

Craniofacial resection incorporating the anterior cranial fossa floor has in the past been associated with significant morbidity and mortality due to cerebrospinal fluid (CSF) fistula and resultant intracranial infection. In our RMH series of 82 patients (see also Danks et al 1994), there have been no cases of CSF fistula requiring repair or mortality but we have had one case of infection (a superficial facial cellulitis). There has also been one case of postoperative tension pneumocephalus, requiring reoperation and temporary tracheostomy. We will emphasize certain technical points that have been crucial in achieving these results. The patient is under the care of the neurosurgical department. Preoperative nasal swabs are taken to guide perioperative antibiotics, which are vigorously employed, including 36 h of preoperative intranasal soframycin, intra- and postoperative intravenous prophylaxis with flucloxacillin, amoxicillin and metronidazole, and intraoperative topical antibiotic irrigation using flucloxacillin and amoxicillin; in the latter 3 years of the series, cephalothin has replaced the combination of flucloxacillin and amoxicillin. An intraoperative lumbar drain and neurosurgical anesthetic techniques are employed to ensure adequate brain relaxation. The head is positioned in moderate extension in a three-pin headrest to allow gravity to assist with brain retraction and exposure of the anterior cranial fossa floor. A bicoronal scalp flap is positioned well posteriorly to allow a large pericranial flap, based upon the supraorbital and supratrochlear vessels of both sides to be reflected inferiorly. A low free bifrontal bone flap is cut just above the supraorbital ridges. We do not employ the approach via a shell-shaped craniotomy through the frontal sinus (Cheesman et al 1986), nor do we incorporate the superior orbital margin in our craniotomies (Sekhar et al 1992) as we have not encountered complications from brain retraction, which only needs to be light due to the CSF drainage. The dura is dissected from the anterior cranial fossa floor using magnification and a head light for adequate visualization. Involved dura is resected and then grafted with temporalis fascia or fascia lata. All dural tears are meticulously closed with 5–0 polypropylene; the integrity of the dural closure is the key to preventing CSF leaks. *En bloc* tumor resection is then performed in conjunction with a lateral nasal approach performed by the ear, nose, and throat (ENT) surgeon and the tumor is passed out inferiorly via that incision. Frozen section examination of the surgical margins or any suspicious looking areas is very useful in guiding the resection and assessing resectability.

After the resection, liberal antibiotic irrigation is used before and after suturing the pericranial flap to the margin of the bony defect to hold it firmly to the skull base (Fig. 39.7). No graft is used on the nasal side of this vascularized pericranial flap as the nasal epithelium covers this gradually over a 3–4-week period. Lumbar CSF drainage is ceased when the pericranial flap is sutured in place. The pericranial flap technique (Johns et al 1981; Horowitz et al 1984; Danks et al 1994) is crucial in achieving satisfactory results with low morbidity; this is confirmed by an analysis

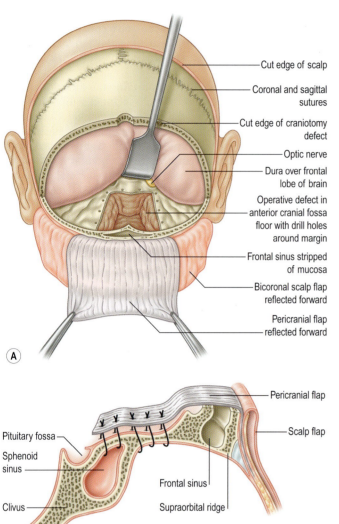

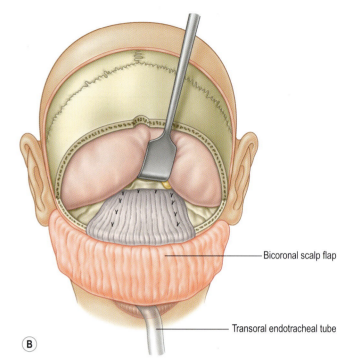

Figure 39.7 The pericranial flap is designed and positioned to close the defect in the anterior cranial fossa floor. (A) The defect in the anterior cranial fossa floor following the *en bloc* removal of the tumor. Fine holes are drilled around the margins of this defect for suturing down the pericranial flap. (B) Midsagittal section of the operative field showing the pericranial flap being sutured into position around the bony defect. (C) The pericranial flap in position sutured to the margins of the operative defect, and covering a wide area of the anterior cranial fossa floor beyond that. Fibrin glue is used to seal the edges of the flap.

of the published series of craniofacial resection with and without this technique. There was a 4–10-fold reduction in the rate of CSF fistula, intracranial infection, and operative mortality in those series employing this technique over those using other techniques for cranial base reconstruction (Table 39.4).

Craniotomy without a second stage resection from below has been reported by a group which also had performed craniofacial resection for PNC (McCutcheon et al 1996); the former group tended to have a greater number of local complications including frontal lobe retraction injuries and postoperative hematomas, thought to be due to the more limited exposure. This technique also had worse results in terms of survival, because of the lack of *en bloc* resection.

In cases where orbital exenteration is required, the dura of the optic nerve is closed to prevent CSF leak. The eyelids are sutured together and the orbital cavity is filled by transposition of the temporalis muscle; this local flap is more convenient than a microvascular free flap; however, a free

Table 39.4 Pericranial flaps in craniofacial resection

	Pericranial flap not used[a]	Pericranial flap used[b]	Current RMH series (82 patients)
No. in series (n)	3	5	1
CSF fistula (%)	16	2	0
Intracranial infection (%)	13	5	0
Mortality (%)	6	2	0

[a]Terz et al (1980); Ketcham & Van Buren (1985); Cheesman et al (1986).
[b]Sundaresan & Shah (1988); Blacklock et al (1989); Snyderman et al (1990); Danks et al (1994); Sekhar et al (1992).

flap is required if substantial facial skin needs to be sacrificed due to tumor involvement.

In our series of 82 patients, there have been no significant complications other than one case of tension pneumocephalus requiring re-exploration, five cases of non-fatal thromboembolism (three deep vein thromboses and two cases of pulmonary embolism), and one case of postoperative facial cellulitis. Reported complications of craniofacial resection include CSF fistula and infections such as meningitis, intracranial abscess, or bone flap infection (Bebear et al 1992; Catalano et al 1994; Kraus et al 1994; McCaffrey et al 1994; McCutcheon et al 1996). Other complications may occur due to brain retraction causing frontal lobe edema, hemorrhage, or epilepsy, but correct positioning of the head, minimization of brain retraction, and careful technique can eliminate these problems. Intracranial aerocele may occur due to excessive lumbar drainage late in the operation and postoperatively. The eye may be damaged due to exposure to the air or alcoholic skin preparation or by pressure; we use ointment and then suture the eyelids closed before skin preparation and are vigilant to prevent pressure on the orbital structures throughout the operation. Damage to the optic nerve may occur due to dissection at the orbital apex damaging that structure; this may lead to the dreaded complication of bilateral blindness if the other orbit is exenterated.

The benefit of craniofacial surgery over traditional approaches has been clearly established in the literature. There are five published series assessing the 5-year results of craniofacial resection and radiotherapy in advanced (T4) SCC (Terz et al 1980; Ketcham & van Buren 1985; Sundaresan & Shah 1988; Bridger et al 1991; Danks et al 1994). The 5-year survival was in the range of 50–70%. A similar number of series employing conventional non-craniofacial surgery and radiotherapy for such tumors gave a 5-year survival of 7–25% (Lavertu et al 1989; Sisson et al 1989; Tsujii et al 1989; Anniko et al 1990; Logue & Slevin 1991). For adenocarcinoma of the ethmoid sinus, two series employing craniofacial surgery and radiotherapy had 5-year survivals of 78% and 83%, respectively (Bridger et al 1991; Danks et al 1994), compared with 25–46% for transnasofacial surgery and radiotherapy (Ellingwood & Million 1979; Parsons et al 1988; Sisson et al 1989). In the above comparisons, there was a much higher ratio of recurrent to untreated tumors in the craniofacial series; thus the therapeutic advantage from a craniofacial approach is possibly even greater than these figures suggest. Our updated RMH series had a 63% incidence of recurrent PNC proceeding to craniofacial resection (52 recurrent cases in 82 patients). For esthesioneuroblastoma, good results are achievable by radical surgical resection and radiotherapy, with 77–100% 5-year control (O'Connor et al 1989; Beitler et al 1991; Lund 2003); this is clearly better than the results with single modality treatment (Fig. 39.8).

In recent years, the major addition to the surgical armamentarium has been the advent of endoscopic approaches. These approaches are now routinely used to resect sellar tumors, and even some tumors extending anteriorly into the skull base. Large paranasal sinus tumors with significant extension into the frontal sinuses or anterior skull base would not be appropriate for a purely endoscopic approach, requiring a craniotomy, however, a number of case reports describe endoscopic-assisted approaches (Tripathy et al 2009; Folbe et al 2009). Hatano et al (2009) described an endoscopic-assisted approach where a transnasal endoscope placement provided illumination from below, while the neurosurgeon resected tumor from the craniotomy (Hatano et al 2009). This is currently the most common technique we use

in our institution for those tumors based mainly in the ethmoid and frontal sinuses, without significant orbital or maxillary extension. The addition of a transfacial incision extends the more limited view available with a transnasal endoscopic approach if necessary. The largest series in the USA of endoscopic resection for PNC was recently reported by the group from the MD Anderson Cancer Center in Texas (Hanna et al 2009). A total of 120 patients underwent the procedure, 77.5% by a purely endoscopic and 22.5% by a combined cranio-endoscopic approach. The purely endoscopic group had less extensive disease. The overall complication rate was 11% with a CSF leak rate of 3%. The 5-year disease-specific survival was 87% and this did not differ between the two groups. This study demonstrated that for selected patients, in expert hands, the endoscopic approach can offer comparable surgical and oncologic outcomes to traditional craniofacial resection. A few small series have reported the use of this technique for esthesioneuroblastoma as well (Castelnuovo et al 2007; Yuen et al 2005; Unger et al 2005; Liu et al 2003).

Radiotherapy

Several studies have compared patient groups treated with surgery alone with similar groups given additional postoperative radiotherapy (Gabriele et al 1986; Kenady 1986; Wustrow et al 1989; Anniko et al 1990; Lund et al 1998). All but the series of Wustrow et al (1989) found that adjuvant radiotherapy gave significant improvement in outcome. A recent large series compared the effect on survival of administering radiotherapy before or after craniofacial resection and no statistically significant difference was found (Lund et al 1998). It appears widely accepted in the literature that postoperative radiotherapy offers additional benefit to the patient after radical tumor resection. Several series have suggested that many PNCs can be cured by radical high dose radiotherapy combined with sub-radical surgery or even surgical biopsy only (Ellingwood & Million 1979; Bush & Bagshaw 1982; Parsons et al 1988; Tsujii et al 1989; Karim et al 1990; Haylock et al 1991). There are no series that have compared different radiotherapy dosages in a controlled manner, but comparison between series suggests that doses to 60–80 Gy produce an improved outcome compared with lower doses. In the three series employing the higher dosage, there was a 5-year survival averaging 56%, compared with those series where 45–55 Gy was given, where the 5-year survival averaged 37%. One series employing high-dose radiotherapy used vigorous orbital shielding to try to limit ocular toxicity but this group suffered a high rate of orbital relapses leading to a 5-year survival of only 37% (Bush & Bagshaw 1982). The literature indicates that radical radiotherapy can give results similar to those achieved by simple transnasal surgery and radiotherapy combined, but the results are still marginally inferior to those series that have employed radical craniofacial surgery to achieve as complete a tumor resection as possible. Furthermore, comparison of two similar groups of patients treated in Toronto by either radiotherapy alone or radiotherapy and surgery revealed better results in the combined therapy group (51% vs 40% 5-year survival) (Beale & Garrett 1983). Unfortunately, many

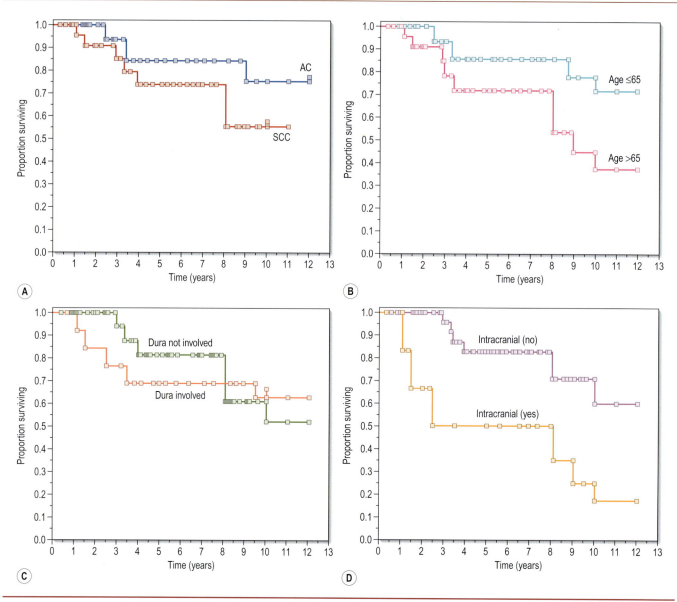

Figure 39.8 Actuarial survival curves from the RMH series of 82 patients showing the survival for patients with (A) adenocarcinoma (AC) and squamous cell carcinoma (SCC); (B) by age; (C) by dural involvement, and (D) by intracranial extension of tumor.

patients suffer significant morbidity following radical radiotherapy, particularly dry eyes, but the most serious morbidity is damage to the visual apparatus; optic nerve or retinal damage to the ipsilateral eye occurs in 25–100% of cases (Midena et al 1987), while frank blindness occurs in 7–22%. Several authors have claimed that blindness is inevitable if the orbit is radically treated, although this may be delayed for up to 5 years; such morbidity is defended by the argument that orbital exenteration would otherwise be necessary to control tumor spread; the dreaded complication of bilateral blindness occurred in 2–8% of cases (Bush & Bagshaw 1982; Parsons et al 1988; Logue & Slevin 1991). Osteoradionecrosis occurred in a similar number in these series but was up to 17% in one series (Bush & Bagshaw 1982). Transient central nervous system disturbances occurred in up to 10% of cases but no long-term sequelae were detected.

Sinonasal side-effects are common after RT radiotherapy for PNC (Kamel et al 2004).

Reduction in morbidity can be achieved by the use of immobilizing shells and three-dimensional CT-guided computerized treatment planning systems to deliver precise differential dosimetry to the tumor and surrounding important structures (Tsujii et al 1989; Karim et al 1990); both of these series also claimed a modest improvement in disease control attributable to this technique. Newer radiotherapy techniques may offer some advantages. Conformal RT and intensity-modulated RT (IMRT) have been shown to enable dose reduction to the local at-risk structures (pituitary gland, optic pathway, and brain, etc.) (Mock et al 2004; Huang et al 2003). The radiation dose is usually a minimum of 60 Gy. However, improvement in local control has not been clearly shown (Padovani et al 2003). Other radiotherapy techniques, such as intraoperative high-dose-rate brachytherapy has been reported as feasible (Nag et al 2004).

Proton beam therapy has been evaluated for the treatment of esthesioneuroblastoma in a few centers. In the Massachusetts Eye and Ear Infirmary series of 10 patients treated with craniofacial resection followed by proton beam irradiation ± chemotherapy, there was an excellent 90% 5-year disease-free survival (Nichols et al 2008). Similar results were obtained by another group in Japan (Nishimura et al 2007). The rate of serious adverse effects in these series was quite low. Obviously, the apparent benefits of this radiation modality are mitigated by its cost and availability.

A number of papers have favored preoperative radiotherapy as routine (Klintenberg et al 1984; Cheesman et al 1986) but the results did not offer clearly significant improvements. However, the authors felt that this technique did allow them to better preserve the orbital contents in some cases. The morbidity of craniofacial resection subsequent to radiotherapy did not appear worse than in other series using similar techniques (Cheesman et al 1986). Pre- and postoperative radiotherapy were compared at one center and no difference in outcome or morbidity was evident (Sisson et al 1989). Preoperative radiotherapy does allow observation of changes in tumor histology to document the effectiveness of the treatment, e.g., in 6 of 19 patients with adenocarcinoma treated with preoperative radiotherapy, no tumor could be found at operation 6 weeks later (Klintenberg et al 1984); none of these patients developed recurrence on prolonged follow-up. A substantial number of other tumors in this series exhibited large areas of tumor necrosis, emphasizing that adenocarcinoma is significantly radiosensitive.

Among cases of SCC, combined preoperative radio- and chemotherapy produced elimination of all viable tumor in 34 of 86 cases on the basis of histopathology (Konno et al 1980). Esthesioneuroblastoma appears to be more sensitive than other PNC to both radio- and chemotherapy (Morita et al 1993; Irish et al 1997). Preoperative combination therapy for this tumor has shown good response rates (see below).

In summary, it is certainly widely accepted that radiotherapy is of major benefit in the treatment of PNC. The most commonly held view is that radiotherapy should be given after radical surgical resection of the tumor. To achieve maximal effect, the radiotherapy needs to be given in high dosage, of the order of 60–80 Gy. CT-guided computer-assisted three-dimensional treatment planning appears to offer benefits in terms of reduced morbidity and possibly improved outcomes.

Chemotherapy

Chemotherapy has not been widely used in the primary treatment of PNC. However, regimens containing *cis*-platinum and 5FU have a beneficial effect; such treatments have been pioneered in Japan, where intra-arterial and topical routes have been combined with intravenous therapy. Treatment regimens have evolved over many years prompted by two factors: the relatively high incidence of PNC in Japan, and the realization that the mean 5-year survival treated by surgery and radiotherapy was only 35% (Knegt et al 1985). Maximal combination therapy using preoperative radiotherapy, intra-arterial 5FU, and intravenous bromodeoxyuridine combined with surgery, achieved results of 55–50% 5-year survival (Sato et al 1970; Konno et al 1980). Subsequently, the intra-arterial 5FU therapy was replaced by repeated applications of topical 5FU with maintenance of these good results (Sakai et al 1983; Knegt et al 1985; Inuyama et al 1989). In another Japanese series, the use of preoperative intra-arterial *cis*-platinum and peplomycin was felt to be the major factor in improving the 5-year survival rate from 22% to 55%, despite a reduction in the rate of radical maxillectomy from 50% to 18% (Inuyama et al 1989). Another series found no improvement in patients treated with intra-arterial 5FU, although the patients who received 5FU received lower doses of radiotherapy than the control group, severely confounding the results of this study (Tsujii et al 1989). A very careful prospective study was performed in Rotterdam based on this Japanese work (Knegt et al 1985); a vigorous surgical internal decompression of the PNC was performed via an anterior maxillectomy but without removing orbital periosteum or dura, even if involved. The cavity was then packed, internally débrided thrice weekly, and topical 5FU applied to the walls of the cavity before re-packing; this was continued over several weeks depending on the progress and appearance of the cavity. Radiotherapy of 4 Gy was administered preoperatively followed by 10 Gy over 1 week postoperatively. The 5-year survival in cases of SCC and undifferentiated maxillary sinus carcinoma was 52%. In 20 cases of ethmoid adenocarcinoma, a 100% 5-year disease-free survival was achieved even though dura and/or periorbita were involved, although not penetrated, in many cases. The treatment mortality was 1% due to one case of postoperative pulmonary embolism but there were no cases of major morbidity. The treatments were well tolerated, although the tumor debridement was painful during the 1st week but not subsequently. Knegt and co-workers' (1985) conclusions were appropriately cautious but they suggested that their less aggressive treatment, which did not disturb the patient's appearance, could achieve results equal to or better than conventional combined radical surgery and high dose radiotherapy. Three American series studying the use of chemotherapy have concentrated on salvage treatment of massive recurrent SCCs (Rooney et al 1985; LoRusso et al 1988; Lee et al 1989); 90% of the cases demonstrated significant response to treatment and 45% of tumors resolved completely on radiologic criteria, producing a mean survival of over 21 months. These authors all employed several courses of chemotherapy, based on cisplatin and 5FU, and all patients had radiotherapy but did not have additional surgery. One study tested different protocols and found that a 5-day infusion of cisplatin and 5FU gave significantly better results than other regimens tested (Rooney et al 1985). A dramatic response to chemotherapy was reported in one case of transitional cell carcinoma treated with cisplatin, methotrexate, and bleomycin (Sooriyachi et al 1984).

The use of superselective intra-arterial injections of high dose cisplatin with concomitant radiotherapy has been reported in 47 patients with advanced paranasal sinus cancer with a 5-year OS of 69% (Homma et al 2009).

Esthesioneuroblastoma appears to be relatively chemo-sensitive (O'Connor et al 1989). A review of 12 patients with high-grade, Kadish Stage C tumors treated at the Mayo Clinic between 1976 and 2003 showed a significant improvement in overall survival for those that received adjuvant chemo-therapy post-surgery (35 months), compared with those that did not (10.5 months) (Porter et al 2008).

The role of neo-adjuvant therapy has received some enthusiasm based on the experience at the University of Virginia and of others (Kim et al 2004; Turano et al 2010; Resto et al 2000). Patients with tumors stage Kadish C were treated with preoperative chemotherapy and radiotherapy, followed by craniofacial resection (Loy et al 2006). In the University of Virginia series of 34 patients, two-thirds showed a reduction in tumor burden and in the responder group there was a lower disease-related mortality with on overall 5-year survival of 81% (Polin et al 1998). Another series reported an 89% response rate to two courses of cis-platin and etoposide (VP-16) (Bhattacharyya et al 1997). In one further study, a regimen of induction chemotherapy consisting of cisplatin and 5FU resulted in an 87% clinical response and 30% complete response, as assessed at the time of surgery (Lee et al 1999). A non-platinum based com-bination of irinotecan plus docetaxel has also been reported (Kiyota et al 2008). These various treatment regimens, although promising, have not been standardized and await validation in large multicenter trials.

In conclusion, there is evidence to suggest that chemo-therapy based on *cis*-platinum and 5FU improve results in the treatment of PNC. However, the exact timing and selec-tion of appropriate patients is not clear at the current time and deserves closer examination.

Other adjuvant therapies

Molecular targeted therapies have transformed the thera-peutic landscape for many cancers in the modern era. An exponential growth in knowledge regarding the molecular pathways that drive the cancer cell has led to an explosion of novel drugs at every level of the pipeline from 'bench to bedside'. These drugs are generally either monoclonal antibody-based agents or small-molecule kinase inhibitors, but their ultimate effect is to switch off key oncogenic pro-teins within the cell. Squamous cell carcinomas are well recognized to over-express large amounts of epidermal growth factor receptor (EGFR), a membrane protein that drives cell proliferation, invasion and inhibits apoptosis, therefore treatments for this type of cancer are often focused on this protein. For instance, cetuximab is a monoclonal antibody against EGFR that is FDA approved for use in colorectal cancer and has been shown to improve survival together with radiotherapy in advanced head and neck SCC (Bonner et al 2010; Mehra et al 2008). Although no specific studies have focused on the use of these agents in the rare paranasal sinus cancers, these tumors could benefit in the future from the advent of targeted drugs toward tumors of this histological type in other anatomical locations.

There is a paucity of knowledge, to date, about molecu-lar pathways in the rarer PNCs. Esthesioneuroblastoma commonly expresses the apoptotic pathway molecule Bcl-2

and this may predict response to neoadjuvant chemother-apy, as well as worse survival (Kim et al 2008). In addition, this tumor, similarly to pediatric neuroblastomas, expresses Trk-A, Trk-B, GRP78 and p75NRT neurotropin receptors, however they have not been shown to have a clear prognos-tic correlation (Weinreb et al 2009). Bortezomib, a protea-some inhibitor, sensitized esthesioneuroblastoma cells to TRAIL-induced apoptosis *in vitro* (Koschny et al 2009). In clinical studies, sunitinib, a PDGFR inhibitor has been used as palliative therapy in late stage esthesioneuroblastoma (Preusser et al 2010). The next few years will hopefully provide further insights into the potential for these agents as adjuvant therapies for paranasal sinus cancers.

There is one case report of adoptive immunotherapy in combination with radiotherapy causing cellular differentia-tion of an adenoid cystic carcinoma into normal appearing bone (Sato et al 1990). The immunotherapy involved intra-arterial injection of lymphokine-activated killer cells and intravenous recombinant interleukin-2. Gene therapy using many different strategies has also been trialled in diverse tumor types (Culver et al 1992). It is hoped that practical applications will result from this work to allow better treat-ment of PNC.

Patterns of failure

Prevention of local recurrence is the major challenge facing those who treat patients with PNC. Traditional limits to resection have been the common sites of recurrence in earlier series; these sites include the floor of the anterior cranial fossa, particularly the olfactory groove, the orbit, and the pterygopalatine fossa. More distant recurrence may occur due to extension of tumor along nerves such as the trigeminal or vidian nerves, particularly well documented with adenoid cystic carcinoma (Pandolfo et al 1989). Spread to local lymph nodes is uncommon at presentation (8%) and occurs in a further 5–10% of cases in long-term follow-up. Generally, this form of recurrence is adequately treated by radical neck dissection and radiotherapy (Konno et al 1980). Distant metastases to bone, lung, and liver occur in a similar proportion of patients (5–10%); however, in the sub-group with anaplastic carcinoma, distal metastases occur in up 50% of cases within 1 year (Konno et al 1980; Lund 1983). Cervical nodal metastasis and distant metastasis is a strong negative prognostic factor in recurrent esthesioneuroblast-oma (Dias et al 2003). Local radiotherapy to symptomatic metastases and systemic chemotherapy have a role in the management of these problems. Intracranial metastases are rare, although we noted two cases of cerebellar metastasis in our initial experience of 45 cases (Murphy et al 1991); these were treated by local excision and neuraxis radiotherapy.

Treatment of recurrent disease

Recurrent disease can be effectively treated in many cases. Many of the series discussing advanced disease include a high proportion of recurrent cancers. The patient should be assessed fully by clinical examination, CT and MRI, chest

X-ray and other tests as appropriate. Interpretation of postoperative scans can be difficult as the healing tissues used in reconstruction may exhibit contrast enhancement that may simulate tumor recurrence (Som et al 1986). Radical or palliative surgical resection may be appropriate; craniofacial resection has a major role in cases where there is involvement of the anterior cranial fossa floor. In the large craniofacial series, including our own, over half of the patients treated with a craniofacial resection had recurrent disease. Despite that, a high proportion (50–70%) have enjoyed long-term disease control and probable cure. If previous craniofacial resection has been performed the pericranium may not be available for reconstruction. Frontal galeal flaps (Snyderman et al 1990) or a microvascularized free flap of omentum (Yamaki et al 1991) or other donor material (Sekhar et al 1992) can be used for reconstruction. Many patients will already have received radiotherapy and may only be able to receive limited further therapy. Chemotherapy with cis-platinum and 5FU-based regimens has a demonstrable effect on these tumors, as already discussed. Palliative sub-total surgical resections can be of value in the slower growing tumor types such as adenocarcinoma, adenoid cystic carcinoma, and transitional cell carcinoma, and may provide surprisingly long periods of tumor control.

Management outcome

The management outcomes differ widely between series but, as discussed above, it is often difficult to compare series due to the many differences in the groups of patients. Nonetheless, on review of many series, several broad patterns emerge, as discussed in the preceding section.

Treatment by conventional non-craniofacial surgery and radiotherapy gives a 5-year survival of approximately 35% in series including all grades of tumor (Knegt et al 1985); such treatment yields only a 7–25% 5-year survival in patients with T4 disease (Lavertu et al 1989; Sisson et al 1989; Tsujii et al 1989; Anniko et al 1990; Logue & Slevin 1991). In series employing craniofacial resection, about 50–70% of patients with T4 SCC were alive and free of disease at 5 years (Terz et al 1980; Ketcham & van Buren 1985; Sundaresan & Shah 1988; Bridger et al 1991; Danks et al 1994). In a recent international collaborative study of outcomes following craniofacial surgery, there was a surgical postoperative mortality of 4.5% and complication rate of 33% (Ganly et al 2005).

Of 38 patients with SCC in the current RMH series, there was a 75% 5-year survival; the figures are somewhat better for adenocarcinoma, with 30 patients enjoying an 85% 5-year survival. In earlier series, there has been a 25–46% 5-year survival for conventional therapy and 78–83% 5-year survival for craniofacial series (Bridger et al 1991; Danks et al 1994); there is a greater tendency for delayed recurrence in this tumor type, resulting in more late recurrences after the 5-year period.

The Peter MacCallum Cancer Institute in Melbourne, Australia, reported its experience with PNC in 60 patients (32, SCC; 25, adenocarcinoma) between 1991 and 2000 (Porceddu et al 2004). Local recurrence was the commonest cause of failure. The 5-year local control rate was 49% and

overall survival was 40%. The authors noted that the proximity to neural and orbital structures was often a limiting factor in the extent of resection possible.

Multimodality therapy employing chemotherapy by various routes, preoperative radiotherapy, and non-craniofacial surgery has produced approximately 70% 5-year survival for the overall group (Sato et al 1970; Konno et al 1980), a treatment which also enjoys the advantage of a lower rate of disfiguring surgery. One group achieved the spectacular result of 100% 5-year disease-free survival employing multimodality therapy based on topical 5FU in adenocarcinoma.

With respect to esthesioneuroblastoma, Dulguerov performed a meta-analysis of studies between 1990 and 2000 (Dulguerov et al 2001). Hyams grade III–IV and cervical lymphadenopathy were associated with poorer survival. Five-year survival rates were 65% for surgery plus radiotherapy and 51% for radiotherapy and chemotherapy. Rates for surgery or radiotherapy alone were worse, emphasizing the benefit of multi-modality treatment in this tumor. However, the exact role of chemotherapy is still unclear.

Despite the serious nature of PNC and the restrictions placed on treatment by the important surrounding structures, at least temporary disease control can be achieved in the majority of patients and many patients have a long period of relief from the tumor. There remain many challenges in developing more effective therapies and refining their application to improve the results of present therapies.

Key points

- Almost all PNC adenocarcinoma, and approximately one-half of SCC, relate to prolonged exposure to hardwood.
- Late presentation of PNC can be diminished by vigorous examination of all adult patients with sinonasal complaints of >6 weeks, including biopsy of suspicious areas.
- CT and MRI are essential and complementary investigations in the assessment of PNC.
- Involvement of the upper nasal cavity by PNC and, particularly, the cribriform plate and fovea ethmoidalis (i.e., floor of anterior cranial fossa) mandates craniofacial resection rather than a purely endonasal/endosinus approach.
- Involvement of sphenoid sinus or anterior cranial fossa floor by PNC are adverse predictors for survival.
- We reserve orbital exenteration for when a bony orbital wall is breached by PNC and when complete tumor resection is felt to be achievable.
- The key to avoidance of postoperative CSF leak after craniofacial resection is obvious but cannot be understated – the dura must be fastidiously repaired and closed watertight; the pericranial flap over the anterior cranial fossa floor is a physical, not watertight, support.
- Radiotherapy is recognized as a valuable adjuvant to craniofacial resection, probably in higher dosages (e.g., 60–80 Gy) but the optimal timing (pre- or postoperative) and dosage are yet to be adequately determined.
- Other adjunctive therapies need to be studied and considered as there have been many reports of the benefits of chemotherapy, particularly based on cis-platinum and 5FU.
- Better treatment of PNC will come with improved understanding of its molecular biology.

REFERENCES

Acheson, E.D., Cowdell, R.H., Hadfield, E., et al., 1968. Nasal cancer in woodworkers in the furniture industry. BMJ 2, 587–596.

Acheson, E.D., Winter, P.D., Hadfield, E., et al., 1982. Is nasal adenocarcinoma in the Buckinghamshire furniture industry declining? Nature 299, 263–265.

Acheson, E.D., Cowdell, R.H., Jolles, B., 1970. Nasal cancer in the Northamptonshire boot and shoe industry. BMJ 1, 385–393.

Anniko, M., Franzen, L., Lofroth P.O., 1990. Long-term survival of patients with paranasal sinus carcinoma. Otorhinolaryngology 52, 187–193.

Beale, F.A., Garrett P.G., 1983. Cancer of the paranasal sinuses with particular reference to maxillary sinus cancer. J. Otolaryngol. 12, 377–382.

Bebear, J.P., Darrouzet, V., Stoll, D., 1992. Surgery of the anterior skull base: total ethmoidectomy for malignant ethmoidal tumors. Isr. J. Med. Sci. 28, 169–172.

Beitler, J.J., Fass, D.E., Brenner, H.A., et al., 1991. Esthesioneuroblastoma: is there a role for elective neck treatment? Head Neck 13, 321–326.

Bhattacharyya, N., Thornton, A.F., Joseph, M.P., et al., 1997. Successful treatment of esthesioneuroblastoma and neuroendocrine carcinoma with combined chemotherapy and proton radiation. Results of 9 cases. Arch. Otolaryngol. Head Neck Surg. 123, 34–40.

Bilsky, M.H., Kraus, D.H., Strong, E.W., et al., 1997. Extended anterior craniofacial resection for intracranial extension of malignant tumors. Am. J. Surg. 174, 565–568.

Blacklock, J.B., Weber, R.S., Lee, Y.Y., et al., 1989. Transcranial resection of tumors of the paranasal sinuses and nasal cavity. J. Neurosurg. 71, 10–15.

Bonner, J.A., Harari, P.M., Giralt, J., et al., 2010. Radiotherapy plus cetuximab for locoregionally advanced head and neck cancer: 5-year survival data from a phase 3 randomised trial, and relation between cetuximab-induced rash and survival. Lancet Oncol. 11, 21–28.

Bridger, G.P., Mendelsohn, M.S., Baldwin, M., et al., 1991. Paranasal sinus cancer. Aust. N. Z. J. Surg. 61, 290–294.

Bush, S.E., Bagshaw M.A., 1982. Carcinoma of the paranasal sinuses. Cancer 50, 154–158.

Castelnuovo, P., Bignami, M., Delu, G., et al., 2007. Endonasal endoscopic resection and radiotherapy in olfactory neuroblastoma: our experience. Head Neck 29, 845–850.

Catalano, P.J., Hecht, C.S., Biller, J.F., et al., 1994. Craniofacial resection: an analysis of 73 cases. Arch. Otolaryngol. Head Neck Surg. 120, 1203–1208.

Cheesman, A.D., Lund, V.J., Howard D.J., 1986. Craniofacial resection for tumors of the nasal cavity and paranasal sinuses. Head Neck Surg. 8, 429–435.

Culver, K.W., Ram, Z., Wallbridge, S., et al., 1992. In vivo gene transfer with retroviral vector-producer cells for treatment of experimental brain tumors. Science 256, 1550–1552.

Danks, R.A., Kaye, A.H., Millar, H., et al., 1994. Cranio-facial resection in the management of cancer of the paranasal sinuses. J. Clin. Neurosci. 1 (2), 111–117.

Derdeyn, C.P., Moran, C.J., Wippold, F.J. 2nd, et al., 1994. MRI of esthesioneuroblastoma. J. Comput. Assist. Tomogr. 18, 16–21.

Dias, F.L., Sa, G.M., Lima, R.A., et al., 2003. Patterns of failure and outcome in esthesioneuroblastoma. Arch. Otolaryngol. Head Neck Surg. 129, 1186–1192.

Doll, R., Morgan, L.G., Speizer F.E., 1970. Cancer of the lung and nasal sinuses in nickel workers. Br. J. Cancer 24, 623–632.

Dulguerov, P., Jacobsen, M.S., Allal, A.S., et al., 2001. Nasal and paranasal sinus carcinoma: are we making progress? A series of 220 patients and a systematic review. Cancer 92, 3012–3029.

Egedahl, R.D., Coppock, E., Homik, R., 1991. Mortality experience at a hydrometallurgical nickel refinery in Fort Saskatchewan, Alberta between 1954 and 1984. J. Soc. Occup. Med. 41, 29–33.

Ellingwood, K.E., Million R.R., 1979. Cancer of the nasal cavity and ethmoid/sphenoid sinuses. Cancer 43, 1517–1526.

Franklin C.I.V., 1982. Adenocarcinoma of the paranasal sinuses in Tasmania. Australas. Radiol. 26, 49–52.

Fatterpekar, G.M., Delman B.N., Som, P.M., 2008. Imaging the paranasal sinuses: where we are and where we are going. Anat. Rec. (Hoboken) 291, 1564–1572.

Folbe, A., Herzallah, I., Duvvuri, U., et al., 2009. Endoscopic endonasal resection of esthesioneuroblastoma: a multicenter study. Am. J. Rhinol. Allergy. 23, 91–94.

Frierson, H.F. Jr., Mills, S.E., Fechner, R.E., et al., 1986. Sinonasal undifferentiated carcinoma. An aggressive neoplasm derived from schneiderian epithelium and distinct from olfactory neuroblastoma. Am. J. Surg. Pathol. 10, 771–779.

Fukuda, K., Shibata, A., 1985. Demographic correlation between occupation and maxillary sinus cancer mortality in Japan. Kurume Med. J. 32, 151–155.

Fukuda, K., Shibata, A., Harada, K., 1987. Squamous cell cancer of the maxillary sinus in Hokkaido, Japan: a case-control study. Br. J. Ind. Med. 44, 263–266.

Gabriele, P., Besozzi, M.C., Pisani, P., et al., 1986. Carcinoma of the paranasal sinuses. Results with radiotherapy alone or with a radiosurgical combination. Radiol. Med. (Torino) 72, 210–214.

Gallo, O., Di Lollo, S., Graziani, P., et al., 1995. Detection of Epstein-Barr virus genome in sinonasal undifferentiated carcinoma by use of in situ hybridization. Otolaryngol. Head Neck Surg. 112, 659–664.

Ganly, I., Patel, S.G., Singh, B., et al., 2005. Craniofacial resection for malignant paranasal sinus tumors: Report of an International Collaborative Study. Head Neck 27, 575–584.

Gruber, G., Laedrach, K., Baumert, B., et al., 2002. Esthesioneuroblastoma: irradiation alone and surgery alone are not enough. Int. J. Radiat. Oncol. Biol. Phys. 54, 486–491.

Hadfield, E.H., MacBeth R.G., 1971. Adenocarcinoma of ethmoids in furniture workers. Ann. Otol. Rhinol. Laryngol. 80, 699–703.

Hanna, E., Demonte, F., Ibrahim, S., et al., 2009. Endoscopic resection of sinonasal cancers with and without craniotomy: oncologic results. Arch. Otolaryngol. Head Neck Surg. 135, 1219–1224.

Har-El, G., Hadar, T., Krespi, Y.P., et al., 1988. An analysis of staging systems for carcinoma of the maxillary sinus. Ear Nose Throat J. 67, 511–520.

Hatano, A., Nakajima, M., Kato, T., et al., 2009. Craniofacial resection for malignant nasal and paranasal sinus tumors assisted with the endoscope. Auris. Nasus. Larynx. 36, 42–45.

Hayes, R.B., Gerin, M., Raatgever, J.W., et al., 1986. Woodrelated occupations, wood dust exposure, and sinonasal cancer. Am. J. Epidemiol. 124, 569–577.

Hayes, R.B., Kardaun, J.W., de Bruyn, A., 1987. Tobacco use and sinonasal cancer: a case-control study. Br. J. Cancer 56, 843–846.

Haylock, B.J., John, D.G., Paterson I.C., 1991. The treatment of squamous cell carcinoma of the paranasal sinuses. Clin. Oncol. (R. Coll. Radiol.) 3, 17–21.

Homma, A., Oridate, N., Suzuki, F., et al., 2009. Superselective high-dose cisplatin infusion with concomitant radiotherapy in patients with advanced cancer of the nasal cavity and paranasal sinuses: a single institution experience. Cancer 115, 4705–4714.

Horowitz, J.D., Persing, J.A., Nichter, L.S., et al., 1984. Galealpericranial flaps in head and neck reconstruction. Am. J. Surg. 148, 489–497.

Huang, D., Xia, P., Akazawa, P., et al., 2003. Comparison of treatment plans using intensity-modulated radiotherapy and three-dimensional conformal radiotherapy for paranasal sinus carcinoma. Int. J. Radiat. Oncol. Biol. Phys. 56, 158–168.

Hyams, V.J., Batsakis, J.G., Micheals, L., 1988. Tumors of the upper respiratory tract and ear, second ed. Armed Forces Institute of Pathology, Washington, DC.

Inuyama, Y., Kawaurs, M., Toji, M., et al., 1989. Intra-arterial chemotherapy of maxillary sinus carcinoma. Gan. To. Kagaku. Ryoho. 16, 2688–2691.

Irish, J., Dasgupta, R., Freeman, J., et al., 1997. Outcome and analysis of the surgical management of esthesioneuroblastoma. J. Otolaryngol. 26, 1–7.

Ironside, P., Matthews, J., 1975. Adenocarcinoma of the nose and paranasal sinuses in woodworkers in the State of Victoria, Australia. Cancer 36, 1115–1124.

Giles, G., Farrugia, H., Silver, B., et al., 1992. Cancer in Victoria, 1982–1987. Anti-Cancer Council of Victoria, Melbourne.

Johns, M.E., Winn, H.R., McLean, W.C., et al., 1981. Pericranial flap for the closure of defects of craniofacial resections. Laryngoscope 91, 952–959.

Kadish, S., Goodman, M., Wang, C.C., 1976. Olfactory neuroblastoma. A clinical analysis of 17 cases. Cancer 37, 1571–1576.

Kairemo, K.J., Jekunen, A.P., Kestila, M.S., et al., 1998. Imaging of olfactory neuroblastoma – an analysis of 17 cases. Auris. Nasus. Larynx. 25, 173–179.

Kamel, R., Al-Badawy, S., Khairy, A., et al., 2004. Nasal and paranasal sinus changes after radiotherapy for nasopharyngeal carcinoma. Acta Otolaryngol. 124, 532–535.

Kanno, K., Morokuma, Y., Tateno, T., et al., 2005. Olfactory neuroblastoma causing ectopic ACTH syndrome. Endocr. J. 52, 675–681.

Karim, A.B.M.F., Kralendonk, J.H., Njo, K.H., et al., 1990. Ethmoid and upper nasal cavity carcinoma: treatment, results and complications. Radiother. Oncol. 19, 109–120.

Kenady, D.E., 1986. Cancer of the paranasal sinuses. Surg. Clin. N. Am. 66, 119–131.

Ketcham, A.S., Van Buren, J., 1985. Tumors of the paranasal sinuses: a therapeutic challenge. Am. J. Surg. 150, 406–413.

Ketcham, A.S., Chretien, P.B., Van Buren, J.M., et al., 1973. The ethmoid sinuses: a reevaluation of surgical resection. Am. J. Surg. 126, 469–476.

Kim, D.W., Jo, Y.H., Kim, J.H., et al., 2004. Neoadjuvant etoposide, ifosfamide, and cisplatin for the treatment of olfactory neuroblastoma. Cancer 101, 2257–2260.

Kim, H., Kong, I.G., Lee, C.H., et al., 2008. Expression of Bcl-2 in olfactory neuroblastoma and its association with chemotherapy and survival. Otolaryngol. Head Neck Surg. 139, 708–712.

Kiyota, N., Tahara, M., Fujii, S., et al., 2008. Nonplatinum-based chemotherapy with irinotecan plus docetaxel for advanced or metastatic olfactory neuroblastoma: a retrospective analysis of 12 cases. Cancer 112, 885–891.

Klintenberg, C., Olofsson, J., Hellquist, H., et al., 1984. Adenocarcinoma of the ethmoid sinuses. A review of 28 cases with special reference to wood dust exposure. Cancer 54, 482–488.

Knegt, P.P., de Jong, P., van Anfrl, J.G., et al., 1985. Carcinoma of the paranasal sinuses. Results of a prospective pilot study. Cancer 56, 57–62.

Konno, A., Togawa, K., Inoue, S., 1980. Analysis of the results of our combined therapy for maxillary cancer. Acta Otolaryngol. Suppl. 372, 1–16.

Koschny, R., Holland, H., Sykora, J., et al., 2009. Bortezomib sensitizes primary human esthesioneuroblastoma cells to TRAIL-induced apoptosis. J. Neurooncol. 97 (2), 171–185.

Kraus, D.H., Shah, J.P., Arbit, E., 1994. Complications of craniofacial resection for tumors involving the anterior skull base. Head Neck 16, 307–312.

Lavertu, P., Roberts, J.K., Kraus, D.H., et al., 1989. Squamous cell carcinoma of the paranasal sinuses: The Cleveland Clinic Experience 1977–1986. Laryngoscope 99, 1130–1136.

Lee, M.M., Vokes, E.E., Rosen, A., et al., 1999. Multimodality therapy in advanced paranasal sinus carcinoma: superior long-term results. Cancer J. Sci. Am. 5, 219–223.

Lee, Y.Y., Dimery, I.W., Van Tassell, P., et al., 1989. Superselective intra-arterial chemotherapy of advanced paranasal sinus tumors. Arch. Otolaryngol. Head Neck Surg. 115, 503–511.

Liu, J.K., O'Neill, B., Orlandi, R.R., et al., 2003. Endoscopic-assisted craniofacial resection of esthesioneuroblastoma: minimizing facial incisions – technical note and report of 3 cases. Min. Invasive Neurosurg. 46, 310–315.

Logue, J.P., Slevin N.J., 1991. Carcinoma of the nasal cavity and paranasal sinuses: an analysis of radical radiotherapy. Clin. Oncol. (R. Coll. Radiol.) 3, 84–89.

LoRusso, P., Tapazoglou, E., Kish, J.A., et al., 1988. Chemotherapy for paranasal sinus carcinoma. A 10-year experience at Wayne State University. Cancer 62 (1), 1–5.

Loy, A.H., Reibel, J.F., Read, P.W., et al., 2006. Esthesioneuroblastoma: continued follow-up of a single institution's experience. Arch. Otolaryngol. Head Neck Surg. 132, 134–138.

Luce, D., Leclerc, A., Mame, M.J., et al., 1991. Sinonasal cancer and occupation: a multicenter case-control study. Rev. Epidemiol. Sante Publique 39, 7.

Lund, V.J., 2003. Olfactory neuroblastoma: past, present, and future? Laryngoscope 113 (3), 502–507.

Lund, V.J., 1983. Malignant tumors of the nasal cavity and paranasal sinuses. Otolaryngology 45, 1.

Lund, V.J., Howard, D.J., Wei, W.I., et al., 1998. Craniofacial resection of tumors of the nasal cavity and paranasal sinuses – a 17-year experience. Head Neck 20, 97–105.

Lund, V.J., Lloyd G.A.S., Howard, D.J., et al., 1996. Enhanced magnetic resonance imaging and subtraction techniques in the postoperative evaluation of craniofacial resection for sinonasal malignancy. Laryngoscope 106, 553–558.

Maroldi, R., Farina, D., Battaglia, G., et al., 1997. MR of malignant nasosinusal neoplasms: frequently asked questions. Eur. J. Radiol. 24, 181–190.

McCaffrey, T.V., Olsen, K.D., Yohanan, J.M., et al., 1994. Factors affecting survival of patients with tumors of the anterior skull base. Laryngoscope 104, 940–945.

McCutcheon, I.E., Blacklock, J.B., Weber, R.S., et al., 1996. Anterior transcranial (craniofacial) resection of tumors of the paranasal sinuses: 1997 surgical technique and results. Neurosurgery 38, 471–480.

Mehra, R., Cohen, R.B., Burtness, B.A., 2008. The role of cetuximab for the treatment of squamous cell carcinoma of the head and neck. Clin. Adv. Hematol. Oncol. 6, 742–750.

Midena, E., Segato, T., Piermarocchi, S., et al., 1987. Retinopathy following radiation therapy of paranasal sinus and nasopharyngeal carcinoma. Retina 7, 142.

Millar, H.S., Petty, P.G., Hueston J.T., 1973. A combined intracranial and facial approach for excision and repair of cancer of the ethmoid sinuses. Aust. N. Z. J. Surg. 43, 179.

Mills, S., Freison, H., 1985. Olfactory neuroblastoma: a clinicopathologic study of 21 cases. Am. J. Surg. Pathol. 9, 317–327.

Miyamoto, R.C., Gleich, L.L., Biddinger, P.W., et al., 2000. Esthesioneuroblastoma and sinonasal undifferentiated carcinoma: impact of histological grading and clinical staging on survival and prognosis. Laryngoscope 110, 1262–1265.

Mock, U., Georg, D., Bogner, J., et al., 2004. Treatment planning comparison of conventional, 3D conformal, and intensity-modulated photon (IMRT) and proton therapy for paranasal sinus carcinoma. Int. J. Radiat. Oncol. Biol. Phys. 58, 147–154.

Mohtashamipur, E., Norpoth, K., Luhmann, F., 1989. Cancer epidemiology of woodworking. J. Cancer Res. Clin. Oncol. 115, 503.

Morita, A., Ebersold, M.J., Olsen, K.D., et al., 1993. Esthesioneuroblastoma: prognosis and management. Neurosurgery 32, 706–715.

Muir, C.S., Nectoux, J., 1980. Descriptive epidemiology of malignant neoplasms of nose, nasal cavities, middle ear and accessory sinuses. Clin. Otolaryngol. 5, 195.

Muir, C., Waterhouse, J., Mack, T., et al., 1987. Cancer incidence in five continents, fifth ed. IARC, Lyon.

Murphy, M.A., Kaye, A.H., Hayes I.P., 1991. Intracranial metastasis from carcinoma of the paranasal sinus. Neurosurgery 28, 890.

Nag, S., Tippin, D., Grecula, J., et al., 2004. Intraoperative high-dose-rate brachytherapy for paranasal sinus tumors. Int. J. Radiat. Oncol. Biol. Phys. 58, 155–160.

Nichols, A.C., Chan, A.W., Curry, W.T., et al., 2008. Esthesioneuroblastoma: the Massachusetts eye and ear infirmary and Massachusetts general hospital experience with craniofacial resection, proton beam radiation, and chemotherapy. Skull Base 18, 327–337.

Nishimura, H., Ogino, T., Kawashima, M., et al., 2007. Proton-beam therapy for olfactory neuroblastoma. Int. J. Radiat. Oncol. Biol. Phys. 68, 758–762.

Nishioka, K., Masuda, Y., Yanagi, E., et al., 1989. Cytologic diagnosis of the maxillary sinus re-evaluated. Laryngoscope 99, 842.

O'Connor, T.A., McLean, P., Juillard, G.J., et al., 1989. Olfactory neuroblastoma. Cancer 63, 2426.

Olsen J.H., 1987. Epidemiology of sinonasal cancer in Denmark, 1943–1982. Acta Pathol. Microbiol. Immunol. Scand. 95, 171.

Padovani, L., Pommier, P., Clippe, S.S., et al., 2003. Three-dimensional conformal radiotherapy for paranasal sinus carcinoma: clinical results for 25 patients. Int. J. Radiat. Oncol. Biol. Phys. 56, 169–176.

Pandolfo, I., Gaeta, M., Blandino, A., et al., 1989. MR imaging of perineural metastasis along the vidian nerve. J. Comput. Assist. Tomogr. 13, 498.

Parsons, J.T., Mendenhall, W.M., Mancuso, A.A., et al., 1988. Malignant tumors of the nasal cavity and ethmoid and sphenoid sinuses. Int. J. Radiat. Oncol. Biol. Phys. 14, 11.

Perry, C., Levine, P.A., Williamson, B.R., et al., 1988. Preservation of the eye in paranasal sinus cancer surgery. Arch. Otolaryngol. Head Neck Surg. 114, 632.

Pickuth, D., Heywang-Kobrunner S.H., 1999. Imaging of recurrent esthesioneuroblastoma. Br. J. Radiol. 72, 1052–1057.

Polin, R.S., Sheehan, J.P., Chenelle, A.G., et al., 1998. The role of preoperative adjuvant treatment in the management of esthesioneuroblastoma: the University of Virginia experience. Neurosurgery 42, 1029–1037.

Porceddu, S., Martin, J., Shanker, G., et al., 2004. Paranasal sinus tumors: Peter MacCallum Cancer Institute experience. Head Neck 26, 322–330.

Porter, A.B., Bernold, D.M., Giannini, C., et al., 2008. Retrospective review of adjuvant chemotherapy for esthesioneuroblastoma. J. Neurooncol. 90, 201–204.

Preusser, M., Hutterer, M., Sohm, M., et al., 2010. Disease stabilization of progressive olfactory neuroblastoma (esthesioneuroblastoma) under treatment with sunitinib mesylate. J. Neurooncol. 97 (2), 305–308.

Rankow, R.M., Conley, J., Fodor, P., 1974. Carcinoma of the maxillary sinus following thorotrast instillation. J. Maxillofac. Surg. 2, 119.

Ratech, H., Burke, J.S., Blayney, D.W., et al., 1989. A clinicopathologic study of malignant lymphomas of the nose, paranasal sinuses, and hard palate, including cases of lethal midline granuloma. Cancer 64, 2525.

Resto, V.A., Eisele, D.W., Forastiere, A., et al., 2000. Esthesioneuroblastoma: the Johns Hopkins experience. Head Neck 22, 550–558.

Robin, P.E., Powell, D.J., Stansbie J.M., 1979. Carcinoma of the nasal cavity and paranasal sinuses: incidence and presentation of different histological types. Clin. Otolaryngol. 4, 431.

Rooney, M., Kish, J., Jacobs, J., et al., 1985. Improved complete response rate and survival in advanced head and neck cancer after three-course induction therapy with 120-hour 5-FLT infusion and cisplatinum. Cancer 55, 1123.

Rosai, J., 1981. Ackerman's surgical pathology, sixth ed. Mosby, St Louis.

Roush G.C., 1979. Epidemiology of cancer of the nose and paranasal sinuses: current concepts. Head Neck Surg. 2, 3.

Sakai, S., Ebihara, T., Ono, I., et al., 1983. A comparison of AJC and JJC proposals on TNM classification of maxillary sinus carcinoma. Arch. Otorhinolaryngol. 237, 139.

Sato, M., Yoshida, H., Kaji, R., et al., 1990. Induction of bone formation in an adenoid cystic carcinoma of the maxillary sinus by adoptive immunotherapy involving intra-arterial injection of lymphokine-activated killer cells and recombinant interleukin-2 in combination with radiotherapy. J. Biol. Response Modi. 9, 329–334.

Sato, Y., Morita, M., Takahashi, H., et al., 1970. Combined surgery, radiotherapy and regional chemotherapy in carcinoma of the paranasal sinuses. Cancer 25, 571.

Sekhar, L.N., Nanda, A., Sen, C.N., et al., 1992. The extended frontal approach to tumors of the anterior, middle and posterior skull base. J. Neurosurg. 76, 198.

Shimizu, H., Hozawa, J., Saito, H., et al., 1989. Chronic sinusitis and woodworking as risk factors for cancer of the maxillary sinus in northeast Japan. Laryngoscope 99, 58.

Sisson, G.S., Toriumi, D.M., Atiyah R.A., 1989. Paranasal sinus malignancy: a comprehensive update. Laryngoscope 99, 143.

Snyderman, C.H., Janecka, I.P., Seckhar, L.N., et al., 1990. Anterior skull base reconstruction: role of galeal and pericranial flaps. Laryngoscope 100, 607.

Som, P.M., Lawson, W., Biller, H.F., et al., 1986. Ethmoid sinus disease: CT evaluation in 400 cases. Radiology 159, 605.

Sooriyachi, G.S., Skuta, G.L., Busse J.M., 1984. Transitional cell carcinoma of the nasal passages: dramatic response to chemotherapy. Med. Pediatr. Oncol. 12, 50.

Sundaresan, N., Shah J.P., 1988. Craniofacial resection for anterior skull base tumors. Head Neck. Surg. 10, 219.

Terz, J.J., Young, H.F., Lawrence, W., 1980. Combined craniofacial resection for locally advanced carcinoma of the head and neck: carcinoma of the paranasal sinuses. Am. J. Surg. 140, 618.

Tripathy, P., Dewan, Y., 2009. Endoscopic-assisted microscopic decompression of adenoid cystic carcinoma of paranasal sinus extending to the sella: a case report and review of literature. Neurol. India 57, 197–199.

Tsujii, H., Kamada, T., Matsuoka, Y., et al., 1989. The value of treatment planning using CT and an immobilizing shell in radiotherapy for paranasal sinus carcinomas. Int. J. Radiat. Oncol. Biol. Phys. 16, 243.

Turano, S., Mastroianni, C., Manfredi, C., et al., 2010. Advanced adult esthesioneuroblastoma successfully treated with cisplatin and etoposide alternated with doxorubicin, ifosfamide and vincristine. J. Neurooncol. 98 (1), 131–135.

Unger, F., Haselsberger, K., Walch, C., et al., 2005. Combined endoscopic surgery and radiosurgery as treatment modality for olfactory neuroblastoma (esthesioneuroblastoma). Acta Neurochir. (Wien) 147, 595–601; discussion 601–602.

Waldron, J., Witterick, I., 2003. Paranasal sinus cancer: caveats and controversies. World J. Surg. 27, 849–855.

Waterhouse, J., Muir, C., Correa, P., et al., 1976. Cancer incidence in five continents, third ed. IARC, Lyon.

Wax, M.K., Yun, K.J., Wetmore, S.J., et al., 1995. Adenocarcinoma of the ethmoid sinus. Head Neck 17, 303–311.

Weinreb, I., Goldstein, D., Irish, J., et al., 2009. Expression patterns of Trk-A, Trk-B, GRP78, and p75NRT in olfactory neuroblastoma. Hum. Pathol. 40, 1330–1335.

Willatt, D.J., Morton, R.P., McCormick, M.S., et al., 1987. Staging of maxillary cancer. Which classification? Ann. Otol. Rhinol. Laryngol. 96, 137–141.

Wills, J.H., 1982. Nasal carcinoma in woodworkers: a review. J. Occup. Med. 24, 526.

Wustrow, J., Rudert, H., Diercks, M., et al., 1989. Squamous epithelial carcinoma and undifferentiated carcinoma of the inner nose and paranasal sinuses. Strahlenther. Onkol. 165, 468.

Yamaki, T., Uede, T., Tano-oka, A., et al., 1991. Vascularized omentum graft for the reconstruction of the skull base after removal of a nasoethmoidal tumor with intracranial extension: case report. Neurosurgery 28, 877.

Yu, J., Koch, C.A., Patsalides, A., et al., 2004. Ectopic Cushing's syndrome caused by an esthesioneuroblastoma. Endocr. Pract. 10, 119–124.

Yu, T., Xu, Y.K., Li, L., et al., 2009. Esthesioneuroblastoma methods of intracranial extension: CT and MR imaging findings. Neuroradiology 51, 841–850.

Yuen, A.P., Fan, Y.W., Fung, C.F., et al., 2005. Endoscopic-assisted cranionasal resection of olfactory neuroblastoma. Head Neck 27, 488–493.

Esthesioneuroblastoma: management and outcome

Jeremy L. Fogelson, Michael J. Link, Kerry D. Olsen, Eric J. Moore,
Caterina Giannini, Robert L. Foote and Jan C. Buckner

40

Introduction

Esthesioneuroblastoma (olfactory neuroblastoma) is an uncommon tumor originating in the upper nasal cavity. Berger and Luc first reported this tumor in the French literature in 1924. Schall and Lineback are credited with initially describing this tumor in the English literature in 1951. This tumor accounts for 1–5% of all malignant neoplasms of the nasal cavity (Stewart et al 1988). Advances in skull base surgery and neuroimaging have resulted in increased awareness and therapeutic strategies to treat esthesioneuroblastoma. More recently, endoscopic approaches are being employed either independently or in conjunction with craniotomy in the surgical management (Devaiah et al 2003; Zafereo et al 2008). Because of the rarity of this tumor, few practitioners have had an opportunity to witness the effects of various treatment options for it. A systematic approach to the evaluation of management outcomes is difficult, because most series have limited numbers of patients entered over a long period, during which diagnostic and therapeutic capabilities varied immensely.

Pathogenesis

Although esthesioneuroblastoma is the term used most commonly to describe this tumor, other names have been used by various authors, including olfactory neuroblastoma, olfactory neural neoplasm, olfactory esthesioneuroblastoma, and neuroendocrine carcinoma (Christiansen et al 1974).

The tumor is a round-cell tumor, probably of neural crest origin, thought to arise from olfactory neuroepithelium cells high in the nasal cavity. Microscopically, the tumors may show a spectrum of neuronal and epithelial differentiation (Taraszewska et al 1998; Hirose et al 1995). This broad histological spectrum has made the histogenesis of this tumor a point of controversy. Immunocytochemical studies suggest that esthesioneuroblastoma is a primitive neural tumor but fail to support the hypothesis that it is a member of the peripheral neuroectodermal tumor family (Nelson et al 1995). There are no known risk factors for the development of an esthesioneuroblastoma. There has been a single case report of an esthesioneuroblastoma developing in a kidney transplant recipient, but the role of immunosuppression in the development of this tumor is unknown (Oliveras et al 1997). There has never been a report of a familial form of the tumor.

Diagnosis

In a review of 49 patients who received their initial evaluation and treatment at the Mayo Clinic, the ages of the patients at diagnosis ranged from 3 to 78 years old (mean 48 years old). There was a bimodal peak of presentation in the 2nd and 5th decades of life (Morita et al 1993). In the MD Anderson series, there was a unimodal peak in the 4th and 5th decade (Diaz et al 2005). There was a slight male predominance (27 male and 22 female patients) (Morita et al 1993). Most of the patients in this series presented to otolaryngologists because of symptoms suggestive of nasal obstruction or epistaxis (Table 40.1). The time from the onset of symptoms to diagnosis can range from months to as long as 10 years. A physical examination may reveal proptosis or signs of obstructed nasal sinuses, but there is no unique history or physical finding specific for this tumor. Evaluation of the nasal cavity often shows a fleshy, lobulated mass, which in some cases may be friable and prone to hemorrhage.

Unusual presentations have been reported, including an esthesioneuroblastoma that caused inappropriate secretion of antidiuretic hormone (al Ahwal et al 1994), and another case that presented with Cushing's syndrome that went into remission with treatment of the tumor and recurred when the tumor recurred (Arnesen et al 1994). The tumor does have the capability to metastasize. Synchronous cervical lymph node metastases occur with an incidence of between 17% and 48% (Davis & Weisser 1992). Intracranial and leptomeningeal infiltration is also possible and usually portends a poor prognosis (McElroy et al 1998; Louboutin et al 1994). Hematogenous metastases are unusual at presentation, but may occur subsequently at the time of relapse in bone, bone marrow, lung or skin (Stewart et al 1988). There has even been a case of a cardiac metastasis from an esthesioneuroblastoma (Chatterjee et al 1997).

Computed tomography (CT) and magnetic resonance imaging (MRI) scans delineate the lesion as a tumor with its epicenter usually just below the cribriform plate. Coronal CT usually reveals bony destruction of the ethmoid sinuses and cribriform plate. MRI scanning, particularly in the coronal and sagittal plane, is optimal to display the intracranial extension of the tumor, as well as the intranasal component (Fig. 40.1). After gadolinium, there is usually homogeneous enhancement. The differential diagnosis includes meningioma, squamous cell carcinoma, juvenile angiofibroma, adenoid cystic carcinoma, lymphoma, rhabdomyosarcoma, melanoma, and sinonasal undifferentiated carcinoma

Table 40.1 Presenting symptoms of esthesioneuroblastoma in 49 patients

Symptoms	Patients (n)
Nasal obstruction	29
Epistaxis	22
Nasal mass	5
Loss of sense of smell	4
Headache	4
Excessive tearing	2
Nasal discharge	2
Proptosis	2
Mental change	2
Neck mass	2
Face pain	1
Facial mass	1
Diplopia	1

Reproduced from Morita A, Ebersold MJ, Olsen KD, et al. (1993) Esthesioneuroblastoma: Prognosis and management. Neurosurgery 32:706–715.

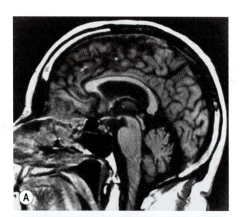

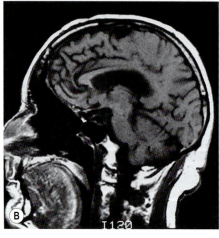

Figure 40.1 Magnetic resonance scans from a patient with a large esthesioneuroblastoma. (A) Preoperative scan shows tumor extending through cribriform plate. (B) Postoperative scan has no evidence of residual tumor.

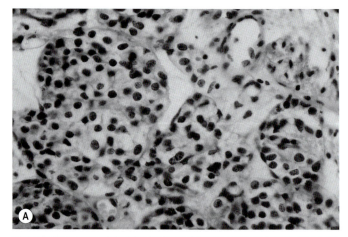

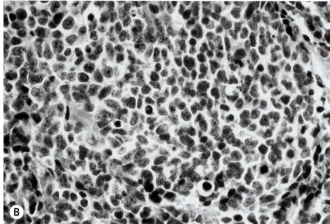

Figure 40.2 Photomicrograph of representative cases of esthesioneuroblastoma. (A) Hyams grade II. Note lobular arrangements of uniform cells with little cytoplasm and occasional Homer Wright rosettes. (B) Hyams grade IV. Cellular tumor with atypical cells in dense chromatin; no apparent rosette is noted.

(SNUC). Screening for recurrence or metastasis may be aided by using 111In-labeled octreotide as reported by Ramsay et al (1996) since most tumors express somatostatin receptors. Other authors report 111In-labeled bleomycin complex may be a useful imaging agent for detection and possibly also for treatment and assessing response to treatment (Jekunen et al 1996). The role of radionuclide imaging in a large number of tumors remains to be seen.

Outpatient biopsy via a transnasal route is often performed. This may be aided by fiberoptic endoscopy (Homer et al 1997). The light microscopic features of esthesioneuroblastoma include a lobular architecture, sheets of neoplastic cells, an intercellular neurofibrillary background, round or oval nuclei with poorly-defined cytoplasm, and occasional pseudorosettes or rosettes (Fig. 40.2) (Obert et al 1960). Electron microscopy reveals intracytoplasmic neurosecretory granules and neuritic processes with microtubules and neurofilaments (Fig. 40.3) (Taxy & Hidvegi 1977). These tumors show immunoreactivity for synaptophysin, class III β-tubulin, S-100 protein and chromogranin A in the majority of cases (Hirose et al 1995). Aberrant p53 hyperexpression is also detected in the majority of cases (Papadaki et al 1996; Hirose et al 1995). The Ki-67 labeling index varied from 0 to 43.8% with a mean of 7.4% in the study by Hirose et al (1995) and from 3% to 42%, with a mean of 16% in the study by Tatagiba et al (1995).

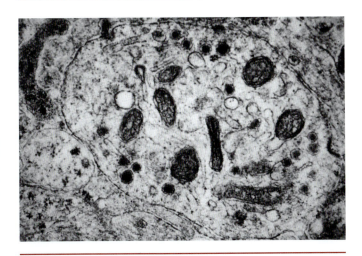

Figure 40.3 Electron microscopic findings of esthesioneuroblastoma. Dense core vesicles are noted within cytoplasm, and cell processes are noted.

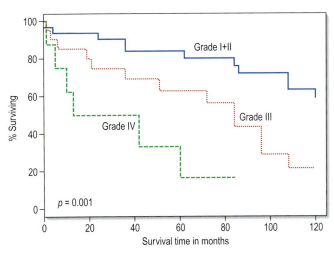

Figure 40.4 Survival rate based on Hyams grade of 78 patients treated at Mayo Clinic. There was a statistically significant decreased survival in patients with higher Hyams grade tumors.

Table 40.2 Modified Kadish staging of esthesioneuroblastoma

Stage	Finding
A	Tumor confined to nasal cavity
B	Tumor confined to nasal cavity and paranasal sinuses
C	Tumor extent beyond nasal cavity and paranasal sinuses, including involvement of cribriform plate, base of skull, orbit, or intracranial cavity
D	Tumor with metastasis to cervical lymph nodes or distant sites

Reproduced from Morita A, Ebersold MJ, Olsen KD, et al. (1993) Esthesioneuroblastoma: Prognosis and management. Neurosurgery 32:706–715.

Staging and grading

Kadish et al (1976) have developed a staging system that has been modified by Morita et al (1993) (Table 40.2). This is based on the anatomic extension of the tumor beyond the nasal cavity. The majority of tumors in the series reported by Morita et al (1993) were Kadish stage C at presentation, and this has been confirmed in multiple other series (Loy et al 2006; Bachar et al 2008; Diaz et al 2005). In a recent review of patients treated in Toronto, tumor stage correlated with both overall survival as well as progression-free survival. However, tumor grade did not affect recurrence rates (Bachar et al 2008). In contrast, review of the Mayo Clinic experience suggests that both tumor grade, and stage, are important prognostic factors (Fig. 40.4). The rarity of this tumor makes it difficult for any institution to report treatment advances with a consistent protocol, or to relate definite prognostic factors. Stage and grade, as well as age, sex and adjuvant therapy will need to be continuously scrutinized in the hopes of arriving at the best treatment strategy for future patients.

Treatment

Controversies remain regarding the optimal treatment for esthesioneuroblastoma. Advances in skull base surgery complimented by improved imaging techniques have made it possible to achieve gross total resection of almost all tumors. With Kadish stage A, and some stage B lesions, an isolated endoscopic approach may be possible. Conversely, we feel stage C and D lesions require a transcranial approach to achieve the best chance of negative histologic margins at the time of initial resection, combined with either transfacial or endoscopic approach. Some centers may be able to achieve equally good resection with a purely endoscopic approach (Devaiah & Andreoli 2009) but we have found this difficult, particularly with sampling all areas of concern at the conclusion of the operation (Levine 2009). Additionally, we have found reconstruction of the large skull base defect is much more formidable through a purely endoscopic operation. However, a recent case report by Zanation et al (2009) demonstrates that even vascularized pericranial flaps may be done with combined open and endoscopic techniques. The following is a discussion of the literature experience with treating esthesioneuroblastoma, and a detailed review of our experience at Mayo Clinic.

Radiotherapy and chemotherapy

Radiotherapy has been advocated as a primary treatment alone (Ahmad & Fayos 1980; Elkon et al 1979), as a preoperative adjuvant (Eden et al 1994; Loy et al 2006) and as a postoperative adjuvant (Morita et al 1993; Chao et al 2001) in the treatment of esthesioneuroblastoma. Likewise, the role of chemotherapy has begun to change. Once thought to be primarily a postoperative adjuvant, or as a salvage therapy for local and distant failures, some authors report good success with chemotherapy as a first-line treatment strategy (Bhattacharyya et al 1997), and others use chemotherapy as a neoadjuvant treatment (Loy et al 2006).

Gueda et al (1994) reported on five of seven patients treated at their institution with radiotherapy alone, and two patients treated with radiotherapy following resection. The dose used was >60 Gray (Gy) in all cases. They reported no complications and no local or regional recurrences with follow-up ranging from 6 months to 12 years. Two patients died of disease within 1 month of treatment; one of distant metastases and one of meningeal carcinomatosis. Elkon et al (1979) concluded from a review of 97 patients that single modality therapy, including radiotherapy alone, was comparable to multimodality treatment in local tumor control. Koka et al (1998) also concluded that there was no difference in their 40 patients with regards to survival or local control comparing single therapy (surgery or radiotherapy) versus the multimodality treatment of surgery and radiotherapy. Interestingly, they noted the incidence of neck failure was 0% in those patients who received elective radiotherapy to the first station cervical nodes, compared to 19% neck failure in patients who did not have this radiotherapy (Koka et al 1998). Slevin et al (1996) treated nine patients with resection followed by 50 Gy radiotherapy with less favorable results, with one patient developing a local recurrence and three patients dying of metastatic disease. Three patients had ocular complications of radiotherapy, resulting in blindness in two. Chao et al (2001) reported on 25 patients, and demonstrated that resection combined with radiotherapy yielded the best treatment outcome, and recommend both modalities, even in Kadish A and B lesions, with negative marginal resections.

Loy et al (2006) reported on the use of preoperative radiotherapy for stage A and B tumors, with a median dose of 50 Gy, and stage C tumors were treated with a chemotherapy regimen of cyclophosphamide and vincristine with or without doxorubicin followed by radiotherapy and resection. Preoperative radiotherapy and/or chemotherapy has the theoretical advantages of improving tumor resectability by shrinkage of the tumor, decreasing local tumor dissemination and distant metastasis at the time of operation by tumor cell sterilization, and reducing the risk of radiotherapy-associated complications by using moderate doses (50 Gy). We have been concerned about potential wound-healing complications after preoperative radiotherapy. Therefore, we have traditionally favored the use of postoperative radiotherapy. The rate of local tumor control (14 of 16 tumors) and low complication rate in light of the proportion of patients with high stage (15 of 16 stage C) and high grade (6 of 16) tumors has been encouraging using this regimen (Foote et al 1993).

When radiotherapy is used, it is important for the patient to be immobilized daily with a thermoplastic face mask and customized head and neck rest during treatment to optimize the reproducibility, precision and accuracy of each treatment. Imaging devices (kV or MV X-rays and cone beam CT), combined with robotic treatment tables with 6° of movement, allow submillimeter positioning accuracy using bony anatomy, soft tissue anatomy and/or gold fiducial markers. An oral dental prosthesis can be fabricated to displace the tongue, floor of the mouth, and mandible inferiorly away from the radiotherapy beams and to fill the oral cavity with tissue equivalent material. Preoperative diagnostic CT and/or MR images can be fused with the radiotherapy simulation CT images or diagnostic CT and/or MR images can be obtained with the patient immobilized in the treatment position following CT simulation and fused for tumor volume delineation and treatment planning. This set of images is utilized for computerized radiotherapy treatment planning and dosimetry calculations. We have found intensity modulated radiotherapy (IMRT) provides optimal delivery of the prescribed treatment dose to the tumor volume, while minimizing dose to surrounding normal tissues including the lens, retina, lacrimal gland, optic nerves and chiasm, pituitary, brain, brain stem, mastoid air cells, middle and inner ear structures, parotid glands and oral cavity. Review of preoperative imaging studies, the operative note, and the pathology report, helps to determine the treatment volume to be irradiated. This volume typically includes the preoperative tumor volume plus a margin of 3–20 mm, depending upon the location of adjacent critical normal structures. The immediately adjacent retropharyngeal lymph nodes are also included. Care is taken to limit the dose per fraction to <200 cGy (ideal dose, 180 cGy) to the retina, optic nerve, optic chiasm, and brain stem. In our experience, the optimal postoperative adjuvant dose for negative margins is 55.8 Gy over 6–6.5 weeks. When treatment involves radiotherapy for positive margins or radiotherapy alone or combined with chemotherapy for gross unresectable disease, doses of 63–70 Gy over 7–8 weeks using a combination of IMRT and radiosurgery are utilized. We require that ≥95% of the treatment volume receives the prescribed dose. We attempt to limit the maximum dose within the treatment volume to ≤110% of the prescribed dose. The minimum dose allowed to the treatment volume is ≥93% of the prescribed dose, or ≥98% of the treatment volume should receive ≥92% of the prescribed dose. Less than 5% of normal tissues outside of the treatment volume is allowed to receive the prescribed dose and ≤1% or ≤1 cc of normal tissues outside of the treatment volume is allowed to receive ≥110% of the prescribed dose. In order to minimize nausea and vomiting, the volume of brain stem that receives 30 Gy (V30) is limited to ≤33%. The maximum dose allowed to the brain stem is 52 Gy. The mean dose allowed to the retina is ≤30 Gy with V50 ≤1% and V40 ≤50%. The maximum optic nerve and chiasm dose is ≤50 Gy or V55 ≤1%. The mean dose allowed to the lacrimal glands is ≤10 Gy with a maximum dose ≤30 Gy. The maximum dose allowed to the brain is ≤56 Gy or V60 ≤1%. The mean dose allowed to the parotid glands is ≤26 Gy or V30 ≤50% for either parotid gland and/or ≥20 cc combined volume of both parotid glands ≤20 Gy. For the mastoid air cells and structures of the middle and inner ear (tympanic membrane, ossicles, cochlea, semicircular canals and proximal eustachian tube) the mean dose allowed is 30 Gy with a maximum dose of 45 Gy. For the oral cavity, the mean dose allowed is ≤30 Gy with V50 ≤20% and V60 ≤1%. For unresectable tumors, the maximum dose allowed to the mandible is ≤70 Gy or V75 ≤1% or ≤1 cc. In postoperative cases the maximum dose to the mandible is ≤66 Gy.

When there is pathological evidence of parotid or cervical adenopathy, the dissected side of the neck is treated to 60 Gy in 30 fractions of 2.0 Gy each and the contralateral side of the neck, if undissected, is treated to 54 Gy in 30 fractions of 2.0 Gy each. When the cervical lymphatics (levels II through V) are treated the maximum dose allowed to the brachial plexus is <66 Gy and the volume of the brachial plexus allowed to receive ≥60 Gy, (V60) is ≤5%. The mean dose to the pharyngeal constrictors is <45–62 Gy, or V50 ≤33% and V60 ≤15%. The mean dose allowed to the larynx is 35 Gy with V50 ≤33% and V60 <10%. The mean dose allowed to the esophagus is 30 Gy, with V40 ≤20%, and V54 ≤15%. The mean dose allowed to the submandibular glands is <39 Gy.

One of the most interesting advancements in the treatment of esthesioneuroblastoma concerns the use of preoperative chemotherapy. Bhattacharyya et al (1997) reported nine patients treated with cisplatin and etoposide initially. Chemotherapy responders (eight of the nine patients) were treated with combined photon and stereotaxic fractionated proton radiotherapy totaling approximately 68 Gy to the primary site, whereas the single non-responder was treated with surgical resection, followed by postoperative radiotherapy. Of the eight patients who responded to chemotherapy, there were no recurrences with a mean follow-up of 14 months. Notably, there were two patients who subsequently underwent surgery and no tumor was discovered in the pathology specimen, suggesting tumor response to chemotherapy without radiographic response. While this is encouraging, the follow-up is short. Others have also reported finding no tumor in surgical specimens after patients have undergone preoperative radiotherapy (Polonowski et al 1990; Levine et al 1986). Polin et al (1998) reviewed the University of Virginia experience using vincristine and cyclophosphamide pre and postoperatively in stage C tumors in addition to craniofacial resection and preoperative radiotherapy. Of the 16 patients who received preoperative chemotherapy, five had a substantial response, two had a partial response, five had no response, one progressed and data was not available for the remaining three patients. Patients with response to neoadjuvant therapy demonstrated a significantly lower rate of disease-related mortality (Polin et al 1998).

Chemotherapy has traditionally been employed to treat advanced stage disease. Goldsweig and Sundaresan (1990) reviewed 25 cases from the English literature and reported one additional case. In their review, 19 of 20 patients given chemotherapy alone for recurrent or metastatic disease improved. In the Mayo Clinic experience, treating 10 patients with advanced stage disease with primarily a platinum-based regimen, Hyams grade once again determined both prognosis and response to adjuvant chemotherapy. The only tumor regression resultant from chemotherapy was observed in patients with high-grade tumors. This occurred in two of four patients and response was short-lived (McElroy et al 1998). In the series reported by Koka et al (1998) eight of 40 patients received chemotherapy using a variety of combinations. The response of tumor to chemotherapy did not significantly influence the survival when the patients underwent surgery. Not surprisingly, a significantly better survival was noted in patients with complete regression of tumor when chemotherapy was employed prior to definitive radiotherapy for a locally advanced or unresectable tumor compared with patients who had no response (Koka et al 1998). In a recent review by Porter et al (2008) of 12 patients with Kadish C and Hyams grade III or IV tumors, six received adjuvant chemotherapy (AC) after craniofacial resection, and six did not. Median time to relapse for patients who did not receive AC was 10.5 months, compared with those who did, at 35 months. However, this is a small sample size and a major confounder, in that more of the patients who received AC also received adjuvant radiotherapy (five of six,

compared with only two of six in the non-AC group.) Also, the adjuvant therapy was not randomized, so it is possible that performance status played a role as a selection bias.

Undoubtedly, preoperative chemotherapy is going to play a greater role in the initial treatment of esthesioneuroblastoma as more experience is acquired. The response to chemotherapy may also begin to have a greater role in deciding further treatment for advanced stage and high-grade tumors.

Surgery

Resection of esthesioneuroblastoma has played a major role in the treatment of this tumor for the past four decades. The superiority of craniofacial resection as opposed to attempted transfacial or transcranial resection alone for local tumor control, seems well established, and complication rates have been acceptable (Lund et al 1998; Shah et al 1997; Loy et al 2006). Levine et al (1986) found survival improved from 37.5% to 82% when craniofacial resection and preoperative radiotherapy replaced limited resection.

Between 1951 and 1990, 38 (78%) of 49 patients at the Mayo Clinic underwent gross total resection with or without radiotherapy and seemed to have better survival and disease-free survival rates than those who had partial resection or biopsy with radiotherapy alone. Patient selection may have biased the outcome however, because gross total resection may not have been attempted or accomplished in patients who had extremely extensive tumors. Local recurrence in this series developed in 12 (55%) of the 22 patients who had total resection alone but in only three (19%) of the 16 who had total resection, followed by radiotherapy (Morita et al 1993). Some surgeons advise to perform prophylactic resection of the cervical lymph nodes. Ferlito et al (2003) reviewed the literature and concluded that a neck dissection should be performed in patients with modified Kadish stage B or greater, although we have not adopted this practice.

We also feel that surgery for recurrent disease is very effective in controlling tumor. Of the 16 patients who had initial salvage treatment for local recurrence, local tumor control was obtained in seven (43%). The 5-year survival rate was 82% after salvage treatment for local recurrence (Morita et al 1993). Seven of ten patients with neck lymph node metastases underwent radical neck dissection. Radiotherapy was also given to four patients. Two patients had radiotherapy alone, and one did not have any treatment. Neck dissection in combination with radiotherapy appeared to offer the most favorable outcome in this group (Morita et al 1993). Figure 40.5 demonstrates the overall survival. Figures 40.4 and 40.6 demonstrate how tumor grade and stage influenced survival in the Mayo Clinic series.

Surgical technique

Unlike many other skull-base tumors, which require extensive dissection to reach the lesion, tumors in the region of the cribriform plate are easily accessible from both below, via a lateral rhinotomy, transethmoidal approach, and above utilizing a frontal craniotomy.

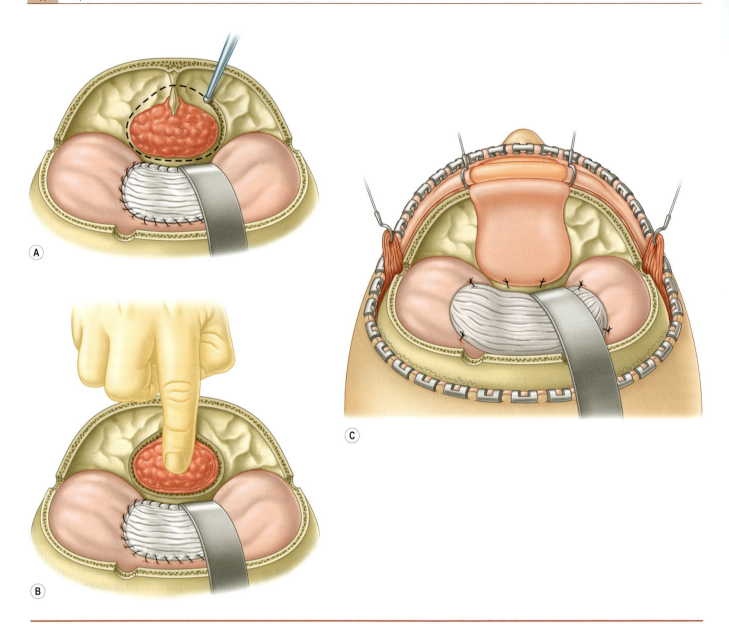

Figure 40.8 (A) Osteotomies are performed on the floor of the frontal fossa surrounding the tumor. (B) After the ENT surgeon dissects the tumor with the endonasal approach, the two teams work together to deliver the specimen through the nose. (C) Fibrin glue is placed over the dural repair, and the remaining fascia lata graft is tacked to the dura overlapping the margins. Tack holes are made posteriorly on the planum sphenoidale and the vascularized pericranial flap is swung in and tacked posteriorly to repair the floor of the frontal fossa. After visualizing the placement of the nasal packing from the cranial incision, further fibrin glue is placed over the pericranium and the wound is closed.

evidence of obvious tumor within the maxillary sinus with direct inspection the mucosa is removed and sent for pathologic examination.

The rhinotomy incision is then extended around the nasal ala, and the soft tissues are separated from the pyriform aperture with cautery up to the level of the nasal bone. The attachments of the upper lateral cartilage to the nasal bone are divided to the midline. Generally, it is unnecessary to split the upper lip and elevate the tissues off the maxilla in the labial-gingival sulcus. If the tumor involves the maxilla, however, a partial, total, or extended maxillectomy can be performed after dividing the upper lip through the philtral crest.

The anterior periosteum is separated from the nasal bones up to the midline. Depending on the extent of involvement of the contralateral ethmoid maxillary complex and nasal bone, the elevation can continue across to the opposite side, freeing the orbit from the lamina papyracea through the single rhinotomy incision.

A periosteal elevator frees the nasal tissues from the posterior portion of the frontal process of the maxilla and nasal bone. The frontal process of the maxilla is removed with a rongeur up to the lacrimal bone. A Kerrison punch is used to continue the opening to the inferior portion of the frontal sinus. The nasal soft tissues at the midline of the nose are divided with cautery up to the roof of the nose and across to the ethmoid area. This exposure permits complete inspection of the superior nasal cavity.

The bone connecting the maxillary sinus to the inferior and anterior ethmoid complex is then removed. The amount of bone divided is dictated by the tumor's extent. Tumor involvement of the nasal septum can be determined by direct inspection. The septum is divided anterior or caudally to the tumor and extended posteriorly to the choanae. The remaining posterior septum is now attached in the cribriform area and to the rostrum of the sphenoid.

Utilizing the previous bone cuts made from above, the tumor can then be pushed down from above and delivered into the nasal cavity (Fig. 40.8B). Multiple frozen sections are obtained from the margins to determine whether additional tissue should be removed and also to determine the status of the tumor margins.

Some tumors also extend into the orbit. An ophthalmologic surgeon then may continue with the portion of the dissection relative to the orbit or orbital contents. This may involve dissecting tumor from the extraocular muscles or, for some very aggressive tumors, exenteration of the orbit.

After hemostasis has been achieved, fibrin glue is placed over the dural repair. Then the remainder of fascia lata is placed against the dura to cover the dural repair. The graft must extend beyond the extent of any previous dural openings. It is tacked in place to prevent migration. This provides the first barrier to repair the frontal fossa and helps insure a watertight closure even if a tiny dural defect persists after dural repair. The pericranium is then carefully dissected from the galea, leaving it vascularized at its base. Any defects are repaired with Prolene suture. Tack-holes are created in the residual planum sphenoidale with a 2 mm burr and the pericranial flap is swung in and tacked to the planum (Fig. 40.8C). The nasal cavity is then packed with well-lubricated nasal packing gauze, while directly visualizing from the intracranial compartment to ensure there is no mass effect on the brain. Further fibrin glue is applied to adhere the fascial graft to the pericranial graft.

The cranial bone flap is then secured in place using burr hole covers, and the scalp is closed in the usual manner over a closed suction drainage system. The suction may have an air leak as it is in continuity with the pharynx, thus we also rely on a snug head dressing for 3 days to minimize subgaleal fluid collections. The patient receives antibiotics while the nasal packs are in place. The nasal packs are usually removed on the seventh postoperative day. This allows ample time for the fascial and pericranial graft to seal to the underlying dura. We have not had problems with spinal fluid leaks when the above-described techniques were followed.

Complications

The surgical complication rate is relatively low (Table 40.3) (Loy et al 2006). Although the published series (Morita et al 1993) has a higher wound complication rate, a subset of 22 patients were operated upon with our current technique as described above. The only spinal fluid leak (4.5%) occurred in a patient whose fascia free graft did not extend far enough laterally to cover a small dural rent over the medial orbital roof. Meticulous attention must be paid to such detail or

Table 40.3 Complications of treatment for esthesioneuroblastoma in 50 patients

Category	Patients n	(%)	Complications
CNS	10	20	1 Increased ICP, 3 pneumocephalus, 1 transient stroke syndrome, and 5 CSF leaks
Orbital	9	18	3 Epiphora, 2 radiation-induced cataracts, 1 radiation keratopathy, 2 transient fourth cranial nerve palsy, and 1 periorbital cellulitis
Systemic	8	16	1 Hyponatremia, 1 temporary respiratory arrest, 2 abdominal wound seroma, 2 DI, 1 pulmonary embolus, and 1 hypothyroidism
Chemotoxic	5	10	1 Acute myocardial infarction, 1 bilateral vocal cord palsy, 1 peripheral neuropathy, 1 herpes zoster, and 1 digit paresthesia
Infectious	3	6	2 Infected bone flaps and 1 epidural abscess

CNS, central nervous system; CSF, cerebrospinal fluid; DI, diabetes insipidus; ICP, intracranial pressure. (Reproduced from Table 2 in Loy AH, Reibel JF, Read PW, et al. (2006) Esthesioneuroblastoma: Continued Follow-up of a Single Institution's Experience. Arch Otolaryngol Head Neck Surg 132: 134–138. With permission from the American Medical Association. Copyright © American Medical Association, All rights reserved.)

reoperation to repair the problem will be necessary. Lund et al (1998) reported only eight CSF leaks in a series of 209 (3.8%) patients treated with craniofacial resection for a variety of pathologies; only four of these required reoperation.

The most bothersome complication has been skin breakdown. Anything short of a vascularized free tissue transfer graft to this area in our experience has a high likelihood of failure if the patient has already received radiotherapy. In two cases, the patients elected not to proceed with any major reconstructive procedure. It is our suspicion that this occurs more commonly in patients who are treated with preoperative radiotherapy.

In general, the surgical procedure is well tolerated, and the patient responds postoperatively in much the manner of patients who have a sinus procedure. Usually the patient is alert, awake, and talking by the evening of operation, and the next day, the patient is allowed to walk about the hospital room and corridor.

Results

The results of various treatment series are difficult to compare because the numbers of patients are often small and treatment methods have been variable over long periods of time. In reviewing 50 patients treated from 1976 to 2004 at the University of Virginia, Loy et al (2006) found a 5- and 15-year disease free survival of 86.5 and 82.6%, respectively. Diaz et al (2005) reported 5- and 10-year overall survival of 89% and 81%, and progression free survival at 5 and 10 years of 69% and 38%, respectively, in 30 patients. A total of 39 patients reviewed by Bachar et al (2008) had 82.6% disease free survival at 5 years, and 5- and 10-year overall survival of 87.9% and 69.2%, respectively.

One of the most striking features of esthesioneuroblastoma is the ability for late recurrence and late metastases. Eden et al (1994) noted median time to first recurrence of 21.5 months and 39% of first recurrences were ≥5 years after diagnosis. Likewise, the first recurrences developed later than 5 years in 8 of 19 (42%) patients, with local recurrence in the series reviewed by Morita et al (1993). In reviewing the literature, Shaari et al (1996) noted a highly variable onset of central nervous system metastases in 17 patients, ranging from 1–228 months after initial diagnosis. Careful long-term follow-up is necessary for all patients with esthesioneuroblastoma (Fig. 40.9).

Various authors have tried to determine prognostic factors that might help guide treatment and predict outcome. Some feel tumor stage is most predictive of outcome (Eden et al 1994; Polin et al 1998; Bachar et al 2008). Koka et al (1998) reported the presence of cervical lymph node metastases at diagnosis was the only significant risk factor for survival. In contrast, Eden et al (1994) did not find neck status at presentation to be predictive. Dulguerov and Calcaterra (1992) found negative prognostic factors to be age >50 years at presentation, female sex, tumor recurrence, and metastasis. A meta-analysis by Dulguerov et al (2001) demonstrated that both cervical metastasis at the time of presentation, as well as Hyams grading, were significant poor prognosticators. Polin et al (1998) also found advanced age was predictive of decreased disease-free survival. Central nervous system or leptomeningeal metastases appear to have a particularly poor prognosis with survival generally <2 years (Shaari et al 1996). In our review of the Mayo series, Hyams grade I and II tumors had a 5- and 10-year overall survival of 83% and 60%, whereas the survival of grade III and IV tumors were 48% and 19%, respectively. Kadish stage A and B tumors had an overall survival of 84% and 60% at 5 and 10 years, whereas modified Kadish C and D tumors overall survival was 60% and 36%, respectively. These are statistically significant differences in survival in a series of 74 patients, and we believe grade and stage are important prognosticators (Figs 40.4, 40.6).

Conclusion

Due to the rarity of esthesioneuroblastoma, its variability of histologic grade, clinical stage and biologic behavior, definite treatment recommendations are difficult. At this time, we recommend attempted gross total removal with negative tumor margins as the goal for all cases. Typically, this should be accomplished with a craniofacial resection, with either transnasal or assisted endonasal techniques. It may be possible to utilize an endoscopic-only technique in some Kadish A and B tumors. For low-grade and low-stage tumors we feel this is the optimal treatment and we usually withhold adjuvant therapy if we are confident the resection margins are free of tumor. We recommend yearly follow-up with MRI scanning for at least the first 5 years, and then every other year indefinitely. For low-grade and low-stage tumors with close margins (<5 mm) (e.g., adjacent to the cavernous carotid artery), we recommend postoperative radiotherapy to a dose of 55.8 Gy. We recommend this same dose of postoperative radiotherapy for all stages of high-grade tumors with negative or close margins. If the tumor margins are positive or there is gross residual or unresectable disease, the dose is increased to 63 Gy (microscopically positive margins) to 70 Gy (gross residual unresectable disease) and we also consider postoperative chemotherapy, using a platinum-based regimen. When cervical lymph node disease is present, we usually perform neck dissection at the time of initial operation, or when cervical node disease develops if it is not present when the initial tumor resection is performed. We then include the cervical lymph nodes in the postoperative radiotherapy treatment volume, regardless of initial tumor grade. Koka et al (1998) provide compelling evidence to include the first station cervical nodes in the initial radiotherapy treatment volume, in that this significantly reduced the incidence of neck failure in their series.

Aggressive therapy is also indicated for recurrent disease, and in most cases, is as effective as the initial treatment for controlling tumor. We also believe aggressive therapy is warranted for distant metastases, usually radiotherapy and chemotherapy, although survival is usually <1 year. Our colleagues at UVA recommend preoperative radiotherapy, as well as chemotherapy for Kadish stage C patients, and continue to demonstrate excellent results (Loy et al 2006). The report of Bhattacharyya et al (1997) was intriguing in regards to the role of chemotherapy as an initial therapy for esthesioneuroblastoma, being successful in eight of nine patients with short-term follow-up, however, these results have not been duplicated. This may be the preferable way to treat initially unresectable, bulky tumors. In our series of patients treated with adjuvant chemotherapy (AC), with or without radiotherapy, AC patients had a longer average time to recurrence (Porter et al 2008). However, we await further reports. We prefer to defer radiotherapy in all cases until the postoperative period to try and prevent wound-healing problems following surgery. Unfortunately, we do not believe there will ever be randomized trials for the treatment of esthesioneuroblastoma. Continued reported

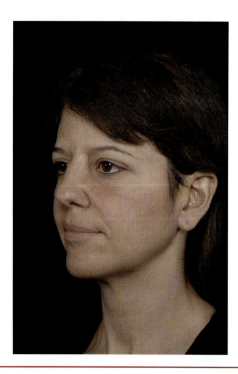

Figure 40.9 Acceptable cosmetic results after a left lateral rhinotomy, and bicoronal incision above the hairline for a craniofacial resection.

series will have to be carefully examined to try and decide optimal treatment and prognosis.

REFERENCES

Ahmad, K., Fayos, J.V., 1980. Role of radiation therapy in the treatment of olfactory neuroblastoma. J. Radiat. Oncol. Biol. Phys. 6, 349–352.

al Ahwal, M., Jha, N., Nabholtz, J.M., et al., 1994. Olfactory neuroblastoma: report of a case associated with inappropriate antidiuretic hormone secretion. J. Otolaryngol. 23, 437–439.

Arnesen, M.A., Scheithauer, B.W., Freeman, S., 1994. Cushing's syndrome secondary to olfactory neuroblastoma. Ultrastruct. Pathol. 18, 61–68.

Bachar, G., Goldstein, D.P., Shah, M., et al., 2008. Esthesioneuroblastoma: The Princess Margaret Experience. Head Neck 30, 1607–1614.

Berger, L., Luc, R., 1924. L'Esthesioneuroeitheliome olfactif. Bulletin de l'Association Francaise pour l'etude du Cancer 13, 410–421.

Bhattacharyya, N., Thornton, A.F., Joseph, M.P., et al., 1997. Successful treatment of esthesioneuroblastoma and neuroendocrine carcinoma with combined chemotherapy and proton radiation. Arch. Otolaryngol. Head Neck Surg. 123, 34–40.

Chao, K.S.C., Kaplan, C., Simpson, J.R., et al., 2001. Esthesioneuroblastoma: The impact of treatment modality. Head Neck 23, 749–757.

Chatterjee, T., Muller, M.F., Meier, B., 1997. Cardiac metastasis of an esthesioneuroblastoma. Heart 77, 82–83.

Christiansen, T.A., Duvall, A.J., III, Rosenberg, Z., et al., 1974. Juvenile nasopharyngeal angiofibroma. Trans. Am. Acad. Ophthalmol. Otolaryngol. 78, ORL140–ORL147.

Davis, R.E., Weisser, M.C., 1992. Esthesioneuroblastoma and neck metastases. Head Neck 14, 477–482.

Devaiah, A.K., Andreoli, M.T., 2009. Treatment of esthesioneuroblastoma: A 16 year meta-analysis of 361 patients. Laryngoscope 119, 1412–1416.

Devaiah, A.K., Larsen, C., Tawfik, O., et al., 2003. Esthesioneuroblastoma: endoscopic nasal and anterior craniotomy resection. Laryngoscope 113, 2086–2090.

● Diaz, E.M., Johnigan, R.H., Pero, C., et al., 2005. Olfactory neuroblastoma: The 22-year experience at one comprehensive cancer center. Head Neck 27 (2), 138–149.

Dulguerov, P., Allal, A.S., Calcaterra, M., 2001. Esthesioneuroblastoma: A meta-analysis and review. Lancet. Oncol. 2, 683–690.

Dulguerov, P., Calcaterra, M., 1992. Esthesioneuroblastoma: The UCLA experience 1970–1990. Laryngoscope 102, 843–848.

Eden, B.V., Debo, R.F., Larner, J.M., et al., 1994. Esthesioneuroblastoma. Cancer 73, 2556–2562.

Elkon, D., Hightower, S.I., Lim, M.L., et al., 1979. Esthesioneuroblastoma. Cancer 44, 1087–1094.

Ferlito, A., Rinaldo, A., Rhys-Evans, P.H., 2003. Contemporary clinical commentary: esthesioneuroblastoma: an update on management of the neck. Laryngoscope 113, 1935–1938.

Foote, R.L., Morita, A., Ebersold, M.J., et al., 1993. Esthesioneuroblastoma: the role of adjuvant radiation therapy. Int. J. Radiat. Oncol. Biol. Phys. 27, 835–842.

Goldsweig, H.G., Sundaresan, N., 1990. Chemotherapy of recurrent esthesioneuroblastoma: Case report and review of the literature. Am. J. Clin. Oncol. 13, 139–143.

Gueda, F., Van Limbergen, E., Van den Bogaert, W., 1994. High dose level radiation therapy for local tumor control in esthesioneuroblastoma. Eur. J. Cancer Clin. Oncol. 30A, 1757–1760.

Hirose, T., Scheithauer, B.W., Lopes, B.S., et al., 1995. Olfactory neuroblastoma. An immunohistochemical, ultrastructural, and flow cytometric study. Cancer 76, 4–19.

Homer, J.J., Jones, N.S., Bradley, P.J., 1997. The role of endoscopy in the management of nasal neoplasia. Am. J. Rhinol. 11, 41–47.

Jekunen, A.P., Kairemo, K.J.A., Lehtonen, H.P., et al., 1996. Treatment of olfactory neuroblastoma. Am. J. Clin. Oncol. 19, 375–378.

Kadish, S., Goodman, M., Wang, C.C., 1976. Olfactory neuroblastoma: A clinical analysis of 17 cases. Cancer 37, 1571–1576.

Koka, V.N., Julieron, M., Bourhis, J., et al., 1998. Aesthesioneuroblastoma. J. Laryngol. Otol. 112, 628–633.

Levine, P.A., 2009. Would Dr. Ogura approve of endoscopic resection of esthesioneuroblastomas? an analysis of endoscopic resection data vs. that of craniofacial resection. Laryngoscope 119, 3–7.

Levine, P.A., McClean, W.C., Cantrell, R.W., 1986. Esthesioneuroblastoma: the University of Virginia experience: 1960–1985. Laryngoscope 96, 742–746.

Link, M.J., Converse, L.D., Lanier, W.L., 2008. A new technique for single-person fascia lata harvest. Neurosurgery 63, ONS 359–361.

Louboutin, J.P., Maugard-Louboutin, C., Fumoleau, P., 1994. Leptomeningeal infiltration in esthesioneuroblastoma: report of two cases with poor prognosis. Eur. Neurol. 34, 236–238.

● Loy, A.H., Reibel, J.F., Read, P.W., et al., 2006. Esthesioneuroblastoma: Continued follow-up of a single institution's experience. Arch. Otolaryngol. Head Neck Surg. 132, 134–138.

Lund, V.J., Howard, D.J., Wei, W.I., et al., 1998. Craniofacial resection for tumors of the nasal cavity and paranasal sinuses – A 17-year experience. Head Neck 20, 97–105.

McElroy, E.A., Buckner, J.C., Lewis, J.E., 1998. Chemotherapy for advanced esthesioneuroblastoma: The Mayo Clinic Experience. Neurosurgery 42, 1023–1028.

Mertz, J.S., Pearson, B.W., Kern, E.B., 1983. Lateral rhinotomy: indications, technique, and review of 226 patients. Arch. Otolaryngol. 109, 235–239.

● Morita, A., Ebersold, M.J., Olsen, K.D., et al., 1993. Esthesioneuroblastoma: Prognosis and management. Neurosurgery 32, 706–715.

Nelson, R.S., Perlman, E.J., Askin, F.B., 1995. Is esthesioneuroblastoma a peripheral neuroectodermal tumor? Hum. Pathol. 26, 639–641.

Obert, G.J., Devine, K.D., McDonald, J.R., 1960. Olfactory neuroblastomas. Cancer 13, 205–215.

Oliveras, A., Puig, J.M., Lloveras, J., 1997. Esthesioneuroblastoma developing in a kidney transplant recipient. Transpl. Int. 10, 85–86.

Papadaki, H., Kounelis, S., Kapadia, S.B., et al., 1996. Relationship of p53 gene alterations with tumor progression and recurrence in olfactory neuroblastoma. A. J. Surg. Pathol. 20, 715–721.

Polin, R.S., Sheehan, J.P., Chenelle, A.G., et al., 1998. The role of preoperative adjuvant treatment in the management of esthesioneuroblastoma: The University of Virginia experience. Neurosurgery 42, 1029–1037.

Polonowski, J.M., Brasnu, D., Roux, F.X., et al., 1990. Esthesioneuroblastoma: complete tumor response after induction chemotherapy. Ear. Nose Throat J. 69, 743–746.

• **Porter, A.B., Bernold, D.M., Giannini, C., et al.**, 2008. Retrospective review of adjuvant chemotherapy for esthesioneuroblastoma. J. Neurooncol. 90, 201–204.

Ramsay, H.A., Kairemo, K.J., Jekunen, A.P., 1996. Somatostatin receptor imaging of olfactory neuroblastoma. J. Laryngol. Otol. 110, 1161–1163.

Schall, L.A., Lineback, M., 1951. Primary intranasal neuroblastoma. Ann. Otol. Rhinol. Laryngol. 60, 221–229.

Shaari, C.M., Catalano, P.J., Sen, C., et al., 1996. Central nervous system metastases from esthesioneuroblastoma. Otolaryngol. Head Neck Surg. 114, 808–812.

Shah, J.P., Kraus, D.H., Bilsky, M.H., et al., 1997. Craniofacial resection for malignant tumors involving the anterior skull base. Arch. Otolaryngol. Head Neck Surg. 123, 1312–1317.

Slevin, N.J., Irwin, C.J.R., Banerjee, S.S., et al., 1996. Olfactory neural tumours – the role of external beam radiotherapy. J. Laryngol. Otol. 110, 1012–1016.

Stewart, F.M., Frieson, H.F., Levine, P.A., et al., 1988. Esthesioneuroblastoma. In: **Williams, C.J., Krikorian, J.G., Grenn, M.R., et al.** (Eds.), Textbook of uncommon cancer. John Wiley, Chichester, pp. 631–652.

Taraszewska, A., Czorniuk-Sliwa, A., Dambska, M., 1998. Olfactory neuroblastoma (esthesioneuroblastoma) and esthesioneuroepithelioma: histologic and immunohistochemical study. Folia Neuropathologica 36, 81–86.

Tatagiba, M., Samii, M., Dankoweit-Timpe, E., et al., 1995. Esthesioneuroblastomas with intracranial extension. Proliferative potential and management. Arquivos de Neuro-Psiquiatria 53, 577–586.

Taxy, J.B., Hidvegi, D.F., 1977. Olfactory neuroblastoma: an ultrastructural study. Cancer 39, 131–138.

• **Zafereo, M.E., Fakhri, S., Prayson, P.B.**, 2008. Esthesioneuroblastoma: 25-year experience at a single institution. Otolaryngol. Head Neck Surg. 138, 452–458.

Zanation, A.M., Snyderman, C.H., Carrau, R.L., 2009. Minimally invasive endoscopic pericranial flap: a new method for endonasal skull base reconstruction. Laryngoscope 119, 13–18.

Primary central nervous system lymphoma

Mark A. Rosenthal and Samar Issa

41

Introduction

The descriptive term 'primary central nervous system lymphoma' encompasses a number of distinct pathologic and clinical entities. Historically, the disease has been described under a variety of synonyms including reticulum sarcoma, microgliomatosis, perivascular sarcoma, perithelial sarcoma, adventitial sarcoma, primary cerebral lymphoma, and others. Current nomenclature divides 'primary central nervous system lymphoma' into: non-Hodgkin lymphoma (NHL) or Hodgkin disease and patients who are immuno-competent or immunosuppressed. In addition, there are a number of rare diseases that may fall under the umbrella of 'primary central nervous system lymphoma'. The categories of primary central nervous system lymphoma are listed in Box 41.1.

The first formal description of primary central nervous system lymphoma was ascribed to Bailey in 1929, although he suggested that probable cases were reported in the late nineteenth century (Bailey 1929). Primary central nervous system lymphoma has been the focus of numerous small studies and case reports ever since this initial observation. The disease was seen as a rare and lethal curiosity until the introduction of radiotherapy, when significant gains in survival and symptom relief were obtained.

The last three decades have seen an unprecedented increase in the number of cases of primary central nervous system lymphoma that can not be explained solely by the HIV epidemic. Concurrently, our understanding of primary central nervous system lymphoma biology has improved dramatically and therapeutic gains have been achieved with the introduction of chemotherapy.

Primary central nervous system lymphoma (PCNSL)

Incidence and prevalence

Historically, lymphoma involving the central nervous system (CNS) was considered a rare phenomenon, representing <3% of all CNS tumors with about half of these lymphomas confined entirely to the CNS. Thus, primary central nervous system lymphoma (PCNSL), that is, lymphoma confined to the CNS, represented approximately 0.85–1.5% of all CNS

tumors (Jellinger et al 1975; Zimmerman 1975; Houthoff et al 1978; Freeman et al 1986). In large autopsy series, the diagnosis of PCNSL in patients dying from all causes was extremely low. In one series of 6000 consecutive autopsies performed between 1960 and 1975 only nine cases (0.0015%) of PCNSL were recorded (Reznik 1975). PCNSL represented between 0.007–0.7% of all lymphoma cases and accounted for approximately 0.01% of extra nodal lymphomas (Freeman et al 1972; Henry et al 1974; Liang et al 1989; Aozasa et al 1990).

There has, however, been a re-focus on primary central nervous system lymphoma due to an increase in incidence. The rise in incidence can be directly attributed to at least two known factors: the acquired immune deficiency syndrome (AIDS) epidemic and the extensive use of immunosuppressive therapy. However, the most perplexing aspect of PCNSL is an unexplained increase in the incidence of this disease in non-immunosuppressed patients in a similar manner to the increase in systemic NHL. Eby et al (1988) drew attention to this phenomenon in 1988, reporting a three-fold increase in the incidence of PCNSL between the years 1973–1975 and 1982–1984. The increase appeared to equally affect males and females, both young and old. At the Massachusetts General Hospital there was an increase in hospital admissions for PCNSL compared with admissions for other brain tumors. Prior to 1977, patients with PCNSL represented 3.3% of the hospital's primary intracerebral neoplasm cases. In the subsequent years to 1989, this rose to 6.3% of primary intracerebral neoplasms. The frequency of cases has risen from 2.1 per year (1958–82) to five per year (1983–89). There has been no apparent change in median age, sex incidence or tumor location despite this increase in PCNSL in immunocompetent patients (Hochberg & Miller 1988).

Other studies have also suggested an increased incidence of PCNSL in immunocompetent patients. O'Sullivan et al (1991) documented a rapid rise in the number of PCNSL cases seen in South-East Scotland, and a similar increase was suggested in West Scotland and Yorkshire (Murphy et al 1989; Adams & Howatson 1990). At Memorial Sloane-Kettering Cancer Center, the incidence of PCNSL in apparently immunocompetent patients as a percentage of all gliomas rose from 0.9% prior to 1984 to 15.4% since 1985 (DeAngelis 1991a). Corn et al (1997) projected that the incidence rate of PCNSL (excluding never married males) would

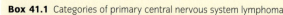

Box 41.1 Categories of primary central nervous system lymphoma

NON-HODGKIN LYMPHOMA

Primary central nervous system lymphoma

- Immunocompetent
- Immunosuppressed
  - AIDS related
  - Organ transplant related
  - Congenital
  - Therapeutic

HODGKIN DISEASE

OCULAR LYMPHOMA

MYCOSIS FUNGOIDES

LYMPHOMATOID GRANULOMATOSIS

MALIGNANT ANGIOENDOTHELIOSIS

rise from 30 per 10 million population in 1992 to 51.1 per 10 million population in the year 2000.

There are a number of confounding issues despite this apparent increased incidence. These include population age shifts, observed increases in the incidence of brain tumors (Greig et al 1990) and NHL (DeVita et al 1997), improvements in the accuracy of histologic diagnosis, changes in nosology, improved radiologic diagnostic techniques and increased physician awareness. In addition, immunosuppressive regimens, transplantation and human immunodeficiency virus (HIV) infection may have covertly influenced incidence figures despite the best efforts of investigators to exclude them. While it is difficult to refute some influence, these issues do not fully explain the increase in incidence of PCNSL in apparently immunocompetent patients (Baumgartner et al 1990; O'Sullivan et al 1991; Desmeules et al 1992).

Interestingly, there is accumulating evidence that the rise in PCNSL has plateaued or may have declined (Kadan-Lottick 2002). Further, the incidence of AIDS-related PCNSL has fallen due to the introduction of antiretroviral therapies (Haldorsen et al 2008).

Age distribution

The median age at presentation in patients with primary central nervous system lymphoma depends on the underlying cause. Primary central nervous system lymphoma in immunocompetent patients usually arises in the 7th decade – median age of onset 60 years. According to Murray's extensive literature review of 693 PCNSL cases, the median age at diagnosis was 64 years, with most patients aged between 40 and 75 years (Murray et al 1986). The age range in this series was 2 months to 90 years. More recent series have reported median ages at diagnosis ranging from 48–58 years (Hochberg & Miller 1988; Socie et al 1990; Neuwelt et al 1991; DeAngelis et al 1992a; Rosenthal et al 1993; Tomlinson et al 1995; Glass et al 1996; Trans-Tasman Radiation Oncology Group 1996; Cher et al 1996; Brada et al 1998; Wagner et al 1998). Reports of PCNSL in childhood are rare and are usually associated with inherited or acquired immunosuppression (Helle et al 1984; Epstein et al 1988; Kai et al 1998).

In contrast to immunocompetent patients with PCNSL, the median age at presentation is much lower in patients who are immunosuppressed. The median age at onset in renal transplant patients is approximately 37 years (Schneck & Penn 1971; Morrison et al 1991) and in AIDS patients approximately 39 years (Snider et al 1983; So et al 1986; Beral et al 1991). In AIDS patients the relative frequency of PCNSL is equal across all age groups (Beral et al 1991). Thus the lower median age at presentation represents the incidence of age-related AIDS cases rather than an intrinsic feature of PCNSL in AIDS patients.

Sex distribution

The distribution of primary central nervous system lymphoma between the sexes is also dependent on the underlying predisposing disease. Thus for PCNSL in immunocompetent patients, only a slight male preponderance has been noted in most large series. Murray et al recorded a male: female ratio of 1.5:1 among the 693 cases reviewed. More recent reports of PCNSL estimate the male: female ratio as ranging between 1:1 and 4:1 (Hochberg & Miller 1988; Brada et al 1990; Socie et al 1990; Neuwelt et al 1991; DeAngelis et al 1992a; Rosenthal et al 1993; Tomlinson et al 1995; Glass et al 1996; Trans-Tasman Radiation Oncology Group 1996; Cher et al 1996; Brada et al 1998; Wagner et al 1998). This slight male predominance mirrors the male predominance noted in systemic lymphomas (DeVita et al 1997).

As a consequence of the AIDS epidemic, a higher ratio of males is developing primary central nervous system lymphoma. Large series of AIDS-related PCNSL (AR-PCNSL) suggest a male: female ratio of approximately 17:1. The relative risk of developing PCNSL in female AIDS patients appears to be lower than for male AIDS patients, with an estimated risk for females of 0.66 in comparison to males (Beral et al 1991). The reason for this discrepancy has not been elucidated.

Racial, national, and geographic factors

The incidence of PCNSL in immunocompetent patients is too low to clearly define a particular racial, national or geographic character. Cases of PCNSL have been reported from centers around the world and the larger series have been reported from most Western countries including the USA, United Kingdom, France, Italy, and Australia as well as Japan. In contrast, there is a clear country to country variation in the incidence and character of systemic NHL (DeVita et al 1997). In immunocompetent patients with either PCNSL or systemic NHL there is no apparent difference in the incidence of disease between whites, African-Americans or Asians.

Beral et al reviewed 538 cases of AR-PCNSL and suggested that Hispanic and white groups have a higher relative risk of developing the disease compared with African-Americans. The relative risks of developing AR-PCNSL for Hispanics, whites and African-Americans were 1.08, 1.0 and 0.61, respectively ($p < 0.05$) (Beral et al 1991).

The incidence of AR-PCNSL is directly linked to the prevalence of HIV infection within a community. Thus, it is not surprising that the incidence of AR-PCNSL is highest in major cities in the USA, with the largest single-institution series reporting AR-PCNSL coming from centers in Los Angeles, San Francisco, and New York (So et al 1986; Baumgartner et al 1990; Goldstein et al 1991). Despite this concentration of cases, AR-PCNSL may arise in any community where HIV infection is present. The relative risk of an AIDS patient developing AR-PCNSL or for that matter AIDS-related systemic lymphoma is not influenced by state of residence or place of birth (Beral et al 1991).

Family history, genetic factors and predisposition to lymphoma

There are no reported cases of familial PCNSL among immunocompetent patients. However, there are a number of factors that may predispose a person to developing lymphoma and, more specifically, PCNSL. Some of these factors are listed below.

1. Congenital immunodeficiency syndromes
   a. Wiskott–Aldrich syndrome
   b. Ataxia-telangiectasia
   c. Severe combined immunodeficiency
   d. X-linked lymphoproliferative syndrome
   e. Chediak–Higashi syndrome
   f. Swiss-type agammaglobulinemia
2. Acquired immunodeficiency syndromes
   a. HIV-associated syndromes
   b. Acquired humoral/cellular deficiencies
3. Immunosuppressive therapy
4. Autoimmune disease
   a. Systemic lupus erythematosus
   b. Rheumatoid arthritis
   c. Sjögren's syndrome
   d. Inflammatory bowel disease
   e. Hemolytic anemia
5. Infectious mononucleosis
6. Infections
   a. HTLV-I
   b. Epstein–Barr virus
7. Miscellaneous
   a. Celiac disease
   b. Previous malignancy
   c. Chemotherapy
   d. Radiation.

There is strong evidence that patients who are immunodeficient are at higher risk of developing systemic lymphoma. Similarly, the risk of PCNSL also appears to be increased in immunodeficient patients. In addition, conditions which result in chronic and low grade antigenic stimulation may predispose to the development of lymphoma, and a number of such conditions have been directly linked to the development of both systemic lymphoma and PCNSL (Riggs & Hagemeister 1988).

It is difficult to be dogmatic about a definite role for these conditions in the development of PCNSL. However, some congenital immunodeficiency syndromes are clearly associated with an increased risk of developing PCNSL. The Wiskott–Aldrich syndrome, for example, has a strong link

with PCNSL; of 78 cases of cancer in Wiskott–Aldrich syndrome patients reported to the Immunodeficiency Cancer Registry, 17.9% had PCNSL (Model 1977; Hutter & Jones 1981; Filopovich et al 1987). This represented 24% of the 59 cases of lymphoma reported in these patients. In comparison, there are no reported cases of PCNSL in patients with ataxia-telangiectasia syndrome, despite 67 cases of systemic lymphoma being recorded in these patients (Filopovich et al 1987).

There is little opportunity to determine the true role that some other conditions play in the pathogenesis of PCNSL. PCNSL has been described in association with Sjögren's syndrome (Talal & Bunim 1964), Immunoglobulin A deficiency (Gregory & Hughes 1973), hyperimmunoglobulin E syndrome (Bale et al 1977), rheumatoid arthritis (Good et al 1978), immune thrombocytopenic purpura (Vogel et al 1968), sarcoidosis (Trillet et al 1982), Kleinfelter's syndrome (Liang et al 1990a), and in patients undergoing immunosuppressive therapy for systemic lupus erythematosus (Lipsmeyer 1972; Woolf & Conway 1987), vasculitis (Jellinger et al 1979) and post-liver transplantation (Kim et al 2009). Cases of PCNSL have also been described in association with progressive multifocal leukoencephalopathy (PML). This rare association may occur in immunosuppressed patients suffering from AIDS, leukemia (GiaRusso & Koeppen 1978) or following renal transplantation (Ho et al 1980). At least one case of PCNSL in association with PML has been described in an immunocompetent patient (Liberski et al 1982).

PCNSL has also been reported as a second malignancy occurring many years after therapy for Hodgkin disease (Yang et al 1986; Miller et al 1989; Davenport et al 1991), systemic small cell lymphocytic lymphoma (Weissman et al 1990), systemic chronic lymphatic leukemia (Richter's syndrome) (O'Neill et al 1989; Ng et al 1991) and cancer of the colon, breast and thyroid, respectively (DeAngelis 1991b). PCNSL has also been described in association with a low-grade astrocytoma (Giromini et al 1981), hepatocellular carcinoma, meningioma and squamous cell carcinoma (Yamasaki et al 1992; Ildan et al 1995). PCNSL has been reported after whole brain irradiation for a low-grade glioma (Stein et al 1995).

An association may exist between PCNSL and prior malignancy for three reasons. First, there may be an underlying and inherent predisposition to cancer. Second, the lymphoma may have resulted as a complication of chemotherapy or irradiation used as therapy for the initial cancer. Finally, patients may be immunologically compromised in association with tumors such as Hodgkin disease, thus predisposing them to second malignancies.

Association with Epstein–Barr virus

The role of the Epstein–Barr virus (EBV) in the pathogenesis of PCNSL in immunocompetent patients has been under increased scrutiny as investigative techniques have improved. Initial reports using the techniques of restriction digests and in situ hybridization record that, in immunocompetent patients, between 5% and 38% of PCNSL tumors contained EBV (Hochberg et al 1983; Murphy et al 1990; Rouah et al 1990; Bignon et al 1991; MacMahon et al 1991; Geddes et al 1992). Using the more sensitive technique of the polymerase chain reaction (PCR), 7 of 13 patients (54%) with PCNSL had EBV incorporated into the tumor genome (DeAngelis et al 1992b). In contrast, Camilleri-Broët et al (1998) detected no evidence of EBV by *in situ* hybridization in 71 patients with PCNSL. At least one case of PCNSL has been reported in a patient who was selectively immunodeficient to the Epstein–Barr virus (Pattengale et al 1979). Corboy et al (1998) demonstrated human herpes virus 8 DNA in 56% of PCNSL cases. There did not appear to be a significant difference in detection of this virus between PCNSL and AR-PCNSL. In contrast, human herpes virus 6 was not detected in PCNSL specimens (Liedtke et al 1995).

The role of Epstein–Barr virus infection in the pathogenesis of AR-PCNSL has also been explored. Camilleri-Broët et al (1997) documented EBV by PCR in almost all of 51 cases of AR-PCNSL. Similarly, in another study, *in situ* hybridization revealed that AR-PCNSL tumors from 21 patients all expressed the EBV early region protein (EBER) and 45% expressed the latent membrane protein (MacMahon et al 1991). The former is indicative of latent infection and the latter is known to have oncogenic properties (Wang et al 1985).

Interestingly, none of nine AIDS patients with other CNS pathology expressed the early region protein (MacMahon et al 1991). A number of smaller studies have also demonstrated a very high frequency of EBV expression in AR-PCNSL (Katz et al 1986; Rosenberg et al 1986; Bashir et al 1989; DeAngelis et al 1992b). Also of note is that only about 40% of patients with systemic AR-NHL have evidence of EBER expression (Subar et al 1988; Meeker et al 1991; Levine 1992). The implication from all these studies is that AIDS-related PCNSL may be directly associated with EBV infection.

Multiple biopsies from different sites in AIDS-related NHL demonstrate single clonal EBV genomic terminus fusion configurations detected at each individual site. This suggests that all tumor cells at that site were infected with a single form of the EBV genome. However, comparisons of sites demonstrated different configurations, suggesting a multiclonal origin of the lymphoma (Cleary et al 1988). Based on Southern blotting techniques, AR-PCNSL are usually monoclonal tumors whereas systemic AR-NHL is frequently polyclonal in nature (Meeker et al 1991).

The role of Epstein–Barr virus remains uncertain in the genesis of post-transplant primary central nervous system lymphoma, although at least one case of post-transplant systemic lymphoma was associated with seroconversion for the Epstein–Barr virus capsid antigen and nuclear antigen (Walker et al 1989). As the Epstein–Barr virus appears to have an established role in the pathogenesis of AR-PCNSL, it would be surprising if the mechanisms were any different for cases of PCNSL arising from other immunodeficient states such as organ transplantation. More recent data have suggested that EBV may play a role in the genesis of PCNSL in immunosuppressed elderly patients. (Kleinschmidt-DeMasters et al 2008).

Sites of predilection

The typical sites of predilection in PCNSL have been well documented. In Murray's series, there was sufficient

Table 41.1 Site of primary central nervous system lymphoma in 434 cases

Location	n	(%)
Supratentorial		
Frontal	60	14
Temporal	34	8
Parietal	32	7.5
Deep nuclei	30	7
Occipital	11	2
Pineal	1	<1
Site not specified	63	15
Infratentorial		
Cerebellum	49	11
Brainstem	10	2
Spinal cord	2	<1
Multiple sites	142	33.5

Adapted from Murray K, Kun L, Cox J 1986 Primary malignant lymphoma of the central nervous system. Results of treatment of 11 cases and review of the literature. Journal of Neurosurgery 65: 600–607.

Table 41.2 Frequency of symptoms at presentation

Symptom	Percentage of cases
Personality change	24
Cerebellar signs	21
Headache	15
Seizures	13
Motor dysfunction	11
Visual changes	8

Adapted from Hochberg F H, Miller D C 1988 Primary central nervous system lymphoma. Journal of Neurosurgery 68: 835–853.

information in 434 cases to determine tumor location (Table 41.1). In his analysis the majority of patients develop a solitary supratentorial tumor (52.1%) but a significant minority has multiple tumor sites (33.5%). The most common sites are: frontal lobe, temporal lobe, parietal lobe, deep nuclei, occipital lobe, cerebellum, and brainstem (Murray et al 1986). Primary leptomeningeal disease has been reported in approximately 8% of PCNSL cases (LaChance et al 1991). Rare examples of dural PCNSL have been described (Jazy et al 1980, Lehrer & McGarry 1968) as has chiasmal PCNSL (Cantore et al 1989).

Presenting features

There are no pathognomonic presenting symptoms or signs in PCNSL. Despite this, typical presenting features have been well described and these features are simply manifestations of the typical disease sites in PCNSL (Table 41.2). In a review of 248 patients, Bataille et al (2000) documented that 70% had focal neurological deficits, 43% had neuropsychiatric symptoms and 33% had symptoms consistent with raised intracranial pressure. The high frequency of frontal lobe involvement results in a common mode of presentation as memory loss, forgetfulness and altered affect. Up to 10–15% of patients with PCNSL present with a seizure (Hochberg & Miller 1988; Tomlinson et al 1995).

Similarly, the signs associated with the presentation of PCNSL can be related to the anatomic site of disease. Thus the most common signs include: motor and sensory deficits, altered visual acuity, diminished visual fields, papilledema, and confusion. Careful analysis of cognitive function frequently reveals significant deficits (Neuwelt et al 1986). In view of the incidence of multiple lesions, it is not surprising that many patients present with a constellation of symptoms and signs. The symptoms and signs at presentation in AR-PCNSL and PCNSL arising in immunodeficient patients do not appear to be different from those in immunocompetent patients with PCNSL. The median time from commencement of symptoms to diagnosis is about 2–3 months although in some cases the time to diagnosis may be as long as 2 years. Some studies have reported a prodrome of respiratory or gastrointestinal illness although this may be incidental (Hochberg & Miller 1988).

Despite the usual manner of presentation, PCNSL initially may manifest itself as an unusual symptom or sign. Within the literature there are reports of PCNSL presenting as pure optic ataxia (Ando & Moritake 1990), steroid responsive optic neuropathy (Purvin & van Dyk 1984), diabetes insipidus (Patrick et al 1989; Layden et al 2009), chronic subdural hematoma (Reyes et al 1990), fever of unknown origin (Salih et al 2009), benign intracranial hypertension (Kori et al 1983), narcolepsy (Onofri et al 1992), parkinsonism and trigeminal neuropathy (Kuntzer et al 1992) and dementia (Carlson 1996). We have seen one patient admitted to a psychiatric ward with a paranoid psychosis before a diagnosis of PCNSL was suggested by a routine CT scan and confirmed at biopsy. PCNSL has been suggested as the most common cause of the rare phenomenon of tumor-induced central neurogenic hyperventilation. The mechanism of action in such cases may be anatomic or humoral. Importantly, patients may respond to therapy, including those patients being mechanically ventilated at the time of diagnosis (Pauzner et al 1989).

The differential diagnosis of PCNSL is extensive. It includes all possible causes of solitary and multiple cerebral mass lesions in immunocompetent and immunosuppressed patients. These include other primary brain tumors, secondary carcinomas and infections. PCNSL may mimic multiple sclerosis, particularly in patients with nonspecific radiologic findings who have a prolonged response to corticosteroid administration. However, the prolonged dependence on corticosteroids should encourage consideration of PCNSL as the possible diagnosis (Ruff et al 1979; DeAngelis 1990).

Imaging diagnosis

Magnetic resonance (MR) imaging is now the radiologic investigation of choice for PCNSL (Fig. 41.1). Despite typical appearances, the findings cannot be construed as diagnostic. The lesions are usually hypointense to isointense on T1-weighted imaging and isointense to hyperintense on T2-weighted images (Schwaighofer et al 1989; Zimmerman 1990; Roman-Goldstein et al 1992; Johnson et al 1997). Higher signal intensity can be achieved following an intravenous injection of gadolinium-DTPA (Zimmerman 1990). The lesions may be multiple and are generally sharply demarcated with a small rim of surrounding edema. The lesions are frequently large, with >75% being >2 cm in diameter but, surprisingly for the size of the lesions, the mass effect may be relatively small (Schwaighofer et al 1989). There appears to be a correlation between the

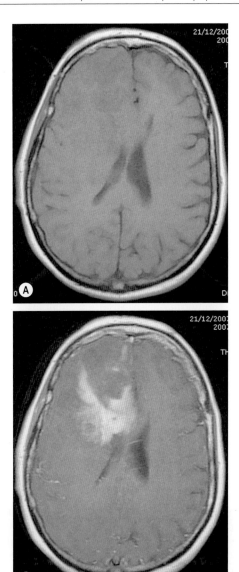

Figure 41.1 (A) T1-weighted non-contrast MRI scan. (B) T1-gadolinium-enhanced MRI scan of the same patient showing PCNSL.

hyperintensity noted on T2-weighted MR appearances and central tumor necrosis (Johnson et al 1997). Differentiation of PCNSL from high grade glioma may be enhanced by the use of dynamic susceptibility contrast-enhanced perfusion magnetic resonance imaging and spectroscopy (Liao et al 2008; Toh et al 2008; Zacharia et al 2008)

Contrast-enhanced computed tomographic (CT) of the brain was previously the standard radiologic technique in the imaging of PCNSL in immunocompetent patients. Although typical appearances have been well described (Enzmann et al 1979; Spillane et al 1982; Thomas & MacPherson 1982; Mendenhall et al 1983; Jack et al 1988; Zimmerman 1990), a definitive diagnosis cannot be made from the scan alone. In one study where experienced radiologists were asked to diagnose a number of solitary brain lesions as seen on CT scan, the diagnosis of PCNSL was correctly made in only 16.7% of cases (Heimans et al 1990).

Characteristically, there is a hyperdense or isodense mass in the cerebrum with associated mild to moderate edema. Multifocal disease is observed in 30–45% of CT scans. The sensitivity of CT scans in PCNSL is very high, with <5% of scans being falsely negative. The site of the lesion is also typical but not diagnostic, with most PCNSL tumors arising in the periventricular region particularly involving the corpus callosum, thalamus and basal ganglia. This is in contrast with secondary cerebral NHL which has a propensity to involve subdural, subarachnoid and epidural spaces as well as the spinal cord (Brant-Zawadzki & Enzmann 1978; Thomas & MacPherson 1982; Zimmerman 1990). There is an excellent correlation between radiologic appearance and pathologic findings with respect to site and extent of macroscopic disease (Thomas & MacPherson 1982; Lee et al 1986; Jack et al 1988).

PCNSL in immunocompetent patients may be confused radiologically with other disease processes. Even the 'typical' appearance may be misdiagnosed as a meningioma, particularly if the lymphoma arises in an unusual site such as the cranial vault (Thomson & Brownell 1981; Agbi et al 1983). PCNSL may also be confused with any other intracranial pathology that produces solitary or multiple enhancing lesions on CT scanning. However, other pathology such as metastatic carcinoma, gliomas or intracerebral infections is suggested by the presence of hypodense lesions, ring enhancement, calcification, hemorrhage or cyst formation (Jenkins & Colquhoun 1998). PCNSL may also appear as a diffuse cerebral infiltration (Furusawa et al 1998).

CT and MR scans are sensitive indicators of the disease. The response to treatment is rapid in PCNSL and, as a consequence, the CT and MR scan appearances may resolve rapidly once therapy is instituted (Schwaighofer et al 1989). Similarly CT and MR scanning may detect relapse early, even prior to a recrudescence of symptoms.

Cerebral angiography has little if any role to play in the diagnosis of PCNSL. Historically, angiography was frequently used as a method of investigation; however, the findings in PCNSL were non-specific. Some studies described avascular masses (Cassady & Wilner 1967; Enzmann et al 1979; Ashby et al 1988a), others described increased capillary circulation (Enzmann et al 1979; Spillane et al 1982) or vessel irregularity (Leeds et al 1971), while others still described no abnormal vascularity (Tallroth et al 1981). No angiographic study demonstrated consistent findings that would suggest a diagnosis of PCNSL. Less invasive modalities such as CT and MR offer more information in PCNSL without the attendant risks of cerebral angiography.

Other imaging techniques remain experimental. ^{123}I-IMP single-photon emission computerized tomography (SPECT) has had a limited role in the diagnosis of brain tumors as sensitivity does not surpass that of CT and MR scans. Usually brain tumors appear as low-density defects, however, in three patients with PCNSL there was high uptake in the delayed image (Ohkawa et al 1989; Kitanaka et al 1992). This result points towards a degree of specificity that may assist in the diagnosis of primary central nervous system lymphoma.

The role of positron emission tomography (PET) in the evaluation of primary central nervous system lymphoma requires further study. There are promising but limited data

regarding the sensitivity and specificity of PET in this disease (Kuwabara et al 1988; Rosenfeld et al 1992; Sawataishi et al 1992; Mohile et al 2008).

Laboratory diagnosis

A careful analysis of the cerebrospinal fluid (CSF) may be diagnostic of primary central nervous system lymphoma (Matsuda et al 1981; Schmitt-Graff & Pfitzer 1983; Lai et al 1991). Concerns regarding raised intracranial pressure may prevent lumbar puncture being performed in some of the patients (Murray et al 1986). In those for whom lumbar puncture is not contraindicated, cytocentrifugation techniques & flow cytometry may increase the cellular yield 60-fold (Hansen et al 1974; Bromberg et al 2007).

The main abnormality in the CSF of patients with PCNSL is a monomorphic population of abnormal lymphocytes consistent with the International Working Formulation descriptions of intermediate and high-grade lymphomas (Rosenberg et al 1982). Immunohistochemistry may assist in the diagnosis by the demonstration of monoclonality. The CSF protein is usually markedly elevated, the CSF glucose is low, and a pleocytosis is found in about 40% of patients (Matsuda et al 1981; Lai et al 1991).

Murray et al (1986) collected information from 12 studies and found that 10% of patients undergoing lumbar puncture had positive CSF cytology at initial presentation. Uncommonly, the initial diagnosis of PCNSL has been made on the basis of CSF cytology alone without cerebral CT scan changes (Schmitt-Graff & Pfitzer 1983; Lai et al 1991). However, more recent data suggest that the incidence of CSF detected disease is higher. Further, examination of CSF with flow cytometry may also assist in the diagnosis of PCNSL (Bromberg et al 2007).

There are no other serum or CSF markers of disease specific for patients with PCNSL. CSF β_2-microglobulin may be a useful marker of occult CNS disease in patients with systemic NHL (Hansen et al 1992) but its role in the management of PCNSL remains to be elucidated. CSF platinum is depleted in PCNSL although this is not specific to this disease. In contrast to leukemia involving the CNS, lymphoma does not result in depletion of CSF manganese (El-Yazigi et al 1990). Finally, CSF protein biomarker identification (proteomic analysis of CSF) may provide improved diagnostic accuracy (Roy et al 2008).

Gross morphologic features

Primary central nervous system lymphoma has pathologic features comparable with the spectrum of systemic lymphoma. However, the macroscopic appearance of PCNSL may vary considerably between patients. Most commonly, PCNSL appears as a solitary, bulky and irregular mass merging into the surrounding edematous brain tissue (Fig. 41.2). The cut surface is yellow-white and granular, and the tumor soft. There may be areas of focal necrosis or hemorrhage but cystic change is rare (O'Neill et al 1987). Multiple lesions occur in up to 30% of patients. On other occasions there may only be poorly-defined expansion of tissue with loss of intrinsic markings (Adams & Howatson 1990).

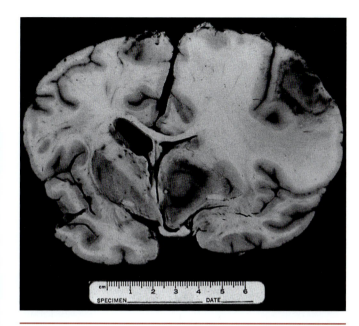

Figure 41.2 Coronal section of brain demonstrating multifocal primary central nervous system lymphoma with associated mass effect.

Table 41.3 Histopathologic classification of NHL according to a working formulation

Grade	Histologic sub-type
Low grade	
A.	Small lymphocytic, consistent with chronic lymphocytic leukemia; plasmacytoid.
B.	Follicular, predominantly small cleaved cell; diffuse areas, sclerosis.
C.	Follicular, mixed, small cleaved and large cell; diffuse areas, sclerosis.
Intermediate grade	
D.	Follicular predominantly large cell; diffuse areas; sclerosis.
E.	Diffuse small cleaved cell.
F.	Diffuse mixed small and large cell; sclerosis; epithelioid component.
G.	Diffuse large cell; cleaved cell, noncleaved cell, sclerosis.
High grade	
H.	Large cell, immunoblastic; plasmacytoid, clear cell, polymorphous, epithelioid component.
I.	Lymphoblastic; convoluted cell, nonconvoluted cell.
J.	Small noncleaved; Burkitt's follicular area.

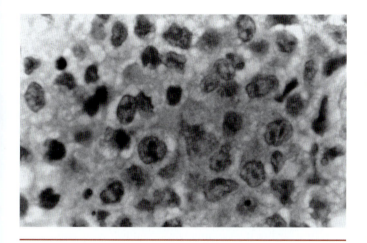

Figure 41.3 High power photomicrograph demonstrating the typical appearance of primary central nervous system lymphoma (large cell type).

Table 41.4 Frequency of PCNSL histopathologic sub-types

Histologic sub-type	Patients (*n* = 61)	
	n	(%)
Large cell immunoblastic	24	39.3
Diffuse large cell	15	24.7
Small cleaved cell	11	18
Large cell (not specified)	6	9.8
Small noncleaved	5	8.2

Adapted from Hochberg F H, Miller D C 1988 Primary central nervous system lymphoma. Journal of Neurosurgery 68: 835–853.

Histopathologic features

Microscopic examination usually demonstrates tumor infiltration well beyond the macroscopic margin. Angiotropism is an important and distinctive histopathological feature (Fig. 41.3). The tumor invades along perivascular spaces with perivascular cuffing and vessel wall infiltration. This cuffing is most prominent at the tumor margin and for a distance beyond (Ashby et al 1988a; Murphy et al 1989). In advanced tumors, there may be a loss of the perivascular relationship (O'Neill et al 1987). There may be an associated astrocytic reaction accompanied by the presence of body macrophages (Ashby et al 1988a). In contrast to gliomas and metastatic tumors, PCNSL does not produce a significant degree of endothelial proliferation in the tumor or adjacent brain.

Multiplication of involved blood vessel basement membranes may be observed (Henry et al 1974). The periphery of the tumor is typically composed of a T-lymphocyte infiltrate with some occasional T-cells seen throughout the tumor itself (Murphy et al 1989). The presence of reactive astrocytes has been described and may mimic a low-grade astrocytoma (Kepes 1987; Adams & Howatson 1990). Demyelinative leukoencephalopathy in association with PCNSL has been noted to occur (Lach et al 1985). This is manifested by large areas of severe myelin loss in proximity to the tumor.

The tumor itself is described and classified according to the International Working Formulation criteria (Rosenberg et al 1982) (Table 41.3). The most common histologic sub-types are diffuse large cell lymphoma and diffuse immunoblastic lymphoma. Higher-grade lymphomas, including Burkitt's lymphoma, have frequently been described but there are no reported cases of follicular sub-types in PCNSL. Many authors have noted the pleomorphic histologic appearance of PCNSL (Taylor et al 1978; Murphy et al 1989). Table 41.4 shows histopathologic sub-types of PCNSL arising in immunocompetent patients from a single institution (Hochberg & Miller 1988).

Diffuse large cell lymphoma is characterized by large lymphoid cells containing abundant cytoplasm, prominent nucleoli and dense nuclear chromatin (Fig. 41.3), while the small non-cleaved cell Burkitt's lymphomas are characterized by uniform cells of moderate size with round to oval nuclei. The nuclei contain numerous and prominent nucleoli and a coarse chromatin pattern; mitoses are frequently seen. The classic 'starry-sky' appearance is notable but not pathognomonic. In comparison, cells of non-Burkitt's small non-cleaved cell lymphoma are typically smaller in size and are more pleomorphic with occasional giant forms and bizarre cell types. Similarly, the prominence and number of nucleoli and the pattern of nuclear chromatin are more varied (DeVita et al 1997).

EM appearance

The electron microscopic (EM) appearance of PCNSL is no different from the appearances described for the sub-types of systemic NHL. The most notable features are tumor cells containing few organelles, abundant free ribosomes, large nucleoli and scant cytoplasm. There is an absence of junctional devices (Hirano 1975; Ishida 1975; Houthoff et al 1978).

Immunological markers

Analysis of tumor cell surface immunoglobulins in PCNSL was initiated in the late 1970s and rapidly found a place in assisting the histopathologists (Taylor et al 1978). Staining for monoclonal B- and T-cell antigens has been performed on frozen and paraffin sections, confirming that almost all cases of PCNSL are of B-cell origin and only rare cases of T-cell lymphoma have been described (Marsh et al 1983; Murphy et al 1989; Aozasa et al 1990; Grant & von Deimling 1990; Camilleri-Broët et al 1998; Dulai et al 2008). In a number of studies, PCNSL were demonstrably B-cell tumors with typical immunoglobulin rearrangements suggesting monoclonality (Smith et al 1988; Albrecht et al 1992). These findings are consistent with those seen in systemic B-cell lymphomas. In addition, the B-cell immunophenotype may be associated with the relatively poor outcome of PCNSL compared with systemic lymphoma (Camilleri-Broët et al 2007).

Molecular genetics

Gene expression profile studies have previously demonstrated that large B cell lymphomas can be subdivided into at least three molecular sub-types, activated B-cell-like type (ABC), germinal center B-cell-like type (GCB) and type 3; these sub-types have been associated with distinct clinical outcomes (Camilleri-Broët et al 2000, 2006).

A multitude of molecular abnormalities have been described in PCNSL. A relationship between the expression of activated P-STAT-6 and outcome in patients treated with high dose methotrexate based chemotherapy has been documented (Rubenstein et al 2006). Bulky tumors with strong expression of activated P-STAT-6 were associated with resistance to methotrexate, suggesting a correlation with IL-4 signaling and tumor aggressiveness. Nevertheless, while the activation marker of phospho P-STAT-6 is related to outcome, no molecular markers have been demonstrated to reproducibly correlate with favorable outcome. There is some speculation that BCL-6 expression has been associated with outcome in this disease, however, few studies showed a positive correlation (Braatan et al 2003; Levy et al 2008), one study showed negative correlation (Chang

et al 2003). Cady et al (2008) observed frequent rearrangements of Chromosome 6 (q22) and BCL6 in PCNSL and suggested a correlation with poorer prognosis. The B cell attracting chemokine CXCL13, has been found to be expressed by the malignant lymphoid cells and the vascular endothelium in PCNSL tumors (Smith et al 2003; Smith et al 2007). Adhesion molecules and matrix metalloproteinases may also play a role in the pathogenesis of PCNSL (Kinoshita et al 2008). These molecular observations may be important and could lead to the development of targeted therapies in PCNSL.

Prognosis

A prognostic index has been developed through the International Extranodal Lymphoma Study Group (Ferreri et al 2003). The index recognizes five factors associated with poorer risk: age >60 years, performance status 2–4, elevated serum LDH, high CSF protein and tumor located in deep regions of the brain. Patients with 0 or 1, 2 or 3, or 4 or 5 of these factors had respective 2-year survivals of 80%, 48%, and 15%.

General management plan

The principles concerning the management of PCNSL revolve around obtaining a histologic diagnosis, ensuring that the disease is confined to the brain, excluding an underlying predisposing illness and instituting definitive therapy.

In order to identify the extent of local disease and to exclude systemic NHL, patients with primary central nervous system lymphoma require appropriate 'staging' investigations. The usual sequence of events is a CT or MR scan followed by a biopsy proving primary central nervous system lymphoma. Having identified the presence of primary central nervous system lymphoma, the delineation of local disease extent requires an examination of the vitreous humor and the CSF. Thus slit lamp examination of the eye and CSF analysis (unless contraindicated) should be performed.

The need to exclude systemic disease is debated by some authors. Hochberg & Miller (1988) argued that none of 66 cases of PCNSL in their institution had systemic disease and therefore further investigations were unnecessary and costly. However, concurrent cerebral and systemic lymphoma has been described, and cases have been reported where the cerebral component predates the systemic component in disseminated NHL (Johnson et al 1984; Haerni-Simon et al 1987; Liang et al 1989; Ferreri et al 1996). Whether this represents distant relapse of the cerebral tumor or progression of concurrent, albeit covert, systemic disease, is difficult to prove. Despite this, most centers at present would perform routine staging investigations in order to exclude systemic disease.

Routine staging includes: a full clinical examination, complete blood count with white cell differentiation and platelet count, serum creatinine, urea and electrolytes, liver function tests, erythrocyte sedimentation rate and lactate dehydrogenase. In addition, the patient should undergo a unilateral bone marrow aspiration and trephination, chest X-ray, and chest, abdominal and pelvic computerized tomographic scans. Testing for evidence of HIV infection is highly recommended.

Although a number of reports have documented the rare phenomenon of spontaneous regression (Weingarten et al 1983; Sugita et al 1988; Weissman et al 1990), primary central nervous system lymphoma has a rapid, relentless and ultimately fatal course if untreated.

If PCNSL is suspected, then the institution of corticosteroid therapy should be delayed until a definitive biopsy has been performed unless cerebral herniation is imminent. The immediate introduction of corticosteroids prior to diagnosis is tempting in the face of symptoms and focal intracerebral lesions. However, the early use of corticosteroids may make histologic assessment difficult due to the exquisite sensitivity of PCNSL to the drug. In fact, radiologic disappearance of the tumor can occur rapidly after the commencement of corticosteroids (Singh et al 1982; Vaquero et al 1984; Hochberg & Miller 1988; DeAngelis 1990; Pirotte et al 1997; Heckman 1998). This response is due to tumor cell lysis rather than the resolution of cerebral edema (Baxter et al 1971; Gametchu 1987). As a consequence of this rapid lysis, cerebral biopsies may be non-diagnostic and may delay or misdirect definitive therapy (Singh et al 1982; Vaquero et al 1984; DeAngelis 1991a). Once the diagnosis has been established, initial therapy with corticosteroids usually consists of dexamethasone at doses of 16–24 mg/day.

Surgical management

It is clear that a definitive diagnosis of PCNSL can only be made from histologic and cytologic examination. The method of biopsy needs to consider both operative risk and the success for obtaining satisfactory specimens allowing accurate diagnosis. The goal of surgery in PCNSL is to obtain tissue for diagnosis with minimum morbidity.

In past years, the diagnostic approach to PCNSL was one of craniotomy with tumor excision or debulking. However, when Murray et al (1986) reviewed the outcome of the 85 patients who underwent surgery alone as reported in the literature to 1986, there was no difference in median survival time as defined by the extent of surgical resection. Moreover, the median survival time for the surgically debulked patients was 1 month, with only one patient surviving beyond 3 years. The recognition that extensive surgery had a very limited role in PCNSL prompted the use of stereotactic biopsy as a means of obtaining tissue for diagnosis.

Stereotactic biopsy of intracranial lesions has an established role in obtaining an accurate histologic diagnosis without the attendant risks of craniotomy (Apuzzo et al 1987; O'Neill et al 1987; Namiki et al 1988; Feiden et al 1990; Sherman et al 1991). Feiden et al (1990) demonstrated that stereotactic brain biopsy is an excellent means of obtaining tissue in order to establish the diagnosis of PCNSL. In 34 patients undergoing stereotactic biopsy, 25 had a clear-cut histologic diagnosis of PCNSL, with the remaining nine having appearances highly suggestive of PCNSL. In a study by Sherman et al (1991), all but one of 15 patients with primary central nervous system lymphoma was diagnosed with tissue obtained from CT-guided stereotactic brain biopsy. In 12 of the 14 patients, sufficient material was obtained to classify the lymphoma according to the working formulation.

Radiotherapy

PCNSL is a radiosensitive tumor with clinical response rates of up to 80%. Not surprisingly, this high response rate translates into increased median survival times in PCNSL patients receiving radiotherapy compared with patients who receive no therapy or surgery alone. In 1974, Henry and colleagues reviewed the survival of 83 patients with PCNSL and reported a median survival time of 3.3 months in untreated patients, 4.6 months in patients treated with surgical excision alone, and, in 21 patients receiving irradiation, a median survival of 15.2 months (Henry et al 1974).

Subsequent reports of radiation therapy confirmed these findings. Berry & Simpson (1981) reported a median survival of 10 months in 21 patients receiving cranial irradiation. Importantly, they documented rapid and sustained clinical improvement in 14 patients. Other studies document median survival times between 14.5 and 40.8 months in those patients receiving cranial irradiation alone for PCNSL (Leibel & Sheline 1987).

Whole brain radiotherapy alone as treatment for PCNSL rarely produces long-term survivors, despite the high response rate and apparent improvement in median survival time. Only a few examples of long-term survival have been documented following cranial radiotherapy (Sagerman et al 1967; Littman & Wang 1975; Leibel & Sheline 1987). When the results of eight separate series reporting radiotherapy alone in patients with PCNSL are combined, the 1-year survival is 66% and the 2-year survival is 43%, with a 5-year survival of only 7% (Leibel & Sheline 1987).

The dose and volume of irradiation required for disease control have not been clearly defined. Murray et al (1986) reviewed dose response in 198 cases. Dose to the primary tumor was: <40 Gy (14.0%), 40–50 Gy (23.1%), >50 Gy (14.3%), and in 38.6%, the dose was not recorded. The median survival of the 54 patients receiving doses of 50 Gy or more to the primary tumor was 17 months compared with a median survival of 15 months in the 144 patients who received <50 Gy. Actuarial 5-year survival was 42.3% and 12.8%, respectively, a statistically significant value of $p < 0.05$. The conclusion from this study was that there was a demonstrable dose-response relationship, resulting in improved longer-term survival in those patients receiving 50 Gy or more to the primary tumor (Murray et al 1986).

Other studies have suggested a similar trend, with increasing doses of radiotherapy associated with delayed time to treatment failure (Berry & Simpson 1981; Michalski et al 1990). An RTOG study attempted to optimize irradiation by delivering 40 Gy to the whole brain with a 20 Gy boost to the tumor plus a 2 cm margin. The results were disappointing, with a median survival from diagnosis of only 12.2 months for the 41 patients enrolled (Nelson et al 1992). Laperriere et al (1998) examined accelerated radiotherapy and documented a median survival of 17 months in a small group of patients. This was considered a disappointing result and was coupled with significant neurotoxicity.

The most appropriate volume of irradiation, like dosage, remains disputed and undefined. Older series point to the incidence of spinal relapse as reason to irradiate the entire neuraxis (Sagerman et al 1967; Rampen et al 1980; Mendenhall et al 1983). The incidence of spinal relapse as the first site of progression has been estimated in older studies to be between 4% and 25% of cases.

Murray et al (1986) estimated that between 1967 and 1985, 6.5% of patients relapsed with positive CSF cytology or overt spinal cord disease. He assessed the radiation volume for 308 patients who were part of his large 1986 review. The volume irradiated included whole brain in 124 patients (40.30%), local tumor in 16 patients (5.2%), and the entire neuraxis in 16 patients (5.2%). Treatment volume was not specified in 152 cases (49.3%). There was no clear relationship between the volume irradiated and survival outcome.

Invariably, patients with spinal relapse also develop cerebral relapse and it is this that creates the most significant problems rather than the spinal disease. Even if one still contends that preventing spinal relapse warrants spinal irradiation, it is clear that the current regimens of intrathecal or intravenous chemotherapy may be adequate for prophylaxis against occult spinal disease. Other arguments against spinal irradiation include the extension of radiation toxicities to other sites and the possibility that spinal irradiation may compromise spinal and pelvic marrow reserve, thus making chemotherapy less tolerable. It is therefore not surprising that the notion of prophylactic spinal irradiation has diminished with time.

While many authors have advocated larger volumes of irradiation, one review, combining data from seven studies, suggested an improved survival time in those patients who received less radiotherapy. Those patients who received radiotherapy to the primary tumor alone had a median survival of 39.4 months compared with 25.3 months in those patients who received whole brain irradiation. As the study rightly points out, this finding may simply represent a bias in patient selection, with those receiving smaller fields representing patients with less extensive tumors (Leibel & Sheline 1987).

Delineation of the current trends in radiotherapy is complicated by the incorporation of chemotherapy into treatment regimens. The dose, volume and timing of radiotherapy vary between studies. In general, most centers irradiate the whole brain to a dose of at least 45 Gy, including a boost to the tumor site, and do not routinely include spinal irradiation. Despite such recommendations, there is no scientific basis for a dogmatic approach when it comes to radiation dose and volume in the therapy of PCNSL.

Complications of radiotherapy

There is increasing evidence regarding toxicity of whole brain irradiation at least at 45 Gy, with a reproducible rate of severe neurotoxicity in up to 50% of all patients (Correa et al 2004) and in at least 75% of patients aged ≥60 years or older (Abrey et al 1998; Blay 1998) that develops within 1 year of completion of irradiation. As a consequence, there is currently a move away from using radiotherapy as first-line treatment in patients >60 years of age.

The complications of cranial irradiation in general have been well described and include acute toxicities such as nausea and vomiting, headache, and local skin reactions. Chronic complications include cerebral necrosis, cataract formation, and cognitive impairment (Leibel & Sheline 1987; Johnson et al 1990). There are no complications of cranial irradiation that are typical or specific to PCNSL. Acute exacerbations of symptoms or signs due to edema associated with the initiation of irradiation have not been described in PCNSL. Radiation necrosis may be indistinguishable from recurrent tumor due to its predilection for the sites commonly involved in PCNSL such as the corpus callosum, basal ganglia, thalamus and deep white matter. As a consequence, focal necrosis may require biopsy for a definitive diagnosis (Merchut et al 1985).

Chemotherapy

Currently, there is no consensus on the optimal treatment of primary central nervous system lymphoma (PCNSL). This is partly due to the lack of randomized clinical trials related to the small numbers and patient heterogeneity. Unlike systemic diffuse large B cell lymphoma, the median survival of patients with PCNSL has not improved over the previous decades (Panageas et al 2005).

Early reports documented the use of intrathecal or intravenous methotrexate as therapy for disease that had recurred following radiotherapy (Herbst et al 1976; Ervin & Canellos 1980) or in patients with systemic disease with intracranial involvement (Pitman & Frei 1977; Skarin et al 1977). Durable complete responses were noted.

Methotrexate-based therapies represent the most effective regimens in the treatment of PCNSL (Blay et al 1998). Radiotherapy alone was the standard of care until the mid-1980s when emerging data showed that the addition of high dose methotrexate to the radiation therapy treatment protocols for PCNSL improved survival (Ferreri et al 1995; Reni et al 1997) but the inclusion of radiotherapy in these treatment protocols continued to cause problems with its long-term adverse effects on cognitive function (Abrey et al 1998; Ferreri et al 2003).

Subsequently, there have been a number of reports demonstrating the value of single agent high-dose IV methotrexate in the treatment of PCNSL. Batchelor et al (2003) reported a response rate of 74%, progression free survival of 12.8 months, and median survival of 55.4 months in their landmark NABBT study; radiotherapy was not used as part of the treatment regimen.

Response rates to MTX-based combination chemotherapy are very high, with most series documenting complete response rates of between 60% and 100%, and the majority achieving response rates >80% but with higher rate of treatment associated mortality and morbidity (Sandor et al 1998).

An apparent plateau in survival has been reached with the current therapy using high-dose methotrexate-based regimens plus whole brain irradiation. This approach results in a median survival of approximately 40 months with a 22% 5-year survival (Abrey et al 1998).

Studies are also exploring the potential role of lower doses of whole brain irradiation as a mean to consolidate methotrexate with good progression free survival and reduced long-term toxicity resulting from the radiotherapy (Shah et al 2007).

There is established evidence for the importance of the use of anti CD-20 monoclonal antibody in combination with CHOP (cyclophosphamide, doxorubicin, vincristine, and prednisone) chemotherapy in the treatment of patients with systemic large B cell lymphoma with a significant improvement in progression free and overall survivals in both elderly and young patients (Coiffier et al 2002; Pfreundschuh et al 2006). There is no evidence of overlapping toxicity with the co-administration of rituximab and high dose methotrexate (Rubenstein et al 2003). As CD20 positive large B cell is the most common sub-type of PCNSL, the use of Rituximab is logical. While penetration of this macromolecule into the CNS is limited, there are several facts that support its use.

During the first month of treatment of PCNSL, the tumor is associated with an abnormal vasculature lacking a normal blood brain barrier; this early compromise occurs as a result of tumor cell angiotropism (Fig. 41.4) and by the elaboration of cytokines that lead to increased permeability (Rubenstein et al 2002). Rituximab can reproducibly be detected in the CSF of patients with PCNSL who are treated systemically with this drug (Rubenstein et al 2003; Stern 2005). Rituximab has been recently added to some treatment protocols with encouraging preliminary results (Shah et al 2007). A randomized trial will be required to confirm these results.

One approach in the treatment of PCNSL is blood brain barrier (BBB) disruption. The aim of such therapy is to improve tumor penetration by chemotherapeutic drugs and monoclonal antibodies including rituximab and as a consequence improve their efficacy. In the setting of PCNSL, BBB permeability may only be modest and non-uniform (Neuwelt et al 1982; Rapoport 1988; Blasberg et al 1990). In addition, as the tumor responds to chemotherapy, the integrity of the BBB may be restored and, as a consequence, the access of systemically delivered drugs to the tumor may be diminished. Neuwelt et al (1991) utilized intra-arterial mannitol to disrupt the BBB in patients with PCNSL and followed this with a year-long protocol consisting of methotrexate, cyclophosphamide, procarbazine, and dexamethasone (Neuwelt et al 1991). Patients did not receive cranial radiotherapy as part of their primary therapy. The median survival of 44.5 months for the 17 patients undergoing this therapy compared very favorably with a concurrent cohort of 11 patients who underwent RT alone and who had a median survival of

17.8 months ($p = 0.039$). The procedure nevertheless is physiologically stressful, associated with significant acute toxicities including strokes and is contraindicated in the presence of a mass effect.

Toxicity of chemotherapy

The acute and chronic toxicities of chemotherapeutic agents have been well-documented (Chabner & Lango 1996). The type and severity of toxicity is dependent on the drug regimen, and most side-effects can be predicted. Acute side-effects include myelosuppression, mucositis, alopecia, and nausea and vomiting. These toxicities are usually self-limiting and are rarely severe in the context of treating PCNSL.

Long-term side-effects have been more keenly considered in view of the advances in treating PCNSL with the resultant improvements in disease-free and overall survival. Chronic side-effects may impinge significantly on a patient's quality of life. Long-term sequelae of chemotherapy include secondary malignancy (secondary to alkylating agents), anthracycline-induced cardiomyopathy, pulmonary fibrosis, and infertility in younger patients (Chabner & Lango 1996).

When treating PCNSL, a major concern is the effect of therapy on cognitive function. Cranial irradiation may result in major or minor deteriorations in cognitive function, and post-irradiation intrathecal methotrexate results in a higher incidence of leukoencephalopathy with consequent neuropsychological impairment (Allen et al 1980; Sheline et al 1980; Crossen et al 1992; Wagner et al 1998). To a lesser degree, mental state deterioration may occur with other single agent or combination regimens in conjunction with radiotherapy (Turrisi 1980; Johnson et al 1990; Correa et al 2004; Correa et al 2008).

The incidence of thromboembolism may be increased in PCNSL. A retrospective review of 55 patients recorded 10 cases (18%) of thromboembolic complications including two instances of pulmonary embolism (Thorin & DeAngelis 1991). In one series of 12 patients, one fatal case of pulmonary embolism was documented (Rosenthal et al 1993). The cause of thrombotic disease in these patients is no doubt multifactorial and stems particularly from typical postoperative risks, the hypercoagulable state associated with malignancy and the prothrombotic effects of some chemotherapeutic agents (Lazzato & Schafer 1990).

This is a worrisome complication for the clinician due to the risk of intracerebral bleeding occurring with anticoagulant therapy. This risk may be increased in patients with PCNSL due to the highly vascular and vasocentric characteristics of this tumor. Despite this theoretical risk, no intracerebral bleeding complications appear to have occurred in those patients treated for thrombotic disease (Thorin & DeAngelis 1991).

Advances in chemotherapy and supportive care

New approaches to the primary therapy of de novo PCNSL are expanding. In particular, there is increasing interest in agents such as rituximab and temozolomide that have demonstrable activity in this disease (Omuro et al 2007; Pfreundschuh et al 2006). Similarly, high-dose chemotherapy with autologous hematopoietic stem cell transplantation has been evaluated as first-line treatment in PCNSL (Brevet et al 2005;

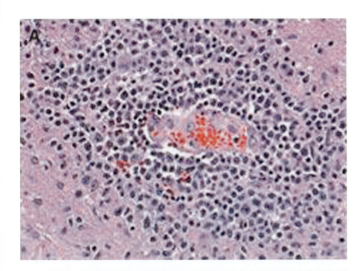

Figure 41.4 Angiotropism in PCNSL.

Illerhaus et al 2006). A variety of strategies using high dose methotrexate, alone or in combination in induction followed by BEAM or thiotepa in conditioning have emerged. The largest study enrolled 30 patients (Illerhaus et al 2006). The induction regimen included HDMTX, Ara-C and Thiotepa, the conditioning consisted of thiotepa, BCNU and WBRT. The response rate was 65%, and after 63 months F/U the 3-year OS was 87%. The treatment related mortality was 3%.

Despite the high response rates (64–82%) in the published data; the overall survival is still low and ranges between 55% and 87%. The treatment related mortality is as high as 26%.

Management of associated phenomena

One of the striking radiologic features of PCNSL is the relative lack of edema and mass effect despite large tumor masses. Thus associated phenomena such as raised intracranial pressure and hydrocephalus are uncommon. Even if present, rapid resolution of such complications occurs due to the exquisite sensitivity of PCNSL to steroids, chemotherapy and radiotherapy.

In the uncommon circumstance, where the histologic diagnosis is known and associated complications mandate urgent intervention, definitive therapy should be introduced immediately. The choice of irradiation or chemotherapy in such circumstances should be predicated by availability, experience and personal prejudice rather than documented superior efficacy of one modality over the other in this situation. Corticosteroids will add to the acute resolution of symptoms.

In the very rare circumstance where a histologic diagnosis has not been made and associated complications mandate urgent intervention, the introduction of parenteral corticosteroids results in rapid tumor lysis and may negate the need for any further acute treatment. A biopsy of the lesion should be performed as soon as possible following recovery in order to obtain a histologic diagnosis.

Patterns of failure

The majority of patients with PCNSL eventually relapse. In a review of older series, the reported relapse rates ranged from between 60% and 80% (Loeffler et al 1985). With the advent of chemotherapy as part of primary therapy, more recent series have documented a lower relapse rate of between 0% and 50% but with considerably shorter follow-up (Gabbai et al 1989; Shibamoto et al 1990; Socie et al 1990; Neuwelt et al 1991; DeAngelis et al 1992a; Rosenthal et al 1993; Tomlinson et al 1995; Glass et al 1996; Trans-Tasman Radiation Oncology Group 1996; Cher et al 1996; Brada et al 1998; Wagner et al 1998).

Relapse can be separated into four typical sites: intracerebral, spinal, ocular and systemic. Many authors would argue that the patterns of relapse are, to an extent, determined by the type of initial therapy. Thus patients receiving whole brain irradiation alone may be more susceptible to spinal and systemic relapse than those who receive adjunctive spinal irradiation or chemotherapy. However, the incidence of spinal and systemic relapse is so low when compared

with intracerebral failure that such assertions remain unproven in the face of such small patient numbers.

Reviews of large series of patients prior to the routine introduction of chemotherapy document the main site of relapse as intracerebral. Up to 90% of relapses are confined to the brain. Nelson et al (1992) combined data from a number of series and noted that spinal cord relapse occurred in only 4% of 254 patients, and the incidence of distant systemic relapse was 7%.

A number of distant sites of relapse have been reported. These include the mediastinum, lung, kidney, testis, and myocardium (Benjamin & Case 1980; Loeffler et al 1985). Systemic 'relapse' may in truth represent progression of what always was systemic disease rather than distant relapse of PCNSL. Older studies did not have the luxury of CT or MR scans in order to detect small volume systemic disease; as a consequence, what was called PCNSL with systemic relapse may have been systemic NHL with intracerebral disease as its initial manifestation. Despite this semantic concern, it should be possible to document the sequence of PCNSL followed by systemic relapse through thorough staging at initial diagnosis.

There are no clearly documented variables that significantly alter prognosis in PCNSL. Pollack et al (1989) performed a multivariate analysis for prognostic factors on a series of PCNSL patients. Their findings suggested that prolonged survival was associated with age <60 years, good performance status, and presence of hemispheric tumor alone, therapy that included cranial radiotherapy to a dose of at least 40 Gy and the addition of chemotherapy. These data must be seen in the light of being based on only 27 patients and over a 10-year period. On the other hand, when Neuwelt et al (1991) analyzed their survival data, the only significant variable appeared to be performance status.

Blay et al (1998) performed a multivariate analysis in order to assess prognostic factors influencing the survival of 53 immunocompetent patients with PCNSL. The findings suggested that the following features resulted in a longer survival: CSF protein <0.6 g/L, good performance status and treatment with high dose methotrexate. This study is replicated by a large retrospective analysis of 226 patients in whom the prognostic factors on multivariate analysis included: age, performance status, CSF protein and treatment with high dose methotrexate (Wagner et al 1998). Tomlinson et al (1995) performed a multivariate analysis on 89 patients with PCNSL and proposed four unfavorable prognostic factors: age >60 years, history of cancer in 1st-degree relatives, focal deficit and ependymal contact. Interestingly, the use of chemotherapy was not associated with a survival benefit.

Data from studies of other intracerebral tumors and systemic NHL may lead to intuitive assumptions as to the outlook for a particular patient with PCNSL. In patients with systemic NHL, unfavourable prognostic features include increasing age, poor performance status, elevated LDH, aggressive histologic sub-types, disease extent, and failure to achieve a complete response following primary therapy (Shipp et al 1992). One may reasonably consider that these criteria are likely to influence prognosis in patients with PCNSL, however, it remains unresolved whether these criteria can truly be applied to PCNSL.

Management of recurrent disease

There are no clear guidelines as to second-line therapy, either for relapsed or resistant disease (Reni et al 1999). Previously, patients would be treated with cranial irradiation primarily and if disease recurred or persisted, chemotherapy could be instituted as second-line therapy. However, as most patients now receive chemotherapy primarily, the options for second-line therapy are reduced in the setting of relapsed disease. High-dose WBRT, is associated with a good response rate but a poor overall survival. Nguyen and colleagues documented a response rate in 20/27 patients given WBRT following relapse, but the survival was 10.9 months (Nguyen et al 2005). Other studies have demonstrated that salvage WBRT may provide significant disease control (Hottinger et al 2007; Plotkin et al 2004).

Reinduction with chemotherapy using HDMTX, CVP or novel chemotherapeutic agents, such as temozolomide and topotecan, has been attempted. The most effective strategy was using single agent HDMTX (≥ 3 g/m^2) by Plotkin et al (2004); 20 of 22 patients responded, overall survival following first relapse was 61.9 months. Soussain et al (2008) published encouraging results using salvage chemotherapy and autologous peripheral stem cell transplantation, while others have reported small studies and case reports of salvage therapies, including temozolomide or intrathecal rituximab (Enting et al 2004; Reni et al 2007; Rubenstein et al 2008).

Management outcome

Long-term survival with PCNSL was rare prior to the advent of routine chemotherapy treatment. In 1986, Murray and colleagues documented 56 of 693 cases (8%) who had survived longer than 3 years; of these only 21 (3%) had survived for more than 5 years. The longest survival time was 16.5 years in an infant diagnosed at age 2 months.

Since the introduction of chemotherapy, the long-term outlook for patients with PCNSL has improved. Recent chemotherapy series recorded disease-free survival of between 40% and 100% over periods of time ranging from 4 months to 5 years (Table 41.5). In most of these studies, the median survival is at least 2 years, with one long-term follow-up study documenting a median survival of 42 months and a 5-year survival of 22.3% (Abrey et al 1998). Although these findings are promising, nearly 50% of long-term survivors relapse between 5 and 12.5 years after diagnosis (Murray et al 1986). Thus, the frequency of late relapse in PCNSL dictates that care must be taken before an individual is pronounced cured or a particular regimen is said to be curative.

Aids-related primary central nervous system lymphoma (AR-PCNSL)

In the early 1980s, an increase in aggressive NHL was linked to risk groups for AIDS (Ziegler et al 1982; Ziegler et al 1984; Ross et al 1985). Shortly after, a definitive relationship between AIDS and NHL was established and, in 1985, disseminated high-grade lymphoma and PCNSL were included in the Centers for Disease Control (CDC) definition of AIDS (Centers for Disease Control 1985). Currently, NHL accounts for approximately 3% of newly diagnosed AIDS cases and represents the second most common malignancy in AIDS patients following Kaposi's sarcoma. The relative risk of developing NHL in AIDS patients is 60 times greater than in the normal population and, in patients under 20 years, the relative risk rises to a 360-fold increase (Beral et al 1991; DeWeese et al 1991; Rabkin et al 1991).

AIDS-related NHL (AR-NHL) has a typical but not pathognomonic clinicopathological pattern. These typical

Table 41.5 Response rate, progression-free survival and overall survival with different treatment regimens for primary central nervous system (CNS) lymphoma

Study	Patients (n)	Regimen	Response rate (CR+PR) (%)	Median PFS (months)	Median OS (months)
Radiotherapy alone					
Nelson et al 1992	41	40 Gy WBRT with 20 Gy boost	NA[a]	NA	12.1
Shibamoto et al 2005	132	40 Gy WBRT	NA	NA	18
Chemo-radiotherapy					
Abrey et al 2000	52	MPV (MTX 3.5 g/m^2), cytarabine (3 g/m^2) IT MTX $\pm$ 45 Gy WBRT	94	NA	60
Ferreri et al 2001	13	MPV (MTX 3 g/m^2) + 36–45 Gy WBRT with boost	92	NA	≥ 25
DeAngelis et al 2002	102	MPV (MTX 2.5 g/m^2) + IT MTX + 36–45 Gy WBRT	94	24	36.9
Poortmans et al 2003	52	MTX (3 g/m^2)/teniposide/carmustine + IT MTX + IT cytarabine + 30 Gy WBRT with 10 Gy boost	81	NA	46
Omuro et al 2005	17	MTX (1 g/m^2)/thiotepa/procarbazine + IT MTX + 41.4 Gy WBRT with 14.4 Gy boost	88	18	32
Multidrug chemotherapy without radiotherapy					
Abrey et al 2000[b]	22	MPV (MTX 3.5 g/m^2), cytarabine (3 g/m^2), IT MTX	NA	NA	33
Pels et al 2003	65	MTX (5 g/m^2) + cytarabine (3 g/m^2) + ifosfamide/vinca-alkaloids/ cyclophosphamide + IT MTX + IT cytarabine	71	21	50
Hoang-Xuan et al 2003[b]	50	MTX (1 g/m^2) + lomustine/procarbazine + IT MTX + IT cytarabine	71	21	50
Single agent MTX					
Batchelor et al 2003	25	MTX (8 g/m^2)	74	12.8	≥ 22.8
Herrlinger et al 2005	37	MTX (8 g/m^2)	35	10	25

Adapted from DeAngelis 2006.
PFS, progression-free survival; OS, overall survival; IT, intrathecal; MPV, methotrexate, procarbazine, vincristine; MTX, methotrexate; NA, not available; PFS, progression-free survival; WBRT, whole-brain radiotherapy; [a]After excluding patients with disease progression during radiotherapy, 26 patients were assessed by CT: 62% had a complete response (CR), 19% an almost CR and 19% a partial response; [b]Patients over age 60.

features of AR-NHL differ from NHL in the general population on a number of accounts, including the frequency of presentations with disseminated or extranodal disease and the markedly increased proportion of high-grade NHL. Concurrent CNS involvement is more common in AR-NHL and has been described in up to 50% of AIDS patients with NHL. Finally, there is a significant increase of PCNSL in AIDS patients (Snider et al 1983; Ziegler et al 1984; Gill et al 1985; Monfardini et al 1990; Beral et al 1991; Hamilton-Dutoit et al 1991).

AIDS-related primary central nervous system lymphoma (AR-PCNSL) has rapidly become a significant clinical problem. In 1988, Levy and colleagues (1985) reviewed 1286 adults with AIDS and found that PCNSL was the presenting diagnosis in 0.6% of these patients and a further 1.9% eventually developed PCNSL. Baumgartner et al (1990) estimated that, by 1986, AR-PCNSL had become more common than PCNSL in immunocompetent patients and that, by 1991, AR-PCNSL would be more common than low-grade astrocytomas and almost as common as meningiomas. The number of AIDS patients who develop intracerebral NHL may in fact be much higher. A number of cases occur after the initial diagnosis of AIDS and as a consequence may not be reported to centers collating epidemiologic data such as the Centers for Disease Control. In addition, up to 84% of AR-PCNSL are only diagnosed at autopsy (MacMahon et al 1991).

Of 2824 cases of AR-NHL diagnosed among the 97 258 cases of AIDS who were reported to the Centers for Disease Control prior to July 1989, 548 were PCNSL (19.4%) (Beral et al 1991). The relative risk of developing PCNSL in AIDS patients was at least 1000 times greater than in the normal population. Other centers have reported similar findings, reporting that PCNSL represented between 18% and 42% of all NHL cases in their own series of HIV-infected patients (Ziegler et al 1982; Monfardini et al 1988; Formenti et al 1989; Ioachim et al 1991).

Gail et al (1991) predicted that between 8% and 27% of US lymphoma cases in 1992 would occur as a result of HIV infection. The reasons for this are two-fold. First, the absolute number of HIV-infected patients continues to increase and, second, prolonged survival with the use of antiretroviral agents and better control of opportunistic infections renders an HIV-infected patient more likely to develop lymphoma.

A number of studies suggest that the risk of developing NHL increases with time. Pluda et al (1990) assessed the risk of developing NHL in patients receiving zidovudine antiviral therapy. After 24 months of therapy, the probability of developing lymphoma was 12% while at 3 years the actuarial probability was 29%. In comparison, a study of 1030 patients treated with zidovudine noted a much smaller rise in the risk of developing NHL (3.2% at 2 years) (Moore et al 1991). Although the absolute risk of developing lymphoma is difficult to ascertain there appears no doubt that the longer an HIV-infected patient lives, the more likely he or she is to develop NHL. One can only speculate as to whether a comparable increase will occur in the incidence of AR-PCNSL.

The influence of new therapeutic strategies such as the use of protease inhibitors has clearly altered the natural history of HIV-related illness. These agents have reduced the morbidity and mortality associated with AIDS. Specifically, the incidence of opportunistic infections and AIDS related

malignancy have declined (Palella et al 1998). Their influence on the incidence of AR-PCNSL remains uncertain at this time.

Presentation

The clinical features of AR-PCNSL closely resemble those of PCNSL in immunocompetent patients (Gill et al 1985; So et al 1986; Formenti et al 1989; Baumgartner et al 1990; Goldstein et al 1991). The most striking differences include the much younger age at presentation and the poor outcome in AR-PCNSL. Other features that may distinguish the two entities are the higher incidence of B symptoms and poorer performance status in those with AR-PCNSL (Diamond et al 1990; Remick et al 1990). The incubation period between HIV infection and development of lymphoma is approximately 50 months, a similar period to the AIDS-defining opportunistic infections (Beral et al 1991). The means of acquiring HIV infection does not appear to influence the risk of developing AR-PCNSL (Beral et al 1991).

The frequent presence of concurrent or alternative intracerebral pathology makes diagnosis difficult. Central nervous system disease is a frequent manifestation of AIDS, with significant neurologic symptoms developing in 40% of AIDS patients at some point in their disease. Up to 10% of AIDS patients present with a neurologic disorder as the initial manifestation of their disease (Snider et al 1983; Moskowitz et al 1984; Levy et al 1985) and autopsy studies reveal the presence of CNS pathology in 55–95% of AIDS patients (Moskowitz et al 1984; Levy et al 1985).

Radiology

The CT scan appearance of AR-PCNSL may be quite different to that of PCNSL occurring in non-immunosuppressed patients. Typically, the lesions are large and centrally hypodense with ring or target enhancement and have associated edema with mild mass effect (Sze et al 1987; Poon et al 1989). Lee et al (1986) demonstrated a consistent correlation between the ring enhancement and central hypodensity with the pathologic appearance of central necrosis and preservation of viable tumor cells at the periphery. In 30–40% of cases, the disease is multicentric, with multiple lesions seen on CT or MR scans (Lee et al 1986; Sze et al 1987; Poon et al 1989). One study suggests that a focal enhancing mass with subependymal spread and hyperattenuation on non-enhanced CT scan were the most reliable features in distinguishing AR-PCNSL and toxoplasmosis (Dina 1991). Despite such observations and the dramatic appearances on CT scan, AR-PCNSL cannot be confidently diagnosed by scan alone.

The use of CT scans in the imaging of AR-PCNSL is associated with a small but significant incidence of false negative findings. A number of studies have reported normal CT scans in patients who have demonstrable disease on MR imaging or at autopsy (So et al 1986; Levy et al 1985; Sze et al 1987). In one study, 7% of AR-PCNSL not seen on CT scans was diagnosed at autopsy shortly afterwards (Ciricillo & Rosenblum 1990). The MR scan appearance in patients with AR-PCNSL is also nonspecific. Typical findings are poorly defined regions of reduced intensity on T1-weighted images that become high intensity on T2-weighted images

(Sze et al 1987). Magnetic resonance imaging is more sensitive than CT scanning in locating intracranial lesions later identified at autopsy (Jarvik et al 1988; Ramsay & Geremia 1988; Ciricillo & Rosenblum 1990; Kupfer et al 1990). Despite its apparent increased sensitivity, MR imaging may still provide rare false negative results (Kupfer et al 1990).

The ability to diagnose AR-PCNSL by CT or MR scans is complicated by the presence of concurrent intracranial pathology. Intracranial toxoplasmosis, for example, also appears on CT and MR scans as multiple, bilateral ring or nodular enhancing lesions with mild to moderate edema and mass effect. These lesions are frequently located at the corticomedullary junction and basal ganglia, as are the lesions of AR-PCNSL (Lee et al 1986; Poon et al 1989; Kupfer et al 1990). Although CT and MR scans are regarded as nonspecific, solitary lesions are more likely to represent AR-PCNSL while multiple lesions are more typical of toxoplasmosis. In one study of 17 solitary lesions on MR scan, 12 (71%) were PCNSL compared with 34% of multiple lesions (Ciricillo & Rosenblum 1990).

Confusingly, multiple lesions may represent dual pathology (Levy et al 1985) and most authors caution against making scan-based diagnoses and encourage biopsy of the lesion if the clinical situation warrants such a procedure. Thus, the CT and MR scan appearances of AR-PCNSL are not only at variance with the appearances of PCNSL in non-immunosuppressed patients but also are essentially indistinguishable from toxoplasmosis and in some circumstances other intracranial pathology. Despite this, newer studies show promise in distinguishing between these two entities using perfusion MR or Thallium-201 SPECT scans (Ernst et al 1998; Kessler et al 1998). Interestingly, recent data document a significant fall in the incidence of cerebral toxoplasmosis in these patients and a three fold rise in AR-PCNSL between 1991 and 1996 (Ammassari et al 1998).

When AIDS-related systemic lymphoma spreads to the CNS, it predominantly involves meningeal invasion rather than parenchymal disease. In these circumstances CT and MR scans are usually unhelpful. On the rare occasions when systemic disease also involves the cerebral parenchyma, the CT and MR scan appearances are the same as for AR-PCNSL (Sze et al 1987). Other sites of disease have been recorded including epidural lesions resulting in cord compression (Snider et al 1983; Ziegler et al 1984).

Laboratory diagnosis

CSF analysis is rarely helpful in the diagnosis of AR-PCNSL. Many studies report non-specific findings such as an elevated protein level, pleocytosis and hypoglycorrhachia. However, it is rare to demonstrate diagnostic cytological abnormalities, despite cytocentrification and immunohistochemical techniques (So et al 1986).

Pathology

HIV infection itself may be considered as a prelymphomatous state. HIV infection causes B-cell activation resulting in elevated levels of serum immunoglobulins and circulating immune complexes (Schnittman et al 1986). B-cell proliferation occurs as a response to the mitogenic properties of HIV with or without the release of cytokines such as interleukin

6 and 10 or in an antigen-specific manner (Benjamin et al 1991; Pluda et al 1991; Bower 1992; Roithmann & Andrieu 1992). Other factors may also be involved in the pathogenesis of AIDS-related NHL including p53 mutations (Gaidano et al 1991) and secondary non-random chromosomal abnormalities of band 13q34 (Berger et al 1989). There is no evidence to suggest that HIV itself may be directly responsible for the malignant transformation of B lymphocytes. The molecular components of HIV have not been demonstrated in AIDS-related NHL, either by Southern blot analysis or polymerase chain reaction (Levine 1992).

AR-PCNSL may involve any region of the brain. Most commonly the disease involves the cerebral hemispheres, cerebellum and brainstem. Concurrent leptomeningeal involvement has been frequently described, in contrast with non-AR-PCNSL where meningeal involvement is rare (Gill et al 1985; So et al 1986). The macroscopic appearance of the disease is indistinguishable from non-AR-PCNSL, however the tumor is more commonly multicentric and frequently larger in size and with lesions >3 cm in diameter being recorded (Gill et al 1985; MacMahon et al 1991).

In AR-PCNSL, the most common pathologic sub-types are immunoblastic and diffuse large B cell lymphomas, with a smaller percentage of Burkitt's lymphomas (Gill et al 1985; So et al 1986; Baumgartner et al 1990; Goldstein et al 1991; MacMahon et al 1991; Raphael et al 1991; Levine 1992). Some authors have noted the pleomorphic nature of these tumors, with a spectrum of cell type varying between small-cleaved cells to large immunoblasts (So et al 1986). As a consequence, it may not be possible to accurately define the Working Formulation Classification for a particular tumor.

The spectrum of pathologic sub-types in AR-PCNSL distinguishes it from systemic AR-NHL, in which 80–90% of tumors is high-grade with almost 30% being Burkitt's lymphoma (Kaplan et al 1989; Hamilton-Dutoit et al 1991; Roithmann & Andrieu 1992). This compares to an expected incidence of high-grade tumors in non-AIDS systemic NHL of 10–15% (Rosenberg et al 1982). In systemic AR-NHL, tumors are uncommonly of intermediate grade and only rare examples of low-grade tumors have been reported (Levine 1992).

Immunohistochemical studies have demonstrated that AR-PCNSL are B-cell-derived tumors (So et al 1986; Roithmann & Andrieu 1992). T-cell systemic NHL has been described in AIDS patients but their incidence does not appear to be increased beyond the expected values for non-AIDS populations. Similarly, there have been occasional cases reported of mycosis fungoides, lymphoblastic lymphoma, HTLV-1-associated T-cell leukemia and T-cell lymphoma but there is no apparent increase in incidence in AIDS patients (Levine 1992). There is no evidence that these uncommon tumors are disproportionately represented in AR-PCNSL.

Burkitt's lymphoma accounts for one-third of AIDS-related systemic NHL (Ziegler et al 1984; Bower 1992; Roithmann & Andrieu 1992) and between 20% and 50% of AR-PCNSL (So et al 1986; Baumgartner et al 1990). It differs from the other AR-NHL sub-types in two ways. First, it may arise at all stages of the disease, including patients with normal levels of helper lymphocytes (CD4 cells). In one study, the median CD4 cell count at diagnosis was 266 (range

28–1198) compared with other AIDS-related NHLs, such as diffuse large B cell lymphoma, where the median figure was significantly less at 112 (range 0–1125) (Roithmann et al 1991). Second, Burkitt's lymphoma in AIDS patients more commonly arises as the first manifestation of the AIDS syndrome than other classifications of NHL (Boyle et al 1990; Roithmann et al 1991).

The typical chromosomal translocation t(8,14) is present in almost all AIDS-related Burkitt's lymphomas, although the less common translocations of t(2,8) and t(8,22) have also been described (Whang-Peng et al 1984; Roithmann & Andrieu 1992). Further analysis of trans-location breakpoints demonstrates that in most cases of AIDS-related NHL, the breakpoints occur within the first exon of the *myc* gene on chromosome 8 and the switch region lying between joining regions of the immunoglobulin H gene on chromosome 14. These molecular findings define AIDS-related Burkitt's lymphoma as typical of the sporadic form of this disease rather than the endemic form found in Africa (Subar et al 1988; Shiramizu et al 1991).

Management plan

The management of AR-PCNSL is determined primarily by the status of the patients' AIDS. Institution of highly active anti-retroviral therapy (HAART) may result in effective therapy (Aboulafia et al 2007). However, in patients who are already on HAART, the management of AR-PCNSL requires an acknowledgement that therapy is palliative, not curative. It is therefore paramount to carefully consider the patient's performance status and likely outcome from any concurrent AIDS-related illness. The aims of therapy should be to alleviate symptoms. As a consequence of therapy, some patients may live longer.

Extending survival should not be at the expense of a patient's quality of life although there are no clear-cut guidelines to distinguish the patients who should be treated aggressively from those in whom such treatment is inappropriate. Despite these caveats, it is clear that a patient presenting with PCNSL, a normal CD4 count and an otherwise excellent performance status needs to be approached differently from a moribund patient with PCNSL and end-stage concurrent opportunistic infections.

Radiotherapy

Radiotherapy as treatment for AR-PCNSL has been addressed by a number of studies (Table 41.6). Cranial irradiation regularly provides clinical and radiologic responses in these patients; however, response duration is brief, with a median survival <5 months overall and in some studies <3 months (Rosenblum et al 1988; Formenti et al 1989; Baumgartner et al 1990; DeWeese et al 1991; Goldstein et al 1991; Donahue et al 1995). More recent studies still recommend WBRT as the standard of care for AR-PCNSL (Newell et al 2004).

No adequate dose-response studies have been performed, thus the dose administered varies between studies and remains speculative. Some studies have attempted to assess the efficacy of different doses of radiotherapy in the setting of AR-PCNSL but the findings are inconsistent. In some studies, higher doses of irradiation resulted in an

Table 41.6 Radiotherapy in AIDS-related PCL

Study author	Year	Cases (n)	Dose (rads)	Median survival (months)
Donahue et al	1995	32	3000	2.1
Goldstein et al	1991	17	3500	2.4
DeWeese et al	1991	7	3000	2.2
Baumgartner et al	1990	55	4000	3.9
Formenti et al	1989	10	4200	5.5
Rosenblum et al	1988	7	4057	3.1

Adapted from DeWeese et al (1991).

apparent prolongation of survival (Formenti et al 1989). Other studies have suggested that survival was dependent on performance status at presentation and that patients with good performance status were selected to receive higher doses of radiotherapy (Goldstein et al 1991).

In view of the palliative nature of this therapy, irradiation should be given over as short a period as possible. Thus some authors have reasonably recommended that patients with poor performance status should receive 30 Gy over 2 weeks (Cooper 1989) or even a more rapid fractionation of 20–25 Gy over 1 week (Goldstein et al 1991). In patients with excellent performance status and no concurrent opportunistic infections, it may be reasonable to treat with higher doses in more protracted fractionation regimens.

Comparisons between AR-PCNSL and PCNSL in non-immunocompromised patients suggest that the AIDS patients have fewer responses to irradiation, less satisfactory symptom relief and significantly shorter survival times (Formenti et al 1989; DeWeese et al 1991). Some authors have even questioned the benefit of such time-consuming and ineffective therapy in patients with such a poor prognosis (DeWeese et al 1991).

Chemotherapy

Chemotherapy has rarely been used in the treatment of AR-PCNSL. Although the addition of systemic or intrathecal chemotherapy may complement cranial irradiation, there is no evidence for its efficacy in this disease. In the face of severe immunodeficiency associated with AIDS, the additional immunodeficiency burden created by chemotherapy may limit its use. Chemotherapy may be indicated in the subset of patients with excellent performance status, relatively normal levels of helper T cells and those who have no evidence of concurrent opportunistic infections.

Survival

Despite attempts to treat these patients, the prognosis is very poor. In one review of 247 patients with AR-PCNSL, the median survival was <3 months, with a longest reported survival time of 28 months (Remick et al 1990). Patients die from either uncontrollable progression of lymphoma or as a consequence of other AIDS-related illnesses, such as opportunistic infections (So et al 1986; Formenti et al 1989). However, the introduction of HAART has significantly improved outcomes in this patient group (Haldorsen et al 2008; Newell 2004).

Other categories of primary central nervous system lymphoma

Transplantation-related PCNSL

The association between immunosuppression and the development of non-Hodgkin lymphoma was first recognized in renal transplant patients (Schneck & Penn 1971; Penn & Starzl 1972; Hoover & Fraumeni 1973; Barnett & Schwartz 1974). Systemic NHL is the most common post-transplant malignancy excluding non-melanoma skin cancers and carcinoma in situ of the cervix and has been described in all manner of organ transplantations (Hanto et al 1981; Penn 1987; Nalesnik et al 1988). In renal transplantation series, there is a 28–50-fold increase in expected cases of systemic NHL when compared with populations matched for age and sex (Hoover & Fraumeni 1973; Kinlen et al 1979; Riggs & Hagemeister 1988), while in cardiac transplantation series, the incidence of systemic NHL post transplant has been estimated at between 3.5% and 4.6% (Weintraub & Warnke 1982; Gratten et al 1990). The frequency of post-transplant NHL relates to the organ type and the degree of immunosuppression required to prevent rejection (Aisenberg 1991). Reports have noted the peculiarities of these lymphomas, in particular the frequency of PCNSL, the monotonous appearance of high- and intermediate-grade lymphomas and the rarity of Hodgkin lymphoma.

Historically, PCNSL constituted approximately 25% of all transplant-related lymphomas and, in a further 10% of patients; the CNS was involved as part of a systemic lymphomatous process, usually as leptomeningeal disease (Riggs & Hagemeister 1988). Some studies recorded even higher percentages of PCNSL, with nearly 50% of post-transplant lymphomas being of cerebral origin (Schneck & Penn 1971; Hoover & Fraumeni 1973). This represented a marked increase in the risk of developing PCNSL in transplant patients compared with the normal population. One estimate put this as a 350-fold increase in risk (Penn 1981). For PCNSL, the median time from transplantation to the diagnosis of lymphoma ranged from 5.5–46 months (Schneck & Penn 1971; Hoover & Fraumeni 1973; Hochberg & Miller 1988). In one series, the time to develop PCNSL was shorter than for systemic lymphoma, with median times of 16.5 months and 30.4 months, respectively (Schneck & Penn 1971).

The introduction of cyclosporin A into standard post-transplant immunosuppressive regimens has resulted in significant changes to the pattern of post-transplant lymphomas. First, the incidence of extranodal disease has dropped and, furthermore, cerebral involvement is markedly reduced compared with the incidence seen with older immunosuppressive regimens. In Penn's study of transplant recipients receiving cyclosporin A immunosuppressive therapy, only 3% of the post-transplant lymphomas were confined to the brain. Some authors have postulated that the incidence of post-transplant lymphomas following immunosuppression with cyclosporin A is dose-dependent and the reason for the apparent fall in incidence is a result of using lower 'standard' doses of cyclosporin A and improved monitoring of plasma levels (Gratten et al 1990).

The second feature of cyclosporin A immunosuppression is the shorter time to the development of lymphoma than occurred with older regimens. In one such study, the median time to the development of lymphoma was only 12 months, compared with 44 months in those treated without cyclosporin A (Penn 1987).

Most reported post-transplant lymphomas are of B-cell origin, although the lymphomas are frequently multiclonal and polymorphic (Hanto et al 1981; Weintraub & Warnke 1982; Nalesnik et al 1988) and while the true method of tumor evolution has not been elucidated, a common theory suggests that multiple malignant monoclonal lymphomas develop from an initial polyclonal proliferation of B-cells (Penn 1981; Cleary et al 1988; Riggs & Hagemeister 1988; Aisenberg 1991). On the other hand, some authors have suggested that these tumors can be divided into polymorphic diffuse B-cell hyperplasias and polymorphic diffuse B-cell lymphomas (Frizzera et al 1981; Hanto et al 1981, 1982).

There has been much speculation about which factors contribute to the development of lymphoma and, more specifically, PCNSL in transplant patients. There is no clear pathogenic mechanism; however it appears that a combination of decreased immune surveillance and chronic antigenic stimulation may play a role. Other factors may have an influence including the prolonged use of azathioprine and the cause of end-organ failure, at least in cardiac transplantation (Anderson et al 1978; Weintraub & Warnke 1982; Riggs & Hagemeister 1988). The incidence of post-transplant systemic lymphoma does not appear to be influenced by the sex of the donor or recipient, the use of antithymocyte globulin, number of rejection crises, donor-host histocompatibility or in cases of renal transplantation, the cause of end-organ failure (Riggs & Hagemeister 1988). It is difficult to know how one may best apply these findings to aid in the identification of risk factors for the development of post-transplant PCNSL.

Treatment of transplantation-related PCNSL

It is not clear what constitutes the best therapeutic approach to transplant-related PCNSL. Historically, this disease had a very poor outlook, with almost all patients dying of progressive lymphoma within a few months (Schneck & Penn 1971). In accordance with the approach to systemic transplant-related lymphoma, therapeutic options include radiotherapy and chemotherapy, a reduction in immunosuppression and the introduction of antiviral agents (Hanto et al 1982; Starzl et al 1984; Nalesnik et al 1988; Locker & Nalesnik 1989). Logically, therapy should at least be comparable with current treatments for PCNSL in non-immunosuppressed patients with the addition of a reduction in immunosuppressive therapy. The efficacy of treatment regimens in patients with transplant-related PCNSL is not well documented and as a result no regimen can be considered superior.

Secondary central nervous system lymphoma

Central nervous system lymphoma may be secondary to systemic lymphoma. Large studies of patients with systemic lymphoma reveal that between 7% and 29% of patients develop clinical or pathologic evidence of cerebral involvement (Haerni-Simon et al 1987; Liang et al 1989; Haddy et al 1991). Almost all cases are associated with relapsed or progressive systemic disease; isolated CNS relapse is not only very rare but is usually followed soon after by systemic relapse (Johnson et al 1984; Haerni-Simon et al 1987; Liang et al 1989).

Based on data from retrospective multivariate analyses, a number of factors have been suggested to predict a higher incidence of CNS relapse. These include unfavorable histology (Burkitt's and lymphoblastic NHL), elevated LDH, stage IV disease, and the presence of 'B' symptoms (fever, weight loss, sweats). Specific sites of systemic involvement may also be associated with an increased risk of developing cerebral disease. These sites include testis, bone marrow, bone, orbit, peripheral blood and paranasal sinuses (Johnson et al 1984; Perez-Soler et al 1986; Haerni-Simon et al 1987; Liang et al 1989, 1990b).

The site of disease in secondary central nervous system lymphoma is almost invariably the meninges of the brain or spinal cord, with involvement of the cerebral parenchyma less common. As a consequence, the presenting symptoms and signs of secondary central nervous system lymphoma reflect this feature. Thus patients develop headache, meningism, cranial nerve palsies, mental state alterations, sensory and motor deficits and nerve root palsies (Haerni-Simon et al 1987; Liang et al 1989; Zimmerman 1990).

The radiologic appearances of secondary central nervous system lymphoma are identical to those of PCNSL except for sites of disease. MR scanning, with or without gadolinium contrast enhancement, may provide improved resolution with respect to meningeal disease and should be considered in the evaluation of a patient with suspected secondary cerebral or spinal lymphoma, particularly if the CT scan is unrewarding. Other investigative modalities such as myelography are not as sensitive as MR scanning in the detection of meningeal disease (Zimmerman 1990).

The majority of cases of secondary cerebral NHL are high grade lymphomas or diffuse large B cell lymphoma according to the Working Formulation criteria. Secondary involvement of the brain occurs in <2% of low-grade lymphomas. Up to 50% of patients have positive CSF cytology due to the propensity of secondary central nervous system lymphoma to involve the meninges (Young et al 1979; Haerni-Simon et al 1987; Liang et al 1989).

The management of secondary cerebral NHL requires the consideration of both cerebral and systemic components of the relapsed disease. There are no studies that adequately define optimal therapy, and treatment should be individualized according to the clinical situation. For a patient with a good performance status and in whom an aggressive treatment approach may be warranted, therapy should at least include combination systemic chemotherapy and some form of therapy to treat the cerebral disease. While it would be reasonable to base the therapy of the cerebral component on that used for PCNSL within a particular institution, consideration of the frequency of meningeal involvement suggests that intrathecal chemotherapy may be the best alternative.

The role of CNS prophylaxis in patients at high risk of developing secondary cerebral NHL is less well-defined than for acute lymphocytic leukemia, which also has a propensity to intracerebral involvement. Standard management practice in high grade systemic NHL is to include some form of CNS prophylaxis such as intrathecal methotrexate in high risk patients. In a recent study by Bernstein et al (2009), they evaluated incidence, natural history and risk factors for CNS relapse in patients with aggressive non-Hodgkin Lymphoma. The efficacy of CNS prophylaxis, in patients with aggressive NHL in the SWOG 8516, a randomized trial reported in 1993 was assessed. After 20 years follow-up, the cumulative incidence of CNS relapse was 2.8% versus 55.0% for non-CNS relapse.

All patients with CNS relapse died within 1 year; 16/25 patients developed CNS relapse while on chemotherapy treatment for their systemic NHL or 1 month post-treatment; 11/25 had isolated CNS relapse; 10/25 had systemic and CNS relapses. The 2-year survival rate was 0% versus 30% ($p < 0.0001$) and median survival 2.2 months versus 9 months (non-CNS relapses). The number of extranodal sites and the International Prognostic Index were predictive of CNS relapse. Assuming CNS relapse is 6%, reduced to 2% with prophylaxis, we will need to treat 960 patients to benefit 40. Hence, high risk patients with high to high/intermediate IPI score at diagnosis should have CSF evaluation, if the CNS is involved then CNS treatment rather than prophylaxis. There was no significant benefit of CNS prophylaxis in patients with BM involvement at diagnosis; however, given the small number of events, the power of this analysis is limited. Overall survival in patients with secondary central nervous system lymphoma appears to be less than for PCNSL. Less than 15% of patients survive 1 year after the diagnosis of secondary cerebral NHL (Young et al 1979; Haerni-Simon et al 1987; Liang et al 1989). These authors have also recognized the fact that many of the former die of progressive systemic disease rather than from their CNS disease. It may be that CNS disease per se simply represents extensive systemic disease and that this is responsible for the poor prognosis rather than an intrinsic feature of secondary cerebral NHL (Haddy et al 1991).

Hodgkin disease

Intracerebral Hodgkin disease (HD) remains a very rare entity. Unlike non-Hodgkin lymphoma, there is no apparent increase in its incidence. Reflecting the rarity of the disease, the medical literature contains only a limited number of small series and single case reports.

Almost all cases of intracranial HD are associated with relapsing systemic disease. Large historical series of HD patients document the rarity of intracerebral involvement. A review from the Christie Hospital reported only two definite cases of cerebral disease in 1339 HD patients (Todd 1967). On available evidence, the incidence of intracranial HD accompanying systemic disease ranges from 0.2–0.5% (Todd 1967; Cuttner et al 1979; Sapozink & Kaplan 1983; Blake et al 1986; Hair et al 1991). In the setting of systemic disease, intracranial disease stems either from hematogenous metastases or direct meningeal infiltration.

Primary intracranial HD has been sporadically reported (Schricker & Smith 1955; Ashby et al 1988b; Clark et al 1992; Camilleri-Broët et al 1998). Isolated intracranial HD is so rare that <20 cases have been published in the literature. Many of the cases were reported prior to improved staging and immunohistochemical techniques and as a result may have had unrecognized systemic disease or alternate histologies such as NHL.

The paucity of data predicates against clear definitions of epidemiologic factors, specific sites of predilection, histologic sub-types and approaches to management. The histologic sub-type varies according to reports. All sub-types are represented, although nodular sclerosing HD has been most frequently reported in the recent literature (Sapozink & Kaplan 1983; Ashby et al 1988; Clark et al 1992). Symptoms and signs of intracranial HD represent local tumor effects, commonly expressed as cranial nerve palsies, headache and long tract motor disturbances. There have been no reported cases of the classic 'B' symptoms of fever, sweats or loss of weight in primary intracerebral HD.

The diagnosis of primary intracerebral HD cannot be made by CT or MR scan. Although the CT scan usually demonstrates a solitary lesion the appearance may be confused with other intracranial lesions including gliomas, metastases and meningiomas. Examination of CSF should be routine despite the limitations of diagnosing HD by cytologic methods. Diagnostic Reed–Sternberg cells have been recognized in the CSF of some patients with intracerebral HD (Billingham et al 1975; Cuttner et al 1979).

The most likely scenario in the diagnosis of intracranial HD is as an unexpected finding at craniotomy or stereotactic brain biopsy. The surgeon may be alerted by the well-circumscribed and homogeneous appearance of the tumor. Fresh tissue should accompany formalin-fixed specimens so as to provide adequate tissue for immunohistochemical studies. Once the diagnosis of intracerebral HD has been made, the most important aspect of management is the need to exclude systemic disease. Routine staging should include the investigations listed previously for cerebral non-Hodgkin lymphoma.

Intracerebral HD has been described in at least one patient who was seropositive for the human immunodeficiency virus (Hair et al 1991). HD is not currently recognized as an AIDS-defining illness, however an increasing number of HIV-associated HD cases have been reported, particularly in intravenous drug users, and sero-testing should be considered in 'at risk' patients (Roithmann et al 1990; Ames et al 1991; Ree et al 1991).

The treatment of patients with intracerebral HD accompanying systemic relapse should include therapy for both intracranial and systemic components. Treatment decisions must necessarily be individualized according to the clinical situation. Empirically, however, treatment should include irradiation of intracranial disease in addition to definitive systemic chemotherapy.

A recent study published by Gerstner et al (2008) collected data on 16 patients, the largest number to date, with meningeal or parenchymal CNS-HD confirmed by histopathology (15) or CSF (1). Eight patients presented with CNS-HL at diagnosis, two of whom had isolated CNS disease; eight patients developed CNS-HL at relapse. Median overall survival 60.9 months from first diagnosis of HL (systemic or CNS) and 43.8 months from diagnosis of CNS-HL. Although a majority of patients have died, long-term survival is possible in patients who achieve a complete response to treatment, particularly those who present with CNS involvement or involvement of the CNS is the sole site of relapsed disease. The treatment was variable and included radiotherapy and chemotherapy.

In view of its rarity, the standard and optimal therapy of primary intracerebral HD has not been defined. Surgical excision, radiotherapy and chemotherapy have been used in isolation or in combination as treatment for this disease (Ashby et al 1988b; Clark et al 1992). In primary disease with a solitary focus, the most common approach has been surgical excision followed by cranial irradiation. Descriptive accounts of surgery in these patients suggests that the tumor mass is well encapsulated and can be removed in its entirety. Postoperative whole brain irradiation with a tumor dose to 40–45 Gy has been recommended and may confer an added survival benefit. There is no evidence that systemic or intrathecal chemotherapy adds to surgery or radiotherapy in the treatment of primary intracerebral HD.

Long-term outcome for patients with intracranial HD is difficult to determine from reported cases. Among the rare cases of primary intracranial HD, complete responses and long-term survival have been described (Ashby et al 1988b; Clark et al 1992). Similarly, in those patients with concurrent intracerebral and systemic disease, aggressive combination therapy may result in complete responses and long-term survival.

Intraocular lymphoma

Intraocular lymphoma is a rare condition affecting those in their 6th or 7th decades (Grimm et al 2008). Typically, the disease presents with a painless reduction in acuity in one or both eyes and the disease may affect the vitreous, retina or subretinal space. The ocular findings include retinal and sub-retinal infiltrates, vitreous cells and retinal detachments. The majority of patients have bilateral ocular disease (Margolis et al 1980; Rockwood et al 1984; Strauchen et al 1989; Maiuri 1990).

The diagnosis is established by vitreous aspiration or biopsy (Strauchen et al 1989), with subsequent cytologic or histologic assessment – sensitivity 80–95%. Ultrasound of the eye is frequently abnormal but remains non-specific (Ursea et al 1997). Most reported cases are large cell NHL of B-cell origin (Kaplan et al 1980). Immunoglobin gene rearrangements can be detected through PCR techniques (Shen et al 1998). Up to 60–80% of patients with ocular lymphoma have concurrent primary central nervous system lymphoma, while <25% have associated systemic disease (Vogel et al 1968; Margolis et al 1980; Rockwood et al 1984). In general, the ocular symptoms precede symptoms attributable to the cerebral disease (Maiuri 1990).

In contrast to PCNSL, ocular lymphoma may not respond to steroids (Margolis et al 1980). Treatment often incorporates binocular irradiation, prophylactic cranial irradiation and adjunctive intravenous single agent or combination chemotherapy (Strauchen et al 1989; Soussain et al 1996). Therapeutic levels of cytosine arabinoside (Ara-C) or methotrexate have been recorded within the vitreous following intravenous and sub-conjunctival administration (Rootman et al 1983; Baumann et al 1986; Strauchen et al 1989; Fishburne et al 1997). This therapeutic approach frequently results in complete or partial responses; however, most patients eventually relapse and die. Over 50% of relapses occur within the central nervous system, with rare cases of systemic relapse being reported (Baumann et al 1986).

Mycosis fungoides

Mycosis fungoides, a cutaneous T-lymphocyte lymphoma, may disseminate to the CNS as well as to other internal organs (Zonenshayn et al 1998). This rare complication is associated with advanced disease and may be diagnosed by stereotactic biopsy or by the presence of typical tumor cells in the CSF. Treatment with cranial irradiation and chemotherapy may have a palliative effect and prolong survival; however long-term survival has not been reported (Zackheim et al 1983; Hallahan et al 1986; Lindae et al 1990).

Lymphomatoid granulomatosis

Lymphomatoid granulomatosis (LG) is now recognized as an angiocentric, angiodestructive lymphoproliferative disorder that frequently progresses to lymphoma. Investigators have documented T-cell clonality and, in some cases, an association with Epstein–Barr virus (Donner et al 1990; Mittal et al 1990). Although the disease commonly involves the lungs and skin, the CNS is involved in up to 20% of cases (Hogan et al 1981) and there are a few reported cases of LG isolated to the CNS (Kokinen et al 1977; Schmidt et al 1984; Kleinschmidt-DeMasters et al 1992). CNS involvement with LG has been reported in patients with HIV infection (Anders et al 1989; Ioachim 1989).

The sites of CNS involvement appear random and, as a consequence, presenting symptoms and signs vary. Focal neurologic deficits result from solitary lesions whilst multifocal disease may present with a constellation of CNS features. There have also been rare descriptions of diffusely infiltrating disease resulting in dementia (Kleinschmidt-DeMasters et al 1992).

Historically, LG was considered as a relatively benign tumor and therapy consisted of low doses of cyclophosphamide and prednisolone. However, increasingly it appears that the disease may run an aggressive course and many authors now advocate an aggressive approach towards therapy utilizing combination chemotherapy regimens and irradiation (Lipford et al 1988; Jenkins & Zaloznik 1989; Nair et al 1989).

Malignant angioendotheliosis (intravascular lymphomatosis)

Malignant angioendotheliosis is an unusual intravascular lymphoma that has a predilection for the CNS. The derivation of the neoplastic cells has been questioned since the first description of the disease in 1959 (Pfleger & Tappeiner 1959). There appears no doubt that the cell of origin is a lymphocyte, based on recent immunocytochemical, histologic and molecular evidence (Otrakji et al 1988; Clark et al 1991; Fredericks et al 1991).

More than 60 cases have been described within the literature and a pattern of the disease is apparent. Most patients are elderly and present with cerebral disease manifested by a progressive cognitive decline as a consequence of small vessel occlusion. Focal neurologic deficits may occur in tandem with a global decline or as an isolated feature. The diagnosis of malignant angioendotheliosis may be suggested by the clinical presentation and the MR scan appearance; however, the majority of cases are only diagnosed at autopsy (Fredericks et al 1991; Smadja et al 1991; Williams et al 1998).

Untreated, the disease progresses inexorably over weeks or months, with a median survival of only 9.5 months (Smadja et al 1991). The recognition that malignant angioendotheliosis is a lymphoma has prompted the use of cranial irradiation and combined chemotherapy regimens with some success (Fredericks et al 1991; Smadja et al 1991).

Key points

- PCNSL is a disease of the elderly except when resulting from HIV infection.
- PCNSL has typical radiological appearances.
- PCNSL is usually a B cell high-grade non-Hodgkin lymphoma.
- Corticosteroids may mask the illness and delay the diagnosis.
- PCNSL is highly responsive to radiotherapy or chemotherapy.
- The optimal treatment regimen has not been established.
- Relapses are common.
- AIDS-related PCNSL has a significantly worse median survival than non-AIDS PCNSL.

REFERENCES

Aboulafia, D.M., Puswella, A.L., 2007. Highly active antiretroviral therapy as the sole treatment for AIDS-related primary central nervous system lymphoma: a case report with implications for treatment. AIDS Patient Care STDS 12, 900–907.

Abrey, L.E., DeAngelis, L.M., Yahalom, J., 1998. Long-term survival in primary central nervous system lymphoma. J. Clin. Oncol. 16, 859–963.

Abrey, L.E., Yahalom, J., DeAngelis L.M., 2000. Treatment for primary CNS lymphoma: the next step. J. Clin. Oncol. 18, 3144–3150.

Adams, J., Howatson, A.G., 1990. Primary central nervous system lymphomas: review of 70 cases. J. Clin. Pathol. 43, 544–547.

Agbi, C.B., Bannister, C.M., Turnbull, I.W., 1983. Primary cranial vault lymphoma mimicking a meningioma. Neurochirurgia 26, 130–132.

Aisenberg, A.C., 1991. Malignant lymphoma. Biology, natural history and treatment. Lea & Febiger, Philadelphia.

Albrecht, S., Bruner, J.B., SeGall, G.K., 1992. Immunoglobulin heavy chain rearrangements in primary brain lymphomas. Proc. Am. Assoc. Cancer Res. 33 (Abstract), 1493.

Allen, J.C., Rosen, G., Mehta, B.M., et al., 1980. Leukoencephalopathy following high-dose IV methotrexate chemotherapy with leucovorin rescue. Cancer TreatRep. 64, 1261–1273.

Ames, E.D., Conjalka, M.S., Goldberg, A.F., et al., 1991. Hodgkin disease and AIDS: Twenty-three new cases and a review of the literature. Hematol. Oncol. Clin. North Am. 5, 343–356.

Ammassari, A., Scoppettuolo, G., Murri, R., et al., 1998. Changing patterns in focal brain lesion-causing disorders in AIDS. J. Acquir. Immune. Defic. Syndr. Hum. Retrovirol. 18, 365–371.

Anders, K.H., Latta, H., Chang, B.S., 1989. Lymphomatoid granulomatosis and malignant lymphoma of the central nervous system in the acquired immunodeficiency syndrome. Hum. Pathol. 20, 326–334.

Anderson, J.L., Fowles, R.E., Bieber, C.P., et al., 1978. Idiopathic cardiomyopathy, age, and suppressor-cell dysfunction as risk determinants of lymphoma after cardiac transplantation. Lancet ii, 1174–1177.

Ando, S., Moritake, K., 1990. Pure optic ataxia associated with a right parieto-occipital tumor. J. Neurol. Neurosurg. Psychiatry 53, 805–806.

Aozasa, K., Ohsawa, M., Yamabe, H., et al., 1990. Malignant lymphoma of the central nervous system in Japan: Histologic and immunohistologic studies. Int. J. Cancer 45, 632–636.

Apuzzo, M.L., Chandrasoma, P.T., Cohen, D., et al., 1987. Computed imaging stereotaxy: experience and perspective related to 500 procedures applied to brain masses. J. Neurosurg. 20, 930–937.

Ashby, M.A., Bowen, D., Bleehen, N.M., et al., 1988a. Primary lymphoma of the central nervous system: experience at Addenbrooke's Hospital, Cambridge. Clin. Radiol. 39, 173–181.

Ashby, M.A., Barber, P.C., Holmes, A.E., et al., 1988b. Primary intracranial Hodgkin disease. A case report and discussion. Am. J. Surg. Pathol. 12, 29–299.

Bailey, P., 1929. Intracranial sarcomatous tumors of leptomeningeal origin. Arch. Surg. 18, 1359–1402.

Bale, I.F., Wilson, J.F., Hill, H.R., 1977. Fatal histiocytic lymphoma of the brain associated with hyperimmunoglobulinemia-E and recurrent infections. Cancer 39, 2386–2390.

Barnett, L.B., Schwartz, E., 1974. Cerebral reticulum cell sarcoma after multiple renal transplants. J. Neurol. Neurosurg. Psychiatry 37, 966–970.

Bashir, R.M., Harris, N.L., Hochberg, F.H., et al., 1989. Detection of Epstein-Barr virus in CNS lymphoma by in-situ hybridisation. Neurology 39, 813–817.

Bataille, B., Delwail, V., Menet, E., et al., 2000. Primary intracerebral malignant lymphoma: a report of 248 patients. J. Neurosurg. 92, 261–266.

Batchelor, T., Carson, K., O'Neill, A., et al., 2003. Treatment of primary CNS lymphoma with methotrexate and deferred radiotherapy: A report of NABTT 96–07. J. Clin. Oncol. 21, 1044–1049.

Baumann, M.A., Ritch, P.S., Hande, K.R., et al., 1986. Treatment of intraocular lymphoma with high dose Ara C. Cancer 57, 1273–1275.

Baumgartner, J.E., Rachlin, J.R., Beckstead, I.H., et al., 1990. Primary central nervous system lymphomas: natural history and response to radiation therapy in 55 patients with acquired immunodeficiency syndrome. J. Neurosurg. 73, 206–211.

Baxter, J.D., Harris, A.W., Tomltins, G.M., et al., 1971. Glucocorticoid receptors in lymphoma cells in culture: relationship of glucocorticoid killing activity. Science 171, 189–191.

Benjamin, D., Knobloch, T.J., Abrams, J., et al., 1991. Human B cell IL-10: B cell lines derived from patients with AIDS and Burkitt's lymphoma constitutively secrete large quantities of IL-10. Blood 78, A384a.

Benjamin, I., Case, M.E., 1980. Primary reticulum-cell sarcoma (microglioma) of the brain with massive cardiac metastasis. J. Neurosurg. 53, 714–716.

Beral, V., Peterman, T., Berkelman, R., et al., 1991. AIDS-associated non-Hodgkin lymphoma. Lancet 337, 805–809.

Berger, R., La Coniat, M., Devve, J., et al., 1989. Secondary non-random chromosomal abnormalities of band 13q34 in Burkitt's lymphoma-leukaemia. Genes Chrom. Cancer 1, 115–118.

Bernstein, H., Unger, J.M., LeBlanc, M., 2009. Natural History of CNS Relapse in Patients With Aggressive Non-Hodgkin Lymphoma: A 20-Year Follow-Up Analysis of SWOG 8516—The Southwest Oncology Group. J. Clin. Oncol. 27, 114–119.

Berry, M.P., Simpson, W.J., 1981. Radiation therapy in the management of primary malignant lymphoma of the brain. Int. J. Radiat. Oncol. Biol. Physics 7, 55–59.

Bignon, Y.J., Clavelou, P., Ramos, F., et al., 1991. Detection of Epstein-Barr virus sequences in primary brain lymphoma without immunodeficiency. Neurology 41, 1152–1153.

Billingham, M.E., Rawlinson, D.G., Berry, P.F., et al., 1975. The cytodiagnosis of malignant lymphomas and Hodgkin Disease in cerebrospinal, pleural and ascitic fluids. Acta Cytol. 19, 547–556.

Blake, P.R., Carr, D.H., Goolden, A.W.G., 1986. Intracranial Hodgkin disease. Br. J. Radiol. 59, 41–46.

Blasberg, R.G., Groothuis, D., Molnar, P., 1990. A review of hyperosmotic blood-brain barrier disruption in seven experimental tumor models. In: Johansson, B.B., Widner, C.O. (Eds.), Pathophysiology of the blood-brain-barrier. Elsevier, New York, pp. 197–220.

Blay, J.Y., Conroy, T., Cheveau, C., et al., 1998. High dose methotrexate for the treatment of primary central nervous system lymphomas: analysis of survival and late neurologic toxicity in a retrospective series. J. Clin. Oncol. 16, 864–871.

Bower, M., 1992. The biology of HIV-associated lymphomas. Br. J. Cancer 66, 421–423.

Boyle, M.J., Swanson, C.E., Turner, J.J., et al., 1990. Definition of two distinct types of AIDS-associated non-Hodgkin lymphoma. Br. J. Haematol. 76, 506–512.

Braatan, K.M., Betensky, R.A., De Leval, A., et al., 2003. BCL-6 expression predicts improved survival in patients with primary central nervous system lymphoma. Clin. Cancer Res. 9, 1063–1069.

Brada, M., Dearnaley, D., Horwich, A., et al., 1990. Management of primary central nervous system lymphoma with initial chemotherapy: preliminary results and comparison with patients treated with radiotherapy alone. Int. J. Radiat. Oncol. Biol. Physics 18, 787–792.

Brada, M., Hjiyiannakis, D., Hines, F., et al., 1998. Short intensive primary chemotherapy and radiotherapy in sporadic primary CNS lymphoma (PCNSL). Int. J. Radiat. Oncology Biol. Physics 40, 1157–1162.

Brant-Zawadzki, M., Enzmann, D.R., 1978. Computed tomographic brain scanning in patients with lymphoma. Radiology 129, 67–71.

Brevet, M., Garidi, R., Gruson, B., et al., 2005. First-line autologous stem cell transplantation in primary CNS lymphoma. Eur. J. Haematol. 75, 288–292.

Bromberg, J.E., Breems, D.A., Kraan, J., et al., 2007. CSF flow cytometry greatly improves diagnostic accuracy in CNS hematologic malignancies. Neurology 68, 1674–1679.

Cady, F.M., O'Neill, B.P., Law, M.E., et al., 2008. Del (6) (q22) and Bcl6 re-arrangements in primary CNS lymphoma are indicators of an aggressive clinical course. J. Clin. Oncol. 26, 4814–4819.

Camilleri-Broët, S., Davi, F., Feuillard, J., et al., 1997. AIDS-related primary brain lymphomas: histopathologic and immunohistochemical study of 51 cases, the French Study group for HIV-Associated Tumors. Hum. Pathol. 28, 367–374.

Camilleri-Broët, S., Martin, A., Moreau, A., et al., 1998. Primary central nervous system lymphoma in 72 immunocompetent patients: pathologic findings and clinical correlations. Groupe Ouest Est d'etude des Leucenies et Autres Maladies du Sang. Am. J. Clin. Pathol. 110, 607–612.

Camilleri-Broët, S., Camparo, P., Mokhtari, K., et al., 2000. Overexpression of BCL-2, BCL-X, and BAX in primary central nervous system lymphomas that occur in immunosuppressed patients. Mod. Pathol. 13, 158–165.

Camilleri-Broët, S., Crinière, E., Broët, P., et al., 2006. A uniform activated B-cell-like immunophenotype might explain the poor prognosis of primary central nervous system lymphomas: analysis of 83 cases. Blood 107, 190–196.

Camilleri-Broët, S., Criniere, E., Broet, P., et al., 2007. A uniform activated B-cell like immunophenotype might explain the poor prognosis of primary central nervous system lymphomas: analysis of 83 cases. Blood 107, 190–196.

Cantore, G.P., Raco, A., Artico, M., et al., 1989. Primary chiasmatic lymphoma. Clin. Neurol. Neurosurg. 91, 71–74.

Carlson, B.A., 1996. Rapidly progressive dementia caused by nonenhancing primary lymphoma of the central nervous system. Am. J. Neuroradiol. 17, 1695–1697.

Cassady, J.R., Wilner, H., 1967. The angiographic appearance of intracranial sarcomas. Radiology 88, 258–263.

Centers for Disease Control, 1985. Revision of the case definition of acquired immunodeficiency syndrome for national reporting United States. MMWR 34, 373–375.

Chabner, B.A., Lango, D.L. (Eds)., 1996. Cancer chemotherapy and biotherapy. Principles and practice. Lippincott-Raven, Philadelphia, PA.

Chang, C.C., Kampalath, B., Schultz, C., et al., 2003. Expression of p53, c-Myc, or Bcl-6 suggests a poor prognosis in primary central nervous system diffuse large B-cell lymphoma among immunocompetent individuals. Arch. Pathol. Lab. Med. 127, 208–212.

Cher, L., Glass, J., Harsh, G.R., et al., 1996. Therapy of primary central nervous system lymphoma with methotrexate-based chemotherapy and deferred radiotherapy: preliminary results. Neurology 46, 1757–1759.

Ciricillo, S.F., Rosenblum, M.L., 1990. Use of CT and MR imaging to distinguish intracranial lesions and to define the need for biopsy in AIDS patients. J. Neurosurg. 73, 720–724.

Clark, W.C., Dohan, F.C., Moss, T., et al., 1991. Immunocytochemical evidence of lymphocytic derivation of neoplastic cells in malignant angioendotheliomatosis. J. Neurosurg. 74, 757–762.

Clark, W.C., Callihan, T., Schwartzberg, L., et al., 1992. Primary intracranial Hodgkin lymphoma without dural attachment. Case report. J. Neurosurg. 76, 692–695.

Cleary, M.L., Nalesnik, M.A., Shearer, W.T., et al., 1988. Clonal analysis of transplant-associated lymphoproliferations based on the structure of the genomic termini of the Epstein-Barr Virus. Blood 72, 349–352.

Coiffier, B., Lepage, E., Briere, J., et al., 2002. CHOP chemotherapy plus rituximab compared with CHOP alone in elderly patients with diffuse large-B-cell lymphoma. N. Engl. J. Med. 346, 235–242.

Cooper, J.S., 1989. Radiation therapy and the treatment of patients with AIDS. In: Radiation oncology: rationale, techniques, results. CV Mosby, Baltimore, MD, pp. 762–776.

Corboy, J.R., Garl, P.J., Kleinschmidt-DeMasters, B.K., 1998. Human herpesvirus 8 DNA in CNS lymphomas from patients with and without AIDS. Neurology 50, 335–340.

Corn, B.W., Marcus, S.M., Topham, A., et al., 1997. Will primary central nervous system lymphoma be the most frequent brain tumor diagnosed in the year 2000? Cancer 79, 2409–2413.

Correa, D.D., DeAngelis, L.M., Shi, W., et al., 2004. Cognitive functions in survivors of primary central nervous system lymphoma. Neurology 62, 548–555.

Correa, D.D., Rocco-Donovan, M., DeAngelis, et al., 2008. Prospective cognitive follow-up in primary CNS lymphoma patients treated with chemotherapy and reduced dose radiotherapy. J. Neurooncol. 91, 315–321.

Crossen, J.R., Goldman, D.L., Dahlborg, S.A., et al., 1992. Neuropsychological assessment outcomes of nonacquired immunodeficiency syndrome patients with primary central nervous system lymphoma before and after blood-brain barrier disruption chemotherapy. Neurosurgery 30, 23–29.

Cuttner, J., Meyer, R., Huang, Y.P., 1979. Intracerebral involvement in Hodgkin Disease. A report of 6 cases and review of the literature. Cancer 43, 1497–1506.

Davenport, R.D., O'Donnell, L.R., Schnitzer, B., et al., 1991. Non-Hodgkin lymphoma of the brain after Hodgkin disease. Cancer 67, 440–443.

DeAngelis, L.M., 1990. Primary central nervous system lymphoma imitates multiple sclerosis. J. Neurooncol. 9, 177–181.

DeAngelis, L.M., 1991a. Primary central nervous system lymphoma: A new clinical challenge. Neurology 41, 619–621.

DeAngelis, L.M., 1991b. Primary central nervous system lymphoma as a secondary malignancy. Cancer 67, 1431–1435.

DeAngelis, L.M., Yahalom, J., Thaler, H.T., et al., 1992a. Combined modality therapy for primary CNS lymphoma. J. Clin. Oncol. 10, 635–643.

DeAngelis, L.M., Wong, E., Rosenblum, M., et al., 1992b. Epstein-Barr virus in Acquired Immune Deficiency Syndrome (AIDS) and non-AIDS primary central nervous system lymphoma. Cancer 70, 1607–1611.

DeAngelis, L.M., Seiferheld, W., Schold, S.C., et al., 2002. Combination chemotherapy and radiotherapy for primary central nervous system lymphoma: Radiation Therapy Oncology Group Study 93-10. J. Clin. Oncol. 15, 4643–4648.

DeAngelis, L.M., 2006. American Society of Hematology Education program book. Proc. Am. Soc. Haem.

Desmeules, M., Mikkelsen, T., Mao, Y., 1992. Increasing incidence of primary malignant brain tumors: influence of diagnostic methods. J. Nat. Cancer Inst. 84, 442–445.

DeVita, V.T., Jaffe, E.S., Mauch, P., et al., 1997. Lymphocytic lymphomas. In: DeVita, V.T., Hellman, S., Rosenberg, S.A. (Eds.), Cancer principles and practices of oncology. Lippincott, Philadelphia, PA.

DeWeese, T.L., Hazuka, M.B., Hommel, D.J., et al., 1991. AIDS-related non-Hodgkin lymphoma: the outcome and efficacy of radiation therapy. Int. J. Radiat. Oncol. Biol. Physics 20, 803–808.

Diamond, C., Remick, S., Migliozzi, J., et al., 1990. Primary central nervous system lymphoma (PCNSL) in patients with and without acquired immunodeficiency syndrome (AIDS). Proc. Am. Soc. Clin. Oncol. 9 (Abstract), 367.

Dina, T.S., 1991. Primary central nervous system lymphoma versus toxoplasmosis in AIDS. Radiology 179, 823–828.

Donahue, B., Sullivan, J.W., Cooper, J.S., 1995. Additional experience of empiric radiotherapy for presumed human immunodeficiency virus-associated primary central nervous system lymphomas. Cancer 76, 328–332.

Donner, L.R., Dobin, S., Harrington, D., et al., 1990. Angiocentric immunoproliferative lesion (lymphomatoid granulomatosis). A cytogenetic, immunophenotypic, and genotypic study. Cancer 65, 249–254.

Dulai, M.S., Park, C.Y., Howell, W.D., et al., 2008. CNS T-cell lymphoma: an under-recognised entity? Acta Neuropathol. 115, 345–356.

Eby, N.L., Grufferman, S., Flannelly, C.M., et al., 1988. Increasing incidence of primary brain lymphoma in the US. Cancer 62, 2461–2465.

El-Yazigi, A., Kanaan, I., Martin, C.R., et al., 1990. Cerebrospinal fluid content of manganese, platinum, and strontium in patients with cerebral tumors, leukemia and other noncerebral neoplasms. Oncology 47, 385–388.

Enting, R.H., Demopoulos, A., DeAngelis, L.M., et al., 2004. Salvage therapy for primary CNS lymphoma with a combination of rituximab and temozolomide. Neurology 63, 901–903.

Enzmann, D.R., Krikorian, J., Norman, D., et al., 1979. Computed tomography in primary reticulum cell sarcoma of the brain. Radiology 130, 165–170.

Epstein, L.G., DiCarlo, F.J., Joshi, V.V., et al., 1988. Primary lymphoma of the central nervous system in children with Acquired Immunodeficiency Syndrome. Pediatrics 82, 355–363.

Ernst, T.M., Chang, L., Witt, D., et al., 1998. Cerebral toxoplasmosis and lymphoma in AIDS: perfusion MR imaging experience in 13 patients. Radiology 208, 663–669.

Ervin, T., Canellos, G.P., 1980. Successful treatment of recurrent primary central nervous system lymphoma with high-dose methotrexate. Cancer 45, 1556–1557.

Feiden, W., Bise, K., Steude, U., 1990. Diagnosis of primary cerebral lymphoma with particular reference to CT-guided stereotactic biopsy. Virchows Arch. Pathol. Anat. Histopathol. 417, 21–28.

Ferreri, A.J., Blay, J.-Y., Reni, M., et al., 2003. Prognostic scoring system for primary CNS lymphomas: The International Extranodal Lymphoma Study Group experience. Jo. Clin. Oncol. 21, 266–272.

Ferreri, A.J., Reni, M., Zoldan, M.C., et al., 1996. Importance of complete staging in non-Hodgkin lymphoma presenting as a cerebral lesion. Cancer 77, 827–833.

Ferreri, A.J., Reni, M., Bolognesi, A., et al., 1995. Combined therapy for primary central nervous system lymphoma in immunocompetent patients. Eur. J. Cancer 31, 2008–2012.

Ferreri, A.J., Reni, M., Dell'Oro, S., et al., 2001. Combined treatment with high-dose methotrexate, vincristine and procarbazine, without intrathecal chemotherapy, followed by consolidation radiotherapy for primary central nervous system lymphoma in immunocompetent patients. Oncology 60, 134–140.

Filopovich, A.H., Heinitz, K.I., Robison, L.L., et al., 1987. The Immunodeficiency Cancer Registry. A research source. Am. J. Pediatr. Hematol. Oncol. 9, 183–184.

Fishburne, B.C., Wilson, D.J., Rosenbaum, J.T., et al., 1997. Intravitreal methotrexate as an adjunctive treatment of intraocular lymphoma. Arch. Ophthalmol. 115, 1152–1156.

Formenti, S.C., Gill, P.S., Lean, E., et al., 1989. Primary central nervous system lymphoma in AIDS. Results of radiation therapy. Cancer 63, 1101–1107.

Fredericks, R.K., Walker, F.O., Elster, A., et al., 1991. Angiotropic intravascular large-cell lymphoma (malignant angioendotheliomatosis): report of a case and review of the literature. Surg. Neurol. 35, 218–223.

Freeman, C., Berg, J.W., Cutier, S., 1972. Occurrence and prognosis of extranodal lymphomas. Cancer 29, 252–260.

Freeman, C.R., Shustik, C., Brisson, M., et al., 1986. Primary malignant lymphoma of the central nervous system. Cancer 58, 1104–1111.

Frizzera, G., Hanto, D.W., Gajl-Peczalska, K.J., et al., 1981. Polymorphic diffuse B-cell hyperplasias and lymphomas in renal transplant recipients. Cancer Res. 41, 4262, A279.

Furusawa, T., Okamoto, K., Ito, J., et al., 1998. Primary central nervous system lymphoma presenting as diffuse cerebral infiltration. Radiat. Med. 16, 137–140.

Gabbai, A.A., Hochberg, F.H., Linggood, R.M., et al., 1989. High-dose methotrexate for non-AIDS primary central nervous system lymphoma. J. Neurosurg. 70, 190–194.

Gaidano, G., Ballerini, P., Gong, J.Z., et al., 1991. P53 mutations in human lymphoid malignancies: association with Burkitt lymphoma and chronic lymphocytic leukemia. Proc. Nat. Acad. Sci. 88, 5413–5417.

Gail, M.H., Pluda, J.M., Rabkin, C.S., et al., 1991. Projections of the incidence of non-Hodgkin lymphoma related to Acquired Immunodeficiency Syndrome. J. Nat. Cancer Inst. 83, 695–701.

Gametchu, B., 1987. Glucocorticoid receptor-like antigen in lymphoma cell membranes: correlation to cell lysis. Science 236, 456–461.

Geddes, J.F., Bhattacharjee, M.B., Savage, K., et al., 1992. Primary central nervous system lymphoma: a study of 47 cases probed for Epstein-Barr virus genome. J. Clin. Pathol. 45, 587–590.

GiaRusso, M.H., Koeppen, A.H., 1978. Atypical progressive multifocal leukoencephalopathy and primary cerebral malignant lymphoma. J. Neurol. Sci. 35, 391–398.

Gill, P.S., Levine, A.M., Meyer, P.R., et al., 1985. Primary central nervous system lymphoma in homosexual men. Clinical, immunologic, and pathologic features. Am. J. Med. 78, 742–748.

Giromini, D., Peiffer, I., Tzonos, T., 1981. Occurrence of a primary Burkitt type lymphoma of the central nervous system in an astrocytoma patient. Acta Neuropathol. 54, 165–167.

Glass, J., Shustik, Hochberg, F.H., et al., 1996. Therapy of primary central system lymphoma with preirradiation methotrexate, cyclophosphamide, doxorubicin, vincristine and dexamethasone. J. Neurooncology 30, 257–265.

Goldstein, J.D., Dickson, D.W., Moser, F.G., et al., 1991. Primary central nervous system lymphoma in Acquired Immune Deficiency Syndrome. A clinical and pathological study with results of treatment with radiation. Cancer 67, 2756–2765.

Good, A.E., Russo, R.H., Schnitzer, B., et al., 1978. Intracranial histiocytic lymphoma with rheumatoid arthritis. J. Rheumatol. 5, 75–78.

Grant, J.W., von Deimling, A., 1990. Primary T-cell lymphoma of the central nervous system. Arch. Pathol. Lab. Med. 114, 24–27.

Gratten, M.T., Moreno-Cabral, C.E., Starnes, V.A., et al., 1990. Eight-year results of cyclosporine-treated patients with cardiac transplants. J. Thoracic. Cardiovasc. Surg. 99, 500–509.

Gregory, M.C., Hughes, J.T., 1973. Intracranial reticulum cell sarcoma associated with Immunoglobulin A deficiency. J. Neurol. Neurosurg. Psychiatry 36, 769–776.

Greig, N.H., Ries, L.G., Yancik, R., et al., 1990. Increasing annual incidence of primary malignant brain tumors in the elderly. J. Nat. Cancer Inst. 82, 1621–1624.

Grimm, S.A., McCannel, C.A., Omuro, A.M., et al., 2008. Primary CNS lymphoma with intraocular involvement: International PCNSL Collaborative Group Report. Neurology 21, 1355–1360.

Haddy, T.B., Adde, M.A., Magrath, I.T., 1991. CNS involvement in small noncleaved-cell lymphoma: is CNS disease per se a poor prognostic sign. J. Clin. Oncol. 9, 1973–1982.

Gerstner, E.R., Abrey, L.E., Schiff, D., et al., 2008. CNS Hodgkin lymphoma. Blood 112, 1658–1661.

Haerni-Simon, G., Suchaud, J.P., Eghbali, H., et al., 1987. Secondary involvement of the central nervous system in malignant non-Hodgkin lymphoma. Oncology 44, 98–101.

Hair, L.S., Rogers, J.D., Chadburn, A., et al., 1991. Intracerebral Hodgkin disease in a Human Immunodeficiency Virus-seropositive patient. Cancer 67, 2931–2934.

Haldorsen, I.S., Krakenes, J., Goplan, A.K., et al., 2008. AIDS-related primary central nervous system lymphoma: a Norwegian national survey 1989–2003. BMC Cancer 8, 225.

Hallahan, D., Greim, M., Greim, S., et al., 1986. Mycosis fungoides involving the central nervous system. J. Clin. Oncol. 4, 1638–1644.

Hamilton-Dutoit, S.J., Pallesen, G., Franzmann, M.B., et al., 1991. AIDS-related lymphoma. Histopathology, immunophenotype and association with Epstein-Barr virus as demonstrated by in situ nucleic acid hybridisation. Am. J. Pathol. 138, 149–163.

Hansen, H.H., Bender, R.A., Shelton, B.I., 1974. Use of the cytocentrifuge and CSF. Acta Cytol. 18, 251–262.

Hansen, P.B., Kjeldsen, L., Dalhoff, K., et al., 1992. Cerebrospinal fluid beta-2-microglobulin in adult patients with acute leukemia or lymphoma: a useful marker in early diagnosis and monitoring of CNS involvement. Acta Neurol. Scand 85, 224–227.

Hanto, D.W., Frizzera, G., Purtilo, D.T., et al., 1981. Clinical spectrum of lymphoproliferative disorders in renal transplant recipients and evidence for the role of Epstein-Barr Virus. Cancer Res. 41, 4253, A261.

Hanto, D.W., Frizzera, G., Gajl-Peczalska, K.J., et al., 1982. Epstein-Barr virus induced B-cell lymphoma after renal transplantation. N. Engl. J. Med. 306, 913–918.

Heckman, J.G., Bockhorn, J., Stolte, M., et al., 1998. An instructive false diagnosis: steroid-induced complete remission of a CNS tumor- probably lymphoma. Neurosurg. Rev. 21, 48–51.

Heimans, I.J., De Visser, M., Polman, C.H., et al., 1990. Accuracy and interobserver variation in the interpretation of computed tomography in solitary brain lesions. Arch. Neurol. 47, 520–523.

Helle, T.L., Britt, R.H., Colby, T.V., 1984. Primary malignant lymphomas of the central nervous system. Clinicopathological study of experience at Stanford. J. Neurosurg. 60, 94–103.

Henry, J.M., Heffner, R.R., Dillard, S.H., et al., 1974. Primary malignant lymphomas of the central nervous system. Cancer 34, 1293–1302.

Herbst, K.D., Corder, M.P., Justice, G.R., 1976. Successful therapy with methotrexate of a multicentric lymphoma of the central nervous system. Cancer 38, 1476–1478.

Herrlinger, U., Küker, W., Uhl, M., et al., 2005. NOA-03 trial of high-dose methotrexate in primary central nervous system lymphoma: final report. Ann. Neurol. 57, 843–847.

Hirano, A., 1975. A comparison of the fine structure of malignant lymphoma and other neoplasms in the brain. Acta Neuropathol. Suppl. 6, 141–145.

Ho, K., Garancis, J., Paegle, R.D., et al., 1980. Progressive multifocal leukoencephalopathy and malignant lymphoma in a patient with immunosuppressive therapy. Acta Neuropathol. 52, 81–83.

Hoang-Xuan, K., Taillandier, L., Chinot, O., et al., 2003. Chemotherapy alone as initial treatment for primary CNS lymphoma in patients older than 60 years: a multicenter phase II study (26952) of the European Organization for Research and Treatment of Cancer Brain Tumor Group. J. Clin. Oncol. 15, 2726–2731.

Hochberg, F.H., Miller, D.C., 1988. Primary central nervous system lymphoma. J. Neurosurg. 68, 835–853.

Hochberg, F.H., Miller, G., Schooley, R.T., et al., 1983. Central-nervous-system lymphoma related to Epstein-Barr virus. N. Engl. J. Med. 309, 745–748.

Hogan, P.J., Greenberg, M.K., McCarty, G.E., 1981. Neurological complications of lymphomatoid granulomatosis. Neurology 31, 619–620.

Hoover, R., Fraumeni, J.F., 1973. Risk of cancer in renal-transplant recipients. Lancet 14, 55–57.

Hottinger, A.F., DeAngelis, L.M., Yahalom, J., et al., 2007. Salvage whole brain radiotherapy for recurrent or refractory primary CNS lymphoma. Neurology 69, 1178–1182.

Houthoff, H.J., Poppema, S., Ebels, E.J., Elema, I.D., 1978. Intracranial malignant lymphomas. A morphologic and immunocytologic study of twenty cases. Acta Neuropathol. 44, 203–210.

Hutter, J.I., Jones, J.F., 1981. Results of thymic epithelial transplant in a child with Wiskott-Aldrich syndrome and central nervous system lymphoma. Clin. Immunol. Immunopathol. 18, 121–125.

Ildan, F., Bagdatoglou, H., Boyar, B., et al., 1995. Combined occurrence of primary central nervous system lymphoma and meningioma. Neurosurg. Rev. 18, 45–48.

Illerhaus, G., Marks, R., Ihorst, G., et al., 2006. High-dose chemotherapy with autologous stem-cell transplantation and hyperfractionated radiotherapy as first-line treatment of primary CNS lymphoma. J. Clin. Oncol. 24, 3865–3870.

Ioachim, H.L., 1989. Lymphomatoid granulomatosis versus lymphoma of the brain and central nervous system in the acquired immunodeficiency syndrome. Hum. Pathol. 20, 1222–1224.

Ioachim, H.L., Dorsett, B., Cronin, W., et al., 1991. Acquired immunodeficiency syndrome associated lymphomas: Clinical, pathological, immunologic and viral characteristics of 111 cases. Hum. Pathol. 22, 659–673.

Ishida, Y., 1975. Fine structure of primary reticulum cell sarcoma of the brain. Acta Neuropathol. Suppl. 6, 147–153.

Jack, C.R., O'Neill, B.P., Banks, P.M., et al., 1988. Central nervous system lymphoma: histologic types and CT appearance. Radiology 167, 211–215.

Jarvik, J.G., Hesselink, J.R., Kennedy, C., et al., 1988. Acquired immunodeficiency syndrome. Magnetic resonance patterns of brain involvement with pathologic correlation. Arch. Neurol. 45, 731–736.

Jazy, F.K., Shehata, W.M., Tew, J.M., et al., 1980. Primary intracranial lymphoma of the dura. Arch. Neurol. 37, 528–529.

Jellinger, K., Radaskiewicz, T.H., Slowik, F., 1975. Primary malignant lymphomas of the central nervous system in man. Acta Neuropathol. Suppl. 6, 95–102.

Jellinger, K., Kothbauer, P., Weiss, R., et al., 1979. Primary malignant lymphoma of the CNS and polyneuropathy in a patient with necrotising vasculitis treated with immunosuppression. J. Neurol. 220, 259–268.

Jenkins, C.N., Colquhoun, I.R., 1998. Characterisation of primary intracranial lymphoma by computed tomography: an analysis of 36 cases and a review of the literature with particular reference to calcification haemorrhage and cyst formation. Clin. Radiol. 53, 528–534.

Jenkins, T.R., Zaloznik, A.J., 1989. Lymphomatoid granulomatosis. A case for aggressive therapy. Cancer 64, 1362–1365.

Johnson, B.A., Fram, E.K., Johnson, P.C., et al., 1997. The variable MR appearance of primary lymphoma of the central nervous system: comparison with histopathologic features. Am. J. Neuroradiol. 18, 563–572.

Johnson, B.E., Patronas, N., Hayes, W., et al., 1990. Neurologic, computed cranial tomographic, and magnetic resonance imaging abnormalities in patients with small-cell lung cancer. Further follow-up of 6- to 13-year survivors. J. Clin. Oncol. 8, 48–56.

Johnson, G.J., Oken, M.M., Anderson, J.R., et al., 1984. Central nervous system relapse in unfavourable-histology non-Hodgkin lymphoma: is prophylaxis indicated? Lancet 22, 685–687.

Kadan-Lottick, N.S., Skluzarek, M.C., Gurney, J.G., 2002. Decreasing incidence rates of primary central nervous system lymphoma. Cancer 95, 193–202.

Kai, Y., Kuratsu, J., Ushio, Y., 1998. Primary malignant lymphoma of the brain in childhood. Neurol. Medico-Chirurgica 38, 232–237.

Kaplan, I.I., Meredith, T.A., Aaberg, M., et al., 1980. Reclassification of intraocular reticulum cell sarcoma (histiocytic lymphoma); immunologic characterization of vitreous cells. Arch. Ophthalmol. 89, 707–710.

Kaplan, L.D., Abrams, D.I., Feigel, E., et al., 1989. AIDS-associated non-Hodgkin lymphoma in San Francisco. J. Am. Med. Assoc. 261, 719–727.

Katz, B.Z., Andiman, W.A., Eastman, R., et al., 1986. Infection with two genotypes of Epstein-Barr virus in an infant with AIDS and lymphoma of the central nervous system. J. Infect. Dis. 153, 601–604.

Kepes, J.I., 1987. Astrocytomas: Old and newly recognized variants, their spectrum and morphology and antigen expression. Can. J. Neurol. Sci. 14, 109–121.

Kessler, L.S., Ruiz, A., Donovan Post, M.J., et al., 1998. Thallium-201 brain SPECT of lymphoma in AIDS patients: pitfalls and technique optimization. Am. J. Neuroradiol. 19, 1105–1109.

Kim, M.S., Lee, J.I., Kim, W.S., et al., 2009. Primary central nervous system lymphoma after liver transplantation treated by radiosurgery combined with fractionated radiotherapy. J. Clin. Neurosci. 16, 583–585.

Kinlen, U., Sheil, A.G.R., Peto, J., et al., 1979. Collaborative United Kingdom–Australasian study of cancer in patients treated with immunosuppressive drugs. BMJ 2, 1461–1466.

Kitanaka, C., Eguchi, T., Kokubo, T., 1992. Secondary malignant lymphoma of the central nervous system with delayed high uptake on ^{123}1-IMP single-photon emission computerized tomography. J. Neurosurg. 76, 871–873.

Kleinschmidt-DeMasters, B.K., Damek, D.M., Lillehei, K.O., et al., 2008. Epstein Barr virus associated primary CNS lymphomas in elderly patients on immunosuppressive medications. J. Neuropathol. Exp. Neurol. 67, 1103–1111.

Kleinschmidt-DeMasters, B.K., Filley, C.M., Bitter, M.A., 1992. Central nervous system angiocentric, angiodestructive T-cell lymphoma (lymphomatoid granulomatosis). Surg. Neurol. 37, 130–137.

Kinoshita, M., Izumoto, S., Hashimoto, N., et al., 2008. Immunohistochemical analysis of adhesion molecules and matrix metalloproteinases in malignant CNS lymphomas and CNS intravascular lymphomas. Brain Tumour Pathol. 25, 73–78.

Kokinen, E., Billman, J.K., Abell, M.R., 1977. Lymphomatoid granulomatosis clinically confined to the CNS. Arch. Neurol. 34, 782–784.

Kori, S.H., Devereaux, M., Roessmann, U., 1983. Unusual presentations of CNS lymphoma. Neurol. 33 (Suppl. 2), A127.

Kuntzer, T., Bogousslavsky, I., Rilliet, B., et al., 1992. Herald facial numbness. Eur. J. Neurol. 32, 297–301.

Kupfer, M.C., Zee, C., Colletti, P.M., et al., 1990. MRI evaluation of AIDS-related encephalopathy: Toxoplasmosis vs lymphoma. Magn. Res. Imag. 8, 51–57.

Kuwabara, Y., Ichiya, Y., Otsuka, M., et al., 1988. High [18F] FDG uptake in primary cerebral lymphoma: A PET study. J. Comput. Assist. Tomogr. 12, 47–48.

Lach, B., Atack, E., Hylton, D., 1985. Clinical and pathological analysis of primary lymphomas of the brain: association of tumors with demyelinative leukoencephalopathy. J. Neuropathol. Exp. Neurol. 44, 309.

LaChance, D.H., O'Neill, B.P., Macdonald, D.R., et al., 1991. Primary leptomeningeal lymphoma: report of 9 cases, diagnosis with immunocytochemical analysis, and review of the literature. Neurology 41, 95–100.

Lai, A.P., Wierzbicki, A.S., Notman, P.M., 1991. Immunocytological diagnosis of primary cerebral non-Hodgkin lymphoma. J. Clin. Pathol. 44, 251–253.

Laperriere, N.J., Wong, C.S., Milosevic, M.F., et al., 1998. Accelerated radiation therapy for primary lymphoma of the brain. Radiother. Oncol. 47, 191–195.

Layden, B.T., Dubner, S., Toft, D.J., et al., 2009. Primary CNS lymphoma with bilateral symmetric hypothalamic lesions presenting with panhypopituitarism and diabetes insipidus. Pituitary Jan. 3 [Epub ahead of print].

Lazzato, G., Schafer, A.I., 1990. The prethrombotic state in cancer. Sem. Oncol. 17, 147–149.

Lee, Y., Bruner, J.M., van Tassel, P., et al., 1986. Primary central nervous system lymphoma: CT and pathologic correlation. Am. J. Radiol. 147, 747–752.

Leeds, N.E., Rosenblatt, R., Zimmetman, H.M., 1971. Focal angiographic changes of primary central nervous system lymphoma with pathologic correlation. Radiology 99, 595–599.

Lehrer, H., McGarry, P., 1968. Meningeal lymphosarcoma as a primary intracranial lesion. South Med. J. 61, 115–159.

Leibel, S.A., Sheline, G.E., 1987. Radiation therapy for neoplasms of the brain. J. Neurosurg. 66, 1–22.

Levine, A.M., 1992. Acquired Immunodeficiency Syndrome-related lymphoma. Blood 80, 8–20.

Levy, R.M., Bredesen, D.E., Rosenblum, M.L., 1985. Neurological manifestations of the acquired immunodeficiency syndrome (AIDS): experience at UCSF and review of the literature. J. Neurosurg. 62, 475–495.

Levy, O., Deangelis, L.M., Filippa, D.A., et al., 2008. Bcl-6 predicts improved prognosis in primary central nervous system lymphoma. Cancer 112, 151–156.

Liang, R.H.S., Woo, E.K.W., Yu, Y., et al., 1989. Central nervous system involvement in non-Hodgkin lymphoma. Eur. J. Clin. Oncol. 25, 703–710.

Liang, R., Woo, E., Ho, F., et al., 1990a. Klinefelter's syndrome and primary central nervous system lymphoma. Med. Pediatr. Oncol. 18, 236–239.

Liang, R., Chiu, E., Lake, S.L., 1990b. Secondary central nervous system involvement by non-Hodgkin lymphoma: the risk factors. Hematol. Oncol. 8, 141–145.

Liao, W., Liu, Y., Wang, X., et al., 2008. Differentiation of primary central nervous system lymphoma and high-grade glioma with dynamic susceptibility contrast-enhanced perfusion magnetic resonance imaging. Acta Radiol. 19, 1–9.

Liberski, P.P., Alwasiak, I., Wegrzyn, Z., 1982. Atypical progressive multifocal leucoencephalopathy and primary cerebral lymphoma. Neuropatol. Polska. 20, 413–419.

Liedtke, W., Trubner, K., Schwechheimer, K., 1995. On the role of human herpes virus 6 in viral latency in nervous tissue and in primary central nervous system lymphoma. J. Neurol. Sci. 134, 184–188.

Lindae, M.L., Lay, J., Abel, E.A., et al., 1990. Mycosis fungoides with CNS involvement: neuropsychiatric manifestations and complications of treatment with intrathecal methotrexate and whole-brain irradiation. J. Dermatol. Surg. Oncol. 16, 550–553.

Lipford, E.H., Margolick, J.B., Longo, D.L., et al., 1988. Angiocentric immunoproliferative lesions: a clinicopathologic spectrum of post-thymic T-cell proliferations. Blood 72, 1674–1681.

Lipsmeyer, E.A., 1972. Development of primary central nervous system lymphoma in a patient with systemic lupus erythematosus treated with immunosuppression. Arthr. Rheumat. 15, 183–186.

Littman, P., Wang, C.C., 1975. Reticulum sarcoma of the brain. A review of the literature and a study of 19 cases. Cancer 35, 1412–1420.

Locker, J., Nalesnik, M., 1989. Molecular genetic analysis of lymphoid tumors arising after organ transplantation. Am. J. Pathol. 135, 977–987.

Loeffler, I.S., Ervin, T.J., Mauch, P., et al., 1985. Primary lymphomas of the central nervous system: patterns of failure and factors that influence survival. J. Clin. Oncol. 3, 490–494.

MacMahon, F.M.F., Glass, J.D., Hayward, S.D., et al., 1991. Epstein-Barr virus in AIDS-related primary central nervous system lymphoma. Lancet 338, 969–973.

Maiuri, F., 1990. Visual involvement in primary non-Hodgkin lymphomas. Clin. Neurol. Neurosurg. 92, 119–124.

Margolis, L., Fraser, R., Lichter, A., et al., 1980. The role of radiation therapy in the management of ocular reticulum cell sarcoma. Cancer 45, 688–692.

Marsh, W.L., Stevenson, D.R., Long, H.J., 1983. Primary leptomeningeal presentation of T-cell lymphoma. Report of a patient and review of the literature. Cancer 51, 1125–1131.

Matsuda, M., McMurria, H., VanHale, P., et al., 1981. CSF findings in primary lymphoma of the CNS. Arch. Neurol. 38, 397.

Meeker, T.C., Shiramiza, B., Kaplan, L., et al., 1991. Evidence for molecular sub-types of HIV-associated lymphoma: division into peripheral monoclonal, polyclonal and central nervous system lymphoma. AIDS 5, 669–674.

Mendenhall, N.P., Thar, T.L., Agee, O.F., et al., 1983. Primary lymphoma of the central nervous system. Computerized tomography scan characteristics and treatment results for 12 cases. Cancer 52, 1993–2000.

Merchut, M.P., Haberland, C., Naheedy, M.H., et al., 1985. Long survival of primary cerebral lymphoma with progressive radiation necrosis. Neurology 35, 552–556.

Michalski, J.M., Garcia, D.M., Kase, E., et al., 1990. Primary central nervous system lymphoma: analysis of prognostic variables and patterns of treatment failure. Radiology 176, 855–860.

Miller, D.C., Knee, R., Schoenfeld, S., et al., 1989. Non-Hodgkin lymphoma of the central nervous system after treatment of Hodgkin disease. Am. J. Clin. Pathol. 91, 481–485.

Mittal, K., Neri, A., Feiner, H., et al., 1990. Lymphomatoid granulomatosis in the acquired immunodeficiency syndrome. Evidence of Epstein-Barr virus infection and B-cell clonal selection without myc rearrangement. Cancer 65, 1345–1349.

Model, L.M., 1977. Primary reticulum cell sarcoma of the brain in Wiskort-Aldrich syndrome. Arch. Neurol. 34, 633–635.

Mohile, N.A., DeAnngelis, L.M., Abrey, L.E., 2008. Utility of brain FDG-PET in primary CNS lymphoma. Clin. Adv. Haematol. Oncol. 6, 818–820.

Monfardini, S., Tirelli, U., Vaccher, F., et al., 1988. Malignant lymphomas in patients with or at risk for AIDS in Italy. J. Nat. Cancer Inst. 80, 855–860.

Monfardini, S., Vaccher, F., Foa, R., et al., 1990. AIDS-associated non-Hodgkin lymphoma in Italy: intravenous drug users versus homosexual men. Ann. Oncol. 1, 203–211.

Moore, R.D., Kessler, H., Richman, D.D., et al., 1991. Non-Hodgkin lymphoma in patients with advanced HIV infection treated with Zidovudine. J. Am. Med. Assoc. 265, 2208–2211.

Morrison, V., Gruber, S., Peterson, B., 1991. Therapy and outcome of post-transplant lymphomas. Proc. Am. Assoc. Cancer Res. 32, abstract 1137.

Moskowitz, L.B., Hensley, G.T., Chan, J.C., et al., 1984. The neuropathology of Acquired Immune Deficiency Syndrome. Arch. Pathol. Lab. Med. 108, 867–872.

Murphy, J.K., O'Brien, C.J., Ironside, J.W., 1989. Morphologic and immunophenotypic characterisation of primary brain lymphomas using paraffin-embedded tissue. Histopathology 15, 449–460.

Murphy, J.K., Young, L.S., Bevan, I.S., et al., 1990. Demonstration of Epstein-Barr virus in primary brain lymphoma by in situ DNA hybridisation in paraffin wax embedded tissue. J. Clin. Pathol. 43, 220–223.

Murray, K., Kun, L., Cox, J., 1986. Primary malignant lymphoma of the central nervous system. Results of treatment of 11 cases and review of the literature. J. Neurosurg. 65, 600–607.

Nair, S.D., Joseph, M.G., Catton, G.F., et al., 1989. Radiation therapy in lymphomatoid granulomatosis. Cancer 64, 821–824.

Nalesnik, M.A., Jaffe, R., Starzl, T.F., et al., 1988. The pathology of posttransplant lymphoproliferative disorders occurring in the setting of Cyclosporin A-prednisolone immunosuppression. Am. J. Pathol. 133, 173–192.

Namiki, T.S., Nichols, P., Young, T., et al., 1988. Stereotaxic biopsy diagnosis of central nervous system lymphoma. Am. J. Clin. Pathol. 90, 40–45.

Nelson, D.F., Martz, K.L., Bonner, H., et al., 1992. Non-Hodgkin lymphoma of the brain: Can high dose, large volume radiation therapy improve survival? Report on a prospective trial by the Radiation Oncology Group (RTOG): RTOG 8315. Int. J. Radiat. Oncol. Biol. Phys. 23, 9–17.

Neuwelt, E.A., Barnett, P.A., Bigner, D.D., et al., 1982. Effects of adrenal cortical steroids and osmotic blood-brain opening on methotrexate delivery to gliomas in the rodent: the factor of the blood-brain barrier. Proc. Nat. Acad. Sci. (USA) 79, 4420–4423.

Neuwelt, E.A., Howieson, J., Frenkel, F.P., et al., 1986. Therapeutic efficacy of multiagent chemotherapy with drug delivery enhancement by blood-brain barrier modification in glioblastoma. Neurosurgery 19, 573–582.

Neuwelt, F.A., Goldman, D.L., Dahlborg, S.A., et al., 1991. Primary CNS lymphoma treated with osmotic blood-brain barrier disruption: prolonged survival and preservation of cognitive function. J. Clin. Oncol. 9, 1580–1590.

Newell, M.E., Hoy, J.F., Cooper, S.G., et al., 2004. Human immunodeficiency virus related primary cerebral lymphoma: factors influencing survival in 111 patients. Cancer 100, 2627–2636.

Ng, K., Nash, J., Woodcock, B.E., 1991. High grade lymphoma of the cerebellum: a rare complication of chronic lymphatic leukaemia. Clin. Lab. Haematol. 13, 93–97.

Nguyen, P.L., Chakravarti, A., Finkelstein, D.M., et al., 2005. Results of whole-brain radiation as salvage of methotrexate failure for immunocompetent patients with primary CNS lymphoma. J. Clin. Oncol. 23, 1507–1513.

Ohkawa, S., Yamadori, A., Mori, E., et al., 1989. A case of primary malignant lymphoma of the brain with high uptake of ^{123}I-IMP. Neuroradiology 31, 270–272.

Omuro, A.M., DeAngelis, L.M., Yahalom, J., Abrey, L.E., 2005. Chemoradiotherapy for primary CNS lymphoma: an intent-to-treat analysis with complete follow-up. Neurology 64, 69–74.

Omuro, A.M., Taillandier, L., Chinot, O., et al., 2007. Temozolomide and methotrexate for primary central nervous system lymphoma in the elderly. J. Neurooncol. 85, 207–211.

O'Neill, B.P., Kelly, P.J., Earle, J.D., et al., 1987. Computer-assisted stereotaxic biopsy for the diagnosis of primary central nervous system lymphoma. Neurology 37, 1160–1164.

O'Neill, B.P., Haberman, T.M., Banks, P.M., et al., 1989. Primary central nervous system lymphoma as a variant of Richter's syndrome in two patients with chronic lymphocytic leukemia. Cancer 64, 1296–1300.

Onofri, M., Curatola, L., Ferracci, F., et al., 1992. Narcolepsy associated with primary temporal lobe B-cell lymphoma in a HLA D-negative subject. J. Neurol. Neurosurg. Psychiatry 55, 852–853.

O'Sullivan, M.G., Whittle, I.R., Gregor, A., et al., 1991. Increasing incidence of CNS primary lymphoma in south-east Scotland. Lancet 338, 895–896.

Otrakji, C.L., Voigt, W., Amador, A., et al., 1988. Malignant angioendotheliosis - a true lymphoma: a case of intravascular malignant lymphomatosis studied by Southern BWT hybridisation analysis. Hum. Pathol. 19, 475–478.

Palella, F.J., Delaney, K.M., Moorman, A.C., et al., 1998. Declining morbidity and mortality among patients with advanced human immunodeficiency virus infection. N. Engl. J. Med. 338, 853–860.

Panageas, K.S., Elkin, E.B., DeAngelis, L.M., et al., 2005. Trends in survival from primary central nervous system lymphoma, 1975–1999: a population based analysis. Cancer 104, 2466–2472.

Patrick, A.W., Campbell, I.W., Ashworth, B., et al., 1989. Primary cerebral lymphoma presenting with cranial diabetes insipidus. Postgrad. Med. J. 65, 771–772.

Pattengale, P.K., Taylor, C.R., Panke, T., et al., 1979. Selective immunodeficiency and malignant lymphoma of the central nervous system. Possible relationship to the Epstein-Barr virus. Acta Neuropathol. 48, 165–169.

Pauzner, R., Mouallem, M., Sadeb, M., et al., 1989. High incidence of primary cerebral lymphoma in tumor-induced central neurogenic hyperventilation. Arch. Neurol. 46, 510–512.

Pels, H., Schmidt-Wolf, I.G., Glasmacher, A., et al., 2003. Primary central nervous system lymphoma: results of a pilot and phase II study of systemic and intraventricular chemotherapy with deferred radiotherapy. J. Clin. Oncol. 21, 4489–4495.

Penn, I., 1981. Depressed immunity and the development of cancer. Clin. Exp. Immunol. 46, 459–474.

Penn, I., 1987. Cancers following cyclosporine therapy. Transplantation 43, 32–35.

Penn, I., Starzl, T.F., 1972. Malignant tumors arising de novo in immunosuppressed organ transplant patients. Transplantation 14, 407–417.

Perez-Soler, R., Smith, T.L., Cabanillas, F., 1986. Central nervous system prophylaxis with combined intravenous and intrathecal methotrexate in diffuse lymphoma of aggressive histologic type. Cancer 57, 971–977.

Pfleger, L., Tappeiner, J., 1959. Zur Kenntnis der systemisierten Endotheliomatose der cutanen Blutgefasse (reticuloendotheliose?) Hautarzt. 10, 359–363.

Pfreundschuh, M., Trümper, L., Osterborg, A., et al., 2006. CHOP-like chemotherapy plus rituximab versus CHOP-like chemotherapy alone in young patients with good-prognosis diffuse large-B-cell lymphoma: a randomised controlled trial by the MabThera International Trial (MInT) Group. Lancet Oncol. 7, 379–391.

Plotkin, S.R., Betensky, R.A., Hochberg, F.H., et al., 2004. Treatment of relapsed central nervous system lymphoma with high-dose methotrexate. Clin. Cancer Res. 10, 5643–5646.

Pirotte, B., Levivier, M., Goldman, S., et al., 1997. Glucocorticoid-induced long-term remission in primary cerebral lymphoma: case report and review of the literature. J. Neurooncology 31, 63–69.

Pitman, S.W., Frei, E., 1977. Weekly methotrexate-calcium leucovorin rescue: effect of alkalinization on nephrotoxicity; pharmacokinetics in the CNS; and use in CNS non-Hodgkin lymphoma. Cancer Treat Rep. 61, 695–701.

Pluda, J.M., Yarchoan, R., Jaffe, E.S., et al., 1990. Development of non-Hodgkin lymphoma in a cohort of patients with severe Human Immunodeficiency Virus (HIV) infection on long-term antiretroviral therapy. Ann. Int. Med. 113, 276–282.

Pluda, K.M., Venzon, D., Tosato, G., et al., 1991. Factors which predict for the development of non-Hodgkin lymphoma (NHL) in patients with HIV infection receiving antiviral therapy. Blood 78 (no. 10) abstract, 1129.

Pollack, I.F., Lunsford, L.D., Flickinger, J.C., et al., 1989. Prognostic factors in the diagnosis and treatment of primary central nervous system lymphoma. Cancer 63, 939–947.

Poon, T., Matoso, I., Tchertkoff, V., et al., 1989. CT features of primary cerebral lymphoma in AIDS and non-AIDS patients. J. Comp. Assist. Tomogr. 13, 6–9.

Poortmans, P.M., Kluin-Nelemans, H.C., Haaxma-Reiche, H., et al., 2003. High-dose methotrexate-based chemotherapy followed by consolidating radiotherapy in non-AIDS-related primary central nervous system lymphoma: European Organization for Research and Treatment of Cancer Lymphoma Group Phase II Trial 20962. J. Clin. Oncol. 15, 4483–4488.

Purvin, V., Van Dyk, H.J., 1984. Primary reticulum cell sarcoma of the brain presenting as steroid-responsive optic neuropathy. J. Clin. Neurol. Ophthalmol. 4, 15–23.

Rabkin, C.S., Biggar, R.J., Horm, J.W., 1991. Increasing incidence of cancers associated with the Human Immunodeficiency virus epidemic. Int. J. Cancer 47, 692–696.

Rampen, F.H.J., van Andel, J.G., Sizoo, W., et al., 1980. Radiation therapy in primary non-Hodgkin lymphomas of the CNS. Eur. J. Cancer 16, 177–184.

Ramsay, R.G., Geremia, G.K., 1988. CNS complications of AIDS: CT and MR findings. Am. J. Radiol. 151, 449–454.

Raphael, J., Gentilhomme, O., Tulliez, M., et al., 1991. Histopathologic features of high grade non-Hodgkin lymphomas in acquired immunodeficiency syndrome. Arch. Pathol. Lab. Med. 115, 15–20.

Rapoport, S.I., 1988. Osmotic opening of the blood-brain barrier. Ann. Neurol. 24, 677–684.

Ree, H.J., Strauchen, J.A., Khan, A.A., et al., 1991. Human Immunodeficiency Virus-associated Hodgkin disease. Cancer 67, 1614–1621.

Remick, S.C., Diamond, C., Migliozzi, J.A., et al., 1990. Primary central nervous system lymphoma in patients with and without the acquired immune deficiency syndrome. A retrospective analysis and review of the literature. Medicine. 69, 345–360.

Reni, M., Ferreri, A.J.M., Villa, E., 1999. Second line treatment for primary central nervous system lymphoma. Br. J. Cancer 79, 530–534.

Reni, M., Ferreri, A.J., Garancini, M.P., et al., 1997. Therapeutic management of primary central nervous system lymphoma in immunocompetent patients: results of a critical review of the literature. Ann. Oncol. 8, 227–234.

Reni, M., Zaja, F., Mason, W., et al., 2007. Temozolomide as salvage treatment in primary brain lymphomas. Br. J. Cancer 96, 864–867.

Reyes, M.G., Homsi, M.F., Mangkornkanong, M., et al., 1990. Malignant lymphoma presenting as a chronic subdural hematoma. Surg. Neurol. 33, 35–36.

Reznik, M., 1975. Pathology of primary reticulum cell sarcoma of the human central nervous system. Acta Neuropathol. Suppl. 6, 91–94.

Riggs, S., Hagemeister, F.B., 1988. Immunodeficiency states: A predisposition to lymphoma. In: Fuller, L.M., Sullivan, M.P., Hagemeister, F.B., et al. (Eds) Hodgkin disease and non-Hodgkin lymphomas in adults and children. Raven Press, New York, pp. 451–478.

Rockwood, E.J., Zakov, Z.N., Bay, J.W., 1984. Combined malignant lymphoma of the eye and CNS (reticulum-cell sarcoma). Report of three cases. J. Neurosurg. 61, 369–374.

Roithmann, S., Andrieu, J.M., 1992. Clinical and biological characteristics of malignant lymphomas in HIV-infected patients. Eur. J. Cancer 28, 1501–1508.

Roithmann, S., Tourani, J.M., Andrieu, J.M., 1990. Hodgkin Disease in HIV-infected intravenous drug abusers. N. Engl. J. Med. 323, 275–276.

Roithmann, S., Toledano, M., Tourani, J.M., et al., 1991. HIV-associated non-Hodgkin lymphomas: Clinical characteristics and outcome. The experience of the French Registry of HIV-associated tumors. Ann. Oncol. 2, 289–295.

Roman-Goldstein, S.M., Golgman, D.L., Howieson, J., et al., 1992. MR of primary CNS lymphoma in immunologically normal patients. AJNR Am. J. Neuroradiol. 13, 1207–1213.

Rootman, J., Gudauskas, G., Kumi, C., 1983. Subconjunctival versus intravenous cytosine arabinoside: effect of route of administration and ocular toxicity. Invest. Ophthalmol. Vis. Sci. 24, 1607–1611.

Rosenberg, N.L., Hochberg, F.H., Miller, G., et al., 1986. Primary central nervous system lymphoma related to Epstein-Barr virus in a patient with acquired immune deficiency syndrome. Ann. Neurol. 20, 98–102.

Rosenberg, S.A., Berard, C.W., Byron, W., et al., 1982. National Cancer Institute sponsored study of classifications of non-Hodgkin lymphomas. Summary and description of a working formulation for clinical usage. Cancer 49, 2112–2135.

Rosenblum, M.L., Levy, M.R., Bredesen, D.E., et al., 1988. Primary central nervous system lymphomas in patients with AIDS. Ann. Neurol. 23 (Suppl.), 13–16.

Rosenfeld, S.S., Hoffman, J.M., Coleman, R.E., et al., 1992. Studies of primary central nervous system lymphoma with fluorine-18-fluorodeoxyglucose positron emission tomography. J. Nucl. Med. 33, 532–536.

Rosenthal, M.A., Sheridan, W.P., Green, M.D., et al., 1993. Primary cerebral lymphoma: an argument for the use of adjunctive systemic chemotherapy. Aust. N. Z. J. Surg. 63, 30–32.

Ross, R., Dworsky, R., Paganini-Hill, A., et al., 1985. Non-Hodgkin lymphomas in never married men in Los Angeles. Br. J. Cancer 52, 785–787.

Rouah, E., Rogers, B.B., Wilson, D.R., et al., 1990. Demonstration of Epstein-Barr virus in primary central nervous system lymphomas by the polymerase chain reaction and in situ hybridisation. Hum. Pathol. 21, 545–550.

Roy, S., Josephson, S.A., Fridlyand, J., et al., 2008. Protein biomarker identification in the CSF of patients with CNS lymphoma. J. Clin. Oncol. 26, 96–105.

Rubenstein, J.L., Combs, D., Rosenberg, J., et al., 2003. Rituximab therapy for CNS lymphomas: targeting the leptomeningeal compartment. Blood 101, 466–468.

Rubenstein, J., Ferreri, A.J., Pittaluga, 2008. Primary lymphoma of the central nervous system: epidemiology, pathology and current approaches to diagnosis, prognosis and treatment. Leuk. Lymphoma 49, 43–51.

Rubenstein, J., Fischbein, N., Aldape, K., et al., 2002. Hemorrhage and VEGF expression in a case of primary CNS lymphoma. J. Neurooncol. 58, 53–56.

Rubenstein, J.L., Fridlyand, J., Shen, A., et al., 2006. Gene expression and angiotropism in primary CNS lymphoma. Blood 107 (9), 3716–3723.

Ruff, R.L., Petito, C.K., Rawlinson, D.G., 1979. Primary cerebral lymphoma mimicking multiple sclerosis. Arch. Neurol. 36, 598.

Sagerman, R.H., Cassady, J.R., Chang, C.H., 1967. Radiation therapy for intracranial lymphoma. Radiology 88, 552–554.

Salih, S.B., Saeed, A.B., Alzahrani, M., et al., 2009. Primary CNS lymphoma presenting as fever of unknown origin. J. Neurooncol. 93, 401–404.

Sandor, V., Stark-Vancs, V., Pearson, D., et al., 1998. Phase II trial of chemotherapy alone for primary CNS and intraocular lymphoma. J. Clin. Oncol. 16, 3000–3006.

Sapozink, M.D., Kaplan, H.S., 1983. Intracranial Hodgkin disease. A report of 12 cases and review of the literature. Cancer 1301–1307.

Sawataishi, J., Mineura, K., Sasajima, T., et al., 1992. Effects of radiotherapy determined by 11 C-methyl-L-methionine positron emission tomography in patients with primary cerebral malignant lymphoma. Neuroradiology 34, 517–519.

Schmidt, B.J., Meagher-Villemure, K., Del Carpio, J., 1984. Lymphomatoid granulomatosis with isolated involvement of the brain. Ann. Neurol. 15, 478–481.

Schmitt-Graff, A., Pfitzer, P., 1983. Cytology of the cerebrospinal fluid in primary malignant lymphomas of the central nervous system. Acta Cytologica 27, 267–272.

Schneck, S.A., Penn, I., 1971. De-novo brain tumours in renal-transplant recipients. Lancet i, 983–986.

Schnittman, S.M., Lane, H.C., Higgins, S.E., et al., 1986. Direct polyclonal activation of human B lymphocytes by the acquired deficiency syndrome virus. Science 233, 1084–1086.

Schricker, J.L., Smith, D.E., 1955. Primary intracerebral Hodgkin disease. Cancer 8, 629–633.

Schwaighofer, B.W., Hesselink, J.R., Press, G.A., et al., 1989. Primary intracranial CNS lymphoma: MR manifestations. AJNR Am. J. Neuroradiol. 10, 725–729.

Shah, G.D., Yahalom, J., Correa, D.D., et al., 2007. Combined immunohistochemistry with reduced whole brain radiotherapy for newly diagnosed primary CNS lymphoma. J. Clin. Oncol. 25, 4730–4735.

Sheline, G.E., Wara, W.M., Smith, V., 1980. Therapeutic irradiation and brain injury. Int. J. Radiat. Oncol. Biol. Phys. 6, 1215–1228.

Shen, D.F., Zhuang, Z., LeHoang, P., et al., 1998. Utility of microdissection and polymerase chain reaction for the detection of immunoglobulin gene rearrangement and translocation in primary intraocular lymphoma. Ophthalmology 105, 1664–1669.

Sherman, M.E., Erozan, Y.S., Mann, R.B., et al., 1991. Stereotactic brain biopsy in the diagnosis of malignant lymphoma. Am. J. Clin. Pathol. 95, 878–883.

Shibamoto, Y., Tsutsui, K., Dodo, Y., et al., 1990. Improved survival rate in primary intracranial lymphoma treated by high-dose radiation and systemic vincristine-doxorubicin-cyclophosphamide-prednisolone chemotherapy. Cancer 65, 1907–1912.

Shipp, M., Harrington, D., Anderson, J., et al., 1992. Development of a predictive model for aggressive lymphoma: The International NHL Prognostic Factors Project. Proc. Am. Soc. Clin. Oncol. Abstract 1084.

Shiramizu, B., Barriga, F., Neequaye, J., et al., 1991. Patterns of chromosomal breakpoint locations in Burkitt's lymphoma: relevance to geography and Epstein-Barr virus association. Blood 7, 1516–1526.

Singh, A., Strobos, R.J., Singh, B.M., et al., 1982. Steroid-induced remissions in CNS lymphoma. Neurology 32, 1267–1271.

Skarin, A.T., Zuckerman, K.S., Pitman, S.W., et al., 1977. High-dose methotrexate with folinic acid rescue in the treatment of advanced non-Hodgkin lymphoma including CNS involvement. Blood 50, 1039–1047.

Smadja, D., Mas, J., Fallet-Bianco, C., et al., 1991. Intravascular lymphomatosis (neoplastic angioendotheliosis) of the central nervous system: case report and literature review. J. Neurooncol. 11, 171–180.

Smith, W.J., Garson, J.A., Bourne, S.P., et al., 1988. Immunoglobulin gene rearrangement and antigenic profile confirm B cell origin of primary cerebral lymphoma and indicate a mature phenotype. J. Clin. Pathol. 41, 128–132.

Smith, J.R., Braziel, R.M., Paoletti, S., et al., 2003. Expression of B-cell attracting chemokine1 (CXCL13) by malignant lymphocytes and vascular endothelium in primary central nervous system lymphoma. Blood 101, 815–821.

Smith, J.R., Falkenhagen, K.M., Coupland, S.E., et al., 2007. Malignant B cells from patients with primary central nervous system lymphoma express stromal cell-derived factor-1. Am. J. Clin. Pathol. 127, 633–641.

Snider, W.D., Simpson, D.M., Aronyk, K.F., et al., 1983. Primary lymphoma of the nervous system associated with Acquired Immune-deficiency Syndrome. N. Eng. J. Med. 308, 45.

So, Y.T., Beckstead, J.H., Davis, R.L., 1986. Primary central nervous system lymphoma in Acquired Immune Deficiency Syndrome: A clinical and pathological study. Ann. Neurol. 20, 566–572.

Socie, G., Piprot-Chauffat, C., Schlienger, M., et al., 1990. Primary lymphoma of the central nervous system. An unresolved therapeutic problem. Cancer 65, 322–326.

Soussain, C., Hoang-Xuan, K., Taillandier, L., et al., 2008. Intensive chemotherapy followed by hematopoietic stem-cell rescue for refractory and recurrent primary CNS and intraocular lymphoma: Societe Francaise de Greffe de Moelle Osseuse-Therapie Cellulaire. J. Clin. Oncol. 26, 2512–2518.

Soussain, C., Merle-Beral, H., Reux, I., et al., 1996. A single center study of 11 patients with intraocular lymphoma treated with conventional chemotherapy followed by high dose chemotherapy and autologous bone marrow transplantation in 5 cases. Leuk. Lymphoma 23, 339–345.

Spillane, J.A., Kendall, B.F., Moseley, I.F., 1982. Primary central nervous system lymphoma: clinical radiological correlation. J. Neurol. Neurosurg. Psychiatry 45, 199–208.

Starzl, T.F., Nalesnik, M.A., Porter, K.A., et al., 1984. Reversibility of lymphomas and lymphoproliferative lesions developing under cyclosporin-steroid therapy. Lancet 1, 583–587.

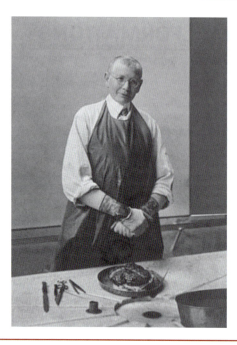

Figure 42.1 Jakob Erdheim (1874–1937).

Embryology

The origin of craniopharyngiomas remains controversial. Several observations indicate that they are derived from Rathke's pouch epithelium. Two theories have been proposed, both linking the origin of these tumors to small rests of ectoderm.

The first hypothesis relates the development of craniopharyngiomas to the embryogenesis of the adenohypophysis (Samii & Tatagiba 2001). In week 4, the roof of the primitive oral cavity or stomodeum develops a rostral invagination lined by epithelial cells of ectodermal origin. This is situated anterior to the buccopharyngeal membrane and is known as Rathke's pouch. Simultaneously, the infundibulum forms a downward growth of neuroepithelium from the floor of the diencephalon (Fig. 42.2).

During the 2nd month of development, these come into contact. The neck of Rathke's pouch then attenuates, eventually separating from the oral epithelium. The remaining Rathke's vesicle then applies itself against the front of the infundibulum. The anterior wall of the vesicle develops into a glandular, pseudostratified columnar epithelium, normally representing the primordium of the adenohypophysis that gives rise to the pars distalis, pars tuberalis and pars intermedia. The cavity, reduced to a narrow cleft, usually involutes. The path along which the Rathke's pouch migrates constitutes the craniopharyngeal duct. Erdheim (1904) proposed that craniopharyngiomas originate from ectoblastic epithelial rests along the craniopharyngeal duct and in the pars distalis and tuberalis (see also Samii & Tatagiba 2001).

If parts of Rathke's pouch fail to develop into the adenohypophysis, as per normal, they may differentiate into either tooth primordia (giving rise to adamantinomatous craniopharyngioma) or into oral mucosa (giving rise to papillary craniopharyngioma). The occasional occurrence of mixed

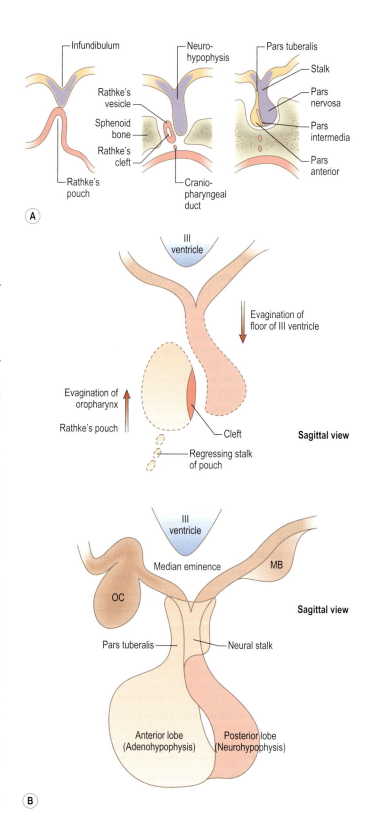

Figure 42.2 Schematic drawing of the development of Rathke's pouch and the hypophysis. OC = optic chiasm, MB = mammilliary body.

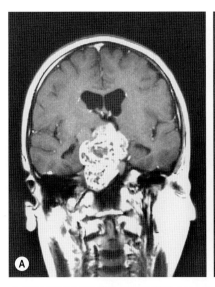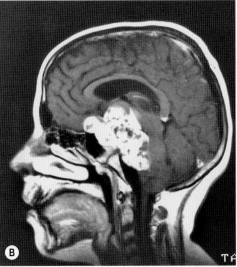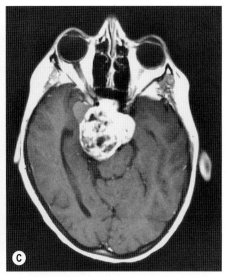

Figure 42.3 (A) Coronal, (B) sagittal and (C) axial T1-weighted gadolinium enhanced MRI sections showing a large hyperintense typical craniopharyngioma mass extending into the anterior and posterior fossa, the third ventricle and compressing the right temporal lobe. (With permission from Samii, M. and Tatagiba, M., Craniopharyngioma, in Brain tumors: an encyclopedic approach A.H. Kaye and E.R. Laws (Jr.), Editors. Churchill Livingstone, 2001. p. 945–964. With permission of Elsevier.)

tumors with features of both craniopharyngioma and Rathke's cleft cyst, support this theory (Janzer et al 2000). Contrary to this hypothesis is evidence that these hypophyseal cell rests, supposedly ectoblastic remnants from embryogenesis, are present in only 3% of neonates (Goldberg & Eshbaugh 1960), do not show any proof of neoplastic transformation, and occur more frequently with age (Luse & Kernohan 1955). It has also been noted that Rathke's cleft cysts and craniopharyngiomas, although both considered to arise from the embryonic rests of Rathke's pouch, appear different histologically (Samii & Tatagiba 2001).

The second hypothesis concerning the pathogenesis of craniopharyngiomas suggests that the residual squamous epithelium found in the adenohypophysis and anterior infundibulum undergoes metaplasia. As squamous cell rests occur more frequently with each passing decade and are rarely found in children, it was thus suggested that craniopharyngiomas arise from metaplasia of mature components of the anterior pituitary rather than embryonic remnants (Samii & Tatagiba 2001; Hunter 1955). The theory of a dual origin is supported by craniopharyngiomas having a biphasic age incidence with the so-called 'childhood' (adamantinomatous) craniopharyngioma arising from the embryonic remnants and the 'adult' (papillary squamous) craniopharyngioma from metaplastic foci of adenohypophyseal cells (Adamson et al 1990). Russell and Rubinstein (1989) have suggested that the frequency of both tumor types in pathology specimens of craniopharyngiomas represents a single group of tumors ranging from a purely childhood type, through a mixed variety to the adult type.

Surgical anatomy

Craniopharyngiomas present as part of a wide spectrum with regard to a number of characteristics (Thapar & Laws

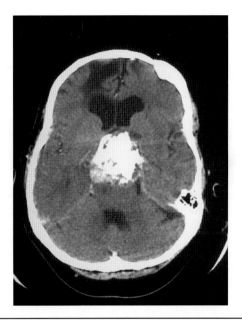

Figure 42.4 Axial CT scan of craniopharyngioma showing extensive calcification.

1995). They can vary in size from being microscopic to extensive lesions comprising a large percentage of the intracranial volume (Fig. 42.3).

Almost all have both cystic and solid components in varying combinations (Fahlbusch et al 1999). Calcification is found on microscopic examination in approximately half of adult craniopharyngiomas and in almost all pediatric cases (Fig. 42.4) (Sung et al 1981).

Craniopharyngiomas vary from being well circumscribed to being grossly invasive and may cause an intense glial reaction in surrounding brain. This reaction is particularly dense around small papillary projections towards the hypothalamus. Some surgeons maintain that traction on this glial attachment will invariably lead to hypothalamic injury and preclude safe total resection of the tumor (Kempe 1968), while others maintain that this 'glial envelope' often provides a safe plane facilitating cleavage without damaging neural tissue (Sweet 1980).

As well as being adherent to the hypothalamus, craniopharyngiomas are usually also adherent to major arteries at the skull base, including small perforators originating from the anterior communicating vessels, the posterior communicating artery, branches from the anterior choroidal artery and thalamo-perforating vessels (Symon & Sprich 1985; Samii & Bini 1991). Tumor adherence to vessels is one of the primary reasons for incomplete tumor resection (Fahlbusch et al 1999). Attempted radical dissection has been associated with weakening of the adventitia of blood vessels by injury to the vasa vasorum. This may result in fusiform dilatation of the internal carotid artery and the potential for delayed catastrophic hemorrhage (Sutton et al 1991). The above factors, tumor within the third ventricle, size and the presence of hydrocephalus, all play an important role in determining the extent of resection (Fahlbusch et al 1999; Chakrabarti et al 2005).

The blood supply of the anterior part of the tumor is supplied by perforators from the anterior communicating artery and proximal anterior cerebral artery. The lateral part of the tumor receives branches from the posterior communicating artery. The intrasellar component is supplied by the intracavernous meningohypophyseal arteries. Of great surgical significance is that craniopharyngiomas never receive blood supply from the posterior cerebral and basilar arteries unless the anterior blood supply from the lower hypothalamus and floor of the third ventricle is absent (Pertuiset 1975).

Cystic components are identified in 54–94% of all craniopharyngiomas but are found in 99% of pediatric craniopharyngiomas (Gottfried & Couldwell 2008). From a histological point of view, craniopharyngiomas can vary from having columnar to cuboidal to respiratory to squamous epithelium. Their cyst contents vary from being clear fluid to viscid then 'purulent' with cholesterol crystals, flakes and calcific and keratinized debris (Fig. 42.5).

Approximately 5–15% are truly intrasellar (Fahlbusch et al 1999; Harwood-Nash 1994). On average, another 25% present as a suprasellar mass, 30% extend anteriorly to involve the frontal lobes, 25% grow laterally into the middle cranial fossa and 20% grow posteriorly and inferiorly encroaching on the brainstem and extending into the cerebellopontine angle. The degree of vertical extension of tumor is classified into five grades.

Intrasellar craniopharyngiomas may expand, compressing the pituitary gland and cause endocrinopathies before compressing the optic chiasm. More frequently the tumor grows pushing the diaphragma upward, potentially breaking through and extending in any direction. In relation to the optic chiasm, the tumor may extend anteriorly (prechiasmatic) in the direction of the subfrontal spaces. These tumors are frequently cystic and can achieve a large size before being diagnosed. When the tumor grows posterior to the chiasm (retrochiasmatic), it displaces the pituitary stalk

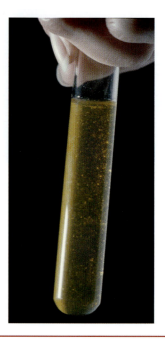

Figure 42.5 Test-tube filled with the typical fluid contents of a cystic craniopharyngioma. Cyst contents range from 'machinery oil' to shimmering cholesterol laden fluid as demonstrated.

anteriorly and the chiasm forwards and upwards, making the optic nerve appears falsely prefixed (pseudo-prefixity). Cystic retrochiasmatic craniopharyngiomas may reach enormous size by expanding into the posterior fossa along the petroclival area. The tumor may also displace the chiasm upwards (sub-chiasmatic) and the stalk posteriorly. Retro- and sub-chiasmatic craniopharyngiomas are frequently solid tumors. They usually grow into the third ventricle causing compression of the hypothalamus and obstruction of the foramina of Munro. Further extension upward causes the ventricular floor to attenuate allowing the tumor to protrude into the ventricle. The tumor may also expand laterally causing compression of the temporal lobe.

Craniopharyngiomas may arise directly from the floor of the third ventricle but this is unusual (Sipos & Vajda 1997). This is essentially a retrochiasmatic tumor but it may extend anteriorly to the prechiasmatic space, superiorly to the lumen of the third ventricle, posteriorly to the interpeduncular and prepontine cisterns, and laterally to the basal ganglia and temporal lobes (Samii & Tatagiba 2001).

Their microanatomic disposition might be either extra-arachnoid or subarachnoid and extrapial or intrapial. This wide variation in pathology and behavior once again underscores the fact that management of craniopharyngiomas needs to be very much individualized for each patient and is not suited to the occasional surgeon (Laws 1994; Epstein 1994; Ciric & Cozzens 1980).

Importantly, the position of the optic chiasm relative to the tumor can usually be extrapolated from the position of the anterior communicating artery on preoperative midsagittal MRI. This is critical in determining the optimal and safest approach. One third are sub-chiasmatic, 20%

prechiasmatic and 10–15% intrasellar (Pang 1993). The size of the lateral ventricles usually allows determination of the anatomical relationship of a craniopharyngioma to the third ventricle or its remnants and to plan an appropriate surgical approach to avoid transgressing the hypothalamus (Steno et al 2004; Honegger & Tatagiba 2008).

Incidence and prevalence

Due to their relatively low incidence and except for isolated centers worldwide, surgical experience consequently remains relatively sparse for these unique tumors. Craniopharyngiomas account for 1.2–4.6% of all intracranial tumors, corresponding to 0.5–2.5 new cases per million population per year (Janzer et al 2000; Choux et al 1991; Russell & Rubinstein 1989; Adamson et al 1990; Zulch 1986; Bunin et al 1998). They formed 4.6% of Cushing's series of 2000 intracranial tumors. They affect patients of all age groups but guided by a bimodal age distribution, they have a peak incidence among children 5–14 years old and a second peak incidence among adults 50–74 years old (Samii & Tatagiba 2001; Ture & Krisht 1999; Karavitaki & Wass 2008). They comprise 5–10% of intracranial tumors in children and 56% of sellar and suprasellar tumors and are consequently considered a tumor of childhood which is technically incorrect as they are more frequent in adults. Although there are studies indicating that craniopharyngiomas are male predominant, more recent studies show that craniopharyngiomas have no sex predilection (Ture & Krisht 1999; Karavitaki & Wass 2008). They are more frequent in Japanese children with an incidence of 5.25 cases per million in the pediatric age group in Africa (18%) and in the Far East (16%) (Choux et al 1991; Zulch 1986). They are the most common non-epithelial intracerebral neoplasm in children, accounting for 5–10% of intracranial tumors in this age group (Janzer et al 2000). There have been isolated reports of neonatal and intrauterine cases (Bunin et al 1998).

Familial history and genetics

Familial incidence is exceptional and only rare cases of craniopharyngiomas occurring in siblings, cousins and children of affected parents have been reported (Vargas et al 1981; Combelles et al 1984; Wald et al 1982). They occur sporadically and no definite genetic relationship has been reported in their pathogenesis (Rienstein et al 2003). Rienstein and colleagues demonstrated that a sub-set of adamantinous craniopharyngiomas were monoclonal in origin – presumably due to chromosomal defects on specific loci. Several genetic abnormalities have been observed including translocation, deletion and an increase in DNA copies (Rienstein et al 2003; Górski et al 1992; Karnes et al 1992). All adamantinous craniopharyngiomas express beta-catenin. Some harbor beta-catenin mutations affecting exon 3 that activates the Wnt signalling pathway resulting in mitogenic stimulation – a process implicated in the formation of several neoplasms (Kato et al 2004; Sekine et al 2002). In contrast, mutations of p53 suppressor gene and the gsp or gip oncogene have not been demonstrated (Karavitaki & Wass 2008).

Genetic studies have also shown conflicting results (Gottfried & Couldwell 2008). One study showed no chromosomal abnormalities amongst 20 adamantinomatous and nine papillary craniopharyngiomas (Rickert & Paulus 2003). Another study revealed that six of nine tumors had genomic alterations, with three having six or more abnormalities – mostly chromosomal gains (Rienstein et al 2003).

Presentation

The presentation of craniopharyngiomas is largely determined by their site of origin, size and direction of growth but remains consistently various combinations of endocrine dysfunction, visual failure, cognitive disturbances and raised intracranial pressure. Due to their predilection for the pituitary stalk, although not altogether statistically correct, the 'classical' presentation of a craniopharyngioma is that of a suprasellar mass with calcification, manifesting with visual failure, hypopituitarism and diabetes insipidus. Frequently, however, their presentation is more subtle and often much delayed, with diabetes insipidus occurring in about 15% preoperatively. Although the duration of symptoms prior to diagnosis ranges from 1 week to 30 years (Karavitaki et al 2006), there is generally a 12–24-month interval between the onset of clinical symptoms and clinical detection (Samii & Samii 1995). Early diagnosis is favorable as it warrants prompt treatment that leads to better clinical outcomes. Hence early recognition of clinical features is an essential part of patient management.

Increased intracranial pressure (ICP)

Craniopharyngiomas are indolent neoplasms and have a relatively slow growth rate in comparison with other brain malignancies. This together with their extra-axial location make it possible for them to stay asymptomatic until they are relatively large (Ture & Krisht 1999; Carmel 1995). Many craniopharyngiomas will eventually become big enough to impede the CSF circulation at the foramina of Munro and result in obstructive hydrocephalus (Fig. 42.6).

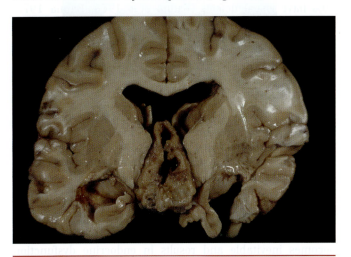

Figure 42.6 Pathological coronal specimen demonstrating a large craniopharyngioma extending into the third ventricle with obstruction of the foramina of Munro and hydrocephalus.

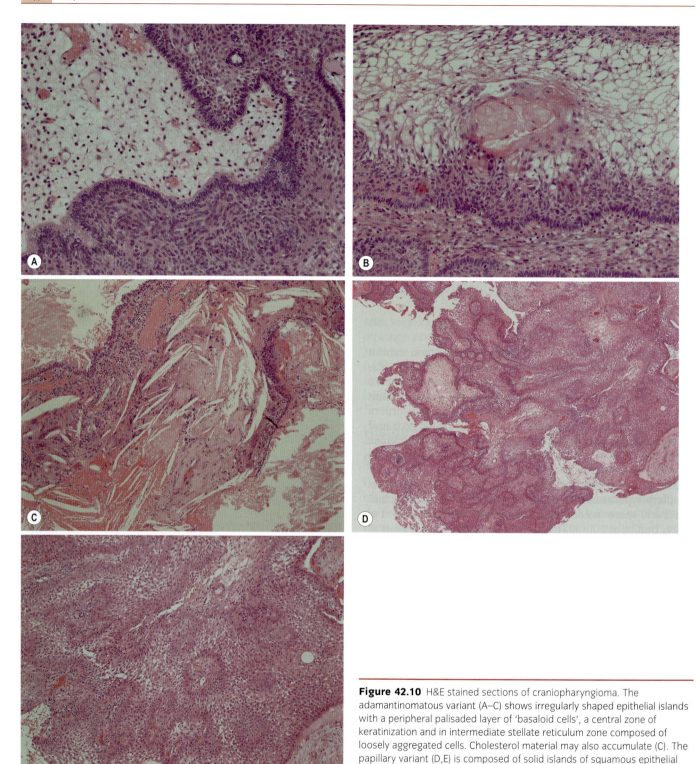

Figure 42.10 H&E stained sections of craniopharyngioma. The adamantinomatous variant (A–C) shows irregularly shaped epithelial islands with a peripheral palisaded layer of 'basaloid cells', a central zone of keratinization and in intermediate stellate reticulum zone composed of loosely aggregated cells. Cholesterol material may also accumulate (C). The papillary variant (D,E) is composed of solid islands of squamous epithelial cells with less prominent central keratinization. Cyst formation is unusual in this variant. (Courtesy of Michael Gonzales.)

papillary projections into the hypothalamus appear as islands of epithelium, but on investigation, are not suggestive of malignancy.

Individual craniopharyngioma cells vary greatly on electron microscopy but show a relatively uniform pattern with desmosomes, tonofibrils and microvilli (Samii & Tatagiba 2001). The initial phase of calcification is due to calcification and the deposition of hydroxyapatite by small membrane bound vesicles and tonofibrils (Sato et al 1986). Szeifert and colleagues (1991) demonstrated secretory activity in microcysts and some epithelial cells. Anaplastic changes have been seen in aggressive tumors (Liszczak et al 1978). Malignant degeneration is exceedingly rare, if ever previously seen on histology (Figs 42.9, 42.10).

Molecular markers and immunohistochemistry

The identification of molecular markers for craniopharyngiomas has been initiated but as yet, no clinical application established (Gottfried & Couldwell 2008). In tissue culture, a sub-set of craniopharyngiomas with strong insulin-like growth factor 1 (IGF-1) receptor expression have shown growth arrest with IGF-1 receptor inhibitors (Ulfarsson et al 2005). The expression of p-glycoprotein, somatostatin receptors and oestrogen receptors has been reported with unknown significance (Thapar et al 1994). It is, however, appreciated that the incidence of recurrence is higher for patients negative for these receptors, due to loss of differentiation (Izumoto et al 2005). Pituitary hormones (Szeifert & Pasztor 1993), β-hCG (Tachibana et al 1994) and chromogranin A (Yamada et al 1995) may also be expressed with CSF β-hCG levels being elevated in patients with craniopharyngiomas.

Monoclonal antibody MIB-1 has been used to study proliferation in craniopharyngiomas. Nishi et al (1999) suggested that tumors with a lower MIB-1 labeling index (LI) have less chance of recurring, with an MIB-1 LI >7% being a useful predictor for recurrence. A clear relationship between MIB-1 LI and tumor biology has not been established by other authors (Dickey et al 1999) perhaps because of proliferative heterogeneity between regions (Janzer et al 2000). An elevated K_i-67 index is associated with a high possibility of tumor recurrence (Izumoto et al 2005).

Surgical management

Craniopharyngiomas are benign midline tumors with a propensity for local recurrence. Ideally, total surgical removal is therefore arguably the management of choice (Samii & Tatagiba 2001; Fahlbusch et al 1999; Yaşargil et al 1990; Di Rocco et al 2006; Van Effenterre & Boch 2002). Despite this, their optimal management remains very controversial with ongoing debate about both natural history and therapy (Thapar et al 2003).

With advances in microsurgical and endoscopic techniques, complete resection rates have increased from 69–90% with 'acceptable' mortality and morbidity (Honegger et al 1992; Chakrabarti et al 2005; Gottfried & Couldwell 2008), although some authors may not fully appreciate and underestimate the adverse neuroendocrine and cognitive effects of surgery in children. However, complete resection becomes even more important in children, especially those <3 years because of the additional morbidity of radiotherapy in the first years of life (Regine et al 1993). The chances of a recurrence-free survival is also diminished if a craniopharyngioma is diagnosed in early childhood (Honegger et al 1999). Some single center studies have demonstrated no difference in total resection rates between adults and children (Fahlbusch et al 1999), while other studies have demonstrated a higher success rate for total resection in children (Honegger et al 1999; Weiner et al 1994).The assessment of completeness of resection may be problematic, as small remnants of tumor can remain even if both the postoperative CT and MRI demonstrate no radiological evidence of tumor. A policy of aggressive surgical resection is, however, not always feasible or may come at an unacceptable cost to the patient – the consequences of hypothalamic damage being

devastating. On the other hand, hypopituitarism with diabetes insipidus due to sacrifice of the pituitary stalk while preserving the hypothalamus, could be acceptable if it facilitates a total removal as endocrine replacement therapy is able to maintain decent quality of life (Honegger et al 1999). The primary surgical objective should be decompression of the optic and ventricular pathways regardless of whether a total or sub-total resection occurs (Gottfried & Couldwell 2008). The pituitary stalk is identifiable by the delicate striate pattern of the portal vasculature. Prolonged microdissection of involved stalk and potential traction on the hypothalamus should be avoided. It is preferable to section the stalk as far distally as possible as frequently diabetes insipidus can be averted (Samii & Tatagiba 2001; Jane et al 2002).

Two schools of thought have emerged regarding surgical therapy with one group advocating that aggressive resection offers the best chance of recurrence-free survival with another advocating sub-total resection and adjuvant radiotherapy (Laws 1994; Duff et al 2000; Baskin & Wilson 1986). Surgical experience with respect to both judgment and technical ability plays a major role (Epstein 1994). Tumors >4 cm in size, recurrent tumors, supradiaphragmatic location, hypothalamic involvement, hydrocephalus, poor cleavage planes and adherence to blood vessels, are adverse prognostic factors with regard to radical resection (Honegger & Tatagiba 2008; Yaşargil et al 1990; Weiner et al 1994; Duff et al 2000). Special consideration must be given to primarily cystic lesions. Stereotactic drainage with instillation of chemotherapeutic agents or radioisotopes can be considered.

The decision and rationale regarding the optimal neurosurgical microsurgical approach to a craniopharyngioma should be based on an interpretation of the clinical findings, radiological investigations in conjunction with an understanding of the pathological anatomy and embryology of these lesions (Laws 1994). Broadly speaking, for neurosurgical resection of intracranial tumors, four criteria are taken into consideration; the shortest route to the tumor, minimizing trauma to surrounding structures, exposure and the flexibility of the approach to facilitate resection (Samii & Tatagiba 2001). Table 42.1 provides gross total resection rates from important surgical series (Maartens & Kaye 2009).

Surgical approaches

See Figure 42.11.

Craniotomy approaches

Frontotemporal approach

This approach, more commonly known as the pterional approach and advocated by Yaşargil, is probably the simplest and most widely used approach (Yaşargil et al 1990). It facilitates the shortest transcranial approach to tumors in the suprasellar cistern. It is best suited for tumors that have pushed the chiasm anteriorly as it enables surgical access inferior to the chiasm. As it is a lateral approach, it can be combined with a subfrontal approach for access to both anterior and posterior aspects of the tumor (Fig. 42.12).

It is furthermore very versatile, facilitating prechiasmatic access, opticocarotid triangle access, access lateral to the carotid, superior to the carotid bifurcation and also

Table 42.1 Selection of important surgical series

Publication	Year	Cases (n)	Adults (%)	Preferred approach	Total removal (%)	Early mortality (%)	Follow-up (%)	Recurrence (%)
Baskin & Wilson	1986	74	62	Subfrontal → transsphenoidal	9.5	3	48	14
Yaşargil et al	1990	144	51	Pterional	90	9	NA	7
Symon et al	1991	50	80	Transtemporal	60	4	30	10
Maira et al	1995	57	88	Transsphenoidal → pterional	75	0	78	0
Fahlbusch et al	1999	168	80	Pterional → transsphenoidal → bifrontal	49 prim	0.7 prim, 10 rec	65	11
Van Effenterre & Boch	2002	122	76	Pterional	59	2.5	84	13
Chakrabarti et al	2005	86	NA	Transsphenoidal	84	0	>60	7
Di Rocco et al	2006	54	0	Pterional	78	3.7	104	7
Shi et al	2006	284	80	Pterional → bifrontal	84	4.2	25	14
Zuccaro	2005	153	15 days to 21 years		69	NA	192	0
Gardner et al	2008	16	100	Endoscopic endonasal	50	0	34	31
Shi et al	2008	309	83.8	Pterional (68.3%)	89.3	3.9	25	13.7

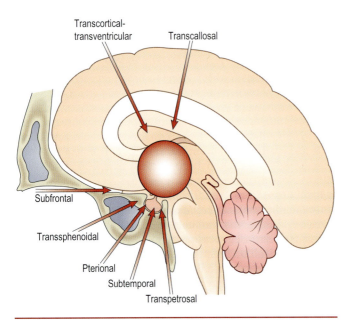

Figure 42.11 Schematic drawing of the most commonly used approaches for craniopharyngiomas.

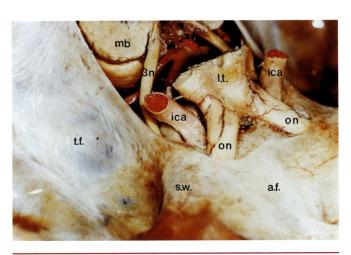

Figure 42.12 Anatomic dissection of the view through the frontolateral approach. The brain tissue has been removed above the level of the third ventricle and the midbrain. Note that the view is less lateral than via a pterional approach and less medial than via the bifrontal approach. 3n, third cranial nerve; a.f., anterior fossa; ica, internal carotid artery; l.t., lamina terminalis; mb, midbrain; on, optic nerve; s.w., sphenoid wing; t.f., temporal fossa. (With permission from Samii, M. and Tatagiba, M., Craniopharyngioma, in Brain tumors: an encyclopedic approach A.H. Kaye and E.R. Laws (Jr.), Editors. Churchill Livingstone, 2001. p. 945–964. With permission of Elsevier.)

access to intraventricular tumors via the lamina terminalis. For tumors with more suprasellar and intraventricular extension the exposure can be extended into the orbitozygomatic approach enhancing the exposure and allowing for a steeper angle of approach for access to the hypothalamic and suprasellar regions.

A limitation of the pterional approach is difficulty visualizing tumor through the lamina terminalis in the third ventricle on the side of the approach, with dissection of the tumor remnant from the hypothalamus being problematic (Fig. 42.13).

Midline subfrontal approach

This approach involves cranialization of the frontal sinus and mobilization of the olfactory tracts from the undersurface of the frontal lobes with the associated respective risks of CSF fistula, infection and anosmia. Midline approaches may allow easier orientation and earlier identification of important structures such as the carotid arteries, optic nerves and chiasm and the pituitary stalk. As craniopharyngiomas

enlarge, they frequently displace the hypothalamus and optic chiasm superiorly creating a large space for the dissection and exposure of important neurovascular structures, particularly after tumor enucleation. Large retrochiasmatic tumors with anterior extension furthermore attenuate the lamina terminalis, which can be fenestrated for access into the third ventricle (Samii & Tatagiba 2001).

Due to their embryonic relationship to the diencephalon, craniopharyngiomas do not derive any blood supply from the basilar or posterior cerebral arteries. They are furthermore well separated from the posterior vessels and midbrain by Liliequist's membrane. A variation of the subfrontal approach, avoiding the difficulties associated with a transfrontal craniotomy, is a true interhemispheric access but this may necessitate division of the anterior communicating artery (Shibuya et al 1996).

Tumor extending caudally into the pituitary fossa or sphenoid sinus is obscured by this approach. Curettage

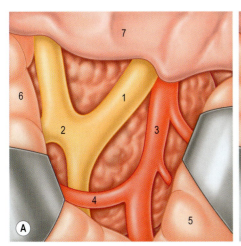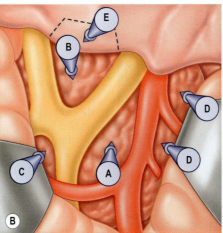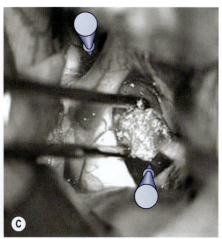

Figure 42.13 Schematic drawing of a right-sided pterional approach showing anatomical structures and surgical corridors. (A) 1. optic nerve, 2. optic chiasm, 3. right internal carotid artery, 4. right anterior cerebral artery (A1), 5. temporal lobe being retracted, 6. frontal lobe being retracted. 7. tuberculum sella. (B) shows a drawing of the surgical corridors. A. between right optic nerve and optic chiasm medially and the internal carotid artery laterally. B. prechiasmatic, C. retrochiasmatic, D. lateral to the right internal carotid artery, E. through the tuberculum sella. (From Honegger, J., Tatagiba, M., 2008. Craniopharyngioma surgery. Pituitary 11, 361–373, with permission Springer Science+Business Media, London.)

using a 70° scope or drilling away the tuberculum sella has been advocated (Alvarez-Garijo et al 1998) but in our opinion it is best to stage the procedure with an endonasal transsphenoidal approach resection with a skull base repair to avoid postoperative CSF fistulas (Fig. 42.14).

Transcallosal approach
The transcallosal approach is advocated for primarily intraventricular craniopharyngiomas (Fukushima et al 1990). The difficulty with this approach is that identification of the optic chiasm may be difficult and preservation of the pituitary stalk impossible. Its use has generally been reserved for giant tumors and possibly in staged procedures (Fig. 42.15).

Many lesions previously regarded as amenable to transcallosal approaches are now being resected via extended transsphenoidal approaches. Primarily basal craniopharyngiomas – especially those with post-fixed chiasms and extending into the third ventricle are also more accessible via sub-frontal translamina terminalis approaches (Samii & Tatagiba 2001). A detailed operative atlas is available (Apuzzo 1998). Care must also be taken not to damage the fornix, anterior commissure, choroid plexus, choroidal arteries, and internal cerebral veins (Samii & Tatagiba 2001).

Transcortical approach
The use of a transcortical-transventricular approach becomes tempting for cases with ventriculomegaly and tumor extending to the dorsal surface of the frontal lobe (Yaşargil et al 1990). Difficulty with ipsilateral dissection and increased postoperative morbidity, such as injury to the floor of the third ventricle, seizures and porencephalic cysts, have restricted its use (Samii & Tatagiba 2001).

Sub-temporal approach
This approach has been used for retrochiasmatic and predominantly unilateral lesions. It requires division of the tentorium to access the posterior aspects of the tumor. Care must be taken to avoid damage to the 4th nerve at the tentorial margin. If the tumor extends into the posterior fossa, it may be combined with a transpetrosal approach (Hakuba et al 1985). Frequently, the tumor can be reduced from the posterior fossa as this extension is usually soft and does not derive a blood supply from the basilar artery (Samii & Tatagiba 2001).

Transsphenoidal approaches
Up until very recently, most patients with craniopharyngiomas were thought to require a transcranial resection of one form or another (Samii & Tatagiba 2001; Fahlbusch et al 1999; Pang 1993; Samii & Samii 1995; Laws 1987). There is, however, an expanding proportion of patients in which the transsphenoidal approach represents an alternative, if not superior, option (Fahlbusch et al 1999; Laws 1994). When deciding on an optimal surgical approach to craniopharyngiomas, several factors need to be taken into consideration:

- Is the sella enlarged and where did the lesion arise?
- Is the lesion predominantly cystic or solid?
- Is there a major calcified component?
- Can the position of the chiasm be determined?
- Is hypopituitarism present?
- How large is the tumor?
- What degree of lateral extension is there?
- Has there been prior surgical therapy or irradiation?
- What is the relationship of the third ventricle and hypothalamus to the tumor?

When craniopharyngiomas arise above the diaphragma, the sella turcica will appear normal with regard to its size and content. Approximately one-third of craniopharyngiomas arise from below the diaphragma sella (Honegger & Tatagiba 2008). When they arise here, they produce progressive

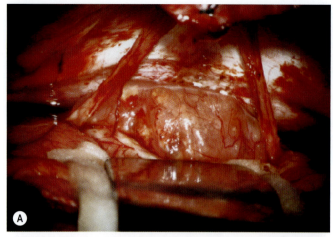

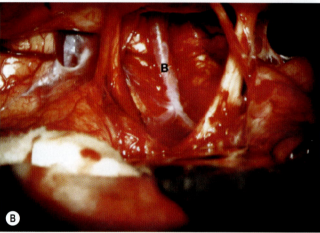

Figure 42.14 (A) Intraoperative photograph of a prechiasmatic craniopharyngioma via a subfrontal approach. (B) After tumor resection from within the third ventricle through the lamina terminalis. The basilar artery (B) is demonstrated with the brainstem behind. (With permission from Samii, M. and Tatagiba, M., Craniopharyngioma, in Brain tumors: an encyclopedic approach A.H. Kaye and E.R. Laws (Jr.), Editors. Churchill Livingstone, 2001. pp. 945–964. With permission of Elsevier).

enlargement of the sella, a radiological feature seen in 30–60% in previously reported series and presumptive evidence of the intrasellar origin (Laws 1980; König et al 1986; Hardy 2007; Hardy & Lalonde 1976). This anatomical origin has important implications regarding the optimal surgical strategy and is by far the most important consideration when selecting an approach. As the tumor enlarges, the diaphragma stretches over it. This occurs even with considerable suprasellar expansion. The advantage this pattern of growth has is that although the dorsal tumor capsule may virtually fuse with the diaphragma – the craniopharyngioma does not extend through it. The diaphragma therefore remains an effective barrier against pial invasion. This prevents the craniopharyngioma arising in the sella from having intimate attachments to rostral intracranial contents above the diaphragma – in particular the optic chiasm, basal vasculature and hypothalamus. It also prevents mutual vascularization of the tumor and the optic apparatus. Accordingly, tumors of intrasellar origin remain almost invariably 'extra-arachnoid' and 'extrapial' in disposition

(Thapar et al 2003). These features of the pathologic anatomy of infradiaphragmatic craniopharyngiomas theoretically permit complete resection transsphenoidally if the surgeon is prepared to resect the diaphragma and risk the potential of a postoperative CSF fistula and meningitis (Laws 1980; Laws 1994).

It is also critical to be aware that the same principles do not necessarily apply to the lateral capsule of the intrasellar component of a craniopharyngioma. This may be densely adherent to the medial wall of the cavernous sinus which may also be deficient, adversely affecting resectability. Dissection between the lateral wall of the tumor capsule and the cavernous sinus runs the risk of precipitating hemorrhage from the cavernous sinus, injuring the cavernous internal carotid artery, false aneurysm formation or traumatizing cranial nerves within the sinus.

An expanded sella is also extremely advantageous in allowing the surgeon sufficient room and maneuverability to effectively manipulate transsphenoidal instrumentation during a resection. Nowadays, however, sellar enlargement should not be regarded as an absolute prerequisite for transsphenoidal surgery (Honegger et al 1992). Until only very recently, and before the advent of extended transsphenoidal approaches, it was considered at best challenging and at worst inadvisable, proceeding in the presence of a normal sized sella. In important craniopharyngioma surgical series reported over the last 20 years, the use of the transsphenoidal approach has varied between 10–79% (Honegger & Tatagiba 2008). To a certain extent, this variation is explained by individual surgical preferences, experience and training, particularly with respect to extended transsphenoidal approaches (Kaptain et al 2001). A comprehensive description of transsphenoidal surgical techniques can be reviewed (Maartens & Kaye 2009).

Extended transsphenoidal surgery

The transsphenoidal approach was initially advocated primarily for lesions arising in the sella, with or without suprasellar extension with the resection technique predicated on an intracapsular removal. Not infrequently, total tumor resection is prevented by invasion into adjacent structures, fibrous consistency (Hashimoto et al 1986) or the adherence of the tumor to structures such as the hypothalamus, the optic nerves and chiasm. Maneuvers designed to increase intracranial pressure in order to reduce suprasellar lesions into the operative field are thus not universally effective (Kaye & Rosewarne 1990).

Early experience with extended transsphenoidal surgical approaches evolved in the process of attempting to achieve gross total removal of craniopharyngiomas (Kaptain et al 2001). The simultaneous development of modern micro-instrumentation, microsurgery air drills, frameless stereotaxy, micro-Doppler ultrasound, the operating microscope, precision ultrasonic aspirators and the endoscope, has extended the role of this approach still further (Couldwell et al 2004).

During the past two decades, other innovative methods of exposing the anterior fossa cranial base have been described. In this respect, the transsphenoidal approach is 'extended' to gain access to lesions of the parasellar and

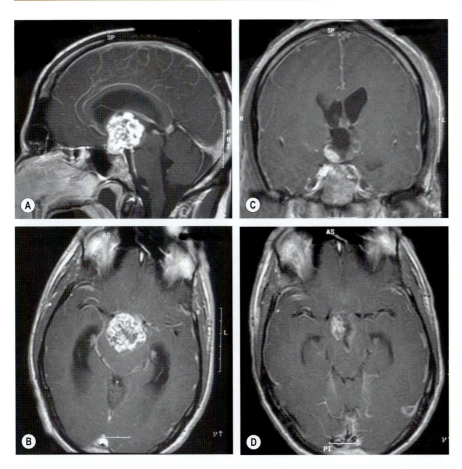

Figure 42.15 (A–D) Large predominantly solid craniopharyngioma extending into the third ventricle (A,B). This was resected via staged procedures. The majority of the lesion was initially resected via a transcallosal approach (C,D) and subsequently the intrasellar residuum via a transsphenoidal approach.

Table 42.2 Outcome of primary transsphenoidal surgery for craniopharyngiomas

Study	n	'Total' resection		Operative mortality		Hypopituitarism (new onset)		Diabetes insipidus (new onset)		Visual recovery		Recurrence rate (%)	Mean follow-up period
		n	%	n	%	n	%	n	%	n	%		
Laws 1980	14	13/14	93	1/14	7	N/A		2/13	15	45	80	0	3 years
Landolt & Zachman 1991	14	N/A		1/14	7	11/14	79	5/10	50	N/A		8	12 years
Honegger et al 1992	19	15/19	79	0			~9	8/15	57	7/8	88	0	3 years
Maira et al 1995	35	23/35	66	0		1/35	3	4/35	11	14/14	100	0	6 years
Ganslandt et al 1999	50	38/50	76	0		16/35	46	19/26	73				
Abe et al 1999	11	3/11	27	0		3/11	27	7/11	64	0			37.4 months
Chakrabarti et al 2005	68	61/68	90	0		4/61	6.6	54/62	87			4.9	Minimum 5 years

clival regions (Jane et al 2002; Kaptain et al 2001; Hashimoto et al 1986; Couldwell & Weiss 1998; Hashimoto & Kikuchi 1990; Kouri et al 2000; Mason et al 1997). In the hands of experienced transsphenoidal surgeons, craniopharyngiomas arising above the diaphragma of predominantly solid composition and even with significant calcification, are now being successfully resected transsphenoidally, providing an alternative to craniotomy.

This approach has numerous advantages, although it requires the expertise of an experienced transsphenoidal surgeon. Its main advantage is that midline exposure is achieved without requiring any brain retraction enabling one to expose the tumor face-on. The exposure provided, albeit via a narrower corridor, is often wider than the exposure provided via pterional and frontal craniotomy approaches using the surgical corridors in the region of the optic chiasm, nerves and internal carotid arteries. It has the added advantage of facilitating a dissection along the axis of the tumor, not around blind corners, with the tumor/brain interface under direct vision facilitating classic microdissection. It also avoids dissecting across the long axis of the optic nerves. It does not require an enlarged sella and is not so critically restricted by the position of the chiasm in the same way as a transcranial approach. It also facilitates rapid debulking of the tumor enabling mobilization of the tumor capsule. See Table 42.2 for a review of the literature.

When craniopharyngiomas arise within the sella turcica, they usually compress, are densely adherent to or can even invade the pituitary gland hence the reason most such patients present with hypopituitarism. If they do not have pituitary dysfunction prior to surgery, many will develop hypopituitarism following removal of an entirely intrasellar lesion. For this reason, transsphenoidal surgery is ideally suited as the primary approach for patients with evidence of pituitary dysfunction. When pituitary function is intact, usually with suprasellar lesions, it is often easier to preserve function via a craniotomy (Oskouian et al 2006).

Transsphenoidal-transsellar-transdiaphragmatic approach

This approach is utilized for craniopharyngiomas with intrasellar components and suprasellar extension. Usually, while undertaking the transsphenoidal resection of a sellar lesion, preserving the integrity of the tumor capsule, an intracapsular approach is preferred whenever possible, to avoid complications resulting from the disruption of the diaphragma sella or from entering the cavernous sinus. In the transsphenoidal-transsellar-transdiaphragmatic approach, once the sellar portion of the tumor has been removed, the suprasellar component is excised by transgressing the tumor capsule and diaphragma to enter the subarachnoid space. The diaphragma is often inseparable from a craniopharyngioma and in order to obtain a complete resection, needs to be excised, deliberately creating a large CSF fistula. This approach is used for the removal of both craniopharyngiomas (Laws 1980; Fahlbusch et al 1999; Maira et al 1995), and pituitary adenomas (Hashimoto et al 1986).

Transsphenoidal-transtuberculum sellae approach

Frequently, craniopharyngiomas are situated in the suprasellar cistern in relation to the pituitary stalk. In 1987, Weiss described an innovative technique for accessing purely suprasellar tumors. This variation or 'extension' of the transsphenoidal approach facilitated access to such lesions by a more rostral approach with removal of the tuberculum sellae and the planum sphenoidale. The underlying dura is then widely opened after careful ligation and division of the intercavernous sinus. This exposes the chiasmal cistern and permits a supradiaphragmatic view of the contents of the basal cisterns (Kouri et al 2000; Mason et al 1997; Weiss 1987). Following dural opening, extra-arachnoid dissection is performed once the pituitary gland has been carefully identified and protected. The arachnoid is opened using sharp dissection and the dissection taken further implementing general principles of microsurgery. The capsule of the tumor is delineated and cauterized with sharp bipolar electrocoagulation. Capsular feeders can be identified, coagulated and cut sharply. The tumor is subsequently debulked, allowing the capsule to be carefully mobilized. Circumferential dissection of the capsule is undertaken and extracapsular feeders controlled as they are encountered (Dumont et al 2006).

The intentional disruption of the integrity of the subarachnoid space is contrary to customary practice of transsphenoidal surgery and magnifies the potential for postoperative CSF rhinorrhea and meningitis. The incidence of these complications ranges from 2% to 6.5% for CSF leak and 0.4–2% for meningitis in transsphenoidal series where extra-capsular resection is not an objective of surgery (Kaptain et al 2001).

Additional indications

The transsphenoidal approach has additional applications, even with regard to suprasellar craniopharyngiomas.

Cystic suprasellar craniopharyngiomas

Transsphenoidal drainage of large, predominantly cystic craniopharyngiomas is an extremely useful, perhaps underutilized, minimally invasive strategy that may confer considerable benefit. This is particularly useful to alleviate pressure symptoms, mainly on the optic chiasm. It is also useful following multiple re-procedures, in the presence of hydrocephalus due to obstruction of the foramina of Munro, as a palliative procedure, or as a precursor to transcranial resection of the more solid component or capsule of the tumor, allowing it to retract from the hypothalamus (Fahlbusch et al 1999). This approach allows the aspiration and drainage of a tumor cyst under direct vision.

Honegger et al (1992), from a series of 32 craniopharyngiomas resected transsphenoidally in which the sella was of normal size in 18, asserted that the cystic components of a craniopharyngioma could be removed regardless of the size of the pituitary fossa. If a large cystic component is present and no CSF fistula has been demonstrated, then it is even possible to secure a short length of silastic tubing within the collapsed craniopharyngioma cyst to permit chronic drainage into the postnasal space.

Often by draining a large suprasellar cystic component, the tumor capsule is frequently able to be mobilized and reduced into the operative field, permitting complete transsphenoidal resection in a surprising number of cases (Chakrabarti et al 2005). On the other hand, tumors with a solid suprasellar component are unlikely to simply descend to within reach of resection of a conventional transsphenoidal approach. Heavily calcified tumors are even more resistant in this respect.

Combined approaches

The surgical management strategy for difficult complex craniopharyngiomas may often be best resolved by considering two approaches (Fig. 42.11). These can be either undertaken simultaneously or at separate sittings (Fahlbusch et al 1999; Di Rocco et al 2006; Yaşargil 1984), and are required in approximately 10% of cases (Fahlbusch et al 1999; Maira et al 1995; Yaşargil et al 1990). Craniopharyngiomas having both supradiaphragmatic and infradiaphragmatic components may require both transcranial and transsphenoidal approaches. Complex large craniopharyngiomas with extensions into different intracranial compartments may require multiple different surgical approaches and therapeutic strategies (Fig. 42.3). The introduction of extended transsphenoidal approaches and endoscopic approaches has reduced the frequency with which combined approaches are utilized, benefiting patients.

Endoscopic techniques

The introduction of the endoscope, either as an assist to the microsurgical approach or as a purely endoscopic approach, has extended the scope of transsphenoidal procedures considerably and endoscopic techniques appear to be slowly gaining acceptance (Jho & Carrau 1997; Jho & Alfieri 2001; Cappabianca et al 2002).

The endoscope has the major advantage of panoramic views allowing identification of structures in the lateral walls of the sphenoid sinus and thereby maximizing exposure. It offers the further advantage of angled views facilitating resection under direct vision of suprasellar and lateral extensions of tumors, albeit at the expense of some loss of depth perception. In the past few years, series utilizing endoscopic techniques for resection of craniopharyngiomas have been published with results comparable with the best microsurgical series (de Divitiis et al 2007a,b; Gardner et al 2008; Cavallo et al 2008; Frank et al 2006).

Radiotherapy

Radiotherapy plays an important role in the management of craniopharyngiomas. The long-term profound neurocognitive effects of radiotherapy, particularly in children, resulted in radiotherapy being reserved for children older than 5 years, but at least older than 3 years, for whom surgery became the main and often only consideration. The appreciation of often disastrous outcomes of aggressive surgical resections during the 1970s and 1980s (Symon & Sprich 1985; Yaşargil et al 1990; De Vile et al 1996; Duff et al 2000; Hoffman et al 1992; Shapiro et al 1979) led to a resurgence of interest in radiotherapy, that was further intensified by the development of more sophisticated delivery modalities.

External beam irradiation

Numerous studies have reported the efficacy of fractionated radiotherapy for the treatment of craniopharyngiomas (Karavitaki et al 2005; Regine et al 1993; Hetelekidis et al 1993; Rajan et al 1993; Manaka et al 1985; Varlotto et al 2002). Radiotherapy alone provides 10-year recurrence rates ranging between 0% and 23% (Fahlbusch et al 1999; Karavitaki et al 2005; De Vile et al 1996; Duff et al 2000; Hetelekidis et al 1993; Rajan et al 1993). Recurrence-free survival rates vary but are considerably enhanced for patients having undergone sub-total resections averaging 80% at 10 years follow-up. Varlotto et al (2002) reported 24 patients with craniopharyngioma undergoing radiotherapy. The control rates at 10 and 20 years were 89% and 54%, respectively.

Generally, the optimal dose advocated is between 50 and 65 Gy in fractionated doses. The fractionation into doses of 180–200 cGy/day permits an overall larger total radiation dose and is better tolerated by the brain thus sparing normal tissue within the radiation field. The protective effect of fractionation is enhanced by the addition of conformational fields. Complications such as radiation necrosis, optic neuritis, dementia, radiation vasculopathy, hypothalamic-pituitary dysfunction, radiation induced tumors and decreased IQ in the young, have all been reported. Irradiation of cystic craniopharyngiomas also has the potential of causing a transient increase in the size of the cystic component before involution ensues, often necessitating urgent surgical intervention (Constine et al 1989).

Internal irradiation (brachytherapy)

Stereotactic implantation of β-emitting radioisotopes was first described by Leksell & Linden in 1952. Different β-emitting and λ-emitting isotopes have subsequently been used; namely yttrium-90, phosphorous-32, rhenium-186 and gold-198, with yttrium now being the most common. None has an ideal biological or physical profile, namely a pure β-emitter, a short half-life and a tissue penetrance limited to the cyst wall (Blackburn et al 1999). Theoretically, they are said to facilitate delivery of higher radiation doses to the cyst lining than can be achieved by external beam radiotherapy, damaging the secretory epithelial lining, leading to elimination of fluid production and eventually cyst involution. The target radiation dose for the cyst wall is approximately 200–250 Gy (Van den Berge et al 1992; Lunsford et al 1994).

In a meta-analysis of four studies, Karavitaki and Wass (2008) demonstrated complete or partial cyst involution in 71–88% of cases with administration of radiation doses of 200–267 Gy with between 3.1 and 11.9 years' follow-up. Stabilization was observed in 3–19% cases and an increase in size in 5–10% cases. New cyst formation or an increase of the solid component was observed in 6.5–20% cases (Karavitaki & Wass 2008; Van den Berge et al 1992; Pollock et al 1995; Voges et al 1997; Hasegawa et al 2004). Surprisingly the overall recurrence and survival rates of brachytherapy do not compare with external beam radiotherapy (Voges et al 1997). The difficulty is that the thickness to the tumor capsule cannot be measured from MRI and consequently the radiation dose to the adjacent visual pathway is unpredictable, resulting in visual impairment or blindness in over 30% of patients (Van den Berge et al 1992).

Stereotactic radiosurgery

Stereotactic radiosurgery (SRS) delivers multiple convergent beams of ionizing radiation all intersecting at a target lesion. Due to the sharp dose fall-off beyond the target area, collateral neural or vascular damage is minimized (Backlund et al 1989). It can be delivered by the GammaKnife or a linear accelerator (Suh & Gupta 2006). Its limitations are with lesions approaching or >3 cm and lesions in close proximity to the optic chiasm which can only tolerate a radiation dose of 8–10 Gy (Leber et al 1998). It is consequently a therapeutic option for selected small residual or recurrent craniopharyngiomas (Chiou et al 2001). Experience has shown it not to be the panacea anticipated – the outcomes remaining inferior to conventional fractionated external beam radiotherapy (Honegger & Tatagiba 2008). In four studies of 164 patients using radiation doses ranging between 8 and 20 Gy and giving mean tumor margin doses of 10 Gy, a reduction in tumor size was observed in 58–79% of patients (Chiou et al 2001; Mokry 1999; Chung et al 2002; Kobayashi et al 2005). In the largest series of 98 consecutive patients, tumors were treated with a maximal dose of 21.8 Gy and a tumor margin dose of 11.5 Gy using a mean of 4.5 isocenters. Final overall response rates were as follows: complete response 19.4%; partial response 67.4%; tumor control 79.6%; and tumor progression 20.4%. The actuarial 5- and 10-year survival rates were 94.1 and 91%, respectively. The progression-free survival rates were 60.8 and 53.8%, respectively. Deterioration both in vision and endocrinological functions were documented as side-effects in six patients (6.1%) (Kobayashi et al 2005).

Stereotactic radiotherapy

This modality uses stereotactically-guided fractionated ionizing radiation. Its advantage is that it can be utilized for lesions >3 cm in size or for lesions adjacent to important neural structures (Kalapurakal et al 2000). In a study of 14 children with recurrent craniopharyngioma, if radiotherapy was used for first or second recurrence, the 5-, 10-, and 15-year relapse-free survival was 100%, 83%, and 83%, respectively, compared with 67%, 0%, and 0%, respectively, for surgery alone.

Chemotherapy

Intracystic bleomycin therapy

Bleomycin is a chemotherapeutic agent used against epithelial tumors (Samii & Tatagiba 2001). Considering that craniopharyngiomas are thought to have epithelial origin, it was first tested against craniopharyngioma tissue culture in 1974 (Kubo et al 1974). Its use is said to be indicated in selected cases of predominantly cystic craniopharyngiomas, especially cystic recurrence and particularly in young children where radiotherapy is best delayed or avoided. It is administered via a stereotactically positioned catheter connected to a subcutaneous Ommaya reservoir. Although experience is limited, initial results appear to be encouraging. In 1989, Broggi et al reported involution of craniopharyngioma cysts in 13 of 18 patients treated with stereotactic intracystic bleomycin instillation. In the follow-up ranging from 3–12 years, at least a 50% decrease in cystic tumor size was observed in 64–86% of children (Takahashi et al 2005; Hader et al 2000). In a study of 24 craniopharyngiomas treated with intracystic bleomycin, Mottolese and colleagues (2001) observed complete tumor resolution in nine patients and a decrease in cyst size of between 50–70% in 15. At a median of 5 years follow-up, there had been no recurrence. In 1996, Cavalheiro observed regression of calcification after bleomycin treatment. More recent experience with longer follow-up has shown that although the response rate is initially high, the rate of regression free survival is poor (Hukin et al 2007; Frank et al 1995). Bleomycin therapy is furthermore associated with serious complications related to its toxicity and hypothalamic damage following instillation after sub-total resection, ischemic attacks, peritumoral edema, cranial nerve palsies, including blindness and death related to leakage into the CSF space, have all been observed (Samii & Tatagiba 2001; Honegger & Tatagiba 2008; Mottolese et al 2001).

Interferon-α might prove to be an alternate agent for bleomycin with negligible CSF toxicity. Heideman et al (1997) investigated its efficacy in nine patients with cystic craniopharyngiomas. At a mean of just under 2 years follow-up the tumors had disappeared in seven patients and two had reduced in size.

Differential diagnosis

The principle radiological differential diagnosis for sellar region tumors with or without extension into the suprasellar cistern is a pituitary tumor or, if cystic, a Rathke's cleft cyst.

Adamantinous-type craniopharyngiomas intermittently appear similar histologically to xanthogranulomas of the sellar region. Degeneration within adamantinomatous craniopharyngiomas replicates many xanthogranuloma features; namely hemosiderin deposition, cholesterol clefts, macrophages (xanthoma cells), chronic inflammation and necrotic

debris. Xanthogranulomas, however, tend not to occur in young patients, are usually sellar based, smaller, more easily resectable and tend to have greater associated endocrine deficits (Paulus et al 1999). Sometimes craniopharyngiomas and epidermoid cysts cannot be differentiated on histology because of similarities in keratin deposition (Russell & Rubinstein 1989). The differentiation between a craniopharyngioma and a Rathke's cleft cyst can sometimes be difficult because of squamous differentiation that the epithelial lining of a Rathke's cleft cyst might undergo (Crotty et al 1995). Usually, extensive ciliation and mucin production are more characteristic of a Rathke's cyst as well as the expression of cytokeratin 8 and 20 (Ulfarsson et al 2005).

Recurrence

Despite their histologically benign nature, the recurrence rate for craniopharyngiomas remains high and a dilemma in their management. Their anatomical location, consistency, pial 'invasion' with adherence to the hypothalamus and vascular structures and the frequency of cyst formation, make complete resection difficult with a propensity for recurrence. Apparent 'total' macroscopic resection can be very misleading. Almost all studies report that the surgeon's impression of a complete removal through the operating microscope to be an unreliable predictor (Hoffman et al 1992). Even low-field strength intraoperative MRI, has been shown to be an unreliable in this regard (Nimsky et al 2003). Nowadays, assessment of resection should be based on the gold standard of quality gadolinium enhanced postoperative MRI imaging, but this may fail to show small tumor fragments.

The recurrence rate for craniopharyngiomas varies between 0 and 28% (Fahlbusch et al 1999; Maira et al 1995; Symon & Sprich 1985; Chakrabarti et al 2005; Yaşargil et al 1990; Di Rocco et al 2006; Van Effenterre & Boch 2002; Baskin & Wilson 1986; Shi et al 2006) and averages at about 10%. Reports of recurrence rates of up to 33% following gross total resection have been noted. In contrast, 63–90% of tumors sub-totally removed subsequently increase in size (Gottfried & Couldwell 2008). Adjuvant radiotherapy reduces this recurrence rate to 30% (Samii & Tatagiba 2001). In a review of radiation therapy for pediatric craniopharyngiomas, Kalapurakal reported the 10-and 20-year progression-free survival rates following limited surgery with radiation therapy to be superior to those achieved by primary surgery alone with a significantly lower incidence of panhypopituitarism (Kalapurakal 2005; Kalapurakal et al 2000). They also concluded that for children with recurrence after radical resection, the use of three-dimensional conformal radiotherapy or fractionated stereotactic radiotherapy resulted in very good local control with a low incidence of complications. They went on to advise that in young children with stable small recurrences, a policy of close surveillance could be adopted allowing for the brain to mature and ideally puberty negotiated before beginning radiotherapy and that the use of secondary surgery for recurrent tumors was associated with a low cure rate and a high risk of complications (Kalapurakal et al 2000). In the Erlangen series (1999) the recurrence-free survival rates were 86.9% and 81.3% at 5 and 10 years, respectively (Honegger et al 1999). When their surgeons reported sub-total resection, the rate for recurrence free survival for radical sub-total resection was 48.8% and for sub-total resection as low as 15.6% at 10 years' follow-up (Honegger & Tatagiba 2008). In Yaşargil's series of 144 patients reporting macroscopic resection in 90%, the recurrence rate was 7% (Yaşargil et al 1990). It is accepted that although unpredictable, the extent of surgical resection remains the most significant predictor of recurrence (Weiner et al 1994).

Although the pathogenesis of recurrence is not always understood, various theories have been proposed. Craniopharyngiomas, particularly the adamantinomatous variety seen more commonly in children, have microscopic fingerlike projections that 'invade' through the pia of the surrounding hypothalamus. This apparent 'invasion' on histology is in fact islets of tumor cells surrounded by neural tissue as opposed to true invasion. The higher recurrence rate in children is thought to arise from remnants at the apex of these projections – particularly within the hypothalamus (Adamson et al 1990). While it is generally accepted that the recurrence rate in the papillary squamous variety seen more exclusively in adults is reduced, not all studies have demonstrated a difference between the two varieties (Karavitaki et al 2005; Weiner et al 1994; Duff et al 2000).

There also appears to be the ability for craniopharyngiomas to 'seed' along the tract of the approach to a craniopharyngioma (Rangoowanski & Piepgras 1991; Barloon et al 1988) and there has been an isolated case report of a rapidly progressive craniopharyngioma recurrence during pregnancy (Maniker & Krieger 1996).

It is well recognized that surgery for recurrent craniopharyngiomas has considerably higher associated morbidity and mortality (Matson & Crigler 1969; Yaşargil et al 1990; Katz 1975). In a paper investigating morbidity and mortality in a series of 158 transsphenoidal re-procedures for a combination of pituitary adenomas and craniopharyngiomas, Laws (1992) recorded mortality and morbidity rates of 2.5% and 29%, respectively. This contrasts with the usually quoted figures of 0.5% mortality and 2.2% morbidity for primary transsphenoidal surgery (Thapar & Laws 1995; Laws 1992). Sweet (1988) noted that one of eight patients died when an attempt at radical removal was made at repeat surgery following an initial less extensive resection. Yaşargil et al (1990) also noted greatly increased mortality from re-procedures. In his series that included both adults and children, the mortality rate for primary resections was 9% (11 of 125 patients), whereas the mortality rate for re-procedures was three-fold, at 32.5% (13 of 40 patients). Frequently, recurrent craniopharyngiomas that have been operated on before transcranially cannot be resected without inflicting significant neurological or neuroendocrine deficits. It may be useful in settings such as this to be able to utilize an alternate approach, for example a transsphenoidal approach via the skull base following a craniotomy in order to palliate (Fig. 42.15). This may be achieved conservatively through either aspiration of a dominant cystic component or sub-total tumor resection, aiming simply to decompress the optic chiasm, preserve vision and prevent hydrocephalus.

The chances of a complete resection in the face of previous surgery appear significantly diminished (Kalapurakal et al 2000). In Fahlbusch's experience, this was 53.4% for re-procedures and 85.7% for primary transsphenoidal resections (Laws 1980; Fahlbusch et al 1999; Landolt & Zachmann 1991). A multidisciplinary approach involving neurosurgical, endocrine, and radiotherapy input is therefore advocated for the management of recurrence and as outlined above, alternate treatment modalities exist if the tumor is not safely amenable to redo surgery.

Outcome

Craniopharyngiomas are associated with significant long-term morbidity (Karavitaki & Wass 2008; Pereira et al 2005), particularly in children and adolescents. This morbidity is attributable to either the primary tumor, recurrence or the sequelae of management. In various combinations and to various degrees, this includes visual failure, hypopituitarism, cognitive decline, hypopituitarism, diabetes insipidus, epilepsy, and hypothalamic syndrome. Appropriately, the issues related to outcome and quality-of-life have been increasingly emphasized – if necessary at the expense of total resection (Carpentieri et al 2001; Cavazzuti et al 1983; Dekkers et al 2006; Honegger et al 1998; Riva et al 1998). While it is appreciated that some patients present with impaired performance, no longer is it acceptable to consider patients in whom total resection has been achieved at the expense of hypothalamic damage with adipsic diabetes insipidus as a success (Yaşargil et al 1990; Hoffman et al 1977). It is prudent when treating a patient with a craniopharyngioma to rather consider 'managing' as opposed to 'curing', as there are a considerable number of therapeutic strategies to utilize ranging from conservative to radical. Nevertheless, it is still best to consider the feasibility of a total resection at the first surgical sitting as this remains the best opportunity for and provides the best chance of long-term remission (Yaşargil et al 1990). Recently there has been a trend towards more aggressive extended transsphenoidal resection of craniopharyngiomas, which appears to confer a better associated quality-of-life and cognitive outcome (Fig. 42.16) (Fahlbusch et al 1999; Maira et al 1995; Symon & Sprich 1985; Yaşargil et al 1990).

In a consecutive series of 54 patients undergoing surgery for craniopharyngiomas with long-term follow-up, Pereira et al (2005) described a long-term cure rate of 82% and a recurrence rate of 18%. Visual field evaluation improved or stabilized in 74%. The long-term rate of hypopituitarism was high at 89% and in addition, the long-term cardiovascular, neurological, and psychosocial morbidities were 22%, 49%, and 47%, respectively (Pereira et al 2005). In a meta-analysis of published series, the spectrum of 5- and 10-year survival rates were 58–100% and 24–100% for total resection; 37–71% and 31–52% for sub-total excision; and 69–95% and 62–84% for sub-total resection and postoperative radiotherapy (Heideman et al 1997).

It is both intuitive and evident that the incidence of hypopituitarism is greater after total resection as opposed to sub-total resection (Sklar 1994b; Thomsett et al 1980). Furthermore, it is becoming evident that the effects of radiotherapy on the hypothalamic-pituitary axis combined with sub-total resection may also not be as harmful as total resection. Multiple endocrinopathies occur in 84–97% of patients following treatment (Gottfried & Couldwell 2008; Poretti et al 2004; Stripp et al 2004).

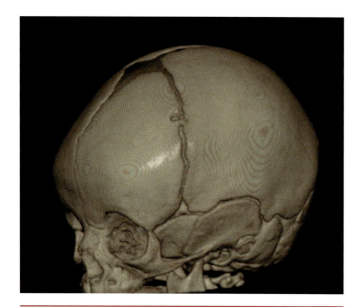

Figure 43.3 Three-D reconstruction of head CT with left frontal coronal dermoid.

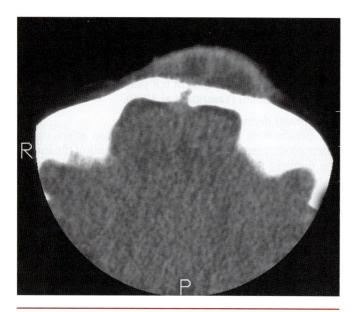

Figure 43.4 Frontal dermoid. A 12-month-old infant with 4-week history of soft painless swelling above the bridge of the nose. No neurologic deficit. (Axial CT brain, non-contrast.)

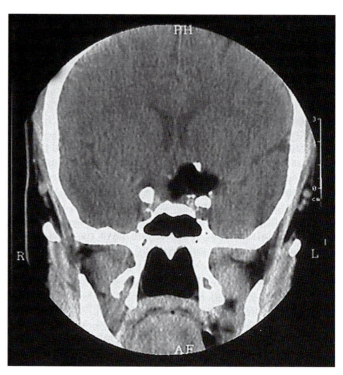

Figure 43.5 Suprasellar dermoid. Middle-aged female presenting with visual acuity and field dysfunction. (Low density lesion on a non-contrast coronal CT brain scan.)

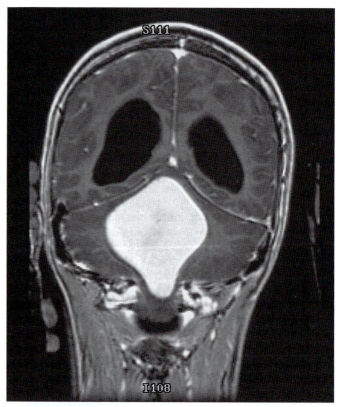

Figure 43.6 Fourth ventricular dermoid. Young female presenting with raised ICP symptoms and unsteadiness and signs consistent with a posterior fossa lesion and failure of upgaze. T1-weighted MR image showing a hyperintense lesion in the fourth ventricle.

dysfunction. These lesions can occasionally cause pituitary dysfunction, resulting in diabetes insipidus (Tan 1972).

One-third of the lesions arise in the fourth ventricle (Fig. 43.6) (Sweet 1940; Guidetti & Gagliardi 1977) and thus present with headaches from raised intracranial pressure, ataxia, and incoordination. The posterior fossa dermoid is more likely to be associated with a dermal sinus (Schijman et al 1986) and thus predispose the patient to a bacterial meningitis (Matson & Ingraham 1951).

Dermoids of the medial petrous bone present with facial paresis, hemifacial spasm, and trigeminal neuralgia. They must be differentiated from a cholesteatoma or chronic middle ear disease.

Chemical meningitis from leakage of the contents of a dermoid may cause an aseptic meningitis (Ulrich 1964; Berger & Wilson 1985) and occasionally can be catastrophic (Greenfield 1932). The aseptic meningitis can occur spontaneously or iatrogenically following surgery. These patients can present with all the signs and symptoms of an infective meningitis: headache, photophobia, and neck stiffness. They will have an abnormal CSF picture, yet no infective organism is identified. Patients who develop hydrocephalus are more likely to do so from bouts of aseptic meningitis rather than the mass lesion.

Intraventricular tumors are rare but have been documented. These patients are more likely to present with dementia or psychiatric disturbance. The presentation has been attributed to demyelination (Bailey 1920) and possibly a consequence of multiple episodes of aseptic meningitis and hydrocephalus.

Liu et al (2008) found ruptured dermoid cysts causing headache, epilepsy or hydrocephalus. Patients had subarachnoid or intraventicular fat droplets and represented 0.18% of all surgically treated CNS tumors over a 12-year period, at their institute.

Occasionally, a patient may present with recurrent bacterial meningitis. In such a case, it is vital to perform a thorough search for a dermal sinus or skin punctum, which may represent the communication with an intracranial dermoid.

It is extremely rare for a dermoid to develop intratumoral haemorrhage, with probably only three reported cases in the literature (Chen et al 2005).

Intracranial epidermoid

Like the dermoid cyst, intracranial epidermoids also present primarily with headache and epilepsy, however most of these lesions are lateral and thus the rest of the clinical picture is different.

Parasellar lesions are more likely to present with epilepsy or cranial nerve dysfunction involving the cavernous sinus; most common is facial sensory disturbance rather than an ophthalmoplegia.

The cerebellopontine angle lesions present with ataxia, nystagmus, and lower cranial nerve dysfunction. The commonest presentation is from involvement of the trigeminal nerve causing facial pain, of the facial nerve resulting in spasm, and of the vestibulocochlear nerve resulting in hearing difficulty. Swallowing can certainly be affected with involvement of glossopharyngeal and vagus nerves (Fig. 43.7).

Spinal dermoid and epidermoid

As with the cranial counterparts, most patients have a long history; back pain associated with variable leg pain is the commonest presentation. The conus tends to be the commonest site for dermoids of the spinal canal and thus, patients have a mixed myeloradiculopathy and are very likely to have sphincteric dysfunction. Rarely can an intraspinal dermoid rupture, resulting in fat droplets in the intracranial CSF space (Goyal et al 2004).

Radicular pain with lower motor neuron signs of weakness and hyporeflexia are most likely to be present if the lesion is primarily in the cauda equina. These patients are less likely to have sphincteric disturbance.

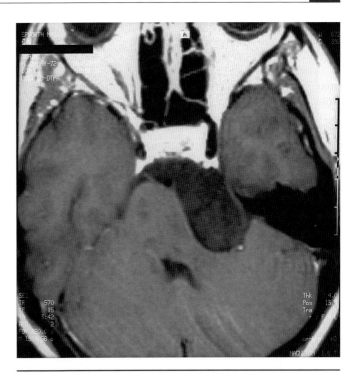

Figure 43.7 Cerebellopontine angle epidermoid. Young female presenting with atypical facial pain and facial sensory dysfunction but no other neurologic deficit. Axial T1-weighted MR image revealed a hypointense lesion in the left cerebellopontine angle.

Most lesions are separate from cutaneous lesions such as a hairy patch, sinus, or punctum; however, in the cauda equina region the dermoid is more likely to have a dermal sinus or tract and thus predisposes the patient to an infective meningitis. A third of the lesions are also likely to be associated with spina bifida or diastematomyelia.

Epidermal inclusion cysts are not tumors. They can grow to a large size with retention of keratin and sebaceous fluid. These inclusion cysts are attached to skin but mobile within its subcutaneous layer. They have no malignant potential. Their presentation is often from discomfort due to their size, but they can also present with pain, or infection of the scalp. Treatment is by excision of the lesion with its punctum.

Radiologic features

Plain radiology of the skull is most helpful in revealing diploic lesions, which result in an expanded bony table with osteolysis and dense scalloped margins. The first radiologic description of an epidermoid was provided by Cushing in 1922; the radiograph revealed a discrete sharply defined area of osteolysis and a raised hyperdense edge. The laterality of a lesion suggests the pathology – a dermoid being midline or medial and an epidermoid being lateral. There are no other specific local plain radiologic features.

Petrous apex erosion will be evident with a lesion of the petrous. Again, there will be osteolysis with a raised scalloped hyperdense edge and possible involvement of the mastoid air cells.

Computed tomography

Both lesions can resemble an arachnoid cyst on CT because of the low attenuation of the lipid content of the lesion. The

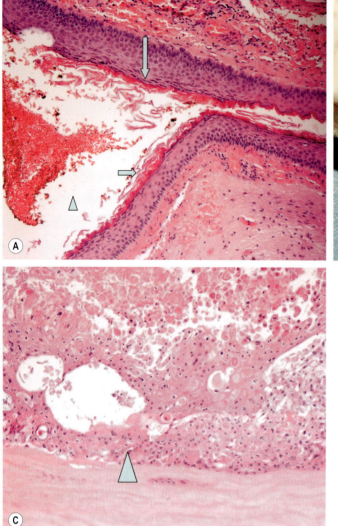

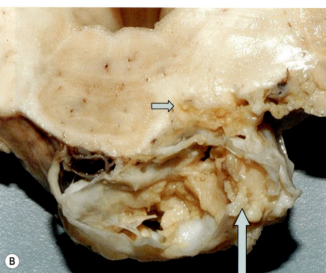

Figure 43.14 (A) Epidermoid cyst. Simple stratified squamous epithelium. The dark granular layer is diagnostic of the epidermoid cyst (long arrow) from which the flakes of keratin (short arrow) within the lumen arise (arrowhead) (H&E ×80). (B) Macroscopic specimen of an epidermoid cyst that recurred showing papillary proliferation (long arrow) and brain stem invasion (short arrow) and (C) histologically squamous cell carcinoma (arrowhead) (H&E ×100). (Courtesy of Dr M Gonzales.)

Significant problems can arise in patients with cerebellopontine and/or posterior fossa mass lesions who present with overt or covert lower cranial nerve dysfunction. They are likely to have subclinical or obvious aspiration, resulting in repeated aspiration pneumonia. The lower cranial nerve dysfunction can also result in nutritional dysfunction and secondary malnutrition that needs to be reversed prior to surgical intervention. Very rarely, a temporary tracheostomy and gastrostomy may be necessary in patients presenting with severe lower cranial nerve palsies who have poor nutrition and respiratory dysfunction (Johnston & Crockard 1995).

Patients with supratentorial lesions will probably benefit from routine anticonvulsant therapy in the perioperative period.

An aseptic meningitis is occasionally seen either spontaneously or after surgery. Aggressive steroid therapy has a major role in the symptomatic treatment and attenuation of the effects of this meningitic process. In patients with a dermal sinus, pyogenic meningitis must be suspected, appropriately investigated, and managed with organism-sensitive antibiotics.

Surgical management

The aim is total surgical excision of the lesion but this philosophy has to be modulated according to the size, location, and clinical presentation. The lesions grow slowly and the size is proportional to the rate of turnover of epithelium (Alvord 1977). Thus, small incidental lesions can be monitored safely.

Scalp lesions can be excised completely. Recurrence of the lesion is unusual. Extension through the bone needs to be treated by excision of the bony margin and definitive treatment of the intracranial lesion.

Diploic lesions must be removed completely by curettage and excision of the margin of bone or a craniectomy around the lesion using a high speed drill. The dura should be excised if involved and a duraplasty performed. The bony defect will require a cranioplasty. An infected lesion may preclude the placement of a cranioplasty until the infection has settled.

Intradural lesions are often difficult to remove completely as their adherence to adjacent nerves and vessels may make this impossible (Berger & Wilson 1985). Tytus reported 50% total removal of intradural lesions (Penny-backer & Tytus 1956). It is easy to empty the contents of the cyst, and an attempt should be made to excise the part of the capsule that is not adherent to adjacent nerves or blood vessels. The remaining capsule is likely to re-grow at the rate of turnover of epidermal or dermal cells. Thus, clinically symptomatic recurrence from the lesion is rare.

During the time when these lesions were first treated surgically, the mortality was up to 70% (Bailey 1920; Sweet 1940; Guidetti & Gagliardi 1977). This was attributed to an attempt at total excision in all patients. An acceptance by surgeons of a maximal but incomplete removal of the cyst wall has dramatically reduced the mortality and morbidity. Despite the adherence of the capsule to surrounding structures, maximal dissection of the wall is possible in a large number of patients (Yaşargil et al 1989). A judicious surgical approach to excision of brain stem lesions is important, in view of the high risk with radical surgery compared to its benign course (Caldarelli et al 2001).

The surgical approach is dependent upon location. Most of the anterior fossa lesions are approached via the pterional approach. A middle fossa lesion can be reached via a subtemporal extension of the pterional approach. Posterior fossa lesions are best approached via the suboccipital approach for midline lesions and the retrosigmoid approach for cerebellopontine angle lesions. Spinal lesions are removed via a laminectomy. The role of endoscopic removal is continuing to evolve.

Postoperative aseptic meningitis is common and is a result of spilling of the contents of the lesion into the CSF circulation. The initial meningitic response may be masked by the perioperative use of steroids; however, as the steroids are decreased the meningitis may flare up. The patient will need postoperative steroids for a longer period, tapered over 3–4 weeks (Berger & Wilson 1985). Long-term control with stereotactic radiosurgery has been reported in seven patients (Kida et al 2006). There is no defined role for postoperative radiotherapy or chemotherapy in the treatment of dermoid or epidermoid tumors but is intermittently used in recurrent tumours and those that have undergone malignant change (Bretz et al 2003).

Results

The operative mortality following excision of an intracranial dermoid or epidermoid has fallen from 70% during the 1930s (Bailey 1920; Sweet 1940; Guidetti & Gagliardi 1977) to 10% in the 1970s (Guidetti & Gagliardi 1977). Since the 1970s, the mortality and morbidity has continued to decline with improvements in imaging, surgical technique, and equipment. Yaşargil and co-workers (1989) managed to obtain an improvement in 86% of their patients, with a 9% neurologic morbidity and 5% mortality. In this same series, Yaşargil found the rate of septic meningitis to be 19%, and hydrocephalus was present in 19% of the patients (Yaşargil et al 1989).

Complications

The primary complications from management of these lesions are aseptic meningitis, septic meningitis, hydrocephalus, and neurologic dysfunction related to the position of the lesion. The neurologic deficits of concern follow involvement of the lower cranial nerves and subsequent difficulty with swallowing, aspiration pneumonia and death. The posterior fossa lesion also increases the risk of brain stem vascular compromise.

Recurrence

Local recurrence
Both dermoid and epidermoid cysts can re-grow after many years, although symptomatic recurrence is rare. The recurrence potential is related to the volume of capsule that is unresected. This capsule will produce cells at the normal rate of cell transformation (Alvord 1977) and thus a symptomatic recurrence is uncommon. A recurrent tumor is still likely to be benign as malignant change is rare. A tumor that has not recurred at twice the age of presentation plus 9 months is considered a surgical cure (Collin's law).

Malignant change has now been reported in both dermoid and epidermoid cysts.

Dissemination
Dissemination can only occur if there has been rupture of the cyst contents into the CSF spaces. Maravilla (1977) described this pattern of dissemination associated with multiple secondary satellites nodule.

Adjuvant therapy

In view of the benign nature of both dermoid and epidermoid cysts, there is no role for adjuvant therapy. The sebaceous cyst component of a dermoid cyst may occasionally respond to isotretinoin, which is a pharmacologic agent used in the treatment of acne vulgaris. Isotretinoin causes atrophy of the sebaceous glands (Johnston & Crockard 1995).

Neurenteric cyst

Epithelial cysts are those cysts lined by a single layer of epithelium. There are two distinct types of epithelial cysts, depending upon their cell of origin – endodermal or neuroepithelial. The neuroepithelial cysts have historically been described as ependymal (Rilliet & Berney 1981; Ho & Chason 1987), choroidal (Inoue et al 1985; Fukushima et al 1988) and neuroepithelial (Shuangshoti et al 1988). The endodermal cysts refer to colloid (Parkinson & Childe 1952; Shuangshoti et al 1965), enterogenous (Chavda et al 1985; Walls et al 1986; Kak et al 1990), neurenteric (Zalatnai 1987), respiratory epithelium (Schelper et al 1986; Del Bigio et al 1992), and epithelial of endodermal origin (Mackenzie & Gilbert 1991). This characterization is based upon intraoperative observations and light microscopy, however, immunohistochemistry and electron microscopy have an important role in the final diagnosis of these cysts (Elmadbouh et al 1999).

Incidence

Neurenteric cysts are rare lesions comprising 0.01% of all CNS tumours (Itakura et al 1986; Chhang et al 1992) and are three times more common in the spine than in the brain (Osborn et al 2004). About 80 cases of intracranial

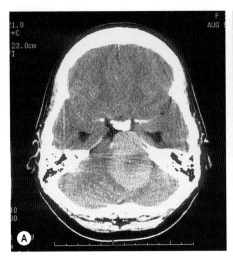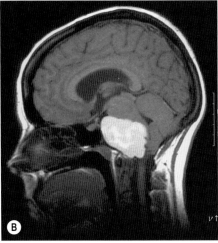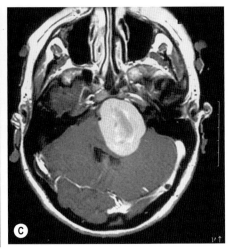

Figure 43.15 Cerebellopontine angle neurenteric cyst. Young female presenting with symptoms and unilateral cerebellar signs. (A) Post-contrast CT brain scan revealed a large cerebellopontine angle non-enhancing hyperdense lesion with hydrocephalus. (B) Sagittal pre-gadolinium T1-weighted MR image and (C) post-gadolinium T1-weighted MR image confirming a large cerebellopontine angle neurenteric cyst, hyperintense to CSF with no enhancement. There is marked distortion of the fourth ventricle yet no associated hydrocephalus.

neurenteric cysts have been reported to date (Bejjani et al 1998; Christov et al 2004; Osborn et al 2004; Preece et al 2006).

Age

Neurenteric cyst lesions can present from birth to the 5th decade, although they are seen primarily in the 4th and 5th decades of life. Agnoli et al (1984) reviewed the literature and noted the age of presentation as 0–10 years in 21%, 10–20 years in 21%, and over 20 years in 58% of the patients.

Sex

There is a slight male predominance of 2:1 (Agnoli et al 1984; Preece et al 2006).

Sites

Most neurenteric cysts occur primarily in the thoracic spine, and thus cause spinal cord compression or tethering. Even although they are most common in the cervicothoracic region, they can occur anywhere from the cerebellopontine angle to the coccyx. Agnoli et al (1984) report that most neurenteric cysts occur between C3 and T12.

Most of the lesions are situated anteriorly within the spinal canal and thus may communicate with a mediastinal or abdominal cyst through a defect in the vertebral body (Harriman 1958). French (1990) reported that the incidence of communication via a vertebral body defect may be up to 80% if the patients present under the age of 10 years, compared to 25% for those over the age of 10 years. The cyst may occasionally be dorsal or within the spinal cord.

The lesions must be suspected in patients with bowel, bladder, or renal abnormalities. These lesions are rare in the posterior fossa or craniovertebral junction but have been reported (Markwalder & Zimmerman 1979; Hirai et al 1981; Anderes 1984; Yoshida et al 1986; Koksel et al 1990; Scaravilli et al 1992). We managed a patient with a

cerebellopontine angle neurenteric cyst, although it did extend down to the midline anteriorly at the foramen magnum (Fig. 43.15). Kachur et al (2004) and Takumi et al (2008) present a patient each with a supratentorial neurenteric cyst presenting with seizures which is a rare presentation for this pathology, while more have been now been reported in the supratentorial compartment (Preece et al 2006).

Clinical presentation

In younger patients, a high index of suspicion is appropriate in patients with a prenatal or postnatal diagnosis of chest, mediastinal, or abdominal cysts, or those with bowel, bladder, or renal abnormalities. The presentation in older patients will be that of a mass lesion at the site of pathology.

Infratentorial cysts present with ataxia, incoordination, or lower cranial nerve dysfunction, involving mainly the trigeminal, facial and cochlear nerves. Features of hydrocephalus tend to occur late. Supratentorial lesions cause headache, seizures or effects from an expanding mass lesion.

Pain is the primary feature of presentation in all the spinal lesions and is often associated with dysesthesia. The motor dysfunction is often late, variable, and fluctuant in its course, thus the most common initial diagnosis is demyelination from multiple sclerosis (Agnoli et al 1984).

A lesion in the cervical spine will have features of a myelopathy with clumsiness of hands, difficulty with fine movement, and a vague disturbance of gait. Clinical examination will reveal a myelopathy, increased tone, hyperreflexia, and a spastic gait. A thoracic lesion will spare the upper limbs and thus present only with a disturbance of gait and spasticity. Sphincter dysfunction occurs late. Lumbosacral lesions are most likely to present with a radiculopathy, and thus hypotonic involvement of the lower limbs. Rarely, the lesion is associated with a dermal sinus tract and the patient may present with an infective meningitis as with dermoid or epidermoid lesions.

Embryology

The first neurenteric cyst was described by Puusepp in 1934 (initially as a teratoma but later confirmed to be a neurenteric cyst) and is also known as an enterogenous cyst, enteric cyst, endodermal cyst, gastro-enterogenous cyst, gastrocytoma, intestinoma, and archenteric cyst (Harris et al 1991; Brooks et al 1993; Eynon-Lewis et al 1998; Kim et al 1999; Osborn et al 2004), reflecting the dilemma of its embryonic origin. The neurenteric connections and its embryology were first alluded to by Feller and Sternberg (1929) and reaffirmed by Cohen and Sledge (1960).

They are essentially of endodermal origin, when the endoderm fuses with the developing notochord during the 3rd week of gestation. The neurenteric canal of Kovalevsky runs from the yolk sac through the Hensen's node (the primitive knot) to the amniotic cavity and thus remnants of this communication must lie caudal to the coccyx. Bremer (1952) suggested that the communication at a higher level, as it occurs clinically, must arise at an earlier stage when the yolk sac is shrinking and that there are lateral forces upon it that push components of the yolk sac dorsally into the developing notochord. Thus, the lesion may be situated anywhere within the transverse axis of the spinal canal, including within the spinal cord, although most are situated ventral to the spinal cord. This theory of Bremer's (1952) may explain the associated midline spinal defect and bony spurs that are seen. The process was expanded upon by Bentley and Smith (1960) to explain the association of neurenteric cysts with lesions in the mediastinum and an anterior meningocele. This does not explain the supratentorial lesions. The midline supratentorial lesions may be explained by inclusion of the endodermal diverticulum – the Seessel pouch – found behind the oropharyngeal membrane (Bejjani et al 1998; Christov et al 2004). There is no good explanation for off-midline supratentorial lesions.

Radiology

Plain radiology of the spine may reveal midline fusion defects that involve the vertebral bodies with or without spina bifida occulta. Plain radiology of the chest may reveal a mediastinal mass, while abdominal ultrasound may reveal an abdominal cyst or renal abnormalities.

MRI has superseded CT myelography and reveals an intradural extramedullary lesion that is iso- or hypointense on a T1 signal and hyperintense on a T2 signal (Fig. 43.16A). The wall does not usually enhance with contrast, although

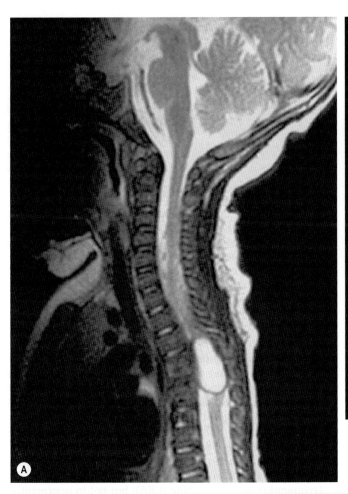
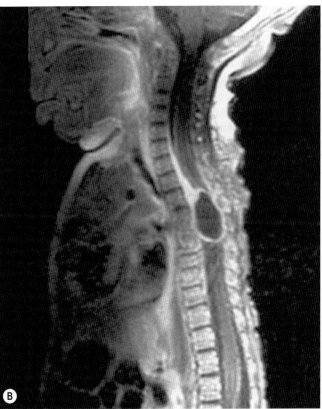

Figure 43.16 Spinal neurenteric cyst. A 2-month-old infant with paraplegia, (A) T2-weighted MR image with high signal intensity lesion and cord compression. Associated vertebral body abnormality present. (B) Post-gadolinium T1-weighted MR image revealed peripheral enhancement of the cyst. Histopathology confirmed this to be a neurenteric cyst with neural tissue and gastric mucosa.

Akins 1996; Vandertop et al 1995; Aggarwal 1999; Nader-Sepahi 2000; Ahmed 2002; Socin 2002; Stoodley 2002; Joshi et al 2005; Partington 2004). Vandertop et al (1995) and Socin et al (2002) postulated an autosomal recessive mode of inheritance, although the later familial cluster reported by Partington (2004) suggested that autosomal dominant transmission was more likely. To date, no specific chromosomal or genetic features have been determined.

It must be stressed that the vast majority of colloid cyst cases have not been associated with any familial characteristics, and therefore at this stage, radiographic screening of asymptomatic relatives would be difficult to justify, except if there has been more than one family member affected.

Theories of embryologic origin

The embryologic derivation of colloid cysts is far from certain. The major theories will be briefly discussed.

Paraphysis/ventricular roof structures

In 1909, Sjovall proposed that these cysts were embryonic remnants derived from the paraphysis (Sjovall 1909; Little & MacCarty 1974), although at that time this embryonal neuroectodermal structure had only been described in lower vertebrates. In 1916, Bailey described the paraphysis in human embryos, and for over 50 years following this description, the term 'paraphysial cysts' was commonly used (Bailey 1916; Parkinson & Childe 1952; Shuangshoti & Netsky 1966; Ciric & Zivin 1975; Kondziolka & Bilbao 1989).

The paraphysis has been described by Kappers (1955) to exist transiently in the human embryo (between a crown-rump length of 17 and 100 mm; approximately 7–14 weeks), having normally completely regressed by the 145-mm stage (Kappers 1955; Palacios et al 1976). It is a midline structure within the diencephalic roof immediately rostral to the telencephalic border, and consists microscopically of low columnar epithelium that differs from the surrounding epithelium by the absence of cilia and blepharoplasts.

The rare descriptions of colloid cysts in the posterior third ventricle, the fourth ventricle, and within leaves of the septum pellucidum (Parkinson & Childe 1952; Shuangshoti & Netsky 1966; Ciric & Zivin 1975; Kondziolka & Bilbao 1989) cast doubt on the paraphysial theory and opened debate as to their histologic origin.

Shuangshoti et al (1965, 1966) have presented a theory that the paraphysis itself represents extraventricular choroid plexus, and that colloid cysts arose either from choroid plexus, ependyma or paraphysis, which were all products of neuroepithelium. Electron microscopic examination of the colloid cyst epithelium has demonstrated both normal and abnormal cilia, and Coxe & Luse (1964) considered this appearance to be suggestive of an ependymal origin.

Kappers (1955) proposed that the more likely origin of colloid cysts is from diencephalic roof ependymal recesses, which pinch off into closed vesicles. Ciric & Zivin (1975) supported the hypothesis of cyst formation by invagination of neuroepithelium from the diencephalic roof. These theories could account for the occurrence of these cysts at sites closely related to the ventricular system other than within the anterior third ventricle.

Respiratory/enterogenous origin

A comparison between the epithelium found in colloid cysts and the pseudostratified epithelium found in Rathke's cleft cysts and suprasellar neuroenteric cysts has been made (Leech & Olafson 1977; Graziani et al 1995). Leech & Olafson (1977) have suggested that the colloid cyst may be derived from respiratory epithelium. Respiratory-type epithelium was also described in one of the 21 cases of colloid cysts examined by Loizou et al (1986), and another case was considered to have the appearance of foregut-type epithelium (Loizou et al 1986). Histologic and immunohistochemical similarities between five colloid cysts and two spinal enterogenous cysts have also been demonstrated by Mackenzie & Gilbert (1991), also supporting an endodermal origin hypothesis.

More recently, Ho & Garcia (1992) have reported the ultrastructural features of four cases of colloid cysts, and demonstrated ciliated cells, non-ciliated cells with microvilli, goblet cells, basal cells, and also junctional complexes between some of the cell types. They considered this to be very similar to normal respiratory epithelium, and also to the lining of intraspinal bronchogenic cysts, and felt that these features were consistent with the hypothesis of an endodermal respiratory origin (Ho & Garcia 1992). Similar ultrastructural findings have been identified in six pediatric colloid cysts (Macaulay 1997).

Another ultrastructural study of 13 colloid cysts has been reported, which confirms the ultrastructural similarity between the colloid cyst epithelium and the epithelium from Rathke's cleft cysts and enterogenous cysts and also follicular cysts from the normal pituitary gland. This study also supported the enterogenous origin of colloid cysts (Lach & Scheithauer 1992).

Theories based on immunohistochemical markers

Mucin-secreting cells have been commonly demonstrated in the cyst epithelium (Mosberg & Blackwood 1954; Kondziolka & Bilbao 1989). There is disagreement as to whether or not mucin-containing cells are found in the choroid plexus ependyma, being demonstrated by Shuangshoti & Netsky (1966) but not by Kondziolka & Bilbao (1989).

PAS-positive material was found in the cyst epithelium in 11 of the 12 specimens studied by Kondziolka & Bilbao (1989), but was not found by them in choroid plexus. They also reported that, unlike choroid plexus (Kasper et al 1986), the colloid cyst epithelium had no reaction to intermediate filament antibodies to vimentin and neurofilament, or to Bodian's silver preparation (Kondziolka & Bilbao 1989). Positivity to the epithelial membrane antigen had been noted in two separate studies (Perentes & Rubinstein 1987; Kondziolka & Bilbao 1989) and has not been demonstrated in choroid plexus epithelium (Kondziolka & Bilbao 1989). Negativity of the colloid cyst epithelium for vimentin is in contrast to immature glial tissue, and GFAP negativity is in contrast to mature glial tissue. Kondziolka & Bilbao (1989) considered that these immunohistochemical findings were consistent with the theory that the colloid cyst was derived from primitive neuroectoderm involved in the formation of the tela choroidea, and was inconsistent with the derivation of colloid cyst from either choroid plexus or ependyma.

Immunohistochemical studies of 11 colloid cysts performed by Kuchelmeister & Bergmann (1992) have confirmed the different profiles of colloid cyst epithelium, choroid plexus epithelium and ependyma. However, their conclusion was that the most likely derivation was of a non-neuroepithelial origin.

Sites of predilection

More than 99% of reported cases of colloid cysts have occurred within the third ventricle, almost all in the anterior half. The cyst typically has an attachment to the roof of the third ventricle immediately dorsal to the foramen of Monro, although adhesions to the lateral walls of the third ventricle and the floor of the third ventricle are not infrequent. Rare cases of colloid cysts occurring in the posterior third ventricle have been reported (Shuangshoti & Netsky 1966; Kondziolka & Bilbao 1989), and there have been individual case reports of colloid cyst in the septum pellucidum (Ciric & Zivin 1975), in the vellum interpositum (Hingwala 2008) and in the fourth ventricle (Parkinson & Childe 1952; Kchir et al 1992). A single case of an intracerebral cystic lesion in the right frontoparietal region that had histopathological features of a colloid cyst has been reported (Campbell & Varma 1991). A case has also been reported of an intrasellar cystic lesion with radiographic and histologic features of a colloid cyst (Sener & Jinkins 1991).

Presenting features

As has been mentioned, many colloid cysts are asymptomatic and are diagnosed at the time of CT or MR scanning for an unrelated condition.

A classic clinical presentation for colloid cyst has long been described, and is characterized by paroxysmal headache associated with changes in head position (Bull & Sutton 1949; Kelly 1951; Yenermen et al 1958; Palacios et al 1976). It was generally considered that such symptoms were due to a pedunculated midline cyst within the third ventricle that was capable of altering position with head movement, and therefore intermittently obstructing either the foramen of Monro or the aqueduct of Sylvius. However, such presentations are not common, nor is the corresponding pathologic entity of a highly mobile cyst (Bull & Sutton 1949; Kelly 1951; Yenermen et al 1958; Little & MacCarty 1974; Palacios et al 1976). Kelly (1951) has made the point that, as well as being rare, the classic presentation is by no means pathognomonic of colloid cysts, and he found that patients presenting in this manner were in fact more likely to have other tumor types. He found that in his series of cases, the most frequent presenting symptom apart from headache was sudden weakness in the lower limbs, causing falling without unconsciousness (Kelly 1951). The association of obstruction of the third ventricle with these sudden drop attacks, although recognized in the more recent literature, has been reported relatively infrequently.

Progressive headache associated with raised intracranial pressure is a common presentation Little & MacCarty (1974) noted that in these patients, the relatively long history of the headaches suggested a benign lesion, although acute presentation with raised intracranial pressure is not uncommon. The presentation of a colloid cyst with headache and papilledema, but no localizing neurological signs, was well recognized by Dandy (1933).

A review of three pre-CT era series of 121 symptomatic colloid cysts found an 88% incidence of significant headaches, and >25% of the cases deteriorating to coma or sudden death (Young 1997; Pollock 2000).

As would be expected, patients presenting with the symptom of headache not infrequently exhibit the other manifestations of raised intracranial pressure, such as vomiting, altered conscious state, and papilledema. Patients presenting with paroxysmal headaches not uncommonly have associated transient diplopia and blurred vision (Batnitzky et al 1974). It should be noted that these presentations, due to acute hydrocephalus, are in no way different from the presentation for any other cause of acute hydrocephalus. Isolated symptoms over 1 month of relatively minor headache have preceded sudden death due to acute hydrocephalus in a 13-year-old with a colloid cyst (Aronica et al 1998).

Patients with colloid cysts can also present with a progressive or fluctuating dementia, often in the absence of headaches or papilledema. This was first described by Riddoch (1936) and has been since confirmed by other authors (Grossiord 1941; Kelly 1951; Yenermen et al 1958; Ojemann 1971; Little & MacCarty 1974). The progressive dementia is frequently associated with gait disturbance and urinary incontinence, and thus has the same clinical presenting features as 'normal pressure hydrocephalus' (Adams et al 1965; Ojemann 1971; Little & MacCarty 1974). Indeed, three of the cases in the original series describing normal pressure hydrocephalus had lesions in the anterior part of the third ventricle (Adams et al 1965). It is necessary to consider third ventricular lesions in patients presenting with the clinical syndrome of normal pressure hydrocephalus, as those patients with third ventricular lesions have a risk of sudden neurological deterioration, particularly following lumbar puncture (Little & MacCarty 1974). A case report of colloid cyst presenting with Korsakoff syndrome has recently been reported in the Russian literature (Konovalov et al 1998).

Neuropsychological assessment of patients with tumors within the third ventricle finds a significant incidence of deficits in the areas of memory, executive function, and manual speed and dexterity (Friedman 2003). It is important to recognize that a sizable proportion of colloid cyst patients with impaired memory and impaired new learning ability are not aware of these problems (Moorthy 2006), and formal neuropsychological evaluation is recommended prior to elective treatment. Neurosurgeons tend to understandably focus on the well recognized neuropsychological impairments which may be associated with surgical removal of colloid cysts, although these deficits are by no means invariable and surgery may actually improve some preoperative impairments in some cases (Friedman 2003; Moorthy 2006).

The most catastrophic event associated with colloid cysts of the third ventricle is sudden death. This has been well recognized in the literature (Grossiord 1941; Cairns & Mosberg 1951; Kelly 1951; Little & MacCarty 1974; Ryder et al 1986; Williams & Tannenberg 1997; Büttner 1997). Ryder et al (1986) analyzed 52 cases of colloid cyst reported in the literature as having suffered sudden death, and found that neither the tumor size, the degree of ventricular dilatation as assessed on CT scan, nor the duration of symptoms prior to the patient's collapse could be reliably used to indicate the risk of sudden neurological deterioration or death. That review noted that while many of the cases of sudden death could be attributed to acute hydrocephalus, this was not always present. They postulated that reflex effects involving cardiovascular centers near the third ventricle might also have played a role in these patients (Ryder et al 1986).

The risk of neurological deterioration is high for symptomatic colloid cysts (Young 1997; Pollock 2000; De Witt Hamer 2002). The actual incidence of sudden death with asymptomatic colloid cysts is unknown. The absence of strong predictive factors for the development of symptoms has resulted in there being a neurosurgical tendency to recommend treatment in young patients for larger colloid cysts.

Imaging diagnosis

Walter Dandy (1922, 1933) first indicated that it was impossible to diagnose colloid cysts on clinical grounds alone and introduced ventriculography for their accurate diagnosis. The pathognomonic ventriculographic findings associated with colloid cysts were described at length by Bull & Sutton (1949); as late as 1974, Little and McCarty considered ventriculography to be still the most reliable diagnostic study for the demonstration of third ventricular lesions. Pneumoencephalography could also be used for the diagnosis of third ventricle lesions, but could not be considered the procedure of choice as it was less accurate than ventriculography (Taveras & Wood 1964; Batnitzky et al 1974; Little & MacCarty 1974) and also had a significant risk of neurological deterioration in patients with raised intracranial pressure (Bull & Sutton 1949; Batnitzky et al 1974).

Plain X-rays of the skull are of no particular value in the diagnosis of colloid cyst, although they may show nonspecific signs of chronically raised intracranial pressure, as was found in 17 of the 25 cases studied by Batnitzky et al (1974) and in seven of the 38 cases reported by Little and MacCarty (1974). There is only one reported example of a colloid cyst with calcifications visible on skull X-rays (Palacios et al 1976), and calcification seen in the region of the third ventricle would suggest a diagnosis other than colloid cyst (Taveras & Wood 1964; Batnitzky et al 1974). The plain skull X-rays may also show posterior inferior displacement of the calcified pineal, and although this is well recognized it is by no means pathognomonic or common (Davidoff & Dyck 1935; Bull & Sutton 1949; Yenermen et al 1958; Little & MacCarty 1974).

Radionucleotide brain scanning, other than possibly showing some evidence of hydrocephalus, will not aid in the diagnosis of colloid cysts. This study is usually normal (Batnitzky et al 1974; Little & MacCarty 1974). Cerebral angiography, although not providing a definitive diagnosis,

may give useful indications as to the possibility of colloid cyst (Batnitzky et al 1974; Little & MacCarty 1974).

Hydrocephalus may be recognized on angiography by outward bowing of the thalamostriate veins in the frontal venous phase and also the increased sweep of the pericallosal artery in the lateral arterial phase. In the presence of a colloid cyst, the internal cerebral vein has been commonly described as showing an anterior hump, with flattening and depression in its posterior two-thirds (Batnitzky et al 1974; Little & MacCarty 1974). Since the introduction of high resolution CT scanning, the most valuable role of angiography in the study of a third ventricular lesion is the exclusion of a cerebral aneurysm.

CT and MRI technology has now made the previously mentioned radiographic investigations largely obsolete in the investigation of colloid cysts. The characteristic CT appearance of a colloid cyst is of a rounded or ovoid lesion, typically 5–25 mm in diameter, lying in the region of the anterior third ventricle adjacent to and just behind the foramen of Monro (Lee et al 1979; Ganti et al 1981). The lesions are usually homogeneous, although occasionally a central lucency has been demonstrated (Ganti et al 1981). Most commonly the colloid cyst is hyperdense on precontrast CT scanning (Figs 44.1, 44.2). Review of the reported series of colloid cysts investigated with CT scan reveals a total of 144 cases, 100 of which were hyperdense on CT scan (69.4%), 34 isodense (23.6%), and 10 (6.9%) hypodense (Sackett et al 1975; Guner et al 1976; Osborn & Wing 1977; Ganti et al 1981; Zilkha 1981; Powell & Torrens 1983; Rivas & Lobato 1985; Donauer et al 1986; Hall & Lunsford 1987; Mohadjer et al 1987; Abernathey et al 1989; Kondziolka & Bilbao 1989; Musolino et al 1989). The cyst wall sometimes enhances following intravenous contrast injection, occurring in two of the 17 cases reported by Hall & Lunsford (1987) and eight of the 14 cases reported by Ganti et al (1981). There is one reported case of a colloid cyst having a CT appearance of a ring-enhancing lesion (Bullard et al 1982). The high density on pre-contrast CT scan is thought to be due to the proteinaceous contents of

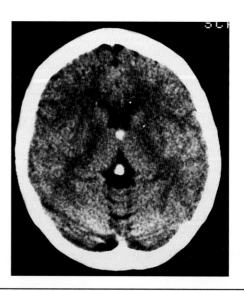

Figure 44.1 Hyperdense colloid cyst; axial CT scan.

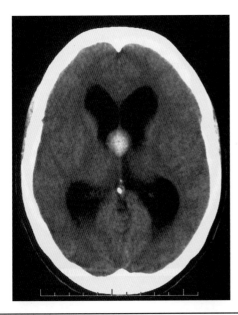

Figure 44.2 Hyperdense colloid cyst causing obstructive hydrocephalus; axial CT scan.

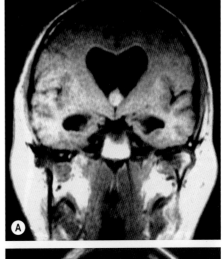

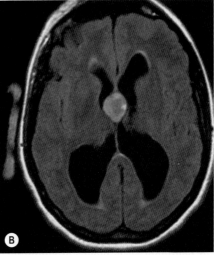

Figure 44.3 High signal colloid cyst on (A) coronal and (B) axial T1-weighted MR scan (TR 500).

the cyst, and possibly also due to hemosiderin (Ganti et al 1981). The CT appearance of a hyperdense colloid cyst has also been correlated with the degree of calcium within the colloid cyst content (Sackett et al 1975; Ganti et al 1981; Kondziolka & Lunsford 1991). Donaldson and Simon (1980) determined the elemental composition of the contents of a hyperdense colloid cyst with atomic emission spectometry, and found calcium, sodium and magnesium to be the predominant radiodense ions. Microscopic calcification in the cyst wall is a not infrequent histopathological finding, and may contribute to increased radiodensity on CT scanning. Actual calcification demonstrated on any radiographic investigation is uncommon (Taveras & Wood 1964; Batnitzky et al 1974; Ganti et al 1981; Yuceer et al 1996), being noted in two of the 17 CT scans reported by Hall and Lunsford (1987).

Multiplanar MR scanning clearly demonstrates the anatomical location of the rounded cyst in the anterior aspect of the third ventricle adjacent to the foramen of Monro. MRI is also able to differentiate between the colloid cyst and an aneurysm of the basilar tip, which may occasionally be indistinguishable on CT scan. Earlier reports have incorrectly stated that the colloid cyst has a high signal on both T1- and T2-weighted images (Kjos et al 1985; Hall & Lunsford 1987; Symon & Pell 1990; Mamourian et al 1998). Of the eight cases of colloid cysts imaged with MRI scan reported by Kondziolka and Lunsford (1991), at a short relaxation time two had a low signal; three were isointense, and three had a high signal intensity, and on the long relaxation time two had a low signal intensity, two were isointense, and four had a high signal intensity (Figs 44.3–44.6).

The radiodensity of the colloid cyst on CT scan has been shown to correlate with the viscosity of the cyst contents, with the hypodense and isodense cysts being less viscous, and relatively more liquid (Powell & Torrens 1983; Rivas & Lobato 1985; Kondziolka & Lunsford 1991; Urso

et al 1998). Kondziolka and Lunsford (1991) found that the MRI scanning technique failed to predict the viscosity of the cyst contents, and in this respect they considered CT scan to be superior. However, Pollock's comparison of symptomatic and asymptomatic colloid cysts not only identified high T2 signal as characteristic of increased fluid content (and therefore lower viscosity) but also that high T2 signal found more frequently in symptomatic colloid cysts, leading him to postulate that those cysts may be more likely to enlarge rapidly and become symptomatic (Pollock 2000).

Laboratory diagnosis

Hematologic and biochemical analysis of blood, CSF analysis, and other laboratory tests are of no diagnostic value for patients with colloid cysts. Lumbar puncture poses a significant risk to any patient with a third ventricular lesion, and is absolutely contraindicated in the presence of obstructive hydrocephalus.

thalamostriate vein) and the suprachoroidal approach (opening the ependymal taenia fornicis which lies between the superomedial choroid plexus and the fornix and thus poses less risk to the thalamostriate vein) (Wen 1998; Yasargil & Abdulrauf 2008). The extent that the transchoroidal approach can be safely extended posteriorly is limited by the junction of the anterior septal vein and internal cerebral vein (Türe 1997; Yasargil & Abdulrauf 2008), and the transchoroidal extension of the exposure adds significant risk (including those of infarction in the basal ganglia, mutism, and hemiparesis) to those already associated with a standard transforaminal excision. Therefore, although these techniques are very useful in selected cases and neurosurgeons treating colloid cysts need proficiency in their application, they are not recommended routinely (Apuzzo & Litofsky 1993; Yasargil & Abdulrauf 2008). Even large colloid cysts can be readily collapsed after puncture and aspiration and the capsule can usually be delivered through even a relatively small foramen, these additional techniques are rarely required for colloid cyst excision (Symon & Pell 1990).

The major advantages of the transcallosal approach are that it is technically more advantageous than the transcortical approach in the absence of hydrocephalus, and it gives ready access to either foramen of Monro (Yasargil et al 1990). Also, unlike the transcortical exposure, a transcallosal approach allows an interforniceal approach for lesions situated more posteriorly in the third ventricle. This has been described by Apuzzo and co-workers (1987, 1993) as being division of the midline forniceal raphe allowing access through the roof of the third ventricle between the two forniceal bodies. In this procedure, having opened the septum pellucidum, the midline forniceal raphe is identified at the site of the septum attachment on the dorsal fornix, and is then opened starting at the foramen of Monro and extending posteriorly 1–2 cm (but not more than 2 cm to avoid injuring the hippocampal commissure) (Apuzzo et al 1987, 1993; Amar 2004; Yasargil & Abdulrauf 2008). A more limited variation of the interforniceal approach involves less opening of the forniceal raphe, with the exposure being limited anteriorly by the posterior aspect of the anterior commissure and posteriorly by the posterior aspect of the foramen of Monro (Siwanuwatn 2005). It must however be remembered that the potential complications or the interforniceal approach include memory loss and hemiparesis (Apuzzo & Litofsky 1993). As discussed above, a transforaminal resection is usually adequate for the majority of colloid cysts (Hall & Lunsford 1987; Yasargil et al 1990; Yasargil & Abdulrauf 2008) and further exposures should be performed only when definitely required.

Significant neuropsychological deficits have not been reported in the uncomplicated cases of transcallosal approach to third ventricular tumors (Jeeves et al 1979; Winston et al 1979; Hall & Lunsford 1987; Friedman 2003), although careful neuropsychometric testing may reveal some deficit (European Association Neurosurgical Societies, EANS 1990). The transcallosal approach is considered to entail less risk of epilepsy than the transcortical approach (Jeeves et al 1979; Hall & Lunsford 1987), although actual statistical evidence for this is lacking and post-operative seizures are well recognized (EANS 1990; Horn 2007). The transcallosal approach does carry a risk of venous infarction, which has been associated with division of large bridging cortical veins running into the superior sagittal sinus and with prolonged cortical retraction (Shucart & Stein 1978; Hall & Lunsford 1987; Horn 2007). Cortical retraction may also cause contralateral leg weakness, and the pericallosal arteries are at risk of damage with this procedure. However, with good microsurgical technique the risk of these complications should be minimal. Yasargil et al (1990) have reported a series of 18 cases with 17 good results, one fair result, no specific postoperative technical complications, but one death two weeks postoperatively from a pulmonary embolus. More recently a detailed critical analysis of a series of 27 transcallosal resections of colloid cysts from the Barrow institute found a 44% incidence of complications, including new seizures in two cases, venous infarction with significant deficit in one case, infections in five cases, residual cyst (not requiring reoperation) in one case, reoperation in three cases (two for fractured ventricular drainage catheter and one for epidural hematoma) the need for VP shunt in five cases (Horn 2007). The routine use of postoperative ventricular drainage catheters in these cases obviously was associated with two of the three re-operations, and may have contributed to the infection rate (Horn 2007).

Transcortical approach

This procedure employs a right frontal craniotomy and a small cerebrotomy through the middle frontal gyrus to approach the frontal horn of the lateral ventricle (Fig. 44.9). McKissock (1951) recommended excision of a conical block of cortex and underlying white matter to expose the frontal horn; however, most surgeons would now employ a smaller

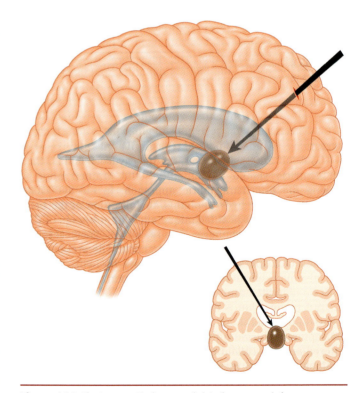

Figure 44.9 The transcortical approach (similar approach for open transcortical or endoscopic resection).

linear cerebrotomy (Symon & Pell 1990; Charalampaki et al 2006). The approach to the frontal of the lateral ventricle is calculated using the same landmarks that would typically be used for a frontal ventricular puncture. Indeed, a useful technique is to pass a ventricular catheter into the ventricle, and use micro-suction to dissect through the white matter around the catheter to make the formal ventricular approach

Stereotactic anatomical localization allows the most accurate and direct approach to the lateral ventricle and ensures that the cerebrotomy tract is pointed directly at the foramen of Monro, and is strongly recommended. Indeed it would now be difficult to justify not using frameless stereotaxy, if available, for the transcortical approach. Kondziolka and Lunsford (1996) reported excellent results in a series of 20 cases of colloid cyst resected with a stereotactically-guided microsurgical transcortical approach utilizing small (10–20 mm) cerebrotomy. Six (30%) of these patients did not have preoperative hydrocephalus. Although one patient had a temporary hemiparesis due to a small contusion in the head of the caudate, all patients made complete recovery, and only one patient had a single postoperative seizure.

The foramen of Monro is approached and the colloid cyst delivered in the same manner as the transcallosal approach. The use of stereotactic techniques in planning and accurately executing the approach has the obvious advantages.

The transchoroidal approaches described above can also be readily performed through a transcortical exposure if required. However, the option of an interforniceal approach, which is possible through the a transcallosal approach, is not possible when using the transcortical exposure.

For the same reasons described above with the transcallosal exposure, when reforming the transcortical approach a pellucidotomy should be routine performed and the retractor tips should not be allowed to retract on the ventricular wall.

Obvious neuropsychological consequences of a small right frontal cerebrotomy (uncomplicated) have not been reported. The main concern with this approach is the risk of epilepsy, which is in the order of 5% (McKissock 1951; Little & MacCarty 1974; Hall & Lunsford 1987). The major technical disadvantage of this procedure is that it is difficult to perform in the absence of hydrocephalus, some dilatation of the lateral ventricle allowing for improved access, and it is only possible to approach the cyst through one foramen of Monro.

The most common use of this approach currently is when used in an endoscopically assisted minimally invasive open-resection (Charalampaki et al 2006). The use of the endoscope in conjunction with microsurgical technique provides excellent light and visualization through a narrow corridor, and using the angled endoscope it allows viewing 'around the corner'. Recent improvements in endoscope design and instrumentation are now such that complete endoscopic resection alone is usually feasible, with progression to the endoscopically assisted open transcortical procedure being used when technical issues preclude complete removal or complications arise (Schroeder & Gaab 2002; Longatti et al 2006; Bergsneider 2007; Horn 2007; Greenlee 2008).

Endoscopic surgery

Endoscopic surgery for colloid cysts follows the same transcortical path to the foramen of Monro as does the open transcortical operation. It has the major advantages that it can be performed through a small burr hole, and requires a smaller cortical incision, and arguably offers improved illumination and visualization. Stereotactic localization will allow optimal trajectory to the foramen of Monro, and is now routinely used in most cases, and is essential in the cases without hydrocephalus (Apuzzo et al 1987; Caemart & Calliauw 1990; Hellwig et al 2003). Using the endoscope, the colloid cyst may be directly punctured and aspirated, and part of the wall may be coagulated by diathermy or laser technique. In an increasing proportion of cases, gentle traction on the cyst wall using forceps in a working channel, combined with coagulation and endoscopic microsurgical techniques, allows complete endoscopic excision of the cyst wall (Abdou & Cohen 1998; Schroeder & Gaab 2002; Longatti et al 2006; Bergsneider 2007; Horn 2007; Greenlee 2008). Complete endoscopic resection of the colloid cyst was achieved in 29/35 cases reported by Greenlee (2008) and in 10/19 cases reported by Horn (2007). Although the procedure can be performed under local anaesthetic (Powell & Torrens 1983; Auer et al 1988; Caemart & Calliauw 1990; Ostertag 1990), most surgeons would routinely recommend general anaesthesia for these cases.

The major disadvantage with the endoscopic procedure is that at the removal, the whole wall of the colloid cyst often requires significant traction (and therefore risking hemorrhage particularly from the choroid plexus on the roof on the third ventricle) and, like the transcortical open approach, the inability to access the opposite foramen of Monro should this be required. This results in a somewhat lower rate of complete cyst removal by the endoscopic technique, with the comparative series reported by Horn (2007) having a complete excision in 53% of endoscopic and 94% of transcallosal cases. The major advantage of endoscopic treatment is that it is less invasive, requires no retraction, does not pose a risk to the bridging veins or pericallosal vessels, and has a lower risk of seizures. Horn (2007) reported a total complication rate of 75% (21/28) of endoscopic and 56% (15/27) of transcallosal cases. However, with the exception of a higher incidence of VP shunting following transcallosal cases (19% vs 7%), they found no significant difference in the overall complication rates for the two procedures (Horn 2007). Three cases (11%) of neurological deficit were found following both the transcallosal (one venous infarct and two new seizures) and endoscopic (two significant memory impairments and one hemiparesis from internal capsule injury) procedures (Horn 2007).

Even if the cyst wall is not completely excised in an endoscopic procedure, the cyst can usually be punctured under direct vision, removing part of the cyst wall and aspirating the cyst and coagulating the residual wall. Two series of 15 cases each have been reported, and in each series, only 12 cysts could be completely aspirated (Ostertag 1990; Decq et al 1998). In each series, there were three cases where only partial aspiration was possible due to the viscosity of the contents, but in each case, the patient's symptoms were relieved. The only complication in either series was one case of meningitis (Ostertag 1990). None of the cysts re-collected, although the follow-up period was relatively short (<5 years). Of the seven patients who were not shunted prior to the procedure, none required postoperative shunts (Ostertag 1990).

The septum pellucidum can also be fenestrated endoscopically, and this is recommended for the same reasons as described above in relation to open surgical approaches.

It should be noted that endoscopy and open microsurgical techniques are not necessarily competitive techniques, but have complimentary roles. The endoscope can assist visualization in open microsurgical colloid cyst resections. Although endoscopic assistance is not required in most transcallosal or transcortical cases, it can by virtue of its angled view, occasionally be invaluable in identifying a small residual area of cyst wall (usually attached to the third ventricular roof), not visible under the operating microscope. Similarly, proficiency in the microsurgical approaches is required following failed or complicated endoscopic procedures.

Stereotactic aspiration of colloid cysts

Gutierrez-Lara et al (1975) first described aspiration of colloid cysts without resection using a free-hand method in 1975. Application of stereotactic localization for aspiration of four colloid cysts was then reported by Bosch et al (1978). Because of the simplicity, relatively low risk, and wide availability of stereotaxy, stereotactic (CT-guided) aspiration of colloid cysts was widely advocated in the 1980s (Bosch et al 1978; Rivas & Lobato 1985; Donauer et al 1986; Hall & Lunsford 1987; Mohadjer et al 1987; Musolino et al 1989; Kondziolka & Lunsford 1991). The initial success of the stereotactic aspiration related largely to the viscosity of the cyst contents, and this has been found to have some correlation with the radiodensity of the cyst on CT scans (Kondziolka & Lunsford 1991; Pollock 2000). Kondziolka & Lunsford (1991) reported 22 patients treated with stereotactic aspiration of the colloid cyst as the primary treatment. Of those, 11 patients had a satisfactory result: the cyst was not apparent on postoperative imaging studies in three cases; seven had a small residual cyst; and one had >30% of the original cyst volume but had relief of CSF obstruction. Eleven (50%) of the patients required further procedures (endoscopic aspiration, shunting procedures or open operation). There was no significant morbidity or mortality from the stereotactic aspiration, regardless of whether this was considered successful or not (Kondziolka & Lunsford 1991). The same authors subsequently reported an expansion of this series (total 25 cases) in 1994; and still found that endoscopic aspiration alone was successful in only 52%, and that 12 of the 25 cases required further procedures (Kondziolka & Lunsford 1994). Similarly, Hall & Lunsford (1987) reported seven cases of CT-guided stereotactic aspiration, with six of these having ventricular patency as shown on post-aspiration ventriculography, and one failed aspiration requiring open resection of the tumor. They also found no complications related to stereotactic aspiration. Large size of the cyst does not contraindicate stereotactic aspiration, and Kondziolka & Lunsford (1991) found that size of the cyst related to successful aspiration only insofar as very small cysts were more difficult to puncture.

Although most series report minimal morbidity associated with stereotactic aspiration of colloid cysts, Mathiesen et al (1993) reported a series of 26 aspirations in 16 patients with colloid cysts, and found temporary memory deficit and confusion following three procedures and one case of postoperative central pain syndrome. However, of even more importance, is that this paper has questioned the long-term durability of the procedure, with 11 of the 26 procedures having recurrences from 6 to 15 years following aspiration (Mathiesen et al 1993). The stereotactic aspiration is only somewhat less invasive than an endoscopic procedure, and endoscopy allows visualization avoiding the small risk of vascular damage, which attends blind stereotactic cyst puncture (Ostertag 1990). Therefore, the role of aspiration should be generally restricted to those few patients requiring treatment and in whom an endoscopic or open procedure is not possible, and the need for long-term follow-up of these patients is emphasized.

Adjuvant therapy

As colloid cysts are benign lesions and produce symptoms by virtue of their mass, surgical therapy (aspiration, excision and/or CSF diversion) is the only recognized form of effective treatment at present. There is no place for radiotherapy or other adjuvant therapy in the treatment of these cysts.

Long-term prognosis

Following the successful outcome of microscopic or endoscopic complete resection of a colloid cyst the patient should be considered cured, although in a small number of these cases, the patient may still require CSF diversion. A small amount of residual cyst wall can result in recurrence of the cyst, although this is also infrequent. The required long-term follow-up data for these cases is, as yet, not available.

> **Key points**
>
> - Colloid cysts are benign congenital lesions in the third ventricle.
> - Most colloid cysts present in adults with hydrocephalus or as coincidental findings on CT or MRI scans.
> - The risk of sudden death is probably small, but is well reported, and requires that treatment be undertaken in all symptomatic cases. Even in asymptomatic cases, particularly in younger patients, treatment should still be recommended and, in those cases where treatment is not undertaken, radiographic and clinical monitoring must be diligently followed.
> - Current recommended treatment options include microsurgical resection (transcortical or transcallosal) or endoscopic aspiration/resection.
> - Stereotactic aspiration is a low risk procedure, but long-term recurrence rates are high.

REFERENCES

Abdou, M.S., Cohen, A.R., 1998. Endoscopic treatment of colloid cysts of the third ventricle. Technical note and review of the literature. J. Neurosurg. 89 (6), 1062–1068.

Abernathey, C.D., Davis, D.H., Kelly, P.J., 1989. Treatment of colloid cysts of the third ventricle by stereotaxic microsurgical laser craniotomy. J. Neurosurg. 70, 195–200.

Adams, R.D., Fisher, C.M., Hakim, S., et al., 1965. Symptomatic occult hydrocephalus with 'normal' cerebrospinal-fluid pressure: a treatable syndrome. N. Engl. J. Med. 273, 117–126.

Aggarwal, A., Corbett, A., Graham, J., 1999. Familial colloid cyst of the third ventricle. J. Clin. Neurosci. 6 (6), 520–522.

Ahmed, S.K., Stanworth, P.A., 2002. Colloid cyst of the third ventricle in identical twins. Br. J. Neurosurg. 16 (3), 303–307.

Akins, P.T., Roberts, R., Coxe, W.S., et al., 1996. Familial colloid cyst of the third ventricle: case report and review of associated conditions. Neurosurgery 38, 392–395.

Amar, A.P., Ghosh, S., Apuzzo, M.L., 2004. Ventricular tumors. In: Winn, H.R. (Ed.), Youmans neurological surgery. WB.Saunders, Philadelphia, PA, pp 1237–1263.

Antunes, J.L., Louis, K.M., Ganti, S.R., 1980. Colloid cysts of the third ventricle. Neurosurgery 7, 450–455.

Apuzzo, M.L., Chi-Shing Zee, Breeze, R.E., 1987. Anterior and mid-third ventricular lesions: a surgical overview. In: Apuzzo, M.L. (Ed.), Surgery of the third ventricle. Williams & Wilkins, Baltimore, MD, pp 520–522.

Apuzzo, M.L., Litofsky, N.S., 1993. Surgery in and around the anterior third ventricle. In: Apuzzo, M.L. (Ed.), Brain surgery. Churchill Livingstone, New York, pp 541–579.

Aronica, P.A., Ahdab-Barmada, M., Rozin, L., et al., 1998. Sudden death in an adolescent boy due to colloid cyst of the third ventricle. Am. J. Forens. Med. Pathol. 19 (2), 119–122.

Auer, L., Holzer, P., Ascher, P.W., et al., 1988. Endoscopic neurosurgery. Acta Neurochir. (Wien) 90, 1–14.

Bailey, P., 1916. Morphology of the roof plate of the fore-brain and the lateral choroid plexuses in the human embryo. J. Compar. Neurol. 26, 79–120.

Batnitzky, S., Sarwar, M., Leeds, N.E., et al., 1974. Colloid cysts of third ventricle. Radiology 112, 327–341.

Bergsneider, M., 2007. Complete microsurgical resection of colloid cysts with a dual-port endoscopic technique. Neurosurgery 60 (Suppl.), 33–43.

Bosch, D.A., Rahn, T., Backlund, E.O., 1978. Treatment of colloid cysts of the third ventricle by stereotaxic aspiration. Surg. Neurol. 9, 15–18.

Brun, A., Egund, N., 1973. The pathogenesis of cerebral symptoms in colloid cysts of the third ventricle: a clinical and pathoanatomical study. Acta Neurol. Scand. 49, 525–535.

Buchsbaum, H.W., Colton, R.P., 1967. Anterior third ventricular cysts in infancy. Case report. J. Neurosurg. 26, 264–266.

Bull, J.W.D., Sutton, D., 1949. The diagnosis of paraphysial cysts. Brain 72, 487–518.

Bullard, D.E., Osbourne, D., Cook, W.A., 1982. Colloid cyst of the third ventricle presenting as a ring-enhancing lesion on computed tomography. Neurosurgery 11, 790–791.

Büttner, A., Winkler, P.A., Eisenmenger, W., et al., 1997. Colloid cysts of the third ventricle with fatal outcome: A report of two cases and review of the literature. Int. J. Legal. Med. 110, 260–266.

Caemart, J., Calliauw, L., 1990. A note on the use of a modern endoscope. In: Symon, L., Calliauw, L., Cohadon, F., et al. (Eds.), Advances and technical standards in neurosurgery, vol 17. Surgical techniques in the management of colloid cysts of the third ventricle. Springer-Verlag, Wien, pp 149–153.

Cairns, H., Mosberg, W.H. Jr., 1951. Colloid cysts of the third ventricle. Surg. Gynecol. Obstet. 92, 545–570.

Cameron, A.S., Archibald, Y.M., 1981. Verbal memory deficit after left fornix removal: A case report. Int. J. Neurosci. 12, 201.

Campbell, D.A., Varma, T.R., 1991. An extraventricular colloid cyst: Case report. Br. J. Neurosurg. 5, 519–522.

Carmel, P.W., 1985. Tumors of the third ventricle. Acta Neurochir. 75, 136–146.

Chan, R.C., Thompson, G.B., 1983. Third ventricular colloid cysts presenting with acute neurological deterioration. Surg. Neurol. 19, 258–362.

Charalampaki, P., Filippi, R., Welschehold, S., et al., 2006. Endoscope-assisted removal of colloid cysts of the third ventricle. Neurosurg. Rev. 29 (1), 72–79.

Ciric, I., Zivin, I., 1975. Neuroepithelial (colloid) cysts of the septum pellucidum. J. Neurosurg. 43, 69–73.

Coxe, W.S., Luse, S.A., 1964. Colloid cyst of the third ventricle. An electron microscope study. J. Neuropathol. Exp. Neurol. 23, 431–445.

Dandy, W.E., 1922. Diagnosis, localization and removal of tumors of the third ventricle. Bull. Johns Hopkins 33, 188–189.

Dandy, W.E., 1933. Benign tumors of the third ventricle of the brain: Diagnosis and treatment. Charles C. Thomas, Springfield, IL.

Davidoff, L.M., Dyck, C.M., 1935. Congenital tumors of the third ventricle, their diagnosis by encephalography and ventriculography. Bull. Neurol. Inst. New York 4, 221–263.

Decq, P., Le Guerinel, C., Brugieres, P., et al., 1998. Endoscopic management of colloid cysts. Neurosurgery 42, 1288–1294.

De Witt Hamer, P.C., Verstegen, M.J., De Haan, R.J., et al., 2002. High risk of acute deterioration in patients harboring symptomatic colloid cysts of the third ventricle. J. Neurosurg. 96, 1041–1045.

Donaldson, J.O., Simon, R.H., 1980. Radiodense ions within a third ventricular colloid cyst. Arch. Neurol. 37, 246.

Donauer, E., Moringlane, J.R., Ostertag, C.B., 1986. Colloid cysts of the third ventricle. Open operative approach or stereotactic aspiration. Acta Neurochir. (Wien) 83, 24–30.

Dott, N.M., 1938. Surgical aspects of the hypothalamus. In: Clark, W.E., Beattie, J., Riddoch, G., et al. (Eds.), The hypothalamus: morphological, functional, clinical and surgical aspects. Oliver & Boyd, Edinburgh, pp 131–185.

European Association Neurosurgical Societies (EANS), 1990. A short critique of the variety of approaches to handle colloid cysts. In: Symon, L., Calliauw, L., Cohadon, F., et al. (Eds.), Advances and technical standards in neurosurgery, vol 17. Surgical techniques in the management of colloid cysts of the third ventricle. Springer-Verlag, Wien, pp 153–155.

Ferrand, B., Pecker, J., Javalet, A., et al., 1971. Le kyste colloide du troisième ventricule. Etude anatomo-pathologique et pathogenique. Ann. Anat. Pathol. 16, 429–450.

Ferry, D.J., Kemp, L.G., 1968. Colloid cyst of the third ventricle. Military Med. 773, 734–737.

Friedman, M.A., Meyers, C.A., Sawaya, R., 2003. Neuropsychological effects of third ventricle tumor surgery. Neurosurgery 52, 791–798.

Ganti, S.R., Antunes, J.L., Louis, K.M., et al., 1981. Computed tomography in the diagnosis of colloid cysts of the third ventricle. Radiology 138, 385–391.

Gardner, W.J., Turner, M., 1937. Neuroepithelial cysts of the third ventricle. Arch. Neurol. Psychiatry 38, 1055–1061.

Gemperlein, J., 1960. Paraphyseal cysts of the third ventricle. Report of two cases in infants. J. Neuropathol. Exp. Neurol. 19, 133–134.

Graziani, N., Dufour, H., Figarella-Branger, D., et al., 1995. Do the suprasellar neuroenteric cysts, the Rathke cleft cyst and the colloid cyst constitute the same entity? Acta Neurochir. 133 (3–4), 174–180.

Greenwood, J. Jr., 1949. Paraphysial cysts of the third ventricle with report of 8 cases. J. Neurosurg. 6, 153–159.

Greenlee, J.D., Teo, C., Ghahreman, A., et al., 2008. Purely endoscopic resection of colloid cysts. Neurosurgery 62 (Suppl. 1), 51–56.

Grossiord, A., 1941. Le kyste colloide du troisième ventricule. These de Paris, No 216.

Guner, M., Shaw, M.D.M., Turner, J.W., et al., 1976. Computed tomography in the diagnosis of colloid cysts. Surg. Neurol. 6, 345–348.

Gutierrez-Lara, F., Patino, R., Hakim, S., 1975. Treatment of tumors of the third ventricle. A new and simple technique. Surg. Neurol. 3, 323–325.

Hall, W.A., Lunsford, L.D., 1987. Changing concepts in the treatment of colloid cysts. An 11-year experience in the CT era. J. Neurosurg. 66, 186–191.

Hellwig, D., Bauer, B., Schulte, M., et al., 2003. Neuroendoscopic treatment for colloid cysts of the third ventricle: The experience of a decade. Neurosurgery 52, 525–533.

Hingwala, D.R., Sanghvi, D.A., Shenoy, A.S., et al., 2008. Colloid cyst of the velum interpositum: a common lesion at an uncommon site. Surg. Neurol. 72 (2), 182–184.

45

Metastatic brain tumors

Raymond Sawaya, Rajesh K. Bindal, Frederick F. Lang, and Dima Suki

Introduction

Brain metastases are neoplasms that originate in tissues outside the central nervous system and spread secondarily to the brain. These tumors are a common complication of systemic cancer and an important cause of morbidity and mortality in cancer patients. They are the most common intracranial tumors and their incidence may be rising. This chapter deals with epidemiology, pathology, clinical features and diagnostic techniques, and methods of treatment of brain (parenchymal) metastases.

Epidemiology

There are three sources of epidemiologic data on brain metastases: epidemiologic studies, clinical studies, and autopsy series. Epidemiologic data from large patient populations by definition represent the best type of evidence. Unfortunately, inadequate ascertainment of tumor pathology and under-reporting of cases are limiting factors in many studies. In a national survey for intracranial neoplasms (Walker et al 1985), only 20% of the metastatic cases diagnosed during 1973 and 1974 were verified by tissue examination. Neuro-surgical series reporting patients with brain tumors have suffered from major selection biases and confounding problems. For example, metastatic tumors were largely under-represented in these series because of the widespread notion that therapy for brain metastases was not beneficial.

Autopsy studies (Table 45.1) have commonly been used to estimate the incidence of brain metastases for a given primary disease. These studies, however, were generally performed at referral centers and relied on nonrandomly selected groups of patients who happened to be autopsied. For the above reasons, there are major fluctuations in the reported epidemiologic data on brain metastases. Nevertheless, although a precise estimate is difficult to obtain, the existing body of evidence has helped to identify useful epidemiologic trends and different risk groups.

Epidemiologic trends

The incidence of brain metastases was estimated at 2.8–11.1/100 000 individuals in earlier epidemiologic studies of large populations in the USA, Iceland, and central Finland (Fogelholm et al 1984; Guomundsson 1970; Percy et al 1972; Walker et al 1985). It is currently estimated that over 100 000 patients will develop brain metastases per year in the USA alone (Landis et al 1998; Patchell 2003) (Table 45.2). Brain metastases are now considered to be the most common intracranial tumors, significantly outnumbering primary brain tumors (Posner 1995; Walker et al 1985; Wingo et al 1995). This trend is increasing (Johnson & Young 1996; Posner & Chernik 1978; Gloeckler Ries et al 2003; Levin et al 2001), relative to earlier population studies (incidence ratio of metastatic to primary tumors from the above population-based studies ranged from 30% to 90%) and earlier neurosurgical series (ratio of metastatic to primary tumors is much lower and ranges from 3% to 25%) (Arseni & Constantinescu 1975; Christensen 1949; Cushing 1932; Elkington 1935; Livingston et al 1948; Meagher & Eisenhardt 1931; Paillas & Pellet 1975; Petit-Dutaillis et al 1956; Richards & McKissock 1963; Simionescu 1960; Stortebecker 1954; Zulch 1957).

Between one-quarter and one-fifth of patients with cancer have brain metastases at autopsy (Cairncross & Posner 1983; Posner & Chernik 1978; Takakura et al 1982). This prevalence at autopsy translates into 112 960–141 200 cancer patients per year who will die with brain metastases, based on 1998 estimates from the American Cancer Society of 564 800 cancer deaths (Landis et al 1998), an increase over previous estimates. A true increase could have resulted from an increased incidence of lung cancer and melanoma, improved cancer treatment for the primary cancer, and an aging patient population. An apparent increase could have resulted from a more adequate representation of brain metastases in more recent neurosurgical series, advances in neuroimaging techniques, and routine staging that assesses the central nervous system.

Table 45.1 Autopsy data on frequency of brain metastases in patients dying of cancer

Investigators	Histology of primary cancer	Autopsies (n)	Patients with brain metastases (%)
Galluzzi & Payne (1956)	Lung	647	26
Newman & Hansen (1974)	Lung	247	23
Takakura et al (1982)	Lung	747	36
Sorensen et al (1988)	Adeno	87	44
Burgess et al (1979)	SCLC	177	40
Hirsch et al (1982)	SCLC	87	50
Cox & Komaki (1986)	Squamous	123	13
	Adeno	129	54
	SCLC	82	45
	Large	54	52
All lung cancer		2380	32
Takakura et al (1982)	Breast	526	21
Tsukada et al (1983)	Breast	1044	18
Lee 1983[a]	Breast	3846	22
All breast cancer		5416	21
Takakura et al (1982)	Melanoma	49	49
Amer et al (1978)	Melanoma	53	68
de la Monte et al (1983)	Melanoma	56	64
Lee (1980)[a]	Melanoma	553	46
All melanoma		711	48
Takakura et al (1982)	GI	773	6
Saitoh et al (1982)	Renal	1828	10
Takakura et al (1982)	Renal	199	17
All renal cancer		2027	11

[a]Literature review.
Adeno, lung adenocarcinoma; Large, large cell lung carcinoma; SCLC, small cell lung carcinoma; Squamous, squamous cell lung carcinoma.

Table 45.2 Estimated number of patients developing brain metastases each year in the USA

Primary site	Deaths (n)[a]	Frequency of brain metastases (%)	Patients with brain metastases (n)
Lung	160 100	32[b]	51 232
Breast	43 900	21[b]	9219
Skin	7300	48[b]	3504
Colon	47 700	6[b]	2862
Kidney	11 600	11[b]	1276
Liver and pancreas	41 900	5	2095
Prostate	39 200	6	2352
Leukemia	21 600	8	1728
Sarcoma	5700	15	855
Female genital	27 100	2	542
Lymphoma	26 300	5	1315
Thyroid	1200	17	204
Others	131 200	19	24 928
Total	564 800	19	107 312

[a]Data from Landis SH, Murray T, Bolden S, et al. Cancer statistics, 1998. CA Cancer J Clin 1998;48(1): 6–29.
[b]Values estimated from Table 45.1; remaining frequencies estimated from data in (Takakura et al 1982).

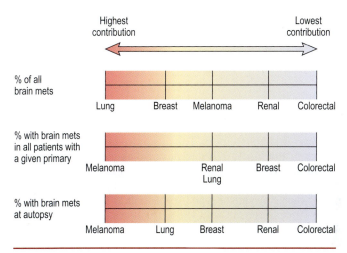

Figure 45.1 Relative contributions of the most common primary cancers to brain metastasis. mets, metastases.

Risk groups

Type of primary cancer

Although virtually any malignancy can metastasize to the brain, the incidence of brain metastases varies dramatically from one type of cancer to another (Jemal et al 2003; Jemal et al 2004; Landis et al 1999; Patchell 2003). Lung, breast, melanoma, renal, and colon cancers account for most brain metastases (Table 45.2, Fig. 45.1). Primary lung tumors rank first, accounting for 30–60% of all brain metastases (Baker 1942; Baker et al 1951; Chang et al 1992; Lang & Slater 1964; Le Chevalier et al 1985; MacGee 1971; Markesbery et al 1978; Sundaresan & Galicich 1985; Takakura et al 1982; Zimm et al 1981). Of all patients with lung cancer, 18–65% will develop brain metastasis (Abrams et al 1950; Burt et al 1992; Nugent et al 1979; Takakura et al 1982), and the actual histological nature of the primary tumor is very important in determining metastatic frequency. Indeed, more than 40% of patients with small cell lung cancer and lung adenocarcinoma have brain metastases at autopsy, a prevalence of more than twice that found in the other types of lung carcinoma such as squamous cell carcinoma (Cox & Komaki 1986; Sen et al 1998; Takakura et al 1982).

Breast cancer ranks second in metastasizing to the brain, with 10% to 30% of all brain metastases among women originating from primary breast tumors (Baker 1942;

Baker et al 1951; Lang & Slater 1964; Markesbery et al 1978; Takakura et al 1982; Tsukada et al 1983; Vieth & Odom 1965; Zimm et al 1981). A total of 20–30% of patients with breast cancer will develop a brain metastasis (Abrams et al 1950; Aronson et al 1964; Chason et al 1963; Cifuentes & Pickren 1979; Posner 1995; Tsukada et al 1983). Nevertheless, in a large population-based study by Barnholtz-Sloan et al (2004), only 5.1% (95% CI = 4.9–5.3) of breast cancer patients with a single primary developed brain metastases.

Melanoma ranks third in tendency to metastasize to the brain; among patients with brain metastases, approximately 5–21% will have melanoma as the primary tumor (Chason et al 1963; Lang & Slater 1964; Le Chevalier et al 1985; Markesbery et al 1978; Posner 1980b; Sundaresan & Galicich 1985; Zimm et al 1981). Interestingly, malignant melanoma, which represents only 4% of all cancers (Landis et al 1998), has the highest propensity of all systemic malignant tumors to metastasize to the brain (Amer et al 1978;

Chason et al 1963; Pickren et al 1983). The incidence of brain metastases among patients with malignant melanoma varies from 6% to 43% in clinical series (Amer et al 1979; Atkinson 1978; McNeer & das Gupta 1965) and 12–90% in autopsy series (Amer et al 1978; Chason et al 1963; Madajewicz et al 1984; Pickren et al 1983), and in a recent large, population-based study of brain metastasis incidence from single primary cancers (Barnholtz-Sloan et al 2004), the incidence proportion percentage was 6.9% (95% CI = 6.3–7.4).

Patients with renal and colon cancers frequently experience metastasis of these tumors to the brain. In the Barnholtz-Sloan population-based study (Barnholtz-Sloan et al 2004), patients with a single renal cell cancer primary had a brain metastasis incidence proportion percentage of 6.5% (95% CI = 5.9–7.1). Metastases to the brain are more rarely found from other types of cancers such as sarcoma and genitourinary primaries (Anderson et al 1992; Bloch et al 1987; Castaldo et al 1983; Dauplat et al 1987; Lewis 1988; Martínez-Mañas et al 1998; Stein et al 1986; Steinfeld & Zelefsky 1987; Taylor et al 1984). In 10–15% of cases, patients with no known history of cancer present with symptoms caused by a brain metastasis from an undiagnosed primary malignancy (Soffietti et al 2002). Although the frequency of such presentation varies (Khansur et al 1997), in most of these instances, the patients are suspected to suffer from lung cancer (Khansur et al 1997; van den Bent 2001).

Patient age

Figure 45.2 is a histogram of the incidence of brain metastases based on age, an incidence that is similar to that of primary systemic tumors. The incidence of brain metastases peaks in the 5th to 7th decades (Takakura et al 1982) and tends to decline thereafter (Graus et al 1983; Takakura et al 1982). The age group at risk for brain metastasis development varies by cancer type (Aronson et al 1964; de la Monte et al 1988; Sorensen et al 1988; Takakura et al 1982). There is a lower incidence of brain metastases in children than in

adults, with frequencies ranging from 6% to 13% (Graus et al 1983; Posner & Chernik 1978; Posner 1980b, 1992, 1995; Tasdemiroglu & Patchell 1997; Vannucci & Baten 1974). The most common cause of childhood brain metastases is leukemia, followed by lymphoma (Takakura et al 1982); osteogenic sarcoma and rhabdomyosarcoma are the most frequent causes of solid brain metastases among children <15 years old, whereas germ cell tumors are the most frequent producers of solid brain metastases for patients 15–21 years old (Graus et al 1983).

Patient sex

Although brain metastases occur at a similar frequency among men and women, some differences are seen in the types of primary cancer responsible for the brain metastases in the two sexes. Lung cancer is the most common source of brain metastasis in males, whereas breast cancer is the most common source in females (Takakura et al 1982; Walker et al 1985). This difference is largely a result of the different incidences of these primary cancers in the sexes. The incidence of brain metastasis from a given primary appears to be the same regardless of the sex of the patient, except in patients with melanoma and lung cancer. Men with melanoma are more likely than women to develop brain metastases. It has been suggested that this difference is because melanoma in men is more likely to develop on the head, neck, or trunk in those with outdoor occupations and more consequent solar exposure of those regions. Melanoma primaries in these locations are more likely to spread to the brain (Amer et al 1978; Robinson et al 1987). Women with lung cancer show a significantly higher incidence of brain metastases than men (Barnholtz-Sloan et al 2004). This difference could stem from the fact that the incidence of primary lung cancer is rising in women (Weir et al 2003).

Pathology

Despite their varied sites of origin, the macroscopic appearance of brain metastases has many similarities (Russell & Rubinstein 1971). Tumors are generally spheroid and well-demarcated from brain tissue. Cut surfaces tend to be pinkish-gray, granular, and soft (Fig. 45.3). Tumors are

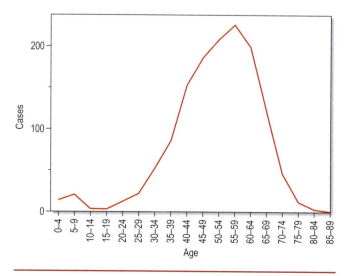

Figure 45.2 Histogram of the incidence of brain metastasis based on age. (Reproduced with permission from Takakura K, Sano K, Hojo S, et al. Metastatic Tumors of the Central Nervous System. New York: Igaku-Shoin, Japan; 1982).

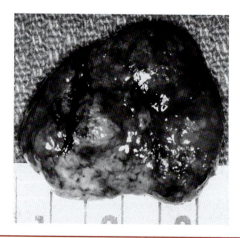

Figure 45.3 Gross pathological specimen of a lung carcinoma metastatic to the brain.

often surrounded by an extensive zone of edema. The extent of this edema does not correlate with the size of the tumor nodule. Large tumors very often have a central region of necrosis resulting in a softened or even liquified, pus-like core. They also tend to be flattened along the brain surface or even elongated along white-matter fiber tracts. Metastases are most often located at the junction of the gray and white matter of the brain, where it is postulated that the tumor emboli are trapped in the cerebral vasculature. The microscopic histological appearance of these metastases is similar to that of other systemic metastases. It is interesting to note that although most metastases appear well-demarcated from surrounding brain tissue on gross examination, microscopically these tumors may have a somewhat infiltrative appearance (Henson & Urich 1982; Stortebecker 1954). This has been noted for tumors of various histological types, such as small cell (Takakura et al 1982) and epidermoid (Paillas & Pellet 1975; Sundaresan & Galicich 1985) lung cancer, melanoma (Kaye 1992), and colon carcinoma (Sundaresan & Galicich 1985). This infiltration is not as extensive as that of malignant gliomas, but it may still play an important role in recurrence after surgical excision. Why some metastases may appear infiltrative whereas others do not, and why malignant primary brain tumors are far more infiltrative than metastatic tumors, is poorly understood.

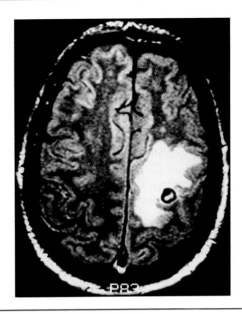

Figure 45.4 A T2-weighted magnetic resonance (MR) image of a left parietal renal carcinoma metastasis (dark ring, 1 cm in diameter) surrounded by an extensive zone of edema (white area).

Blood–brain barrier

The nature of the blood–brain barrier is changed in metastatic brain tumors. It is well known that blood vessels formed by neoplasms are often defective, even in systemic tumors. In the brain, tumor-induced blood vessels have increased permeability and an imperfect blood–brain barrier. Capillary endothelial cells in metastatic brain tumors display characteristics found in blood vessels of systemic neoplasms, including gap junctions and membrane fenestration, with these characteristics being most common in the center of the tumor (Long 1979). This lack of a blood–brain barrier presumably results in an increased capillary permeability to serum proteins and other large molecular weight compounds in the blood. Experimental evidence suggests that tumor angiogenesis and increased permeability begin when a tumor exceeds 1 mm in size (Hasegawa et al 1983). This fact is taken advantage of in contrast-enhanced computed tomography (CT) and magnetic resonance (MR) imaging studies. Tumors show enhancement on radiographs owing to their preferential uptake of contrast agents, presumably as a result of a defective blood–brain barrier.

The often extensive edema surrounding brain metastases is generally thought to arise from tumor-induced alterations in the blood–brain barrier; these allow fluids and proteins to leak out of blood vessels into brain tissue, causing what is termed vasogenic edema. This edema is largely confined to the extracellular space of the white matter of the brain. Interestingly, the size of the lesion itself often does not correlate with the extent of peritumoral edema (Fig. 45.4), and the exact relationship between tumors and extent of edema is poorly characterized. The disrupted blood–brain barrier in metastases also has important implications for chemotherapy, which will be discussed in the corresponding section.

Localization and number

The cerebrum is the site of localization of 80–85% of all brain metastases, the cerebellum is the site of 10–15%, and the brain stem is the site of 3–5% (Delattre et al 1988; Haar & Patterson 1972; Takakura et al 1982). There is a rough tendency for the overall distribution of brain metastases to correspond to the relative size and blood flow of regions in the brain; however, there are exceptions to this. Cerebral metastases have an increased tendency to occur at the temporo-parieto-occipital junction, where the terminal branches of the middle cerebral artery are located (Delattre et al 1988; Kindt 1964). It is estimated that the weight of the cerebrum is nine times that of the cerebellum (Ask-Upmark 1956); however, the relative frequency of metastasis to the cerebellum and brain stem is higher than is predicted by their relative weights. The reasons for this are unclear. The relative distribution of metastases may also vary with the tumor histology (Graf et al 1988), but this phenomenon is also poorly characterized. Some reports suggest that the rate of posterior fossa metastasis may be higher for pelvic and gastrointestinal tumors (Cascino et al 1983b; Delattre et al 1988; Takakura et al 1982), a phenomenon that may be caused by propagation via Batson's venous plexus (Batson 1942).

The relative frequency of single or multiple metastases varies with the type of primary tumor. Melanoma has the highest tendency to produce multiple lesions, followed by lung and breast primaries. Metastases from colon primaries present with multiple tumors 50% of the time (Cascino et al 1983b), whereas those from renal cancer usually present with only one lesion (Decker et al 1984; Gay et al 1987). Table 45.3 shows the percentage of patients with multiple brain metastases in various studies. Overall, autopsy studies

The use of radiosensitizers might be expected to increase the response of brain metastases to WBRT. Earlier studies showed no indication that they are effective in improving response rates (Aiken et al 1984; Buckner 1992; DeAngelis et al 1989a; Komarnicky et al 1991). However, a recent phase III clinical trial (Mehta et al 2003; Meyers et al 2004) studied the use of motexafin gadolinium (MGd), an oxidative drug that sensitizes tumor cells to radiation. In this randomized trial, although MGd increased the time to progression of neurological disease in some patients and improved the neurocognitive function in the subset of patients with lung cancer, it had no effect on overall survival time.

Subsequently, Suh et al (2006) performed a phase III trial of the use of Efaproxiral, a noncytotoxic radiosensitizer, as an adjuvant to WBRT in 515 patients with multiple brain metastases. Although overall survival times were not significantly different between groups who did or did not receive Efaproxiral, patients in the breast cancer subset who received the radiosensitizer showed a 13% improved response rate ($p = 0.01$) and survived longer.

Dose fractionation

Various dose fraction schemes have been examined in the literature. The criteria for defining the best dose fraction regimen include: (1) high initial response rate, (2) short hospital stay, (3) long duration of response, and (4) minimal radiation-induced complications. The best fractionation regimen gives optimal results for all four criteria. Survival is at best a crude measure of the effectiveness of WBRT because 50–75% of patients die from systemic disease and not from the brain metastases. The Radiation Therapy Oncology Group (RTOG) has performed many studies to determine the effectiveness of various treatment schedules. These studies have indicated that 30 Gy delivered in 10 fractions over 2 weeks resulted in a rate and length of palliation equivalent to more protracted and higher dose schedules (Borgelt et al 1980; Gelber et al 1981; Kurtz et al 1981). Use of ultra-rapid fractionation, with 10–12 Gy delivered in one or two doses, gave an equivalent rate of initial improvement, but this palliation lasted for a shorter length of time (Borgelt et al 1981). More recently, the RTOG has completed a randomized phase III study comparing the results of accelerated hyperfractionation with those from the standard dose scheme (30 Gy in 10 days) (Murray et al 1997). Patients with unresected brain metastases were treated either with 32 Gy in 20 fractions over 10 treatment days (1.6 Gy twice daily) followed by a boost of 22.4 Gy in 14 fractions (total of 54.4 Gy) or with the standard regimen. Because this randomized comparison was unable to demonstrate any improvement in survival relative to the standard treatment schedule, most cancer centers continue to treat brain metastasis patients with 30 Gy in 10 fractions.

Prophylactic cranial irradiation

As previously discussed, lung cancers having adenocarcinoma and small cell histologies tend to metastasize to the brain quite often and quite early in the disease course. Because lung cancer patients who develop clinically evident brain metastases undoubtedly had the first seeding occur some time earlier, it has been proposed that many patients may already have had early seeding of the brain at the time of detection of the primary cancer. Micrometastatic seeds of <1–3 mm in diameter are not detectable by CT or MR imaging. Additionally, radiation therapy is most effective against smaller tumors. These facts have been used to justify the use of prophylactic cranial irradiation (PCI), in which the brain is irradiated soon after the initial diagnosis of lung cancer, before any evidence of brain metastasis develops. PCI has been used most commonly for small cell lung cancer but has also been used for lung adenocarcinoma. In theory, small undetectable lesions are destroyed, and the patient is spared the pain and short life expectancy accompanying the development of brain metastases. Both quality and length of life should be increased, but the results have been mixed.

Many studies of the role of PCI in patients with lung cancer have shown that the incidence of brain metastases is indeed lower with the use of PCI (Cox & Komaki 1986; Jacobs et al 1987; Kristjansen & Pedersen 1989; Lishner et al 1990; Rosenstein et al 1992; Rusch et al 1989; Russell et al 1991). One study demonstrated a statistically significant increase in life span with PCI (Rosenstein et al 1992), but the authors examined a patient group with only limited stage small cell lung cancer, patients in whom prevention of brain metastasis would be expected to play a more important role than in patients with advanced stage disease. Significant neurotoxicity has been reported in patients receiving PCI (Fleck et al 1990; Johnson et al 1990; Laukkanen et al 1988). The concurrent use of chemotherapy with PCI is likely to result in substantially increased neurotoxicity (Turrisi 1990); however, delaying PCI until after delivery of systemic chemotherapy may reduce its effectiveness (Lee et al 1987).

The Prophylactic Cranial Irradiation Overview Collaboration Group reported a meta-analysis in which data on 987 patients having SCLC in complete remission were collected in seven trials that randomized patients to receive PCI or no PCI (Auperin et al 1999). The main endpoint of the study was survival. The risk of death in the treatment group relative to the control group was 0.84 ($p = 0.01$), corresponding to a 5.4 percent increase in the rate of survival at 3 years (15.3% in the control group vs 20.7% in the treatment group). PCI also decreased the relative risk (RR) of recurrence or death to 0.75 ($p < 0.001$) and decreased the cumulative incidence of brain metastasis RR to 0.46 ($p < 0.001$). Larger doses of radiation led to greater decreases in the risk of brain metastasis, according to an analysis of four total doses (8 Gy, 24–25 Gy, 30 Gy, and 36–40 Gy) (p for trend = 0.02), but the effect on survival did not differ significantly according to the dose. Critics of PCI point to the neurocognitive impairment seen in patients who have undergone PCI. Yet, the two largest trials in this meta-analysis used neuropsychological tests to evaluate most patients before, during, and after treatment, and neurocognitive impairment was often detected at initial diagnosis, but no deterioration was found after PCI (Arriagada et al 1995; Gregor et al 1997). This meta-analysis makes a strong case for including PCI as standard treatment for all patients who have SCLC in complete remission.

To minimize neurological toxicity, PCI should not be given concurrently with chemotherapy (Carney 1999). Although the optimal sequencing and dose of PCI to maximize reduction in the incidence of brain metastases while minimizing toxicity has not yet been determined, there is some indication that 30–36 Gy in 2–3 Gy per fraction or a biologically equivalent dose may produce a better outcome than a lower dose or less aggressive fractionation regimen (Suwinski et al 1998).

Recently, a multicenter phase III randomized trial (EORTC 09993–22993) determined that in patients with extensive SCLC and any response to prior chemotherapy, PCI significantly reduces the risk of brain metastasis and doubles the 1-year survival rate (Slotman et al 2007). After undergoing 4–6 cycles of chemotherapy that induced a response of their SCLC, 286 patients were randomized to either receive PCI ($n = 143$) or to be observed ($n = 143$). The cumulative risk of brain metastases within 1 year was 14.6% in the irradiation group (95% CI, 8.3–20.9) and 40.4% in the control group (95% CI, 32.1–48.6; $p < 0.001$). Moreover, 27.1% of the patients receiving PCI were alive after 1 year, compared with 13.3% of the patients not undergoing PCI. Cranial irradiation was generally well tolerated, and side effects did not significantly influence patients' self-assessment of their global health status. These results bolster support for the extension of PCI to the management of patients with widespread SCLC, in addition to those with more limited disease.

Complications

Despite its noninvasive character, WBRT is not a treatment modality that is completely free of morbidity. Complications from radiation therapy are classified as acute or late, depending on the onset interval after therapy. These complications are generally a function of the total dose used, the size of the fractions, and the total time over which radiation is administered.

Side effects occurring immediately are referred to as acute and include dry desquamation, hair loss, headaches, nausea, lethargy, otitis media, and brain edema leading to increased ICP. A 'somnolence syndrome' of increased fatigue can also appear 1–4 months after treatment. These symptoms are generally transient; however, complications such as dermatitis, alopecia, and otitis media have been known to persist for months after irradiation.

Because very few patients treated with WBRT alone survive for longer than 1 year, long-term radiation effects are not a very important consideration for them. Yet, patients undergoing surgery for brain metastases often survive significantly longer than 1 year. Late effects can be far more serious than acute complications. There have been numerous reports of serious, debilitating side effects, including radiation necrosis, atrophy, leukoencephalopathy, and neurological deterioration with dementia (DeAngelis et al 1989b; DeAngelis et al 1989c; Lee et al 1986; Sundaresan et al 1981; Sundaresan & Galicich 1985).

One report indicated that 11% of 1-year survivors developed severe radiation-induced dementia (DeAngelis et al 1989b), whereas another indicated that 50% of 2-year survivors were so affected (Sundaresan & Galicich 1985). Nevertheless, Patchell and Regine (2003) have suggested that the frequency of long-term neuropsychological side effects of WBRT in adult brain metastasis patients may have been overestimated. Although five of 47 patients (11%) in the study by DeAngelis et al (1989b) experienced dementia 1 year after WBRT for nonrecurrent brain metastases, all five received either abnormally high daily radiation fractions (3–6 Gy) not currently in use, or were given cell radiation-sensitizing agents, potentially increasing damage to normal tissue. Yet, none of the 15 patients who were treated with more modern fractionation schemes (<3 Gy per fraction) had dementia at 1 year. Moreover, Langer and Mehta (2005) have recently shown that the risk of neurological decline induced by recurrent disease outweighs the potential long-term effects of WBRT regarding loss of neurocognitive function after WBRT.

Certain factors such as increased dose per fraction, increased total dose, reirradiation, and concurrent use of chemotherapy are associated with increased development of late radiation-induced complications. Because neurocognitive decline remains a possible complication of WBRT, it may be reasonable to consider administering WBRT in daily fractions of 1.8–2 Gy to a total of 40–45 Gy in order to reduce long-term sequelae in patients with a more favorable prognosis.

Surgery

Surgical excision has been performed in patients with brain metastases, since the turn of the twentieth century. Results were often discouraging owing to the crude techniques available at the time for localization and surgical removal. Some early neurosurgeons, such as Grant (1926), felt that surgery was not warranted in patients with brain metastases because of extensive operative mortality and morbidity and poor postoperative survival. With improvement in imaging and localization techniques and operative procedures, complication rates have fallen dramatically and survival times have risen. Currently, surgery is accepted as an important part of the management of select patients with brain metastases. Results of retrospective studies (and four prospective randomized studies) on such patients treated surgically are presented in Table 45.6. Series examining heterogeneous groups of patients now report median survival times of 10–20 months (Bindal et al 1996; Bindal et al 1993; Ferrara et al 1990; Patchell et al 1990; Patchell et al 1998; Pieper et al 1997; Sundaresan & Galicich 1985).

The rationale behind surgical excision is simple. Complete excision of a tumor immediately eliminates the effects of increased ICP and the direct irritation that these tumors cause, providing a large degree of palliation. If all tumor cells can be removed in a patient with a solitary brain metastasis, the possibility of a complete cure exists. This is admittedly a rare occurrence as microscopic metastases are often present, either systemically or in the brain. Even so, in a patient with limited systemic disease, elimination of the brain metastasis can significantly prolong survival. Diagnostic tissue is also obtained to confirm the diagnosis of metastasis. This is important because some patients with a clinical diagnosis of metastasis may in fact have nonmetastatic lesions.

Determination of whether or not a patient is a surgical candidate has already been discussed. It is obvious that a lesion in an inaccessible location cannot be surgically removed. What makes a lesion unresectable is, however, somewhat ill-defined. Lesions located in the brain stem fall into this category, but cases of successful operation on selected patients with such lesions have been reported

Table 45.6 Results of surgical treatment of patients with brain metastases

Investigators	Tumor histology	Patients (n)	Postoperative mortality (%)	Median survival time (months)	1-year survival (%)
Lang & Slater (1964)	Mixed	208	22	4	20
Vieth & Odom (1965)	Mixed	155	15	<6	14
Haar & Patterson (1972)	Mixed	167	11	<6	22
White et al (1981)	Mixed	122	6	7	30
Sundaresan & Galicich (1985)	Mixed	125	6	12	50
Ferrara et al (1990)	Mixed	100	6	13	>50
Patchell et al (1990)	Mixed	23[a]	NS	40 weeks	NS
Vecht et al (1993)	Mixed	63[a]	NS	12	NS
Bindal et al (1993)	Mixed	30[b]	3	6	23
		26[c]	4	14	55
Bindal et al (1995)	Mixed	48[d]	0	12[e]	NS
Bindal et al (1996)	Mixed	62	0	16.4	58
Mintz et al (1996)	Mixed	41[a]	NS	5.6	12.2
Patchell et al (1998)	Mixed	95[a]	NS	48 weeks	NS
O'Neill et al (2003)	Mixed	74	NS	NS	62
Burt et al (1992)	Lung	185	3	14	55
Wronski et al (1995)	Lung	231	3	11	46
Koutras et al (2003)	NSCLC	32	NS	17	53
Oredsson et al (1990)	Melanoma	40	18	8	NS
Stevens et al (1992)	Melanoma	45	NS	9	NS
Wronski & Arbit (2000)	Melanoma	91	NS	6.7	36.3
Wronski et al (1996)	Renal	50	10	12.6	51
Badalament et al (1990)	Renal	22	9	21	NS
Wronski et al (1997a)	Breast	70	NS	16.2	53
Pieper et al (1997)	Breast	63	5	16	62
Wronski & Arbit (1999)	Colon	73	4	8.3	31.5

[a]Prospective, randomized study. [b]Patients had multiple brain metastases, some lesions remaining after surgery (see text). [c]Patients had multiple brain metastases, all lesions surgically removed. [d]Surgery for recurrent metastases. [e]From time of reoperation.
NS, not stated; NSCLC, non-small cell lung carcinoma.

(Tobler et al 1986). Lesions located deep within the brain parenchyma have also traditionally been considered unresectable, but with the use of intraoperative ultrasound and stereotactic approaches, these lesions are now accessible (Kelly et al 1988; Rubin & Chandler 1990) (Fig. 45.7). Other lesions considered inaccessible include those located in the internal capsule, thalamus, and basal ganglia; however, each lesion must be considered individually, and few generalizations can be made. Ultimately, the level of risk of postoperative morbidity a patient is willing to accept is of utmost importance in determining resectability. The location of an accessible lesion is important with respect to potential postoperative deficits or complications. Lesions located in or near the motor cortex and Broca's area require particular care for obvious reasons. Lesions located in the visual cortex can produce temporary or permanent visual deficits. For all of these lesions, careful pre- and intraoperative localization is vital; techniques such as cortical mapping can be useful to minimize damage to vital areas (Landy & Egnor 1991).

Many authors have indicated that the presence of multiple lesions is a strong contraindication to surgery. This is despite the fact that no study prior to 1993 had ever specifically analyzed the role of surgery in the management of these patients. Bindal and coworkers (1993) retrospectively evaluated the results of surgery in patients with multiple lesions. This study indicated that surgery can play a very important role in managing these patients. In this study, 56 patients who underwent surgery for multiple brain metastases were analyzed. These patients were divided into two groups: those who had one or more lesions remaining after

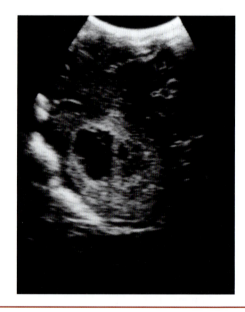

Figure 45.7 Intraoperative ultrasound image of a large metastatic lung carcinoma located 3 cm below the surface of the brain.

surgery (Group A, n = 30) and those who had all lesions removed (Group B, n = 26). Patients having all lesions removed were matched to a group of patients undergoing surgery for a single lesion (Group C, n = 26). The type of primary tumor, presence or absence of systemic disease, and time from first diagnosis of cancer to diagnosis of brain

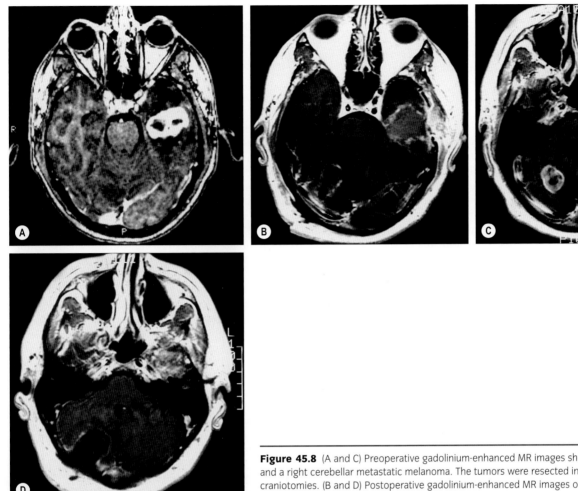

Figure 45.8 (A and C) Preoperative gadolinium-enhanced MR images showing a left temporal and a right cerebellar metastatic melanoma. The tumors were resected in two consecutive craniotomies. (B and D) Postoperative gadolinium-enhanced MR images of the same patient showing a gross-total resection of both tumors.

metastasis were matched. The median survival time was 6 months for patients in Group A, 14 months for those in Group B, and 14 months for those in Group C. There was a significant difference in survival between both Groups A and B and Groups A and C. Additionally, no difference was detected in recurrence or neurological improvement rates between Groups B and C. This study indicates that surgery for patients with multiple metastatic lesions is just as effective as surgery for a single lesion if all metastases can be removed (Fig. 45.8). Patients in whom all lesions cannot be surgically excised may also be surgical candidates in some circumstances. If a patient has one or two highly symptomatic, debilitating, or life-threatening lesions, resection of these lesions can produce greater and more rapid palliation of symptoms than might be achieved by radiation alone, and can possibly extend survival.

Prognostic factors

Certain prognostic factors have been identified in patients who are surgical candidates. These factors can be used to determine which patients might have a better or worse life expectancy after surgery. It must be stressed that patients who are otherwise considered surgical candidates will usually still survive longer than non-surgical candidates, regardless of unfavorable prognostic factors. Therefore,

patients who are otherwise considered surgical candidates should not be denied surgery for these reasons. Prognostic factors include status of systemic disease, extent of neurological deficit, length of time between the first diagnosis of cancer and the diagnosis of brain metastasis, location of the lesion, and type of primary tumor (Burt et al 1992; Galicich et al 1980; Sundaresan & Galicich 1985; White et al 1981; Winston et al 1980; Yardeni et al 1984). In addition, increasing age and male sex have been associated with reduced survival time in patients with brain metastases (Patchell et al 1990; White et al 1981; Winston et al 1980). Among these variables, the most important factors influencing survival are the status of the systemic cancer and the extent of neurological impairment.

The status of the systemic disease is important because most patients undergoing surgery for brain metastasis eventually succumb to the systemic disease, often without any recurrence of the brain metastasis. For this reason, patients with no systemic disease at the time of surgery are expected to survive considerably longer than patients with detectable cancer. Of course, even these patients often have microscopic systemic cancer that only becomes clinically evident at a later time. Patients with limited or no systemic cancer in whom the brain metastasis can be effectively controlled have a chance of becoming long-term survivors.

Extent of neurological deficit is also a strong indicator of postoperative survival. Studies that stratify patients in terms of extent of neurological deficit consistently show that increased neurological deficit is strongly associated with decreased postoperative survival (Gaspar et al 1997). The most important goal of surgery in patients with severe neurological deficits is palliation. Often, excision of a lesion can dramatically reduce symptoms and greatly improve the quality of life for these patients.

The time from first diagnosis of cancer to diagnosis of brain metastasis is also considered to be an important prognostic indicator. A short interval may be considered a rough indicator of the biological aggressiveness of the neoplastic cells. These tumors may have a greater predilection for overall metastasis or, perhaps, a greater affinity for the brain itself. Regardless of which factor is responsible, the prognosis is poorer than that of patients for whom this interval is longer. This indicator is not as important as the previous two factors, however, and it is most valuable when compared within a specific tumor histological category. When comparing latent interval and survival time among patients with varying primaries, the effect of tumor histology on survival can obscure results. For example, although melanoma has, on average, the longest time interval between diagnosis of the primary and diagnosis of brain metastases, patients with brain metastases from melanoma often have the poorest median expected survival time.

The location of the brain metastasis is also a potential prognostic indicator. Studies of large patient series sometimes give survival breakdowns between patients with supratentorial and infratentorial lesions. Patients with infratentorial lesions often survive for a shorter interval than those with supratentorial lesions. The reasons for this are not clear. Patients with cerebellar lesions are at increased risk for development of leptomeningeal carcinomatosis, and this may contribute to the poorer prognosis (DeAngelis et al 1989c; Kitaoka et al 1990; Suki et al 2008).

The type of primary tumor is also considered an indicator of survival. As Table 45.6 suggests, patients with melanoma have consistently poorer survival after surgery than do patients with other types of cancer. The fact that melanoma appears to have a very high propensity to spread to the brain may mean that these patients have a greater chance of harboring small, undetectable lesions at time of surgery. These lesions may become evident later, giving the appearance of a recurrence at a site distant to the site of surgery. The relative radioresistance of melanoma would make microscopic lesions less likely to be eradicated by postoperative WBRT. The very unpredictable course of melanoma also may result in a patient with apparently limited systemic disease developing widespread metastases soon after craniotomy. The few studies that report survival after surgical excision of brain metastases from kidney cancers suggest that the prognosis is relatively good for these patients. The effect of the histological nature of the primary tumor on survival is poorly defined, however, as very few studies contain sufficient numbers of patients to statistically examine differences in prognosis owing to this factor. Lang and Sawaya (1998) have summarized survival data from 46 brain metastasis surgery series in the post-CT era according to primary tumor type. They found that patients who had brain metastases from melanoma and colon cancer primaries experienced the shortest survival times, whereas those with metastatic lung, breast, and kidney carcinomas lived the longest.

Recurrence

Failure of surgical therapy for a brain metastasis presents in two different ways. The tumor may reappear in the site of a previous resection (local), new metastases may appear at a different site (distant), or patients may have both local and distant recurrences. Recurrence occurs in 30–40% of all patients undergoing surgery. Local recurrence occurs in 5–15% of patients, distant recurrence occurs in 10–20%, and 5–10% have both local and distant recurrence (Bindal et al 1993; Bindal et al 1995; Patchell et al 1990; Sundaresan & Galicich 1985). Local recurrence is usually caused by incomplete removal of all neoplastic cells during an operation. Although the goal of almost all modern operations is gross-total removal of tumor, sometimes residual tumor is left in the tumor bed owing to invasiveness of the tumor or its proximity to vital tissue such as eloquent brain or major blood vessels. This residual tumor may be detectable on immediate postoperative contrast CT or MR images; however, even if no visible tissue is left and the postoperative scan appears to indicate complete resection, microscopic amounts of tumor may remain. The use of postoperative radiation or chemotherapy may not eradicate these cells, which will survive and multiply to form a detectable local recurrence. Distant recurrences are caused by new seeding of the brain from the systemic neoplasm, from the release of neoplastic cells into the bloodstream during surgical excision, or from pre-existing undetected microscopic lesions that grow to detectable size.

Bindal and coworkers (1995) performed a retrospective study of outcomes for 48 patients with recurrent brain metastases who underwent surgery at The University of Texas MD Anderson Cancer Center (MD Anderson) between January 1984 and April 1993. They found neurological improvement in 75% of patients after surgery and observed no operative morbidity or mortality. The median survival time reported for patients after reoperation was 11.5 months, and 2- and 5-year survival rates were 26% and 17%, respectively. These results agree with those of an earlier study of reoperation for brain metastases (Sundaresan et al 1988) and suggest that reoperation for recurrent brain metastases can extend the survival and improve the quality of life of properly selected patients.

Postoperative WBRT

The role of postoperative WBRT as adjuvant treatment has not yet been clearly defined. Theoretically, postoperative WBRT is expected to destroy microscopic residual cancer cells at the site of resection and at other locations in the brain if they exist. This should reduce the recurrence rate, prolonging survival and sparing the patient the anguish of reoperation. Although most authors recommend postoperative WBRT, only five retrospective studies have specifically examined this issue (DeAngelis et al 1989c; Dosoretz et al 1980; Hagen et al 1990; Skibber et al 1996; Smalley et al 1987). Four of these studies have demonstrated that recurrence rate is, indeed, reduced by adjuvant WBRT (DeAngelis et al 1989c; Hagen et al 1990; Skibber et al 1996; Smalley et al 1987). Only two of these studies indicated that survival was also significantly extended for patients receiving WBRT (Skibber et al 1996; Smalley et al 1987). Both of these examined the results of WBRT on patients with no evidence of systemic disease. The patients in the study by Smalley et al were operated on between 1972 and 1982, and it is unclear whether all patients were evaluated with CT scanning. Without such evaluation, it is obvious that many patients suspected of having had single metastases would, in fact, harbor multiple lesions. In such patients there would be an obvious advantage to receiving adjuvant WBRT. The other three studies showed no increase in survival.

It is likely that adjuvant WBRT does, indeed, reduce the incidence of brain recurrence. Survival is not necessarily extended, however, because the status of the systemic disease is the most important indicator of survival in surgically treated patients. It is interesting to note that the only study that failed to detect any beneficial effect of WBRT (Dosoretz et al 1980), either in terms of reducing recurrence or extending survival, also examined patients with no evidence of systemic disease at the time of craniotomy. The most important argument against the routine use of postoperative WBRT involves the significant risk of radiation-induced dementia and other long-term neurotoxicity, as discussed in the section on complications from radiation therapy. One of the most important benefits of surgical excision of brain metastases is the significant chance some patients have of becoming long-term survivors. If these patients are neurologically crippled by WBRT given at the time of craniotomy, the value of surgery is greatly diminished.

Patchell and coworkers (1998) have reported the results of a randomized prospective trial examining the benefits of adjunctive WBRT in the surgical treatment of single brain metastases. After surgery, patients were randomly assigned to either observation or to treatment with 50.4 Gy over a 5.5-week interval, and patients were stratified according to extent of disease and primary tumor type. The patient group receiving WBRT showed a striking reduction in tumor recurrence relative to the observation group (18% vs 70%, respectively) and experienced less local recurrence at the surgical site as well. Nevertheless, the KPS scores for the patients undergoing WBRT declined at the same rate as for those in the surgery only (observation) group, raising the possibility that the toxicity of WBRT offsets its beneficial effects. In addition, overall patient survival was not improved by adjunctive WBRT. An unexplained result was that among patients who died from systemic disease, those not receiving WBRT survived longer, which may indicate an adverse effect of WBRT on the ability to survive systemic disease, either by altering the patients' immune response or lowering their Karnofsky performance. The authors concluded WBRT to be a valuable adjunct to neurological outcome and tumor control; yet, the lack of overall survival improvement, the use of higher than standard radiation doses (50 rather than 30 Gy), and the potential for radiation toxicity leave some unresolved concerns as to the best recommendations for treatment of patients with single brain metastases. At MD Anderson, there has been an evolving tendency to avoid WBRT after initial resection of a single brain metastasis,

based on the presumption that local or distant recurrences can be treated surgically or radiosurgically. WBRT is reserved for patients who develop multiple synchronous lesions that are too numerous to treat by the foregoing modalities.

Complications

Operative complications must always be considered in a discussion of surgical therapy. Operative mortality is most often defined as death within 30 days of operation. Causes of death in this time period are often related to: (1) herniation owing to edema and increased intracranial pressure, (2) hemorrhage at the operative site or in other metastatic foci, (3) uncontrolled systemic cancer, or (4) thromboembolic phenomena such as pulmonary embolism. Because death from uncontrolled systemic cancer is not related to events in the brain, the rate of postoperative mortality is not entirely due to the neurosurgical operation. Other, generally non-fatal complications include hematomas, wound infections, pseudomeningocele formation, and surgery-induced neurological impairment. Although these can potentially be quite serious, often they are transient events without long-term importance. Complications such as hematomas, infections, and pseudomeningocele formation occur in 8–9% of all patients undergoing craniotomies for brain metastasis (Bindal et al 1993). An estimated 10% of patients will develop clinically evident thromboembolic complications such as deep vein thrombosis or pulmonary embolism (Constantini et al 1991; Sawaya et al 1992).

Early neurosurgical studies conducted around the middle of the twentieth century reported very high rates of complications. The unsophisticated radiographic methods available and the limited ability to control brain herniation resulted in high operative mortality and morbidity rates that were a hallmark of surgery in that period. Mortality was generally in the 15–50% range (Horwitz & Rizzoli 1982). With the gradual introduction of advances such as the use of corticosteroids and modern anesthesia, the advent of CT and MR imaging, the use of the operating microscope, and the development of intraoperative ultrasonography, stereotactic localization, and cortical mapping, operative mortalities and morbidities have steadily declined (Cabantog & Bernstein 1994). Almost all studies of patients treated after the mid-1970s show an operative mortality of <10%. Recent studies often report an operative mortality rate of 3% or less. Surgical mortality has been reported to vary with the extent of removal of the brain metastasis. Investigators comparing results of gross-total removal and partial removal of brain metastases have reported that gross-total removal of a metastasis gives the lowest rate of operative mortality. Patients undergoing partial resection may have a doubled risk of 30-day mortality (Haar & Patterson 1972). Therefore, the goal of any operation should be gross-total tumor removal, whenever possible. Surgical morbidity is more difficult to quantify owing to the somewhat subjective nature of determination. Morbidity is defined as an increase in postoperative neurological deficits. Many studies indicate that morbidity is generally ≤5% (Bindal et al 1993; Brega et al 1990; Patchell et al 1990; Sundaresan & Galicich 1985). The average major neurological deficit rate reported within 30 days after surgery in a series of 194 patients undergoing resection of brain metastases at MD Anderson was 6%

(Sawaya 1999). It is important to distinguish between transient and permanent morbidity. Whereas transient morbidity can be considered to be a relatively unimportant factor, the same cannot be said of severe, permanent surgically-induced deficits.

Leptomeningeal disease (LMD) is a relatively rare but serious complication of metastatic brain disease. A recent study at MD Anderson considered whether 260 patients with brain metastases in the posterior fossa who underwent conventional resection were more at risk for LMD than those (119 patients) undergoing SRS (Suki et al 2008). Although there was no significant difference in the risk for LMD in patients undergoing en bloc tumor resection or SRS, piecemeal tumor resection (137 cases) was associated with a significantly higher risk of LMD than en bloc resection (123 cases, $p = 0.006$) or SRS ($p = 0.006$). A similar study at MD Anderson that focused on the impact of surgery on leptomeningeal dissemination of supratentorial metastases appears to show the same results of significantly increased risk of LMD with piecemeal resection relative to en bloc resection ($p = 0.009$) or SRS ($p < 0.001$) (Suki et al 2009). These studies represent the first time it has been shown that the way a brain tumor is resected can affect its dissemination, and they warrant further assessment of the role of resection for brain metastases in a controlled prospective setting.

Stereotactic radiosurgery

The technique of SRS was first developed in Sweden in 1951 by Leksell. It was originally used primarily to treat functional disorders of the brain by ablating specific sites. Since then, many other potential uses have been developed, especially for arteriovenous malformations, acoustic neuromas, and Cushing's disease. Other applications of SRS include treatment of primary and metastatic brain tumors. The radiosurgical system developed by Leksell has become known as the Gamma Knife. Subsequently, other radiosurgical systems have been developed, requiring a modification of the linear accelerator (LINAC).

SRS refers to the use of small, well-collimated beams of ionizing radiation to ablate intracranial lesions. All stereotactic systems have the ability: (1) to accurately locate and immobilize an intracranial target in three-dimensional space, (2) to produce sharply collimated beams of radiation with a steep dose gradient at the beam edge, and (3) to target the beams accurately, minimizing radiation exposure to surrounding brain tissue. The radiation dose is usually delivered in a single fraction. Hypofractionation has a more lethal effect on tissue than is possible by delivery of the same dose of radiation in many fractions. The use of numerous beams of radiation converging on the target site results in a high dose of radiation delivery to the tumor site. This dose falls rapidly away from the target in a ratio dependent on the size of the target. With a small target, surrounding brain tissue receives a smaller radiation dose than with a large target.

The main advantage of SRS with regard to brain metastasis lies primarily in its ability to treat lesions that are not amenable to surgical resection, and secondarily, in its non-invasive nature, with fewer attendant risks and a shorter hospital stay. Brain metastases are particularly well suited for treatment by SRS because: (1) metastases are often

spherical with margins showing contrast enhancement on CT or MR images; (2) they are generally small (<3 cm in diameter) when first detected; (3) normal brain parenchyma is circumferentially displaced by the lesion, reducing the chance of damaging normal brain tissue, and (4) brain metastases tend to be well demarcated and minimally invasive (Alexander & Loeffler 1992; Alexander et al 1995). Recurrent brain metastases and lesions located in unreachable regions of the brain are the ones that are often selected for radiosurgical procedures (Fig. 45.9).

A limitation of SRS is its inability to provide histological verification that a lesion identified radiologically is truly a metastasis. It is now known that from 4.3% to 11% of patients with verified systemic disease and a brain lesion radiographically consistent with a metastasis, actually have non-metastatic disease (Patchell et al 1990; Voorhies et al 1980). Another problem is that whereas traditional surgery removes

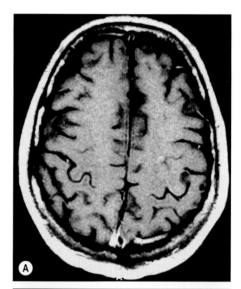

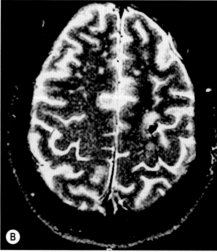

Figure 45.9 (A) A gadolinium-enhanced MR image of the patient shown in Figure 45.5, indicating a nearly complete eradication of the tumor two months after stereotactic radiosurgery. (B) A T2-weighted MR image of the patient shown in Figure 45.4, indicating the virtual disappearance of the zone of edema.

Table 45.7 Results of stereotactic radiosurgery in patients with brain metastases

Investigators	Radiation source	Lesions treated (n)/ tumor histology	Local control (%)	Median follow-up (months)	Median survival time (months)
Bindal et al (1996)	LINAC	31/mixed	61	6.5	7.5
Auchter et al (1996)	LINAC	122/mixed	86	28.4 (123 weeks)	13 (56 weeks)
Cho et al (1998)	LINAC	48/mixed	89	8	9.8
Gerosa et al (2002)	GK	1307/mixed	93	14[a]	13.5
Vesagas et al (2002)	GK	174/mixed	85	8.4	8.4
Andrews et al (2004)	GK/LINAC	269/mixed[b]	82	NS	6.5 (mean survival time)
Shehata et al (2004)	GK	468/mixed	97	7	8.2
Aoyama et al (2006)	NS	247/mixed	89 (no WBRT); 73 (w/WBRT)	7.8	8 (no WBRT); 7.5 (w/WBRT)
Muacevic et al (2008)	GK	31/mixed[c]	97	NS	10.3
Jawahar et al (2004)	GK	91/lung	72	18	7
Sheehan et al (2002)	GK	627/NSCLC	96	NS	10, adenocarcinoma; 7, not adenocarcinoma
Combs et al (2004)	LINAC	103/breast	9 months	NS	15
Muacevic et al (2004b)	GK	197/breast	94	8.3	10
Noel et al (2002)	LINAC	61/melanoma	84	12.6[a]	8
Herfarth et al (2003)	LINAC	122/melanoma	81 at 1 year	9.4[a]	10.6
Selek et al (2004)	LINAC	153/melanoma	49	6	25.2%[d]
Muacevic et al (2004a)	GK	376/RCC	94	NS	11.1
Noel et al (2004)	LINAC	65/RCC	93	14	11
Sheehan et al (2003)	GK	146/RCC	96	NS	15

[a]Mean follow-up time. [b]Patients were randomized to receive either WBRT plus an SRS boost or WBRT alone. [c]Patients were randomized to receive either SRS alone or resection plus WBRT. [d]Percent surviving at 1 year.
GK, Gamma Knife; LINAC, modified linear accelerator; NS, not stated; NSCLC, non-small cell lung carcinoma; RCC, renal cell carcinoma; SRS, stereotactic radiosurgery; WBRT, whole-brain radiation therapy.

a tumor in one stroke, with SRS there is a delay before its effects can reverse symptoms. Additionally, because brain metastases frequently cause significant amounts of edema, treatment with SRS may necessitate higher steroid doses for longer intervals than traditional surgery would, thus increasing the rate of steroid complications and dependence.

The results of SRS in patients with metastatic brain tumors are shown in Table 45.7. Median survival time is sometimes not reported, owing to the relatively short follow-up times given in many studies. The results presented indicate that SRS is definitely superior to WBRT alone in prolonging survival. Whether surgical resection or SRS is better at treating brain metastases that are ≤3 cm in maximum diameter, is still very controversial. To put this in perspective, we will review three retrospective studies and two prospective trials comparing SRS with conventional surgery for the treatment of single brain metastases.

In a multi-institutional retrospective study, Auchter and coworkers (1996) analyzed results for patients with single cerebral metastases who were treated with SRS plus WBRT, but who would have been eligible for surgical resection. From a database of 533 patients with brain metastases who were treated with SRS and WBRT, 122 patients were identified who met the criteria for surgical resection established in the earlier prospective randomized study of Patchell and coworkers (1990), including having a surgically resectable single brain metastasis, no prior surgical or radiation treatment, an age of no less than 18 years, independent functional status (KPS score ≥70), a non-radiosensitive tumor, and no urgent need for surgery. The outcome for these 122 patients was compared with that for the series of patients treated by surgery and WBRT in the randomized trials of Patchell and coworkers (1990) and Noordijk and coworkers (1994) (note: Noordijk et al reported the same study population and results as Vecht and coworkers 1993). For SRS plus

WBRT, the actuarial median survival was 56 weeks compared with 40 (Patchell et al 1990) and 43 weeks (Noordijk et al 1994), respectively, after surgery plus WBRT. Fewer local recurrences occurred in patients undergoing SRS plus WBRT (14%) than were seen in those treated with surgery and WBRT (20%) (Patchell et al 1990). Moreover, after SRS 'no treatment-related deaths or major acute toxicity' were reported (Auchter et al 1996). These results led the authors to conclude that SRS followed by WBRT was as good as, if not superior to, traditional surgery followed by WBRT.

Another retrospective study comparing the results of SRS with surgery, in matched sets of patients, was conducted at MD Anderson (Bindal et al 1996). Between August 1991 and March 1994, 31 consecutive patients with new brain metastases who were treated with SRS were retrospectively matched with 62 consecutive patients whose metastases were treated surgically. The two patient groups were matched with respect to age, sex, histological nature of primary tumor, extent of systemic disease, pretreatment KPS score, interval between diagnosis of primary tumor and brain metastasis, and number of brain metastases. The median survival period was 16.4 months for the surgically treated group and 7.5 months for the radiosurgical group, and the difference was statistically significant by both univariate ($p = 0.0041$) and multivariate ($p = 0.0009$) analyses. The local recurrence rate for surgically treated patients was 13%, whereas 39% of radiosurgically treated patients experienced local progression. Similarly, the complication rate was lower in the surgical group (5%), than in the radiosurgical group (23%). Based on these results, in contrast to the conclusions of Auchter and coworkers (1996), Bindal et al (1996) concluded that surgery was superior to SRS in clinically similar patients in terms of survival, local recurrence, and morbidity. They thus favored using surgery instead of SRS for treatment of single brain metastases.

In a third study of this type, Cho and coworkers (1998) described a series of 225 patients with single brain metastases who were treated with either WBRT alone, SRS followed by WBRT, or surgery plus WBRT. All three patient groups had similar distributions for prognostic factors such as age, sex, location of metastasis, and KPS score; however, there was more extracranial disease in the group undergoing SRS plus WBRT than in the surgically treated group. Both the radiosurgical and surgical groups had the same actuarial median survival time, and patients in both groups survived substantially longer than patients receiving WBRT alone. These authors concluded that 'given that stereotactic radiosurgery is minimally invasive, is able to treat lesions in surgically inaccessible locations, and is potentially more cost-effective than surgery, it is a reasonable and potentially more attractive alternative than surgery in the management of single brain metastases' (Cho et al 1998).

Recently, Muacevic et al (2008) compared surgery plus WBRT with SRS alone in a randomized prospective study (Table 45.7) that treated patients with single small brain metastases (≤ 3 cm in maximum diameter). Owing to poor patient accrual, there were only 33 patients in the surgery group and 31 patients in the SRS group. No significant differences were found between the two groups with respect to patient survival interval, neurological death rate, or freedom from local tumor recurrence; however, patients undergoing SRS experienced significantly more distant tumor recurrences than those in the surgery group. Patients in the surgery plus WBRT group experienced significantly more early or late grade 1 or 2 complications than those in the SRS group. The authors concluded that SRS alone is as effective as surgery plus WBRT in controlling local tumor recurrence but that SRS salvage treatment may be necessary to curb distant recurrence in the absence of adjuvant WBRT.

An additional prospective study with both randomized and nonrandomized arms that compared patients treated for single brain metastases with either conventional surgery or SRS has been completed at MD Anderson (Lang et al 2008). In the randomized arm, 30 patients received surgical resection and 29, SRS. In the nonrandomized arm, 89 patients chose surgery and 66 chose SRS. In the nonrandomized cohort, follow-up of patients who were eligible for randomization was identical to that in the randomized arm. It was possible to compare tumor recurrence rates (but not overall survival times) using multivariate analyses that took into account both randomized and nonrandomized groups (and compensated for confounding covariates: age, sex, WBRT treatment, primary tumor type, extent of disease, tumor volume and location, KPS score, and RPA class). Contrary to the findings of Muacevic et al (2008), the analyses showed that patients receiving SRS experienced significantly more local recurrences than those undergoing conventional surgery and found no differences in distant recurrence between the two groups.

Although there is still much debate over the relative advantages and disadvantages of surgery and SRS in treating brain metastases, at MD Anderson we base our decision on which modality to recommend according to the size and location of the metastasis and its clinical presentation. Tumors that are >3 cm in maximum diameter are almost always surgically resected, whereas small lesions (<1–2 cm

in maximum diameter) that are deeply located are treated with SRS. The patient's symptoms dictate the treatment for lesions amenable to either therapy. Asymptomatic patients may be treated with SRS, whereas surgery is more often used for lesions that cause symptoms. This approach may be modified, depending on the patient's medical condition or his systemic disease status.

Stereotactic radiosurgery plus WBRT

The use of WBRT as an adjuvant to SRS is controversial. A primary reason for the use of SRS alone to treat brain metastases is to avoid the neurocognitive side effects of WBRT. Several single-institution retrospective reviews of patients with newly diagnosed brain metastases managed initially with SRS alone have noted an increased risk of failure of intracranial tumor control compared with patients receiving SRS plus WBRT (Chidel et al 2000; Sneed et al 1999; Sneed et al 2002). In contrast, a retrospective study by Hasegawa and colleagues (2003) of 121 patients with brain metastases managed with SRS alone showed a local tumor control rate of 87%. The authors concluded that SRS alone as initial therapy had controlled brain metastases well enough that WBRT was unnecessary in the initial treatment of selected patients with one or two tumors and controlled primary cancer. This conclusion was supported by other retrospective studies (Chidel et al 2000; Joseph et al 1996; Pirzkall et al 1998; Sneed et al 1999). Moreover, a retrospective, multi-institutional study in which 268 patients were treated with SRS alone and 301 patients received WBRT in addition to SRS showed no significant difference in survival rate (Sneed et al 2002).

In a prospective controlled trial (RTOG 95–08), patients with no more than three unresected brain metastases were randomized to treatment with WBRT alone ($n = 164$) or WBRT with an SRS boost ($n = 167$) (Andrews et al 2004). Patients were stratified according to the number of brain metastases and the status of their extracranial cancer. The overall survival times were similar in both treatment arms. Univariate analysis showed a survival advantage for patients with a single brain metastasis who received the SRS boost (6.5 months) relative to those who did not (4.9 months; $p = 0.039$). Patients in the SRS arm of the study had better KPS scores at the 6-month follow-up visit than those not receiving SRS. Multivariate analysis of the two study arms showed that survival improved in patients receiving the SRS boost who had RPA class 1 status ($p < 0.0001$) or a favorable histological tumor type ($p = 0.0121$).

In a more recent phase III study by Aoyama et al (2006), 132 patients with 1–4 brain metastases (<3 cm in maximum diameter) were treated with either SRS alone ($n = 67$) or SRS plus WBRT ($n = 65$). Although the addition of WBRT to SRS did not increase survival time, it significantly reduced the number of recurrent brain metastases. No gross neurologic or neurocognitive functional differences were observed by omitting WBRT. Yet, these workers concluded that as long as the patient's brain tumor status is frequently monitored, WBRT is not necessary and could be safely omitted.

Subsequently, Patchell et al (2006a,b) noted that exactly the opposite conclusion could be drawn from this study. Although Aoyama et al (2006) indicated that the main reason for omitting WBRT was to avoid adverse long-term neuro-toxic effects, they had actually found no differences between patients treated with or without WBRT in terms of neurological or neurocognitive functioning, radiation-induced adverse effects, or survival times. Thus, their study really offered strong support for using WBRT as an up-front treatment for brain metastases, as WBRT appeared to significantly reduce the number of recurrent brain metastases without demonstrable neurotoxic effects. Moreover, Patchell et al (2006b) showed that the study by Aoyama et al (2006) was statistically underpowered to demonstrate a meaningful survival benefit of WBRT + SRS over SRS alone, or even whether these treatments were equivalent.

Thus, although some retrospective and prospective randomized studies suggest that WBRT will improve tumor control in the brain, they do not demonstrate a survival advantage. Better assessment of survival and freedom from brain tumor progression in patients with brain metastases awaits additional prospective randomized trials comparing the use of SRS with and without WBRT.

Prognostic factors

The histological nature, size, and invasiveness of the metastatic lesion are the most important factors in determining the success of SRS in controlling it. Earlier studies suggested that the response of a lesion to SRS depended on the radiosensitivity of the tumor, with melanoma responding least well and germ cell tumors demonstrating excellent response (Alexander & Loeffler 1992). Yet, more recent studies that have included larger sample sizes indicate that SRS is effective against metastases from tumors resistant to conventional radiation therapy, including melanoma (Alexander et al 1995; Alexander & Loeffler 1996). This result may be a consequence of the small size of the metastases that are typically treated with SRS. Generally, lesions that are ≤3 cm in diameter (volume ≤10–12 cm³) are considered the best radiosurgical targets (Kondziolka & Lunsford 1993; Sturm et al 1991), and the intense concentration of radiation beams focused on such a small target is apparently sufficient to overcome radioresistance. Size is important in that large metastases cannot be treated very safely because a greater zone of normal brain tissue surrounding the lesion will receive a potentially toxic amount of radiation. Invasiveness of tumors is important because tumor cells located beyond the sphere of treatment will receive a significantly lower dose of radiation and may survive. These cells might continue to grow into a new lesion located just peripherally to the site of treatment. This has been reported in some studies (Alexander & Loeffler 1992). Improvement in technique will probably reduce the rate of peritumoral growth.

Recurrence

Radiosurgical studies generally report a rate of local control of 85–95% at 1 year, a level that exceeds the 80% local control rate expected with surgical excision. In truth, these figures are difficult to compare because recurrence is a function of the length of follow-up of a patient. Many SRS studies have very limited follow-up times. Most studies report that the majority of deaths in these patients are the result of systemic disease or distant brain recurrence and are not due to local failure of treatment. It is important to remember that

local control for SRS is defined as complete elimination, shrinkage, or stabilization of a tumor, whereas for surgery, local control is defined as complete elimination without local recurrence of any kind at any time in the patient's life. For SRS, failure of local control is defined as continued growth of a lesion at any time in the patient's life (Fig. 45.10). Often, tumor shrinkage continues over a period of months after the treatment date, as dead tumor cells continue to be removed from the treated lesion. In SRS studies that have sufficient follow-up periods, the actual local control rate is in the 62–65% range.

Complications

Most studies evaluating the outcomes of patients treated with SRS for metastatic brain disease focus on treatment efficacy, with few mentioning treatment-related complications. A study by Nedzi and coworkers (1991) identified variables associated with the development of significant complications. A total of 40 primary and 24 metastatic tumors were treated, and complications were associated with increases in the following five variables: (1) tumor dose inhomogeneity, (2) maximum tumor dose, (3) number of isocenters, (4) maximum normal tissue dose, and (5) tumor volume. It is interesting to note, however, that not a single patient with a metastatic tumor developed significant complications. This is probably because metastatic tumors generally are small and homogeneously treated with only one isocenter per lesion.

Complications from SRS stem from the delivery of a high single fraction dose of radiation. By design, the large number of converging radiation beams result in normal brain tissue receiving only a limited amount of radiation that is well within the tolerable range. Nevertheless, brain parenchyma immediately surrounding the tumor may receive an excessive amount of radiation. This can result in chronic complications that may require long-term steroid administration or may include radiation necrosis, which sometimes requires reoperation (Kondziolka & Lunsford 1993; Sturm et al 1991; Vecil et al 2005). Radiation necrosis has been estimated to occur in 3% of patients. The percentage of patients developing necrosis may be underestimated because such necrosis is easily mistaken for recurrent tumor on CT or MR images. The risk of developing radiation necrosis is increased in patients with large metastases (>3 cm in diameter) and in patients who have previously received extensive WBRT (>40 Gy) (Adler et al 1992). The additional complications of nausea and vomiting have been noted in patients receiving a dose of over 275 cGy to the area postrema, and these patients should be treated with prophylactic antiemetics (Alexander et al 1989).

Williams and coworkers (2009) have conducted the largest study to date that specifically addresses complications of SRS for brain metastases. The series included 273 patients undergoing SRS for one or two brain metastases, with a total of 316 lesions treated. Whereas many studies reporting complications from SRS for brain metastases include patients who have undergone other treatments including WBRT (either prior to or concurrently with SRS), which may confound analysis of the impact of SRS on treatment-related complications, this study included no patients undergoing WBRT or resection prior to SRS. The

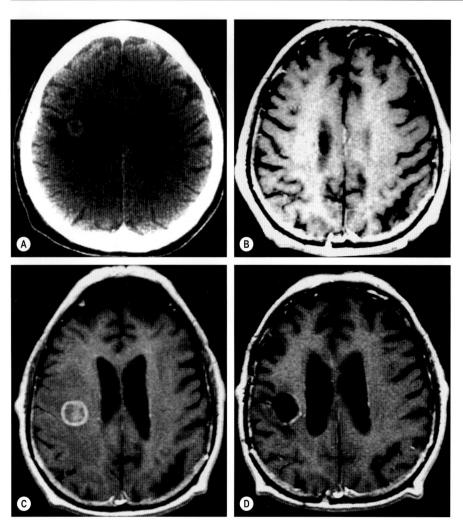

Figure 45.10 (A) A CT scan of the head showing a right subcortical metastatic lung carcinoma in a patient previously treated with whole-brain radiation therapy. (B) A gadolinium-enhanced MR image obtained 3 months after stereotactic radiosurgery showing marked reduction in the size of the tumor. (C) A gadolinium-enhanced MR image taken 5 months after stereotactic radiosurgery shows significant regrowth of the tumor. (D) A gadolinium-enhanced MR image taken 5 months after resection of the recurrent metastatic tumor shows no further recurrence.

authors reported a higher rate of complications (40% for new complications) than has generally been reported in the literature, with 14% of them noted as severe (RTOG ≥3). In the multivariate analysis, progressing primary cancer ($p < 0.001$), tumor location in eloquent cortex ($p < 0.001$), and lower (<15 Gy) SRS dose ($p = 0.04$) were significantly associated with new complications overall; moreover, new neurological complications were significantly associated with a tumor location in eloquent cortex ($p < 0.001$) and progressing primary cancer ($p = 0.03$). Thus, patients with lesions in brain regions controlling eloquent functions are at a significantly increased risk for SRS treatment-related complications, and both clinicians and patients should be aware of this possibility.

Chemotherapy

There are obvious theoretical advantages in the use of chemotherapy to treat patients with brain metastases. Chemotherapy can treat the whole brain, unlike surgery or SRS, which provide only focal treatment. Additionally, systemic sites of cancer can be concurrently treated. Unfortunately,

the value of chemotherapy in the management of these patients is limited. Many explanations have been offered for the apparent ineffectiveness of chemotherapy for brain metastases, including: (1) the presence of the blood–brain barrier, (2) the relatively drug-resistant nature of cancers that metastasize to the brain, (3) the fact that brain metastases frequently occur in patients in whom chemotherapy has failed, and (4) the fact that suboptimal chemotherapeutic agents were often used in past trials (Bernardo et al 2002; Buckner 1991; Greig 1984; Siegers 1990).

Most tumors with a known propensity to metastasize to the brain are not considered chemosensitive. The results of chemotherapy in these patients have been mixed (Cascino et al 1983a; Dvorak et al 2004; Lange et al 1990; Ushio et al 1991). Of all primary tumors known to metastasize to the brain in significant numbers, small cell lung, breast, and germ cell tumors are the only ones considered relatively chemosensitive. There is evidence that chemotherapy does, indeed, have significant effects on brain metastases from these cancers. Chemotherapy for brain metastases from germ cell tumors is considered standard therapy. Its effectiveness, either in conjunction with surgery and WBRT or as the sole treatment, has been well documented (Spears et al 1992). The effectiveness of chemotherapy on metastases of small cell lung and breast cancers is less well defined. Chemotherapy in these patients has been reported to give response rates for brain metastases that are very similar to those seen for systemic cancer in these patients (Boogerd et al 1992; Lange et al 1990; Rosner et al 1983; Seute et al 2006; Twelves et al 1990). This seems to indicate that the blood–brain barrier has minimal effect in complicating chemotherapy for brain metastasis. It has even been suggested that chemotherapy should be made standard treatment for patients developing brain metastases from small cell lung cancer (Twelves & Souhami 1991).

It has not been conclusively determined whether chemotherapy gives better results than could be obtained by WBRT alone or how useful chemotherapy is as an adjunct to WBRT. However, a phase III study of teniposide administration in SCLC patients treated with or without WBRT (Postmus et al 2000) showed a higher response rate of brain metastases and a longer time to progression in the WBRT cohort (although survival was poor and similar in both groups). Moreover, although the use of temozolomide as a single therapeutic agent produces a low response rate in treatment of brain metastases from different primary cancers (Abrey & Christodoulou 2001; Adonizio et al 2002; Agarwala et al 2004), the combination of temozolomide and WBRT has been shown to be synergistic (Antonadou et al 2002; Hofmann et al 2006; Verger et al 2005).

In these studies, despite the improvement seen in brain metastasis response rates with this combination therapy, there is little corresponding improvement in the survival of patients, because they generally succumb to progression of their systemic metastases. Until stronger evidence of the effectiveness of chemotherapeutic agents emerges, the role of chemotherapy will remain undefined, and its use in patients with brain metastases from cancers other than small cell lung and germ cell tumors must remain experimental.

Conclusion

The brain metastasis represents by far the most common type of intracranial tumor. Most patients develop such metastases in the setting of advanced systemic disease and require only palliative care. Nevertheless, the need to effectively treat brain metastases is becoming increasingly important as advances in the treatment of systemic disease result in an increasing number of patients developing brain metastases in the setting of limited systemic disease. For many such patients, surgery or SRS provide the best therapy, but results are still not encouraging as even patients with the best prognostic indicators often die within 18–24 months. Unfortunately, few therapies with more promise have appeared on the horizon. Until superior treatment modalities are developed, the judicious use of available techniques for treatment of patients with limited systemic disease provides the best opportunity for palliation and extended survival.

Acknowledgments

We thank David M. Wildrick, PhD, for reviewing this chapter.

Key points

- It is currently estimated that over 100 000 patients will develop brain metastases per year in the USA alone.

- Lung, breast, melanoma, renal, and colon cancers are responsible for most brain metastases.

- Brain metastases show enhancement on radiographs owing to their preferential uptake of contrast agents as a result of a defective blood–brain barrier. This disruption of the blood–brain barrier results in the often extensive edema surrounding metastases.

- The relative frequency of single or multiple brain metastases varies with the type of primary tumor. Melanoma has the highest tendency to produce multiple lesions, followed by lung and breast primaries. Patients with brain metastases from colon primaries present with multiple tumors 50% of the time, whereas those who have renal cancer usually present with only one lesion.

- The percentage of patients with multiple lesions as demonstrated on MR imaging is likely to be higher than is indicated by CT scans.

- Up to two-thirds of all brain metastases are symptomatic at some time during life. Symptoms have two main etiologies: increased intracranial pressure and focal irritation or destruction of neurons.

- Contrast-enhanced MR imaging is the single best tool for radiographic evaluation of patients with suspected brain metastasis. On T1 imaging, metastases appear as loci of increased signal intensity, whereas peritumoral edema appears as a region of decreased signal intensity. In T2 images, tumors often have decreased intensity whereas edema appears with increased intensity, allowing better appreciation of the presence and extent of edema.

- Some 89–93% of patients with a history of cancer who present with a single supratentorial lesion have a brain metastasis.

- A diagnosis of brain metastasis cannot be made with certainty unless the primary tumor or (other) systemic metastases are found and histologically confirmed or a biopsy of the brain lesion is performed.

- As a general rule, patients who are not expected to die from their systemic disease within 3–4 months are evaluated for more aggressive therapy because, in such individuals, treatment with WBRT and corticosteroids alone is unlikely to provide adequate palliation for the duration of the patient's life, and more aggressive therapy may also be able to prolong life significantly.

- Survival time of patients undergoing surgery for recurrent brain metastases has been shown to be negatively affected by the presence of systemic disease ($p = 0.008$), a KPS score of $\leq$70 ($p = 0.008$), a time to recurrence of <4 months ($p = 0.008$), being $\geq$40 years old ($p = 0.051$), and having a primary tumor type of breast cancer or melanoma ($p = 0.028$).

- Although survival cannot be significantly extended by the use of corticosteroids alone, they play an important part in reducing the often debilitating symptoms of brain metastasis.

- Whole-brain radiation therapy (WBRT) is the most widely used method for treating brain metastasis and is the method of choice for treating patients with advanced systemic disease, who constitute the majority of patients having metastatic brain tumors.

- Numerous reports of serious, debilitating side effects of WBRT have surfaced, including radiation necrosis, atrophy, leukoencephalopathy, and neurological deterioration with dementia, especially in patients who survive for longer than 1 year. Yet, the risk of neurological decline induced by recurrent disease may outweigh the potential long-term effects of WBRT on loss of neurocognitive function. For surgically treated patients with a good prognosis, a more protracted course using smaller doses per fraction is indicated, if WBRT is to be given at all.

- Surgery for patients with multiple metastatic lesions (up to three tumors) is just as effective as surgery for a single lesion, if all metastases can be removed.

- The most important factors influencing survival of patients with brain metastases are the status of the systemic disease and the extent of the neurological impairment.

- A randomized prospective trial considering the effects of adjunctive WBRT in the surgical treatment of single brain metastases has now shown that this adjunct significantly reduces recurrence but does not improve survival. At MD Anderson, WBRT is reserved for patients who develop multiple synchronous lesions that are too numerous to treat by surgery or stereotactic radiosurgery.

- To date, the literature on the respective roles of surgery and stereotactic radiosurgery for patients with single brain metastases that are amenable to either treatment primarily consists of retrospective studies that fail to provide definitive evidence favoring either treatment. Two recent prospective randomized trials comparing the two modalities with respect to such lesions have had poor patient accrual and have failed to show a survival advantage for either modality; however, in the absence of adjuvant WBRT, tumor recurrence rates appear to be higher with SRS than with surgical resection. At M.D. Anderson, the decision on which modality to recommend is based on the size and location of the metastasis and its clinical presentation.

REFERENCES

- **Abrams**, **H.L.**, **Spiro**, **R.**, **Goldstein**, **N.**, 1950. Metastases in carcinoma: analysis of 1000 autopsied cases. Cancer 3 (1), 74–385.

Abrey, **L.E.**, **Christodoulou**, **C.**, 2001. Temozolomide for treating brain metastases. Semin. Oncol. 28 (Suppl), 34–42.

Adler, **J.R.**, **Cox**, **R.S.**, **Kaplan**, **I.**, et al., 1992. Stereotactic radiosurgical treatment of brain metastases. J. Neurosurg. 76 (3), 444–449.

Adonizio, **C.S.**, **Babb**, **J.S.**, **Maiale**, **C.**, et al., 2002. Temozolomide in non-small-cell lung cancer: preliminary results of a phase II trial in previously treated patients. Clin. Lung Cancer 3 (4), 254–258.

- **Agarwala**, **S.S.**, **Kirkwood**, **J.M.**, **Gore**, **M.**, et al., 2004. Temozolomide for the treatment of brain metastases associated with metastatic melanoma: a phase II study. J. Clin. Oncol. 22 (11), 2101–2107.

Aiken, **R.**, **Leavengood**, **J.M.**, **Kim**, **J.H.**, et al., 1984. Metronidazole in the treatment of metastatic brain tumors. Results of a controlled clinical trial. J. Neurooncol. 2 (2), 105–111.

Alexander, **E. 3rd**, **Siddon**, **R.L.**, **Loeffler**, **J.S.**, 1989. The acute onset of nausea and vomiting following stereotactic radiosurgery: correlation with total dose to area postrema. Surg. Neurol. 32 (1), 40–44.

Alexander, **E. 3rd**, **Loeffler**, **J.S.**, 1992. Radiosurgery using a modified linear accelerator. Neurosurg. Clin. N. Am. 3 (1), 167–190.

- **Alexander**, **E. 3rd**, **Moriarty**, **T.M.**, **Davis**, **R.B.**, et al., 1995. Stereotactic radiosurgery for the definitive, noninvasive treatment of brain metastases. J. Natl. Cancer Inst. 87 (1), 34–40.

Alexander, **E. 3rd**, **Loeffler**, **J.S.**, 1996. Treatment of intracranial metastases: Surgery vs. radiosurgery. In: **Al-Mefty**, **O.**, **Origitano**, **T.C.**, **Harkey**, **H.L.** (Eds.), Controversies in Neurosurgery. Thieme, New York, pp. 49–54.

Allan, **S.**, **Cornbleet**, **M.**, 1990. Brain metastases in melanoma. In: **Rumke**, **P.** (Ed.), Therapy of advanced melanoma. Karger, Basel, pp. 36–52.

Amer, **M.H.**, **Al-Sarraf**, **M.**, **Baker**, **L.H.**, et al., 1978. Malignant melanoma and central nervous system metastases: incidence, diagnosis, treatment and survival. Cancer 42 (2), 660–668.

Amer, **M.H.**, **Al-Sarraf**, **M.**, **Vaitkevicius**, **V.K.**, 1979. Clinical presentation, natural history and prognostic factors in advanced malignant melanoma. Surg. Gynecol. Obstet. 149 (5), 687–692.

Anderson, **R.S.**, **el-Mahdi**, **A.M.**, **Kuban**, **D.A.**, et al., 1992. Brain metastases from transitional cell carcinoma of urinary bladder. Urology 39 (1), 17–20.

- **Andrews**, **D.W.**, **Scott**, **C.B.**, **Sperduto**, **P.W.**, et al., 2004. Whole brain radiation therapy with or without stereotactic radiosurgery boost for patients with one to three brain metastases: phase III results of the RTOG 9508 randomized trial. Lancet 363 (9422), 1665–1672.

Antonadou, **D.**, **Paraskevaidis**, **M.**, **Sarris**, **G.**, et al., 2002. Phase II randomized trial of temozolomide and concurrent radiotherapy in patients with brain metastases. J. Clin. Oncol. 20 (17), 3644–3650.

- **Aoyama**, **H.**, **Shirato**, **H.**, **Tago**, **M.**, et al., 2006. Stereotactic radiosurgery plus whole-brain radiation therapy vs stereotactic radiosurgery alone for treatment of brain metastases: a randomized controlled trial. JAMA 295 (21), 2483–2491.

Aronson, **S.M.**, **Garcia**, **J.H.**, **Aronson**, **B.E.**, 1964. Metastatic neoplasms of the brain: their frequency in relation to age. Cancer 17, 558–563.

Arriagada, **R.**, **Le Chevalier**, **T.**, **Borie**, **F.**, et al., 1995. Prophylactic cranial irradiation for patients with small-cell lung cancer in complete remission. J. Natl. Cancer Inst. 87 (3), 183–190.

Arseni, **C.**, **Constantinescu**, **A.I.**, 1975. Considerations on the metastatic tumours of the brain with reference to statistics of 1217 cases. Schweiz. Arch. Neurol. Psychiatry 117, 179–195.

Ask-Upmark, **E.**, 1956. Metastatic tumors of the brain and their localization. Acta Med. Scand. 154 (1), 1–9.

Atkinson, **L.**, 1978. Melanoma of the central nervous system. Aust. N Z J. Surg. 48 (1), 14–16.

Auchter, **R.M.**, **Lamond**, **J.P.**, **Alexander**, **E.**, et al., 1996. A multi-institutional outcome and prognostic factor analysis of radiosurgery for resectable single brain metastasis. Int. J. Radiat. Oncol. Biol. Phys. 35 (1), 27–35.

Auperin, **A.**, **Arriagada**, **R.**, **Pignon**, **J.P.**, et al., 1999. Prophylactic cranial irradiation for patients with small-cell lung cancer in complete remission. Prophylactic Cranial Irradiation Overview Collaborative Group. N. Engl. J. Med. 341 (7), 476–484.

Badalament, **R.A.**, **Gluck**, **R.W.**, **Wong**, **G.Y.**, et al., 1990. Surgical treatment of brain metastases from renal cell carcinoma. Urology 36 (2), 112–117.

Baker, **A.B.**, 1942. Metastatic tumors of the nervous system. Arch. Pathol. Lab. Med. 34, 495–537.

Baker, **G.S.**, **Kernohan**, **J.W.**, **Kiefer**, **E.J.**, 1951. Metastatic tumors of the brain. Surg. Clin. North Am. 31 (4), 1143–1145.

- **Barnholtz-Sloan**, **J.S.**, **Sloan**, **A.E.**, **Davis**, **F.G.**, et al., 2004. Incidence proportions of brain metastases in patients diagnosed (1973 to 2001) in the Metropolitan Detroit Cancer Surveillance System. J. Clin. Oncol. 22 (14), 2865–2872.

Batson, **O.**, 1942. The role of the vertebral veins in metastatic processes. Ann. Intern. Med. 16, 38–45.

Bernardo, **G.**, **Cuzzoni**, **Q.**, **Strada**, **M.R.**, et al., 2002. First-line chemotherapy with vinorelbine, gemcitabine, and carboplatin in the treatment of brain metastases from non-small-cell lung cancer: a phase II study. Cancer Invest. 20 (3), 293–302.

- **Bindal**, **A.K.**, **Bindal**, **R.K.**, **Hess**, **K.R.**, et al., 1996. Surgery versus radiosurgery in the treatment of brain metastasis. J. Neurosurg. 84 (5), 748–754.

- **Bindal**, **R.K.**, **Sawaya**, **R.**, **Leavens**, **M.E.**, et al., 1993. Surgical treatment of multiple brain metastases. J. Neurosurg. 79 (2), 210–216.

• Bindal, R.K., Sawaya, R., Leavens, M.E., et al., 1995. Reoperation for recurrent metastatic brain tumors. J. Neurosurg. 83 (4), 600–604.

Black, P., 1979. Brain metastasis: current status and recommended guidelines for management. Neurosurgery 5 (5), 617–631.

Bloch, J.L., Nieh, P.T., Walzak, M.P., 1987. Brain metastases from transitional cell carcinoma. J. Urol. 137 (1), 97–99.

Boogerd, W., Dalesio, O., Bais, E.M., et al., 1992. Response of brain metastases from breast cancer to systemic chemotherapy. Cancer 69 (4), 972–980.

Borgelt, B., Gelber, R., Kramer, S., et al., 1980. The palliation of brain metastases: final results of the first two studies by the Radiation Therapy Oncology Group. Int. J. Radiat. Oncol. Biol. Phys. 6 (1), 1–9.

Borgelt, B., Gelber, R., Larson, M., et al., 1981. Ultra-rapid high dose irradiation schedules for the palliation of brain metastases: final results of the first two studies by the Radiation Therapy Oncology Group. Int. J. Radiat. Oncol. Biol. Phys. 7 (12), 1633–1638.

Brega, K., Robinson, W.A., Winston, K., et al., 1990. Surgical treatment of brain metastases in malignant melanoma. Cancer 66 (10), 2105–2110.

Breneman, J.C., Sawaya, R., 1991. Cerebral radiation necrosis. In: Barrow, D. (Ed.), Perspectives in neurological surgery. Quality Medical, St Louis, MO, pp. 127–140.

Broadbent, A.M., Hruby, G., Tin, M.M., et al., 2004. Survival following whole brain radiation treatment for cerebral metastases: an audit of 474 patients. Radiother. Oncol. 71 (3), 259–265.

Buchsbaum, J.C., Suh, J.H., Lee, S.Y., et al., 2002. Survival by radiation therapy oncology group recursive partitioning analysis class and treatment modality in patients with brain metastases from malignant melanoma: a retrospective study. Cancer 94 (8), 2265–2272.

• Buckner, J., 1992. Surgery, radiation therapy, and chemotherapy for metastatic tumors to the brain. Curr. Opin. Oncol. 4 (3), 518–524.

Buckner, J.C., 1991. The role of chemotherapy in the treatment of patients with brain metastases from solid tumors. Cancer Metastasis. Rev. 10 (4), 335–341.

Burgess, R.E., Burgess, V.F., Dibella, N.J., 1979. Brain metastases in small cell carcinoma of the lung. JAMA 242 (19), 2084–2086.

Burt, M., Wronski, M., Arbit, E., et al., 1992. Resection of brain metastases from non-small-cell lung carcinoma. Results of therapy. Memorial Sloan-Kettering Cancer Center Thoracic Surgical Staff. J. Thorac. Cardiovasc. Surg. 103 (3), 399–410.

Cabantog, A.M., Bernstein, M., 1994. Complications of first craniotomy for intra-axial brain tumour. Can. J. Neurol. Sci. 21 (3), 213–218.

Cairncross, J.G., Kim, J.H., Posner, J.B., 1980. Radiation therapy for brain metastases. Ann. Neurol. 7 (6), 529–541.

Cairncross, J.G., Posner, J.B., 1983. The management of brain metastases. In: Walker, M.D., (Ed.), Oncology of the Nervous System. Martinus Nijhof, Boston, MA, pp. 341–377.

Cannady, S.B., Cavanaugh, K.A., Lee, S.Y., et al., 2004. Results of whole brain radiotherapy and recursive partitioning analysis in patients with brain metastases from renal cell carcinoma: a retrospective study. Int. J. Radiat. Oncol. Biol. Phys. 58 (1), 253–258.

Carney, D.N., 1999. Prophylactic cranial irradiation and small-cell lung cancer. N. Engl. J. Med. 341 (7), 524–526.

Cascino, T.L., Byrne, T.N., Deck, M.D., et al., 1983a. Intra-arterial BCNU in the treatment of metastatic brain tumors. J. Neurooncol. 1 (3), 211–218.

Cascino, T.L., Leavengood, J.M., Kemeny, N., et al., 1983b. Brain metastases from colon cancer. J. Neurooncol. 1 (3), 203–209.

Castaldo, J.E., Bernat, J.L., Meier, F.A., et al., 1983. Intracranial metastases due to prostatic carcinoma. Cancer 52 (9), 1739–1747.

Chang, D.B., Yang, P.C., Luh, K.T., et al., 1992. Late survival of non-small cell lung cancer patients with brain metastases. Influence of treatment. Chest 101 (5), 1293–1297.

Chao, J., Phillips, R., Nickson, J., 1954. Roentgen-ray therapy of cerebral metastases. Cancer 7 (4), 682–689.

Chason, J., Walker, F., Landers, J., 1963. Metastatic carcinoma in the central nervous system and dorsal root ganglia. Cancer 16, 781–787.

Chidel, M.A., Suh, J.H., Reddy, C.A., et al., 2000. Application of recursive partitioning analysis and evaluation of the use of whole brain radiation among patients treated with stereotactic radiosurgery for newly diagnosed brain metastases. Int. J. Radiat. Oncol. Biol. Phys. 47 (4), 993–999.

Cho, K.H., Hall, W.A., Lee, A.K., et al., 1998. Stereotactic radiosurgery for patients with single brain metastasis. J. Radiosurg. 1 (2), 79–85.

Choi, K.N., Withers, H.R., Rotman, M., 1985. Intracranial metastases from melanoma. Clinical features and treatment by accelerated fractionation. Cancer 56 (1), 1–9.

Christensen, E., 1949. Intracranial carcinomatous metastases in a neurosurgical clinic. Acta Psychiatr. Neurol. 24, 353–361.

Cifuentes, N., Pickren, J.W., 1979. Metastases from carcinoma of mammary gland: an autopsy study. J. Surg. Oncol. 11 (3), 193–205.

Combs, S.E., Schulz-Ertner, D., Thilmann, C., et al., 2004. Treatment of cerebral metastases from breast cancer with stereotactic radiosurgery. Strahlenther. Onkol. 180 (9), 590–596.

Constantini, S., Kornowski, R., Pomeranz, S., et al., 1991. Thromboembolic phenomena in neurosurgical patients operated upon for primary and metastatic brain tumors. Acta Neurochir. (Wien) 109 (3–4), 93–97.

Cox, J.D., Komaki, R., 1986. Prophylactic cranial irradiation for squamous cell carcinoma, large cell carcinoma, and adenocarcinoma of the lung: indications and techniques. In: Mountain, C.F., Carr, D.T. (Eds.), Lung cancer: current status and prospects for the future, vol. 28. Year Book Medical, Chicago, IL, pp. 233–237.

Cushing, H., 1932. Notes upon a series of two thousand verified cases with surgical-mortality percentages pertaining thereto. Charles C Thomas, Springfield, IL.

Dauplat, J., Nieberg, R.K., Hacker, N.F., 1987. Central nervous system metastases in epithelial ovarian carcinoma. Cancer 60 (10), 2559–2562.

Davis, P.C., Hudgins, P.A., Peterman, S.B., et al., 1991. Diagnosis of cerebral metastases: double-dose delayed CT vs contrast-enhanced MR imaging. AJNR Am. J. Neuroradiol. 12 (2), 293–300.

de la Monte, S.M., Moore, G.W., Hutchins, G.M., 1983. Patterned distribution of metastases from malignant melanoma in humans. Cancer Res. 43 (7), 3427–3433.

de la Monte, S.M., Hutchins, G.M., Moore, G.W., 1988. Influence of age on the metastatic behavior of breast carcinoma. Hum. Pathol. 19 (5), 529–534.

DeAngelis, L.M., Currie, V.E., Kim, J.H., et al., 1989a. The combined use of radiation therapy and lonidamine in the treatment of brain metastases. J. Neurooncol. 7 (3), 241–247.

• DeAngelis, L.M., Delattre, J.Y., Posner, J.B., 1989b. Radiation-induced dementia in patients cured of brain metastases. Neurology 39 (6), 789–796.

DeAngelis, L.M., Mandell, L.R., Thaler, H.T., et al., 1989c. The role of postoperative radiotherapy after resection of single brain metastases. Neurosurgery 24 (6), 798–805.

Debevec, M., 1990. Management of patients with brain metastases of unknown origin. Neoplasma 37 (5), 601–606.

Decker, D.A., Decker, V.L., Herskovic, A., et al., 1984. Brain metastases in patients with renal cell carcinoma: prognosis and treatment. J. Clin. Oncol. 2 (3), 169–173.

Delattre, J.Y., Krol, G., Thaler, H.T., et al., 1988. Distribution of brain metastases. Arch. Neurol. 45 (7), 741–744.

Dhopesh, V.P., Yagnik, P.M., 1985. Brain metastasis: analysis of patients without known cancer. South Med. J. 78 (2), 171–172.

DiStefano, A., Yong Yap, Y., Hortobagyi, G.N., et al., 1979. The natural history of breast cancer patients with brain metastases. Cancer 44 (5), 1913–1918.

Dosoretz, D.E., Blitzer, P.H., Russell, A.H., et al., 1980. Management of solitary metastasis to the brain: the role of elective brain irradiation following complete surgical resection. Int. J. Radiat. Oncol. Biol. Phys. 6 (12), 1727–1730.

Dvorak, J., Melichar, B., Zizka, J., et al., 2004. Complete response of multiple melanoma brain metastases after treatment with temozolomide. Onkologie. 27 (2), 171–174.

Eden, E.A., Muggia, J.M., Hiesiger, E.M., et al., 1990. Plasma carcinoembryonic antigen as an indicator of cerebral metastases. J. Neurooncol. 8 (3), 281–287.

Elkington, J.S., 1935. Metastatic tumors of the brain. Proc. R. Soc. Med. 28 (8), 1080–1096.

Ferrara, M., Bizzozzero, L., Talamonti, G., et al., 1990. Surgical treatment of 100 single brain metastases. Analysis of the results. J. Neurosurg. Sci. 34 (3–4), 303–308.

Fidler, I.J., 1989. Origin and biology of cancer metastasis. Cytometry 10 (6), 673–680.

Fidler, I.J., 1991. Cancer metastasis. Br. Med. Bull. 47 (1), 157–177.

• Fidler, I.J., 1997. Molecular biology of cancer: invasion and metastasis. In: DeVita, V.T. Jr., Hellman, S., Rosenberg, S.A. (Eds.), Cancer: principles and practice of oncology. JB Lippincott, Philadelphia, pp. 135–152.

Flaschka, G., Desoye, G., 1987. CEA plasma levels in patients with intracranial tumours. Neurochirurgia 30 (1), 5–7.

Fleck, J.F., Einhorn, L.H., Lauer, R.C., et al., 1990. Is prophylactic cranial irradiation indicated in small-cell lung cancer? J. Clin. Oncol. 8 (2), 209–214.

Fleckenstein, K., Hof, H., Lohr, F., et al., 2004. Prognostic factors for brain metastases after whole brain radiotherapy. Data from a single institution. Strahlenther. Onkol. 180 (5), 268–273.

Fogelholm, R., Uutela, T., Murros, K., 1984. Epidemiology of central nervous system neoplasms: a regional survey in central Finland. Acta Neurol. Scand. 69 (3), 129–136.

Galicich, J.H., Sundaresan, N., Arbit, E., et al., 1980. Surgical treatment of single brain metastasis: factors associated with survival. Cancer 45 (2), 381–386.

Galluzzi, S., Payne, P., 1956. Brain metastases from primary bronchial carcinoma: a statistical study of 741 necropsies. Cancer 10 (3), 408–414.

Gamache, F.W., Posner, J.B., Patterson, R.H., 1982. Metastatic brain tumors. In: Youmans, J. (Ed.), Neurological surgery, vol. 5. WB Saunders, Philadelphia, PA, pp. 2872–2898.

• Gaspar, L., Scott, C., Rotman, M., et al., 1997. Recursive partitioning analysis (RPA) of prognostic factors in three Radiation Therapy Oncology Group (RTOG) brain metastases trials. Int. J. Radiat. Oncol. Biol. Phys. 37 (4), 745–751.

Gay, P.C., Litchy, W.J., Cascino, T.L., 1987. Brain metastasis in hypernephroma. J. Neurooncol. 5 (1), 51–56.

Gelber, R.D., Larson, M., Borgelt, B.B., et al., 1981. Equivalence of radiation schedules for the palliative treatment of brain metastases in patients with favorable prognosis. Cancer 48 (8), 1749–1753.

Gerosa, M., Nicolato, A., Foroni, R., et al., 2002. Gamma knife radiosurgery for brain metastases: a primary therapeutic option. J. Neurosurg. 97 (Suppl.), 515–524.

Giannone, L., Johnson, D.H., Hande, K.R., et al., 1987. Favorable prognosis of brain metastases in small cell lung cancer. Ann. Intern. Med. 106 (3), 386–389.

Ginsberg, L.E., Lang, F.F., 1998. Neuroradiologic screening for brain metastases–can quadruple dose gadolinium be far behind? AJNR. Am. J. Neuroradiol. 19 (5), 829–830.

Gloeckler Ries, L.A., Reichman, M.E., Lewis, D.R., et al., 2003. Cancer survival and incidence from the Surveillance, Epidemiology, and End Results (SEER) program. Oncologist 8 (6), 541–552.

Graf, A.H., Buchberger, W., Langmayr, H., et al., 1988. Site preference of metastatic tumours of the brain. Virchows. Arch. 412 (5), 493–498.

Grant, F.C., 1926. Concerning intracranial malignant metastases: Their frequency and the value of surgery in their treatment. Ann. Surg. 84 (5), 635–646.

Graus, F., Walker, R.W., Allen, J.C., 1983. Brain metastases in children. J. Pediatr. 103 (4), 558–561.

Graus, F., Rogers, L., Posner, J., 1985. Cerebrovascular complications in patients with cancer. Medicine 64 (1), 16–35.

Gregor, A., Cull, A., Stephens, R.J., et al., 1997. Prophylactic cranial irradiation is indicated following complete response to induction therapy in small cell lung cancer: results of a multicentre randomised trial. United Kingdom Coordinating Committee for Cancer Research (UKCCCR) and the European Organization for Research and Treatment of Cancer (EORTC). Eur. J. Cancer 33 (11), 1752–1758.

Greig, N.H., 1984. Chemotherapy of brain metastases: current status. Cancer Treat Rev. 11 (2), 157–186.

Guerrieri, M., Wong, K., Ryan, G., et al., 2004. A randomised phase III study of palliative radiation with concomitant carboplatin for brain metastases from non-small cell carcinoma of the lung. Lung Cancer 46 (1), 107–111.

Guomundsson, K.R., 1970. A survey of tumors of the central nervous system in Iceland during the 10-year period 1954–1963. Acta Neurol. Scand. 46 (4), 538–552.

Haar, F., Patterson, R.H. Jr., 1972. Surgery for metastatic intracranial neoplasm. Cancer 30 (5), 1241–1245.

Hagen, N.A., Cirrincione, C., Thaler, H.T., et al., 1990. The role of radiation therapy following resection of single brain metastasis from melanoma. Neurology 40 (1), 158–160.

Hardy, J., Smith, I., Cherryman, G., et al., 1990. The value of computed tomographic (CT) scan surveillance in the detection and management of brain metastasis in patients with small lung cancer. Br. J. Cancer 62 (4), 684–686.

Hasegawa, H., Ushio, Y., Hayakawa, T., et al., 1983. Changes of the blood–brain barrier in experimental metastatic brain tumors. J. Neurosurg. 59 (2), 304–310.

Hasegawa, T., Kondziolka, D., Flickinger, J.C., et al., 2003. Brain metastases treated with radiosurgery alone: an alternative to whole brain radiotherapy? Neurosurgery 52 (6), 1318–1326.

Hazle, J.D., Jackson, E.F., Schomer, D.F., et al., 1997. Dynamic imaging of intracranial lesions using fast spin-echo imaging: differentiation of brain tumors and treatment effects. J. Magn. Reson. Imaging 7 (6), 1084–1093.

Healy, M.E., Hesselink, J.R., Press, G.A., et al., 1987. Increased detection of intracranial metastases with intravenous Gd-DTPA. Radiology 165 (3), 619–624.

Hendrickson, F.R., 1975. Radiation therapy of metastatic tumors. Semin. Oncol. 2 (1), 43–46.

Hendrickson, F.R., 1977. The optimum schedule for palliative radiotherapy for metastatic brain cancer. Int. J. Radiat. Oncol. Biol. Phys. 2, 165–168.

Henson, R.A., Urich, H., 1982. Cancer and the nervous system. Blackwell, London.

Herfarth, K.K., Izwekowa, O., Thilmann, C., et al., 2003. Linac-based radiosurgery of cerebral melanoma metastases. Analysis of 122 metastases treated in 64 patients. Strahlenther. Onkol. 179 (6), 366–371.

Hildebrand, J., 1973. Early diagnosis of brain metastases in an unselected population of cancerous patients. Eur. J. Cancer 9 (9), 621–626.

Hirsch, F.R., Paulson, O.B., Hansen, H.H., et al., 1982. Intracranial metastases in small cell carcinoma of the lung: correlation of clinical and autopsy findings. Cancer 50 (11), 2433–2437.

Hofmann, M., Kiecker, F., Wurm, R., et al., 2006. Temozolomide with or without radiotherapy in melanoma with unresectable brain metastases. J. Neurooncol. 76 (1), 59–64.

Horwitz, N.H., Rizzoli, H.V., 1982. Postoperative complications of intracranial neurological surgery. Williams & Wilkins, Baltimore, MD.

Jacobs, L., Kinkel, W.R., Vincent, R.G., 1977. 'Silent' brain metastasis from lung carcinoma determined by computerized tomography. Arch. Neurol. 34 (11), 690–693.

Jacobs, R.H., Awan, A., Bitran, J.D., et al., 1987. Prophylactic cranial irradiation in adenocarcinoma of the lung. A possible role. Cancer 59 (12), 2016–2019.

Jawahar, A., Matthew, R.E., Minagar, A., et al., 2004. Gamma knife surgery in the management of brain metastases from lung carcinoma: a retrospective analysis of survival, local tumor control, and freedom from new brain metastasis. J. Neurosurg. 100 (5), 842–847.

Jemal, A., Murray, T., Samuels, A., et al., 2003. Cancer statistics, 2003. CA Cancer J. Clin. 53 (1), 5–26.

Jemal, A., Tiwari, R.C., Murray, T., et al., 2004. Cancer statistics, 2004. CA Cancer J. Clin. 54 (1), 8–29.

Johnson, B.E., Patronas, N., Hayes, W., et al., 1990. Neurologic, computed cranial tomographic, and magnetic resonance imaging abnormalities in patients with small-cell lung cancer: further follow-up of 6- to 13-year survivors. J. Clin. Oncol. 8 (1), 48–56.

• Johnson, J.D., Young, B., 1996. Demographics of brain metastasis. Neurosurg. Clin. N. Am. 7 (3), 337–344.

Joseph, J., Adler, J.R., Cox, R.S., et al., 1996. Linear accelerator-based stereotaxic radiosurgery for brain metastases: the influence of number of lesions on survival. J. Clin. Oncol. 14 (4), 1085–1092.

Kamby, C., Soerensen, P.S., 1988. Characteristics of patients with short and long survivals after detection of intracranial metastases from breast cancer. J. Neurooncol. 6 (1), 37–45.

Kaye, A.H., 1992. Malignant brain tumors. In: Little, J.R., Awad, I.A. (Eds.), Reoperative neurosurgery. Williams & Wilkins, Baltimore, MD, pp. 49–76.

Kelly, P.J., Kall, B.A., Goerss, S.J., 1988. Results of computed tomography-based computer-assisted stereotactic resection of metastatic intracranial tumors. Neurosurgery 22 (1 Pt 1), 7–17.

Khansur, T., Routh, A., Hickman, B., 1997. Brain metastases from unknown primary site. J. Miss. State Med. Assoc. 38 (7), 238–242.

Kindt, G., 1964. The pattern of location of cerebral metastatic tumors. J. Neurosurg. 21, 54–57.

Kitaoka, K., Abe, H., Aida, T., et al., 1990. Follow-up study on metastatic cerebellar tumor surgery–characteristic problems of surgical treatment. Neurol. Med. Chir. (Tokyo) 30 (8), 591–598.

Klos, K.J., O'Neill, B.P., 2004. Brain metastases. Neurologist 10 (1), 31–46.

Knauth, M., Forsting, M., Hartmann, M., et al., 1996. MR enhancement of brain lesions: increased contrast dose compared with magnetization transfer. AJNR. Am. J. Neuroradiol. 17 (10), 1853–1859.

Koehler, P.J., 1995. Use of corticosteroids in neuro-oncology. Anti-Cancer Drugs 6 (1), 19–33.

Kofman, S., Garvin, J., Nagamani, D., et al., 1957. Treatment of cerebral metastases from breast carcinoma with prednisolone. JAMA 163 (16), 1473–1476.

Komarnicky, L.T., Phillips, T.L., Martz, K., et al., 1991. A randomized phase III protocol for the evaluation of misonidazole combined with radiation in the treatment of patients with brain metastases (RTOG-7916). Int. J. Radiat. Oncol. Biol. Phys. 20 (1), 53–58.

Kondziolka, D., Lunsford, L.D., 1993. Brain metastases. In: Apuzzo, M.L. (Ed.), Brain surgery: complication avoidance and management, Vol 1. Churchill Livingstone, New York, pp. 615–641.

Koutras, A.K., Marangos, M., Kourelis, T., et al., 2003. Surgical management of cerebral metastases from non-small cell lung cancer. Tumori. 89 (3), 292–297.

Kristjansen, P.E., Pedersen, A.G., 1989. CNS therapy in small-cell lung cancer. In: Hansen, H.H. (Ed.), Basic and clinical concepts of lung cancer. Kluwer Academic, Boston, MA, pp. 275–298.

Kurtz, J.M., Gelber, R., Brady, L.W., et al., 1981. The palliation of brain metastases in a favorable patient population: a randomized clinical trial by the Radiation Therapy Oncology Group. Int. J. Radiat. Oncol. Biol. Phys. 7 (7), 891–895.

Kurup, P., Reddy, S., Hendrickson, F.R., 1980. Results of re-irradiation for cerebral metastases. Cancer 46 (12), 2587–2589.

Landis, S.H., Murray, T., Bolden, S., et al., 1998. Cancer statistics, 1998. CA Cancer J. Clin. 48 (1), 6–29.

Landis, S.H., Murray, T., Bolden, S., et al., 1999. Cancer statistics, 1999. CA Cancer J. Clin. 49 (1), 9–31.

Landy, H.J., Egnor, M., 1991. Intraoperative ultrasonography and cortical mapping for removal of deep cerebral tumors. South Med. J. 84 (11), 1323–1326.

Lang, E.F., Slater, J., 1964. Metastatic brain tumors: results of surgical and nonsurgical treatment. Surg. Clin. North Am. 44, 865–872.

Lang, F.F., Sawaya, R., 1998. Surgical treatment of metastatic brain tumors. Semin. Surg. Oncol. 14 (1), 53–63.

Lang, F.F., Suki, D., Maor, M., et al., 2008. Conventional surgery versus stereotactic radiosurgery in the treatment of single brain metastases: a prospective study with both randomized and non-randomized arms. American Association of Neurological Surgeons Meeting, Article 48938.

Lange, O.F., Scheef, W., Haase, K.D., 1990. Palliative radio-chemotherapy with ifosfamide and BCNU for breast cancer patients with cerebral metastases. A 5-year experience. Cancer Chemother. Pharmacol. 26 (Suppl): S78–S80.

Langer, C.J., Mehta, M.P., 2005. Current management of brain metastases, with a focus on systemic options. J. Clin. Oncol. 23 (25), 6207–6219.

Lassman, A.B., DeAngelis, L.M., 2003. Brain metastases. Neurol. Clin. 21 (1), 1–23, vii.

Laukkanen, E., Klonoff, H., Allan, B., et al., 1988. The role of prophylactic brain irradiation in limited stage small cell lung cancer: clinical, neuropsychologic, and CT sequelae. Int. J. Radiat. Oncol. Biol. Phys. 14 (6), 1109–1117.

Le Chevalier, T., Smith, F.P., Caille, P., et al., 1985. Sites of primary malignancies in patients presenting with cerebral metastases. A review of 120 cases. Cancer 56 (4), 880–882.

Lee, J.S., Umsawasdi, T., Barkley, H.T. Jr., et al., 1987. Timing of elective brain irradiation: a critical factor for brain metastasis-free survival in small cell lung cancer. Int. J. Radiat. Oncol. Biol. Phys. 13 (5), 697–704.

Lee, Y.T., 1980. Malignant melanoma: pattern of metastasis. CA Cancer J. Clin. 30 (3), 137–142.

Lee, Y.T., 1983. Breast carcinoma: pattern of metastasis at autopsy. J. Surg. Oncol. 23 (3), 175–180.

Lee, Y.Y., Nauert, C., Glass, J.P., 1986. Treatment-related white matter changes in cancer patients. Cancer 57 (8), 1473–1482.

Leeds, N.E., Sawaya, R., Van Tassel, P., et al., 1992. Intracranial hemorrhage in the oncologic patient. Neuroimaging Clin. N. Am. 2, 119–2136.

Leksell, L., 1951. The stereotaxic method and radiosurgery of the brain. Acta Chir. Scand. 102 (4), 316–319.

Levin, V.A., Leibel, S.A., Gutin, P.H., 2001. Neoplasms of the central nervous system. In: De Vita, V.T. Jr., Hellman, S., Rosenberg, S.A. (Eds.), Cancer: principles and practice of oncology. Lippincott Williams & Wilkins, Philadelphia, PA, pp. 2100–2160.

Lewis, A.J., 1988. Sarcoma metastatic to the brain. Cancer 61 (3), 593–601.

Liotta, L., Stetler-Stevenson, W., 1989. Principles of molecular cell biology of cancer: cancer metastasis. In: DeVita, V.T. Jr., Hellman, S., Rosenberg, S.A. (Eds.), Cancer: principles and practice of oncology. JB Lippincott, Philadelphia, PA, pp. 98–115.

Lishner, M., Feld, R., Payne, D.G., et al., 1990. Late neurological complications after prophylactic cranial irradiation in patients with small-cell lung cancer: the Toronto experience. J. Clin. Oncol. 8 (2), 215–221.

Livingston, K.E., Horrax, G., Sachs, E. Jr., 1948. Metastatic brain tumors. Surg. Clin. North Am. 28, 805–810.

Long, D.M., 1979. Capillary ultrastructure in human metastatic brain tumors. J. Neurosurg. 51 (1), 53–58.

Lutterbach, J., Bartelt, S., Ostertag, C., 2002. Long-term survival in patients with brain metastases. J. Cancer Res. Clin. Oncol. 128 (8), 417–425.

MacGee, E.E., 1971. Surgical treatment of cerebral metastases from lung cancer. The effect on quality and duration of survival. J. Neurosurg. 35 (4), 416–420.

Madajewicz, S., Karakousis, C., West, C.R., et al., 1984. Malignant melanoma brain metastases. Review of Roswell Park Memorial Institute experience. Cancer 53 (11), 2550–2552.

Magilligan, D.J. Jr., Duvernoy, C., Malik, G., et al., 1986. Surgical approach to lung cancer with solitary cerebral metastasis: twenty-five years' experience. Ann. Thorac. Surg. 42 (4), 360–364.

Mahmoud-Ahmed, A.S., Suh, J.H., Lee, S.Y., et al., 2002. Results of whole brain radiotherapy in patients with brain metastases from breast cancer: a retrospective study. Int. J. Radiat. Oncol. Biol. Phys. 54 (3), 810–817.

Mandell, L., Hilaris, B., Sullivan, M., et al., 1986. The treatment of single brain metastasis from non-oat cell lung carcinoma. Surgery and radiation versus radiation therapy alone. Cancer 58 (3), 641–649.

Markesbery, W.R., Brooks, W.H., Gupta, G.D., et al., 1978. Treatment for patients with cerebral metastases. Arch. Neurol. 35 (11), 754–756.

Sze, G., Milano, E., Johnson, C., et al., 1990. Detection of brain metastases: comparison of contrast-enhanced MR with unenhanced MR and enhanced CT. AJNR. Am. J. Neuroradiol. 11 (4), 785–791.

Sze, G., Johnson, C., Kawamura, Y., et al., 1998. Comparison of single- and triple-dose contrast material in the MR screening of brain metastases. AJNR. Am. J. Neuroradiol. 19 (5), 821–828.

Takakura, K., Sano, K., Hojo, S., et al., 1982. Metastatic tumors of the central nervous system. Igaku-Shoin, New York.

Tasdemiroglu, E., Patchell, R.A., 1997. Cerebral metastases in childhood malignancies. Acta Neurochir. (Wien) 139 (3), 182–187.

Taylor, H.G., Lefkowitz, M., Skoog, S.J., et al., 1984. Intracranial metastases in prostate cancer. Cancer 53 (12), 2728–2730.

Tobler, W.D., Sawaya, R., Tew, J.M. Jr., 1986. Successful laser-assisted excision of a metastatic midbrain tumor. Neurosurgery 18 (6), 795–797.

Trillet, V., Catajar, J.F., Croisile, B., et al., 1991. Cerebral metastases as first symptom of bronchogenic carcinoma. A prospective study of 37 cases. Cancer 67 (11), 2935–2940.

Tsukada, Y., Fouad, A., Pickren, J.W., et al., 1983. Central nervous system metastasis from breast carcinoma. Autopsy study. Cancer 52 (12), 2349–2354.

Turrisi, A.T., 1990. Brain irradiation and systemic chemotherapy for small-cell lung cancer: dangerous liaisons? J. Clin. Oncol. 8 (2), 196–199.

Twelves, C.J., Souhami, R.L., 1991. Should cerebral metastases be treated by chemotherapy alone? Ann. Oncol. 2 (1), 15–17.

Twelves, C.J., Souhami, R.L., Harper, P.G., et al., 1990. The response of cerebral metastases in small cell lung cancer to systemic chemotherapy. Br. J. Cancer 61 (1), 147–150.

Ushio, Y., Arita, N., Hayakawa, T., et al., 1991. Chemotherapy of brain metastases from lung carcinoma: a controlled randomized study. Neurosurgery 28 (2), 201–205.

van den Bent, M.J., 2001. The diagnosis and management of brain metastases. Curr. Opin. Neurol. 14 (6), 717–723.

Vannucci, R.C., Baten, M., 1974. Cerebral metastatic disease in childhood. Neurology 24 (10), 981–985.

• Vecht, C.J., Haaxma-Reiche, H., Noordijk, E.M., et al., 1993. Treatment of single brain metastasis: radiotherapy alone or combined with neurosurgery? Ann. Neurol. 33 (6), 583–590.

• Vecil, G.G., Suki, D., Maldaun, M.V. et al., 2005. Resection of brain metastases previously treated with stereotactic radiosurgery. J. Neurosurg. 102 (2), 209–215.

Verger, E., Gil, M., Yaya, R., et al., 2005. Temozolomide and concomitant whole brain radiotherapy in patients with brain metastases: a phase II randomized trial. Int. J. Radiat. Oncol. Biol. Phys. 61 (1), 185–191.

Vesagas, T.S., Aguilar, J.A., Mercado, E.R., et al., 2002. Gamma knife radiosurgery and brain metastases: local control, survival, and quality of life. J. Neurosurg. 97 (Suppl.), 507–510.

Vieth, R.G., Odom, G.L., 1965. Intracranial metastases and their neurosurgical treatment. J. Neurosurg. 23 (4), 375–383.

Voorhies, R.M., Sundaresan, N., Thaler, H.T., 1980. The single supratentorial lesion. An evaluation of preoperative diagnostic tests. J. Neurosurg. 53 (3), 364–368.

Walker, A.E., Robins, M., Weinfeld, F.D., 1985. Epidemiology of brain tumors: the national survey of intracranial neoplasms. Neurology 35 (2), 219–226.

Weir, H.K., Thun, M.J., Hankey, B.F., et al., 2003. Annual report to the nation on the status of cancer, 1975–2000, featuring the uses of surveillance data for cancer prevention and control. J. Natl. Cancer Inst. 95 (17), 1276–1299.

Weiss, L., Grundmann, E., Torhorst, J., et al., 1986. Haematogenous metastatic patterns in colonic carcinoma: an analysis of 1541 necropsies. J. Pathol. 150 (3), 195–203.

White, K.T., Fleming, T.R., Laws, E.R. Jr., 1981. Single metastasis to the brain. Surgical treatment in 122 consecutive patients. Mayo. Clin. Proc. 56 (7), 424–428.

• Williams, B.J., Suki, D., Fox, B.D., et al., 2009. Stereotactic radiosurgery for metastatic brain tumors: a critical and comprehensive review of complications. Neurosurgery 111 (3), 439–448.

Wingo, P.A., Tong, T., Bolden, S., 1995. Cancer statistics, 1995. CA Cancer J. Clin. 45 (1), 8–30.

Winston, K.R., Walsh, J.W., Fischer, E.G., 1980. Results of operative treatment of intracranial metastatic tumors. Cancer 45 (10), 2639–2645.

Wronski, M., Arbit, E., 1999. Resection of brain metastases from colorectal carcinoma in 73 patients. Cancer 85 (8), 1677–1685.

Wronski, M., Arbit, E., 2000. Surgical treatment of brain metastases from melanoma: a retrospective study of 91 patients. J. Neurosurg. 93 (1), 9–18.

Wronski, M., Arbit, E., Burt, M., et al., 1995. Survival after surgical treatment of brain metastases from lung cancer: a follow-up study of 231 patients treated between 1976 and 1991. J. Neurosurg. 83 (4), 605–616.

Wronski, M., Arbit, E., McCormick, B., et al., 1997a. Surgical treatment of 70 patients with brain metastases from breast carcinoma. Cancer 80 (9), 1746–1754.

Wronski, M., Arbit, E., Russo, P., et al., 1996. Surgical resection of brain metastases from renal cell carcinoma in 50 patients. Urology 47 (2), 187–193.

Wronski, M., Maor, M.H., Davis, B.J., et al., 1997b. External radiation of brain metastases from renal carcinoma: a retrospective study of 119 patients from the MD Anderson Cancer Center. Int. J. Radiat. Oncol. Biol. Phys. 37 (4), 753–759.

Yardeni, D., Reichenthal, E., Zucker, G., et al., 1984. Neurosurgical management of single brain metastasis. Surg. Neurol. 21 (4), 377–384.

Yuile, P.G., Tran, M.H., 2002. Survival with brain metastases following radiation therapy. Australas. Radiol. 46 (4), 390–395.

Zimm, S., Wampler, G.L., Stablein, D., et al., 1981. Intracerebral metastases in solid-tumor patients: natural history and results of treatment. Cancer 48 (2), 384–394.

Zulch, K.J., 1957. Brain tumors. Their biology and pathology. Springer, New York.

Page numbers followed by "f" indicate figures, "t" indicate tables, and "b" indicate boxes.